Kidney
Transplantation

5th Edition

Kidney Transplantation

Principles and Practice

PETER J. MORRIS
Ph.D., F.R.C.S.

University of Oxford
Nuffield Department of Surgery
John Radcliffe Hospital
Headington, Oxford
England

W.B. SAUNDERS COMPANY
A Harcourt Health Sciences Company
Philadelphia London New York St. Louis Sydney Toronto

W.B. SAUNDERS COMPANY
A Harcourt Health Sciences Company

The Curtis Center
Independence Square West
Philadelphia, Pennsylvania 19106

Library of Congress Cataloging-in-Publication Data

Kidney transplantation / [edited by] Sir Peter J. Morris.—5th ed.

p. ; cm.

Includes bibliographical references and index.

ISBN 0–7216–8297–9

1. Kidneys—Transplantation.   I. Morris, Peter J.   [DNLM: 1. Kidney
  Transplantation.   2. Kidney Failure—surgery. WJ 368 K46 2001]

RD575.K53 2001   617.4'610592—dc21   00–059542

Acquisitions Editor: Richard Lampert
Project Manager: Edna Dick
Production Manager: Norman Stellander
Illustration Specialist: Robert Quinn
Book Designer: Karen O'Keefe Owens

KIDNEY TRANSPLANTATION: Principles and Practice   ISBN 0–7216–8297–9

Printed in the United States of America.

Last digit is the print number: 9   8   7   6   5   4   3   2   1

Contributors

GREGORY A. ABRAHAMIAN, M.D.
Department of Surgery, Harvard Medical School;
Transplantation Unit, Massachusetts General Hospital,
Boston, Massachusetts, United States.
Antilymphocyte Globulin and Monoclonal Antibodies

GEETA BAJAJ, M.D.
Professor and Chairman, Department of Pediatrics, State
University of New York at Stony Brook, Stony Brook, New
York, United States.
Renal Transplantation in Children

JOHN M. BARRY, M.D.
Professor of Surgery, School of Medicine, The Oregon
Health Sciences University; Head, Division of Abdominal
Organ Transplantation and Director, Renal Transplantation,
Staff Surgeon, Doernbecher Children's Hospital, The Oregon
Health Sciences University, Portland, Oregon, United States.
Surgical Techniques of Renal Transplantation

CRISTINA BORDEA, M.D.
Clinical Research Fellow, Nuffield Department of Surgery,
University of Oxford, John Radcliffe Hospital, Oxford,
England.
*Nonmalignant and Malignant Skin Lesions in Renal Transplant
Patients*

J.D. BRIGGS, M.B., F.R.C.P.
Honorary Clinical Senior Lecturer, Glasgow University;
Consultant Nephrologist, Western Infirmary, Glasgow,
Scotland.
The Recipient of a Renal Transplant

M. BUNCE, Ph.D.
Tissue Typing Laboratory, Formerly Clinical Scientist,
Oxford Transplant Centre, Oxford Radcliffe Hospital,
Oxford, England
*HLA Typing, Matching and Cross matching in Renal
Transplantation*

J. COHEN, M.Sc., F.R.C.P., F.R.C.(Path)
Professor and Chairman, Department of Infectious Diseases
and Microbiology, Imperial College School of Medicine;
Honorary Consultant Physician, Hammersmith Hospital,
London, England.
Infectious Complications After Renal Transplantation

ROBERT B. COLVIN, M.D.
Benjamin Castleman Professor of Pathology, Harvard
Medical School; Chief, Department of Pathology,
Massachusetts General Hospital, Boston, Massachusetts,
United States.
Pathology of Kidney Transplantation

A. BENEDICT COSIMI, M.D.
Claude E. Welch Professor of Surgery, Harvard Medical
School; Visiting Surgeon and Chief, Transplantation Unit,
Massachusetts General Hospital, Boston, Massachusetts,
United States.
*The Donor and Donor Nephrectomy; Antilymphocyte Globulin
and Monoclonal Antibodies*

D. CRANSTON, M.B.Ch.B., D.Phil., F.R.C.S.
Honorary Senior Lecturer in Surgery, University of Oxford;
Consultant Urological and Transplant Surgeon, Oxford
Kidney Unit, Churchill Hospital, Oxford, England.
Urological Complications After Renal Transplantation

**ABDALLAH S. DAAR, D.Phil.(Oxon), F.R.C.P.(Lon), F.R.C.S.
(Lon, Edin)**
Professor of Surgery, Sultan Qaboos University, Sultanate of
Oman; Hunterian Professor, Royal College of Surgeons of
England (2000), Muscat, Sultanate of Oman.
*Renal Transplantation in Developing Countries; Ethics in
Transplantation: Allotransplantation and Xenotransplantation*

MARGARET J. DALLMAN, D.Phil.
Professor of Immunology, Department of Biology, Imperial
College of Science, Technology and Medicine, London,
England.
Immunology of Graft Rejection

MICHAEL DONAGHY, M.A., D.Phil., F.R.C.P.
Reader in Clinical Neurology, University of Oxford;
Honorary Civilian Consultant in Neurology to the Army,
Consultant Neurologist, Radcliffe Infirmary, Oxford,
England.
Neurological Complications

**JOHN B. DOSSETOR, B.M.B.Ch.(Oxon), Ph.D., F.R.C.P.(UK),
F.R.C.S.**
Professor Emeritus (Medicine and Bioethics), University of
Alberta, Edmonton, Canada.
*Ethics in Transplantation: Allotransplantation and
Xenotransplantation*

JOHAN W. DE FIJTER, M.D., Ph.D.
Associate Professor of Medicine, Leiden University Medical
Center; Senior Physician, Department of Nephrology,
Leiden University Medical Center, Leiden, The Netherlands.
Chronic Renal Transplant Rejection

RICHARD N. FINE, M.D.
Professor and Chairman, Department of Pediatrics, State
University of New York at Stony Brook, Stony Brook, New
York, United States.
Renal Transplantation in Children

**PATRICIA M. FRANKLIN, B.Sc(Hons), R.G.N. Apr.D.P.
Counselling**
Clinical Nurse Specialist and Psychologist in
Transplantation, Oxford Transplant Centre, Churchill
Hospital, Headington, Oxford, England.
*Psychological Aspects of Kidney Transplantation and Organ
Donation*

AMY L. FRIEDMAN, M.D.
Assistant Professor, Department of Surgery, Yale University
School of Medicine; Assistant Professor, Staff, Yale New
Haven Hospital, New Haven, Connecticut, United States.
Renal and Pancreas Transplantation for Diabetic Nephropathy

ELI A. FRIEDMAN, B.S., M.D.
Distinguished Teaching Professor, Department of Medicine,
State University of New York Downstate Medical Center;
Chief, Division of Renal Disease, University Hospital of
Brooklyn, Brooklyn, New York, United States.
Renal and Pancreas Transplantation for Diabetic Nephropathy

PETER J. FRIEND, M.A., M.B., B.Chir., F.R.C.S., M.D.
Professor of Transplantation, University of Oxford; Oxford
Radcliffe Hospital NHS Trust, John Radcliffe Hospital,
Oxford, England.
Renal Xenotransplantation

SUSAN V. FUGGLE, M.Sc., D.Phil.
University Research Lecturer, University of Oxford; Director
of Clinical Transplant Immunology, Oxford Transplant
Centre, Oxford Radcliffe Hospital, Oxford, England.
Immunohistology of the Transplanted Kidney

DEREK W.R. GRAY, D.Phil., F.R.C.P., F.R.C.S.
Professor of Experimental Surgery, University of Oxford;
Honorary Consultant in Transplantation, John Radcliffe
Hospital NHS Trust, Oxford, England.
*Vascular and Lymphatic Complications After Renal
Transplantation*

DAVID HAMILTON, Ph.D., F.R.C.S.
Consultant Surgeon, Western Infirmary, Glasgow, Scotland.
Kidney Transplantation: A History

J. HOPKIN, M.D., M.Sc., M.A., F.R.C.P.
Professor of Experimental Medicine, University of Wales
Swansea; Honorary Consultant Physician, Swansea NHS
Trust, Singleton Hospital, Swansea, Wales.
Infectious Complications After Renal Transplantation

DAVID HUGHES, B.Sc., M.Sc., Ph.D.(Lon.)
Clinical Scientist, Nuffield Department of Surgery, Oxford
Radcliffe Hospital, Headington, Oxford, England.
Fine-Needle Aspiration Cytology of the Transplanted Kidney

BARRY D. KAHAN, Ph.D., M.D.
Professor and Director, Division of Immunology and Organ
Transplantation, Department of Surgery, The University of
Texas Medical School, Houston, Texas, United States.
Sirolimus

STUART J. KNECHTLE, M.D.
Professor of Surgery, Division of Organ Transplantation,
University of Wisconsin Medical School; Professor of
Surgery, University of Wisconsin Hospital and Clinics,
Madison, Wisconsin, United States.
Early Course of the Patient with a Kidney Transplant

DICKEN S.C. KO, M.D., F.R.C.S.(C)
Instructor in Surgery and Instructor in Urology, Harvard
Medical School; Assistant Surgeon, Massachusetts General
Hospital, Boston, Massachusetts, United States.
The Donor and Donor Nephrectomy

DICKEN D.H. KOO, M.Sc., D.Phil.
Postdoctoral Scientist, Nuffield Department of Surgery,
University of Oxford, John Radcliffe Hospital, Oxford,
England.
Immunohistology of the Transplanted Kidney

ADAM KOPELAN, M.D.
Transplant Fellow, University of Chicago, Chicago, Illinois,
United States.
Tacrolimus Therapy in Renal Transplantation

SANJAY KULKARNI, M.D.
Transplant Fellow, University of Chicago, Chicago, Illinois,
United States.
Tacrolimus Therapy in Renal Transplantation

J. KURTZ, M.A., M.B., B.Chir(Cambridge, UK)
Consultant Virologist, Public Health Laboratory,
Birmingham Heartlands Hospital, Birmingham, England.
Infectious Complications After Renal Transplantation

D. LITTLE, M.D., B.Sc., F.R.C.S.(Urol)
Teaching Consultant, Royal College of Surgeons of Ireland;
Consultant Transplant Surgeon and Urologist, Beaumont
Hospital, Dublin, Ireland.
Urological Complications After Renal Transplantation

VERNON C. MARSHALL, M.B.B.S., F.R.A.C.S., F.A.C.S.
Professor Emeritus of Surgery, Monash University,
Melbourne, Australia.
Renal Preservation

PHILIP D. MASON, B.Sc., Ph.D., M.B.B.S., F.R.C.P.
Honorary Senior Lecturer, Oxford University; Consultant
Nephrologist, Oxford Kidney Unit, Churchill Hospital,
Oxford, England.
Chronic Renal Failure: Renal Replacement Therapy

TIMOTHY H. MATHEW, M.B.B.S., F.R.A.C.P.
Associate Professor, School of Medicine, University of
Adelaide; Director, Renal Unit, The Queen Elizabeth
Hospital, Woodville, South Australia, Australia.
Mycophenolate Mofetil

CHANTAL MATHIEU, M.D., Ph.D.
Associate Professor of Internal Medicine (Endocrinology),
Catholic University Leuven; Associate Professor,
Department of Endocrinology, U.Z. Gasthuisberg, Leuven,
Belgium.
Other Forms of Immunosuppression

SHAMILA MAUIYYEDI, M.D.
Instructor, Department of Pathology, Harvard Medical
School; Assistant in Pathology, Massachusetts General
Hospital, Boston, Massachusetts, United States.
Pathology of Kidney Transplantation

ROBERT A. MONTGOMERY, M.D., D.Phil.
Assistant Professor of Surgery, Johns Hopkins University
School of Medicine; Transplantation Surgeon, Johns
Hopkins Hospital, Baltimore, Maryland, United States.
The Laparoscopic Donor Nephrectomy

M. RAFIQUE MOOSA, F.C.P.
Principal Specialist, Nephrologist and Lecturer, Department
of Internal Medicine, University of Stellenbosch; Head of
Renal Unit, Tygerberg Hospital, Cape Town, South Africa.
Renal Transplantation in Developing Countries

PETER J. MORRIS, PhD., F.R.C.S.
Nuffield Professor of Surgery, Oxford University, Oxford
Radcliffe Hospital, Oxford, England.
*Surgical Techniques of Renal Transplantation; Azathioprine and
Steroids; Cyclosporine; Results of Renal Transplantation*

SVETLOZAR N. NATOV, M.D.
Assistant Professor of Medicine, Tufts University School of Medicine; Staff Physician, New England Medical Center, Boston, Massachusetts, United States.
Liver Disease Among Renal Transplant Recipients

MICHAEL L. NICHOLSON, M.D., F.R.C.S.
Professor of Surgery, University of Leicester; Honorary Consultant Surgeon, Leicester General Hospital, Leicester, England.
Access for Renal Replacement Therapy

C. PALLIS, M.D.
Emeritus Reader in Neurology, Royal Postgraduate Medical School, Imperial College, Hammersmith Hospital, London, England.
Brain Stem Death: The Evolution of a Concept

LEENDERT C. PAUL, M.D., Ph.D.
Professor of Medicine, Leiden University Medical Center; Director, Department of Nephrology, Leiden University Medical Center, Leiden, The Netherlands.
Chronic Renal Transplant Rejection

BRIAN J.G. PEREIRA, M.D., M.B.A.
Professor of Medicine, Tufts University School of Medicine; Senior Vice President, New England Medical Center, Boston, Massachusetts, United States.
Liver Disease Among Renal Transplant Recipients

JACQUES PIRENNE, M.D., Ph.D.
Professor, Transplant Surgery, Catholic University Leuven; Head, Abdominal Transplant Surgery, U.Z. Gasthuisberg, Leuven, Belgium.
Other Forms of Immunosuppression

JOHN D. PIRSCH, M.D.
Professor of Medicine and Surgery, Division of Organ Transplantation, University of Wisconsin Medical School; Director of Medical Transplantation Service, University of Wisconsin Hospital and Clinics, Madison, Wisconsin, United States.
Early Course of the Patient with a Kidney Transplant

LLOYD E. RATNER, M.D.
Associate Professor and Director, Renal Transplantation, Johns Hopkins University School of Medicine, Baltimore, Maryland, United States.
The Laparoscopic Donor Nephrectomy

C.J. RUDGE, F.R.C.S.
Consultant Surgeon, Department of Renal Medicine and Transplantation, The Royal London Hospital, London, England.
Transplantation and the Abnormal Bladder

CHRISTINE RUSSELL, M.B.B.S., F.R.A.C.S.
Honorary Senior Lecturer, University of Oxford; Consultant Surgeon, Oxford Transplant Centre, Churchill Campus, Oxford Radcliffe Hospital, Oxford, England.
Cyclosporine

JOHN W. SEAR, M.A., Ph.D., F.F.A.R.C.S., F.A.N.Z.C.A.
Reader in Anaesthetics and Honorary Consultant Anaesthetist, Nuffield Department of Anaesthetics, University of Oxford; John Radcliffe Hospital, Oxford, England.
Anesthesia for Patients Undergoing Renal Transplantation

A.G.R. SHEIL, M.B.B.S., M.A.(Oxon), B.Sc.(Oxon), F.R.C.S., F.R.A.C.S., F.A.C.S.
Professor of Surgery (in the Field of Transplantation), University of Sydney; Head, Department of Transplantation Surgery, Royal Prince Alfred Hospital, Sydney, Australia.
Cancer in Dialysis and Transplant Patients

YVO W.J. SIJPKENS, M.D.
Assistant Professor of Medicine, Leiden University Medical Center; Physician, Department of Nephrology, Leiden University Medical Center, Leiden, The Netherlands.
Chronic Renal Transplant Rejection

BOB SOIN, M.A., M.B., B.Chir., F.R.C.S.
Specialist Registrar, Nuffield Department of Surgery, University of Oxford; Oxford Transplant Centre, Oxford Radcliffe Hospital, Oxford, England.
Renal Xenotransplantation

BRUCE G. SOMMER, M.D.
Professor and Interim Chair, Surgery, SUNY Downstate Medical Center; Chief, Division of Transplantation, University Hospital of Brooklyn, Brooklyn, New York, United States.
Renal and Pancreas Transplantation for Diabetic Nephropathy

CRAIG J. TAYLOR, Ph.D.
Consultant Clinical Scientist, Tissue Typing Laboratory, Addenbrooke's NHS Trust (Cambridge University Teaching Hospitals Trust), Cambridge, England.
The HLA System and Nomenclature

C.R.V. TOMSON, M.A., B.M., B.Ch., D.M.
Consultant Nephrologist, Southmead Hospital, Bristol, England.
Cardiovascular Complications After Renal Transplantation

VANESSA A. VENNING, D.M.(Oxon), F.R.C.P.(UK)
Consultant Dermatologist, The North Hampshire Hospital, Hampshire, England.
Nonmalignant and Malignant Skin Lesions in Renal Transplant Patients

MARK WAER, M.D., Ph.D.
Professor of Medicine, University of Leuven; Medical Director, University Hospital, Leuven, Belgium.
Other Forms of Immunosuppression; Total Lymphoid Irradiation

ABDUL AZIZ WALELE, F.C.P.
Specialist, Renal Unit, Department of Internal Medicine, University of Stellenbosch and Consultant Nephrologist, Tygerberg Hospital, Cape Town, South Africa. Currently Nephrology Fellow, Division of Nephrology, University of Toronto and Sunnybrook Health Science Centre, Toronto, Canada.
Renal Transplantation in Developing Countries

K.I. WELSH, BSc., M.A., Ph.D.
Formerly Director, Tissue Typing, Oxford Transplant Centre, Oxford Radcliffe Hospital, Oxford England.
HLA Typing, Matching and Crossmatching in Renal Transplantation

STEVEN A. WHITE, M.B.Ch.B., F.R.C.S.(Eng), M.D.
Lecturer in Surgery, Department of Surgery, University of Leicester; Honorary Specialist Registrar, Leicester General Hospital, Leicester, England.
Access for Renal Replacement Therapy

CHRISTOPHER G. WINEARLS, D.Phil., M.B.Ch.B.(Cape Town), F.R.C.P.(Lon)
Honorary Senior Lecturer in Medicine, Oxford University; Consultant Nephrologist, Oxford Kidney Unit, Churchill Hospital, Oxford Radcliffe Hospital, Oxford, England.
Chronic Renal Failure: Renal Replacement Therapy

FENELLA WOJNAROWSKA, M.Sc., F.R.C.P., D.M.
Professor of Dermatology, University of Oxford; Consultant Dermatologist, Churchill Hospital, Oxford Radcliffe Hospital, Oxford, England.
Nonmalignant and Malignant Skin Lesions in Renal Transplant Patients

KATHRYN J. WOOD, D.Phil.
Professor of Immunology, Nuffield Department of Surgery, University of Oxford, Oxford, England.
Approaches to the Induction of Tolerance

E. STEVE WOODLE, M.D.
Professor of Surgery and Director, Division of Transplantation, University of Cincinnati College of Medicine, Cincinnati, Ohio, United States.
Tacrolimus Therapy in Renal Transplantation

Preface to the Fifth Edition

In the Preface to the previous edition I predicted that a fifth edition would be necessary in due course to keep abreast with this ever-advancing discipline. However, I am not sure that I realized how much would have happened in the six years since the fourth edition. The current edition has been expanded yet again to 43 chapters with many new authors and includes new chapters on laparoscopic donor nephrectomy, liver complications after renal transplantation, chronic rejection, access surgery and even now a chapter on xenotransplantation of the kidney. Equally important, the development of new immunosuppressive agents has required individual chapters on the new immunosuppressive agents—mycophenolate mofetil, tacrolimus and sirolimus—which were all covered in one chapter in the last edition, as well as a chapter dealing with other newer agents still in development. The chapter on antilymphocyte agents also illustrates the advances in the use of monoclonal antibodies in therapy over the last few years. Other developments since the last edition have been the widespread adoption of DNA typing methods for HLA and more sophisticated crossmatching techniques.

Virtually all the previous chapters have been extensively rewritten and updated such that this edition represents the state-of-the-art in renal transplantation at this moment in time. However, the continuing developments in immunosuppression, both with immunosuppressive drugs and antilymphocyte agents, will no doubt change our approach to this over the coming years. Furthermore, I am hopeful that the chapter on approaches to the induction of tolerance will be accompanied by an additional chapter in the next edition describing clinical trials of some of these approaches. One of the new chapters covers chronic rejection, which does present a major problem in renal transplantation with no treatment available at this point in time. But again by the next edition I hope that there will be some means of both preventing and treating the changes of chronic allograft rejection.

However, who knows what the next edition will bring? Currently, the fifth edition illustrates the continuing progress in all aspects of renal transplantation. Graft survival figures at one year of around 85% to 90% in increasingly higher risk patients is a monument to the work of the scientists and clinicians who have made this possible.

Peter J. Morris

Preface to the First Edition

Renal transplantation is now an accepted treatment of patients in end-stage renal failure. A successful transplant restores not merely life but an acceptable quality of life to such patients. The number of patients in end-stage renal failure in the Western World who might be treated by hemodialysis and transplantation is considerable and comprises some 30–50 new patients/million of population. Unfortunately in most, if not all, countries the supply of kidneys for transplantation is insufficient to meet the demand. Furthermore, hemodialysis facilities are usually inadequate to make up this deficit so that many patients are still dying of renal disease who could be restored to a useful and productive life. Nevertheless, few of us would have imagined even 10 years ago that transplantation of the kidney would have become such a relatively common procedure as is the case today, and indeed well over 30,000 kidney transplantations have been performed throughout the world.

Transplantation of the kidney for the treatment of renal failure has been an attractive concept for many years. As long ago as 1945, three young surgeons at the Peter Bent Brigham Hospital in Boston, Charles Hufnagel, Ernest Landsteiner and David Hume, joined the vessels of a cadaver kidney to the brachial vessels of a young woman who was comatose from acute renal failure due to septicemia. The kidney functioned for several days before it was removed, and the woman regained consciousness. Shortly afterwards, the woman's own kidneys began to function and she made a full recovery. The advent of the artificial kidney at that time meant that this approach to the treatment of acute renal failure was no longer necessary, but attention was soon given to the possibility of transplanting kidneys to patients with end-stage renal failure who were requiring dialysis on the newly developed artificial kidney to stay alive.

Although the first experimental kidney transplants in animals were reported first in Vienna by Dr. Emerich Ulmann in 1902 and then in 1905 by Dr. Alexis Carrel in the United States, the problem of rejection was not mentioned by either author. Later in 1910, Carrel did discuss the possible differences between an autograft and a homograft. The vascular techniques developed by Carrel for the anastomosis of the renal vessels to the recipient vessels are still used today. But in 1923, Dr. Carl Williamson of the Mayo Clinic clearly defined the difference between an autografted and homografted kidney and even published histological pictures of a rejecting kidney. Furthermore, he predicted the future use of tissue matching in renal transplantation.

It is unfortunate that the lower animals, such as the dog, do not possess a blood grouping like that of man. In the future it may be possible to work out a satisfactory way of determining the reaction of the recipient's blood serum or tissues to those of the donor and the reverse; perhaps in this way we can obtain more light on this as yet relatively dark side of biology.

The recognition that allogeneic tissues would be rejected was further established in later years by Drs. Gibson and Medawar, who treated burn patients with homografts in Glasgow during the Second World War. Indeed, it was the crash of a bomber behind the Medawars' house in Oxford during the early years of the war that first stimulated his interest in transplantation, especially of skin.

In his address at the opening of the new Oxford Transplant Unit in 1977, Sir Peter Medawar recounted this event.

Early in the war, an R.A.F. Whitley bomber crashed into a house in North Oxford with much serious injury and loss of life. Among the injured was a young man with a third degree burn extending over about 60% of his body. People burned as severely as this never raised a medical problem before: they always died; but the blood transfusion services and the control of infection made possible by the topical use of sulphonamide drugs now made it possible for them to stay alive. Dr. John F. Barnes, a colleague of mine in Professor H. W. Florey's School of Pathology, asked me to see this patient in the hope that being an experimental biologist I might have some ideas for treatment. With more than half his body surface quite raw, this poor young man was a deeply shocking sight; I thought of and tried out a number of ingenious methods, none of which worked, for ekeing out his own skin for grafting, trying to make one piece of skin do the work of ten or more. The obvious solution was to use skin grafts from a relative or voluntary donor, but this was not possible then and it is not possible now.

I believe I saw it as my metier to find out why it was not possible to graft skin from one human being to another, and what could be done about it. I accordingly began research on the subject with the Burns Unit of the Glasgow Royal Infirmary, and subsequently in the Zoology Department in Oxford. If anybody had then told me that one day, in Oxford, kidneys would be transplanted from one human being to another, not as a perilous surgical venture, but as something more in the common run of things, I should have dismissed it as science fiction; yet it is just this that has come about, thanks to the enterprise of Professor Morris and his colleagues.

Nevertheless in 1951, David Hume in Boston embarked on a series of cadaver kidney transplants in which the kidney was placed in the thigh of the recipient. All but one of these kidneys were rejected within a matter of days or weeks, the one exception being a patient in whom the kidney functioned for nearly 6 months and enabled the patient to leave the hospital! This event provided hope for the future as no immunosuppressive therapy had been used in this patient. At this time, the problems of rejection of kidney allografts in the dog were being clearly defined by Dr. Morton Simonsen in Copenhagen and Dr. William Dempster in London, but in 1953, a major boost to transplantation research was provided by the demonstration, by Drs. Rupert Billingham, Lesley Brent and Peter Medawar, that tolerance to an allogeneic skin graft in an adult animal could be produced by injecting the fetus with donor strain tissue, thus confirming experimentally the clonal selection hypothesis of Burnet and Fenner in the recognition of self and non-self. The induction of specific unresponsiveness of a host to a tissue allograft has remained the ultimate goal of transplant immunologists ever since.

Then in 1954, the first kidney transplant between identical twins was carried out successfully at the Peter Bent Brigham Hospital which led to a number of further successful identical twin transplants in Boston and elsewhere in the world over the next few years.

There still remained the apparently almost insoluble problem of rejection of any kidney other than an identical-twin kidney. The first attempts to suppress the immune response to a kidney allograft employed total body irradiation of the recipient and were carried out by Dr. Merril's group in Boston, two groups in Paris under the direction of Drs. Kuss and Hamburger, respectively, and by Professor Shackman's group in London. Rejection of a graft could be suppressed by irradiation, but the complications of the irradiation were such that this was really an unacceptable approach, although an occasional relatively long-term acceptance of a graft provided encouragement for the future.

Then came the discovery by Drs. Schwartz and Dameshek in 1959 that 6-mercaptopurine could suppress the immune response of rabbits to human serum albumin. Shortly afterwards, they showed that the survival of skin allografts in rabbits was significantly prolonged by the same drug. This event ushered in the present era of renal transplantation, for very quickly Roy Calne in London and Charles Zukoski working with David Hume in Virginia showed that this same drug markedly prolonged the survival of kidney allografts in dogs. And indeed, 6-mercaptopurine was first used in a patient in Boston in 1960. Elion and Hitchings of the Burroughs Wellcome Research Laboratories in New York State then developed azathioprine, which quickly replaced 6-mercaptopurine in clinical practice as it was less toxic. With the addition of steroids, the standard immunosuppressive therapy of today was introduced to the practice of renal transplantation in the early sixties.

Not that this meant the solution of the problems of renal transplantation for this combination of drugs was dangerous and mortality was high in those early years. But there was a significant number of long-term successful transplants, and as experience grew, the results of renal transplantation improved. Another major area of endeavor in renal transplantation at that time was directed at the study of methods of matching donor and recipient for histocompatibility antigens with the aim of lessening the immune response to the graft and so perhaps allowing a decrease in the immunosuppressive drug therapy. Although this aim has only been achieved to any great extent in siblings who are HLA identical, tissue typing has made a significant contribution to renal trans-

plantation, perhaps best illustrated by the recognition in the late sixties that the performance of a transplant in the presence of donor-specific presensitization in the recipient leads to hyperacute or accelerated rejection of the graft in most instances. Nevertheless, the more recent description of the Ia-like system in man (HLA-DR) may have an important impact on tissue typing in renal transplantation. The present decade also has seen an enormous effort directed at immunological monitoring in renal transplantation and at attempts to induce experimental specific immunosuppression. We have solved most of the technical problems of renal transplantation; we have been left with the problem of rejection and the complications arising from the drug therapy given to prevent rejection.

Although the contributions in this book cover all aspects of renal transplantation, certain subjects, as for example immunological monitoring before transplantation, transplantation in children and cancer after renal transplantation, have received considerable emphasis as they do represent developing areas of great interest, and I must take responsibility for this emphasis. For in the seventies we have seen many of the principles and practice of renal transplantation become established and the areas of future investigation become more clearly defined. With an ever-increasing demand for renal transplantation, more and more people in many different disciplines, doctors (surgeons, physicians, pathologists, virologists, immunologists), nurses, scientists and ancillary staff are becoming involved in renal transplantation either in the clinic or in the laboratory. It is to these people I hope this book will be of value.

Oxford, November 1978   Peter J. Morris

Contents

Color plates follow front matter.

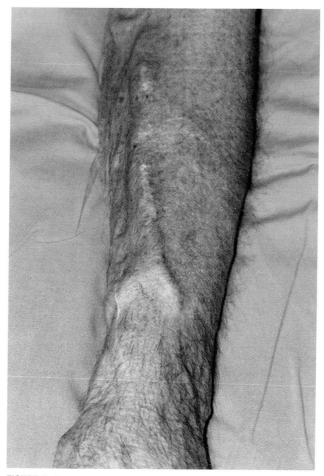

FIGURE 5–4

An established Brescia-Cimino radiocephalic arteriovenous fistula.

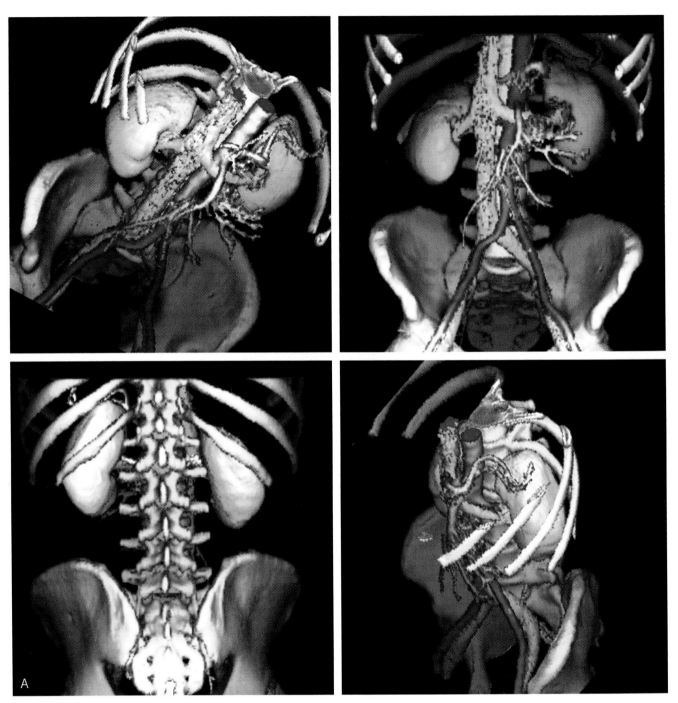

FIGURE 7–2A

3D reconstructed images of renal CT angiography. Images reconstructed with bony structures. (Top images—anterior view; bottom images—posterior/oblique views.)

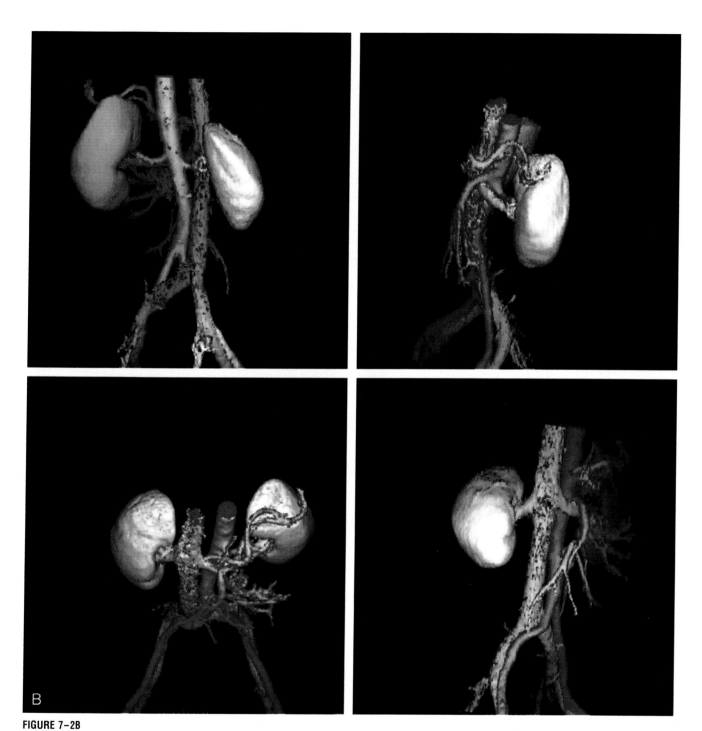

FIGURE 7–2B

Images reconstructed without bony structures. (Top images—posterior/oblique view demonstrating early bifurcation of right renal artery; bottom images—anterior view demonstrating orientation of left renal vein and superior mesenteric artery.)

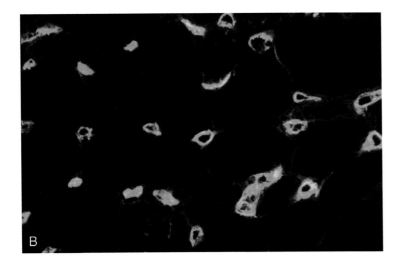

FIGURE 24–5B

Acute humoral rejection. Immunofluorescence microscopy: widespread bright staining of peritubular capillaries with C4d (monoclonal antibody), a marker of acute humoral rejection, that strongly correlates with presence of circulating donor-specific antibody. (Strepavidin-FITC, 400×.)

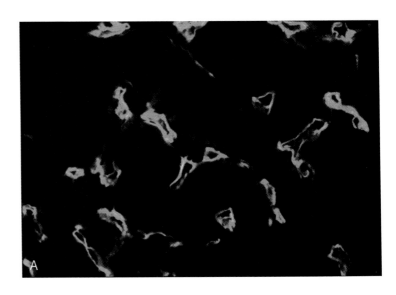

FIGURE 24–9A

Chronic humoral rejection. Immunofluorescence microscopy: peritubular capillaries with bright and diffuse staining for C4d (monoclonal antibody), indicating activation of the classical complement pathway, triggered by "humoral" antidonor antibodies. (Strepavidin-FITC, 400×.)

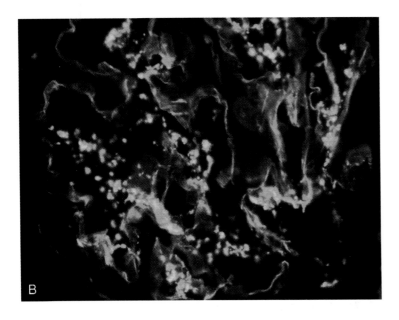

FIGURE 24–21B

Recurrent dense deposit disease. Immunofluorescence microscopy: staining for C3 shows broad linear ribbon-like deposits along with GBM and blob-like deposits in the mesangium (mesangial rings). (IF, C3-FITC, 400×.)

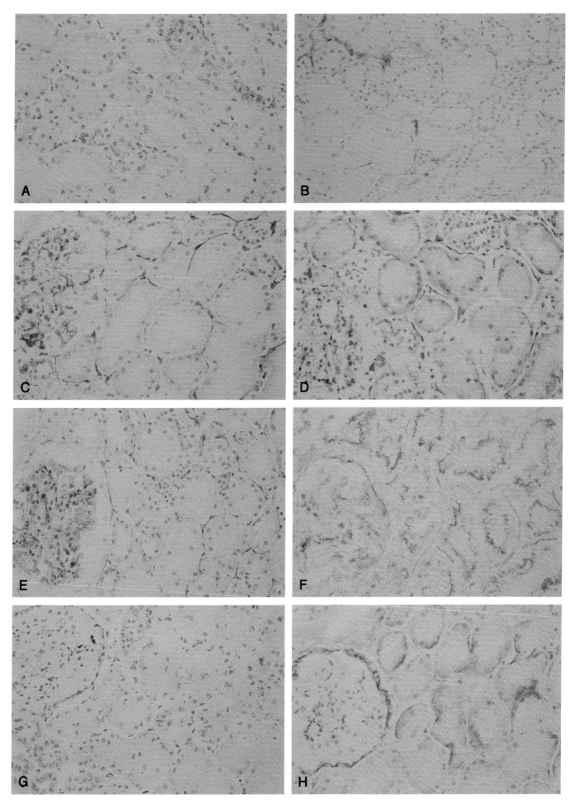

FIGURE 25–2

Differences in adhesion molecule and HLA-DR antigen expression between cadaveric and living related donor (LRD) kidneys. All biopsies were stained with monoclonal antibodies using an indirect immunoperoxidase technique. (A) LRD kidney stained for E-selectin demonstrating negative expression and (B) a cadaveric kidney with high levels of E-selectin on the intertubular capillaries. (C) LRD kidney with no tubular expression of HLA-DR antigens and (D) a cadaveric kidney with strong expression of HLA-DR antigens on the proximal tubules. (E) Intercellular adhesion molecule-1 (ICAM-1) was absent on the tubules of all LRD kidneys whereas (F) tubular ICAM-1 was detected at high levels in a proportion of the cadaver kidneys. (G) None of the LRD kidneys expressed tubular vascular cell adhesion molecule-1 (VCAM-1), whereas (H) a proportion of the cadaveric kidneys expressed high levels of proximal tubular VCAM-1. (Original magnification ×250). Reproduced with permission from the International Society of Nephrology (Koo, *et al.*, 1999).

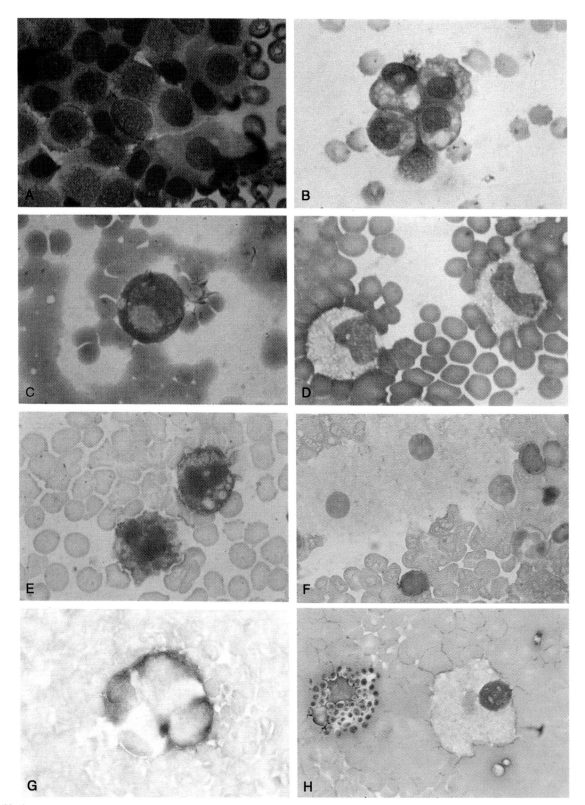

FIGURE 26–1

Cells sampled from human renal allografts using fine-needle aspiration biopsy may include (A) well-preserved tubule epithelial cells associated with good graft function or (B) tubule cells with swollen, vacuolated cytoplasm that are more characteristic of acute tubular necrosis. Typical of cells seen during acute cellular rejection are (C) a lymphoblast with deeply basophilic cytoplasm and a prominent peri-nuclear halo, (D) macrophages, (E) CD14-labeled macrophages, (F) Fas-ligand labeled lymphocytes with faintly-labeled tubule cells, (G) ICAM-1–labeled tubule cells, (H) kidney tubule cells in an FNAB sample taken in a case of early fungal pyelonephritis at 7 days posttransplantation; one cell is laden with *Candida glabrata*. (A–D & H = May-Grünwald-Giemsa stain; E–G = alkaline phosphatase anti-alkaline phosphatase monoclonal antibody labeling. Magnification ×800.)

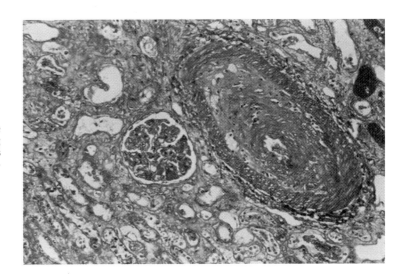

FIGURE 27-1

Photomicrograph of a renal transplant removed because of chronic rejection. There is extensive intimal thickening with narrowing of the vascular lumen, glomerulosclerosis with expansion of the mesangial matrix, interstitial fibrosis and tubular atrophy. Trichrome staining.

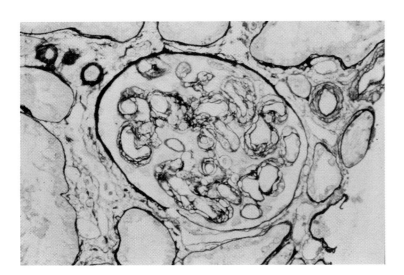

FIGURE 27-2

Photomicrograph of a renal transplant with transplant glomerulopathy. There is splitting of the glomerular basement membrane. Silver-methenamine staining.

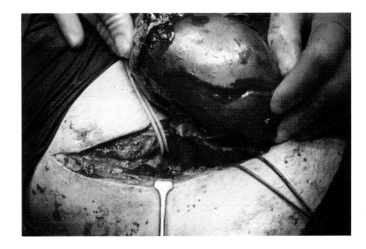

FIGURE 28-3

Photograph taken at operation for acute renal vein thrombosis. An early capsule rupture is present.

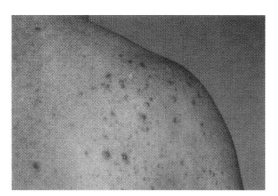

FIGURE 34-1

Steroid acne showing monomorphic inflamed lesions with few comedones.

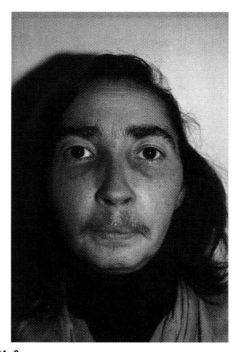

FIGURE 34-3

Hypertrichosis in a 35-year-old woman on cyclosporine alone 3 months after transplantation.

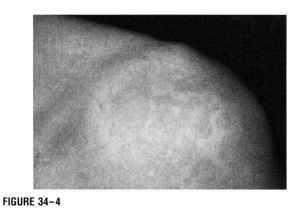

FIGURE 34-4

Pityriasis versicolor: pigmented macular lesions with superficial scaling over the shoulder region.

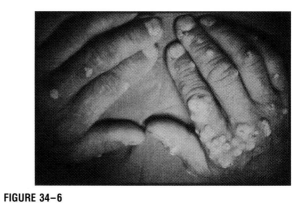

FIGURE 34-6

Extensive common warts on the hands of a renal-transplant recipient.

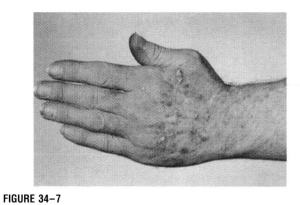

FIGURE 34-7

"Transplant hand." Sun-damaged skin on the hand of a renal transplant recipient showing solar keratosis.

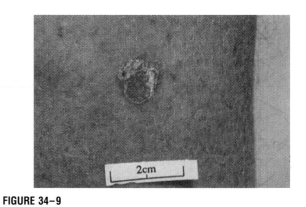

FIGURE 34-9

Typical annular lesion of porokeratosis showing the distinctive keratotic edge and slightly atrophic center.

Kidney Transplantation: A History

David Hamilton

Introduction

The modern period of transplantation began in the late 1950s, but two earlier periods of interest in clinical and experimental transplantation were the early 1950s and the first two decades of the twentieth century (see Hamilton, 1982, for a bibliography of the history of organ transplantation, and Table 1–1 for a summary of landmarks in kidney transplantation).

Early Experiments

The reasons for the interest in transplantation in the early part of the twentieth century were that experimental and clinical surgical skills were rapidly advancing and many of the pioneering surgeons took an interest in vascular surgical techniques as part of their broad familiarity with the advance of all aspects of surgery. Payr's demonstration of the first workable, although cumbersome, methods of vascular suturing led to widespread interest in organ transplantation in Europe. Many centers were involved, notably Vienna, Bucharest and Lyon. The first successful experimental organ transplant was reported by Ullmann in 1902. Emerich Ullmann (1861–1937) (Fig. 1–1) had studied under Edward Albert before obtaining a position at the Vienna Medical School, then at its height. His article shows that he managed to autotransplant a dog kidney from its normal position to the vessels of the neck, which resulted in some urine flow. The animal was presented to a Vienna medical society on March 1, 1902, and caused considerable comment (Ullmann, 1902). At this time Ullmann was Chief Surgeon to the Spital der Baumhertigen Schwestern, and his experimental work was done in the Vienna Physiology Institute under Hofrath Exner. Exner's son Alfred had already tried such a transplant without success. In the same year, another Vienna physician, Alfred von Decastello, physician assistant at the 2nd Medical Clinic, carried out dog-to-dog kidney transplants at the Institute of Experimental Pathology (von Decastello, 1902).

Ullmann and von Decastello had used Payr's method, and later in 1902 Ullmann demonstrated a dog-to-goat kidney transplant that, to his surprise, passed a little urine for a while. Neither Ullmann nor von Decastello continued with this work, although von Decastello was noted for his work on blood groups, and Ullmann published extensively on bowel and biliary surgery.

In Lyon, the department headed by Mathieu Jaboulay (1860–1913) had a major influence (Fig. 1–2). In his research laboratories, his assistants Carrel, Briau and Villard worked on improved methods of vascular suturing, leading to Carrel's famous article credited with establishing the modern method of suturing (Carrel, 1902). Carrel left to work in the United States, and in the next 10 years he published extensively on organ grafting, successfully carrying out autografts of kidneys in cats and dogs and showing that allografts

eventually failed after functioning briefly. For this work he was awarded a Nobel Prize in 1912.

Human Kidney Transplants

Jaboulay, Carrel's teacher, had carried out the first recorded human kidney transplant in 1906 (Jaboulay, 1906), although Ullmann later claimed an earlier attempt in 1902 (Ullmann, 1914). Jaboulay was later to be better known for his work on thyroid and urological surgery but, doubtless encouraged by the success of Carrel and others in his laboratory, he carried out two xenograft kidney transplants using a pig and goat as donors, transplanting the organ to the arm or thigh of patients with chronic renal failure. Each kidney worked for only 1 hour. This choice of an animal donor was acceptable at that time in view of the many claims in the surgical literature for success with xenograft skin, cornea or bone.

More is known of the second and third attempts at human kidney transplantation. Ernst Unger (1875–1938) (Fig. 1–3) had a thorough training in experimental work and set up his own clinic in 1905 in Berlin, being joined there by distinguished colleagues. He continued with experimental work

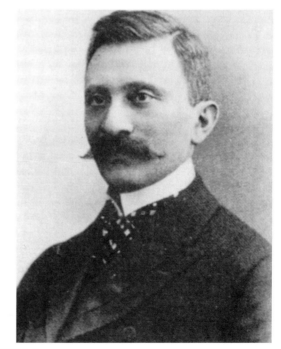

FIGURE 1–1

Emerich Ullmann (1861–1937) in 1902 carried out the first experimental kidney transplants in dogs. (Courtesy of The Vienna University, Institute for the History of Medicine.)

TABLE 1–1

LANDMARKS IN KIDNEY TRANSPLANTATION

1902	First successful experimental kidney transplant (Ullman, 1902)
1906	First human kidney transplant—xenograft (Jaboulay, 1906)
1933	First human kidney transplant—allograft (Voronoy, 1936)
1950	Revival of experimental kidney transplantation (Dempster, 1953; Simonsen, 1953)
1950–53	Human kidney allografts without immunosuppression, in Paris (Dubost *et al.*, 1951; Küss *et al.*, 1951; Servelle *et al.*, 1951) and Boston (Hume *et al.*, 1955)
1953	First use of live related donor, Paris (Michon *et al.*, 1953)
1954	First transplant between identical twins, Boston (Murray *et al.*, 1958)
1958	First description of leukocyte antigen Mac (Dausset, 1958)
1959–62	Radiation used for immunosuppression, in Boston (Murray *et al.*, 1960) and Paris (Hamburger *et al.*, 1959; Küss *et al*, 1960)
1960	Effectiveness of 6-MP in dog kidney transplants (Calne, 1960; Zukoski *et al.*, 1960)
1960	Prolonged graft survival in patient given 6-MP after irradiation (Küss *et al.*, 1962)
1962	First use of tissue matching to select a donor and recipient (Hamburger *et al.*, 1962; Terasaki *et al.*, 1965 Dausset, 1980)
1966	Recognition that positive crossmatching leads to hyperacute rejection (Kissmeyer-Nielson *et al.*, 1966; Terasaki *et al.*, 1965)
1967	Creation of Eurotransplant (van Rood, 1967)
1967	Development of kidney preservation (Belzer *et al.*, 1967)
1973	Description of the transfusion effect (Opelz *et al.*, 1973)
1978	First clinical use of cyclosporine (Calne *et al.*, 1978)
1978	Application of matching for HLA-DR in renal transplantation (Ting and Morris, 1978)
1987	First of new wave of immunosuppressive agents appears (tacrolimus)
1995	Transgenic pigs produced (Bogaerde and White [1997])

6-MP = mercaptopurine.

and by 1909 reported successful transplantation of the kidneys *en masse* from a fox terrier to a boxer dog. The urine output continued for 14 days, and the animal was presented to two medical societies. By 1910 Unger had performed more than 100 experimental kidney transplants. On December 10, 1909, Unger attempted a transplant using a stillborn child's kidney grafted to a baboon. No urine was produced. The animal died shortly after the operation, but postmortem ex-

amination showed that the vascular anastomosis had been successful. This success and the new knowledge that monkeys and humans were serologically similar led Unger to attempt, later in the same month, a monkey-to-human transplant (Unger, 1909). The patient was a young girl dying of renal failure, and the kidney from a pig ape was sutured to the thigh vessels. No urine was produced. Unger's report concluded that there was a biochemical barrier to trans-

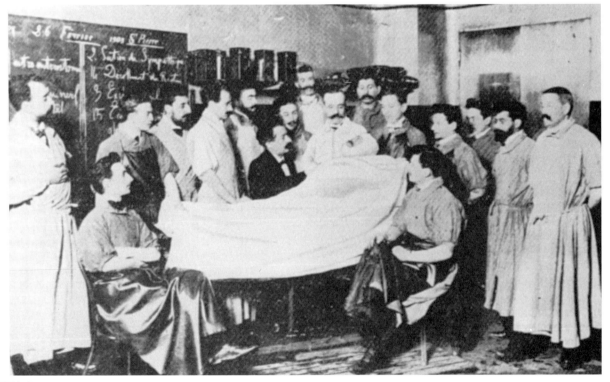

FIGURE 1–2

Mathieu Jaboulay (1860–1913) and his surgical team at Lyon in 1903. Until his death in a rail accident, he made numerous surgical contributions and encouraged Alexis Carrel's work on vascular anastomosis. In 1906, Jaboulay reported the first attempt at human kidney transplantation.

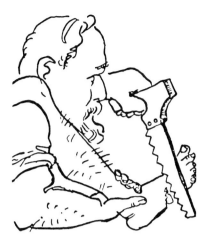

FIGURE 1–3

A contemporary cartoon of Ernst Unger (1875–1938) at work at the Rudolf Virchow Hospital, Berlin. (Courtesy of the Rudolf Virchow Hospital.)

plantation, a view mistakenly advocated by the basic science of the day; his main contributions thereafter were in esophageal surgery. (For a biography of Unger, see Winkler, 1982.)

These early experiments established that kidney transplants were technically possible. Methods of study of renal function were then primitive, for without routine measurement of blood urea and without any radiological methods, subtle studies of transplant function were impossible. This, plus the uncertainty of the mechanism of allograft rejection, led to a diminished interest in organ transplantation after about 10 years of activity. By the start of World War I, interest in organ transplantation had almost ceased and was not resumed in the European departments of surgery after the war. Carrel had switched his attention to studies of tissue culture. Interest elsewhere was also low, and in Britain and the United States scarce research funds were being applied to fundamental biochemistry and physiology rather than applied projects of clinical relevance. Transplantation immunology faded away, after this bright start in the capable surgical hands of Carrel, plus Murphy's sound grasp of immunosuppression and Landsteiner's awareness of the serological detection of human antigens, all of whom worked at the Rockefeller Institute in New York.

In 1914 in a remarkable lecture to the International Surgical Society, Carrel did anticipate the future development of transplantation. His colleague, J. B. Murphy, at the Rockefeller Institute, had found that radiation or benzol treatment would increase the "take" of tumor grafts in rats, and Carrel realized the potential of these findings:

It is too soon to draw any definite conclusions from these experiments. Nevertheless it is certain that a very important point has been acquired with Dr. Murphy's discovery that the power of the organism to eliminate foreign tissue was due to organs such as the spleen or bone marrow, and that when the action of these organs is less active a foreign tissue can develop rapidly after it has been grafted (Carrel, 1914).

It is not possible to foresee whether or not the present experiments of Dr. Murphy will lead directly to the practical solution of the problem in which we are interested.

The surgical side of the transplantation of organs is now completed, as we are now able to perform transplantations of organs with perfect ease and with excellent results from an anatomical standpoint. But as yet the methods cannot be applied to human surgery, for the reason that homoplastic transplantations are almost always unsuccessful from the standpoint of the functioning of the

organs. All our efforts must now be directed toward the biological methods which will prevent the reaction of the organism against foreign tissue and allow the adapting of homoplastic grafts to their hosts.

The Middle Years

Until the revival of interest in transplantation in the 1950s, the 1930s and 1940s were a stagnant period in clinical science. The great European surgical centers had declined, and in North America only at the Mayo Clinic was there a cautious program of experimental transplantation without building on Carrel's work, notably failing to make attempts at immunosuppression. In transplantation circles, such as they were, there was not even the confidence to counter the vivid claims of Voronoff to rejuvenate human patients via monkey gland grafts, and the endless reports of successful human skin grafts were not examined critically.

The main event of this period was an isolated and little known event—the first human kidney allograft. It was performed in the Ukraine by the Soviet surgeon Yu. Yu. Voronoy (Voronoy, 1936). The surgeon was an experienced investigator, and he eventually performed six such transplants up to 1949. Voronoy (1895–1961) trained in surgery at Kiev under the distinguished Professor V. N. Shamov and there obtained experience with serological methods of blood transfusion, then in their developmental stage. He used these methods to detect complement-fixing antibodies after testis slice transplants, and later he had some success with the same methods applied to kidney grafts (Fig. 1–4). In 1933, Voronoy transplanted a human kidney of blood group B to a patient of blood group O suffering from acute renal failure as a result of mercuric chloride poisoning. The donor kidney was obtained from a patient dying as a result of a head injury and was transplanted to the thigh vessels under local anesthetic: the warm time for the kidney was about 6 hours. There was a major mismatch for blood groups, and despite a modest exchange transfusion, the kidney never worked. The patient died 2 days later; at postmortem the donor vessels were patent. By 1949, Voronoy reported six such transplants, although no substantial function had occurred in any. (For a biography of Voronoy, see Hamilton and Reid, 1984.)

Post–World War II

The sounder basis of transplantation immunology, which followed Medawar's pioneer studies during World War II, led to a new interest in human transplantation. In 1946, a human allograft kidney transplant to arm vessels under local anesthetic was attempted by Hufnagel, Hume and Landsteiner at the Peter Bent Brigham Hospital in Boston. The brief period of function of the kidney may have helped the patient's recovery from acute renal failure; it marked the beginning of that hospital's major interest in transplantation and dialysis (Moore, 1964).

In the early 1950s, the interest in experimental and clinical kidney transplantation increased. With a growing certainty that immunological mechanisms were involved, the destruction of kidney allografts could be reinvestigated. Simonsen, then an intern in Ålborg in Denmark, persuaded his surgical seniors to teach him some vascular surgery, and, using dog kidney transplants, he reported on the mechanism of kidney rejection (Simonsen, 1953). Dempster in London also reexamined this question (Dempster, 1953). Both workers found that the pelvic position of the kidney was preferable to a superficial site, and both concluded that an immunological mechanism was responsible for failure. Dempster found that radia-

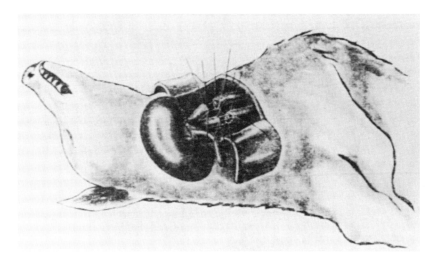

FIGURE 1–4

Yu. Yu. Voronoy (1895–1961) had experience with dog allografts before carrying out the first human kidney allograft in 1933 at Kherson in the Ukraine. His experimental animal model is shown here.

tion, but not cortisone, delayed rejection. Both workers considered that a humoral mechanism of rejection was likely.

In the early 1950s, two groups simultaneously started human kidney transplantation. In Paris, with encouragement from the nephrologist Jean Hamburger, the surgeons Küss (five cases), Servelle (one case) and Dubost (one case) reported on kidney allografts without immunosuppression in human patients, placing the transplant in the now-familiar pelvic position (Dubost *et al.*, 1951; Küss *et al.*, 1951; Servelle *et al.*, 1951). The Paris series included a case reported by Hamburger of the first live related kidney transplant, the donor being the mother of a boy whose solitary kidney had been damaged in a road accident. The kidney functioned immediately but rejected abruptly on the 22nd day (Michon *et al.*, 1953). In the United States, the Chicago surgeon Lawler had been the first to attempt such an intraabdominal kidney allograft in 1950; he met with the intense public interest and professional skepticism that was to characterize innovative transplantation thereafter. A series of nine cases, closely studied, was recorded from Boston, using the thigh position of the graft, and for the first time hemodialysis had been used in preparing the patients, employing Merrill's skill with the early Kolff/Brigham machine. David Hume (Fig. 1–5) reported on this Boston experience in 1953. Modest but unexpected survival of the kidney was obtained in some of these cases and served to encourage future careful empirical surgical adventures, despite advice from scientists to wait for elegant solutions. Although small doses of adrenocorticotropic hormone (ACTH) or cortisone were used, it was thought that the endogenous immunosuppression of uremia was responsible for these results rather than the drug regimen. Many of Hume's tentative conclusions from this short series were confirmed later, notably that prior blood transfusion might be beneficial, that blood group matching of graft and donor might be necessary, and that host bilateral nephrectomy was necessary for control of posttransplant blood pressure (Hume *et al.*, 1955). The first observation of recurrent disease in a graft was made, and accelerated arteriosclerosis in the graft vessels was noted at postmortem. Other cases were reported from Chicago, Toronto and Cleveland in the early 1950s, but because no sustained function was achieved, interest in clinical and experimental renal allograft transplantation waned, despite increasing knowledge of basic immunological mechanisms in the laboratory.

The technical lessons learned from the human allograft attempts of the early 1950s allowed confidence in the surgical methods, and in Boston, on December 23, 1954, the first transplant of a kidney from one twin to another suffering

from renal failure was performed. From then on, many such cases were transplanted successfully in Boston (Murray *et al.*, 1958). Although sometimes seen now merely as a technical triumph, valuable new findings emerged from this series. Some had predicted that in the short-term the activity of the inactive bladder could not be restored and that in the long-term human kidney grafts would decline in vitality as a result of denervation or ureteric reflux. Others were convinced that a single kidney graft could not restore biochemical normality to an adult and that in any case the existing changes caused by chronic renal failure were not reversible. All these gloomy predictions were neutralized by the success of the twin kidney transplants, and the greatest triumph came when one such recipient became pregnant and had a normal infant, delivered cautiously by cesarean section, with the anxious transplanters in attendance. Many of the twin recipients are still alive today, although the good results were tempered by failures caused by the prompt return of glomerulonephritis in some transplanted kidneys. This complication was later abolished by immunosuppression. Other

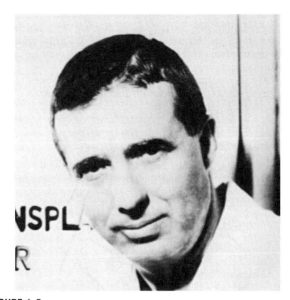

FIGURE 1–5

David M. Hume (1917–1973) pioneered human kidney transplantation at the Peter Bent Brigham Hospital, Boston, and the Medical College of Virginia. He died in an air crash at the age of 55.

lessons learned were that the hazard of multiple donor renal arteries provided a need for pretransplant angiography of the kidneys in living donors, although it still was not thought necessary to perfuse or cool the donor organ. Lastly, there was the first airing of the legal aspects of organ donation, particularly the problem of consent in young, highly motivated related donors. (For an account of this period, see Murray *et al.*, 1976.)

Immunosuppression and the Modern Era

In 1948, the first patients crippled with rheumatoid arthritis were given the Merck Company's cortone at the Mayo Clinic, and intense worldwide interest in the pharmacological actions of adrenal cortical hormones followed. Careful studies by Medawar's group in the early 1950s suggested a modest immunosuppressive effect of cortisone, but when Medawar shortly afterward showed profound, specific and long-lasting graft acceptance via the induction of tolerance, the weak steroid effect was understandably sidelined and thought to be of no clinical interest. Induction of tolerance in adult animals (rather than newborns) was then accomplished by lethal irradiation and bone marrow infusion, and with this strong lead from the laboratory, it was natural that the first attempts at human immunosuppression for organ transplants were with preliminary total body irradiation and allograft bone marrow rescue. These procedures were carried out in Paris, Boston and elsewhere in the late 1950s. This regimen was too difficult to control, and graft-versus-host disease was inevitable. It was found unexpectedly that sublethal irradiation alone in human patients was quite immunosuppressive, however, and this approach was used up to 1962, the year of the first general availability of azathioprine (Imuran). In Boston, 12 cases were treated in this way, but with only one long-term survival in a man receiving his transplant from his nonidentical twin (Murray *et al.*, 1960). In Paris, similar success was obtained with sibling grafts (Hamburger *et al.*, 1959; Küss *et al.*, 1960). These isolated kidney survivals after a single dose of radiation gave further hope and showed again that the immunology of humans, dogs and mice is different. These cases also showed that if a human organ could survive the initial crucial rejection period, it could be protected or adapted to the host in some way, possibly shielded by new endothelium, by enhancement or, as suggested later, by microchimeric tolerance induced by mobile cells in the graft.

Chemical Immunosuppression

In 1958, at the New England Medical Center, attempts were made at human bone marrow transplantation for aplastic anemia and leukemia. To enable the marrow grafts to succeed, irradiation to the recipient was used. Results were poor, and mortality was high. Dameshek and Schwartz looked for alternatives to irradiation and reasoned that an anticancer drug such as 6-mercaptopurine (6-MP) or methotrexate might be of use for immunosuppression in their patients. (For an account of this period, see Schwartz, 1976.) Their important paper in 1959, showing a poor immune response to foreign protein in rabbits treated with 6-MP (Schwartz and Dameshek, 1959), was noticed by Roy Calne, then a surgeon in training at the Royal Free Hospital, London. Calne had been disappointed at the failure of irradiation to prolong kidney allograft survival in dogs, and like the others looking for an alternative, he found that 6-MP was successful (Calne, 1960). Zukoski and colleagues in Richmond found the same effect (Zukoski *et al.*, 1960).

In 1960, Calne visited Boston for a period of research, and Hitchings and Elion of Burroughs Wellcome, then at Tuckahoe, provided him with new derivatives of 6-MP. Of these, BW57-322 (later known as azathioprine [Imuran]) proved to be more successful in dog kidney transplants and less toxic than 6-MP (Calne *et al.*, 1962).

In 1960–1961, 6-MP was used in many human kidney transplants. In London at the Royal Free Hospital, three cases were managed in this way but without success, although one patient receiving a live related transplant died of tuberculosis rather than rejection (Hopewell *et al.*, 1964). In Boston, no lasting human kidney function was obtained, but in Paris Küss and associates reported one prolonged survival of a kidney from a nonrelated donor when 6-MP was used together with intermittent prednisone in a recipient who had also received irradiation as the main immunosuppressive agent (Küss *et al.*, 1962; Fig. 1–6). This case was the first success for chemical immunosuppression.

This change in approach, giving lifelong, risky medication with toxic drugs, although an obvious development in retrospect, was accepted with reluctance because it meant leaving

FIGURE 1–6

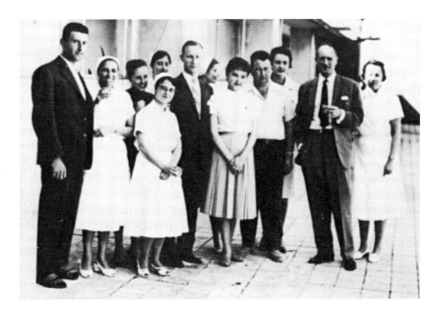

R. Küss (right) and M. Legrain (center) in 1960 with their first long-term kidney transplant survivor. The patient and her brother-in-law donor (center right) are shown with the staff of the unit at the Hôpital Foch. Immunosuppression with irradiation and 6-mercaptopurine was used. (Courtesy of Prof. M. Legrain.)

aside, at least in the short term, the hopes from the work of the transplantation immunologists for the elegant, specific, one-shot, nontoxic tolerance regimen. Many thought that entry into this new paradigm was only a temporary diversion.

In 1961, azathioprine became available for human use, and the dosage was difficult to judge at first. The first two Boston cases using the drug did not show prolonged survival of the grafts, but in April 1962 the first extended successes with human kidney allografts were obtained (Murray *et al.*, 1963). Shortly afterward, at the bedside rather than in the laboratory, it was discovered that steroids, notably prednisolone, when given with azathioprine had a powerful synergistic effect. The regular use of both together became a standard regimen after reports by Starzl *et al.* (1963) and Goodwin *et al.* (1962), and this combined therapy continued to be the routine immunosuppressive method despite many other suggested alternatives, until azathioprine was displaced by cyclosporine much later. Use of the combined immunosuppression and the increasing use of live related donors (rather than occasional twin or free or cadaveric kidneys), along with the remarkably good results reported in 1963 from Denver (Starzl *et al.*, 1963) and Richmond (Hume *et al.*, 1963), greatly encouraged the practice of transplantation. (For an account of this period, see Starzl, 1978.)

A Time of Optimism

The mid-1960s was a period of great optimism. The rapid improvement in results seemed to indicate that routine success was at hand. Looking to the future, calculations were made that suggested that enough donor organs would be available in the future if all large hospitals cooperated, and such donations did start to come from outside the transplantation pioneer hospitals. Transplantation societies were set up and specialist journals started. The improvements in regular dialysis treatment meant an increasing pool of patients in good health suitable for transplantation, and this allowed for better and planned preparation for transplantation. With a return to dialysis being possible, heroic efforts to save a rejected kidney were no longer necessary. Management of patients improved in many aspects, and the expected steroid long-term effects were met and managed. The need for cooling of donor organs was belatedly recognized, many tests of viability were announced, and transport of organs between centers began. Bone disease and exotic infections were encountered and treated, but the kidney units were afflicted by a hepatitis B epidemic in the mid-1960s, which affected their morale and status. The narrow age limit for transplantation was widened, and in Richmond the first experience with kidney grafts in children was obtained. Recipients of kidney transplants reentered the normal business of life and became politicians, professors, pilots and fathers and mothers of normal children. Other good news in the United States came when the federal government accepted the costs of regular dialysis and transplantation in 1968. There were always unexpected findings, usually reported from the pioneer units with the longest survivors. Cautiously, second kidney transplants were performed at Richmond when a first had failed; these did well, and the matter became routine. Chronic rejection and malignancy first were reported in kidney transplant recipients from Denver. As a result of the optimism, experimental heart transplantation started, the first human livers were grafted, and there was a revival of interest in xenotransplantation. Although the attempts of Reemtsma *et al.* (1964), Hume (1964) and Starzl (quoted in Starzl, 1978) at transplantation with chimpanzee or baboon kidneys ultimately failed, rejection did not occur immediately, and the cases were studied closely and described.

In the search for better immunosuppression, there was great excitement when laboratory studies by Woodruff and Medawar produced a powerful immunosuppressive antilymphocyte serum, and production of a version suitable for human use started. Initial results were favorable, but the antilymphocyte serum had an unspectacular role thereafter, supplanted from 1975 onward by the production of monoclonal antibodies. Hopes for another biological solution to transplantation were raised in 1969 when French and Batchelor found an enhancing serum effect in the new experimental model of rat kidney transplantation made possible by the development of microsurgical methods, but it proved impossible to mimic the effect in humans.

Tissue Typing

The greatest hopes resided in the evolution of tissue typing methods, which entered routine use in 1962 (Dausset, 1980; Hamburger *et al.*, 1962; Fig. 1–7). The increasing identification of the antigens of the HLA system seemed to promise excellent clinical results in the future from close matching made possible when choosing from a large pool of patients. Sharing of kidneys in Europe started in 1967 at van Rood's suggestion, and in North America, Amos and Terasaki set up similar sharing schemes on both coasts of the United States. Others followed throughout the world, and these organizations not only improved the service, but also soon gathered excellent data on kidney transplant survival. The need to transport kidneys within these schemes encouraged construction of perfusion pumps designed to increase the survival of organs and the distance they could be transported (Belzer *et al.*, 1967). Much work on perfusion fluids was done until the final intracellular type of fluid devised by Collins in 1969 allowed a simple flush and chill to suffice for prolonged storage (Collins *et al.*, 1969). Although the hopes for typing were not fully realized, such schemes had other benefits in obtaining kidneys when urgently required for patients with rarer blood groups, for children or for the highly sensitized. Such patients had been recognized by the new lymphocytotoxicity testing using a crossmatch between donor cells and recipient serum. First noted by Terasaki *et al.* (1965) and described in more detail by Kissmeyer-Nielsen and colleagues in 1966, such pretransplant testing explained cases of

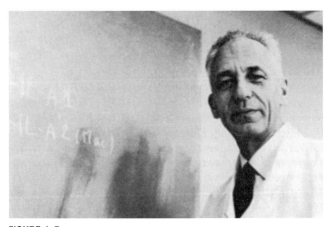

FIGURE 1–7

Jean Dausset first described an antigen MAC, later known as HL-A2, defined by a number of antisera from multitransfused patients and which later was shown to be part of the major histocompatibility complex in humans (HLA).

sudden failure and led to a marked diminution in hyperacute rejection (Kissmeyer-Nielsen *et al.*, 1966).

The 1970s Plateau

The 1970s was a period of consolidation of improvements in data collection, such as the valuable European Dialysis and Transplant Association (EDTA) surveys, and increased sophistication in HLA typing methods and organ-sharing schemes. Cadaveric organ procurement generally increased as a result of wider involvement of the public and medical profession, although the number of patients waiting for transplantation persistently exceeded the organs available, and donation declined transiently during times of public concern over transplantation issues. Governments took initiatives to increase donations; in Britain the Kidney Donor Card was introduced in 1971, becoming a multidonor card 10 years later. In hospital practice, methods of resuscitation and intensive care improved, and the concept of *brain death* was established to prevent prolonged, pointless ventilation, but its immediate application to transplantation provoked controversy. Despite many new claims for successful methods of immunosuppression, trials of splenectomy, thymectomy and thoracic duct drainage and a new look at cyclophosphamide, no agent except antithymocyte globulin became established in routine use.

Although patient survival after kidney transplantation continued to rise, the 1970s did not show the expected increase in cadaveric graft survival. Some groups reported decreased survival figures, and this paradox was solved, in part, by the demonstration that blood transfusion during regular dialysis, which had been discouraged because of the risk of sensitization, was beneficial to the outcome of kidney transplantation (Opelz *et al.*, 1973), an observation made some years earlier by Morris *et al.* (1968).

The 1970s ended with two innovations that revived hopes of reaching the goal of routine, safe and successful kidney transplantation. Ting and Morris (1978) reported the successful clinical application of HLA-DR matching, and Calne et al. (1978) revived memories of the excitement of the early days of the use of azathioprine by introducing into clinical practice the first serious rival to it in 20 years, cyclosporine, which had been discovered to be a powerful immunosuppressive agent by Borel (1976). It replaced the earlier drug regimens and was the dominant agent in use until the 1990s. Transplantation had grown to a sufficiently large clinical service that it was worth the attention of the pharmaceutical companies, and in the 1990s steady production of new agents occurred—tacrolimus, mycophenolate mofetil, rapamycin, sirolimus, brequinar and others.

The improved results of transplantation meant that the procurement of organs became a more dominant issue. Comparisons of transplantation practice throughout the world showed remarkable differences in attitudes to use of live related donors and cadaveric organs, depending on religion and cultural traditions. Kidney transplantation had started as a difficult surgical and scientific challenge confined to a few academic centers in the developed world, but its success had led to the technique becoming a routine service in all parts of the world (reviewed by Burdick *et al.*, 1999). In some nations not sharing Western attitudes, the donor shortage meant the appearance of undesirable commercial developments in renal transplantation, such as the purchase of kidneys from living unrelated donors (Morris, 1987; discussed in more detail in Chapter 41).

Waiting for Xenografts

As the demand for kidney transplants continued to exceed supply, other initiatives appeared and included study of na-tions and areas with high donation rates (such as Spain), the regulated use of properly motivated unrelated individuals, and a return to use of *marginal* cadaveric kidneys, notably from non–heart beating donors. As all attempts to increase donor supply fell short of the ever-rising target, the radical alternative of the use of animal organs was examined afresh. Profound immunosuppression alone was ineffective, and at first methods of removing natural antibody from recipient plasma were tried to deal with the hyperacute phase of xenograft organ rejection. Although the traditional hopes for xenografting of human patients had assumed that concordant species such as the monkey would be used, a new strategy using genetic engineering methods first used knock-out mice, which lacked the antibody attachment site, and then a line of transgenic pigs, a distant species discordant with humans with a modified endothelium that reduced the complement-mediated immediate reaction (reviewed by van den Bogaerde and White, 1997; see also Chapter 42). These new hopes for xenografts raised old fears among the public and legislators, notably regarding disease transmission, and although this had been a familiar problem in human-to-human transplantation and had been met regularly and dealt with, governments sought to discourage xenograft transplants until reassurances were obtained.

Conclusion

Kidney transplantation was the first of the organ transplant services to develop because of availability of live donors and the crucial backup of dialysis. When radical new ideas are to be tested, pioneers will still turn to kidney transplantation. Kidney transplantation is where it all started, with good reason, and it will always be a test bed for major innovation.

In the early 1990s, Murray was awarded the Nobel Prize in Medicine for his pioneer work in renal transplantation (Murray, 1992) and in the development of many new immunosuppressive agents, both drugs and monoclonal antibodies. The future promises to be exciting. Nowhere is the excitement of the past reflected better than in the recollections of 35 of the pioneers of transplantation gathered together by Terasaki (1991).

REFERENCES

Belzer, F. O., Ashby, B. S. and Dunphy, J. S. (1967). 24-Hour and 72-hour preservation of canine kidneys. *Lancet* **2**, 536.

Bogaerde, J. van den and White, D. J. G. (1997). Xenogeneic transplantation. *Br. Med. Bull.* **53**, 904.

Borel, J. F. (1976). Comparative study of in vitro and in vivo drug effects on cell mediated cytotoxicity. *Immunology* **31**, 631.

Burdick, J. F., DeMeester, J. and Koyama, I. (1999). Understanding Organ Procurement and the Transplant Bureaucracy. *In Transplantation*, (L. C. Ginns, A. B. Cosimi and P. J. Morris, eds.), Blackwell, Boston, pp 875–894.

Calne, R. Y. (1960). The rejection of renal homografts: inhibition in dogs by 6 mercapto-purine. *Lancet* **1**, 417.

Calne, R. Y. (1981). The development of immunosuppressive therapy. *Transplant. Proc.* **13**, 44.

Calne, R. Y., Alexandre, G. P. J. and Murray, J. E. (1962). The development of immunosuppressive therapy. *Ann. N. Y. Acad. Sci.* **99**, 743.

Calne, R. Y., White, D. J. G., Thiru, S., *et al.* (1978). Cyclosporin A in patients receiving renal allografts from cadaver donors. *Lancet* **2**, 1323.

Carrel, A. (1902). La technique operatoire des anastomoses vasculaires et la transplantation des visceres. *Lyon Med.* **98**, 859.

Carrel, A. (1914). The transplantation of organs. *N.Y. Med. J.* **99**, 389.

Collins, G. M., Bravo-Shugarman, M. and Terasaki, P. I. (1969). Kidney preservation for transportation: initial perfusion and 30 hours' ice storage. *Lancet* **2**, 1219.

Dausset, J. (1958). Iso-leuco-anticorps. *Acta Haematol. (Basel)* **20**, 156.

Dausset, J. (1980). The challenge of the early days of human histocompatibility. *Immunogenetics* **10**, 1.

Decastello, A. von (1902). Experimentelle nierentransplantation. *Wien Klin. Wochenschr.* **15**, 317.

Dempster, W. J. (1953). The homotransplantation of kidneys in dogs. *Br. J. Surg.* **40**, 447.

Dubost, C., Oeconomos, N., Vaysse, J., Hamburger, J., Nenna, A. and Milliez, P. (1951). Resultants d'une tentative de greffe renale. *Bull. Soc. Med. Hop. Paris* **67**, 1372.

French, M.E. and Batchelor, J.R. (1969). Immunological enhancement of rat kidney grafts. *Lancet* **2**, 1103.

Goodwin, W. E., Mims, M. M. and Kaufman, J. J. (1962). Human renal transplant III: technical problems encountered in six cases of kidney homotransplantation. *Trans. Am. Assoc. Genitourin. Surg.* **54**, 116.

Hamburger, J., Vaysse, J., Crosnier, J., *et al.* (1959). Transplantation of a kidney between non-monozygotic twins after irradiation of the receiver: good function at the fourth month. *Presse Med.* **67**, 1771.

Hamburger, J., Vaysse, J., Crosnier, J., Auvert, J., Lalanne, Cl. M. and Hopper, J. (1962). Renal homotransplantation in man after radiation of the recipient. *Am. J. Med.* **32**, 854.

Hamilton, D. (1982). A history of transplantation. *In Tissue Transplantation*, 2nd ed. (P. J. Morris, ed.), p. 1, Churchill Livingstone, Edinburgh.

Hamilton, D. and Reid, W. A. (1984). Yu. Yu. Voronoy and the first human kidney allograft. *Surg. Gynecol. Obstet.* **159**, 289.

Hopewell, J., Calne, R. Y. and Beswick, I. (1964). Three clinical cases of renal transplantation. *Br. Med. J.* **1**, 411.

Hume, D. M. (1964). Discussion. *Ann. Surg.* **160**, 409.

Hume, D. M., Magee, J. H., Kauffman, H. M., Rittenbury, M. S. and Prout, G. R. (1963). Renal homotransplantation in man in modified recipients. *Ann. Surg.* **158**, 608.

Hume, D. M., Merrill, J. P., Miller, B. F. and Thorn, G. W. (1955). Experiences with renal homotransplantation in the human: report of nine cases. *J. Clin. Invest.* **34**, 327.

Jaboulay, M. (1906). Greffe de reins au pli du coude par soudure arte. *Bull. Lyon Med.* **107**, 575. (For a biography of Jaboulay, see *Biogr. Med. Paris* (1936). **10**, 257.)

Kissmeyer-Nielsen, F., Olsen, S., Peterson, V. P. and Fjeldborg, O. (1966). Hyperacute rejection of kidney allografts. *Lancet* **2**, 662.

Küss, R., Legraine, M. and Mathe, G., *et al.* (1960). Prémices d'une homotransplantation rénale de souer à frère non jumeaux. *Presse Med.* **68**, 755.

Küss, R., Legraine, M., Mathe, G., Nedey, R. and Camey, M. (1962). Homologous human kidney transplantation. *Postgrad. Med. J.* **38**, 528.

Küss, R., Teinturier, J. and Milliez, P. (1951). Quelques essais de greffe du rein chez l'homme. *Mem. Acad. Chir.* **77**, 755.

Michon, L., Hamburger, J., Oeconomos, N., *et al.* (1953). Une tentative de transplantation renale chez d'homme. *Presse Med.* **61**, 1419.

Moore, F. D. (1964). *Give and Take: The Development of Tissue Transplantation*, p. 1, W. B. Saunders, Philadelphia.

Morris, P. J. (1987). Problems facing the Society today. *Transplant. Proc.* **19**, 16.

Morris, P. J., Ting, A. and Stocker, J. (1968). Leucocyte antigens in renal transplantation I: the paradox of blood transfusions in renal transplantation. *Med. J. Aust.* **2**, 1088.

Murray, J. E. (1992). Human organ transplantation: background and consequences. *Science* **256**, 1411.

Murray, J. E., Merrill, J. P., Dammin, G. J., *et al.* (1960). Study of transplantation immunity after total body irradiation: clinical and experimental investigation. *Surgery* **48**, 272.

Murray, J. E., Merrill, J. P. and Harrison, J. H. (1958). Kidney transplantation between seven pairs of identical twins. *Ann. Surg.* **148**, 343.

Murray, J. E., Merrill, J. P., Harrison, J. H., Wilson, R. E. and Dammin, G. J. (1963). Prolonged survival of human kidney homografts by immunosuppressive drug therapy. *N. Engl. J. Med.* **268**, 1315.

Murray, J. E., Tilney, N. L. and Wilson, R. E. (1976). Renal transplantation: a twenty-five year experience. *Ann. Surg.* **184**, 565.

Opelz, G., Sengar, D. P. S., Mickey, M. R. and Terasaki, P. I. (1973). Effect of blood transfusions on subsequent kidney transplants. *Transplant. Proc.* **5**, 253.

Reemtsma, K., McCracken, B. H., Schlegel, J. U., *et al.* (1964). Renal heterotransplantation in man. *Ann. Surg.* **160**, 384.

Rood, J. J. van (1967). *Histocompatibility Testing, 1967*, p. 451, Munkgaard, Copenhagen.

Schwartz, R. S. (1976). *In Design and Achievements in Chemotherapy* (G. H. Hitchings, ed.), Burroughs Wellcome, Research Triangle Park, Durham, N.C.

Schwartz, R. and Dameshek, W. (1959). Drug-induced immunological tolerance. *Nature* **183**, 1682.

Servelle, M., Soulié, P., Rougeulle, J., Delahaye, G. and Touche, M. (1951). Greffe d'une reine de supplicie a une malade avec rein unique congenital, atteinte de nephrite chronique hypertensive azotemique. *Bull. Soc. Med. Hop. Paris* **67**, 99.

Simonsen, M. (1953). Biological incompatibility in kidney transplantation in dogs: serological investigations. *Acta Pathol. Microbiol. Scand.* **32**, 1.

Starzl, T. E. (1978). Personal reflections in transplantation. *Surg. Clin. North Am.* **58**, 879.

Starzl, T. E., Marchioro, T. L. and Waddell, W. R. (1963). The reversal of rejection in human renal homografts with subsequent development of homograft tolerance. *Surg. Gynecol. Obstet.* **117**, 385.

Terasaki, P. I. (1991). *History of Transplantation: Thirty-five Recollections*, UCLA Tissue Typing Laboratory, Los Angeles.

Terasaki, P. I., Marchioro, T. L. and Starzl, T. E. (1965). *In Histocompatibility Testing*. (D.B. Amos and J.J. van Rood, eds.) p. 83, National Academy of Sciences, Washington.

Ting, A. and Morris, P. J. (1978). Matching for B-cell antigens of the HLA-DR (D-related) series in cadaver renal transplantation. *Lancet* **1**, 575.

Ullmann, E. (1902). Experimentelle Nierentransplantation. *Wien Klin. Wochenschr.* **15**, 281. (For a biography of Ullmann, see Lesky, E. (1974). Die erste Nierentransplantation: Emerich Ullmann (1861–1937). *Munch. Med. Wochenschr.* **116**, 1081.)

Ullmann, E. (1914). Tissue and organ transplantation. *Ann. Surg.* **60**, 195.

Unger, E. (1909). Nierentransplantation. *Berl. Klin. Wochenschr.* **1**, 1057.

Voronoy, Yu. Yu. (1936). Sobre el bloqueo del aparato reticulo-endothelial. *Siglo Med.* **97**, 296.

White, O.J.G., Langford, A., Cozzi, E.E., and Young, V. (1995). Production of pigs transgenic for human DAF. Xenotransplantation **2**, 213.

Winkler, F. A. (1982). Ernst Unger: a pioneer in modern surgery. *J. Hist. Med. Allied Sci.* **37**, 269.

Zukoski, C. F., Lee, H. M. and Hume, D. M. (1960). The effect of 6-mercaptopurine on renal homograft survival in the dog. *Surg. Forum* **11**, 47.

Immunology of Graft Rejection
Margaret J. Dallman

Introduction

For patients with renal failure, transplantation remains the treatment of choice. In most cases, this procedure entails the use of an organ from a genetically disparate individual (see Table 2–1 for terminology) and inevitably results in a response both of the host and in the graft. Some of these responses occur as a result of the trauma associated with organ harvest, perfusion and surgery, whereas others involve specific recognition by the immune system of antigenic differences between donor and recipient. The cumulative effect of these events is a destructive response that, if uncontrolled, leads to loss of the transplant, as originally highlighted by workers such as Little and Tyzzer (1916). The immunological nature of tissue rejection as originally suggested by Gorer (1938) was firmly established more than 50 years ago by Medawar (Gibson and Medawar, 1943; Medawar, 1944, 1945) after the demonstration that the rejection process in humans and rodents displays marked specificity and memory for donor tissue and is accompanied by infiltration with leukocytes.

Understanding of the immune system has evolved considerably, and as a consequence we now are able to describe more fully the molecular and cellular events that result in graft rejection. With such knowledge has come an impressive range of new, primarily biological agents including antibodies and fusion proteins that are targeted to specific aspects of the immune response in an attempt to deliver better and more selective immunosuppression. Many of these agents are currently in clinical use or trial, complementing current favorites such as cyclosporine, FK506 and steroids. Despite this wealth of immunosuppressive agents, clinically detectable acute rejection is common and may damage the graft such that slowly deteriorating renal function accompanied by the histological changes of chronic rejection occurs (see Chapters 24 and 27). Current use of immunosuppressive agents is relatively unsophisticated in that we have little means by which we can tailor therapy to individual patients. An ability to do just this remains a major challenge in transplantation and is likely to be achieved only when we can develop an entire profile of the evolution of the immune response after transplantation and understand all of the parameters that control immunity. Developing new methods to trace the emerging response and to predict its outcome remains an important goal.

This chapter describes the molecular and cellular events of the immune response that are understood, and it assumes a basic level of knowledge of the cells and molecules involved in immune responses. The reader is referred to other books and reviews for general descriptions of the immune system (Halloran et al., 1993; Janeway et al., 1999).

Trauma of Transplantation

The response to a transplant occurs in a series of relatively well-defined stages as laid out in Figure 2–1, the first of which involves the severe physical assault that the graft undergoes during harvest from the donor and transplantation into the recipient. This involves cooling the kidney to lower its metabolic rate; perfusion with preservation solution, which is designed to reduce cold-induced cell swelling and prevent loss of potassium from the cell; storage for sometimes long periods, which results in pH changes and the accumulation of toxic products, and the surgical procedures required for transplantation to the recipient. All of these events sensitize the organ to reperfusion injury when the organ is warmed rapidly on revascularization in the recipient. The use of superoxide dismutase, which has antioxidant action and may limit the effects of free radicals released at this time, has been shown to be beneficial in the clinical setting (Land et al., 1994). During and shortly after the ischemic and reperfusion periods, a variety of genes become activated, and inflammatory cells begin to infiltrate the graft. The induction of several soluble proteins or cytokines (or transcripts of cytokines), such as interleukin (IL)-6 and IL-1, can be shown at early time points after transplantation even of syngeneic grafts in which there is no antigenic difference between donor and recipient and in which an immune response is not generated (Dallman et al., 1991a; Tono et al., 1992). Probably as a result of this induction together with an up-regulated expression of adhesion proteins on the vascular endothelium and other cells of the graft (Koo et al., 1998), an early infiltrate of inflammatory cells including macrophages develops (McLean et al., 1997). These early events alone do not result in graft rejection and, as noted, are observed in syngeneic grafts. Their influence on early graft function and later importance in acute and chronic rejection are unclear, however.

The specific immune response to a graft occurs in two main stages. In the first, the afferent arm, donor antigens are presented to the recipient T lymphocytes, which become activated, proliferate and differentiate further while sending signals for growth and differentiation to a variety of other cells. In the second stage, or efferent arm, effector leukocytes are recruited into the organ where they can wreak the havoc that results in tissue destruction.

Presentation of Antigen to Recipient T Lymphocytes

ANTIGENS THAT STIMULATE GRAFT REJECTION

The histocompatibility antigens determine the outcome of tissue allografts between different members of the same species. In all vertebrate species, histocompatibility antigens can be divided into a single major histocompatibility complex or system (MHC) and numerous minor histocompatibility (miH) systems. Incompatibility for either MHC or miH antigens between donor and recipient leads to an immune response against the graft, but more vigorous rejection occurs in the face of MHC differences. In a nonsensitized recipient,

TABLE 2–1

TRANSPLANT TERMINOLOGY

Autograft (autologous transplant)	Transplantation of an individual's own tissue to another site (e.g., the use of a patient's own skin to cover third-degree burns or a saphenous vein femoropopliteal graft)
Isograft (syngeneic or isogeneic transplant)	Transplantation of tissue between genetically identical members of the same species (e.g., kidney transplant between identical twins or grafts between mice of the same inbred strain)
Allograft (allogeneic transplant)	Transplantation of tissue between genetically nonidentical members of the same species (e.g., cadaveric renal transplant or graft between mice of different inbred strains)
Xenograft (xenogeneic transplant)	Transplantation of tissue between members of different species (e.g., baboon kidney into a human)

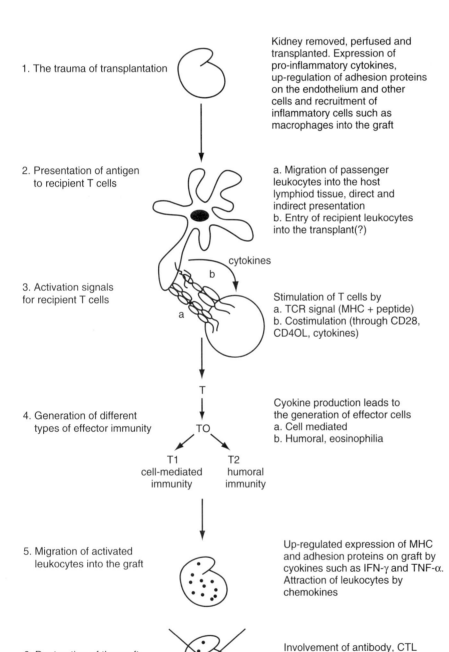

1. The trauma of transplantation

Kidney removed, perfused and transplanted. Expression of pro-inflammatory cytokines, up-regulation of adhesion proteins on the endothelium and other cells and recruitment of inflammatory cells such as macrophages into the graft

2. Presentation of antigen to recipient T cells

a. Migration of passenger leukocytes into the host lymphiod tissue, direct and indirect presentation
b. Entry of recipient leukocytes into the transplant(?)

cytokines
b

3. Activation signals for recipient T cells

a

Stimulation of T cells by
a. TCR signal (MHC + peptide)
b. Costimulation (through CD28, CD4OL, cytokines)

T
TO

4. Generation of different types of effector immunity

Cyokine production leads to the generation of effector cells
a. Cell mediated
b. Humoral, eosinophilia

T1
cell-mediated
immunity

T2
humoral
immunity

5. Migration of activated leukocytes into the graft

Up-regulated expression of MHC and adhesion proteins on graft by cyokines such as IFN-γ and TNF-α. Attraction of leukocytes by chemokines

6. Destruction of the graft

Involvement of antibody, CTL macrophages, cytokines and eosinophiils

FIGURE 2–1

The evolution of the immune response after kidney transplantation. TCR = T-cell receptor; MHC = major histocompatibility complex; IFN = interferon; TNF = tumor necrosis factor; CTL = cytotoxic T cell.

rejection of MHC-compatible organ grafts may not occur or may be delayed, although there is evidence that multiple miH differences alone can result in cardiac allograft rejection in mice as rapidly as that seen with transplantation across a full MHC barrier (Peugh et al., 1986). It is a different matter with bone marrow, however, in which transplants between HLA-identical siblings may be rejected or cause graft-versus-host disease because of a disparity between host and donor in only a limited number of minor antigens (Goulmy, 1985).

Major Histocompatibility Antigens

There is substantial similarity between the MHC in different species with respect to immunogenetics and protein structure, although the order of genes within the complex varies among different species (Fig. 2–2). The genes within the MHC are divided into class I, class II and class III types (Campbell and Trowsdale, 1993; Klein et al., 1981); the human MHC (HLA) is described more fully in Chapter 10 and Chapter 43. Major histocompatibility class I proteins (Fig. 2–3) are cell surface glycoproteins composed of two chains, the heavy chain (molecular weight approximately 45 kd), which is highly polymorphic and encoded within the MHC by a class I gene, and a nonvariable light chain, β_2-microglobulin (molecular weight approximately 12 kd), which is encoded at another chromosomal location. In contrast to the heavy chain, β_2-microglobulin is not anchored in the membrane so that it may be exchanged for, or stabilized by, β_2-microglobulin from the surrounding fluid. Major histocompatibility class I proteins are expressed on most nucleated cells albeit at variable levels and are, in general, responsible for activating T cells bearing the CD8 surface protein (CD8+ cells; see later). Major histocompatibility class II proteins are encoded entirely within the MHC and are also membrane anchored glycoproteins. They are composed of two chains of similar molecular weight (alpha chain, molecular weight approximately 35 kd; beta chain, molecular weight approximately 28 kd). These chains primarily stimulate T cells bearing the CD4 surface protein (CD4+ cells). The tissue distribution of class II proteins is far more restricted than that of class I, being ex-

pressed constitutively only by B lymphocytes, dendritic cells and some endothelial cells. During an immune or inflammatory response, however, many other cell types, with a few exceptions, may be induced to express MHC class II proteins (Dallman et al., 1982; Fellous et al., 1982; Fuggle et al., 1986; Lampert et al., 1981; Mason et al., 1981; de Waal et al., 1983; Wong et al., 1984).

Major histocompatibility class I and II proteins form a similar three-dimensional structure at the cell surface (see Fig. 2–3 for a ribbon diagram of HLA-A2). Within this structure is a groove flanked by two alpha helices, and the amino acids in this groove show the highest degree of polymorphism within a species. During the synthesis and transport of MHC class I and class II proteins to the cell surface, they become associated with small peptides that fit into the groove. The groove of MHC class I has a rather closed structure, allowing peptides no longer than about 8 to 10 amino acids in size to be accommodated, whereas that of MHC class II has a more open structure permitting the ends of the peptides to flop out of the groove, allowing it to accommodate peptides of at least 13 and often many more amino acids in length. A major difference between proteins of the two MHC classes is in the origin of these peptides, which are acquired primarily (although not exclusively) from the intracellular environment in the case of class I and extracellular environment in the case of class II (Fig. 2–4). The combination of MHC and peptide is recognized by the antigen receptor (T-cell receptor [TCR]) on the T cell. In a pathogen-free immune system, the peptides contained within the MHC proteins originate largely from self-proteins, and many may be derived from the MHC proteins themselves. It is only when a foreign pathogen invades or a graft is in place that the MHC proteins become loaded with foreign peptides. The ability to extract peptides from within MHC proteins (Rammensee et al., 1993; Rotzschke et al., 1991) has begun to indicate the types of peptides that are generated from antigens and that reside within the MHC groove. It is becoming possible to predict from the protein sequence of an antigen which peptides will be recognized in the context of different MHC antigens. It is possible, with a knowledge of the MHC and

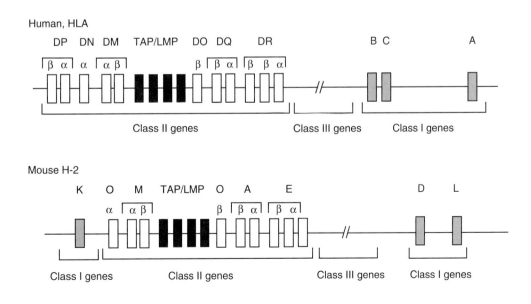

FIGURE 2–2

Genomic organization of HLA and H-2 regions. The order of genes in the MHC of human (HLA) and mouse (H-2). Many people have, in addition to those shown, an extra HLA-DR beta gene whose product can pair with HLA-DR alpha, and consequently many people have four possible class II products from each chromosome. See Figure 2–4 legend for an explanation of HLA-DNα and HLA-DOβ. TAP = transporters associated with antigen processing; LMP = proteosome components.

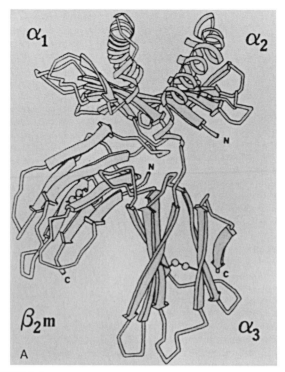
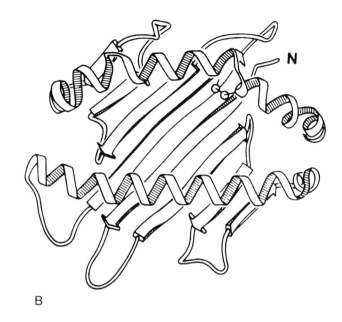

FIGURE 2–3

Ribbon diagrams of HLA-A2. The structure of the human MHC complex class I antigen HLA-A2. The peptide groove is clearly visible lying between the two alpha helices. (A) Side view. (B) Bird's eye, or the T cell's, view. MHC class II proteins have a similar structure, although the ends of the groove are less closely associated allowing the peptide to extend beyond the constraints of the groove.

peptide sequences, to predict which amino acids in the peptide will be associated with the floor and sides of the groove and which will be in contact with the TCR.

Several other proteins encoded within the MHC aid the assembly and loading of class I and II proteins with their peptides. One type of class II protein, HLA-DM, does not appear on the cell surface but plays a role in exchanging the CLIP peptide for the antigenic peptide in class II proteins before they emigrate to the cell surface (Roche, 1995). The *LMP* (proteosome components) and *TAP* (transporters associated with antigen processing) genes also lie within the class II region of the MHC and are involved in processing and loading of peptides for MHC class I presentation. Understanding of such antigen processing and presentation pathways has increased (Belich and Trowsdale, 1995; Cresswell, 1994; Germain and Margulies, 1993; Grey and Chestnut, 1985; Monaco, 1992, 1993, 1995), and this, together with the structural resolution of MHC and TCR proteins (Bjorkman, 1997;

Bjorkman *et al.*, 1987; Garcia *et al.*, 1996; see Fig. 2-3), represents some of the most important advances in immunology in the 1990s.

Data from experiments performed between congenic strains of animals in which only MHC class I or II antigens differ in donor and recipient show that both are important in graft rejection, although frequently grafts with only MHC class I disparities reject more slowly than grafts with class II only or class I and class II differences (Klein *et al.*, 1977; Rosenberg, 1993). Mice with disrupted expression of either β_2-microglobulin (in which surface expression of the whole class I protein is largely prevented, class I$^{-/-}$ mice) or class II genes (class II$^{-/-}$ mice) have been generated and used as recipient (see later) or donor in transplantation experiments. The literature regarding this work is complex. In many studies a lack of class I or class II antigens alone on donor tissue has little effect on graft survival (Auchincloss *et al.*, 1993; Dierich *et al.*, 1993; Henretta *et al.*, 1995; Li and Faustman,

FIGURE 2–4

Antigen processing and presentation in the MHC class I and II pathways. (A) Processing of endogenous antigens occurs primarily by way of the class I pathway. Peptides are produced and loaded into MHC class I proteins as shown in steps 1 through 4. During the synthesis of MHC class I proteins (steps A through C), the alpha chain is stabilized by calnexin before β_2-microglobulin binds. Folding of the MHC class $1/\beta_2$-microglobulin remains incomplete, but the complex is released by calnexin to bind with the chaperone proteins, tapaisin and calreticulin. Only when the TAP transporter delivers peptide to the MHC class $1/\beta_2$-microglobulin can folding of this complex be completed and transport to the cell membrane occur (steps 5, 6). (B) Processing of exogenous antigens occurs primarily by way of the class II pathway. Antigens are taken up into intracellular vesicles where acidification aids their degradation into peptide fragments (steps 1, 2). Vesicles containing peptides fuse with trans-Golgi, containing CLIP-MHC class II complexes (step 3). DM aids removal of CLIP and loading of peptide before the class II peptide complex is displayed on the cell surface (steps 4, 5). MHC class II proteins are synthesized in the endoplasmic reticulum where peptide binding is prevented by invariant chain. Invariant chain is cleaved leaving the CLIP peptide still in place (steps A, B) before fusing with acidified vesicles containing peptide. In B lymphocytes and epithelial cells of the thymus, an atypical class II protein, HLA-DO, is expressed that is a dimer of HLA-DNα and HLA-DOβ. It, similar to HLA-DM, is not expressed at the cell surface and inhibits the action of HLA-DM. Its precise role is unknown. TAP = transporters associated with antigen processing; ER = endoplasmic reticulum; MHC = major histocompatibility complex; ATP = adenosine triphosphate; CLIP = class II associated invariant chain peptide; β_2m = β-2-microglobulin.

The Class I pathway

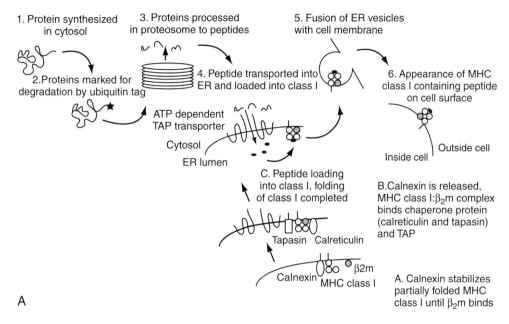

1. Protein synthesized in cytosol

2. Proteins marked for degradation by ubiquitin tag

3. Proteins processed in proteosome to peptides

4. Peptide transported into ER and loaded into class I

ATP dependent TAP transporter

Cytosol

ER lumen

5. Fusion of ER vesicles with cell membrane

6. Appearance of MHC class I containing peptide on cell surface

Inside cell Outside cell

C. Peptide loading into class I, folding of class I completed

Tapasin Calreticulin

Calnexin MHC class I $\beta 2m$

B. Calnexin is released, MHC class I:β_2m complex binds chaperone protein (calreticulin and tapasin) and TAP

A. Calnexin stabilizes partially folded MHC class I until β_2m binds

A

The Class II pathway

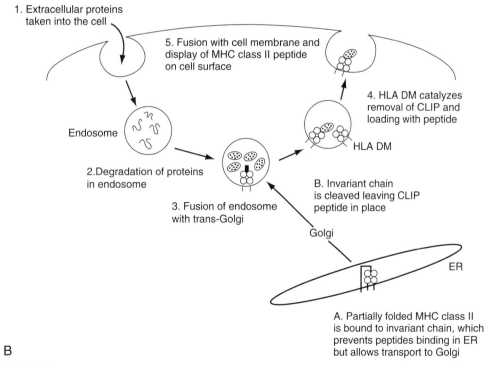

1. Extracellular proteins taken into the cell

Endosome

2. Degradation of proteins in endosome

3. Fusion of endosome with trans-Golgi

5. Fusion with cell membrane and display of MHC class II peptide on cell surface

4. HLA DM catalyzes removal of CLIP and loading with peptide

HLA DM

B. Invariant chain is cleaved leaving CLIP peptide in place

Golgi

ER

A. Partially folded MHC class II is bound to invariant chain, which prevents peptides binding in ER but allows transport to Golgi

B

FIGURE 2–4

See legend on opposite page

1993; Mannon *et al.*, 1995). In other experiments, graft survival may be prolonged or permanent when donor tissue lacks either class I (Henretta *et al.*, 1995; Markmann *et al.*, 1992) or class II only (Campos *et al.*, 1995; Henretta *et al.*, 1995) or both class I and II antigens (Campos *et al.*, 1995; Mannon *et al.*, 1995; Osorio *et al.*, 1993). It is clear from all of this work that results vary when different types of grafts are used, probably reflecting a greater or lesser involvement of the different T-cell subsets ($CD4^+$ and $CD8^+$; see later; Campos *et al.*, 1995; Henretta *et al.*, 1995). The interpretation of some of these apparently straightforward experiments is complicated, however, by the suggestion that grafts from class $I^{-/-}$ mice may be reconstituted in their expression of class I by serum β_2-microglobulin in the recipient or may express residual cell surface class I protein in the absence of β_2-microglobulin (Lee *et al.*, 1997; Li and Faustman, 1993).

One notable feature of MHC protein that makes it quite unlike any other region of the chromosome and the feature that creates serious problems for the transplant clinician is the high degree of polymorphism in the class I and II cell surface proteins that it encodes. It is likely that this extensive polymorphism has evolved as a product of immune defense mechanisms against infection (Klein *et al.*, 1981). Certain species that have limited polymorphism at class I or class II loci can be devastated by infections that in closely related species with a polymorphic MHC are cleared without difficulty (O'Brien *et al.*, 1985). With two alleles at each MHC locus, most people can express six different MHC class I proteins and eight different MHC class II proteins (see Fig. 2–2). Combined with the polymorphism at this locus, this means that for transplantation between unrelated individuals MHC-identical donors and recipients are extremely uncommon, and even when they are found, miH antigens are almost undoubtedly different. It is only realistically possible clinically to graft tissue that is both MHC and miH antigen identical between monozygotic twins; this is why immunosuppression is needed routinely in clinical transplantation.

As described earlier, there are several genes within the class II and class I regions that do not encode classic MHC proteins. In addition to the genes mentioned previously, some of these encode nonclassic MHC proteins that are similar in structure to classic MHC proteins but that are nonpolymorphic. These may have antigen presenting capacity for specialized antigens, such as lipids (e.g., mycolic acid and lipoarabinomannan from mycobacterium) or peptides of different sequence but with common characteristics (e.g., with *N*-formylated amino termini).

The class III region of the MHC is large and contains many uncharacterized genes (Campbell and Trowsdale, 1993). The genes that have been characterized encode proteins with a variety of different functions, and although they themselves do not stimulate T cells in the same way as class I and II proteins, many have important activities in generating and influencing immunity. For example, tumor necrosis factor TNF-α and TNF-β are encoded in the class III region, and a marker of TNF-α polymorphism that associates with high TNF production has been found in heart transplant patients (Turner *et al.*, 1995).

Minor Histocompatibility Antigens

Although the highest degree of genetic polymorphism within a species lies within the MHC, many other loci encode proteins with a lower degree of variability, and from genetic studies it has been clear that such proteins can act as transplantation antigens. They have been termed *minor histocompatibility antigens*, although their structure and distribution was for many years elusive. Although T cells could recognize

and respond to cells from MHC-identical individuals, it was almost impossible to raise antibodies against the antigens involved, making biochemical characterization difficult. The knowledge that T cells recognize small peptides from antigens, together with the resourceful application of molecular techniques, allowed the characterization of the prototypic miH antigen, the male antigen or H-Y (Scott *et al.*, 1995; Wang *et al.*, 1995). From such work, it is clear not only that miH antigens are a composite of peptides from low-polymorphic or nonpolymorphic proteins, presented in the MHC groove, but also that the so-called H-Y antigen is derived from a group of proteins encoded on the Y chromosome (Greenfield *et al.*, 1996; Scott *et al.*, 1995, 1997; Wang *et al.*, 1995). The former finding explains why it has been difficult to raise antibodies to miH antigens because antibodies most frequently recognize conformational determinants on proteins, and peptides bound within the MHC groove may not be accessible for recognition by the antibody-producing B lymphocyte.

Minor histocompatibility antigens may play a prominent role in graft rejection in a recipient who is given an MHC-compatible graft but in whom preexisting sensitization to miH antigens exists. This situation can be demonstrated in the rat and mouse (Fabre and Morris, 1975; Peugh *et al.*, 1986) and probably explains the occurrence of rejection episodes (which rarely result in graft loss) in renal transplants performed between HLA-identical siblings. Multiple miH differences have been shown to represent an immunogenic stimulus equivalent to that of the MHC in a nonsensitized recipient of a cardiac allograft in the mouse (Peugh *et al.*, 1986), but it is difficult to gather similar data in clinical transplantation. Polymorphic tissue–specific antigens also may be common, and such systems have been shown for mouse skin (Steinmuller and Wachtal, 1980) and rat kidney (Hart and Fabre, 1980). In the rat, incompatibility for kidney antigens alone is not capable of causing rejection of a renal allograft, even when the recipient has been presensitized. An endothelial-monocyte antigenic system has been shown in humans, and it has been suggested that cells sensitized to these antigens can cause graft damage (Cerrilli *et al.*, 1977; Paul *et al.*, 1979). More miH antigens are being characterized, and this whole area has been reviewed extensively by others (Simpson, 1998; Simpson *et al.*, 1998).

DONOR PASSENGER LEUKOCYTES AND DIRECT ANTIGEN PRESENTATION

Immunization with MHC antigen in the form of a soluble membrane extract or in liposomes may not produce an immune response (Welsh *et al.*, 1977), whereas integrated cell surface MHC proteins may be highly immunogenic. Presentation of MHC class I antigen on cells that do not express class II antigens (e.g., red cells in the rodent or platelets) does not produce a good primary immune response (Batchelor *et al.*, 1978; Fisher *et al.*, 1985; Rollinghoff and Wagner, 1975), suggesting that MHC class II antigens must be present on the immunizing cells for an immune response to be generated. It seems that in some cases presentation of incompatible class I antigens in the absence of class II antigen may not only fail to evoke a primary immune response, but also may initiate a state of active suppression or tolerance (see Chapter 23).

The level of immunogenicity of MHC proteins varies considerably with the cell type on which they are found. Cells with the characteristics of bone marrow–derived leukocytes were found throughout the body in nonlymphoid as well as in lymphoid tissues (Daar *et al.*, 1983; Hart and Fabre, 1981a). The nonlymphoid *passenger leukocytes*, which clearly are not macrophages, migrate rapidly out of a tissue after transplantation to the recipient lymphoid organs where they are able to interact with and stimulate the host immune response (Larsen *et al.*, 1990a, 1990b). Such passenger leukocytes have the characteristics of immature dendritic cells (Reis e Sousa *et al.*, 1993), which on migration mature rapidly into antigen-presenting cells that are particularly potent in their ability to stimulate T lymphocytes (Steinman, 1991; Steinman and Witmer, 1978; Steinman *et al.*, 1983). Mature dendritic cells express a high level of MHC class I and II antigens and as such are able to stimulate CD4[+] and CD8[+] T lymphocytes. These cells have many additional features (see later—costimulation) that make them uniquely powerful in stimulating naive (previously unactivated) T cells, earning them the title of *professional* antigen-presenting cells. Because T cells are central to the rejection of foreign transplants—animals deprived of T cells through genetic mutation or through experimental manipulation are unable to reject grafts (Hall *et al.*, 1978; Rolstad and Ford, 1974; Rygaard, 1974)—it made sense that these migrant dendritic cells were central to the activation of the recipient immune system in response to a transplant.

Many experimental transplantation systems have been used to dissect the role of the dendritic cell in graft rejection. Such experiments have been essentially of two types. In the first type of experiment, grafts have been depleted of their own passenger leukocytes by irradiation or tissue culture of the graft or by exchange with dendritic cells of recipient type (Emma and Jacobs, 1981; Guttman *et al.*, 1969; Lafferty *et al.*, 1976; Steinmuller and Hart, 1971; Stuart *et al.*, 1971). The latter situation is achieved by placing grafts in immunosuppressed animals of recipient origin or in an F1 hybrid recipient (in which rejection will not occur) and allowing the replacement of passenger leukocytes by cells of recipient type to result from the natural turnover of bone marrow–derived cells. Such grafts transplanted into a secondary recipient may show prolonged survival, which was taken originally to suggest that donor dendritic cells were critical to the initiation of rejection. This interpretation is complicated by the fact that we now know that long-term surviving grafts in this type of situation may contain leukocytes with an immunoregulatory function, however, and it may be these leukocytes that allow prolonged survival of the graft in the second host. In the second type of experiment, induction of a rejection episode in long-term surviving grafts has been attempted using passenger leukocytes of tissue donor origin (Lechler and Batchelor, 1982).

In all of these studies, the presence or origin of the passenger leukocyte may influence graft survival, but clear data implicating the dendritic cell as the primary or only stimulus of graft rejection in all donor-recipient pairs are lacking. One must interpret these experimental data with some caution when considering clinical transplantation rejection because although in rodents often the only cell within the graft to express MHC class II antigens is the passenger leukocyte, in humans vascular endothelial cells constitutively express these proteins (Frelinger *et al.*, 1979; Fuggle *et al.*, 1983; Hart and Fabre, 1981b; Katz *et al.*, 1979) and as such also may stimulate the rejection. There are data to suggest that this is the case (Hughes *et al.*, 1990; Page *et al.*, 1994a, 1994b; Pober and Cotran, 1991; Rose, 1997, 1998).

Despite the caveats mentioned with the previously described experiments, it generally has become accepted that presentation of donor MHC by donor dendritic cells does provide a major stimulus to the T cells of the recipient by so-called direct antigen presentation (Fig. 2–5A) and that this largely is responsible for the stimulation of acute graft rejection. This suggestion is somewhat counterintuitive when one considers that the T-cell repertoire is skewed (by positive

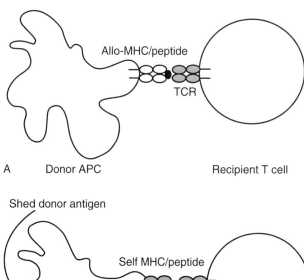

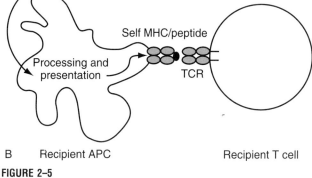

FIGURE 2–5

Direct and indirect pathways of antigen presentation. Sensitization of the recipient can occur by antigen presentation delivered through passenger leukocytes or dendritic cells of donor origin (direct antigen presentation, A) or recipient origin (indirect antigen presentation, B). APC = antigen presenting cell; MHC = major histocompatibility complex; TCR = T cell receptor.

selection of T cells in the thymus) toward recognition of peptide in the context of self-MHC proteins. It is clear experimentally, however, that allogeneic MHC/peptide complexes provide a strong stimulus to the immune system, and a high frequency—1 to 10%—of all T cells respond to any allogeneic MHC. The allogeneic MHC contains peptides derived from the donor tissue originating mainly from normal nonpolymorphic proteins (Rotzschke *et al.*, 1991) or the MHC itself (Golding and Singer, 1984; Parham *et al.*, 1987). In the context of self-MHC, the former type of peptide would not induce an immune response because the body would be tolerant of them.

When the MHC is allogeneic (i.e., when a graft is placed into an MHC-disparate recipient), the sum of the MHC + nonpolymorphic peptide may now be recognized as not-self and stimulate a T cell. The real job of such T cells is not to respond to alloantigen but to eliminate invading organisms. Their ability to respond to alloantigen is due to an inconvenient cross-reactivity of their receptor for self-MHC + foreign peptide with allogeneic MHC + self-peptide. For many T cells that have respectable reactivity with a foreign peptide + self-MHC, it is possible to show cross-reactivity on one or more alloantigens. Also, different peptides from the same proteins may be displayed by the foreign MHCs and self-MHCs because of the different peptide-binding capacities of each MHC groove. Peptides normally not displayed in self-MHC do not have an opportunity to induce tolerance in the recipient and may induce an immune response when presented on allogeneic MHC proteins. Alloreactive cytotoxic T lymphocytes (CTLs) induced by direct antigen presentation are able to recognize a wide spectrum of different peptide-MHC aggregates and empty MHC molecules, as elegantly shown by Rotzshe et al. (1991). The most likely explanation for the unusually high number of T cells that react to any given allogeneic MHC is that many different self-peptides are derived from the graft, and the combination of these with the allogeneic MHC stimulates many different T-cell clones in the recipient (Dorling and Lechler, 1996).

INDIRECT ANTIGEN PRESENTATION

The fact that elimination from the graft of passenger leukocytes does not abrogate rejection completely suggested that there is a second route to sensitization of the recipient that requires antigen presentation by a class II–expressing cell. As alluded to, in humans the endothelium that bears MHC class II antigens may provide such a route, but also it has become apparent that foreign, graft-derived antigens (of MHC or non-MHC origin) can be presented to the recipient immune system by its own dendritic cells in the process of indirect antigen presentation (Butcher and Howard, 1982; Fangmann et al., 1992; Golding and Singer, 1984; Liu et al., 1992; Rock et al., 1983; Sherwood et al., 1986; Fig. 2–5B). This represents the process by which normal antigens are displayed to the host on an antigen-presenting cell. From what we understand about antigen processing and presentation (see Fig. 2–4), it seems likely that most allogeneic MHC peptides are presented in the context of class II MHC antigens because it is this pathway that deals with proteins exogenous to the cell. There is some crossover between class II and class I pathways, however, such that allogeneic MHC peptides also may be presented in the context of self-class I antigens (Pfeiffer et al., 1995; Malaviya et al., 1996). Fangmann and coworkers in a straightforward experiment showed that indirect presentation may have a practical significance in transplantation responses (Fangmann et al., 1992). They showed that peptides derived from rat class I antigens were able to immunize animals via the indirect pathway for accelerated rejection of a subsequent skin graft carrying the class I antigens from which the peptides were derived. Further information on this issue comes from experiments in which skin grafts from class II$^{-/-}$ mice are transplanted onto normal mice. Antigen-presenting cells from these grafts do not directly stimulate CD4$^+$ cells because of the absence of class II antigen, but graft rejection still occurs and is CD4$^+$ cell dependent. In this case, the CD4$^+$ cells are presumed to have been stimulated by indirect presentation of donor alloantigens on self-MHC (Auchincloss et al., 1993; Lee et al., 1994, 1997). The most recent experiments addressing this issue involve antigen-presenting cells from the recipient or host that are disabled by genetic manipulation such that they no longer express costimulatory molecules, which are one of the hallmarks of professional antigen-presenting cells (B7$^{-/-}$ mice; Mandelbrot et al., 1999). The nature of these costimulatory proteins is described in more detail later in this chapter; the interesting observations of these workers were that the absence of B7 on donor cells had no effect on the kinetics of vascularized heart allograft rejection. Absence of such proteins on the cells of the recipient had a dramatic effect, however, and allowed long-term survival of normal, B7-expressing hearts, data that were taken by the authors to suggest that in this mouse model, costimulation provided by recipient antigen-presenting cells is much more important in the initiation of graft rejection than is that provided by donor antigen-presenting cells. The simplest interpretation is that indirect presentation is playing a more important role than direct presentation in this model, although the possibility that it is simply costimulation provided by recipient antigen-presenting cells that is

important rather than antigen presentation and costimulation cannot be discounted completely.

One problem arises if recipient T cells are stimulated via indirect antigen presentation and that is one of MHC restriction in the effector cell population. The problem arises when the cytotoxic T cell, once stimulated with self-MHC and allogeneic peptide, comes to lyse its target cell—in the case of graft rejection, this is the foreign transplanted tissue, which does not express self-MHC molecules. This problem is overcome if the foreign MHC on the target cell appears to be identical to the degraded foreign MHC in association with self insofar as the T cell is concerned or if the effector arm of the immune response is activated via direct antigen presentation (e.g., cytotoxic T cells reactive with allogeneic MHC class I) or does not involve MHC restriction (e.g., macrophages, delayed-type hypersensitivity [DTH]).

Some workers have long believed that indirect antigen presentation plays the dominant role in acute rejection (Auchincloss and Sultan, 1996), and the evidence appears to be accumulating in favor of this suggestion. Indirect antigen presentation also can provide the continuing antigenic stimulus required for chronic graft rejection (Cramer et al., 1989; Shirwan, 1999), whereas because donor dendritic cells are lost quickly from the graft, direct antigen presentation always has assumed a lesser or absent role in this process.

ACTIVATION OF DENDRITIC CELLS

So far this chapter has concentrated on the role that dendritic cells (or other antigen-presenting cells) play in activating T lymphocytes. T lymphocyte–dendritic cell interactions are reciprocal, however, and it is becoming increasingly clear that T cells control the maturation (Shreeder et al., 1999) and functional phenotype (Rissoan et al., 1999) of dendritic cells. Ligation of CD40 on dendritic cells by CD154 (CD40 ligand) on the T cell results in the up-regulation of the B7 proteins, which, in turn, may affect the T cell further.

Another important feature of dendritic cells and macrophages and other cells of the innate immune system is that although they do not have such a vast range of antigen receptors with the level of fine specificity as do T cells and B cells, they have pattern recognition receptors that recognize common features on pathogens (Medzhitov and Janeway, 1997). The role of these receptors in activating macrophages to a state of cytotoxicity is not in doubt, but it has been suggested that they are less important for the dendritic cell. For dendritic cells, other signals produced from within the body, such as those from stressed or necrotic cells, may assume greater significance (Galluchi et al., 1999).

Although this chapter has concentrated on the role of dendritic cells in activating the immune response, it is becoming increasingly apparent that there are (functional) subsets of dendritic cells and that some of these populations may be critical in the induction of tolerance. This view is becoming widely held, and the consequences of this for the regulation of transplantation responses is increasingly a focus of attention (Thomson and Lu, 1999).

ENTRY OF NAIVE RECIPIENT LYMPHOCYTES INTO GRAFT TISSUE

Naive lymphocytes normally recirculate from blood into lymphoid tissues without entering peripheral tissues and as such are unlikely to become activated in the graft. After small bowel transplantation, however, recipient-derived leukocytes including T lymphocytes migrate in large numbers into the mesenteric lymph nodes and Peyer's patches of the graft, generating a marked cytokine response within 24 hours of grafting (Ingham-Clark *et al.*, 1990; Kim *et al.*, 1991; Toogood *et al.*, 1997). This situation may represent normal homing of such cells because the small bowel is so rich in lymphoid tissue. It is likely that these T cells, if not already activated, may become so within the transplant, which is rich in mature dendritic cells. The extent to which naive T cells enter other types of transplants and become activated *in situ* is less clear—neither do the cells express those adhesion proteins normally associated with homing to peripheral tissues, nor are the dendritic cells within the graft mature.

Activation of Recipient T Cells

T-lymphocyte activation, central to the immune response to a transplant, is a complex process. Much information has been accumulated in this area, and although the antigen signal delivered to the T cell through the TCR/CD3 complex (Fig. 2–6) is absolutely required for activation, T cells also receive many other signals via cell surface receptors without which they do not become fully able to initiate a productive immune response. It is becoming increasingly clear that the contact between antigen-presenting cells and T lymphocytes (and other cells of the immune system) involves supramolecular organization of receptors and ligands into microdomains, or immune synapses, which exhibit reproducible patterns of the receptor-ligand pairs. For instance, it has been shown that adhesion molecules cluster with TCRs on the lymphocyte (Monks *et al.*, 1998). In the T cell–antigen presenting cell synapse, MHC protein initially accumulates in a ring around adhesion proteins but on interaction with the TCR moves to a central patch (Grakoui *et al.*, 1999). This is a newly emerging area of immunology, and it is likely that increased knowledge in this area will help in predicting more accurately the outcome of intercellular interactions.

T-CELL RECEPTOR SIGNALS

Without an interaction of the TCR with its cognate antigen, T cells remain in a quiescent or resting state and can recirculate through the lymphoid tissues for many years (Gowans, 1959; Butcher and Picker, 1996). Most T cells bear a TCR composed of two similar chains, the alpha and beta chains, which are complexed with several more proteins, the γ, δ, ε, and ζ chains of the CD3 complex. The TCR confers specificity of antigen/MHC binding (see Fig. 2–5), whereas the ζ chains of the CD3 complex transduce signals of activation to the T cell. Many intracellular signaling pathways are activated, resulting in *de novo* expression of a range of genes, including those encoding cytokines and new cell surface proteins. The signaling pathways are increasingly well characterized and have been described fully elsewhere (Cantrell *et al.*, 1998; van Leeuwen and Samuelson, 1999). They form the target of many immunosuppressive drugs (Brazelton and Morris, 1996; Gummert *et al.*, 1999; Morris, 1991, 1993).

SECOND OR COSTIMULATORY SIGNALS

The fate of a CD4$^+$ T cell once in receipt of a TCR signal appears to depend critically on whether or not it secures other so-called costimulatory or second signals. Without these second signals, a T cell may become anergic or unresponsive (Jenkins and Schwartz, 1987; Jenkins *et al.*, 1987; Schwartz, 1990, 1997), a state that also may result in an ability to prevent the activation of its neighboring T cells (Frasca *et al.*, 1997; Lombardi *et al.*, 1994). The fact that deprivation of second signals results in such an unresponsive and regulatory fate for T cells has attracted enormous interest because it has implications in preventing graft rejection. There are many cell surface proteins on a T cell that potentially contribute to its activation in this way (see Fig. 2–5). CD4 and CD8 proteins act by binding to class II and class I on the antigen-presenting cell. CD4 and CD8 are linked to intracellular proteins, which are involved in transducing further signals to the T cell. A series of additional proteins on the T-cell surface, such as CD54, CD2, CD11a/CD18 and CD5, act largely to increase the affinity of interaction between the T cell and its antigen-presenting cell, although they also may transduce further signals to the T cell.

Interest in the area of T-cell costimulation has centered on the CD28 pathway (Chambers and Allison, 1997; Harding *et al.*, 1992; June *et al.*, 1987; Lenschow *et al.*, 1996b). CD28 is a homodimeric glycoprotein that is present on the surface of T cells and that interacts with two counterreceptors, CD80 and CD86 (the B7 proteins), which may be expressed on the surface of antigen-presenting cells. CD80 and CD86 are simi-

FIGURE 2–6

APC–T cell protein interactions that are required for T lymphocyte activation. Many cell surface proteins are involved in the interactions of T cells with their antigen presenting cells (APC). The interactions often may be bidirectional and affect both APC and T cell.

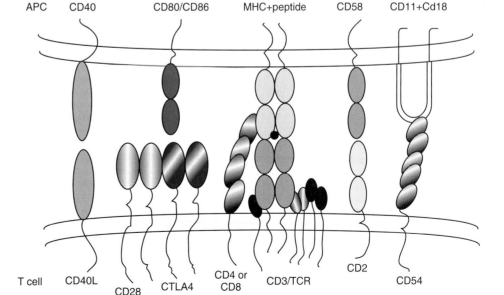

lar in structure, and although they have different patterns of expression and bind with distinct affinities to CD28 (Larsen et al., 1994; Lenschow et al., 1994; Linsley et al., 1994; Morton et al., 1996), both appear to provide a costimulatory signal to T cells by ligating CD28. CD86, expressed constitutively at low level by professional antigen-presenting cells such as dendritic cells and up-regulated rapidly after interaction with the T cell, has a low affinity for CD28, whereas CD80 is expressed with slower kinetics, only after interaction of an antigen-presenting cell with the T cell, and has an approximately 10-fold greater binding affinity for CD28 than does CD80 (van der Merwe et al., 1997). The result of ligation of CD28 by either CD86 or CD80 appears to be increased cytokine synthesis and proliferation after signaling through as yet incompletely defined intracellular pathways (Lindsten et al., 1989; Rudd, 1996; Rudd et al., 1994; Thompson et al., 1989; Ward, 1999). The reason for the apparent redundancy in expression of the costimulatory proteins CD80 and CD86 is not known, but it is possible that they may have subtly different roles in the development of immunity or interact differentially with CD28 and the homologous protein CTLA-4, thereby having different roles in regulation of T-lymphocyte responses. CTLA-4 is expressed by T cells after activation and, although structurally related to CD28, appears to be critically involved in resolving T-cell immunity (Karandiker et al., 1996; Tivol et al., 1995; Walunas et al., 1994). CTLA-4 also binds to CD80 and CD86, not only showing a higher affinity for CD80 than for CD86, but also showing a higher affinity for both than does CD28. The integration of signals resulting from all of these interactions is complex and remains poorly understood (Chambers and Allison, 1997).

The requirement of CD28 signals for CD4+ T cells in secondary immune responses or for CD8+ T cells is less clear. The prevailing view for CD4+ cells is that if they have not been stimulated recently by antigen (i.e., they have developed into memory cells), they will require costimulation for reactivation, and recently activated cells have been shown to be costimulation dependent (Hamel et al., 1998; Marelli-Berg et al., 1999a). Experimentally it can be shown that in certain situations virus-reactive CD8+ cells require neither costimulation through CD28 nor CD28-dependent help (Kudig et al., 1996; Zimmerman et al., 1997). To achieve this, however, they may require massive TCR stimulation (e.g., provided by a replicating virus), a situation that infrequently may occur during other immune responses. Even for CD4+ cells, overwhelming stimulation through the TCR may obviate the requirement for CD28-mediated costimulation.

Mice with a disrupted cd28 gene have impaired immune responses but can reject skin grafts, albeit in a somewhat delayed fashion (Kawai et al., 1996). Work showing that there are other receptor-ligand pairs that can provide a similar type of costimulation to T cells (including homologues of the B7 proteins) suggests that this latter result is due to redundancy in the immune system (Abbas and Sharpe, 1999). The severe phenotype of CTLA-4$^{-/-}$ mice, in which animals die from lymphoproliferative disorder shortly after birth, suggests that there is less redundancy in this aspect of immune regulation.

Blocking the CD28 pathway in normal animals may have dramatic effects on the generation of immune responses and may result in prolonged graft survival or tolerance of grafts (Lenschow et al., 1992; Pearson et al., 1994; Turka et al., 1992). The most widely used reagent for this purpose has been CTLA-4-Ig, which potentially blocks all CD28 and CTLA-4-B7 interactions. The fact that CTLA-4 seems to provide an essential signal in the resolution of immune responses indicates this is unlikely to be the optimal strategy, however, and reagents that effectively block only CD28-B7 interactions (and

perhaps those between the other costimulatory receptor ligand pairs) should be sought. The potential for blocking this route of immunity in the treatment of transplant patients remains exciting.

On activation T cells express another cell surface protein, CD154 (CD40 ligand, gp39). Interaction of this protein with its counterreceptor, CD40, appears to be critical for the activation of B cells, dendritic cells, and monocytes. Larsen et al. (1996a) showed that blocking this interaction could prolong graft survival in a mouse cardiac transplant model. Even more impressive, however, are more recent data from this group showing that combined blocking of CD28 and CD40 interactions can induce permanent survival of allogeneic skin grafts in mice with no long-term deterioration of graft integrity (Larsen et al., 1996b). Curiously, tolerance to the graft antigens could not be shown in these mice despite the excellent survival of the transplant itself. Other groups have now taken up this approach, always with dramatic effects on the regulation of immunity. Kidney graft rejection in monkeys can be prevented completely with antibodies to CD154 (Kirk et al., 1999). Similar antibodies have been developed for use in the clinical setting and are in trials. The first antibody of this type to have been used clinically has now been withdrawn, however, because of its side effects.

CYTOKINES

In addition to the large number of cell-cell–based interactions required for T-cell activation, important signals are delivered through the binding of soluble proteins, the cytokines, to specific cell surface cytokine receptors. Cytokines such as IL-1 and IL-12, derived primarily from antigen-presenting cells, seem to sensitize T cells, through up-regulating the expression of receptors for other cytokines to the proliferative and differentiative effects of the (primarily) T cell–derived cytokines such as IL-2 and IL-4. A whole cascade of cytokines are produced that amplify immune and inflammatory processes after transplantation (see later; reviewed extensively in Dallman, 1995; Dallman and Clark, 1992; Nickerson et al., 1994; Picotti et al., 1997; Strom et al., 1996).

INITIATION OF THE IMMUNE RESPONSE—CD4+ AND CD8+ CELLS

As described in the previous sections, the interaction of the T cell with antigen-presenting cells plays a fundamental role in initiation of the immune response. The consequences of this interaction include proliferation and differentiation of the so-called helper T cells with the concomitant production of growth and differentiation factors (or cytokines) that are required by other cells so that a potent effector response can be mounted. In many cases, these helper T cells bear the CD4 surface protein, but in certain situations CD8+ cells are able to respond in the absence of CD4+ cells and themselves meet all of the requirements of a helper T cell (Rosenberg, 1993; Sprent et al., 1986). That CD4+ cells frequently are required to initiate graft rejection has been shown by many workers in a variety of experimental systems (Dallman et al., 1982; Gurley et al., 1983; Hall et al., 1983; Loveland et al., 1981; Lowry et al., 1983), although depending on the mismatch between donor and recipient, CD8+ cells may be additionally required or may act independently of CD4+ cells (Rosenberg, 1993; Rosenberg et al., 1986, 1987; Sprent et al., 1986; Tilney et al., 1984). Investigation of the effects of CD4+ and CD8+ cells in transplantation responses has included the use of knock-out mice that are deprived of these populations through genetic manipulation. Mice lacking class I or II antigens are severely depleted of CD8+ or CD4+ cells, as are mice in which either the *cd4* or *cd8* gene has been disrupted (Apasov and Sitkovsky, 1994; Dalloul *et al.*, 1996a, 1996b; Dierich *et al.*, 1993; Krieger *et al.*, 1996; Lamouse-Smith *et al.*, 1993; Mannon *et al.*, 1995; Schilham *et al.*, 1993). The effects on graft rejection of a lack of CD4 or CD8 cells produced in this manner have not been predictable and often depend on the nature of the mismatch between donor and recipient. Furthermore, despite an apparent depletion of CD8$^+$ cells in class I$^{-/-}$ mice, CD8$^+$ CTLs can be generated in large numbers after transplantation and may be involved in the rejection process (Apasov and Sitkovsky, 1994; Lee *et al.*, 1994; Schilham *et al.*, 1993). The results of such experiments basically are consistent with previous ideas in this area—CD4$^+$ cells seem normally to initiate graft rejection, but there are experimental models (usually when there is a dominant or sole MHC class I mismatch) in which CD8$^+$ cells are also required for rejection to proceed with normal kinetics or may act independently of the CD4$^+$ cell.

Generation of Different Types of Effector Immunity

T1 AND T2 DRIVEN IMMUNITY

After stimulation of the immune system, a response develops in which either humoral or cell-mediated immunity may be seen to dominate (Katsura, 1977; Parish, 1972), and it has become clear that cytokines play a determining role in this process (Del Prete *et al.*, 1991; McKnight *et al.*, 1991; Mosmann and Moore, 1991; Mosmann *et al.*, 1986, 1989; Fig. 2–7). The cells (and the cytokines they produce) that drive a cell-mediated response have been called *Th1* and those driving humoral immunity *Th2*. It has been shown that the helper and cytotoxic T-cell populations diverge in their cytokine production, and so here I refer to T1 and T2 populations.

Early on during an immune response, many T cells appear to make a wide range of cytokines. Only after continued antigenic stimulation can clear divergence of cytokine production be observed, and it is the view of some workers that we have through the T1/T2 paradigm oversimplified the view of the immune response (Kelso, 1995). Nevertheless, this paradigm has been extremely useful in extending understanding of immunity and is discussed here. Interferon (IFN)-γ is the prototypic cytokine of T1 cells, and a predominance of this population results in the appearance of cell-mediated immunity involving the generation of specific CTLs and activated macrophages. T2 cells make cytokines such as IL-4, IL-5 and IL-6, which are critical for the induction of humoral immunity (and for immunoglobulin isotype switching) and eosinophilia. Exactly how a T1-dominated or T2-dominated reponse is determined is uncertain, but the local cytokine milieu (Gajewski and Fitch, 1988; Gajewski *et al.*, 1989; Hsieh *et al.*, 1992, 1993; Swain *et al.*, 1990, 1991), involvement of antigen-presenting cells other than dendritic cells (Macatonia *et al.*, 1993a, 1993b) and the type of CD28 signal delivered (i.e. either through CD80 or CD86 [Freeman *et al.*, 1995; Kuchroo *et al.*, 1995; Lenschow *et al.*, 1996a; Ranger *et al.*, 1996]) have all been suggested as important factors.

Interest of the transplantation community has focused particularly on the possibility that although a T1-driven response may inevitably be damaging and result in graft rejection, a T2-driven response may not have this effect and may be associated with the induction of tolerance to a graft (reviewed in Dallman, 1993, 1995; Nickerson *et al.*, 1994; Picotti *et al.*, 1997; Strom *et al.*, 1996). Many groups have found that tolerance or reduced donor-directed reactivity is associated with a decrease in the prolonged expression of the T1-associated cytokines, IL-2 and IFN-γ (Alard *et al.*, 1993; Bugeon *et al.*, 1992; Burdick and Clow, 1990; Dallman *et al.*, 1991b; Mohler and Streilein, 1989; Takeuchi *et al.*, 1992). It has been tempting to speculate that this decrease is accompanied by or even due to the expansion of regulatory T2 cells (Takeuchi *et al.*, 1992). There is some evidence that the expression of cytokines such as IL-4, IL-5 and IL-10 is preserved during the development of tolerance (Dallman *et al.*, 1993; Gorczynski, 1992; Sayegh *et al.*, 1995; Takeuchi *et al.*, 1992). Cells other than T2 lymphocytes can produce such cytokines, however, meaning that their detection does not necessarily infer the presence or action of the T2 population. As described in the following sections, an immune response to a transplant is complex; humoral and a variety of cellular mechanisms can effect graft destruction, and it is likely that any type of immunity, T1 or T2 driven, would result in graft rejection. Clones of T lymphocyte that have T2-like properties are as capable of initiating graft rejection as are clones of T1 cells (VanBuskirk *et al.*, 1996; Zelenika *et al.*, 1998), and it has been suggested that T2 cells drive chronic graft rejection (Shirwan, 1999). In models of true tolerance, rather than prolonged graft survival, a rapid shutdown of cytokine production may be observed (Josien *et al.*, 1995; Pearson *et al.*, 1994).

Several groups have tried to assess the role of key cytokines by performing experiments in which their overexpression or absence is tested. Two groups have shown that tolerance can be induced using reagents that block CD28 signaling in IL-4$^{-/-}$ mice (Lakkis *et al.*, 1997; Nickerson *et al.*, 1996). An important additional finding from these studies was that tolerance was induced more easily in homozygous IL-4$^{-/-}$ mice than in heterozygous IL-4$^{+/-}$ mice (Nickerson *et al.*, 1996), the implication being that the presence of IL-4 itself can be damaging to the graft. In other experiments, it was shown, again using knock-out mice, that neither IL-2 nor IFN-γ is required for rejection (Konieczny *et al.*, 1996; Saleem *et al.*, 1996; Steiger *et al.*, 1995; Strom *et al.*, 1996), but it has been shown more recently that both are required for tolerance induction (Dai and Lakkis, 1999). Interpretation of these experiments can be complicated by the fact that cytokines often can substitute each others' function, and it is unclear whether or not the phenotype of knock-out mice reflects accurately the importance of these cytokines in normal mice.

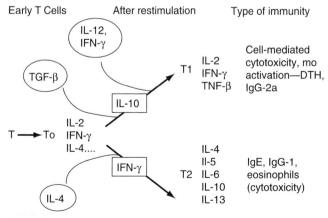

FIGURE 2–7

T1/T2 cell differentiation and immunity. Cytokines produced by T cells and that influence their divergence to T1 and T2 subsets are shown. Cytokines that may positively (circled) or negatively (in squares) regulate divergence of the T1 and T2 cells are shown. DTH = delayed-type hypersensitivity; mo = macrophage; IL = interleukin; IFN = interferon; TNF = tumor necrosis factor.

For instance, IL-15 can substitute many of the actions of IL-2 and IL-13 for IL-4. In the experiments described earlier, IL-15 transcripts were found in grafts put into the IL-2$^{-/-}$ mice and IL-13 transcripts in those transplanted into IL-4 knockout mice. The fact that IL2$^{-/-}$ or IFN-$\gamma^{-/-}$ mice were unable to become tolerant suggests a nonredundant role for these cytokines in the induction of tolerance, a finding that a few years ago not many people would have predicted.

An alternative method of investigation has been used by several groups in experiments in which cytokines have been injected or overexpressed in animal transplant models in an attempt to deviate the immune system toward a T1 or T2 response. Paradoxically, given the aforementioned data, injection of IL-2 or IFN-γ can prevent the induction of tolerance (Bugeon et al., 1992; Dallman et al., 1991b). Injection or overexpression of IL-4 cannot induce tolerance (Mueller et al., 1997), however, and although this treatment may prolong graft survival marginally (Dallman et al., unpublished), it may inhibit tolerance induction (Nickerson et al., 1996).

The most rational conclusion from all of these studies is that an effector immune response driven by either T1 or T2 cells is damaging, although in some cases that driven by T2 cells may be less detrimental acutely than that driven by T1 cells. T2 cells may be the primary drivers of chronic rejection. The individual actions of certain cytokines still are not fully understood, but it would appear, given the data on IL-2 and IFN-γ, that such cytokines may assume different functions depending on the timing or perhaps location of their expression.

Migration of Activated Leukocytes into the Graft

To enter a site of inflammation or immune response, leukocytes must migrate across the vascular endothelium. This migration process is controlled by the elaboration of cell attractants or chemokines and by cell-cell interactions between the leukocyte and the endothelium. Activated and memory cells bear adhesion proteins, chemokine receptors, and addressins, which allow homing to and migration into peripheral tissues (Mackay, 1993a, b).

CELL-CELL INTERACTIONS

The adhesion of leukocytes to the endothelium is a complex multistep process that involves a series of interactions between the surface of the leukocyte and the endothelial cell or its extracellular matrix (reviewed in Butcher and Picker, 1996; Kirby, 1996). The proteins involved fall into three groups—the selectins and members of the integrin and immunoglobulin (Ig) superfamilies. Initial interaction and rolling of leukocytes along the endothelium allows the leukocyte to sample the endothelial environment while maintaining its ability to detach and travel somewhere else. This step is largely controlled by the selectins, although, for example, α4 integrins also may play a role at this stage. Under the correct conditions, this interaction leads to signaling to the leukocyte, slowing down and arresting the rolling process and allowing extravasation. These latter stages are regulated mainly by the integrins and adhesion proteins of the Ig superfamily.

The expression of many adhesion proteins involved in these interactions is up-regulated by proinflammatory cytokines. Ischemic damage alone results in increased expression of several cytokines, and of these, IL-1 up-regulates the expression of members of the selectin family (Collins et al., 1995; Pober et al., 1986). Other adhesion proteins, such as

ICAM-1 and VCAM-1 of the Ig superfamily and E-selectin (endothelial-specific selectin), are known to be up-regulated by the type of cytokines also induced after the trauma of transplantation. Before an immune response has been generated, the graft becomes attractive to circulating leukocytes, although as previously mentioned, naive lymphocytes tend not to home into nonlymphoid sites. Antigen-activated lymphocytes have an altered recirculation pattern, however, and migrate into extralymphoid sites (Butcher, 1986; Mackay, 1993b; Picker and Butcher, 1992). They may show tissue-selective homing and show preference for sites in which they are most likely to reencounter their specific antigen (Santamaria-Babi et al., 1995). The process seems to be facilitated further by recognition by the T cell of MHC class II/peptide complexes on the vascular endothelium (Marelli-Berg et al., 1999b). This process is likely to result in the accumulation of antigen-specific lymphocytes within the site of inflammation, in this case the graft.

One practical aspect with respect to transplantation is that it may be possible to hide the proteins involved in leukocyte extravasation, thereby slowing or preventing the rejection process. Blocking the adhesion proteins by using antibodies or by inhibiting their expression has been attempted in experimental and clinical transplantation (Cosimi et al., 1990; Haug et al., 1993; Heagy et al., 1984; Hourmant et al., 1996). In general, cocktails of antibodies are more potent than single antibodies (Iwata et al., 1996; Yang et al., 1995), although the results are variable, and in one case a combination of antibodies to ICAM-1 and LFA-1 has been shown to result in accelarated rejection of rat cardiac allografts (Morikawa et al., 1994).

CHEMOKINES

Several chemokines—small soluble proteins, similar to cytokines—have been identified and form two major groups based on their structure: the CXC or alpha chemokines, which primarily attract neutrophils and T cells, and the CC or beta chemokines, which attract T cells, monocytes/macrophages, dendritic cells, natural killer (NK) cells and some polymorphs (Oppenheim et al., 1991, 1996). The CXC chemokines include IL-8 and IFN-γ–inducible protein, and the CC chemokines include macrophage inflammatory protein-1α/β (MIP-1α/β), RANTES and macrophage chemoattractant protein-1 (MCP-1). Initial excitement surrounding the involvement of chemokines in extravasation of leukocytes has been tempered somewhat by the finding that chemokine receptors are expressed at low levels by resting leukocytes (Bacon and Schall, 1996). Nevertheless, they play a role in increasing the weak initial binding of leukocytes to the endothelium and in directing the migration of activated leukocytes across a gradient toward the source of the chemokine. Transplantation studies have suggested that chemokines are important in not only the development of graft infiltrates (DeVries et al., 1999; Fairchild et al., 1997; Grandaliano et al., 1997), but also reperfusion injury (Lentsch et al., 1998). The indications are that they act not only as attractants for various leukocyte populations, but also by augmenting the effector functions of leukocytes within the graft (Koga et al., 1999).

Destruction of the Graft

The immune system generates many different effector mechanisms depending on the challenge it meets. In certain infections, a single mechanism appears to be essential for the clearance of the organism, and the absence of that mechanism renders the host susceptible to disease. For example, in the clearance of lymphocyte choriomeningitis virus infections in mice, cytotoxic cells are absolutely required, and disabling this arm of immunity by disrupting the perforin gene leads to death of infected animals (Kagi *et al.*, 1995). As seen in more detail subsequently, most of the known effector mechanisms of the immune system are capable of damaging a graft such that the obliteration of any single effector mechanism has little beneficial effect on graft survival. This is most likely to be the reason that it is so difficult to prevent graft rejection without disabling the central components of the immune system.

SPECIFICITY OF REJECTION

The nature of tissue destruction during rejection reveals a lot about the processes involved; that is, graft destruction can show fine specificity for cells carrying donor alloantigens. The elegant studies of Mintz and Silvers (1967, 1970) showed an exquisite specificity of donor cell lysis in experiments using allophenic mice as tissue donors. Such allophenic, or tetraparental, mice are bred by fusing the embryos from mice of two different genetic origins. The tissues of the resulting mosaic offspring are made up of patches of cells from each parental type. Mintz and Silvers performed experiments using mice with different coat colors, and when skin from an allophenic donor was grafted to mice of either parental origin only the cells of nonidentical type were rejected, leaving cells of recipient type intact and capable of hair growth. These studies have been repeated and extended in experiments performed by Rosenberg and Singer (1992); in this work, an initial large inflammatory/immune response was observed, but this resolved, remarkably leaving cells only of the recipient genotype in place. In a different type of experiment, Sutton *et al.* (1989) showed that transplantation of an intimate mixture of allogeneic and syngeneic pancreatic islets resulted in destruction only of the allogeneic cells, with no evidence of bystander damage to the syngeneic islets. It is difficult to imagine how an essentially nonspecific effector mechanism, such as that involved in DTH lesions, could mediate graft rejection in the exquisitely specific manner observed in these experiments.

Bystander destruction of tissue may, however, be observed after specific immune responses to foreign antigens (Rubin and Tolkoff Rubin, 1984). Snider and Steinmuller (1987) have shown that destruction of bystander tissue may occur in the immune response to miH antigens. In their experiments, cytotoxic T-cell clones reactive with a variety of minor antigens (e.g., H-Y and Epa-1 antigens) were injected intradermally together with their specific antigen into a syngeneic animal, which did not express that antigen. As a result, ulcerating skin lesions developed that were radiosensitive, suggesting the involvement of a nonspecific, host-derived effector mechanism in the tissue destruction. In the experiments described earlier using donor material from tetraparental animals, if most cells in the graft were allogeneic to the recipient, the overwhelming inflammatory response led to destruction of the entire tissue.

From these experiments, we can conclude that antigen-specific and antigen-nonspecific effector mechanisms may be involved in graft destruction. In both types of experiment, the initial damage was mediated in a specific fashion—it was only when this initiated a massive inflammatory response that the nonspecific elements resulted in tissue destruction. The various effector systems that can damage tissue are described subsequently, and their roles in hyperacute, acute, and chronic rejection are discussed.

ANTIBODY

Antibody may cause tissue damage not only through the fixation of complement, but also through the activity of K cells in antibody-dependent cellular cytotoxicity (ADCC). In the latter case, the antibody acts as a bridge between the target tissue and the effector cell, activating the lytic machinery of the K cell and resulting in tissue damage (Perlmann and Holm, 1969). Many different leukocytes appear to be capable of K-cell activity, but although ADCC activity may be recovered from grafts (Tilney *et al.*, 1975), its role in graft rejection has not been investigated fully.

Patients who have been exposed to MHC antigens through transplant, blood transfusions or pregnancy often develop antibodies reactive with those MHC antigens. These preformed antibodies can cause *hyperacute* rejection, a process in which the organ fails immediately after revascularization (Kissmeyer-Nielsen *et al.*, 1966; Morris and Ting, 1982; Patel and Terasaki, 1969; Williams *et al.*, 1968). Histologically, it may be seen that this process is accompanied by deposition of antibody and complement and the accumulation of polymorphonuclear leukocytes within the graft (Williams *et al.*, 1968). Hyperacute rejection is now largely a thing of the past since the introduction of pretransplant screening by the crossmatch test for antibodies directed toward donor antigens. The conventional crossmatch test detects, however, not only harmful MHC-directed cytotoxic antibodies, but also harmless autoantibodies (Ting and Morris, 1977, 1981). In most cases, it is now possible to distinguish autoreactive from alloreactive antibodies, and it has become possible to transplant an increasing number of patients across an apparent positive crossmatch, but in whom the reactivity is due to autoantibodies. Of interest is that liver transplantation appears to be an exception to the rules regarding transplantation across a positive crossmatch. Liver transplants are carried out with little regard to the immune system and are performed successfully not only across positive crossmatches, but also without any MHC matching of donor and recipient (Powelson and Cosimi, 1999).

Many of the changes associated with acute rejection, including arteriolar thrombosis, interstitial hemorrhage and fibrinoid necrosis of the arteriolar walls, may result from the deposition of antibody and fixation of complement (Dunnill, 1984). The appearance of donor-specific antibody does not necessarily accompany graft rejection, however, and its presence may be compatible with unimpaired graft function (Baldwin *et al.*, 1991; Ting and Morris, 1978). At least experimentally, however, acute rejection of MHC class I incompatible rat kidney grafts is associated with and can be initiated by donor-specific antibody (Gracie *et al.*, 1990).

Donor-specific antibodies also may be found in the circulation, and immunoglobulin deposits may be seen in vessel walls during chronic rejection, but it is not clear whether or how the presence of such antibodies may be causally related to graft dysfunction (Taylor *et al.*, 1991; Yilmaz *et al.*, 1992). Experimentally, there is considerable evidence that antibody can mediate many of the vascular changes associated with chronic rejection. For example, mice with severe combined immunodeficiency develop such lesions when infused with preformed donor-specific antibody (Russell *et al.*, 1994).

An area of increasing interest is that of xenotransplantation, in which the use of animal donors is being considered for human transplantation. Many problems are associated with this approach none the least of which is the presence in the circulation of humans of antibodies that react with the cells of many animal species including the pig, which currently is the animal of choice as a donor in xenotransplantation. These antibodies show a predominant reactivity to sugars on cell surface proteins, which as a result of the activity of the α-1,3-galactosyltransferase gene are present in pigs (and many other species) but not in humans (Cooper *et al.*, 1993; Galili *et al.*, 1984, 1985; Parker *et al.*, 1994; Sandrin *et al.*,

1993). Such natural antibodies result in hyperacute rejection of pig tissue by the human (Auchincloss and Sachs, 1998; Platt, 1999, and see Chapter 42).

CELLULAR MECHANISMS

The involvement of cell-mediated mechanisms usually is invoked in acute or chronic graft rejection, but although hyperacute rejection almost always has been attributed to antibody, in certain situations a rapid rejection may occur when the role of antibody has been excluded. In these situations, a cellular mechanism of rejection has been implicated (Kirkman et al., 1979).

Natural Killer Cells

Natural killer cells do not need prior exposure to antigen to become lytic to target cells (although it is clear that their activity can be increased by certain cytokines) and as such provide a primary defense mechanism. Natural killer cells may be recovered from the blood or spleen, for example, and are able to lyse NK-sensitive targets, which tend to be of tumor origin (Herberman et al., 1979). Although clearly a potent source of cytotoxic activity, a role for the NK cell in organ graft rejection remains to be established. Several laboratories using different experimental models have found that grafts survive indefinitely in the presence of demonstrable NK effector activity (Armstrong et al., 1987; Bradley et al., 1985; Mason and Morris, 1984). However, natural killer cells clearly have been shown to be involved in the rejection of bone marrow transplants (Murphy et al., 1987a, 1987b). The method of target cell recognition employed by the NK cell is increasingly understood (Colonna et al., 1993; Leibson, 1995; Long and Wagtmann, 1997), and the nature of the immune synapse between effector and target cell is the subject of some interest (Davis et al., 1999). In contrast to T cells, the interaction with MHC on a target cell may result in the delivery of a negative signal to the NK cell, preventing the activation of its lytic machinery. The absence of self-class I MHC antigens triggers the NK cell to attack its target, a finding that is consistent with the observation that NK cells are important in the rejection of bone marrow cells that express little or no class I antigen (Bix et al., 1991). This fact is important to remember in any approach that considers the removal or blocking of donor MHC antigen as a strategy to overcome rejection of allogeneic or xenogeneic graft rejection.

Specific Cytotoxic T Cell

In cell culture systems, MHC-mismatched lymphocytes proliferate and produce cytokines in response to one another in the mixed lymphocyte reaction. The resulting cytokine production allows the differentiation of precursor CTLs into effector cells that lyse target cells bearing the mismatched MHC antigens (Hayry and Defendi, 1970; Hodes and Svedmyr, 1970). The fact that a powerful yet antigen-specific response is generated rapidly in mixed lymphocyte reaction has made the CTL a prime suspect as the central effector mechanism of acute graft rejection.

Considerable evidence suggests that CTLs may be involved in graft rejection. First, CTLs may be recovered from allografts that are undergoing rejection, but they are present only at low levels in grafts of animals that have been treated with cyclosporine to prevent rejection (Bradley et al., 1985; Mason and Morris, 1984). Second, cloned populations of CTLs are capable of causing the type of tissue damage associated with rejection (Engers et al., 1982; Tyler et al., 1984). Third, most class I MHC antigen-directed CTLs express the CD8 protein, and graft rejection often may be delayed in the absence of CD8$^+$ cells (Cobbold et al., 1984; Lowry et al., 1983; Madsen et al., 1987, 1988; Tilney et al., 1984).

Conversely, graft destruction may occur in the absence of demonstrable CTL activity, and the presence of such cells within a graft may not always lead to graft destruction. The male-specific miH antigen, H-Y, first was detected by the rejection of male skin grafts by female mice of the same strain, but there is not always a clear correlation between rejection and the presence or absence of CTLs (Hurme et al., 1978a, 1978b). In other experiments, the presence of cytotoxic effector cells has been shown within a graft that is not rejected (Armstrong et al., 1987; Dallman et al., 1987). Rats given a donor-specific preoperative blood transfusion may retain a subsequent renal allograft indefinitely, but cells extracted from such grafts show high and persistent donor-specific CTL activity. The simple conclusion from these studies is that CTLs cannot always reject grafts, although the possibility that the action of these CTLs may be blocked in the graft itself or that the activity of CTLs in cell culture does not accurately reflect their potential in the animal must be considered. These results remain intriguing, however, and provide direct evidence of the presence of cytotoxic effector cells within an organ graft that is not ultimately rejected. CTLs are able to kill their targets through the elaboration of perforins and granzymes, through activation of the Fas death pathway, or through secretion of the cytokine TNF-α. Their involvement in graft rejection has been questioned further by the finding that mice deficient in perforin (perforin knockouts) are able to reject tumor (Walsh et al., 1996), skin (Selvaggi et al., 1996) and organ (Schulz et al., 1995) grafts, even when the grafts are resistant to Fas-mediated and TNF-α-mediated killing (Walsh et al., 1996). In the experiments of Schulz and colleagues, however, grafts mismatched only at the class I MHC are rejected more slowly in perforin knockout mice, indicating that, in this situation at least, cytotoxic cells are important in rejection (Schulz et al., 1995).

As alluded to earlier, even if CTLs themselves do not mediate the tissue damage that ultimately results in graft loss, they still may be important in generating the destructive response to the graft. Through the elaboration of high levels of IFN-γ and other cytokines or chemokines, they are able to recruit and activate cells involved in DTH lesions, initiating acute or chronic rejection.

Macrophages and Delayed-Type Hypersensitivity Reactions

T cells initiate a DTH reaction (Loveland and McKenzie, 1982), which involves an essentially nonspecific effector phase (as described by Koch in 1891 in the tuberculin skin reaction—see Florey and Jennings, 1970), characterized by an infiltrate of lymphocytes and cells of the monocyte/macrophage lineage. Damage occurs in a tissue during a DTH reaction through the elaboration of various noxious substances, including reactive nitrogen and oxygen intermediates and TNF-α. Support for the role of DTH reactions in acute graft rejection comes from the studies on rejection of H-Y disparate grafts. In situations in which the cytotoxic cell response does not correlate with graft rejection, the generation of DTH reactions to H-Y antigens follows closely the ability of female mice to reject male skin (Liew and Simpson, 1980). In addition, irradiated rats reconstituted with CD4 cells may reject heart grafts in the absence of a detectable CTL response within the transplant (Lowry et al., 1983).

The high level of inflammatory mediators and the type of changes within grafts undergoing chronic rejection suggest a role for activated macrophages in this process (Chen et al.,

1996; Hayry *et al.*, 1993; Paul and Benediktsson, 1993; Paul *et al.*, 1996). Cytokines such as IL-1, TNF-α, transforming growth factor (TGF)-β and platelet-derived growth factor (PDGF) lead to smooth muscle proliferation, and TGF-β and PDGF result in an increased synthesis of extracellular matrix proteins. These cytokines are products of activated macrophages and may result in the atherosclerotic and fibrotic changes associated with chronic graft failure.

Cytokines

The primary role of cytokines in an immune response to a graft is to initiate proliferation, differentiation and homing of leukocytes in the generation of immunity. However, certain cytokines also may directly damage tissue acutely or chronically. As described earlier, TNF-α, produced by CTLs and macrophages, may damage a graft, and blocking the effects of TNF with neutralizing antibodies can prolong organ graft survival (Bolling *et al.*, 1992; Imagawa *et al.*, 1990, 1991). The rather minimal effects of these antibodies, however, suggest that the TNFs may not contribute centrally to graft rejection or that once neutralized other effector mechanisms take over. Islets appear to be particularly susceptible to damage mediated by proinflammatory cytokines, such that these may be a more important component in the rejection of islet transplants (Mandrup-Poulsen *et al.*, 1986, 1989; Rabinovitch *et al.*, 1988; Wolf *et al.*, 1989).

Eosinophils

It has been recognized for some years that acute and chronic kidney allograft rejection are associated with a varying level of eosinophilia (Foster *et al.*, 1989; Kormendi and Amend, 1988; Nolan *et al.*, 1995), but the significance of this in terms of its contribution to rejection has not been acknowledged widely. In an experimental model of acute mouse cardiac allograft rejection in which the depletion of CD8$^+$ T lymphocytes results in a dominant T2 response, rejection appears to be mediated by eosinophils (Chan *et al.*, 1995). In another model, in which acute rejection of MHC class II disparate mouse skin grafts was studied, IL-5-dependent infiltration with eosinophils was observed. In this model, when Fas/FasL interactions were absent, neutralizing antibodies to IL-5 blocked eosinophilia and rejection, implicating the eosinophil as an effector cell in this system (LeMoine *et al.*, 1999). In another experimental model of skin allograft rejection, the same group has shown a role for IL-5 and eosinophilia in chronic rejection, but in this system, not all of the pathology could be attributed to eosinophils (LeMoine *et al.*, 1999b).

Target Cells of Destructive Immunity

Damage to the vascular endothelium, which may express class I and class II MHC antigens, is likely to result in rapid cell necrosis and graft loss (Kauntz *et al.*, 1963). The predominantly vascular changes that occur during rejection of an organ graft suggest that this is the case (Dvorak *et al.*, 1979; Laden and Sinclair, 1971; Porter *et al.*, 1964). It is possible that parenchymal cells also may be targets for tissue destruction, but this is more likely to be secondary to the initial attack on endothelium. The increase in expression of class I and class II MHC antigens after transplantation could increase susceptibility of endothelium and parenchymal cells to destruction. The marked arterial changes seen as a manifestation of acute and chronic rejection also suggest the importance of the endothelium as the main target of the response, and in the case of chronic rejection the fibrotic changes seen histologically could be due, in large part, to ischemia resulting from gradual vascular obliteration.

Privileged Sites

Tissue allografts placed in certain sites may evoke a weak immune response, and the grafts may survive for prolonged periods or indefinitely (Billingham and Silvers, 1971). The anterior chamber of the eye, the cornea, the brain and the testis all show immune privilege either in that transplantation of tissue into these sites evokes a reduced immune response or in that they themselves seem to have low immunogenicity. The classic privileged site experimentally is the cheek pouch of the Syrian hamster, in which a skin allograft survives indefinitely, provided that the host has not been specifically sensitized against donor histocompatibility antigens (Billingham and Silvers, 1964).

These sites have in common to a greater or lesser extent a lack of or abnormal lymphatic drainage, which seems to play such an important role in sensitization of the host against a free graft such as skin. Although there are undoubtedly well-documented privileged sites in many species, it does appear that no site is uniformly privileged for all grafts, even in the same species. Nevertheless, the experimental work in this area has defined clearly the important physiological role of lymphatics draining the site of implantation of free tissue allografts.

As indicated previously, a vascularized graft that often behaves as a privileged tissue is the liver. Calne and colleagues first showed that outbred pigs often failed to reject orthotopic liver allografts (Calne *et al.*, 1969); kidney allografts transplanted at the same time and that normally are rejected also show prolonged survival. In certain strain combinations in the rat in which an orthotopic liver allograft is not rejected, the liver allograft has been shown to abrogate an existing state of sensitization of the host against donor histocompatibility antigen (Kamada *et al.*, 1981). Although HLA matching and crossmatching have been shown to be of some benefit in liver transplantation (Doyle *et al.*, 1996; Powelson and Cosimi, 1999), usually the urgency with which the graft is required precludes the use of matching, yet these grafts survive well. The reasons for the refractoriness to immune rejection displayed by liver grafts are not fully understood and may be, in part, due to the size and enormous capacity for regeneration displayed by the liver. The immune response to liver transplants also differs from that to other grafts, however, and spontaneous tolerance can develop in several rat and all mouse strain combinations. An understanding of this phenomenon may help workers design new strategies of tolerance induction (Farges *et al.*, 1994, 1995; Kamada, 1988; Kamada and Wight, 1984).

Fas ligand (FasL) in binding to Fas, the so-called death receptor, on the surface of cells, initiates the apoptotic pathway in the Fas$^+$ cells. It has been suggested that overexpression of FasL on certain tissues affords them immune privilege (Bellgrau *et al.*, 1995; Griffith *et al.*, 1995; Niederkorn, 1999), and in some workers' hands, engineering tissues to overexpress FasL has allowed their prolonged survival in an allogeneic recipient (Gainer *et al.*, 1998; Lau *et al.*, 1996; Li and Faustman, 1993). This approach is thought to work by destroying the Fas$^+$ leukocytes that would otherwise mediate tissue damage, although this type of experiment has not always been successful, and overexpression of FasL on islet cells itself results in their death (Lau and Stoeckert, 1997).

Chronic Rejection

Although chronic rejection has been mentioned at various points in this chapter, most of what has been said refers to the acute processes that occur rapidly after transplantation. (See Chapter 27 for a more complete discussion of chronic rejection.) That these may influence the likelihood of more chronic changes seems reasonable, although accumulating evidence in favor of this suggestion has not been easy (Basadonna *et al.*, 1993; Tesi *et al.*, 1993; Tullius *et al.*, 1998). As better immunosuppression reduces the loss of organ allograft to acute rejection, with the steady attrition of grafts as time passes, chronic rejection becomes more evident; currently the greatest loss of kidney grafts is to chronic rather than acute rejection.

As described in the previous section, multiple effector mechanisms are thought to contribute to the immunological aspects of chronic graft rejection. It has become apparent that other factors are involved in this process, however, which have nothing to do with the immune response. The development of experimental models of chronic allograft rejection has increased knowledge of the possible causative mechanisms and pointed to therapies that might prevent the development of the obliterative arterial changes of chronic rejection in the future (reviewed in Hayry *et al.*, 1993; Paul and Benediktsson, 1993). An inflammatory cellular infiltrate is always seen, comprising macrophages and T cells, but the phenotypic composition of the cells is no different from that seen in acute rejection. The T cells comprise CD4 and CD8 cells, with usually a predominance of the former (Cramer *et al.*, 1992; Demetris *et al.*, 1989; Duijvestijn and Van Breda Vriesman, 1991; Hancock *et al.*, 1993).

Because of the predominant vascular nature of chronic rejection, alloantibody has been long thought to play a role in the development of this process, and the demonstration of donor-specific alloantibodies in patients with chronic rejection of cardiac allografts (Rose *et al.*, 1989) and the deposition of immunoglobulin in graft vessel walls of chronically rejected organs (Busch *et al.*, 1971; Rossen *et al.*, 1971) would be compatible with that concept. It is also possible, however, to show immunoglobulin and complement deposition in organs that show no evidence of rejection so that the role of antibody remains uncertain.

The graft arteriosclerosis seen in chronic rejection is concentric and affects all graft arteries, and this forms the basis of a working hypothesis for the development of chronic rejection prepared by Hayry *et al.* (1993). It is suggested that low-grade damage to the graft endothelium, with possibly loss of endothelium, allows platelet deposition on the arterial wall and the production of a variety of growth factors, which, in turn, cause proliferation of smooth muscle cells in the media of the arterial wall and their subsequent invasion of the intima. This response to injury hypothesis first proposed for atherosclerosis (Ross and Glomset, 1976) has been tested in an experimental model in the rat using an aortic allograft by Hayry and colleagues (Mennander *et al.*, 1991). These grafts undergo an initial acute inflammatory reaction in the adventitia, which subsides and is followed by gradual migration of proliferating muscle cells from the vascular media to the intima and the appearance of intimal fibrosis. Once induced, this allograft arteriosclerosis is not reversible by transplanting the aortic allograft into a syngeneic recipient. The development of the chronic arterial lesion could be due to cytokines (IL-1, IL-6, TNF, IFN-γ), growth factors (PDGF, TGF-β) and lipid mediators of inflammation (eicosamoids and platelet activation factor). These molecules have all been shown in models of chronic allograft rejection, but this does not mean that they are the cause of the changes observed. The demonstration that a particular somatostatin analogue, lanreotide, which down-regulates the production of several growth factors, prevents smooth muscle proliferation and the development of arteriosclerosis in the aortic allograft model

does suggest that these growth factors may be important effector molecules in the development of the chronic lesion (Hayry *et al.*, 1993).

The causes of chronic rejection are immunological and nonimmunological (Orosz and Pelletier, 1997), with the immunological causes being important and the primary target of the immunological response being the endothelium. Nonimmunological causes are attracting increasing attention, but a full discussion of these is outside the scope of this chapter.

Conclusion

The immune response to a tissue allograft is a complex phenomenon, in the manner by which allogeneic histocompatibility antigen is recognized and in the response to this recognition, which generally results in graft damage. In the recognition of antigen, the dendritic cell, be it of donor or recipient origin, plays a central role, whereas the effector arm is mediated by cells and by antibody. The hierarchy of importance of all the effector mechanisms described is affected by the type and nature of the graft, the incompatibility between donor and recipient and the type of immunosuppression used. Because all potential effector mechanisms can cause graft damage, adequate immunosuppression usually appears to require disabling of the immune system at a central point. The consequence of this requirement is that patients become susceptible to infection, are at increased risk of cancer and suffer the other side effects of long-term immunosuppression. The only true solution to this problem is the development of an effective strategy for the induction donor-specific tolerance in the recipient. Although this is straightforward in rodents, it remains an elusive goal in humans.

REFERENCES

Abbas, A. K. and Sharpe, A. H. (1999). T-cell stimulation: an abundance of B7s. *Nat. Med.* **5**, 1345.

Alard, P., Lantz, O., Perrot, J. Y., *et al.* (1993). A possible role for specific 'Anergy' in immunologic hyporeactivity to donor stimulation in human kidney allograft recipients. *Transplantation* **55**, 277.

Apasov, S. G. and Sitkovsky, M. V. (1994). Development and antigen specificity of CD8+ cytotoxic T lymphocytes in beta 2-microglobulin-negative, MHC class 1-deficient mice in response to immunization with tumor cells. *J. Immunol.* **152**, 2087.

Armstrong, H. E., Bolton, E. M., McMillan, I., *et al.* (1987). Prolonged survival of actively enhanced rat renal allografts despite accelerated cellular infiltration and rapid induction of both class I and class II MHC antigens. *J. Exp. Med.* **165**, 891.

Auchincloss, H., Lee, R., Shea, S., *et al.* (1993). The role of "indirect" recognition in intiating rejection of skin grafts from major histocompatibility complex class II-deficient mice. *Proc. Natl. Acad. Sci. U. S. A.* **90**, 3373.

Auchincloss, H. and Sachs, D. H. (1998). Xenogeneic transplantation. *Annu. Rev. Immunol.* **16**, 433.

Auchincloss Jr., H. and Sultan, H. (1996). Antigen processing and presentation in transplantation. *Curr. Opin. Immunol.* **8**, 681.

Bacon, K. B. and Schall, T. J. (1996). Chemokines as mediators of allergic inflammation. *Int. Arch. Allergy Immunol.* **109**, 97.

Baldwin, W. M. I., Pruitt, S. K. and Sanfilippo, F. (1991). Alloantibodies: basic and clinical concepts. *Transplant. Rev.* **5**, 100.

Basadonna, G., Matas, A., Gillingham, K., *et al.* (1993). Does early vs late rejection affect renal transplant graft loss to chronic rejection? *Transplant. Proc* **25**, 910.

Batchelor, J. R., Welsh, K. I. and Burgos, H. (1978). Transplantation antigens per se are poor immunogens within a species. *Nature* **273**, 54.

Belich, M. P. and Trowsdale, J. (1995). Proteosome and class I antigen processing and presentation. *Mol. Biol. Rep.* **21**, 53.

Bellgrau, D., Gold, D., Selawry, H., *et al.* (1995). A role for CD95 ligand in preventing graft rejection. *Nature* **377**, 630.

Billingham, R. and Silvers, W. K. (1971). *Immunobiology of Transplantation*, p. 64, Prentice-Hall, Englewood Cliffs, N.J.

Billingham, R. E. and Silvers, W. K. (1964). *Proc. R. Soc. Biol.* **161**, 168.

Bix, M., Liao, N. S., Zijlstra, M., *et al.* (1991). Rejection of class I MHC-deficient haemopoietice cells by irradiated MHC-matched mice. *Nature* **349**, 329.

Bjorkman, P. J. (1997). MHC restriction in three dimensions: a view of the T cell receptor/ligand interactions. *Cell* **89**, 167.

Bjorkman, P. J., Saper, M. A., Samraoni, B., *et al.* (1987). Structure of the human class I histocompatibility antigen, HLA-A2. *Nature* **329**, 506.

Bolling, S., Kunkel, S. L. and Lin, H. (1992). Prolongation of cardiac allograft survival in rats by anti-TNF and cyclosporin combination therapy. *Transplantation* **53**, 283.

Bradley, J. A., Mason, D. W. and Morris, P. J. (1985). Evidence that rat renal allografts are rejected by cytotoxic T cells and not by non-specific effectors. *Transplantation* **39**, 169.

Brazelton, T. R. and Morris, R. E. (1996). Molecular mechansisms of action of new xenobiotic immunosuppressive drugs: tacrolimus (FK506), sirolimus (rapamycin) mycophenolate mofetil and leflunomide. *Curr. Opin. Immunol.* **8**, 710.

Bugeon, L., Cuturi, M.-C., Hallet, M.-M., *et al.* (1992). Peripheral tolerance of an allograft in adult rats—characterization by low interleukin-2 and interferon-γ mRNA levels and by strong accumulation of major histocompatibility complex transcripts in the graft. *Transplantation* **54**, 219.

Burdick, J. F. and Clow, L. W. (1990). Rejection of primarily vascularized heart grafts III: depression of the interleukin 2 mechanism early after grafting. *Transplantation* **50**, 476.

Busch, G. J., Galvanek, E. and Reynolds, E. S. (1971). Human renal allografts: analysis of lesions in long-term survivors. *Hum. Pathol.* **2**, 253.

Butcher, E. C. (1986). The regulation of lymphocyte traffic. *Curr. Top. Microbiol. Immunol.* **128**, 85.

Butcher, E. C. and Picker, L. J. (1996). Lymphocyte homing and homeostasis. *Science* **272**, 60.

Butcher, G. W. and Howard, J. C. (1982). Genetic control of transplant rejection. *Transplantation* **34**, 161.

Calne, R. Y., Sellse, R. A., Pena, J. R., *et al.* (1969). Induction of immunological tolerance by porcine liver allografts. *Nature* **223**, 472.

Campbell, R. D. and Trowsdale, J. (1993). Map of the human major histocompatibility complex. *Immunol. Today* **14**, 349.

Campos, L., Naji, A., Deli, B. C., *et al.* (1995). Survival of MHC-deficient mouse heterotopic cardiac allografts. *Transplantation* **59**, 187.

Cantrell, D., Bluestone, J., Vivier, E., *et al.* (1998). Signalling through the TCR. *Res. Immunol.* **149**, 866.

Cerrilli, J., Holliday, J. E., Koolemans-Beynen, A., *et al.* (1977). Immunologic evaluation of renal allograft recipients. *Transplant. Proc.* **9**, 1815.

Chambers, C. A. and Allison, J. P. (1997). Co-stimulation in T cell responses. *Curr. Opin. Immunol.* **9**, 396.

Chan, S. Y., DeBruyne, L. A., Goodman, R. E., *et al.* (1995). In vivo depletion of CD8+ T cells results in Th2 cytokine production and alternate mechanisms of allograft rejection. *Transplantation* **59**, 1155.

Chen, J., Myllarniemi, M., Akyurek, L. M., *et al.* (1996). Identification of differentially expressed genes in rat aortic allograft vasculopathy. *Am. J. Pathol.* **149**, 597.

Cobbold, S. P., Jayasuriya, A., Nash, A., *et al.* (1984). Therapy with monoclonal antibodies by elimination of T cell subsets in vivo. *Nature* **312**, 548.

Collins, T., Read, M. A., Neish, A. S., *et al.* (1995). Transcriptional regulation of endothelial cell adhesion molecules: NF-kappa B and cytokine-inducible enhancers. *FASEB J.* **9**, 899.

Colonna, M., Brooks, E. G., Falco, M., *et al.* (1993). Generation of allospecific natural killer cells by stimulation across a polymorphism of HLA-C. *Science* **260**, 1121.

Cooper, D. K. C., Good, A. H., Koren, E., *et al.* (1993). Identification of α-galactosyl and other carbohydrate epitopes that are bound by human anti-pig antibodies: relevance to discordant xenografting in man. *Transpl. Immunol.* **1**, 198.

Cosimi, A. B., Conti, D., Delmonico, F. L., *et al.* (1990). In vivo effects of monoclonal antibody to ICAM-1 (CD54) in nonhuman primates with renal allografts. *J. Immunol.* **144**, 4604.

Cramer, D. V., Qian, S., Harnaha, J., *et al.* (1989). Cardiac transplantation in the rat I: the effect of histocompatibility differences on graft arteriosclerosis. *Transplantation* **47**, 414.

Cramer, D. V., Wu, G. D., Chapman, F. A., *et al.* (1992). Lymphocyte subsets and histopathologic changes associated with the development of heart transplant arteriosclerosis. *J. Heart Lung Transplant.* **11**, 458.

Cresswell, P. (1994). Assembly, transport and function of MHC class II molecules. *Annu. Rev. Immunol.* **12**, 259.

Daar, A. S., Fuggle, S. V., Hart, D. N. J., *et al.* (1983). Demonstration and phenotypic characterisation of HLA-DR positive interstitial dendritic cells widely distributed in human connective tissue. *Transplant. Proc.* **XV (Suppl 1)**, 311.

Dai, Z. and Lakkis, F. G. (1999). The role of cytokines, CTLA-4 and costimulation in transplant tolerance and rejection. *Curr. Opin. Immunol.* **11**, 504.

Dallman, M. J. (1993). Cytokines as mediators of organ graft rejection and tolerance. *Curr. Opin. Immunol.* **5**, 788.

Dallman, M. J. (1995). Cytokines and transplantation: Th1/Th2 regulation of the immune response to solid organ transplants in the adult. *Curr. Opin. Immunol.* **7**, 632.

Dallman, M. J. and Clark, G. J. (1992). Cytokine and their receptors in transplantation. *Curr. Opin. Immunol.* **3**, 729.

Dallman, M. J., Larsen, C. P. and Morris, P.J. (1991a). Cytokine gene transcription in vascularised organ grafts—analysis using semi-quantitative polymerase chain reaction. *J. Exp. Med.* **174**, 493.

Dallman, M. J., Mason, D. W. and Webb, M. (1982). Induction of Ia antigens on murine epidermal cells during the rejection of skin allografts. *Eur. J. Immunol.* **12**, 511.

Dallman, M. J., Shiho, O., Page, T. H., *et al.* (1991b). Peripheral tolerance to alloantigen results from altered regulation of the interleukin 2 pathway. *J. Exp. Med.* **173**, 79.

Dallman, M. J., Wood, K. J., Hamano, K., *et al.* (1993). Cytokines and peripheral tolerance to alloantigen. *Immunol. Rev.* **133**, 5.

Dallman, M. J., Wood, K. J. and Morris, P. J. (1987). Specific cytotoxic T cells are found in the non-rejected kidneys of blood transfused rats. *J. Exp. Med.* **165**, 566.

Dalloul, A. H., Chmouzis, E., Ngo, K., *et al.* (1996a). Adoptively transferred CD4+ lymphocytes from CD8−/− mice are sufficient to mediate rejection of MHC class II or class I disparate skin grafts. *J. Immunol.* **156**, 411.

Dalloul, A. H., Ngo, K. and Fung-Leing, W.-P. (1996b). CD4-negative cytotoxic T cells with a T cell receptor alpha/beta intermediate expression in CD8-deficient mice. *Eur. J. Immunol.* **26**, 213.

Davis, D. M., Chui, I., Fassett, M., *et al.* (1999). The human natural killer cell synapse. *Proc. Natl. Acad. Sci. U. S. A.* **96**, 15062.

Del Prete, G. F., De Carli, M., Mastromauro, C., *et al.* (1991). Purified protein derivative of Mycobacterium tuberculosis and excretory-secretory antigen(s) of Toxocara canis expand in vitro human T cells with stable and opposite (type 1 T helper or type 2 T helper) profile of cytokine production. *J. Clin. Invest.* **88**, 346.

Demetris, A. J., Zerbe, T. and Banner, B. (1989). Morphology of solid organ allograft arteriopathy: identification of proliferating intimal cell populations. *Transplant. Proc.* **21**, 3667.

DeVries, M. E., Ran, L. and Kelvin, D. (1999). On the edge: the physiological and pathophysiological role of chemokines during inflammatory and immunological responses. *Semin. Immunol.* **11**, 95.

Dierich, A., Chan, S. H., Benoist, C., *et al.* (1993). Graft rejection by T cells not restricted by conventional major histocompatibility complex molecules. *Eur. J. Immunol.* **23**, 2725.

Dorling, A. and Lechler, R. I. (1996). The passenger leucocyte, dendritic cell and antigen-presenting cell (APC). *In Transplantation Biology: Cellular and Molecular Aspects*, (N. L. Tilney, T. B. Strom and L. C. Paul, eds.), p. 355, Lippincott-Raven, Philadelphia.

Doyle, H. R., Marino, I. R., Morelli, F., *et al.* (1996). Assessing risk in liver transplantation—special reference to the significance of a positive crossmatch. *Ann. Surg.* **224**, 168.

Duijvestijn, A. M. and Van Breda Vriesman, P. J. C. (1991). Chronic renal allograft rejection: selective involvement of the glomerular endothelium in humoral immune reactivity and intravascular coagulation. *Transplantation* **52**, 195.

Dunnill, M. S. (1984). Histopathology of rejection in renal transplantation. *In Kidney Transplantation: Principles and Practice*, 2nd ed., (P. J. Morris, ed.), p. 355, Grune & Stratton, New York.

Dvorak, H. F., Mihm, M. C. J., Dvorak, A. M., *et al.* (1979). Rejection of first-set skin allografts in man—the microvasculature is the critical target of the immune response. *J. Exp. Med.* **150**, 322.

Emma, D. A. and Jacobs, B. B. (1981). Prolongation of skin allograft survival following donor irradiation and organ culture explanation. *Transplantation* **31**, 138.

Engers, H. D., Glasebrooke, A. L. and Sorenson, G. D. (1982). Allogeneic tumour rejection induced by the intravenous injection of Lyt-2+ cytolytic T lymphocyte clones. *J. Exp. Med.* **156**, 1280.

Fabre, J. W. and Morris, P. J. (1975). Studies on the specific suppression of renal allograft rejection in presensitised rats. *Transplantation* **19**, 121.

Fairchild, R. L., VanBuskirk, A. M., Kondo, T., *et al.* (1997). Expression of chemokine genes during rejection and long-term acceptance of cardiac allografts. *Transplantation* **63**, 1807.

Fangmann, J., Dalchau, R. and Fabre, J. W. (1992). Rejection of skin allografts by indirect allorecognition of donor class I major histocompatibility complex peptides. *J. Exp. Med.* **175**, 1521.

Farges, O., Morris, P. J. and Dallman, M. J. (1994). Spontaneous acceptance of liver allografts in the rat: analysis of the immune response. *Transplantation* **57**, 171.

Farges, O., Morris, P. J. and Dallman, M. J. (1995). Spontaneous acceptance of rat liver allografts is associated with an early down regulation of intragraft IL-4 mRNA expression. *Hepatology* **21**, 767.

Fellous, M., Nir, U., Wallach, D., *et al.* (1982). Interferon-dependent induction of mRNA for the major histocompatibility antigens in human fibroblasts and lymphoblastoid cells. *Proc. Natl. Acad. Sci. U. S. A.* **79**, 3082.

Fisher, M., Chapman, J. R., Ting, A., *et al.* (1985). Alloimmunisation to HLA antigens following transfusion with leucocytes poor and purified platelet suspensions. *Vox. Sang.* **49**, 331.

Florey, H. W. and Jennings, M. A. (1970). *In General Pathology*, 4th ed., (H. W. Florey, ed.), p. 124, Lloyd-Luke, London.

Foster, P., Sankary, H. N. and Hart, M. (1989). Blood and graft eosinophilia as predictors of rejection in human liver transplantation. *Transplantation* **47**, 72.

Frasca, L., Carmichael, P., Lechler, R., *et al.* (1997). Anergic T cells effect linked suppression. *Eur. J. Immunol.* **27**, 3191.

Freeman, G. J., Boussiotis, V. A., Anumanthan, A., *et al.* (1995). B7-1 and B7-2 do not deliver identical costimulatory signals, since B7-2 but not B7-1 preferentially costimulates the initial production of IL-4. *Immunity* **2**, 523.

Frelinger, J. G., Hood, L., Hill, S., *et al.* (1979). Mouse epidermal Ia molecules have a bone marrow origin. *Nature* **282**, 321.

Fuggle, S., McWhinnie, D. L., Chapman, J. R., *et al.* (1986). Sequential analysis of HLA-Class II antigen expression in human renal allografts. *Transplantation* **42**, 144.

Fuggle, S. V., Errasti, P., Daar, A. S., *et al.* (1983). Localisation of major histocompatibility complex (HLA-ABC and DR) antigens in 46 kidneys: differences in HLA-DR staining of tubules among kidneys. *Transplantation* **35**, 385.

Gainer, A. L., Suarez-Pinzon, W. L., Min, W. P., *et al.* (1998). Improved survival of biolistically transfected mouse islet allografts expressing CTLA4-Ig or soluble Fas ligand. *Transplantation* **66**, 194.

Gajewski, T. F. and Fitch, F. W. (1988). Anti-proliferative effect of IFN-γ in immune regulation I: IFN-γ inhibits the proliferation of TH2 but not TH1 murine helper T lymphocyte clones. *J. Immunol.* **140**, 4245.

Gajewski, T. F., Schell, S. R., Nau, G., *et al.* (1989). Regulation of T cell activation: differences among T-cell subsets. *Immunol. Rev.* **111**, 79.

Galili, U., Macher, B. A., Buchler, J., *et al.* (1985). Human natural anti-α-galactosyl IgG II: the specific recognition of α (1-3)-linked galactosyl residues. *J. Exp. Med.* **162**, 573.

Galili, U., Rachmilewitz, E. A., Peleg, A., *et al.* (1984). A unique natural human IgG antibody with anti α-galactosyl specificity. *J. Exp. Med.* **160**, 1519.

Galluchi, S., Lolkema, M. and Matzinger, P. (1999). Natural adjuvants: endogenous activators of dendritic cells. *Nat. Med.* **5**, 1249.

Garcia, K. C., Degano, M., Stanfield, R. L., *et al.* (1996). An αβ T cell receptor structure at 2.5A and its orientation in the TCR-MHC complex. *Science* **274**, 209.

Germain, R. N. and Margulies, D. H. (1993). The biochemistry and cell biology of antigen processing and presentation. *Annu. Rev. Immunol.* **11**, 403.

Gibson, J. M. and Medawar, P. B. (1943). The fate of skin homografts in man. *J. Anat.* **77**, 299.

Golding, H. and Singer, A. (1984). Role of accessory cell processing and presentation of shed H-2 alloantigens in allospecific cytotoxic T lymphocyte responses. *J. Immunol.* **133**, 597.

Gorczynski, R. M. (1992). Immunosuppression induced by hepatic portal venous immunization spares reactivity in IL-4 producing T lymphocytes. *Immunol. Lett.* **33**, 67.

Gorer, P. A. (1938). The antigenic basis of tumour transplantation. *J. Pathol. Bacteriol.* **47**, 231.

Goulmy, E. (1985). Class I restricted human cytotoxic T lymphocytes directed against minor transplantation antigens and their role in organ transplantation. *Prog. Allergy* **36**, 44.

Gowans, J. L. (1959). The recirculation of lymphocytes from blood to lymph in the rat. *J. Physiol.* **146**, 54.

Gracie, J. A., Bolton, E. M., Porteous, C., *et al.* (1990). T cell requirements for the rejection of renal allografts bearing an isolated class I disparity. *J. Exp. Med.* **172**, 1547.

Grakoui, A., Bromley, S. K., Sumen, C., *et al.* (1999). The immunological synapse: a molecular machine controlling T cell activation. *Science* **285**, 221.

Grandaliano, G., Gesualdo, L., Ranieri, E., *et al.* (1997). Monocyte chemotactic peptide-1 expression and monocyte infiltration in acute renal transplant rejection. *Transplantation* **63**, 414.

Greenfield, A., Scott, D., Pennisi, D., *et al.* (1996). An H-YDb epitope is encoded by a novel mouse Y chromosome gene. *Nat. Genet.* **14**, 474.

Grey, H. M. and Chestnut, R. (1985). Antigen processing and presentation to T cells. *Immunol. Today* **6**, 101.

Griffith, T. S., Brunner, T., Fletcher, S. M., *et al.* (1995). Fas ligand-induced apoptosis as a mechanism of immune privilege. *Science* **270**, 1189.

Gummert, J. F., Ikonen, T. and Morris, R. E. (1999). Newer immunosuppressive drugs: a review. *J. Am. Soc. Nephrol.* **10**, 1366.

Gurley, K. E., Lowry, R. P. and Clarke-Forbes, R. D. (1983). Immune mechanisms in organ allograft rejection II: T helper cells, delayed type hypersensitivity and rejection of renal allografts. *Transplantation* **36**, 401.

Guttman, R. D., Lindquist, R. R. and Ockner, S. A. (1969). Renal transplantation in the inbred rat. *Transplantation* **8**, 472.

Hall, B. M., DeSaxe, I. and Dorsch, S. E. (1983). The cellular basis of allograft rejection in vivo: restoration of first set rejection of heart grafts by T helper cells in irradiated rats. *Transplantation* **36**, 700.

Hall, B. M., Dorsch, S. and Roser, B. (1978). The cellular basis of allograft rejection in vivo. *J. Exp. Med.* **148**, 878.

Halloran, P. F., Broski, A. P., Batiuk, T. D., *et al.* (1993). The molecular immunology of acute rejection: an overview. *Transpl. Immunol.* **1**, 3.

Hamel, M. E., Noteboom, E. and Kruisbeek, A. M. (1998). Non-responsiveness of antigen-experienced CD4 T cells reflects more stringent co-stimulatory requirements. *Immunology* **93**, 366.

Hancock, W. H., Whitley, W. D., Tullius, S. G., *et al.* (1993). Cytokines, adhesion molecules and the pathogenesis of chronic infection in rat renal allografts. *Transplantation* **56**, 643.

Harding, F. A., McArthur, J. G., Gross, J. A., *et al.* (1992). CD28-mediated signalling co-stimulates T cells and prevents induction of anergy in T-cell clones. *Nature* **356**, 607.

Hart, D. N. and Fabre, J. W. (1980). Kidney-specific alloantigen system in the rat: characterisation and role in transplantation. *J. Exp. Med.* **151**, 651.

Hart, D. N. and Fabre, J. W. (1981a). Demonstration and characterisation of Ia positive dendritic cells in the interstitial connective tissues of the rat heart and other tissues, but not brain. *J. Exp. Med.* **154**, 347.

Hart, D. N. J. and Fabre, J. W. (1981b). Major histocompatibility complex antigens in rat kidney, ureter and bladder. *Transplantation* **31**, 318.

Haug, C. E., Colvin, R. B., Delmonico, F. L., *et al.* (1993). A phase I trial of immunosuppression with anti-ICAM-1 (CD54) mAb in renal allograft recipients. *Transplantation* **55**, 766.

Hayry, P. and Defendi, V. (1970). Mixed lymphocyte cultures produce effector cells: model in vitro for allograft rejection. *Science* **168**, 133.

Hayry, P., Mennander, A., Raisanen-Sokolowski, A., *et al.* (1993). Pathophysiology of vascular wall changes in chronic allograft rejection. *Transplant. Rev.* **7**, 1.

Heagy, W., Waltenbaugh, C. and Martz, E. (1984). Potent ability of anti-LFA-1 monoclonal antibody to prolong allograft survival. *Transplantation* **37**, 520.

Henretta, J., Araneda, D., Pittman, K., *et al.* (1995). Marked prolongation of incompatible class I deficient heart allografts: paradoxical effects between primarily and secondarily vascularized allografts. *Transplant. Proc.* **27**, 1303.

Herberman, R. B., Djeu, J. Y., Kay, H. D., *et al.* (1979). Natural killer cells: characteristics and regulation of activity. *Immunol. Rev.* **44**, 43.

Hodes, R. J. and Svedmyr, E. A. J. (1970). Specific cytotoxicity of H-2-incompatible mouse lymphocytes following mixed culture in vitro. *Transplantation* **9**, 470.

Hourmant, M., Bedrossian, J., Durand, D., *et al.* (1996). A randomized multicenter trial comparing leukocyte function-associated antigen-1 monoclonal antibody with rabbit antithymocyte globulin as induction treatment in first kidney transplantations. *Transplantation* **62**, 1565.

Hsieh, C. S., Heimberger, A. B., Gold, J. S., *et al.* (1992). Differential regulation of T helper phenotype development by interleukins 4 and 10 in an alpha beta T-cell-receptor transgenic system. *Proc. Natl. Acad. Sci. U. S. A.* **89**, 6065.

Hsieh, C. S., Macatonia, S. E., Tripp, C. S., *et al.* (1993). Development of Th1 CD4 + T cells through IL-12 produced by Listeria-induced macrophages. *Science* **260**, 547.

Hughes, C. C., Savage, C. O. and Pober, J. S. (1990). The endothelial cell as a regulator of T-cell function. *Immunol. Rev.* **117**, 85.

Hurme, M., Chandler, P. R., Hetherington, C. M., *et al.* (1978a). Cytotoxic T cell responses to H-Y: correlation with the rejection of syngeneic male skin grafts. *J. Exp. Med.* **147**, 768.

Hurme, M., Hetherington, C. M., Chandler, P. R., *et al.* (1978b). Cytotoxic T cell responses to H-Y: mapping of the Ir genes. *J. Exp. Med.* **147**, 758.

Imagawa, D. K., Millis, J. M., Olthoff, K. M., *et al.* (1990). The role of tumor necrosis factor in allograft rejection II: evidence that antibody therapy against tumor necrosis factor-alpha and lymphotoxin enhances cardiac survival in rats. *Transplantation* **50**, 189.

Imagawa, D. K., Millis, J. M., Seu, P., *et al.* (1991). The role of tumor necrosis factor in allograft rejection III: evidence that anti-TNF antibody therapy prolongs allograft survival in rats with acute rejection. *Transplantation* **51**, 57.

Ingham-Clark, C. L., Cunningham, A. J., Crane, P. W., *et al.* (1990). Lymphocyte infiltration patterns in rat small-bowel transplants. *Transplant. Proc.* **22**, 2460.

Iwata, T., Kamei, Y., Esaki, S., *et al.* (1996). Immunosuppression by anti-ICAM-1 and anti-LFA-1 monoclonal antibodies of free and vascularized skin allograft rejection. *Immunobiology* **195**, 160.

Janeway, C. A., Walport, M., Travers, P., *et al.* (1999). *Immunobiology: The Immune System in Health and Disease*, 4th ed., Current Biology Ltd., London, U.K.

Jenkins, M. K., Pardoll, D. M., Mizuguchi, J., *et al.* (1987). Molecular events in the induction of a nonresponsive state in interleukin 2-producing helper T-lymphocyte clones. *Proc. Natl. Acad. Sci. U. S. A.* **84**, 5409.

Jenkins, M. K. and Schwartz, R. H. (1987). Antigen presentation by chemically modified splenocytes induces antigen-specific T cell unresponsiveness in vitro and in vivo. *J. Exp. Med.* **165**, 302.

Josien, R., Pannetier, C., Douillard, P., *et al.* (1995). Graft infiltrating T helper cells CD45RC phenotype and TH1/TH2-related cytokines in donor specific transfusion-induced tolerance in adult rats. *Transplantation* **60**, 1131.

June, C. H., Ledbetter, J. A., Gillespie, M. M., *et al.* (1987). T cell proliferation involving the CD28 pathway is associated with cyclosporine-resistant interleukin 2 gene expression. *Mol. Cell. Biol.* **7**, 4472.

Kagi, D., Seiler, P., Pavlovic, J., *et al.* (1995). The roles of perforin- and Fas-dependent cytotoxicity in protection against cytopathic and non-cytopathic viruses. *Eur. J. Immunol.* **25**, 3256.

Kamada, N. (1988). *Experimental Liver Transplantation.* CRC Press, Boca Raton, Fla.

Kamada, N., Davies, H. and Roser, B. (1981). Reversal of transplantation of immunity by liver grafting. *Nature* **292**, 840.

Kamada, N. and Wight, D. G. D. (1984). Antigen-specific immunosuppression induced by liver transplantation in the rat. *Transplantation* **38**, 217.

Karandiker, N., Vanderlugt, C. L., Walunas, T. L., *et al.* (1996). CTLA-4: a negative regulator in autoimmune disease. *J. Exp. Med.* **184**, 783.

Katsura, Y. (1977). Cell-mediated and humoral immune responses in mice III: dynamic balance between delayed-type hypersensitivity and antibody response. *Immunology* **32**, 227.

Katz, S. I., Tamaki, K. and Sachs, D. H. (1979). Epidermal Langerhans cells are derived from cells originating in bone marrow. *Nature* **282**, 324.

Kauntz, S. L., Williams, M. A., Williams, P. L., *et al.* (1963). Mechanism of rejection of homotransplantated kidneys. *Nature* **199**, 257.

Kawai, K., Shahinian, A., Mak, T. W., *et al.* (1996). Skin allograft rejection in CD28-deficient mice. *Transplantation* **61**, 352.

Kelso, A. (1995). Th1 and Th2 subsets: paradigms lost? *Immunol. Today* **16**, 374.

Kim, P. C., Levy, G. A., Koh, I., *et al.* (1991). Immunologic basis of small intestinal allograft rejection. *Transplant. Proc.* **23**, 830.

Kirby, J. A. (1996). Function of leucocyte adhesion molecules during allograft rejection. In *Transplantation Biology: Cellular and Molecular Aspects*, (N. L. Tilney, T. B. Strom and L. C. Paul, eds.), Lippincott-Raven Publishers, Philadelphia.

Kirk, A. D., Burkly, L. C., Batty, D. S., *et al.* (1999). Treatment with humanized monoclonal antibody against CD154 prevents acute renal allograft rejection in nonhuman primates. *Nat. Med.* **5**, 686.

Kirkman, R. L., Colvin, R. B., Flye, M. W., *et al.* (1979). Transplantation in miniature swine. *Transplantation* **28**, 24.

Kissmeyer-Nielsen, F., Olsen, S., Peterson, V. P., *et al.* (1966). Hyperacute rejection of kidney allografts associated with pre-existing humoral antibodies against donor cells. *Lancet* **2**, 662.

Klein, J., Chiang, C. L. and Hauptfeld, V. (1977). Histocompatibility antigens controlled by the I region of the Murine H-2 complex. *J. Exp. Med.* **145**, 450.

Klein, J., Juretic, A., Baxevanis, C. N., *et al.* (1981). The traditional and a new version of the mouse H-2 complex. *Nature* **291**, 455.

Koga, S., Novick, A. C., Toma, H., *et al.* (1999). CD8 + T cells produce RANTES during acute rejection of murine allogeneic skin grafts. *Transplantation* **67**, 854.

Konieczny, B. T., Saleem, S., Lowry, R. P., *et al.* (1996). Vigorous cardiac allograft rejection in IFN gamma knockout mice. Proceedings of the *15th Annual Meeting of the American Society of Transplant Physicians*, p. 170.

Koo, D. D., Welsh, K. I., Roake, J. R., *et al.* (1998). Ischemia/reperfusion injury in human kidney transplantation: an immunohistochemical analysis of changes after reperfusion. *Am. J. Pathol.* **153**, 557.

Kormendi, F. and Amend, W. J. C. (1988). The importance of eosinophil cells in kidney allograft rejection. *Transplantation* **45**, 537.

Krieger, N. R., Yin, D.-P. and Fathman, C. G. (1996). CD4 + but not CD8 + cells are essential for allorejection. *J. Exp. Med.* **184**, 2013.

Kuchroo, V. K., Das, M. P., Brown, J. A., *et al.* (1995). B7.1 and B7.2 costimulatory molecules activate differentially the Th1/Th2 developmental pathways: application to autoimmune disease. *Cell* **80**, 707.

Kudig, T., Shahinian, A., Kawai, K., *et al.* (1996). Duration of TCR stimulation determines co-stimulatory requirement of T cells. *Immunity* **5**, 41.

Laden, A. M. K. and Sinclair, R. A. (1971). Thickening of arterial intima in rat cardiac allografts. *Am. J. Pathol.* **63**, 69.

Lafferty, K. J., Bootes, A., Dart, G., *et al.* (1976). Effect of organ culture on the survival of thyroid allografts in mice. *Transplantation* **22**, 138.

Lakkis, F. G., Konieczny, B. T., Saleem, S., *et al.* (1997). Blocking the CD28-B7 T cell costimulation pathway induces long term cardiac allograft acceptance in the absence of IL-4. *J. Immunol.* **158**, 2443.

Lamouse-Smith, E., Clements, V. K. and Ostrand-Rosenberg, S. (1993). Beta 2M − / − knockout mice contain low levels of CD8 + cytotoxic T lymphocyte that mediate specific tumor rejection. *J. Immunol.* **151**, 6283.

Lampert, I. A., Suitters, A. J. and Chisholm, P. M. (1981). Expression of Ia antigen on epidermal keratinocytes in graft-versus-host disease. *Nature* **293**, 149.

Land, W., Schneeberger, H., Schleibner, S., *et al.* (1994). The beneficial effect of human recombinant superoxide dismutase on acute and chronic rejection events in recipients of cadaveric renal transplants. *Transplantation* **57**, 211.

Larsen, C. P., Alexander, D. Z., Hollenbaugh, D., *et al.* (1996a). CD40-gp39 interactions play a critical role during allograft rejection: suppression of allograft rejection by blockade of the CD40-gp39 pathway. *Transplantation* **61**, 4.

Larsen, C. P., Elwood, E. T., Alexander, D. Z., *et al.* (1996b). Long term acceptance of skin and cardiac allografts after blocking CD40 and CD28 pathways. *Nature* **381**, 434.

Larsen, C. P., Morris, P. J. and Austyn, J. M. (1990a). Migration of dendritic leucocytes from cardiac allografts into host spleens: a novel pathway for initiation of rejection. *J. Exp. Med.* **171**, 307.

Larsen, C. P., Ritchie, S. C., Hendrix, R., *et al.* (1994). Regulation of immunostimulatory function and costimulatory molecule (B7-1 and B7-2) expression on murine dendritic cells. *J. Immunol.* **152**, 5208.

Larsen, C. P., Steinman, R. M., Witmer-Pack, M., *et al.* (1990b). Migration and maturation of Langerhans cells in skin transplants and explants. *J. Exp. Med.* **172**, 1483.

Lau, H. T. and Stoeckert, C. J. (1997). FasL—too much of a good thing? Transplanted grafts of pancreatic islet cells engineered to express Fas ligand are destroyed not protected by the immune system. *Nat. Med.* **3**, 727.

Lau, H. T., Yu, M., Fontana, A., *et al.* (1996). Prevention of islet allograft rejection with engineered myoblasts expressing FasL in mice. *Science* **273**, 109.

Lechler, R. I. and Batchelor, J. R. (1982). Restoration of immunogenicity to passenger cell-depleted kidney allografts by the addition of donor strain dendritic cells. *J. Exp. Med.* **155**, 31.

Lee, R. S., Grusby, M. J., Glimcher, L. H., *et al.* (1994). Indirect recognition by helper cells can induce donor-specific cytotoxic T lymphocytes in vivo. *J. Exp. Med.* **179**, 865.

Lee, R. S., Grusby, M. J., Laufer, T. M., *et al.* (1997). CD8+ effector cells responding to residual class I antigens, with help from CD4+ cells stimulated indirectly cause rejection of "major histocompatibility complex-deficient" skin grafts. *Transplantation* **63**, 1123.

Leeuwen van, J. E. and Samelson, L. E. (1999). T cell antigen-receptor signal transduction. *Curr. Opin. Immunol.* **11**, 242.

Leibson, P. J. (1995). MHC-recognising receptors: they're not just for T cells anymore. *Immunity* **3**, 5.

Le-Moine, A., Flamand, V., Demoor, F. X., *et al.* (1999a). Critical roles for IL-4, IL-5 and eosinophils in chronic skin allograft rejection. *J. Clin. Invest.* **103**, 1659.

Le-Moine, A., Surquin, M., Demoor, F. X., *et al.* (1999b). IL-5 mediates eosinophilic rejection of MHC class II-disparate skin allografts in mice. *J. Immunol.* **163**, 3778.

Lenschow, D. J., Herold, K. C., Rhee, L., *et al.* (1996a). CD28/B7 regulation of Th1 and Th2 subsets in the development of autoimmune diabetes. *Immunity* **5**, 285.

Lenschow, D. J., Sperling, A. I., Cooke, M. P., *et al.* (1994). Differential up-regulation of the B7-1 and B7-2 costimulatory molecules after Ig receptor engagement by antigen. *J. Immunol.* **153**, 1990.

Lenschow, D. J., Walunas, T. L. and Bluestone, J. A. (1996b). CD28/B7 system of T cell co-stimulation. *Annu. Rev. Immunol.* **14**, 233.

Lenschow, D. J., Zeng, Y., Thistlethwaite, J. R., *et al.* (1992). Long-term survival of xenogeneic pancreatic islet grafts induced by CTLA4Ig. *Science* **257**, 789.

Lentsch, A. B., Yoshidome, H., Cheadle, W. G., *et al.* (1998). Chemokine involvement in hepatic ischemia/reperfusion injury in mice: roles for macrophage inflammatory protein-2 and KC [corrected and republished article originally printed in *Hepatology* (1998). **27(2)**, 507]. *Hepatology* **27**, 1172.

Li, X. and Faustman, D. (1993). Use of donor beta 2-microglobulin-deficient transgenic mouse liver cells for isografts, allografts and xenografts. *Transplantation* **55**, 940.

Liew, F. Y. and Simpson, E. (1980). Delayed type hypersensitivity to H-Y: characterisation and mapping of Ir genes. *Immunogenetics* **11**, 255.

Lindsten, T., June, C. H., Ledbetter, J. A., *et al.* (1989). Regulation of lymphokine messenger RNA stability by a surface-mediated T cell activation pathway. *Science* **244**, 339.

Linsley, P. S., Greene, J. L., Brady, W., *et al.* (1994). Human B7-1 (CD80) and B7-2 (CD86) bind with similar avidities but distinct kinetics to CD28 and CTLA-4 receptors. *Immunity* **1**, 793.

Little, C. C. and Tyzer, E. E. (1916). Further experimental studies on the inheritance of susceptibility to a transplantable tumour carcinoma (JWA) of the Japanese Waltzing mouse. *J. Med. Res.* **33**, 393.

Liu, Z., Braunstein, N. S. and Suciu, F. N. (1992). T cell recognition of allopeptides in context of self-MHC. *J. Immunol.* **148**, 35.

Lombardi, G., Sidhu, S., Batchelor, R., *et al.* (1994). Anergic T cells as suppressor cells in vitro. *Science* **264**, 1587.

Long, E. O. and Wagtmann, N. (1997). Natural killer cell receptors. *Curr. Opin. Immunol.* **9**, 344.

Loveland, B. E., Hogarth, P. M., Ceredig, R., *et al.* (1981). Delayed type hypersensitivity and allograft rejection in the mouse: correlation of effector cell phenotype. *J. Exp. Med.* **153**, 1044.

Loveland, B. E. and McKenzie, I. F. C. (1982). Cells mediating graft rejection in the mouse. *Immunology* **46**, 313.

Lowry, R. P., Gurley, K. E. and Clarke-Forbes, R. D. (1983). Immune mechanisms in organ allograft rejection: 1. delayed type hypersensitivity and lymphocytotoxicity in heart graft rejection. *Transplantation* **36**, 391.

Macatonia, S. E., Doherty, T. M., Knight, S. C., *et al.* (1993a). Differential effect of IL-10 on dendritic cell-induced T cell proliferation and IFNγ production. *J. Immunol.* **150**, 3755.

Macatonia, S. E., Hsieh, C.-S., O'Garra, A., *et al.* (1993b). Dendritic cells and macrophages are required for Th1 development of CD4+ T cells from alpha beta TCR transgenic mice: IL-12 substitution for macrophages to stimulate IFN-gamma production is IFN-gamma-dependent. *Int. Immunol.* **5**, 1119.

Mackay, C. R. (1993a). Homing of naive, memory and effector lymphocytes. *Curr. Opin. Immunol.* **5**, 423.

Mackay, C. R. (1993b). Immunological memory. *Adv. Immunol.* **53**, 217.

Madsen, J. C., Peugh, W. N., Wood, K. J., *et al.* (1987). The effect of anti-L3T4 monoclonal antibody treatment on first set rejection of murine cardiac allografts. *Transplantation* **44**, 849.

Madsen, J. C., Superina, R. A., Wood, K. J., *et al.* (1988). Induction of immunological unresponsiveness using recipient cells transfected with donor MHC genes. *Nature (Lond.)* **332**, 161.

Malaviya, R., Twesten, N. J., Ross, E. A., *et al.* (1996). Mast cells process bacterial Ags through a phagocytic route for class I MHC presentation to T cells. *J. Immunol.* **156**, 1490.

Mandelbrot, D. A., Furukawa, Y., McAdam, A. J., *et al.* (1999). Expression of B7 molecules in recipient, not donor mice determines the survival of cardiac allografts. *J. Immunol.* **163**, 3753.

Mandrup-Poulsen, T., Bendtzen, K., Nerup, J., *et al.* (1986). Affinity-purified human interleukin I is cytotoxic to isolated islets of Langerhans. *Diabetologia* **29**, 63.

Mandrup-Poulsen, T., Helqvist, S., Molvig, J., *et al.* (1989). Cytokines as immune effector molecules in autoimmune endocrine diseases with special reference to insulin-dependent diabetes mellitus. *Autoimmunity* **4**, 191.

Mannon, R. B., Nataraj, C., Kotzin, B. L., *et al.* (1995). Rejection of kidney allografts by MHC class 1-deficient mice. *Transplantation* **59**, 746.

Marelli-Berg, F. M., Barroso-Herrera, O. and Lechler, R. I. (1999a). Recently activated T cells are costimulation-dependent in vitro. *Cell. Immunol.* **195**, 18.

Marelli-Berg, F. M., Frasca, L., Weng, L., *et al.* (1999b). Antigen recognition influences transendothelial migration of CD4+ T cells. *J. Immunol.* **162**, 696.

Markmann, J. F., Bassiri, H., Desai, N. M., *et al.* (1992). Indefinite survival of MHC class I-deficient murine pancreatic islet allografts. *Transplantation* **54**, 1085.

Mason, D. W., Dallman, M. J. and Barclay, A. N. (1981). Graft-versus-host disease induces expression of Ia antigen in rat epidermal cells and gut epithelium. *Nature* **293**, 150.

Mason, D. W. and Morris, P. J. (1984). Inhibition of the accumulation, in rat kidney allografts, of specific- but not nonspecific-cytotoxic cells by cyclosporine. *Transplantation* **37**, 46.

McKnight, A. J., Barclay, A. N. and Mason, D. W. (1991). Molecular cloning of rat interleukin 4 cDNA and analysis of the cytokine repertoire of subsets of CD4+ T cells. *Eur. J. Immunol.* **21**, 1187.

McLean, A. G., Hughes, D., Welsh, K. I., *et al.* (1997). Patterns of graft infiltration and cytokine gene expression during the first 10 days of kidney transplantation. *Transplantation* **63**, 374.

Medawar, P. B. (1944). Behaviour and fate of skin autografts and skin homografts in rabbits. *J. Anat.* **78**, 176.

Medawar, P. B. (1945). A second study of the behaviour and fate of skin homografts in rabbits. *J. Anat.* **79**, 157.

Medzhitov, R. and Janeway, C. A. J. (1997). Innate immunity: the virtues of a nonclonal system of recognition. *Cell* **91**, 295.

Mennander, A., Tisala, S., Paavonen, T., *et al.* (1991). Chronic rejection of rat aortic allograft II: administration of cyclosporine induces accelerated allograft arteriosclerosis. *Transpl. Int.* **4**, 173.

Merwe van der, P. A., Bodian, D. L., Daenke, S., *et al.* (1997). CD80 (B7-1) binds both CD28 and CTLA-4 with a low affinity and very fast kinetics. *J. Exp. Med.* **185**, 393.

Mintz, B. and Silvers, W. K. (1967). "Intrinsic" immunological tolerance in allophenic mice. *Science* **158**, 1484.

Mintz, B. and Silvers, W. K. (1970). Histocompatibility antigens on melanoblasts and hair follicle cells. *Transplantation* **9**, 497.

Mohler, K. M. and Streilein, J. W. (1989). Differential expression of helper versus effector activity in mice rendered neonatally tolerant of class II MHC antigens. *Transplantation* **47**, 633.

Monaco, J. J. (1992). Major histocompatibility complex-linked transport proteins and antigen processing. *Immunol. Res.* **11**, 125.

Monaco, J. J. (1993). Structure and function of genes in the MHC class II region. *Curr. Opin. Immunol.* **5**, 17.

Monaco, J. J. (1995). Pathways for the processing and presentation of antigens to T cells. *J. Leukoc. Biol.* **57**, 543.

Monks, C. R., Freiberg, B. A., Kupfer, H., *et al.* (1998). Three-dimensional segregation of supramolecular activation clusters in T cells. *Nature* **395**, 82.

Morikawa, M., Tamatani, T., Miyasaka, M., *et al.* (1994). Cardiac allografts in rat recipients with simultaneous use of anti-ICAM-1 and anti-LFA-1 monoclonal antibodies leads to accelerated graft loss. *Immunopharmacology* **28**, 171.

Morris, P. J. and Ting, A. (1982). Studies of HLA-DR with relevance to renal transplantation. *Immunol. Rev.* **66**, 103.

Morris, R. E. (1991). Rapamycin: FK506's fraternal twin or distant cousin? *Immunol. Today* **12**, 137.

Morris, R. E. (1993). New small molecule immunosuppressants for transplantation: review of essential concepts. *J. Heart Lung Transplant.* **12**, S275.

Morton, P. A., Fu, X.-T., Stewart, J. A., *et al.* (1996). Differential effects of CTLA-4 substitutions on the binding of human CD80 (B7-1) and CD86 (B7-2). *J. Immunol.* **156**, 1047.

Mosmann, T. R., Cherwinski, H., Bond, M. W., *et al.* (1986). Two types of murine helper T cell clone: 1. definition according to profiles of lymphokine activities and secreted proteins. *J. Immunol.* **136**, 2348.

Mosmann, T. R. and Coffman, R. L. (1989). TH1 and TH2 cells: different patterns of lymphokine secretion lead to different functional properties. *Annu. Rev. Immunol.* **7**, 145.

Mosmann, T. R. and Moore, K. W. (1991). The role of IL-10 in crossregulation of TH1 and TH2 responses. *Immunoparasitol. Today* **12**, A49.

Mueller, R., Davies, J. D., Krahl, T., *et al.* (1997). IL-4 expression by grafts from transgenic mice fails to prevent allograft rejection. *J. Immunol.* **159**, 1599.

Murphy, W. J., Kumar, V. and Bennett, M. (1987a). Acute rejection of murine bone marrow allografts by natural killer cells and T cells: differences in kinetics and target antigens recognized. *J. Exp. Med.* **166**, 1499.

Murphy, W. J., Kumar, V. and Bennett, M. (1987b). Rejection of bone marrow allografts by mice with severe combined immune deficiency (SCID): evidence that NK cells can mediate the specificity of marrow graft rejection. *J. Exp. Med.* **165**, 1212.

Nickerson, P., Steurer, W., Steiger, J., *et al.* (1994). Cytokines and the Th1/Th2 paradigm in transplantation. *Curr. Opin. Immunol.* **6**, 757.

Nickerson, P., Zheng, X.-X., Steiger, J., *et al.* (1996). Prolonged islet allograft acceptance in the absence of interleukin 4 expression. *Transpl. Immunol.* **4**, 81.

Niederkorn, J. Y. (1999). The immune privilege of corneal allografts. *Transplantation* **67**, 1503.

Nolan, C. R., Saenz, K. P., Thomas, C. A., *et al.* (1995). Role of eosinophils in chronic vascular rejection in renal allografts. *Am. J. Kidney Dis.* **26**, 634.

O'Brien, S. J., Roelke, M. E., Marker, L., *et al.* (1985). Genetic basis for species vulnerability in the cheetah. *Science* **227**, 1428.

Oppenheim, J. J., Wang, J. M., Chertov, O., *et al.* (1996). The role of chemokines in transplantation. *In Transplantation Biology: Cellular and Molecular Aspects*, (N. L. Tilney, T. B. Strom and L. C. Paul, eds.), p. 187, Lippincott-Raven Publishers, Philadelphia.

Oppenheim, J. J., Zacharie, C. O. C., Mukaida, N., *et al.* (1991). Properties of the proinflammatory supergene 'intercrine' cytokine family. *Annu. Rev. Immunol.* **9**, 617.

Orosz, C. G. and Pelletier, R. P. (1997). Chronic remodeling pathology in grafts. *Curr. Opin. Immunol.* **9**, 676.

Osorio, R. W., Ascher, N. L., Jaenisch, R., *et al.* (1993). Major histocompatibility complex class 1 deficiency prolongs islet allograft survival. *Diabetes* **42**, 1520.

Page, C. S., Holloway, N., Smith, H., *et al.* (1994a). Alloproliferative responses of purified CD4+ and CD8+ T cells to endothelial cells in the absence of contaminating accessory cells. *Transplantation* **57**, 1628.

Page, C. S., Thompson, C., Yacoub, M., *et al.* (1994b). Human endothelial stimulation of allogeneic T cells via a CTLA-4 independent pathway. *Transpl. Immunol.* **2**, 342.

Parham, P., Clayberger, C., Zorn, S. L., *et al.* (1987). Inhibition of alloreactive cytotoxic T lymphocytes by peptides from the OL2 domain of HLA-A2. *Nature* **325**, 625.

Parish, C. (1972). The relationship between humoral and cell-mediated immunity. *Transplant. Rev.* **13**, 35.

Parker, W., Bruno, D., Holzknecht, Z. E., *et al.* (1994). Characterization and affinity isolation of xenoreactive human natural antibodies. *J. Immunol.* **153**, 3791.

Patel, R. and Terasaki, P. I. (1969). Significance of the positive crossmatch test in kidney transplantation. *N. Engl. J. Med.* **280**, 735.

Paul, L. C. and Benediktsson, H. (1993). Chronic transplant rejection: magnitude of the problem and pathogenetic mechanism. *Transplant. Rev.* **7**, 96.

Paul, L. C., Claas, H. J., Van Es, A., *et al.* (1979). Accelerated rejection of a renal allograft associated with pretransplantation antibodies directed against donor antigens on endothelium and monocytes. *N. Engl. J. Med.* **300**, 1258.

Paul, L. C., Saito, K., Davidoff, A., *et al.* (1996). Growth factor transcripts in rat renal transplants. *Am. J. Kidney Dis.* **28**, 441.

Pearson, T. C., Alexander, D. Z., Winn, K. J., *et al.* (1994). Transplantation tolerance induced by CTLA-4 Ig. *Transplantation* **57**, 1701.

Perlmann, P. and Holm, G. (1969). Cytotoxic effects of lymphoid cells in vitro. *Adv. Immunol.* **11**, 117.

Peugh, W. N., Superina, R. A., Wood, K. J., *et al.* (1986). The role of H-2 and non-H-2 antigens and genes in the rejection of murine cardiac allografts. *Immunogenetics* **23**, 30.

Pfeiffer, C., Stein, J., Southwood, S., *et al.* (1995). Altered peptide ligands can control CD4 T lymphocyte differentiation in vivo. *J. Exp. Med.* **181**, 1569.

Picker, L. J. and Butcher, E. C. (1992). Physiological and molecular mechanisms of lymphocyte homing. *Annu. Rev. Immunol.* **10**, 561.

Picotti, J. R., Chan, S. Y., VanBuskirk, A. M., *et al.* (1997). Are Th2 helper T lymphocytes beneficial, deleterious, or irrelevant in promoting allograft survival? *Transplantation* **63**, 619.

Platt, J. L. (1999). Prospects for xenotransplantation. *Paediatr. Transplant.* **3**, 193.

Pober, J. S. and Cotran, R. S. (1991). Immunologic interactions of T lymphocytes with vascular endothelium. *Adv. Immunol.* **50**, 261.

Pober, J. S., Gimbrone, Jr., M. A., Lapierre, L. A., *et al.* (1986). Overlapping patterns of activation of human endothelial cells by interleukin 1, tumour necrosis factor and immune interferon. *J. Immunol.* **137**, 1893.

Porter, K. A., Calne, R. Y. and Zukoski, C. F. (1964). Vascular and other changes in 200 renal homotransplants treated with immunosuppressive drugs. *Lab. Invest.* **13**, 810.

Powelson, J. A. and Cosimi, A. B. (1999). Liver transplantation. *In Transplantation*, (L. C. Ginns, A. B. Cosimi and P. J. Morris, eds.), p. 324, Boston, Blackwell Science.

Rabinovitch, A., Pukel, C. and Baquerizo, H. (1988). Interleukin-1 inhibits glucose-modulated insulin and glucagon secretion in rat islet monolayer cultures. *Endocrinology* **122**, 2393.

Rammensee, H.-G., Falk, K. and Rotzschke, O. (1993). Peptides naturally presented by MHC class I molecules. *Annu. Rev. Immunol.* **11**, 213.

Ranger, A. M., Das, M. P., Kuchroo, V. K., *et al.* (1996). B7-2 (CD86) is essential for the development of IL-4 producing cells. *Int. Immunol.* **8**, 1549.

Reis e Sousa, C., Stahl, P. D. and Austyn, J. M. (1993). Phagocytosis of antigens by Langerhans cells in vitro. *J. Exp. Med.* **178**, 509.

Rissoan, M.-C., Soumelis, V., Kadowaki, N., *et al.* (1999). Reciprocal control of T helper cell and dendritic cell differentiation. *Science* **283**, 1183.

Roche, P. A. (1995). HLA-DM: an in vivo facilitator of MHC class II peptide loading. *Immunity* **3**, 259.

Rock, K. L., Barnes, M. C., Germain, R. N., *et al.* (1983). The role of Ia molecules in the activation of T lymphocytes II: Ia-restricted recognition of allo-K/D antigens is required for class I MHC-stimulated mixed lymphocyte responses. *J. Immunol.* **130**, 457.

Rollinghoff, M. and Wagner, H. (1975). Secondary cytotoxic allograft response in vitro. *Eur. J. Immunol.* **5**, 875.

Rolstad, B. and Ford, W. L. (1974). Immune responses of rats deficient in thymus-derived lymphocytes to strong transplantation antigens. *Transplantation* **17**, 405.

Rose, E. A., Smith, C. R., Petrossian, G. A., *et al.* (1989). Humoral immune responses after cardiac transplantation: correlation with fatal rejection and graft atherosclerosis. *Surgery* **106**, 203.

Rose, M. L. (1997). Role of endothelial cells in allografts rejection. *Vasc. Med.* **2**, 105.

Rose, M. L. (1998). Endothelial cells as antigen-presenting cells: role in human transplantation. *Cell. Mol. Life Sci.* **54**, 965.

Rosenberg, A. S. (1993). The T cell populations mediating rejection of MHC class I disparate skin grafts in mice. *Transpl. Immunol.* **2**, 93.

Rosenberg, A. S., Mizuochi, T., Sharrow, S. O., *et al.* (1987). Phenotype, specificity and function of T cell subsets and T cell interactions involved in skin allograft rejection. *J. Exp. Med.* **165**, 1296.

Rosenberg, A. S., Mizuochi, T. and Singer, A. (1986). Analysis of T cell subsets in rejection of Kᵇ mutant skin allograft differing at class I MHC. *Nature* **322**, 829.

Rosenberg, A. S. and Singer, A. (1992). Cellular basis of skin allograft rejection: an in vivo model of immune-mediated tissue destruction. *Annu. Rev. Immunol.* **10**, 333.

Ross, R. and Glomset, J. A. (1976). The pathogenesis of atherosclerosis. *N. Engl. J. Med.* **295**, 369.

Rossen, R. D., Butler, W. T., Reisberg, M. A., *et al.* (1971). Immunofluorescent localisation of human immunoglobulin on tissues from cardiac allograft recipients. *J. Immunol.* **106**, 171.

Rotzschke, O., Falk, K., Faath, S., *et al.* (1991). On the nature of peptides involved in T cell alloreactivity. *J. Exp. Med.* **174**, 1059.

Rubin, R. H. and Tolkoff Rubin, N. E. (1984). The problem of cytomegalovirus infection in transplantation. *Prog. Transplant.* **1**, 89.

Rudd, C. E. (1996). Upstream-downstream: CD28 cosignalling pathways and T cell function. *Immunity* **4**, 527.

Rudd, C. E., Janssen, O., Cai, Y.-C., *et al.* (1994). Two-step TCRζ/CD3-CD4 and CD28 signalling in T cells: SH2/SH3 domains, protein-tyrosine and lipid kinases. *Immunol. Today* **15**, 225.

Russell, P. S., Chase, C. M., Winn, H. J., *et al.* (1994). Coronary atherosclerosis in transplanted mouse hearts II: importance of humoral immunity. *J. Immunol.* **152**, 5135.

Rygaard, J. (1974). Skin grafts in nude mice. *Acta Pathol. Microbiol. Scand.* **82**, 93.

Saleem, S., Konieczny, B. T., Lowry, R. P., *et al.* (1996). Acute rejection of vascularized heart allografts in the absence of IFNγ. *Transplantation* **62**, 1908.

Sandrin, M. S., Vaughan, H. A., Dabkrowski, P. L., *et al.* (1993). Anti-pig IgM antibodies in human serum react predominantly with Gal(α1-3)Gal epitopes. *Proc. Natl. Acad. Sci. U. S. A.* **90**, 11391.

Santamaria-Babi, L. F., Moser, R., Perez-Soler, M. T., *et al.* (1995). Migration of skin-homing T cells across cytokine-activated human endothial cell layers involves interaction of the cutaneous lymphocyte-associated antigen (CLA), the very late antigen-4 (VLA-4) and the lymphocyte function-associated antigen-1 (LFA-1). *J. Immunol.* **154**, 1543.

Sayegh, M. H., Akalin, E., Hancock, W. W., *et al.* (1995). CD28-B7 blockade after alloantigenic challenge in vivo inhibits Th1 cytokines but spares Th2. *J. Exp. Med.* **181**, 1869.

Schilham, M. W., Fung-Leung, W. P., Rahemtulla, A., *et al.* (1993). Alloreactive cytotoxic T cells can develop and function in mice lacking both CD4 and CD8. *Eur. J. Immunol.* **23**, 1299.

Schulz, M., Schuurman, H.-J., Joergensen, J., *et al.* (1995). Acute rejection of vascular heart allografts by perforin-deficient mice. *Eur. J. Immunol.* **25**, 474.

Schwartz, R. H. (1990). A cell culture model for T lymphocyte clonal anergy. *Science* **248**, 1349.

Schwartz, R. H. (1997). T cell clonal anergy. *Curr. Opin. Immunol.* **9**, 351.

Scott, D. M., Ehrmann, I. E., Ellis, P. S., *et al.* (1995). Identification of a mouse male-specific transplantation antigen, H-Y. *Nature* **376**, 695.

Scott, D. M., Ehrmann, I. E., Ellis, P. S., *et al.* (1997). Why do some females reject males? The molecular basis for male-specific graft rejection. *J. Mol. Med.* **75**, 103.

Selvaggi, G., Ricordi, C., Podack, E. R., *et al.* (1996). The role of the perforin and Fas pathways of cytotoxicity in skin graft rejection. *Transplantation* **62**, 1912.

Sherwood, R. A., Brent, L. and Rayfield, L. S. (1986). Presentation of allo-antigens by host cells. *Eur. J. Immunol.* **16**, 569.

Shirwan, H. (1999). Chronic allograft rejection: do the Th2 cells preferentially induced by indirect alloantigen recognition play a dominant role? *Transplantation* **68**, 715.

Shreeder, V., Moodycliffe, A. M., Ullrich, S. E., *et al.* (1999). Dendritic cells require T cells for functional maturation in vivo. *Immunity* **11**, 625.

Simpson, E. (1998). Minor transplantation antigens: animal models for human host-versus-graft, graft-versus-host and graft-versus-leukemia reactions. *Transplantation* **65**, 611.

Simpson, E., Roopenian, D. and Goulmy, E. (1998). Much ado about minor histocompatibility antigens. *Immunol. Today* **19**, 108.

Snider, M. E. and Steinmuller, D. (1987). Non-specific tissue destruction as a consequence of cytotoxic T lymphocyte interaction with antigen-specific target cells. *Transplant. Proc.* **19**, 421.

Sprent, J., Schaeffer, M., Lo, D., *et al.* (1986). Properties of purified T cell subsets II: in vivo class I vs class II H-2 differences. *J. Exp. Med.* **163**, 998.

Steiger, J., Nickerson, P. W., Steurer, W., *et al.* (1995). IL-2 knockout recipient mice reject islet cell allografts. *J. Immunol.* **155**, 489.

Steinman, R. M. (1991). The dendritic cell system and its role in immunogenicity. *Annu. Rev. Immunol.* **9**, 271.

Steinman, R. M., Gutchinov, B., Witmer, M. D., *et al.* (1983). Dendritic cells are the peripheral stimulators of the primary mixed leukocyte reaction in mice. *J. Exp. Med.* **157**, 613.

Steinman, R. M. and Witmer, M. D. (1978). Lymphoid dendritic cells are potent stimulators of the primary mixed leucocyte reaction in mice. *Proc. Natl. Acad. Sci. U. S. A.* **75**, 5132.

Steinmuller, D. and Hart, E. A. (1971). Passenger leukocytes and induction of allograft immunity. *Transplant. Proc.* **3 (Suppl 1)**, 673.

Steinmuller, D. and Wachtal, S. S. (1980). Passenger leukocytes and induction of allograft immunity. *Transplant. Proc.* **12**, 100.

Strom, T. B., Roy-Chadhury, P., Manfro, R., *et al.* (1996). The Th1/Th2 paradigm and the allograft response. *Curr. Opin. Immunol.* **8**, 688.

Stuart, F. P., Bastien, E., Holter, A., *et al.* (1971). Role of passenger leukocytes in the rejection of renal allografts. *Transplant. Proc.* **3 (Suppl 1)**, 461.

Sutton, R., Gray, D. W., McShane, P., *et al.* (1989). The susceptibility of rejection and the absence of susceptibility of pancreatic islet B cells to nonspecific immune destruction in mixed strain islets grafted beneath the renal capsule in the rat. *J. Exp. Med.* **170**, 751.

Swain, S. L., Huston, G., Tonkonogy, S., *et al.* (1991). Transforming growth factor-β and IL-4 cause helper T cell precursors to develop into distinct effector helper cells that differ in lymphokine secretion pattern and cell surface phenotype. *J. Immunol.* **147**, 2991.

Swain, S. L., Weinberg, A. D., English, M., *et al.* (1990). IL-4 directs the development of TH2-like helper effectors. *J. Immunol.* **145**, 3796.

Takeuchi, T., Lowry, R. P. and Konieczny, B. (1992). Heart allografts in murine systems. *Transplantation* **53**, 1281.

Taylor, D. O., Ibrahim, H. M., Tolman, D. R., *et al.* (1991). Accelarated coronary arteriosclerosis in cardiac transplantation. *Transplant. Rev.* **5**, 165.

Tesi, R. J., Elkhammas, E.A., Henry, M. L., et al. (1993). Acute rejection episodes: best predictor of long-term primary cadaveric renal transplant survival. *Transplant. Proc.* **25**, 901.

Thompson, C. B., Lindsten, T., Ledbetter, J. A., *et al.* (1989). CD28 activation pathway regulates the production of multiple T-cell-derived lymphokines/cytokines. *Proc. Natl. Acad. Sci. U. S. A.* **86**, 1333.

Thomson, A. W. and Lu, L. (1999). Dendritic cells as regulators of immune reactivity: implications for transplantation. *Transplantation* **68**, 1.

Tilney, N. L., Kupiec-Weglinski, J. W., Heidecke, C. D., *et al.* (1984). Mechanisms of rejection and prolongation of vascularised organ allografts. *Immunol. Rev.* **77**, 185.

Tilney, N. L., Strom, T. B., MacPherson, S. G., *et al.* (1975). Surface properties and functional characteristics of infiltrating cells harvested from acutely rejecting cardiac allografts in inbred rats. *Transplantation* **20**, 323.

Ting, A. and Morris, P. J. (1977). Renal transplantation and B cell crossmatches with autoantibodies and alloantibodies. *Lancet* **2**, 1095.

Ting, A. and Morris, P. J. (1978). Reactivity of autolymphocytotoxic antibodies from dialysis patients with lymphocytes from chronic lymphocytic leukemia (CLL) patients. *Transplantation* **25**, 31.

Ting, A. and Morris, P. J. (1981). Positive-crossmatch transplants—safe or not. *Transplant. Proc.* **13**, 1544.

Tivol, E. A., Borriello, F., Schweitzer, A. N., *et al.* (1995). Loss of CTLA-4 leads to massive lymphoproliferation and fatal multiorgan tissue destruction, revealing a critical negative regulatory role of CTLA-4. *Immunity* **3**, 541.

Tono, T., Moden, M., Yoshizaki, K., *et al.* (1992). Biliary interleukin 6 levels as indicators of hepatic allograft rejection in rats. *Transplantation* **53**, 1195.

Toogood, G. J., Rankin, A. M., Tam, P. K. H., *et al.* (1997). The immune response following small bowel transplantation II: a very early cytokine response in the gut associated lymphoid tissue. *Transplantation* **63**, 1118.

Tullius, S. G., Nieminen, M., Bechstein, W. O., *et al.* (1998). Contribution of early acute rejection episodes to chronic rejection in a rat kidney retransplantation model. *Kidney Int.* **53**, 465.

Turka, L. A., Linsley, P. S., Lin, H., *et al.* (1992). T-cell activation by the CD28 ligand B7 is required for cardiac allograft rejection in vivo. *Proc. Natl. Acad. Sci. U. S. A.* **89**, 11102.

Turner, D. M., Grant, S. C., Lamb, W. R., *et al.* (1995). A genetic marker of high TNF-alpha production in heart transplant recipients. *Transplantation* **60**, 1113.

Tyler, J. D., Galli, S. J., Snider, M. E., *et al.* (1984). Cloned LyT-2+ cytolytic T lymphocytes destroy allogeneic tissue in vivo. *J. Exp. Med.* **159**, 234.

VanBuskirk, A. M., Wakely, M. E. and Orosz, C. G. (1996). Transfusion of polarised TH2-like cell populations into SCID mouse cardiac allograft recipients results in acute allograft rejection. *Transplantation* **62**, 62.

Waal de, R. M. W., Bogman, M. J. J., Mass, C. N., *et al.* (1983). Variable expression of Ia antigens on the vascular endothelium of mouse skin allografts. *Nature (Lond.)* **303**, 426.

Walsh, C. M., Hayashi, F., Saffron, D. C., *et al.* (1996). Cell-mediated cytotoxicity results from, but may not be critical for, primary allograft rejection. *J. Immunol.* **156**, 1436.

Walunas, T. L., Lenschow, D. J., Bakker, C. Y., *et al.* (1994). CTLA-4 can function as a negative regulator of T cell activation. *Immunity* **1**, 405.

Wang, W., Meadows, L. R., den Haan, J. M. M., *et al.* (1995). Human H-Y: a male-specific histocompatibility antigen derived from the SMCY protein. *Science* **269**, 1588.

Ward, S. G. (1999). The complexities of CD28 and CTLA-4 signalling: PI3K and beyond. *Arch. Immunol. Ther. Exp. Warsz.* **47**, 69.

Welsh, K. I., Burgos, H. and Batchelor, J. R. (1977). The immune response to allogeneic rat platelets: Ag-B antigens in matrix form lacking Ia. *Eur. J. Immunol.* **7**, 267.

Williams, G. M., Hume, D. M., Hudson, R. P. J., *et al.* (1968). "Hyperacute" renal homograft rejection in man. *N. Engl. J. Med.* **279**, 611.

Wolf, B. A., Hughes, J. H., Florholmen, J., *et al.* (1989). Interleukin-1 inhibits glucose-induced Ca2+ uptake by islets of Langerhans. *FEBS Lett.* **248**, 35.

Wong, G. H. W., Clark-Lewis, I., Harris, A. W., *et al.* (1984). Effect of cloned interferon-γ on expression of H-2 and Ia antigens on cell lines of hemopoietic, lymphoid, epithelial, fibroblastic and neuronal origin. *Eur. J. Immunol.* **14**, 52.

Yang, H., Issekutz, T. B. and Wright, Jr., J. R. (1995). Prolongation of rat islet allograft survival by treatment with monoclonal antibodies against VLA-4 and LFA-1. *Transplantation* **60**, 71.

Yilmaz, S., Taskinen, E., Paavonen, T., *et al.* (1992). Chronic rejection of rat renal allograft I: histological differentiation between chronic rejection and cyclosporin nephrotoxicity. *Transpl. Int.* **5**, 85.

Zelenika, D., Adams, E., Mellor, A., *et al.* (1998). Rejection of H-Y disparate skin grafts by monospecific CD4+ Th1 and Th2 cells: no requirement for CD8+ T cells or B cells. *J. Immunol.* **161**, 1868.

Zimmerman, C., Seiler, P., Lane, P., *et al.* (1997). Antiviral immune responses in CTLA4 transgenic mice. *J. Virol.* **71**, 1802.

Chronic Renal Failure: Renal Replacement Therapy

Christopher G. Winearls • Philip D. Mason

Introduction

Renal replacement therapy (RRT) is a general term describing the various substitution treatments available for severe acute and end-stage chronic renal failure, including dialysis (hemodialysis and peritoneal dialysis), hemofiltration, and renal transplantation. The development, widespread application and refinement of these therapies are among the triumphs of medicine in the second part of the 20th century. Until the 1950s, renal failure had been as surely lethal as metastatic cancer. All types of RRT are incomplete solutions, however, providing an extension of life but restoring neither full life expectancy nor quality of life.

Nephrologists have come to view the need to institute RRT as an admission of failure to prevent renal disease, control its pathology or halt its progression. This is a harsh judgment but reinforces the point that the outcome after RRT is started can be improved by careful planning and the care provided in the pre–end-stage phase of the illness. Management includes measures directed against the cause, the progression and the consequences of the loss of renal excretory and endocrine function (Walker, 1997). The choice of treatment options and the order in which they are adopted should be made well in advance of the point at which end-stage renal failure (ESRF) is reached. The aim is to provide the treatment that allows the longest and best-quality extension of useful and enjoyable life. Ideally the choice of dialysis modality or the transplantation option should be made with patients after they have been able to consider the advantages and disadvantages of each. Engaging patients at an early stage in their management also should reduce the risk of noncompliance.

Renal replacement therapy programs have been victims of their own success, growing more rapidly than their budgets and placing a strain on the health care resources of the wealthiest countries. In 1997, the cost in the United States was $15.6 billion, 75% of which was a charge on the federal government. Even if the numbers of new patients starting RRT remain constant, the total costs escalate each year as the numbers of patients in programs accumulate and survival improves. This situation is illustrated for the Oxford Regional RRT Program in Figure 3–1. The pressure has been compounded by the fact that the elderly, who have a higher incidence of ESRF than individuals younger than 65 years of age and previously were excluded, can be treated successfully, albeit at a higher cost because of comorbid conditions. The challenge for nephrologists and transplant surgeons is to provide the most appropriate RRT of the highest quality for the individual patient at the lowest possible cost. Quality standards and guidelines have been set by a number of organizations (e.g., The British Transplantation Society, 1998; The National Kidney Foundation, 1997; The Renal Association, 1997).

Definition and Timing Referral

End-stage renal failure (formerly called terminal renal failure) is the degree of irreversible loss of renal function that is incompatible with life (i.e., when the glomerular filtration rate is <5 ml/min). (The earlier stages are listed in Table 3–1.) Patients in the last three stages should be under the care of physicians trained in nephrology. Although those in the first or mild stage should be assessed by a nephrologist, care can be shared safely with a family practitioner or general physician (internist). There is still a problem with avoidable late referral of patients known to have renal failure (Obrador and Pereira, 1998). This problem is explained, in part, by a failure to recognize the nonlinear relationship between plasma creatinine and glomerular filtration rate (Fig. 3–2). A plasma creatinine of 400 µmol/L is erroneously understood to imply that a patient is only 40% of the way to a need for dialysis at a creatinine of 1,000 µmol/L. About 30% of pa-

TABLE 3–1

SEVERITY OF RENAL FAILURE

| Degree of Renal Failure | Glomerular Filtration Rate (ml/min) | Representative Creatinine (µmol/L) | | Symptoms and Signs |
		Males	Females	
Mild	30–50	~170	~150	None except hypertension
Moderate	16–29	~300	~250	Few: anemia, hypertension, early osteodystrophy
Severe	5–15	~500	~350	Anorexia, pruritus, poor concentration, dyspnea, anemia, pericarditis, pulmonary edema
End-stage	<5	>900	~600	All of the above plus fits, coma, acidosis, hyperkalemia, cardiac arrhythmias

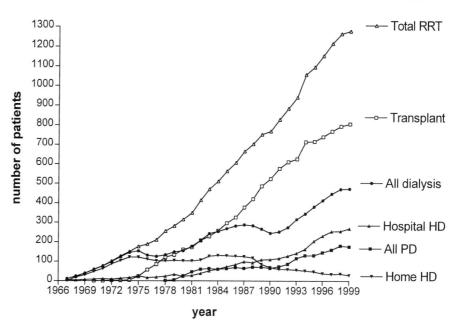

FIGURE 3–1

The accumulation of patients in the Oxford Regional Replacement Program, 1966–1999. HD = hemodialysis; PD = peritoneal dialysis.

tients starting RRT in the United Kingdom see a nephrologist fewer than 12 weeks before they start RRT. In some cases, this situation is unavoidable—the patients may have had a truly silent illness or an acute presentation of an irreversible renal injury (e.g., myeloma, anti–glomerular basement membrane disease or cortical necrosis). The consequences for patients of late presentation are many: they suffer a huge psychological shock, which makes coming to terms with a chronic illness difficult; they have to rely on temporary vascular access; they often lose their jobs because of the sudden, prolonged absence from work. These patients will have suffered the complications of renal failure untreated, and although renal anemia can be reversed, renal osteodystrophy

and hypertensive damage to the heart cannot be. Patients may die from the complications of the acute uremic emergency. These patients have a worse prognosis (Innes *et al.*, 1992). The cost of initiating dialysis in patients with ESRF presenting late is much higher than for those in whom an elective start is made (Jungers *et al.*, 1993).

Prevalence and Incidence

The point prevalence of all chronic renal failure (whatever the definition) is impossible to ascertain because many patients are unaware of its presence. A prospective study conducted in Britain that involved ascertainment through hospital biochemistry laboratories revealed a point prevalence of acute and chronic renal failure (creatinine, >150 µmol/L, 1.7 mg/dl) of 2,058 adults per million of population (pmp) (Feest *et al.*, 1992). Many of these patients had only temporary derangements in renal function or already were undergoing treatment. About 600 pmp have established chronic renal failure not requiring RRT, however. Precise information is available for the prevalence and incidence of ESRF from various national and international registries. Examples are given in Table 3–2.

The discrepancies between the United States and Japan and the United Kingdom and Australia are explained largely by the prevalence of causes of renal failure, especially diabetes and hypertension and their severity. Both conditions are common in black Americans, who compose approximately 20% of the population. Although the same pattern is seen in Asians and Afro-Caribbeans in the United Kingdom and Aboriginals in Australia, there are fewer subjects from the at-risk ethnic groups in these countries. The effect of age is dramatic. In the United States, the incidence of ESRF is 12-fold higher in individuals older than 65 years than in individuals aged 20 to 44 years. In England and the United States, 50% of patients starting dialysis are 65 years old or older.

Acceptance criteria for RRT are more stringent in the United Kingdom than in the United States, but this cannot account for the threefold difference in incidence. Estimates of incidence of ESRF in the United Kingdom made from rigorous population surveys relying on biochemical data for

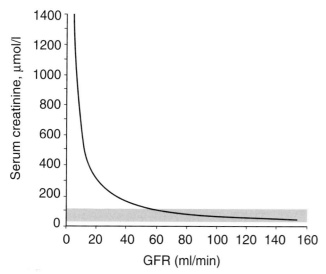

FIGURE 3–2

The relationship between plasma creatinine concentration and glomerular filtration rate (GFR). Depending on the baseline creatinine concentration (determined by the individual's muscle mass and meat intake), it is possible for renal function to decrease by 50% before the creatinine rises above the normal range. The shaded area is the normal serum creatinine range.

TABLE 3–2

INCIDENCE AND PREVALENCE OF END-STAGE RENAL FAILURE

Country	Year	Incidence*	Prevalence†	Transplant‡	Source
U.S.	1997	287	1,105	28%	USRDS Annual Report, 1999
England	1995	82	476	52%	Roderick et al., 1998
Japan	1994	192	1,150	Not given	Shinzato et al., 1997
Australia	1997	79	530	47%	ANZDATA Registry Report, 1998

*Number of new patients per 1 million population per year starting renal replacement therapy.
†Number of patients with end-stage renal disease relying on renal replacement therapy.
‡Percentage on renal replacement therapy maintained by a functioning transplant.

ascertainment were of approximately 80 pmp (<80 years old) per year. Nephrologists in the United Kingdom generally accept any patient with ESRF expected to survive at least 3 months out of the hospital. Patients with terminal illness, dementia and severe comorbid disease and patients reliant on full-time nursing care are seldom started on dialysis. Few patients who would benefit from dialysis are excluded.

The prevalence of ESRF (i.e., the numbers of patients alive on dialysis or relying on a functioning transplant) varies according to the incidence in the country and ease of access to treatment now and historically (see Table 3–2). Prevalence is highest in the wealthiest countries of the developed world and lowest in the poorest. The incidence of renal failure is higher in the poorest countries so that the imbalance in provision is greater than statistics suggest.

The numbers of patients on RRT have yet to reach a steady-state. This will occur when the number of new patients accepted into programs is balanced by the number of deaths. This situation is illustrated by the trends in the Oxford RRT Program, which serves a population of 1.8 million and has an acceptance rate of 80 new patients pmp per year (140 patients). There are approximately 90 deaths in program patients each year, accounting for a net increase of 50 patients, or 4% growth (see Fig. 3–1).

Etiology

A consideration of the causes of ESRF is relevant to the problem of RRT as a whole. What are the prospects for reducing the incidence of ESRF by early diagnosis and treatment of the diseases that lead to it? With the exception of analgesic nephropathy and tuberculosis, none can be prevented. The best one can hope for in the future is that it will be possible to arrest renal injury in diseases such as diabetes, glomerulonephritis and reflux nephropathy and delay the progression of others. Protein-restricted diets have proved disappointing, as shown in the Modification of Diet in Renal Disease (MDRD) study (Klahr et al., 1994), but angiotensin-converting enzyme inhibitors seem to have a useful and class-specific effect on progression as shown in the Ramipril Efficacy in Nephropathy (REIN) study (Ruggenenti et al., 1999).

For most patients, establishing the cause of renal failure is simple and usually is revealed by the history. There is no difficulty, for example, in attributing the cause of renal failure to diabetes, adult polycystic kidney disease, radiologically proven reflux nephropathy and obstruction, biopsy-proven glomerulonephritis or systemic diseases, such as systemic lupus erythematosus, amyloidosis and myeloma. The problem arises in patients with little past medical history, contracted kidneys on ultrasound and bland urine deposits. Renal vascular disease, chronic cholesterol embolism to the kidneys, chronic interstitial nephritis caused by drugs and

silent glomerulonephritis probably account for many of these cases. If the cause cannot be established by standard clinical methods, it should not be pursued relentlessly because the implications for treatment are minimal. Biopsy of small kidneys is dangerous and rarely reveals a specific diagnosis or alters management. If interstitial tuberculosis is suspected, a biopsy for a single core of tissue for histology and culture is justifiable.

Transplant surgeons prefer to know the cause of renal failure in potential kidney transplant recipients. This is because diagnoses such as focal segmental glomerular sclerosis (FSGS), anti-glomerular basement membrane disease, myeloma, amyloid and dense deposit disease, a form of membranoproliferative glomerulonephritis, alter the decision about whether or when to proceed to renal transplantation. Also, surgeons can anticipate particular problems (e.g., infection in patients with reflux nephropathy and recurrence of disease in the transplanted kidney).

The major causes of ESRF are described in the national registries and reveal intriguing differences in the pattern of causes in different age groups, between race groups in the same country and between countries (e.g., diabetes is three times more common in the United States than in Australia and Europe). Differences in hypertension and glomerulonephritis may be related to the choice of labels by nephrologists in the United States and Europe. It is unlikely that cystic disease is less common in the United States; rather the lower percentage incidence is explained by the larger number of patients treated and the high prevalence of diabetes (Table 3–3). Other and rarer causes are listed in Table 3–4.

The incidence of diseases that cause ESRF in patients older than age 65 is similar to that in the population as a whole, but there are important differences. Many more patients are never diagnosed (20% in Europe), and they are more likely to suffer from acquired obstructive uropathy, amyloidosis, myeloma and renal vascular disease.

Treatment

Ideally patients with ESRF should be offered the modality that suits them practically and psychologically. In practice, economic and cultural pressures, the limit in donor supply and medical prejudices dictate what treatment patients receive. Although patients should be able to choose their modality, they have to accept that they will move between treatments because of failure and complications.

The aim should be to transplant all patients in whom the risk is equivalent to or less than that of remaining on dialysis treatment. Patients should be allowed to choose between hemodialysis and continuous ambulatory peritoneal dialysis (CAPD). Home dialysis is encouraged for patients with appropriate home circumstances, patients with partners who can act as helpers and patients who are unlikely to receive a

TABLE 3–3

COMMON CAUSES OF END-STAGE RENAL FAILURE REQUIRING RENAL REPLACEMENT THERAPY*

Cause	England and Wales, 1995	United States, 1993–1997	Australia, 1997	Japan, 1994
Glomerulonephritis	12.4	12.9	34	39.8
Diabetes	13.8	40.3	21	31.2
Cystic disease	5.9	3.4	6	2.6
Hypertension	7.8	27	12	6.2
Pyelonephritis (including reflux nephropathy)	9.1	4.2	6	†
Analgesic nephropathy	†	†	5	†
Unknown	17	4.0	6	†
Missing	15.7	3.5		
Miscellaneous	18.1	4.7	10	†

*Given diagnosis: percentage of patients entering renal replacement therapy programs. See Table 3–2 for sources.
†Data not given.

transplant, often because they are highly sensitized. In-center dialysis is provided as close to the patient's home as possible by the use of satellite hemodialysis facilities. Ideally, no patient should have to journey more than 20 miles for treatment.

In the United Kingdom and Australia, most patients with ESRF are maintained with functioning renal transplants, and home hemodialysis is still an option, but the pattern is changing (Fig. 3–3). Hemodialysis and peritoneal dialysis use is split 70:30. The situation is different in the United States and Japan, where most patients are treated by in-center hemodialysis. These countries also rely less on CAPD because of the wide availability of hemodialysis (Table 3–5).

Dialysis
GENERAL ASPECTS

The aims of dialysis are to control all symptoms of uremia, ensure adequate nutrition, maintain plasma potassium at less than 6.5 mmol/L before dialysis, control hypertension, avoid pulmonary edema, maintain plasma phosphate at less than 2 mmol/L and maintain albumin at greater than 35 g/L. A protein catabolic rate of 1 g/kg/d and a clearance constant (Kt/V) of greater than or equal to 1.2 per dialysis for thrice-weekly hemodialysis and greater than or equal to 2.0 per week (including residual renal function) for peritoneal dialysis are usual. Dialysis provides the equivalent of only 6 to 10 ml/min of glomerular filtration rate so that there are many consequences of chronic renal failure for which additional measures are needed.

Hypertension and Fluid and Electrolyte Balance

Hypertension is common in dialysis patients and usually is related to expansion of the extracellular fluid volume caused by positive sodium and water balance. Patients find it difficult to stick to target dry weights and frequently run at greater than 2 kg probably in response to thirst. Dietary sodium restriction is essential, but ultrafiltration by dialysis is needed to a greater or lesser extent in all patients. Antihypertensive drugs have to be used with care because of the risks of aggravating hypotension during dialysis. This is a particular problem with β-blockers. Excessive water intake leads to dilutional hyponatremia. Dialysis removes about 60 mmol of potassium a day so that dietary restriction is essential. Hyperkalemia has effects on cardiac muscle (arrhythmias) and on skeletal muscle (weakness and ultimately paralysis). A persistent metabolic acidosis usually indicates insufficient dialysis and the need for an increase in hours of hemodialysis or the daily volume of peritoneal dialysis fluid.

Hematopoiesis and Immunity

Anemia accounts for many of the symptoms attributed to the general effects of uremia—fatigue, breathlessness and

TABLE 3–4

OTHER CAUSES OF CHRONIC RENAL FAILURE

Metabolic	Cystinosis, oxalosis, nephrocalcinosis, cystinuria, hyperuricemia
Vascular	Renovascular disease, scleroderma, HUS, postpartum, cholesterol emboli
Dysproteinemias	Amyloid, myeloma, cryoglobulinemia, light-chain deposition disease
Hereditary	Alport's syndrome, Fabry's disease, tuberous sclerosis, sickle cell disease
Vasculitis	Wegener's granulomatosis, microscopic polyangiitis, PAN, SLE
Malignancy	Hypernephroma, lymphoma
Structural	Congenital and acquired abnormalities of the urinary tract (e.g., associated with spina bifida, spinal cord injury, other obstruction, medullary cystic disease)
Miscellaneous	AIDS nephropathy, postbone marrow and solid organ transplantation

HUS = hemolytic-uremic syndrome; PAN = periarteritis nodosa; SLE = systemic lupus erythematosus; AIDS = acquired immunodeficiency syndrome.

TABLE 3–5

INTERNATIONAL COMPARISON OF DISTRIBUTION OF MODALITIES OF RENAL REPLACEMENT TREATMENT

Country, Year	Transplant (%)	Hemodialysis (%)	Peritoneal Dialysis (%)
England, 1995*	53	25§	22
Australia, 1997†	47	37‖	16
U.S., 1997‡	28	62.9¶	8.7

*Roderick et al., 1998.
†ANZDATA Report, 1998.
‡USRDS Annual Data Report, 1999.
§3% on home hemodialysis.
‖6% on home hemodialysis.
¶0.6% on home hemodialysis.

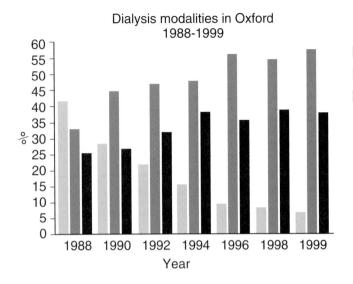

FIGURE 3–3

Changes in percentage of patients on dialysis modalities in Oxford, 1988–1999. HD = hemodialysis; PD = peritoneal dialysis.

loss of stamina. Approximately 80% of dialysis patients now receive treatment with recombinant human erythropoietin (epoetin) administered subcutaneously in doses of approximately 100 units/kg/wk, with most achieving hemoglobin concentrations of greater than 10 g/dl. In the United States, hemodialysis patients receive epoetin intravenously, which is less economical than the subcutaneous route. Although there is likely to be some specific effect of uremia on the bone marrow, this effect can be overridden by doses of erythropoietin that are only slightly higher than estimates of physiological replacement. Patients who fail to respond to erythropoietin usually are found to be iron deficient or bleeding or to have foci of infection and inflammation. Oral iron supplements are inadequate in most patients so that regular intravenous administration of iron saccharate (50–100 mg/wk) is likely to become routine. Aluminum overload is now rare. Side effects of epoetin are few but include hypertension, which may be associated rarely with seizures; a high incidence of vascular access failure, especially Gore-Tex grafts and occasional hyperkalemia. The results of renal transplantation are unchanged. Stopping blood transfusions has a varying effect on the level of sensitization to histocompatibility antigens (reviewed in Muirhead, 1997). Production of platelets is normal, but their function is abnormal (see under Hemostasis).

Granulocyte function, but not production, is impaired, explaining the frequency and severity of bacterial infection (e.g., with *Staphylococcus aureus*). Infections are the second major threat to the lives of patients with renal failure. Cell-mediated immunity is depressed in chronic renal failure, which explains the failure to clear hepatitis B infection and the higher risk of reactivating tuberculosis and varicella zoster. *Clostridium difficile* is endemic in most renal units so that patients frequently develop diarrhea or pseudomembranous colitis after treatment with broad-spectrum antibiotics such as cephalosporins.

Calcium, Phosphate and the Skeleton

Changes in calcium and phosphate homeostasis occur early in renal failure as a result of phosphate retention and reduced production of the active form of vitamin D, 1,25-dihydroxycholecalciferol, the production of which depends on the action of the renal enzyme 1α-hydroxylase. The relative deficiency of 1,25-dihydroxycholecalciferol and hypocalcemia cause an increase in the secretion of parathyroid hormone (PTH) by the parathyroid glands, which eventually become hyperplastic and autonomous. Although the increased concentration of PTH enhances phosphate excretion, it increases bone turnover by disturbing the balance between osteoblast and osteoclast activity. The structure of bone becomes disorganized, and bones become subject to fracture. Calcium concentrations rise in response to the action of PTH on the bone, and when the phosphate concentration is also high, deposits of calcium phosphate form in soft tissues and blood vessels.

Nutrition and Metabolism

Malnutrition is common in dialysis patients and is caused by inappropriate dietary restrictions, anorexia, acidosis and insulin resistance and is aggravated by intercurrent infections. It manifests as loss of muscle mass and hypoalbuminemia. Hypercholesterolemia and hypertriglyceridemia are common and may contribute to the excessive risk of cardiovascular disease (see Chapter 30).

Hemostasis

Dialysis patients have a bleeding diathesis, which is, in part, a consequence of abnormal platelet function but is aggravated by the need for heparin during dialysis, and many patients also are taking aspirin and oral anticoagulants. The manifestations of this abnormal platelet function are nosebleeds, heavy menstrual periods, occult gastrointestinal blood and a tendency to ooze from incisions. Careful attention to surgical hemostasis is required.

Skin

Itching is a variable and unpredictable symptom in dialysis patients and is aggravated by heat and stress. Its pathogenesis is understood poorly but may be related to histamine release and a high calcium (Ca) $\times$ inorganic phosphate (P_i) product (>6.25 mmol^2/L^2, >70 mg^2/dl^2). Treatment with antihistamines and moisturizing skin lotions sometimes helps.

Neurological and Musculoskeletal Manifestations

Uremic encephalopathy usually manifests as subtle cognitive impairment and is an indication for increasing dialysis dose. Coma and seizures are rare except in noncompliant patients who skip treatments. An asymmetrical distal poly-neuropathy is common in patients with ESRF. The symptoms are those of dysesthesia—a prickling or burning sensation and rarely footdrop. *Restless legs* especially at night are a nuisance and may respond to clonazepam, 500 μg, at night. An autonomic neuropathy is variable in its effects—manifesting mostly as sexual dysfunction and sluggish car-diovascular reflexes during hemodialysis. Median nerve com-pression in the carpal tunnel, caused by β_2-microglobulin amyloid, is a specific form of uremic mononeuropathy. Most hemodialysis patients develop it within 10 years of starting treatment. Surgical release is effective but may need re-peating. Gout and pyrophosphate cause crystal arthritis and β_2-microglobulin amyloid deposits in the synovium of large joints, causing severe disability. Severe hyperparathyroidism can present with a proximal myopathy making arising from a chair difficult.

Endocrine Abnormalities

There are diverse abnormalities in hormone production, control, protein binding, catabolism and tissue effects in dial-ysis patients. The most obvious examples are those of the vitamin D–PTH axis and erythropoietin caused by damage to the endocrine function of the kidney, but thyroid hormone, growth hormone and the sex hormones are also affected. Women usually are infertile, and men often have erectile dysfunction. Sildenafil (Viagra) has proved effective but should be used with caution in patients with heart disease and not at all by patients taking nitrates for angina.

Psychological Problems

The psychological problems of dialysis patients, usually anxiety and depression, are the predictable and understand-able consequences of loss of health, control and pleasure. Psychological problems are greatest in patients with the most to lose—the young and ambitious—and are relatively minor in the elderly, who are grateful that they have a treatable illness and not an immediately lethal one. There is a rela-tively high risk of suicide.

When should dialysis be started in a patient with ESRF? When dialysis facilities are not limited, the usual threshold is at a glomerular filtration rate of less than 10 ml/min, but some patients have uremic symptoms at levels of renal function higher than this. It is probably better to start earlier to prevent malnutrition. Difficulty in maintaining fluid and acid-base balance, a potassium level less than 6.5 mmol/L, refractory hypertension or deteriorating intellectual perfor-mance are all indications for starting dialysis regardless of the level of renal function. If a patient monitored in a renal clinic presents with pericarditis, pulmonary edema or periph-eral neuropathy, dialysis has been delayed too long.

HEMODIALYSIS

Hemodialysis (reviewed by Mallick and Gokal, 1999) is theoretically simple, relying on the diffusion of solutes across a semipermeable membrane down a concentration gradient. This process and the removal of fluid are enhanced by the creation of a pressure gradient across the semipermeable membrane leading to ultrafiltration. In practice, this requires a dialysis filter with a surface area of 1 to 2 m², now conve-niently packaged in hollow-fiber or flat-plate dialyzers; a blood flow of 200 to 350 ml/min and a countercurrent flow of dialysate, generated by a proportioning machine, of 500 ml/min. The dialysis machine generates the dialysate by adding concentrated dialysate to dialysis water, warming it,

checking its conductivity and pumping it through the dial-ysis filter and to waste. The machine pumps the blood from the patient through the dialysis filter and returns it via a venous bubble trap with an air-detector alarm to prevent air embolism. It adds heparin by continuous infusion and generates a transmembrane pressure to allow ultrafiltration of 1 to 4 L plasma water per treatment. Modern dialysis machines can be programmed to alter the sodium concentra-tion and the rate of ultrafiltration to make dialysis as smooth as possible. Dialysis prescription is altered by choice of dial-ysis filter, surface area, blood flow, dialysate constituents and hours and frequency of dialysis. Bicarbonate-buffered dialysate is preferred to acetate but requires slightly more sophisticated equipment to generate.

There is no certain method of quantitating how much dialysis to give a patient. Although more is likely to be better (Charra et al., 1992), patients resist the requirement for dialysis of more than 5 hours three times a week. With high blood flows and high flux dialyzers, it is possible to reduce dialysis hours to 2.5 hours three times a week, but fluid balance in such patients is more difficult to control. Measures of dialysis adequacy developed from the National Coopera-tive Dialysis Study (NCDS) showed that time, averaged urea concentrations and protein catabolic rate correlated with patient outcome (Lowrie et al., 1981). From these data, the *Kt/V* term emerged as a predictive parameter. *K* is the clear-ance of the dialyser, *t* is the time on dialysis and *V* is the volume of distribution of urea (equivalent to the total body water). A detailed description of the measurement of this term is beyond the scope of this chapter. The current consen-sus is that the minimum target should be 1.2 per dialysis for patients receiving three treatments per week.

An expensive alternative to hemodialysis is hemodiafil-tration, which involves the ultrafiltration of fluid across a hemofilter device and direct infusion of sterile replacement solution resembling plasma without the proteins. This ap-proach is tolerated better by patients with unstable cardiovas-cular systems and may provide better clearances, especially of high-molecular-weight solutes. The cost of this treatment can be reduced by reuse (see later).

The key to adequate hemodialysis is reliable vascular ac-cess (see Chapter 5). Poorly functioning access inevitably leads to poor dialysis and increases morbidity. Reliance on central access exposes patients to the risk of bacterial infec-tion, which may mean, at best, replacement of the catheter and, at worst, metastatic infection or death.

The organization and management of hemodialysis units is a major exercise. The aim is to use the capital equipment and staff in the most economical way. Dialysis units generally should have not less than 10 stations running two to three shifts a day, 6 days a week, with one nurse or dialysis technician being responsible for two to three dialysis patients at a time. Although dialysis filters can be reused, the cleaning process is labor intensive. This practice reduces the per-treatment cost, especially when the higher cost high flux membranes are being used. An important consideration is the production of large volumes of water in the generation of dialysate. Tap water is purified by filtration to remove bacteria, softening to remove calcium and reverse osmosis to remove other contaminating substances including metals and nitrites. Ideally, such water should be pyrogen-free. This con-dition is essential if high flux treatments are being used.

Patients who are hepatitis B antigen positive should be dialyzed in isolation and on dedicated dialysis machines. Hepatitis B vaccinations are recommended and are most ef-fective if administered before ESRF develops. Universal pre-cautions are said to be sufficient to prevent spread of human immunodeficiency virus and hepatitis C. The incidence of the latter is decreasing as a result of reduced transfusion since the introduction of erythropoietin and screening of blood for the virus.

Complications

Several complications are common during long-term hemodialysis sessions. Hypotension occurs in 30% of dialyses and most commonly is secondary to intravascular hypovolemia. It is more common when large volumes of fluid have to be removed after excessive gains between dialyses. It also occurs more often if the patients eat on dialysis and may be more frequent with acetate (versus bicarbonate) dialysate. Hypotension usually responds to lying the patient flat or head-down, stopping ultrafiltration or giving a volume of normal saline. Muscle cramps (approximately 5–20% dialyses) often accompany hypotension, an excessively low target weight or the use of a low sodium dialysate. Correction of these or the administration of a hypertonic solution (saline or glucose) usually is effective treatment. Regular sufferers may be helped by prophylactic quinine sulfate. Nausea, vomiting and headache also are fairly common during hemodialysis. Mild chest and back pains may be related to complement activation by the dialysis membrane and are less common with *biocompatible* membranes. Pyrogen or microbial contamination of the dialysate occasionally may occur. Patients developing fever and/or rigors on dialysis must be examined carefully for evidence of infection of dialysis access; blood cultures are taken, and patients are treated with broad-spectrum antibiotics.

PERITONEAL DIALYSIS

Peritoneal dialysis is the process by which solutes, buffer, waste products and fluid are exchanged between the blood in the peritoneal capillaries and the solution infused into the peritoneal cavity. This exchange takes place across the peritoneal barrier, which comprises the vessel wall, the interstitium and the mesothelial cells, but considerable absorption of solutes and water also occurs via the peritoneal lymphatics. The amount of substances exchanged depends on the vascularity of the peritoneum; the blood flow; the permeability of the barrier; the volume and frequency of the fluid instilled and the osmotic gradient generated by the glucose, polymer or amino acid concentration of the solution.

Dialysis Adequacy

The efficacy of peritoneal dialysis can be altered only by changes in the volume and frequency of exchanges. Weekly creatinine clearance and urea clearance (measured using the weekly Kt/V) are used to assess adequacy of peritoneal dialysis but remain controversial in the absence of an adequate controlled study. The much-quoted CANUSA study prospectively followed 680 patients after starting CAPD (Canada-USA [CANUSA] Peritoneal Dialysis Study Group, 1996). Although survival was related to Kt/V (5% increase in relative risk of death for every 0.1 decrease in Kt/V), this reduced over time as a result of the loss of residual renal function with no change in dialysis clearance. A larger study also found a correlation with residual function but not dialysis clearance, and currently there is no evidence that increasing peritoneal dialysis dose reduces morbidity or mortality. Most circumstantial data suggest that more dialysis is better, and the current consensus is that the target should be a Kt/V (dialysis and residual renal function) of 2.1 per week. V is estimated from height, weight, age and sex, but the ideal body weight should be used to avoid inaccuracies in obese or fluid-overloaded patients. A creatinine clearance of 60 L/1.73 m^2 also has been suggested as a target, but this is virtually impossible in patients with no residual renal function. As residual renal function reduces, it may become impossible to achieve target clearance even with larger and more exchanges, especially for larger patients, and transfer to hemodialysis is necessary.

Intermittent Peritoneal Dialysis

About 40 to 48 hours of intermittent peritoneal dialysis are performed per week, either as two 20- to 24-hour sessions or four 10- to 12-hour sessions. During each session, dialysis fluid is cycled rapidly (e.g., 2 L every half hour) so that the dwell period is short. This means that the concentration gradient is kept steep so that the rate of removal of waste products is kept high to compensate for the shorter time that dialysis is being performed. The treatment is best performed using an automatic cycling machine that can be set to instill and drain fluid every half hour. Intermittent peritoneal dialysis is a good treatment for those who are unable to participate in their own management, who have residual renal function and who do not become fluid overloaded. It is labor intensive and if performed in the hospital requires two bed days per week for each patient. The risk of infection is low because only two connections and disconnections of the peritoneal dialysis catheter are made each week. Cycling machines save a huge amount of nursing time, but only if they are simple to set up and reliable in operation. Responding to a frequently alarming machine test tries the patience of patient and caregiver alike, and exasperation may lead to abandonment of the technique.

Continuous Cycling Peritoneal Dialysis

Continuous cycling peritoneal dialysis is similar to intermittent peritoneal dialysis except that treatment is performed every night and the exchanges are less rapid. This is a good treatment for children and the elderly because it can be set up at home by a caregiver and allowed to run automatically overnight. With improvements in automated peritoneal dialysis machines, continuous cycling peritoneal dialysis is becoming popular with patients who need their days free to work.

Continuous Ambulatory Peritoneal Dialysis

Continuous ambulatory peritoneal dialysis is the most widely used form of peritoneal dialysis and relies on the prolonged dwell phase to make up for the lower frequency of exchanges. Dialysis is continuous, exchanges following one another, usually without interruption. To deliver sufficient dialysis, three to five 1.5- to 3-L exchanges are performed every 24 hours. The usual routine starts in the morning with the drainage of the overnight dialysis fluid and is followed by the installation of the first bag of dialysate of the day. The next change is before lunch, the next late afternoon, and the last immediately before bed. If patients have a tendency to absorb fluid from the overnight exchange, they should drain out and cap off the catheter overnight and start dialysis on a dry peritoneum in the morning. The volume of dialysate instilled depends on the abdominal capacity of the patient (1.5 L for small adults and children, 2 L for regular-sized adults and 3 L for large men). The *glucose concentration* depends on the amount of ultrafiltration required to keep the extracellular fluid volume constant. To generate a higher volume, *strong bags* of 3.86% glucose are provided, usually as the first exchange of the day and never overnight.

Practical Considerations

For all types of peritoneal dialysis, a properly placed peritoneal dialysis catheter is required (see Chapter 5). The intraperitoneal tip should be in the pelvis, free from the omentum. The internal cuff must be watertight and sewn outside the peritoneum. The track should be diagonal, and the catheter should emerge away from the belt-line with the external cuff 2 cm from the skin exit site. The major dialyzer companies provide delivery of a selection of dialysis solutions. They vary in volume, osmotic strength and calcium concentration.

The key issue in peritoneal dialysis is the avoidance of infection introduced at the time of connection of the dialysis bag to the transfer set, which is attached to the peritoneal dialysis catheter. Many different connection systems have been designed to reduce the risk of introducing infection. Originally the connection was made by spiking the port of the peritoneal dialysis bag, but this required dexterity and strength. Luer-Loks are now used, and the connection can be made by an automatic mechanical device, after which it is subjected to ultraviolet light. This is particularly helpful for patients with weak hands, such as those with rheumatoid arthritis, or reduced visual acuity. The most reliable way to avoid introducing infection is to use the so-called Y-set. This allows the transfer set to be flushed with about 30 ml of sterile fluid from the full bag at the beginning of each exchange so that bacteria introduced at the time of the connection of the new bag are flushed to waste and are not infused into the peritoneal cavity. This system is more complex, requiring instillation of antiseptic into the transfer set between exchanges. It is also more expensive but probably pays for itself because of the lower incidence of infection (Maiorca *et al.*, 1983).

Indications for and Advantages of Peritoneal Dialysis

Peritoneal dialysis has major advantages over hemodialysis, but there are many limitations and drawbacks, too. It is a legitimate alternative to hemodialysis when the facilities for the latter are limited and is the modality used by 15% of patients worldwide (about 40% in the United Kingdom). It is 25% cheaper than hemodialysis in that it does not require an expensive dialysis machine and large numbers of technically expert trained nursing staff. With CAPD, a nurse can supervise approximately 30 CAPD patients. The outpatient nature of the treatment is an important consideration—patients are kept away from the hospital, are not constrained by their dialysis slots, can travel and can vacation more easily. The treatment becomes expensive if beset by complications, such as peritonitis, that require hospital admission and expensive antibiotics, such as vancomycin and ciprofloxacin. Continuous ambulatory peritoneal dialysis is particularly useful in patients experiencing practical difficulties with hemodialysis, for example, vascular access problems or cardiovascular instability. It has social advantages for children and mothers of young children (Table 3–6).

The disadvantages are the problems of peritoneal infection, the absorption of glucose leading to weight gain, and the amount of time required to go through the disciplined exercise of performing an exchange. This discipline is too much for some patients who like to limit their obligation to renal failure to three 4-hour hemodialysis sessions a week. Younger patients, especially women, are embarrassed by the catheter and dislike the discomfort and appearance of holding 2 L of fluid in the abdomen.

TABLE 3–6

SUITABILITY OF PATIENTS FOR CONTINUOUS AMBULATORY PERITONEAL DIALYSIS

Especially Suitable	To Be Avoided
Children	Large-frame men
Awaiting a scheduled transplant	Obese patients
Young, blood group A	Hernias
Poor vascular access	Poor personal hygiene
Diabetes	Obliterated peritoneal space
Serious cardiac disease	Full-time peripatetic jobs
Live a long distance from hemodialysis center	

Indications and Implications for Transplantation

In Oxford, CAPD is recommended for patients presenting late with renal failure and without vascular access, smaller frame patients with residual function and patients unable to tolerate the cardiovascular stress of hemodialysis. Patients in whom the wait for renal transplant should be short, for example, blood group A candidates on the cadaveric waiting list or those in whom a living related donor transplant has been arranged before the ESRF can be held on CAPD, avoiding vascular access procedures that would be used only short-term.

After transplantation, provided that graft function is adequate, the peritoneal dialysis catheter can be capped off and left. The catheter should be removed at about 3 months, by which time most renal transplants have *declared* themselves. If the graft fails within 3 months, the catheter needs to be flushed to remove debris and fibrin. Infection occasionally is introduced at this first exchange after a break (see also subsequent section on dialysis posttransplant).

Complications
Loss of Ultrafiltration

A proportion of patients (10–30% by 5 years but increasing with time) retain fluid after more than 4 hours dwell and have poor ultrafiltration even with more hypertonic fluid. It occurs transiently after peritonitis and is more likely to become a chronic problem after multiple attacks. Patients present with fluid overload, and it is important to exclude poor compliance with dialysis or excessive fluid intake. The problem is due to rapid transport of solutes including glucose and can be assessed using the peritoneal equilibration test, which involves instilling a standard solution and measuring glucose, urea and creatinine concentrations in fluid and blood samples over the following 4 hours. Rapid transport is referred to as type 1 failure. Low ultrafiltration associated with slow transport, known as type 2 failure, is associated with loss of surface area, usually as a result of sclerosing peritonitis, which may follow *S. aureus* peritonitis.

In the early stages, reduced ultrafiltration can be managed by using shorter dwell times and leaving the peritoneum dry overnight. The use of an overnight solution of icodextrin (a glucose polymer) that is osmotically active but too large to be absorbed is an alternative strategy. When fluid retention occurs during the daytime exchanges, even with medium or strong bags, the only option to avoid abandoning peritoneal dialysis is to convert the patient to ambulatory peritoneal dialysis, sometimes with additional daytime icodextrin.

Peritonitis

Peritonitis is a potentially serious problem and one of the most common complications of peritoneal dialysis. Its average incidence is one episode per 24 to 36 patient months. The incidence of peritonitis is reduced using the Y-set.

About 55% of cases are due to gram-positive organisms, 15% are due to gram-negative organisms, and about 20% are *culture negative. Staphylococcus epidermidis* is the most common cause, and this agent usually causes a relatively mild peritonitis, which responds promptly to treatment. *S. aureus* causes a severe peritonitis with marked systemic features, including high fever and frequently hypotension. Response to antibiotics is less good, and the catheter has to be removed more often than in peritonitis resulting from other organisms. Sclerosing peritonitis, which carries a high morbidity and mortality, may develop. *Pseudomonas* accounts for approximately 5% of cases and is similarly difficult to clear, often necessitating catheter removal.

Peritonitis usually presents as cloudy bags (apparent with >50 leukocytes/μl) and abdominal pain, but the latter may precede the former by one exchange or 1 to 2 days. There may be fever (approximately 50%), nausea and vomiting (approximately 30%) and, when severe, hypotension. Abdominal tenderness with peritonism is the major clinical finding. The effluent peritoneal fluid usually contains greater than 100 leukocytes (>50% neutrophils) per μl (normally <10/μl, although the number may be higher after a *dry period* (e.g., during the day in patients on ambulatory peritoneal dialysis). Peritonitis may be present with lower cell counts, however. Cloudy bags are occasionally due to macrophages and/or eosinophils and are not associated with peritonitis.

The diagnosis is made in the presence of any two of the following: abdominal pain, cloudy bags or the presence of bacteria on Gram stain. A variety of regimens are successful, for example, intraperitoneal vancomycin, 2 g (1 g if <60 kg), left to dwell for 4 hours and repeated after 7 days, and oral ciprofloxacin. Unless patients are ill, they are generally treated as outpatients (approximately 80%). The appropriate antibiotic is continued when the results of the microbiology are available, but both antibiotics are continued in the case of culture-negative peritonitis. If the patient fails to respond within 48 hours and is unwell, gentamicin, 4 mg/L in alternate bags, should be substituted to cover for gram-negative organisms. Further delay in response should raise the possibility of fungal peritonitis. Occasionally (<5%), peritonitis is secondary to intraabdominal disease, such as diverticulitis, appendicitis or perforated viscus, and if suspected laparotomy is indicated.

Patients with recurrent episodes of peritonitis from the same organism may have persistent infection of the catheter or its track or may be due to the buildup of a biofilm on the catheter that provides protection for bacteria from antibiotics. This buildup can be treated by removal of the peritoneal dialysis catheter with a rest on hemodialysis and later placement of a fresh catheter or by removal and replacement at the same operation. Recurrent peritonitis may be due to poor technique, and this should be reassessed carefully.

Exit Site and Tunnel Infection

Nearly half of all exit sites are colonized by *S. aureus*, and this organism causes greater than 50% of all exit site infections and usually is associated with nasal carriage. Prevention is the best strategy by careful education regarding daily washing, drying, avoiding forceful removal of scabs and avoiding tugging the catheter by careful tethering. Treatment of infection should be guided by microbiology, but because staphylococci are common, 2 weeks of flucloxacillin is often first-line treatment. Recurrence may be treated effectively by adding rifampicin to flucloxacillin. Sometimes the outer cuff

extrudes, and shaving this may cure the problem, but catheter replacement may be necessary, especially if there is evidence of a tunnel infection or recurrent peritonitis. The prophylactic use of mupirocin nasal ointment is associated with a lower incidence of exit site infections (and peritonitis in some studies), but there is a concern about the emergence of resistance, especially when used in hospitals.

Anatomical Complications

The presence of abdominal fluid increases intraabdominal pressure and predisposes to the development of hernias, which are relatively common (10–15% of all peritoneal dialysis patients and higher in patients with polycystic kidneys). Although often asymptomatic, prompt repair is essential because they inevitably enlarge, and there is the risk of obstruction and/or strangulation. Acid reflux, indigestion, a feeling of fullness and delayed gastric emptying also are more common than in patients on hemodialysis.

Scrotal or labial edema occurs when fluid leaks from the peritoneum to subcutaneous tissues. This condition usually occurs soon after insertion of the Tenckhoff catheter and spontaneously settles after resting for a few weeks. Occasionally, patients have a congenital communication between the pleura (usually right) and peritoneum resulting in a hydrothorax (diagnosed by measuring the glucose concentration in the pleural fluid), which precludes peritoneal dialysis.

Pain on draining fluid into the abdomen is relatively common early on but usually settles. This pain can be reduced by ensuring the fluid is at body temperature and may be improved by slowing the inflow rate. It is important to exclude peritonitis. For a few, the pain remains a problem preventing CAPD. For some of these patients, the use of bicarbonate-based fluids (rather than lactate) may be helpful. Other problems include back pain and diaphragmatic stenting in patients with severe pulmonary disease.

Metabolic Complications

The peritoneal fluid contains high concentrations of glucose. It has been estimated that 200 g of glucose (more with many high concentration bags and during peritonitis) may be absorbed daily, equivalent to 800 kcal. This absorption may cause obesity, hyperglycemia, hyperinsulinemia and type II diabetes. The glucose load stimulates fat synthesis, and hypertriglyceridemia is common. Cholesterol levels also rise during the first year on CAPD. Albumin levels often are low. The explanation is multifactorial, including losses in the fluid and malnutrition because of poor appetite, especially during and after peritonitis.

About 25% of CAPD patients are hypokalemic, and they may need potassium supplements. A few need a stringent low-potassium diet. Many patients using 2.5- to 3-L bags run high bicarbonate levels, which may be dangerous, especially if the patient develops an additional respiratory alkalosis. Alkalosis has been associated with lethargy, nausea and headaches. It is difficult to deal with in the absence of commercially available solutions with lower lactate concentrations.

Choice and Planning for the Individual Patient

Patients with chronic renal failure are never cured. The illness takes on the characteristics of a career with many changes in treatment likely to occur within the remaining lifetime. This requirement for different modalities of RRT, each with its liabilities to complications and failure, means that a coordinated and multidisciplinary approach is required from the outset. This approach requires not only cooperation between clinicians but also a formidable degree of planning.

The first issue to settle is whether the patient is suitable for renal transplantation. There are few contraindications, and none is absolute. In patients older than age 65, the decision has to be based on an overall assessment of the patient's fitness and ability to withstand surgery and immunosuppression. This is necessarily subjective. Availability of kidneys also influences policy.

The best first option is a pre–end-stage transplant from a living related donor because this avoids the need for an initial period of dialysis and the creation of permanent vascular access. It also enables planning of transplantation that avoids major disruption to the life of young patients at a crucial stage in their education or career. Nephrologists should emphasize the much longer survival of living related donor transplants, the lower morbidity and the reduced doses of immunosuppression. Although it must be acknowledged that the transplants ultimately may fail, families of young patients should be reminded of the benefits of 10 years of dialysis-free life in the early years after the development of ESRF, which would allow completion of education, establishment of a career and having a family.

If living related donor transplantation is not possible, the next best option is to put the patient forward for a pre–end-stage cadaver donor transplant, if possible. Apart from avoiding dialysis, this option allows the patient to spend a longer period in the recipient pool; because there is less urgency, the patient can wait for a better-matched kidney. Some nephrologists object to this policy on the grounds that it is unfair to patients already on dialysis who may have waited a long time for a transplant. Given the shortage of cadaver kidneys and the superior survival of well-matched grafts, this objection can be rejected. Another objection to pre–end-stage transplantation is that it removes the experience of dialysis so that the advantages of transplantation are not appreciated. Perhaps it is believed that the memory of the limitations and discipline of dialysis treatment would ensure compliance with immunosuppressive medication. This is a puritanical view that should not shape policy for most patients. There are some patients who are ambivalent about transplantation, however, and, especially if they have few uremic symptoms, would be difficult to persuade to have a preemptive transplant. If noncompliance is the fear, one has to remember that such patients would be more difficult to persuade to adhere to the dietary and fluid restrictions of dialysis. The final objection is based on the belief that pre–end-stage patients are more immunologically competent than those already on dialysis and so are more likely to reject their first graft. There are no data to support this opinion, and at Oxford, patients transplanted pre–end-stage have done as well as those transplanted from dialysis (Roake et al., 1996).

The only disadvantage of pre–end-stage transplantation is the occasional need to perform a dialysis immediately preoperatively to ensure that the plasma potassium concentration is safe for surgery and to obviate the need for early postoperative dialysis to reduce the plasma potassium concentration or control fluid overload. If graft function is delayed and the combination of hypotension and cyclosporine stops the residual renal function and the patient has no vascular access, an acute dialysis catheter has to be inserted. This procedure carries a small risk. It is emotionally difficult for patients transplanted pre–end-stage if the transplant fails and the need to start regular dialysis is precipitated. These patients need extra support and reminding that dialysis was imminent anyway and that when they are fit another transplant will be possible.

If dialysis is necessary before transplantation can be performed, the best holding treatment depends on the length of time waiting for a graft. If the patient is fit, is not sensitized and is blood group A or if a living related donor is available, CAPD is a good holding treatment because it avoids the need for creating permanent or temporary vascular access. Occasionally, such patients would be held on hemodialysis using a temporary internal jugular or subclavian vein catheter, but this should be discouraged because of the risks of infection and the development of subclavian vein stenosis, which may exclude the arm from future arteriovenous fistula formation. If hemodialysis is required, a tunneled dialysis catheter, such as the twin Tesio catheter system, is the best option (see Chapter 5). If the wait for a transplant is indeterminate, the dialysis treatment has to be chosen after consideration of the patient's preference, social considerations such as distance from the dialysis center and ease with which vascular access can be created.

Dialysis Posttransplant

The need for dialysis after transplantation depends on the degree of early graft function, which, in turn, depends on many factors related to the donor organ (see Chapter 14). During any period when graft function is absent or compromised, it is essential to modify doses of drugs for which the predominant route of excretion is the kidney. Particular care is required for aminoglycoside antibiotics (see Chapter 31), certain muscle relaxants (see Chapter 13) and opiates, the active metabolites of which accumulate in renal failure. These drugs are listed in Bennett et al. (1994), and important examples are listed in Table 3–7.

HEMODIALYSIS

Hemodialysis should be performed as for any postoperative patient (i.e., as remote from the surgical procedure as is safe for the control of potassium and fluid balance). In practice, this is usually more than 24 hours after the operation. The danger is hemorrhage from the operation wound and biopsy sites, but in practice the risks are small with short dialyses, thorough flushing of dialysis lines and filters with heparinized saline and low loading doses of heparin, minimum maintenance heparin and reversal with protamine at the end of dialysis. If the patient is actively bleeding, dialysis is possible without heparin at all, provided that the lines have been flushed adequately and the blood flow kept greater than 250 ml/min. For the patient with an unstable cardiovascular system, hemofiltration is preferable. Fluid balance is simple, but continuous heparinization is required. The usual vascular access should be used for hemodialysis, but fistulae should not be used for continuous treatments lasting more than 4 hours. Dislodgment of needles would lead to catastrophic hemorrhage, and so femoral or internal jugular dialysis catheters should be used. The choice of dialyser membrane may be important. Prospective studies show that patients with *acute renal failure* dialyzed with bioincompatible, usually cuprophane, membranes have a lower survival rate, a higher risk of sepsis and a more prolonged period of acute renal failure than those treated with biocompatible membranes (polymethyl methacrylate or polyacrylonitrile). These findings have not been universally accepted or reproduced in the setting of posttransplant dialysis. The use of biocompatible filters that are expensive should not be considered obligatory (reviewed by Jacobs, 1997).

TABLE 3–7

DRUGS TO BE USED WITH CARE IN RENAL FAILURE

Drug Class and Specific Drugs	Comment
Antimicrobial	
Aminoglycosides	Reduce dose, ototoxic
Acyclovir	Reduce dose
Cephalosporins	Reduce dose
Co-trimoxazole	Reduce dose
Ethambutol	Reduce dose, retinal toxicity
Ganciclovir	Reduce dose
Nitrofurantoin	Avoid, neuropathy
Penicillins	Avoid high doses, fits
Vancomycin	Reduce dose, ototoxic
Anesthetic	
Pancuronium	Avoid, prolonged paralysis
Gallamine	Avoid, prolonged paralysis
Opiates	Reduce dose, prolonged effect
Suxamethonium	Increases plasma potassium concentrations
Gastrointestinal	
Metoclopramide	Be aware of extrapyramidal effects
H_2 antagonists	Reduce dose
Magnesium salts	Monitor magnesium concentration
Cardiac	
Digoxin	Reduce dose and frequency
β-blockers	May need to reduce dose
Spironolactone	Avoid, hyperkalemia
ACE inhibitors	Monitor creatinine and potassium
Clofibrate	Avoid, muscle injury
Oral hypoglycemics	
Chlorpropamide	Avoid, hypoglycemia
Tolbutamide	Reduce dose
Biguanides	Avoid, lactic acidosis

ACE = angiotensin-converting enzyme.

Vascular access needs particular care in the postoperative phase. Periods of hypotension predispose to collapse and thrombosis of fistulae and Gore-Tex grafts, especially those with preexisting stenoses. The accesses must be explored and flow restored as soon as possible, not only for their immediate use, but also for the long-term should the graft fail. Rehabilitation of patients with failed renal transplants is prolonged greatly if they lose their vascular access as well.

It is reasonable to dialyze patients to above their so-called dry weight in the postoperative period. This approach avoids the hypotension that may delay the graft *opening up* and even predispose to thrombosis of the anastomosis. The exception is before the administration of anti–T cell agents, which may predispose to pulmonary edema (see Chapter 20).

CONTINUOUS AMBULATORY PERITONEAL DIALYSIS

Peritoneal dialysis can be performed safely after the transplant procedure, provided that the peritoneum has not been breached; the risk can be minimized by draining the peritoneum before surgery. It is a gentle treatment in the postoperative period and avoids the need for heparinization, which is required for hemodialysis. If clear fluid does leak from the transplant wound, it can be shown to be peritoneal dialysis fluid by measuring the glucose concentration. Peritoneal dialysis should be stopped immediately, the peritoneum drained and hemodialysis used to support the patient. Peritoneal dialysis can be reinstituted at about 7 days but should be with low volumes or preferably using a cycling machine that allows low volumes and no dwell time. Patients should not be transplanted during an episode of peritonitis, however, because the risk of leaking peritoneal dialysis fluid onto the graft site is too great. A balanced decision has to be made if a well-matched graft is offered to a patient whose episode of peritonitis is resolving.

Return to Dialysis After Transplant Failure

The return to dialysis after transplantation is a difficult period for the patient and the nephrologist. Not only are there understandable emotional difficulties, but also there are frequently physical problems. Early graft failure is less traumatic for the patient who has not enjoyed independence from dialysis. Immunosuppression, particularly steroid doses, should be reduced rapidly and the patient returned to the usual dialysis schedule. Grafts that fail early usually are removed surgically, but the need for this often is precipitated by the reduction in immunosuppression. Patient survival is affected adversely by graft failure (Cattran and Fenton, 1993).

Patients whose long-term grafts have failed present more complex problems. The temptation to maintain a failing graft should be resisted because it is better for the patient to be established on dialysis than to suffer the continual effects of uremia and immunosuppression (Cattran and Fenton, 1993). The physician has to discuss with the patient the appropriate modality, which may be different from that employed before transplantation. Often home dialysis is no longer acceptable, or vascular access difficulties may mean that CAPD is more appropriate. If the graft is failing slowly, vascular access should be fashioned before dialysis is required again. These patients frequently have many side effects from immunosuppression, such as osteoporosis, skin atrophy and malignancy, hyperglycemia, hypertension and secondary hyperparathyroidism. Although prednisolone should be withdrawn gradually, this needs to be done over a 3- to 4-month period. Even then the patient is at risk of hypoadrenalism and should be warned that he or she will require an increased dose of steroids to cover any intercurrent illness. It is reasonable to perform a short Synacthen test if there is doubt about the adrenal status to ensure that withdrawal has been effected safely.

Conservative measures to control the effect of renal failure as graft function declines should be instituted early. These measures include phosphate control by diet and with binders such as calcium acetate, prescription of vitamin D analogues (one α-hydroxyvitamin D, or 1,25-dihydroxyvitamin D, calcitriol), mild protein, sodium and potassium restriction and recombinant human erythropoietin if the hemoglobin runs less than 10 g/dl.

Results

The most useful and informative way to consider the results of RRT is to describe survival after starting, regardless of the modality first used. Because patients may experience one or both forms of dialysis and transplantation and the choice of first modality depends on factors that also influence prognosis, direct comparisons of CAPD, hemodialysis and transplantation are difficult. Overall the survival rate of transplant recipients is higher than for dialysis patients because of the exclusion of high-risk and elderly patients.

Some support for the belief that survival is better in patients receiving a transplant than in those who are eligible but remain on dialysis comes from a report of an analysis of the United States Renal Data System (USRDS) data (Wolfe *et al.*, 1999). The long-term mortality was 48 to 82% lower among transplant recipients than patients on the waiting list. Although there was a higher earlier mortality, the benefits were seen particularly in the younger patients (20–39 years old).

Opinion on the difference between CAPD and hemodialysis is divided. Most data fail to show a significant difference in survival in patients receiving CAPD or hemodialysis, but there are contradictory reports suggesting reduced mortality and morbidity with both. Data from the USRDS suggest that CAPD patients have a 19% higher mortality than patients treated by hemodialysis, especially in older patients and diabetics (Bloembergen et al., 1995). Patients with poor cardiac function do better on CAPD, however. Home hemodialysis patients have the lowest mortality figures, and this is not entirely explained by selection bias. The hemodialysis membrane also may have an effect. USRDS data suggest that mortality is significantly lower in patients dialyzed using modified cellulose and synthetic membranes compared with standard cellulose dialyzers. High flux dialysis has been suggested to reduce morbidity and mortality further; this is currently being studied in a prospective trial (Depner et al., 1999).

MODALITY SUCCESS

Comparisons of methods are difficult because hemodialysis is rarely impossible, whereas CAPD frequently cannot be used, but if there are difficulties with CAPD, patients can be switched to hemodialysis. One must expect a proportion of CAPD patients to fail (i.e., CAPD is unsuccessful or proves unsatisfactory), and this number will increase with time. The usual reasons are recurrent peritonitis, inadequate dialysis as residual renal function declines and loss of ultrafiltration. In some patients, failure may result from practical problems of repeated exchanges, hernias, rectal prolapse, peritoneopleural leaks or rarely the development of sclerosing peritonitis. The reported technique survival, which does not distinguish between failure resulting from complications and successful transplantation, varies widely but for the European Dialysis and Transplant Association (EDTA) registry is 23% at 5 years (Mallick et al., 1995). In a few patients, hemodialysis becomes impossible because of vascular access failure. The only solution is peritoneal dialysis or transplantation with the first available crossmatch-negative graft.

QUALITY OF LIFE

Quality of life is the most difficult aspect of RRT to quantitate, especially because there are big differences in the ages and other circumstances of patients being managed by the various modalities. Employment is an important criterion by which the quality of life or outcome of RRT can be judged, and in this respect transplant recipients are at an advantage. The other advantages of transplantation hardly need listing. There is no doubt that the quality of life of a transplant patient with minimal complications is far greater than that of even the most well-adjusted hemodialysis patient. The advantages are less clear-cut if comparison is made between an independent home hemodialysis patient and a transplant patient who suffers major complications of immunosuppres-

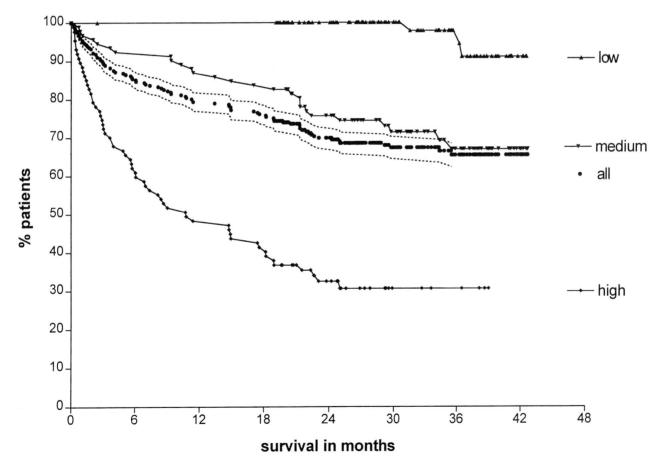

FIGURE 3–4

Comparison of actuarial survival of all patients starting renal replacement treatment in Oxford in 1996–1997 according to their risk group (Khan et al., 1996). Of the 281 patients, 102 were low risk, 92 were medium risk and 87 were high risk.

sion. The ANZDATA Registry is one of the few that examines the issue of quality of life systematically. The 1998 report showed that 85% of transplant recipients were judged to have a normal quality of life in that they were able to carry on normal activities with only minor symptoms (Disney *et al.*, 1998). Only 44% of dialysis patients were in this category; however, 83% of dialysis patients were self-caring; 9% required considerable or special assistance.

MORTALITY

Survival on dialysis depends on the patient's age at which dialysis is started and the presence of comorbid conditions such as diabetes. For example, in 1996, the 1-year mortality in the United States for the age groups 20 to 44, 45 to 64, 65 to 74 and older than 75 was 10.1%, 17.3%, 29.8% and 46%. In a study comparing various European centers, the 2-year survival in low-risk, medium-risk and high-risk groups was 86 to 100%, 59 to 79% and 27 to 70% (Khan *et al.*, 1996). Mortality is always higher in diabetics. Figure 3–4 shows the Oxford dialysis mortality data.

Survival of patients with a chronic disease should be considered in a longer time frame. In the United States, the 5- and 10-year survivals of the 1987 cohort of patients aged 50 to 54 were 47% and 23%. Another way to express survival is to describe the average remaining life years for a particular age group. These are tabulated in the USRDS report. For example, for all white men with ESRF aged 50 to 54, it is 7.1 years; for those on dialysis, it is 5.2 years. For the non-ESRF population, the figure is 27.3 years. These figures reinforce the need to improve RRT and tackle the causes of accelerated cardiovascular disease in renal failure patients.

REFERENCES

Bennett, W. M., Aronoff, G. R., Golper, T. A., Morrison, G., Brater, D. C. and Singer, I. (1994). *Drug Prescribing in Renal Failure*, American College of Physicians, Philadelphia.
Bloembergen, W. E., Port, F. K., Mauger, E. A., *et al.* (1995). A comparison of mortality between patients treated with hemodialysis and peritoneal dialysis. *J. Am. Soc. Nephrol.* 6, 177.
Burton, P. R. and Walls, J. (1987). Selection-adjusted comparison of life-expectancy of patients on continuous ambulatory peritoneal dialysis, haemodialysis, and renal transplantation. *Lancet* 1, 1115.
Canada-USA (CANUSA) Peritoneal Dialysis Study Group. (1996). Adequacy of dialysis and nutrition in continuous peritoneal dialysis: association with clinical outcomes. *J. Am. Soc. Nephrol.* 7, 198.
Cattran, D. C. and Fenton, S. S. (1993). Contemporary management of renal failure: outcome of the failed allograft recipient. *Kidney Int.* 41(Suppl.), S36.
Charra, B., Calemard, E., Ruffet, M., *et al.* (1992). Survival as an index of adequacy of dialysis. *Kidney Int.* 41, 1286.
Depner, T., Beck, G., Daugirdas, J., Kusek, J. and Eknoyan, G. (1999). Lessons from the Hemodialysis (HEMO) Study: an improved measure of the actual hemodialysis dose. *Am. J. Kidney Dis.* 33, 142.
Disney, A. P. S, Russ, G. R., Walker, R., Collin, J., Herberrt K. and Kerr, P. (eds.). (1998). *ANZDATA Registry Report 1998. Australia and New Zealand Dialysis and Transplant Registry,* Adelaide, South Australia.
Feest, T. G., Mistry, C. D., Grimes, D. S. and Mallick, N. P. (1990).

Incidence of advanced chronic renal failure and the need for end-stage renal replacement treatment. *B. M. J.* 301, 897.
Feest, T. G., Round, A., Hamad, S., Mistry, C. D., Grimes, D. and Mallick, N. P. (1992). Prospective study of severe acute renal failure in an unselected population. *Nephrol. Dial. Transplant.* 7, 553.
Innes, A., Rowe, P. A., Burden, R. P. and Morgan, A. G. (1992). Early deaths on renal replacement therapy: the need for early nephrological referral. *Nephrol. Dial. Transplant.* 7, 467.
Jacobs, C. (1997). Current trends in dialysis therapy. *Kidney Int.* 62(Suppl), S93.
Jungers, P., Zingraff, J., Albouze, G., *et al.* (1993). Late referral to maintenance dialysis: detrimental consequences. *Nephrol. Dial. Transplant.* 8, 1089.
Khan, I. H., Campbell, M. K., Cantarovich, D., *et al.* (1996). Survival on renal replacement therapy in Europe: is there a 'centre effect'? *Nephrol. Dial. Transplant.* 11, 300.
Klahr, S., Levey, A. S., Beck, G. J., *et al.* (1994). The effects of dietary protein restriction and blood-pressure control on the progression of chronic renal disease: modification of Diet in Renal Disease Study Group. *N. Engl. J. Med.* 330, 877.
Lowrie, E.G., Laird, N. M., Parker, T. F., and Sargent, J. A. (1981). Effect of haemodialysis prescription on patient morbidity: report from the National Cooperative Dialysis Study. *N. Engl. J. Med.* 305, 1176.
Maiorca, R., Cantaluppi, A., Cancarini, G. C., *et al.* (1983). Prospective controlled trial of a Y-connector and disinfectant to prevent peritonitis in continuous ambulatory peritoneal dialysis. *Lancet* 2, 642.
Mallick, N. P. and Gokal, R. (1999). Haemodialysis. *Lancet* 353, 737.
Mallick, N. P., Jones, E. and Selwood, N. (1995). The European (European Dialysis and Transplantation Association–European Renal Association) Registry. *Am. J. Kidney Dis.* 25, 176.
Muirhead, N. (1997). Renal disease II: the clinical impact of recombinant human erythropoietin. *J. R. Coll. Physicians Lond.* 31, 125.
National Kidney Foundation (1997). Dialysis outcomes quality initiative (DOQI). National Kidney Foundation, New York.
Obrador, G. T. and Pereira, B. J. G. (1998). Early referral to the nephrologist and timely initiation of renal replacement therapy: a paradigm shift in the management of patients with chronic renal failure. *Am. J. Kidney Dis.* 31, 398.
Roake, J. A., Cahill, A. P., Gray, C. M., Gray, D. W. and Morris, P. J. (1996). Pre-emptive cadaveric renal transplantation—clinical outcome. *Transplantation* 62, 1411.
Roderick, P. J., Ferris, G. and Feest, T. G. (1998). The provision of renal replacement therapy for adults in England and Wales: recent trends and future directions. *Q. J. M.* 91, 581.
Ruggenenti, P., Perna, A., Gherardi, G., *et al.* (1999). Renoprotective properties of ACE-inhibition in non-diabetic nephropathies with non-nephrotic proteinuria. *Lancet* 354, 359.
Shinzato, T., Nakai, S., Akiba, T., *et al.* (1997). Current status of renal replacement therapy in Japan: results of the annual survey of the Japanese Society for Dialysis Therapy. *Nephrol. Dial. Transplant.* 12, 889.
The British Transplantation Society (1998). *Towards Standards for Organised Tissue Transplantation in the United Kingdom.* British Transplantation Society, London.
The Renal Association (1997). *Treatment of Adult Patients with Renal Failure: Recommended Standards and Audit Measures,* 2nd. ed. Royal College of Physicians, London.
U.S.R.D.S. 1999 Annual Data Report. (1999). *Am. J. Kidney Dis.* 34(Suppl 1), S9.
Walker, R. (1997). General management of end-stage renal disease. *B. M. J.* 315, 1429.
Wolfe, R. A., Ashby, V. B., Milford, E. L., *et al.* (1999). Comparison of mortality in all patients on dialysis, patients on dialysis awaiting transplantation, and recipients of a first cadaveric transplant [see comments]. *N. Engl. J. Med.* 341, 1725.

The Recipient of a Renal Transplant
J. D. Briggs

Patient Selection

The selection criteria for dialysis and transplantation are now much less restrictive than in the past. This change is due to many factors, especially safer surgery and anesthesia and more effective immunosuppression. The reduction in acute rejection after the introduction of cyclosporine, tacrolimus and mycophenolate mofetil has led to a reduction in the total steroid dose, and this has made an important contribution to the reduction in morbidity and mortality. Consequently, patients who, in the past, would have been considered as carrying too high a risk of failure or death are now being accepted for transplantation. This higher risk group includes older patients and patients with comorbid disease (e.g., diabetes mellitus). The availability of more potent immunosuppression and more sophisticated HLA typing and crossmatching allows the acceptance of patients previously considered as having a high risk of immunological failure, such as patients who are highly sensitized to HLA antigens. The process of selection takes into account the type of renal disease and the results of a detailed examination, in particular for comorbid disease or complications of the renal failure and, when indicated, of the lower urinary tract.

TYPES OF RENAL DISEASE

The commonest group of renal diseases in patients selected for a transplant is glomerulonephritis, followed by reflux nephropathy or other type of interstitial nephritis, diabetes mellitus, polycystic kidneys and renal vascular disease. The relative frequency of these diseases in renal allograft recipients in the United Kingdom is shown in Table 4–1. In the United States and Scandinavia, diabetes mellitus has become the major cause of end-stage renal failure leading to transplantation. Since the 1970s, the main change in the acceptance rate of patients with different causes of end-stage renal disease has been an increase in patients with diabetes mellitus as a result of not only the increasing prevalence of diabetes in the Western world but also a greater willingness to accept patients with comorbid disease as well as increasingly older patients.

Glomerulonephritis

Recurrence of glomerulonephritis after transplantation has been described with all the common histological types. The subject has been reviewed comprehensively by Mathew (1991), Ramos and Tisher (1994) and Kotanko *et al.* (1997); the incidence of recurrence from the analysis of Mathew is summarized in Table 4–2. Although the recurrence rates are high for some types of glomerulonephritis, the short-term failure rates are low. Within the first 5 years, the overall failure rate from recurrence of glomerulonephritis is less than 2% even in the 15- to 24-year-old age group, the age range in which the incidence of glomerulonephritis in native kidneys is highest (Raine *et al.*, 1992).

There is as yet little information available from longer term studies. Analysis of the United Kingdom Transplant Support Service Authority database shows that of the 16,606 renal transplants carried out between 1984 and 1993, only 114 had failed from recurrence of disease by the end of 1998 (J. D. Briggs, unpublished, 1999). This represented a failure rate from this cause of less than 1%, whereas failure from recurrence accounted for only 2% of all failures of transplants carried out during that period. One has to accept the proviso, however, that because of difficulty in accurately diagnosing recurrent disease, there is likely to be underreporting in registry data. The frequency and severity of recurrence are so variable among the various forms of glomerulonephritis that one has to take note of the type of glomerulonephritis when assessing the risk of graft loss from recurrence. The risk of recurrent disease rarely would constitute a contraindication to transplantation, but in certain instances, as discussed subsequently, it could be an adverse factor.

Focal Segmental Glomerulosclerosis. In adults with no additional risk factors, the recurrence rate of focal segmental glomerulosclerosis (FSGS) is 10 to 15%, whereas in children younger than 5 years old it is 50%. In patients younger than 15 years whose native kidney disease progressed to end-stage renal failure within 3 years and in whom the native kidney biopsy showed mesangial expansion, the recurrence rate is 80 to 100% (Kotanko *et al.*, 1997). Loss of a first graft from recurrent FSGS leads to a likelihood of recurrence in the second graft in 75 to 85% of patients (Artero *et al.*, 1992; Stephanian *et al.*, 1992). Recurrent FSGS is the least benign of the commoner types of recurrent glomerulopathy and overall leads to graft failure in 40 to 50% of patients (Artero *et al.*, 1992). One has to consider carefully whether to perform more than one regraft in patients whose first graft is lost from recurrent disease and question the use of living donor grafts in patients with a high risk of recurrence of FSGS.

Membranous Nephropathy. Membranous nephropathy occurs *de novo* in 2% of renal allografts, but in patients

TABLE 4–1

PRIMARY RENAL DISEASE*

Type	% of Total
Glomerulonephritis	24
Reflux nephropathy/interstitial nephritis	16
Adult polycystic kidneys	14
Diabetes mellitus	11
Renal vascular disease	9
Miscellaneous/unknown	27

*These figures were taken from the database of the United Kingdom Transplant Support Services Authority (UKTSSA) and are for patients receiving transplants in the United Kingdom in the period 1990–1998. Diabetes mellitus represents the commonest cause of end-stage renal failure in patients transplanted in the United States and Scandinavia.

TABLE 4–2

RECURRENCE OF GLOMERULONEPHRITIS IN RENAL ALLOGRAFTS

Type of Glomerulonephritis	Approximate Frequency of Recurrence %
Focal segmental glomerulosclerosis	30
Membranous nephropathy	10
Mesangiocapillary type I	20–30
Mesangiocapillary type II	95
IgA nephropathy	50
Henoch-Schönlein purpura	80
Anti–glomerular basement membrane nephritis	5
Idiopathic crescentic glomerulonephritis	?

Data from Mathew (1991).

with this condition as their primary renal disease, recurrence is relatively common. Cosyns and associates have described a series of 30 patients with a recurrence rate of 29% at 3 years and a graft failure rate among those with recurrence of 38% and 52% at 5 and 10 years (Cosyns et al., 1998). This is one of the types of renal disease in which recurrence is less benign than in most of the others.

Mesangiocapillary Glomerulonephritis Type I. Mesangiocapillary glomerulonephritis type I is one of the less common types of glomerulonephritis, and although the recurrence rate usually quoted is 20 to 30% (Kotanko et al., 1997), this is based on small patient numbers and is probably an overestimate. A European Renal Association (ERA) Registry survey showed a graft failure rate from recurrence of 6% among 564 patients (Briggs and Jones, 1999a) so that on the combined basis of the recurrence and failure rates, there seldom would be an argument against transplantation.

Mesangiocapillary Glomerulonephritis Type II. Because mesangiocapillary glomerulonephritis type II is an uncommon disease, most series are small. Almost all studies have documented a high recurrence rate, however, between 70% and 100%, and with recurrence taking place early, usually within the first few months. Andresdottir and colleagues calculated the failure rate resulting from recurrence from all published series to be 16% (Andresdottir et al., 1999), which agrees well with the figure of 19% from the ERA Registry (Briggs and Jones, 1999a). The high recurrence rate would make one approach live donor transplantation with caution.

IgA Nephropathy. In most countries, IgA nephropathy is now the commonest type of glomerulonephritis and is by far the commonest type to recur in renal allografts. Berger (1988) reported a recurrence rate of 53% in a study of renal transplant patients who underwent routine biopsies, although proteinuria and/or hematuria was often mild or absent. Recurrence of this disease may follow a more benign course than does recurrence of most other types of glomerulonephritis, however. For example, the graft survival rate in an ERA Registry study of recurrent IgA nephropathy was 91% at 2 years compared with 43% for recurrent mesangiocapillary glomerulonephritis type II and 35% in patients younger than 15 years old with recurrent FSGS (Briggs and Jones, 1999a). Patient and graft survival rates are higher in IgA nephropathy patients than in most other primary renal disease groups, and this fact together with the low rate of graft loss in the presence of recurrent disease makes these patients good candidates for renal transplantation. There is evidence that the recurrences that occur relatively early after transplantation are likely to lead to graft failure (Clarkson et

al., 1999). In contrast to this general rule, there also is evidence of a genetic predisposition to IgA nephropathy, and this has raised the question of whether kidneys from living related donors should be accepted for these patients. The answer is that the use of live donor kidneys probably is justified for primary grafts, although probably not for regrafts if the first graft has failed from recurrence.

Henoch-Schönlein Nephritis. Because Henoch-Schönlein nephritis occurs predominantly in children, most of the experience relates to this age group. Meulders and coworkers reported a recurrence rate of 35% and graft loss from recurrence of 11% at 5 years posttransplant (Meulders et al., 1994). The ERA Registry reported a higher loss from recurrent disease, however, 33% at 2 years (Briggs and Jones, 1999a). The report of Hasegawa et al. (1987) was of concern in that it documented recurrent disease in 9 of 12 recipients of live donor kidneys with two graft losses but no recurrence in cadaver kidney recipients. Henoch-Schönlein nephritis shares with IgA nephropathy the predisposition toward frequent recurrence.

Anti–Glomerular Basement Membrane Disease. The article still quoted for the recurrence rate of anti–glomerular basement membrane disease as shown by the deposition of linear IgG along the glomerular basement membrane is that of Wilson and Dixon (1973), who found such deposition in 55% of cases. Only a quarter of renal transplant patients with Goodpasture's syndrome develop clinical evidence of recurrent disease (Kotanko et al., 1997), however, and an ERA Registry analysis found that recurrence was responsible for 5 of the 37 (14%) grafts that failed in a series of 190 patients with Goodpasture's syndrome (Briggs and Jones, 1999b). This same analysis found that 5-year graft survival after transplantation in Goodpasture's syndrome patients was 44%, whereas it was 58% in patients with standard primary renal disease,* and this difference was not statistically significant. Cameron (1982) suggested that recurrence could be reduced to less than 5% if dialysis were continued for at least 6 to 12 months before transplantation to allow the anti–glomerular basement membrane antibody to subside, and it is almost certainly preferable to delay transplantation until the antibody has disappeared from the blood.

Idiopathic Crescentic Glomerulonephritis. There is reassuring evidence from three large series that only 20 patients from among 1,240 (1.6%) with idiopathic crescentic glomerulonephritis developed recurrent disease (Kotanko et al., 1997).

In conclusion, clinically evident recurrent disease is a relatively uncommon complication in most patients with glomerulonephritis who receive renal transplants. When recurrence does become manifest, it often pursues a benign course leading to graft loss only after a number of years. The risk of graft failure from recurrent disease needs to be considered only infrequently when recommending whether a patient should go on to the transplant waiting list. The risk of recurrent disease is seldom a contraindication but in a few patients may be considered as an adverse factor. The main group of patients in this category are children with FSGS, particularly if a first graft already has been lost from recurrent disease. More than one graft lost from recurrent membranous nephropathy should make one proceed to a further transplant with caution, but this is an uncommon circumstance. One should be cautious about the use of a live donor kidney in a patient with Henoch-Schönlein nephritis.

---

*Standard primary renal disease consists predominantly of glomerulonephritis, interstitial nephritis, toxic nephropathies and cystic kidney disease.

Hereditary Disease

Retrospective studies have shown no difference in patient or graft survival when patients with polycystic kidneys are compared with patients with other primary renal diseases (Hadimeri et al., 1997). The mean age of patients with polycystic kidneys, however, usually is higher (Tzardis et al., 1989). It now is common policy to leave the native kidneys in situ unless they are causing abdominal discomfort, are grossly enlarged or are the site of persistent infection or recurrent, troublesome bleeding. In a review of their experience, Tzardis and colleagues found no disadvantage in this policy, with a need for removal of the native kidneys after transplantation in only 3.6% of patients (Tzardis et al., 1990). It is common for one of a large pair of kidneys to be removed before transplantation, however, to make space for a subsequent transplant.

In Alport's syndrome, the glomerular basement membrane characteristically lacks the so-called Goodpasture antigen. A number of patients with this syndrome have been described who developed crescentic glomerulonephritis after transplantation in association with the presence in the serum of glomerular basement membrane antibody, presumably as a response to the Goodpasture antigen in the donor kidney (Oliver et al., 1991). In two series with a combined total of 53 patients with Alport's syndrome reported by Quérin et al. (1986) and Peten et al. (1991), no cases of posttransplant crescentic nephritis occurred, although linear deposition of IgG commonly was found in graft biopsy samples. Similarly, Gobel and coworkers found the occurrence of crescentic glomerulonephritis to be rare despite some cases of deposition of antibody along the glomerular basement membrane (Gobel et al., 1992). Although when crescentic glomerulonephritis occurs this has a serious effect on the graft, it should not be a deterrent to transplantation in Alport's syndrome in view of its low incidence.

The final hereditary disease to mention is tuberous sclerosis. The kidney commonly is the site of angiomyolipoma and/or cysts, and renal cell carcinoma has been described. Bilateral nephrectomy before or at the time of transplantation has been advocated because of the risk of neoplasia. Monitoring by computed tomography scan is recommended posttransplant in patients whose own kidneys remain in situ (Balligand et al., 1990).

Metabolic Disease

Diabetes Mellitus

When one considers the two types of diabetes mellitus together, they constitute in some countries the commonest cause of chronic renal failure and are approaching that position in other countries. For example, the 1998 Annual Report from the United States Renal Data System (USRDS, 1998) showed that 39% of treated end-stage renal failure patients were diabetic, 14% having type I diabetes and 25% having type II. Although most studies have documented a higher mortality in diabetic renal allograft recipients than in nondiabetics (Munson et al., 1992; Rischen-Vos et al., 1992), this has not invariably been so, particularly in the more recent past. For example, Ekberg and Christensson (1996) have found no higher mortality in diabetics than in nondiabetics in the period since 1988, in contrast to the 16-year period before that. Although it is illogical to define an upper age limit in the selection of diabetic patients for transplantation, few older than age 65 years are sufficiently free of vascular disease to experience long-term survival. In contrast to the often reduced patient survival, graft survival is good in the diabetic recipient, provided that one excludes those who die

with functioning grafts when calculating graft survival (Ekberg and Christensson, 1996; McMillan et al., 1990).

The commonest contraindication to transplantation in diabetic patients is vascular disease of a degree that is too advanced to be amenable to effective therapy or that has resulted in severe and irreversible end-organ damage. The commonest examples are extensive cerebrovascular disease and severe cardiac dysfunction resulting from coronary artery disease. Blindness from retinopathy and the presence of neuropathy are not regarded as contraindications to transplantation. The assessment of cardiovascular disease before transplantation is discussed later in this chapter, and this is especially important in diabetic patients.

Although early transplantation is advantageous to all renal failure patients, this applies particularly to the diabetic. Hemodialysis carries an increased complication rate in the form of intraocular hemorrhage precipitated by heparin administration and vessel access thrombosis as a consequence of the often widespread vascular disease. Also, continuous ambulatory peritoneal dialysis may be complicated by poor blood glucose control resulting from the glucose load contained in the dialysis fluid.

It was inevitable that reports would appear describing the occurrence of diabetic nephropathy in the allograft (Maryniak et al., 1985), but graft failure from this cause usually has been thought likely only after a prolonged posttransplant interval. The report by Hariharan et al. (1996) documents well-established diabetic glomerulosclerosis shown by transplant biopsy in 14 renal allograft recipients after a mean interval of 97 months from the time of the transplant. This report indicates the need for larger scale studies of the incidence and time of development of diabetic glomerulosclerosis in the renal allograft. The interval between transplantation and a significant degree of graft dysfunction resulting from diabetic glomerulosclerosis is clearly long enough, however, that one never would look on this complication as an argument against renal transplantation in diabetes mellitus.

Enthusiasm for pancreatic transplantation continues to grow as the success rate of the procedure increases. In a report from the International Pancreas Transplant Registry, pancreas graft survival at one year was 83% when performed at the same time as a kidney transplant and was not far behind the survival of the kidney (Gruessner and Sutherland, 1999; Table 4–3). Table 4–3 shows that pancreas graft survival is better when combined with a renal allograft than is the case with a pancreas transplant alone. Selection of patients for a simultaneous pancreas and kidney transplant is along similar lines as for a renal allograft alone but with stricter criteria in particular regarding cardiovascular disease, in view of the higher morbidity of the procedure (Stratta et al., 1992). Cardiovascular assessment is discussed later in this chapter.

Hyperoxaluria

Hyperoxaluria is a rare inborn error of metabolism that is inherited as an autosomal recessive trait and is characterized

TABLE 4–3

PANCREAS TRANSPLANT SURVIVAL

Type of Transplant	1-Year Survival (%)		
	Patient	Pancreas Graft	Kidney Graft
Simultaneous kidney/pancreas	94	83	90
Pancreas after kidney	95	71	
Pancreas alone	95	64	

Data from Gruessner and Sutherland, 1999.

by increased synthesis of oxalate and glycolate. The consequences are recurrent urolithiasis, nephrocalcinosis and widespread tissue deposition leading especially to severe bone and vascular disease. The early reports of the outcome after transplantation were discouraging mainly owing to the severe vascular disease to which these patients are prone and to early oxalate deposition in the allograft.

A more optimistic account was given by Scheinman et al. (1984), who recorded continuing function of 7 of 10 grafts from live donors after 1 to 9 years. These investigators placed considerable emphasis on measures to prevent oxalate deposition in the graft, such as prolonged preoperative dialysis and maintenance of an effective diuresis after the operation with administration of pyridoxine, phosphate and magnesium solutions. There now is little doubt, however, that the preferred treatment option is combined hepatic and renal transplantation or hepatic transplantation alone at a stage of the disease before advanced renal damage has occurred. A prolonged period of dialysis should be avoided in these patients in view of the likely development of severe vascular disease from oxalate arteriopathy. In a collected series of 13 combined liver and kidney transplants performed between 1984 and 1989, a 1-year graft survival of 77% was achieved, which is much better than prior success rates with kidney-only grafts (Watts et al., 1991). There now is little role for isolated renal transplantation in the treatment of hyperoxaluria.

Cystinosis

In cystinosis, the results of transplantation are as good or possibly better than in other renal diseases (Ehrich et al., 1991). Because cystinotic nephropathy is due to an intrinsic lysosomal transport defect of the tubular cell, a renal allograft removes the lysosomal cystine load by restoring the normal transport system. Transplantation is the treatment of choice for children with this condition. There is a strong case for early transplantation in view of the slow but inexorable progression of the disease leading to severe stunting of growth, followed by multiple organ damage, including visual impairment, hypothyroidism, other endocrine dysfunction, myopathy and sometimes dementia. Although deposition of cystine occurs in the transplanted kidney, there is no evidence so far of any significant adverse effect on renal function in the transplant recipient (Langlois et al., 1981).

Fabry's Disease

Fabry's disease is a rare inherited disorder resulting from deficiency of α-galactosidase, a lysosomal enzyme; it is characterized clinically by recurrent episodes of limb pain and fever, skin papules, premature vascular disease and renal failure. The concept of renal transplantation is attractive in that, in theory, it should restore the missing enzyme, but there is no good evidence that this occurs in practice. A high mortality after transplantation was reported by Maizel et al. (1981), but more recently an ERA Registry analysis showed similar mortality to that in patients with the common types of renal disease (Tsakiris et al., 1996). The limb pain has tended to persist after transplantation. Further experience is required in particular to determine if the mortality can be reduced by transplantation at an earlier stage before the vascular disease has become too advanced.

Amyloidosis

A higher mortality has been reported in patients with amyloidosis after renal transplantation than in a group of

patients with glomerulonephritis, the 5-year patient survival figures being 66% and 86%, respectively (Heering et al., 1998). Graft survival was also lower in the amyloidosis group, the comparable 5-year figures being 55% and 63%. Primary amyloidosis recurs in the transplant after an interval, as does the secondary type unless the disease responsible for it has been eradicated (Cameron, 1983). Graft failure from recurrence has not been reported within the first 10 years, however. Despite the higher mortality, patient and graft survival are sufficiently good for transplantation to be preferable to continuing dialysis for patients who are in reasonable health, are free of active infection and have adequate cardiac function.

Gout

Average graft survival usually is achieved in gouty nephropathy. One problem is that bone marrow depression is probable if azathioprine and allopurinol are given concurrently. In patients who require maintenance allopurinol, azathioprine is contraindicated, but cyclosporine, tacrolimus and mycophenolate mofetil can be used (see Chapter 15).

Porphyria

Chronic renal failure is a recognized, although uncommon, complication of acute porphyria (Laiwah et al., 1983), and treatment by transplantation has been reported in four patients, all of whom had functioning grafts at the time of reporting (Nunez et al., 1987). In view of evidence from animal studies that there is a risk of cyclosporine precipitating an acute attack, these authors advise against its use in patients with porphyria. In my own unit, however, we have used cyclosporine without precipitating an attack, and I am unaware of adverse reports from other centers. I recommend that cyclosporine be used to achieve satisfactory graft survival.

Obstructive Uropathy

Obstructive uropathy is an important cause of renal failure, particularly in the younger patient, and it accounted for 26% of renal allograft recipients younger than 12 years of age in a series from Los Angeles (Warshaw et al., 1980). The graft survival rate in this series and in subsequent analyses, such as the one by Cairns et al. (1991), was comparable to that in patients with normal lower urinary tracts. Such an outcome was observed regardless of whether the ureter was placed in the patient's own bladder or in an intestinal conduit. The pretransplant assessment of patients with abnormal lower urinary tracts is discussed later in this chapter, and their management is discussed in more detail in Chapter 12.

Toxic Nephropathy
Analgesics

Disney (1981) reported poorer patient survival after transplantation in patients with analgesic nephropathy than in patients with the commoner causes of renal failure, and this finding was confirmed in an ERA Registry analysis (Briggs and Jones, 1999b). In this latter analysis, however, the poorer survival was thought to be related to the presence of older patients in the analgesic nephropathy group. By contrast, in a large series from Germany, patient and graft survival were as good in the analgesic nephropathy group as in those with other renal diseases (Schwarz et al., 1992). Uroepithelial carcinoma was found in 3.7% of the analgesic nephropathy group of Schwarz et al. (1992), compared with 0.3% among patients with other renal diseases. Also in the ERA Registry analysis (Briggs and Jones, 1999b), neoplasia accounted for 17% of deaths in analgesic nephropathy patients compared with 6% in the group with the common types of renal disease, and this higher incidence was, in part, due to more uroepithelial tumors. Pretransplant evaluation should include assessment of the urinary tract to exclude the presence of this type of tumor. It was reassuring that in the analysis of Schwarz *et al.* (1992) patient compliance in the analgesic nephropathy group was satisfactory in two respects: Blood cyclosporine levels were comparable to those in other patients, indicating reasonable adherence to the immunosuppressive regimen, and few had detectable analgesic drug in urine samples. One further recognized problem in patients with analgesic nephropathy is the high incidence of vascular disease.

Narcotics

In a small group of eight patients with a long history of intravenous opiate abuse, excellent graft survival was achieved (Ross *et al.*, 1983). Noncompliance is likely to be a problem in some of these patients, however. Although still relatively uncommon, this cause of renal failure is likely to be detected with increasing frequency as the incidence of opiate abuse rises. A problem that complicates the management of some of these patients is the presence of human immunodeficiency virus (HIV) infection. The suitability for transplantation of patients with HIV infection is discussed later.

Multisystem Diseases
Systemic Lupus Erythematosus

There is now considerable experience with renal transplantation in patients with systemic lupus erythematosus (SLE), and the results are encouraging. Earlier reports showed patient and graft survival rates that were not significantly worse than those of patients with other renal diseases (Goss *et al.*, 1991). There is widespread agreement that many patients with SLE are suitable for transplantation, and the main point of controversy is the policy for patients whose serological tests for SLE are still positive at the time of assessment for transplantation. On the basis of their experience, Goss and associates do not consider positive serological test results to be a contraindication to transplantation, and there is no clear evidence in the literature to contradict this view (Goss *et al.*, 1991). An ERA Registry report containing 539 SLE patients has confirmed these encouraging earlier reports because it showed almost identical patient and graft survival as in patients with standard primary renal diseases (Briggs and Jones, 1999b). One point that works in favor of the SLE patient is the tendency for the disease to enter an inactive or less active phase after the development of renal failure, a process to which the immunosuppressive effect of uremia may contribute (Ziff and Helderman, 1983). In view of the natural history of SLE, it is not surprising that lupus nephritis may recur in the allograft. In practice, clinical manifestations of recurrence have been uncommon in most series, although among 16 transplant recipients who underwent biopsies in the study of Nyberg *et al.* (1992), pathological evidence of lupus nephritis was found in 7. Six of these seven patients were experiencing a benign course at the time of the report, but this study differs from others in the larger number of routine biopsies performed. It may be that in long-term studies an increasing incidence of recurrence of lupus nephritis will be found on biopsy, but the large ERA Registry series

reported by Briggs and Jones (1999b) was reassuring in that there were no recorded cases of graft loss because of recurrent disease among the 539 patients.

Vasculitis

The three types of vasculitis usually associated with renal failure are polyarteritis nodosa, microscopic polyarteritis and Wegener's granulomatosis. All carry a high mortality rate resulting either from the aggressive nature of the disease or from complications of the immunosuppressive therapy used in their treatment. If irreversible renal failure results but is followed by resolution of the active phase of the disease, the prognosis with renal replacement therapy can approach the average for other types of renal disease.

The largest published series is contained in the ERA Registry report of Briggs and Jones (1999b), which documented 112 patients with polyarteritis and 115 with Wegener's granulomatosis who received renal allografts. Patient and graft survival at 3 years were poorer in the patients with polyarteritis; patient survival was 77% in comparison with patients who had standard primary renal disease, in whom it was 91%, whereas the comparable graft survival figures were 60% and 69%. This 9% difference could be accounted for by the greater number of deaths with functioning grafts in the polyarteritis group. Three of the 23 graft failures in the patients with polyarteritis were due to disease recurrence. By contrast, neither patient nor graft survival in the 115 patients with Wegener's granulomatosis was significantly poorer than in patients with standard primary renal disease, and there were no recorded failures because of recurrent disease in the former group. In two cases of recurrence of Wegener's granulomatosis in the graft described by Kuross *et al.* (1981) and Aunsholt and Ahlbom (1989), remission followed a change in immunosuppression with the introduction of cyclophosphamide. Overall the outcome of renal transplantation in vasculitis has been encouraging, although the opportunity for a transplant exists only for the relatively small number of patients whose general health is restored to a reasonable level while they remain dialysis dependent. Testing for antineutrophil antibody (ANCA) is a useful measurement of disease activity (Lockwood, 1986), and preferably transplantation should be delayed until the disease is judged to be relatively inactive on the basis of this test and clinical assessment. In some patients, evidence of disease activity persists while the patient remains dialysis dependent, however, and this should not preclude transplantation because one can have a reasonable expectation that the immunosuppressive therapy will prevent a major flare of the primary disease posttransplant.

Progressive Systemic Sclerosis

Few patients with progressive systemic sclerosis survive and retain a sufficient degree of well-being on dialysis to be considered for a renal transplant. In an ERA Registry analysis, 625 patients with this progressive systemic sclerosis from throughout Europe were recorded as being accepted for dialysis over a 20-year period (Tsakiris *et al.*, 1996). Only 28 underwent renal transplantation, and their 3-year graft survival rate was 44% compared with 60% for patients with standard primary renal disease. Renal transplantation has a role in only a small percentage of patients with progressive systemic sclerosis.

Hemolytic Uremic Syndrome

Hemolytic uremic syndrome accounts for about 5% of the patients on long-term dialysis in childhood but only about

0.2% among adults. The epidemic type is seen mainly in children and usually follows gastroenteritis caused by a vero-toxin-producing bacteria. The sporadic type is seen in children and adults. When acute renal failure occurs in hemolytic uremic syndrome, it is usually reversible, but in a few patients renal function fails to recover, leading to the need for continuation of dialysis. Consideration for transplantation can follow and usually is preferable to long-term dialysis in view of the preponderance of young patients, but there is a risk of graft loss because of recurrence of hemolytic uremic syndrome. A meta-analysis showed four factors to predispose to recurrence: older age, the use of calcineurin inhibitors, the use of live donor kidneys and a short time interval between onset of the disease and the time of reaching dialysis dependency (Ducloux et al., 1998). Older age and a shorter interval to end-stage renal failure tend to be associated with the sporadic type. The most important influence on possible recurrence is probably the sporadic as opposed to the epidemic form of the disease. Renal transplantation is worthwhile for most patients with hemolytic uremic syndrome, but the use of live donor kidneys should probably be avoided in patients with the sporadic type because of the risk of graft loss from recurrent disease. If graft failure does occur as a consequence of recurrent disease, calcineurin inhibitors probably should be avoided at the time of a second graft because they have been implicated as cofactors in the mechanism of hemolytic uremic syndrome recurrence.

Tumors

Primary Renal Tumors

Three types of primary renal tumor in the potential recipient have to be considered. First, there are symptomatic renal carcinomas, recurrence of which is common. In a retrospective study of 203 renal allograft recipients, 59 developed recurrences after the transplant (Penn, 1995). Of these, 34 patients (60%) had been treated for their primary disease less than 2 years before the transplant, 18 (31%) between 2 and 5 years before, and 5 (9%) more than 5 years before. An interval of at least 2 years between treatment of the tumor and transplantation should be advised strongly, whereas a longer interval, such as 4 or 5 years, increases the degree of safety. The second type of primary renal tumor is Wilms' tumor. Penn's retrospective analysis (1995) included 76 patients, among whom recurrence developed in 11, and in 10 of these the interval between treatment and transplantation was 24 months or less. With this type of tumor, a 2-year interval provides a reasonable degree of safety. A third type of renal cell carcinoma may develop as a sequela to the acquired renal cystic disease that frequently occurs in the kidneys of patients with long-standing renal failure. In this setting, the incidence of renal cell carcinoma is 50 times higher than in the general population (MacDougall et al., 1987). Although this still represents a low incidence, surveillance of native kidneys by ultrasound before transplantation is a worthwhile precaution with the addition of a computed tomography scan if indicated. In this context, the finding of Mallofré and colleagues was reassuring: They found 22 renal adenomas but no carcinomas on pathological examination of 72 kidneys affected by acquired renal cystic disease (Mallofré et al., 1992).

Paraproteinemias

The term *paraproteinemias* covers a spectrum of disease, the commonest subgroup being myeloma but including light-chain nephropathy and Waldenström's macroglobulinemia. Neither dialysis nor transplantation is indicated for patients with progressive disease unresponsive to therapy. There are a few patients, however, in whom remission can be induced and whose prognosis is good enough to make transplantation potentially worthwhile. Bumgardner and coworkers reported 13 patients with functioning grafts in 6 patients at the time of reporting (Bumgardner et al., 1990).

AGE

The age range within which renal transplantation is being performed continues to broaden, and the lower end extends down to the first year of life (see Chapter 39). Graft and patient survival rates can be as good for infants 6 to 12 months old as for older children (Samuel et al., 1986), but the younger infants may be treated better initially by dialysis. Transplantation has additional advantages over dialysis for the child in comparison with adults, such as better growth in the prepubertal period and the psychological benefit of freedom from dialysis.

At the other end of the age range, there is no well-defined or widely agreed on upper age limit. In the young adult transplant recipient, patient survival is better than with dialysis treatment. The younger patient has the potential to achieve a high level of fitness after a transplant, in contrast to the much lower potential with dialysis. In the older recipient, few studies have been reported comparing survival on dialysis and after transplantation. The single-center study by Fauchald et al. (1988) showed higher survival in older transplant recipients in comparison with patients selected for transplantation but remaining on the waiting list. Encouraging survival rates have been reported in other single-center series and in registry data. For example, 5-year patient survival rates of 68% and 80% were recorded in patients older than age 60 years in two single-center series (Cantarovich et al., 1994; Tesi et al., 1994), whereas the comparable figure from a European Renal Association (ERA) registry report was almost as good at 67% (Berthoux et al., 1996a). Graft loss often is lower in older compared with younger patients because of a reduced rate of irreversible acute rejection (Tesi et al., 1994). The most crucial factor in the selection of the older patient for transplantation is the degree of cardiovascular disease. If the detailed assessment that is described in the next section suggests absence of severe vascular disease or cardiac dysfunction, older patients can be selected for transplantation with the expectation of an acceptable survival rate. Although it would not be appropriate to set an upper age limit for transplantation, the older patient may have lower priority in the current context of demand for donor kidneys exceeding the supply. Consequently the number of patients older than age 70 receiving transplants will remain small. The ethical issues involved are considered further in Chapter 41.

MISCELLANEOUS FACTORS AFFECTING SELECTION

There is a variation between centers in the percentage of dialysis patients who are placed on transplant waiting lists. This variation influences the prospects of the individual patient being given the opportunity to have a transplant. In the United States, several studies have shown that gender and race may influence selection for transplantation, and in the study of Soucie et al. (1992), women and blacks were found to be less likely to be selected than men and whites. Efforts currently are being made in many countries to improve the equity of access to donor kidneys and to eliminate the inequalities of distribution that have been highlighted in studies such as that of Soucie et al. (1992). Shortage of organs has been shown to be a deterrent to selection for transplantation, particularly when combined with adverse medical factors in the individual patient. A questionnaire to transplant physicians and surgeons has suggested that around 25% more patients would be selected for transplantation if there were an adequate supply of donor organs (McMillan and Briggs, 1995).

General Assessment

In view of the high prevalence of comorbid disease in patients with chronic renal failure, careful assessment is important before the patient's name is placed on the transplant waiting list. Although the cardiovascular system is the most important to investigate, others include the gastrointestinal tract and a thorough search for infection also is necessary. When a urological abnormality is known or suspected, assessment of this aspect is essential. A good review of the assessment process has been prepared by the American Society of Transplant Physicians (Kasiske *et al.*, 1995).

Usually the assessment process begins with a medical appraisal and preliminary counseling by the dialysis physician. If this appraisal does not reveal any of the contraindications or major adverse factors discussed in the following section, the patient can be referred to the transplant center for more detailed assessment. Any further medical evaluation that is required probably can best be decided on jointly by the transplant physician and surgeon. They can provide counseling, although the transplant coordinator is well placed to fulfill this role. The assessment process should not cease when the patient is accepted as suitable for transplantation and his or her name goes onto the waiting list. With the current shortage of donor organs, several years or longer may pass before a suitable donor organ becomes available. By this time, the recipient could have developed significant comorbid disease, which might contraindicate transplantation or confer high risk in relation to the operation or the patient's subsequent course. Regular review is necessary of all patients on the transplant waiting list, and this should probably be done annually. Although it is distressing if a patient on the waiting list has to be told that he or she no longer is well enough to undergo a transplant, that end result is preferable to death resulting from preexisting comorbid disease after the transplant, which in the case of cadaveric transplantation has to be carried out as an emergency.

CARDIOVASCULAR SYSTEM

Despite the wide variation in the prevalence of cardiovascular disease in different populations and in countries around the world, it is the experience in virtually all renal centers that cardiovascular disease is the commonest cause of death before and after renal transplantation (see Chapter 30). Screening for cardiovascular disease is the most important component in the assessment of the renal transplant candidate. This screening is especially important in higher risk groups, such as older patients and patients with diabetes mellitus. One can divide the assessment into five aspects: coronary artery disease, left ventricular hypertrophy and function, blood pressure, cerebrovascular disease and peripheral vascular disease.

Coronary Artery Disease

One should look at coronary artery disease in two ways—first at the presence of risk factors for atheroma and second at the condition of the coronary arteries themselves. Virtually all renal failure patients have one or more risk

factors and how far one takes the search for coronary artery disease depends, in part, on the number and degree of the risk factors. The most important are shown in Table 4–4. The other main determinant that influences the extent of investigation is whether there is a history indicative of coronary artery disease, such as a past history of a myocardial infarction or current history of angina. All potential recipients should have an electrocardiogram (ECG); the presence of atrial fibrillation, a ventricular arrhythmia, Q waves, ST-T segment changes or left bundle-branch block are indications for further investigation. When age, the clinical history, the combination of risk factors or the ECG indicates the need for further investigation, the next question is which test should follow. There is a consensus that a noninvasive test should be used initially, but there is no unanimity as to which one. An exercise ECG is fairly reliable, provided that the patient can reach target heart rate levels, but with dialysis patients this often is not possible. Thallium imaging has been assessed in many studies, with conclusions varying from useful (Boudreau *et al.*, 1990) to ineffective (Marwick *et al.*, 1990). Although it is at an earlier stage of evaluation, dobutamine stress echocardiography also has shown promise (Bates *et al.*, 1996). I suggest that when further investigation is indicated, the patient should have an exercise ECG, and if the target heart rate cannot be reached, a dobutamine stress echocardiogram or thallium scan should be performed, the choice depending on the relative level of expertise in the local department of cardiology. Coronary angiography is indicated in the presence of an abnormality of one of these screening tests.

Left Ventricular Hypertrophy and Function

Echocardiography provides a useful assessment of left ventricular hypertrophy and left ventricular function in the potential transplant candidate. It is not necessary in every patient but should be widely used. If clinical and/or echocardiographic assessment indicate a major degree of cardiac failure, renal transplantation is indicated only if combined with cardiac transplantation. If the supply of organs permits, this approach will be used increasingly in the future in patients with combined cardiac and renal failure, although the necessary availability of organs is unlikely in the short-term. Left ventricular hypertrophy may begin to develop soon after the onset of chronic renal disease and is present in 74% of patients by the time of starting dialysis (Foley *et al.*, 1995). Most patients being assessed for renal transplantation have left ventricular hypertrophy, and it would constitute a contraindication to a transplant only if accompanied by the presence of established left ventricular failure. Nonetheless, it is an adverse factor, and its degree correlates with patient survival (McGregor *et al.*, 1998; Silberberg *et al.*, 1989). Measures that can lessen the degree of left ventricular hypertrophy

TABLE 4–4

MAIN RISK FACTORS FOR ATHEROMA

Age >40 years (men)
Age >50 years (women)
Diabetes mellitus
Smoking
Hypertension
Family history
Elevated serum triglyceride
Elevated serum cholesterol
Low HDL cholesterol
Elevated LDL cholesterol

HDL = high-density lipoprotein; LDL = low-density lipoprotein.

in the period before transplantation are discussed later in this chapter.

Blood Pressure

Most potential renal transplant recipients are hypertensive, the main determining factors being the type of primary renal disease and the degree of damage to the major arteries. Although several factors contribute to left ventricular hypertrophy, poor blood pressure control probably is the most important, and assessment of blood pressure control should form part of the patient evaluation before transplantation. It is appreciated that the ideal target blood pressure level should be 130/70 mm Hg, although such levels frequently are not achieved. Studies have shown that systolic blood pressure is at least as important as the diastolic level because it correlates better with left ventricular hypertrophy than does the diastolic blood pressure. Clinic values correlate with the degree of left ventricular hypertrophy much less well than 24-hour recordings (Tucker *et al.*, 1997).

Cerebrovascular and Peripheral Vascular Disease

A history of stroke or transient ischemic attacks is common in patients with renal failure because many of these patients possess risk factors. Transplantation is contraindicated in the presence of severe residual disability after a stroke but not by the history of a stroke *per se*. If there have been transient ischemic attacks in the past, duplex scanning of the carotid arteries is indicated as part of the pretransplant assessment.

Peripheral vascular disease of a degree sufficient to produce ischemic toes or feet or exercise pain in the legs is fairly common in renal failure patients, especially in patients with diabetes. It usually is a feature of fairly advanced vascular disease and is seen mainly in patients who are known also to have myocardial ischemia. Ischemic limbs *per se* pose no major problems for renal transplantation surgery, but because they often are markers for advanced vascular disease, their presence often indicates a high-risk patient who at the end of the assessment process may be considered unsuitable for transplantation. It is important to exclude significant disease in the iliac arteries, which may make implantation difficult. This assessment can be achieved by duplex scanning or arteriography of the aortoiliac system.

UROLOGICAL ASSESSMENT

A precise diagnosis of the cause of the renal failure should be made if possible in all patients being assessed for a renal transplant. There should be enquiry with regard to urinary symptoms; if the patient still passes urine, recent urine culture reports should be obtained. If the primary disease involves only the kidneys and the urine is sterile, further urological assessment is not required. In particular, routine voiding cystourethrography has a low yield of worthwhile information and is indicated only in the setting of suspected urological disorders (Glazier *et al.*, 1996; Shandera *et al.*, 1993).

Some common diseases that require pretransplant urological assessment are listed in Table 4–5. The most useful investigations are cystoscopy, urodynamic studies and voiding cystourethrography. Cystoscopy enables the bladder to be inspected, and, if necessary, a catheter can be introduced for retrograde pyelography. Next the voiding cystourethrogram shows the bladder size and efficiency of emptying and the presence of ureteric reflux. Urodynamic studies include a cystometrogram, which provides evidence of bladder func-

TABLE 4–5

CONDITIONS REQUIRING PRETRANSPLANT UROLOGICAL ASSESSMENT

Ureteropelvic stricture
Vesicoureteric reflux
Neurogenic bladder
Bladder neck obstruction
Posterior urethral valves

tion and sensation; urine flow measurements to assess the characteristics of micturition; electromyography of the urethral sphincter and urethral pressure profiles. After this assessment, a decision can be made as to whether or not urological surgery is required before transplantation (see Chapter 12).

MALIGNANT DISEASE EXCLUDING PRIMARY RENAL TUMORS

Penn (1993) has divided tumors occurring before transplantation into three groups—those with low, intermediate and high recurrence rates (Table 4–6). Penn recommends that no waiting time is necessary in the case of incidentally discovered renal carcinomas, *in situ* carcinomas of organs in which there is a small single focus of tumor (such as the prostate and uterus) and low-grade bladder cancers and basal cell cancers of the skin. At the other end of the scale are the tumors that have a high recurrence rate and in which a delay of several years (i.e., 3–5 years) is recommended, such as symptomatic renal tumors; colorectal, breast and prostate cancers and malignant melanoma. In between are most other tumors, and with these a 2-year interval is sufficient to avoid recurrence in most patients. The more frequently encountered ones include most bladder, testicular, uterine and thyroid cancers.

LIVER DISEASE

Hepatitis B remains a problem in some countries, although in others, for example, the United Kingdom, preventive measures have led to a low incidence of patients positive for hepatitis B. (See also Chapter 32 for an extensive discussion of liver disease.) Even in low-incidence countries, active immunization should be carried out, preferably before the start of hemodialysis, to protect the patient from cross-infection once on renal replacement therapy. Patients who are already hepatitis B positive are at risk of progressive liver disease after transplantation, and it is thought that this is due to a stimulatory effect of immunosuppressive therapy on virus replication. The adverse effect of transplantation on liver disease tends to occur beyond 2 years rather than in the early stages (Katkov and Rubin, 1991). These patients are

TABLE 4–6

RECURRENCE RATE OF PREEXISTING TUMORS

Low Recurrence Rate	Intermediate Recurrence Rate	High Recurrence Rate
Incidental renal	Breast	Symptomatic renal
Uterine cervix	Wilms' tumor	Nonmelanoma skin
Thyroid	Colon	Bladder
Testicular	Prostate	Melanoma
Lymphoma	Body of uterus	Sarcoma

high risk with regard to the possibility of developing hepatocellular carcinoma as well as cirrhosis. In a group of 26 hepatitis B surface antigen–positive patients receiving renal allografts, 42% developed cirrhosis and 54% died of liver failure during a mean follow-up period of 82 months (Rao et al., 1991). In view of the high mortality from liver failure, there must be serious doubt as to the suitability for transplantation of patients with established liver disease. In some cases, however, a good quality of life can follow for 10 years or more. I suggest that hepatitis B–positive recipients should be regarded as higher risk but suitable for renal transplantation, provided that liver histology shows a relatively mild degree of hepatic damage. Liver histology is much more useful in assessing suitability for transplantation than are clinical or biochemical criteria (Rao et al., 1991).

Hepatitis C is much commoner than hepatitis B and more often gives rise to the need to decide whether a patient is suitable for renal transplantation. In countries such as the United Kingdom where hepatitis B is uncommon, 5% of patients in dialysis units are hepatitis C positive, but their liver disease usually follows a more benign course after transplantation than does liver disease in patients with hepatitis B infection. Although hepatitis C–positive patients in some studies have had a higher mortality after renal transplantation than patients who are hepatitis C negative (Bouthot et al., 1997), in others no mortality difference has been found (Kliem et al., 1996). Hepatitis C–positive patients who receive a renal transplant have been reported to have a better survival than those who are hepatitis C positive and remain on dialysis (Knoll et al., 1997). Although most reports suggest that hepatitis C infection is not a major adverse factor for renal transplantation, the analysis of Pereira et al. (1995) is of concern because it showed a mortality of 41% after transplantation in hepatitis C–positive patients compared with 15% in those who were hepatitis C negative, with a high risk of death from infection in the former group. There were probably more patients in this study with a history of established liver disease pretransplant than in most other studies, however. Patients with hepatitis C infection usually can be advised to opt for a renal transplant with the exception of the few with well-established liver disease as judged by histological criteria.

There are causes of liver disease other than hepatitis B and C, although these are uncommon in the dialysis population. When such cases arise, the decision regarding suitability for renal transplantation should depend mainly on the degree of liver damage rather than its cause, and liver biopsy forms an important part of the assessment of these patients.

HLA TYPING AND ANTIBODY TESTING

In addition to determining the HLA antigens at the A, B, C, DR and DQ loci, the serum of the patient awaiting transplantation should be screened regularly for HLA antibodies. (See also Chapter 10 for a further discussion of HLA matching and crossmatching.) Antibodies often appear transiently after events such as blood transfusion and rejection of a previous kidney transplant, and testing for HLA antibodies after such events is recommended.

Patients who become highly sensitized to HLA antigens usually present a problem in the finding of a crossmatch-negative donor kidney. National donor organ exchange programs increase the prospects of obtaining such a kidney considerably, however, although sometimes after a long wait; being highly sensitized should never be considered as a contraindication to placement on the transplant waiting list. Once a suitable kidney is found, graft survival is only slightly less or the same as in the nonsensitized patient as a result of

the availability of highly effective immunosuppressive therapy, more sensitive crossmatching and more accurate HLA typing.

One can attempt to remove HLA antibodies before transplantation, and good graft survival in the short-term has been reported using extracorporeal immunoadsorption by means of staphylococcal protein A columns (Palmer et al., 1989). The experience of Hiesse et al. (1992) has been less encouraging, however, and this approach has been largely abandoned. It is hoped that the present low rate of graft loss from acute rejection, the abandonment of deliberate blood transfusion and the widespread use of erythropoietin in dialysis patients with a consequent reduction in transfusion requirements will lead to fewer highly sensitized patients in the future.

PREVIOUS TRANSPLANT

Loss of a renal allograft from rejection often used to be followed by a lower survival rate for a subsequent graft. More recent analyses have shown, however, that although this applies if the first graft failed within 3 months (Mahoney et al., 1996), overall, survival rates of second grafts are now within a few percentage points of those for first grafts (Cho and Cecka, 1994). Previous graft loss from rejection would become a contraindication to a further transplant only in the occasional patient in whom it had occurred two or three times and each time within months of the transplant.

When early irreversible rejection leads to graft failure or when infection occurs in or around the graft, removal of the kidney is indicated. It is much less certain whether late graft failure needs to be followed by graft nephrectomy in the absence of symptoms. It could be argued on theoretical grounds that removal of a source of foreign antigen might be beneficial in the prevention of further sensitization, but in practice there is no evidence of benefit. In contrast, Douzdjian and colleagues, in a retrospective study, found higher levels of preformed cytotoxic antibody in patients whose failed primary grafts had been removed (Douzdjian et al., 1996). Also it was found in this study that transplant nephrectomy did not influence the early graft function rate, the frequency of acute rejection or graft survival after retransplantation. In a proportion of patients after graft failure and withdrawal of immunosuppression, subsequent acute rejection with discomfort over the graft or less frequently a swollen tender kidney leads to the need for nephrectomy. In the absence of this complication, routine transplant nephrectomy no longer is considered to be necessary.

INFECTION

Infection should be looked for in such sites as the urinary and respiratory tracts. Frequently or persistently positive urine cultures indicate the need for full urological evaluation. If such evaluation reveals no anatomical abnormality, transplantation can proceed with careful observation of urine samples thereafter and appropriate antibiotic therapy. Chronic respiratory infection, for example, in the form of bronchiectasis, is an adverse factor. In such instances, the decision for or against renal transplantation has to be made on an individual patient basis, but there is no doubt that even patients with fairly quiescent disease are at much higher than average risk of a life-threatening exacerbation of infection as a result of immunosuppression. Now it often is assumed that bacterial infection can almost always be treated successfully with antibiotic therapy, but in the immunosuppressed patient this is not true. Dental caries should be treated to reduce the risk of dental abscess after transplantation.

Active tuberculosis should be excluded in patients with a history of the disease or radiological evidence of a previous silent primary infection. In this context, the skin reaction to tuberculin often gives false-negative results in dialysis patients owing to suppression of the immune response by the uremia. In patients with pulmonary tuberculosis, culture of the sputum or laryngeal swabs also may yield negative results, and sometimes reliance has to be placed mainly on serial chest radiographs.

In patients on continuous ambulatory peritoneal dialysis, catheter exit site infection should, if possible, be eradicated, as should infection around synthetic vascular access grafts in those on hemodialysis. Such eradication may require removal of the catheter or graft.

The serum should be tested for antibody to cytomegalovirus. The absence of previous infection with this virus exposes the patient to the risk of a primary infection should a kidney be transplanted from a cytomegalovirus-positive donor, and this is associated with significant morbidity and mortality and sometimes renal allograft dysfunction. The development of an effective vaccine is a possible solution for the future, but no vaccine is yet available. At present, one solution is to use only kidneys from cytomegalovirus-negative donors for seronegative recipients. This approach adds further difficulty to the already complicated problem of trying to match up the donor and recipient from the viewpoint of HLA and other relevant factors, however. An alternative way of dealing with the cytomegalovirus-positive donor/cytomegalovirus-negative recipient combination is to give prophylactic antiviral therapy after the transplant; this approach often prevents cytomegalovirus-related disease. As far as recipient evaluation is concerned, the important point is to know the patient's cytomegalovirus status before the transplant. A similar mismatch for Epstein-Barr virus as for cytomegalovirus predisposes the recipient to posttransplant lymphoproliferative disorder, and it is worth establishing the recipient's Epstein-Barr virus status before the transplant.

Recipients who are seronegative for the varicella-zoster virus are at risk of a fulminant form of varicella if exposed to the virus posttransplant. It is worth identifying these patients before the transplant by testing for IgG antibody to varicella in those who do not give a clear history of chickenpox. In patients lacking IgG antibody, immunization against varicella should be carried out before transplantation. Should this immunization be omitted and the seronegative patient be exposed to the varicella virus after transplantation, specific varicella immunoglobulin should always be given in view of the high risk of fulminating varicella infection.

All potential recipients should be tested for HIV infection. Although one third of HIV carriers may experience prolonged survival after renal transplantation (Rubin, 1993), the consensus view is that until more effective therapy for HIV infection is available, these patients should not be considered as candidates for renal transplantation.

BONE DISEASE

The main types of renal osteodystrophy that are encountered in dialysis patients are secondary hyperparathyroidism, osteomalacia or its equivalent, rickets, in children and osteoporosis. Transplantation has a beneficial effect on osteodystrophy by increasing 1,25-dihydroxycholecalciferol synthesis and lowering serum phosphorus levels. Despite this effect, three types of bone disease may follow transplantation that can be ameliorated by appropriate action before the transplant: persistent hyperparathyroidism with hypercalcemia, osteoporosis and bone necrosis. The last of these has become uncommon since the introduction of low-dose steroid regi-

mens (Davidson *et al.*, 1985). With regard to hyperparathyroidism, this should be treated during the dialysis phase with 1,25-dihydroxycholecalciferol or 1α-hydroxycholecalciferol and a phosphorus-binding agent, the aim of the latter being to avoid serum phosphorus levels greater than 1.5 mmol/L. The preferred group of binding agents are those containing calcium, such as calcium carbonate or acetate. Parathyroidectomy is indicated in the dialysis patient in the presence of severe hyperparathyroidism unresponsive to medical therapy. The operation can consist of total or subtotal parathyroidectomy. With the latter procedure, a small portion of one gland can be left in the neck or tissue implanted in a subfascial position in the forearm or thigh. Although this procedure often avoids the need for permanent vitamin D replacement, it is likely to be followed by a recurrence of hyperparathyroidism should the patient not receive a renal transplant. Consequently, there has been a shift toward the use of total parathyroidectomy unless transplantation is likely to take place within 1 year.

Osteoporosis usually is not a clinically apparent problem in dialysis patients because its effects are overshadowed by hyperparathyroidism and/or osteomalacia. There is limited scope for treatment during the dialysis phase because bisphosphonates are not advised in renal failure, but hormone replacement therapy may be worthwhile in women of the appropriate age group.

GASTROINTESTINAL DISEASE

Since the introduction of H_2-receptor antagonists together with the use of low-dose steroids, the high frequency of peptic ulcer disease that was encountered previously after renal transplantation has fallen markedly. If dyspepsia is present in the dialysis patient, it should be investigated and followed by appropriate treatment, and enquiry regarding dyspeptic symptoms always should be made at the time of assessment for renal transplantation. If symptoms are present, endoscopy should be carried out and the *Helicobacter pylori* status of the patient established. Before placement on the transplant waiting list, *H. pylori* eradication and/or treatment with an H_2-receptor antagonist or proton-pump inhibitor should be initiated when the endoscopy findings indicate the need. A history of peptic ulcer that has not responded fully to treatment may be an indication for steroid-free immunosuppression after transplantation.

Cholelithiasis is common in renal failure (Badalamenti *et al.*, 1994). Ultrasound examination always should be performed in the presence of symptoms that could indicate the presence of gallstones. Vigilance regarding the possibility of cholelithiasis is important in view of the high risk associated with cholecystitis and pancreatitis in the immunosuppressed patient. A past history of pancreatitis is not a contraindication to transplantation, but it is an important risk factor, and in this setting careful pretransplant assessment is important together with consideration of steroid-free immunosuppression.

With the increase in older transplant recipients, diverticulitis is encountered more commonly. Awareness of the presence of diverticulosis is helpful in the evaluation of abdominal pain in the posttransplant patient. This awareness is important in view of the paucity of abdominal signs that one often finds despite major pathology when the immunosuppressed patient develops an acute abdomen. This comment also applies to other abdominal complications.

PSYCHOSOCIAL ASPECTS

Psychosocial problems are among the most difficult to evaluate, in part because of the lack of objective criteria (see

Chapter 40). Dependence on drugs or alcohol that has not responded to treatment almost always is considered a contraindication to transplantation. Major psychotic illness also is considered a contraindication, whereas milder psychotic illness is an adverse factor but not a contraindication. Noncompliance with treatment, in particular with immunosuppressive therapy, is relatively common after renal transplantation, especially in teenagers and young adults; in a comprehensive review, Colón and associates quote noncompliance rates of 5 to 43% (Colón et al., 1991). Graft loss is a common sequela, and the question of a second transplant requires careful consideration if noncompliance was an important factor in the loss of a first graft. In this context, the report of Troppmann et al. (1995) offers some encouragement in that no evidence of noncompliance after a second transplant was found among 14 patients whose first grafts were lost after noncompliance. The number of patients in this study is small, however. A reasonable policy would be to offer a second transplant to a patient whose first graft was lost after noncompliance, provided that there were no factors that would make further noncompliance especially likely. A third transplant in a persistently noncompliant patient often would not be justified.

MISCELLANEOUS FACTORS

Chronic obstructive pulmonary disease is an adverse factor and should be evaluated thoroughly. Obesity, which is particularly a problem in some patients on continuous ambulatory peritoneal dialysis, is associated with an increased complication rate, and this is reflected in various ways in the transplant recipient. Modlin and colleagues reported a 5-year survival rate of 67% in obese patients, which was significantly lower than the figure of 89% in their nonobese group, with cardiac disease being the main cause of death in the obese patients compared with infection in the nonobese (Modlin et al., 1997). The obese group also had a much higher incidence of posttransplant diabetes mellitus. Other reported adverse effects of obesity are a higher frequency of delayed graft function, wound complications and immunological graft loss (Pirsch et al., 1995). Moderate obesity (body mass index >30) is an adverse factor for renal transplantation, and gross obesity (body mass index >35) is a contraindication.

It is not surprising that smokers have poorer survival than nonsmokers after transplantation, and Cosio and associates have shown cigarette smoking to have an adverse effect of similar degree to the presence of diabetes mellitus (Cosio et al., 1999). Smokers should be strongly encouraged to stop when being counseled at the time of evaluation for renal transplantation.

CONTRAINDICATIONS

Some of the circumstances in which renal transplantation carries a higher than average risk have been discussed. In addition, there are a group of comorbid illnesses or other factors that render transplantation inadvisable, and they are listed in Table 4–7.

Preparation for Transplantation
DIALYSIS

Most patients are treated by hemodialysis before transplantation, although in some countries a substantial minority receive continuous ambulatory peritoneal dialysis. There is no evidence that the type of dialysis has any influence on the outcome of the transplant (Evangelista et al., 1985). While

TABLE 4–7
CONTRAINDICATIONS TO TRANSPLANTATION

Disseminated malignancy
Refractory cardiac failure
Chronic respiratory failure
Advanced hepatic disease
Extensive vascular disease: coronary, cerebral or peripheral
Severe congenital urinary tract abnormality, e.g., exstrophy of the bladder
Chronic infection, unresponsiveness to treatment
Human immunodeficiency virus infection
Persistent coagulation disorder
Severe mental retardation
Psychosocial problems: severe psychosis, alcoholism or drug addiction

awaiting a cadaver transplant, a high percentage of patients require a period of dialysis, and in the past some analyses suggested that graft survival was superior in those on dialysis for longer periods (Brynger et al., 1985). Several more recent studies, including that of Katz et al. (1991), have failed to show any advantage to graft outcome from previous dialysis. The patient in advanced renal failure may be debilitated and have other risk factors for surgery, such as poor blood pressure and biochemical control. In this setting, a limited period of dialysis may fulfill a useful role in improving well-being and control of the uremia before transplantation. An extension of the period of dialysis beyond a few weeks is useful only as a holding measure until a suitable kidney becomes available.

Preemptive renal transplantation (i.e., without a previous period of dialysis) accounts for only a small percentage of transplants (approximately 7% in an ERA Registry analysis; Berthoux et al., 1996b). There is a wide variation among countries, however, and this approach is used more widely in children and in the setting of live donors. Preemptive transplantation carries no disadvantage, provided that the state of health of the potential recipient is good enough in the absence of a period of dialysis to allow transplantation without undue risk. On the contrary, it has the benefits of reduced cost and avoidance of the inconvenience of dialysis and the risk of its complications (Vanrenterghem and Verberckmoes, 1998). A higher incidence of noncompliance has been presented as an argument against preemptive transplantation (Katz et al., 1991), but a more recent study showed no evidence of this (Roake et al., 1996). There are good reasons for encouraging preemptive transplantation when possible.

BLOOD TRANSFUSION

The report by Opelz et al. (1973) that nontransfused patients had poorer graft survival led to a decade of deliberate transfusion protocols. During the 1980s, the transfusion effect became less apparent, however, and consequently deliberate transfusion disappeared from the regimens of most transplant units. The subsequent prospective study reported by Opelz and coworkers is of interest in that it showed better graft survival in deliberately transfused patients, but this report is not likely to lead to a resurgence of interest in deliberate blood transfusion (Opelz et al., 1997). Another relevant fact is that with the advent of erythropoietin there is now much less need to transfuse to maintain an adequate hemoglobin level. No evidence exists that the higher hemoglobin value of the erythropoietin-treated transplant recipient has any major disadvantage to graft outcome (Linde et al.,

1992). The use of erythropoietin (Vasquez and Pollak, 1996) and a higher hematocrit at the time of transplantation (Schmidt et al., 1993) both have been reported to be associated with higher frequencies of delayed graft function, however. Donor-specific transfusion for live donor transplantation persisted in some units beyond the demise of third-party transfusion in cadaver transplantation, but it too is rarely practiced now.

OPERATIONS BEFORE TRANSPLANTATION

Bilateral Nephrectomy

In the early days of transplantation, bilateral nephrectomy was performed routinely in many centers (Russell and Winn, 1970). There has been a steady decline in the frequency of this procedure, and currently it is seldom needed. Hypertension used to be the commonest indication, but drug therapy combined with dialysis usually can control blood pressure adequately. Occasionally the development of severe hypertension after transplantation leads to a decision to perform bilateral nephrectomy, but the blood pressure response to this procedure often is disappointing (Midtvedt et al., 1996).

Polycystic kidneys often shrink considerably in size after successful transplantation. Removal of such kidneys before transplantation occasionally is required if one or both are of massive size or if they are the site of persistent infection. If size is the only indication, it usually is sufficient to remove only one kidney to leave space for the allograft. There is no evidence that routine removal of polycystic kidneys has any beneficial effect on the outcome of the transplant (Tzardis et al., 1990).

Other indications for nephrectomy include persistent infection, for example, as the result of calculi, hydronephrosis or other urological disease. If accompanied by ureteric reflux and hydroureter, the ureter should be removed as well. Nephrectomy is indicated for bilateral renal tumors. Sanfilippo and coworkers reported reduced graft loss from rejection in patients with bilateral nephrectomy, but this report has not been confirmed, and the evidence is not strong enough to constitute an indication for nephrectomy (Sanfilippo et al., 1984). In the few patients who do require bilateral nephrectomy, the subsequent increase in blood transfusion requirements, which used to be an important disadvantage, is no longer an issue in view of the availability of erythropoietin.

With regard to surgical technique, bilateral posterior or loin incisions have a lower morbidity and mortality rate than an anterior approach and generally are preferred (Novick et al., 1980). In this series, the mortality was zero. An anterior transperitoneal approach usually is required for the removal of large polycystic kidneys. A laparoscopic technique also is an option (Doublet et al., 1997), whereas an alternative to surgery is embolization of the kidneys; this technique has been used particularly in the setting of poorly controlled hypertension (Thompson et al., 1984).

Urological Operations

An anatomically abnormal lower urinary tract should not be a deterrent to renal transplantation. Initially, cystoscopy and urodynamic studies can establish the degree of scarring and trabeculation of the bladder and its capacity and ability to empty. Thereafter the decision can be made as to whether corrective or other surgery is required before the transplant. When adequate bladder function is associated with an obstructive lesion, such as posterior urethral valves or prostatic hypertrophy, correction of the obstruction can be followed by implantation of the transplant ureter into the patient's own bladder. Even in the absence of preexisting bladder disorders, the capacity of some bladders and their ability to void diminish after initiation of dialysis. This change sometimes may be important because reduced graft survival has been found in association with bladders that have a capacity of less than 100 ml (Kashi et al., 1994). If the bladder capacity is inadequate, it can be increased before the transplant by ileocecocystoplasty.

In the presence of a neurogenic bladder with an inability to void, implantation of the transplant ureter into the bladder is the preferred procedure with self-catheterization several times a day after the transplant. In patients who already have a urinary diversion into a conduit, the bladder still should be assessed because it may be suitable with or without cystoplasty despite trabeculation, scarring or prolonged defunctionalization (Stephenson et al., 1984).

Previously, implantation of the transplant ureter into an established or newly created ileal conduit probably was performed more often than necessary. It is only in a small proportion of patients that the bladder could not be used or had to be removed in the past. If required, the conduit should be created before transplantation. A variety of techniques have been suggested, using ileum or sigmoid colon (see Chapter 12). In most cases, preparatory investigation and, if necessary, surgery enable use to be made of the patient's bladder, although sometimes with the need for self-catheterization after the transplant, and an intestinal conduit needs to be considered only for a relatively small proportion of patients. Regardless of whether the patient's own bladder or a conduit is used, the outcome after transplantation in patients with abnormal lower urinary tracts can be as good as in patients with healthy bladders (Cairns et al., 1991; Griffin et al., 1994).

Vesicoureteral reflux is the commonest lower urinary tract abnormality encountered in potential transplant recipients, constituting 47% of such abnormalities in the series of Cairns et al. (1991). Although the presence of such reflux seldom is considered sufficient indication for nephroureterectomy, it does predispose the patient to posttransplant bacteriuria and infection in the native kidneys. In this setting, the endoscopic injection of polytetrafluoroethylene (Teflon) into the submucosa at the ureteral orifice has been found to correct reflux in 65% of cases (Sironvalle et al., 1992). Whether this technique will prove to be of benefit in the long-term still has to be determined.

Splenectomy

Although prospective trials of pretransplant splenectomy in the past showed improved allograft survival without an increased mortality rate (Mozes et al., 1983; Stuart et al., 1980), other retrospective analyses have reported a higher posttransplant mortality rate (Rai et al., 1977; Schofer et al., 1986). The reports showing benefit were from the precyclosporine era, and in the current setting of effective immunosuppressive therapy there is no indication for splenectomy as a preparation for transplantation.

PATIENT COUNSELING

Although transplantation has the potential to restore good health, this benefit does not apply to all recipients. In particular, those with significant comorbid illness may not experience any benefit to their well-being, although they are released from the tedium of dialysis. The potential exists for complications and death as a result of the operation and/or the immunosuppression. Some of the side effects of immunosuppressive drugs can be distressing, such as the hirsutism of cyclosporine and the obesity that is, in part, due to steroids. The patient should know what to expect with regard to the operation and postoperative period, for example, the possibility of delayed graft function and readmission for diagnosis and treatment of rejection episodes. Counseling is required to cover all these points. This counseling can be accomplished satisfactorily in one or more sessions involving the transplant surgeon and/or physician and the transplant coordinator or senior nurse. Such sessions are particularly important for patients who are dialyzed in renal units other than the one in which they will receive the transplant. These sessions provide the opportunity not only for the patient to meet the transplant team and to receive counseling, but also for the transplant team to ensure that the patient is a suitable candidate from medical and other points of view.

PREOPERATIVE PREPARATION

Recipient of a Cadaver Kidney

A typical preoperative workup includes a biochemical profile, complete blood count, coagulation screen, blood transfusion crossmatch, chest radiograph and ECG. In the patient with known or suspected cardiac dysfunction, an echocardiogram is useful, although in the setting of established cardiovascular disease, detailed assessment should have preceded placement on the transplant waiting list. With hemodialysis patients, preoperative dialysis may be required to reduce the serum potassium to a safe level (i.e., <5.5 mmol/L). In the absence of hyperkalemia, lowering the blood urea or serum creatinine level seldom is necessary. Avoidance of fluid depletion is important to ensure against occult oligemia and consequent suboptimal perfusion of the transplanted kidney after completion of the vascular anastomoses. Oligemia usually can be avoided by adjustment of the body weight during any preoperative dialysis to a level 1 to 2 kg above the patient's estimated dry body weight. The central venous pressure should be measured at the beginning of the operation and fluid infused to bring the central venous pressure up to within the range of 5 to 15 cm H_2O. Management of the patient on continuous ambulatory peritoneal dialysis is easier because fluid balance usually is more stable and hyperkalemia is less common.

Infection in particular in the chest or urinary tract or at vessel access or peritoneal catheter exit sites should be looked for and an antibiotic given if there is evidence of infection. In the absence of infection, prophylactic antibiotic therapy is not essential, although in some transplant centers broad-spectrum antibiotic therapy is given with the premedication.

There is no evidence that beginning immunosuppressive therapy before surgery has any benefit. Theoretical grounds exist for suggesting that preoperative cyclosporine might impair perfusion of the newly vascularized transplant and increase the likelihood of delayed renal function. A reasonable policy is to give intravenous prednisolone during the operation followed by the first dose of the remaining immunosuppressive therapy during the subsequent 24 hours.

Recipient of Live Donor Kidney

Being an elective procedure, live donor transplantation has the advantage of allowing more thorough preparation. In addition to the measures just discussed, the risk of respiratory infection can be lessened by preoperative avoidance of smoking and by physiotherapy. Although immunosuppression sometimes is started a few days before the operation, this is not of proven value. Finally, there is the opportunity to carry out a final crossmatch with donor lymphocytes at least a few days before the transplant, avoiding the distress

of an unexpected positive crossmatch and cancellation of the procedure at the last minute.

REFERENCES

Andresdottir, M. B., Assmann, K. J. M., Hoitsma, A. J., Koene, R. A. P. and Wetzels, J. F. M. (1999). Renal transplantation in patients with dense deposit disease: morphological characteristics of recurrent disease and clinical outcome. *Nephrol. Dial. Transplant.* **14**, 1723.

Artero, M., Biavia, C., Amend, W., Tomlanovich, S. and Vincenti, F. (1992). Recurrent focal glomerulosclerosis: natural history and response to therapy. *Am. J. Med.* **92**, 375.

Aunsholt, N. A. and Ahlbom, G. (1989). Recurrence of Wegener's granulomatosis after kidney transplantation involving the kidney graft. *Clin. Transplant.* **3**, 159.

Badalamenti, S., De Fazio, C., Castelnovo, C., *et al.* (1994). High prevalence of silent gallstone disease in dialysis patients. *Nephron* **66**, 225.

Balligand, J.-L., Pirson, Y. and Squifflet, J.-P. (1990). Outcome of patients with tuberous sclerosis after renal transplantation. *Transplantation* **49**, 515.

Bates, J. R., Sawada, S. G., Segar, D. S., *et al.* (1996). Evaluation using dobutamine stress echocardiography in patients with insulin dependent diabetes mellitus before kidney and/or pancreas transplantation. *Am. J. Cardiol.* **77**, 175.

Berger, J. (1988). Recurrence of IgA nephropathy in renal allografts. *Am. J. Kidney Dis.* **12**, 371.

Berthoux, F. C., Jones, E. H. P., Mehls, O. and Valderrabano, F. (1996a). Transplantation report 1: renal transplantation in recipients aged 60 years or older at time of grafting. *Nephrol. Dial. Transplant.* **11(Suppl. 1)**, 37.

Berthoux, F., Jones, E. H. P., Mehls, O. and Valderrabano, F. (1996b). Transplantation report 2: pre-emptive renal transplantation in adults aged over 15 years. *Nephrol. Dial. Transplant.* **11(Suppl. 1)**, 41.

Boudreau, R. J., Strony, J. T., du Cret, R. P., et al. (1990). Perfusion thallium imaging of Type I diabetes patients with end-stage renal disease: comparison of oral and intravenous dipyridamole administration. *Radiology* **175**, 103.

Bouhot, B. E., Murthy, B. V. R., Schmid, H., Levey, A. S. and Pereira, B. J. G. (1997). Long-term follow-up of hepatitis C virus infection among organ transplanted recipients: implications for policies on organ procurement. *Transplantation* **63**, 849.

Briggs, J. D. and Jones, E. (1999a). Recurrence of glomerulonephritis following renal transplantation. *Nephrol. Dial. Transplant.* **14**, 564.

Briggs, J. D. and Jones, E. (1999b). Renal transplantation for uncommon diseases. *Nephrol. Dial. Transplant.* **14**, 570.

Brynger, H., Brunner, F. P., Challah, S., et al. (1985). Influence of pretransplant dialysis on survival of first cadaveric renal transplants. *Transplant. Proc.* **17**, 2798.

Bumgardner, G. L., Matas, A. J., Payne, W. D., et al. (1990). Renal transplantation in patients with paraproteinaemias. *Clin. Transplant.* **4**, 399.

Cairns, H. S., Leaker, B., Woodhouse, C. R. J., et al. (1991). Renal transplantation into abnormal lower urinary tract. *Lancet* **338**, 1376.

Cameron, J. S. (1982). Glomerulonephritis in renal transplants. *Transplantation* **34**, 237.

Cameron, J. S. (1983). Effect of recipient's disease on the results of transplantation (other than diabetes mellitus). *Kidney Int.* **23(Suppl. 14)**, 24.

Cantarovich, D., Baatard, R. and Baranger, T. (1994). Cadaveric renal transplantation after 60 years of age: a single centre experience. *Transplant. Int.* **7**, 33.

Cho, Y. W. and Cecka, J. M. (1994). Cadaver-donor renal retransplants. *In Clinical Transplants 1993*, (P. I. Terasaki and J. M. Cecka, eds.), p. 469, UCLA Tissue Typing Laboratory, Los Angeles.

Clarkson, A. R., Elias, T. J., Faull, R. J. and Bannister, K. M. (1999). Immunoglobulin A nephropathy and renal transplantation. *Transplant. Rev.* **13**, 174.

Colón, E. A., Popkin, M. K., Matas, A. J. and Callies, A. L. (1991). Overview of noncompliance in renal transplantation. *Transplant. Rev.* **5**, 175.

Cosio, F. G., Falkenhain, M. F., Pesavento, T. E., *et al.* (1999). Patient survival after renal transplantation II: the impact of smoking. *Clin. Transplant.* **13**, 336.

Cosyns, J. P., Couchoud, C., Pouteil-Noble, C., Squifflet, J. P. and Pirson, Y. (1998). Recurrence of membranous nephropathy after renal transplantation: probability, outcome and risk factors. *Clin. Nephrol.* **50**, 144.

Davidson, J. K., Tskaris, D., Briggs, J. D. and Junor, B. J. R. (1985). Osteonecrosis and fractures following renal transplantation. *Clin. Radiol.* **36**, 27.

Disney, A. P. (1981). *Fourth report of the Australian and New Zealand Dialysis and Transplant Registry,* p. 21, Australian Kidney Foundation, Adelaide.

Doublet, J. D., Peraldi, M. N., Monsaint, H., *et al.* (1997). Retroperitoneal laparoscopic nephrectomy of native kidneys in renal transplant recipients. *Transplantation* **64**, 89.

Douzdjian, V., Rice, J. C., Carson, R. W., Gugliuzza, K. K. and Fish, J. C. (1996). Renal retransplants: effect of primary allograft nephrectomy on early function, acute rejection and outcome. *Clin. Transplant.* **10**, 203.

Ducloux, D., Rebibou, J.-M., Semhoun-Ducloux, S., *et al.* (1998). Recurrence of hemolytic uremic syndrome in renal transplant recipients. *Transplantation* **65**, 1405.

Ehrich, J. H. H., Brodehl, J., Byrd, D. J., *et al.* (1991). Renal transplantation in 22 children with nephropathic cystinosis. *Pediatr. Nephrol.* **5**, 708.

Ekberg, H. and Christensson, A. (1996). Similar treatment success rate after renal transplantation in diabetic and nondiabetic patients due to improved short- and long-term diabetic patient survival. *Transplant. Int.* **9**, 557.

Evangelista, J. B., Bennett-Jones, D., Cameron, J. S., *et al.* (1985). Renal transplantation in patients treated with haemodialysis and short term and long term continuous ambulatory peritoneal dialysis. *B. M. J.* **291**, 1004.

Fauchald, P., Albrechtsen, D., Leivestad, T., *et al.* (1988). Renal replacement therapy in elderly patients. *Transplant. Int.* **1**, 131.

Foley, R. N., Parfrey, P. S., Harnett, J. D., *et al.* (1995). Clinical and echocardiographic disease in patients starting end-stage renal disease therapy. *Kidney Int.* **47**, 186.

Glazier, D. B., Whang, M. I. S., Geffner, S. R., *et al.* (1996). Evaluation of voiding cystourethrography prior to renal transplantation. *Transplantation* **62**, 1762.

Gobel, J., Olbricht, C. J., Offner, G., *et al.* (1992). Kidney transplantation in Alport's syndrome: long-term outcome and allograft anti-GBM nephritis. *Clin. Nephrol.* **38**, 299.

Goss, J. A., Cole, B. R., Jendrisak, M. D., *et al.* (1991). Renal transplantation for systemic lupus erythematosus and recurrent lupus nephritis. *Transplantation* **52**, 805.

Griffin, P. J. A., Stephenson, T. P., Brough, S. and Salaman, J. R. (1994). Transplanting patients with abnormal lower urinary tracts. *Transplant. Int.* **7**, 288.

Gruessner, A. C. and Sutherland, D. E. R. (1999). Analysis of US and non-US pancreas transplants as reported to the International Pancreas Transplant Registry and to the United Network for Organ Sharing. *In Clinical Transplants 1998*, (J. M. Cecka and P. I. Terasaki, eds.), p. 53, UCLA Tissue Typing Laboratory, Los Angeles.

Hadimeri, H., Nordén, G., Friman, S. and Nyberg, G. (1997). Autosomal dominant polycystic kidney disease in a kidney transplant population. *Nephrol. Dial. Transplant.* **12**, 1431.

Hariharan, S., Smith, R. D., Viero, R. and First, M. R. (1996). Diabetic nephropathy after renal transplantation. *Transplantation* **62**, 632.

Hasegawa, A., Kawamura, T. and Ito, H. (1987). Fate of renal grafts with recurrent Henoch-Schönlein nephritis in children. *Transplant. Proc.* **21**, 2130.

Heering, P., Hetzel, R., Grabensee, B. and Opelz, G. (1998). Renal transplantation in secondary systemic amyloidosis. *Clin. Transplant.* **12**, 159.

Hiesse, C., Kriaa, F., Rousseau, P., *et al.* (1992). Immunoadsorption of anti-HLA antibodies for highly sensitized patients awaiting renal transplantation. *Nephrol. Dial. Transplant.* **7**, 944.

Kashi, S. H., Wynne, K. S., Sadek, S. A. and Lodge, J. P. A. (1994). An evaluation of vesical urodynamics before renal transplantation and its effect on renal allograft function and survival. *Transplantation* **57**, 1455.

Kasiske, B. L., Ramos, E. L. and Gaston, R. S. (1995). The evaluation of renal transplant candidates: clinical practice guidelines. *J. Am. Soc. Nephrol.* **6**, 1.

Katkov, W. N. and Rubin, R. H. (1991). Liver disease in the transplant recipient: etiology, clinical impact, and clinical management. *Transplant. Rev.* **5**, 200.

Katz, S. M., Kerman, R. H., Golden, D., *et al.* (1991). Preemptive transplantation—an analysis of benefits and hazards in 85 cases. *Transplantation* **51**, 351.

Kliem, V., Van Den Hoff, U. and Brunkhorst, R. (1996). The long-term course of hepatitis C after kidney transplantation. *Transplantation* **62**, 1417.

Knoll, G. A., Tankersley, M. R., Lee, J. Y., Julian, B. A. and Curtis, J. J. (1997). The impact of renal transplantation on survival in hepatitis C-positive end-stage renal disease patients. *Am. J. Kidney Dis.* **29**, 608.

Kotanko, P., Pusey, C. D. and Levy, J. B. (1997). Recurrent glomerulonephritis following renal transplantation. *Transplantation* **63**, 1045.

Kuross, S., Davin, T. and Kjellstrand, C. M. (1981). Wegener's granulomatosis with severe renal failure: clinical course and results of dialysis and transplantation. *Clin. Nephrol.* **16**, 172.

Laiwah, A. C. Y., Mactier, R., McColl, K. E. L., Moore, M. R. and Goldberg, A. (1983). Early onset chronic renal failure as a complication of acute intermittent porphyria. *Q. J. M.* **52**, 92.

Langlois, R. P., O'Regan, S., Pelletier, M. and Robitaille, P. (1981). Kidney transplantation in uremic children with cystinosis. *Nephron* **28**, 273.

Linde, T., Wahlberg, J., Wikström, B. and Danielson, B. G. (1992). Outcome of renal transplantation in patients treated with erythropoietin. *Clin. Nephrol.* **37**, 260.

Lockwood, C. M. (1986). New advances in understanding the treatment of glomerulonephritis. *Clin. Nephrol.* **26(Suppl. 1)**, 76.

MacDougall, M. L., Welling, L. W. and Wiegmann, T. B. (1987). Renal adenocarcinoma and acquired cystic disease in chronic haemodialysis patients. *Am. J. Kidney Dis.* **9**, 166.

Mahoney, R. J., Norman, D. J., Colombe, B. W., Garavoy, M. R. and Leeber, D. A. (1996). Identification of high- and low-risk second kidney grafts. *Transplantation* **61**, 1349.

Maizel, S. E., Simmons, R. L., Kjellstrand, C. and Fryd, D. S. (1981). Ten-year experience in renal transplantation for Fabry's disease. *Transplant. Proc.* **13**, 57.

Mallofré, C., Almirall, J. and Campistol, J. M. (1992). Acquired renal cystic disease in HD: a study of 82 nephrectomies in young patients. *Clin. Nephrol.* **37**, 297.

Maryniak, R. K., Mendoza, N., Clyne, D., *et al.* (1985). Recurrence of diabetic nodular glomerulosclerosis in a renal transplant. *Transplantation* **39**, 35.

Marwick, T. H., Steinmuller, D. R., Underwood, D. A., *et al.* (1990). Ineffectiveness of SPECT thallium imaging as a screening technique for coronary artery disease in patients with end-stage renal failure. *Transplantation* **49**, 100.

Mathew, T. H. (1991). Recurrent disease after renal transplantation. *Transplant. Rev.* **5**, 31.

McGregor, E., Jardine, A. G., Murray, L. S., *et al.* (1998). Preoperative echocardiographic abnormalities and adverse outcome following renal transplantation. *Nephrol. Dial. Transplant.* **13**, 1499.

McMillan, M. A. and Briggs, J. D. (1995) Survey of patient selection for cadaveric renal transplantation in the United Kingdom. *Nephrol. Dial. Transplant.* **10**, 855.

McMillan, M. A., Briggs, J. D. and Junor, B. J. R. (1990). Outcome of renal replacement treatment in patients with diabetes mellitus. *B. M. J.* **301**, 540.

Meulders, Q., Pirson, Y., Cosyns, J. P., Squifflet, J.-P. and van Ypersele de Strihou, C. (1994). Course of Henoch-Schönlein nephritis after renal transplantation. *Transplantation* **58**, 1179.

Midtvedt, K., Hartmann, A., Bentdal, Ø., Brekke, I. B. and Fauchald, P. (1996). Bilateral nephrectomy simultaneously with renal allografting does not alleviate hypertension 3 months following living-donor transplantation. *Nephrol. Dial. Transplant.* **11**, 2045.

Modlin, C. S., Flechner, S. M., Goormastic, M., *et al.* (1997). Should obese patients lose weight before receiving a kidney transplant? *Transplantation* **64**, 599.

Mozes, M. F., Spigos, D. G., Thomas, P. A., Jr., *et al.* (1983). Antilymphocyte globulin and splenectomy or partial splenic embolisation: evidence for a synergistic beneficial effect on cadaver renal allograft survival. *Transplant. Proc.* **15**, 613.

Munson, J. L., Bennett, W. M., Barry, J. M. and Norman, D. J. (1992). A case control study of renal transplantation in patients with Type I diabetes. *Clin. Transplant.* **6**, 306.

Novick, A. C., Ortenburg, J. and Braun, W. E. (1980). Reduced morbidity with posterior surgical approach for pre-transplant bilateral nephrectomy. *Surg. Gynecol. Obstet.* **151**, 773.

Nunez, D., Williams, P. F., Herrick, A. L., *et al.* (1987). Renal transplantation for chronic renal failure in acute porphyria. *Nephrol. Dial. Transplant.* **2**, 271.

Nyberg, G., Blohmé, I., Persson, H., *et al.* (1992). Recurrence of SLE in transplanted kidneys: a follow-up transplant biopsy study. *Nephrol. Dial. Transplant.* **7**, 1116.

Oliver, T. B., Gouldesbrough, D. R. and Swainson, C. P. (1991). Acute crescentic glomerulonephritis associated with antiglomerular basement membrane antibody in Alport's syndrome after second transplantation. *Nephrol. Dial. Transplant.* **6**, 893.

Opelz, G., Sengar, D. P. S., Mickey, M. R., *et al.* (1973). Effect of blood transfusions on subsequent kidney transplants. *Transplant. Proc.* **5**, 253.

Opelz, G., Vanrenterghem, Y., Kirste, G., *et al.* (1997). Prospective evaluation of pre-transplant blood transfusions in cadaver kidney recipients. *Transplantation* **63**, 964.

Palmer, A., Taube, D., Welsh, K., *et al.* (1989). Removal of anti-HLA antibodies by extracorporeal immunoadsorption to enable renal transplantation. *Lancet* **7**, 10.

Penn, I. (1993). The effect of immunosuppression on pre-existing cancers. *Transplantation* **55**, 742.

Penn, I. (1995). Primary kidney tumors before and after renal transplantation. *Transplantation* **59**, 480.

Pereira, B. J. G., Wright, T. L., Schmid, C. H. and Levey, A. S. (1995). The impact of pre-transplantation hepatitis C infection on the outcome of renal transplantation. *Transplantation* **60**, 799.

Peten, E., Pirson, Y., Cosyns, J.-P., *et al.* (1991). Outcome of thirty patients with Alport's syndrome after renal transplantation. *Transplantation* **52**, 823.

Pirsch, J. D., Armbrust, M. J., Knechtle, S. J., *et al.* (1995). Obesity as a risk factor following renal transplantation. *Transplantation* **59**, 631.

Quérin, S., Noël, L. H., Grünfeld, J.-P., *et al.* (1986). Linear glomerular IgG fixation in renal allografts: incidence and significance in Alport's syndrome. *Clin. Nephrol.* **25**, 134.

Rai, G. S., Wilkinson, R., Taylor, R. M. R., *et al.* (1977). Adverse effect of splenectomy in renal transplantation. *Clin. Nephrol.* **9**, 194.

Raine, A. E. G., Margreiter, R., Brunner, F. P., *et al.* (1992). Report on management of renal failure in Europe. XXII, 1991. *Nephrol. Dial. Transplant.* **7(Suppl. 2)**, 7.

Ramos, E. L. and Tisher, C. C. (1994). Recurrent diseases in the kidney transplant. *Am. J. Kidney Dis.* **24**, 142.

Rao, K. V., Kasiske, B. L. and Anderson, W. R. (1991). Variability in the morphological spectrum and clinical outcome of chronic liver disease in hepatitis B-positive and B-negative renal transplant recipients. *Transplantation* **51**, 391.

Rischen-Vos, J., van der Woude, F. J., Tegzess, A. M., *et al.* (1992). Increased morbidity and mortality in patients with diabetes mellitus after kidney transplantation as compared with non-diabetic patients. *Nephrol. Dial. Transplant.* **7**, 433.

Roake, J. A., Cahill, A. P., Gray, C. M., Gray, D. W. R. and Morris, P. J. (1996). Pre-emptive renal transplantation—clinical outcome. *Transplantation* **62**, 1411.

Ross, G., Jr., Weinstein, S., Dutton, S. and Whittier, F. C. (1983). Renal transplantation in the end-stage renal disease of drug abuse. *J. Urol.* **129**, 14.

Rubin, R. H. (1993). Infectious disease complications of renal transplantation. *Kidney Int.* **44**, 221.

Russell, P. S. and Winn, H. J. (1970). Transplantation. *N. Engl. J. Med.* **282**, 896.

Samuel, K. S., So, S., Mauer, M., *et al.* (1986). Current results in pediatric renal transplantation in the University of Minnesota. *Kidney Int.* **30(Suppl. 19)**, 25.

Sanfilippo, F., Vaughn, W. K. and Spees, E. K. (1984). The association of pretransplant native nephrectomy with decreased renal allograft rejection. *Transplantation* **37**, 256.

Scheinman, J. I., Najarian, J. S. and Mauer, S. M. (1984). Successful strategies for renal transplantation in primary oxalosis. *Kidney Int.* **25**, 804.

Schmidt, R., Kupin, W., Dumler, F., Venkat, K. K. and Mozes, M. (1993). Influence of the pretransplant haematocrit level on early graft function in primary cadaveric renal transplantation. *Transplantation* **55**, 1034.

Schofer, F. S., London, W. T., Lyons, P., *et al.* (1986). Adverse effect of splenectomy on the survival of patients with more than one kidney transplant. *Transplantation* **42**, 473.

Schwarz, A., Offermann, G. and Keller, F. (1992). Analgesic nephropathy and renal transplantation. *Nephrol. Dial. Transplant.* **7**, 427.

Shandera, K., Sago, A., Angstadt, J., Peretsman, S. and Jaffers, G. (1993). An assessment of the need for the voiding cystourethrogram for urologic screening prior to renal transplantation. *Clin. Transplant.* **7**, 299.

Silberberg, J. S., Barre, P. E., Prichard, S. S. and Sniderman, A. D. (1989). Impact of left ventricular hypertrophy on survival in end-stage renal disease. *Kidney Int.* **36**, 286.

Sironvalle, M. S., Gelet, A., Martin, X., *et al.* (1992). Endoscopic treatment of vesicoureteric reflux prior to renal transplantation. *Transplant. Int.* **5**, 231.

Soucie, J. M., Neylan, J. F. and McClellan, W. (1992). Race and sex differences in the identification of candidates for renal transplantation. *Am. J. Kidney Dis.* **19**, 414.

Stephanian, E., Matas, A. J., Mauer, S. M., *et al.* (1992). Recurrence of disease in patients re-transplanted for focal segmental glomerulosclerosis. *Transplantation* **53**, 755.

Stephenson, T. P., Salaman, J. R., Stone, A, R., *et al.* (1984). Urinary tract reconstruction before renal transplantation. *Transplant. Proc.* **16**, 1340.

Stratta, R. J., Taylor, R. J., Wahl, T. O., *et al.* (1992). Recipient selection and evaluation for vascularised pancreas transplantation. *Transplantation* **55**, 1090.

Stuart, F. P., Reckard, C. R., Ketel, B. L. and Schulak, J. A. (1980). Effect of splenectomy on first cadaver kidney transplants. *Ann. Surg.* **192**, 553.

Tesi, R. J., Elkhammas, E. A., Davies, E. A., Henry, M. L. and Ferguson, R. M. (1994). Renal transplantation in older people. *Lancet* **343**, 461.

Thompson, J. F., Fletcher, E. W. L., Wood, R. F. M., *et al.* (1984). Control of hypertension after renal transplantation by embolisation of host kidneys. *Lancet* **2**, 424.

Troppmann, C., Benedetti, E., Gruessner, R. W. G., *et al.* (1995). Retransplantation after renal allograft loss due to noncompliance. *Transplantation* **59**, 467.

Tsakiris, D., Simpson, H. K. L., Jones, E. H. P., *et al.* (1996). Rare diseases in renal replacement therapy in the ERA-EDTA Registry. *Nephrol. Dial. Transplant.* **11(Suppl. 7)**, 4.

Tucker, B., Fabbian, F., Giles, M., *et al.* (1997). Left ventricular hypertrophy and ambulatory blood pressure monitoring in chronic renal failure. *Nephrol. Dial. Transplant.* **12**, 724.

Tzardis, P. J., Gruessner, R. W. G., Matas, A. J., *et al.* (1989). Renal transplantation in patients with polycystic kidney disease: a single-center experience. *Clin. Transplant.* **3**, 325.

Tzardis, P. J., Gruessner, R. W. G., Matas, A. J., *et al.* (1990). Fate of native polycystic kidneys left in situ after renal transplantation. *Clin. Transplant.* **4**, 309.

United States Renal Data System (USRDS) (1998). 1998 Annual Data Report. *Am. J. Kidney Dis.* **32(Suppl. 1)**, 538.

Vanrenterghem, Y. and Verberckmoes, R. (1998). Pre-emptive kidney transplantation. *Nephrol. Dial. Transplant.* **13**, 2466.

Vasquez, E. M. and Pollak, R. (1996). Effect of pre-transplant erythropoietin therapy on renal allograft outcome. *Transplantation* **62**, 1026.

Warshaw, B. L., Edelbrock, H. H., Ettenger, R. B., *et al.* (1980). Renal transplantation in children with obstructive uropathy. *J. Urol.* **123**, 737.

Watts, R. W. E., Danpure, C. J., De Pauw, L., *et al.* (1991). Combined liver-kidney and isolated liver transplantation for primary hyperoxaluria Type I: the European experience. *Nephrol. Dial. Transplant.* **6**, 502.

Wilson, C. B. and Dixon, F. J. (1973). Antiglomerular basement membrane antibody induced glomerulonephritis. *Kidney Int.* **3**, 74.

Ziff, M. and Helderman, J. H. (1983). Dialysis and transplantation in end-stage lupus nephritis. *N. Engl. J. Med.* **308**, 218.

Access for Renal Replacement Therapy
Michael L. Nicholson • Steven A. White

Introduction

The provision of long-term vascular and peritoneal access usually is the responsibility of the renal transplant surgeon. The demand for vascular access surgery is great, and this is becoming an increasingly important area of specialist surgical interest. The aim is to provide the patient with a reliable vascular access site that will be suitable for long-term catheterization. Even for the most straightforward operations, the best results can be achieved only by surgeons with a high level of technical skill and the necessary experience to choose the right procedure in each case. The temptation to relegate vascular access procedures to junior surgeons should be resisted.

Many developments have occurred in the field of vascular access surgery, many of which have come about in response to the increasing number of patients with inadequate forearm veins or previous failure of simpler vascular access operations, such as a wrist arteriovenous fistula (AVF). The judicious use of long-term central venous catheters, upper arm fistulae and prosthetic grafts has been required. There have been improvements in fistula surveillance to diagnose failing access procedures as well as the use of interventional radiology for treatment.

Historical Development of Vascular Access Surgery

In 1960, Quinton, Dillard and Scribner described the external arteriovenous shunt (Fig. 5–1) and opened the era of repeated hemodialysis for end-stage renal disease. The technique had many disadvantages, however. External shunts were inconvenient for the patient and were prone to infection and thrombosis, which often required many revision procedures. This procedure has largely been consigned to history. The introduction of the Brescia-Cimino internal radiocephalic AVF in 1966 was the next major advance and solved many of the problems associated with external shunts. This operation has been so successful that it remains the first-choice procedure for dialysis vascular access. The number of patients with inadequate forearm veins or previously failed radiocephalic AVF increased, and the 1970s saw the introduction of various elbow AVF. Prosthetic graft fistulae for dialysis followed; these have been favored more in the United States than in Great Britain, Europe and Australasia.

Planning Vascular Access

Patients with end-stage renal failure are living much longer and may need to be maintained on dialysis for many decades. Careful planning is a key feature of vascular acccess surgery. The importance of protecting the venous system of chronic renal failure patients cannot be overemphasized. The veins of the forearm and antecubital fossa must not be used for venesection or for intravenous catheterization. These procedures should be confined, as far as possible, to the veins on the dorsum of the hand. Most medical and nursing staff working in renal units understand this issue. Staff working outside the renal unit may be less well informed, and the importance of preserving the arm veins should be emphasized to all dialysis patients so that they are in a position to take some responsibility for their own veins. The central veins are equally important, and every effort must be made to avoid direct catheterization of the subclavian vein. Temporary vascular access catheters placed through this route may be complicated by subclavian stenosis, which may complicate or preclude subsequent ipsilateral access operations.

There are a few general rules relating to the planning of vascular access. Arm vessels should be used in preference to the legs, and the nondominant arm should be used first. This rule is especially important in patients who needle their own fistula during home hemodialysis. Distal sites should be used first because this allows the greatest possible length of vascular conduit and preserves proximal sites for the future. When possible, the AVF should be created preemptively. This approach requires careful judgment and the use of a reciprocal creatinine plot to estimate when individual patients will reach end-stage disease.

In most renal failure patients, progression to end-stage disease occurs over a prolonged and carefully monitored period. This situation allows plenty of time to make a choice between continuous ambulatory peritoneal dialysis (CAPD) and hemodialysis, and if the latter is chosen, it should be possible to plan and provide access to the circulation well in advance of need. Nonetheless, a significant minority of new patients present acutely in end-stage disease and need some form of temporary vascular access while a more long-term plan is made.

The Brescia-Cimino radiocephalic fistula is the first choice for hemodialysis access. If a radiocephalic AVF fails in the longer term, it usually is because of the development of intimal hyperplasia at or near the anastomosis. In some cases, the patient still has usable forearm veins that can be anastomosed to the radial artery at a more proximal site or to the ulnar artery. In patients with unsuitable forearm veins or failed wrist fistulae in both arms, the best option is a brachiocephalic fistula. If this option is not possible, the next choice should be the brachiobasilic AVF using transposed vein. Prosthetic AVF grafts are best created using expanded polytetrafluoroethylene (e-PTFE) but should not be used until all the native arm veins, including both basilic veins, have been used or deemed to be unsuitable. Patients with failed secondary and tertiary access procedures may be suitable for long-term management using tunneled cuffed central venous catheters.

An increasing number of patients who need vascular access surgery develop central venous stenoses or occlusions, including lesions in the superior vena cava. These patients present some of the most challenging vascular access problems. Interventional radiology is an important adjunct to

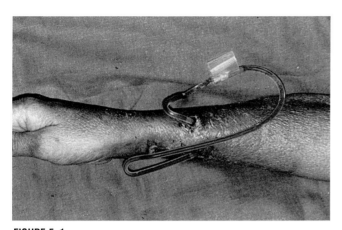

FIGURE 5–1

A Scribner shunt.

management because some central venous lesions can be treated successfully by percutaneous transluminal angioplasty with or without stenting. Only when all potential upper limb procedures fail should the legs be considered for vascular access using a prosthetic graft AVF.

Temporary Vascular Access

Approximately 40% of end-stage renal failure patients present acutely and require some form of temporary vascular access. The procedure of choice is percutaneous catheterization of the superior vena cava through the subclavian or the internal jugular veins. The subclavian approach was the most popular for many years, but it is now recognized that this approach is associated with a significant risk of subclavian venous stenosis (Fig. 5–2), which may make subsequent definitive vascular access in the ipsilateral limb more difficult. The reported incidence of venous stenosis after subclavian catheterization can be 50% (Koo *et al.*, 1996). The risk is higher when the procedure is difficult and becomes complicated by hematoma formation. The point where the subcla-

vian vein runs between the first rib and the clavicle is the commonest site of injury. Stenosis is commoner in the left subclavian vein and when multiple catheterizations have been performed.

In view of these considerations, the internal jugular vein has been advocated as the site of choice for all temporary vascular catheters. Adoption of this site along with the use of soft Silastic catheters and short catheterization periods has been effective in reducing the venous complications of temporary hemodialysis access dramatically (Canaud *et al.*, 1986, Cappello *et al.*, 1989). The disadvantage of jugular catheters is that they remain visible, and patients may find this unacceptable.

Vascular access catheters usually can be placed under local anesthesia. The Seldinger technique is used, and the procedure usually is straightforward. Many well-designed double-lumen temporary vascular access catheters are available commercially. Their drawbacks include thrombosis, displacement and infection, all of which may occur quickly after placement.

An alternative strategy can be employed in patients presenting with acute or chronic renal failure requiring long-term hemodialysis. A temporary vascular catheter can be placed in a femoral vein to allow hemodialysis over a short period. As soon as the patient is stabilized, a tunneled, cuffed venous catheter (e.g., Perma-Cath) *(see later discussion)* is placed in the internal jugular vein. For patient comfort, this procedure is best performed under general anesthesia, but it can be performed using local anesthesia, which may be necessary in the patient too ill for general anesthetic due to cardiac or pulmonary disease. Because internal jugular Perma-Caths can function for a number of months or years, this policy allows for a period of careful investigation and planning for long-term definitive vascular access.

Long-Term Vascular Access

Long-term vascular access may be provided by autogenous AVF, arteriovenous grafts, and long-term central venous catheters.

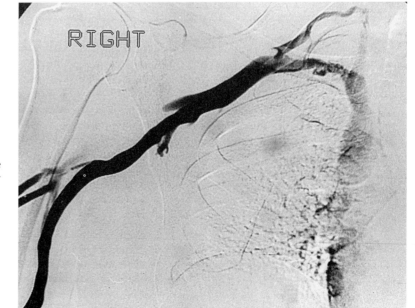

FIGURE 5–2

A venogram shows central venous stenosis at the junction of the right subclavian and right brachiocephalic veins.

Requirements of a Successful Arteriovenous Fistula for Hemodialysis

The ideal AVF has the following features:

1. A blood flow of at least 200 ml/min
2. A large diameter, which facilitates venipuncture
3. Sufficient length to allow two needles to be inserted
4. Creation by a simple and quick operation, preferably under local anesthesia
5. A good long-term patency rate

The veins of the arm can be catheterized easily and repeatedly, but their blood flow is too low to support hemodialysis. The opposite is true for peripheral arteries, which have a higher blood flow but are too small to allow repeated percutaneous catheterization. The creation of an AVF produces an arterialized venous channel, which yields the combined advantages of large diameter and high blood flow. A small anastomosis between the radial artery and cephalic vein leads to arterialization of much of the venous system of the arm, and this has profound hemodynamic consequences. Immediately after creation of a radiocephalic AVF, the radial artery blood flow increases 10-fold to a level of 200 to 400 ml/min. The flow rate increases further over the next 2 to 4 weeks, after which it plateaus. The underlying mechanism is a loss of the downstream resistance in the arterioles and capillary bed. To achieve these dramatic flows, the artery must dilate as well as the vein. Although failure of maturation of a radiocephalic AVF may be due to an inadequate vein, it also can be due to an atheromatous or frankly calcified artery that is unable to dilate. The vessels of diabetic patients often fall into this category.

Preoperative Assessment

The three requirements for a successful AVF in the arm are:

1. A good arterial inflow
2. A suitable superficial vein
3. A patent subclavian and axillary venous system

The first two of these requirements usually are assessed clinically, but the third requires radiological investigation. The radial and ulnar arteries can be palpated at the wrist to assess the pulse volume and to identify overt atheromatous disease, such as calcification. Allen's test usually is described as a method of establishing the patency of the palmar arches, but it also can provide a subjective assessment of the arterial inflow to the hand and define dominance of the radial or ulnar artery. The veins of the forearm can be assessed by simple inspection and palpation after placing a tourniquet around the upper arm. The cephalic vein is the one most often used for AVF creation, and for success it needs to be patent from the wrist to the antecubital fossa and have a diameter of at least 3 mm (Reilly et al., 1982). The patency of the vein can be established easily by lightly percussing it at the wrist and feeling for a transmitted wave at the elbow. A good-caliber cephalic vein at the wrist may divide quickly into many small branches in the forearm, and this relatively common anatomical variation may preclude successful AVF formation (Haimov, 1987).

Assessment of the patency of the major venous drainage of the upper limb is particularly important. The only overt clinical signs of stenosis or occlusion in the axillary and subclavian venous system are prominent collateral veins around the shoulder and chest, and associated arm swelling. Most venous stenoses and some occlusions are clinically si-

lent, and the venous drainage of the arm can be assessed properly only by performing a duplex ultrasound scan or a contrast venogram. Logistical and financial constraints usually dictate that these investigations are performed selectively, but it is wise to perform some form of imaging in any patient who has previously had an ipsilateral temporary subclavian vascular catheter.

Anesthesia

Patients with end-stage renal failure commonly display comorbid conditions, such as cardiovascular disease and diabetes, and may be a poor risk for general anesthesia. Almost any vascular access procedure can be performed using a local anesthetic. For simple operations such as wrist fistulae, local infiltration of 1% lignocaine (lidocaine) usually suffices. The addition of epinephrine is also helpful in reducing the oozing that commonly occurs in renal patients as a result of qualitative platelet dysfunction. Regional anesthesia can be achieved by local anesthetic blocks, and these techniques are ideal for more extensive operations such as elbow AVFs and forearm prosthetic loop grafts. These methods also block the sympathetic nervous system, which has the advantage of inhibiting vasospasm. An alternative for more extensive operations is to use simple local anesthetic infiltration and to ask the anesthetist to supplement this with boluses of a short-acting sedative, such as propofol (see Chapter 13).

Surgical Technique

Vascular access surgery requires attention to detail and an immaculate surgical technique. The basic principles of vascular anastomosis must be adhered to. The vessels are anastomosed using a fine continuous nonabsorbable monofilament suture with eversion of the edges to ensure a smooth transition between the two intimal surfaces. There must be no tension between the anastomosed vessels, and the sutures must pick up all layers of the arterial wall to avoid the creation of a subintimal flap. Because suture placement is so crucial, optical magnification using surgical telescopes is an advantage, and good-quality microvascular instruments should be available.

Autogenous Arteriovenous Fistulae
WRIST ARTERIOVENOUS FISTULAE

The radiocephalic AVF is the first-choice procedure in vascular access surgery. This operation is straightforward and can be performed under local anesthesia as an outpatient procedure. It has a low complication rate and excellent long-term patency rates. The original operation described by Brescia and colleagues in 1966 was a side-to-side radial artery–to–cephalic vein AVF formed close to the wrist joint (Figs. 5–3 and 5–4). The main variant, a side of artery–to–end of vein fistula, is preferred by many surgeons because there is a lower incidence of venous hypertension in the hand (Fig. 5–5). Radiocephalic AVF have a primary patency rate of approximately 80% at 2 years (Enzler et al., 1996; Jensen et al., 1990; Reilly, 1982).

A radiocephalic fistula can be fashioned in the anatomical snuffbox (Rassat et al., 1969). This is a greater technical challenge because the vessels are of smaller diameter, but the advantage of this site is that it maximizes the length of cephalic vein available for venipuncture. If the cephalic vein or radial artery at the wrist is found to be unsuitable or thrombosed, an AVF can be fashioned by anastomosing the

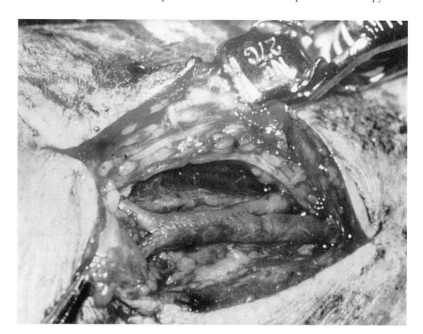

FIGURE 5–3

Operative photograph of a completed side-to-side radiocephalic arteriovenous fistula.

basilic vein to the ulnar artery. The awkward medial position of the basilic vein can make venipuncture difficult, and this operation should not be performed after a failed radiocephalic fistula because there is a theoretical risk of ischemia to the hand.

Surgical Technique for Radiocephalic Arteriovenous Fistula

The radial artery and cephalic vein are exposed at the wrist using an S-shaped, longitudinal or transverse incision depending on how close together the vessels are and to a certain extent on the surgeon's personal preference. Hemostasis is achieved using diathermy, which should be in bipolar mode if the patient is awake. The lateral skin flap is elevated

to expose the cephalic vein, which is mobilized over a distance of approximately 3 cm, taking care to preserve the sensory dorsal branch of the radial nerve. The radial artery is sought just lateral to the flexor carpi radialis muscle and exposed by dividing the transverse fibers of the deep fascia of the forearm over the pulse. Only 2 cm of artery needs to be mobilized by ligating and dividing any small branches. The cephalic vein and radial artery may be anastomosed in a side-to-side or an end-to-side arrangement. We prefer the end-to-side arrangement in which the spatulated end of the divided cephalic vein is anastomosed to the side of the radial artery using a continuous monofilament 6–0 or 7–0 vascular suture. After controlling the artery with Silastic vessel slings or miniature vascular clamps, a short arteriotomy is made. The length of the arteriotomy depends on the diameter of the cephalic vein and radial artery but usually is in the region of 5 mm. Systemic anticoagulation with heparin is unnecessary and unwise in renal patients, who tend to have

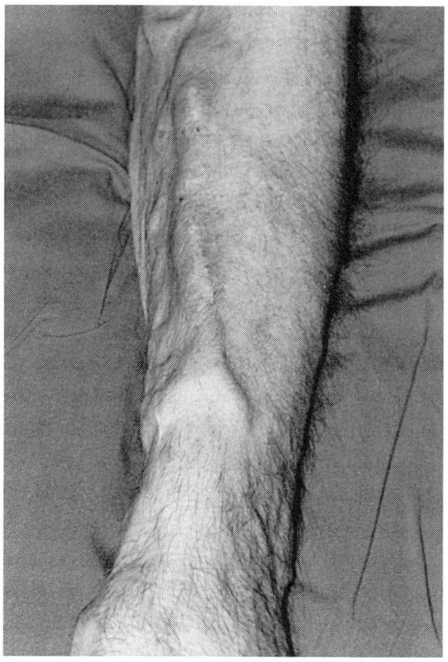

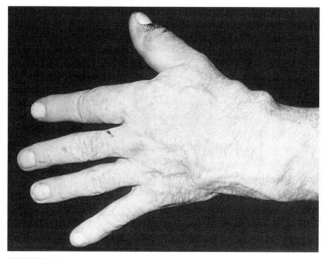

FIGURE 5–4

An established Brescia-Cimino radiocephalic arteriovenous fistula (see color plate).

FIGURE 5–5

Venous hypertension in the thumb secondary to a side-to-side radiocephalic arteriovenous fistula.

a functional platelet disorder, but the proximal and distal radial artery can be filled locally with heparinized saline solution. For a side-to-side anastomosis, the vessels are mobilized sufficiently to allow them to be held together over a distance of 2 cm, and the cephalic vein is not divided. Both vessels are opened by equal-length longitudinal incisions, and the side-to-side anastomosis is again completed using a fine monofilament suture. At clamp release, the flow should be high enough to produce an obvious thrill in the cephalic vein. The causes of an absent thrill include systemic hypotension, adventitial bands that kink the venous run-off, and technical errors in constructing the anastomosis. It is also possible that the radial artery and/or the cephalic vein are too small to support a high flow. If there is any doubt, the anterior wall suture line should be taken down to look for an intimal flap or other technical error.

ELBOW FISTULAE

Many patients referred for vascular access have either inadequate forearm veins or a previously failed wrist fistula. The principal choice for secondary vascular access in this situation is between an upper arm AVF using autogenous vessels or a prosthetic graft AVF. Autogenous elbow fistulae have proved to be more popular in European countries than in the United States, where prosthetic grafts have tended to be favored for secondary access.

Brachiocephalic Arteriovenous Fistulae

Brachiocephalic AVF probably are the best option when it is not possible to form a wrist fistula in either arm. The direct brachiocephalic AVF was first described by Cascardo et al. in 1970, and the first large series was reported by Someya et al. in 1976. The operation usually is straightforward to perform and can be carried out under local anesthesia. The side of artery–to–end of vein configuration usually is preferred. A side-to-side anastomosis may be possible if the cephalic vein and brachial artery are close enough, but as with radiocephalic fistulae this arrangement may give rise to venous hypertension in the hand. The main disadvantage of brachiocephalic fistulae is that they produce a relatively short length of arterialized vein. The procedure may not be suitable for the arms of obese patients. Several technical variations of the brachiocephalic fistula are possible depending on the venous anatomy in the antecubital fossa. When present, the median

cubital vein may be anastomosed directly to the brachial artery, and this technique has the advantage of arterializing the cephalic and the basilic venous systems. Alternatively, the deep perforating branch of the median cubital vein can be anastomosed to the brachial artery (Gracz et al., 1977). The long-term results of brachiocephalic AVFs are good, with secondary cumulative patency rates approximately 80% at 3 years (Bender et al., 1995) and 70% at 4 years (Elcheroth et al., 1994). Elbow fistulae can have high flow rates, and hemodynamic complications, such as steal syndrome and high-output cardiac failure, occur more commonly than in wrist fistulae. To avoid these complications, the length of the brachial arteriotomy should be limited to a maximum of 7 mm.

Brachiobasilic Arteriovenous Fistula with Vein Transposition

Only a short section of the basilic vein at the elbow is superficial, and most of the vein is protected under the deep fascia. If the basilic vein is left in this anatomical position and anastomosed to the brachial artery, only a short length of vein is available for venipuncture. A much longer conduit can be created by dissecting the basilic vein from its bed and transposing it into a more convenient subcutaneous position down the middle of the upper arm. This procedure was first reported by Cascardo et al. (1970) and Dagher et al. (1976). The operation is best performed under general anesthesia because of the extensive incision required. This incision runs along the median aspect of the arm from the antecubital fossa to the axilla, but staged incisions with short skin bridges also can be used. The medial cutaneous nerve of the forearm usually is closely applied to the basilic vein and needs to be preserved carefully during dissection. The vein is then transposed into its new position using a subcutaneous tunneling device and anastomosed end of vein to side of brachial artery (Figs. 5–6 and 5–7).

The subfascial position of the basilic vein means that it is protected from venipuncture, and this usually ensures that it is of good quality and diameter. The operation may be performed as a tertiary procedure after failed wrist and brachiocephalic fistulae, but it also is particularly useful as a primary procedure in small children and slender women. The formation of the brachiobasilic AVF does not compromise the arm for future prosthetic grafting, and the operation probably has been underused.

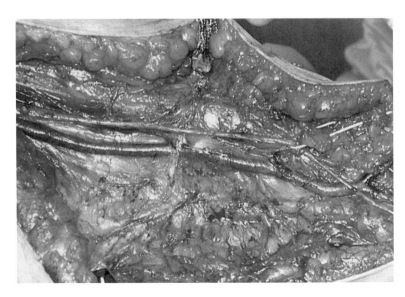

FIGURE 5–6

Operative photograph of the extensive incision required to dissect the left basilic vein free from its subfascial bed. The medial cutaneous nerve of the forearm runs parallel to the basilic vein.

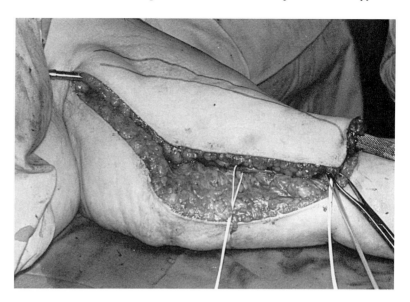

FIGURE 5–7

Operative photograph shows the use of a Kelly-Wick tunneling device to create the transposition tunnel of a left brachiobasilic arteriovenous fistula.

The 1- and 2-year functional patency rates are approximately 50 to 80% (Butterworth *et al.*, 1998; Coburn and Carney, 1994; Elcheroth *et al.*, 1994; Murphy *et al.*, 2000). The disadvantage of the brachiobasilic fistula lies in the extensive incision required. Postoperative analgesia can be improved by administering boluses of a long-acting local anesthetic such as bupivacaine via an epidural catheter placed directly into the axillary sheath at the time of surgery (Butterworth *et al.*, 1997).

GRAFT ARTERIOVENOUS FISTULAE

In Europe and Australasia, graft AVF usually are reserved for patients with previous multiple access failures. In contrast, many centers in the United States favor prosthetic grafts as primary or secondary access procedures. Graft AVF can be constructed under local or regional anesthesia with a short inpatient stay. The graft material is tunneled subcutaneously between a suitable artery and vein and anastomosed to these using an end-to-side technique. The choice of graft material is between biological materials, such as autogenous long saphenous vein, and prosthetic materials, of which ePTFE is preferred.

The use of autogenous saphenous vein is attractive in principle but has been limited by the variable quality of this vein. This variable quality has been reflected by the relatively poor patency rates of 20 to 66% at 2 years (Koo *et al.*, 1996; May *et al.*, 1980; Valenta *et al.*, 1985). The extensive dissection of the long saphenous vein can be performed only under general anesthesia, and the procedure is not cost-effective because the patient needs to be hospitalized for several days because of the leg incision. In view of these disadvantages, the long saphenous vein is used rarely in vascular access surgery. Other biological materials, including human umbilical vein and bovine carotid artery, have not been found to be successful. Although these materials handle well, they are associated with high incidences of infection, rupture and false aneurysm formation, and overall patency rates are poor (Garvin *et al.*, 1982; Karkow *et al.*, 1986; Wilson *et al.*, 1988).

Expanded polytetrafluoroethylene is the most popular prosthetic graft material in access surgery. It is easy to handle, is of predictably high quality and is available in a wide range of sizes. The expected 2-year graft patency rate using e-PTFE is approximately 60%. The disadvantages of e-PTFE are its expense and higher complication rates than autogenous AVF.

A further disadvantage of PTFE is the need to wait for 6 weeks before venipuncture because the PTFE wall is not self-sealing and perigraft fibrosis must develop before the graft can be punctured safely. Of particular concern is the overall infection rate of 11 to 35% (Ready and Buckels, 1995) compared with 2 to 3% for autogenous fistulae (Marx *et al.*, 1990). Thrombosis and intimal hyperplasia at the venous anastomosis are commoner with prosthetic graft materials than autogenous vessels. Newer graft materials such as stretch PTFE have improved compliance and elastic recoil, and these properties may reduce the incidence of intimal hyperplasia and permit earlier venipuncture. It remains to be seen whether or not such innovations will translate into better long-term graft patency rates.

Choice of Procedure

Many variations of prosthetic interposition grafts have been used, including loop, straight or J-shaped configurations. Forearm graft AVF can take their arterial inflow from the brachial or radial artery, and any of the antecubital fossa veins can be used for the outflow. The most popular configuration is a loop graft between the brachial artery and the basilic vein. This configuration is favored by many surgeons because its full length facilitates the rotation of needle sites, reducing the risk of thrombosis, infection and false aneurysm formation. In the absence of suitable veins in the antecubital fossa, a graft AVF can be placed between the brachial artery and the axillary vein. These vessels can be exposed through two short incisions, and the operation can be performed under local anesthesia. This technique appears to be an effective tertiary or quaternary vascular access procedure with 1-year primary and secondary patency rates of approximately 70 and 90% (Polo *et al.*, 1995). A brachiojugular graft fistula may be performed in patients with exhausted arm and axillary veins (Polo *et al.*, 1990). Interposition loop grafts can be placed in the leg with anastomosis to the common femoral artery and vein in the groin. In this site, there is a susceptibility to infection, particularly in diabetic patients. An alternative method that avoids the groin involves exposure of the superficial femoral artery and femoral vein in the midthigh where they run in the adductor canal. This is a clean area and allows a graft to be positioned in a loop configuration in the lower thigh.

FISTULA MATURATION AND VENIPUNCTURE

Over a period of several weeks, the venous outflow of an autogenous fistula becomes arterialized, developing a degree of dilatation and thickening of the vessel wall. The time when a new AVF can first be punctured varies and requires some judgment. Hematoma and early thrombosis are potential complications if a fistula is punctured before it has matured sufficiently. A conservative approach is to leave all fistulae for a period of 6 weeks, but in patients with good-quality veins a new AVF can be punctured successfully after only 2 weeks. The development of a fistula may be aided by exercising the arm, possibly with a tourniquet in place; the rationale is that increased arm blood flow improves fistula maturation, but there are no studies of the effectiveness of such a policy.

In the longer term, persistent venipuncture in exactly the same spot can weaken the vessel wall and may lead to false aneurysm formation. In the same way, the skin over a prosthetic graft may be eroded, leaving the graft exposed and infected. Rotation of the venipuncture site is advisable in autogenous and prosthetic AVF. This advice often is ignored, and there may be considerable pressure from the patient to use the same venipuncture sites repeatedly because the skin here becomes numb with time, and venipuncture becomes more comfortable.

Long-Term Venous Catheters

A subgroup of patients who require hemodialysis do not have any suitable arm or leg vessels, and in this situation a long-term central venous catheter (a Perma-Cath; Figs. 5–8 and 5–9) is placed. The preferred vessel for introduction is the internal jugular vein, which can be approached easily through a transverse incision centered over the lower part of the sternomastoid muscle. The tip of the catheter should be placed at the junction of the superior vena cava and the right atrium. When the catheter tip is placed in the right atrium itself, there is the danger of a thrombus developing around the tip because of the lower flow at this point. Catheters introduced through the left internal jugular vein have a tendency to abut the caval wall and are not as successful as catheters placed on the right. An alternative is to place a cuffed catheter in the subclavian vein by cutting down on the cephalic vein in the deltopectoral groove. The main problem with long-term central venous catheters is that they tend to thrombose. This situation may respond to thrombolysis using streptokinase or recombinant tissue plasminogen activator, but a catheter also may need to be replaced. This replacement usually can be performed over a guidewire placed through the nonfunctioning catheter. It is wise to consider long-term anticoagulation with warfarin in patients who are maintained purely on a central venous catheter.

Complications of Arteriovenous Fistula and Graft Formation

HEMORRHAGE

If hemorrhage occurs in the first 24 hours postoperatively, it is usually due to a technical error with the anastomosis or a slipped ligature. Generalized oozing resulting in hematoma formation is commoner and is related to the functional platelet disorder associated with uremia (Remuzzi, 1988). The synthetic vasopressin analogue, DDAVP, can be used as a specific prophylactic measure in uremic patients who have additional risk factors for bleeding and in whom extensive surgery is planned. DDAVP releases stored factor VIII, von Willebrand factor, from the endothelium into the circulation and by promoting platelet adhesion and aggregation restores the bleeding time to normal (Mannucci, 1988). The desired effect on the bleeding time is relatively short acting with a return to the pretreatment value after 8 hours.

Late hemorrhage from an AVF can occur after venipuncture or as a complication of aneurysm formation and infection. In the emergency situation, this can be controlled by firm pressure over the bleeding point, but surgical exploration may then be required.

THROMBOSIS

Thrombosis may occur in the first 24 hours postoperatively. Although thrombosis may result from preoperative overdialysis leading to dehydration or intraoperative hypotension, a technical error should be suspected. Immediate reexploration is indicated because it may be possible to salvage the situation by thrombectomy using a Fogarty catheter and subsequent refashioning of the anastomosis.

Thrombosis is the commonest cause of AVF failure in the long-term. In this situation, thrombosis usually is due to an underlying stenosis that develops gradually. The type of access and the site of thrombosis are important determinants of outcome. If a radiocephalic or brachiocephalic AVF thromboses in a localized manner at or close to the anastomosis, the runoff usually remains patent because it has many natural tributaries that maintain some venous flow. This situation can be remedied by refashioning the arteriovenous anastomosis at a more proximal site. In contrast, when a brachiobasilic AVF thromboses, it is usual for the whole vein to clot by propagation of thrombus. This clotting is a direct result of the fact that all the tributaries of the venous outflow will have been ligated during the creation of this type of AVF.

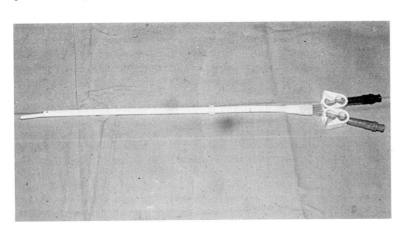

FIGURE 5–8

A cuffed double-lumen Silastic catheter for long-term central venous access.

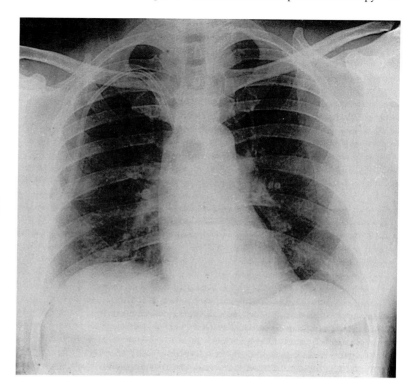

FIGURE 5–9

Chest radiograph shows a right-sided Perma-Cath introduced through a vascular stent that has been used to treat a central venous stenosis.

The only hope of salvage in this situation is to perform an immediate thrombectomy before the clot organizes. AVFs also can thrombose at venipuncture sites as a result of poor technique leading to hematoma formation or undue postcatheterization compression to control bleeding.

Advances in the Treatment of Access Thrombosis

Interventional radiological techniques are being used increasingly in the treatment of thrombosed vascular access conduits. Pulse-spray catheters, which originally were designed for thrombolysis in patients with peripheral vascular disease, can be used with equal success in patients with thrombosed vascular access (Bookstein and Saldinger, 1985). The catheter is introduced into the clotted segment, and the thrombus is dissolved by intralesional spray infusion of agents such as streptokinase, urokinase or recombinant tissue plasminogen activator. Percutaneous access thrombectomy also has been performed using balloon catheters (Beathard, 1994; Trerotola et al., 1994). After successful thrombolysis or thrombectomy, any underlying stenotic lesion can be identified by angiography, then treated by percutaneous transluminal angioplasty with or without endoluminal stenting. The immediate success rate of this type of procedure may be 90% (Pattynama et al., 1995; Valji et al., 1995). Restenosis is frequent, however, and may require repeated angioplasty.

Surgical thrombectomy is the alternative treatment, and many new technologies have been introduced. The standard surgical thrombectomy technique uses a conventional Fogarty balloon catheter. Although this technique is effective in removing soft new thrombus, it is less successful when older, adherent clot is present. Two new catheters, the adherent clot catheter and the graft thrombectomy catheter, are more effective in removing densely adherent thrombotic material. Angioscopy, which allows direct visualization of luminal surfaces and the identification of retained thrombus, also may prove to be helpful in treating the thrombosed vascular access conduit.

INFECTION

Although vascular access procedures are essentially clean operations, patients with end-stage renal failure are more susceptible to infection for many reasons. Uremia is associated with a reduction in the chemotactic, phagocytic and bacteriocidal actions of neutrophils as well as defects in T cell– and B cell–mediated immune responses (Haag-Weber and Hörl, 1993). Patients with renal disease have a 70% incidence of nasal, throat and skin colonization by *Staphylococcus aureus* compared with 15% in the general population (Yu et al., 1986). In view of these considerations, prophylactic antibiotics are essential when prosthetic materials such as e-PTFE are being used to create a graft AVF. The staphylococcal species found in renal patients have a high resistance to flucloxacillin, and the best choice of antibiotic is vancomycin.

Wound infection after a vascular access procedure must be treated seriously because there is a risk of massive secondary hemorrhage. The patient must be hospitalized until the situation has resolved completely. Relatively minor infections presenting with erythema and swelling can be managed by elevation and intravenous antibiotic therapy. If frank pus is present, the wound should be explored under general anesthesia, drained of all pus and thoroughly irrigated with saline or antibiotic solution. If the vascular anastomosis is directly infected, the risk of serious secondary hemorrhage is high, and the safest course of action is to ligate the fistula. Early infection associated with prosthetic graft material presents a particularly serious management problem. Superficial cellulitis can be treated by high-dose intravenous antibiotics, but for purulent infections the prosthetic graft must be removed.

ANEURYSM FORMATION

False and true aneurysms (Fig. 5–10) may occur in vascular access conduits. False aneurysms occur most commonly at venipuncture sites that have been overused. The incidence is 10% for PTFE grafts compared with 2% for autogenous

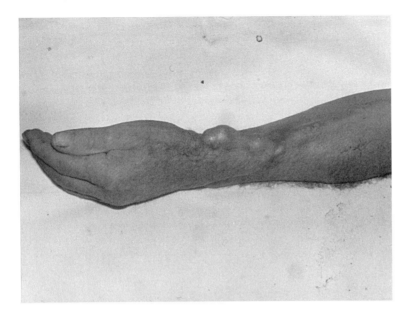

FIGURE 5–10

A true aneurysm of a left radiocephalic arteriovenous fistula.

AVFs (Zibari *et al.*, 1988). Treatment is by resection and restoration of the AVF by direct end-to-end anastomosis or by the placement of a short PTFE bridge graft. True aneurysmal dilatation of autogenous arterialized veins is relatively common. In many cases, no action is required, but if the overlying skin becomes thin and evidence of progressive expansion exists, corrective surgery is indicated. Localized aneurysms can be resected and continuity restored by direct end-to-end anastomosis. Alternatively, if the whole length of an arterialized segment of vein becomes aneurysmal, the AVF may have to be ligated.

VASCULAR STEAL SYNDROMES

A vascular steal is diagnosed when there is hypoperfusion of the limb (usually the arm) distal to the arteriovenous anastomosis. This hypoperfusion occurs most commonly after procedures involving the brachial artery and in patients with generalized arteriosclerosis and diabetes. The patient complains of a cold, weakened hand, and there may be pain and paresthesiae. The incidence of this complication can be reduced by careful attention to detail during the formation of AVF. Total fistula flow and steal can be limited by reducing the anastomotic length to 75% or less of the proximal arterial diameter; in most patients, this translates into an arteriotomy length of approximately 5 mm. Steal syndromes also can be caused by preexisting arterial lesions and must be investigated by an angiographic study from the aortic arch to the digital vessels. This study may show a distal stenosis that may be amenable to treatment by percutaneous transluminal angioplasty. Mild steal syndromes can be expected to improve spontaneously over a period of weeks, but in more severe cases further surgery is required to limit the fistula flow. This limitation of flow can be achieved by a crescent-shaped plication suture placed in the vein or graft just beyond the anastomosis (Rivers *et al.*, 1992). An elegant, albeit more complicated, alternative is to ligate the artery distal to the AVF anastomosis, then to perform a saphenous vein bypass from the proximal artery to a point beyond the ligature (Schanzer *et al.*, 1992). If these interventions are unsuccessful and in cases in which there are clinical signs of severe hand ischemia, the fistula should be ligated.

Arteriovenous Fistula Surveillance

The aim of fistula surveillance is to detect stenotic lesions before frank thrombosis occurs and to allow treatment of the failing fistula rather than the failed fistula (Schwab *et al.*, 1988). Methods of surveillance include regular clinical examination, monitoring of venous pressures during dialysis and measurement of urea recirculation (Schwab *et al.*, 1988). The failing fistula is characterized by rising venous pressures and poor flow, sometimes accompanied by a decrease in the palpable thrill or audible bruit. Color flow Doppler examination is another alternative for the detection of intimal hyperplasia; flow rates of less than 500 ml/min should arouse suspicion of venous or graft stenosis (Strauch *et al.*, 1992). Venous stenoses that are detected by surveillance can be confirmed by contrast fistulography and treated by procedures such as percutaneous angioplasty (Beathard, 1993), endoluminal stent placement (Beathard, 1993) or surgical revision (Etheredge *et al.*, 1983). The establishment of fistula surveillance programs has been shown to reduce significantly the incidence of vascular access thrombosis and to improve long-term patency rates (Nardi and Bosch, 1988; Schwab *et al.*, 1988).

Peritoneal Dialysis

Approximately 16% of the worldwide dialysis population are maintained on peritoneal dialysis, 85% of whom are on CAPD. In the United Kingdom, 51% of the dialysis population use peritoneal dialysis (Westman, 1993) compared with 9% in the United States (Winchester *et al.*, 1993). The concept behind peritoneal dialysis is straightforward. The peritoneal membrane is composed of endothelium, interstitium and mesothelium and can act as an efficient semipermeable membrane (Dobbie *et al.*, 1990). The total surface area of the peritoneal membrane is approximately 2.0 m². Infusing a hypertonic dialysate fluid into the peritoneal cavity allows ultrafiltration of solutes (urea and creatinine) and electrolytes (potassium). To remain reliable and functional, the important surgical considerations of this system are care and maintenance of the appropriate delivery system and the peritoneal cavity.

PERITONEAL DIALYSIS DELIVERY SYSTEMS AND CATHETERS

Peritoneal dialysis is a closed loop system comprising dialysate fluid, a delivery system and an indwelling peritoneal catheter (Fig. 5–11). Fluid is infused under gravity from a reservoir of dialysate contained in a plastic bag (Oreopoulos *et al.*, 1976). Luer-Lok or rotating safe lock devices have been devised to connect the dialysate with the delivery system for ease of connection and sterility.

The Italian Y delivery systems (Buoncristiani *et al.*, 1980) are the commonest. The single branch of the Y is connected to the indwelling peritoneal catheter in the patient by way of an inert titanium connector. The upper two branches are

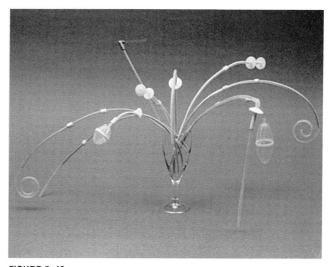

FIGURE 5–12

An assortment of peritoneal dialysis catheters.

connected to the dialysis reservoir and an empty bag. This configuration allows complete drainage of any contaminating dialysate fluid before infusion of sterile, fresh fluid through the indwelling delivery catheter (*flush before fill*) (see Fig. 5–11). Several randomized controlled trials have shown the superiority of various Y systems in reducing the incidence of infective complications when compared with conventional peritoneal dialysis systems (Churchill *et al.*, 1989; Maiorca *et al.*, 1983).

CATHETER SELECTION

Ideally CAPD catheters should be soft, flexible, atraumatic, radiopaque and relatively inert. Several different types of catheter are well recognized (Fig. 5–12), but the Tenckhoff catheter remains the most popular (Tenckhoff and Schechter, 1968). The original Silastic Tenckhoff design was a straight, 5-mm external diameter tube, with two Dacron cuffs (Tenckhoff and Schechter, 1968) and a perforated intraperitoneal segment. Many variations of the Tenckhoff device are available, including catheters with single Dacron cuffs and curled intraperitoneal ends. Curled catheters may result in lower rates of catheter migration when compared with the straight variety (Lye *et al.*, 1996; Rottemburg *et al.*, 1981).

CATHETER INSERTION

Not all patients are suitable for peritoneal dialysis. Severe peritoneal adhesions, previous sclerosing peritonitis and inflammatory bowel disease are absolute contraindications. Obesity, advanced age, lumbosacral osteoarthritis, abdominal hernias, stomas and chronic obstructive pulmonary disease are relative contraindications. Severe colonic diverticular disease may increase the translocation of gut organisms, and there is a strong association between diverticular disease and gram-negative peritoneal dialysis peritonitis. Although peritoneal dialysis can be performed in patients with abdominal wall stomas, there is also a predisposition to infection (Ribot *et al.*, 1982). Abdominal wall hernias (Fig. 5–13) may enlarge in patients receiving CAPD and should be repaired at the time of catheter insertion or at a later date.

CONTINUOUS AMBULATORY PERITONEAL DIALYSIS CATHETER INSERTION

A variety of techniques for catheter insertion have been described, including open under direct vision (surgical), per-

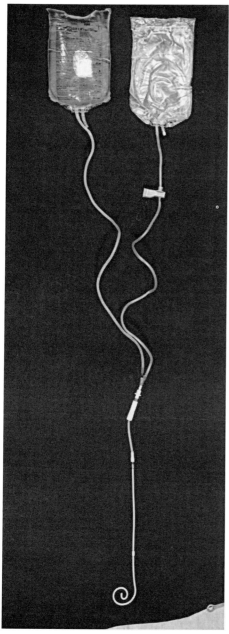

FIGURE 5–11

Peritoneal dialysis delivery system and catheter. A Y delivery system. The dialysate reservoir (left bag) and collecting bag (right) with a titanium connecter to the curled, single-cuffed Tenckhoff catheter.

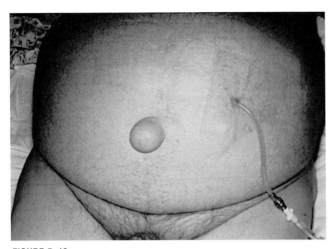

FIGURE 5–13

A reducible umbilical hernia protruding because of increased intraabdominal pressure from the infusion of peritoneal dialysis fluid.

cutaneous (blind) (Bierman *et al.*, 1985), peritoneoscopic (Cruz and Faber, 1989) and laparoscopic (Mutter *et al.*, 1994). Open and closed techniques can be performed with local or general anesthesia, the choice of which may be dictated by preexisting comorbidity, such as ischemic heart disease.

In the open surgical technique, the catheter is introduced through a small vertical infraumbilical incision placed in the midline or through a more lateral approach with the preperitoneal cuff positioned in the rectus abdominis muscle. Before positioning, the catheter should be flushed and immersed in sterile saline because wet cuffs stimulate more rapid ingrowth compared with dry, air-containing cuffs (Poirer *et al.*, 1986). A small incision is made in the peritoneum and the CAPD tube is inserted using blunt forceps or a metal stylet placed through the catheter lumen. The tip of the CAPD tube must be placed in the rectovesical pouch in males and the rectovaginal pouch in females (Fig. 5–14). The peritoneum is closed around the cuff to create a watertight seal. The linea alba or rectus sheath is closed using a continuous nonabsorbable suture (e.g., nylon). The extraperitoneal segment of the catheter is tunneled subcutaneously and brought out at a conveniently placed exit site. At the end of the procedure, the catheter should be flushed to ensure free inward and outward flow of dialysate fluid.

The percutaneous technique of peritoneal dialysis tube insertion requires a dilator introduced over a guidewire to develop a track into the peritoneal cavity (Bierman *et al.*, 1985). This track allows the introduction of a sheath through which the peritoneal dialysis tube can be inserted. In the peritoneoscopic technique, the peritoneal dialysis tube is also introduced through a single infraumbilical stab incision, but a 2.2-mm telescope is introduced first to inspect the peritoneal cavity (Adamson *et al.*, 1992; Pastan *et al.*, 1991). The laparoscopic method of insertion is a similar approach that requires a 10-mm trocar for insertion of the camera and usually two further 5-mm ports for the instruments used to manipulate the peritoneal dialysis tube into the pelvis (Amerling and Cruz, 1993; Brownlee and Elkhairi, 1997; Diaz-Buxo, 1991).

COMPLICATIONS

Peritonitis

Peritonitis is the most frequent complication of peritoneal dialysis and is an important cause of mortality (Chan *et al.*,

1981; Pollock *et al.*, 1989). Peritoneal dialysis peritonitis usually is caused by a single organism, with gram-positive bacteria such as *S. aureus*, *Staphylococcus epidermidis* or *Streptococcus* species accounting for 60 to 80% of all cases. Incidence rates in the United Kingdom and United States range from 0.5 to 1.4 episodes per patient per year (Bailie and Eisele, 1992). At least 60% of patients suffer an episode of peritonitis in the first year (Swartz, 1987), and at least a quarter culminate in catheter failure (Nicholson *et al.*, 1990). Some cases are caused by specific intraabdominal pathology, such as a perforated peptic ulcer or complicated diverticular disease. Fungal peritonitis also may occur and is particularly difficult to eradicate. Yeasts can gain access to the peritoneal cavity through the catheter or vagina. *Candida albicans* accounts for 75% of cases and is the commonest pathogen.

The first indications of peritonitis are abdominal pain in the presence of a cloudy effluent, containing greater than 100 cells × 10^6/L (85% polymorphonuclear cells) (Vas, 1983). Clinical signs usually are mild if the causative organism is a coagulase-negative staphylococcus. Routine investigations include an abdominal radiograph to check the catheter position and an erect chest radiograph to detect free gas, although a pneumoperitoneum is common in patients with peritoneal dialysis (Kiefer *et al.*, 1993). Dialysate fluid must be sent for culture but can be negative in 48% of patients with clinical signs suggestive of peritoneal dialysis peritonitis (von Graevenitz and Amsterdam, 1992). Blood cultures are rarely of value in mild cases (von Graevenitz and Amsterdam, 1992). Intraperitoneal antibiotics are the mainstay of treatment, which in many cases can be completed on an outpatient basis. The preferred regimen is gentamicin, 10 mg/2-L bag qds (every 8 hours), and vancomycin, 50 mg/2-L bag qds, for 5 to 10 days, although some centers advocate a cephalosporin instead of vancomycin. *Pseudomonas* species are particularly difficult organisms to treat (Craddock *et al.*,

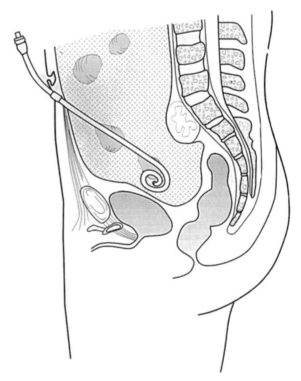

FIGURE 5–14

Correct anatomical positioning of the peritoneal dialysis catheter in the pelvis.

1987), and higher doses of gentamicin, 15 mg/2-L bag, in combination with oral ciprofloxacin, 750 mg twice a day, may be required for 3 to 4 weeks.

In cases of resistant or recurrent peritonitis that does not respond to 5 to 10 days of treatment, an exploratory laparotomy or laparoscopy should be performed with a view toward removing the tube. It may be possible to replace the tube once the episode has resolved. In selected cases, it is possible to replace the tube immediately (Paterson et al., 1986), but this strategy should be used with caution and is contraindicated in cases of fungal, pseudomonal, and mycobacterial peritonitis (Morton et al., 1987).

Catheter Obstruction

Catheter obstruction may be due to luminal or extrinsic obstructions and usually presents as a failure of outward fluid drainage. The presence of clotted blood and fibrin in the early postoperative period can be treated effectively by flushing the tube with heparin, urokinase or streptokinase (Palacious et al., 1982). Peritoneal dialysis catheter snaring by the omentum is a relatively common cause of catheter obstruction (Fig. 5–15) with reported rates of 15 to 32% (Reissman et al., 1998). This complication always requires a further operation and catheter exchange. Some surgeons advocate prophylactic omentectomy during open catheter insertion (Reissman et al., 1998), but the effectiveness of this maneuver has never been tested by a randomized trial. Extrinsic compression may be caused by bladder distention or a loaded sigmoid colon. Significant intraabdominal adhesions from previous abdominal surgery also can obstruct outflow.

Catheter Tip Migration

Long intraperitoneal catheter segments predispose to omental wrapping and tip migration out of the pelvic sump into the upper abdomen. Twardowski (1990) suggests that the incidence of catheter migration is 20%, but only 20% of these are obstructive. In most cases, the catheter needs to be repositioned at a further open or laparoscopic operation (Korten et al., 1983; Mutter et al., 1994). Repositioning using

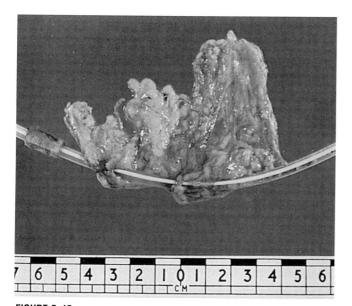

FIGURE 5–15
Catheter obstruction caused by omental wrapping.

a guidewire manipulated under radiological guidance also has been advocated (Jacques et al., 1980).

Peritoneal Dialysis Fluid Leaks

Peritoneal dialysis fluid leaks are relatively common, with rates of 7 to 24% being reported (Gloor et al., 1983; Mallonga et al., 1982; Nicholson et al., 1990). The two common sites for peritoneal dialysis fluid leaks are around the catheter insertion site and through a patent processus vaginalis. The point of leakage may cause diagnostic difficulty because the two most important causes both present with swelling in the subcutaneous tissues of the lower abdomen and scrotum. The best investigation for this situation is an abdominal computed tomography scan performed after an intraperitoneal injection of radiological contrast media (Twardowski et al., 1990). Leaks occurring in the early postoperative period are managed best by small volume exchanges or by resting the catheter and instituting temporary hemodialysis for 6 weeks. Late pericatheter leaks usually require catheter replacement, and scrotal leaks may respond to hernia repair.

Exit Site and Tunnel Infections

Exit site and tunnel infections are major sources of morbidity because they often lead to peritonitis and catheter removal (Piraino et al., 1996). An exit site infection has been defined broadly by Pierratos (1984). A healthy exit site is dry (Fig. 5–16A) without signs of inflammation such as redness, tenderness, scab or crust (Fig. 5–16B). Rates of exit site infections are 0.05 to 1.02 episodes per patient per year (Gupta et al., 1996; Piraino et al., 1996; Vogt et al., 1987). The commonest causal microorganism is S. aureus, but gram-negative enteric bacteria, S. epidermidis and mixed organisms may also be responsible. Nasal carriage of S. aureus is associated with a fourfold increased risk of developing an exit site infection (Luzar et al., 1990).

Double-cuffed catheters originally were thought to minimize exit site and tunnel infections by protecting the subcutaneous tunnel from colonization with skin commensals. Randomized controlled trials (Diaz-Buxo and Geissinger, 1984; Kim et al., 1984) have yet to show any difference between rates of infection. Exit site infections usually respond to treatment with appropriate intravenous or intraperitoneal antibiotics, but persistent and severe infections may resolve only if the peritoneal dialysis tube is exchanged and resited.

RENAL TRANSPLANT ISSUES

When a peritoneal dialysis patient receives a successful renal transplant, the peritoneal dialysis tube can be removed, but the timing of removal requires some judgment. In most cases, transplant recipients have their dialysis catheter removed during the first 2 to 3 months posttransplant. Earlier removal is an alternative when good early allograft function is expected, for example, after a live donor transplant. In contrast, the peritoneal dialysis catheter must be protected in patients who need to continue dialysis in the posttransplant period as a result of delayed graft function. Every effort must be made not to breach the peritoneum at the time of kidney implantation because this may lead to a peritoneal dialysis leak and the need for temporary hemodialysis. There is also a theoretical risk of serious peritransplant infection if peritoneal dialysis fluid leaks through into the transplant bed.

Active peritoneal dialysis peritonitis is an absolute contraindication to transplantation, but it may be safe to proceed with the operation if the patient has had several days of treatment with intraperitoneal antibiotics and the bags are

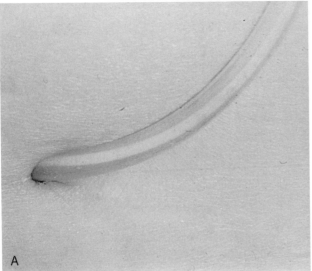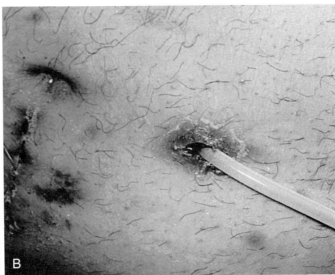

FIGURE 5–16

A pristine exit site of a peritoneal catheter (A) compared with an exit site showing primary infection (B).

clear (Ryckelynck *et al.*, 1984). Previous studies have high-lighted the risks of infection after renal transplantation. The incidence of peritonitis can be 35% (O'Donoghue *et al.*, 1992; Rubin *et al.*, 1987; Tsakiris *et al.*, 1985), but it usually is not life-threatening. Management strategies should include antibiotics and peritoneal lavage, and in resistant cases there should be a low threshold for catheter removal and conver-sion to hemodialysis. Patients receiving peritoneal dialysis at the time of transplantation have been shown to have significantly higher rates of infection compared with patients receiving hemodialysis (Passalacqua *et al.*, 1999). This risk appears to be reduced when patients convert to hemodialysis and peritoneal dialysis is discontinued just before trans-plantation (Passalacqua *et al.*, 1999). The risks can be reduced significantly if the catheter is removed within the first week of transplantation (Passalacqua *et al.*, 1999). Skin and enteric flora (e.g., *Escherichia coli*, enterococcus) are the commonest organisms that cause infection in patients having peritoneal dialysis after renal transplantation.

Studies comparing differences in graft survival rates be-tween patients receiving peritoneal dialysis or hemodialysis are contradictory. Some report no difference between either (Gokal *et al.*, 1981; Tsakiris *et al.*, 1985), whereas others have found improved graft survival in hemodialysis patients (Gu-illou *et al.*, 1984). It also has been suggested that rejection rates are 50% higher in peritoneal dialysis patients (Cardella, 1980; Gelfand *et al.*, 1984; Gokal *et al.*, 1981). A more recent study involving more than 9,000 renal transplant recipients has shown no difference between peritoneal dialysis or he-modialysis in terms of acute rejection rates (Bleyer *et al.*, 1999). There is also controversy over the relationship between the type of dialysis and rates of delayed graft function (Bleyer *et al.*, 1999; Weight *et al.*, 1998).

REFERENCES

Adamson, A. S., Kellecher, J. P., Snell, M. E. and Hulme, B. (1992). Endoscopic placement of of CAPD catheters: a review of 100 procedures. *Nephrol. Dial. Transplant.* **7**, 855.

Amerling, R. and Cruz, C. (1993). A new laparoscopic method for implantation of peritoneal catheters. *Am. J. Kidney Dis.* **39**, 787.

Bailie, G. R. and Eisele, G. (1992). Continuous ambulatory peritoneal dialysis: a review of its mechanics, advantages, complications and areas of controversy. *Ann. Pharmacother.* **26**, 1409.

Beathard, G. A. (1993). Gianturco self-expanding stent in the treat-ment of stenosis in dialysis access grafts. *Kidney Int.* **43**, 872.

Beathard, G. A. (1994). Mechanical versus pharmacomechanical thrombolysis for the treatment of thrombosed dialysis access grafts. *Kidney Int.* **45**, 1401.

Bender, M. H., Bruyninckx, C. M. and Gerlag, P. G. (1995). The Gracz arteriovenous fistula evaluated: results of the brachiocephalic el-bow fistula in hemodialysis angio-access. *Eur. J. Vasc. Endovasc. Surg.* **10**, 294.

Bierman, M., Kasperbauer, J., Kisek, A., *et al.* (1985). Peritoneal cathe-ter survival and complications in end stage renal disease. *Perit. Dial. Bull.* **5**, 229.

Bleyer, A. J., Burkart, J. M., Russell, G. B. and Adams, P. L. (1999). Dialysis modality and delayed graft function after cadaveric renal transplantation. *J. Am. Soc. Nephrol.* **10**, 154.

Bookstein, J. J. and Saldinger, E. (1985). Accelerated thrombolysis: in vitro evaluation of agents and methods of administration. *Invest. Radiol.* **20**, 731.

Brescia, M. J., Cimino, J. E., Appel, E. and Hurrwich, B. J. (1966). Chronic hemodialysis using venipuncture and a surgically cre-ated arteriovenous fistula. *N. Engl. J. Med.* **275**, 1089.

Brownlee, J. and Elkhairi, S. (1997). Laparoscopic assisted placement of peritoneal dialysis catheter: a preliminary experience. *Clin. Nephrol.* **47**, 122.

Buoncristiani, V., Bianchi, P., Cozzari, M., *et al.* (1980). A new safe simple connection system for CAPD. *Int. J. Nephrol. Urol. Androl.* **1**, 50.

Butterworth, P. C., Doughman, T. M., Wheatley, T. J. and Nicholson, M. L. (1998). Arteriovenous fistula using transposed basilic vein. *Br. J. Surg.* **85**, 653.

Butterworth, P. C., Swanevelder, J., Doughman, T., Wheatley, T. J. and Nicholson, M. L. (1997). Postoperative regional analgesia following basilic vein transposition for vascular access. *Br. J. Surg.* **84**, 561.

Canaud, B., Beraud, J. J., Joyeux, H. and Mion, C. (1986). Internal jugular vein cannulation using 2 Silastic catheters: a new, simple, and safe long-term vascular access for extracorporeal treatment. *Nephron* **43**, 133.

Cappello, M., De Pauw, L., Bastin, G., *et al.* (1989). Central venous access for haemodialysis using the Hickman catheter. *Nephrol. Dial. Transplant.* **4**, 988.

Cardella, C. J. (1980). Renal transplantation in patients on peritoneal dialysis. *Perit. Dial. Bull.* **1**, 12.

Cascardo, S., Acchiardo, S., Beven, E. G., Popowniak, K. L. and Nakamoto, S. (1970). Proximal arteriovenous fistulae for haemo-dialysis when radial arteries are unavailable. *Proc. Eur. Dial. Trans-plant. Assoc.* **7**, 42.

Chan, M. K., Baillod, R. M., Chuah, P., *et al.* (1981). Three years experience of continuous ambulatory peritoneal dialysis. *Lancet* **1**, 1409.

Churchill, D. N., Taylor, D. W., Vas, S. I., *et al.* (1989). Peritonitis in continuous ambulatory peritoneal dialysis (CAPD): a multi-center randomised clinical trial comparing y-connector disinfectant system to standard systems. *Perit. Dial. Int.* **9**, 159.

Coburn, M. C. and Carney, W. I., Jr. (1994). Comparison of basilic vein and polytetrafluoroethylene for brachial arteriovenus fistula. *J. Vasc. Surg.* **20**, 896.

Craddock, C. F., Edwards, R. and Finch, R. G. (1987). Pseudomonas peritonitis in continuous ambulatory peritoneal dialysis: laboratory predictors of treatment failure. *J. Hosp. Infect.* **10**, 179.

Cruz, C. and Faber, M. (1989). Peritoneoscopic implantation of catheters for peritoneal dialysis: effect of functional survival and incidence of tunnel infection. *Perit. Dial. Int.* **9A**, 35.

Dagher, F. J., Gleber, R. L. and Ramos, E. J. (1976). The use of the basilic vein and brachial artery as an a-v fistula for long term hemodialysis. *J. Surg. Res.* **20**, 373.

Diaz-Buxo, J. A. (1991). Mechanical complications of chronic peritoneal dialysis catheters. *Semin. Dial.* **4**, 106.

Diaz-Buxo, J. A. and Geissinger, W. T. (1984). Single cuff versus double cuff Tenckhoff catheter. *Perit. Dial. Bull.* **4**, S100.

Dobbie, J. W., Lloyd, J. K. and Gall, C. A. (1990). Categorisation of ultrastructural changes in peritoneal mesothelium, stroma and blood vessels in uremia and CAPD patients. *Adv. Perit. Dial.* **6**, 3.

Elcheroth, J., de Pauw, L. and Kinnaert, P. (1994). Elbow arteriovenous fistula for chronic haemodialysis. *Br. J. Surg.* **81**, 982.

Elcheroth, J., de Pauw, L. and Kinneart, P. (1995). Elbow arteriovenous fistulas for chronic haemodialysis: authors' reply. *Br. J. Surg.* **82**, 137.

Enzler, M. A., Rajmon, T., Lachat, M. and Largiader, F. (1996). Long term function of vascular access for hemodialysis. *Clin. Transplant.* **10**, 511.

Etheredge, E. E., Haid, S. D., Maeser, M. N., Sicard, G. A. and Anderson, Ch. B. (1983). Salvage operations for malfunctioning tetrapolyfluoroethylene hemodialysis access grafts. *Surgery* **94**, 464.

Garvin, P. J., Castaneda, M. A. and Codd, J. E. (1982). Etiology and management of bovine graft aneurysms. *Arch. Surg.* **117**, 281.

Gelfand, M., Kois, J., Quillan, B., *et al.* (1984). CAPD yields inferior transplant results compared to haemodialysis. *Perit. Dial. Bull.* **4(Suppl.)**, S26.

Gloor, H. J., Nichols, W. K., Sorkin, M. I., *et al.* (1983). Peritoneal access and related complications in continuous ambulatory peritoneal dialysis. *Am. J. Med.* **74**, 593.

Gokal, R., Ramos, J. M., Veitch, P. S., *et al.* (1981). Renal transplantation in patients in continuous peritoneal dialysis. *Proc. Eur. Dial. Transplant. Assoc.* **18**, 222.

Gracz, K. C., Ing, T. S., Soung, L. S., Armbruster, K. F. W., Seim, S. K. and Merkel, F. K. (1977). Proximal forearm fistula for maintenance hemodialysis. *Kidney Int.* **11**, 71.

Graevenitz von, A. and Amsterdam, D. (1992). Microbiological aspects of peritonitis associated with continuous ambulatory peritoneal dialysis. *Clin. Microbiol. Rev.* **5**, 36.

Guillou, P. J., Will, E. J., Davison, A. M. and Giles, G. R. (1984). CAPD: a risk factor for renal transplant. *Br. J. Surg.* **71**, 878.

Gupta, B., Bernardini, J. and Piraino, B. (1996). Peritonitis associated with exit site and tunnel infections. *Am. J. Kidney Dis.* **28**, 415.

Haag-Weber, M. and Hörl, W. H. (1993). Uremia and infection: mechanisms of impaired cellular host defence. *Nephron* **63**, 125.

Haimov, M. (1987). The peripheral subcutaneous arteriovenous fistula. In *Vascular Access: A Practical Guide*, (M. Haimov, ed.), p. 41, Future Publishing, New York.

Hobson, R. W., Croom, R. D. and Swan, K. G. (1973). Hemodynamic consequences of chronic experimental arteriovenous fistulas. *J. Surg. Res.* **14**, 483.

Jaques, P., Richey, W. and Mandel, S. (1980). Tenckhoff peritoneal dialysis catheter: cannulography and manipulation. *A. J. R. Am. J. Roentgenol.* **135**, 83.

Jensen, B. V., Vestersgaard Anderston, T. B. and Nielsen, P. H. (1990). Arteriovenous shunts used in hemodialysis: a retrospective study of the results in 86 patients treated during a 5-year period. *Ugeskr. Laeger.* **152**, 2169.

Karkow, W. S., Cranley, J. J., Cranley, R. D., Hafner, C. D. and Ruoff, B. A. (1986). Extended study of aneurysm formation umbilical vein grafts. *J. Vasc. Surg.* **4**, 489.

Kiefer, T., Schenk, U., Weber, J., Hubel, E. and Kulmann, U. (1993). Incidence and significance of pneumoperitoneum in continuous ambulatory peritoneal dialysis. *Am. J. Kidney Dis.* **22**, 30.

Kim, D., Burke, D., Igatt, S., *et al.* (1984). Single or double cuff peritoneal catheters? A prospective comparison. *Trans. Am. Soc. Artif. Intern. Organs* **30**, 232.

Koo Seen Lin, L. C. and Burnapp, L. (1996). Contemporary vascular access surgery for chronic haemodialysis. *J. R. Coll. Surg. Edinb.* **41**, 164.

Korten, G., Arendt, R., Brugmann, E. and Klein, B. (1983). Relocation of a peritoneal catheter without surgical intervention. *Perit. Dial. Bull.* **3**, 46.

Luzar, M. A., Coles, G. A., Faller, B., *et al.* (1990). Staphylococcus aureus nasal carriage in continuous ambulatory peritoneal dialysis patients a link to infection. *N. Engl. J. Med.* **322**, 505.

Lye, W. C., Kour, N. W., Straaten van der, J. C., Leong, S. O. and Lee, E. J. C. (1996). A prospective comparison of the swan neck, coiled and straight Tenckhoff catheters in patients on CAPD. *Perit. Dial. Int.* **16(Suppl. 1)**, S333.

Maiorca, R., Cantaluppi, A., Cancarini, G. C., *et al.* (1983). Prospective controlled trail of a Y connector and disinfectant to prevent peritonitis in continuous ambulatory dialysis. *Lancet* **2**, 642.

Mallonga, E. T., Coerorden van, T., Boeschoten, E. W., Southwood, J. and Krediet, R. (1982). Surgical problems in continuous ambulatory peritoneal dialysis (CAPD). *Neth. J. Surg.* **34**, 117.

Mannucci, P. M. (1988). Desmopressin: a nontransfusional form of treatment for congenital and acquired bleeding disorders. *Blood* **72**, 1449.

Marx, A. S., Landmann, J. and Harder, F. H. (1990). Surgery for vascular access. *Curr. Probl. Surg.* **27**, 1.

May, J., Harris, J. and Fletcher, J. (1980). Long-term results of saphenous vein graft arteriovenous fistulas. *Am. J. Surg.* **140**, 387.

Morton, A. R., Waldek, S. and Holmes, A. M. (1987). Removal and replacement of Tenckhoff catheters. *Lancet* **1**, 229.

Murphy, G. J., White, S. A., Knight, A. J., *et al.* (2000). Long-term results of arteriovenous fistula using transposed autologous basilic vein. *Br. J. Surg.* **87**, 819.

Mutter, D., Marichal, J. F., Heibel, F., Marescaux, J. and Hannedouche, T. (1994). Laparoscopy: an alternative to surgery in patients treated with continuous ambulatory peritoneal dialysis. *Nephron* **68**, 334.

Nardi, L. and Bosch, J. (1988). Recirculation: review, techniques for measurement and ability to predict hemoaccess stenosis before and after angioplasty. *Blood Purification* **6**, 85.

Nicholson, M. L., Donnelly, P., Burton, P., *et al.* (1990). Factors influencing peritoneal catheter survival in continuous ambulatory peritoneal dialysis. *Ann. R. Coll. Surg. Engl.* **72**, 368.

O'Donoghue, D., Manos, J., Pearson, R., *et al.* (1992). Continuous ambulatory peritoneal dialysis and renal transplantation: a ten year experience in one center. *Perit. Dial. Int.* **12**, 242.

Oreopoulos, D. G., Izatt, S., Zellerman, G., Karanicolas, S. and Matthews, R. E. (1976). A prospective study of the effectiveness of three permanent peritoneal catheters. *Proc. Clin. Dial. Forum* **6**, 96.

Palacious, M., Schley, W. and Dougherty, J. S. (1982). Use of streptokinase to clear peritoneal catheters. *Dial. Transplant.* **1**, 172.

Passalacqua, J. A., Wiland, A. M., Fink, J. C., Bartlett, S. T., Evans, D. A. and Keay, S. (1999). Increased incidence of postoperative infections associated with peritoneal dialysis in renal transplant recipients. *Transplantation* **68**, 535.

Pastan, S., Gassensmith, C., Manatunga, A. K., Copley, J. B., Smith, E. J. and Hamburger, R. J. (1991). Prospective comparison of peritoneoscopic and surgical implantation of CAPD catheters. *Am. J. Kidney Dis.* **37**, 154.

Paterson, A. D., Bishop, M. C., Morgan, A. G. and Burden, R. P. (1986). Removal and replacement of Tenckhoff catheter at a single operation: successful treatment of resistant peritonitis in continuous ambulatory peritoneal dialysis. *Lancet* **2**, 1245.

Pattynama, P. M., Baalen van, J., Verburgh, C. A., Pijl van der, J. W. and Schultze Kool, L. J. (1995). Revascularisation of occluded haemodialysis fistulae with the Hydrolyser thrombectomy catheter: description of the technique and report of six cases. *Nephrol. Dial. Transplant.* **10**, 1224.

Pierratos, A. (1984). A peritoneal dialysis glossary. *Perit. Dial. Bull.* **1**, 2.

Piraino, B. (1996). Management of catheter related infections. *Am. J. Kidney Dis.* **27**, 754.

Poirer, V. L., Daly, B. D. T., Dasse, K. A., Haudenschild, C. C. and Fine, R. E. (1986). Elimination of tunnel infection. *In Frontiers in Peritoneal Dialysis. Proceedings of the III International Symposium on Peritoneal Dialysis Washington, D.C., 1984*, (J. F. Maher and J. F. Winchester, eds.), p. 210, Field, Rich and Assoc, New York.

Pollock, C. A., Ibels, L. S., Caterson, R. J., Mahony, J. F., Waugh, D. A. and Cocksedge, B. (1989). Continuous ambulatory peritoneal dialysis: eight years of experience at a single centre. *Medicine (Baltimore)* **68**, 293.

Polo, J. R., Sanabia, J., Garcia-Sabrido, J. L., Luno, J., Menarguez, C. and Echenagusia, A. (1990). Brachio-jugular polytetrafluoroethylene fistulas for hemodialysis. *Am. J. Kidney Dis.* **5**, 465.

Polo, J. R., Tejedor, A., Polo, J., Sanabia, J., Calleja, J. and Gomez, F. (1995). Long-term follow-up of 6–8 mm brachioaxillary polytetrafluoroethylene grafts for haemodialysis. *Artif. Organs* **19**, 1181.

Quinton, W. E., Dillard, D. H. and Scribner, B. H. (1960). Cannulation of blood vessels for prolonged hemodialysis. *Trans. Am. Soc. Artif. Intern. Organs.* **6**, 104.

Rassat, J. P., *et al.* (1969). Artero-venous fistula in the anatomical snuff-box. *J. Urol. Nephrol.* **75**, 482.

Ready, A. R. and Buckels, J. A. C. (1995). Management of infection: vascular access surgery in hemodialysis. *In Vascular Access Principles and Practice*, (S. E. Wilson, ed.)

Reilly, D. T., Wood, R. F. M. and Bell, P. R. F. (1982). Five-year prospective study of dialysis fistulae: problem patients and their treatment. *Br. J. Surg.* **69**, 549.

Reissman, P., Lyass, S., Shiloni, E., Rivkind, A. and Berlatzky, Y. (1998). Placement of a peritoneal dialysis catheter with routine omentectomy—does it prevent obstruction of the catheter? *Eur. J. Surg.* **164**, 703.

Remuzzi, G. (1988). Bleeding in renal failure. *Lancet* **1**, 1205.

Ribot, R., Goldblat, C. and Bocchino, C. (1982). Intermittent peritoneal dialysis in a patient with a colostomy. *Perit. Dial. Bull.* **2**, 98.

Rivers, S. P., Scher, L. A. and Veith, F. J. (1992). Correction of steal syndrome secondary to hemodialysis access fistulas: a simplified quantitive technique. *Surgery* **112**, 593.

Rottemburg, J., Dominque, J., Lantehan von, M., Issad, B. and Shahat, Y. E. (1981). Straight or curled Tenckhoff peritoneal catheter for continuous ambulatory peritoneal dialysis (CAPD). *Perit. Dial. Bull.* **1**, 123.

Ryckelynck, J. P., Verger, C., Pierre, D., Sabatier, J. C., Faller, B. and Beaud, J. M. (1984). Early post-transplantation infections in CAPD patients. *Perit. Dial. Bull.* **4**, 40.

Schanzer, H., Skladany, M. and Haimov, M. (1992). Treatment of angioaccess-induced ischaemia by revascularization. *J. Vasc. Surg.* **16**, 861.

Schwab, S. J., Quarles, D., Middleton, J. P., *et al.* (1988). Hemodialysis-associated subclavian vein stenosis. *Kidney Int.* **33**, 1156.

Schwab, S. J., Raymond, J. R., Saeed, M., *et al.* (1989). Prevention of haemodialysis fistula thrombosis: early detection of venous stenoses. *Kidney Int.* **36**, 707.

Someya, S., Bergan, J. J., Kahan, B. D., Yao, S. T. and Ivanovich, P.

(1976). An upper arm A-V fistula for haemodialysis patients with distal access failures. *Trans. Am. Soc. Artif. Intern. Organs* **22**, 398.

Strauch, B. S., O'Coneel, R. S., Geody, K. L., Grundlehner, M., Yakub, N. and Tietjen, D. P. (1992). Forecasting thrombosis of vascular access with doppler color flow imaging. *Am. J. Kidney Dis* **19**, 554.

Swartz, R. D. (1987). Chronic peritoneal dialysis: mechanical and infectious complications. *Nephron* **40**, 29.

Tenckhoff, H. and Schechter, H. (1968). A bacteriologically safe peritoneal access device. *Trans. Am. Soc. Artif. Intern. Organs* **14**, 181.

Trerotola, S. O., Lund, G. B., Scheel, Jr., P. J., Savader, S. J., Venbrux, A. C. and Osterman, Jr., F. A. (1994). Thrombosed dialysis access grafts: percutaneous mechanical declotting without urokinase. *Radiology* **191**, 721.

Tsakiris, D., Bramwell, S., Briggs, J., and Junor, B. J. R. (1985). Transplantation in patients undergoing CAPD. *Perit. Dial. Bull.* **5**, 161.

Twardowski, Z. J. (1990). Malposition and poor drainage of peritoneal catheters. *Semin. Dial.* **3**, 57.

Twardowski, Z. J., Tully, R. J., Ersoy, F. F. and Dedhia, N. M. (1990). Computerized tomography with and without intraperitoneal contrast for determination of intraabdominal fluid distribution and diagnosis of complications in peritoneal dialysis patients. *A.S.A.I.O. Trans.* **36**, 95.

Valenta, J., Bilek, J. and Opatrny, K. (1985). Autogenous saphenis vein graft as secondary vascular access for hemodialysis. *Dial. Transplant.* **14**, 567.

Valji, K., Bookstein, J. J., Roberts, A. C., Oglevie, S. B., Pittman, C. and O'Neill, M. P. (1995). Pulse-spray pharmacomechanical thrombosed hemodialysis access grafts: long-term experience and comparison of original and current techniques. *A. J. R. Am. J. Roentgenol.* **164**, 1495.

Vas, S. (1983). Microbiological aspects of CAPD. *Kidney Int.* **23**, 88.

Vogt, K., Binswanger, U., Buchmann, P., *et al.* (1987). Catheter related complications during continuous ambulatory peritoneal dialysis (CAPD): a retrospective study on sixty-two double cuff Tenckhoff catheters. *Am. J. Kidney Dis.* **10**, 47.

Weight, S. C., Horsburgh, T., Harris, K. P. G., Khurshid, M., Bell, P. R. F. and Nicholson, M. L. (1998). Delayed graft function and allograft survival: does the type of post transplant dialysis influence outcome? *Nephrol. Dial. Transpl.* **13**, 2427.

Westman, J. (1993). *World-wide Dialysis Update*, annual survey by Baxter Healthcare Inc., Deerfield, Ill.

Wilson, S. E., Owens, M. L., Ozeran, R. S. and Rosental, J. L. (1988). Vascular grafts (bridge fistulas) for haemodialysis. *In Vascular Access Surgery*, (S. E. Wilson, ed.), p. 243, Year Book Medical Publishers, Chicago.

Winchester, J. F., Rotellar, C., Goggins, M., *et al.* (1993). Transplantation in peritoneal dialysis and hemodialysis. *Kidney Int.* **43(Suppl. 40)**, 101.

Yu, V. L., Goetz, A., Wagener, M., *et al.* (1986). Staphylococcus aureus nasal carriage and infection in patients on hemodialysis. *N. Engl. J. Med.* **315**, 91.

Zibari, G. B., Rohr, M. S., Landrenau, M. D., *et al.* (1988). Complications from permanent haemodialysis vascular access. *Surgery* **104**, 681.

Brain Stem Death: The Evolution of a Concept

C. Pallis

Introduction

There is only one kind of human death: the irreversible loss of the capacity for consciousness combined with the irreversible loss of the capacity to breathe (and hence to sustain a spontaneous heart beat). Death, thus conceived, can arise from primary catastrophes within the head. Or it can be the intracranial consequence of extracranial events, such as circulatory arrest. Such arrest will prove lethal only if it lasts long enough for the brain stem to die. All death, in this perspective, is brain stem death—for the key functions that define a human being as an independent biological unit (the capacity to be conscious and the capacity to breathe) are subserved by the brain stem.

This chapter presents the evidence for these conclusions. A failure to define death is identified as a main cause of inconclusive discussions about brain death. It is argued that if the brain stem is dead, the brain as a whole cannot function and that if the brain has permanently lost the ability to function, the individual is dead. The evolution of the concept of brain stem death is described. It is shown how a dead (i.e., irreversibly nonfunctioning) brain stem can be diagnosed at the bedside, without resorting to complicated investigations. Finally, it is demonstrated that a dead brain stem (whatever its philosophical or legal status) predicts inevitable asystole within a short while.

Although the concept of "brain death" is important to those involved in organ transplantation, it was not invented for their benefit. The original account of *coma dépassé* (Mollaret and Goulon, 1959) discussed the implications of a dead brain in some detail but did not speculate about organ transplantation. Ten years had to pass before the renal transplant rate, in the entire United Kingdom, was to exceed one/week (Jennett, 1981). If transplantation were superseded tomorrow by better methods of treating end-stage renal failure, brain death would still, unfortunately, occur in large numbers of patients wherever intensive care units are established. The subject clearly has wide implications.

What Do We Mean by Death?

Unless death is defined, the decision that a person is "dead" cannot be verified by any amount of scientific investigation or by any particular combination of tests. This is because technical data can never answer purely conceptual questions. When we ask, "What is it that is so essential to the nature of humans that its loss is called 'death'?" we should realize (1) that there are several possible answers, (2) that these will vary according to cultural context and (3) that the question itself is essentially philosophical or moral, not medical or scientific (Veatch, 1972). Criteria of death—and *ipso facto* arguments about better criteria—must be related to

some overall concept of what death means. The tests we carry out and the decisions we make should be logically derived from the explicit conceptual and philosophical premises.

Whereas the functions of the lungs and heart can be taken over by machines, those of the brain cannot. An individual can therefore be dead only when the brain is dead. This emphasis on the brain is very old, not radically new as is sometimes thought. It has been unconsciously perceived for centuries, if not millennia, by people with little or no knowledge of physiology. Our ancestors were hanging and decapitating one another long before William Harvey had shown that circulation existed. Figure 6–1 illustrates the general relation between the brain and the heart. It depicts a public execution in a Bangkok square in the early 1930s. The head has been severed, but jets of blood from the carotid and vertebral arteries show that the heart is still beating. Would anyone describe the victim (as distinct from some of his organs) as still alive? As we think the implications through, we are taking the first step toward understanding brain death. It is "physiological decapitation."

We can go further. We can be more specific about which parts of the brain relate most relevantly to various concepts of death. The capacity for consciousness is an *upper* brain stem function, dependent on alertness (i.e., on an intact ascending reticular-activating system). It is "represented" in the tegmental parts of the midbrain and rostral pons, where small, strategically situated lesions cause permanent coma.

The *capacity* for consciousness (a brain stem function) is not the same as the *content* of consciousness (a hemisphere function) but is an essential precondition of the latter. If there is no functioning brain stem, there can be no meaningful or integrated activity of the cerebral hemispheres, no cognitive or affective life, no thoughts or feelings and no social interaction with the environment—nothing that might legitimize our adding the adjective *sapiens* to the noun *Homo*. The capacity for consciousness is perhaps the nearest we can get to giving a biological flavor to the notion of "soul."

The capacity to breathe spontaneously is also a brain stem function, and apnea is a crucial sign of a nonfunctioning *lower* brain stem. Alone, of course, it does not imply death (patients with bulbar poliomyelitis are clearly not dead). Although irreversible apnea has no strictly philosophical dimension, it is useful to include it in any concept of death. This is mainly because of its cultural associations.* It has

---

*The words that stand for "soul" are in many languages the same as those for "breath": *nephesh* in Hebrew, *ruach* in Aramaic, *pneuma* in Greek, *spiritus* in Latin, *nafas* and *nefs* in Arabic and *ghost* in the old English sense. All these had the primary meaning of breath. The Bible of Jews and Christians was fairly explicit concerning the association: "and the Lord had fashioned man of dust of the earth, and instilled in his nostrils the breath of life, and man became a living creature" (Genesis 2:7). No early religious source mentions heart beat or pulse in the determination of death.

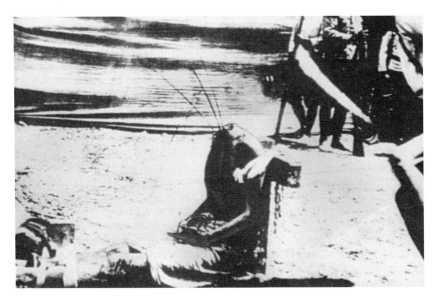

FIGURE 6–1

A public execution in a Bangkok square in the early 1930s. The head has been severed, but jets of blood from the carotid and vertebral arteries show that the heart is still beating. Would anyone describe the victim (as distinct from some of his organs) as still alive? This is anatomical decapitation. Brain death has been described as "physiological decapitation."

been argued (Pallis, 1986) that the irreversible loss of the capacity for consciousness (from destruction of the reticular formation) and "irreversible apnea" (from destruction of respiratory mechanisms in the lower brain stem) are merely the secular equivalents—expressed in the language of modern neurophysiology—of older concepts, prevalent in those cultures that identified death with either the "departure of the soul" from the body and/or the loss of the "breath of life."

Much ground has been covered (both technologically and conceptually) over the last 20 years. Those with a sense of history (and with available time) will enjoy exploring how far we have indeed traveled. In 1966, Wolstenholme and O'Connor collected some seminal discussion documents on the subject. These describe the then prevailing views and highlight the pioneering vision of Dr. G. P. S. Alexandre (of Louvain, Belgium). At a time when most of today's leading transplant surgeons were proclaiming their reluctance to "accept a person as being dead as long as there was a heartbeat," Alexandre was arguing that organs could legitimately be taken from human "heart-lung preparations." The proceedings of this symposium can be contrasted with other texts (Lamb, 1988; Pallis, 1987) seeking to explore in greater depth (and even to correlate) the philosophical and physiological meanings of death.

From Brain Death to Brain Stem Death

Modern technology, in its attempts to save human life, has created many new problems. Brain death is one of them and from its inception the subject has been bedeviled by controversy. The challenges have been clinical, conceptual, ethical and terminological. Unrelated matters ("allowing to die") and extraneous considerations (such as transplantation) have often caught the public eye but obscured the central issue.

Arguments about brain death have highlighted tensions between science and ethics (should one ventilate to asystole?), between enthusiasts (what new test should we use?) and skeptics (what exactly are we testing for, anyway?) and between physicians practicing in different environments (how would a hostile lawyer see all this?). These controversies can be understood only in a historical context. They will not abate. They will, in fact, increase as intensive care facilities develop in new areas of the world and as the people there seek to incorporate into their culture the meaning of a

dead brain in a body whose heart is still kept beating. The basic issues are not difficult and, if approached systematically, can be grasped readily.

Two early accounts of brain death are first given, which epitomize much of what was to follow. Angiographic and electrophysiological attempts to identify a dead brain are then reviewed. It is suggested that both approaches pursue unsuccessfully an unachievable end (the demonstration of the death of all cells in the brain) and that this objective is, moreover, inappropriate because only part of it (the death of the brain stem) is related to a meaningful overall concept of death.

FIRST ACCOUNTS: FIRST CONTROVERSIES

Early in 1959, a group of neurosurgeons from Lyons (France) described a condition they termed "death of the nervous system" (Wertheimer *et al.*, 1959; Jouvet, 1959). It was seen in patients with structural brain lesions (usually traumatic) and was most likely to occur when the trauma had been complicated at a later time by respiratory arrest. It was characterized by persistent apneic coma, absent brain stem and tendon reflexes and an electrically silent brain. The patients looked like cadavers, but had a regular pulse as long as artificial respiration was maintained. Disconnection from the ventilator produced no respiratory response. The relevant neurons in the brain stem were dead because they were "incapable of responding to their most potent habitual stimulus: hypercapnia." The authors equated the condition with the heart-lung preparation of the physiologists.

Persistence with resuscitatory efforts, it was argued, was justifiable in this context only if there was some chance that neural function would return. However, the death of the nervous system could be ascertained only if it was properly looked for. The scalp electroencephalogram (EEG) was only a distant echo of what might be going on below. What was needed was an exploration, in depth, by means of "fine, sterile, bipolar electrodes, passed through burr-holes in the direction of the median thalamic structures." As the probes are advanced from cortex to midline, strong electrical stimuli (up to 140 V) should be delivered at varying frequencies. These should produce no motor responses. Direct stimulation of the sciatic nerves—and of the thalamus itself—should also be resorted to and produce no recordable trace at scalp level.

All these procedures were actually carried out. There were

no responses, and the authors concluded that, in their patients, both diencephalon and cortex were dead. They suggested that in this kind of clinical context, and if efforts at resuscitation had proved unsuccessful over 18–24 hours, negative electrical tests (repeated at intervals of 2–3 hours) amounted to unequivocal evidence of the "irreversible death of the central nervous system." Disconnection from the respirator was warranted. The authors did not address the issue of whether the patients (as distinct from their nervous system) were alive or dead at the time.

Some months later, a much fuller account of the same condition was published by two Parisian neurologists (Mollaret and Goulon, 1959). They called it *coma dépassé* (a state beyond coma). Twenty of their 23 patients were suffering from various structural intracranial lesions and the other 3 from the neurological sequelae of cardiorespiratory arrest. The account was a masterpiece of clinical observation and enlightened speculation. It stressed the disintegration not only of all "relational" responses between the individual and the outside world but also of basic internal homeostatic mechanisms (the patients were poikilothermic, developed diabetes insipidus and their blood pressure could be maintained for a while only with pressor amines). The EEG was "flat" and unresponsive to external stimuli. Even recording from the thalamus or neighboring areas could not tell one with certainty that all brain cells were dead. Could not a few neurons be surviving somewhere? The authors spoke of the difficulties in tracing the "ultimate frontiers of life," but were not prepared to equate *coma dépassé* with death. Unlike Jouvet (1959), they did not advocate withdrawal of ventilatory support. The state of *coma dépassé* was both a revelation (of the capacities of modern resuscitation and intensive care units) and a ransom (because of what the maintenance of patients in this state imposed on others).

Both accounts were written 30 years ago, but their dissonance is strangely modern. In both cases the facts observed at the bedside implied the death of the nervous system as a whole. What did this, in turn, imply concerning the status of the patients? Neither group had discussed the meaning of death, and it is not surprising that they reached different conclusions as to what, in practice, should be done. Similar dilemmas, with somewhat similar roots, were to plague both the angiographic and the neurophysiological approaches to the subject. An increasing mass of technical data proved difficult to interpret. It was not always clear to what question the facts were to provide the answer. Difficulties increased when people began to realize that some of the questions themselves, when identified, were conceptually ill-founded. Advancement proved possible only when sensible and clinically relevant problems were addressed in acceptable philosophical contexts.

THE ANGIOGRAPHIC APPROACH

The basic idea was very simple. If one could demonstrate a total and sustained absence of cerebral blood flow, it followed that every nerve cell in the brain would be dead. That meant a dead patient. What happened to the heart—and when—was as irrelevant as what happened to the circulation in a case of decapitation. The proof that the brain was dead could be made a straightforward down-to-earth technical matter.

Since the early 1950s, neuroradiologists and neurosurgeons have repeatedly demonstrated the phenomenon of "cerebral circulatory arrest" (or "blocked cerebral circulation"). This angiographic finding was common in apneic and comatose patients dying from the effects of head injury, intracranial hemorrhage or other structural brain lesions (Riisehde

and Ethelberg, 1953; Gros *et al.*, 1959; Lofstedt and von Reis, 1959; Lecuire *et al.*, 1962; Heiskanen, 1964; Bergquist and Bergström, 1972). Its basis was intracranial hypertension of such severity that it interfered with cerebral perfusion. Both cerebral edema and the mechanical effects of tentorial pressure cones were pathologically important. In such patients, apnea had catastrophic effects on an already compromised cerebral circulation. The physical signs seen in such cases were those of *coma dépassé*. Some 50% of patients with fatal head injuries probably go through such a phase before the heart stops (Jennett, 1981). A decade or two ago attempts to show a "blocked" cerebral circulation were widely resorted to in the search for "objective evidence" of brain death.

By an irony of fate, it was technical problems that were to prove the undoing of this approach. There were problems in moving respirator-dependent patients to x-ray departments for invasive procedures. Fears were expressed about hypotension, bradycardia and the possible effects of introducing hypertonic contrast material into partially obstructed vessels. Carotid angiography occasionally revealed a blocked circulation, and vertebral injection still revealed some flow (Heiskanen, 1964; Bücheler *et al.*, 1970; Vlahovitch *et al.*, 1971; Rosenklint and Jørgensen, 1974). Four-vessel angiography was therefore required: not once, but twice—because the death of an organ could be considered as proved only if that organ had remained deprived of its blood flow during a period that exceeded its ability to survive circulatory arrest (Brock *et al.*, 1969). The Swedish code was to recommend just that (Ingvar and Widén, 1972). Anxieties began to be voiced. The objective, after all, was to diagnose brain death, not cause it.

Other problems emerged. Angiography began to yield an unacceptably high proportion of disturbing results. A blocked cerebral circulation was shown to be compatible with the persistence, for a short while, of some EEG activity (Brock *et al.*, 1969; Ashwal and Schneider, 1979). Bricolo *et al.* (1972) mentioned six patients with vascular "nonfilling" *and* silent EEGs who had "clear signs of cerebral life." "No-flow" situations were demonstrated that proved reversible after evacuation of subdural hematomas (Bricolo *et al.*, 1972), the emergency removal of a very large tumor (Riishede and Ethelberg, 1953, case 5), tapping the ventricles (Riishede and Ethelberg, 1953, case 2; Pribram, 1961; Bricolo *et al.*, 1972) or a cyst (Gros *et al.*, 1959, case 3) or following the combined effects of hyperventilation and mannitol (Bricolo *et al.*, 1972).

More sophisticated technology stepped into the breach. Attempts were made to assess cerebral blood flow by noninvasive means. The clinical diagnosis of brain death would be confirmed by mobile γ-probes placed over the head (Goodman *et al.*, 1969) or over the head and femoral artery (Korein *et al.*, 1977) as the "patients" were given bolus intravenous injections of the radioisotope technetium 99m sodium pertechnetate. Many technical difficulties were laboriously overcome.

The main shortcoming of the radioisotopic techniques is that they do not enable one to ascertain circulation in the posterior fossa (Kricheff *et al.*, 1978). "If the physician wished to include brain stem death in his diagnosis" (perversely, most physicians did), "he would have to use additional criteria" (Korein *et al.*, 1977). These would presumably be clinical, because the EEG does not relate to brain stem function. Back to square one. Because the vertebrobasilar circulation is as vital to the continuation of life as that of the coronaries, one wonders why so much effort was spent in investigations that missed the central point.

Computed tomography (CT) scanning (after intravenous contrast injection) has been advocated to demonstrate absent cerebral blood flow in brain-dead individuals (Arnold *et al.*, 1981; Handa *et al.*, 1982). The technique is noninvasive, and it has been claimed that flow through the vertebrobasilar system can be assessed readily provided the appropriate "slices" are selected. The lower limits of cerebral blood flow detectable by CT scanning are not yet known.

The results were published of a major study (Jørgensen, 1974b) covering three intensive care units in Copenhagen, which was seeking to correlate the clinical, electroencephalographic and angiographic features of brain death. By 1981, the author's experience of comatose and apneic patients encompassed some 600 cases. He was able to conclude (Jørgensen, 1981) that certain crucial *clinical* signs (persistent apnea and persistently absent brain stem reflexes), when encountered in patients with primary intracranial lesions or in patients "successfully" resuscitated from cardiac arrest, were sufficient to make a diagnosis of irreversible loss of brain stem function. Asystole was then inevitable. "Sooner or later" all such patients developed a blocked cerebral circulation or an isoelectric EEG. In other words, although angiography provided a pathophysiological explanation for the neurological signs in such cases, it added nothing of diagnostic or prognostic significance. At some possible cost to the patient, it gave confidence (to those who lacked it) in the prognostic significance of the physical signs.

Further objections to the angiographic diagnosis of brain death (this time based on the interests of the potential recipients of organs from such sources) have been voiced. Weibull *et al.* (1987) confirmed the transient nephrotoxic effect of iodinated contrast media and showed how the outcome of renal transplantation from brain-dead donors differed significantly in two Swedish centers, according to whether the kidneys were removed within 2 hours, or only some 24 hours after the angiographic demonstration of a blocked cerebral circulation. Delayed removal of the kidneys enhanced the "take rate." In each group of ex-patients, the kidneys were harvested only after disconnection from ventilatory support (as currently required by Swedish law).

THE ELECTROPHYSIOLOGICAL APPROACH

Here too, the basic idea was very simple. If the brain was electrically silent (as assessed by EEG) and if reversible causes for such a state of affairs (such as hypothermia or drug intoxication) had been excluded, the brain must be dead. The longer the period of electrical silence, the greater the likelihood that it would prove permanent.

The main argument about the EEG is conceptual, not technical. To what overall concept of death does the EEG criterion (of electrocerebral silence) relate? Whether they realize it or not, the advocates and the detractors of the EEG are pursuing different objectives related to different concepts of death. The former are seeking to diagnose the biological "death of the whole brain"—that is, the death of most, if not all, brain cells. With this particular objective in mind, the scalp EEG may be considered relevant (provided one remembers that it is quite incapable of achieving the desired end). Those who claim that the EEG is irrelevant are seeking to diagnose death of the brain as a functional unit (death of the "brain as a whole"). They do this by concentrating on what allows the brain to function as a unit: the brain stem. In pursuit of this different objective, the EEG is indeed irrelevant. Recording an EEG from the scalp is not testing a brain stem function.

The earliest attempts to define electrical parameters of brain death in deeply comatose patients were those of Jouvet (1959). Others were to follow. Schwab *et al.* (1963) stated that the EEG "should show flat lines, without any rhythms in all leads, over a 30 minute period." Hamlin (1964) suggested "flat lines with no rhythms in any leads for at least 60

minutes, with no EEG response to auditory or somatic stimuli." Terminological disputes, partly reflecting stricter specifications of the conditions under which the record was to be taken, broke out. References to a "flat" EEG were clearly insufficient. More than mere "low voltage" was required. The scalp EEG had to reflect "electrocerebral silence" (Arfel *et al.*, 1963), be "isoelectric" (Kimura *et al.*, 1968), "equipotential" (Pampiglione and Harden, 1968) or "isopotential" (Bickford *et al.*, 1971).

By 1968, great emphasis was being put on the gains. The EEG had to be flat at "gains of 10 μV/mm to 5 μV/mm" (Rosoff and Schwab, 1968). By the following year, the EEG requirements had escalated. An *ad hoc* Committee of the American Electroencephalographic Society (Silverman *et al.*, 1969) was recommending that there should be "no cerebral activity over 2 μV" and prescribing nine strict specifications for the recordings. Some time later, in a meticulously conducted study from a leading electrophysiological laboratory, it was found that at really high amplifications (0.1–0.3 μV mm^{-1}) the "EEG was never isoelectric" (Jørgensen and Brodersen, 1971; Jørgensen, 1974a). After all known sources of extracerebral interference had been identified and subtracted from the EEG, one was left with a situation in which one could never be certain whether or not "noise" (activity created in the measuring circuit) might be masking very low voltage signals of cortical origin. Meanwhile, awkward cases continued to be described in which thalamic probing had shown persistent neuronal discharges in the presence of an "isoelectric" EEG (Carbonell *et al.*, 1963; Visser, 1969; Jonkman, 1969). Was a return to Jouvet (1959) on the horizon?

It is against this background of shifting definitions that one has to seek to assess the significance of the isoelectric EEG.* As will be emphasized, the question of context is all important.

THE REVERSIBLE ISOELECTRIC EEG

A great deal has been published concerning the significance of an isoelectric EEG in cases of drug intoxication (Goulon *et al.*, 1967; Haider *et al.*, 1971) or severe hypothermia. Severe metabolic upsets (hypoglycemia, uremia) may also profoundly (and reversibly) affect the EEG, the changes again being most marked in the presence of hypoxia. Most codes of practice dealing with brain death warn against diagnosing the condition of such contexts.

Circulatory arrest is probably the most common (and certainly an insufficiently stressed) cause of a reversible isoelectric EEG. For obvious reasons, EEGs are seldom recorded on patients suffering from cardiac arrest. If the arrest occurs during EEG monitoring, the record will very promptly become isoelectric. On reestablishment of the circulation, an isoelectric EEG will, for a while, still be found in as many as 30% of patients (Jørgensen and Malchow-Møller, 1981). These authors reported on 125 such patients who were serially monitored (both clinically and electrically) over several hours. In the 37 who subsequently regained consciousness, the cranial nerve reflexes always returned before any change in the isoelectric EEG. The return of any kind of EEG activity could be delayed for as long as 8 hours. Failure of certain cranial nerve reflexes to reappear was an early prognostic sign of considerable value. As the authors drily put it, "Any patient with a reversible circulatory arrest . . . who presents cranial nerve areflexia for as long as it takes to record an

---

*A shortcut to the assessment of many early publications is a quick glance at the voltage calibrations on the published traces. If there are none or if the illustrations suggest low gain settings, there can be no guarantee that the record was in fact "isoelectric."

EEG or to check the intracerebral circulation will have the diagnosis of brain death confirmed."

Two queries are particularly relevant when discussing the EEG diagnosis of brain death.

Do patients with irremediable structural brain damage ever survive with an isoelectric EEG? The answer is yes. A number of cases have now been recorded where anoxia devastated the cerebral cortex but allowed some brain stem functions to persist (Bennett *et al.*, 1971; Brierley *et al.*, 1971; Pollack and Kellaway, 1978; Cranford and Smith, 1979; Keane, 1979). The same state of affairs has been reported following trauma (Bricolo *et al.*, 1972), streptococcal meningitis (Pollack and Kellaway, 1978) and herpes simplex encephalitis (Pollack and Kellaway, 1978). Some children with hydranencephaly may be in a similar state. Patients in this group will be in a persistent vegetative state, not coma, because usually they open their eyes. Most will breathe spontaneously. Because their brain stems are still functioning, they may live for weeks, months or years.

Do patients with irremediable structural brain damage and clinical signs of brain stem death (apneic coma and absent brain stem reflexes) ever show any residual EEG activity? Again, the answer is yes, but this does not imply that the "patient as a whole" or even that the "brain as a whole" is still alive. When the brain stem dies, the patient sustains the "irreversible loss of the capacity for consciousness" and the "irreversible loss of the capacity to breathe" that I have equated with death (see Introduction). Such minimal EEG activity that may persist for a short while is doomed to extinction (Goulon, 1966; Lindgren *et al.*, 1968; Gaches *et al.*, 1970; Lévy-Alcover and Babinet, 1970; Mohandas and Chou, 1971; Walker and Molinari, 1975; Rappaport *et al.*, 1978; Ayim and Clark, 1979; Hicks and Torda, 1979; Ashwal and Schneider, 1979; Powner and Fromm, 1979; Jennett *et al.*, 1981; Caronna and Plum, 1982). Its persistence may raise false hopes among relatives and even some physicians. It is a question of attitude (rather than of physiology) whether it is ever warranted to record EEGs to reassure relatives, if one knows (and they do not), that such records can only show steady deterioration. Because they have dead brain stems, these "beating-heart cadavers" all soon develop asystole.

Those who hold that minimal residual EEG activity is of some significance in the context of a dead brain stem should reassess their aims. Are they really seeking to track down the last gasping neuron in the cranial cavity? If so, are they prepared to follow the path traced for them by Jouvet (1959; see Introduction)?

Table 6–1 (Pallis, 1981) summarizes the respective prognostic implications, in terms of cardiac function, of an isoelectric EEG and of clinical signs of brain stem death in patients with structural brain damage. No drug-induced cases are included in the totals. It will be seen that the crucial issue is not the EEG but the clinical state of the brain stem. Other arguments concerning the EEG are examined by Pallis (1983a).

BRAIN STEM AUDITORY AND SHORT-LATENCY SOMATOSENSORY EVOKED POTENTIALS

Other electrophysiological approaches to the diagnosis of brain death have been evaluated (Starr, 1976; Chatrian, 1986). Brain stem auditory evoked potentials (BAEPs) provide a useful way of ascertaining function of the auditory pathway from the cochlea to the thalamus. It has been shown (Starr, 1977) that the elicitation of BAEPs may help differentiate the syndrome of apneic coma with absent brain stem reflexes due to drugs (in which the various BAEP waves are preserved) from the identical syndrome due to structural brain disease (where all but the first of the BAEP waves are abolished).

The practical applications of this differentiation are limited. Most patients in whom brain stem death is likely to be diagnosed will have sustained a head injury, an intracranial hemorrhage or an anoxic cerebral insult. Other means (such as taking a clinical history) are available for making these diagnoses. Patients who are comatose and apneic for unknown reasons (or as a result of drug intoxication) will fail to meet both the "preconditions" and "exclusions" requirements for a diagnosis of brain stem death *(vide infra)*. The problem of multiple factors contributing to the clinical state is discussed later. The context, as always, is paramount.

Short-latency somatosensory evoked potentials (in response to electrical median nerve stimulation) may be recorded from the cervicomedullary junction in patients fulfilling clinical criteria of brain death but are not recordable from the parietal cortex (Chiappa *et al.*, 1980; Goldie *et al.*, 1981; Mauguière *et al.*, 1982).

THE CLINICAL APPROACH

In 1968, the *Ad Hoc* Committee of the Harvard Medical School published its report, "A definition of irreversible coma." The words conveyed something of the flavor of *coma dépassé* and no exception could be made. "Irreversible coma" was explicitly stated to be the equivalent of the "brain death syndrome." Unfortunately, the same words were later to be used by others quite inaccurately to refer to a very different condition, namely to a "state in which all functions attributed to the cerebrum are lost, but certain vital functions such as respiration, temperature and blood pressure regulation may be retained" (American Collaborative Study, 1977). This was clearly not "irreversible coma" in the sense the Harvard group had used the terms. It was the "syndrome in search of a name," which Jennett and Plum had meticulously described as early as 1972 and which they had called the "persistent vegetative state." This state is not in fact coma at all: affected patients open their eyes for long periods and exhibit sleep-wake alternations in the EEG. Such terminological ambiguities enshrined in the final (1977) report of the American Collaborative Study (the very body set up to investigate

TABLE 6–1

PROGNOSTIC SIGNIFICANCE OF ISOELECTRIC ELECTROENCEPHALOGRAM (EEG) AND OF APNEIC COMA WITH ABSENT BRAIN STEM REFLEXES IN PATIENTS WITH STRUCTURAL BRAIN DAMAGE

No. of Cases	Brain Stem Areflexia	Apnea	EEG	Asystole Within Days
>1000	All	All	"Isoelectric"	All
147	All	All	Some residual activity	All
16	None	None	"Isoelectric"	None

Reproduced with permission from Pallis (1981).

TABLE 6–2

HARVARD CRITERIA FOR IRREVERSIBLE COMA*

1. Unreceptivity and unresponsivity
2. No movements (observe for 1 hour)
3. Apnea (3 min off respirator)
4. Absence of elicitable reflexes
5. 1968: isoelectric EEG of "great confirmatory value" (at 5 μV mm⁻¹)
   1969: EEG "not essential"

*All these tests shall be repeated at least 24 hours later with no change. EEG = electroencephalogram.

brain death) were to generate much confusion and vitiate much writing on the subject.

The Harvard Committee listed a number of criteria (Table 6–2) for the identification of "irreversible coma," a condition that "should be evident in all cases from clinical examination alone." Although there was wide personal experience among its medical members, the Committee published no evidence that comas of the type it specified were invariably irreversible. In particular, there was no information about what happened if ventilation was continued. The Committee warned of the pitfalls of hypothermia and drug intoxication but did not otherwise specify the contexts in which "irreversible coma" could be diagnosed. It accepted potentially reversible metabolic encephalopathies (for instance those associated with uremia) as possible causes of irreversible coma. It suggested (on the basis of some questionable comments concerning thalamic and basal ganglionic function in deeply unconscious patients) that "irreversible coma" was synonymous with brain death. It further proposed that this condition be accepted as "a new criterion of death." It did not seek to legitimize this identification, nor did it define what it meant by death. In its attempts to document apnea, it proposed methods that relied on a hypoxic (rather than a hypercarbic) stimulus to breathing. Finally, it linked the question of brain death to the issue of organ transplantation. The authors rightly concluded that more than medical problems were involved. There were moral, ethical, religious and legal issues. The Committee saw itself as preparing the way for "better insights" into such problems, as well as for "better law than is currently applicable." Cadmus-like, it had sown dragon's teeth on the Harvard campus. Many warriors would arise to fight about these matters.

The main conclusions of the report proved to be well founded and, as empirical evidence accumulated, began gradually to be accepted. The process has been described elsewhere (Pallis, 1983a). Damaging claims that doctors do not really know what would happen if they maintained ventilation after having diagnosed brain death (and that such diagnoses were therefore self-fulfilling prophecies) cannot be substantiated. Over 1,800 cases ventilated to asystole have in fact been published (Table 6–3), and these must comprise only a small minority of those observed over the years

TABLE 6–3

NONDRUGGED PATIENTS DIAGNOSED AS BRAIN-DEAD BY CLINICAL CRITERIA AND MAINTAINED ON VENTILATOR

Series	Year	Patients Accepted	Silent EEGs/ EEGs Obtained	Survivors
Löfstedt and von Reis	1959	97	2/2	0
Heiskanen	1964	19	0/0	0
Goulon	1966	1	0/1	0
Lindgren et al.	1968	35	27/35	0
Becker et al.	1970	15	6/?*	0
Gaches et al.	1970	69	2/69	0
Mohandas and Chou	1971	25	3/9	0
Ingvar and Widén	1972	26	26/26	0
Ouaknine	1975	42	32/32	0
Walker and Molinari	1975	141	130/141	0
Rappaport et al.	1978	3	0/1	0
Ayim and Clark	1979	30	3/10	0
Hicks and Torda	1979	21	18/20	0
Ashwal and Schneider	1979	5	0/5	0
Kaste et al.	1979	12	?/8*	0
Powner and Fromm	1979	182	164/182	0
Namazie	1980	10	2/2	0
Jennett et al.	1981	326	67/70	0
Jørgensen	1981	70	Not stated*	0
Caronna and Plum	1982	34	1/10	0
Rowland et al.	1983	10	0/0	0
Goulon	1984	23	23/23	0
Nishimura and Sugi	1984	12	Not stated†	0
Ogata et al.	1986	45	Not stated†	0
Yoshioka et al.	1986	16	Not stated†	0
Hung and Tsai	1986	41	Not stated†	0
Takeuchi et al.	1987	552	464/467	0
		1862	964/1106	0

*EEG = electroencephalogram.
†Excluded from totals (data incomplete).
Note: The number of cases from each reported series accepted for tabulation is often smaller than the totals mentioned in the references themselves. All the patients developed asystole, but all did not, in my opinion, fulfill adequate clinical criteria of brain death (some of the series included cases of drug intoxication). An additional 92 cases from two further series (Ibe, 1971; Korein and Maccario, 1971) have not been included (although clinically brain stem dead and ventilated to asystole) because it was impossible to ascertain the exact proportion due to structural brain disease. The table deliberately (and grossly) underrepresents the relevant material.

throughout the world. The type of coma identified by the clinical criteria of the Harvard group is indeed irreversible. Asystole usually develops within hours or days (Lindgren *et al.*, 1968; Jørgensen, 1973; Jennett *et al.*, 1981). The implications would seem to be the same in children as in adults (Rowland *et al.*, 1983; Crone, 1983). Caution is needed with neonates (Volpe, 1987). The question of alleged survivors has been dealt with elsewhere (Pallis, 1983a).

THE SHIFT TO BRAIN STEM–BASED CRITERIA

A major conceptual advance occurred when two Minneapolis neurosurgeons (Mohandas and Chou, 1971) made the challenging suggestion that "in patients with known and irreparable intracranial lesions" irreversible damage to the brain stem was the "point of no return." This was what had to be established "beyond reasonable doubt." The loss of function of the brain stem was in nearly all instances the infratentorial consequence of catastrophic supratentorial events (i.e., the result of an untreatable pressure cone)—a point often missed by those who criticize the concept of brain stem death without appreciating the usual pathogenesis of brain stem failure.

The Minnesota criteria (Table 6–4) became widely known and were to inspire much later work, particularly in the United Kingdom. The novelty of the approach consisted in (1) the specification of etiological preconditions, (2) the explicit emphasis on the brain stem, (3) the awareness of the irrelevance of retained reflexes below the level of the lesion (only brain stem reflexes had to be absent) and (4) the conclusion that if the signs of a dead brain stem were met, the value of the EEG was "extremely questionable." The authors unfortunately refrained from entitling their paper "Brain stem death," but that is undoubtedly what they had described.

Meanwhile, further evidence was accumulating that stressed the links between brain stem function and the capacity for consciousness. Well-documented clinicopathological studies circumscribed the relevant area of the brain stem to the tegmentum of the mesencephalon and rostral pons (Kemper and Romanul, 1967; Chase *et al.*, 1968; Wilkus *et al.*, 1971). Massive involvement of this area caused deep unconsciousness and, when associated with similar involvement of the lower brain stem (causing sustained apnea), was lethal. It was also shown that brain stem injury in humans could massively reduce cerebral blood flow and cerebral oxidative metabolism (Ingvar and Sourander, 1970). These findings were later confirmed (Heiss and Jellinger, 1972; Hass and Hawkins, 1978). Imperceptibly, the scene was being set for a major clinical breakthrough.

In November 1976, the *British Medical Journal* and *Lancet*

TABLE 6–4
"MINNESOTA" CRITERIA*

1. "Known but irreparable intracranial lesion"
2. No spontaneous movement
3. Apnea (4 min)
4. Absent brain stem reflexes
   pupillary
   corneal
   ciliospinal
   vestibuloocular
   oculocephalic
   gag
5. "All findings unchanged for at least 12 hours"

*Electroencephalogram is not mandatory.

TABLE 6–5
DIAGNOSIS OF BRAIN DEATH—THE "UK CODE"*

1. Preconditions
   comatose patient, on a ventilator
   positive diagnosis of cause of coma
      (irremediable structural brain damage)
2. Exclusions
   primary hypothermia (<35° C)
   drugs
   severe metabolic or endocrine disturbances
3. Tests
   absent brain stem reflexes
   apnea (strictly defined)

*1976: Repetition "customary." 1981: Tests "should be repeated."

published a memorandum ("The diagnosis of brain death") endorsed by the Conference of Royal Colleges and Faculties of the United Kingdom. It was the product of long discussions involving specialists in many fields (including clinical neurophysiologists, lawyers and coroners). The recommendations became known as the UK code (Table 6–5).

The main emphasis of this code is that the question of *context* is all important. Unless strict preconditions have been fulfilled, and certain entities excluded, a diagnosis of brain death cannot even be considered. This point has seldom been grasped by those criticizing the code. The scheme outlined is scientifically sound and clinically straightforward, although terminological problems remain. The memorandum is entitled "The diagnosis of brain death," yet however stringent, the tests proposed are basically tests of brain stem function. The document states that "permanent functional death of the brain stem constitutes brain death." This is unexceptionable, if taken to mean that death of the brain stem prevents any kind of functioning of the "brain as a whole." The title of the document remains, however, open to misunderstanding.

In January 1979, the Conference published a further memorandum entitled "Diagnosis of death" that it considered "an addendum to the original report." This concluded "that the identification of brain death meant that the patient was dead, whether or not the function of some organs, such as the heart beat, was still maintained by artificial means." Death was clearly identified as "an irreversible state," the achievement of which was usually a process rather than an event. The problem of defining death was not addressed.

In July 1981, important developments took place in the United States. The President's Commission for the Study of Ethical Problems in Medicine and Biochemical and Behavioral Research submitted a report ("Defining death") to the President, Congress and the relevant departments of government. The report described accurately the UK Code and contained the statement that "if the brain stem completely lacks function, the brain as a whole cannot function." Among the appendices to the Report were "Guidelines for the determination of death" (1981) drawn up by a large panel of medical consultants to the Commission. These guidelines were very similar to the British ones. A "Uniform Determination of Death Act" was also proposed. A critique of some of its formulations has been published elsewhere (Pallis and Prior, 1983; Pallis, 1983a).

Those who criticize the use of purely clinical criteria for diagnosing death on neurological grounds (Allen and Burkholder, 1978; Molinari, 1978; Bennett, 1981; Molinari, 1982) center their arguments on (1) the persistence of some EEG activity in a proportion of cases, and (2) the reversibility of some clinical signs in some instances. Both objections can readily be met (Pallis, 1983a). The occasional persistence of minimal EEG activity is not denied, but those who consider it significant do not tell us what it signifies. They refrain from spelling out their concept of death and explaining to us how the declining activity of a few neuronal aggregates relates to their concept. It is certainly of no relevance if death of the "human organism as a whole" is defined as the "irreversible loss of the capacity for consciousness, combined with the irreversible loss of the capacity to breathe" (both of which are brain stem functions). For those reluctant to venture onto philosophical ground, and ready to accommodate criteria unrelated to any concept, I reiterate that the transient persistence of the EEG does not influence cardiac prognosis, which is solely determined by the state of the brain stem. The argument about the reversibility of clinical signs is of a different order. It centers on case selection. If reversible causes of brain stem dysfunction (such as drug intoxication or the immediate effects of cerebral anoxia) are not rigorously excluded before a diagnosis of brain death is even entertained, the diagnosis will clearly prove wrong in a proportion of cases. That is why sensibly constructed clinical codes stress (1) preconditions, (2) exclusions and (3) the importance of time to testing. As explained in the next section, the neurological signs have never been shown to be reversible when elicited on patients who have been through such very strict selection.

The Clinical Diagnosis of Brain Stem Death

A clinical diagnosis of brain stem death involves three steps. These are as follows:

1. Ascertaining that certain preconditions have been met;
2. Ensuring that reversible causes of a nonfunctioning brain stem (such as primary hypothermia, drug intoxication or severe metabolic disturbance) have been excluded;
3. Establishing (by clinical, bedside tests) that the comatose patient is genuinely apneic and that the brain stem reflexes are absent.

The aim of specifying preconditions and exclusions is a great deal more subtle than is immediately apparent. It is to guarantee that the actual tests for brain stem death are only carried out on the right patients. Before being tested, every patient has to pass, so to speak, through a tight double filter. It is only if the preconditions and exclusions have been strictly complied with that the finding—at the end of the trail—of apneic coma with absent brain stem reflexes implies irreversible loss of brain stem function (i.e., a dead brain stem).

PRECONDITIONS

The patient must be comatose and on a ventilator. The cause of the coma must be firmly established and it must be structural brain damage (for discussion see Pallis, 1983a). About 50% of the cases of brain stem death diagnosed in the United Kingdom are caused by overwhelming head injury. The history is clear, and there is no reason to believe that antecedent factors are affecting brain function, other than recent alcohol intake in some patients (Jennett, 1981). A further 30% of patients have suffered subarachnoid hemorrhage, and the history, physical signs and cerebrospinal fluid changes will be characteristic. Most of the remaining cases will involve intracranial lesions such as cerebral abscess or tumor, meningitis or encephalitis. Varying proportions will be caused by hypoxic encephalopathy: over 50% in the series reported by Jørgensen (1974b) but only 11.4% in a report from Pittsburgh (Jastremski et al., 1978).

The patient must have been maintained on a ventilator for long enough to ascertain that the brain damage is *irremediable*. A judgment to this effect should not be made on purely theoretical grounds (although the visualization of massive brain destruction is strong *prima facie* evidence of irreversibility). The condition should be considered irremediable only after vigorous efforts have been made to remedy it. These efforts may be of various kinds, ranging from the evacuation of intracranial hematomas to control of cerebral edema. They will certainly involve proper attention to cerebral perfusion (maintenance of an adequate blood pressure, reduction of intracranial hypertension), the restoration of a normal arterial oxygen tension and the correction of any obvious metabolic disturbances. Cardiovascular instability (defined as a systolic arterial pressure of less than 100 mg Hg for more than 1 hour or the presence of potentially fatal arrythmias) occurred in 45% of patients in one large series (Grenvik et al., 1978), and the authors warned of the potentiating effects of such findings on brain dysfunction. The application of therapeutic measures will take time: the passage of time is one of the essential considerations in determining that a lesion is irremediable. Brain stem death is a diagnosis that can be made only in an intensive care unit, and it is quite inappropriate to seek to make it in an emergency department.

An unhurried approach is the best safeguard against premature or unjustified suspicions of brain stem death. For how long should a comatose patient with a structural lesion be ventilated before it can be decided that the precondition of an irremediable lesion has been met? This varies from case to case. In most cases, 12 hours are sufficient, although the time may be as short as 6 hours or as long as 24 hours or more. Various clinical scenarios have been graphically described (Jennett and Hessett, 1981) and are worth recapitulating. The "times to testing" suggested (Table 6-6) are for guidance only. In each case it will be up to the physician in charge to determine whether longer periods may be necessary. The general philosophy should be that the potential recipient of organs may be in a hurry but that the donor never is.

EXCLUSIONS

Drug intoxication, primary hypothermia and certain metabolic and endocrine disturbances may cause profound—but

TABLE 6–6

EXAMPLES OF OBSERVATION PERIODS ON VENTILATOR BEFORE TESTING FOR BRAIN STEM DEATH

Apneic Coma Caused By	"Time to Testing" (hours)
Major intracranial surgery	4
Second subarachnoid bleed (in hospital) in patient with angiographically proven aneurysm	
Spontaneous intracranial hemorrhage (without hypoxic brain damage from respiratory arrest)	>6
Head injury (without secondary brain damage from hypoxia, intracranial hematoma or shock)	6–12
Brain hypoxia (respiratory obstruction, drowning, cerebral hypoperfusion)	12–24
Any of the above (when additional drug intoxication suspected and no screening facilities available)	50–100

potentially reversible—depression of brain stem function. It is on this potential reversibility that the UK Code bases its recommendation that patients with these conditions should not be considered for a diagnosis of brain stem death.

The question of drug intoxication is often misunderstood. Undiagnosed patients (even if comatose and apneic) do not "make the short list" for a diagnosis of brain stem death. They fall at the first hurdle: the need for a positive diagnosis of structural brain damage. Should it become established that such patients are comatose from depressant drug poisoning, an additional reason will have emerged why they should not be tested for brain stem death—namely, that they are suffering from a functional (i.e., potentially reversible) disturbance. The tightness of the "double filter" will now be appreciated.

Problems occasionally arise when it is suspected that the patient's state is due to the combined effects of trauma and drugs. In practice, trauma plus significant drug intoxication, other than alcohol, is rare. Common sense and clinical judgment are required. The circumstances are crucial. A depressed elderly person living alone who is found unconscious at the foot of the stairs with a fractured skull presents a different diagnostic problem from the rock climber who has slipped and sustained a similar fracture. A boxer knocked out in a ring and later lapsing into coma (or a hospital patient having a second subarachnoid bleed) is easier to assess than the drunk who has fallen and been knocked out when lurching out of a bar. Alcohol is a common (but transient) cause of diagnostic problems. The depressant effect of acute alcoholic intoxication seldom lasts more than 6–8 hours. Persisting coma implies an urgent need for further evaluation.

When intoxication has been established as complicating head injury, no testing for brain stem death is warranted until the effects of the intoxication have fully worn off. In this context, it is important to keep in mind the approximate plasma half-lives of various coma-producing drugs (Table 6–7) and to remember that, as clearance proceeds, blood concentrations may fail to accurately reflect brain concentrations. When toxicological facilities are not available—and there can be a few major centers with facilities for ventilatory support for head-injured patients but no access to a drug screening center—it is reasonable to allow about 3 days to elapse for the situation to resolve. Some patients may develop asystole during this period (and their kidneys lost to transplantation), but this is a small price to pay for avoiding error.

TABLE 6–7
COMA: DURATION OF DRUG EFFECTS

Alcohol Metabolism (Zero-Order Kinetics): 10 ml h^{-1}	Plasma Half-lives (hours)
Aspirin	0.25–0.30
Pentazocine	2
Paracetamol	2–4
Diphenhydramine	4–10
Imipramine	8–24
Morphine	10–60
Nortriptyline	15–93
Methadone	18–97
Pentobarbitone	20–35
Chlorpromazine	23–37
Phenytoin*	24 (mean)
Carbamazepine	24–48
Diazepam and active metabolites	24–96
Phenobarbitone	50–140

*Prolonged at high concentrations.

Complex neurological deficits may be produced when cardiac or respiratory arrest have developed in the course of severe, accurately diagnosed, drug-induced coma. No accurate assessment of the respective contributions of each insult to the brain is immediately possible. The passage of time will again help resolve matters.

Anesthetists sometimes unwittingly cause problems for their colleagues. Neurologists are still called to intensive care units to assess whether patients (who have met the preconditions and whose coma is clearly not due to drugs) have a dead brain stem only to discover that the patients are under the influence of therapeutically administered substances designed to block neuromuscular transmission. The wise physician called to the intensive care unit will always look at the treatment sheet before embarking on tests to establish brain stem death.

CLINICAL TESTING

The objective is to determine if the brain stem reflexes are absent and whether or not there is total apnea. If such a state can be demonstrated and *preconditions and exclusions have been rigorously observed*, a legitimate conclusion can be drawn: the brain stem has irreversibly ceased to function. It is dead. Whereas time and skill may be necessary to establish that the preconditions have been met, clinical testing is relatively straightforward and does not take long to perform.

Brain Stem Reflexes

Testing the brain stem reflexes enables the functional integrity of the brain stem to be probed in a unique way. No other area of the brain can be investigated so thoroughly. The tests look for the presence or absence of responses, not for gradations of function. They do not depend on elaborate machinery, on the vagaries of maintenance or on the around-the-clock presence of super-specialists. They provide a mutually reinforcing battery of checks: the determination of death does not rely on a single procedure or on the assessment of a single function.

The UK Code specifies that five brain stem reflexes be tested (Fig. 6–2). All should be absent.

No Pupillary Response to Light. Despite earlier writings (Mollaret and Goulon, 1959; *Ad Hoc* Committee of the Harvard Medical School, 1968; Inter-Agency Committee on Irreversible Coma and Brain Death, 1975) the pupils are not invariably dilated when the brain stem is dead. Bilateral mydriasis was present in 45 of 63 patients studied serially by Jørgensen (1973) and unilateral mydriasis was encountered in five additional cases. This common finding contrasts strikingly with what can be seen in any mortuary, where the pupils are usually in the mid-position. The difference may well be owing to the fact that, in the mortuary, the spinal cord is dead as well as the brain stem, whereas in ventilated patients with a dead brain stem "life" may persist in spinal sympathetic ("pupillodilator") centers. The important point is that there should be no pupillary response to really bright light (a reaction mediated exclusively through the brain stem). It is advisable to darken the room for this test. Proper medical torches, with new batteries, should be used. Old household torches, ophthalmoscopes or auroscopes are inadequate sources of light.

Widely dilated, unresponsive pupils may be caused by atropine administered in the course of cardiac resuscitation. The effects may persist for several hours. Errors may also arise when topical mydriatics have been instilled (to facilitate fundoscopy) and the fact has not been recorded in the notes. Preexisting ocular or neurological disease may account for

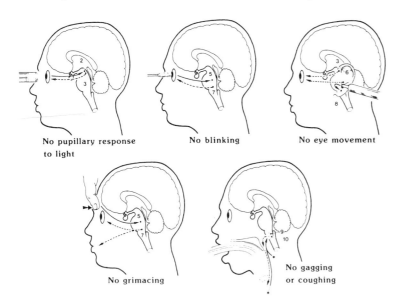

No pupillary response to light

No blinking

No eye movement

No grimacing

No gagging or coughing

FIGURE 6–2

The United Kingdom code specifies that five brain stem reflexes must be absent in the presence of total apnea before a diagnosis of brain stem death can be made.

the pupils failing to respond to light, as may local damage to the globe or nerves to the eye sustained during craniofacial injury, although such factors seldom affect both eyes.

No Corneal Reflexes. When brain stem death is suspected, much firmer pressure is justified than in conscious patients. Delicate dabbing with a wisp of cotton wool does not provide an adequate stimulus. A sterile throat swab is more suitable.

No Vestibuloocular Reflexes. The "caloric tests" require wax-free external auditory canals, verified with an auroscope before testing. The UK Code recommends irrigation on each side with 20 ml of ice-cold water. More may be used if the examiner thinks the whole volume has not been directed at the tympanum. The stimulus should elicit no movement whatsoever in either eye within 1 min of completion of the test. In deeply unconscious patients with some residual brain stem function, there may be deviation of one or both eyes towards the irrigated ear. Downward deviation of the eyes in response to unilateral caloric testing is occasionally a sign of depressant drug poisoning (Simon, 1978).

The central mechanisms responsible for the vestibuloocular reflexes may be impaired or suppressed by drugs including sedatives, anticholinergics, anticonvulsants and tricyclic antidepressants. End-organ disease or end-organ poisoning from antibiotics such as gentamicin occasionally block the vestibuloocular reflexes on their afferent side.

No Motor Response, Within the Cranial Nerve Distribution, to Adequate Stimulation of Any Somatic Area. In practice this means there should be no grimacing in response to painful stimuli, applied either to the trigeminal fields (firm supraorbital pressure) or to the limbs (the side of a pencil pressed firmly down against the patient's fingernail or toenail is the most appropriate stimulus; pinprick should not be used). Iatrogenic neuromuscular blockade is the main pitfall.

No Gag Reflex or Reflex Response to Bronchial Stimulation by Suction Catheter Passed Down the Trachea. Testing will require momentary disconnection from the ventilator. Both reflexes can be tested if the patient has had a tracheotomy. If the patient is tolerating an endotracheal tube, extubation is not necessary to test the gag reflex. Experienced nursing staff will usually be the first to spot that the responses to tracheal or bronchial suction have first lessened and then ceased.

Apnea

Apnea is established by showing that no respiratory movements occur during disconnection from the ventilator for long enough to ensure that the arterial carbon dioxide tension (Pa_{CO_2}) rises to a level (6.65 kPa or 50 mm Hg) capable of driving any respiratory center neurons that may still be alive. Two problems will be apparent immediately: how to prevent hypoxia during the disconnection and how to ensure that the Pa_{CO_2} does in fact build up to the appropriate level.

Hypoxia is prevented by a combination of preoxygenation (before disconnection) and diffusion oxygenation (during disconnection). If the patient is made to breathe 100% O_2 for 10 min before the test, very high starting levels of arterial oxygen tension (Pa_{O_2}) are achieved. These are reinforced by the endotracheal delivery of O_2 by catheter (at 6 L min^{-1}) while the patient is off the ventilator. The physiological basis of these procedures is well established (Enghoff et al., 1951; Frumin et al., 1959; Payne, 1962).

During disconnection the Pa_{CO_2} will rise as a result of endogenous metabolism. This rise will exceed the somewhat conservative estimate of 2 mm Hg min^{-1} (0.27 kPa min^{-1}) mentioned in the UK Code (Milhaud et al., 1978; Schafer and Caronna, 1978; Ropper et al., 1981). Provided the starting Pa_{CO_2} was 30 mm Hg (4 kPa) or more, the crucial level of 50 mm Hg (6.65 kPa) will have been achieved by the end of a 10-min disconnection period. The easiest way of ensuring an appropriate starting level of Pa_{CO_2} is to make the patient breathe 5% CO_2 in 95% O_2 for 5 min before testing. This procedure, which should always be resorted to when there are no facilities for blood gas analysis, will raise the starting Pa_{CO_2} to at least 40 mm Hg (5.3 kPa). At the end of the disconnection period of 10 min, the Pa_{CO_2} will have reached a level such that any respiratory neurons able to respond to a hypercarbic stimulus will be fired.

Possible pitfalls should be kept in mind. Neuromuscular blockade has been mentioned. Posthyperventilation apnea may be seen in patients who have been overventilated before testing. The error will not occur if ventilation is slowed down for a while before disconnection, if the patient is made to breathe 5% CO_2 before disconnection (as described), or if the blood gases have been monitored. Patients with chronic obstructive airways disease (who depend on an anoxic stimulus to breathing) and patients with acute lung pathology (who remain hypoxemic after breathing oxygen) are not really suitable for this test.

WHO TESTS? RETESTING, AND THEN?

Unnecessary anguish and distress to relatives and nurses may be caused by insensitive or thoughtless handling of brain-dead patients. Inadequate or conflicting statements (or a failure to explain anything whatsoever about what is happening) often prove to be the basis for sensationalization of the issue by the media and for a great deal of ill-informed talk about "pulling the plug," "discontinuing life support" and so on (Pallis, 1983b). A correct approach should make it abundantly clear (both to relatives and to a wider public) that in the act of disconnection "the doctor is not withdrawing treatment and allowing someone to die, but ceasing to do something useless to someone who is already dead" (Jennett and Hessett, 1981).

The UK Code now recommends that the tests should be carried out by two medical practitioners who "have expertise in this field." One should be a consultant and the other a consultant or senior resident (Robson, 1981). When transplantation is envisaged, neither of the doctors should be associated with potential recipients. In practice, those doctors often are anesthetists, neurologists or intensive care physicians. One survey showed that in the United Kingdom, 45% of brain-dead kidney donors came from nonteaching hospitals without neurosurgical facilities (Jennett and Hessett, 1981).

Practice in various parts of the world differs considerably. Some countries specify the required specialty of the doctors making the diagnosis, others do not. Some specify how long he or she should have been qualified. The number of people required at the bedside may vary from one to four and at times includes nonmedical personnel such as coroners, magistrates or judges. The various approaches provide interesting insights for the cultural anthropologist.

Virtually all codes urge that testing be carried out twice. The UK Code stresses that this is to ensure that there has been no observer error. This is entirely praiseworthy, although no properly documented case has been published where the diagnosis of brain stem death has been revised after repeat testing. In my opinion, retesting usually has an additional purpose. It ensures that the nonfunctioning of the brain stem is not just a single observation at one point in time, but that it has persisted. For how long? For a period several hundred-fold that during which brain stem neurons could survive the total ischemia of a nonperfused brain. At Hammersmith Hospital, we like to separate our tests by 2–3 hours, which is more than enough to ensure that the findings are irreversible. Over the years, it has become widely recognized that the more time spent in ascertaining the irremediable nature of the structural brain damage causing the coma, the less important the interval between tests.

As soon as they have completed their first examination, the physicians concerned should write down their findings in the patient's notes, or on special checklists provided. The entry should confirm that a disconnection test for apnea has been performed. It is advised that the $PaCO_2$ be estimated at the end of the disconnection period and the result recorded. It is sound and helpful to perform the disconnection test as the last of the tests of brain stem function.

After the first clinical testing, the patient is reconnected to the ventilator. If second testing confirms a dead brain stem, death should be declared, the relatives notified and a further appropriate entry made in the notes. Legally, a patient is deemed to be dead when a doctor (using accepted criteria)

TABLE 6–8
DECLARATION OF BRAIN STEM DEATH

1. Have the preconditions been met?
   Is the patient comatose and on a ventilator?
   Is there a positive diagnosis of structural brain damage?
   Have all possible attempts been made to remedy it?
2. Has proper attention been given to the necessary "exclusions" (drug intoxication, primary hypothermia, major metabolic disturbances)?
3. The patient having been on the ventilator for several hours, have each of two clinical examinations revealed:
   absent brain stem reflexes
   persistent apnea (disconnection test)?
4. If so, the patient can be declared dead, even if the heart is still beating?
5. Once the patient has been declared dead, the respirator is ventilating a cadaver. It is no longer a "life-support system."
6. The patient is dead when the brain stem is declared dead, not when the cadaver is disconnected from the respirator and the heart stops beating.
7. Neither electroencephalography nor angiography is necessary for a diagnosis of brain stem death.

declares him or her to be dead. A death certificate can then be issued, which is a good way of making it clear that any continued ventilation (to allow organ donation) does not constitute "life" (Table 6–8).

If organ donation is not envisaged, there is no need to reconnect the cadaver to the ventilator. The second test for apnea will have merged with permanent disconnection. If transplantation is planned, the "beating-heart cadaver" should be reconnected to the ventilator. The operation can then be carried out at the convenience of the surgical team. Only in exceptional cases should artificial ventilation have to be maintained for more than 12 hours after a declaration of brain stem death. The main consideration is to ensure that the potential recipients receive organs in as good a condition as possible. The administration of pressure agents or antibodies may have to be continued.

To minimize the risk of possible later misunderstandings, all disconnections are best performed by doctors, not nurses. There are no logical reasons for this recommendation, but the whole subject is one in which irrational behavior is still occasionally encountered.

Vasopressin and the Brain-Dead Donor

The management of the brain-dead kidney donor entails attention to gas exchange, blood pressure maintenance and fluid balance (Luksza, 1979; Cooper et al., 1982). The central question remains unanswered, however: why does cardiac function, adequate a few hours earlier, gradually and inexorably decline?

Diabetes insipidus seems to be an almost constant feature of brain death. It is caused by decreased antidiuretic hormone (ADH) production, resulting from hypothalamic injury. The polyuria may result in dehydration, hypernatremia, hyperosmolality and hypokalemia. It has been suggested (Blaine et al., 1984) that in the brain dead there is a general defect of extracellular homeostasis, related to the loss of sensitive feedback mechanisms located above the foramen magnum.

In addition to its effects on the renal tubule, vasopressin (ADH) is probably the most potent vasoconstrictor known. There is experimental evidence (Cowley et al., 1974) that the sensitivity of the vasculature to vasopressin may be enhanced if certain baroceptor feedback mechanisms are inoperative (as would be the case if their reflex arcs were destroyed in the brain stem). A group of Japanese investigators (Yoshioka *et al.*, 1986) demonstrated the dramatic effect of synthetic arginine vasopressin on brain-dead patients. Administered by continuous infusion at rate of 1–2 units h^{-1} (285 ± 45 μU kg^{-1} min^{-1}), ADH potentiated the effect of epinephrine and ensured prolonged hemodynamic maintenance. There were striking effects on total peripheral resistance and mean arterial pressure, and the mean time to asystole was increased from less than 2 days to over 3 weeks. The finding, if substantiated, will have profound effects on transplantation practice. It will also have another repercussion. It will reinforce the proposition made at the beginning of this chapter that brain stem death is death in its own right, whatever the cardiac prognosis.

Conclusion

It is pointless to maintain ventilatory and circulatory functions by artificial means when there is no longer a working brain for oxygenated blood to irrigate. The individual can and should be considered dead if the brain as a whole has irreversibly and permanently ceased to function. Attempts to diagnose such a state of affairs have followed various routes. The alternatives posited by the French accounts of more than 40 years ago (Jouvet, 1959; Mollaret and Goulon, 1959) should now be reexamined and resolved. Efforts to establish the death of the last surviving intracranial neuron (whether by the angiographic demonstration of a "blocked" cerebral circulation or by electroencephalographic means) are today known to provide answers of doubtful validity to what is widely felt to be the wrong question.

In striking contrast, a diagnosis of a dead brain stem can be made on clinical criteria alone. Brain stem death is the physiological core of brain death and the substratum of its cardinal signs (apneic coma and absent brain stem reflexes). A permanently nonfunctioning brain stem relates to an acceptable overall concept of death (the "irreversible loss of the capacity for consciousness" combined with the "irreversible loss of the capacity to breathe") and has well-established prognostic implications of inevitable asystole.

REFERENCES

Ad Hoc Committee of the Harvard Medical School (1968). A definition of irreversible coma. *J. A. M. A.* **205**, 337.

Allen, N. and Burkholder, J. (1978). Clinical criteria of brain death. *Ann. N.Y. Acad. Sci.* **315**, 70.

American Collaborative Study (1977). An appraisal of the criteria of cerebral death: a summary statement. A collaborative study. *J.A.M.A.* **237**, 982.

Arfcl, G., Fischgold, H. and Weiss, J. (1963). *In Problèmes de Base en Electroencephalographie*, (H. Fishgold *et al.*, eds.), Masson, Paris.

Arnold, H., Kuhne, D. and Rohr, W. (1981). Contrast bolus technique with rapid CT scanning. A reliable diagnostic tool for the determination of brain death. *Neuroradiology* **22**, 129.

Ashwal, S. and Schneider, S. (1979). Failure of electroencephalography to diagnose brain death in comatose children. *Ann. Neurol.* **6**, 512.

Ayim, E. N. and Clark, G. P. M. (1979). Brain death: experience in an intensive care unit. *East Afr. Med. J.* **56**, 571.

Becker, D. P., Robert, C. M., Nelson, J. R. and Stern, W. E. (1970). An evaluation of the definition of cerebral death. *Neurology* **20**, 459.

Bennett, D. R. (1981). Brain death. *Lancet* **1**, 106.

Bennett, D. R., Nord, N. M., Roberts, T. S. and Mavor, H. (1971). Prolonged "survival" with flat EEG following cardiac arrest. *Electroencephalogr. Clin. Neurophysiol.* **30**, 94.

Bennett D. R., Hughes J. R., Korein J., *et al.* (1976). *An Atlas of Electroencephalography in Coma and Cerebral Death*, p. 1, Raven Press, New York.

Bergquist, E. and Bergström, K. (1972). Angiography in cerebral death. *Acta Radiol.* **12**, 283.

Bickford, R. G., Sims, J. K., Billinger, T. W., and Aung, M. L. (1971). *Trauma* **12**, 61.

Blain, E. M., Tallman, R. D., Frolicher, D., Jordan, M. A., Bluth, L. L. and Howie, M. B. (1984). Vasopressin supplementation in a porcine model of brain-dead potential organ donors. *Transplantation* **38**, 459.

Bricolo, A., Dalle Ore, G., Da Pian, R., Benati, A. and Turella, G. (1972). *In Present Limits of Neurosurgery*, (Fusek and Kune, eds.), Avicenum, Prague.

Brierley, J. B., Graham, D. I., Adams, J. H. and Simpson, J. A. (1971). Neocortical death after cardiac arrest. A clinical neurophysiological and neuropathological report of two cases. *Lancet* **2**, 560.

Brock, M., Schurmann, K. and Hadjidimos, A. (1969). Cerebral blood flow and cerebral death. *Acta Neurochir.* **20**, 195.

Bücheler, E., Kaufer, C. and Dux, A. (1970). Cerebral angiography to determine brain death. *Fortschr. Gieb. Rontgenstr. Nuklearmed. Erganzuugsbaud.* **113**, 278.

Carbonell, J., Carrascosa, G., Diersen, S., Obrador, S., Oliveros, J. C. and Sevillano, M. (1963). Some electrophysiological observations in a case of deep coma secondary to cardiac arrest. *Electroencephal ogr. Clin. Neurophysiol.* **15**, 520.

Caronna, J. J. and Plum F. (1982). *In The Diagnosis of Stupor and Coma*, (F. Plum and J. B. Posner, eds.), F. A. Davis, Philadelphia.

Chase, T. N., Moretti, I. and Prensky, A. L. (1968). Clinical and electroencephalographic manifestations of vascular lesions of the pons. *Neurol. Minneap.* **18**, 357.

Chatrian, G. E. (1986). *In Electrodiagnosis in Clinical Neurology*, (M. Aminoff, ed.), Churchill Livingstone, Edinburgh.

Chiappa, K. H., Choi, S. K. and Young, R. R. (1980). *Prog. Clin. Neurophysiol.* **7**, 264.

Conference of Medical Royal Colleges and Their Faculties in the UK. (1976). Diagnosis of brain death. *Br. Med. J.* **2**, 1187.

Conference of Medical Royal Colleges and Their Faculties in the UK. (1979). Diagnosis of brain death. *Br. Med. J.* **1**, 322.

Cooper, D. K., de Villiers, J. C. and Smith, L. S. (1982). Medical, legal and administrative aspects of cadaveric organ donation in the RSA. *S. Afr. Med. J.* **62**, 933.

Cowley, A. W., Monos, E. and Guyton, A. C. (1974). Interaction of vasopressin and the baroreceptor reflex system in the regulation of arterial blood pressure in the dog. *Circ. Res.* **34**, 505.

Cranford, R. E. and Smith, H. L. (1979). Some critical distinctions between brain death and the persistent vegetative state. Ethics Sci. Med. **6**, 199.

Crone, R. K. (1983). Brain death. *Am. J. Dis Child.* **137**, 545.

Crow, H. J. and Winter, A. (1969). Serial electrophysiological studies (EEG, EMG, ERG, evolved responses) in a case of 3 months' survival with flat EEG following cardiac arrest. *Electroencephalogr. Clin. Neurophysiol.* **27**, 332.

Enghoff, H., Holmdahl, M. H. and Risholm, M. (1951). Diffusion respiration in man. *Nature*, **168**, 830.

Frumin, M. J., Epstein, R. M. and Cohen, G. (1959). Apneic oxygenation in man. *Anaesthesiology* **20**, 789.

Gaches, J., Caliscan, A., Findji, F. and Le Beau, J. (1970). Irreversible coma and brain death. Study of 71 cases. *Sem. Hop. Paris* **46**, 1487.

Goldie, W. D., Chiappa, K. H., Young, R. R. and Brooks, E. B. (1981). Brainstem in brain death. *Neurology* **31**, 248.

Goodman, J. M., Mishkin, F. S. and Dyken, M. (1969). Determination of brain death by isotope angiography. *JAMA* **209**, 1869.

Goulon, M. (1966). *Marseille Chir.* 18th year. p. 18.

Goulon, M. (1984). *Int. Crit. Care Dig.* **3**, 23.

Goulon, M., Novailhat, F., Levy-Alcover, M. and Dordain, G. (1967). Toxic coma with autonomic consideration, with a favorable outcome. *Rev. Neurol.* **116**, 297.

Grenvik, A., Powner, D. J., Snyder, J. V., Jastremski, M. S., Babcock, R. A. and Loughhead, M. G. (1978). Cessation of therapy in terminal illness and brain death. *Crit. Care Med.* **6**, 284.

Gros, C., Vlahovitch, B. and Roilgen, A. (1959). Les arrêts circulatoires dans l'hypertension intra-cranienne suraigue. *Presse Med.* **67**, 1065.

Guidelines for the determination of death. Report of the medical consultants on the diagnosis of death to the President's Commission for the Study of Ethical Problems in Medicine and Biomedical and Behavioral Research. (1981). *J. A. M. A.* **246**, 2184.

Halder, I., Matthew, H. and Oswald, I. (1971). Electroencephalographic changes in acute drug poisoning. *Electroencephalogr. Clin. Neurophysiol.* **30**, 23.

Hamlin, H. (1964). Life or death by EEG. *J. A. M. A.* **190**, 112.

Handa, J., Matsuda, M., Matsuda, I. and Nakasu, S. (1982). Dynamic computed tomography in brain death. *Surg. Neurol.* **17**, 417.

Hass, W. K. and Hawkins, R. A. (1978). Bilateral reticular formation lesions causing coma: their effects on regional cerebral blood flow, glucose utilization and oxidative metabolism. *Ann. N.Y. Acad. Sci.* **315**, 105.

Heiskanen, O. (1964). Cerebral circulatory arrest caused by acute increase of intracranial pressure. *Acta Neurol. Scand.* **40(suppl. 7)**, 1.

Heiss, W. D. and Jellinger, K. (1972). Cerebral blood flow and brain stem lesion. *Z. Neurol.* **203**, 197.

Hicks, R. G. and Torda, T. A. (1979). The vestibulo-ocular (caloric) reflex in the diagnosis of cerebral death. *Anaesth. Intensive Care* **7**, 169.

Hung, T. P. and Tsai, T. T. (1986). *J. Formos. Med. Assoc.* **85**, 514.

Ibe, K. (1972). Clinical and pathophysiological aspects of the intravital brain death. *Electroencephalogr. Clin. Neurophysiol.* **30**, 272.

Ingvar, D. H. and Sourander, P. (1970). Destruction of the reticular core of the brain stem. A patho-anatomical follow-up of a case of coma of three years' duration. *Arch. Neurol.* **23**, 91.

Ingvar, D. H. and Widen, L. (1972). Brain death. Summary of a symposium. *Lakartidningen* **69**, 3804.

Inter-Agency Committee on Irreversible Coma and Brain Death. (1975). *Trans. Am. Neurol. Assoc.* **100**, 280.

Jastremski, M., Powner, D., Snyder, J., Smith, J. and Grenvik, A. (1978). Problems in brain death determination. *Forensic Sci.* **11**, 201.

Jennett, B. (1981). Brain death. *Br. J. Anaesth.* **53**, 1111.

Jennett, B. and Hessett, C. (1981). Brain death in Britain as reflected in renal donors. *Br. Med. J.* **283**, 359.

Jennett, B. and Plum, F. (1972). Persistent vegetative state after brain damage. A syndrome in search of a name. *Lancet* **1**, 734.

Jennett, B., Gleave, J. and Wilson, P. (1981). Brain death in three neurosurgical units. *Br. Med. J.* **282**, 533.

Jonkman, E. J. (1969). Cerebral death and the isoelectric EEG. *Electroencephalogr. Clin. Neurophysiol.* **27**, 215.

Jørgensen, E. O. (1973). Spinal man after brain death. The unilateral extension-pronation reflex of the upper limb as an indication of brain death. *Acta Neurochir.* **28**, 259.

Jørgensen, E. O. (1974a). Technical contribution. Requirements for recording the EEG at high sensitivity in suspected brain death. *Electroencephalogr. Clin. Neurophysiol.* **36**, 65.

Jørgensen, E. O. (1974b). Clinical note. EEG without detectable cortical activity and cranial nerve areflexia as parameters of brain death. *Electroencephalogr. Clin. Neurophysiol.* **36**, 70.

Jørgensen, E. O. (1981). Brain death—retrospective surveys. *Lancet* **1**, 378.

Jørgensen, E. O. and Brodersen, P. (1971). Criteria of death. The value of cliniconeurologic examination of cerebral circulation for the assessment of brain death. *Nord Med* **86**, 1549.

Jørgensen, E. O. and Malchow-Møller, A. (1981). A natural history of global and critical brain ischaemia. *Resuscitation* **9**, 133.

Jouvet, M. (1959). Electrosubcorticographic diagnosis of death of the central nervous system during various types of coma. *Electroencephalogr. Clin. Neurophysiol.* **11**, 805.

Kaste, M., Hillbom, M. and Palo, J. (1979). Diagnosis and management of brain death. *Br. J. Med.* **1**, 525.

Keane, J. R. (1979). Blinking to sudden illumination. A brain stem reflex present in neocortical death. *Arch. Neurol.* **36**, 52.

Kemper, T. L. and Romanul, F. C. A. (1967). State resembling akinetic mutism in basilar artery occlusion. *Neurology* **17**, 74.

Kimura, J., Gerber, H. W. and McCormick, W. F. (1968). The isoelectric electroencephalogram. Significance in establishing death in patients maintained on mechanical respirators. *Arch. Intern. Med.* **121**, 511.

Korein, J., Braunstein, P., George, A., *et al.* (1977). Brain death. I. Angiographic correlation with the radioisotopic bolus technique for evaluation of critical deficit of cerebral blood flow. *Ann. Neurol.* **2**, 195.

Kricheff, I. I., Pinto, R. S., George, A. E., Braunstein, P. and Korein, J. (1978). Angiographic findings in brain death. *Ann. N. Y. Acad. Sci.* **315**, 168.

Lamb, D. (1988). *In* Mortal Philosophy and Contemporary Problems, (Royal Institute of Philosophy Series, J. D. G. Evans, ed.), Cambridge University Press, Cambridge.

Lecuire, J., de Rougemont, J., Descotes, J. and Jouvet, M. (1962). Data concerning cerebral circulatory arrest (value of the atropine test). *Neurochirurgie* **8**, 158.

Lévy-Alcover, M. and Babinet, P. (1970). Chronologic relation between onset of the clinical picture of final coma and persistence of minimal EEG activity: 9 cases. *Rev. Neurol.* **122**, 411.

Lindgren, S., Petersen, I. and Zwetnow, N. (1968). Prediction of death in serious brain damage. *Acta Chir. Scand.* **134**, 405.

Löfstedt, S. L. and von Reis, G. (1959). *Opusula. Med.* **4**, 345.

Luksza, A. R. (1979). Brain dead kidney donor: selection, care and administration. *Br. Med. J.* **1**, 1316.

Mauguière, F., Grand, C., Fischer, C. and Courjon, J. (1982). Aspects of early somatosensory and auditory evoked potentials in neurologic comas and brain death. *Rev. Electroencephalogr. Neurophysiol.* **12**, 280.

Milhaud, A., Riboulot, M. and Gayet, H. (1978). Disconnecting tests and oxygen uptake in the diagnosis of total brain death. *Ann. N. Y. Acad. Sci.* **315**, 241.

Mohandas, A. and Chou, S. N. (1971). Brain death. A clinical and pathological study. *Neurosurgery* **35**, 211.

Molinari, G. F. (1978). Review of clinical criteria of brain death. *Ann. N. Y. Acad. Sci.* **315**, 62.

Molinari, G. F. (1982). Brain death, irreversible coma and words doctors use. *Neurology* **32**, 400.

Mollaret, P. and Goulon, M. (1959). The depassed coma (preliminary memoir). *Rev. Neurol.* **101**, 3.

Namazie, M. (1980). Diagnosis and management of brain death. *Med. J. Malaysia* **34**, 363.

Nishimura, N. and Sugi, T. (1984). Circulatory support with sympathetic amines in brain death. *Resuscitation* **12**, 25.

Ogata, J., Yutani, C., Imakita, M. and Ueda, H. (1986). Autolysis of the granular layer of the cerebellar cortex in brain death. *Acta Neuropathol. (Ber)* **70**, 75.

Ouaknine, G. E. (1975). Bedside procedures in the diagnosis of brain death. *Resuscitation* **4**, 159.

Pallis, C. (1981). Prognostic value of brain stem lesion. *Lancet* **1**, 379.

Pallis, C. (1983a). ABC of brain stem death [booklet]. *Br. Med. J.*, p. 1.

Pallis, C. (1983b). Letter. *The Times*, 28 March 1983.

Pallis, C. (1986). *Encyclopaedia Britannica* **16**, 1030.

Pallis, C. (1987). Brain stem death—the evolution of a concept. *Med. Leg. J.* **55(Part 2)**, 84.

Pallis, C. and Prior, P. F. (1983). Guidelines for the determination of death. *Neurology* **33**, 251.

Pampiglione, G. and Harden, A. (1968). Resuscitation after cardiocirculatory arrest. Prognostic evaluation of early electroencephalogical findings. *Lancet* **1**, 1261.

Payne, J. P. (1962). Apneic oxygenation in anaesthetised man. *Acta Anaesth. Scand.* **6**, 129.

Pollack, M. A. and Kellaway, P. (1978). Cortical death with preservation of brain stem function: correlation of clinical, electrophysiologic and CT scan findings in 3 infants and 2 adults with prolonged survival. *Trans. Am. Neurol. Assoc.* **103**, 36.

Powner, D. J. and Fromm, G. H. (1979). The electroencephalogram in the determination of brain death. *N. Engl. J. Med.* **300**, 502.

President's Commission for the Study of Ethical Problems in Medicine and Behavioral Research (1981). *Whistleblowing in Biomedical Research: Policies and Procedures for Responding to Reports of Misconduct*, p. 1, U.S. Government Printing Office, Washington D. C.

Pribram, H. F. W. (1961). Angiographic appearances in acute intracranial hypertension. *Neurology* **11**, 10.

Rappaport, Z. H., Brinker, R. A. and Rovit, R. L. (1978). Evaluation of brain death by contrast-enhanced computerized cranial tomography. *Neurosurgery* **2**, 230.

Riishede, J. and Ethelberg, S. (1953). Angiographic changes in sudden and severe herniation of brain stem through tentorial incisure; report of 5 cases. *Arch. Neurol. Psychiat.* **70**, 399.

Robson, J. G. (1981). Brain death. *Lancet* **2**, 364.

Ropper, A. H., Kennedy, S. K. and Russell, L. (1981). Apnea testing in the diagnosis of brain death. Clinical and physiological observations. *Neurosurgery* **55**, 942.

Rosenklint, A. and Jørgensen, P. B. (1974). Evaluation of angiographic methods in the diagnosis of brain death. Correlation with local and systemic arterial pressure and intracranial pressure. *Neuroradiology* **7**, 215.

Rosoff, S. D. and Schwab, R. S. (1968). The EEG in establishing brain death. A 10-year report with criteria and legal safeguards in the 50 states. *Electroencephalogr. Clin. Neurophysiol.* **24**, 283.

Rowland, T. W., Donnelly, J. H., Jackson, A. H. and Jamroz, S. B. (1983). Brain death in the pediatric intensive care unit. A clinical definition. *Am. J. Dis. Child.* **137**, 547.

Schafer, J. A. and Caronna, J. J. (1978). Duration of apnea needed to confirm brain death. Clinical and physiological observations. *Neurol. Minneap.* **28**, 661.

Schwab, R. S., Potts, F. and Bonazzi, A. (1963). EEG as an aid in determining death in the presence of cardiac activity (ethical, legal and medical aspects). *Electroencephalogr. Clin. Neurophysiol.* **15**, 147.

Silverman, D., Saunders, M. G., Schwab, R. S. and Masland, R. L. (1969). Cerebral death and the electroencephalogram. Report of the *ad hoc* committee of the American Electroencephalographic Society on EEG criteria for determination of cerebral death. *J. A. M. A.* **209**, 1505.

Simon, R. P. (1978). Forced downward ocular deviation. Occurrence during oculovestibular testing in sedative drug-induced coma. *Arch. Neurol.* **35**, 456.

Starr, A. (1976). Auditory brain-stem responses in brain death. *Brain* **99**, 543.

Starr, A. (1977). *In* Progress in Clinical Neurophysiology, Vol. 2, (J. E. Desmedt, ed.), Karger, Basel.

Takeuchi, K., Takeshita, H., Takakura, K., *et al.* (1987). Evolution of criteria for determination of brain death in Japan. *Acta Neurochir.* **87**, 93.

Veatch, R. M. (1972). Brain death: welcome definition—or dangerous judgment? *Hastings Center Rep.* **11**, 10.

Visser, S. L. (1969). Two cases of isoelectric EEGs ("apparent exceptions proving the rule"). *Electroencephalogr. Clin. Neurophysiol.* **27**, 215.

Vlahovitch, B., Frerebeau, P., Kuhner, A., Billet, M. and Gros, C. (1971). Angiographies under pressure in brain death with encephalic circulatory arrest. *Neurochirurgie* **17**, 81.

Volpe, J. J. (1987). Brain death determination in the newborn. *Pediatrics* **80**, 293.

Walker, A. E. and Molinari, G. F. (1975). Criteria of cerebral death. *Trans. Am. Neurol. Assoc.* **100**, 29.

Weibull, H., Bergqvist, D., Alment, T., *et al.* (1987). Is cerebral angiography of organ donors dangerous in kidney transplantation? *Lakartidningen* **84**, 128.

Wertheimer, P., Jouvet, M. and Descotes, J. (1959). *Presse Med.* **67**, 87.

Wilkus, R. J., Harvey, F., Ojemann, L. M. and Lettich, E. (1971). Electroencephalogram and sensory evoked potentials. Findings in an unresponsive patient with pontine infarct. *Arch. Neurol.* **24**, 538.

Wolstenholme, G. E. W. and O'Connor, M. (1966). *Ethics in Medical Progress* (Ciba Foundation Symposium), p. 1, J and A Churchill, London.

Yoshioka, T., Sugimoto, H., Uenishi, M., *et al.* (1986). Prolonged hemodynamic maintenance by the combined administration of vasopressin and epinephrine in brain death: a clinical study. *Neurosurgery* **18**, 565.

The Donor and Donor Nephrectomy
Dicken S. C. Ko • A. Benedict Cosimi

Introduction

Donor selection for allografting of a nonpaired vital organ, such as the heart, is necessarily limited to cadaveric or possibly xenogeneic sources. In contrast, because of the presence in most normal persons of two kidneys—each with a physiological reserve capable of providing four to five times the minimal required function—renal transplantation has become an accepted medical procedure using cadaveric and living related or unrelated volunteers as organ sources. Each of these donor categories presents unique ethical, legal and social implications (Spital, 1991; Woo, 1992; Youngner *et al.*, 1985) that must be addressed carefully to protect not only the health and rights of the recipient but also those of the donor.

Of equal importance are the medical aspects of donor evaluation and the technical features of the nephrectomy procedure, which now include minimally invasive approaches (Ratner *et al.*, 1995). The initial functional capacity of the transplanted kidney is largely independent of immunological factors; however, it is highly dependent on the efficacy of donor preparation and procurement techniques in preventing ischemic injury. This situation has become more complicated as retrieval of extrarenal organs from the same cadaver donor has become commonplace. As a result, it has been necessary to adapt the surgical procedures to develop combination procurement techniques that provide equal protection for the extrarenal organs as well as the kidneys (Starzl *et al.*, 1984).

Another area of consideration that had been primarily of historical interest involves efforts to modify or reduce the graft's antigenicity by treatment of the organ donor or the kidney itself. For allografts, this approach is presumed to be directed toward removal of *passenger leukocytes* that may be involved with initiation of the host's immune response (see Chapter 2). As discussed subsequently, clinical trials using these approaches have been inconclusive and are no longer being pursued. With the increasing enthusiasm over the potential use of organs from nonhuman donors (xenografts), such manipulations are being evaluated again, now primarily by production of transgenic animals expressing, for example, human complement regulators or other chimeric molecules (Fodor and Squinto, 1995; see Chapter 42).

Living Kidney Donor
JUSTIFICATION

The first successful renal transplant (between monozygotic twins) was performed in 1954. This experience emphasized that in situations in which no histoincompatibilities exist, the allograft can restore normal function completely for indefinite periods of time. With the development of increasingly effective immunosuppressive regimens, this observation was extended successfully to less compatible intrafamilial donors and eventually to unrelated donors.

Among the many reasons that may be cited for the continued use of the living related donor, the most important has been the more favorable results that can be achieved with a physiologically perfect kidney that is also biologically matched. The morbidity and mortality after cadaver donor transplantation were so great until the early 1980s that many dialysis patients were hesitant to consider transplantation unless a related donor was available (Freeman, 1985). With the introduction of calcineurin inhibitors, monoclonal and polyclonal antibody immunosuppression and other new immunosuppressives into clinical regimens, the gap in graft survival between living related and cadaveric renal transplantation narrowed considerably. This change historically had led some groups to conclude that living related donor renal transplantation might no longer be justified (Starzl, 1987). Living related donor grafts still have a 10 to 12% better survival rate at 1 year and a significantly higher probability of function thereafter, however (Cecka and Terasaki, 1998). Most transplant units continue to recommend family members as suitable organ donors (Delmonico *et al.*, 1990; Dunn *et al.*, 1986; Leivestad *et al.*, 1986; see Chapter 39).

Because the improved results using intrafamilial donors were believed to be directly related to the degree of histocompatibility between donor and recipient, living unrelated donors were initially not thought to provide any biological advantage over cadaver donors. The experience of using living unrelated kidneys in transplantation has shown that these organs have a graft survival profile that, in fact, approaches that of related donors (Terasaki *et al.*, 1995). Such encouraging results have led most groups routinely to include in the donor pool two HLA haplotype mismatched related donors (Kaufman *et al.*, 1989) and genetically unrelated but emotionally linked volunteers (Spital, 1994). Between 1988 and 1996, the number of living unrelated donor transplants in the United States increased from 4.1 to 14.2% of living donors (First, 1998).

Even with the current widespread application of calcineurin inhibitors and monoclonal and polyclonal antibody immunosuppression, there is a persisting biological advantage of living donor kidneys (living related donor or living unrelated donor) over cadaver donor allografts. Although short-term graft survival after transplantation from both donor sources is excellent, the 5-year success rate of greater than 80% that can be attained using living donor kidneys exceeds by 10 to 15% any reported cadaver donor results.

Another justification for using living donors is that the operation can be specifically planned, limiting waiting time on dialysis. This aspect is relevant for economic reasons. Because successful transplantation allows more complete patient rehabilitation (Evans *et al.*, 1985), this approach proves to be approximately one third as expensive as long-term dialysis (Iglehart, 1993). Of greater importance is the ability to perform the transplant when the recipient is in optimal medical condition. This ability is particularly pertinent for diabetic patients, whose condition may deteriorate rapidly on dialysis. Finally, there is the risk that the patient may develop antibody to HLA antigens (see Chapter 10) during prolonged dialysis, especially if intermittent blood transfusions are required. As a result of such allosensitization, a negative crossmatch donor kidney becomes increasingly difficult, and sometimes impossible, to find.

The final reason for the continued expansion of living donor transplantation is the insufficient supply of cadaver donor organs required to fulfill the needs of renal failure victims awaiting transplantation (Cohen et al., 1998). Because the results of kidney transplantation have improved dramatically since the 1980s, increasing numbers of patients are being placed on waiting lists. The supply of kidneys has increased minimally, however (Evans et al., 1992; Peters et al., 1996). A flow chart outlining the projected need for donor organs, if a goal of no net yearly increase in numbers of patients on dialysis is set, is presented in Figure 7–1. For each 1 million of the population, approximately 75 to 80 renal transplants would have to be performed annually to keep pace with the more than 100 new patients diagnosed with end-stage renal disease and previous transplant recipients whose allografts eventually fail. Even in areas with outstanding cadaver donor retrieval rates (Cohen, 1985; Sollinger et al., 1986) or with less stringent criteria for donor selection (Kauffman et al., 1997), the number of potential recipients greatly exceeds the supply of donor kidneys. A steadily growing population of patients is being maintained on dialysis in most areas of the world.

Despite these compelling reasons for using living donors, the procedure could not be justified if unacceptable morbidity or mortality were to be incurred by the donor. In general, a specific medical treatment is selected on the basis of a balance in favor of its intended good over the potential adverse effects. The concept of removal of an organ for transplantation is unique among major surgical procedures, however, in that it seems to expose the healthy donor to the risks of surgery solely for the benefit of another person. This concept has been evaluated carefully not only by the medical profession but also by the courts and by life insurance carriers. Some courts have ruled in favor of donation, even by a minor, on the grounds that the donor would not only benefit psychologically and spiritually from the act of charity, but also might be psychologically harmed if prevented from donating, at little risk, when the life of a close relative is at stake (Masden-Harrison, 1957; see Chapters 40 and 41).

With the extension of minimally invasive techniques to living kidney donation (discussed in detail in Chapter 8), the potential adverse impact of the operation has become less significant. The major advantages to the donor are decreased morbidity of the surgery and quicker return to normal daily activities, including earlier return to work. It was thought initially that removal of a kidney for transplantation using laparoscopy might be harmful to the donor organ because the warm ischemic interval may be prolonged. Incorporation

of Endocatch (U.S. Surgical Corp., Norwalk, CT) and hand-assisted (Handport [Smith & Nephew, Inc., Andover, MA] or Pneumosleeve [LifeQuest Medical, Inc., Roswell, GA]) devices enables shortening of ishemic times to intervals comparable to those of open donor nephrectomies. The results for laparoscopically removed kidneys are now comparable to those achieved after transplantation of organs procured through the classic open incision (Ratner et al., 1997).

What is the risk to the healthy potential renal donor? The immediate postoperative complications are detailed subsequently. Because of the unusually careful follow-up on thousands of renal donors, in addition to the extensive information available from other unilaterally nephrectomized cases (Narkun-Burgess et al., 1993), the long-term risks can be assessed precisely (Johnson et al., 1997). Survival studies indicate that the 5-year life expectancy of a unilaterally nephrectomized 35-year-old male donor is 99.1% compared with 99.3% normal expectation (Merrill, 1964); this has been compared with the risk incurred in driving a car 16 miles every working day. The quality of life after kidney donation has been reported in 979 patients who had donated a kidney for transplantation (Johnson et al., 1997). Most of the responders had an excellent quality of life. Multivariate analysis of those who did not respond favorably identified the following two factors for negative psychosocial outcome: relatives other than first degree and recipients who died within 1 year of transplantation. In an updated survey of major life insurance companies, it was found that 100% now accept applications from kidney donors after nephrectomy, assuming the remaining renal function is normal (Spital, 1988). Of the companies, 94% do not consider the otherwise healthy donor to be at increased risk for shortened survival or medical problems; only 2% indicated they would raise the premium for such a person.

Based on studies of extensive renal ablation in rats, it has been shown that glomerular hyperfiltration in the remaining kidney tissue can produce progressive sclerosis and deterioration in renal function (Brenner et al., 1982). Concern had been raised that healthy human donors might develop hypertension and renal dysfunction years after unilateral nephrectomy. Follow-up studies of hundreds of living donors for 20 years have been unable, however, to identify any convincing evidence of long-term functional abnormalities associated with unilateral nephrectomy (Anderson et al., 1985; Bay and Hebert, 1987; Najarian et al., 1992).

In view of these considerations, living donors continue to represent a significant proportion of the total donor pool. The percentage of transplanted kidneys obtained from this source varies, accounting for nearly all renal transplants in areas where cadaver donor transplantation is unavailable but for less than 5% in other areas. In the United States, approximately 27% of transplanted kidneys are currently obtained from living donors (Table 7–1).

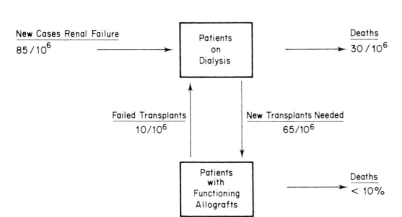

FIGURE 7–1

Flow chart depicts the annual renal transplant rate required to maintain a stable dialysis population. An estimated total of 75 to 80 transplants per 1 million population is projected if previous failed allografts and new cases of renal failure are included.

TABLE 7–1

WORLDWIDE ANNUAL RATES OF KIDNEY TRANSPLANTATION (FROM 1997)*

Donor	Canada	Eurotransplant	France	Greece	Japan	Portugal	Spain	Switzerland	United Kingdom and Ireland	United States
CD†	23.4	26.7	27.5	5.6	1.4	38.2	46.5	26.1	26.0	23.3
LRD†	9.5	2.7	1.2	7.8	3.6	0.6	0.4	7.6	2.8	8.6
%LRD	28.9	9.2	4.3	58.2	73.4	1.6	1.1	22.5	9.7	27.0

*Compiled from ITCS transplant statistics Europe, 1997.
†Per 1 million inhabitants, per country.
CD = cadaveric donors; LRD = living related donors.

MEDICAL EVALUATION AND SELECTION OF THE POTENTIAL LIVING DONOR

From the preceding discussion, it can be concluded that the patient and donor should be presented with the proposed transplant with a spirit of reasonable expectation of benefit compared with acceptably limited risks. All potential donors are first screened for emotional stability and motivation as well as blood group ABO typing (see Chapters 10 and 40). Incompatibility of ABO between donor and recipient typically has resulted in irreversible rejection so that observance of major blood group compatibility usually is practiced. Because of the extreme shortage of donor kidneys, especially for blood group O recipients, this requirement has been constantly reassessed. Several groups have reported successful results after transplantation of blood group A_2 kidneys into group O recipients (Nelson et al., 1998). Approximately 20% of blood group A persons are subtyped as A_2. The highly successful transplantation of A_2 kidneys into group O recipients has been explained by the low expression of A determinants in A_2 kidneys compared with A_1 kidneys. A_1 kidneys have been transplanted successfully into O recipients after elimination of ABO isoagglutinins by plasmapheresis and splenectomy of the recipient (Alexandre and Squifflet, 1988).

Potential donors remaining after the initial screening process are evaluated meticulously and repeatedly to confirm excellent general health and bilateral renal function. Typical evaluations performed (Kasiske et al., 1996) are listed in Table 7–2. Many of the studies are directed toward detection of unsuspected extrarenal pathology. This medical evaluation may reveal significant but treatable problems of which the donor was unaware. In our experience, for example, we have detected early breast, lung and renal cell carcinomas in

TABLE 7–2

EVALUATION OF POTENTIAL LIVING DONORS

Family conference with transplant-dialysis team
ABO blood group, tissue typing, leukocyte crossmatch, ± mixed lymphocyte culture
History, physical examinations, serial blood pressure determinations
Full blood count, coagulation profile, blood urea nitrogen, serum creatinine and clearance, fasting blood sugar glucose, cytomegalovirus antibody, human immunodeficiency virus antibody, hepatitis B and C testing, cholesterol, triglycerides, calcium, phosphorus, urine analysis, urine culture, 24-hour urine protein
Chest radiograph, intravenous pyelogram or ultrasound
Electrocardiogram
Aortogram or digital subtraction angiography and/or three-dimensional computed tomography

asymptomatic potential donors. All of these patients are alive without evidence of disease after appropriate treatment for their cancer. Commoner abnormalities include hypertension, chemical diabetes and unsuspected anemia. This intensive medical evaluation may exclude the volunteer as a donor, but it also accounts for the typically uncomplicated operative procedure and postnephrectomy recovery period. The remaining studies are concerned with the quality of renal function and the clarification of any anatomical abnormalities in either kidney. It must be determined that the nondonated kidney is normal. This determination is especially relevant when the renal failure in the potential donor's relative has resulted from causes that may be hereditary (e.g., diabetes, polycystic disease or hypertension). In the case of diabetes, further evaluation including glucose or cortisone-glucose tolerance tests may be undertaken to identify any subclinical evidence of diabetes. Because of the hereditary nature of polycystic renal disease, cadaver donors usually are preferred for these patients. If an intrafamilial donor is considered, selection may be limited to relatives beyond the third decade of life, in whom latent polycystic disease can be ruled out by the absence of a spongelike nephrogram after rapid injection renal tomography (Hatfield and Pfister, 1972). New genetic tests for the *PKD1* gene and various mutations are available to determine the existence of such genetic predisposition for the development of autosomal dominant polycystic kidney disease. Because most studies have identified an increased incidence of hypertension in first-degree relatives of patients with renal failure, potential donors from this pool should be rejected if they have slight hypertension (Hakim et al., 1984).

Final selection of the donor, if several medically suitable relatives are available, is made on the basis of histocompatibility testing—an HLA-identical sibling being the ideal choice (see Chapter 10). If serological testing identifies several equally compatible family members (e.g., parent, several haploidentical siblings), the person whose cells produce the least stimulation of host cells in mixed lymphocyte culture may be preferred for renal donation. Selection also may be determined on the basis of age (avoiding elderly volunteers or minors if possible) or on less objective factors, such as the special social obligations of a particular family member. If the only suitable donor has not attained the age of majority, it is necessary in the United States to present the medical facts to a court of law so that the necessity and advisability of using that person can be scrutinized.

Throughout this process, at least some unavoidable family pressure to donate must exist despite the physician's attempts to ensure that the final decision is voluntary, reasoned and based on full awareness of relevant information. Scrutiny of the decision process of intrafamilial donors has revealed that most donors make an immediate decision when first contacted, and this decision precedes the acquisition of further scientific data required for truly *informed consent*. Long-term follow-up of intrafamilial donors indicates that they continue to believe they made a correct and an informed decision and would do it again if the opportunity were available (Simmons and Anderson, 1985). These observations do not diminish the responsibilities of the renal transplant team to supply all relevant medical facts to the potential donor, but they emphasize the complicated nature of this particular decision process.

Even more complex is the decision to proceed with transplantation from a genetically unrelated living donor. Because it was presumed that living unrelated donor allografts would have comparable survival to cadaveric donor organs, it was initially proposed that living unrelated donor kidneys should be chosen only in exceptional cases (Brahams, 1989). As noted earlier, however, it is now clear that living unrelated donor kidneys provide significant physiological and consequently long-term survival advantages and are being accepted with increasing frequency. Most centers continue to require that a stable emotional relationship between donor and recipient exist and that donation for monetary compensation not be allowed (Childress, 1996; Quinibi, 1997). In practice, living unrelated donor transplantation occurs most frequently in husband and wife pairs; some spouses have expressed the belief that they have "a right to donate" (Spital, 1991).

For the potential living donor who has been identified by

these criteria, the classic gold standard aortogram historically has been the final diagnostic study scheduled. The optimal study for evaluation of kidney donors has become a subject of debate in the last few years as newer, more sensitive multiplanar simulation technologies have become available using computed tomography (CT) and magnetic resonance imaging (MRI). The ability to visualize data obtained with CT or MRI in a three-dimensional laboratory carefully reconstructing the images isolating artery, veins or parenchymal structures has immensely assisted surgical planning, in particular, with laparoscopic donor nephrectomies (Fig. 7–2).

Despite the increasing availability of these noninvasive modalities and their lower risk potential for kidney donor patients, inadequate definition of the exact status of the renal arteries or the question of a suspected intrarenal lesion may still necessitate an angiogram. The aortogram may be the only study that leads to the decision against accepting a particular donor; for example, when unilateral fibromuscular dysplasia is shown. CT or MRI with three-dimensional reconstruction has not been able to identify reliably the more subtle forms of this lesion. Alternatively, some groups recommend digital subtraction angiography, which can be accomplished through peripheral venipuncture, avoiding some of the costs and morbidity of the aortogram. Although it is technically reasonable to transplant a kidney with multiple arteries, a kidney with a single artery is preferable. When either kidney is shown to be satisfactory, the left is usually

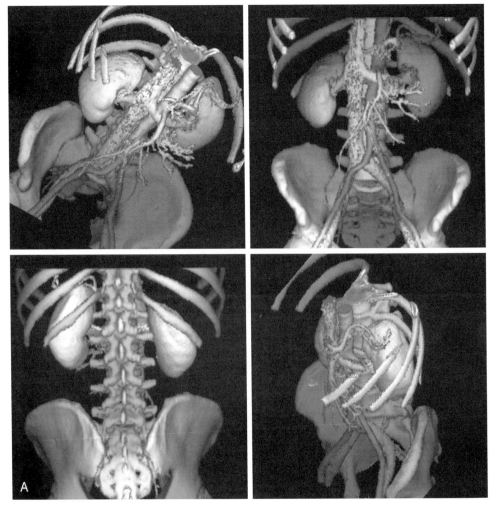

FIGURE 7–2

Three-dimensional reconstructed images of renal computed tomography angiography. (A) Images reconstructed with bone structures (top images—anterior view; bottom images—posterior/oblique views) (see color plate).

chosen because the longer renal vein contributes to the technical ease of the nephrectomy and subsequent transplant.

TECHNIQUE OF OPEN LIVING DONOR NEPHRECTOMY

The technical details of donor nephrectomy vary among different centers—some favor an anterior transperitoneal approach, whereas others favor the loin approach. Many centers have embarked on laparoscopic living donor nephrectomy as the standard for anatomically suitable living related donors and living unrelated donors (see Chapter 8). If an open approach is to be performed, the procedure described herein and in Figure 7–3 is our preferred technique. We emphasize the important principles of (1) adequate exposure; (2) careful handling of the tissues, especially during periarterial dissection to limit vascular spasm; (3) preservation of adequate perihilar and periureteral fat to ensure adequate vascularity and to limit the possibility of subsequent ureteral necrosis and (4) maintenance of active diuresis that makes prompt posttransplantation function more likely.

After induction of general endotracheal anesthesia, the donor is placed in the lateral position with the table flexed to extend the presenting flank (Fig. 7–3A). The incision is made anterior to and extending over the 11th or 12th rib. The latissimus dorsi muscle posteriorly and external oblique muscle anteriorly are divided. This step exposes the periosteum and permits the subperiosteal removal of the rib (Fig. 7–3B), if necessary for adequate exposure. We have found

that in nonobese patients, removal of the rib generally is not required, which results in less postoperative discomfort. The internal oblique and transverse abdominis muscles are divided with the underlying transversalis fascia to enter the retroperitoneal space. Care is taken to avoid entering the pleural or peritoneal cavities (Fig. 7–3C). The paranephric fat and Gerota's fascia, lying in the central part of the wound, are entered. The presenting surface of the kidney is dissected free of the underlying perinephric fat. No dissection is done in the renal hilus to protect the blood supply to the ureter. The renal vein is dissected to its junction with the vena cava, the adrenal and gonadal tributaries being ligated and divided (Fig. 7–3D). The renal artery is skeletonized at its origin from the aorta after lifting the kidney from its bed and rotating it anteriorly (Fig. 7–3E). The ureter is freed, with its investing vessels and fat, down to or below the pelvic brim, then transected. The kidney is now mobilized except for its vascular connections. A brisk diuresis should be evident from the cut ureter, mannitol and furosemide plus adequate crystalloid solutions having been infused during dissection of the kidney.

If the transperitoneal approach is used, which is the practice, for example, in Oxford, a transverse incision is made beneath the costal margin on the side of the kidney to be removed. On the left side, the spleen, pancreas and splenic flexure of the colon are mobilized and retracted to the right to expose the kidney, renal vessels, aorta and ureter. On the right side, the duodenum and hepatic flexure of the colon are mobilized and reflected to the left to expose the kidney,

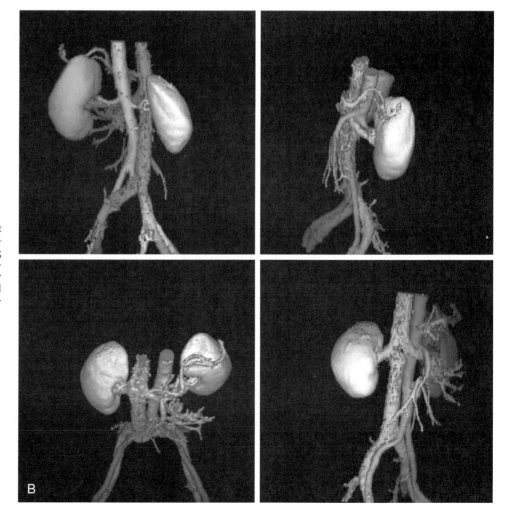

FIGURE 7–2 (Continued)

(B) Images reconstructed without bone structures (top images— posterior/oblique views showing early bifurcation of right renal artery; bottom images—anterior view showing orientation of left renal vein and superior mesenteric artery) (see color plate).

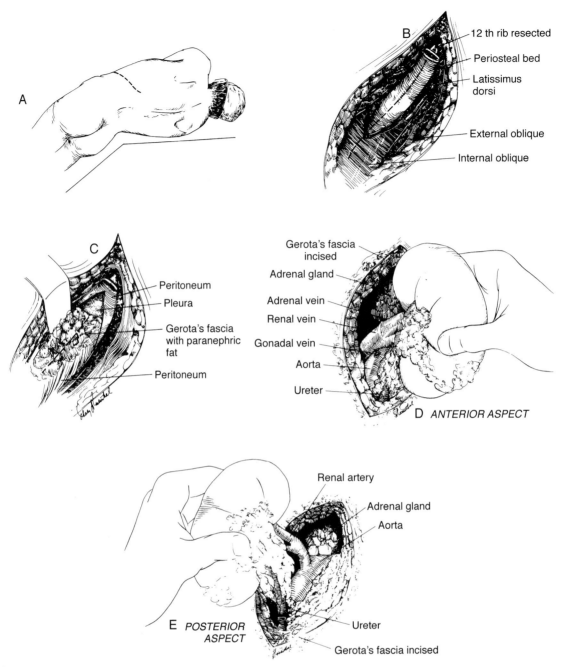

FIGURE 7–3

Living donor nephrectomy. (A–C) In this patient, the kidney is approached through the bed of the 12th rib. Care is taken to avoid entering the pleural or peritoneal cavities. (D) The renal vein is dissected to the vena cava, ligating and dividing the gonadal and adrenal branches. (E) The renal artery is approached by lifting the kidney anteriorly. Gentle dissection continues down to the aorta. The ureter is divided at or below the pelvic brim, carefully preserving the periureteral vascular supply.

inferior vena cava, renal vessels and ureter. Dissection then proceeds much as outlined previously.

Once urinary output from the skeletonized kidney is ensured, the renal artery and vein are clamped and divided, taking care to leave a sufficient cuff of the retained donor vessel to allow secure repair. Although some surgeons prefer to anticoagulate the donor systemically before clamping the vessels, most omit this step and simply perfuse the excised kidney with a chilled, heparinized electrolyte solution. Increasing the osmolarity of the perfusate with mannitol is believed by some to protect the kidney further from ischemic

damage. The use of more complex and more expensive preservation solutions (see Chapter 9) is not required for living donor kidneys, which typically are reimplanted with only a brief cold ischemic interval. The wound is closed without drains, and the patient is returned to the recovery room, where a chest radiograph is obtained to exclude the possibility of pneumothorax.

POSTOPERATIVE CARE AND COMPLICATIONS

The evidence now available indicates that patients undergoing clean contaminated procedures, such as unilateral nephrectomy, can benefit from prophylactic antibiotics (Wenzel, 1992). We routinely administer a first-generation cephalosporin for 24 hours, beginning 1 hour before surgery. Nasogastric tubes usually are not required. Bladder catheters, if present, usually are removed in the immediate postoperative period. Graded resumption of oral alimentation is necessary because these patients may exhibit a more prolonged ileus than might be anticipated after retroperitoneal surgery. This ileus may be the result of the rather extensive periaortic dissection and consequent autonomic nerve disruption. Nevertheless, most of these patients are ready for discharge from the hospital in 3 to 4 days and for return to employment by 3 to 4 weeks if unusually strenuous physical labor is not involved. Urine culture, renal function and a complete blood count are reassessed before discharge. The patient then has follow-up evaluations at increasing intervals.

The perioperative mortality rate for kidney donors is estimated to be 0.03% (Kasiske et al., 1996). Approximately 20 deaths have been reported after living donor allograft donation over 35 years (Jones et al., 1993). Other complications of the renal donor procedure are generally minimal and easily remedied (Blohme et al., 1992; Dunn et al., 1986; Johnson et al., 1997; Spital et al., 1986; Weinstein et al., 1980). The current overall complication rate is approximately 2% (Bia et al., 1995). The more commonly observed problems and their approximate incidence, compiled from these reports and from our own experience with more than 800 patients, are listed in Table 7–3.

Occasionally a complication occurs during the preoperative evaluation, most likely related to the aortogram, which

TABLE 7–3

COMPLICATIONS OF LIVING DONORS

Procedure Complications	Incidence (>2,000 Cases) (%)
Aortogram	
Prolonged discomfort	<1
Femoral thrombosis or aneurysm	<1
Intraoperative	
Splenic laceration	<1
Pancreatic injury, pseudocyst	<1
Nephrectomy wound	
Prolonged discomfort	3.2
Infection	2.1
Hernia	<1
Hematoma	<1
Pulmonary	
Atelectasis	13.5
Pneumothorax or pneumomediastinum	3.2
Pneumonitis or pleural effusion	4.3
Urinary Tract	
Infection	4.5
Retention	3.0
Acute tubular necrosis	<1
Late proteinuria	3.0
Other	
Prolonged ileus	5.2
Thrombophlebitis with or without pulmonary embolus	1.9
Peripheral nerve palsy	1.1
Hepatic dysfunction (late)	<1
Acute depression	<1
Hypertension (late)	15.0*

*Similar to general population (Levey et al., 1986).

is now being used less frequently. Such complications include localized hematoma formation, femoral artery thrombosis or false aneurysm formation at the arterial puncture site or, more rarely, reaction to the radiographic dye, such as an allergic response or acute tubular necrosis. Most complications occur in the perioperative period, with atelectasis, urinary retention or infection, wound problems and prolonged bowel dysfunction accounting for most complications. These conditions typically are reversible by the time the patient is discharged from the hospital. One of the most dangerous complications is thrombophlebitis with possible life-threatening pulmonary embolus. The cause of the approximately 20 known deaths in a worldwide experience estimated to be greater than 100,000 donor operations most commonly has been pulmonary embolus. Single fatal cases of hepatitis, myocardial infarction and depression, leading to alcoholism and death in an automobile accident, have been reported.

Longer term morbidity should be minimal. Endogenous creatinine clearance rates rapidly approach 70 to 80% of the preoperative level, and reports of late renal failure have been extremely rare. An important factor is the exclusion during the selection process of pathology or potential pathology in the donors. As part of a continuing study at Massachusetts General Hospital of the long-term impact of kidney transplantation on the patient and family, 70 adults who had donated a kidney to a close relative between 1963 and 1975 have been studied for the perceptions of the effect of that donation on their lives. No long-term medical problems related to the nephrectomy were identified. As mentioned earlier, in describing how they had come to donate a kidney, more than 50% reportedly made their decision to donate instantaneously and believed that as a result of donation their relationship with the recipient had been strengthened. Approximately one third of the donors reported a positive change in their outlook on life, often citing increased appreciation of their own health. In cases in which the allograft had failed, many donors reported initially a sense of anger and frustration. Ultimately, however, they claimed a sense of worthwhile accomplishment and belief that they would pursue the same course again. Representing a wide variety of occupations, the donors agreed almost universally that their earning capacity and ability to carry out their occupational responsibilities were not adversely affected by the donation.

The immediate and long-term morbidity of nephrectomy is sufficiently low to make the risk acceptable for fully informed, genetically or emotionally related donors for patients with chronic renal disease. The worsening donor shortage and the remarkably successful results currently being reported after transplantation from genetically unrelated living donors have encouraged some centers to consider donation from altruistic strangers (Spital, 1994).

Cadaver Kidney Donor

If a suitable living donor is not available, most patients with end-stage renal failure should be considered for cadaveric renal transplantation, not only because transplantation is more cost-effective but also because true rehabilitation seldom is achieved on long-term dialysis (Evans et al., 1985). Although the long-term success rates remain inferior to those achieved with intrafamilial transplantation, projections indicate that cadaver donor allografts currently have a 1-year graft survival rate of greater than 85% and graft half-life (time to loss of 50% of currently surviving grafts) has improved to at least 10 years (Cecka and Terasaki, 1998). Nonliving donors present the advantage that any morbidity of the nephrectomy experienced by living donors, however small, is absent. Present methods of preservation may permit 72 hours of maintenance of the cadaver donor kidney in a condition sufficiently viable to allow return of function after revascularization (see Chapter 9). Opportunities are present for evaluation of the physiological and bacteriological condition of the donor kidney and for pursuing histocompatibility selection after the organ is removed from the cadaver. Because of these factors and the increasingly widespread establishment of the definition of brain death guidelines that allow removal of organs that are more likely to be physiologically healthy, cadaver donor renal allografts continue to account for approximately 75% of reported transplants. The total number is limited only by the unsolved worldwide problem of persisting barriers to organ donation (Cohen et al., 1998).

MEDICAL AND NEUROLOGICAL EVALUATION OF THE POTENTIAL CADAVER KIDNEY DONOR

The ideal donor is typically a young, previously healthy individual who has sustained a fatal head injury or cerebrovascular accident. The generally accepted criteria for initial screening of potential donors are listed in Table 7–4. Historically, it has been thought that kidneys from elderly donors may not be suitable because of the known physiological deterioration in organ function with age (Kaplan et al., 1975). The urgent need for more transplantable organs has prompted a reevaluation of this concept, however (Kauffman et al., 1997). As a result, recovery of usable kidneys from selected donors in their 60s or 70s, although rare, has been accomplished. Implantation of two kidneys (each with >15% glomerulosclerosis) from the same older donor, to provide more nephron mass for one recipient, has been performed with good success. Transplantation of kidneys from small pediatric donors also is possible, although the technical aspects are more exacting. When kidneys are obtained from a pediatric donor less than 3 years of age, most groups recommend en bloc transplantation of both organs into a single adult recipient.

Maintenance of renal blood flow and function with adequate hydration, after irreversibility of brain damage is established, is important. Minor terminal elevations of blood urea nitrogen and creatinine levels are not unusual and do not necessarily exclude the donor.

A major concern for the donor team is the risk of transmitting infection with the allograft into an immunosuppressed

recipient (see Chapters 31 and 32). Donor infections that can adversely affect the recipient are divided into two categories. Particularly dangerous infections that antedate the terminal illness include active hepatitis B (hepatitis B surface antigen positive), human immunodeficiency virus (HIV), encephalitis of unknown causes, Jakob-Creutzfeldt disease and active tuberculosis. Any evidence of these illnesses in a thorough history of risk factors or rapid serological tests should reclassify these potential donors as high risk and usually precludes organ donation.

A more controversial issue relates to the donor found to be positive for hepatitis C. Some retrospective studies have recommended that because this virus also is highly transmissible by the allograft, transplantation of kidneys from positive donors should not be performed (Pereira and Levey, 1997; see Chapter 32). Others have challenged this conclusion, however (Kliem et al., 1996). Current policy regarding these donors varies among different transplant groups. Because approximately 5% of all organ donors test positive for hepatitis C virus, establishing this as a medical contraindication would result in a severe reduction of the number of available organs for transplantation (Pereira and Levey, 1997). Many centers have adopted a more flexible policy with which hepatitis C virus–positive kidneys are selectively targeted for recipients with a more limited life expectancy, during which chronic hepatitis is unlikely to develop (Fishman et al., 1996).

Cytomegalovirus also can be transmitted with the allograft to a previously uninfected recipient and occasionally produces a serious primary infection (Rubin et al., 1985). With the current availability of effective antiviral agents, such as ganciclovir, most groups now accept allocation of a kidney from a cytomegalovirus-seropositive donor, even for a seronegative recipient (Patel et al., 1996).

The more difficult category of infections to evaluate includes new conditions that complicate the donor's terminal care. Any potential donor with unequivocal systemic sepsis is eliminated from consideration. In contrast, catheter-related urinary tract infection, pneumonitis or a history of treated central line–related septic episodes is commonly discovered during evaluation of the donor. Use of kidneys from such donors, even if terminal blood cultures were positive, has not been found to transmit bacterial infection to recipients treated with appropriate antibiotics (Freeman, 1985). Attempts also are made to rule out significant organ contamination by culturing perfusate and transport media. Frequently, such cultures turn positive (Spees et al., 1982). Most such positive cultures are with nonvirulent skin flora, however, and these results have correlated poorly with the occurrence of posttransplant allograft infection. In contrast, the occasional instances in which surveillance cultures have yielded Staphylococcus aureus, Candida or gram-negative organisms, particularly Pseudomonas aeruginosa, have been associated with serious posttransplant infection (Rubin and Cosimi, 1989). These kidneys usually should be discarded.

The procurement of cadaver donor organs for transplantation has naturally raised new moral and legal issues, the most significant of which is to establish when death occurs (Youngner et al., 1985). The phenomenon of irreversible coma, or brain death, which has been recognized with increasing clarity by neurologists and neurosurgeons, has presented a set of circumstances that are of great potential benefit to patients needing organ allografts (see Chapter 6). The concept and definition of brain death do not depend in any way on transplantation. The discontinuation of respiratory support and other extraordinary therapy for patients who have been declared dead after careful assessment of brain function should be considered a humane and necessary act

TABLE 7–4
RECOMMENDED CRITERIA FOR INITIAL SCREENING OF POTENTIAL CADAVER DONORS

Maximum age 70 years; marginal donors to age 80 years
No history of
  Untreated hypertension
  Diabetes mellitus
  Malignancy other than primary brain tumor or nonmelanoma skin cancer
No evidence of
  Primary renal disease
  Generalized viral or bacterial infection
Acceptable urinalysis (minor abnormalities attributable to acute illness ignored)
Preterminal urine output >0.5 ml/kg/h
Normal blood urea nitrogen and creatinine (except for terminal elevations)
Warm ischemia time <60 minutes
Negative serologic assays for hepatitis B, human immunodeficiency virus; acceptability of hepatitis C remains controversial

without regard to the possibility of such a person serving as an organ donor. The philosophical argument about the definition of death has arisen not because of transplantation but because of technical innovations that can now artificially maintain, for indefinite periods, the historically recognized vital functions of respiration and circulation. After extensive assessment of such patients, neurologists and neurosurgeons universally have agreed that once functional death of the brain stem occurs, there is no chance for partial recovery, and artificial support should be withdrawn.

To avoid conflict of interest, the declaration of death must always be the responsibility of that patient's physician with any assistance he or she may request. It is done with the full understanding of the family in every case. When organ donation is involved, the permission of the family and, if necessary, of the medical examiner is then secured. The transplantation team is available for consultation with the family and the responsible physician but is not involved with medical decisions regarding the donor's therapy or chances of recovery.

Before the acceptance of brain death as a clear definition of the termination of human life, organs were routinely recovered after the donor's death had been determined by the absence of heartbeat and respiratory activity (non–heart beating donors [NHBD]). The NHBD are considered less desirable because the viability of the organs is affected by the cessation of cardiorespiratory function, in contrast to donors with brain death, in whom organ perfusion is interrupted under controlled conditions that minimize ischemia. Organs procured from NHBD may experience significant periods of warm ischemia before the rapid infusion of preservation fluids as the surgeon awaits cessation of the donor's heartbeat. Unless kidneys are recovered from NHBD in carefully orchestrated situations, they may have a high rate of delayed function. Selective use of *ex vivo* machine preservation of the removed allograft may lessen the risk of dysfunction by identifying and discarding kidneys that have suffered irreversible ischemic injury. Even with this approach, some of these renal allografts may never function, and consequently the hospital stay of recipients of NHBD organs may be prolonged significantly. The proportion of NHBD today continues to represent less than 1% of all organ donors as reported by United Network for Organ Sharing (UNOS).

One of the major problems with the use of NHBD is related to the period of asystole that is required to ensure the patient can be declared brain dead. Kootstra (1997) has suggested that 10 minutes should lapse before allowing any interventions, such as initiation of organ preservation approaches. With this policy, there is a clear transition from the medical care of the patient to the recovery of organs from the cadaver (Kootstra, 1997). Kootstra acknowledges that the 10-minute period of asystole likely prohibits the recovery of organs other than the kidneys. In other institutions, different protocols have been accepted to increase the potential opportunity for multiple organ procurement. These protocols may permit the declaration of death 2 minutes after the cessation of cardiorespiratory activity. These variations in approach have fostered ethical controversy about the validity of death declaration. In the United States, this controversy stimulated establishment of a Committee on Medical and Ethical Issues in Maintaining the Viability of Organs for Transplantation, by the Institute of Medicine of the National Academy of Sciences. After discussing in depth the complete testimonials from patient families, medical providers, transplant surgeons and other experts in the field, the Institute of Medicine released its report in December 1997, fully supporting the NHBD process. The report recommends that all transplant organizations adopt a consistent approach that respects the wishes of the patients and families and addresses all the specific issues surrounding NHBD at each medical center as the protocols are being developed (Institute of Medicine, 1997). In a society of growing health awareness, increased use of health care proxies and advanced directives and a public reluctance for prolonging extraordinary life-sustaining measures, there may be an opportunity to increase the number of NHBD. Clinical conditions have become recognized in which complete irreversible brain injury may have occurred without fulfilling the criteria for brain death. With the family's approval, a joint decision with the physician may be made, concluding that withdrawal of life-sustaining support is the optimal, compassionate care for these patients. Non–heart-beating organ donation may then provide the families with an important consolation, while increasing the number of organs available for transplantation.

TECHNIQUE OF CADAVER DONOR NEPHRECTOMY

The most commonly practiced procurement technology today continues to retrieve viable organs for transplantation from brain-dead patients who are maintained in stable physiological balance by artificial support. This approach gives rise to the term *heart-beating* cadaver donor. These donors are brought to the operating room where organ procurement is undertaken under semielective conditions while employing the usual sterile precautions of any aseptic surgical procedure. The donor may require large volumes of intravenous fluids to restore blood volume, which typically has been severely depleted by premortem attempts to decrease brain swelling and achieve neurological resuscitation. Diuretics, mannitol and vasopressors are administered as needed to promote diuresis during the nephrectomy procedure. Some groups systemically heparinize the donor and administer vasoactive agents, such as phenoxybenzamine or phentolamine, to combat vasospasm in the kidneys. Other donor pretreatment modalities, such as possible immunomodulating measures, are seldom employed but are discussed here.

In situations in which the criteria for brain death have been fulfilled but the concept of heart-beating donation has not been accepted or in which there is irreversible brain injury but not fulfilling the criteria of brain death, respiratory support is discontinued in the operating room (termed *controlled* NHBD). After cardiac function ceases, the donor is declared dead, and the surgical procedure is expeditiously undertaken (Kootstra, 1997). The kidneys must be removed and chilled more rapidly than in the heart-beating donation procedure to minimize ischemic damage to the retrieved organs. The goal is to limit the warm ischemic period, whenever possible, to less than 30 minutes.

In an effort to increase further the number of kidneys available for transplantation, interest also has been revived in the possible procurement of organs from donors who are dead on arrival or who die after unsuccessful cardiorespiratory resuscitation (*uncontrolled* NHBD). Several studies have confirmed that significant numbers of patients succumb in emergency departments or intensive care units without brain death being declared (Daemen *et al.*, 1997). Presumably, suitable allografts could be salvaged from such potential donors if reliable methods could be identified to control the ischemic damage that occurs shortly after death. Current approaches include combined *in situ* kidney flushing and core body cooling by femoral artery and peritoneal catheters placed at the bedside immediately after cardiac arrest (Kootstra, 1997; Paprocki *et al.*, 1992). The NHBD can then be transported to the operating room for bilateral nephrectomy.

REMOVAL OF KIDNEYS ALONE

If only the kidneys are to be removed, bilateral nephrectomy is accomplished through a long midline incision. The objective is to take both kidneys with the full length of the renal artery and vein, preferably on aortic and vena caval cuffs. This approach limits the possibility of injuring accessory vessels, which are present in 12 to 15% of normal kidneys. The technique we prefer entails *en bloc* removal of both kidneys with an intact segment of aorta and inferior vena cava to allow early *in situ* cooling of the kidneys. This approach reduces the time required for the nephrectomies because the fine dissection necessary for identification and isolation of the artery and vein can be performed after the kidneys are removed. With this technique, the risk of damaging accessory vessels is essentially eliminated. Continuous perfusion of the kidneys, if this preservation technique is used, usually can be provided via the aorta, avoiding direct renal artery cannulation and the possibility of intimal injury. Multiple arteries can be left on a cuff of aorta, giving the transplant surgeon the option of using a single Carrel patch anastomosis for a simpler reimplantation procedure.

On entering the donor's abdomen, rapid exploration excludes the presence of unsuspected sepsis, neoplasia or other important pathology. The small bowel and mesentery are retracted to the right, and the posterior parietal peritoneum is incised over the great vessels and through the ligament of Treitz. The peritoneal incision is extended around the right colon so that the bowel can be retracted upward and to the left (Fig. 7–4A). The duodenum and pancreas are retracted superiorly. The proximal aorta is freed to above the celiac axis, dividing and ligating the superior mesenteric artery (Fig. 7–4B).

Tapes or large silk sutures are passed around the distal aorta and vena cava just above the iliac bifurcations. Because only the kidneys are being removed, the proximal aorta also is encircled, enabling isolation of the renal circulation. After achieving proximal aortic, distal aortic and distal caval occlusion, preservation of the kidneys *in situ* is begun by perfusion with chilled University of Wisconsin solution, Euro-Collins

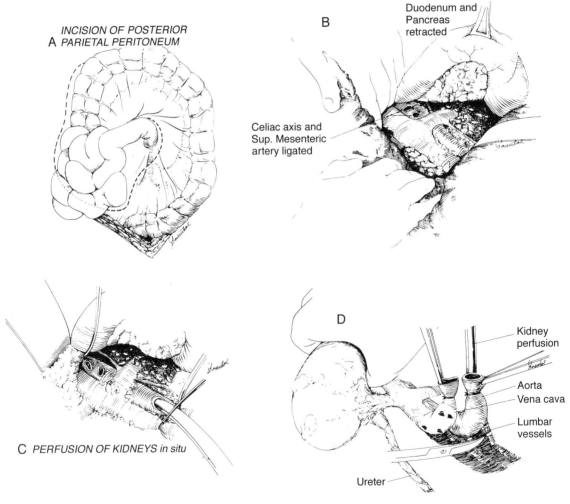

FIGURE 7–4

Cadaver donor nephrectomy without other organ retrieval. (A) After widely opening and exploring the peritoneal cavity, the small bowel is retracted to expose the posterior parietal peritoneum, which is incised. This allows retraction of the bowel superiorly and to the left. (B) The duodenum and pancreas are retracted superiorly to obtain exposure of the proximal aorta and vena cava. The superior mesenteric and celiac trunks are ligated and divided several centimeters above the level of the left renal vein crossing the aorta. (C) After ligation of the proximal and distal aorta and the distal vena cava, perfusion of the kidneys is begun through the intravenous tubing that has been introduced into the distal aorta. (D) Isolation of the kidneys and ureters has been completed (left kidney not shown). The distal aorta and vena cava are transected, and the lumbar vessels posteriorly are clamped and divided, allowing removal of the entire block of tissue while cold perfusion continues.

solution or Ringer's lactated solution containing mannitol (18 g/L) and heparin (20,000 units/L) infused through sterile intravenous tubing that has been placed directly into the aorta. The perfusate is allowed to return to the donor circulation via the proximal vena cava (Fig. 7–4C). The kidneys are generally cool and pale after rapid infusion of 500 to 600 ml of perfusate, but the perfusion is continued at a slower rate throughout the remainder of the procedure.

The final mobilization of the kidneys is undertaken within the plane of Gerota's fascia in a more leisurely manner. Care is taken to free and section the ureters as far down toward the bladder as possible and to avoid dissection within the renal hilus. The distal aorta and vena cava are divided, and the entire block is lifted anteriorly to expose the lumbar vessels posteriorly (Fig. 7–4D). Once the proximal aorta and vena cava have been divided, the block consisting of both kidneys and ureters, aorta and inferior vena cava can be lifted out of the abdomen and placed immediately into a basin of cooled perfusion solution. A more complete dissection and assessment of the anatomy of the renal vessels can then be undertaken. Before closure of the abdominal incision, specimens of donor lymph nodes and spleen are removed for subsequent histocompatibility and other immunological studies.

REMOVAL OF KIDNEYS WITH OTHER ORGANS

The more typical situation involves multiple-organ procurement from the same donor. Acceptable donors for heart, liver or pancreas transplantation are younger (generally <70 years old) and hemodynamically more stable than some donors from whom kidneys alone can be retrieved. For example, kidneys suitable for transplantation can be salvaged from a donor after cardiac function has ceased, whereas multiple-organ procurement is seldom accomplished from the NHBD cadaver.

The successful undertaking of multiple-organ recovery requires careful coordination among three surgical teams to ensure that there is no compromise in viability of any transplantable organ. It is crucial to have anesthesia support to monitor and maintain cardiovascular integrity of the donor during the extensive dissection, which may take 1 to 3 hours. Although the details differ, depending on the combination of organs to be removed, certain common principles prevail, including wide exposure, dissection of each organ to its vascular connection while the heart is still beating, placement of catheters for *in situ* cooling and removal of organs while perfusion continues, usually in the order of heart, lungs, liver, kidneys and pancreas (Van Buren and Barakat, 1994).

The organs are exposed through a midline incision extending from suprasternal notch to the pubis (Fig. 7–5A). If the heart is to be retrieved, it is usually partially mobilized as the first maneuver so that it can be removed quickly at any later stage should vascular instability occur during the dissection of the other organs. The preparatory steps for cardiectomy require opening of the pericardium, mobilization of the superior vena cava and separation of the aorta from the pulmonary artery. Dissection is then undertaken to mobilize the liver and/or pancreas. If the pancreas is not to be used, the splenic and superior mesenteric arteries may be ligated and/or divided (Fig. 7–5B). The common bile duct is transected, and the gallbladder is incised and flushed with cold saline to prevent biliary autolysis. The portal vein is dissected to the confluence of the splenic and superior mesenteric veins where a catheter can be placed into the splenic vein for subsequent rapid portal perfusion (see Fig. 7–5B). Alternatively, the inferior mesenteric vein is used for the

placement of the portal vein catheter. Isolation of the liver is completed by mobilizing the vena cava posteriorly.

If the pancreas is to be transplanted, the spleen is mobilized, the short gastric vessels are divided and the spleen and pancreas are retracted to the right (Fig 7–5C). The body and tail of the pancreas are then carefully dissected free. Although now used infrequently, this mobilization can terminate at the junction of the splenic and superior mesenteric veins, where the pancreas can be transected for segmental transplantation. More commonly, the entire pancreas and a segment of duodenum can be mobilized for pancreaticoduodenal transplantation.

The kidneys and major abdominal vessels are next exposed by retracting the right colon and small bowel to the left and lifting the mobilized duodenum anteriorly (Fig. 7–5D). The kidneys are elevated from the retroperitoneum, and the distal aorta and vena cava are completely freed. The donor is heparinized and mannitol infused, after which a perfusion catheter is placed in the aorta and a venous drainage catheter in the vena cava (Fig. 7–5E).

Initial organ cooling usually is begun via the previously placed portal vein catheter (see Fig. 7–5B). When the donor core temperature falls to about 30°C or if hemodynamic instability occurs, the aorta is cross-clamped at the diaphragm, and the aortic flush is begun for rapid cooling of the abdominal organs. Precise coordination among the retrieval teams is required at this critical stage. Cardioplegic infusion into the ascending aorta is begun, and cardiectomy and pneumonectomy are performed first. The liver is removed next. Finally the remaining mobilization of the kidneys is undertaken. Care is taken to free and section the ureters as far down toward the bladder as possible and to avoid dissection within the renal hilus. The distal aorta and vena cava are divided, and the entire block is lifted anteriorly to expose the lumbar vessels posteriorly. These vessels are divided after being doubly clamped with vascular clips (Fig. 7–5F). Once these vessels are controlled, the block consisting of both kidneys and ureters, aorta and inferior vena cava can be lifted out of the abdomen and placed immediately into a basin of cooled perfusion solution. A more complete dissection and assessment of the detailed anatomy of the renal vessels can then be undertaken.

In donors from whom whole pancreaticoduodenal procurement is included, we advise removing this organ block after the kidneys have been taken from the field to avoid possible contamination from the transected duodenum. Although it had been believed that total removal of the pancreas is anatomically incompatible with simultaneous retrieval of the liver, currently most groups routinely procure both organs from the same donor and use vascular grafts for pancreatic rearterialization in the recipients (Yang *et al.*, 1991). Before closure of the abdominal incision, specimens of donor lymph nodes and spleen are removed for subsequent histocompatibility and other immunological studies. Most groups have concluded that the immediate and long-term functional results observed in transplanted kidneys obtained from multiple organ donors are comparable to those in procedures involving donor nephrectomy alone (McMaster, 1984).

Donor Pretreatment for Renal Transplantation

Despite continuing improvements in the pharmacotherapeutic regimens administered to renal allograft recipients, the intensity and lack of specificity of the immunosuppression produced remain a source of long-term morbidity. Among those approaches that have been employed attempting to reduce the need for recipient immunosuppression has been

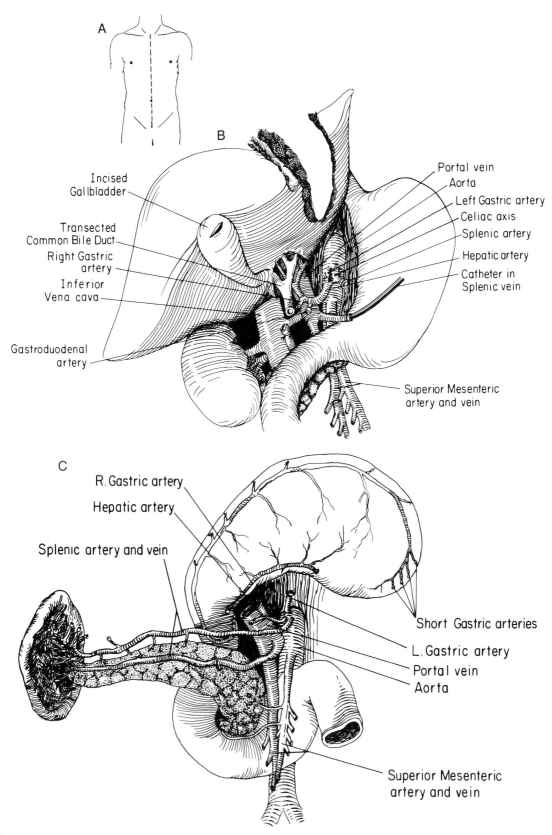

FIGURE 7–5

Cadaver donor multiple organ retrieval. (A) The chest and abdominal cavities are entered through a long midline incision. After general evaluation of the organs to be procured and initial mobilization of the heart, the liver dissection is completed. (B) The splenic vein is catheterized for portal perfusion. The gastroduodenal and splenic arteries are divided if the pancreas is not to be used. (C) For pancreas retrieval, dissection is begun from the left, retracting the spleen and pancreas to the right, carefully preserving the splenic artery and vein. For simplicity, the superior mesenteric vessels are depicted as separate from the pancreas, but they remain closely adherent to the posterior pancreas.

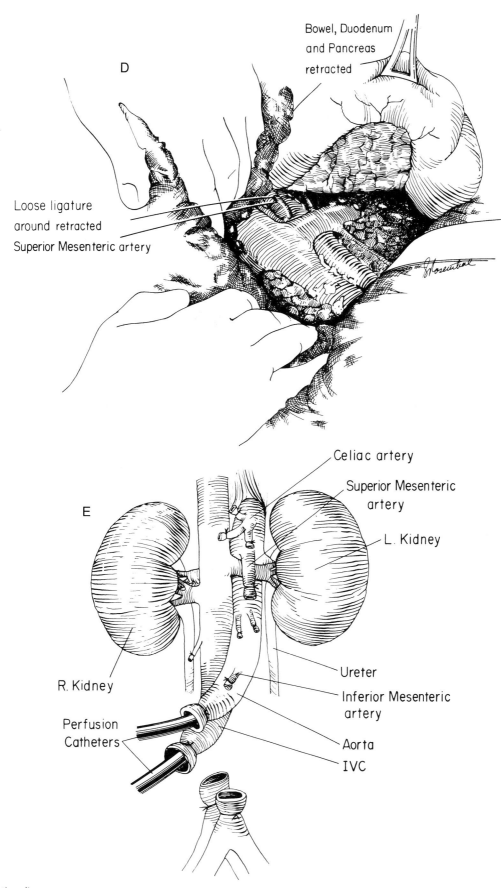

D

Bowel, Duodenum
and Pancreas
retracted

Loose ligature
around retracted
Superior Mesenteric artery

E

Celiac artery

Superior Mesenteric
artery

L. Kidney

R. Kidney

Ureter

Inferior Mesenteric
artery

Aorta

IVC

Perfusion
Catheters

FIGURE 7–5 *(Continued)*

(D) Returning to the right side, the duodenum and pancreas are retracted exposing the superior mesenteric artery. (E) Mobilization of the kidneys and ureters from the retroperitoneum is completed, and the distal vena cava and aorta are catheterized. For illustrative purposes, the bowel, which remains attached via the mesenteric vessels, is not shown in this figure.

Illustration continued on following page

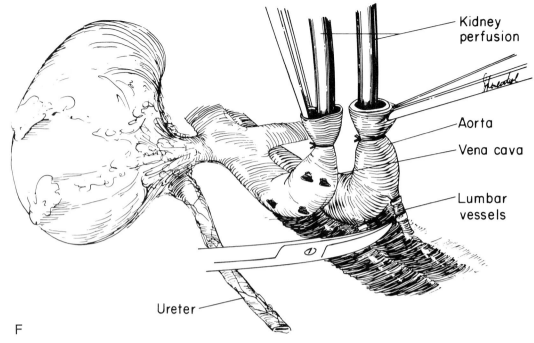

FIGURE 7–5 *(Continued)*

(F) After cooling and removal of the heart and liver, the kidneys are removed by lifting the entire tissue block (left kidney not shown) anteriorly, while clamping and dividing the lumbar vessels posteriorly.

the institution of maneuvers designed to modulate graft immunogenicity. Because an important source of antigen for the inductive phase of allograft immunity resides in the bone marrow–derived mononuclear cells (passenger leukocytes or dendritic cells) contained within the graft (Ricordi *et al.,* 1992), depletion of these cells by donor or allograft pretreatment might provide a means of reducing the allogeneic stimulus. Therapeutic efforts to accomplish this goal have included the use of antilymphocyte sera, cytotoxic drugs and monoclonal antibody perfusion of kidneys before transplantation (Taube *et al.,* 1987; Zincke *et al.,* 1978). Significantly better results have been observed after transplantation of the pretreated kidneys in some reports, but the lack of randomized control data limited the interpretation of these early trials. Concurrently controlled studies have not defined a beneficial effect of donor pretreatment for kidney transplantation (Jeffery *et al.,* 1978). More encouraging observations have been provided from evaluation of these approaches in transplantation of pancreatic islets (Faustman and Coe, 1991; Ricordi *et al.,* 1992). In these studies, rejection of xenogeneic tissue has been circumvented by masking, before transplantation, donor class I histocompatibility antigens or tissue-specific epitopes with F(ab′)₂ antibody fragments. Inconsistent results reported in these trials suggest that passenger leukocytes are not the sole source of immunogen within a graft and that complete absence of passenger leukocytes may only delay the onset of rejection without preventing it. The true relevance of the interstitial dendritic cells for clinical transplantation and the degree of improved graft survival that might be achieved if these cells could be removed effectively remain the object of continuing experimental and clinical studies (see Chapter 2 for further discussion). With the exception of small bowel transplantation, in which the donor may receive a dose of monoclonal anti–T cell therapy during donor procurement, there are currently no active clinical protocols being employed for donor pretreatment.

Xenogeneic Kidney Donor

The need for kidneys is growing steadily, whereas organ donation has leveled off or decreased in some regions. This situation has resulted in a rapidly escalating demand for medical and economic resources to support long-term peritoneal dialysis or hemodialysis programs. Because the supply of such resources is limited, constant efforts must be made to improve the efficacy and increase the number of transplants performed. The latter is determined primarily by the number of donor organs available.

Nonhuman (xenogeneic) donors represent a possible alternative source of transplantable organs (see Chapter 42). Beginning in the early 1900s, several isolated attempts were made to transplant kidneys from various animal donors into patients with renal failure. If a successful approach to the use of such organs could be established, an unlimited pool of donors free of most of the legal and moral issues associated with the use of human organs could be made available. The major obstacle to such an approach has been the in-

TABLE 7–5

CLINICAL RENAL XENOGRAFTS IN THE MODERN ERA

Report	No.	Donor	Longest Survival
Reemtsma *et al.,* 1964	12	Chimpanzee	9 months
	1	Monkey	10 days
Starzl *et al.,* 1964	6	Baboon	2 months
Hitchcock *et al.,* 1964	1	Baboon	5 days
Hume, 1964	1	Chimpanzee	1 day
Traeger *et al.,* 1965	3	Chimpanzee	48 days
Goldsmith, 1965, in Millard *et al.,* 1985	2	Chimpanzee	4 months
Cortesini *et al.,* 1969	1	Chimpanzee	31 days

TABLE 7–6
CLINICAL LIVER AND HEART XENOGRAFTS IN THE MODERN ERA

Organ	Report	No.	Donor	Longest Survival
Liver	Starzl et al., 1966	1	Chimpanzee	1 day
	Starzl, 1969	2	Chimpanzee	2 days
	Bertoye, 1969	1	Baboon	1 day
	Leger et al., 1970	1	Baboon	3 day
	Marion et al., 1970	1	Baboon	1 day
	Pouyet and Berard, 1971	1	Baboon	1 day
	Motin, 1971, in Dubernard et al., 1974	1	Baboon	3 day
	Starzl et al., 1974	3	Chimpanzee	14 days
	Starzl et al., 1993b	2	Baboon	70 days
	Makowa et al., 1995	1	Pig	1 day
Heart	Hardy et al., 1964	1	Chimpanzee	2 hours
		1	Baboon	6 hours
	Cooley et al., 1968	1	Sheep	0
	Ross, 1969	1	Pig	0
	Marion, 1969	1	Chimpanzee	4 hours
	Barnard et al., 1977	1	Chimpanzee	4 days
	Bailey et al., 1985	1	Baboon	20 days
	Czaplicki et al., 1992	1	Pig	1 day

creased intensity of the rejection response elicited by the more diverse genetic relationship between donor and recipient. The complete inadequacy of conventional immunosuppression in controlling concordant xenogeneic (chimpanzee or baboon donor) responses in humans has been emphasized in the clinical trials performed over three decades.

Since the early 1960s, approximately 50 primarily vascularized xenografts have been transplanted from animals to humans (Tables 7–5 and 7–6). Initial studies by Reemtsma et al. (1964) indicated that prompt renal function with diuresis could be achieved in patients after chimpanzee renal transplantation. Despite intensive immunosuppression, however, most of these grafts failed within 2 months. The 9-month survival of one of them has continued to intrigue investigators in this field. Evaluation of baboon donors also was pursued during this early era (Starzl et al., 1964). Graft survival in these human recipients ranged from 19 to 60 days, during which multiple vigorous rejection episodes were encountered.

With the introduction of cyclosporine and tacrolimus into the immunosuppressive armamentarium, renewed interest in the potential of xenografts was stimulated. Although laboratory models using these agents have suggested many promising approaches, no successful xenogeneic transplant to humans has been achieved whether using concordant or discordant (pig) donors. Combined immunosuppression with tacrolimus, steroids, cyclophosphamide and prostaglandin provided survival for only 70 days in a baboon liver recipient (Starzl et al., 1993a). The intensity of such suppression resulted in numerous life-threatening infectious episodes and ultimate fatal disseminated *Aspergillus* infection. A subsequent baboon-to-human liver transplant by the same group also failed in the early postoperative period, leading most investigators to conclude, at that point, that further human trials were not warranted until more effective methods to control the xenogeneic immune response could be identified. For several reasons, there is renewed interest in the possibility that xenotransplantation could provide the solution for the shortage of human donor organs. The first reason for this enthusiasm is the increasingly successful use of genetic engineering to produce transgenic animals expressing recombinant molecules designed to moderate the immune response

(Bhatti et al., 1999; Schmoeckel et al., 1998; Waterworth et al., 1998; Zaidi et al., 1998). Another reason for the renewed optimism regarding xenotransplantation has been the demonstration in preclinical primate models that tolerance of allografts can be produced without the need for long-term immunosuppression (Kawai et al., 1995; Kirk et al., 1999). The concept of transplanting genetically modified animal organs into recipients conditioned with tolerance-inducing protocols has led to the prediction that pig-to-human transplantation studies may be initiated within the next 5 years. Should such studies be accomplished successfully, the entire field of transplantation will be not only radically expanded, but also forced to address a new series of ethical, economic and resource allocation issues.

ACKNOWLEDGMENT

This work was supported in part by the Helen and George Burr Research and Educational Fund.

REFERENCES

Alexandre, G. P. J. and Squifflet J. P. (1988). Significance of the ABO antigen system. *In Organ Transplantation and Replacement*, (G. J. Cirelli, ed.), p. 230, J. B. Lippincott, Philadelphia.
Anderson, C. F., Velosa, J. A., et al. (1985). The risks of unilateral nephrectomy: status of kidney donors 10 to 20 years postoperatively. *Mayo Clin. Proc.* **60**, 367.
Bailey, L. L., Nehlsen-Cannarella, S. L., et al. (1985). Baboon-to-human cardiac xenotransplantation in a neonate. *J. A. M. A.* **254**, 3321.
Barnard, C. N., Wolpowitz, A., et al. (1977). Heterotopic cardiac transplantation with a xenograft for assistance of the left heart in cardiogenic shock after cardiopulmonary bypass. *S. Afr. Med. J.* **52**, 1035.
Bay, W. H. and Hebert, L. A. (1987). The living donor in kidney transplantation. *Ann. Intern. Med.* **106**, 719.
Bertoye, A. (1969). Essais de traitement de certaines insuffisances hepatiques graves par greffe hepatique heterologue. *Lyon Med.* **222**, 245.
Bhatti, F. N., Schmoeckel, M., et al. (1999). Three-month survival of HDAFF transgenic pig hearts transplanted into primates. *Transplant. Proc.* **31**, 958.
Bia, M. J., Ramos, E. L., et al. (1995). Evaluation of living renal donors: the current practice of US transplant centers. *Transplantation* **60**, 322.
Blohme, I., Fehrman, I., et al. (1992). Living donor nephrectomy: complication rates in 490 consecutive cases. *Scand. J. Urol. Nephrol.* **26**, 149.
Brahams, D. (1989). Kidney for sale by live donor. *Lancet* **1**, 285.
Brenner, B. M., Meyer, T. W., et al. (1982). Dietary protein intake and the progressive nature of kidney disease: the role of hemodynamically mediated glomerular injury in the pathogenesis of progressive glomerular sclerosis in aging, renal ablation, and intrinsic renal disease. *N. Engl. J. Med.* **307**, 652.
Cecka, J. M. and Terasaki, P. I. (1998). The UNOS Scientific Renal Transplant Registry—1998. *Clin. Transplant.* 1.
Childress, J. (1996). The gift of life: ethnical issues in organ transplantation. *Bull. Am. Coll. Surg.* **81**, 8.
Cohen, B. (1985). Organ donor shortage: European situation and possible solutions. *Scand. J. Urol. Nephrol.* **92(Suppl.)**, 77.
Cohen, B., McGrath, S. M., et al. (1998). Trends in organ donation. *Clin. Transplant.* **12**, 525.
Cooley, D. A., Hallman, G. L., et al. (1968). Human heart transplantation: experience with twelve cases. *Am. J. Cardiol.* **22**, 804.
Cortesini, R., Casciani, C., et al. (1969). Heterotransplantation in primates: current state of affairs. *In Infection and Immunosuppression in Subhuman Primates*, (H. Balner, ed.), p. 239, Murksgaard, Copenhagen.
Czaplicki, J., Blonska, B., et al. (1992). The lack of hyperacute xenogeneic heart transplant rejection in a human. *J. Heart Lung Transplant.* **11(2 Pt. 1)**, 393.
Daemen, J. W., Oomen, A. P., et al. (1997). The potential pool of non-heart-beating kidney donors. *Clin. Transplant.* **11**, 149.

Delmonico, F. L., Fuller, T. C. and Cosimi, A. B. (1990). 1,000 renal transplants at the Massachusetts General Hospital: improved allograft survival for high-risk patients without regard to HLA matching. *Clin. Transplant.* **247**, 53.

Dubernard, J. M., Bonneau, M., *et al.* (1974). *Heterografts in Primates.* Fondation Merieux, Villeurbanne.

Dunn, J. F., Nylander, Jr., W. A., *et al.* (1986). Living related kidney donors: a 14-year experience. *Ann. Surg.* **203**, 637.

Evans, R. W., Manninen, D. L., *et al.* (1985). The quality of life of patients with end-stage renal disease. *N. Engl. J. Med.* **312**, 553.

Evans, R. W., Orians, C. E., *et al.* (1992). The potential supply of organ donors: an assessment of the efficacy of organ procurement efforts in the United States. *J. A. M. A.* **267**, 239.

Faustman, D. and Coe, C. (1991). Prevention of xenograft rejection by masking donor HLA class I antigens. *Science* **252**, 1700.

First, M. R. (1998). New solutions to overcome the organ donor shortage. *Graft* **1**, 117.

Fishman, J. A., Rubin, R. H., *et al.* (1996). Hepatitis C virus and organ transplantation. *Transplantation* **62**, 147.

Fodor, W. L. and Squinto, S. P. (1995). Engineering of transgenic pigs for xenogeneic organ transplantation. *Xenotransplantation* **3**, 23.

Freeman, R. B. (1985). Treatment of chronic renal failure: an update. *N. Engl. J. Med.* **312**, 577.

Hakim, R. M., Goldszer, R. C., *et al.* (1984). Hypertension and proteinuria: long-term sequelae of uninephrectomy in humans. *Kidney Int.* **25**, 930.

Hardy, J. D., Kurrus, F. E., *et al.* (1964). Heart transplantation in man: developmental studies and report of a case. *J. A. M. A.* **188**, 1132.

Hatfield, P. M. and Pfister, R. C. (1972). Adult polycystic disease of the kidneys (Potter type 3). *J. A. M. A.* **222**, 1527.

Hitchcock, C. R., Kiser, J. C., *et al.* (1964). Baboon renal grafts. *J. A. M. A.* **189**, 934.

Hume, D. M. (1964). Discussion of Reemtsma paper. *Ann. Surg.* **160**, 384.

Iglehart, J. K. (1993). The American health care system: the End Stage Renal Disease Program. *N. Engl. J. Med.* **328**, 366.

Institute of Medicine. (1997). *Non-Heart Beating Organ Transplantation: Medical and Ethical Issues in Procurement,* National Academy of Sciences, Washington, D.C.

Jeffery, J. R., Downs, A., *et al.* (1978). A randomized prospective study of cadaver donor pretreatment in renal transplantation. *Transplantation* **25**, 287.

Johnson, E. M., Remucal, M. J., *et al.* (1997). Complications and risks of living donor nephrectomy. *Transplantation* **64**, 1124.

Jones, J., Payne, W. D., *et al.* (1993). The living donor—risks, benefits, and related concerns. *Transplant. Rev.* **7**, 115.

Kaplan, C., Pasternack, B., *et al.* (1975). Age-related incidence of sclerotic glomeruli in human kidneys. *Am. J. Pathol.* **80**, 227.

Kasiske, B. L., Ravenscraft, M., *et al.* (1996). The evaluation of living renal transplant donors: clinical practice guidelines. Ad Hoc Clinical Practice Guidelines Subcommittee of the Patient Care and Education Committee of the American Society of Transplant Physicians. *J. Am. Soc. Nephrol.* **7**, 2288.

Kauffman, H. M., Bennett, L. E., *et al.* (1997). The expanded donor. *Transplant. Rev.* **11**, 165.

Kaufman, D. B., Sutherland, D. E., *et al.* (1989). Renal transplantation between living-related sibling pairs matched for zero-HLA haplotypes. *Transplantation* **47**, 113.

Kawai, T., Cosimi, A. B., *et al.* (1995). Mixed allogeneic chimerism and renal allograft tolerance in cynomolgus monkeys. *Transplantation* **59**, 256.

Kirk, A. D., Burkly, L. C., *et al.* (1999). Treatment with humanized monoclonal antibody against CD154 prevents acute renal allograft rejection in nonhuman primates. *Nat. Med.* **5**, 686.

Kliem, V., Hoff, U., van den, *et al.* (1996). The long-term course of hepatitis C after kidney transplantation. *Transplantation* **62**, 1417.

Kootstra, G. (1997). The asystolic, or non-heartbeating, donor. *Transplantation* **63**, 917.

Leger, L., Chapuis, J. P., *et al.* (1970). Greffe heterotopique d'un foie de baboun sur une malade atteinte d'hepatite fulminate. *Chirurgie* **96**, 249.

Leivestad, T., Albrechtsen, D., *et al.* (1986). Renal transplants from HLA-haploidentical living-related donors: the influence of donor-specific transfusions and different immunosuppressive regimens. *Transplantation* **42**, 35.

Levey, A. S., Hou, S., *et al.* (1986). Kidney transplantation from unrelated living donors: time to reclaim a discarded opportunity. *N. Engl. J. Med.* **314**, 914.

Makowa, L., Cramer, D. V., *et al.* (1995). The use of a pig liver xenograft for temporary support of a patient with fulminant hepatic failure. *Transplantation* **59**, 1654.

Marion, P. (1969). Les transplantations cardiaques et les transplantations hepatiques. *Lyon Med.* **222**, 585.

Marion, P., Bertoye, A., *et al.* (1970). Traitement du coma hepatique par transplantation auxiliaire heterologue du foie. *Chirurgie* **96**, 152.

Masden-Harrison (1957). Massachusetts Supreme Judicial Court, Equity Number 68651.

McMaster, P. (1984). Techniques of multiple organ harvesting. *In Progress in Transplantation,* (P. J. Morris and N. L. Tilney, eds.), p. 209, Churchill Livingstone, Edinburgh.

Merrill, J. P. (1964). Moral problems of artificial and transplanted organs. *Ann. Intern. Med.* **61**, 355.

Millard, C., Shumway, N. E., *et al.* (1985). Xenografts: review of the literature and current status. *J. A. M. A.* **254**, 3353.

Najarian, J. S., Chavers, B. M., *et al.* (1992). 20 years or more of follow-up of living kidney donors. *Lancet* **340**, 807.

Narkun-Burgess, D. M., Nolan, C. R., *et al.* (1993). Forty-five year follow-up after uninephrectomy. *Kidney Int.* **43**, 1110.

Nelson, P. W., Landreneau, M. D., *et al.* (1998). Ten-year experience in transplantation of A2 kidneys into B and O recipients. *Transplantation* **65**, 256.

Paprocki, S., Kruk, R., *et al.* (1992). A technique for successful transplantation of organs from non-heartbeating cadaver donors. *Transplantation* **54**, 381.

Patel, R., Snydman, D. R., *et al.* (1996). Cytomegalovirus prophylaxis in solid organ transplant recipients. *Transplantation* **61**, 1279.

Pereira, B. J. and Levey A. S. (1997). Hepatitis C virus infection in dialysis and renal transplantation. *Kidney Int.* **51**, 981.

Peters, T. G., Kittur, D. S., *et al.* (1996). Organ donors and nondonors: an American dilemma. *Arch. Intern. Med.* **156**, 2419.

Pouyet, M. and Berard, P. (1971). Deux cas de transplantation heterologues du foie de babouin au cours d'hepatites aigues malignes. *Lyon Chir.* **67**, 287.

Quinibi, W. (1997). Commercially motivated renal transplantation: results in 540 patients transplanted in India. The Living Non-Related Renal Transplant Study Group. *Clin. Transplant.* **11**, 536.

Ratner, L. E., Ciseck, L. J., *et al.* (1995). Laparoscopic live donor nephrectomy. *Transplantation* **60**, 1047.

Ratner, L. E., Kavoussi, L. R., *et al.* (1997). Laparoscopic assisted live donor nephrectomy—a comparison with the open approach. *Transplantation* **63**, 229.

Reemtsma, K., McCracken, B. H., *et al.* (1964). Renal heterotransplantation in man. *Ann. Surg.* **160**, 384.

Ricordi, C., Ilstad, S. T., *et al.* (1992). Induction of pancreatic islet graft acceptance: the role of antigen presenting cells. *Transplant. Sci.* **2**, 34.

Ross, D. N. (1969). *In Experience with Human Heart Transplantation,* (H. Shapiro, ed.), p. 227, Butterworths, Durban.

Rubin, R. H. and Cosimi A. B. (1989). Therapy, both immunosuppressive and antimicrobial, for the transplant patient in the 1990s. *In Organ Transplantation: Current Clinical and Immunological Concepts,* (L. Brent and R. A. Sells, eds.), p. 71, Bailliere Tindall, London.

Rubin, R. H., Tolkoff-Rubin, N. E., *et al.* (1985). Multicenter seroepidemiologic study of the impact of cytomegalovirus infection on renal transplantation. *Transplantation* **40**, 243.

Schmoeckel, M., Bhatti, F. N., *et al.* (1998). Orthotopic heart transplantation in a transgenic pig-to-primate model [published erratum appears in *Transplantation* 1998 Oct 15; **66(7)**, 943]. *Transplantation* **65**, 1570.

Simmons, R. G. and Anderson C. R. (1985). Social-psychological problems in living donor transplantation. *In Transplantation and Clinical Immunology,* (J. L. Touraine, ed.), p. 47, Elsevier Science Publishers, Amsterdam.

Sollinger, H. W., Kalayoglu, M., *et al.* (1986). Use of the donor specific transfusion protocol in living-unrelated donor-recipient combinations. *Ann. Surg.* **204**, 315.

Spees, E. K., Light, J. A., *et al.* (1982). Experiences with cadaver renal allograft contamination before transplantation. *Br. J. Surg.* **69**, 482.

Spital, A. (1988). Life insurance for kidney donors—an update. *Transplantation* **45**, 819.

Spital, A. (1991). The ethics of unconventional living organ donation. *Clin. Transplant.* **5**, 322.

Spital, A. (1994). Unrelated living kidney donors: an update of attitudes and use among U.S. transplant centers [published erratum appears in *Transplantation* 1994 Jul 27; **58(2)**, 268]. *Transplantation* **57**, 1722.

Spital, A., Spital, M., *et al.* (1986). The living kidney donor: alive and well. *Arch. Intern. Med.* **146**, 1993.

Starzl, T. E. (1969). Orthotopic heterotransplantation. *In Experience in Hepatic Transplantation*, (T. E. Starzl, ed.), p. 408, W.B. Saunders, Philadelphia.

Starzl, T. E. (1987). Living donors: con. *Transplant. Proc.* **19(1 Pt. 1)**, 174.

Starzl, T. E., Fung, J., *et al.* (1993a). Baboon-to-human liver transplantation. *Lancet* **341**, 65.

Starzl, T. E., Hakala, T. R., *et al.* (1984). A flexible procedure for multiple cadaveric organ procurement. *Surg. Gynecol. Obstet.* **158**, 223.

Starzl, T. E., Ishikawa, M., *et al.* (1974). Progress in and deterrents to orthotopic liver transplantation, with special reference to survival, resistance to hyperacute rejection, and biliary duct reconstruction. *Transplant. Proc.* **6(4 Suppl. 1)**, 129.

Starzl, T. E., Marchioro, T. L., *et al.* (1964). Renal heterotransplantation from baboon to man: experience with 6 cases. *Transplantation* **2**, 752.

Starzl, T. E., Marchioro, T. L., *et al.* (1966). Avenues of future research in homotransplantation of the liver with particular reference to hepatic supportive procedures, antilymphocyte serum, and tissue typing. *Am. J. Surg.* **112**, 391.

Starzl, T. E., Tzakis, A., *et al.* (1993b). Human liver transplantation. *Xenotransplantation* **1**, 4.

Taube, D., Welsh, K. I., *et al.* (1987). Pretreatment of human renal allografts with monoclonal antibodies to induce long-term tolerance. *Transplant. Proc.* **19(1 Pt. 3)**, 1961.

Terasaki, P. I., Cecka, J. M., *et al.* (1995). High survival rates of kidney transplants from spousal and living unrelated donors. *N. Engl. J. Med.* **333**, 333.

Traeger, J., Fries, D., *et al.* (1965). Heterotransplantation chez l'homme: premiers resultats. *Proc. Eur. Dial. Transplant. Assoc.* **2**, 214.

Van Buren, C. T. and Barakat, O. (1994). Organ donation and retrieval. *Surg. Clin. North Am.* **74**, 1055.

Waterworth, P. D., Dunning, J., *et al.* (1998). Life-supporting pig-to-baboon heart xenotransplantation. *J. Heart Lung Transplant.* **17**, 1201.

Weinstein, S. H., Navarre, Jr., R. J., *et al.* (1980). Experience with live donor nephrectomy. *J. Urol.* **124**, 321.

Wenzel, R. P. (1992). Preoperative antibiotic prophylaxis. *N. Engl. J. Med.* **326**, 337.

Woo, K. T. (1992). Social and cultural aspects of organ donation in Asia. *Ann. Acad. Med. Singapore* **21**, 421.

Yang, H. C., Gifford, R. R., *et al.* (1991). Arterial reconstruction of the pancreatic allograft for transplantation. *Am. J. Surg.* **162**, 262.

Youngner, S. J., Allen, M., *et al.* (1985). Psychosocial and ethical implications of organ retrieval. *N. Engl. J. Med.* **313**, 321.

Zaidi, A., Schmoeckel, M., *et al.* (1998). Life-supporting pig-to-primate renal xenotransplantation using genetically modified donors. *Transplantation* **65**, 1584.

Zincke, H., Woods, J. E., *et al.* (1978). Immunological donor pretreatment in combination with pulsatile preservation in cadaveric renal transplantation. *Transplantation* **26**, 207.

8

The Laparoscopic Donor Nephrectomy
Robert A. Montgomery • Lloyd E. Ratner

Introduction and Rationale

Laparoscopic live donor nephrectomy originally was designed with the intent of decreasing disincentives to live kidney donation, in an attempt to increase the number of live donor renal transplants performed. Despite the use of numerous strategies to increase cadaveric organ donation, the disparity between organ demand and supply continues to widen. As a result of this widening disparity there has been an increase in waiting time. Concomitant with prolonged waiting times, an increase has occurred in the number of individuals who die while awaiting renal transplantation.

Live donor renal transplantation offers many advantages compared with cadaveric donor transplantation, including ability to perform transplants preemptively before starting dialysis, lower incidence of delayed graft function, shorter hospitalization, decreased incidence of rejection, improved patient and graft survival and lower costs. Despite these advantages, live donor renal transplantation has been an underused option. Logistical and financial disincentives prohibit many individuals from donating kidneys. Lost wages, job security, inability to tend to other responsibilities (e.g., child care), fear of postoperative pain and cosmetic results are all concerns of potential donors (Hiller *et al.*, 1998). It was hypothesized that more people would be willing to donate if some of these disincentives could be decreased through the use of minimally invasive surgical techniques. The advent of laparoscopic cholecystectomy increased profoundly the number of cholecystectomies performed. Clayman and associates showed that laparoscopic nephrectomy performed for disease resulted in less pain, shorter hospitalization and quicker recuperation than open nephrectomy (Clayman *et al.*, 1991).

The first laparoscopic live donor nephrectomy was performed in 1995 (Ratner *et al.*, 1995). The annual number of live donor renal transplants at our institution has nearly tripled since then. Approximately 20% of donors report that they would not have donated if the laparoscopic operation had not been available. Two thirds of donors state that the availability of the laparoscopic operation had a major influence on their decision whether or not to donate. Other centers have reported similar increases in live kidney donation after the adoption of the laparoscopic donor operation.

Preoperative Evaluation

All live kidney donors should undergo thorough surgical, nephrological and psychological evaluations, as has been described previously (Kasiske *et al.*, 1996; see Chapter 7). Patients undergoing laparoscopic live donor nephrectomy do not need any additional screening studies beyond that applied to a potential kidney donor undergoing standard flank operation. The venous anatomy is crucial to the laparoscopic donor operation. We find it useful to obtain three-dimensional spiral computed tomography (CT) scans with intrave-

nous contrast administration (Smith *et al.*, 1998). In addition to providing adequate definition of the arterial anatomy, three-dimensional spiral CT provides excellent depictions of the venous anatomy. It gives superb definition of the renal parenchyma as well as a urography phase. We use this technique in lieu of conventional angiography. Other centers use magnetic resonance angiography as another noninvasive alternative to conventional angiography. Similar to three-dimensional spiral CT, magnetic resonance angiography provides good definition of venous anatomy.

The process of selecting which donor kidney to use involves a different set of criteria when the laparoscopic technique is used. Laparoscopic removal of the right kidney for transplantation is more technically challenging than removal of the left. Use of the endo-gastrointestinal anastomosis stapler to divide the right renal vein can result in loss of approximately 1 to 1.5 cm of renal vein length. This loss may be problematic during the recipient operation. An early series reported that there was a higher allograft thrombosis rate when right kidneys were used. Unless there is a clear benefit to the donor to leave the left kidney *in situ*, the use of the left kidney is preferred. This situation is true in the presence of multiple renal arteries or anomalous renal venous vasculature, such as circumaortic or retroaortic renal veins. Most laparoscopic live donor nephrectomies performed involve the removal of the left kidney. When a right donor nephrectomy is performed, it may necessitate modification of the donor or recipient procedure (Ratner *et al.*, 1999).

The contraindications to laparoscopic donor nephrectomy are the same as those established for open nephrectomy. Because the laparoscopic donor operation is performed through a transperitoneal approach, however, a relative contraindication is prior extensive upper abdominal surgery. In our series of 236 laparoscopic donor nephrectomies, we did not exclude any individual on the basis of anything other than medical or psychological reasons.

The laparoscopic donor nephrectomy is a technically challenging operation. Preoperative assessment of technical difficulty is useful for surgeons with limited experience with this operation. In a study of 41 laparoscopic live donor nephrectomies, we were unable to identify any preoperative demographic, radiological or anatomical parameters that would predict accurately the degree of operative difficulty (Ratner *et al.*, 2000). It is equally likely that a thin patient's operation would be difficult as an obese patient's operation would be easy. Operative difficulty appears to be related to mobility of the mesentery, degree of retroperitoneal fibrosis and laparoscopic working space. At present, these factors are not quantifiable before surgery.

Intraoperative Management

The anesthetic management of patients undergoing a laparoscopic donor nephrectomy can have a profound effect on operative technical difficulty and outcome for the donor and the recipient. To obtain sufficient laparoscopic working space, the patient must be kept completely relaxed, and nitrous oxide must never be used. Trocar sites should be injected with 0.25% bupivacaine to minimize operative and postoperative narcotic requirements. Kuo and colleagues have been successful in limiting hospital stay to 23 hours by using propofol-based anesthesia supplemented with desflurane to limit postoperative nausea (Kuo *et al.*, 1999). In our experience, patient-controlled anesthesia should be avoided postoperatively to minimize nausea and constipation.

The pneumoperitoneum required for laparoscopy necessitates different operative fluid management than that used for the open donor operation. The presence of the pneumoperitoneum results in a reduction in renal blood flow and urine output (London *et al.*, 1998). Experimental data suggest that the effects of this relative hypoperfusion can be abrogated by fluid loading (London *et al.*, 1998). It is not unusual for laparoscopic donors to receive 8 to 10 liters of crystalloid during the procedure. We use the turgor of the renal vein to gauge the adequacy of the intravascular expansion. A brisk diuresis is stimulated throughout the procedure by several bolus administrations of mannitol. Just before removing the kidney, the donor is given intravenous furosemide and heparin. Once the kidney has been removed, protamine is given to reverse the heparin.

Economic Considerations

In a study performed at our institution that looked at the costs of 71 laparoscopic donor nephrectomies compared with 71 open donor nephrectomies, there was no significant difference in hospital cost between the two operations (Sosa *et al.*, 1998). The mean hospital cost for a laparoscopic live donor nephrectomy was $6,454 versus $6,075 for the open operation (P = not significant). Savings resulting from the decreased hospital length of stay (laparoscopic $1,774 versus open $2,411; $P < 0.001$) were largely offset by the added expense of disposable laparoscopic instruments (laparoscopic $2,251 versus open $812; $P < 0.001$). To the donor, however, the shorter recuperative time that the laparoscopic operation affords is economically advantageous. Similarly, because live donor renal transplantation has been shown to be signifi-

cantly cheaper than cadaveric donor transplantation and dialysis (Eggers, 1992), the increase in live donation seen with laparoscopic donor nephrectomy should result in savings overall.

Laparoscopic Donor Nephrectomy Operative Procedure

The donor receives no particular preparation before surgery. The patient is positioned in a modified lateral decubitus position with the hips rotated back and the arms extended above the head in a prayer position. The table is flexed to expand the area between the costal margin and the pelvic brim. A 15-mm Hg pneumoperitoneum is established through a Veress needle inserted in the left iliac fossa along the lateral rectus border. The initial operative field consists of two 12-mm ports and one 5-mm port that are placed (1) just below the umbilicus in the midline, (2) halfway between the umbilicus and the anterior superior iliac spine and (3) in the midline 3 to 4 fingerbreadths below the xiphoid process (Fig. 8–1). The video endoscope is placed in the umbilical port and attached to a robotic arm. The epigastric and lateral ports are the operative ports.

On the left side, using a DeBakey grasper and curved scissors, the descending and sigmoid colon is taken down by dividing the lateral attachments (Fig. 8–2). The colon is reflected medially, exposing Gerota's fascia. Care must be taken not to buttonhole the mesocolon. Much of the dissection can be accomplished bluntly by sweeping the tissue medially and developing a natural plane between the mesocolon and Gerota's fascia (Fig. 8–3).

At this point, we often make a 4- to 5-cm Pfannenstiel incision just above the pubis and carry it down to the level of the peritoneum (see Fig. 8–1). A pursestring suture is placed in the peritoneal tissue around the Endocatch (U.S. Surgical Corp., Norwalk, CT) tube, which is inserted to retract the colon medially. In cases in which one of the other incision sites is used (e.g., presence of a previous midline incision), a fourth 2-mm port can be introduced at the midpoint between the costal margin and the anterior superior iliac spine in the axillary line (see Fig. 8–1). A 2-mm grasper is used to retract the colon medially.

On the right side, the cecum is mobilized and reflected

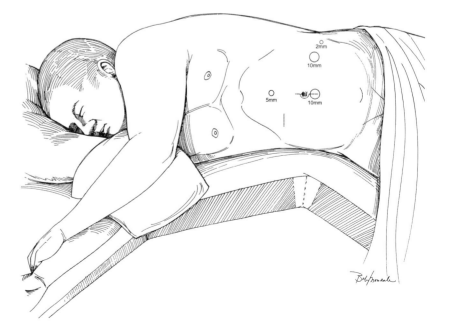

FIGURE 8–1

The patient is placed in a lateral decubitus position, and three laparoscopic ports are introduced.

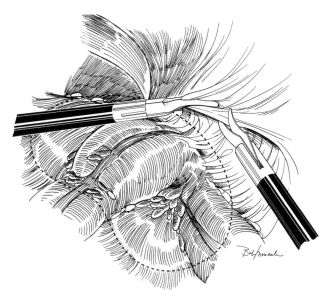

FIGURE 8–2

The lateral attachments to the colon are taken down.

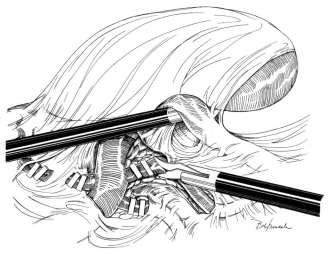

FIGURE 8–4

The renal vein is exposed, and the adrenal gonadal and lumbar branches are divided.

medially. The liver is lifted away from the upper pole of the kidney using a laparoscopic fan blade retractor. The right-sided nephrectomy is technically challenging and has unique problems that are discussed later.

At this point, the renal vein is exposed by tracing the gonadal vein in a cephalad direction or bluntly sweeping the perinephric tissue several centimeters medial to the renal hilum. The renal vein is cleared completely of investing tissue, and the gonadal, lumbar and adrenal branches are clipped and cut (Fig. 8–4). The renal artery lies posterior to the vein and can be exposed by elevating the lower pole of the kidney (Fig. 8–5). Dissection should be conducted medial to the gonadal vein to avoid devascularizing the hilar region. The artery is separated from the surrounding nervous plexus and isolated to the level of the aorta. The plane of dissection is carried along the cephalad border of the vein between the

adrenal gland and the upper pole of the kidney. Vascularized tissue in this region is divided between clips, and the upper pole is shelled out of the envelope of Gerota's fascia. The posterior attachments are lysed by elevating the upper pole and teasing the adherent tissue away.

The DeBakey grasper is inserted medial and posterior to the bundle of tissue containing the ureter. The gonadal vein, ureter and mesoureter are separated from the psoas muscle and dissected free from a point below the lower pole of the kidney to the pelvic inlet (Fig. 8–6). At the juncture where the ureter descends into the pelvis, the individual structures of the bundle are isolated, clipped and cut. The lateral attachments of the mesoureter are cauterized and cut in a caudad to cephalad direction. This plane of dissection is carried along the lateral surface of the kidney, completely mobilizing the kidney except for the renal pedicle.

If the incision has not yet been made, one of the preferred sites is chosen, and the incision is carried down to the level of the peritoneum (see Fig. 8–1). The camera is moved to the

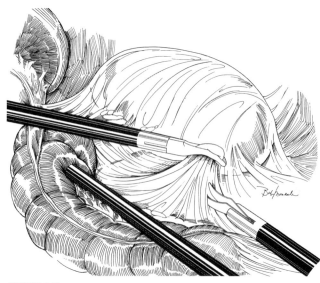

FIGURE 8–3

Gerota's fascia is separated from the mesocolon.

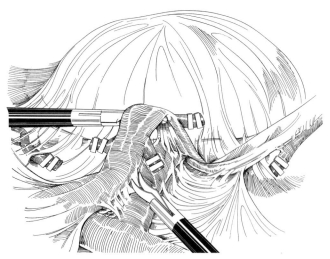

FIGURE 8–5

Posterior to the vein lies the renal artery, which is freed back to the level of the aorta.

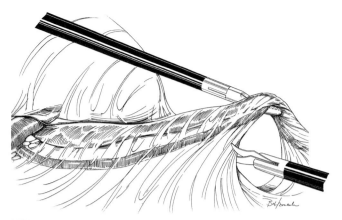

FIGURE 8–6

The mesoureter is isolated from the lower pole to the pelvic inlet, where it is divided.

lateral port. A vascular endo-GIA stapler is used to divide first the artery and then the vein, optimizing the length of both vessels (Fig. 8–7). The Endocatch bag is deployed through either the umbilical port site or the Pfannenstiel incision. The kidney is placed in the bag and is removed by incising the peritoneum at the base of the wound (Fig. 8–8). The fascia is closed with absorbable sutures. The 12-mm port sites are closed with figure-of-eight absorbable sutures aided by the Carter-Thomas instrument. After reestablishing a pneumoperitoneum, the abdomen is inspected for bleeding.

Hand-Assisted Laparoscopic Technique

The hand-assisted variation of the laparoscopic nephrectomy was developed to give surgeons greater tactile feedback and to facilitate the definition of tissue planes. There is some evidence that it may reduce operative time (Slakey *et al.*, 1999) and allow transplant centers that lack advanced laparoscopic expertise to perform the operation safely. Perhaps the most significant advantage occurs during the removal of the kidney, in which the pneumosleeve simply is inverted and

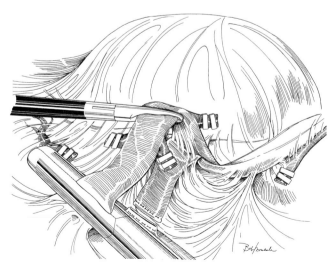

FIGURE 8–7

The kidney is completely mobilized except for its attachment to the renal pedicle, which is divided using the endo-GIA.

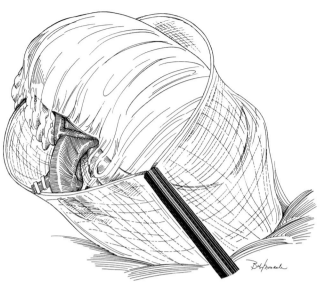

FIGURE 8–8

The kidney is placed in the Endocatch bag and brought through one of the preferred incision sites (see Fig. 8–1).

removed, obviating the need to place the kidney in the Endocatch bag.

We prefer the purely laparoscopic technique because we have found the pneumosleeve to be cumbersome and prone to leakage of gas around the flange. The requirement of a slightly larger incision placed more cephalad in the midline and the additional 12-mm port in the subcostal region may abrogate some of the advantages of the laparoscopic technique. The circumstance in which it may have some advantage occurs when the removal of the right kidney clearly is preferred.

Patient positioning and preparation is essentially unchanged. The pneumosleeve flange is placed below or at the level of the umbilicus, centered on an incision large enough to permit the smooth insertion of the surgeon's hand. Three 12-mm ports are placed in the following positions: (1) lateral to the midpoint between the umbilicus and the anterior superior iliac spine, (2) 4 to 5 fingerbreadths below the xiphoid in the midline and (3) along the lateral rectus border in the subcostal region. The operating surgeon's left hand is placed in the pneumosleeve, and the camera is inserted through the supraumbilical port. The surgeon's hand replaces the DeBakey instrument, but otherwise the content and order of the subsequent steps of the procedure remain unchanged.

The camera is moved to the subcostal port when the vascular pedicle is divided. At this point, the surgeon usually switches to the right hand for retraction. The endovascular stapler is introduced through the supraumbilical port. After the kidney is removed, a pneumoperitoneum can be reestablished by placing a dome over the pneumosleeve flange.

Donor Results

There now is enough collective experience with laparoscopic nephrectomy to show technical feasibility. Centers without advanced laparoscopic expertise have been able to adopt the laparoscopic and hand-assisted techniques. The remaining important questions pertinent to the assessment of any new donor procedure when a reliable operation currently exists include the following: (1) Can it be performed safely? (2) Are there clear advantages for the donor? (3) Does the

TABLE 8–1

DONOR MORBIDITY (n = 100)

	n (%)
Open conversion	0 (0)
Reoperation	1 (1)
Blood transfusion	3 (3)
Bowel injury	1 (1)
Anterior thigh paresthesia	3 (3)
Wound infection	4 (4)
Hernia	1 (1)
Left lower lobe pneumonia	1 (1)

operation produce a kidney that functions well and can be transplanted in the standard manner?

The open live donor nephrectomy procedure has been used successfully with acceptable mortality (0.03%) and morbidity (15–20%) for 40 years (Blohme et al., 1992; Dunn et al., 1986). It will take years of careful monitoring of donor and recipient outcomes to generate results showing parity. This operation is unique among surgical procedures because it places an otherwise healthy individual at risk without clear self-benefit. It also stands alone as an operation that directly affects the outcome of two patients. For these reasons, a higher burden of proof must be assumed in assessing a change in the surgical paradigm.

Safety

We have performed more than 200 laparoscopic donor procedures without a mortality. We are not aware of any donor mortalities associated with this procedure, although it is alleged that they have occurred. The donor morbidity is presented in Table 8–1. A duodenal injury that was not recognized immediately constitutes the only serious complication in our series.

In a retrospective review of the 142 cases at our institution, the laparoscopic donor complication rate was significantly less when compared with the open donor group (9% vs. 22.2%). Complications associated with the extraperitoneal flank incision employed by most centers for the open procedure and that are reduced in the laparoscopic donor cohort include wound infections, hernias, pneumothorax, chronic incision pain and wound diastasis (Blohme et al., 1992; Dunn et al., 1986). Flowers and coworkers in a single-institution study compared their first 70 laparoscopic donors with a historic open nephrectomy group and found comparable morbidity rates (Flowers et al., 1997). Their series included three splenic injuries, which is a complication we have not seen. At centers with a large experience and expertise in advanced laparoscopic techniques, the donor operation can be performed safely and without excess morbidity. Some centers use a transperitoneal approach for the open operation

and claim less morbidity than is seen with the flank approach (see Chapter 7).

Advantages to the Donor

There have been no large randomized prospective studies comparing the laparoscopic technique with the open nephrectomy published to date. Because of our initial compelling results (Ratner et al., 1997a; Schulam et al., 1996) and the public awareness of the procedure, we have not found such a study to be tenable. We tell all patients that this is a new, experimental procedure with results that are unproven. We have not had any patients who have requested the open donor procedure.

One of the criticisms of using historic open nephrectomy results to look at various endpoints is that the two data sets are from different eras. A retrospective review was conducted of 62 contemporaneous donor operations (25 laparoscopic and 37 open) that were performed between January 1995 and December 1996 when both procedures were being performed at our institution (Ratner et al., 1997b). The donor characteristics were comparable between the two groups. All donor functional recuperative parameters that we looked at reached statistical significance and favored the laparoscopic approach (Table 8–2). Other centers in the United States, Australia and Holland have reported similar results (Flowers et al., 1997; Hensman et al., 1999; Ijzermans et al., 1999).

We developed this procedure in response to data that we had collected from prospective donors about perceived disincentives to live donation (Hiller et al., 1998). Many of these disincentives have been addressed by the laparoscopic procedure. Based on the initial series, we conclude that the laparoscopic donor operation is associated with a significant reduction in intraoperative blood loss, time until resumption of oral intake, postoperative pain, length of hospitalization and time to return to normal activities and employment.

Does the Operation Produce a Kidney That Functions Well and Can Be Transplanted in the Standard Manner?

It has been our experience that the laparoscopic operation consistently produces kidneys with adequate lengths of ureters (11.3 ± 2.6 cm), renal veins (4.0 ± 1.4 cm) and renal arteries (3.1 ± 0.8 cm) to perform the recipient operation using standard techniques. The average warm ischemc time, 4.8 ± 1.5 minutes, is well within acceptable limits and has not been associated with increase in delayed graft function.

These results differ from those obtained by Kuo and colleagues, who have had problems with vessel lengths less than 1 cm because of arterial shortening associated with laparoscopic vascular staplers (Kuo et al., 1997). We have not found it necessary to reconstruct multiple arteries using saphenous vein patches. In cases in which two or three

TABLE 8–2

FUNCTIONAL RECUPERATIVE PARAMETERS

	Laparoscopic	Open	P Value
n	25	37	
Length of hospitalization (d)	2.9 ± 1.0	5.5 ± 1.2	< 0.001
Return to normal activities (wk)	1.8 ± 1.5	4.5 ± 0.5	< 0.001
Able to return to work (wk)	3.2 ± 2.1	6.2 ± 3.2	< 0.001

TABLE 8-3
RECIPIENT GRAFT LOSS AND COMPLICATIONS

	First 100 Laparoscopic	Last 100 Laparoscopic	Open (n = 48)
Graft loss	6 (6%)	2 (2%)	4 (8.3%)
Vascular thrombosis	2	1	1
Rejection	1	1	1
HUS	1		1
Cholesterol embolus	1		
Recurrent disease			1
Noncompliance	1		
Deaths	4 (4%)	3 (3%)	1 (2%)
Sepsis	3	1	1
Cardiovascular	1	1	
Hemorrhage		1	
Ureteral complications	10 (10%)	3 (3%)	3 (6.3%)
Urine leak	7	2	1
Ureteral stenosis	3	1	2

HUS = hemolytic-uremic syndrome.

arteries are present, we spatulate each and sew them together side-to-side on the back table. This creates a single orifice, which is then sewn to the recipient iliac artery.

The one problematic vessel is the right renal vein, which has an average length of 2.5 ± 0.7 cm versus 4.7 ± 1.0 cm for the left vein ($P < 0.001$) and which probably was associated with two graft losses early in our experience owing to venous thrombosis. We now try to use the left kidney unless there is a compelling reason to leave the left kidney with the donor. If the right vein is short after the kidney is completely mobilized, we make a transverse rectus splitting incision and apply a Satinsky clamp to the inferior vena cava; this generally produces an additional 1 to 1.5 cm of vein length. Mobilizing the entire right common and external iliac vein with division of the hypogastric vein and lateral transposition also is advisable when the right kidney is used.

In 100 laparoscopic donor nephrectomies at our institution, we have experienced five graft losses (Table 8–3). The two vascular thromboses were associated with superimposed pernicious conditions (hypercoagulable state and severe acute rejection) and were not thought to be technical in

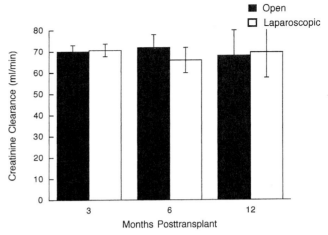

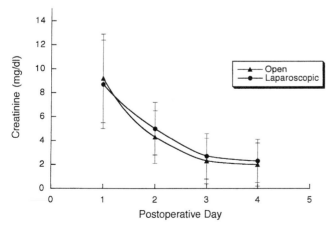

FIGURE 8–9

Early renal function. A comparison of the rate of fall in recipient creatinine between 100 laparoscopic donor nephrectomies and a historic open donor nephrectomy cohort. There is no significant difference between the two groups.

FIGURE 8–10

Renal function during the first year. A comparison of recipient creatinine clearance at 3, 6 and 12 months between 100 laparoscopic donor nephrectomies and a historic open donor nephrectomy group. There is no significant difference between the two groups at any of the time points.

nature. The three deaths in this cohort were due to sepsis, hemorrhage and myocardial infarction.

The incidence of the ureteral complications among our first 100 laparoscopic nephrectomy recipients compared with an open nephrectomy cohort appeared to be higher, although this difference did not reach statistical significance. The University of Maryland group during their initial experience observed the same trend (Philosophe *et al.*, 1999). During a subsequent 100 cases, the number of ureteral complications decreased to a level consistent with the open cohort and previously published data on this subject. We attribute the more recent reduction in the incidence of ureteral complications to more careful surgical technique when dissecting in the hilum and greater familiarity with the nuances of using the Endocatch bag. We no longer carry the hilar dissection beyond the gonadal vein. The ureter is mobilized as part of the ureteral and gonadal bundle. These structures are separated, then clipped at the point where the ureter enters the pelvis. Early renal function as manifested by the rate of fall in serum creatinine is comparable to that observed among recipients procured by open nephrectomy (Fig. 8–9). There was no difference in the need for posttransplant dialysis. The length of hospital stay for the recipient averaged 7.2 ± 4.8 days and was comparable to the open cohort. Likewise, there is no statistical difference in the creatinine clearance at 3, 6 or 12 months (Fig. 8–10). The kidney that is produced by the laparoscopic donor nephrectomy can be transplanted using standard techniques without excess recipient morbidity and has equivalent short-term and long-term function as that achieved by open nephrectomy.

REFERENCES

Blohme, I., Fehrman, I. and Norden, G. (1992). Living donor nephrectomy: complication rates in 490 cases. *Scand. J. Urol. Nephrol.* **26**, 149.

Clayman, R. V., Soper, N. J., Dierks, S. M., *et al.* (1991). Laparoscopic nephrectomy. *N. Engl. J. Med.* **325**, 1110.

Dunn, J. F., Richie, R. E., MacDonell, R. C., *et al.* (1986). Living related kidney donors: a 14-year experience. *Ann. Surg.* **203**, 637.

Eggers, P. (1992). Comparison of treatment costs between dialysis and transplantation. *Semin. Nephrol.* **12**, 284.

Flowers, J. L., Jacobs, S., Cho, E., *et al.* (1997). Comparison of open and laparoscopic live donor nephrectomy. *Ann. Surg.* **226**, 483.

Hensman, C., Lionel, G., Hewett, P. and Rano, M. M. (1999). Laparoscopic live donor nephrectomy: the preliminary experience. *Aust. N. Z. J. Surg.* **69**, 365.

Hiller, J., Sroka, M., Weber, R., *et al.* (1998). Identifying donor concerns to increase live organ donation. *J. Transplant. Coord.* **8**, 51.

Ijzermans, J. N., Berends, F. J., van Riemsdijk, I. C., *et al.* (1999). Laparoscopic donor nephrectomy for kidney transplants from living family members: good preliminary results. *Ned. Tijdschr. Geneeskd.* **143**, 942.

Kasiske, B. L., Ravenscraft, M., Ramos, E. L., *et al.* (1996). The evaluation of living renal transplant donors: clinical practice guidelines. Ad Hoc Clinical Practice Guidelines Subcommittee of the Patient Care and Education Committee of the American Society of Transplant Physicians. *J. Am. Soc. Nephrol.* **7**, 2288.

Kuo, P. C., Bartlett, S. T., Schweitzer, E. J., *et al.* (1997). A technique for management of multiple renal arteries after laparoscopic donor nephrectomy. *Transplantation* **64**, 779.

Kuo, P. C., Plotkin, J. S. and Johnson, L. B. (1999). Is living donor nephrectomy a "23-hr stay" procedure? *Transplantation* **68**, 1064.

London, E., Neuhaus, A., Ho, H., *et al.* (1998). Beneficial effect of volume expansion on the altered renal hemodynamics of prolonged pneumoperitoneum. *American Society of Transplant Surgeons* Abstract 85.

Philosophe, B., Kuo, P. C., Schweitzer, E. J., *et al.* (1999). Laparoscopic versus open donor nephrectomy: comparing ureteral complications in the recipients and improving the laparoscopic technique. *Transplantation* **68**, 497.

Ratner, L., Kavoussi, L., Sroka, M., *et al.* (1997a). Laparoscopic assisted live donor nephrectomy—a comparison with the open approach. *Transplantation* **63**, 229.

Ratner, L. E., Ciseck, L., Moore, R., *et al.* (1995). Laparoscopic live donor nephrectomy. *Transplantation* **60**, 1047.

Ratner, L. E., Fabrizio, M. D., Montgomery, R. A., *et al.* (1999). Technical considerations in the delivery of the kidney during laparoscopic live donor nephrectomy. *J. Am. Coll. Surg.* **189**, 427.

Ratner, L. E., Hiller, J., Sroka, R., *et al.* (1997b). Laparoscopic live donor nephrectomy removes disincentives to live donation. *Transplant. Proc.* **29**, 3402.

Ratner, L. E., Kavoussi, L. R., Chavin, K. D. and Montgomery, R. (1998). Laparoscopic live donor nephrectomy: technical considerations and allograft vascular length. *Transplantation* **65**, 1657.

Ratner, L. E., Smith, P., Montgomery, R. A., *et al.* (2000). Laparoscopic live donor nephrectomy: pre-operative assessment of technical difficulty. (submitted).

Schulam, P. G., Kavoussi, L. R., Cheriff, A. D., *et al.* (1996). Laparoscopic live donor nephrectomy: the initial 3 cases. *J. Urol.* **155**, 1857.

Slakey, D. P., Wood, J. C., Hender, D., *et al.* (1999). Laparoscopic living donor nephrectomy: advantages of the hand-assisted method. *Transplantation* **68**, 581.

Smith, P. A., Ratner, L. E., Lynch, F. C. and Fishman, E. K. (1998). Preoperative evaluation for laparoscopic nephrectomy in the living related renal donor: the role of dual-phase spiral CT angiography with 3D volume rendering. *Radiographics* **18**, 589.

Sosa, J. A., Albini, T. A., Powe, N. R., *et al.* (1998). Laparoscopic vs. open live donor nephrectomy: a multivariate patient outcomes analysis. *American Society of Transplant Physicians* Abstract 332.

Renal Preservation

Vernon C. Marshall

Introduction

Three linchpins support all effective kidney transplantation programs: (1) preservation of viability of the graft between its removal and implantation, (2) avoidance of technical surgical problems and (3) expert recipient care with specifically effective immunosuppression. Good preservation and optimal immunosuppression are interlinked; minimizing preservation damage provides a graft with immediate and normal renal function (see Chapter 25). This graft has clinical advantages in recipient management and is advantageous in reducing immunological challenge at basic cellular and humoral levels. Kidney transplantation from living volunteer donors offers ideal circumstances for organ preservation. The results using living donors, related or unrelated, generally are better than with cadaver donors and reflect these attributes. Cadaver donors still necessarily comprise most sources of kidneys for transplantation, however.

Widespread use of organs from brain-dead cadavers, improved clinical management of cadaver donors before and during organ removal, optimal conditions of preservation and storage and more effective immunosuppression all have contributed to the efficacy of kidney transplantation as the best treatment for end-stage renal failure. A kidney removed from a heart-beating cadaver with minimally impaired renal perfusion until nephrectomy, cold flushed with a preserving solution containing effective impermeable solutes and adjuvants, then stored by simple hypothermia for 1 or more days reliably can be expected to function to sustain life from the moment of implantation. In many centers, these optimal conditions still cannot be met because of cultural and legal prohibition of organ retrieval from brain-dead cadavers.

Worldwide shortage of donors and inability of organ supply to meet demand contribute to pressures to use living donors (related and unrelated) more often. Increasing use of kidneys from less optimal heart-beating cadaver donors and from cadavers presenting after cardiac arrest (the so-called marginal donor) also has occurred. This chapter reviews conditions necessary for optimal preservation for kidneys removed from both the living and the dead as well as strategies for *rescue* of kidney grafts obtained under less than ideal conditions.

Effect of Renal Ischemia

ISCHEMIC INJURY

In organ procurement, it is important to consider normothermic ischemic tolerance because of the disproportionately severe damage that warm ischemia can induce (Fig. 9–1). Sensitivity of different tissues to warm ischemia varies considerably. The brain suffers permanent loss of function within a few minutes. Skin and cornea can tolerate several hours. In limb ischemia, nervous tissue is most sensitive, followed by muscle, skin and bone.

Kidney damage is predictably reversible only if renal warm ischemia is less than 30 minutes (Florack *et al.*, 1986). Complete normothermic renal ischemia in humans, dogs, rabbits and rats for 30 minutes or less causes temporary reversible loss of function. Recovery is rapid after 10 minutes of warm ischemia; recovery can take 1 week or longer after 30 minutes of warm ischemia. The limits of warm ischemic renal tolerance vary among species: In the Sprague-Dawley rat, 60 minutes causes severe loss of function with slow (>2 weeks) recovery, and 90 minutes causes complete, permanent loss of function (Friedman *et al.*, 1954; Jablonski *et al.*, 1983a). In dogs, 2 hours of warm ischemia almost always is fatal unless the contralateral undamaged kidney is left to support the dog for a period. The smaller the animal and the higher the metabolic rate, the more sensitive the kidney is to ischemic damage.

Ischemia involves oxygen and nutrient depletion; continuance of anaerobic metabolism; a buildup of catabolites with the potential to precipitate cell death and obstruction of the vasculature with erythrocytes, leukocytes and platelets. The renal cortex has a high requirement for oxygen. Normothermic ischemia, involving progression from hypoxia to anoxia, results in ultimate cessation of the oxidation of glucose and fatty acids. Anaerobic metabolism (anaerobic glycolysis) continues but can generate only 2 adenosine triphosphate (ATP) molecules per glucose molecule metabolized compared with 38 ATP molecules during aerobic metabolism. Renal ATP is depleted rapidly. Further dephosphorylation of nucleotides and catabolism reduce the energy pool available for rephosphorylation when blood flow is restored. The concentration of ATP or of other nucleotides is not a reliable criterion of cellular viability in the ischemic rat (Trifillis *et al.*, 1984) or dog (Maessen *et al.*, 1989) kidney. The ability of the ischemic cell to resynthesize ATP after reperfusion provides a better determinant of the reversibility of the injury.

The intracellular and intramitochondrial ionic environment is important to cellular viability. The high internal cellular concentration of potassium and magnesium and low intracellular sodium and calcium is maintained, under conditions of normal metabolism, by sodium-potassium-ATPase and calcium-magnesium-ATPase. Both require ATP as fuel. The anoxic ischemic cell no longer can maintain its ionic composition: Sodium, chloride, calcium and water diffuse into the cell along concentration gradients, and potassium and magnesium diffuse out. The cell becomes edematous and swollen; intracellular potassium and magnesium are depleted and cytosolic calcium is increased, activating phospholipase A, an enzyme that lyses cellular and subcellular membranes.

Increased lactate formation resulting from anaerobic glycolysis lowers cellular pH. The falling intracellular pH initially may be cytoprotective, but subsequently increasing acidosis (1) decreases the stability of lysosomal membranes, activating lysosomal lytic enzymes (Wattiaux and Wattiaux-De Conninck, 1984), and (2) disrupts the binding of transition metals (iron, copper) to carrier proteins (transferrin, ferritin).

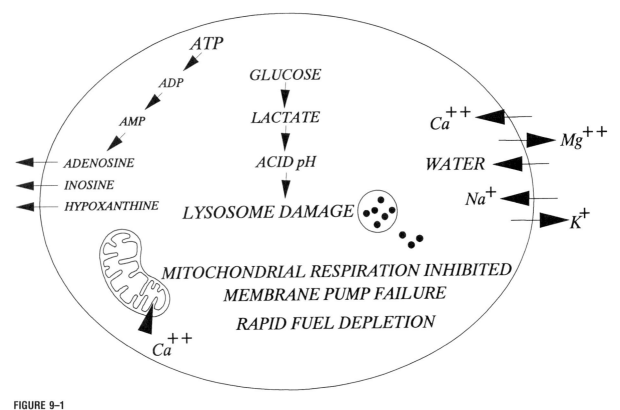

FIGURE 9–1

Effects of warm ischemia and anoxia on renal cellular metabolism (see text).

The free iron generated can propagate the damage caused by the generation of free radicals after reperfusion.

REPERFUSION INJURY

Irreversible damage after ischemia may be a consequence of injury during reperfusion and reoxygenation of the kidney. During the period of warm ischemia, ATP is degraded to adenosine monophosphate (AMP), which is catabolized further to hypoxanthine. This degradation occurs in all ischemic cells: renal cells, blood cells trapped in the vasculature and endothelial cells. Calcium influx has activated cytosolic proteases to produce xanthine, with the formation of superoxide free radical and hydrogen peroxide. Free iron reacts with hydrogen peroxide to form the highly reactive hydroxyl free radical. Naturally occurring free radical scavengers (glutathione, ascorbic acid, tryptophan and histidine) have been depleted after ischemia, increasing the vulnerability of cellular and subcellular membranes to injury by lipid peroxidation (Green *et al.*, 1986). Damage to subcellular membranes profoundly affects the capacity of restoration of homeostasis within the cell. Injury to cellular membranes augments this damage and may have profound rheological effects, particularly affecting vulnerable endothelial cells lining the blood vessels. Erythrocytes, leukocytes and platelets adhere to damaged vasculature. Trapping of erythrocytes in the outer renal medulla has been shown to be related to the duration of warm ischemia (Hellberg *et al.*, 1990). Such trapping causes secondary hypoxia in the renal medulla, predisposing to further preservation injury.

PROTECTION OF THE KIDNEY FROM WARM ISCHEMIC INJURY

Investigations have addressed individual aspects of warm ischemic damage with the following treatments:

1. *Energy sources.* Infusion of ATP–magnesium chloride ($MgCl_2$) (12.5 μmol) before or just after warm ischemia increases tissue ATP concentration (Siegal *et al.*, 1983) and improves kidney function in rats (Chaudry, 1983; Gaudio *et al.*, 1982; Sumpio *et al.*, 1984), dogs and humans (Hirasawa *et al.*, 1983). ATP-$MgCl_2$ may improve microcirculatory flow and reduce cellular edema. Adenosine is a component of the successful University of Wisconsin (UW) solution.

2. *Calcium channel blockers.* These comprise dihydropyridines (e.g., nifedipine), diphenylalkylamines (e.g., verapamil) and benzothiazepines (e.g., diazepam). In some experiments, administration of calcium channel blockers before an ischemic insult has afforded protection in rat, guinea pig and dog kidneys (Hertle and Garthoff, 1985; Papadimitriou *et al.*, 1984; Shapiro *et al.*, 1985). These agents have vasoactive effects, which may help diminish reperfusion injury.

3. *Allopurinol.* Allopurinol, an additive to UW solution, inhibits the oxidation of hypoxanthine to xanthine. It has been found to be effective when infused immediately on reperfusion after 60 minutes of rat renal warm ischemia (Baker *et al.*, 1985); treatment just before ischemia was ineffective (Paller *et al.*, 1984).

4. *Free radical scavengers.* Several agents capable of detoxifying superoxide or hydroxyl free radicals have been tested. Superoxide dismutase was effective when administered before warm ischemia and just before or immediately after reperfusion (Baker *et al.*, 1985; Ouriel *et al.*, 1985; Paller *et al.*, 1984; Ratych *et al.*, 1986). Dimethylthiourea, a hydroxyl radical scavenger, also was effective (Burke *et al.*, 1984; Paller *et al.*, 1984). Catalase, which destroys hydrogen peroxide, is effective only in conjunction with superoxide dismutase and cannot permeate the cell; its effect may be at the vascular level. The beneficial effects of treatment with mannitol (Pavlock *et al.*, 1981), polyethylene glycol (Burke *et al.*, 1983), dimethyl sulfoxide (Kedar *et al.*, 1981, 1983) and phenothi-

azines such as chlorpromazine (Jablonski *et al.*, 1983b) have been attributed to their ability to scavenge free radicals, although these compounds have vasoactive and other properties that may be of direct benefit. The efficacy of Bretschneider's histidine tryptophan ketoglutarate (HTK) solution may be due, in part, to the free radical scavenging ability of histidine, tryptophan and mannitol components. Several other successful renal preservation solutions also contain agents (such as glutathione) with free radical scavenging properties.

5. *Steroids.* Methylprednisolone, another component of UW solution, has the property of stabilizing lysosomes and preventing release of lytic enzymes. Pretreatment with methylprednisolone before 2 hours of renal warm ischemia reduced the mortality in dogs from 80 to 20% (Miller and Alexander, 1973) and from 70 to 0% with 90 minutes of warm ischemia (Chatterjee and Berne, 1975). A direct effect of methylprednisolone pretreatment on the excretion of lysosomal enzymes in the urine after warm ischemia and reperfusion has been shown (Smeesters *et al.*, 1983).

6. *Vasoactive drugs.* Warm ischemia produces vasospasm, and many of the previously mentioned effective agents are vasodilators. Pretreatment with phenoxybenzamine has not been confirmed to be beneficial (Jablonski *et al.*, 1983b). Treatments with practolol and propranolol were inconclusive; results obtained with denervated kidney grafts were different from kidneys exposed *in situ* to warm ischemia (Solez *et al.*, 1977). The vascular endothelial lining cells are more vulnerable to ischemic damage than are the parenchymal cells, a characteristic observed in all vascularized organ grafts (Marshall, 2000).

Despite the efficacy of some of these treatments to mitigate the effects of warm ischemia, warm ischemic times are best kept to the minimum possible. Ultimately the best salvage is rapid cooling of the ischemic-anoxic kidney. Current techniques of multiple organ procurement from heart-beating donors reduce warm ischemia before organ cooling to less than 1 minute. In circumstances in which it is difficult to procure grafts from brain-dead, heart-beating donors, double-balloon, triple-lumen catheters have been used to begin *in situ* cooling soon after cessation of heart beat (Kozaki *et al.*, 1991; Ruers *et al.*, 1986).

Donor Factors in Preservation

Preservation effectively begins with identification and preparation of the renal donor. The state of renal function at the time of kidney removal is important. The significance of factors in the donor is highlighted by the different circumstances of preservation in the living donor compared with the cadaver.

LIVING DONOR

During living donor nephrectomy, blood volume and extracellular fluid volumes are maintained by transfusion; normal homeostatic mechanisms are maintained. Mannitol often is given to ensure a steady diuresis. Renal vascular trauma is avoided as the kidney is mobilized. Kidney cooling starts after only a few seconds of warm ischemia. Total ischemia usually is 15 to 30 minutes and is unlikely to be more than 1 hour if donor and recipient operations are synchronous. Excellent preservation of function is provided by simple ice cooling, enhanced by an intraarterial flush with a cold preserving solution. Unless technical or immunological problems occur, function is immediate and normal. When protection of renal function is required only for the period of extracorporeal cold storage and when this is predictably

fewer than 6 hours (as in transplantation from a live donor), any of several preservation solutions (citrate, Collins, buffered sucrose, Bretschneider, UW, Celsior) provides adequate renal preservation.

CADAVER DONOR

Avoiding ischemic damage to the kidney before removal is crucial when extended preservation times are required. Lessons learned in the living donor can be applied directly to the heart-beating cadaver donor. The donor operation has been described in detail in Chapter 7. Effective preservation necessitates supporting blood and interstitial fluid volumes, maintaining renal perfusion and diuresis until kidney removal, supporting metabolic needs and avoiding vasospasm and nephrotoxins.

Diabetes insipidus is common (40–80%) in brain-dead cadavers (Wijnen and van der Linden, 1991). Hypernatremia and hypokalemia may develop; hypokalemia, if persistent, requires potassium infusion. Desmopressin, 1 to 2 µg intramuscularly, can be given. Arginine vasopressin should be considered if urine output persistently exceeds 300 ml/h and is given intravenously in doses of 0.002 to 0.01 IU h^{-1}. Approximately one third of donors in the Australian National Organ Donor Registry required hormone treatment for diabetes insipidus (Herbertt and Disney, 1991).

Alterations in other circulating hormones, especially in thyroid hormone levels, have been observed (Masson *et al.*, 1990) in brain-dead cadavers. Early reports of a diminished acute tubular necrosis incidence after treatment of brain-dead donors with triiodothyronine and cortisol have not been confirmed by later workers; the place of hormonal supplements in cadaver donors has not been confirmed by controlled clinical trials (Howlett *et al.*, 1989). Hormonal deficits could be of greater significance in liver and heart preservation than in kidney preservation. Donors should be maintained with intravascular volume expansion and dopaminergic renal support as required (approximately two thirds of Australian donors), with goals of a systolic blood pressure maintained at greater than 100 mm Hg and a urinary output maintained at 100 ml/h. Renal vasospasm is common in clinical shock and during donor nephrectomy when handling the renal vessels. Agents to minimize vasospasm should be given before starting the donor operation. Steroids (methylprednisolone), phenothiazines (chlorpromazine) and mannitol have been shown to be effective experimentally in preventing warm ischemic damage (Collins *et al.*, 1980; Pentlow *et al.*, 1979). Additional dopamine, dobutamine, isoproterenol or epinephrine is required for hypotension unresponsive to fluids and steroids; kidneys from such donors may give poorer results (Schneider *et al.*, 1983). Phenoxybenzamine is another vasoactive agent that previously was widely used, but it is less effective than chlorpromazine (Jablonski *et al.*, 1983b). Calcium channel antagonists have been shown to be effective experimentally in reversing acute renal insufficiency and should be considered particularly if norepinephrine or epinephrine has been given to the donor. Prostaglandins, glucagon, propranolol and aprotinin are less commonly used clinically. Each agent has been investigated experimentally with variable results (Godfrey and Salaman, 1978; Halasz, 1982; Santiago-Delphin, 1982). Metaanalysis of trials using prostaglandin E$_1$ has not shown significant value from its administration (Ray, 1998).

Management of a potential cadaver donor can be aided by central venous pressure measurements. Intravenous nutrition may be required if intravenous treatment is prolonged. Infusions of nutrients or adenine nucleotides or precursors may enhance subsequent preservation. Specific nephrotoxins, such as aminoglycoside antibiotics, should be avoided. Systemic acidosis should be corrected; intrarenal acidosis is a limiting factor of preservation by simple ice storage (Chan et al., 1983).

Serious mechanical and metabolic damage can occur during kidney removal, particularly by the inexperienced surgeon. Kidneys now more usually are removed by en bloc techniques, and multiple organs usually are harvested from a single donor. Such techniques are compatible with excellent early kidney function (Rosenthal et al., 1983). Techniques of in situ aortic cold perfusion for multiple organ removal such as described in Chapter 7 are helpful in minimizing warm ischemia and renal vasospasm. Heparin should be given intravenously during donor surgery to minimize risks of clotting.

Recommendations for management of the heart-beating cadaver are summarized as follows:

1. A body temperature of greater than 35°C is a prerequisite for diagnosis of brain death: Hypothermia must be avoided to minimize risks of cardiac irregularities. In situ and in vivo organ cooling are reserved until organ removal.

2. Respiratory, circulatory and metabolic support are given: ventilator with fractional inspired oxygen, 60%; partial pressure of arterial oxygen (PaO$_2$), greater than 13 kPa (100 mm Hg); partial pressure of arterial carbon dioxide (PaCO$_2$), less than 5 kPa (40 mm Hg); central venous pressure, 5 to 15 cm H$_2$O; blood pressure, greater than 100 mm Hg systolic; hematocrit, greater than 30%; intravenous dextrose and electrolyte infusion—4% dextrose in 1/5 normal saline to replace previous hour's urine output plus 1,000 ml in 24 hours for insensible losses; urine output, 60 to 120 ml/h and careful management of diabetes insipidus.

3. Dehydration, systemic infection, nephrotoxic antibiotics, catecholamines, electrolyte disturbance, acidosis, neurogenic pulmonary edema and inadequate nutrition (parenteral feeding if intensive care unit stay >24 hours) are avoided.

4. Pharmacological adjuvants include mannitol, 20 g; dopaminergic (2–5 μg kg^{-1} min^{-1}) renal support; steroids, 1 g; chlorpromazine, 50 mg; heparin, 10,000 U and verapamil, 5 mg, or diltiazem, 10 mg, given before donor nephrectomy.

These points are stressed because it is easier (and better) to improve the function of the kidney before it is removed than subsequently. The state of the kidney at the time of its removal has a greater influence in determining early function than the methods used after kidney removal. Provided that immunological threats are averted, immediate function on reimplantation after 24 to 48 hours' storage can be predicted confidently if warm ischemia is minimal and if the kidneys have been removed and implanted expertly and atraumatically.

Less-than-Ideal Donors

Organs from less-than-ideal, brain-dead donors (elderly, diabetics and hypertensives with normal renal function) are capable of giving good results (Newstead and Dyer, 1992). Careful evaluation, including histological assessment of the removed organs, is mandatory.

Cadaver nephrectomy from brain-dead donors formerly was performed under conditions in which the supporting ventilator was turned off in the operating room; kidney removal did not begin until the heart stopped. These techniques were standard in the 1960s, when cardiac arrest was the necessary criterion of certification of death. After the ventilator was switched off, progressive hypotension and renal circulatory impairment followed. Cardiac arrest occurred after a period varying from a few minutes to 1 hour. During that time, arterial oxygen tensions fell to less than 20

mm Hg (2.6 kPa) with profound metabolic acidosis (Marshall, 1971). Kidneys were removed by rapid mobilization and removal of kidneys in sequence followed by extracorporeal cooling or by en bloc removal of both kidneys after in situ cold flushing. Times of absolute warm ischemia usually were 20 to 40 minutes, and total preservation times were 6 to 24 hours. Most kidneys functioned immediately after transplantation, confirming experimental findings that addition of 30 minutes of warm ischemia to later cold ischemia was compatible with early function after transplantation, provided that total storage times did not much exceed 24 hours, whereas 60 minutes of warm ischemia followed by 24 or 48 hours of cold ischemia approached the limits of tolerance and required machine perfusion preservation to improve early function. These historical clinical data are relevant to current use of donors presenting after cardiac arrest.

Asystolic (Non–Heart-Beating) Cadaver Donors

Cadavers presenting after sudden cardiac arrest provide another potential donor pool, and good results can be obtained under these emergency circumstances. A mechanism of rapid renal cooling is necessary, instituted as soon as possible after irretrievable cardiac arrest has been diagnosed. This cooling most commonly has been by rapid introduction (in the emergency department or ward) of a large double-balloon catheter into the aorta by cutdown onto the femoral artery at the groin, together with insertion of a caval catheter (for venting of perfusate) through the femoral vein. The lower balloon is inflated and the catheter drawn back until the balloon impacts at the aortic bifurcation—the catheter now should be positioned appropriately to perfuse through side holes of visceral aortic branches, including kidneys. The upper balloon is inflated to isolate the aortic segment perfused. Large volumes of chilled balanced electrolyte or preserving solution are infused to establish in situ cooling while preparations are made for nephrectomy in the operating room (see Chapter 7).

Asystolic donors are declared dead by cardiac arrest criteria: The heart has ceased to function and cannot be restored despite vigorous cardiopulmonary resuscitation. After the resuscitation team has certified death, the transplant team restarts cardiac massage and ventilation while preparing introduction of the catheter. The time between cardiac arrest and institution of in situ cooling preferably should not exceed 30 minutes. If immediate cardiopulmonary resuscitation measures were available in cases of sudden death, the allowable interval would be extended to 50 minutes. Using such criteria, the available cadaver donor pool can be increased by about 25%, with acceptable results after transplantation (life-sustaining function in the grafts occurred in ≥90% of grafts; Schlumpf et al., 1992). As expected, delayed function in such grafts is twice as common as in grafts taken from heart-beating cadavers, and the best ultimate renal function remains 10% less than in kidneys from heart-beating cadavers (Kootstra et al., 1992). The effects of warm ischemia and cold ischemia are additive; as a crude guide, 1 minute of warm ischemia has effects similar to 1 hour of cold ischemia.

Other methods of hypothermic kidney protection after cardiac arrest that have been used include total body cooling and intraperitoneal cooling with a peritoneal dialysis catheter (Rapaport et al., 1990). Because external cooling is much slower in reducing core organ temperatures than intraarterial flushing, these means are best used as adjuvants to core cooling with an intraarterial cannula.

Effects of Cold Ischemia

The earliest attempts at tissue and organ preservation used cooling to overcome the detrimental effects of ischemic anoxia. Cooling diminishes metabolic activity and curtails the oxygen demand of the preserved organ. Metabolism still proceeds during hypothermic storage in ice (Burg and Orloff, 1964). Oxygen consumption decreases at an exponential rate with falling temperatures: to 10% normal at 10°C, 5% at 5°C (Harvey, 1959) and 3% at 0°C (Levy, 1959). Simple surface cooling of the kidney allows ischemia to be tolerated for 12 hours (Calne *et al.*, 1963; Collins *et al.*, 1969). Cooling by flushing the kidney with a cold preserving solution provides reliable preservation for 12 to 120 hours, depending on the solution used (Marshall *et al.*, 1991). Continuous perfusion of the kidney with oxygenated plasma-derived or colloid-containing perfusates at 4 to 8°C enables storage for 120 hours, with better early function (Belzer *et al.*, 1967; Schilling *et al.*, 1993), and is useful in the salvage of kidneys from non–heart-beating donors (Kozaki *et al.*, 1991).

The effect of cold is not simply a slowing of all metabolic functions but a discordance in the metabolic processes that occur in concert at 37°C (Fig. 9–2). Cellular homeostasis is not preserved during hypothermia:

1. The degree of inhibition of each enzymic reaction is not identical—key enzymes of glycolysis and fatty acid oxidation are inactivated (Lundstam *et al.*, 1976), whereas the glycerophosphate pathway is cold resistant. Some enzymes undergo irreversible conformational changes in the cold (glyceraldehyde dehydrogenase, lactate dehydrogenase), whereas others are reversible on rewarming (pyruvate kinase, glutamate dehydrogenase, arginosuccinase; Chilson *et al.*, 1965).

2. Transmembrane passive diffusion of ions is not affected appreciably, whereas active transport mechanisms involving Na^+/K^+ and Ca^{++}/Mg^{++} ATPases are inhibited at less than 10°C (Leaf, 1959). Intracellular influx of Na^+, Ca^{++}, Cl^- and water occurs with efflux of K^+ and Mg^{++}. Influx of water causes cellular swelling. Short-term hypothermic changes are readily reversed, but in the long term the damage becomes irreversible. Calcium influx and rising cellular phosphate (from dephosphorylation of ATP and adenosine diphosphate [ADP]) cause additional damage. Sequestration of calcium in the mitochondria, activation of the calcium-calmodulin complex (Anaise *et al.*, 1986) and activation of phospholipase by cytosolic calcium contribute to irreversible damage. Restoration of the ionic milieu is essential for adequate renal function: Glucose and amino acid transport in renal tubules depends on the transmembrane Na^+ gradient.

3. Intracellular pH is not maintained. Anaerobic glycolysis proceeds during cold ischemia at a reduced rate. Lactate accumulates, and the pH continues to fall to a value where glycolysis is inhibited. As described for warm ischemia, acid pH affects the stability of lysosomal membranes with release of lytic enzymes. Tissue free iron is increased at acid pH.

4. Free radical formation still takes place: Lipid peroxidation with release of oxygen and hydroxyl free radicals occurs at 2°C.

5. ATP dephosphorylation proceeds; ADP cannot enter the mitochondrion (Southard *et al.*, 1980) and is dephosphorylated to AMP. Further degradation to inosine, hypoxanthine and xanthine occurs, and these progressively diffuse out of the cell.

6. Membrane lipid fluidity is diminished (Chapman, 1975). Increased membrane *leakiness* resulting from separation of protein and lipid constituents allows influx of molecules normally excluded.

7. Erythrocytes, leukocytes and platelets trapped in the cold kidney tend to aggregate as well as suffering the same hypothermic damage. The removal of these cells by flushing or continuous perfusion with a cold solution improves the efficacy of preservation.

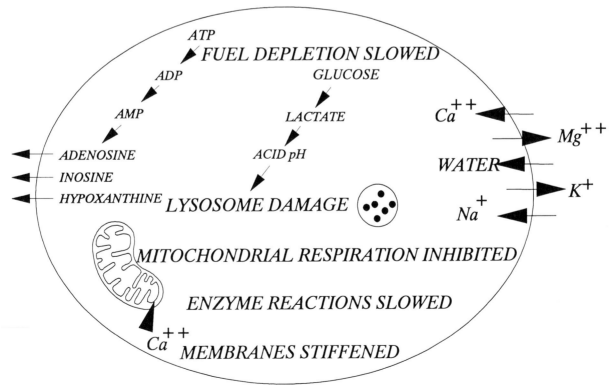

FIGURE 9–2

Effects of cold ischemia: fuel depletion slowed, cellular homeostasis still impaired.

Ischemia exacerbates the effect of cold, accelerating the depletion of energy stores and the influx of Na^+, Ca^{++} and water.

COLD PRESERVATION METHODS

Cold preservation methods have attempted to address some of the aforementioned problems as follows:

1. *Oxygen supply*: Static cold storage cannot supply oxygen, whereas continuous perfusion with asanguineous oxygenated perfusion can provide adequate oxygen for the kidney's low metabolic requirements. Perfusion with oxygenated perfluorochemical emulsions (Fluosols) has been used to improve preservation further. Retrograde venous oxygen persufflation has proved to be a useful adjunct to static preservation but has not gained wide acceptance because of fear of increased endothelial vascular damage.

2. *Metabolic supply*: Glucose often is incorporated in perfusates as a metabolic fuel; amino acids and fatty acids, ATP, adenosine and phosphate also have been added. Complete oxidative phosphorylation may require such additional supplements (Pegg *et al.*, 1981) during perfusion. Adenosine was found to be an essential additive in UW solution (Biguzas *et al.*, 1990b) for static storage; its vasoactive properties may facilitate the flushing procedure.

3. *pH maintenance*: Flushing solutions effective in static cold storage generally have good buffering capacities (e.g., by phosphate, citrate or histidine). Bicarbonate, which generally is used for continuous perfusion, is not as effective in the pH range 7.1 to 7.8; protein in the perfusate can offer additional buffering capacity. The addition of glucose to solutions for static preservation may be counterproductive if lactate production is enhanced and acidosis develops. Such additions can prove effective for continuous perfusion, however, because acid catabolites continually are diluted and leached out of the organ.

4. *Prevention of cellular edema*: The use of solutions containing slowly permeable (mannitol, glucose) or impermeable (sucrose, raffinose) nonelectrolyte solutes helps reduce edema during static and perfusion storage. A further advantage is obtained by replacing the permeable anion, chloride, with an impermeable anion (lactobionate, gluconate). The gradients affecting loss of potassium and magnesium and influx of sodium can be minimized by preserving solutions containing high *intracellular* concentrations of potassium and magnesium and low concentrations of sodium; sodium/potassium ratios in solutions with proven effectiveness for static and perfusion storage can be reversed without significant ill effect.

5. *Modification of cellular calcium*: Diltiazem, a calcium antagonist, attracted attention because it increased renal blood flow (Wagner and Neumayer, 1987) and prevented influx of calcium. In a clinical trial (Puig *et al.*, 1991), the incidence of acute tubular necrosis was reduced from 31 to 16% after diltiazem, 20 mg L^{-1}, was incorporated in Euro-Collins flushout solution, administered during kidney retrieval (0.002 mg kg^{-1} min^{-1}) and to the recipient after transplantation. Another calcium antagonist, verapamil, has similar protective properties (Dawidson and Rooth, 1990). Incorporation of phenothiazines, such as trifluoperazine, into flushing solutions also has been used to inhibit the activation of the calcium-calmodulin complex (Asari *et al.*, 1984) and has improved kidney preservation.

6. *Prevention of free radical damage*: Several strategies have been tested to limit free radical formation after reperfusion of the graft. Allopurinol, a xanthine oxidase inhibitor, has been added to the preserving solution or administered to

donor and recipient (Toledo-Pereyra *et al.*, 1977; Winchell and Halasz, 1989). Its omission from UW solution was found to be deleterious (Biguzas *et al.*, 1990b) to renal function. The free radical scavengers glutathione and ascorbate also have been included in some preserving solutions; the efficacy of such additives may be limited by their instability. Mannitol, polyethylene glycol, histidine and tryptophan also have been used. The iron chelating agent deferoxamine has been an effective additive (656 mg L^{-1}) to the perfusate for machine preservation of dog kidneys for 48 hours with 30 minutes of warm ischemia (Baron *et al.*, 1991).

HYPOTHERMIA IN HIBERNATORS

The effect of hypothermia on enzymes and membranes cannot be manipulated. In nature, such modification is a characteristic of hibernating animals, which can withstand low temperatures for long periods with no damage. During hibernation, brown fat shrinks, urine production ceases, blood ketone concentration rises and glucose concentration falls, pH is maintained and renal K^+/Na^+ ratio is normal. Glomerular filtration ceases, oxygen consumption falls by 98% and tissue ATP is maintained. Kidneys from hibernating squirrels can be preserved for 10 days, compared with 3 days from nonhibernating squirrels (Green *et al.*, 1983). Elucidation of this metabolic shift to increased cold tolerance has potential for the amelioration of the damage resulting from cold sensitivity in organ transplantation but has defied resolution so far. Xenotransplants from hibernators may become a potential future modality.

Techniques of Clinical Preservation

In clinical practice, kidneys first are flushed free of blood with a cold solution, often beginning *in situ* in the heart-beating cadaver. Subsequently, the kidneys are immersed in a cold solution after removal. Thereafter, kidneys are preserved in one of two ways:

1. *Static storage*: The kidneys are immersed in the cold preserving solution and stored at 0° to 4°C to reduce metabolic rates.

2. *Perfusion storage*: The kidneys are continuously perfused with a recirculating volume of preserving solution at 4 to 10°C. This method provides a dilution of toxic metabolic end products as well as reducing metabolic rate by cooling. Such perfusion can provide a more efficient supply of necessary metabolites and of pharmacological adjuvants.

Combinations of simple hypothermia and of perfusion also have been used.

STATIC STORAGE

Cold flushing washes out the blood and enhances cooling rate. Cooling by flushing through the aorta *in situ* can reduce core temperature to less than 10°C in 3 to 5 minutes (Johnson, 1982), compared with 20 minutes for an equivalent reduction by surface cooling (Markland and Parsons, 1963). The preferred storage temperature in rat and dog kidney preservation has been shown to be 0°C rather than 5 or 10°C. Rapid cooling has been shown to be detrimental to rabbit kidneys (Jacobsen *et al.*, 1979), but such rapid rates of cooling are not obtained in larger human kidneys.

The recommended practice for cadaver kidneys is to submerge the organ in iced saline slush after removal from the body and to complete the flush with cold preserving solution at 0 to 4°C until the effluent is clear of blood. The kidney

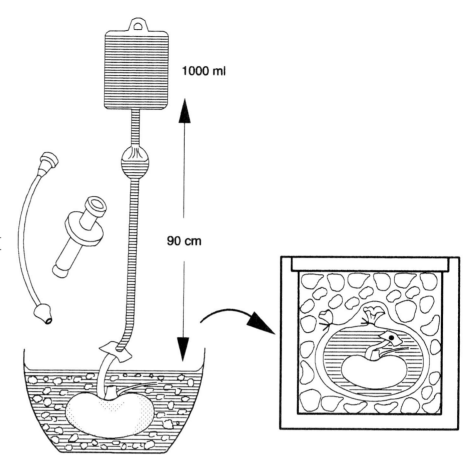

FIGURE 9–3

Techniques of cold flushing with preserving solution followed by static hypothermic storage.

then is surrounded with the perfusing solution, placed in a sterile container (usually double plastic bags) and stored in ice in an insulated container (Fig. 9–3).

A variety of preserving solutions of varying solute composition have been developed in the course of 40 years. Solutions of extracellular electrolyte composition, such as plasma, saline or Hartmann's solution, are unsuitable for prolonged (>12 hours) preservation but often are used to flush cool kidneys *in situ* during multiple organ procurement. They are *not* suitable for cooling kidneys before immediate transfer in living donor transplantation and are not recommended; alternative solutions have been shown to be markedly superior.

Collins-Type Solutions

Prolonged preservation became possible after the development of solutions of intracellular electrolyte composition (Collins *et al.*, 1969, 1972, 1979; Hardie *et al.*, 1977; Sacks *et al.*, 1973; Table 9–1). These solutions minimized cellular edema and the loss of intracellular potassium. Initial function after 72 hours of cold storage was poor, however, and any added warm ischemia markedly diminished the efficacy of these solutions (Halasz and Collins, 1976).

The original Collins' solution had high concentrations of potassium, magnesium, phosphate, sulfate and glucose. Precipitation of magnesium phosphate was a major technical defect. Subsequently, magnesium was omitted from the widely used Euro-Collins solution (Dreikorn *et al.*, 1980; Squifflet *et al.*, 1981; Watkins *et al.*, 1971).

The high concentration of glucose may reduce the efficacy of this preserving solution. Glucose is slowly permeable

across cell membranes, stimulates cellular anaerobic glycolysis and augments tissue acidosis. Rat kidneys preserved with Collins' solution have high tissue concentrations of lactate. Replacement of glucose by mannitol or by sucrose reduces tissue lactate and improves renal function after renal ischemia or transplantation in the rat (Andrews and Bates, 1985; Marshall *et al.*, 1983a, 1985a). Replacement of glucose by mannitol and addition of adenosine significantly improved preservation of dog kidneys when compared with Collins' C2 solution (Bretan *et al.*, 1991). A reduction of postoperative renal failure occurred (from 77 to 15%) when human kidneys were preserved in a Euro-Collins solution in which mannitol was substituted for glucose (Grino *et al.*, 1987).

TABLE 9–1

COLLINS-TYPE FLUSHING SOLUTIONS

	C2	Euro-Collins	Euro-Collins Sucrose
Sodium (mmol L^{-1})	9	10	10
Potassium (mmol L^{-1})	108	108	108
Magnesium (mmol L^{-1})	30	—	—
Bicarbonate (mmol L^{-1})	9	10	10
Chloride (mmol L^{-1})	14	15	15
Phosphate (mmol L^{-1})	47	60	60
Sulfate (mmol L^{-1})	30	—	—
Glucose (mmol L^{-1})	126	180	—
Sucrose (mmol L^{-1})	—	—	180
Osmolality (mmol kg^{-1})	320	340	340
pH (0°C)	7.0	7.3	7.2

Citrate-Based Solutions

Hypertonic citrate solution was developed to overcome some of the limitations of the Collins-type solutions (Marshall *et al.*, 1977; Ross *et al.*, 1976; Table 9–2). This solution also contained high concentrations of potassium and magnesium, but citrate replaced phosphate and mannitol replaced glucose. Citrate provided buffering capacity as well as chelating magnesium to form impermeable solutes.

Isotonic citrate solutions containing less mannitol proved to be as efficient as hypertonic solutions in preserving human kidneys and livers. Rat and dog kidneys preserved with isotonic citrate solution have better function after transplantation than those preserved with the hypertonic solution (Howden *et al.*, 1983).

A high concentration of magnesium is necessary for the efficacy of citrate solutions; only 4% of the magnesium remains unchelated, and magnesium-citrate chelate contributes to the semipermeable solute available physically to maintain cellular integrity. High levels of potassium may minimize loss of cellular potassium. Citrate chelates calcium as well as magnesium and may aid in the extrusion of calcium from the cell as well as the maintenance of pH. Citrate could be replaced by its nonmetabolizable analogue tricarballylate, provided that hepes is added to augment its buffering capacity (Jablonski *et al.*, 1980). Sulfate also is a component of the solution but can be replaced by other anions.

Mannitol is a component of both citrate solutions but can be replaced by sucrose with equal results. Replacement of mannitol with glucose was detrimental: Tissue lactate increased with significant medullary damage and less effective preservation.

Effective buffering of the preserving solutions was an important feature. An acid pH (6.8) was found to be deleterious (Jablonski *et al.*, 1980), whereas pH ranges from 7.1 to 7.8 were equally effective.

Sucrose-Based Solutions

Addition of sucrose to ineffective solutions or replacement of glucose by sucrose improved the efficacy of preserving solutions (Andrews and Bates, 1985; Table 9–3). Simple isomolar sodium phosphate–buffered sucrose solutions provided effective preservation of rat (Marshall *et al.*, 1985a), dog (Lam *et al.*, 1989a), pig (Lodge *et al.*, 1991) and human (Lam *et al.*, 1989b) kidneys. These solutions contained no potassium or magnesium. Addition of gluconate did not improve the efficacy of the solution. Optimal sucrose concentration was around 140 (mmol L^{-1}). Hyperosmolar sucrose-based solutions were less effective than isosmolar solutions.

TABLE 9–2

CITRATE-BASED FLUSHING SOLUTIONS

	Hypertonic Citrate	Isotonic Citrate
Sodium (mmol L^{-1})	78	78
Potassium (mmol L^{-1})	84	84
Magnesium (mmol L^{-1})	40	40
Chloride (mmol L^{-1})	1	1
Citrate (mmol L^{-1})	54	54
Sulfate (mmol L^{-1})	40	40
Glucose (mmol L^{-1})	—	—
Mannitol (mmol L^{-1})	200	100
Osmolality (mmol kg^{-1})	400	300
pH (0°C)	7.1	7.1

TABLE 9–3

SUCROSE-PHOSPHATE FLUSHING SOLUTIONS

	PBS	PBS140
Sodium (mmol L^{-1})	126	92
Phosphate (mmol L^{-1})	82	60
Sucrose (mmol L^{-1})	100	140
Osmolality (mmol kg^{-1})	300	310
pH (0°C)	7.1	7.2

These sucrose solutions provide buffering and impermeant solute only; cooling reduces metabolic requirements, and no other physicochemical attributes can be shown. It seems ineluctable that hypothermia, buffering and impermeable solute constitute important factors in static preservation of kidneys.

Bretschneider's HTK Solution

Bretschneider's HTK solution initially was developed for cardioplegia in cardiac surgery (Table 9–4). Its efficacy was tested experimentally in dog kidneys subjected to warm and cold ischemia (Kallerhoff *et al.*, 1986, 1988) as well as clinically (Isemer *et al.*, 1988). The solution is an excellent buffer, tryptophan and histidine are free radical scavengers and histidine and α-ketoglutarate may have some metabolic benefit. In a multicenter trial by Eurotransplant, primary graft function was rapid using HTK in 74%, with 11% incidence of acute tubular necrosis in the 202 transplants studied (Groenewoud *et al.*, 1990). A subsequent report comparing HTK and Collins' solution in a prospective randomized trial showed that the incidence of delayed graft function was reduced by 13% (from 37% in the Euro-Collins group to 24% in the HTK group), with better creatinine clearances at all times after transplantation in the HTK group (Groenewoud and Thorogood, 1992).

University of Wisconsin Solution

University of Wisconsin solution originally was developed for preservation of the pancreas (Wahlberg *et al.*, 1986, 1987; Table 9–5). Its components included impermeable solutes (lactobionate, raffinose), a colloid (hydroxyethyl starch [HES]), phosphate buffer, other electrolytes (high K$^+$, low Na$^+$) and several other additives (adenosine, allopurinol, glutathione, steroids, insulin). Subsequently, UW was effectively applied to liver (Jamieson *et al.*, 1988), kidney (Ploeg *et al.*, 1988) and heart (Demertzis *et al.*, 1992; Jeevanandam *et al.*, 1992a, 1992b; Stein *et al.*, 1991) preservation. The clinical success of UW solution in liver (Kalayoglu *et al.*, 1988; Todo

TABLE 9–4

BRETSCHNEIDER HTK SOLUTION

Sodium (mmol L^{-1})	15
Potassium (mmol L^{-1})	9
Magnesium (mmol L^{-1})	4
Chloride (mmol L^{-1})	26
Histidine (mmol L^{-1})	198
Tryptophan (mmol L^{-1})	2
α-Ketoglutarate (mmol L^{-1})	1
Mannitol (mmol L^{-1})	30
Osmolality (mmol kg^{-1})	310
pH (0°C)	7.3

TABLE 9–5

UNIVERSITY OF WISCONSIN–BASED SOLUTIONS FOR STATIC HYPOTHERMIC STORAGE AFTER FLUSHING UNIVERSITY OF WISCONSIN SOLUTION

Sodium (mmol L^{-1})	30
Potassium (mmol L^{-1})	125
Magnesium (mmol L^{-1})	5
Sulfate (mmol L^{-1})	5
Lactobionate (mmol L^{-1})	100
Phosphate (mmol L^{-1})	25
Raffinose (mmol L^{-1})	30
Adenosine (mmol L^{-1})	5
Glutathione (mmol L^{-1})	3
Allopurinol (mmol L^{-1})	1
Insulin (U L^{-1})	100
Dexamethasone (mg L^{-1})	8
Trimethoprim-sulfamethoxazole (Bactrim) (ml)	0.5
HES (g L^{-1})	50
Osmolality (mmol kg^{-1})	320
pH	7.4

HES = hydroxyethyl starch.

et al., 1989), pancreas and organ cluster preservation (D'Alessandro *et al.*, 1991a, 1991b) has made it the preferred solution for multiple organ harvest. A multicenter trial in Europe (Ploeg, 1990) comparing UW with Euro-Collins solution for kidney transplantation showed that preservation with UW solution resulted in a more rapid recovery of renal function and less posttransplant dialysis. This difference was accentuated when kidneys were damaged by warm ischemia (Sakagami *et al.*, 1990). In a prospective study with paired cadaveric kidneys (from heart-beating donors), no advantage could be shown of UW over Euro-Collins (Hefty *et al.*, 1992). The use of UW solution for kidney preservation may be preferable for the rescue of grafts obtained from non–heart-beating donors or when long preservation times (>36 hours) are probable. The effect of UW in improving renal hemodynamics and microvasculature (Ueda *et al.*, 1989) and reducing the trapping of erythrocytes in the outer medulla (Jacobsson *et al.*, 1989) may be contributory factors. A key distinction between UW and other solutions could be improved resistance of the microvasculature to ischemia rather than a protective effect on renal parenchyma.

Relative Importance of Components of Flush Storage Preservation Solutions

Apart from impermeable solutes and buffering, UW solution incorporates a variety of additives, including adenosine (ATP precursor, vasodilator), allopurinol (xanthine oxidase inhibitor), glutathione (free radical scavenger), insulin and steroid (membrane stabilizer). The solution has a high concentration of potassium, mimicking intracellular fluid. The relative importance of individual components has been elucidated in many studies. Modifications of the original solution with omission of one or more components have given equivalent preservation of kidney and other organs. Few modifications have been shown to improve preservation markedly, but simplification of the base solution has allowed additional room for other additives.

Colloid Hydroxyethyl Starch. The inclusion of the synthetic colloid HES does not confer any advantage (Baatard *et al.*, 1993; Biguzas *et al.*, 1990a; Schlumpf *et al.*, 1991). Colloid added to flushing solutions has long been known to affect their rheological properties and perhaps to improve the efficiency of vascular washout, but the addition of colloid

is essential only in continuous perfusion storage. Colloid increases the viscosity of the solution; this does not appear to be harmful or helpful in simple flushing, although it slows the rate. Preservation of canine kidneys by simple hypothermic storage was reliably extended to 5 days by a modified HES-free UW solution (Marshall *et al.*, 1991). Omission of colloid in a randomized clinical trial showed equivalent and satisfactory preservation of kidneys with HES-free UW solution. University of Wisconsin solution and its colloid-free modification gave significantly better preservation than did Euro-Collins solution (Baatard *et al.*, 1993).

Electrolytes. Reduction of potassium concentration with reversal of the Na$^+$/K$^+$ ratio (Biguzas *et al.*, 1990a; Moen *et al.*, 1989) to mimic extracellular fluid improves flushing efficacy considerably (potassium is markedly vasoconstrictive) and is just as effective in preservation. A modification without HES and based on sodium lactobionate and sucrose with low K$^+$ has been widely used experimentally and clinically for multiple organ preservation (Collins *et al.*, 1993).

Impermeable Solutes. The great efficacy of UW solution in organ preservation primarily is due to the impermeable anion, lactobionate. Gluconate, also impermeable, can replace lactobionate. Similarly, raffinose can be replaced by sucrose with little detriment.

The introduction of UW solution and its modifications has markedly enhanced preservation of all transplantable organs. It has restored order to the operations of liver and pancreas grafting, it has given more effective heart preservation than previous methods and it has served as a gold standard for all transplantable organs. Although differences among organs in their sensitivity to ischemic damage and in their individual requirements for optimal preservation exist, these are outweighed by the universally protective effects of the major components of UW solution. The original colloid-containing, high-potassium intracellular fluid UW solution and modified HES-free, high-sodium extracellular fluid UW solutions, without some of the original adjuvants and with other additions, have been shown equivalently effective in kidney preservation (Table 9–6).

Oxygen. A limitation of static storage is the oxygen deficit and the inevitable shift to anaerobic metabolism with progressive intracellular acidosis. Early attempts at oxygen provision involved storage of the kidneys hyperbarically to increase the solubility of oxygen in the solution; these did not improve preservation. Preservation was improved by continuously bubbling humidified oxygen through the organ (persufflation) via the renal vessels or ureter (Fischer *et al.*, 1978; Rolles *et al.*, 1984; Ross and Escott, 1979). Retrograde venous persufflation seemed preferable and improved initial function of the revascularized dog kidney, particularly kidneys damaged by warm ischemia. Increased vascular damage with postoperative clotting at the anastomoses was reported in one study (Ross and Escott, 1982). The method has not received major clinical support because of its moderate invasiveness and possible deleterious side effects on vascular endothelium.

Metabolites. Metabolites and their precursors and inhibitors (ATP, adenosine, adenine and allopurinol) have been added with advantage to various solutions. Adenosine, allopurinol and glutathione were found to confer some benefit in preservation of rat kidneys (Biguzas *et al.*, 1990b), but adenosine and allopurinol have been omitted in a clinical trial with no detriment (Baatard *et al.*, 1993).

Steroids. Methylprednisolone often is added as a membrane stabilizer, but its value has not been shown, and the value of insulin has not been shown (Biguzas *et al.*, 1990b). Procaine was added to reduce vasospasm until the demon-

TABLE 9–6

UNIVERSITY OF WISCONSIN–DERIVED SOLUTIONS FOR STATIC HYPOTHERMIC STORAGE AFTER FLUSHING

Solution	Main Constituents
UW solution (Viaspan)	Impermeables—lactobionate 100, raffinose 30 Adjuvants—adenosine 5, glutathione 3, allopurinol 1 Electrolytes ICF Na 30, K 125, Mg 5, PO$_4$ 25 Colloid—yes, HES

HES-free UW	Impermeables—lactobionate 100, raffinose 60
	Adjuvants—adenosine 5, glutathione 3, allopurinol 1
	Electrolytes ICF
	  Na 30, K 125, Mg 5, PO$_4$ 25, or ECF
	  Na 125, K 30, Mg 5, PO$_4$ 25
	Colloid—no
	ICF and ECF equally effective

Sodium lactobionate	Impermeables—lactobionate 100, sucrose 75 Adjuvants—glutathione 3, chlorpromazine 5 Electrolytes ECF Na 150, K 5, Mg 5, PO$_4$ 25 Colloid—no
Celsior	Impermeables—lactobionate, mannitol Adjuvants—glutathione, histidine, glutamate Electrolytes ECF Na 100, K 15, Mg 13, Ca 2.5, Cl 40 Colloid—no

UW = University of Wisconsin; HES, hydroxyethyl starch; ICF, intracellular fluid; ECF, extracellular fluid.

stration that its inclusion in the flushing solution was detrimental (Collins and Halasz, 1975).

Calcium Channel Blockers. The calcium channel blockers diltiazem, verapamil, nifedipine and nisoldipine have been added with variable but encouraging benefit. Trifluoperazine, a calcium calmodulin complex inhibitor, has been shown to improve survival and renal function of dog kidneys after 72 hours of storage in Collins' C2 solution (Asari et al., 1984). The addition of trifluoperazine preserved the cortical microcirculation of the dog kidneys during 72 hours of storage (Anaise et al., 1987). Another calcium antagonist, lidoflazine, improved preservation of rat kidneys (Jacobsson et al., 1992). This compound is different from other calcium antagonists in that it inhibits calcium influx after ischemia or hypoxia and potentiates the vasodilatory properties of adenosine. Another antianginal agent, ranolazine, was found to be beneficial when given to the donor (0.85 mg kg^{-1} plus 0.25 mg kg^{-1} h^{-1}) and included in the flush-out (0.5 mg L^{-1} in PBS140 solution). Recipient treatment had no effect (Lodge et al., 1990). Human atrial natriuretic peptide has been added to Euro-Collins solution to prolong dog kidney preservation to 72 hours (Marumo et al., 1991).

These calcium channel blockers have important effects in immune modulation as well as in preservation. In preservation, they can inhibit calcium-mediated ischemic damage by preventing calcium from entering the cytosol. Immunological effects include inhibition of calcium-mediated lymphocyte proliferation and diminished cyclosporine nephrotoxicity by blocking the vasoconstrictive effects of endothelin and thromboxane A$_2$ on the afferent arteriole.

Free Radical Scavengers (Superoxide Dismutase, Mannitol, Reduced Glutathione). Glutathione is unsta-

ble in solution, which may reduce its efficacy (Astier and Paul, 1989). Preservation-induced endothelial damage is effected by release of cytotoxic oxygen free radicals, such as superoxide and hydroxyl ions, by activation of adhesion molecules promoting leukocyte and platelet adhesion and aggregation and by activation of proinflammatory cytokines (tumor necrosis factor, interleukins and growth factors) and other locally produced messengers causing vasoconstriction and endothelial damage. Various additives combating these effects have been shown to enhance preservation significantly.

Other Agents. Other agents include prostaglandins, β-blockers, angiotensin-converting enzyme inhibitors, pentoxifylline and natriuretic peptide.

1. Prostaglandins are unsaturated fatty acids produced by metabolism of arachidonic acid, along with other eicosanoids (thromboxane and leukotrienes). These agents form rapidly, act locally and are destroyed enzymatically. They are classified as autacoids or prostanoids, to distinguish them from systemic hormones. Prostaglandins participate in and modulate inflammatory responses. Many are vasoconstrictive. Thromboxane is synthesized in platelets; it stimulates platelet aggregation and is a potent vasoconstrictor. Prostacyclin (prostaglandin G$_1$) is vasodilatory and inhibits platelet aggregation. Prostaglandin E$_1$ analogues (e.g., misoprostol, enisoprostol), in a review of more than 200 articles (7 of which were study trials in renal transplant patients comparing prostaglandin E$_1$ with placebo), showed no improvement in the drug over placebo (Ray, 1998).
2. Corticosteroids and nonsteroidal antiinflammatory drugs inhibit formation of arachidonic acid, prostaglandin, and thromboxane.
3. Benzodiazepines (chlorpromazine, trifluoperazine), aprotinin and corticosteroids act as membrane stabilizers.
4. Lazaroids (aminosteroids) inhibit lipid membrane peroxidation.
5. Other cell messenger and adhesion molecules (cyclic AMP and guanosine monophosphate [GMP], interleukins, nitric oxide and endothelin inhibitors) act to inhibit the complement cascade and neutrophil chemotaxis and sequestration.

Agonal or Preservation Injury and the Immune Response

The success rate of organ grafts from brain-dead cadaver donors is consistently inferior to those from living donors, even when live donors are unrelated genetically to the recipient. Irreversible brain injury up-regulates proinflammatory cytokine mediators and MHC class I and II antigens, facilitating host inflammatory and immunological responses. Preservation-induced injury promotes inflammatory responses, which further potentiate immune damage by up-regulation of histocompatibility antigens. Future improvements in preservation solutions and cadaver donor treatments have the challenging potential to minimize or reverse these effects with consequent improved results of transplantation.

Additives to Enhance Endothelial Integrity Further

Other potentially renoprotective agents include bioflavinoids, which are found in various plants and which have antioxidant, antiinflammatory, and tyrosine kinase–inhibiting properties. Two such agents, Quercetin and curcumin, attenuated chemokine induction and reduced renal inflammatory infiltrate in a rat warm ischemia model (Shoskes, 1998).

Glutathione S-transferases (GSTs) are a group of isoenzymes, each with its own distribution in renal tubules. These GSTs are released in extracellular fluid and urine in high concentrations in response to renal injury. Their assay makes it possible to localize injury to different parts of the renal tubule. They may serve as biomarkers for acute renal damage. In humans, ligandin (α GST) is found exclusively in the proximal tubule and II GST in the distal tubule. Their presence in the graft perfusate has been used to monitor viability of kidney grafts from asystolic donors (Kievit *et al.*, 1997).

Additives to flushing or perfusion solutions optimally would include effective immunosuppressive agents. Pretreatment of human renal allografts with monoclonal antileukocyte antibodies has been tested by adding these to the flushing solution before implantation (Taube *et al.*, 1987); initial results suggested improved function and fewer rejection episodes, but this has not been confirmed by later studies.

PERFUSION STORAGE

Carrel and Lindbergh (1938) developed continuous kidney perfusion in a series of classic experiments. Belzer and colleagues preserved kidneys for 3 days by continuous perfusion with oxygenated cryoprecipitated plasma at 8°C (Belzer *et al.*, 1967). Continuous perfusion storage with a recirculating volume of perfusate still provides the most effective renal preservation for the longest time, especially for kidneys damaged by warm ischemia.

Instrumentation

All perfusion storage is carried out in the temperature range 4 to 9°C, and the perfusion circuit must include a heat exchanger to maintain hypothermia. An automatic pump is essential to perfuse the kidneys with the cold perfusate. The original Belzer pump provided physiological pulsatile flow, but nonpulsatile pumps have been equally effective (Toledo-Pereyra, 1982). The commonly used equipment provides non-

physiological pulsatile flow at a pressure of 20 to 60 mm Hg and an average flow of 1 to 6 ml g^{-1} min^{-1}.

Oxygenation is a feature of all perfusion storage circuits. Some systems include a membrane oxygenator (e.g., Belzer, Waters); other systems rely on surface oxygenation (e.g., Gambro) and appear to be equally reliable. A mixture of air or oxygen with added carbon dioxide is essential for membrane oxygenators to maintain pH as well as oxygen tension. Surface oxygenation is possible without added carbon dioxide. The perfusates must pass through a bubble-trap before reaching the kidney (Fig. 9–4).

Blood has no advantages and considerable disadvantages in hypothermic perfusion. Cold blood introduces problems of increased viscosity, resistance to flow, aggregation of platelets and red cells. Cryoprecipitated plasma (Belzer *et al.*, 1967) derived from blood treated with the anticoagulant acid/citrate/glucose, with added magnesium sulfate (5 mmol L^{-1}) and mannitol (28 mmol L^{-1}), provided good preservation for 3 days. The preparation of this perfusate was time-consuming and difficult to standardize, and other plasma-derived solutions were developed, such as plasma protein fraction (Johnson *et al.*, 1972) and silica-gel fraction plasma (Toledo-Pereyra *et al.*, 1977).

The introduction of synthetic stable albumin-based perfusates in 1973 (Claes and Blohme, 1973) replaced earlier perfusates. Variations among preparations obtained from different suppliers may have been related to the fatty acid content of the albumin preparation; high concentrations of octanoate in the perfusate (Cohen *et al.*, 1983) were detrimental to long-term preservation.

The inclusion of an efficient oncotic agent was essential for perfusion storage to prevent vascular collapse and cellular edema. Albumin was shown to be superior to dextrans, gelatin, starch or gum arabic (Belzer *et al.*, 1982a; Hoffman *et al.*, 1982). A special preparation of HES subsequently was shown to be an effective substitute for albumin in the preservation of dog kidneys (Hoffman *et al.*, 1983).

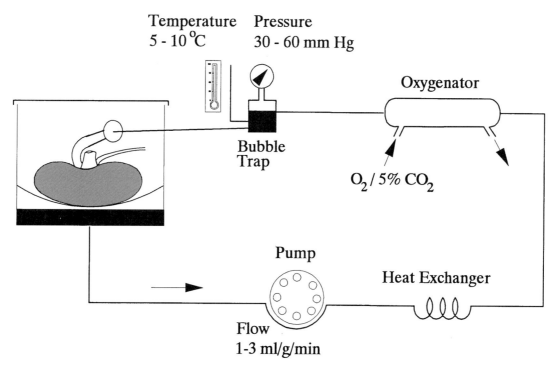

FIGURE 9–4

Techniques of continuous hypothermic perfusion.

In clinical practice, the electrolyte composition of the perfusate was determined empirically and mimicked extracellular composition with added magnesium. Prolonged perfusion allowed albumin to escape into the extravascular space and organ swelling to occur. Increasing perfusate albumin did not overcome this problem of an exploded extracellular fluid space; replacing chloride with less permeable anions, gluconate and phosphate (Southard and Belzer, 1980), improved effectiveness of preservation of dog kidneys. Addition of magnesium and citrate to conventional perfusates (Marshall et al., 1983b) improved preservation of rat and dog kidneys. Solutions of albumin or HES in sodium phosphate–buffered sucrose also were effective. These findings showed that the inclusion of impermeable or semipermeable solutes was beneficial in perfusion storage as well as in static storage.

Plasma-derived perfusates contained variable concentrations of glucose, amino acids and fatty acids. The possible benefit of such metabolites in the perfusate has not been evaluated. Glucose and other metabolic fuels are the usual additives to synthetic perfusates.

Oxygenation of the perfusate usually is employed routinely but may not be necessary for short-term preservation (Belzer et al., 1982b). Little aerobic metabolism seems to occur during hypothermic preservation for 24 hours by either method.

A variety of agents have been added empirically to machine perfusates with little evaluation of their benefit, including methylprednisolone, to improve membrane stability; allopurinol, to inhibit xanthine oxidase and reduce free radical formation; glutathione as a free radical scavenger; glutathione and ascorbic acid, to provide optimal redox potential; insulin; antibiotics and phenoxybenzamine. Successful preservation of kidneys also has been possible in the absence of these additives.

The most significant factors in continuous hypothermic perfusion preservation may comprise dilution and washout of toxic metabolites. Optimal perfusion storage requires an efficient oncotic agent (HES) and buffering capacity; perfusion is enhanced further by agents impermeable to cells (gluconate, sucrose, citrate or raffinose). Oxygen to enhance aerobic metabolism and provision of metabolic fuels and precursors (adenosine, ATP-MgCl$_2$, adenine, phosphate, glucose and fatty acids) are lesser benefits. These latter appear of more importance in prolonged perfusion preservation over several days, and perhaps in rescue of ischemically damaged kidneys.

Limitations of Perfusion Storage

Preservation by perfusion is effective for 3 days and becomes less reliable after 5 days, by which time considerable damage to the vascular endothelium can occur. This damage may be due to hemodynamic effects on the endothelium (Ueda et al., 1989), loss of vital metabolites, derangement of calcium compartmentalization or accumulation of toxic products in the cell and in the perfusate. The restoration of cellular homeostasis becomes more difficult after prolonged periods of hypothermic preservation.

Preservation periods were extended for dog kidneys to 6 days by a 3-hour period of normothermic perfusion (ex vivo or in vitro) at the halfway point (Rijkmans et al., 1984; van der Wijk et al., 1983). These observations were confirmed and extended in dog and rat kidneys; however, the underlying mechanism remained obscure (Gaber et al., 1987; Mayfield et al., 1987). Provided that damage during the period of normothermic perfusion can be avoided, the method provides a means to restore metabolite deficits, reverse cold-inhibited enzyme systems and metabolize accumulated toxic

TABLE 9–7

SOLUTIONS FOR CONTINUOUS PERFUSION STORAGE

	Albumin-Based Solutions	HES-Based (UW) Solutions HES-Gluconate
Sodium (mmol L^{-1})	140	140
Potassium (mmol L^{-1})	25	25
Magnesium (mmol L^{-1})	5	5
Chloride (mmol L^{-1})	40	—
Gluconate (mmol L^{-1})	85	85
Phosphate (mmol L^{-1})	25	25
Glucose (mmol L^{-1})	10	10
Mannitol (mmol L^{-1})	—	—
Albumin (g L^{-1})	37.5	—
HES (g L^{-1})	—	40–50
Glutathione (mmol L^{-1})	3	3
Osmolality (mmol kg^{-1})	305	350
pH (0°C)	7.5	7.1

Note: Further additives sometimes used include insulin 100 IU L^{-1}, hydrocortisone 250 mg L^{-1}, antibiotics (penicillin 6000 IU L^{-1}, ampicillin 1 g L^{-1}), hepes 10 mmol L^{-1}, adenosine 5 mmol L^{-1}, calcium 0.5–1.5 mmol L^{-1}, chlorpromazine 5 mg L^{-1} and a variety of metabolic inhibitors.
HES = hydroxyethyl starch; UW = University of Wisconsin.

products. A period of normothermic perfusion with blood is effective in rescuing kidneys damaged by a period of warm ischemia (Maessen et al., 1989).

The addition of metabolic inhibitors (e.g., quinacrine, a phospholipase inhibitor, and protease inhibitors relevant to mitochondrial function and calcium compartmentalization) may be of value in prolonging kidney preservation to 7 days (McAnulty et al., 1991). Around 1 week has marked the limit of successful kidney preservation by machine perfusion. The UW perfusion solution, containing HES, has formed the basis of such extension of preservation times (Table 9–7).

University of Wisconsin–derived solutions can experimentally preserve kidneys (with minimal warm ischemia) reliably for 5 days by ice storage after a simple flush and for 7 days by continuous machine perfusion. Hypothermic perfusion has no significant advantages experimentally or clinically over static hypothermic storage for 24-hour preservation of kidneys procured with minimal warm ischemia. Hypothermic perfusion currently has its major role in rescuing kidneys removed from marginal donors.

Factors in the Recipient

Management of the donor is manifestly important to subsequent graft function. It has long been suspected that factors in the recipient during operation and after reperfusion may be equally important. Failure of blood flow to return uniformly to all portions of previously ischemic tissues (no reflow phenomenon) is a well-recognized sequela of extended ischemia to organs in situ. This phenomenon has been described after ischemia of kidney, heart, muscle, brain and other tissues (Ratych et al., 1986).

Delayed restoration of blood flow to the renal cortex after reperfusion can contribute significantly to delayed graft function. Reperfusion of the stored kidney, rather than marking a welcome end to the ischemic insult, may serve to exacerbate the effects of ischemia and lead to further cellular damage and acute tubular necrosis.

The extent of cellular preservation damage becomes apparent only on reperfusion of the preserved organ with blood. During this period, cellular equilibrium must be reestablished despite deficits in endogenous cofactors and uneven distribution of extracellular nutrients, oxygen and hormones. Preservation solutions that afford more effective preservation of the microvasculature result in prompt relief of ischemia to all cells in the organs.

In healthy tissues perfused by oxygenated blood under conditions of aerobic metabolism, there is little opportunity for the formation of reactive derivatives of oxygen. Endogenous scavengers can inactivate any such free radicals adequately. During storage, degradation of ATP has produced adenosine, inosine and hypoxanthine. Calcium influx has activated cytosolic proteases to produce xanthine oxidase. Tissue concentrations of free iron have increased as a result of acidosis. On reperfusion, oxygen reacts with hypoxanthine and activated xanthine oxidase to produce the highly reactive superoxide radical. Superoxide can dismutate to hydrogen peroxide, and in the presence of free iron or manganese ion reactive hydroxyl free radical can be formed. Superoxide, hydrogen peroxide and hydroxyl radicals can produce cellular and microvascular injury through lipid peroxidation of cellular and subcellular membranes (Fig. 9–5).

Under normal conditions, active endogenous scavenging mechanisms are available (superoxide dismutase, catalase and glutathione peroxidase) as well as ascorbic acid, glutathione and histidine, α-tocopherol and tryptophan. After storage, these are rapidly depleted, increasing cellular vulnerability. Injury to subcellular membranes impairs cellular recovery of homeostasis. Injury to cellular membranes has a profound effect on intercellular binding, leading to the detachment of endothelial cells from the vasculature and increased adhesion of circulating leukocytes. Leukocytes also produce free radicals when stimulated, and this can compound vascular damage.

Addition of allopurinol (xanthine oxidase inhibitor), glutathione and histidine to preserving solutions and pretreatment of the recipient with allopurinol, superoxide dismutase, catalase and α-tocopherol have improved the function of kidney grafts. Mannitol also may be useful as a free radical scavenger. The benefits of these treatments have varied considerably in different species, possibly reflecting different endogenous conditions.

Damage to the microvasculature has been documented in dog kidneys preserved for 3 days with Euro-Collins solution—this was more apparent in the medulla. Prolonged perfusion storage of the kidney, when unsuccessful, shows major injury to vascular endothelium on scanning electron microscopy. Trapping of erythrocytes in the juxtamedullary zone of the kidney has been shown; the extent of trapping was related to the duration of storage and to the efficacy of preservation. The resulting obstruction of the peritubular capillaries contributed to medullary ischemia—renal function is improved when erythrocyte trapping is reduced by hemodilution of the recipient or pretreatment with allopurinol or superoxide dismutase (Koyama *et al.*, 1985). In severely damaged kidneys, extravasation of blood occurs as well as trapping, and there is increased permeability of the glomerular capillaries, decreased plasma flow and complete obstruction (*no flow*). Increased adherence of neutrophils to damaged endothelium (Klausner *et al.*, 1989) exacerbates the injury by contributing superoxide radical and releasing cytokines (e.g., tumor necrosis factor), which augment neutrophil aggregation and adherence and endothelial damage.

Treatment with calcium antagonists, diltiazem (Neumayer and Wagner, 1987; Puig *et al.*, 1991) and verapamil (Dawidson *et al.*, 1990) has been effective. Infusion of albumin at a high rate (1.2–1.6 g/kg body weight) improved the outcome of cadaveric renal transplantation, decreasing the rate of acute tubular necrosis (Dawidson *et al.*, 1992). This effect may be

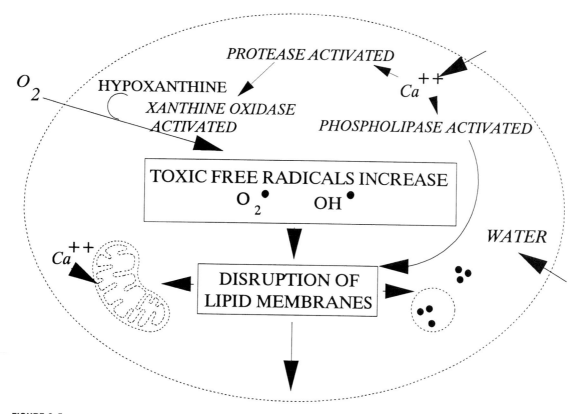

FIGURE 9–5

Free radical production causing reperfusion damage after ischemia.

related to intravascular volume expansion and the possible scavenging effects of albumin.

Vasoconstrictive mechanisms involve prostaglandin synthesis; administration of stable prostacyclin analogues (Kaufman et al., 1987) improved the function of renal and hepatic grafts. The renin/angiotensin system also contributes to vasoconstriction. High plasma renin concentrations can be found in experimental acute tubular necrosis, and salt loading with reduction of renal renin ameliorates acute tubular necrosis. The angiotensin inhibitor saralasin administered before acute tubular necrosis is protective, and the angiotensin-converting enzyme inhibitor captopril improved renal microcirculation and ameliorated renal tubular necrosis after a period of warm ischemia or cold preservation (Anaise et al., 1987; Magnusson et al., 1983).

CYCLOSPORINE, TACROLIMUS AND EARLY GRAFT FUNCTION

Clinical use of cyclosporine has been associated with improved results in transplantation of the kidney and other organs (see Chapter 16). The benefits of cyclosporine are tempered by its cost and the dose-related side effects of nephrotoxicity and hypertension, which complicate its use in kidney transplantation. The renal injury induced by cyclosporine was first recognized by Calne et al. (1979); early oliguria occurred in one third of recipients of cadaver grafts. Subsequently, many clinical protocols have been devised, deferring cyclosporine treatment until adequate function and diuresis have occurred in the cadaver allograft. Other clinical studies on the relationship between cyclosporine and early graft function gave variable results (Kahan et al., 1987); several workers suggested potentiation of cyclosporine-induced nephrotoxicity by prolonged ischemic damage and preservation. Higher rates of early nonfunction were reported with cyclosporine treatment than with azathioprine and steroid immunosuppression. Several randomized clinical trials comparing cyclosporine with other forms of immunosuppression showed delayed function to be commoner and of longer duration with cyclosporine (Canadian Multicentre Transplant Study Group, 1983; Canafax et al., 1986; Novick et al., 1986). The beneficial effects of cyclosporine in diminishing rejection episodes usually outweighed these nephrotoxic effects, however. Nonetheless, delayed administration of cyclosporine until renal function is demonstrably adequate remained a common immunosuppressive mode, for example, in quadruple therapy: initial treatment by antilymphocyte serum (ALS), azathioprine and steroids was followed when function was stable by long-term cyclosporine and steroid treatment. Because cyclosporine is known to affect primarily the early events in the generation of the immune response, there are grounds for using it as an early immunosuppressive, and excellent results have been achieved with such protocols (Chapman and Morris, 1986).

Experimentally the nephrotoxicity of cyclosporine has been studied extensively. Intravenous boluses can cause acute dose-dependent nephrotoxicity (Hirsch et al., 1987) with antinatriuresis at low concentrations and vasoconstriction at high concentrations. The vehicle for intravenous administration also is potentially nephrotoxic, and effective pharmacokinetic monitoring of intravenous cyclosporine given by continuous infusion was shown clinically to lessen the incidence of delayed graft function (Kahan et al., 1987). Cyclosporine nephrotoxicity and ischemic renal damage were shown experimentally to be synergistic in their effects (Jablonski et al., 1986; Khauli et al., 1987). Cyclosporine has been shown experimentally to impair renal cortical mitochondrial function and to impair calcium homeostasis (Strzelecki et al., 1987). It also

has been shown experimentally that verapamil, a calcium channel antagonist, and trifluoperazine, a calcium-calmodulin inhibitor, potentiate the immunological effects of cyclosporine, although not having immunological properties themselves (Tesi et al., 1987), as well as ameliorating to some degree cyclosporine nephrotoxicity. The potential for using these cytoprotective and immune-enhancing agents in preservation solutions and in the recipient during reperfusion to improve early graft function, while providing adequate immunosuppression with lesser doses of cyclosporine, has been used clinically by several groups with benefit.

Calcium antagonists may play a significant role in ameliorating the nephrotoxic effect of cyclosporine. In one clinical study (Tenschert et al., 1991), recipients received diltiazem. The treated patients required less dialysis and were discharged sooner. Verapamil and isradipine have been shown to prevent the impairment of renal blood flow by cyclosporine (Rooth et al., 1987).

TACROLIMUS (FK-506)

Tacrolimus is an immunosuppressive drug that has been shown to be effective in inducing renal allograft acceptance (Starzl et al., 1990), but it does not have a similar nephrotoxic effect to cyclosporine (McCauley et al., 1990) (see Chapter 17). Experimentally, in rat kidneys subjected to 60 minutes of warm ischemia, pretreatment with tacrolimus ameliorated renal injury (Sakr et al., 1992). Concurrently, there was a significant inhibition of the production of tumor necrosis factor, a cytokine that may be a critical early mediator of organ injury.

Freezing and Vitrification

Freezing leads to the separation of pure water, with progressive concentration of solutes in the remaining liquid phase. Freezing normally is lethal to cells. The discovery that certain substances protect against the harmful effects of freezing led to successful long-term storage of a wide range of types of single cells. Red cells, lymphocytes, spermatozoa, fertilized ova and tissue culture cells can be frozen and thawed satisfactorily. Simple tissues such as skin and cornea can be preserved by freezing with cryoprotectant. Freezing of organs, so attractive in concept in approaching true suspended animation and indefinite storage, has not proved feasible (Pegg et al., 1982). Short-term freezing of kidneys causes substantial damage, and organs have never regained normal function (Dietzman et al., 1973; Pegg, 1978; Toledo-Pereyra, 1982).

The low surface area/volume ratio of organs compared with cells makes effective heat exchange a major problem. Cryoprotectants such as glycerol and dimethylsulfoxide require even perfusion throughout the organ. The ideal cryoprotectant should penetrate rapidly and uniformly into cells without excessive osmotic stress, should control the size and rate of ice crystal formation of binding intracellular water and should be nontoxic. Glycerol and macromolecular agents are relatively nontoxic but penetrate slowly, whereas dimethylsulfoxide penetrates rapidly but is nephrotoxic. Combinations of each have been used. The high concentrations needed for adequate cryoprotection usually cause severe organ toxicity and vascular damage. The bulk of whole organs necessitates a relatively low freezing rate. Extracellular ice formation is innocuous when freezing cell suspensions but can disrupt and damage the morphology of whole organs. Heating by microwave ovens has been used to try to limit damage during the thawing process. Matrix designs have been used to investigate combinations of freezing and thawing rates.

The heterogeneity of kidneys is another problem because different cell types differ in their requirements. The vascular system is especially vulnerable, and the attachment of vascular endothelial cells to basement membrane is disrupted by freezing, leading to occlusion after revascularization.

Cooling to subzero temperatures without freezing (supercooling) diminishes problems resulting from ice formation, but the toxicity of cryoprotectants is still excessive. An alternative method of cryopreservation is based on total vitrification of the organ (Fahy, 1982a, 1982b, 1986). In this approach, the organ or tissue first is perfused with a high concentration of cryoprotectants so that on cooling neither intracellular nor extracellular freezing occurs. The solution vitrifies (i.e., solidifies into a glass state) at temperatures of approximately −120°C. This method has been applied successfully to the preservation of viable eight-cell mouse embryos (Rall and Fahy, 1985a, 1985b) and less successfully to pancreatic islets (Rajotte et al., 1985).

Viability Testing and Prediction of Outcome

The ultimate proof of effective kidney preservation is that of sustaining life as an autograft or an allograft. The development of successful preserving regimens has been possible by extensive animal experimentation followed by clinical application. The search for definitive tests of viability that could be applied to each kidney before its implantation has proved to be elusive.

Perfusion characteristics during perfusion storage generally remain satisfactory except for grossly damaged kidneys and are not helpful in excluding all nonviable organs. Analysis of perfusate composition, as a reflection of the kidney's biochemical state, has been used widely to test viability. A variety of metabolites (lactate, glucose and xanthine plus hypoxanthine), potassium, pH and enzymes (lactate dehydrogenase, aspartate-serine transaminase, N-acetyl-D-glycosaminidase and GSTs) have been measured, but there is uneven correlation with ultimate function (Fahy, 1982a). Ligandin (the major organic anion-binding protein in the kidney) has been shown in the perfusate of kidneys that subsequently have acute tubular necrosis.

Biopsy of the preserved kidney for estimation of tissue composition is invasive and not always helpful. Tissue K^+/Na^+ ratios have been shown to relate to the function of human kidneys after transplantation (Sells et al., 1977). Adenine nucleotide concentrations immediately after preservation do not reflect the capacity of the kidney to resynthesize ATP on revascularization and are of little value. Similarly, histological examination of the biopsy is unrewarding because most of the cellular damage becomes apparent only on reperfusion of the organ. Viability of the renal microvasculature is as important as viability of the renal cells, and examination of perfusion characteristics with radioactive labeled microspheres or platelets has been used, as has examination of the endothelium by biopsies.

More organized functions are diminished during hypothermia, but in the past, rewarming the kidney to test its function has been thought likely to damage it irreparably. The demonstration of the helpful effects of brief normothermic perfusion during preservation opened new prospects for using this period for testing function and, more importantly, immunosuppressive modulations. The isolated rat kidney perfused normothermically was an early model for assessing the effectiveness of preservation (Marshall et al., 1982). Paratopic normothermic perfusion from the femoral vessels of donor rabbits has been used similarly by Collins and Halasz (1982). Immunological manipulation of the preserved kidney in the future may be facilitated by normothermic perfusion.

NUCLEAR MAGNETIC RESONANCE

Nuclear magnetic resonance is a novel, completely noninvasive, nondestructive technique of mapping the metabolism and functional anatomy of intact biological systems. The sample of study can be a biopsy fragment, the isolated kidney stored in ice or undergoing hypothermic or normothermic perfusion or the patient and kidney after transplantation. The technique depends on properties of spin and magnetism possessed by certain atomic nuclei—those most commonly used have been ^1H, ^{31}P, ^{13}C and ^{17}O. The nuclei of these atoms can be regarded as tiny bar magnets. When orientated in a powerful magnetic field, a pulse of radio waves causes energy to be absorbed and emitted by the nuclei: These energy signals are detected, amplified and plotted by Fourier analysis, giving spectroscopic fingerprints specific for particular nuclei. Imaging of body water gives anatomical mapping comparable to computed tomography (nuclear magnetic resonance imaging, magnetic resonance imaging). More relevant to kidney preservation are functional spectroscopic metabolic studies on preserved and replanted kidneys. Using ^{31}P spectroscopy (nuclear magnetic resonance spectroscopy, magnetic resonance spectroscopy), phosphocreatine, total adenine nucleotides, ATP, ADP, AMP, inorganic phosphate and intracellular pH can be determined repeatedly on kidneys stored in ice or during perfusion. Intrarenal pH can be observed to fall rapidly and progressively during ischemia to levels as low as pH 6.3. Flushing with preservation solutions before ice storage minimizes the progressive fall in pH, which occurs during 24 hours of ice storage. The effect is particularly marked during the second 12 hours of storage, which is the period during which simple surface cooling begins to be ineffective. Loss of ATP and total adenine nucleotides and subsequent resynthesis also can be followed. Loss of ATP is mirrored by an increase in inorganic phosphate and AMP. Losses of ATP and total adenine nucleotides can be related to subsequent function (Chan et al., 1983).

To apply nuclear magnetic resonance techniques to whole organs or individuals, signals must be available from specifically identifiable parts of a heterogeneous sample. Topical nuclear magnetic resonance is obtained by using a small coil of wire applied to the surface of the tissue. The coil acts intermittently as the exciting signal and as the receiving coil from the local area.

RENAL PRESERVATION

The effectiveness of hypothermic extracorporeal preservation depends on minimizing the effects of hypothermic paralysis of the cell membrane pumps leading to cellular edema, intracellular acidosis and cellular energy depletion. The latter two sequelae can be monitored directly and continuously by ^{31}P nuclear magnetic resonance. Studies in rat, dog and human kidneys have enabled the efficiency of conservation of adenine nucleotide levels, their recovery on reperfusion and intracellular pH to be monitored noninvasively. Relative contributions of oxidative phosphorylation and anaerobic glycolysis during storage and reperfusion can be assessed rapidly and nondestructively. Nuclear magnetic resonance can be combined with monitoring of renal blood flow, oxygen consumption and urine production so that glomerulotubular functions can be assessed separately (Marshall et al., 1985b). Improvement in localization techniques using surface coils enables magnetic resonance imaging to be performed together with magnetic resonance spectroscopy. Loss of ATP and its regeneration on normothermic reperfusion can be quantitated by AMP/inorganic phosphate ratios (normally approximately 1.0), which fall progressively to approximately

0.1 after 72 hours of cold storage. Correlation of these ratios with subsequent function of transplanted kidneys has been reported (Bretan *et al.*, 1987). Regeneration of lost ATP after cold storage by normothermic reperfusion required approximately 2 hours of reperfusion after 24 hours of cold ischemia. Characteristic changes in T_1 and T_2 relaxation times also have been described after acute renal ischemia and reperfusion (Slutsky *et al.*, 1984). Paramagnetic contrast agents can assist in the investigation of vascular ischemia: Using these techniques, falls in relaxation times with prolonged storage correlated well with a loss of capillary integrity. These changes, using a rat kidney model, were used to grade flushing solutions and to show the effectiveness of the addition of a calmodulin inhibitor to the flushing solution (Chin *et al.*, 1986).

Spectroscopic analysis of liver preservation has been used (Bowers *et al.*, 1992; Changani *et al.*, 1999; Moser *et al.*, 1992; Orii *et al.*, 1992). Clinical extension of such noninvasive mapping of biochemical processes in stored, perfused and replanted organs continues.

Impact of Multiple Organ Donor Retrieval on Kidney Transplantation

Criteria for the acceptance of donors for heart, lung and liver transplantation are more restricted than for kidney transplantation (Odom, 1990). Transplanted hearts and livers must function immediately to support life, whereas kidney recipients can be supported by dialysis for a period necessary to recover from acute tubular necrosis. Further restrictions imposed on heart, lung and liver donations relate to the need to match in size the donor and recipient. In areas where active heart, lung, liver and kidney programs coexist, only about 20% of kidney donors used to be suitable as multiple organ donors (Banowsky *et al.*, 1986). However, today some 80% of donors are multiorgan donors in the UK (UKTSSA, personal communication). Specific criteria need to be met to be confident of immediate function of hearts and livers after transplantation. The details of these criteria vary from unit to unit. An example is given in Table 9–8, based on Eurotransplant criteria (Ringe *et al.*, 1985).

Criteria are similarly developed for cadavers for heart and lung donation and pancreas donation. Techniques of multiple organ retrieval are outlined in Chapter 7. In principle, the donor organs are skeletonized. The heart is stopped by infusion of cardioplegic solution and removed first. In sequence, liver, pancreas and kidneys are removed *en bloc* during *in situ* cold perfusion. The principles of preservation of all tissues are broadly similar, with rapid hypothermia the most potent factor. Rapid cooling of organs is initiated by flushing with a cold (0–5°C) electrolyte solution *in situ*; this minimizes the absolute warm ischemic period to minutes. The most successful cold flushing electrolyte solutions for heart, liver, kidney and pancreas are essentially similar, and the elements critical to these solutions have been discussed.

Commonly, 1 L or more of cold buffered electrolyte solution (Hartmann's) is used in a rapid initial flush to start and maintain organ cooling during *en bloc* multiorgan retrieval after induction of cardiac arrest by a cold cardioplegic solution; UW and its variants also are preferred cardioplegics (Drinkwater *et al.*, 1991). Final organ preparation is done as bench surgery after removal while organs are maintained in ice slush. Organs are finally flushed with the definitive organ preservation solution before packing, storage and transport.

Recommendations for Clinical Preservation

Kidney preservation currently is adequate for clinical needs. With the important corollary that significant warm ischemic damage must be absent, static ice storage and perfusion give similarly reliable preservation for 60 hours. Preservation can be extended to 120 hours (5 days) by ice storage and perfusion. Storage into the third, fourth and fifth days is more uniformly reliable with perfusion, as is rescue of kidneys damaged by warm ischemia.

Avoidance of warm ischemia in the donor is of first importance. Optimal preservation starts with identification of a heart-beating cadaver, circulatory support (fluids, mannitol and low-dose dopamine) and membrane stabilization (steroids). Nutritional supplement (ATP-$MgCl_2$) should be provided if the intensive care unit course is prolonged during the workup to organ retrieval. Anticoagulants (heparin), calcium channel blockers (verapamil or diltiazem), xanthine oxidase inhibitors (allopurinol) and vasoprotective agents (chlorpromazine) are best given during or before organ procurement. Organ removal should employ *in situ* cooling with buffered electrolyte or sucrose or UW solutions before an extracorporeal cold flush with UW solution or its simpler

TABLE 9–8

ACCEPTANCE OF MULTIORGAN DONOR

Organ-Specific Criteria	Kidney, Pancreas	Liver	Heart, Lung
Age limits (y)	<65 (70)	<45 (60)	15–35 (45)
Exclusion	Preexisting renal disease, diabetes mellitus	Preexisting hepatobiliary disease, abdominal trauma, intoxication, cardiac arrest	Preexisting cardiovascular disease, chest trauma, high-dose inotropic drugs
Workup required	Serum creatinine, urinalysis, CMV status, HB_sAg negative, AIDS (HIV negative)	ICU course <7 d, SGOT <100 UL^{-1}, bilirubin <17 μmol L^{-1} (<1 mg dl^{-1}), CMV status, HB_sAg negative, AIDS (HIV negative)	ICU course <7 d, ECG, chest radiograph, CMV status, HB_sAg negative, AIDS (HIV negative)
Compatibility required for			
Weight and size	No	Yes	Yes
ABO groups	Yes	Yes	Yes
HLA crossmatch	Yes	Only in sensitized recipients	Only in sensitized recipients

Numbers in parentheses indicate upper age limit. ICU = intensive care unit; CMV = cytomegalovirus; HB_sAg = hepatitis B surface antigen; AIDS = acquired immunodeficiency syndrome; HIV = human immunodeficiency virus; SGOT = serum glutamic-oxaloacetic transaminase; ECG = electrocardiogram.

modifications. Addition of a phenothiazine calcium-calmodulin inhibitor (trifluoperazine) or calcium channel antagonist (diltiazem) to the flushing solution is beneficial and is recommended. Kidneys then can be preserved by static hypothermic storage (most kidneys) or less often by hypothermic perfusion.

Static hypothermic storage is simpler, safer, more economical and in most cases equally effective. A carefully performed cold intraarterial flush combined with surface cooling is required initially in all cases of cadaver nephrectomy. Only rarely is subsequent machine preservation obligatory. After appropriate kidney washout, packaging and cold storage, no further complications or side effects of preservation exist. If renal function in the donor has been satisfactory up to the time of kidney removal and warm ischemia minimal, good early function after transplantation should be possible in almost all kidneys after 24 to 48 hours of storage. Ice storage and machine perfusion give similar results. After 48 hours, static storage becomes marginally less effective than perfusion but still can give effective preservation for periods of 120 hours.

For static storage, Collins' and citrate flushing solutions gave satisfactory results clinically. Citrate is a more stable solution, and the glucose in Collins' solution preferably is replaced by mannitol or sucrose. A simple buffered sucrose solution also is effective. A high-sodium, HES-free, UW solution is optimal for ease of flushing and economy of local manufacture, and a UW-derived solution should be used for multiorgan flushing.

The sole advantage of machine perfusion is its greater effectiveness for preservation times in excess of 48 hours or when there has been a period of warm ischemia. Disadvantages are self-evident: It is far more complex and costly, it introduces (often unnecessarily) potential and actual hazards and it is no more effective for short-term preservation. Inadequate or unskilled perfusion is worse than none. Colloid (HES)-containing UW solutions are best. Modifications have incorporated extra substrates and precursors. Kidneys removed from cadavers after cardiac arrest with inevitable warm ischemia should be considered for perfusion-preservation rescue.

Several historical retrospective studies showed better graft survival with kidneys preserved by static storage (Opelz and Terasaki, 1976, 1982). The groups were not comparable in these studies, and preservation times with perfused kidneys were usually much longer.

Prospective randomized trials comparing perfusion and static storage in matched-donor pairs showed few significant differences between the two methods (Heil et al., 1987; Mendez et al., 1987). Early function and long-term graft survival were similar (Marshall et al., 1977). On economic, immunological and functional grounds, static hypothermic storage is the preferred method for most kidney grafts.

Factors in the recipient during and after the operation of renal transplantation are of major significance. Normothermic ischemia must be minimized during reimplantation. Elaborate techniques are unnecessary; simple surface cooling with packs moistened in ice-saline slush can keep the core temperature at less than 15°C. Revascularization should be expeditious, and times seldom need to exceed 30 to 60 minutes. Anastomoses are performed most simply and safely with optimally procured and prepared organs. The technical aspects of dealing with multiple vessels are described in Chapters 11 and 28. Severe ischemic damage can occur if major anastomoses need revision after reclamping, so it is important to ensure that the anastomoses are performed satisfactorily in the first instance.

Adequate hydration of the recipient is important but often difficult to assess in the functionally anephric, dialyzed patient. Monitoring central venous pressure is common, but the routine administration of 250 ml of 20% mannitol (50 g) intravenously just before revascularization is recommended (Tiggeler et al., 1985; Weimar et al., 1983).

The early use of free radical scavengers or calcium antagonists such as diltiazem in the recipient is now routine clinical practice in many centers, especially when early immunosuppressive treatment with cyclosporine is given. The potentially hypotensive effects of some of these agents must be monitored closely.

Overall, delayed graft function after cadaveric transplantation has an incidence of about 25%, but variation between centers can range from 6 to 50% (Marcen et al., 1998). Delayed function has an adverse effect on graft outcome, is associated with a higher incidence of rejection and increases length of hospital stay. For all these reasons, effective kidney procurement and preservation remain important aspects of global care.

Progress and Prospects

True long-term organ preservation by freezing remains as distant as it was in the 1980s. Paradoxically, progress in cell and tissue freezing over this time has been rapid. *In vitro* fertilization, embryo freezing, thawing and transplantation are now used routinely in clinical practice. The eight-cell embryo is serendipitously tolerant of techniques that its developed organs find uniformly lethal.

Organ preservation has shown significant advances in protection against ischemic damage in the donor and recipient; in improved techniques of multiple organ procurement to the betterment of transplantation programs in general and in improved understanding of the mechanisms, limitations and ancillary benefits of methods of extracorporeal storage. Flushing and perfusing techniques, solutions and adjuvants continue to evolve and to improve. Development of UW solutions has been a major advance in static and perfusion storage of kidneys and all other transplantable organs.

Optimal management of the heart-beating, brain-dead donor sets the stage for good early function in the recipient. Kidney preservation begins with the identification of the potential donor and continues well into the recipient's postoperative period. Preservation techniques can help reverse or ameliorate some of the early nephrotoxic effects of cyclosporine, and effective preservation is more vital in the cyclosporine era than ever before.

It is now clear that irreversible brain injury and subsequent preservation damage up-regulates proinflammatory cytokines and MHC antigens, facilitating host inflammatory and immunological responses. Minimization and amelioration of these effects are important aims of current preservation techniques.

Kidney preservation currently is adequate for clinical needs, providing effective storage for 5 days by static hypothermic storage. Perfusion preservation can extend the limits to 7 days, but its main role is currently in resuscitating kidneys removed from donors after cardiac arrest. Attempts to *rescue* kidneys from less-than-optimal donors are required more frequently, as need for organs continues to outstrip supply. Adjuvant immunosuppression with incorporation of monoclonal antibodies to perfusing solutions has not fulfilled initial promise. The future may see increasing use of therapy through the wider immmunological window that more prolonged preservation can offer. Xenotransplantation may offer fresh prospects of using optimal donor preparation and pretreatment. The kidney xenograft may be best prepared for transplantation immunologically and physiologically while in the heart-beating donor: No artificial oxygenators or pumps have succeeded in matching nature. Xenotransplantation, if widely applied, would minimize the need for extracorporeal preservation and focus attention more on donor management before organ removal.

Organ transplantation was pioneered predominantly in developed countries, but a currently effective global kidney preservation solution for static storage is buffered sucrose, which is adequate for live donor kidney transplantation and for transplantation from heart-beating cadavers in most circumstances. Simpler and more economic modifications of extracellular fluid UW solutions with better flushing properties also are increasingly available.

REFERENCES

Abouna, G. M., Samhan, M. S., Kumar, M. S. A., White, A. G. and Silva, O. S. G. (1987). Limiting factors in successful preservation of cadaveric kidneys with ischaemia time exceeding 50 hours. *Transplant. Proc.* **19**, 2051.

Anaise, D., Lane, B., Waltzer, W. C. and Rapaport, F. T. (1987). The protective effect of calcium inhibitors and of captopril in the renal microcirculation during reperfusion. *Transplantation* **43**, 128.

Anaise, D., Waltzer, W. C. and Rapaport, F. T. (1986). Metabolic requirements for successful extended hypothermic kidney preservation. *J. Urol.* **136**, 345.

Andrews, P. M. and Bates, S. B. (1985). Improving Euro-Collins flushing solution's ability to protect kidneys from normothermic ischemia. *Miner. Electrolyte Metab.* **11**, 309.

Asari, H., Anaise, D., Bachvaroff, R. J., Sato, K. and Rapaport, F. (1984). Preservation techniques for organ transplantation: I. protective effects of calmodulin inhibitors in cold-preserved kidneys. *Transplantation* **37**, 113.

Astier, A. and Paul, M. (1989). Instability of reduced glutathione in commercial Belzer cold storage solution. *Lancet* **2**, 556.

Baatard, R., Pradier, F., Dantal, J., *et al.* (1993). University of Wisconsin versus UW-modified (lacking hydroxyethyl starch) storage solutions: a prospective randomized study in first kidney transplantations. *Transplantation* **55**, 31.

Baker, G. L., Corry, R. J. and Autor, A. P. (1985). Oxygen free radical induced damage in kidneys subjected to warm ischemia and reperfusion. *Ann. Surg.* **202**, 628.

Banowsky, L., Jaffers, G., Singleton, R., Hayes, J. and Nicastro, J. (1986). Multiple organ donation: its impact on the recovery of cadaver kidneys. *J. Urol.* **135**, 1157.

Baron, P., Gomez-Marin, O., Casas, C., *et al.* (1991). Renal preservation after warm ischemia using oxygen free radical scavengers to prevent reperfusion injury. *J. Surg. Res.* **51**, 60.

Barry, J. M., Norman, D. J., Fischer, S. M. and Bennett, W. M. (1984). Prolonged human kidney preservation by intracellular electrolyte flush followed by cold storage. *Am. J. Kidney Dis.* **3**, 293.

Belzer, F. O., Ashby, B. S. and Dunphy, J. E. (1967). 24-hour and 72-hour preservation of canine kidneys. *Lancet* **2**, 536.

Belzer, F. O., Glass, N. R., Sollinger, H. W., Hoffman, R. M. and Southard, J. H. (1982a). A new perfusate for kidney preservation. *Transplantation* **33**, 322.

Belzer, F. O., Hoffman, R. M. and Southard, J. H. (1982b). Aerobic and anaerobic perfusion of canine kidneys with a new perfusate. *In Organ Preservation III: Basic and Applied Aspects*, (D. E. Pegg, I. A. Jacobsen and N. A. Halsz, eds.), p. 253, MTP Press, Lancaster.

Biguzas, M., Jablonski, P., Howden, B. O., *et al.* (1990a). Evaluation of UW solution in rat kidney preservation: I. the effect of hydroxyethyl starch and electrolyte composition. *Transplantation* **49**, 872.

Biguzas, M., Jablonski, P., Howden, B. O., *et al.* (1990b). Evaluation of UW solution in rat kidney preservation: II. the effect of pharmacological additives. *Transplantation* **49**, 1051.

Bowers, J. L., Teramoto, K., Khettry, U. and Clouse, M. E. (1992). ^{31}P NMR assessment of orthotopic rat liver transplant viability. *Transplantation* **54**, 604.

Bretan, P. N., Baldwin, N., Martinez, A., *et al.* (1991). Improved renal transplant preservation using a modified intracellular flush solution (PB-2): characterisation of mechanisms by renal clearance, high performance liquid chromatography, phosphorus-31 magnetic resonance spectroscopy, and electron microscopy studies. *Urol. Res.* **19**, 73.

Bretan, P. N., Jr, Vigneron, D. P., Hricak, H., *et al.* (1987). Assessment of clinical renal preservation by phosphorus-31 magnetic resonance spectroscopy. *J. Urol.* **137**, 146.

Burg, M. B. and Orloff, M. J. (1964). Active cation transport by kidney tubules at 0°C. *Am. J. Physiol.* **207**, 983.

Burke, T. J., Arnold, P. E., Gordon, J. A., Bulger, P. E., Dobyon, D. C. and Schrier, R. W. (1984). Protective effect of intrarenal calcium membrane blockers before or after renal ischemia. *J. Clin. Invest.* **74**, 1830.

Burke, T. J., Arnold, P. E. and Schrier, R. W. (1983). Prevention of ischemic acute renal failure with impermeant solutes. *Am. J. Physiol.* **244**, 646.

Busson, M., Prevost, P., Bignon, J. D., *et al.* (1992). Multifactorial analysis of the outcome of 6430 cadaver kidney grafts. *Transpl. Int.* **5**, 162.

Cacciarelli, T. V., Sumrani, N., DiBendetto, A., Hong, J. H. and Sommer, B. G. (1992). The influence of cold ischaemia and donor age on renal allograft outcome in the cyclosporine era. *Transplant. Proc.* **24**, 2044.

Calne, R. Y., Pegg, D. E., Pryse-Davis, J. and Brown, F. L. (1963). Renal preservation by ice-cooling: an experimental study relating to kidney transplantation from cadavers. *B. M. J.* **2**, 651.

Calne, R. Y., Rolles, K., Thiru, S., *et al.* (1979). Cyclosporine A initially as the only immunosuppressant in 34 recipients of cadaveric organs: 32 kidneys, 2 pancreases and 2 livers. *Lancet* **2**, 1033.

Canadian Multicentre Transplant Study Group. (1983). A randomized clinical trial of cyclosporine in cadaveric renal transplantation. *N. Engl. J. Med.* **309**, 809.

Canafax, D. M., Torres, A., Fryd, D. S., *et al.* (1986). The effects of delayed function on recipients of cadaver renal allografts: a study of 158 patients randomized to cyclosporine or ALG-azathioprine. *Transplantation* **41**, 177.

Carrel, A. and Lindbergh, C. A. (1938). *The Culture of Organs*, Hamish Hamilton, London.

Chan, L., Bore, P. and Ross, B. (1983). Renal preservation. *In International Perspectives in Urology*, (M. Marberger and K. Dreikorn, eds.), p. 323, Williams & Wilkins, Baltimore.

Changani, K. K., Fuller, B. J., Bell, J. D., Taylor-Robinson, S. D., Moore, D. P. and Davidson, B. R. (1999). Improved preservation solutions for organ storage. *Transplantation* **68**, 345.

Chapman, D. (1975). Phase transitions and fluidity characteristics of lipids and cell membranes. *Q. Rev. Biophys.* **8**, 185.

Chapman, J. R. and Morris, P. J. (1986). Long-term effects of short-term cyclosporine. *Transplant. Proc.* **18(Suppl. 1)**, 186.

Chatterjee, S. N. and Berne, T. V. (1975). Failure of 48 hours of cold storage of canine kidneys using Sacks' solution. *Transplantation* **19**, 441.

Chaudry, I. H. (1983). Cellular mechanisms in shock and ischemia and their correction. *Am. J. Physiol.* **245**, 117.

Chilson, O. P., Costello, L. A. and Kaplan, N. O. (1965). Effects of freezing on enzymes. *Fed. Proc.* **24**, S55.

Chin, J. L., Stiller, C. R. and Karlik, S. J. (1986). Nuclear magnetic resonance assessment of renal perfusion and preservation for transplantation. *J. Urol.* **136**, 1351.

Claes, G. and Blohme, I. (1973). Experimental and clinical results of continuous albumin perfusion of kidneys. *In Organ Preservation*, (D. E. Pegg, ed.), p. 51, Churchill-Livingstone, Edinburgh.

Cohen, G. L., Hunt, L. and Johnson, R. W. G. (1983). Octanoate toxicity in 5-day kidney preservation. *Cryobiology* **20**, 731.

Collins, G. M., Bravo-Shugarman, M. and Terasaki, P. I. (1969). Kidney preservation for transportation: initial perfusion and 30 hours' ice storage. *Lancet* **2**, 1219.

Collins, G. M., Hartley, L. C. and Clunie, G. J. (1972). Kidney preservation for transportation: experimental analysis of optimal perfusate composition. *Br. J. Surg.* **59**, 187.

Collins, G. M. and Halasz, N. A. (1975). Composition of intracellular flush solutions for hypothermic kidney storage. *Lancet* **1**, 220.

Collins, G. M., Green, R. D. and Halasz, N. A. (1979). Importance of anion content and osmolarity in flush solutions for 48 to 72 hr hypothermic kidney storage. *Cryobiology* **16**, 217.

Collins, G. M., Green, R. D., Boyer, D. and Halasz, N. A. (1980). Protection of kidneys from warm ischemic injury: dosage and timing of mannitol administration. *Transplantation* **29**, 83.

Collins, G. M. and Halasz, N. A. (1982). A species difference in the efficacy of two intracellular flush solutions. *Transplantation* **33**, 324.

Collins, G. M., Wicomb W., Warren, R. et al. (1993). Canine and cadaver kidney preservation with sodium lactobionate sucrose solution (SLS). *Transplant. Proc.* **25**, 1588.

D'Alessandro, A. M., Kalayoglu, M., Solinger, H. W., Pirsch, J. D., Southard, J. H. and Betzer, F. O. (1991a). Current status of organ preservation with University of Wisconsin solution. *Arch. Pathol. Lab. Med.* **115**, 306.

D'Alessandro, A. M., Reed, A., Hoffmann, R. M., et al. (1991b). Results of combined hepatic, pancreaticoduodenal, and renal procurements. *Transplant. Proc.* **23**, 2309.

Dawidson, I. and Rooth, P. (1990). Effects of calcium antagonists in ameliorating cyclosporine A nephrotoxicity and posttransplant ATN. *In Calcium Antagonists and the Kidney*, (M. Epstein and R. Loutzenhiser, eds.), p. 233, Hanley Belfus, Philadelphia.

Dawidson, I. J. A., Sandor, Z. F., Coorpender, L., et al. (1992). Intraoperative albumin administration affects the outcome of cadaver renal transplantation. *Transplantation* **53**, 774.

Demertzis, S., Wahlers, T., Schafers, H. J., et al. (1992). Myocardial preservation with the UW solution: first European results in clinical heart transplantation. *Transplant. Int.* **5**, 343.

Dietzman, R. H., Rebelo, A. E., Graham, E. F., Crabo, B. G. and Lillehei, R. C. (1973). 48- to 96-hour preservation of canine kidneys by initial perfusion and hypothermic storage using the Euro-Collins solution. *Surgery* **74**, 181.

Dreikorn, K., Horsch, R. and Rohl, L. (1980). 48- to 96-hour preservation of canine kidneys by initial perfusion and hypothermic storage using the Euro-Collins solution. *Eur. Urol.* **6**, 221.

Drinkwater, D. C., Steva, D. G., Permit, L. C. and Laks, H. (1991). Clinical trial of University of Wisconsin solution for cardiac transplantation: preliminary results. *J. Thorac. Cardiovasc. Surg.* **102**, 798.

Fahy, G. (1982a). The effect of cryoprotectant concentration on freezing damage in kidney slices. *In Basic Concepts in Organ Procurement, Perfusion and Preservation*, (L. H. Toledo-Pereyra, ed.), p. 121, Academic Press, New York.

Fahy, G. (1982b). Prevention of toxicity from high concentrations of cryoprotective agents. *In Basic Concepts in Organ Procurement, Perfusion and Preservation*, (L. H. Toledo-Pereyra, ed.), p. 367, Academic Press, New York.

Fahy, G. (1986). Vitrification: a new approach to organ cryopreservation. *Prog. Clin. Biol. Res.* **224**, 305.

Fischer, J. H., Czerniak, A., Hauer, U. and Isselhard, W. (1978). A new simple method for optimal storage of ischemically damaged kidneys. *Transplantation* **25**, 43.

Florack, G., Sutherland, D. E. R., Ascherl, R., Heil, J., Erhardt, W. and Najarian, J. S. (1986). Definition of normothermic ischemia limits for kidney and pancreas grafts. *J. Surg. Res.* **40**, 550.

Friedman, S. M., Johnson, R. I. and Friedman, C. L. (1954). The pattern of recovery of renal function following renal artery occlusion in the dog. *Circ. Res.* **2**, 231.

Gaber, A. O., Yang, H. C., Haag, B. W., et al. (1987). Intermediate normothermic hemoperfusion doubles safe cold preservation of rat kidneys. *Transplant. Proc.* **9**, 1369.

Gaudio, K. M., Taylor, M. R., Chaudry, I. H., Kashgarian, M. and Siegel, N. J. (1982). Accelerated recovery of single nephron function by the postischemic infusion of ATP-MgCl$_2$. *Kidney Int.* **22**, 13.

Godfrey, A. M. and Salaman, J. R. (1978). Trasylol (aprotinin) and kidney preservation. *Transplantation* **25**, 167.

Green, C. J., Fuller, B. J., Ross, B., Marriot, S. and Simpkin, S. (1983). Storage of organs from ground squirrels during and after hibernation. *Proc. Soc. Cryobiol.* **20**, 739.

Green, C. J., Healing, G., Lunec, J., Fuller, B. J. and Simpkin, S. (1986). Evidence of free-radical-induced damage in rabbit kidneys after simple hypothermic preservation and autotransplantation. *Transplantation* **41**, 161.

Grino, J. M., Castelao, A. M., Sabate, I., et al. (1987). Low-dose cyclosporine, ALG, and steroids in first cadaveric renal transplants. *Transplant. Proc.* **19**, 3674.

Groenewoud, A. F., Buchholz, B., Gubernaitis, F., et al. (1990). First results of the multicentre study of HTK protection for kidney transplants. *Transplant. Proc.* **22**, 2212.

Groenewoud, A. F. and Thorogood, J. (1992). A preliminary report of the HTK randomized multicenter study comparing kidney

graft preservation with HTK and EuroCollins solutions. *Transplant. Proc.* **5**, 429.

Halasz, N. A. (1982). Pharmacological factors in organ preservation. *In Organ Preservation III: Basic and Applied Aspects*, (D. E. Pegg, I. Jacobsen and N. A. Halasz, eds.), p. 151, MTP Press, Lancaster.

Halasz, N. A. and Collins, G. M. (1976). Forty-eight-hour kidney preservation: a comparison of flushing and ice storage with perfusion. *Arch. Surg.* **111**, 175.

Hardie, I., Balderson, G., Hamlyn, L., McKay, D. and Clunie, D. (1977). Extended ice storage of canine kidneys using hyperosmolar Collins solution. *Transplantation* **23**, 282.

Harvey, R. B. (1959). Effect of temperature on function of isolated dog kidney. *Am. J. Physiol.* **197**, 181.

Hefty, T., Fraser, S., Nelson, K. and Bennett, W. (1992). Comparison of UW and Euro-Collins solutions in paired cadaveric kidneys. *Transplantation* **53**, 491.

Heil, J. E., Canafax, D. M., Sutherland, D. E. R., Simmons, R. L., Dunniy, M. and Najarian, J. (1987). A controlled comparison of kidney preservation by two methods: machine perfusion and cold storage. *Transplant. Proc.* **19**, 2046.

Hellberg, O. A., Bayati, A., Kallskog, O. and Wolgast, M. (1990). Red cell trapping after ischaemia and long-term kidney damage: influence of haematocrit. *Kidney Int.* **37**, 1240.

Herbertt, K. and Disney, A. P. S. (1991). The Second Annual Report of the National Organ Donor Registry of Australia (ANZDATA Registry), Adelaide, South Australia.

Hertle, L. and Garthoff, B. (1985). Calcium channel blocker nisoldipine limits ischemic damage in rat kidney. *J. Urol.* **134**, 1251.

Hirasawa, H., Odaka, M., Soeda, K., et al. (1983). Experimental and clinical study on ATP-MgCl$_2$ administration for postischemic acute renal failure. *Clin. Exp. Dial. Apheresis* **7**, 37.

Hirsch, S., Besarab, A., Jarrell, B. E., Carabasi, R. D., Cressman, M. D. and Green, P. (1987). Acute nephrotoxicity following intravenous cyclosporin. *Transplant. Proc.* **19**, 1387.

Hoffman, R. M., Southard, J. H. and Belzer, F. O. (1982). The use of oncotic support agents in perfusion preservation. *In Organ Preservation III: Basic and Applied Aspects*, (D. E. Pegg, I. A. Jacobsen and N. A. Halasz, eds.), p. 261, MTP Press, Lancaster.

Hoffman, R. M., Southard, J. H., Lutz, M., Mackety, A. and Belzer, F. O. (1983). Synthetic perfusate for kidney preservation: its use in 72-hour preservation of dog kidneys. *Arch. Surg.* **118**, 919.

Howden, B., Rae, D., Jablonski, P., Marshall, V. C. and Tange, J. (1983). Studies in renal preservation using a rat kidney transplant model. *Transplantation* **35**, 311.

Howlett, T. A., Keogh, A. M., Perry, L., Touzel, R. and Rees, L. H. (1989). Anterior and posterior pituitary function in brain-stem-dead donors. *Transplantation* **47**, 828.

Isemer, F. E., Ludwig, A., Schunck, O., Bretschneider, H. J. and Peiper, H. J. (1988). Kidney procurement with the HTK solution of Bretschneider. *Transplant. Proc.* **20**, 885.

Jablonski, P., Harrison, C., Howden, B. O., et al. (1986). Cyclosporin A and the ischaemic rat kidney. *Transplantation* **41**, 147.

Jablonski, P., Howden B. O., Leslie, E., et al. (1983b). Recovery of renal function after warm ischaemia: 1. the effect of chlorpromazine and phenoxybenzamine. *Transplantation* **35**, 535.

Jablonski, P., Howden, B. O., Marshall, V. C. and Scott, D. F. (1980). Evaluation of citrate flushing solution using the isolated perfused kidney. *Transplantation* **30**, 239.

Jablonski, P., Howden, B. O., Rae, D. A., Birrell, C. S., Marshall, V. C. and Tange, J. (1983a). An experimental model for assessment of renal recovery from warm ischemia. *Transplantation* **35**, 198.

Jacobsen, I. A., Kemp, E. and Buhl, M. R. (1979). An adverse effect of rapid cooling in kidney preservation. *Transplantation* **27**, 135.

Jacobsson, J., Odlind, B., Tufveson, G. and Wahlberg, J. (1992). Improvement of renal preservation by adding lidoflazine to University of Wisconsin solution: an experimental study in the rat. *Cryobiology* **29**, 305.

Jacobsson, J., Tufveson, G., Odlind, B. and Wahlberg, J. (1989). The effect of type of preservation solution and hemodilution of the recipient on postischaemic erythrocyte trapping in kidney grafts. *Transplantation* **47**, 876.

Jamieson, N. V., Sundberg, R., Lindell, S., et al. (1988). Preservation of the canine liver for 24–48 hours using simple cold storage with UW solution. *Transplantation* **46**, 517.

Jeevanandam, V., Auteri, J. S., Sanchez, J. A., et al. (1992b). Cardiac transplantation after prolonged graft preservation with UW solution. *J. Thorac. Cardiovasc. Surg.* **104**, 224.

Jeevanandam, V., Barr, M. L., Auteri, J. S., *et al.* (1992a). University of Wisconsin solution versus crystalloid cardioplegia for human donor heart preservation: a randomized blinded prospective clinical trial. *J. Thorac. Cardiovasc. Surg.* **103**, 194.

Johnson, R. W. G. (1982). The donor kidney. *In Scientific Foundations of Urology*, (G. D. Chisholm and D. I. Williams, eds.), p. 150, William Heinemann, London.

Johnson, R. W. G., Anderson, M., Flear, C. T., Murray, S., Swinney, J. and Taylor, R. M. R. (1972). Evaluation of a new perfusion solution for kidney preservation. *Transplantation* **13**, 270.

Kahan, B. D., Mickey, R., Flechner, S. M., *et al.* (1987). Multivariate analysis of risk factors impacting on immediate and eventual cadaver allograft survival in cyclosporine treated recipients. *Transplantation* **43**, 65.

Kalayoglu, M., Sollinger, W. H., Stratta, R. J., *et al.* (1988). Extended preservation of the liver for clinical transplantation. *Lancet* **2**, 617.

Kallerhoff, M., Blech, M., Isemer, F. E., *et al.* (1988). Metabolic, energetic and structural changes in protected and unprotected kidneys at temperatures of 1°C and 25°C. *Urol. Res.* **16**, 57.

Kallerhoff, M., Blech, M., Kehrer, G., *et al.* (1986). Post-ischaemic renal function after kidney protection with the HTK-solution of Bretschneider. *Urol. Res.* **14**, 271.

Kaufman, R., Anner, H., Kobzik, L., Valeri, C., Shepro, D. and Hechtman, H. (1987). A high plasma prostaglandin to thromboxane ratio protects against renal ischaemia. *Surg. Gynecol Obstet.* **165**, 404.

Kedar, I., Cohen, J., Jacob, E. T. and Ravid, M. (1981). Alleviation of experimental ischemic acute renal failure by dimethyl sulfoxide. *Nephron* **29**, 55.

Kedar, I., Jacob, E. T., Bar-Natan, N. and Ravid, M. (1983). Dimethyl sulfoxide in acute ischemia of the kidney. *Ann. N. Y. Acad. Sci.* **411**, 131.

Khauli, R. B., Strzelecki, T., Kumar, S., Fink, M., Stoff, J. and Menon, M. (1987). Mitochondrial alterations after cyclosporine and ischemia: insights on the pathophysiology of nephrotoxicity. *Transplant. Proc.* **19**, 1395.

Kievit, J. K., Oomen, A. P. A., Janssen, B. K., van Kreel, B. K., Heineman, E. and Kootstra, G. (1997). Viability assessment of non-heart-beating donor kidneys by alpha glutathione S-transferase in the machine perfusate. *Transplant. Proc.* **29**, 1381.

Klausner, J. M., Paterson, I. S., Goldman, G., *et al.* (1989). Postischemic renal injury is mediated by neutrophils and leukotrienes. *Am. J. Physiol.* **256**, F794.

Kootstra, G., Wynen, R. and van Hoof, J. P. (1992). The non-heart beating kidney donor: of any help in developing countries? *Transplant. Proc.* **24**, 2040.

Koyama, I., Bulkley, G. B., William, G. M. and Im, M. J. (1985). The role of oxygen free radicals in mediating the reperfusion injury of cold-preserved ischaemia kidneys. *Transplantation* **40**, 590.

Kozaki, M., Matsuno, N., Tamaki, T. (1991). Procurement of kidney grafts from non-heart-beating donors. *Transplant. Proc.* **23**, 2575.

Lam, F. T., Mavor, A. I. D., Potts, D. J. and Giles, G. R. (1989a). Improved 72-hour renal preservation with phosphate buffered sucrose. *Transplantation* **47**, 767.

Lam, F. T., Ubhi, C. S., Mavor, A. I. D., Lodge, J. P. A. and Giles, G. R. (1989b). Clinical evaluation of PBS140 solution for cadaveric renal preservation. *Transplantation* **48**, 1067.

Leaf, A. (1959). Maintenance of concentration gradients and regulation of cell volume. *Ann. N. Y. Acad. Sci.* **72**, 396.

Levy, M. N. (1959). Oxygen consumption and blood flow in the hypothermic, perfused kidney. *Am. J. Physiol.* **197**, 111.

Lodge, J. P. A., Lam, F. T., Perry, S. L. and Giles, G. R. (1990). Ranolazine—a new drug with beneficial effects on renal preservation. *Transplantation* **50**, 755.

Lodge, J. P. A., Perry, S. L., Skinner, C., *et al.* (1991). Improved porcine renal preservation with a simple extracellular solution—PBS140: comparison with hyperosmolar citrate and University of Wisconsin solution. *Transplantation* **51**, 574.

Lundstam, S., Claes, G., Jonsson, O., *et al.* (1976). Metabolism in the hypothermically perfused kidney: production and utilization of lactate and utilization of acetate in the dog kidney. *Eur. Surg. Res.* **8**, 300.

Maessen, J. G., Van Der Vusse, G. J., Vork, M. and Kootstra, G. (1989).

The beneficial effect of intermediate normothermic perfusion during cold storage of ischaemically injured kidneys. *Transplantation* **47**, 409.

Magnusson, M. O., Rybka, S. J., Stowe, N. T., Novick, A. C. and Straffon, R. A. (1983). Enhancement of recovery in postischemic acute renal failure with captopril. *Kidney Int.* **24**, 324.

Marcen, R., Orofino, L., Pascual, J., *et al.* (1998). Delayed graft function does not reduce the survival of renal transplant allografts. *Transplantation* **66**, 461.

Markland, C. and Parsons, F. M. (1963). Preservation of kidneys for homotransplantation. *Br. J. Urol.* **35**, 457.

Marshall, V. C. (1971). Organ preservation. *In Clinical Organ Transplantation* (R. Y. Calne, ed.), p. 55, Blackwell Scientific, Oxford.

Marshall, V. C. (2000). Organ and tissue preservation for transplantation. *In Oxford Textbook of Surgery*, 2nd ed. (P. J. Morris and W. C. Wood, eds.), Oxford University Press, Oxford (in press).

Marshall, V. C., Howden, B. O., Jablonski, P., Tavanlis, G. and Tange, J. (1985a). Sucrose-containing solutions for kidney preservation. *Cryobiology* **22**, 622.

Marshall, V. C., Howden, B. O., Thomas, A. C., *et al.* (1991). Extended preservation of dog kidneys with modified UW solution. *Transplant. Proc.* **23**, 2366.

Marshall, V. C., Jablonski, P. and Howden, B. O. (1982). Cold storage and machine preservation of kidney: studies in the isolated rat kidney. *In Organ Preservation III: Basic and Applied Aspects*, (D. E. Pegg, I. A. Jacobsen and N. A. Halasz, eds.), p. 231, MTP Press, Lancaster.

Marshall, V. C., Jablonski, P., Howden, B. O., Rae, D. A. and Rigol, G. (1983a). Hypothermic preservation of the rat kidney for transplantation using flushing solutions: effects of glucose. *Cryobiology* **20**, 720.

Marshall, V. C., Jablonski, P., Howden, B. O., Rae, D. A. and Rigol, G. (1983b). Citrate-magnesium solutions improve both flush and pump preservation of the rat kidney. *Cryobiology* **20**, 729.

Marshall, V. C., Ross, B., Smith, M., Bartlett, S. and Freeman, J. (1985b). Organ and tissue preservation for transplantation: monitoring by ^{31}P nuclear magnetic resonance. *Transplant. Proc.* **17**, 1693.

Marshall, V. C., Ross, H., Scott D. F., *et al.* (1977). Preservation of cadaver renal allografts: comparison of ice storage and machine perfusion. *Med. J. Aust.* **2**, 353.

Marumo, F., Masaki, Y., Ida, T., Sato, K. and Ando, K. (1991). Prolongation of the kidney preservation period by simple cold storage up to 72 hours by human atrial natriuretic peptide. *Transplantation* **51**, 982.

Masson, F., Thiciope, M., Latapie, M. J. and Maurett, P. (1990). Thyroid function in brain-dead donors. *Transplant. Int.* **3**, 226.

Mayfield, K. B., Ametani, M., Southard, J. H. and Belzer, F. O. (1987). Mechanism of action of ex-vivo blood rescue in six-day preserved kidneys. *Transplant. Proc.* **19**, 1367.

McAnulty, J. F., Vreugdenhil, P. K., Southard, J. H. and Belzer, F. O. (1991). Improved survival of kidneys preserved for seven days with phospholipase inhibitor. *Transplant. Proc.* **23**, 691.

McCauley, J., Fung, J., Jain, A., Todo, S. and Starzl, T. E. (1990). The effects of FK-506 on renal function after renal transplantation. *Transplant. Proc.* **22**, 17.

Mendez, R., Mendez, R. G., Koussa, N., Cats, S., Gogaerd T. P. and Khetan, U. (1987). Preservation effect on oligo-anuria in the cyclosporine era: a prospective trial with 26 paired cadaveric renal allografts. *Transplant. Proc.* **19**, 2047.

Miller, H. C. and Alexander, J. W. (1973). Protective effect of methyl-prednisolone against ischemic injury to the kidney. *Transplantation* **16**, 57.

Moen, J., Claesson, K., Pienaar, H., *et al.* (1989). Preservation of dog liver, kidney, and pancreas using the Belzer-UW solution with a high-sodium and low potassium content. *Transplantation* **47**, 940.

Moser, E., Holzmueller, P., Reckendorfer, H. and Burgmann, H. (1992). Cold-preserved rat liver viability testing by proton nuclear magnetic resonance relaxometry. *Transplantation* **53**, 536.

Moukarzel, M., Benoit, G., Bensadoun, H., *et al.* (1990). Nonrandomized comparative study between University of Wisconsin cold storage and Euro-Collins solution in kidney transplantation. *Transplant. Proc.* **22**, 2289.

Neumayer, H. H. and Wagner, K. (1987). Prevention of delayed graft function in cadaver kidney transplants by diltiazem: outcome of two prospective, randomized clinical trials. *J. Cardiovasc. Pharmacol.* **10**, 5170.

Newstead, C. G. and Dyer, P. A. (1992). The influence of increased age and age matching on graft survival after first cadaveric renal transplantation. *Transplantation* **54**, 441.

Novick, A. C., Hwei, H. H., Steinmuller, D., *et al.* (1986). Detrimental effect of cyclosporine on initial function of cadaver renal allografts following extended preservation: results of a randomized prospective study. *Transplantation* **42**, 154.

Odom, N. J. (1990). Management of the multiorgan donor. *B. M. J.* **300**, 1571.

Opelz, G. and Terasaki, P. I. (1976). Kidney preservation: perfusion versus cold storage—1975. *Transplant. Proc.* **8**, 121.

Opelz, G. and Terasaki, P. I. (1982). Advantage of cold storage over machine perfusion for preservation of cadaver kidneys. *Transplantation* **33**, 64.

Orii, T., Ohkohchi, N., Satomi, S., Taguchi, Y., Mori, S. and Miura, I. (1992). Assessment of liver graft function after cold preservation using ^{31}P and ^{23}Na magnetic resonance spectroscopy. *Transplantation* **53**, 730.

Ouriel, K., Smedira, N. G. and Ricotta, J. J. (1985). Protection of the kidney after temporary ischaemia: free radical scavengers. *J. Vasc. Surg.* **2**, 49.

Paller, M. S., Hoidal, J. R. and Ferris, T. F. (1984). Oxygen free radicals in ischemic acute renal failure in the rat. *J. Clin. Invest.* **74**, 1156.

Papadimitriou, M., Alexopoulos, E., Vargemezis, V., Sakellariou, G., Kosmidou, I. and Metaxas, P. (1984). The effect of preventive administration of verapamil on acute ischaemic renal failure in dogs. *Transplant. Proc.* **16**, 44.

Pavlock, G. S., Southard, J. H., Lutz, M. F., Belzer, J. B. and Belzer, F. O. (1981). Effects of mannitol and chlorpromazine pretreatment of rabbits on kidney mitochondria following in vivo ischemia and reflow. *Life Sci.* **29**, 2667.

Pegg, D. E. (1978). An approach to hypothermic renal preservation. *Cryobiology* **15**, 1.

Pegg, D. E., Jacobsen, I. A. and Halasz, N. A. (eds.) (1982). *Organ Preservation III: Basic and Applied Aspects*, MTP Press, Lancaster.

Pegg, D. E., Wusterman, M. C. and Foreman, J. (1981). Metabolism of normal and ischemically injured rabbit kidneys during perfusion for 48 hours at 10°C. *Transplantation* **32**, 437.

Pentlow, B. D., Kostakis, A. J., Wall, W. J. (1979). Preservation of ischaemically injured canine kidneys with hypertonic citrate solution. *Transplantation* **27**, 99.

Ploeg, R. J. (1990). Kidney preservation with the UW and Euro-Collins solutions. *Transplantation* **49**, 281.

Ploeg, R. J., Goosens, D., McAnulty, J. F., Southard, J. H. and Belzer, F. O. (1988). Successful 72-hour storage of dog kidneys with UW solution. *Transplantation* **45**, 935.

Pryor, J. P., Keaveny, T. V., Reed, T. W. and Belzer, F. O. (1981). Improved immediate function of experimental cadaver renal allografts by elimination of agonal vasospasm. *Br. J. Surg.* **58**, 184.

Puig, J. M., Lloveras, J., Oliveras, A., Costa, A., Aubia, J. and Masramon, J. (1991). Usefulness of diltiazem in reducing the incidence of acute tubular necrosis in Euro-Collins–preserved cadaveric renal grafts. *Transplant. Proc.* **23**, 2368.

Rajotte, R. V., De Groot, T. H., Ellis, D. K. and Rall, W. F. (1985). Preliminary experiments on vitrification of isolated rat islets of Langerhans. *Cryobiology* **22**, 602.

Rall, W. F. and Fahy, G. M. (1985a). Ice-free cryopreservation of mouse embryos at 196°C by vitrification. *Nature* **313**, 573.

Rall, W. F. and Fahy, G. M. (1985b). Cryopreservation of mouse embryos by vitrification. *Cryobiology* **22**, 603.

Rapaport, F. T., Waltzer, W. C. and Anaise, D. (1990). How can one balance duty to all cultures and ethnic groups with effective procurement and equitable distribution of organs for clinical transplantation? New evidence of the key importance of local primacy for a successful organ donation effort. *Transplant. Proc.* **22**, 1007.

Ratych, R. E., Bulkley, G. B. and Williams, G. M. (1986). Ischemia/reperfusion injury in the kidney. *Prog. Clin. Biol. Res.* **224**, 263.

Ray, J. G. (1998). Prostaglandin E1 analogs do not improve renal function among either transplant or non-transplant patients. *Transplantation* **66**, 476.

Rijkmans, B. G., Buurman, W. A. and Kootstra, G. (1984). Six day canine kidney preservation: hypothermic perfusion combined with isolated blood perfusion. *Transplantation* **27**, 130.

Ringe, B., Neuhaus, P., Pichlmayr, R. and Heigel, B. (1985). Aims and practical application of a multi organ procurement protocol. *Langenbecks Arch. Chir.* **365**, 47.

Rolles, K., Foreman, J. and Pegg, D. E. (1984). Preservation of ischemically injured canine kidneys by retrograde oxygen persufflation. *Transplantation* **38**, 102.

Rooth, P., Dawidson, I., Diller, K. and Taljedal, I. B. (1987). Beneficial effects of calcium antagonist pretreatment and albumin infusion on cyclosporine A induced impairment of kidney microcirculation in mice. *Transplant. Proc.* **19**, 3602.

Rosenthal, J. T., Danovitch, G. M., Wilkinson, A. and Ettenger, R. B. (1991). The high cost of delayed graft function in cadaveric renal transplantation. *Transplantation* **51**, 1115.

Rosenthal, J. T., Denny, D. and Hakal, T. R. (1983). Results from a single kidney procurement center. *J. Urol.* **129**, 1111.

Rosenthal, J. T., Herman, J. B., Taylor, R. J., Broznick, B. and Hakela, T. R. (1984). Comparison of pulsatile machine perfusion with cold storage for cadaver kidney preservation. *Transplantation* **37**, 425.

Ross, H. and Escott, M. L. (1979). Gaseous oxygen perfusion of the renal vessels as an adjunct in kidney preservation. *Transplantation* **28**, 362.

Ross, H. and Escott, M. L. (1982). Renal preservation with gaseous perfusion. *Transplant. Proc.* **13**, 693.

Ross, H., Marshall, V. C. and Escott, M. L. (1976). 72-hour canine kidney preservation without continuous perfusion. *Transplantation* **21**, 498.

Ruers, T. J. M., Vroemen, J. P. A. M. and Kootstra, G. (1986). Non-heart-beating donors: a successful contribution to organ procurement. *Transplant. Proc.* **18**, 408.

Sacks, S. A., Petritsch, P. H. and Kaufman, J. J. (1973). Canine kidney preservation using a new perfusate. *Lancet* **1**, 1024.

Sakagami, K., Takasu, S., Kawamura, T., *et al.* (1990). A comparison of University of Wisconsin and Euro-Collins solutions for simple cold storage in non-heart-beating cadaveric kidney transplantation. *Transplantation* **49**, 824.

Sakr, M., Zetti, G., McClain, C., *et al.* (1992). The protective effect of FK506 pretreatment against renal ischemia/reperfusion injury in rats. *Transplantation* **53**, 987.

Santiago-Delphin, E. A. (1982). Pharmacological principles during organ harvesting. *In Basic Concepts in Organ Procurement, Perfusion and Preservation*, (L. H. Toledo-Pereyra, ed.), p. 73, Academic Press, New York.

Schilling, M., Saunder, A., Southard, J. H. and Belzer, F. O. (1993). Five- to seven-day kidney preservation with aspirin and furegrelate. *Transplantation* **55**, 955.

Schlumpf, R., Candinas, D., Zollinger, A., Keusch, G., Retsch, M., Decurtins, M. and Largiader, F. (1992). *Transplant. Int.* **5**, 424–428.

Schlumpf, R., Morel, P. H., Loveras, J. J., *et al.* (1991). Examination of the role of colloids hydroxyethyl starch, dextran, human albumin, and plasma proteins in a modified UW solution. *Transplant. Proc.* **23**, 2362.

Schneider, A., Toledo-Pereyra, L. H., Zeichner, W. D., *et al.* (1983). Effect of dopamine and pitressin of kidneys procured and harvested for transplantation. *Transplantation* **36**, 110.

Sells, R. A., Bore, P. J., McLaughlin, G. A., Johnson, J. N. and Tyrell, I. (1977). A predictive test of renal viability. *Transplant. Proc.* **9**, 1557.

Shapiro, J. I., Cheung, C., Itabashi, A., Chan, L. and Schrier, R. W. (1985). The effect of verapamil on renal function after warm and cold ischemia in the isolated perfused rat kidney. *Transplantation* **40**, 596.

Shoskes, D. A. (1998). Effect of bioflavinoids quercetin and curcumin on ischaemic renal injury. *Transplantation* **66**, 147.

Siegel, N. J., Avison, M. J., Reilly, H. F., Alger, J. R. and Shulman, R. G. (1983). Enhanced recovery of renal ATP with post ischaemic infusion of ATP-MgCl$_2$ determined by ^{31}P-NMR. *Am. J. Physiol.* **245**, 530.

Slutsky, R. A., Andre, M. P., Mattrey, R. F. and Brahme, F. J. (1984). In vitro magnetic relaxation times of the ischemic and reperfused rabbit kidney: concise communication. *J. Nucl. Med.* **25**, 38.

Smeesters, C., Corman, J., Fassi, J. C., *et al.* (1983). Beneficial effects of methylprednisolone on urinary excretion of lysosomal enzymes in acute renal ischemia. *Can. J. Surg.* **26**, 175.

Solez, K., Freshwater, M. F. and Su, C. T. (1977). The effect of propranolol on postischemic acute renal failure in the rat. *Transplantation* **24**, 148.

Southard, J. H. and Belzer, F. O. (1980). Control of canine kidney cortex slice volume and in distribution of hypothermia by impermeable anions. *Cryobiology* **17**, 540.

Southard, J. H., Senzig, K. A. and Belzer, F. O. (1980). Effects of hypothermia on canine kidney mitochondria. *Cryobiology* **17**, 148.

Squifflet, J. P., Pirson, Y., Gianello, P., *et al.* (1981). Safe preservation of human renal cadaver transplants by Euro-Collins solutions up to 50 hours. *Transplant. Proc.* **13**, 693.

Starzl, T. E., Fung, J., Jordan, M., *et al.* (1990). Kidney transplantation under FK-506. *J. A. M. A.* **264**, 63.

Stein, D. G., Drinkwater D. C., Laks, H., *et al.* (1991). Cardiac preservation in patients undergoing transplantation: a clinical trial comparing UW solution and Stanford solution. *J. Thorac. Cardiovasc. Surg.* **102**, 657.

Strzelecki, T., Khauli, R. B., Kumar, S. and Menon, M. (1987). In vitro effects of cyclosporine on function of rat kidney mitochondria. *Transplant. Proc.* **19**, 1393.

Sumpio, B. E., Chaudry, I. R., Clemens, M. G. and Baue, A. E. (1984). Accelerated functional recovery of isolated rat kidney with ATP-$MgCl_2$ after warm ischemia. *Am. J. Physiol.* **247**, 1047.

Taube, D., Welch, K. I., Bewick, M., *et al.* (1987). Other protocols: pretreatment of human renal allografts with monoclonal antibodies to induce long-term tolerance. *Transplant. Proc.* **19**, 1961.

Tenschert, W., Harfmann, P., Meyer-Moldenhauer, W. H., Arndt, R. and Klosterhalfen, H. (1991). Kidney protective effort of diltiazem after renal transplantation with long cold ischemia time and triple-drug immunosuppression. *Transplant. Proc.* **23**, 1334.

Tesi, R. J., Hong, J., Butt, K. M. H., Jaffe, B. M. and McMillan, M. A. (1987). Effects of cyclosporine on suboptimally procured kidneys. *Transplant. Proc.* **19**, 1382.

Tiggeler, R. C. W. L., Berden, J. H. M., Hoitsma, A. J. and Koene, R. A. P. (1985). Prevention of acute tubular necrosis in cadaveric kidney transplantation by the combined use of mannitol and moderate hydration. *Ann. Surg.* **201**, 246.

Todo, S., Nery, J., Yanaga, J., Podesta, R., Gordon, R. and Starzl, T. E. (1989). Extended preservation of human liver grafts with UW solution. *J. A. M. A.* **261**, 711.

Toledo-Pereyra, L. H. (1982). Kidney perfusion. In *Basic Concepts of Organ Procurement, Perfusion and Preservation for Transplantation*, L. H. Toledo-Pereyra, ed.), p. 183, Academic Press, New York.

Toledo-Pereyra, L. H., Simmons, R. L., Olsen, L. C. and Najarian, J. S. (1977). Clinical effect of allopurinol on preserved kidneys: a randomized double-bind study. *Ann. Surg.* **185**, 128.

Trifillis, A. L., Kahng, M. W., Cowley, R. A. and Trump, B. F. (1984). Metabolic studies of postischemic acute renal failure in the rat. *Exp. Mol. Pathol.* **40**, 155.

Ueda, Y., Todo, S., Inventarza, O., *et al.* (1989). The UW solution for canine kidney preservation: its specific effect on renal hemodynamics and microvasculature. *Transplantation* **48**, 913.

Wagner, K. and Neumayer, H. H. (1987). Influence of the calcium antagonist diltiazem on delayed graft function in cadaveric kidney transplantation: results of a 6-month follow-up. *Transplant. Proc.* **19**, 1353.

Wahlberg, J. A., Love, R., Landegard, L., Southard, J. H. and Belzer, F. O. (1987). 72-hour preservation of the canine pancreas. *Transplantation* **43**, 5.

Wahlberg, J. A., Southard, J. H. and Belzer, F. O. (1986). Development of a cold storage solution for pancreas preservation. *Cryobiology* **23**, 477.

Watkins, G. M., Prentis, N. A. and Couch, N. P. (1971). Successful 24-hour kidney preservation with simplified hyperosmolar hyperkalaemic perfusate. *Transplant. Proc.* **3**, 612.

Wattiaux, R. and Wattiaux-De Conninck, S. (1984). Trapping of mannitol in rat-liver mitochondria and lysosomes. *Int. Rev. Exp. Pathol.* **26**, 85.

Weimar, W., Geerlings, W., Bijnen, A. B., *et al.* (1983). A controlled study on the effect of mannitol on immediate renal function after cadaver donor kidney transplantation. *Transplantation* **35**, 99.

Wijk, van der J., Rijkmans, B. G. and Kootstra, G. (1983). Six-day kidney preservation in a canine model, influence of a one-to-four hour ex-vivo perfusion in interval. *Transplantation* **35**, 408.

Wijnen, R. M. H. and van der Linden, C. J. (1991). Donor treatment after pronouncement of brain death: a neglected intensive care problem. *Transplant. Int.* **4**, 186.

Wilson, D. R., Arnold, P. E., Burke, T. J. and Schrier, R. W. (1984). Mitochondrial calcium accumulation and respiration in ischemic acute renal failure in the rat. *Kidney Int.* **25**, 519.

Winchell, R. J. and Halasz, N. A. (1989). Lack of effect of oxygen-radical scavenging systems in the preserved reperfused rabbit kidney. *Transplantation* **48**, 393.

10

HLA Typing, Matching and Crossmatching in Renal Transplantation

K. I. Welsh • M. Bunce

Introduction

In renal transplantation, the histocompatibility systems currently used in matching algorithms are the ABO blood group system and the HLA system. The donor should be ABO compatible with the recipient because most renal transplants performed across the ABO barrier result in hyperacute or acute rejection. Some exceptions are allowed, and these are discussed in the next section.

The HLA system is the human major histocompatibility complex (MHC), and analogous complexes have been found in all mammalian species. The system is termed *major* because it is the genetic system that encodes the expression of the most important cell-surface antigens recognized as foreign on an allograft toward which the host's rejection response is directed. HLA antigens are involved in numerous other vital functions apart from their role in tissue and organ transplantation, such as in presentation of viral peptide to induce and target the T-cell response; in disease susceptibility and in presentation of processed antigen from bacteria, vaccinations and fungi through the host's T-cell receptors. We discuss only the histocompatibility role of HLA in this chapter.

Many minor histocompatibility systems exist in humans, and their influence on graft rejection may be significant. Such systems are simply amino acid sequence differences (polymorphisms) between donor and recipient that can be presented (as peptide by donor MHC) to recipient T cells and responded to. A few grafts from HLA-identical siblings undergo rejection episodes, which occasionally lead to graft loss, and this reaction is presumed to be against minor histocompatibility systems. It has been shown by Goulmy and colleagues that minor transplantation antigens can be detected by MHC-restricted cytotoxic T cells during graft-versus-host disease (Goulmy et al., 1983). In the mouse, minor histocompatibility systems have been shown to play a definite role in the rejection of vascularized cardiac allografts (Peugh et al., 1986). In theory, any molecule that can differentiate between donor and recipient (i.e., is polymorphic) has the potential of being a minor histocompatibility antigen if, when processed, its peptide repertoire also is different. This potential is realized in all molecules in which the response has the capacity to damage the graft.

ABO Blood Group System

Transplants that are ABO incompatible may be performed inadvertently or deliberately. Nearly all the early ABO-incompatible kidney transplants were performed in error, and most resulted in hyperacute or acute vascular rejection (Glea-

son and Murray, 1967), although some were successful (Starzl et al., 1964). Rejection is assumed to be caused by antibody reacting with blood group A and/or B antigen on the vascular endothelium (Paul et al., 1978).

ABO-incompatible kidney transplants have been performed deliberately from cadaver donors and from living related and living unrelated donors. Brynger and coworkers were the first to report successful outcome of cadaver transplants from blood group A_2 donors to O recipients (Brynger et al., 1982). Similar grafts have been reported by other centers, with varying degrees of success (Alexandre et al., 1991). A substance is identical in blood group A_1 and A_2 persons, but its expression density is much lower in the latter. Although the bulk of this difference is accounted for by the absence from A_2 persons of two of the four specific core chains able to carry A substance (Breimer and Samuelsson, 1986), additional subtlety exists (Rydberg et al., 1990). For example, two kidneys from the same donor were found to have differences in expression of A substance. Welsh and associates found that the recipient's IgM anti-A_2 titer was a crucial factor in determining long-term success; three of four patients with an antibody titer of 1/64 or greater lost their graft, whereas only two of nine grafts failed when the pretransplant titer was less than 1/64 (Welsh et al., 1987). In true A_2 individuals who are nonsecretors, kidney expression of A substance is low, and there is no immunological reason not to use such donors unless the anti-A titer of the recipient is high. This idea may sound a little extreme, but A_2B individuals regularly form anti-A antibodies yet there have been no reported problems with A_1 or A_1B donors into A_2B recipients.

In living donor transplantation, successful ABO-incompatible grafts were achieved in recipients whose pregraft anti-A or anti-B antibodies were removed or the titer decreased by plasmapheresis and recipient splenectomy (Alexandre et al., 1986, 1991) or by immunoadsorption alone (Agishi et al., 1992). In the patients of Alexandre and associates, the titer of isoagglutinins returned to pretransplant levels after some weeks but without any apparent effect on the graft (Alexandre et al., 1986, 1991).

ABO-incompatible transplants can be carried out successfully in selected circumstances as just described even though many cases of hyperacute and acute rejection have been documented. Two factors crucial to the success of the transplantation are the target antigen density and the pretransplant antibody titer, the first easily predictable and the second easily testable. It is possible to genotype for A_1 and A_2 subtypes and secretor status using the same methodology as employed for tissue typing (Procter et al., 1996). The pretransplant antibody titer may be naturally low in some patients, whereas in others, it may be necessary to lower the titer by means of plasmapheresis or immunoadsorption. From the literature quoted, splenectomy and additional humoral immunosuppression (e.g., cyclophosphamide, deoxyspergualin and methotrexate) to supplement cyclosporine may be needed to enhance the likelihood of graft survival in patients who have high anti-A titers or in situations in which donors are not A₂.

Why does the graft reject if antibody to it is present at the time of transplantation yet survive if such antibody appears later? The consensus about antibodies to HLA in recipients is that graft survival is shortened in cases in which antidonor antibodies are found after transplantation. This apparently is not the case for antibodies to blood groups, although the data are sparse. Rydberg (1991) suggests that at least part of the reason is the development of antibodies to glycosyltransferases. Inactivation of enzymes that add the target carbohydrate to the organ is an attractive explanation for graft accommodation seen in these successful ABO-incompatible grafts.

Antibodies to blood group antigens other than ABO can be relevant to transplantation. For example, antibodies directed against the Ii system can cause hyperacute rejection of cooled donor organs. These are discussed in more detail in the sections on crossmatching (Belzer *et al.*, 1971).

HLA System

The HLA complex is composed of at least 12 closely linked loci located on the short arm of chromosome 6 (Fig. 10–1). The exact location of HLA was shown to be Ch6p21 by Francke and Pellegrino (1977) and now is given more exactly as Ch6p21.31. A more detailed genetic map of the Ch6p21.31 class I and class II regions is shown in Figure 10–2. The loci generally considered relevant for solid-organ transplantation are the class I loci *HLA-A* and *HLA-B* along with the HLA class II locus *DRB1*. The less considered loci *HLA-Cw* and the class II loci *DRB1*, *DRB3*, *DRB4*, *DRB5*, *DQB1* and *DPB1* all can be typed for and have relevance in solid-organ transplantation, as discussed in the crossmatching section.

The HLA class I molecules are formed by the association of a glycosylated polypeptide α chain with molecular weight about 45,000 daltons. The α chain is associated noncovalently with β₂-microglobulin, a nonglycosylated peptide with a molecular weight about 12,000 daltons. β₂-Microglobulin has been shown to contact all three heavy-chain extracellular domains, but it is associated most closely with the α3 domain (Bjorkman *et al.*, 1987). In humans, the gene for β₂-microglobulin is located on chromosome 15 (Goodfellow *et al.*, 1975). Although it does not form part of the antigenic site of the class I HLA molecule, β₂-microglobulin is necessary for processing and expression of class I molecules (Krangel *et al.*,

1979). A ribbon diagram of a class I molecule-peptide complex is shown in Figure 10–3.

The HLA class II molecules, DR, DQ and DP, are heterodimers consisting of a 33,000-dalton heavy chain, designated α, and a 28,000-dalton light chain, designated β. The class II α chain is encoded by the *DRA1*, *DQA1* or *DPA1* gene, whereas the class II β chain is encoded by the *DRB1*, *DRB3*, *DRB4*, *DRB5*, *DQB1* or *DPB1* gene. The α chain consists of two glycosylated domains, α1 and α2, stabilized by disulfide bridges. The β chain also consists of two domains, β1 and β2, that are stabilized by disulfide bridges. The α1 domain is glycosylated. The α and β chains are noncovalently bound together to form an antigen receptor similar to the class I antigen receptor but with more flexibility in the types of peptides it may bind.

The HLA antigens are inherited as codominant alleles. Recombination between the loci occurs, and the frequency is about 1% between HLA-A and HLA-B, 0.8% between HLA-B and HLA-DR, about 4% between HLA-DQ and HLA-DP and negligible between HLA-DR and HLA-DQ. The higher frequency of HLA-DQ and HLA-DP recombinants is thought to be due to a recombination hot spot in this area because the loci are known to be close together (see Fig. 10–2). Because the six loci are linked relatively closely, they usually are inherited *en bloc* by the offspring from each parent. The HLA antigens coded for by the genes of one chromosome are termed an *HLA haplotype*, and each individual has two HLA haplotypes. An understanding of the inheritance of HLA haplotypes is important in the discussion of the evidence that HLA is the human MHC. Different DRB haplotypes have different amounts of DR antigens at the cell surface owing to alternative DRB gene arrangements, as shown in Figure 10–4.

HLA NOMENCLATURE

The HLA class I and II loci are highly polymorphic with more than 860 HLA-A, HLA-B, HLA-C, HLA-DRB and HLA-DQB1 antigens currently described. Current lists of alleles can be found on the Internet (www.ebi.ac.uk/imgt/hla/ and www.anthonynolan.com/hig/data.html). The large number of genes and alleles being discovered in the HLA region has necessitated a formal system of nomenclature organized by a World Health Organization committee.

Historically, a standard format for naming HLA antigens was used in which a newly described antigen was given the next available integer prefixed by a *w*. For example, when HLA-Bw67 was discovered, there previously had been 66 identified antigens. The prefix *w* was given to indicate provisional or *workshop* status. When the new antigen had been proved to exist, normally through International Histocompatibility Workshops, the *w* was dropped. If the new antigen

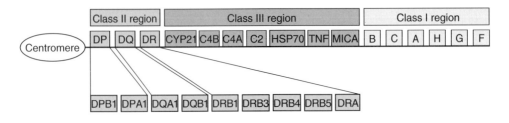

FIGURE 10–1

Diagrammatic representation of the major histocompatibility complex (MHC) shows location and overall organization on the short arm of chromosome 6. The MHC region shown spans approximately 4,000 kb and contains many more genes than shown. The class III region contains the genes for many MHC-related proteins, such as complement factors, tumor necrosis factor, heat-shock proteins and MICA (class I–like molecule).

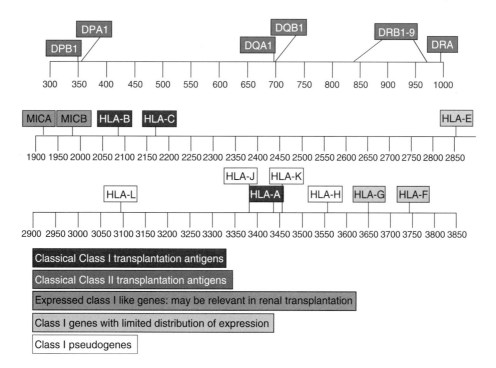

FIGURE 10–2

Chromosomal location of HLA class II and class I genes relevant to transplantation. The scale of the genomic map is in kilobases. The HLA-DR antigens are heterodimers consisting of α and β class II chains, which are encoded by the *DRBA* and *DRB1* genes. The HLA-DQ and HLA-DP antigens also consist of α-β heterodimers. The HLA-DR and HLA-DQ loci are relatively close together so that particular HLA-DR antigens and HLA-DQ antigens generally are found together (e.g., DR3-DQ2 are nearly always found together in linkage dysequilibrium). In contrast, the HLA-DP loci are 500 kb away from HLA-DR with a recombination hot spot between them so that there is less linkage dysequilibrium between HLA-DR and HLA-DP than between HLA-DQ and HLA-DR. Most HLA-DR–identical donor-recipient combinations also are HLA-DQ identical but are not HLA-DP identical. The class I antigens comprise class I α chains stabilized at the cell surface by association with a nonpolymorphic β$_2$-microglobulin chain. HLA-A, HLA-B and HLA-C are the classic transplantation genes. HLA-H, HLA-J, HLA-K and HLA-L are thought to be nonexpressed pseudogenes that may have arisen from HLA-A gene duplication and probably are not relevant in solid-organ transplantation. HLA-E, HLA-F and HLA-G are expressed, but their limited patterns of expression mean they are unlikely to be relevant in solid-organ transplantation. The class I–like MICA and MICB loci are polymorphic, are expressed and may be relevant in transplantation. The genomic map is based on data from the Sanger Centre Internet site (www.sanger.ac.uk/hgp/chr6/mhc.shtml) and Trowsdale (1996).

was deemed to be a split of an existing allele, this could be indicated by the use of parentheses: Bw55(22) indicated that Bw55 was a split of B22. The use of the *w* prefix has been dropped for all antigens except HLA-C and the HLA-B public specificities Bw4 and Bw6. With the increasing amount of sequencing being performed in the 1980s, it became apparent that another nomenclature system was required for the HLA alleles. A standard nomenclature is used now to describe the products of the HLA region so that all sequenced HLA alleles are identified according to the examples given in Table 10–1.

HLA TYPING

Soon after the first solid-organ clinical transplants were performed, it became apparent that some degree of HLA typing was prudent, originally for matching and later as an aid to crossmatching and antibody screening. Many different methods exist for HLA typing, each with advantages and disadvantages. Only two methods are discussed in detail here: the traditional complement-dependent cytotoxicity test (CDC) and the polymerase chain reaction (PCR)–based typing method of allele-specific amplification through sequence-specific primers (PCR-SSP). We selected the latter DNA typing technique because, similar to serology, it can be performed in less than 3 hours and is useful for typing cadaver donors before crossmatching and subsequent transplantation.

Complement-Dependent Cytotoxicity Test

The CDC test, also known as the *serological test*, has been used since the early 1960s (Mittal *et al.*, 1968; Terasaki and McClelland, 1964). The principle of CDC typing and crossmatching is that lymphocytes are lysed by rabbit complement in the presence of antibodies to HLA antigens. Unseparated or separated T lymphocytes are used for class I typing, and B lymphocytes are used for class I and class II typing because HLA-DR, HLA-DQ and HLA-DP antigens are found on B lymphocytes but not normal T lymphocytes. The antibodies to these antigens may be found in the sera of multiply transfused patients and multiparous women. The former source provided Dausset (1958) with antibodies to detect the first HLA antigen (MAC).

The CDC test can provide low-resolution results within 3 hours, which is crucial for reducing cold ischemia times in cadaver donor transplantation. There are drawbacks of CDC, however: Viable lymphocytes are required, the antibodies needed generally are nonrenewable and the technique has limited powers of resolution because of the paucity of antigen-specific alloantisera or monoclonal antibodies. There is strong linkage dysequilibrium between HLA loci, making it difficult, especially with regard to the C locus, to define the individual antibody specificities within typing sera. The problem of serological discrimination of class II antigens, the most important antigens for solid-organ transplantation, led

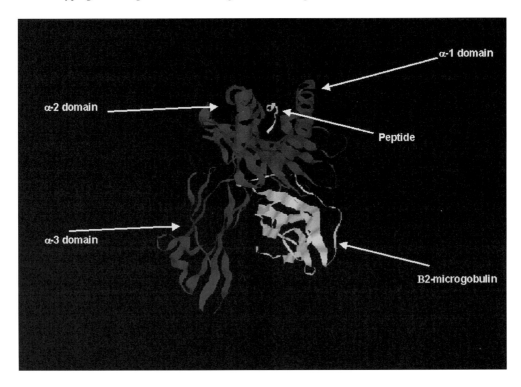

FIGURE 10–3

Ribbon diagram of HLA-B*5301-β_2-microglobulin and peptide complex based on a model by Smith *et al.* (1996) using RasMol 2.6 (download available from www.umass.edu/microbio/rasmol/getras.htm). The α-1 and α-2 domains create helical structures that form the walls of the antigen binding cleft. The α-3 domain interacts with β_2-microglobulin to stabilize the molecule at the cell surface.

to the first comprehensive molecular class II typing system using restriction fragment length polymorphism (RFLP) (Bidwell *et al.*, 1988). The relevance of RFLP was shown by Opelz *et al.* (1993) in the Collaborative Transplant Study and by Mytilineos *et al.* (1990, 1992). These retrospective studies showed that RFLP-defined, HLA-DR–matched renal grafts had improved survival compared with serology-defined, HLA-DR–matched grafts and that serology for class II was inadequate in many typing centers, with an overall discrepancy rate of 25% between serologically defined and RFLP-defined antigens. Restriction fragment length polymorphism had too many drawbacks to be the method of choice for the

TABLE 10–1

HLA NOMENCLATURE

Nomenclature	Refers to
HLA	Identifies the allele as a product of an HLA locus
HLA-A	Identifies the locus
HLA-A*24	Identifies a group of alleles that may be part of the A24 antigen
HLA-A*2402	Identifies a specific HLA allele
HLA-A*24022	Identifies a noncoding change (i.e., A*24022 and A*24021 have different nucleotide sequences but the same amino acids)
HLA-A*2402101	Identifies a noncoding change outside of the mature protein sequence (i.e., in an intron or untranslated region)

Letters may be suffixed to any of the allele names to denote a difference in expression: The letter *N* is used to denote a null (nonexpressed) allele (e.g., A*2411N), whereas *L* is used to denote abnormally low expression (e.g., A*2402102L).

1990s, however, and was replaced rapidly by PCR-based methods.

The development of the PCR (Saiki *et al.*, 1985) allowed the evolution of improved molecular HLA typing techniques. The PCR can generate specific amplified stretches of DNA sequences *in vitro* through repeated cycles of DNA denaturation, annealing of specific primer to a single strand and nucleotide extension from primer pairs using a DNA polymerase.

Techniques for analyzing polymorphisms in amplified DNA can be divided into two basic groups: probe hybridization and direct amplicon analysis. Currently, there are many different PCR-based tissue typing assays (reviewed in Bunce *et al.*, 1997), and it is the decision of individual laboratories which test or combination of tests they use and for which loci they choose to apply the tests. For renal transplantation patients, any combination of molecular tests can be used because the length of time to obtain an HLA genotype is not an issue. Arguably the only realistic method for PCR-based typing of cadaver donors for all relevant loci in less than 3 hours is PCR-SSP.

Polymerase Chain Reaction Using Sequence-Specific Primers

In 1989, two separate groups (Newton *et al.*, 1989; Wu *et al.*, 1989) described a system of PCR in which the specificity of the PCR reaction entailed matching the 3' end of one primer with the target DNA sequence, allowing any point mutation to be identified within one or two PCR reactions. This PCR method was termed *amplification refractory mutation system* or *PCR-SSP*. The PCR-SSP method works because *Taq* polymerase lacks 3' to 5' exonucleolytic proofreading activity (Chien *et al.*, 1976; Tindall and Kunkel, 1988). Such an activity

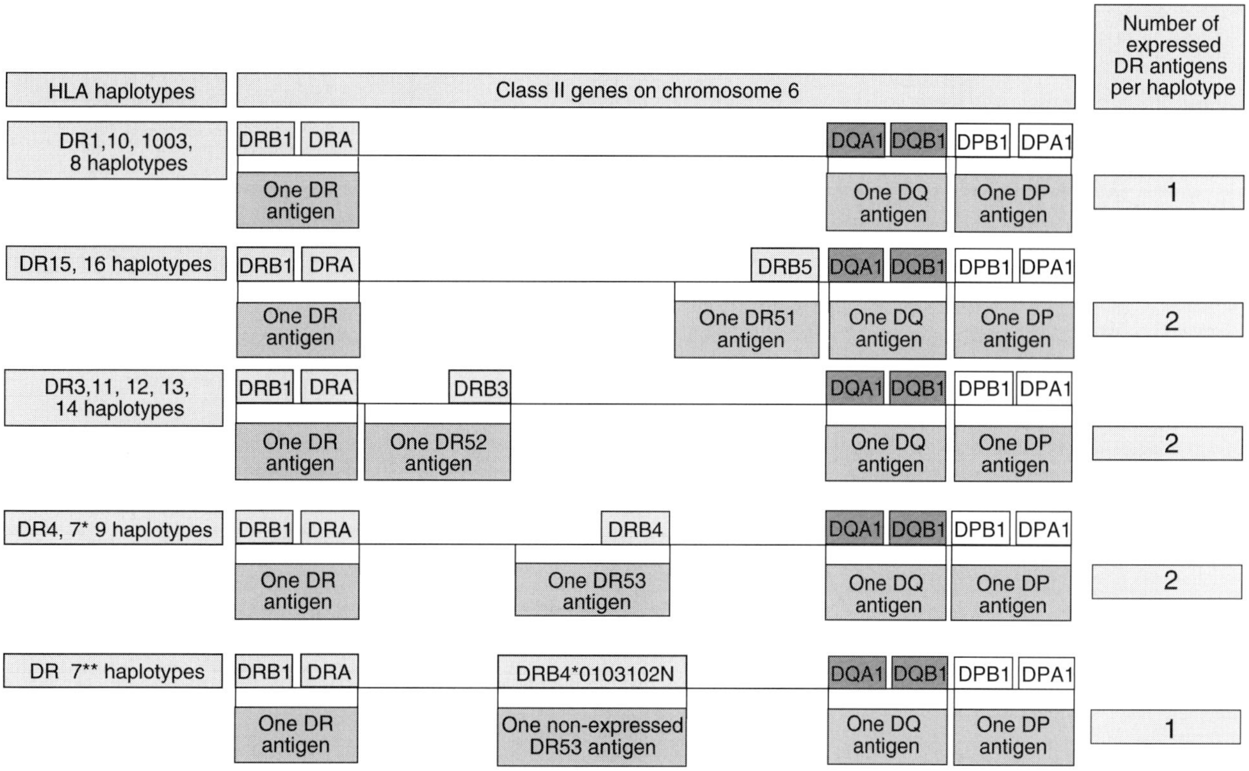

Number of expressed DR antigens per haplotype

HLA haplotypes	Class II genes on chromosome 6		Number of expressed DR antigens per haplotype

HLA haplotypes — Class II genes on chromosome 6

DR1,10, 1003, 8 haplotypes — DRB1 | DRA … DQA1 DQB1 DPB1 DPA1
One DR antigen … One DQ antigen | One DP antigen — **1**

DR15, 16 haplotypes — DRB1 | DRA … DRB5 DQA1 DQB1 DPB1 DPA1
One DR antigen … One DR51 antigen | One DQ antigen | One DP antigen — **2**

DR3,11, 12, 13, 14 haplotypes — DRB1 | DRA … DRB3 … DQA1 DQB1 DPB1 DPA1
One DR antigen … One DR52 antigen … One DQ antigen | One DP antigen — **2**

DR4, 7* 9 haplotypes — DRB1 | DRA … DRB4 … DQA1 DQB1 DPB1 DPA1
One DR antigen … One DR53 antigen … One DQ antigen | One DP antigen — **2**

DR 7** haplotypes — DRB1 | DRA … DRB4*0103102N … DQA1 DQB1 DPB1 DPA1
One DR antigen … One non-expressed DR53 antigen … One DQ antigen | One DP antigen — **1**

FIGURE 10–4

Alternative *DRB* gene arrangements: Depending on the haplotype, most *DRB1* gene products (DR1-18 antigens) are coexpressed with *DRB3*, *DRB4* or *DRB5* gene products (DR antigens DR52, DR53 and DR51). Virtually all DR3, DR11, DR12, DR13 and DR14 antigens are associated with a *DRB3* product (DR52 antigen), which is a heterodimer composed of the *DRA* and *DRB3* genes. Similarly, most DR4-, DR7- or DR9-positive individuals coexpress a DR53 antigen from the *DRB4* gene and DR15- and DR16-positive individuals coexpress a DR51 antigen from the *DRB5* gene. Approximately 30% of DR7 haplotypes are associated with a null nonexpressed version of the *DRB4* gene (shown in figure as the DR7** haplotype). DR1, DR103, DR10 and DR8 haplotypes do not coexpress a second DR antigen. An individual that types as DR11, DR15 would not have two different DR antigens but four—DR11, DR15, DR51 and DR52. The DR51, DR52, DR53 antigens are polymorphic and relevant in solid-organ transplantation because these antigens frequently are the target of recipient alloantibody production.

would correct the mismatched terminal base of an amplification refractory mutation system primer in a mismatched primer-template complex and subsequently permit efficient priming with the *repaired* primer. The PCR-SSP method features multiple PCR reactions in which each reaction is specific for an allele or, more commonly, a group of alleles that correspond to a serologically defined antigen. To type an individual completely at any given locus, multiple PCR-SSP reactions are set up and subjected to PCR under identical conditions. The presence or absence of PCR amplification is detected in a gel-based electrophoresis step with visualization by ethidium bromide incorporation. An example of phototyping is shown in Figure 10–5.

The first PCR-SSP typing system applicable to a single locus was described in 1992 by Olerup and Zetterquist for low-resolution HLA-DRB1 typing. The first PCR-SSP system to enable simultaneous detection of HLA-A, HLA-B, HLA-C, HLA-DRB1, HLA-DRB3, HLA-DRB4, HLA-DRB5 and HLA-DQB1 alleles was described in 1995 (Bunce *et al.*, 1995). This method, known as *phototyping*, has a resolution and accuracy far greater than average serology and takes only 3 hours to complete, making it suitable for genotyping cadaver donors. The development of automatic dispensing equipment and better electrophoresis equipment has facilitated the use of phototyping in many laboratories, and in some laboratories (including our own since September 1994), it has replaced serology completely.

An advantage of PCR-SSP is its flexible resolution; low-resolution typing systems can be upgraded to high resolution by increasing the number of reactions. The phototyping protocols are easily applicable to PCR-SSP reactions used to detect non-HLA polymorphisms, such as cytokines and their receptors. This ability facilitates simultaneous typing of HLA and non-HLA polymorphisms that may be of benefit in renal transplantation.

It is possible to use molecular methods for all tissue typing applications without recourse to serology. However, many molecular typing systems used without serology fail to identify null alleles or expression variants that may cause problems in certain transplant situations, especially in unrelated bone marrow transplantation. Most null alleles are extremely rare (Bunce *et al.*, 1999), although the DR53 null allele (Sutton *et al.*, 1989) is common in many populations. It is possible to devise PCR-SSP reactions to detect known null alleles (Bunce *et al.*, 1999), and the phototyping PCR-SSP method (Bunce *et al.*, 1995) incorporates a PCR-SSP reaction to identify the DR53 null allele (O'Neill *et al.*, 1996; see Fig. 10–4). It is possible to develop PCR-SSP reactions or PCR-SSP probes to detect new null alleles, such as the HLA-A2 null allele A*0215N (Ishikawa *et al.*, 1996), when these null alleles are sequenced. Definition of a new allele requires serology at present, and molecular determination becomes easy when the sequence becomes available. In time, greater sophistication will be required so that new null alleles can be identified by molecular techniques. Clinicians will need to identify low-expression and high-expression variants, cur-

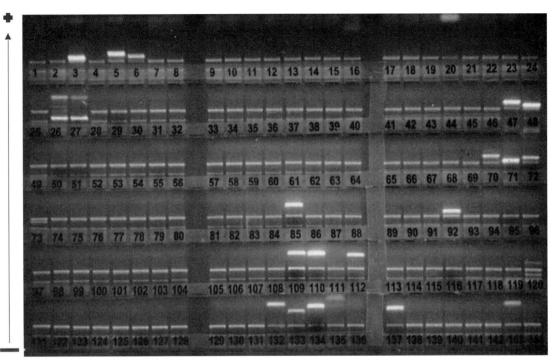

FIGURE 10–5

HLA genotyping using the phototyping method (Bunce *et al.*, 1995). Electrophoretic migration is from bottom to top (− to +). Allele-specific amplicons are shown as intense bands above the 796-bp control: Positive reactions are shown in lanes 3, 5, 6, 26, 27, 47, 48, 70, 71, 72, 85, 92, 109, 110, 112, 132, 133, 134, 137 and 143. When compared with the list of alleles amplified within each reaction, the positive reactions correspond to the HLA alleles A*03, A*23, A*38, B*1518, Cw*04, Cw*0704/11, DRB1*03, DRB1*04, DRB3*02, DRB4*01, DQB1*02 and DQB1*0302/8. To accommodate the ever-increasing number of HLA alleles, the phototyping method now used at the Oxford Transplant Centre uses more than 300 SSP reactions instead of the 144 shown in this figure.

rently observed only with serological or flow cytometry (FC) techniques.

Medium-resolution and high-resolution molecular typing methods have a wider impact on renal transplantation than just allowing accurate typing for matching purposes. The greatest impact is the ability for the transplanter to type accurately antibody screening targets, which, in turn, allows for greater dissection of patients' antibody specificities. Improvements in patients' antibody definition mean that crossmatch outcomes can be predicted more accurately, which should reduce the number of exported kidneys that cannot be used for the proposed recipient because of having an unexpected positive crossmatch. Prolonged cold ischemia time with subsequent damage can be avoided. With accurate typing before retrieval of donor kidneys and accurate antibody screening, it is feasible to transplant in some circumstances without a crossmatch and with a negligible cold ischemia time.

FUNCTION OF HLA ANTIGENS

The basic function of an HLA antigen is to present peptides to T cells. In general, but not exclusively, MHC class I antigens are responsible for aiding with the transport and for the presentation of endogenous peptides (such as those produced after viral invasion), and MHC class II antigens are responsible for the presentation of exogenous peptides, such as those resulting from bacterial breakdown. In general, but again not exclusively, CD8 T cells recognize peptides in the context of class I MHC, whereas CD4 cells recognize peptides in the context of MHC class II.

HLA Matching in Renal Transplantation

EVIDENCE THAT THE HLA SYSTEM IS THE HUMAN MAJOR HISTOCOMPATIBILITY COMPLEX

Most of the evidence that the HLA system is the human MHC comes from skin graft experiments, living related donor kidney transplants and bone marrow transplants. Within a family, the degree of histocompatibility among the members can be determined precisely. Siblings can share two (HLA identical), one (haploidentical) or no HLA haplotypes. Parents and each offspring share one haplotype and are one haplotype disparate.

The most striking proof that HLA is the MHC comes from skin graft experiments in which the immune system of the recipient was not modified by any pretreatment regimen, such as blood transfusions, or by posttransplantation immunosuppression. Ceppellini and coworkers found that skin from HLA-identical sibling donors had a mean survival time of 20 days, whereas haploidentical skin survived a mean of 13.8 days, and skin from siblings with no shared haplotype survived for 12.5 days (Ceppellini *et al.*, 1969). The last-mentioned survival time was similar to that observed with skin from totally unrelated donors (mean of 12.1 days). It was concluded that HLA is the only strong histocompatibility system in humans; if this were not the case, a quarter of the sibling grafts that were HLA mismatched would have been expected to show prolonged survival on the assumption that an MHC other than HLA segregated as a single locus independently of HLA.

In living related donor kidney transplants, an excellent correlation between the number of shared haplotypes and graft outcome has been documented by many transplant centers. In patients treated after transplantation with prednisolone and azathioprine, the reported 1-year graft survival rate was 90 to 95% for HLA-identical siblings, 70 to 80% for haploidentical siblings and parents to children and 60 to 70% when no haplotypes were shared. The results of haploidentical transplants can be improved markedly by pretreating the recipient with donor-specific blood transfusions, a protocol introduced by Salvatierra *et al.* (1981). The use of cyclosporine has led to an increase in graft survival in nontransfused patients as well as in one and two haplotype-disparate donors and recipients. This increase is so striking that most centers no longer practice donor-specific blood transfusions. The influence of HLA on kidney graft survival can be lessened by modifying the host's immune system, but this does not mean that the HLA system is not of prime importance.

Bone marrow transplants usually were carried out only between HLA-identical siblings, and identity usually was determined by serological typing and the mixed lymphocyte culture reaction. Now many centers use DNA typing in place of these two tests for the precise determination of the class II antigens. This strict selection criterion has been used because early transplants with HLA-incompatible siblings failed to implant because of rejection or developed severe, often lethal, graft-versus-host disease.

Despite the importance of the HLA system in clinical transplantation, in HLA-identical sibling combinations, skin grafts in nonimmunosuppressed recipients invariably are rejected, 5 to 10% of kidney grafts undergo rejection by the end of the first year despite immunosuppression and bone marrow transplants can be rejected and cause graft-versus-host disease. These data imply strongly that other histocompatibility antigens must exist in humans, although singly their influence on graft compatibility is not as great as that of the HLA antigens, and they are called *minor histocompatibility antigens*. Rejection through non-HLA antigens most often is described in HLA-identical transplants. Although part of the explanation is undoubtedly that non-HLA antigens are identified more easily in such transplants, it is probable that MHC restriction allows easier response to non-HLA antigens if the donor and recipient are matched. The specificity of such antibodies (e.g., to endothelium, activated endothelium, monocytes, skin and epithelium) is discussed in the section on crossmatching.

HLA MATCHING IN CADAVER DONOR TRANSPLANTATION

The checkered history of serological HLA matching in cadaver donor transplantation was reviewed in the previous editions of this book (Ting and Welsh, 1994). In living related donor transplants, excellent graft survival is seen in combinations in which the recipient and donor are matched for all (identified) HLA loci, as may occur in HLA-identical sibling transplants. For cadavers, matching to this level would be possible only if worldwide sharing were practiced. In most regional and national matching and distribution organizations, only the HLA-A, HLA-B and HLA-DR antigens are matched, and identical matches are achieved in only a relatively small proportion of donor recipient pairs. Although six antigen–matched transplants have been shown to have a better graft survival than transplants with a lesser degree of match (Opelz, 1992; Takemoto *et al.*, 1991), many studies have shown that high success rates can be achieved in *partially matched* grafts, for example, grafts matched for DR antigens only (Ting and Morris, 1978a, 1987) or for HLA-DR and HLA-B antigens (Opelz, 1992). This situation is made possi-

ble by the fact that there is a ranking order in the histocompatibility strengths of the different loci. The HLA-DR antigens are the strongest transplantation antigens, as first shown by Ting and Morris (1978a), followed by HLA-DQ and HLA-B, then HLA-A, HLA-C and HLA-DP; the orders of HLA-DQ and HLA-B are uncertain, as are those of HLA-A, HLA-C and HLA-DP. It is likely that some of these loci have more impact in retransplantation. For example, HLA-DPB mismatches are associated with increased rejection only in retransplants (Mytilineos *et al.*, 1997). An analysis of the United Kingdom data confirmed a significant influence of HLA matching on first cadaver graft outcome using a combination of matching definitions but essentially requiring compatibility at the HLA-DR locus (Morris *et al.*, 1999). Although the effect of HLA-DR matching remains, it has a less convincing effect on graft survival. In Figure 10–6, the United Kingdom data are plotted in a way that stresses that the effect of matching is more important in the first few months after transplantation and that makes it easily comparable to the section in which the relationship between matching and sensitization is discussed.

DEFINING A MATCH

Before defining what is a match, one has to consider what type of HLA typing is available because this has a bearing on what type of matching can be considered. If the typing is low resolution (i.e., serology), it is practical to match in terms of low-resolution matching based on broad antigenic groups. If higher resolution typing is available, it is possible to consider high-resolution matching using immunodominant epitope matching. The broad antigen names used in most national matching schemes mean that low-resolution matching is used in most countries. Broad antigen matching may obscure the subtler effect of matching for splits or epitopes as discussed subsequently. In practical terms, because high-resolution typing is necessary for optimal antibody defini-

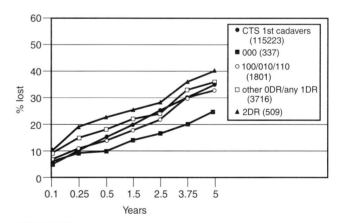

FIGURE 10–6

Two distinct trends are observed in graft survival plots—the first few months, when loss is greater, and a long-term attrition rate, which often is relatively constant. The rather unusual plot of this figure is designed to emphasize this point and to allow direct comparison with the text and form of Figures 10–8 and 10–9. All results from UKT are compared with those produced by the European Collaborative Transplant Study (CTS) for all first cadaver transplants (http://www.ctsorgtransplant.org). In the CTS data, a 5% loss occurs in 0.1 year and a 10% loss occurs in 0.25 year; the plot design reflects this log, then linear relationship between loss and time posttransplant. The 000 mismatched grafts appear to be the only group with improved attrition rates.

tion, many centers have dropped low-resolution typing because maintaining two or more techniques is inefficient.

Low-Resolution Matching

In renal transplantation, virtually all matching studies have confirmed the original findings by Ting and Morris (1978a) that DR matching is more beneficial than class I matching in renal transplantation. Subsequently, kidneys were exchanged between transplant centers on the basis of DR compatibility using low-resolution serological methods that divided the DR antigens into the broad groups DR1 to DR10. When molecular typing became available for class II, it was applied to transplant pairs to identify whether fine specificities or allelic typing improved the HLA-DR matching effect or whether inaccurate serological typing was compromising the observed HLA-DR matching effect. The first application of molecular techniques was by Opelz et al. (1991) in the Collaborative Transplant Study. This study retrospectively used RFLP and identified a better graft survival rate for RFLP-compatible grafts versus serologically typed grafts. This study gave much impetus to the notion that molecular typing was necessary for accurate class II typing because 25% of all serological donor types were found to be incorrect. Opelz and colleagues correlated matching the HLA-DR subgroups DR1 to DR18 with improved graft survival compared with matching for broad HLA-DR specificities DR1 to DR10 (Opelz et al., 1997). The conclusion was that accurate typing and matching of donors and recipients was required for optimal graft survival.

Why is the influence of HLA matching decreasing? The common answer is cyclosporine, but this still begs the original question. The simplest explanation is that an HLA-DR mismatch exerts its greatest influence through its correlation with rejection. There is no question that cyclosporine has reduced the number and severity of rejection episodes and loss of grafts from irreversible rejection. It can be hypothesized that the influence of HLA-DR matching is decreasing because cyclosporine is more efficient than HLA-DR matching in reducing rejection. This hypothesis has two corollaries. First, HLA-DR must exert its effect in the major time period during which acute rejection occurs. A plethora of United Network for Organ Sharing (UNOS), Eurotransplant and Collaborative Transplant Study published data show that the major influence of an HLA-DR mismatch on graft survival occurs well within the first year (see Fig. 10–6). Second, it predicts that rejection-induced graft loss must be no longer significant. To test this prediction we analyzed our data to compare precyclosporine and postcyclosporine 1-year graft survival results (Table 10–2).

Incomplete HLA-DR data were available on 22 transplants before the introduction of cyclosporine and on 2 transplants after its introduction. Graft failure for technical reasons before multiple rejections could occur is a confounder. Rejection data were available on all transplants, but grafts that failed before 7 days were excluded in the postcyclosporine era (22 of 912 grafts). These data were not always available for the precyclosporine grafts, and all are included. These failures were not in any particular HLA-DR match group.

One area of serological matching that has received attention is whether matching for broad or split antigens confers a better chance of success. Generally, matching schemes traditionally have used broad-antigen matching rather than split-antigen matching. For example, the broad antigen A9 is considered matched with either of its splits, A23 and A24; B21 is considered matched with B49 and B50. Opelz (1988), analyzing the data accumulated through the Collaborative Transplant Study, found that split HLA-A and HLA-B antigen matching gave a better correlation with graft survival than broad-antigen matching. Previous studies had not found an advantage of matching for splits (Sanfilippo et al., 1985). Matching for splits rather than broad antigens results in fewer six antigen–matched transplants, but if a better success rate is achieved, the policy is worthwhile. In a large and currently unpublished analysis carried out on the United Kingdom Transplant Service Support Authority (UKTSSA) database, split-antigen matching did show advantage. Centers that introduced the molecular typing necessary for such analysis may have concomitantly lowered their error rates, however.

High-Resolution Matching

The nomenclature used for describing HLA antigen and HLA mismatches disguises the level of amino acid epitope mismatching that may be occurring in transplants. It is possible to have an HLA-identical donor-recipient combination that may be mismatched for many amino acid epitopes (Fig. 10–7A). It also is possible that a donor-recipient combination with a single serologically defined mismatch may have fewer amino acid mismatches than an apparently HLA-identical pair (Fig. 10–7B). It is likely that some amino acid mismatches could be more immunodominant than others. For example, it is to be expected that amino acid substitutions in the α helix of class I or II would be more immunodominant than a substitution in the β-pleated sheet that creates the base of the peptide binding groove (Adorno et al., 1999). Further complexity in amino acid mismatching may be created by the possibility that different amino acids may have different capacity to elicit an immune response. For example, it is likely that amino acids with large side chains, such as tyrosine, would be more immunogenic than others with small side chains. Such complexity in epitope analysis can be resolved only by applying high-resolution typing and more sophisticated computer-based analysis. In time, however, it is hoped that investigators will be able to define a set of rules governing which epitopes are permissible and in which combinations. Various groups already have seen a beneficial effect of matching for epitopes rather than antigens (McKenna et al., 1998; Takemoto and Terasaki, 1991), although these studies were based on serologically defined antigens in which the epitopes are defined using crude cross-reactive groups.

Flexible Mismatching

Various reports suggest that HLA class II genes are the human immune response genes, and as such the class II phenotype of the recipient should contribute to governing which HLA antigens may be responded to. One would expect, from knowledge of differential peptide binding to the MHC, that mismatched HLA antigens after processing would be differentially recognized depending on the MHC class II type of the recipient. Sanfilippo and coworkers showed that patients that reject an HLA-incompatible graft rarely produce antibodies to all the mismatches, suggesting that some mismatches are not recognized by the recipient's immune system (Sanfilippo et al., 1982). Other investigators (Brier-Vriesendorp and Ivanyi, 1986; Young et al., 1997) have shown that T-cell responses to HLA vary. Fuller and Fuller (1999) showed that 73% of patients producing antibody to an HLA-Bw4 epitope expressed either DRB1*01 or DRB1*03 class II alloantigens, suggesting that these alloantigens confer a high risk for Bw4 mismatching. These data taken together suggest that the combinations of donor-recipient phenotypes should be taken into consideration when performing retrospective

TABLE 10–2

INFLUENCE OF GRAFT REJECTION ON CADAVER ALLOGRAFT SURVIVAL*

	Precyclosporine (1974–1985)		Postcyclosporine (1986–1999)	
	Graft no.	*1-year Survival (%)*	*Graft no.*	*1-year Survival (%)*
Total no.	504	65.5	912	83.3
DR matched	155	76.1	397	84.4
DR mismatched	327	60.6	513	82.7
P value for match		0.0008		NS
No rejection	53	81.1	324	86.7
1 or 2 rejections	270	68.5	455	85.1
> 2 rejections	181	56.4	110	80.0
P value for rejection		0.001		NS

*This table includes first grafts and regrafts and excludes patients in whom 1-year follow-up is not available. The changeover point (precyclosporine or postcyclosporine) is reasonably distinct and corresponds to the introduction of triple therapy in Oxford. Eighteen patients were reallocated because they were given cyclosporine in small trials before this time point (they are allocated to the postcyclosporine period), or they were not given it after the changeover (they are allocated to the precyclosporine era). Postcyclosporine immunosuppression has been triple therapy for most recipients. The results indicate that there is no longer a significant relationship between rejection episodes and graft loss at 1 year. Since the introduction of cyclosporine, 1-year graft survival in patients who escape rejection-free has risen by 5%; in patients suffering one or two rejections, it has increased 16.6%, and in patients suffering multiple rejections, it has risen 23.6%.
NS = not significant.

survival studies. These types of study should enable investigators to define a rule set showing which combinations of antigens should be avoided and which epitope mismatches should be avoided. This rule set should lead to matching algorithms designed to take into account the HLA phenotype of the recipients and donors, and kidneys could be allocated by an amino acid mismatch score rather than the number of HLA-A, HLA-B and HLA-DR mismatches.

Value of HLA Matching

Not all transplant centers believe in the value of HLA matching. This is not to say that such centers do not accept that HLA is the MHC, but they question the practicality of HLA matching in cadaver donor programs in which the high polymorphism of the antigens results in a low chance of finding well-matched donors for most recipients. Another important factor is that the need to transport kidneys leads to much longer cold ischemia times. The influence of ischemia time is controversial, but it is apparent that live donor grafts between unrelated unmatched persons do better than expected (see Chapter 39; Kaufman *et al.*, 1993), whereas cadaver grafts with long cold ischemia times (>24 hours) do worse than expected, especially if the recipient is sensitized. The effect of ischemia may be biphasic, with an important effect in the first hour or so, then with little effect until after 24 hours.

Centers that do not have a matching policy often use other means of ensuring graft success. It has been shown that DR mismatching leads to more rejection, but that with modern drugs more rejection need not mean poorer survival. Such centers also use additional immunosuppressive agents, such as antilymphocyte globulin or OKT3, regularly for induction.

A further important point is that absolute definition of antibody responses in transfused, previously transplanted or multiparous women defines which transplant antigens are acceptable as mismatches; this may be the reason why many centers that do not define antibody have a marked HLA matching effect for second and subsequent grafts. Basically, if antibodies have not been defined, possibly because of failure to store samples, there is a need to match to ensure that an anamnestic response would not occur to any given mismatch.

Detection of Sensitization and Crossmatching
CAUSES OF SENSITIZATION AND HIGH SENSITIZATION

Sensitization is indicated by the presence of lymphocyte cytotoxic or binding antibodies in the patient's serum. Sera from patients waiting for solid-organ transplants should be screened for antibodies against a panel of lymphocyte donors on a regular basis and after an immunizing event, such as a blood transfusion. The degree of sensitization depends on the proportion of the test panel against which the serum reacts. The criterion used to define high sensitization varies among laboratories from 50 to 90% panel-reactive antibodies (PRA). Our definition, in common with many other European centers, is 85% or greater PRA. The main causes of sensitization are pregnancies, blood transfusions, failed grafts, bacterial and viral infections and autoimmune diseases. Transfer of intact white cells between individuals by any route as well as the transfer of viable tissue (e.g., heart valves) can induce primary sensitization. Platelets and infection in general cannot induce primary stimulation of an alloresponse but are capable of inducing secondary responses (Welsh *et al.*, 1977).

About 50% of women with two or more pregnancies develop cytotoxic antibodies. These antibodies may be long lasting (≥20 years) or may disappear after a short time (weeks). Blood transfusions can cause sensitization, but the risk of causing high sensitization (>90% PRA) is low even with 20 transfusions unless the patient was pregnant previously (Opelz *et al.*, 1981). Most patients develop antibodies after a rejected graft (Morris *et al.*, 1968), particularly if the graft is rejected early and removed (Sumrani *et al.*, 1992). The appearance of IgM non-HLA lymphocytotoxic antibodies has been associated with viral infections, in particular cytomegalovirus (Jeannet and Stalder, 1978) and systemic lupus erythematosus (Revillard *et al.*, 1979). In most cases, these non-HLA antibodies are autoreactive.

The major cause of high sensitization is a failed graft, particularly if the graft fails early. The intensity of sensitization often is magnified if the graft is removed, immunosuppression is stopped and the patient is transfused at the time of graft nephrectomy. In patients who are to be considered for retransplantation, it is important to collect a serum sample 2 to 4 weeks after failure of the previous graft because it is at this time that the patient is most likely to develop high PRA.

HLA Details
Recipient HLA phenotype: A2,30 B60,15, Cw9,10, DR4,13,52,53, DQ6,7
Donor HLA phenotype: A2,30 B61,15, Cw2,7, DR4,13,52,53, DQ6,7

Recipient genotype: A*0201,*3001, B*1501,*4001, Cw*0303,*0304, DRB1*0401,*1301, DRB4*0101, DRB3*0101, DQB1*0603,*0301
Donor genotype: A*0205,*3002, B*1516,*4002, Cw*0202,*0701, DRB1*0404,*1302, DRB4*0101, DRB3*0301, DQB1*0603,*0301

UKTSSA defined A-B-DR mismatches:	000
Class I amino acid mismatch totals:	21

Recipient HLA-A,B,C Alpha-1 domain

```
              10        20         30         40         50         60         70         80         90
Consensus  GSHSMRYFYT SVSRPGRGEP RFIAVGYVDD TQFVRFDSDA ASPREEPRAP WIEQEGPEYW DRNTQKYKAQ AQTDRESLRN LRGYYNQSEA
A*0201     --------F- ---------- ---------- ---------- ---QR----- ---------- --GE-R-V--H S--H-VD-GT ---------A
A*3001     --------S- ------S--- ---------- ---------- ---QR----- -----R---- --QE-RNV--Q S----VD-GT ---------A
B*1501     --------F- AM-------- ---------- ---------- ----MA---- ---------- --E--I S-TN T--Y------ ----------
B*4001     --------H- AM-------- ---T------ -L-------- T---K----- ---------- --E---S-TN T--Y------ ----------
Cw*0303    ---------- A--------- H--------- ---------- ----G----- -V-------- --------R- -----VS--- ----------
Cw*0304    ---------- A--------- H--------- ---------- ----G----- -V-------- --------R- -----VS--- ----------
```

Donor HLA-A,B,C Alpha-1 domain

```
A*0205     ---------- ---------- ---------- ---------- ---RR----- ---------- -GE-R-V--H S--H-VD-GT ---------A
A*3002     --------S- ------S--- ---------- ---------- ---QR----- -----R---- --QE-RNV--H S-----N-GT ---------A
B*1516     ---F----F- AM-------- ---------- ---------- ----MA---- ---------- --E-RNM--S --Y--N--I  ALR------
B*4002     --------H- ---------- ---T------ -L-------- T---K----- ---------- --E---S-TN T--Y------ ----------
Cw*0202    C--------- A----S---- H--------- ---------- ----G----- -V-------- --------R- -----VN--K ----------
Cw*0701    C-------D- A--------- ---S------ ---------- ----G----- -V-------- ---N--R-- --A--VS--- ---------D
```

Recipient HLA-A,B,C Alpha-2 domain

```
              100       110        120        130        140        150        160        170        180
Consensus  GSHTLQSMYG CDVGPDGRLL RGHDQYAYDG KDYIALNEDL RSWTAADTAA QITQRKWEAA REAEQRRAYL EGECVEWLRR YLENGKDKLE
A*0201     ----V-R--- ----S-W-F- --YH-Y---- ------K--- ------M-- -T-KH----- HV---L---- --T--EW--- ------T-Q
A*3001     ----I-I--- ----S---F- --YE-H---- --------- ------M-- ---Q------ RW---L---- --T--EW--- ------T-Q
B*1501     ------R--- ---------- -----S---- --------- S--------- ---------- -----W---- --L------- -----ET-Q
B*4001     ------R--- ---------- ---N------ ---------- ---------- ---S--L--- -V---L---- ---------- ----------
Cw*0303    R--I I-R--- --V------- --Y------- ---------- ---------- ---------- -----L---- --L------- ---K------
Cw*0304    ---I I-R--- G-L--R--Y- A-Y------- H--A------ ---------- ---------- ---------- --T------- ----------
```

Donor HLA-A,B,C Alpha-2 domain

```
A*0205     ----L-R--- ----S-W-F- --YH-Y---- ------K--- ------M-- -T-KH----- HV---W---- --T--EW--- ------T-Q
A*3002     ----I-I--- ----S---F- --YE-H---- --------- ------M-- ---Q------ RR---L---- --T--EW--- ------T-Q
B*1516     ---W-R--- --L------- -----S---- --------- S--------- ---------- -----L---- --L------- -----ET-Q
B*4002     ---------- ---------- ---N------ ---------- ---------- ---------- -V---L---- ---------- -----ET-Q
Cw*0202    ------R--- --L------- --Y--S---- ---------- ---------- ---------- -----W---- ---------- ----------
Cw*0701    ------R--- --L--R--D- A-Y------- ---------- ---------- ---------- ---------- --T--N--- --A-------
```

A

FIGURE 10–7

The concept of amino acid epitope matching instead of matching for serologically defined antigens is illustrated. A serologically defined antigen such as A2 may be encoded for by any one of approximately 40 different alleles—all with different amino acid epitopes; a serological A2 match between a donor and a recipient may have some amino acid mismatches. (A) A hypothetical situation in which the class I amino acid sequences of a serologically identical but amino acid–mismatched donor-recipient pair are shown as amino acid sequences. The donor amino acid mismatches are shaded and show that in this serologically identical pair there are 21 amino acid mismatches, including 4 in the immunodominant Bw4 epitope of the α helix at positions 77–83.

HLA Details
Recipient HLA phenotype: A2,30 B60,15, Cw9,10, DR4,13,52,53, DQ6,7
Donor HLA phenotype: A2,30 B61,18, Cw2,7, DR4,13,52,53, DQ6,7

Recipient genotype: A*0201,*3001, B*1501,*4001, Cw*0303,*0304, DRB1*0401,*1301, DRB4*0101, DRB3*0101, DQB1*0603,*0301
Donor genotype: A*0205,*3002, B*1801,*4002, Cw*0202,*0701, DRB1*0404,*1302, DRB4*0101, DRB3*0301, DQB1*0603,*0301

UKTSSA defined A-B-DR mismatches: 000
Class I amino acid mismatch totals: 16

Recipient HLA-A,B,C Alpha-1 domain
```
            10        20        30        40        50        60        70        80        90
Consensus GSHSMRYFYT SVSRPGRGEP RFIAVGYVDD TQFVRFDSDA ASPREEPRAP WIEQEGPEYW DRNTQKYKAQ AQTDRESLRN LRGYYNQSEA
A*0201    -------F- ---------- ---------- ---------- --QR------ ---------- -GE-R-V--H S--H-VD-GT ---------A
A*3001    -------S- ------S--- ---------- ---------- --QR------ -----R---- -QE-RNV--Q S----VD-GT ---------A
B*1501    -------F- AM-------- ---------- ---------- ----MA---- ---------- --E--IS-TN T--Y------ ----------
B*4001    -------H- AM-------- ---T------ --L------- -T---K---- ---------- --E---S-TN T--Y------ ----------
Cw*0303   ---------- A--------- H--------- ---------- ----G----- -V-------- --------R- -----VS--- ----------
Cw*0304   ---------- A--------- H--------- ---------- ----G----- -V-------- --------R- -----VS--- ----------
```

Donor HLA-A,B,C Alpha-1 domain
```
A*0205    ---------- ---------- ---------- ---------- --RR------ ---------- -GE-R-V--H S--H-VD-GT ---------A
A*3002    ---------S- ------S--- ---------- ---------- --QR------ -----R---- -QE-RNV--Q S-----N-GT ---------A
B*1801    ---------H- ---------- ----G----- ---------- ----T----- ---------- ------S-TN T--Y------ ----------
B*4002    ---------H- ---------- ---T------ --L------- -T---K---- ---------- --E---S-TN T--Y------ ----------
Cw*0202   C--------- A----S---- H--------- ---------- ----G----- -V-------- --------R- -----VN--K ----------
Cw*0701   C------D- A--------- --S------- ---------- ----G----- -V-------- -----N--R- -A--VS--- --------D
```

Recipient HLA-A,B,C Alpha-2 domain
```
            100       110       120       130       140       150       160       170       180
Consensus GSHTLQSMYG CDVGPDGRLL RGHDQYAYDG KDYIALNEDL RSWTAADTAA QITQRKWEAA REAEQRRAYL EGECVEWLRR YLENGKDKLE
A*0201    ----V-R--- ----S-W-F- --YH-Y---- ------K--- -------M-- -T-KH----- HV---L---- --T--EW--- -------T-Q
A*3001    ----I-I--- ----S---F- --YE-H---- ---------- -------M-- ---Q------ RW---L---- --T--EW--- -------T-Q
B*1501    ------R--- ---------- -----S---- ---------- -S-------- ---------- -----W---- --L------- ------ET-Q
B*4001    ------R--- ---------- ---N------ ---------- ---S--L--- -V--L----- ---------- ---------- ----------
Cw*0303   R--II-R--- --V------- --Y------- ---------- ---------- ---------- -----L---- --L------- --K-------
Cw*0304   ---II-R--- G-L--R--Y- A-Y------- --H--A---- ---------- ---------- ---------- --T------- ----------
```

Donor HLA-A,B,C Alpha-2 domain
```
A*0205    ----L-R--- ----S-W-F- --YH-Y---- ------K--- -------M-- -T-KH----- HV---W---- --T--EW--- -------T-Q
A*3002    ----I-I--- ----S---F- --YE-H---- ---------- -------M-- ---Q------ RR---L---- --T--EW--- -------T-Q
B*1801    ------R--- --L------- -----S---- ---------- -S-------- ---------- -V---L---- --T------- H-----ET-Q
B*4002    ---------- ---N------ ---------- ---------- ---------- -V---L---- ---------- ---------- ------ET-Q
Cw*0202   ------R--- --L------- --Y--S---- ---------- ---------- ---------- -----W---- ---------- ----------
Cw*0701   ------R--- --L--R--D- A-Y------- ---------- ---------- ---------- ---------- --T--N---- --A-------
```

B

FIGURE 10–7 *Continued*

(B) The B15 antigen of the donor is replaced with a B18 antigen, which creates a 0-1-0 serologically defined mismatch, which has five fewer amino acid mismatches than the HLA-identical pair in (A). This difference is principally due to increased compatibility at positions 77–83.

TABLE 10–3

RELATIONSHIP BETWEEN SENSITIZATION STATUS AND TIME ON THE WAITING LIST ANALYZED OVER 10 YEARS

No. in Group	All Patients	Highly Sensitized	Non–Highly Sensitized
827 (All transplants)	300 ± 514 d	1,054 ± 1,133 d	221 ± 308 d
743 (Cadavers only)	308 ± 321 d	1,081 ± 1,154 d	235 ± 309 d

Highly sensitized individuals (those having a panel reactivity of >85%) wait significantly longer for grafts; even with the large standard deviations shown in this table, the *P* values between waiting time are <0.00001.

Should Sensitization Be Considered in Matching Algorithms?

We strongly believe that the answer to the question should sensitization be considered in matching algorithms is *yes*, but this is not a currently accepted concept. The reasons for this proposed consideration are twofold. First, young people may need many grafts throughout their lifetime, and sensitization increases with each failure. In general, the lower the mismatch, the lower the likelihood of possible sensitization. Table 10–3 shows how important sensitization is to the time people have to wait for their grafts in our center. Table 10–4 shows the association between graft number and sensitization.

This tripartite relationship between sensitization, waiting time and graft number is strong, but the attempts to link sensitization status in a more specific way directly to mismatch numbers have been less convincing. This situation is not surprising because of the misleading way in which panel reactivity generally is presented and the markedly different population frequencies of individual HLA antigens coupled with the known rules that govern particular mismatch responsiveness. It can be argued that the data already available are sufficient to force matching to be reevaluated to include sensitization in the algorithm. An additional benefit in terms of the survival of second and subsequent grafts might accrue because, as shown in Figure 10–8, the average graft survival in second and subsequent grafts is poorer. In Oxford and other centers in the United Kingdom with accurate screening, the results are essentially the same. In Figure 10–9, we show that within Europe graft failure rates increase with graft number up to 1 year. Similar to the effect of HLA-DR and the effect of cyclosporine, no further improvement occurs. We include the Oxford retransplant data in Figure 10–9 to show that the effect does not occur in our center.

A reasonable hypothesis can be constructed to explain the difference in survival times between grafts into sensitized and nonsensitized patients that occur in some centers and not others. This hypothesis draws on the fact that all of the difference in survival occurs in the first few months

posttransplant, the period in which most rejection occurs. It simply states that antibody status is a marker for specific T cells, and unless the antibody screening pretransplant is adequate, the chances of vascular and cellular rejection are high. Vascular rejection is ill defined on the Banff criteria. The hypothesis is not easy to test in many centers because for adequate crossmatching or screening involving historical samples, such samples must exist. A survey from the United Kingdom found that one third of United Kingdom centers do not collect regular posttransplant samples (S. Fuggle, 2000, personal communication).

How Would a Matching Algorithm That Takes into Account Sensitization Work?

Certain antigen mismatch combinations are known not to induce antibody response. A simple analysis of these on a large database would validate the hypothesis because they should induce less sensitization and shorter waiting times for subsequent grafts.

IMPORTANCE OF SENSITIZATION AND LYMPHOCYTE CROSSMATCHING

In 1965, Terasaki *et al.* reported a case of a woman who suffered an immediate rejection of a kidney transplanted from her brother. Tests of the recipient's serum collected before transplantation revealed cytotoxic antibodies against the donor's lymphocytes. This was the first report of a possible association between pregraft donor-reactive lymphocytotoxic antibodies and immediate graft rejection. The authors

TABLE 10–4

GRAFT NUMBER INFLUENCES SENSITIZATION STATUS*

	Highly Sensitized (n = 218)	Non–Highly Sensitized (n = 1,361)
First transplant	89	1,215
Second transplant	90	134
Third transplant	30	11
> 3 transplants	9	1
P value between groups	Chi = 355	*P* = <0.00000001

*This association between transplant number and sensitization status is becoming more significant as blood transfusion (a second major source of sensitization) decreases.

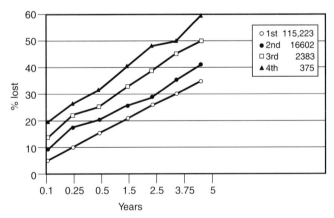

FIGURE 10–8

This graph shows that second and subsequent grafts do progressively worse. It is plotted in such a way as to indicate that effectively all of this difference can be accounted for over the first 5 to 6 weeks posttransplant. After this period, the rate of graft loss is equal in all groups. The raw data were taken from the European Collaborative Transplant Study Internet site (http://www.ctsorgtransplant.org).

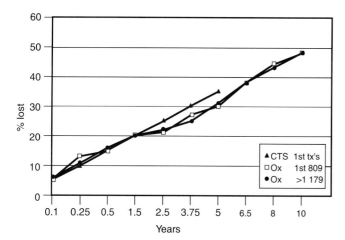

FIGURE 10–9

This graph, plotted in the same way as that for Figure 10–8, compares the first and subsequent (>1) graft survival results in Oxford with those taken from the Collaborative Transplant Study data. We hypothesize that the fact our data are independent of transplant number is an indication of a thorough screening policy (see text) because it is also the case in other United Kingdom centers with similar policies.

stated: "The 'crossmatch' test in which the serum of the prospective recipient is tested with the donor's cells before transplantation is done easily and may be important in preventing a certain number of early rejections."

Reports with the same conclusion subsequently appeared in the literature (Kissmeyer-Nielsen *et al.*, 1966; Patel and Terasaki, 1969; Williams *et al.*, 1968), and by the late 1960s, all laboratories were performing the crossmatch test before transplantation. A positive crossmatch was considered a strict contraindication to transplantation. The screening and crossmatch protocol used by most laboratories from that time until the early 1980s included the following three stages. First, serum samples from all patients on the waiting list were screened periodically for cytotoxic antibodies against a peripheral blood lymphocyte panel using the standard National Institutes of Health technique (30 minutes before and 60 minutes after complement incubation). Second, a pregraft crossmatch was performed against the donor's peripheral blood lymphocytes, spleen or lymph node cells, with a selection of PRA-positive sera and the latest serum using the standard technique. Third, a patient was considered to be crossmatch positive if any serum sample gave a positive crossmatch.

The introduction of crossmatching led to a significant decrease in the incidence of immediate rejection of grafts, but also it meant that many sensitized patients were not transplanted or waited a long time for a transplant (with a negative crossmatch). Since then, studies of sensitization and crossmatching have proceeded in two main directions: to search for more sensitive crossmatch techniques and to determine if some lymphocytotoxic antibody specificities are not damaging to the graft (i.e., clinically irrelevant antibodies).

SENSITIVITY OF PANEL-REACTIVE ANTIBODY SCREENING AND CROSSMATCH TESTS

The search for as well as the use of sensitive crossmatch tests has been prompted by the fact that some grafts suffer early rejection despite a negative standard lymphocytotoxic crossmatch. It is assumed that these rejections are caused by antibodies that are not detected in the standard crossmatch test because they are present in low levels, they do not bind complement *in vitro* or they do not react with lymphocytes but instead with tissue cells. It is relatively easy to find a technique that is more sensitive than the standard cytotoxic method. As the sensitivity of a test increases, however, the rate of false-positive results also increases. The predicament that faces many transplant centers and histocompatibility laboratories in deciding which crossmatch tests to use is how to adjust the balance between tests that are too sensitive and tests that are not sensitive enough. If a test is too sensitive, many patients are denied the opportunity of a successful transplant, and if it is not sensitive enough, early graft rejections are seen.

The philosophies of European and American laboratories vary on sensitive crossmatch tests. In Europe, most laboratories use only the standard cytotoxic method, or some may use a prolonged postcomplement incubation. Few laboratories routinely use antiglobulin augmentation or FC methods. In the United States, the American Society for Histocompatibility and Immunogenetics (ASHI) Standards for Histocompatibility Testing state that "Crossmatching must use techniques documented to have increased sensitivity in comparison with the basic microlymphocytotoxicity test (incubation of cells with antiserum, addition of complement and addition of vital dye)," such as prolonged incubation, washing or augmentation with antiglobulin or FC. Some sensitive screening and crossmatch techniques and their reported clinical relevancy are described.

Prolonged Incubation

With the prolonged incubation test, the postcomplement incubation time is increased to 2 hours from the standard 1 hour. This is the most simple way to increase the sensitivity of the cytotoxic test and the one used by many laboratories, particularly in Europe. The clinical relevance of the weak antibodies detected by prolonged incubation has not been proved, however. These antibodies may not be clinically relevant because Jeannet and colleagues reported 11 of 13 successful transplants performed in the presence of a T-cell crossmatch when the postcomplement incubation was positive at 2 hours but negative at 1 hour (Jeannet *et al.*, 1981).

Wash (Amos) Technique

Washing out the serum after the serum-lymphocyte incubation step and before the addition of complement increases the sensitivity of the test by removing anticomplementary factors in serum, such as immune complexes and immunoglobulin aggregates. The IgM antibodies probably are not detected by this technique because they have a lower affinity and/or avidity than IgG antibodies that enables them to be detached from the cell surface during the wash steps.

Antihuman Globulin Augmentation

The antihuman globulin (AHG) augmentation test differs from the standard test in that an antihuman globulin or anti–κ light chain reagent is added to the serum-lymphocyte mixture after washing out excess serum and before adding complement (Fuller *et al.*, 1978). The extra reactions detected by this method are thought to be predominantly HLA, and along with weak HLA antibodies, it may detect public antibodies not detected by standard cytotoxicity (Fuller, 1991). There is no agreement on the value of this test in predicting grafts that will suffer acute rejection. Some authors concluded from their studies that an AHG-positive crossmatch may be relevant clinically only in recipients of a regraft or in highly sensitized patients but is of little value in nonsensitized and other low-risk patients (Kerman *et al.*, 1991). Gifford and coworkers found that the role of the AHG method has diminished with the currently used posttransplant immunosuppressive strategies that are more potent than those employed previously (Gifford *et al.*, 1986). Similar to the wash method, the AHG method does not detect most IgM antibodies.

Immunomagnetic Bead Isolation of Lymphocytes

Monoclonal antibody–coated immunomagnetic beads rosette around the cells with the greatest antigen density, and after separation these cells are more susceptible to lysis by specific antibodies. The necessary use of fluorescent dyes may help increase the sensitivity. The increased sensitivity of these cells to lysis has resulted in a reduction of the postcomplement incubation times from 2 hours to less than 1 hour for class II typing. Povlsen and associates showed that the immunomagnetic bead separation (IM) technique was more sensitive for crossmatching than the Kissmeyer-Nielsen (KN) technique when the same incubation times were used (Povlsen *et al.*, 1991). The KN-negative and IM-positive crossmatch transplants did not have a worse survival or complication rate than the KN-negative and IM-negative crossmatch transplants. The extra antibodies (that the authors believed were HLA) detected by IM crossmatching may be irrelevant clinically.

Flow Cytometry

Flow cytometry has been reported to have a 30-fold to 250-fold range of greater sensitivity than standard cytotoxicity methods (Garovoy *et al.*, 1983) and a 16-fold greater sensitivity than the AHG method (Thistlethwaite *et al.*, 1986). In our Oxford experience, FACscan analysis is 10-fold to 50-fold more sensitive than standard cytotoxicity methods for detecting IgG antibodies to HLA targets and at least 10-fold less sensitive for the rare IgM antibodies detecting HLA targets. An example of an FC crossmatch is shown in Figure 10–10. We have not used the AHG test. It is probable that this apparent IgG-IgM disparity reflects the effect of FC wash steps on the usually lower IgM affinity plus the much greater ability of IgM to fix rabbit complement.

In 1983, Garovoy *et al.* found that the number of failed grafts was higher in patients transplanted with FC-positive crossmatches than those with FC-negative crossmatches. This finding has been confirmed by others (Iwaki *et al.*, 1987; Mahoney *et al.*, 1990; Talbot *et al.*, 1989). Mahoney *et al.* (1990) found that the FC crossmatch test gave a 16% false-positive rate (12 of 76 FC-positive crossmatch transplants did well) and a 29% false-negative rate (4 of 14 FC-crossmatch negative grafts failed); this may be considered unacceptably high to some people. Lazda *et al.* (1988) found an increase in the incidence of early reversible rejection episodes in FC-positive crossmatch transplants but not an overall lower graft survival. Some studies could not find a benefit of FC crossmatching (Chapman *et al.*, 1985) or found that the test was useful only in immunologically high-risk patients, such as patients having regrafts and highly sensitized patients (Kerman *et al.*, 1990; Mahoney *et al.*, 1990).

The place of FC crossmatching in renal transplantation has not been worked out fully, but today the centers, including our own, that perform the test use it mostly for immunologically high-risk patients. The literature quoted indicates that false-positives are detected by the method, but it is suspected by many that the false-positives are not usually

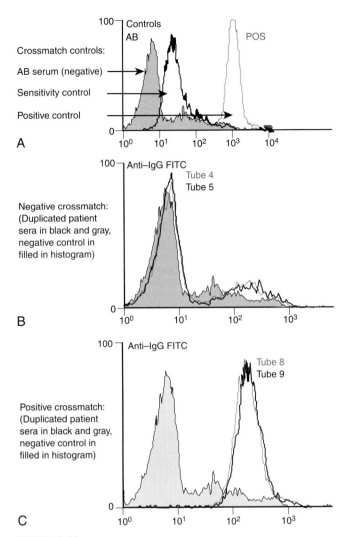

FIGURE 10–10

A flow crossmatch detecting IgG antidonor antibodies. For each crossmatch, donor lymphocytes are incubated with potential recipients' serum samples, unbound antibody is washed off the cells and a FITC-conjugated antihuman IgG second antibody is added. Unbound second antibody is removed by washing, and the cells are assayed in a flow cytometer. For each series of crossmatches, a set of controls are used (A), which includes a negative control (AB serum), a positive control (mixture of HLA multispecific alloantisera) and a $\frac{1}{256}$ dilution of the positive control, which is a sensitivity control. The sensitivity control gives approximately a half-log FACS shift—any antidonor response greater than a half-log shift is considered positive within this system. (B) The FACS profile shows a duplicated patient's serum overlaying the negative control—clearly there is no shift, and the crossmatch is negative. (C) The FACS profile shows a positive crossmatch in which the shift is much greater than the sensitivity control.

antibodies to HLA. In other words, a weak positive on a lymphocyte target in a potential recipient with no history of any type of sensitization is not caused by anti-HLA. In a potential recipient with a history of sensitization, a weak positive stands a much higher chance of being directed against HLA. The use of FC for detecting non-HLA antibodies reactive with monocytes and endothelial cells (i.e., which are relevant to transplantation) also is prudent in highly sensitized recipients and is discussed later.

Even if a technique is more sensitive than the standard

cytotoxicity method, it does not follow that it is detecting clinically relevant antibodies. For example, if an antibody detected is lymphocyte specific, it might have a beneficial effect on graft outcome by clearance of passenger cells from a donor organ. The place of FC still needs further development, and one has to determine more formally whether a sensitive crossmatch technique is needed for all patients or is needed only for immunologically high-risk patients.

Clinically Relevant and Irrelevant Lymphocytotoxic Antibodies

Many variables have been examined alone or in combination in attempts to separate clinically relevant from irrelevant antibodies. Some of these are the specificity of the antibody, the precomplement incubation temperature of the cytotoxic test, the immunoglobulin class of the antibody and the role of old and current sera in crossmatching.

ANTIBODY SPECIFICITY

Two studies published in 1976 were the first to show that not all lymphocytotoxic antibodies are damaging to grafts by documenting successful renal transplantation despite positive crossmatches with pregraft sera. Ettenger *et al.* (1976) reported successful transplantation in seven pediatric patients despite a positive B-cell crossmatch (the T-cell crossmatch was negative in all cases). It was assumed that the specificity of the antibodies was HLA-DR, although studies were not performed to characterize their specificities formally. Cross *et al.* (1976) described nine successful transplants with a positive crossmatch against the donors' unseparated peripheral blood lymphocytes. The percentages killed against each donor ranged from 50 to 80%, which means that the antibodies reacted with T and B cells. The investigators showed that in all cases the antibodies reacted with the patients' own cells (i.e., the antibodies were autoreactive).

On the basis of these and other subsequently published studies, it became evident that lymphocytotoxic antibodies can have different specificities; this is probably the major factor determining whether or not the antibodies cause graft rejection. The specificities we can now detect can be divided into three broad groups: HLA-A, HLA-B, HLA-C; HLA-DR, HLA-DQ and non-HLA.

HLA-A, HLA-B and HLA-C Antibodies

The HLA-A, HLA-B and HLA-C antibodies react with T and B lymphocytes, although weak antibodies may react with B cells alone because these cells have a higher density of class I antigens than T cells (Pellegrino *et al.*, 1978). It is most likely that hyperacute rejections of renal allografts are caused by HLA class I antibodies. Successful transplantation has been seen, however, in the presence of a positive crossmatch owing to class I antibodies but only under certain conditions. The first condition is when the antibody is present in old serum but not in the serum collected just before transplantation (Cardella *et al.*, 1982). This subject is discussed subsequently. A second condition is when the antibody is IgM (Chapman *et al.*, 1986b), which is discussed in the section on immunoglobulin class. Transplanting across peak-positive IgG crossmatches in which the antibody has been proved to be directed against HLA class I has not been successful at Oxford (Taylor *et al.*, 1989). Repeat mismatches involving HLA-A and HLA-B are well known to induce a rapid response if prior sensitization to them has been observed (Welsh *et al.*, 1988), including repeat mismatches for HLA-C (Chapman *et al.*, 1986b).

HLA-DR and HLA-DQ Antibodies

The HLA-DR and HLA-DQ antibodies react with B cells, and HLA-DR antibodies react with activated T cells. The relevance of class II antibodies is unclear for many reasons. First, many transplant centers do not perform a B-lymphocyte crossmatch and transplant solely on the basis of the T-cell result. In these centers, many positive B-cell crossmatch transplants would have been performed, but whether they were class II or non-HLA antibodies is not known. Second, in most published reports on positive B-cell crossmatch transplants, the specificity of the antibody has not been characterized as class II or non-HLA. Class II antigens are found on kidney tissue, such as the endothelium of peritubular capillaries (Daar *et al.*, 1984); one may expect that class II antibodies could cause rejection. Early graft failures in the presence of a positive B-cell crossmatch owing to class II antibodies have been reported (Scornick *et al.*, 1992), but successful grafts also have been reported, even when the antibody was IgG (directed against HLA-DQ) and present at the time of transplantation (Taylor *et al.*, 1987). In this last report, the antibody causing the positive crossmatch had a high titer of 1:128 immediately before transplantation, and the antibody was detected in the serum after transplantation at the same titer. In contrast to the situation with class I antibodies, the immunoglobin isotype of class II antibodies is probably not a reliable predictor of graft outcome (Karuppan *et al.*, 1992; Taylor *et al.*, 1989).

Class II antibodies that react with the donor probably are not an absolute contraindication to transplantation but may represent a relative contraindication in that an overall lower graft survival rate may be expected, particularly in regrafts (Taylor *et al.*, 1989), or a greater number of rejection episodes may occur. Nevertheless, many, if not most, laboratories do not perform B-cell crossmatching routinely and transplant purely on the basis of the T-cell crossmatch result.

Non-HLA Antibodies That Are Not Graft Damaging

Non-HLA antibodies that are not graft damaging can react with T and B lymphocytes or with B lymphocytes alone, and some react with B lymphocytes from chronic lymphocytic leukemia patients (CLL cells), whereas others do not (Ting and Morris, 1978b; Taylor *et al.*, 1991). Despite the different reactivity profiles, the specificity of these antibodies is probably the same (Taylor *et al.*, 1991). The variability in autoantibody reactivity with target cells is a reflection of the titer of the antibody and the sensitivity of the various target cells. The incidence of autoantibodies in renal failure patients has been reported to be 42% (Lobo, 1981), although most centers find a lower incidence and some none at all; perhaps 10 to 15% is a realistic estimate of the frequency of autoantibodies in end-stage renal failure patients. Lymphocytotoxic antibodies of the *auto* type are not a cause of rejection of renal allografts, even if they are present in the serum at the time of transplantation (Taylor *et al.*, 1989). In the cadaver regraft situation, these antibodies may be beneficial to graft survival (Ting and Welsh, 1994).

Non-HLA Antibodies That Are Graft Damaging

The classic example of non-HLA antibodies that are graft damaging is anti-I, a red blood cell cold agglutinin that is directed against a temperature-sensitive carbohydrate target and is invariably IgM unless following a *Mycoplasma* infection. Although each antibody is different in its temperature profile, as a rule these antibodies are totally nonbinding at temperatures greater than 30°C. They are clinically relevant to transplantation only if they bind significantly to a cooled organ. An early report by Belzer *et al.* (1971) showed this fact beautifully. A recipient hyperacutely rejected a donor kidney; the antibody was observed to be anti-I, and so the team retransplanted successfully with the second kidney from the same donor after warming it up before revascularization.

Cold antibody screens are not routine for renal transplant recipients, at least in the United Kingdom, because high-titer anti-I is rare. We have seen three occurrences (one of which was not detected before transplant) in our joint experience of more than 3,000 transplants. A previous *Mycoplasma* infection is the normal trigger point for awareness.

Antibodies to endothelial cells, activated endothelial cells, epithelial cells, donor skin and monocytes all have been described as the likely cause of rapid graft loss posttransplant. Harmer and associates described a cell line (EAhy 926) that can be used to detect at least three types of these non-HLA antibodies (Harmer *et al.*, 1990). It is likely that the antibodies to epithelial cells are a marker for a form of renal allograft loss in children (Harmer *et al.*, 1990). Currently, it appears that cytomegalovirus infections associate with the production of such antibodies, and concurrent cytomegalovirus could explain the Harmer findings. Current methods of confirming cytomegalovirus (i.e., in hours instead of weeks) should make such antibodies irrelevant as surrogate markers in children. In adults, the antibodies are not relevant to renal, cardiac or lung graft survival in adults.

Antibodies to endothelial cells and monocytes are of at least two kinds and bear an undetermined relationship with antibodies to donor skin (Baldwin *et al.*, 1981; Cerilli *et al.*, 1983; Moraes and Stastny, 1977; Paul *et al.*, 1979). It is not known if they all damage grafts or if some are more damaging than others. Antibodies reactive with tumor necrosis factor–activated endothelial cells have been described (Harmer *et al.*, 1990); these antibodies are rare, and it is difficult to conceive how they could cause immediate graft damage. Nevertheless, they are IgG and were observed in association with otherwise unexplainable rapid graft loss.

There is polymorphism in one or more of the targets of antiendothelial-monocyte antibodies and of the closely related or identical antiskin antibodies. It is prudent not to transplant across them if they react at dilution, but how do we test for them? From the literature quoted and from our own experience, it is patients with high-titer anti-HLA-A, anti-HLA-B or broad-panel reactivity who produce antibodies to HLA-DR, HLA-DQ, endothelial cells, monocytes and activated endothelial cells. For most laboratories, setting up the sophisticated screening and crossmatch procedures necessary to detect all of these antibodies is not possible in view of their rarity and because their polymorphisms are not characterized fully. At present, our detection systems usually are limited to flow cytometry crossmatches on spleen T cells, B cells and monocytes in addition to CLL and EAHy prescreening. Table 10–5 outlines the typical reactions found by systems that we have observed.

INCUBATION TEMPERATURE

In the standard cytotoxic test, the precomplement and postcomplement incubation steps are carried out at room temperature (20–25°C). Iwaki and associates introduced the cold and warm tests by changing the precomplement temperatures to 5°C and 37°C (Iwaki *et al.*, 1978). They found that antibodies detected in the cold test (reactivity at 5°C) were non-HLA, IgM and not graft damaging, whereas warm antibodies (reactive at 5°C and 37°C) were usually HLA, IgG and associated with a lower graft survival rate. Data from other laboratories showed that some non-HLA antibodies react at 37°C, but the reactivity is stronger at 5°C (Deierhoi *et al.*, 1983). Just performing the crossmatch at different precomplement incubation temperatures may not be adequate for separating damaging from nondamaging antibodies.

IMMUNOGLOBULIN CLASS

The HLA antibodies are usually but not always IgG, whereas non-HLA antibodies are predominantly IgM. The

TABLE 10–5

REACTIVITY OF TRANSPLANT-RELEVANT ANTIBODIES WITH COMMONLY USED TARGETS AND THEIR ABILITY TO CAUSE HYPERACUTE REJECTION*

Antibody Specificity (Subclass)	T NIH	B NIH	Spleen Flow T, B, M	EaHy (Act) Flow	CLL NIH	CLL Flow	HAR
HLA-A,B (G)	+	+	+ +	−	+	+	+ + +
HLA-A,B (M)	+ +	+ +	+ / −	−	+ +	+	+ / −
HLA-C (G)	+	+	+	−	+	+	+
HLA-C (M)	+	+	−	−	+	+ / −	(−)
HLA-DR (G)	−	+	+ +	−	+	+	+
HLA-DR (M)	−	+	+ / −	−	+ +	+	(−)
TB auto (M)	+	+	−	−	+ / −	−	−
B auto (M)	−	+	−	−	−	−	−
I (4–10C) (M & G)	+	+	+	+ +	+ / −	+ / −	+ +
I (22C) (M & G)	−	−	−	−	−	−	+ +
Endo/mono (G)	−	−	+	+	−	−	+
Activated endo (G)	−	−	−	+	−	−	+
HLA-DQ (G)	−	+	+	−	+	+	−
HLA-DQ (M)	−	+	+ / −	−	+ / −	+	−

*This table outlines the types of reactions that one observes in practice with renal sera. In general, IgG antibodies are detected best by flow cytometry and are harmful to the graft. IgM antibodies are detected best by standard cytotoxicity, but antibodies that are of known relevance to graft survival can be detected by flow cytometry. For IgM, anti-HLA-A,B,C and DR + / − is used to indicate that the situation is unclear and when in parentheses that there is no information. We believe it is prudent not to transplant in the presence of a current positive HLA-DR crossmatch. The antibody to the I antigen is included twice to stress that although it is rare, it escapes detection unless incubations are carried out at lower temperatures. If an anti-I is known to be present in a recipient, prewarming of the donor kidney avoids any problem. Assuming red blood cell compatibility, it can be seen that a positive flow cytometry crossmatch on spleen at 22C and a *cold* crossmatch on TNF-activated EaHy cells, provided that both anti-G and anti-M reagents are used, would detect all the antibodies known to or which might cause hyperacute rejection. EaHy-activated and TNF-activated EaHy do not express class II, and their class I expression is low. In general, they cannot be typed fully using standard serology. Occasional reactions can be seen usually with antibodies to HLA-A9.

CLL = chronic lymphatic leukemia; HAR = hyperacute rejection; EaHy (Act) = activated endothelial cell line.

addition of dithiothreitol (DTT) to the serum before incubation with cells can discriminate between IgM and IgG antibodies (Pirofsky and Rosner, 1974). Donor-reactive IgM HLA class I antibodies, present in old sera but absent in current sera, may be irrelevant clinically (Chapman *et al.*, 1986b).

ROLE OF OLD AND CURRENT SERA IN CROSSMATCHING

Some patients who develop antibodies may lose them with time, or the percentage panel reactivity of the antibody may decrease. Historically, it was the practice of most laboratories to use old peak PRA-positive sera and current sera for crossmatching. If the old peak sera gave a positive crossmatch, the transplant was denied even if the current serum gave a negative crossmatch (termed P + C − crossmatch). This doctrine was challenged in 1982 by Cardella *et al.*, who suggested that old peak PRA-positive sera may not give the clinically relevant crossmatch result, based on their finding of successful transplant outcome with a P + C − T-cell crossmatch. These encouraging results were confirmed by others (Laupacis *et al.*, 1983; Matas *et al.*, 1984). Not all studies have been so encouraging, however; immediately rejected grafts have been reported (Chapman *et al.*, 1986b), and lower overall graft survival rates have been reported (Turka *et al.*, 1989).

Results of a study from the Oxford Transplant Centre suggest that the immunoglobulin class of the antibody may be an important factor in determining graft outcome. In Table 10–6, it is obvious that IgG antibodies are important (12 of 16 grafts failing within 1 month). In marked contrast, IgM HLA class I antibodies often are associated with a successful outcome (5 of 16 failures within the first year). This finding needs to be confirmed by other studies before it can be accepted as established. One characteristic of this Oxford study that distinguishes it from most other studies of P + C − crossmatch transplants is that the precise specificity of the antibody was confirmed as being HLA class I by the cytotoxicity inhibition test (Chapman *et al.*, 1986b). In most other published studies, the specificity of the antibodies was not characterized, but the authors assumed that if the antibody reacted with T and B lymphocytes, it must be HLA class I, a deduction that is not always true. It is likely that in these studies some patients had non-HLA antibodies, which are not graft damaging.

There is no doubt that P + C − crossmatch transplants can be successful, but the conditions under which these transplants can be carried out have not been defined fully. Some of these conditions are the following: How far back in time should one go to select sera for crossmatching? If a patient has clearly defined antibody specificities in old sera, should these be avoided in the graft? Is the immunoglobulin class of the crossmatch-positive sera important? Is the type of posttransplant immunosuppression used important (e.g., cyclosporine, tacrolimus, antithymocyte globulin and OKT3)?

It is the policy of many centers to use only sera collected during the 6 to 12 months pretransplantation for crossmatching. In many of these centers, if a patient has developed specific antibodies, those antigens are avoided in the kidney donor, even if the specificity is found in sera collected years previously (Welsh *et al.*, 1988). Most centers would not perform a transplant in a patient with a positive crossmatch to IgG antibodies, with the exceptions previously discussed. Many centers would perform the transplant if the antibody is IgM, and it is assumed that in most of these cases the specificity of the antibody would be non-HLA. Some but not all transplant centers give prophylactic antithymocyte globulin to immunologically high-risk patients.

Antibodies are stable if frozen but are susceptible to damage during freeze-thaw cycles that occur in some freezers during defrosting (especially if only small volumes are stored) and when the sera are removed for crossmatch purposes. It is important that accurate screening data are available.

Laboratory Protocols Used to Enable Transplantation in Highly Sensitized Patients

Some laboratories employ special protocols to try to determine whether transplantation can occur in a highly sensitized patient. These protocols may differ from laboratory to laboratory. Some protocols are performed as part of the pretransplant workup, autologous crossmatch, screening of sera

TABLE 10–6

OXFORD RESULTS FOR CURRENT NEGATIVE AND PAST POSITIVE IgG CROSSMATCH TRANSPLANTS

No.	Transplant No.	TF	Preg.*	Titer	A	B	DR	RM	No. Days to Failure	Comments
1	1	2	12	16	1	2	2	?	44	
2	1	3		4	2	1	0	n	24	
3	1	4	2	2	1	1	2	y	7	Bw4 pmm
4	3	2		4	0	0	0	?	0	
5	4	2		8	0	0	0	y	0	Cw5 pmm
6	2	13		8	2	1	1	y	0	Cw4 pmm
7	2	6		1	2	0	0	n	9	
8	2	18	3	4	1	1	1	n	28	
9	3	3		8	1	1	1	y	9	Bw4 pmm
10	3	10		32	2	2	2	y	0	Bw6 pmm
11	2	9		2	2	2	0	n	28	
12	2	2		16	1	0	0	n	8	
13	2	7		2	2	2	0	n		Success (1,760)
14	2	8	2	nt	1	1	0	y	0	Bw4 pmm
15	3	21	0	nt	0	1	0	n		Success (375)
16	2	2		nt	2	0	1	n		Success (350)

*Pregnancies that have been responded to are considered as previous transplants.
TF = number of pretransplant transfusions; Preg. = number of pregnancies; nt = not tested; RM = repeat mismatch; y = yes; n = no; pmm = previous mismatch.

against lymphocyte panels from normal donors and CLL cells and screening of sera against panel cells with and without DTT. Other protocols are performed at the time of transplantation: crossmatch with and without DTT treatment of the serum, crossmatch with the AHG method and crossmatch with the FC technique.

DISTINCTION OF HLA FROM NON-HLA ANTIBODIES

Many protocols are used to distinguish HLA from non-HLA antibodies.

Autologous Crossmatch

It is important to perform an autologous crossmatch in patients with high levels of PRA but who do not have a history of sensitization. The crossmatch should be performed with and without DTT to confirm that the autoantibody, if present, is IgM. If a patient has autoantibodies, however, it does not mean that the patient lacks IgM HLA antibodies because sera containing both types of antibodies are found.

Screening of Sera Against Chronic Lymphocytic Leukemia Cells

Most autoantibodies do not react with CLL cells (Ting and Morris, 1978b), although those with a higher affinity and/or avidity may react with CLL cells (Taylor *et al.*, 1991). Non-HLA antibodies that do not react with CLL cells are commoner, and screening sera against a CLL panel is extremely useful in determining whether or not a patient has autoantibodies. When sera also are screened against normal cells, it often is possible to determine that a patient has HLA class I antibodies alone, HLA class II antibodies alone, a mixture of class I and class II antibodies, autoantibodies only or a mixture of HLA and autoantibodies.

Screening of Sera Against K562

Deierhoi and colleagues showed that autoantibodies react with cells of the cell line K562, which lack expression of HLA antigens on their cell surface (Deierhoi *et al.*, 1984). Difficulties in using K562 in the cytotoxic test have led to neglect of this assay.

Screening and Crossmatching Sera with Dithiothreitol

The reactivity of IgM antibodies is inactivated by DTT. By screening sera against panel cells with and without DTT, it is possible to show that sera have IgG antibodies alone, IgM antibodies only or a mixture of IgG and IgM antibodies. If we assume that IgG antibodies are predominantly HLA and IgM antibodies are non-HLA, this technique provides useful information on the transplantability of highly sensitized patients. In these patients, a crossmatch must be performed with and without DTT.

Crossmatching Sera Using Wash, Antihuman Globulin and Flow Cytometry Methods

The IgM antibodies from most patients are not detected in the wash and AHG methods that use wash steps. These antibodies have low-affinity avidity, which allows them to be detached from the cell surface in the wash steps. If a crossmatch is positive in the standard cytotoxic method but negative in the wash and AHG methods, it is highly likely that the antibody is IgM and non-HLA, and a transplant performed should not be subjected to a lesser chance of success than a completely negative crossmatch transplant. The FC method also uses wash steps, and the fluorescein-conjugated second antibody used to detect bound alloantibody usually is against IgG; IgM antibodies are not detected in FC.

USE OF CURRENT SERUM ONLY FOR CROSSMATCHING

Many patients who become highly sensitized lose their antibody in time, particularly if they are not continually immunized by, for example, blood transfusions. We previously discussed the philosophy adopted by many transplant centers; that is, to use sera collected only in the 6 to 12 months pretransplantation for crossmatching, even if the patient had a higher frequency of PRA in an old serum sample. Some centers in addition avoid giving a kidney that has the HLA antigens against which the patient is known to have made antibodies, even if these antibodies were found only in old sera. This means that laboratories need to screen for PRA regularly, particularly after an immunizing event. For patients waiting for a regraft, it is important to obtain and screen a serum collected 2 to 4 weeks after the failed graft because it is at this time that patients are most likely to develop antibodies.

Highly sensitized patients who are continually transfused may not lose their antibodies, and even if not transfused, many remain highly sensitized. Different approaches have been used to decrease the level of PRA before transplantation. Plasmapheresis and immunoadsorption have been used to remove HLA antibodies. Taube *et al.* (1984) first reported the removal of HLA antibodies and prevention of resynthesis by treating patients with a combination of plasmapheresis, cyclophosphamide and prednisolone. In this report of five patients treated while waiting for regrafts, four were transplanted successfully, and one died with a poorly functioning graft. The authors concluded that although the method was successful in removing HLA antibodies, it should be reserved for patients with overwhelming clinical or social reasons for transplantation because of the significant morbidity associated with the treatment.

Plasmapheresis has been used successfully by other groups (Pollack *et al.*, 1979). Palmer *et al.* (1989a, 1989b) reported extracorporeal immunoadsorption on protein A columns to remove IgG HLA antibodies. Ten patients, all of whom had previously lost at least one graft, underwent the procedure; 7 subsequently underwent transplantation, and only one graft was lost because of rejection. Antithymocyte globulin was given prophylactically to these patients, and this may be important in securing a successful graft outcome. Other studies have shown similarly good results (Kupin *et al.*, 1991). In a study by Esnault *et al.* (1990), six patients were treated; only two could undergo transplantation, and both failed. In a further study by Hiesse *et al.* (1992), 15 patients were treated by immunoadsorption with cyclophosphamide and prednisolone, and various effects on antibody production were observed with a high rebound of HLA antibodies. Twelve patients were transplanted; 7 received P−C− well-matched transplants and 6 did well, but 5 patients received a P+C− transplant, and three grafts failed, two owing to hyperacute rejection. These investigators stated that a better definition of patients who might benefit is required.

Palmer and colleagues indicated that not all patients are suited for antibody removal treatment, and only those whose serum contains one main HLA antibody specificity are likely to benefit (this represents about 60% of all highly sensitized patients) (Palmer *et al.*, 1989a, 1989b). The theory is that a highly reactive serum sample contains one main HLA specificity directed at a *private* epitope, and the remainder of the reactivity is due to weaker cross-reactive antibodies. These investigators postulated that plasmapheresis or immunoadsorption removes the cross-reactive antibodies but not the main antibody, and the patient has to be given a kidney that does not have the HLA antigen to which the main specificity is directed. In an article that followed the method of Palmer and associates, with the important extension of trying out the procedure immediately before transplantation (Ross *et al.*, 1993), success has been achieved. The numbers are too small to state that the method improves the chance of graft survival, but it makes implementation easier.

Removal of HLA antibodies by immunoadsorption is a valuable treatment modality that allows successful transplantation of some highly sensitized patients. Immunoadsorption may not be suitable for all highly sensitized patients, and the high cost of the procedure may be a drawback to its general use.

The introduction of recombinant erythropoietin (EPO) to treat anemia in renal failure patients in place of blood transfusions has led to many studies investigating the usefulness of this treatment in lowering HLA antibody levels in highly sensitized patients. Some studies have tested the hypothesis that EPO actively decreases antibody levels, whereas others have looked at whether the cessation of blood transfusions can result in a drop in PRA levels. The results from many studies have been mixed. Koskimies *et al.* (1990) did not find a decline in PRA levels. Grimm *et al.* (1991) found that treatment with EPO led to a reduction in the percent of PRA and the titer of the main HLA-antibody specificity; in addition, these patients developed antiidiotypic antibodies. The authors postulated that the antiidiotypic antibodies might be relevant to the decrease in percent of PRA and successful graft outcome seen in the patients. Antiidiotypic antibodies were not found by Phelan *et al.* (1991), who showed that the decrease in PRA levels in 11 of 54 patients studied mainly was due to a lack of IgM-HLA antibodies with no change in the IgG. Deierhoi and colleagues believed that the reduction in PRA levels seen in their study was due to avoidance of blood transfusions rather than to the specific institution of EPO (Deierhoi *et al.*, 1992).

Treatment with EPO can result in a reduction in PRA levels in some but not all patients, and it is most likely that this reduction is due to avoidance of transfusions. It is unclear which highly sensitized patients may benefit by a decline in PRA. Some variables should be examined. First, the sensitization history of the patient—did the patient become sensitized because of a failed graft, transfusions, pregnancies, a failed graft and transfusions together or other causes? Second, when and for what period was a patient sensitized to each antigen? Third, what was the strength of the antibodies in terms of titer units?

Transplantation Without a Crossmatch

Crossmatching can result in long cold ischemia times, which can affect long-term graft survival and contribute significantly to primary nonfunction. Because it is generally accepted that long cold ischemia time and high sensitization are additive in some way and because crossmatching for high sensitization is more complex, it would be beneficial if crossmatching could be dropped. To circumvent the problem of long crossmatching time, some groups have argued that in certain circumstances the prospective crossmatch is not necessary. It is imperative that patients transplanted without a prospective crossmatch must have a clear history of non-

sensitization to the donor mismatches. This information can come only from a combination of good patient history (pregnancy, infection and transfusion records) and from high-quality, sensitive antibody screening and high-quality genotyping. In practice, well-screened, nontransfused men with a good HLA match do not need crossmatching, with the added benefit of a zero chance of false-positives. For sensitized patients, although no crossmatching would be ideal, it is more difficult to achieve with safety; molecular typing and FACS crossmatching are advantageous in this situation because both can be performed rapidly on donor peripheral blood before organ retrieval. Omitting crossmatching is potentially useful in reducing the cold ischemia times of exported kidneys, especially those that arrive at a transplant center with an already long cold ischemia time.

Regional Sharing of Crossmatch Trays

The chance of finding a kidney donor with a negative crossmatch for a highly sensitized patient is remote but can be improved by increasing the donor pool against which the sera are crossmatched. One such strategy is to send sera from highly sensitized patients to all participating laboratories within an organ-sharing scheme. These sera are crossmatched against all locally procured donors, and if a negative crossmatch is obtained, the kidney is shipped to the appropriate recipient.

Many schemes have been set up, including the Regional Organ Procurement crossmatch tray sharing by the South East Organ Procurement Foundation (Bollinger *et al.*, 1987), the SOS Scheme of the United Kingdom Transplant Service (Bradley *et al.*, 1985), the Highly Immunized Transplant (HIT) Study set up by Opelz in Germany (Schafer *et al.*, 1985) and the Highly Immunized File set up within Eurotransplant. In the early years of the SOS Scheme, no attempt was made to match HLA donors and recipients. An analysis of the early data showed, however, that an HLA-DR–matched graft had a significantly better outcome than an HLA-DR–mismatched graft. The 6-month survival rates of the grafts mismatched for zero, one and two HLA-DR antigens were 64%, 55% and 50%. Subsequent to these findings, kidneys were shipped to a recipient's center only if the crossmatch was negative and the donor was HLA-DR matched.

Definition of Acceptable HLA Mismatches

An approach to increasing the chances of finding a negative crossmatch donor for a highly sensitized patient is to determine the HLA antigens against which the patient has *not* developed antibodies. These antigens together with the patient's own antigens make up the *acceptable mismatches* for that patient. A donor who has any combination of these acceptable mismatches should give a negative crossmatch. With this approach, sera from highly sensitized patients do not have to be shipped to other centers for crossmatching.

Two methods have been used to determine a patient's acceptable mismatches. The first is to use a computer approach to analyze high PRA sera and determine which HLA specificities in a donor should give a negative crossmatch for a given recipient (Barnardo *et al.*, 1997; Duquesnoy *et al.*, 1990; Mickey *et al.*, 1985). The second, which is a novel scheme used by Claas *et al.* (1989), is to screen a serum sample from each highly sensitized patient (>85% PRA) against panel members selected so that only one HLA-A or HLA-B antigen at a time is mismatched with the patient. In the study by Claas *et al.* (1989), more than 40 patients were transplanted with a negative crossmatch and HLA-DR compatibility, and the graft survival at 1 year was greater than 80%. Although successful, this method has two main drawbacks. First, the laboratory must have access to an extremely large pool of panel members. Second, this method is labor intensive in that it takes one technician 2 to 3 weeks to perform a workup of one patient.

Antibody screening strategies that employ a single HLA antigen per screening test are starting to be developed (Barnardo *et al.*, 2000). It is hoped that assays such as this would enable exact determination of antibody specificity unfettered from the problems of multiple antigens and linkage dysequilibrium that plague conventional techniques of antibody screening. Given the utopian scenario of defining antibody specificity exactly, crossmatching may be dropped for most patients, and organ sharing schemes may be used.

Sharing Kidneys Based on HLA Matching

In some regional or national organ-sharing schemes, highly sensitized patients receive priority over non–highly sensitized patients for HLA well-matched kidneys. The supposition is that well-matched kidneys have a better chance of giving a negative crossmatch than poorly matched kidneys. For this scheme to be effective, the antibody specificities possessed by each patient should be listed, and donors with those antigens should not be offered to the patient.

HLA-DR Matching and Prior Sensitization to HLA Class I

HLA-DR matching and prior sensitization to HLA class I are the most important matching and crossmatching factors discussed and have implications besides their direct effect on graft survival. Taylor and coworkers showed that although clinicians no longer see an influence of HLA-DR matching in recipients of first-cadaver grafts, HLA-DR matching is exerting a strong and dose-related effect on the rejection response in sensitized and nonsensitized patients (Taylor *et al.*, 1993). The reason there is no significant correlation with graft survival is simply because modern immunosuppression can overcome this presumed T-cell response with relative ease. For grafts that fail, clinicians have subjected recipients of mismatched grafts to a greater sensitization response. This approach may have subsequent implications in that, for example, we cannot retransplant with a mismatch that has been responded to in the previous graft.

In contrast, we observe an effect of HLA-DR matching on survival figures for regrafts in which most of the recipients are sensitized. We believe that the greater average total magnitude of the responses in regrafts and sensitized patients coupled with the fact that cyclosporine is less potent at blocking secondary responses (especially humoral) explains why more grafts are lost in mismatched recipients. Rejection episodes in sensitized recipients are associated more often with antibodies to MHC class I (Halloran *et al.*, 1992; Martin *et al.*, 1987; Palmer *et al.*, 1989a, 1989b). More accurate screening, more sensitive crossmatches, more attention to matching, avoidance of previous mismatches that have been responded to by an IgG response (Welsh *et al.*, 1988) and additional immunosuppression to counter the increased rejection expected all have contributed to the fact that many centers have equally good graft survival results in sensitized and nonsensitized recipients.

References

Adorno, D., Piazza, A., Canossi, A., *et al.* (1999). The role of DRB1 amino acid residue differences on donor-specific antibody production and acute rejection after cadaveric renal transplant. *J. Biol. Regul. Homeost. Agents* **13**, 32.

Agishi, T., Takahashi, K. and Ota, K. (1992). Comparative evaluation of immunoadsorption and double filtration plasmapheresis for removal of anti-A or -B antibody in ABO-incompatible kidney transplantation. *Transplant. Proc.* **24**, 557.

Alexandre, G. P. J., Latinne, D., Carlier, M., *et al.* (1991). ABO-incompatibility and organ transplantation. *Transpl. Rev.* **5**, 230.

Alexandre, G. P. J., Squifflet, J. P., de Bruyere, M., *et al.* (1986). ABO-incompatible related and unrelated living donor renal allografts. *Transplant. Proc.* **18**, 452.

Baldwin, W., Claas, F. H. J., van Es, L. A. and van Rood, J. J. (1981). Distribution of endothelial-monocyte and HLA antigens on renal vascular endothelial cell antigen system in non-HLA identical renal transplants. *Transplant. Proc.* **13**, 103.

Barnardo, M. C., Bunce, M., Thursz, M. and Welsh, K. I. (1997). Analysis of the molecular epitopes of anti-HLA antibodies using a computer program, OODAS; Object Oriented Definition of Antibody Specificity. *In Genetic Diversity of HLA: Functional and Medical Implications*, Vol. 2, (D. Charron, ed.), p. 132, EDK, Sevres, France.

Barnardo, M. C., Harmer, A. W., Shaw, O. J., *et al.* (2000). Detection of HLA-specific IgG antibodies using single recombinant HLA alleles: the monoLisa assay. *Transplantation* **70**, 531.

Belzer, F. O., Kountz, S. L. and Perkins, H. A. (1971). Red cell cold agglutinins as a cause of failure of renal allotransplantation. *Transplantation* **11**, 422.

Bidwell, J. L., Bidwell, E. A., Savage, D. A., Middleton, D., Klouda, P. T. and Bradley, B. A. (1988). A DNA-RFLP typing system that positively identifies serologically well-defined and ill-defined HLA-DR and DQ alleles, including DRw10. *Transplantation* **45**, 640.

Bjorkman, P. J., Saper, M. A., Samraoui, B., Bennett, W. S., Strominger, J. L. and Wiley, D. C. (1987). Structure of the human Class I histocompatibility antigen, HLA-A2. *Nature* **329**, 506.

Bollinger, R. R., Vaughan, W., Sanfilippo, F., *et al.* (1987). Results of the South-Eastern Organ Procurement Foundation Strategy for transplanting sensitized patients. *Transplant. Proc.* **19**, 1964.

Bradley, B. A., Klouda, P. T., Ray, T. C. and Gore, S. M. (1985). Negative crossmatch selection of kidneys for highly sensitized patients. *Transplant. Proc.* **17**, 2465.

Breimer, M. E. and Samuelsson, B. E. (1986). The specific distribution of glycolipid-based blood group A antigens in human kidney related to A1/A2, Lewis, and secretor status of single individuals. *Transplantation* **42**, 88.

Brier-Vriesendorp, B. S. and Ivanyi, P. (1986). Individual differences in the cytotoxic T-lymphocyte response in man to public HLA determinants. *Cell. Immunol.* **103**, 252.

Brynger, H., Rydberg, L., Samuelsson, B., Blohme, I., Lindholm, A. and Sandberg, L. (1982). Renal transplantation across a blood group barrier—'A2' kidneys to 'O' recipients. *Proc. E. D. T. A.* **19**, 427.

Bunce, M., O'Neill, C. M., Barnardo, M. C., Krausa, P., Browning, M. J., *et al.* (1995). Phototyping: comprehensive DNA typing for HLA-A, B, C, DRB1, DRB3, DRB4, DRB5 and DQB1 by PCR with 144 primer mixes utilising sequence-specific primers (PCR-SSP). *Tissue Antigens* **46**, 355.

Bunce, M., Procter, J. and Welsh, K. I. (1999). A DNA based detection and screening system for identifying HLA class I expression variants by sequence-specific primers. *Tissue Antigens* **53**, 498.

Bunce, M., Young, N. T. and Welsh, K. I. (1997). Molecular HLA typing—the brave new world. *Transplantation* **64**, 1505.

Bushell, A. R., Higgins R. M., Wood, K. J. and Morris, P. J. (1989). HLA-DQ mismatches between donors and recipients in the presence of HLA-DR compatibility do not influence the function or outcome of renal transplants. *Hum. Immunol.* **26**, 179.

Cardella, C. J., Falk, J. A., Nicholson, M. J., Harding, M. and Cook, G. T. (1982). Successful renal transplantation in patients with T-cell reactivity to donor. *Lancet* **2**, 1240.

Ceppellini, R., Mattiuz, P. L., Scudeller, G. and Visetti, M. (1969). Experimental allotransplantation in man: I. the role of the HL-A system in different genetic combinations. *Transplant. Proc.* **1**, 385.

Cerilli, J., Bay, W. and Brasile, L. (1983). The significance of the monocyte crossmatch in recipients of living related HLA identical kidney graft. *Hum. Immunol.* **7**, 45.

Chapman, J. R., Deierhoi, M. H., Carter, N. P., Ting, A. and Morris,

P. J. (1985). Analysis of flow cytometry and cytotoxicity cross-matches in renal transplantation. *Transplant. Proc.* **17**, 2480.

Chapman, J. R., Taylor, C., Ting, A. and Morris, P. J. (1986a). Hyperacute rejection of a renal allograft in the presence of anti-HLA-Cw5 antibody. *Transplantation* **42**, 91.

Chapman, J. R., Taylor, C. J., Ting, A. and Morris, P. J. (1986b). Immunoglobulin class and specificity of antibodies causing positive T cell crossmatches: relationship to renal transplant outcome. *Transplantation* **42**, 608.

Chien, A., Edgar, D. B. and Trela, J. M. (1976). Deoxyribonucleic acid polymerase from the extreme thermophile Thermus aquaticus. *J. Bacteriol.* **127**, 1550.

Claas, F. H. J., Gijbels, Y., van Veen, A., *et al.* (1989). Selection of cross-match negative HLA-A and/or -B mismatched donors for highly sensitized patients. *Transplant. Proc.* **21**, 665.

Cross, D. E., Greiner, R. and Whittier, F. C. (1976). Importance of the autocontrol crossmatch in human renal transplantation. *Transplantation* **21**, 307.

Daar, A. S., Fuggle, S. V., Fabre, J. W., Ting, A. and Morris, P. J. (1984). The detailed distribution of MHC class II antigens in normal human organs. *Transplantation* **38**, 293.

Dausset, J. (1958). Iso-leuco-anticorps. *Acta Haematol.* **20**, 156.

Deierhoi, M. H., Barger, B. O., Hudson, S. L., Shroyer, T. W. and Diethelm, A. G. (1992). The effect of erythropoietin and blood transfusions on highly sensitized patients on a single cadaver renal allograft waiting list. *Transplantation* **53**, 363.

Deierhoi, M. H., Ting, A. and Morris, P. J. (1983). Successful renal transplantation despite warm B cell antibodies. *Transplantation* **36**, 207.

Deierhoi, M. H., Ting, A. and Morris, P. J. (1984). Reactivity of lymphocyte cytotoxic autoantibodies from renal patients with cell line K562. *Transplantation* **38**, 557.

Duquesnoy, R. J., White, L. T., Fierst, J. W., *et al.* (1990). Multiscreen serum analysis of highly sensitized renal dialysis patients for antibodies toward public and private class I HLA determinants: Implications for computer-predicted acceptable and unacceptable donor. *Transplantation* **50**, 427.

Esnault, V., Bignon, J. D., Testa, A., Preud'Homme, J. L., Vergracht, A. and Soulillou, J. P. (1990). Effect of protein A immunoadsorption on panel lymphocyte reactivity in hyperimmunized patients awaiting a kidney graft. *Transplantation* **50**, 449.

Ettenger, R. B., Terasaki, P. I., Opelz, G., *et al.* (1976). Successful renal allografts across a positive cross-match for donor B-lymphocyte alloantigens. *Lancet* **2**, 56.

Festenstein, H., Doyle, P. and Holmes, J. (1986). Long-term follow-up in London Transplant Group recipients of cadaver renal allografts: the influence of HLA matching on transplant outcome. *N. Engl. J. Med.* **314**, 7.

Francke, U. and Pellegrino, M. A. (1977). Assignment of the major histocompatibility complex to a region of the short arm of human chromosome 6. *Proc. Natl. Acad. Sci. U. S. A.* **74**, 1147.

Fuller, T. C. (1991). Monitoring HLA alloimmunization: analysis of HLA alloantibodies in the serum of prospective transplant recipients. *Clin. Lab. Med.* **11**, 551.

Fuller, T. C., Cosimi, A. B. and Russell, P. S. (1978). Use of an antiglobulin-ATG reagent for detection of low levels of alloantibody—improvement of allograft survival in presensitized recipients. *Transplant. Proc.* **10**, 463.

Fuller, T. C. and Fuller, A. (1999). The humoral immune response against an HLA class I allodeterminant correlates with the HLA-DR phenotype of the responder. *Transplantation* **68**, 173.

Garovoy, M. R., Rheinschmidt, M. A., Bigos, M., *et al.* (1983). Flow cytometry analysis: a high technology crossmatch technique facilitating transplantation. *Transplant. Proc.* **15**, 1939.

Gifford, R. R. M., Doran, M. M., Ruth, J. A., Coppage, M. L., Winsett, O. E. and Fish, J. C. (1986). Positive antiglobulin cytotoxicity crossmatch in renal allograft recipients treated with cyclosporine. *Transplantation* **42**, 439.

Gleason, R. E. and Murray, J. E. (1967). Report from the transplant registry: analysis of variables in the function of human kidney transplants: I. blood group compatibility and splenectomy. *Transplantation* **5**, 343.

Goodfellow, P. N., Jones, E. A., Van Heyningen, V., Solomon, E., Bobrow, M., *et al.* (1975). The beta2-microglobulin gene is on chromosome 15 and not in the HL-A region. *Nature* **254**, 267.

Goulmy, E., Gratama, J. W., Blokland, E., Zwann, F. E. and van Rood, J. J. (1983). A minor transplantation antigen detected by MHC-restricted cytotoxic T lymphocytes during graft versus host disease. *Nature* **302**, 159.

Grimm, P. C., Sekiya, N. M., Robertson, L. S., Robinson, B. J. and Ettenger, R. B. (1991). Recombinant human erythropoietin decreases anti-HLA sensitization and may improve renal allograft outcome: involvement of anti-idiotypic antibody. *Transplant. Proc.* **23**, 407.

Halloran, P. F., Schlaut, J., Solez, K. and Srinivasa, N. S. (1992). The significance of the anti-class I response: II. clinical and pathological features of renal transplants with anticlass I-like antibody. *Transplantation* **53,** 550.

Harmer, A. W., Haskard, D., Koffman, C. G. and Welsh, K. I. (1990). Novel antibodies associated with unexplained loss of renal allografts. *Transpl. Int.* **3**, 66.

Hiesse, C., Kriaa, F., Rousseau, P., *et al.* (1992). Immunoadsorption of anti-HLA antibodies for highly sensitized patients awaiting renal transplantation. *Nephrol. Dial. Transplant.* **7**, 944.

Ishikawa, Y., Tokunaga, K., Tanaka, H., *et al.* (1996). HLA-A null allele with a stop codon, HLA-A*0215N, identified in a homozygous state in a healthy adult. *Immunogenetics* **43**, 1.

Iwaki, Y., Cook, D. J., Terasaki, P. I., *et al.* (1987). Flow cytometry crossmatching in human cadaver kidney transplantation. *Transplant. Proc.* **19**, 764.

Iwaki, Y., Terasaki, P. I., Park, M. S. and Billing, R. (1978). Enhancement of human kidney allografts by cold B-lymphocyte cytotoxins. *Lancet* **1**, 1228.

Jeannet, M., Benzonana, G. and Arni, I. (1981). Donor-specific B and T lymphocyte antibodies and kidney graft survival. *Transplantation* **31**, 160.

Jeannet, M. and Stalder, H. (1978). Lymphocytotoxic antibodies in spontaneous cytomegalovirus infection. *Lancet* **1**, 509.

Karuppan, S. S., Lindholm, A. and Moller, E. (1992). Fewer acute rejection episodes and improved outcome in kidney-transplanted patients with selection criteria based on crossmatching. *Transplantation* **53**, 666.

Kaufman, D. B., Matas, A., Arrazola, L., *et al.* (1993). Transplantation of kidneys from zero-haplotype matched sibling donors, and distantly related and unrelated donors in the cyclosporine era. *Transplant. Proc.* **25**, 1530.

Kerman, R. H., Kimball, P. M., van Buren, C. T., *et al.* (1991). Improved renal allograft survival for AHG and DTE/AHG cross-match-negative recipients. *Transplant. Proc.* **23**, 400.

Kerman, R. H., van Buren, C. T., Lewis, R. M., DeVera, V., Baghdahsarian, V. and Kahan, B. D. (1990). Improved graft survival for flow cytometry and antihuman globulin crossmatch-negative retransplant recipients. *Transplantation* **49**, 52.

Kissmeyer-Nielsen, F., Olsen, S., Petersen, V. P. and Fjeldborg, O. (1966). Hyperacute rejection of kidney allografts associated with pre-existing humoral antibodies against donor cells. *Lancet* **1**, 662.

Koskimies, S., Lautenschlager, I., Gronhagen-Riska, C. and Hayry, P. (1990). Erythropoietin therapy and antibody levels of highly sensitized patients awaiting kidney transplantation. *Transplantation* **50**, 707.

Krangel, M. S., Orr, H. T. and Strominger, J. L. (1979). Assembly and maturation of HLA-A and HLA-B antigens in vivo. *Cell* **18**, 979.

Kupin, W. L., Venkat, K. K., Hayashi, H., Mozes, M. F., Oh, H. K. and Watt, R. (1991). Removal of lymphocytotoxic antibodies by pretransplant immunoadsorption therapy in highly sensitized renal transplant recipients. *Transplantation* **51**, 324.

Laupacis, A., Stiller, C. R., Keown, P. A., *et al.* (1983). Renal transplantation across a previously positive crossmatch using cyclosporine immunosuppression. *Transplant. Proc.* **15**, 1919.

Lazda, V. A., Pollack, R., Moses, M. F. and Jonasson, O. (1988). The relationship between flow cytometer crossmatch results and subsequent rejection episodes in cadaver renal allograft recipients. *Transplantation* **45**, 562.

Lobo, P. I. (1981). Nature of autolymphocytotoxins present in renal hemodialysis patients: their possible role in controlling alloantibody formation. *Transplantation* **32**, 233.

Mahoney, R. J., Ault, K. A., Given, S. R., *et al.* (1990). The flow cytometric crossmatch and early renal transplant loss. *Transplantation* **49**, 527.

Martin, S., Dyer, P. A., Mallick, N. P., Gokal, R., Harris, R. and

Joh, R. W. G. (1987). Posttransplant antidonor lymphocytotoxic antibody production in relation to graft outcome. *Transplantation* **43**, 50.

Matas, A. J., Nehlsen-Cannarella, S., Tellis, V. A., Kuemmel, P., Soberman, R. and Veith, F. J. (1984). Successful kidney transplantation with current-sera-negative historical sera-positive T cell crossmatch. *Transplantation* **37**, 111.

McKenna, R. M., Lee, K. R., Gough, J. C., *et al.* (1998). Matching for private or public HLA epitopes reduces acute rejection episodes and improves two-year renal allograft function. *Transplantation* **66**, 38.

Mickey, M. R., Adams, C., Baum, K. A., *et al.* (1985). Increasing donors available to sensitized patients by predicting crossmatch outcome. *Transplant. Proc.* **17**, 52.

Mittal, K. K., Mickey, M. R., Singal, D. P. and Terasaki, P. I. (1968). Serotyping for homotransplantation: 18. refinement of microdroplet lymphocyte cytotoxicity test. *Transplantation* **6**, 913.

Moraes, J. R. and Stastny, P. (1977). Human endothelial cell antigens: molecular independency from HLA expression in blood monocytes. *Transplant. Proc.* **9**, 605.

Morris, P. J., Williams, G. M., Hume, D. M., Mickey, M. R. and Terasaki, P. I. (1968). Serotyping for homotransplantation: XII. occurrence of cytotoxic antibodies following kidney transplantation in man. *Transplantation* **6**, 392.

Morris, P. J., Johnson, R. J., Fuggle, S. V., *et al.* (1999). Analysis of factors that affect outcome of primary cadaveric renal transplantation. *Lancet* **354**, 1147.

Mytilineos, J., Deufel, A. and Opelz, G. (1997). Clinical relevance of HLA-DPB locus matching for cadaver kidney retransplants: a report of the Collaborative Transplant Study. *Transplantation* **63**, 1351.

Mytilineos, J., Scherer, S. and Opelz, G. (1990). Comparison of RFLP-DR beta and serological HLA-DR typing in 1500 individuals. *Transplantation* **50**, 870.

Mytilineos, J., Scherer, S., Trejaut, J., *et al.* (1992). Analysis of discrepancies between serologic and DNA-RFLP typing for HLA-DR in kidney graft recipients. *Transplant. Proc.* **24**, 2478.

Newton, C. R., Graham, A., Heptinstall, L. E., *et al.* (1989). Analysis of any point mutation in DNA: the amplification refractory mutation system (ARMS). *Nucleic Acids Res.* **17**, 2503.

Olerup, O. and Zetterquist, H. (1992). HLA-DR typing by PCR amplification with sequence-specific primers (PCR-SSP) in 2 hours: an alternative to serological DR typing in clinical practice including donor-recipient matching in cadaveric transplantation. *Tissue Antigens* **39**, 225.

O'Neill, C. M., Bunce, M. and Welsh, K. I. (1996). Detection of the DRB4 null gene, DRB4*0101102N, by PCR-SSP and its distinction from other DRB4 genes. *Tissue Antigens* **47**, 245.

Opelz, G. (1988). Importance of HLA antigen splits for kidney transplant matching. *Lancet* **2**, 61.

Opelz, G. (1992). How unusual are the University of Minnesota HLA matching results. *Transplantation* **53**, 694.

Opelz, G., Graver, B., Mickey, M. R. and Terasaki, P. I. (1981). Lymphocytotoxic antibody responses to transfusions in potential kidney transplant recipients. *Transplantation* **32**, 177.

Opelz, G., Mytilineos, J., Scherer, S., *et al.* (1991). Survival of DNA HLA-DR typed and matched cadaver kidney transplants. The Collaborative Transplant Study. *Lancet* **338**, 461.

Opelz, G., Mytilineos, J., Scherer, S., *et al.* (1993). Analysis of HLA-DR matching in DNA-typed cadaver kidney transplants. *Transplantation* **55**, 782.

Opelz, G., Scherer, S. and Mytilineos, J. (1997). Analysis of HLA-DR split-specificity matching in cadaver kidney transplantation: a report of the Collaborative Transplant Study. *Transplantation* **63**, 57.

Palmer, A., Bewick, M., Kennedy, L., Welsh, K. I. and Taube, D. H. (1989a). Anti-HLA antibodies following the transplantation of highly sensitized renal allograft recipients. *Transplant. Proc.* **21**, 766.

Palmer, A., Taube, D., Welsh, K., Bewick, M., Gjorstrup, P. and Thick, M. (1989b). Removal of anti-HLA antibodies by extracorporeal immunoadsorption to enable renal transplantation. *Lancet* **1**, 10.

Patel, R. and Terasaki, P. I. (1969). Significance of the positive crossmatch test in kidney transplantation. *N. Engl. J. Med.* **280**, 735.

Paul, L. C., Claas F. J. H., van Es, L. A. and van Rood, J. J. (1979).

Accelerated rejection of renal allograft associated with pretransplantation antibodies directed against donor antigens on endothelium and monocytes. *N. Engl. J. Med.* **100**, 1258.

Paul, L. C., van Es, L. A., Brutel de la Riviere, G., Eernisse, G. and de Graeff, J. (1978). Blood group B antigen on renal endothelium as the target for rejection in an ABO-incompatible recipient. *Transplantation* **26**, 268.

Pellegrino, M. A., Belvedere, M., Pellegrino, A. G. and Ferrone, S. (1978). B peripheral lymphocytes express more HLA antigens than T peripheral lymphocytes. *Transplantation* **25**, 93.

Peugh, W. N., Superina, R. A., Wood, K. J. and Morris, P. J. (1986). The role of H-2 and non-H-2 antigens and genes in the rejection of murine cardiac allogafts. *Immunogenetics* **23**, 30.

Phelan, D. L., Hibbett, S., Wetter, L., Hanto, D. W. and Mohanakumar, T. (1991). Recombinant erythropoietin: does it really effect sensitization? *Transplant. Proc.* **23**, 409.

Pirofsky, B. and Rosner, E. R. (1974). DTT test: a new method to differentiate IgM and IgG erythrocyte antibodies. *Vox Sang.* **27**, 480.

Ploeg, R. J., Pirsch, J. D., Stegall, M. D., *et al.* (1993). Living unrelated kidney donation: an underutilized resource? *Transplant. Proc.* **25(1 Pt. 2)**, 1532.

Pollack, M. S., Maurer, D., Levine, L. S., *et al.* (1979). Prenatal diagnosis of congenital adrenal hyperplasia (21-hydroxylase deficiency) by HLA typing. *Lancet* **1**, 1107.

Povlsen, J. V., Madsen, M., Rasmussen, A., *et al.* (1991). Clinical applicability of the immunomagnetic beads technique for serological crossmatching in renal transplantation. *Tissue Antigens* **38**, 111.

Procter, J., Crawford, J., Bunce, M. and Welsh, K. I. (1996). A rapid molecular method (PCR-SSP) to genotype for ABO blood group and secretor status and its potential for organ transplants. *Tissue Antigens* **50**, 475.

Revillard, J. P., Vincent, C. and Rivera, S. (1979). Anti-B2-microglobulin lymphocytotoxic autoantibodies in systemic lupus erythematosus. *J. Immunol.* **122**, 614.

Rosenberg, W. M. C., Bushell, A., Higgins, R. M., *et al.* (1992). Isolated HLA-DP mismatches between donors and recipients do not influence the function or outcome of renal transplants. *Hum. Immunol.* **33**, 5.

Ross, C. N., Gaskin, G., Gregor-MacGregor, S., *et al.* (1993). Renal transplantation following immunoabsorption in highly sensitized recipients. *Transplantation* **55**, 785.

Rydberg, L. (1991). *Serological and Immunochemical Studies in ABO Incompatible Blood Transfusion, Renal Transplantation and Blood Group Little p Individuals*, Ph.D. thesis, University of Goteborg, Goteborg, Sweden.

Rydberg, L., Breimer, M. E., Brynger, H. and Samuelsson, B. E. (1990). ABO-incompatible kidney transplantation (A2 to O). *Transplantation* **49**, 954.

Rydberg, L. and Samuelsson, B. E. (1991). Presence of glycosyltransferase inhibitors in the sera of patients with long surviving ABO incompatible (A2 to O) kidney grafts. *Transfus. Med.* **123**, 127.

Saiki, R. K., Scharf, S., Faloona, F., *et al.* (1985). Enzymatic amplification of beta-globin genomic sequences and restriction site analysis for diagnosis of sickle cell anemia. *Science* **230**, 1350.

Salvatierra, O., Amend, W., Vincenti, F., *et al.* (1981). Pretreatment with donor-specific blood transfusions in related recipients with high MLC. *Transplant. Proc.* **13**, 142.

Sanfilippo, F., Vaughan, W. K., Bollinger, R. R. and Spees, E. K. (1982). Comparative effects of pregnancy, transfusion, prior graft rejection on sensitization and renal transplant results. *Transplantation* **34**, 360.

Sanfilippo, F., Vaughan, W. K., Light, J. A. and Lefor, W. M. (1985). Lack of influence of donor-recipient differences in subtypic HLA-A,B antigens (splits) on the outcome of cadaver renal transplantation. *Transplantation* **39**, 151.

Schafer, A. J., Hasert, K. and Opelz, G. (1985). Collaborative transplant study crossmatch and antibody project. *Transplant. Proc.* **17**, 2469.

Scornick, J. C., LeFor, W. M., Cicciarelli, J. C., *et al.* (1992). Hyperacute and acute kidney graft rejection due to antibodies against B cells. *Transplantation* **54**, 61.

Sengar, D. P. S., Couture, R. A., Raman, S. and Jindal, S. L. (1990). Beneficial effect of HLA-DQ compatibility on the survival of cadaveric renal allografts in cyclosporine-treated recipients. *Transplantation* **49**, 1007.

Shaw, S., Johnson, A. H. and Shearer, G. M. (1980). Evidence for a new segregant series of B cell antigens that are encoded in the HLA-D region and that stimulate secondary allogeneic proliferative and cytotoxic responses. *J. Exp. Med.* **152**, 565.

Smith, K. J., Reid, S. W., Harlos, K., *et al.* (1996). Bound water structure and polymorphic amino acids act together to allow the binding of different peptides to MHC class I HLA-B53. *Immunity* **3**, 215.

Starzl, T. E., Marchioro, T. L., Holmes, J. H., *et al.* (1964). Renal homografts in patients with major donor-recipient blood group incompatibilities. *Surgery* **55**, 195.

Sumrani, N., Delaney, V., Hong, J. H., Daskalakis, P. and Sommer, B. G. (1992). The influence of nephrectomy of the primary allograft on retransplantation graft outcome in the cyclosporine era. *Transplantation* **53**, 52.

Sutton, V. R., Kienzle, B. K. and Knowles, R. W. (1989). An altered splice site is found in the DRB4 gene that is not expressed in HLA-DR7,Dw11 individuals. *Immunogenetics* **29**, 317.

Takemoto, S., Carnahan, E. and Terasaki, P. I. (1991). A report of 504 six antigen-matched transplants. *Transplant. Proc.* **23**, 1318.

Takemoto, S. and Terasaki, P. I. (1991). HLA epitopes and graft survival. *In Clinical Transplants 1991*, (P. I. Terasaki, ed.), p. 363, UCLA, Los Angeles.

Talbot, D., Givans, A. L., Shenton, B. K., Stratton, A., Proud, G. and Taylor, R. M. R. (1989). The relevance of a more sensitive crossmatch assay to renal transplantation. *Transplantation* **47**, 552.

Taube, D. H., Williams, D. G., Cameron, J. S., *et al.* (1984). Renal transplantation after removal and prevention of resynthesis of HLA antibodies. *Lancet* **1**, 824.

Taylor, C. J., Chapman, J. R., Fuggle, S. V., Ting, A. and Morris, P. J. (1987). A positive B cell crossmatch due to IgG anti-HLA-DQ antibody present at the time of transplantation in a successful renal allograft. *Tissue Antigens* **30**, 104.

Taylor, C. J., Chapman, J. R., Ting, A. and Morris, P. J. (1989). Characterization of lymphocytotoxic antibodies causing a positive crossmatch in renal transplantation: relationship to primary and regraft outcome. *Transplantation* **48**, 953.

Taylor, C. J., Ting, A. and Morris, P. J. (1991). Production and characterization of human monoclonal lymphocytotoxic autoantibodies from a renal dialysis patient. *Tissue Antigens* **37**, 112.

Taylor, C. J., Bunce, M., Bayne, A. M., *et al.* (1993). Clinical and socioeconomic benefits of serological HLA-DR matching for renal transplantation over three eras of immunosuppression regimens at a single unit. *In Clinical Transplants 1992* (P. I. Terasaki and M. Cecka, eds.), p. 233, UCLA Tissue Typing Laboratory, Los Angeles.

Terasaki, P. I., Marchioro, T. L. and Starzl, T. E. (1965). Sero-typing of human lymphocyte antigens: preliminary trials on long-term kidney homograft survivors. *In Histocompatibility Testing*, (P. S. Russell, H. J. Winn and D. B. Amos, eds.), p. 83, National Academy of Sciences, Washington, D.C.

Terasaki, P. I. and McClelland, J. D. (1964). Microdroplet assay of human serum cytotoxins. *Nature* **204**, 998.

Thistlethwaite, J. R., Buckingham, M. R., Stuart, J. K. and Stuart, F. P. (1986). Detection of presensitization in renal allograft recipients using a flow cytometric immunofluorescence crossmatch. *Transplant. Proc.* **18**, 676.

Tindall, K. R. and Kunkel, T. A. (1988). Fidelity of DNA synthesis by the Thermus aquaticus DNA polymerase. *Biochemistry* **27**, 6008.

Ting, A. and Morris, P. J. (1978a). Matching for B-cell antigens of the HLA-DR series in cadaver renal transplantation. *Lancet* **1**, 575.

Ting, A. and Morris, P. J. (1978b). Reactivity of autolymphocytotoxic antibodies from dialysis patients with lymphocytes from chronic lymphocytic leukemia (CLL) patients. *Transplantation* **25**, 31.

Ting, A. and Morris, P. J. (1987). HLA matching in transfused, cyclosporine-treated patients at Oxford. *In Clinical Transplants 1987*, (P. I. Terasaki, ed.), p. 235, UCLA Tissue Typing Laboratory, Los Angeles.

Ting, A. and Welsh, K. (1994). HLA matching and crossmatching in renal transplantation. *In Kidney Transplantation: Principles and Practice*, 4th ed., (P. J. Morris, ed.), p. 109, WB Saunders, Philadelphia.

Trowsdale, J. (1996). Molecular genetics of HLA class I and class II regions. *In HLA and MHC Genes, Molecules and Function*, (M. Browning and A. McMichael, eds.), p. 23, BIOS Scientific Publishers, Oxford.

Turka, L. A., Goguen, J. E., Carpenter, C. B. and Milford, E. L. (1989). The effect of historical crossmatches and sensitization on renal allograft survival. *Transplant. Proc.* **21**, 696.

Welsh, K. I., Burgos, H. and Batchelor, J. R. (1977). The immune response to allogeneic rat platelets: Ag-B antigens in matrix form lacking Ia. *Eur. J. Immunol.* **7**, 267.

Welsh, K. I., van Dam, M., Bewick, M. E., *et al.* (1988). Successful transplantation of kidneys bearing previously mismatched HLA A and B locus antigens. *Transpl. Int.* **1**, 190.

Welsh, K. I., van Dam, M. and Koffman, C. G. (1987). Transplantation of blood group A2 kidneys into O and B recipients: the effect of pretransplant anti-A titers on graft survival. *Transplant. Proc.* **19**, 4565.

Williams, G. M., Hume, D. M., Hudson, R. P., Morris, P. J., Kano, K. and Milgrom, F. (1968). "Hyperacute" renal-homograft rejection in man. *N. Engl. J. Med.* **279**, 611.

Wu, D. Y., Ugozzoli, L., Pal, B. K. and Wallace, R. B. (1989). Allele-specific enzymatic amplification of beta-globin genomic DNA for diagnosis of sickle cell anemia. *Proc. Natl. Acad. Sci. U. S. A.* **86**, 2757.

Young, N. T., Roelen, D., Bunce, M., Dallman, M. J., Morris, P. J. and Welsh, K. I. (1997). Alloreactive helper T-lymphocyte precursor frequencies correlate with HLA-DRB1 antigen amino acid residue mismatches. *In Genetic Diversity of HLA: Functional and Medical Implications*, Vol. 2, (D. Charron, ed.), p. 501, EDK, Sevres, France.

Surgical Techniques of Renal Transplantation

John M. Barry • *Peter J. Morris*

Introduction

Renal transplantation is a major surgical procedure, which includes a vascular component and a urological component. Although in the past it was common for the general or vascular surgeon to do the vascular component of the implantation and the urologist to do the urological component of the operation, today the entire procedure generally is performed by a transplant surgeon, regardless of his or her background training as a general surgeon, vascular surgeon, or urologist. The recipient, who is uremic and usually being maintained on hemodialysis or peritoneal dialysis, often is a poor-risk patient with comorbid disease (e.g., diabetes, cardiovascular disease). If poorly dialyzed, the recipient has a significant degree of platelet dysfunction with a resultant tendency to bleed. The need for meticulous techniques cannot be stressed enough, bearing in mind that the operation could be the only opportunity that the patient may have to obtain a successful kidney transplant, which can change the quality of the patient's life dramatically.

Preparation of Recipient

The general preparation and selection of recipients for transplantation is discussed in Chapter 4; on admission for transplantation, a careful history and examination are required to ensure that there is no immediate contraindication to major surgery, and particular attention should be paid to the patient's fluid and electrolyte status. The patient may require dialysis before going to surgery because of fluid overload or a high potassium level. Although dialysis may delay surgery by several hours, this should not influence the decision to dialyze the patient before surgery, bearing in mind that if the patient is to receive a cadaver kidney, there is a 20 to 30% chance that there will be delayed graft function.

Immunosuppression, whatever the protocol, usually is begun before the patient goes to surgery. Although there is no hard evidence that this is necessary, the rationale is that a loading dose of cyclosporine or tacrolimus ensures a better blood level in the first 12 hours because most patients are not able to take oral medication in the first 24 hours after surgery.

The use of preventive antibiotics is advised in that although the operation is a clean one, the patient is uremic and will be immunosuppressed, which puts the patient at high risk for wound infection. There is always a possibility of contamination of a cadaver donor kidney, and the combination of a vascular procedure with a urological procedure increases the risk of infection in the vicinity of the vascular anastomosis. An infection of the vascular anastomosis with subsequent secondary hemorrhage is a catastrophic complication, resulting in loss of the kidney, compromise of distal circulation and a threat to life. The case for preventive antibi-

otics is a strong one. In the Oxford Unit, cefuroxime, 1.5 g intravenously, is given with the induction of anesthesia.

After the induction of anesthesia, a central catheter is inserted into the internal jugular vein or into the subclavian vein. Insertion of the catheter is facilitated by the use of duplex ultrasound. Although a central line is not essential intraoperatively, it facilitates management because many patients who have been on long-term hemodialysis are dehydrated and require significant amounts of fluid to maintain a central venous pressure of 7 to 10 cm H_2O. Other aspects of the induction of anesthesia and monitoring during the operative procedure are discussed in Chapter 13.

A balloon catheter is inserted into the bladder with a full aseptic technique (see later) on the operating table. The skin should be prepared carefully in the operating room, first with thorough shaving followed by preparation of the skin of the abdominal wall with an antimicrobial agent such as povidone-iodine (Betadine).

Site

Although traditionally the right iliac fossa was used for implantation of the kidney since the early descriptions (Hume *et al.*, 1963; Kuss *et al.*, 1951; Merrill *et al.*, 1956; Michon *et al.*, 1953; Starzl *et al.*, 1964a), today it is more usual to place the left kidney in the right iliac fossa and the right kidney in the left iliac fossa, other things being equal. This approach places the pelvis and ureter anteriorly, which to some extent facilitates the urological tract reconstruction, particularly if some subsequent urological complication requires surgical intervention. If a continuous ambulatory peritoneal dialysis catheter were emerging from one side of the abdomen, the contralateral side would be chosen. In the presence of polycystic kidneys, one would choose the side of the smaller polycystic kidney, assuming that there was room for the transplanted kidney below the polycystic kidney. Often, one polycystic kidney has to be removed to make room for a transplanted kidney, and this preferably is done as a separate operative procedure before transplantation because a large polycystic kidney is removed more easily as a transperitoneal procedure. It can be done at the time of the transplant procedure, however, through the same extended retroperitoneal approach. In children, in whom the vascular anastomoses of the renal vessels may be to the aorta and vena cava because of the size of the kidney, the right side is the preferred side because the kidney is placed behind the cecum and ascending colon.

Incision

An oblique or curvilinear incision is made in the right lower quadrant of the abdomen beginning almost in the

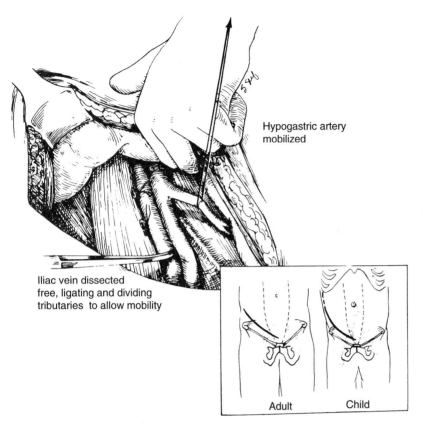

Hypogastric artery
mobilized

Iliac vein dissected
free, ligating and dividing
tributaries to allow mobility

Adult   Child

FIGURE 11–1

Iliac vessels dissected free. (Inset) Incision for adult; incision for child.

midline and curving upward parallel to the inguinal ligament and approximately 2 cm above it and ending just above the anterior superior iliac spine of the iliac crest. In a child or small adult, this incision can be carried up to the costal margin to increase exposure (Fig. 11–1). The external oblique muscle and fascia are divided in the line of the incision and split to the lateral extent of the wound. This incision is carried medially for 2 cm on the rectal sheath to permit retraction or division of part of the rectus muscle for the later exposure of the bladder. To expose the peritoneum, either the internal oblique and transverse muscles are divided with cautery in the line of the incision, or the confluence of the oblique muscles and the rectal sheath is divided medially lateral to the rectal muscle as a pararectal incision, which avoids division of the internal oblique and transversus muscles. The inferior epigastric vessels are ligated and divided, but if there are multiple renal arteries, the inferior epigastric vessels should be preserved in the first instance in case the inferior epigastric artery is required for anastomosis to a lower polar renal artery. Although division of the spermatic cord was advocated in early descriptions of the procedure and was common practice for many years, this should not be done and rarely is required for adequate exposure. The spermatic cord is not cut but freed laterally, which allows it to be retracted medially (Hume, 1968). The round ligament can be divided.

Preparation of Operative Bed

After exposure of the transversalis fascia and peritoneum, the transversalis fascia is divided, and the peritoneum is reflected upward and medially to expose the psoas muscle and the iliac vessels. Depending on whether the internal iliac artery is to be anastomosed to the renal artery of the transplant kidney or whether the renal artery with a cuff of aorta

is to be anastomosed to the external iliac artery, dissection proceeds in the first instance to expose the external, common and internal iliac arteries. The lymphatics that course along and over the vessels must be ligated with a nonabsorbable suture such as silk and divided, rather than cauterized, to prevent the later occurrence of a lymphocele (see Chapter 28). If the internal iliac artery is to be used, it is important to mobilize a length of the common and external iliac arteries so that the internal iliac artery can be rotated laterally without kinking at its origin. Care is taken to inspect the origin of the internal iliac artery, if this is to be used, for any evidence of atheroma, and similarly, any atheromatous disease in the common or external iliac artery should be noted. If there are two or more renal arteries not on a cuff of aorta, the dissection of the internal iliac artery is extended distally to expose the initial branches of the internal iliac artery, some of which may be suitable for anastomosis to individual renal arteries.

Having completed the exposure of the appropriate iliac arteries, dissection of the external iliac vein is begun. If a left kidney with a long renal vein is available, dissection of the external iliac vein alone generally allows a satisfactory anastomosis without tension. If a right kidney, which has a short renal vein, is to be used; or a left kidney, in which a short renal vein has been provided, is to be used or the recipient is obese, the internal iliac vein and usually one or two other quite large tributaries can be ligated with silk and divided (Hume, 1968; Simmons, 1972). This technique allows the common and external iliac veins to be brought well up into the wound, particularly if the internal iliac artery is divided, and this facilitates the performance of a tension-free anastomosis. The peritoneum is further reflected up laterally to prepare the final pocket for the kidney in the parapsoas gutter.

At this stage, a self-retaining retractor is inserted if available. We find the Bookwalter retractor system satisfactory because it provides excellent exposure and allows the assistant to have both hands free to assist with the anastomoses. The vessels are now ready for clamping once the kidney has been prepared and is ready for implantation. Heparin is not administered unless the hemoglobin is greater than 11 g/dl; then a relatively modest dose of heparin should be used (e.g., 2,000 to 4,000 IU depending on the size of the patient).

Vascular clamps are applied to the external iliac artery proximally and distally if an end-to-side anastomosis is to be performed, and if the internal iliac artery is to be used, a vascular clamp is applied to the internal iliac artery at its origin. The vein is clamped proximally and distally with vascular clamps or isolated between tourniquets, or a Satinsky side clamp is used. After division of the internal iliac artery distally, the lumen is flushed out with heparinized saline. Similarly, if the external iliac artery is to be used, an appropriate-sized arteriotomy is made, and again the lumen is flushed out with heparinized saline. The venotomy similarly is flushed out with heparinized saline, and if a valve is present at the site of the venotomy, this should be removed carefully. Before making the arteriotomy or venotomy, the surgeon should visualize mentally the kidney *in situ* in its parapsoas gutter and the course that the renal artery and vein will take to ensure the optimal site for the anastomoses.

Preparation of Kidney

A varying degree of dissection of the kidney is required when it is received in ice. In the case of cadaver kidney, in which usually the kidneys have been removed as part of an *en bloc* procedure, considerable dissection needs to be performed, and this should be done carefully and with a good light on a back table with the kidney in a bowl of ice slush. The dissection of the cadaver kidney usually is done in advance of the transplant procedure in case some anomaly may be present that would preclude going ahead with the transplant. In the dissection, great care must be taken in protecting the blood supply to the ureter, and the so-called golden triangle should not be broached (see Chapter 29).

A kidney from a living donor in general has a single renal artery, but there may be additional arteries. In this case, reconstruction usually is done on the back table, and either the arteries are joined together at their orifices to form a common trunk (Fig. 11–2) or a smaller artery is anastomosed end-to-side to a larger renal artery. It is imperative that a lower polar artery be revascularized because this almost certainly gives rise to the ureteric blood supply. It also is possible to use the epigastric artery to revascularize a lower polar artery, but in general it is preferable to anastomose a lower polar artery to the major renal artery, either end-to-side or as a common trunk. It also is possible to use a portion of saphenous vein as a graft bridge. A small upper polar artery, if thought to be too small to anastomose safely to the major renal artery, may be ligated, provided that it supplies less than one eighth of the kidney (which should be evident on perfusion of the kidney after removal).

A cadaver kidney usually has a renal artery or arteries arising from an aortic patch, and this should be trimmed to an appropriate size and used for anastomosis to the external iliac artery. If two renal arteries are widely separated on the aortic patch, the patch may be divided to allow separate implantation into external iliac artery, or one may be implanted end-to-side and the other to a branch of the internal iliac artery.

If there is more than one renal vein, smaller veins can be

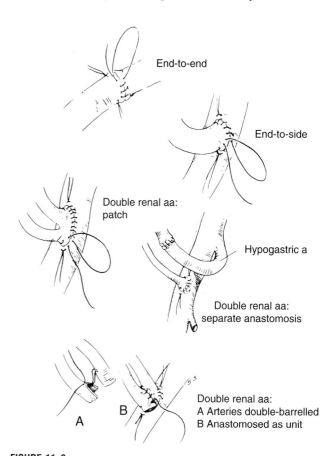

FIGURE 11–2

Some variations of renal artery anastomoses.

ligated, assuming that there is one large renal vein. If two renal veins are of equal size and are not arising from a Carrel patch, there is some risk of subsequent venous infarction if one vein is ligated, and it is then preferable to join the veins to form a common trunk for the subsequent anastomosis. A short right renal vein can be extended with donor inferior vena cava or external iliac vein.

When the kidney finally is prepared and is ready for implantation, a technique that we use in Oxford ensures that the kidney remains cool during the time of the anastomoses. A surgical glove (size 8) is used, the fingers knotted and the ends cut off. The glove is packed partially with crushed ice and the kidney inserted, with care being taken always to have the upper pole of the kidney at the finger end of the glove (*fingers up*). More crushed ice is inserted into the glove, and the glove is tied at its wrist end. A 1.5-cm hole is made over the vessels, which can be brought through this opening in turn. This technique not only keeps the kidney cool during the anastomosis (Roake *et al.*, 1991) but also facilitates handling the kidney because an artery clamp can be placed on the glove itself to allow the kidney to be held in position during the procedure. When the anastomoses are completed, the glove is removed, and the kidney is reperfused.

Revascularization

The question of whether the arterial anastomosis or the venous anastomosis should be done first depends on the final position of the kidney and the ease with which the

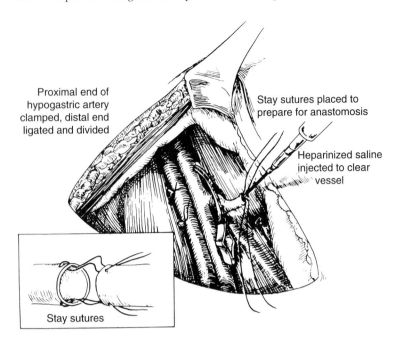

Proximal end of hypogastric artery clamped, distal end ligated and divided

Stay sutures placed to prepare for anastomosis

Heparinized saline injected to clear vessel

Stay sutures

FIGURE 11–3

Hypogastric artery ligated and divided, the lumen flushed with heparinized saline.

second anastomosis may or may not be done. In general, if the renal artery is to be anastomosed to the internal iliac artery, the arterial anastomosis should be done first because this enables the renal vein to be positioned appropriately. If the renal artery is to be anastomosed end-to-side—usually with a cuff of aorta—to the external iliac artery, it is preferable to do the venous anastomosis first, then the end-to-side arterial anastomosis can be positioned correctly.

ARTERIAL ANASTOMOSIS

The internal iliac artery is anastomosed end-to-end to the renal artery using a three-point anastomosis and 6–0 Prolene, as described by Carrel in 1902, or a two-point anastomosis (Fig. 11–3). If there is a disparity between the renal artery and the internal iliac artery, the renal artery being considerably smaller in diameter, the renal artery should be spatulated along one side to broaden the anastomosis. Care should be taken if one side of the renal artery is spatulated to place the spatulation of the renal artery appropriately, taking into consideration the final curve of the internal iliac artery and the renal artery when the kidney will be in its final position (Fig. 11–4). If both arteries are small, at least one third of the anastomosis should be performed with interrupted sutures to allow for expansion. In a child or a small adult with small arteries, the whole anastomosis should be performed with interrupted sutures.

An end-to-side anastomosis of the renal artery to the external iliac artery usually is performed using an appropriately trimmed cuff of aorta attached to the renal artery. An arteriotomy appropriately placed is performed in the external iliac artery, then the anastomosis is carried out with a continuous 6–0 Prolene suture (see Fig. 11–2).

VENOUS ANASTOMOSIS

The renal vein is anastomosed end-to-side usually to the external iliac vein using a continuous 5–0 Prolene suture, with the initial sutures placed at either end of the venotomy (Fig. 11–5). An important aspect of this technique is the placement of an anchor suture at the midpoint of the lateral

wall, which allows the external iliac vein and the renal vein on the lateral side of the anastomosis to be drawn clear of the medial wall of the anastomosis. This technique avoids any possibility of the back wall being caught up in the suture while the medial wall is being sutured. The renal vein may be anastomosed to the external iliac vein lateral or medial to the external iliac artery. This anastomosis depends on the length of the renal vein lateral to the artery, but if the external common iliac vein has been mobilized, as described earlier, usually even with a short vein the venous anastomosis can

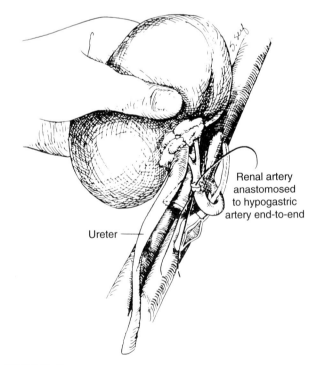

Renal artery anastomosed to hypogastric artery end-to-end

Ureter

FIGURE 11–4

Anastomosis of the renal artery to hypogastric artery.

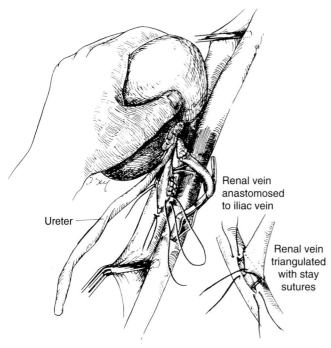

FIGURE 11–5

Vein anastomosis with triangular stay sutures in place.

Ureter

Renal vein anastomosed to iliac vein

Renal vein triangulated with stay sutures

be performed medial to the artery. It is important to ensure, wherever the anastomosis is positioned, that the renal vein is under no tension, and care should be taken that the vein is not twisted before starting the anastomosis. When a small child receives an adult kidney, it is sometimes necessary to shorten the renal vein to prevent kinking, especially when the vein is anastomosed to the inferior vena cava.

Reconstruction of the Urinary Tract

After renal revascularization, the kidney is placed in what will be its final position, and reestablishment of urinary tract continuity begins. Transplantation of the left kidney into the right iliac fossa and the right kidney into the left iliac fossa reverses the normal anterior-to-posterior relationship of the vein, artery and collecting system and positions the renal pelvis and ureter of the kidney transplant so that they are the most medial and superficial of the hilar structures (Merrill *et al.*, 1956). This positioning simplifies primary and secondary urinary tract reconstruction, especially if pyeloureterostomy, ureteroureterostomy or pyelovesicostomy is to be done. The factors that determine the type of urinary tract reconstruction are the length and condition of the donor ureter, the condition of the recipient's bladder or bladder substitute, the condition of the recipient's ureter and the familiarity of the surgeon with the technique.

Suture material is an individual choice. Although urinary tract reconstruction with nonabsorbable sutures has been described (Jaffers *et al.*, 1982; McDonald *et al.*, 1987), it leaves the recipient with the risk of stone formation if the suture material is chronically exposed to urine. Currently available synthetic absorbable sutures have characteristics suitable for the immunocompromised kidney transplant recipient who has the potential for delayed wound healing (Rosen and

McAninch, 1996). *In vivo* strength retention is poorest with natural fibers (plain gut and chromic gut), better with synthetic braided materials (polyglycolic acid and polygalactin), and best with synthetic monofilament materials (polyglyconate and polydioxanone). Monofilament suture has less tissue drag than braided suture, but knot security is better with braided suture. We have found polydioxane to be satisfactory and use 3–0 for bladder closure and 4–0 or 5–0 for ureteric or renal pelvic anastomoses.

URETERONEOCYSTOSTOMY

Ureteroneocystostomy is the usual form of urinary tract reconstruction. Its advantages are (1) it can be done regardless of the quality or presence of the recipient ureter, (2) it is several centimeters away from the vascular anastomoses, (3) the native ureter remains available for the treatment of ureteric complications and (4) native nephrectomy is unnecessary. The goal is to create a 2- to 3-cm submucosal tunnel with muscle backing of the ureter so that when the bladder contracts, there is a valve mechanism to prevent reflux of urine up the ureter (Lich *et al.*, 1961; Paquin, 1959; Politano and Leadbetter, 1958).

The genitalia are prepared with an antiseptic solution, and a lubricated balloon retention catheter is passed into the urinary bladder or bladder substitute. The catheter is connected to a sterile Y-tube system (Kootstra, 1994; Fig. 11–6). This system has a bag filled with an antibiotic solution on one line and a collection bag on the other. With this system, the bladder can be filled, irrigated, drained and refilled during the procedure. It is especially helpful when the bladder is difficult to identify because of pelvic scar tissue, recipient obesity or reduced capacity. After initially accommodating a small volume, the defunctionalized bladder often accepts

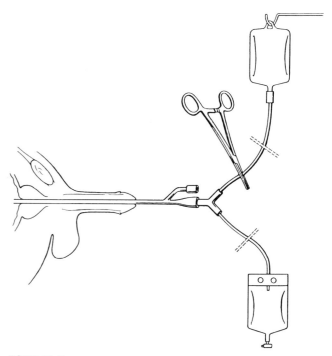

FIGURE 11–6

Y-tube system for rinsing, filling and draining bladder or bladder substitute.

more fluid 1 or 2 hours into the transplantation procedure (Barry *et al.*, 1996).

TRANSVESICAL URETERONEOCYSTOSTOMY

The technique for transvesical ureteroneocystostomy is similar to that described by Merrill and colleagues in the first successful kidney transplant from a twin (Merrill *et al.*, 1956; Fig. 11–7). It is now usually known as the Politano-Leadbetter technique (Politano and Leadbetter 1958). The dome of the bladder is cleared off, and stay sutures or Allis clamps are placed on either side of a proposed vertical midline incision. The urinary bladder is drained, and an incision is made through all layers of the anterior bladder wall. A padded retractor is placed into the dome of the bladder to expose the trigone. A point clear of the native ureter is selected, and a transverse incision is made in the mucosa. A submucosal tunnel is created with a right-angle clamp or Thorek scissors for about 2 cm. The clamp or scissors is punched through the bladder, and the muscular opening is enlarged to accept the kidney transplant ureter. The ureter is drawn under the spermatic cord or round ligament and into the bladder, where it is transected at a length that prevents tension or redundancy. The cut end of the ureter is incised for 3 to 5 mm and approximated to the bladder mucosa with fine absorbable sutures. The inferior suture includes the bladder muscularis to fix the ureter distally and to prevent its move-ment in the submucosal tunnel. The padded retractor is re-moved, and the cystotomy is closed with a single layer of 3–0 absorbable suture, although some surgeons do a two-layer or three-layer closure. The bladder can be refilled to check for leakage, and points of leakage can be repaired with one or two interrupted sutures. Some surgeons use two bladder mucosal incisions about 2 cm apart (Starzl, 1964). When that technique is used, the proximal bladder mucosal incision is closed with a fine absorbable suture.

EXTRAVESICAL URETERONEOCYSTOSTOMY

When compared with the transvesical procedures, the ex-travesical techniques are faster, a separate cystotomy is not required and less ureteric length is necessary. These factors should reduce operating time, bladder spasms and hematuria and improve the probability of adequate distal ureteric blood supply.

Extravesical techniques are based on the procedure de-scribed by Lich *et al.* (1961). Extravesical ureteroneocystos-tomy was adapted for renal transplantation in 1962 (Wood-ruff *et al.*, 1969), and it is well illustrated in a publication by Konnak *et al.* (1972; Fig. 11–8). A subsequent modification was the addition of a stitch to anchor the toe of the spatulated ureter to the bladder to prevent proximal slippage of the ureter in the submucosal tunnel with loss of the antireflux

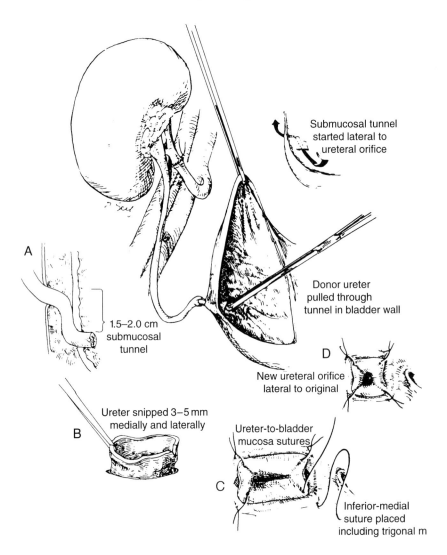

A

1.5–2.0 cm submucosal tunnel

Submucosal tunnel started lateral to ureteral orifice

Donor ureter pulled through tunnel in bladder wall

B Ureter snipped 3–5 mm medially and laterally

C Ureter-to-bladder mucosa sutures

Inferior-medial suture placed including trigonal m

D New ureteral orifice lateral to original

FIGURE 11–7

Transvesical ureteroneocystostomy.

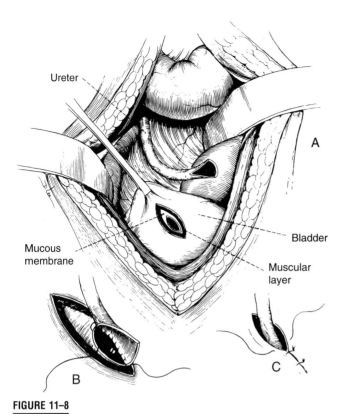

FIGURE 11–8

Extravesical ureteroneocystostomy.

valve and disruption of the ureteric anastomosis (Bradic *et al.*, 1975; de Campos-Freire *et al.*, 1974).

The bladder is distended with an antibiotic solution through the urethral catheter. The lateral surface of the bladder is cleared of fat and the peritoneal reflection, a padded retractor is placed medially, another is placed inferolaterally and a third is placed cephalomedially to hold the peritoneum and its contents out of the way. It is important to place the ureter under the spermatic cord or round ligament to prevent posttransplant ureteric obstruction. A T-shaped or longitudinal oblique incision is made for approximately 3 cm until the bladder mucosa bulges into the incision. The bladder is drained partially, and the mucosa is dissected away from the muscularis to make a submucosal tunnel for the ureter. The bladder mucosa is grasped with atraumatic forceps, the urinary bladder is drained and an incision is made in the mucosa. The ureter is laid in the trough, spatulated and anastomosed to the bladder mucosa with running or interrupted fine absorbable sutures. A horizontal or vertical mattress suture is placed in the toe of the ureter and passed submucosally through the seromuscular layer of the bladder and tied about 5 mm distal to the cystotomy (Fig. 11–9). The seromuscular layer is closed over the ureter with interrupted sutures so that the proximal one or two sutures can be removed if the ureteric lumen has been compromised by the closure.

The *one-stitch* (Shanfield, 1972) and *two-stitch* (MacKinnon *et al.*, 1968) extravesical ureteroneocystostomies are modifications of the Lich procedure in which one or two mattress sutures are placed full thickness through the spatulated ureter and the bladder without an attempt at mucosa-to-mucosa approximation (Fig. 11–10). If the ureter lies too loosely in the partial cystotomy, the seromuscular layer is closed over the ureter with interrupted stitches.

The parallel-incision extravesical ureteroneocystostomy commonly is used in the Oregon program (Barry, 1983; Gibbons *et al.*, 1992; Fig. 11–11). The setup is the same as for a modified Lich procedure. Parallel incisions are made in the lateral bladder about 2 cm apart until the bladder mucosa bulges into both incisions. The bladder is drained partially, and a submucosal tunnel is created between the two incisions. The ureter is drawn through the tunnel, transected, spatulated and anastomosed to the bladder mucosa with interrupted fine absorbable sutures. Sometimes extra stitches are placed between the quadrant sutures to prevent urinary leakage. A vertical or horizontal mattress suture is used to anchor the toe of the ureter to the urinary bladder. This suture is tied about 5 mm distal to the cystotomy. Finally the distal cystotomy is closed with a running fine absorbable suture. The parallel-incision extravesical ureteroneocystostomy has been slightly modified by Caparros and associates by application of the *one-stitch* principle with no suture approximation of the ureteric and bladder mucosa (Caparros *et al.*, 1996).

DOUBLE URETERS

Double ureters can be managed simply by leaving them in their common sheath, trimming them to appropriate length,

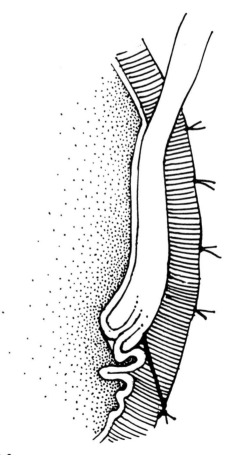

FIGURE 11–9

Mattress suture or two to anchor toe of transplant ureter to full-thickness bladder. This prevents ureteric slippage in the submucosal tunnel.

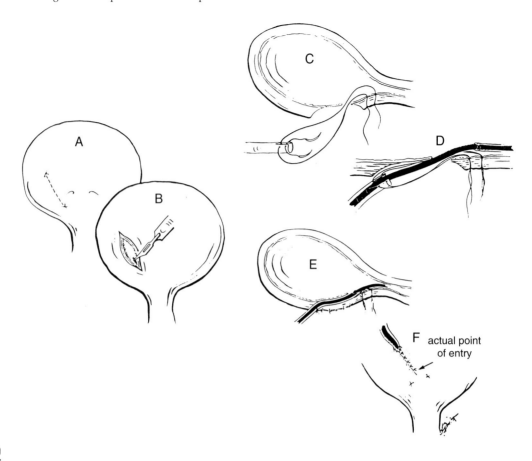

FIGURE 11–10

Extravesical ureteroneocystostomy without mucosa-to-mucosa anastomosis. This also is done without a stent.

spatulating them and either anastomosing the medial edges together with a running fine absorbable suture (Conlin *et al.*, 1994; Prout *et al.*, 1967; Fig. 11–12) or by joining them, one on top of the other, with a single stitch from the toe of the upper one to the heel of the lower one (Barry *et al.*, 1973; Fig. 11–13). The conjoined ureters can be treated as a single ureter by any of the previously described ureteroneocystostomy techniques. The submucosal tunnel needs to be made a bit wider. Others have used a separate ureteroneocystostomy for each of the ureters (Szmidt *et al.*, 1988). These same techniques can be used for the *en bloc* transplantation of pediatric kidneys or the transplantation of two adult kidneys, stacked one on top of the other (Masson and Hefty, 1998), into one recipient. Fjeldborg and Kim (1972) described a pyeloureteric anastomosis in which both renal pelves are joined after dividing the ureters at their ureteropelvic junctions and suturing the posterior walls together, leaving the anterior halves for anastomosis with the recipient ureter (Fig. 11–14).

PYELOPYELOSTOMY

Pyelopyelostomy has been used for orthotopic renal transplantation, usually in the left flank (Gil-Vernet *et al.*, 1989). The native kidney is removed, and the kidney transplant is revascularized with the native renal artery or the splenic artery and the native renal vein. The proximal ureter and renal pelvis of the kidney transplant are opened medially, and the native renal pelvis is anastomosed to the kidney transplant renal pelvis with a running fine absorbable suture. After completion of one wall, a double-pigtail ureteral stent

is passed with or over a wire through the native ureter into the bladder, and the wire is withdrawn to allow the bladder curl to form. Its position in the bladder is confirmed by reflux of bladder irrigant up the stent. The proximal coil is placed in the renal pelvis of the kidney transplant, and the remaining half of the suture line is completed. When compared with ureteroneocystostomy, an advantage of urinary tract reconstruction with the native renal pelvis or ureter is the ease with which subsequent retrograde pyelography, stent placement or ureteroscopy can be accomplished through the normally positioned ureteric orifice.

PYELOURETEROSTOMY AND URETEROURETEROSTOMY

Pyeloureterostomy and ureteroureterostomy usually are done when the transplant ureter's blood supply appears to be compromised, when the urinary bladder is difficult to identify because of pelvic scar, when the bladder does not distend enough for a ureteroneocystostomy or when the surgeon prefers one of them to ureteroneocystostomy (Hamburger *et al.*, 1965; Lawler *et al.*, 1950; Leadbetter *et al.*, 1966). The techniques for ureteropyelostomy and ureteroureterostomy are similar (Fig. 11–15). The posterior, or back wall, anastomosis of the kidney transplant pelvis or ureter to the side or to the spatulated end of the native ureter is completed; a double-pigtail ureteral stent is placed and the anterior suture line is completed. The proximal native ureter is managed by (1) leaving the native kidney *in situ* and using the side of the native ureter for the anastomosis, (2) ipsilateral

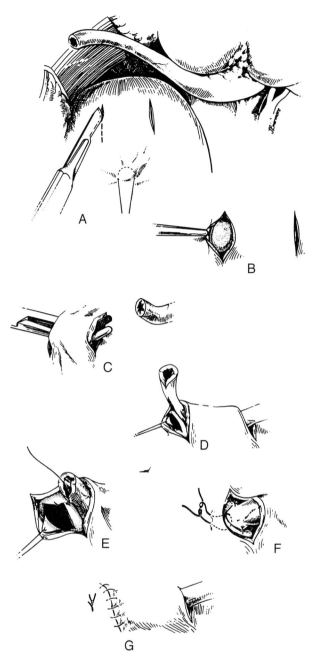

FIGURE 11–11

Parallel incision extravesical ureteroneocystostomy. The adequacy of the submucosal tunnel is judged by pulling the ureter through it.

nephrectomy and proximal ureterectomy or (3) ligation of the proximal ureter with the obstructed native kidney left *in situ*. Although Schiff and Lytton (1981) and Lord *et al.* (1991) have described the safety of native ureteral ligation with kidney transplant urinary tract reconstruction, we prefer to leave the native ureter in continuity with its kidney and to anastomose the pelvis or ureter of the renal transplant to the side of the native ureter. This technique ensures a good blood supply to the native ureter and removes an obstructed, hydronephrotic kidney from the differential diagnosis of a posttransplant problem.

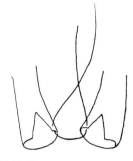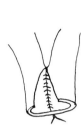

FIGURE 11–12

Management of double ureters to make them into a single ureteric orifice.

PYELOVESICOSTOMY

Pyelovesicostomy has been described by Herwig and Konnak (1973), Bennett (1973) and Firlit (1977) for urinary tract reconstruction when the native ureter and the renal transplant ureter are unsuitable or become so (Fig. 11–16). The bladder must reach the renal pelvis without tension, and a bladder extension with a psoas hitch or Boari flap may be necessary.

URETEROENTEROSTOMY

Ureteroenterostomy into an intestinal conduit or an intestinal pouch has been successful (Hatch *et al.*, 1993; Kelly *et*

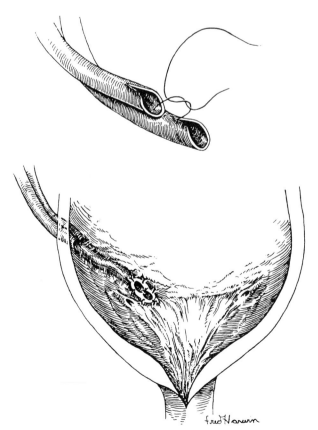

FIGURE 11–13

Alternate method of managing double ureters.

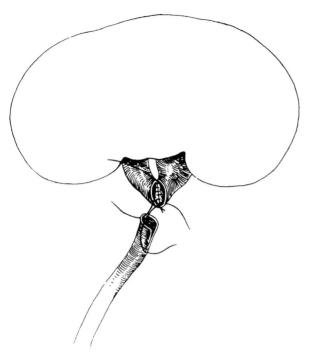

FIGURE 11–14

Management of double ureters by pyelopyelostomy followed by conjoined pyeloureterostomy.

al., 1966). It is performed by slight distention of the conduit or pouch with antibiotic-containing irrigant, then using one of the extravesical ureteroneocystostomy techniques. Successful anastomosis of the transplant ureter to the afferent limb of a Koch pouch has been described (Heritier *et al.*, 1989). If it is difficult to identify the intestinal conduit or pouch because of surrounding intestines, the addition of methylene blue to the irrigant stains the conduit or pouch and makes it easy to find (Whitehead *et al.*, 1972). This topic is discussed more completely in Chapter 12.

URETERIC STENTS

We use ureteric stents when there is concern about urinary leakage or temporary obstruction because of edema, periureteral bleeding or a thickened bladder when pyelopyelostomy, pyeloureterostomy or ureteroureterostomy has been performed or when the ureter has been anastomosed to an intestinal conduit or pouch. The length of the stent is determined by the estimated distance between the renal pelvis of the kidney graft and the bladder or its substitute. The commonest type and size when the transplanted kidney is located in the iliac fossa is a double-pigtail 6F × 12 cm stent. A prophylactic ureteric stent for all kidney transplant ureteroneocystostomies has been shown by Pleass and colleagues in a randomized prospective trial to reduce the incidence of urological complications (Pleass *et al.*, 1995).

MANAGEMENT OF CATHETER AND STENT

The urinary bladder or reservoir catheter usually is removed on the fifth postoperative day after a urine specimen is tested at the bedside for nitrites and sent for bacterial culture and after a single dose of a broad-spectrum antibiotic has been administered. If the urine is shown to be infected,

an antibiotic based on sensitivity results is prescribed for 10 to 14 days. If a stent has been placed, it is removed in the outpatient clinic 6 to 12 weeks later.

Closure

Many units perform a biopsy of the kidney routinely before closure of the wound. This biopsy can be used to provide baseline histology and can provide evidence of ischemic reperfusion injury or early antibody-mediated damage (see Chapters 24 and 25). Methods of closing the wound vary, but in general closure with loop nylon in two layers—internal oblique and transverse muscles followed by external oblique—is common practice, with subcuticular nylon or polygalactin closure of the skin.

The question of drainage is controversial, but if possible drainage should be avoided because of the risk of providing a portal for entry microorganisms. If drainage is required, it should be a closed system of suction drainage, and drains should be removed at the earliest opportunity, when drainage is less than 50 ml/24 hours. The exit site of the drain is cleaned daily with an antimicrobial solution and dressed until the drain is removed.

In the past, a capsulotomy of the transplanted kidney before closure was advocated (Hume, 1968; Shackman *et al.*,

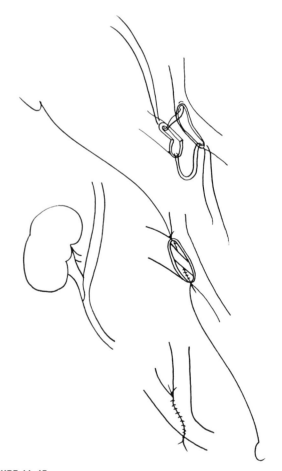

FIGURE 11–15

Pyeloureterostomy and ureteroureterostomy. A double-pigtail stent is placed after the backwall suture line has been completed.

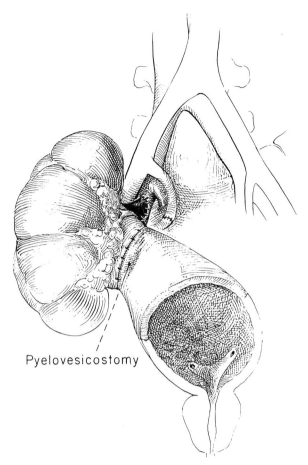

FIGURE 11–16

Pyelovesicostomy.

1963) by carefully splitting the renal capsule at its convex surface from pole to pole but not stripping it. This technique was proposed to prevent ischemic injury when the kidney swells as a result of edema; there is no evidence that this is the case, and this practice has now been abandoned.

Child as Recipient

For older children, the transplant procedure is the same as for adults if their weight is more than 20 kg (Belzer et al., 1972; Fine et al., 1970; Najarian et al., 1971). The skin incision is carried up to the costal margin. The renal vessels are anastomosed end-to-side to the common iliac vessels or aorta and vena cava (Broyer et al., 1981; Calne, 1984).

In smaller children (weight <20 kg), the transperitoneal approach has been described (Starzl et al., 1964b). The abdomen is opened through the midline incision from the xyphoid to the pubis, and the posterior peritoneum is incised lateral to the right colon, which is then reflected medially. The terminal portion of the vena cava is dissected over 3 to 4 cm, ligating and dividing two to three lumbar veins posteriorly. The terminal aorta also is dissected free at its junction with the right common iliac artery. Then a partial occluding clamp is used to isolate the vena cava and aorta, and the renal vein is anastomosed to the vena cava first in an end-to-side technique with sutures of 5–0 monofilament Prolene (Fig. 11–17). The renal artery then is anastomosed to the common iliac or terminal aorta in an end-to-side fashion using 6–0

monofilament Prolene. The renal artery is brought usually in front of the vena cava but at times behind the vena cava (Starzl et al., 1964b). Careful observation of the recipient hemodynamic response on clamping and declamping the vena cava and aorta is required.

The ascending colon is placed back over the anterior surface of the kidney. No fixation is necessary. The ureter is brought down retroperitoneally crossing the common iliac artery at its midpoint and is implanted into the bladder as a ureteroneocystostomy. Najarian and coworkers stated that the ureter should not be brought through the free peritoneal cavity because it may prevent the development of a collateral circulation to the ureter, risking ischemia of the ureteral end (Najarian et al., 1971). The appendix is removed by many surgeons to avoid postoperative appendicitis and/or problems of diagnosis of right-sided abdominal pain in the future (Najarian et al., 1971).

Calne (1963) expressed concern about the development of stenosis of the vascular anastomosis in growing children by the use of continuous sutures. He advised performing at least half of the anastomosis with interrupted sutures in children. This advice may apply when one performs end-to-side anastomosis of the renal artery or the renal vein, but Starzl and colleagues stated that after end-to-side anastomosis, there is little likelihood of the development of relative stenosis as a result of growth of the child (Starzl et al., 1964b).

Child as Donor

When a child's kidney is used as a donor kidney for an adult or child recipient, the surgical technique is essentially the same as has been described. Because of the small size of the renal vessels, however, use of aortic and vena caval patches generally is necessary. Interrupted sutures should be used over at least half the circumference of the anastomosis. When pediatric kidneys are very small, double kidneys are

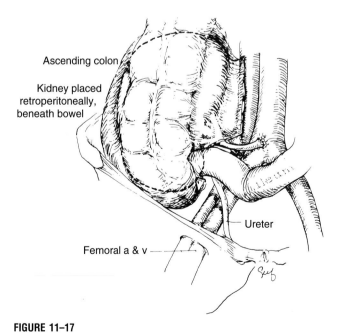

FIGURE 11–17

Renal transplant in small children (<20 kg).

transplanted *en bloc* into adults and bigger children (Dreikorn *et al.*, 1977; Kinne *et al.*, 1974; Lindstrom and Ahonen, 1975; Schneider *et al.*, 1983).

For *en-bloc* transplantation, both kidneys are removed with a segment of aorta and vena cava. The cranial ends of the aorta and vena cava are oversewn. The caudal ends of the aorta and vena cava are anastomosed end-to-side to the iliac vessels. The superior poles of the kidneys are sutured to the sides of the aorta to prevent the torsion or kinking of renal vessel pedicles. Ureters are implanted to the bladder separately using the extravesical approach or are joined together to form a common funnel, as described earlier. Another useful technique is to remove a segment of aorta and vena cava below the renal vessels and to reanastomose these segments to the aorta and vena cava above the renal vessels. This technique allows the kidneys to be placed quite low over the iliac vessels and provides a short distance for the ureters to traverse to the bladder.

Transplant Nephrectomy

Removal of a graft that has undergone chronic rejection and has been in place for many months or years can be extremely difficult and should be performed by an experienced transplant surgeon. The usual approach for the transplant nephrectomy is through the original transplant incision. An abdominal incision may be preferred in small children, particularly if the transplantation was performed intraabdominally. One also may use the abdominal approach to control the iliac artery system in case of a mycotic aneurysm or a perinephric abscess, in which a potential exists for blowout of vessels.

In the early postoperative period, removal of the transplant *in toto* is simple with easy identification of the renal pedicle structures. The long-standing transplanted kidney should be removed subcapsularly to lessen the technical difficulty and the bleeding, however. After deepening the incision sharply to the false capsule, which is incised, the kidney is freed subcapsularly with blunt dissection all around the kidney. The capsule around the hilum has to be incised to get outside it again so as to isolate the pedicle. The pedicle is then mass clamped with a Satinsky clamp and divided to remove the kidney. Most surgeons use 3–0 monofilament Prolene to oversew the vessels as well as for the ligature. One also may dissect the artery and the vein at this time and ligate them separately, but this is difficult, especially if end-to-side anastomoses have been used. Meticulous hemostasis should be obtained with the use of electrocautery. The wound is irrigated with a liberal amount of topical antibiotic solution (10% neomycin solution). It is wise to use prophylactic antibiotics. The wound is closed with a single-layer closure using synthetic monofilament sutures.

If the wound is grossly contaminated or infected, it should be left open with packing, with secondary closure in mind. Insertion of drains should be avoided because it may increase the incidence of infection, and if drains are considered necessary, a closed system of drainage should be used for a short time (Banowsky *et al.*, 1974; Belzer, 1979; Kohlberg *et al.*, 1980; Schweizer *et al.*, 1973).

REFERENCES

Banowsky, L. H., Montie, J. E., Braun, W. E. and Magnusson, M. O. (1974). Renal transplantation III: prevention of wound infections. *Urology* **40**, 656.

Barry, J. M. (1983). Unstented extravesical ureteroneocystostomy in kidney transplantation. *J. Urol.* **129**, 918.

Barry, J. M., Lemmers, M. J., Meyer, M. M., DeMattos, A., Bennett, W. M. and Norman, D. J. (1996). Cadaver kidney transplantation in patients more than 65 years old. *World J. Urol.* **14**, 243.

Barry, J. M., Pearse, H. D., Lawson, R. K. and Hodges, C. V. (1973). Ureteroneocystostomy in kidney transplants with ureteral duplication. *Arch. Surg.* **106**, 345.

Belzer, F. O. (1979). Technical complications after renal transplantation. *In Kidney Transplantation*, 1st ed. (P. J. Morris, ed.), p. 267, Academic Press/Grune & Stratton, London.

Belzer, F. O., Schweizer, R. T., Holliday, M., Potter, D. and Kountz, S. L. (1972). Renal homotransplantation in children. *Am. J. Surg.* **124**, 270.

Bennett, A. H. (1973). Pyelocystostomy in a renal allograft. *Am. J. Surg.* **125**, 633.

Bradic, I., Pasini, M. and Vlatkovic, G. (1975). Antireflux ureteroneocystostomy at the vertex of the bladder. *Br. J. Urol.* **47**, 525.

Broyer, M., Gagnadoux, M. F., Beurton, D., Pascal, B. and Louville, J. (1981). Transplantation in children: technical aspects, drug therapy and problems related to primary renal disease. *Proc. E. D. T. A.* **1**, 313.

Calne, R. Y. (1963). *Renal Transplantation*, p. 1, Williams & Wilkins, Baltimore.

Calne, R. Y. (1965). Technical aspects of cadaveric renal transplantation. *Br. J. Urol.* **37**, 285.

Calne, R. Y. (1984). *Color Atlas of Renal Transplantation*, p. 1, Medical Economics Books, Oradell, N.J.

de Campos-Freire, G., Goes, G. N. and Campos-Freire, J. E. (1974). Extravesical ureteral implantation in kidney transplantation. *Urology* **3**, 304.

Caparros, J., Regalado, R. I., Sanchez-Martin, F. and Villavicencio, H. (1996). A simplified technique for ureteroneocystostomy in renal transplantation. *World J. Urol.* **14**, 236.

Carrel, A. (1902). Le technique operatoire des anastomoses vasculaire et al transplantation des visceres. *Lyon Med.* **98**, 859.

Conlin, M. J., Lemmers, M. J. and Barry, J. M. (1994). Extravesical ureteroneocystostomy for duplicated allograft ureters. *J. Urol.* **152**, 1201.

Dreikorn, J., Rohl, L. and Horsch, R. (1977). The use of double renal transplant from pediatric cadaver donor. *Br. J. Urol.* **49**, 361.

Fine, R. N., Korsch, B. M., Stiles, Q., *et al.* (1970). Renal homotransplantation in children. *J. Pediatr.* **76**, 347.

Firlit, C. F. (1977). Unique urinary diversions in transplantation. *J. Urol.* **118**, 1043.

Fjeldborg, O. and Kim, C. H. (1972). Double ureters in renal transplantation. *J. Urol.* **108**, 377.

Gibbons, W. S., Barry, J. M. and Hefty, T. R. (1992). Complications following unstented parallel incision extravesical ureteroneocystostomy in 1,000 kidney transplants. *J. Urol.* **148**, 38.

Gil-Vernet, J. M., Gil-Vernet, A., Caralps, A., *et al.* (1989). Orthotopic renal transplant and results in 139 consecutive cases. *J. Urol.* **142**, 248.

Hamburger, J., Crosnier, J. and Dormont, J. (1965). Experience with 45 renal homotransplantations in man. *Lancet* **1**, 985.

Hatch, D. A., Belitsky, P., Barry J. M., *et al.* (1993). Fate of renal allografts transplanted in patients with urinary diversion. *Transplantation* **54**, 838.

Heritier, P., Perraud, Y., Relave, M. H., *et al.* (1989). Renal transplantation and Koch pouch: a case report. *J. Urol.* **141**, 595.

Herwig, K. R. and Konnak, J. W. (1973). Vesicopyelostomy: a method for urinary drainage of the transplanted kidney. *J. Urol.* **109**, 955.

Hume, D. M. (1968). Kidney transplantation. *In Human Transplantation* (F. T. Rapaport and J. Dausset, eds.), p. 110, Grune & Stratton, London.

Hume, D. M., Magee, J. H., Kauffman, H. M., Rittenberry, M. S. and Prout, G. R. (1963). Renal homotransplantation in man in modified recipients. *Ann. Surg.* **158**, 608.

Jaffers, G. J., Cosimi, A. B., Delmonico, F. L., *et al.* (1982). Experience with pyeloureterostomy in renal transplantation. *Ann. Surg.* **196**, 588.

Kelly, W. D., Merkel, F. K. and Markland, C. (1966). Ileal urinary diversion in conjunction with renal homotransplantation. *Lancet* **1**, 222.

Kinne, D. W., Spanos, P. K., DeShazo, M. M., Simmons, R. L. and Najarian, J. S. (1974). Double renal transplant from pediatric donors to adult recipients. *Am. J. Surg.* **127**, 292.

Kohlberg, W. I., Tellis, V. A., Bhat, D. J., Driscoll, B. and Veith, F. J.

(1980). Wound infections after transplant nephrectomy. *Arch. Surg.* **115,** 645.

Konnak, J. W., Herwig, K. R. and Turcotte, J. G. (1972). External ureteroneocystostomy in renal transplantation. *J. Urol.* **108,** 380.

Kootstra, G. (1994). Kidney transplantation. *In Atlas of Liver, Pancreas, and Kidney Transplantation* (B. Kremer, C. E. Broelsch and D. Henne-Bruns, eds.), p. 128, Georg Thieme Verlag, Stuttgart.

Kuss, R., Tsenturier, J. and Milliez, P. (1951). Quelgues ess ais de greffos du rein chez l'homme. *Med. Acad. Chir.* **77,** 755.

Lawler, R. H., West, J. W., McNulty, T. H., Clancey, E. J. and Murphey, R. P. (1950). Homotransplantation of the kidney in the human. *J. A. M. A.* **144,** 844.

Leadbetter, G. W., Monaco, A. P. and Russell, P. S. (1966). A technique for reconstruction of the urinary tract in renal transplantation. *Surg. Gynecol. Obstet.* **123,** 839.

Lee, H. M. (1979). Surgical techniques of renal transplantation. *In Kidney Transplantation,* 1st ed. (P. J. Morris, ed.), p. 145, Academic Press/Grune & Stratton, London.

Lich, R., Howerton, L. W. and David, L. A. (1961). Recurrent urosepsis in children. *J. Urol.* **86,** 554.

Lindstrom, B. L. and Ahonen, J. (1975). The use of both kidneys obtained from pediatric donors as en bloc transplant into adult recipients. *Scand. J. Urol. Nephrol.* **29,** 71.

Lord, R. H., Pepera, T. and Williams, G. (1991). Ureteroureterostomy and pyeloureterostomy without native nephrectomy in renal transplantation. *Br. J. Urol.* **67,** 349.

MacKinnon, K. J., Oliver, J. A., Morehouse, D. B. and Taguchi, Y. (1968). Cadaver renal transplantation: emphasis on urological aspects. *J. Urol.* **99,** 46.

Masson, D. and Hefty, T. (1998). A technique for the transplantation of two adult cadaver kidney grafts into one recipient. *J. Urol.* **160,** 1779.

McDonald, J. C., Landreneau, N. D., Hargroder, D. E., Venable, D. D. and Rohr, M. S. (1987). External ureteroneocystostomy and ureteroureterostomy in renal transplantation. *Ann. Surg.* **205,** 428.

Merrill, J. P., Murray, J. E. and Harrison, J. H. (1956). Successful homotransplantation of the human kidney between two identical twins. *J. A. M. A.* **160,** 277.

Michon, L., Hamburger, J., Oeconomos, N., *et al.* (1953). Une tentative de transplantation renale chez l'homme aspects medicaux et abiologiques. *Presse Med.* **61,** 1419.

Najarian, J. S., Simmons, R. L., Tallent, M. B., *et al.* (1971). Renal transplantation in infants and children. *Ann. Surg.* **174,** 583.

Paquin, A. J., Jr. (1959). Ureterovesical anastomosis: the description and evaluation of a technique. *J. Urol.* **82,** 573.

Pleass, H. C., Clark, K. R., Rigg, K. M., *et al.* (1995). Urologic complications after renal transplantation: a prospective randomized trial comparing different techniques of ureteric anastomosis and the use of prophylactic ureteric stents. *Transplant. Proc.* **27,** 1091.

Politano, V. A. and Leadbetter, W. F. (1958). An operative technique for the correction of vesicoureteral reflux. *J. Urol.* **79,** 932.

Prout, G. R., Hume, D. M., Lee, H. M. and Williams, G. M. (1967). Some urological aspects of 93 consecutive renal homotransplants in modified recipients. *J. Urol.* **97,** 409.

Roake, J. A., Toogood, G. J., Cahill, A. P., Gray, D. W. and Morris, P. J. (1991). Reducing renal ischaemia during transplantation. *Br. J. Surg.* **78,** 121.

Rosen, N. A. and McAninch, J. W. (1996). Wound closures and suture techniques in reconstructive procedures. *In Traumatic and Reconstructive Urology* (J. W. McAninch, ed.), p. 49, W. B. Saunders, Philadelphia.

Schiff, M., Jr. and Lytton, B. (1981). Secondary ureteropyelostomy in renal transplant recipients. *J. Urol.* **126,** 723.

Schneider, J. R., Sutherland, D. E. R., Simmons, R. L., Fryd, D. S. and Najarian, J. S. (1983). Long term success with double pediatric cadaver donor renal transplant. *Ann. Surg.* **197,** 439.

Schweizer, R. T., Kountz, S. L. and Belzer, F. O. (1973). Wound complications in recipients of renal transplants. *Ann. Surg.* **1,** 58.

Shackman, R., Dempster, W. J. and Wrong, O. M. (1963). Kidney homotransplantation in the human. *Br. J. Urol.* **35,** 222.

Shanfield, I. (1972). New experimental methods for implantation of ureter in bladder and conduit. *Transplant. Proc.* **4,** 637.

Simmons, R. L. (1972). Technique, complication and results. *In Transplantation* (J. S. Najarian and R. L. Simmons, eds.), p. 445, Lea & Febiger, Philadelphia.

Starzl, T. E. (1964). *Experience in Renal Transplantation,* p. 1, W. B. Saunders, Philadelphia.

Starzl, T. E., Marchioro, T. L., *et al.* (1964a). Technique of renal homotransplantation: experience with 42 cases. *Arch. Surg.* **89,** 87.

Starzl, T. E., Marchioro, T. L., Morgan, W. W. and Waddell, W. R. (1964b). A technique for use of adult renal homografts in children. *Surg. Gynecol. Obstet.* **119,** 106.

Szmidt, J., Karolak, M., Sablinski, T., *et al.* (1988). Transplantation of kidneys with nonvascular abnormalities. *Transplant. Proc.* **20,** 767.

Whitehead, E. D., Narins, D. J. and Morales, P. A. (1972). The use of methylene blue in the identification of the ileal conduit during re-operation. *J. Urol.* **107,** 960.

Woodruff, M. F. A., Robson, J. S., Nolan, B. and MacDonald, M. K. (1969). Renal transplantation in man: experience in 35 cases. *Lancet* **1,** 6.

Transplantation and the Abnormal Bladder

C. J. Rudge

Introduction

A normal bladder acts as a low-pressure, good-volume urinary reservoir that is continent, is sterile and empties freely and completely. An abnormal bladder fails some or all of these criteria and may contribute to the development of end-stage renal failure.

Patients with an abnormal lower urinary tract account for 7.6% of all adult patients on dialysis in Europe and 25% of all children on dialysis. Despite several early reports (Debruyne et al., 1977; Kimbler et al., 1977; Shenasky, 1976) of successful renal transplantation for such patients, there initially was considerable reluctance to consider them as suitable transplant recipients. It is now recognized that acceptable results can be achieved, however, and 6% of greater than 8,000 patients transplanted annually in the United States have end-stage renal failure associated with lower urinary tract abnormalities (Hatch, 1994).

Considerable problems exist in defining the most suitable method of urinary drainage, and the surgery and postoperative management are complex. Many reports suggest that patients with abnormal bladders have inferior graft survival when compared with patients with normal bladders (Castro et al., 1975; Churchill et al., 1988; Reinberg et al., 1988). Others show equivalent results in the two groups (Cairns et al., 1991; Griffin et al., 1994; Hatch, 1994; Hatch et al., 1993; Kreiger et al., 1980; Nguyen et al., 1990; Warshaw et al., 1980). Many studies comparing outcome with a matched control group suggest, however, that although patient and graft survival may be equal, there is a trend toward slightly poorer renal function (Bryant et al., 1991; Crowe et al., 1998; Gonzalez, 1997; Groenwegen et al., 1993).

Most reports describe small numbers of patients, making firm conclusions difficult. Patients with abnormal bladders may be successfully transplanted, despite the higher risk of complications (Hatch, 1994; Hatch et al., 1993; Nguyen et al., 1990). This higher risk requires close cooperation among the urologist, nephrologist, radiologist and transplant surgeon.

Causes of an Abnormal Bladder

Although major congenital abnormalities (e.g., bladder exstrophy) and conditions such as spina bifida that produce a *neuropathic* bladder interfere with normal bladder function, other conditions, apparently more localized and of less significance, may be associated with disturbances of bladder function (Table 12–1). These conditions include posterior urethral valves and vesicoureteral reflux. The diagnosis of *reflux* or of *chronic pyelonephritis* should alert the transplant surgeon to the possibility of abnormal bladder function.

Particular attention has been given to patients with posterior urethral valves. It has been recognized widely that in such patients early successful ablation of the valves still may be associated with progression to end-stage renal failure and that bladder dysfunction may be a significant factor. Ross and colleagues reported 15 patients with posterior urethral valves transplanted using the native bladder whose transplant survival and graft function were equivalent to patients with a normal bladder and suggested that early sepsis and vesicoureteric reflux (before valve ablation) may be the significant factors leading to renal failure (Ross et al., 1994). Similarly, good results have been reported by others (Connelly et al., 1995; Fontaine et al., 1997; Rajagopalan et al., 1994). It also has been reported that although patient and graft survival are equivalent, renal function is worse than in control patients (Bryant et al., 1991; Groenwegen et al., 1993). Gonzalez (1997) emphasized the need for appropriate case-control studies.

Transplantation in association with the prune-belly syndrome was first reported by Shenasky and Whelchel (1976). A specific cause of graft loss in such patients is acute torsion of the allograft, presumably related to the extremely lax abdominal wall musculature (Abbitt et al., 1990; Marvin et al., 1995). Surgical tethering of the kidney is recommended.

It is outside the scope of this chapter to discuss the management of lower tract abnormalities in general. Good medical and surgical management can delay or prevent the development of chronic renal failure. Control of hypertension and an aggressive approach to the diagnosis and management of urinary obstruction and infection are particularly important. The main question for the transplant surgeon is whether the bladder is or can be made suitable for use in draining the transplanted kidney. If the answer is no, urinary diversion is necessary.

Assessment of Bladder Function

A full history is obtained including details of the voiding pattern before development of renal failure. The urinary stream, abdominal compression or straining and continence

TABLE 12–1

CAUSES OF AN ABNORMAL LOWER URINARY TRACT

Bladder exstrophy
Neuropathic bladder (meningomyelocele, spinal cord trauma, neurological disease)
Posterior urethral valves
Prune-belly syndrome
Bladder outflow obstruction (not prostatic)
Tuberculosis
Malignancy
Vesicoureteral reflux

are all relevant (Hatch, 1994). The physical examination should note scars from previous surgery (relevant when planning the transplant procedure) and examination of the site and nature of any urinary diversion.

Preliminary investigations that are mandatory for all patients are measurement of urinary flow rate and ultrasound estimation of the postmicturition urine volume. Urinary flow rate should be greater than 18 to 25 ml/sec, depending on the age of the patient, and the residual volume should be less than 30 ml. These investigations are of such value that in the anuric patient instillation of saline into the bladder, if necessary using a fine suprapubic catheter (Marshall et al., 1982), is worthwhile. Taken together with the history, these investigations identify patients who require further investigation.

Urethrocystoscopy is valuable to exclude urethral stricture and to examine the bladder outlet and mucosa. Biopsy of the bladder, to exclude premalignant change, has been advocated in highly abnormal bladders (Marshall et al., 1982). Complete assessment of bladder function requires a video cystometrogram, although this is indicated only in patients with a significant past history or relevant symptoms (Shandera et al., 1996). This investigation provides information on the behavior of the bladder during filling, including capacity, pressure rise, detrusor response and sensation, and during micturition the mechanism and efficiency of voiding are shown. Further information is obtained by combining urodynamic studies with radioisotope imaging. In the presence of gross vesicoureteral reflux, the urodynamic studies may be difficult to interpret. In the past, bilateral nephroureterectomy has been recommended. If the refluxing bladder has a good capacity and does not generate excessive pressures, however, it may be safe for drainage of the transplanted kidney when major chronic infection is not a problem.

Criteria for a Usable Bladder

There are few published data on which criteria suggest that the bladder is usable. At an Institute of Urology Consensus Conference in 1988, the criteria shown in Table 12–2 were agreed on as a reasonable description of a usable bladder. Houle et al. (1993) suggest that in children a normal bladder fills to 95% of capacity at a pressure less than 20 cm H$_2$O. Also, it has been shown that there is significantly inferior 2-year graft survival in patients whose pretransplant bladder capacity was less than 100 ml compared with patients with a capacity of greater than 100 ml (Kashi et al., 1994).

CAPACITY

A small capacity may be caused by the following:

1. *A thick-walled, scarred bladder.* This can result from multiple previous surgical procedures, chronic infection (e.g., tuberculosis) and long-standing neurogenic detrusor dysfunc-

tion. The bladder is noncompliant and nondistensible. It is not suitable for use after transplantation.

2. *Prolonged oligoanuria.* This can result in a low capacity in patients with a normal bladder initially. The bladder wall is compliant, and the bladder is distensible, however. Such a bladder may be used safely.

Ideally a period of bladder cycling and hydrodistention, using a suprapubic catheter, should be undertaken in preparation for transplantation (MacGregor et al., 1986; Serrano et al., 1996). There are reports of transplantation into an extremely low-capacity bladder (10–50 ml) with restoration of normal capacity and function within weeks of transplantation. It is *potential* rather than actual capacity that is important.

POOR FLOW RATE

If urethral and bladder outlet (including prostatic) obstruction are excluded, a poor flow rate represents inefficient and uncoordinated detrusor function. If the bladder fails to empty completely, even after double micturition, the resulting stasis, infection and functional obstruction are potentially damaging to the transplanted kidney. Intermittent clean self-catheterization (ICSC) is increasingly employed in urological practice. There are many reports of its use by transplant recipients (Barnett et al., 1985; Firlit, 1976; Flechner et al., 1983; Kogan et al., 1986; Schneidman et al., 1984; Stanley et al., 1983). Results are encouraging (Fontaine et al., 1998; Gill et al., 1997), and it appears that anxiety about systemic sepsis in immunosuppressed patients may be unfounded. Flechner et al. (1983) and Barnett et al. (1985) suggest that symptomatic and asymptomatic urinary tract infections are less with ICSC than with transplantation into an ileal conduit, and this finding has been shown to be the case in nontransplant recipients (Ehrlich and Brem, 1982). Gill and colleagues have shown that 52% of patients experience asymptomatic infections, and 22% experience symptomatic infections (Gill et al., 1997). Most investigators recommend long-term low-dose antibiotics, usually trimethoprim-sulfamethoxazole, 1 tablet once or twice daily.

In my experience, it is essential to use ICSC in well-motivated and reasonably competent patients. Failure to perform the technique appropriately may impair renal function seriously (Stanley et al., 1983). Particularly important is the discipline needed to perform ICSC as frequently as it is required. Many patients have high-capacity bladders with little or no sensation of bladder distention. Catheterization occasionally may appear acceptable to the patient with urine volumes of 1 L or more. I have encountered several patients with an anatomically normal transplant ureterovesical anastomosis who had functional ureteric obstruction when the bladder volume exceeded a critical amount. This obstruction presumably was related to distortion of the ureter as it passed through the bladder wall. Frequent ICSC (five or six times daily) may be needed. Occasionally a patient has been advised to leave an indwelling catheter in overnight to prevent overdistention of the bladder.

Whenever possible, the patient should be experienced and satisfied with ICSC before transplantation, primarily to establish that it is feasible and satisfactory. It has been reported as a satisfactory technique in children, including children younger than age 2 years (Hansson et al., 1995).

CONTINENCE

Severe incontinence was an indication for urinary diversion or involved the male patient in wearing a variety of appliances. In 1973, the first Brantley Scott artificial urinary

TABLE 12–2

CRITERIA FOR A USABLE BLADDER*

Good capacity: >300 ml
Low end-filling pressure: <30 cm H$_2$O
Good flow rate: >18–25 ml/s
Absence of systolic detrusor contractions
Continence

*Determined at the Institute of Urology Consensus Conference, 1988.

sphincter (AUS) was introduced, and there have been numerous changes in design since that time to improve the reliability and convenience of the sphincter. The subject was reviewed by Mundy in 1991. There are several case reports of the use of an AUS in transplant recipients. In the first report (Thomalla *et al.*, 1988), an AS 792 was inserted pretransplant; considerable care was taken to avoid the device during the transplant procedure. In the second report (Gelet *et al.*, 1990), an AS 800 was inserted successfully 4 months posttransplant. Although it is possible to insert a small urethral catheter with an AS 800 *in situ* (but *not* with an AS 792), it is advisable to use a suprapubic catheter to avoid the risk of urethral erosion of the cuff of the sphincter. Three patients (out of 23 patients) transplanted into an abnormal lower urinary tract were reported to have had an AUS, although few details were given (Griffin *et al.*, 1994). With increasing experience with the AUS, it is likely that it may be applicable to a number of selected transplant recipients.

There are several relatively simple methods available that may enable the use of a bladder that fails the criteria shown in Table 12–2. It is essential to consider bladder reevaluation in patients who have previously undergone urinary diversion, particularly in the case of patients treated many years ago when diversion was performed for indications that no longer apply (Serrano *et al.*, 1996). Frequently the original indications are obscure. Many of these patients may have a bladder that is acceptable for transplantation. A selected review of the literature (Cerelli *et al.*, 1976; Firlit, 1976; MacGregor *et al.*, 1986; Serrano *et al.*, 1996; Warshaw *et al.*, 1980) shows 91 patients with an existing diversion who were reassessed for transplantation. The native bladder was usable in 75 patients. This review probably exaggerates the scope for using the bladder in a patient with urinary diversion because most of these patients underwent diversion in the 1970s or 1980s. More recent patient selection for diversion has been more selective. The literature review emphasizes that bladder function should be reassessed if the native bladder is *in situ*.

Major Reconstruction

If the bladder remains unusable despite the aforementioned techniques, usually because of low capacity and/or high pressure, there are two options: bladder augmentation or substitution, and urinary diversion.

BLADDER AUGMENTATION OR SUBSTITUTION

Isolated bowel segments, to increase the bladder capacity and decrease the pressure, have become increasingly common. Augmentation cystoplasty involves adding bowel to the existing bladder, whereas substitution cystoplasty is performed when most of the bladder is excised (leaving the trigone and bladder neck) and replaced with bowel. Mitchell and Piser (1987) reviewed 129 children who underwent intestinocystoplasty between 1978 and 1985. In 51 cases, an ileocecal segment was used; in 39, a sigmoid patch; in 33, an ileal patch; and in 6, augmentation with tubular sigmoid colon. The conclusions were that all procedures increased bladder capacity and reduced intravesical pressures. There were problems, attributed to mass unit peristaltic contractions, when tubular colon was used. This segment is the least satisfactory. The investigators concluded that all other procedures were satisfactory, with the type of segment being less important than the size and configuration. Surgical complications developed in 36%. The commonest procedures in the United Kingdom are an ileal patch (*clam*) cystoplasty and a substitution cecocystoplasty or ileocecocystoplasty (using a

detubularized segment of terminal ileum, cecum and ascending colon) (Fig. 12–1). An alternative that is being recommended for use in children is the use of a segment of stomach (Fontaine *et al.*, 1998; Sheldon *et al.*, 1994), which has less metabolic sequelae (in particular, acidosis) than occurs after the use of small or large bowel. A further alternative, applicable only in the presence of gross ureteric dilatation, is bladder augmentation using native ureter—if necessary, combined with transureteroureterostomy to maintain drainage of both native kidneys. This alternative is likely to have minimal metabolic consequences and ensures that the augmented bladder is lined entirely by urothelium (Landau *et al.*, 1997).

There are increasing reports of renal transplantation associated with bladder augmentation or substitution. Marshall *et al.* (1982) first described a single patient who underwent pyeloileocecocystoplasty after renal transplantation, and there have been several additional reports (Alfrey *et al.*, 1997; Barnett *et al.*, 1987; Buerton *et al.*, 1987; Fontaine *et al.*, 1998; Landau *et al.*, 1997; McInerney *et al.*, 1995; Nguyen *et al.*, 1990; Sagalowsky *et al.*, 1989; Sheldon *et al.*, 1994; Thomalla *et al.*, 1989; Zaragoza *et al.*, 1993; and reviewed by Gonzalez, 1997). Most patients had bladder augmentations performed before transplantation. Most investigators used the ileocecal segment, but Thomalla *et al.* (1988) preferred the sigmoid colon, which was anastomosed to the posterocaudal aspect of the intraperitoneal bladder. The anterior surface and pelvic vasculature is left undisturbed for the subsequent transplant. Although augmentation *per se* may be a relatively routine surgical practice, it rarely is adequate without further procedures, such as ICSC (Alfrey *et al.*, 1997).

In the period between bladder augmentation and transplantation, bowel mucus and debris necessitate daily irrigation of the bladder; this maintains distensibility of the bladder. Using this regimen in seven patients, Thomalla *et al.* (1988) reported an increase in mean bladder capacity from 85 to 390 ml and a decrease in intravesical pressure from a mean of 70 to 12 cm H_2O. In one patient, a compliant good-capacity enterocystoplasty became contracted, lost compliance and had an end-filling pressure of 50 cm H_2O during a 10-month anuric period (awaiting transplantation). During this time, the patient ceased bladder cycling. Problems associated with a *dry* augmented bladder are well described (Gonzalez, 1997), and some authors recommended transplantation first followed by subsequent augmentation (McInerney *et al.*, 1995). Others report few problems if augmentation is performed in preparation for transplantation (Fontaine *et al.*, 1998; Zaragoza *et al.*, 1993). In children (Alfrey *et al.*, 1997), it has been suggested that transplantation into an augmented bladder results in numerous problems, including poor bladder emptying, chronic retention, urinary sepsis and failure to comply with ICSC. Alfrey and colleagues recommend use of the native bladder whenever possible or the creation of a short ileal conduit (Alfrey *et al.*, 1997). A further, more serious complication of bladder augmentation is rupture leading to urinary extravasation (Francis and Millar, 1992).

Total reconstruction of the lower urinary tract, using stomach to create a neobladder and appendix or ureter to create a continent, catheterizable perineal urethra, has been reported in two patients with major congenital abnormalities. Five years posttransplantation, both patients were well with good, stable graft function (Sheldon and Welch, 1998).

Surgical Technique of Transplantation

Preoperatively the bladder is irrigated with normal saline to remove any debris. It then is filled with 100 to 200 ml of irrigation solution, and the bladder catheter is clamped. This step aids intraoperative identification of the bladder. The

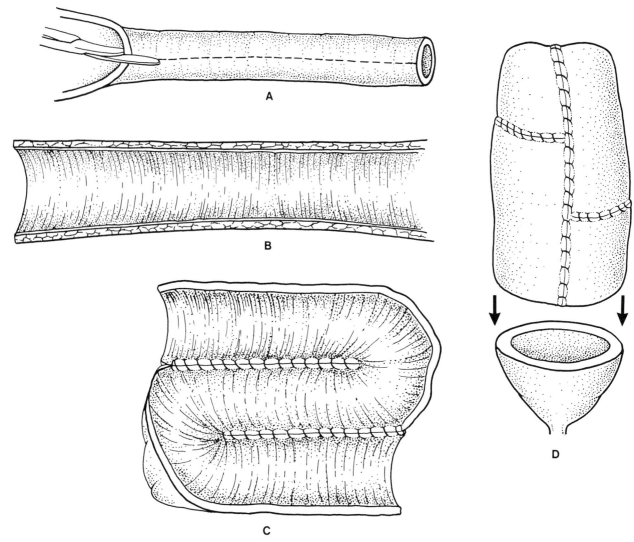

FIGURE 12–1

(A and B) Construction of an enterocystoplasty (semidiagrammatic). A length of ileum with or without cecum and ascending colon (not shown) is isolated and opened along its antimesenteric border. (C and D) The bowel is positioned and sutured as shown to create an appropriate urinary reservoir. This is attached to the bladder (augmentation) or bladder remnant (substitution).

exposure of the iliac vessels may be difficult if extensive scarring from previous surgery exists, but it normally can be performed in the standard extraperitoneal manner. The vascular anastomoses also are performed in the routine way. Several investigators recommend implantation of the transplant ureter into the remaining segment of native bladder if possible (Nguyen *et al.*, 1990; Thomalla *et al.*, 1988), but there also are reports of anastomosis to the augmented bowel segment (Barnett *et al.*, 1987; Nguyen *et al.*, 1990) (Fig. 12–2).

A tunneled Politano-Leadbetter type of anastomosis is done if anastomosing the ureter to the bladder, and a nontunneled direct anastomosis is employed with the bowel. A suprapubic catheter may be more convenient than a urethral catheter because it is advisable to leave the bladder on free drainage for longer (10–14 days) than is usual after routine transplantation. There may be uncertainty about the ability of the patient to void normally. A suprapubic catheter should be clamped but left *in situ* until satisfactory micturition (or ICSC) is achieved.

One minor but irritating problem, not mentioned in the literature but common in my experience, is the difficulty in developing an adequate extraperitoneal space in which the kidney can lie. Peritoneum may be extremely adherent over the iliac fossa and bladder, with dense fibrotic tissue, if the patient has had multiple operations previously. It is worth a little extra time before the vascular anastomoses are performed to consider the likely position of the kidney because this may dictate the site of the anastomoses to prevent tension or angulation of the renal artery and/or vein.

Follow-up and Results

The relatively small number of cases of bladder augmentation or substitution reported in the literature does not allow meaningful long-term results to be discussed. Two main points emerge: (1) Most patients require ICSC and are maintained on long-term prophylactic antibiotic therapy. (2) Satisfactory medium-term transplant function is reported.

In my experience, these patients require close and careful follow-up indefinitely. Anything less than optimal bladder function may produce slowly progressive deterioration in renal function. Churchill and colleagues suggested that in-

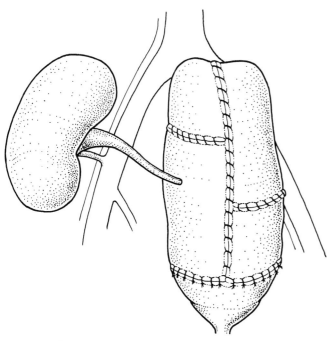

FIGURE 12–2

Transplantation into an enterocystoplasty (semidiagrammatic). The transplant ureter is anastomosed to the bowel segment of a bladder augmentation or substitution.

creased intravesical pressure reduces ureteral transport, causing increased back pressure and reduced renal blood flow (Churchill *et al.*, 1988). The resulting ischemic fibrosis and scarring may be additive to the effects of rejection (Reinberg *et al.*, 1988) and long-term cyclosporine nephrotoxicity.

URINARY DIVERSION

If the bladder is unusable, some form of urinary diversion is necessary. Gleeson and Griffith (1990) reviewed all forms of urinary diversion. Reports of renal transplantation into patients with urinary diversions fall into three main categories: (1) those with a conduit, usually ileal but occasionally colonic; (2) those with a continent urinary reservoir and (3) those with a cutaneous ureterostomy.

Ileal Conduit

After the description by Bricker (1950), the ileal conduit for urinary drainage after cystectomy or for major bladder dysfunction became well established. Kelly *et al.* (1966), Tunner *et al.* (1971) and Markland *et al.* (1972) described renal transplantation in association with an ileal conduit. Since then numerous reports (Gonzalez, 1997; Rudge, 1994) have appeared, although most describe small numbers of patients. It is frequently argued that transplantation into an ileal conduit is inadvisable. If the urinary diversion has been associated with progressive renal dysfunction of the native kidneys, the same would inevitably happen to the transplanted kidney; however, this may not be the case, and Neal and associates describe urodynamic studies of the peristaltic activity in ileal conduits that may predict whether the long-term anatomy and function of native kidneys are likely to be impaired (Neal *et al.*, 1985).

1. Many patients undergo diversion after prolonged bladder dysfunction and have damaged kidneys before diversion.

Progression to renal failure may be the result of prior damage rather than a consequence of the diversion.

2. Progressive deterioration of renal function is exacerbated by repeated infections, minor degrees of urinary obstruction and poor control of hypertension. Careful follow-up of most transplant recipients should minimize these potential problems.

3. Good evidence exists in nontransplant patients that renal function may be maintained for at least 15 years with vigilant supervision and an aggressive approach to the diagnosis and management of complications (Dunn *et al.*, 1979; Pitts and Muecke, 1979; Schwarz and Jeffs, 1975; Shapiro *et al.*, 1975).

Long-term complications of the ileal conduit, apart from upper tract deterioration, include stenosis of the cutaneous stoma, parastomal hernia, pyelonephritis, calculus formation, ureterointestinal stenosis and electrolyte abnormalities. Obstruction at the ureterointestinal anastomosis is the most significant and avoidable cause of progressive upper tract damage (Pitts and Muecke, 1979). Considerable social and psychological effects may result from the need to wear an external urinary collection device. Despite these problems, one review of urinary diversion concluded that "the ileal conduit must be regarded as the gold standard technique of urinary diversion" (Gleeson and Griffith, 1990).

An alternative to the ileal conduit is the colon conduit, which has theoretical advantages in that a ureterocolonic anastomosis that does not reflux may be performed more easily, and the less active peristalsis may produce a lower intraluminal pressure. Results do not support these possible benefits, however, and the colon conduit has not become common practice, although there are reports of transplantation into a colonic conduit (Nguyen *et al.*, 1990; Williams *et al.*, 1980).

Transplantation into an Ileal Conduit

Patients with a Preexisting Conduit. If urinary diversion of the native kidneys has been performed before development of end-stage renal failure and the bladder has been shown to be unusable, renal transplantation should be performed with the existing conduit. The conduit should be assessed before this decision is made because revision of the conduit may be necessary (Lucas *et al.*, 1992). Stomal stenosis must be excluded, and the length and position of the conduit must be defined. Many investigators recommend that the transplanted kidney should be placed in the iliac fossa contralateral to that of the stoma, but this is not an absolute rule (Lucas *et al.*, 1992). In my experience, identification of the distal end of a long-standing loop not positioned with future transplantation in mind may be extremely difficult.

When possible, the transplant is performed in the standard extraperitoneal manner. It has been my practice to consider carefully the eventual position of the kidney and the course of the ureter to the conduit and to implant the kidney *upside down* if this appears more satisfactory (Fig. 12–3). It has been suggested that it may be deleterious for the ureter to drain against gravity (Schick and Tanagho, 1973), but this does not appear to be a problem in practice. After revascularization of the kidney, the ileal conduit is identified by passing a suitable instrument or catheter through the stoma. There appears to be no contraindication to performing the ureteral anastomosis at any convenient site along the length of the conduit, and this often may be identified most easily relatively close to the stoma.

A peritoneal window is made, the conduit is opened and a 1-cm spatulated anastomosis is performed in two layers

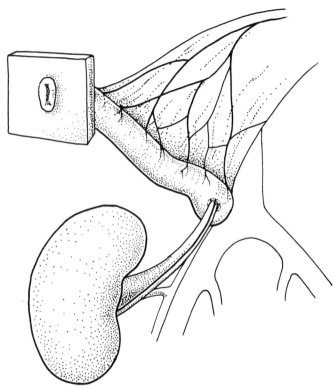

FIGURE 12–3

Transplantation into an ileal conduit (semidiagrammatic). The transplant ureter is anastomosed directly to the ileal conduit. It is the author's preference to transplant the kidney upside down as shown, and it is not essential for the kidney to be in the iliac fossa opposite to the conduit stoma.

over an indwelling ureteral splint brought out through the stoma. The peritoneum should be closed around the conduit, reducing the consequences of a urinary leak. Lucas and colleagues described an alternative skin-level ureterostomy to an isolated, short ileal conduit (Lucas et al., 1992). In a child, it may be necessary to anastomose the renal vessels to the aorta or common iliac artery and inferior vena cava. In this case, the operation is an intraperitoneal procedure. Kreiger and coworkers have found this procedure to be satisfactory (Kreiger et al., 1980).

The ureteral splint is removed 10 to 14 days after the operation. If there is any anxiety about the adequacy of the ureteral anastomosis, radiological contrast medium may be injected through the splint before removal to exclude stenosis and urinary leak.

Creation of a Conduit for Transplantation. A conduit created specifically to drain a future transplant may differ in several respects from that created to drain the native kidneys.

Timing. Most reports recommend that the conduit is created electively before transplantation (Casimir et al., 1977; Glass et al., 1985; Kreiger et al., 1980). Kreiger and associates suggested an increased incidence of complications when nontransplant surgery is performed simultaneously (Kreiger et al., 1980). Levey and coworkers stated that "construction of the conduit at the time of transplantation . . . allows optimal placement of the kidney, ureter and conduit" (Levey et al., 1978). Although cyclosporine A and lower doses of steroids (or no steroids) have reduced the risks of concurrent bowel surgery, the conduit should be constructed at least 2 to 3 months before transplantation.

Position. The ileal conduit may be shorter than is necessary for drainage of the native kidneys: 10 to 15 cm is adequate in most patients, and a short, *preperitoneal* technique also has been described (Lucas et al., 1992). The stoma may be positioned in the right iliac fossa and the conduit brought retroperitoneally across the pelvis to lie close to the left iliac vessels. A single suture of black silk, left long, may help subsequent identification of the end of the conduit. Several reports (Marchioro and Tremann, 1974; Robards et al., 1975) described a technique in which the conduit is positioned as low as possible in the pelvis, and the vascular anastomoses are performed as proximally as possible; the ureter then may drain in a dependent direction to the conduit. With these exceptions, the technique of transplantation is as described.

A single case report described an entirely different surgical approach (Cornejo et al., 1988). An ileal conduit was constructed: the stoma positioned to the left of the navel with the conduit lying vertically in the left iliac fossa. Six months later, a cadaver kidney was transplanted orthotopically after left nephrectomy. The renal artery was anastomosed to the splenic artery and the renal vein to the native renal vein. The ureter was anastomosed end-to-side to the ileal conduit, the proximal third of which had been brought through a window in the posterior parietal peritoneum. The end result was a transplanted kidney lying in the normal anatomical position, with ureteral and conduit peristalsis being dependent.

Complications. Nguyen et al. (1990) reviewed 94 patients in the literature with renal transplantation into an intestinal conduit: 62 complications occurred in 30 patients (31.9%). Several reviews subsequently have reported similar results (Cairns et al., 1991; Hatch, 1994; Hatch et al., 1993). Major problems encountered are the following.

Leakage from the Ureterointestinal Anastomosis. If adequate drainage can be obtained (e.g., percutaneous nephrostomy with or without an internal silastic J-stent), conservative management is indicated for leakage. Reoperation always is difficult and does not guarantee success.

Stricture at the Ureterointestinal Anastomosis. Stricture may be a slow and insidious process, and regular observation using ultrasound or radioisotope imaging is required to detect obstruction before significant renal damage is caused. Exclusion of obstruction is an essential part of the investigation of renal allograft dysfunction, and Stenzel and associates suggested that repeated urinary tract infections almost invariably are associated with obstruction at some site (Stenzel et al., 1974). Antegrade percutaneous nephrostogram may be invaluable in identifying the site and nature of obstruction. It also may allow the passage of a Silastic J-stent or transluminal balloon dilatation of the stricture. Operative repair has been required in most patients, but the increasing sophistication of instruments and techniques for percutaneous surgery may enable less invasive procedures to be performed.

Infection. Recurrent urinary tract infections of clinical significance are relatively infrequent in the well-established transplant recipient with an ileal loop. Acute pyelonephritis mimicking acute rejection has been described (Glass et al., 1985; McLoughlin, 1976). Many reports recommend routine bilateral nephroureterectomy before or at the time of transplantation (MacGregor et al., 1986). Increasing experience suggests that this procedure need not be performed in all patients, although it is advisable to remove grossly diseased and infected kidneys before transplantation. Irrigation of the conduit—with a dilute (0.25%) neomycin solution immediately preoperatively together with a systemic antibiotic—has been recommended by Nguyen et al. (1990). Many authors recommend long-term, low-dose antibiotic prophylaxis, and it has been thought to be particularly appropriate during the treatment of rejection episodes (Hatch *et al.*, 1993).

Calculus Formation. In association with obstruction and infection, calculi have formed in the conduit and the renal pelvis (Cairns *et al.*, 1991; Rattazi *et al.*, 1975).

Pyocystis in the Isolated Bladder. Pyocystis has been well described in nontransplanted patients with an ileal conduit (e.g., 16 of 67 children reported by Dunn *et al.*, 1979) and has been reported in a transplant recipient (Popll *et al.*, 1985). Reinberg and colleagues recommended that in a patient with a urinary diversion and a history of recurrent pyocystis, mucosal cystectomy should be performed before transplantation (Reinberg *et al.*, 1990).

Parastomal Hernias. In one extraordinary report, a patient with a parastomal hernia was observed to have impaired transplant function whenever she became constipated (Stanley *et al.*, 1983).

Results. Nguyen and coworkers assessed the results of transplantation in eight patients with an ileal conduit and two with an enterocystoplasty, compared with seven patients with poor urinary drainage in whom the transplant ureter was implanted into the native bladder (Nguyen *et al.*, 1990). *Normal* transplant recipients, suitably matched for relevant variables, acted as a retrospective control group. No significant difference was found between graft and patient survival in the three groups of patients. Complications were commoner in the group with urinary diversion, however. It was concluded that the native bladder should be used whenever possible. If it is not possible to use the native bladder, an ileal conduit produces equally acceptable graft and patient survival. Follow-up for more than 10 years is available only for a few patients with ileal conduit. All that can be said is that long-term survival is possible.

Continent Urinary Diversion

Attempts to create a continent urinary reservoir, emptied by intermittent self-catheterization through an abdominal stoma, have been made for many years. The subject has been reviewed by Gleeson and Griffith (1990), Cendron and Gearhart (1991) and Woodhouse and MacNeily (1994). Several techniques have been refined and introduced into urological practice: The ileal Kock pouch (Kock *et al.*, 1982; Skinner *et al.*, 1984), the ileocecal mixed augmentation ileum and cecum (Mainz) reservoir (Thuroff *et al.*, 1986) and various forms of colonic reservoir or rectal bladder are the most commonly used. In an assessment of the urodynamic characteristics of the continent ileocecal reservoir, Lowe and Woodside (1990) concluded that using the technique they described—an ileocecal segment with the ileocecal valve acting as an intussuscepted nipple valve (stoma) and an antireflux implantation of the native ureters to the colonic mucosa—satisfactory capacity can be achieved (>500 ml) with acceptable pressures. The reservoir is continent, without reflux and easy to catheterize and produces few fluid or electrolyte abnormalities. Gleeson and Griffith (1990) concluded, however, that "... many operations may be required to perfect the continent stoma. Long-term results using continent reservoirs are awaited."

There are few reports of patients in whom transplants have been drained through a continent Kock pouch (Dawahra *et al.*, 1997; Francis and Millar, 1992; Hatch *et al.*, 1993; Heritier *et al.*, 1989; Marechal *et al.*, 1990). In one of my patients, a continent ileal reservoir is catheterized through a reversed appendiceal conduit constructed according to the Mitrofanoff principle (Mitrofanoff, 1980; Fig. 12–4). In most series, the continent reservoir was created months or years

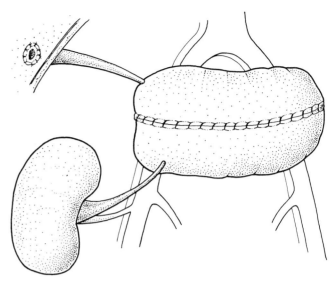

FIGURE 12–4

Transplantation into a continent urinary reservoir using the Mitrofanoff principle (semidiagrammatic). A urinary reservoir is constructed from bowel (see Fig. 12–1). The isolated appendix is reversed, the *cecal* end being brought through the skin as a stoma and the *distal* end being amputated and implanted into the urinary reservoir in a nonrefluxing manner. The patient catheterizes the reservoir through the appendiceal stoma. As with the ileal conduit, the kidney may be transplanted upside down.

before the transplant, and the standard technique was modified in two ways:

1. The afferent limb of the pouch was longer than normal (25 cm rather than 10–15 cm) so that it could cross the abdominal cavity to lie in close proximity to the left iliac vessels—the cutaneous stoma being placed in the right iliac fossa.

2. The pouch was irrigated continuously in the pretransplant period to wash out mucus and to encourage distention of the pouch.

Typically the transplant was performed in the left iliac fossa with direct ureteroileal anastomosis. At reported follow-up, all patients had good renal function. Urinary tract infections had not been a significant problem, and the patients were performing ICSC three to six times daily with a pouch capacity of greater than 500 ml. My patient is 7 years posttransplant with a serum creatinine level of 110 to 120 μmol/L, although renal function deteriorates slightly when she fails to perform ICSC as frequently as advised.

A patient, known to me, who is awaiting transplantation after a modification of the technique just described, has a good-capacity low-pressure bladder with major detrusor failure and is unable to void. After performing ICSC for 4 years, the patient admitted that this was extremely uncomfortable and no longer acceptable. A flap of bladder was fashioned to produce a continent conduit with a stoma in the right iliac fossa. The patient currently passes 2.0 to 2.5 L of urine per day (serum creatinine, 600 μmol/L) and is continent, performing ICSC of the stoma five to six times daily with no difficulty (C. R. J. Woodhouse, personal communication, 1992).

Although it is premature to draw firm conclusions from this extremely limited experience of continent urinary reservoirs, initial results are encouraging. The major advantage that no external urine collection device needs to be worn makes this an attractive option for the patient. Long-term results from nontransplant recipients must be accumulated before the technique can be recommended for extensive use in patients with unusable bladders who are to undergo kidney transplants.

Cutaneous Ureterostomy

In many ways, cutaneous ureterostomy is the least attractive option for urinary diversion. There are reports of 15 patients whose transplants were drained through a cutaneous ureterostomy (Amin *et al.*, 1977; Garrison *et al.*, 1989; Levitt *et al.*, 1979; MacGregor *et al.*, 1986; Santiago-Delpin *et al.*, 1980). In six patients, an end-ureterostomy using the native ureter had been made before the development of renal failure. The transplant was performed in the standard way, with anastomosis of the transplant ureter to the existing ureterostomy. Follow-up was limited, but at least one patient had good stable renal function 3 years posttransplant. Levitt and coworkers identified 20 patients in the literature whose transplants were drained into an ileal conduit (Levitt *et al.*, 1979). Six had cutaneous ureterostomies *in situ* before elective construction of the conduit specifically (and perhaps unnecessarily) in preparation for transplantation. An alternative procedure was described by Amin *et al.* (1977). They created a terminal-loop cutaneous ureterostomy by ligation of the distal end of the transplant ureter, bringing a loop of midureter to the skin surface and making a 1- to 2-cm longitudinal incision in the ureter. Amin and colleagues suggested that this technique may avoid retraction and ischemic stenosis and described three patients, two of whom had successful follow-up evaluations for 2 and 7 years.

The current antipathy to cutaneous ureterostomy in general urological practice and the move toward continent diversion, avoiding the need to wear an external appliance, make the technique less applicable. The simplicity of ureterostomy may have a certain attraction if techniques for more complex procedures are not available, however.

Follow-up and Management

All patients with an abnormal bladder, regardless of the form of urinary drainage, should be monitored more thoroughly than is the case with routine transplant recipients. In addition to the usual long-term complications of transplantation, these patients are at risk of developing impaired renal function resulting from various aspects of bladder dysfunction. Minor degrees of urinary obstruction, which may be urethral, at the bladder neck, at the stoma of a conduit or at the site of the ureteral anastomosis, should be excluded routinely. It also is essential to consider these possibilities as part of the differential diagnosis of allograft dysfunction. For routine follow-up and for investigation of allograft dysfunction, additional tests beyond those standard for all recipients may be indicated (Table 12–3).

Unanswered Questions

I have described the problems that face the transplant surgeon when a patient with an abnormal lower urinary tract is considered for renal transplantation. In addition, I have tried to provide the best available solutions based on published information and my own considerable experience in this area. Many questions remain unanswered and merit discussion.

The most worrisome observation has been the loss of many transplanted kidneys (all with excellent early function

TABLE 12–3

ROUTINE FOLLOW-UP AND ADDITIONAL INVESTIGATIONS IN A RECIPIENT WITH AN ABNORMAL LOWER URINARY TRACT

Every 6 Months
Isotope glomerular filtration rate
Postmicturition bladder ultrasound
Urinary flow rate
Ultrasound of the transplant

Every Year
DTPA isotope scan with furosemide
DMSA isotope scan with tomography
Transplant biopsy

Investigation of Allograft Dysfunction
Urodynamic studies
Antegrade nephrostogram (pressure-flow studies)

during the first 6–12 months) during the second, third and fourth years after transplantation. Despite a policy of intensive investigations, including repeated transplant biopsies, the cause of graft failure remains unclear. The biopsy findings have been consistent, with an appearance of patchy ischemia, fibrosis and atrophy not at all typical of chronic rejection as seen in normal patients, and radioisotope imaging with tomography has shown the development of progressive cortical scars (Cairns *et al.*, 1994). Several pathogenic mechanisms may be involved and may be interlinked, but it is difficult to define the relative importance of the individual factors.

The findings could be explained by some or all of the following:

1. Persistently raised intravesical pressure, with or without vesicoureteral reflux, causing functional impairment of urinary drainage
2. Chronic low-grade urinary tract sepsis or repeated episodes of acute urinary tract infections
3. Long-term cyclosporine–induced vasculopathy, exacerbated by factors 1 and 2
4. Chronic immunological damage, exacerbated by factors 1 and 2

These findings have been most obvious in patients in whom the bladder, although highly abnormal, was deemed usable; they have been less apparent after transplantation into an ileal conduit, and the only very long-term successes reported in the literature are of transplants drained through a conduit. Some of my patients underwent transplantation before the urodynamic criteria agreed to at the Institute of Urology in 1988 (see Table 12–2) became policy. They all had not been studied as thoroughly before transplantation as it is now believed necessary. Several other patients fulfilled the criteria for a usable bladder, however; most underwent augmentation cystoplasty. Further experience is required before it can be concluded that the criteria are incorrect, and at present, I still employ the native bladder using these criteria.

I am now more aggressive in reinvestigating bladder function posttransplantation. It seems likely that ICSC is more important than originally realized and that long-term low-dose antibiotic prophylaxis should be provided more widely. One technical problem that is common in male patients is the many urethral abnormalities (e.g., stricture and false passage) that may follow multiple urological procedures and make ICSC difficult or impossible. The concept of a continent urinary diversion is attractive. Although my own and the published experience is limited, I have many patients with such a diversion approaching end-stage renal failure. I intend to drain these transplants through the diversions. The ileal conduit offers the best-documented long-term success rate, and for a patient who can accept the inconvenience of an external urinary drainage system, a conduit represents a satisfactory option.

Summary

As has been emphasized, the relatively limited experience of surgeons and patients reported in most publications makes it difficult to draw firm conclusions. The publications in this field cover 30 years, and major changes in transplant management during that time make comparisons difficult and pooled data meaningless. Different authors have different criteria to define a usable bladder. Few patients in the past have had thorough urodynamic assessments. A variety of surgical techniques have been used, and follow-up usually is limited. Despite these difficulties, certain general points emerge, as follows:

1. Virtually all patients may be transplanted with a reasonable expectation of success regardless of the underlying urological abnormality. Surgical complications may occur in one third of all patients.

2. Thorough pretransplant assessment of the bladder is essential in patients with a urinary diversion. The native bladder may be usable or be made usable.

3. The main criteria for a usable bladder are an adequate capacity (or potential capacity) and a low end-filling pressure.

4. For a patient with a poor flow rate who fails to empty the bladder, ICSC is safe and effective. Its success depends on a normal urethra and the cooperation of the patient.

5. For an incontinent patient, an AUS is an option to urinary diversion, although experience in transplant recipients is limited.

6. If the bladder has a low capacity along with high pressure, this may be improved by bladder augmentation or substitution using a bowel segment. A clam ileocystoplasty and a cecocystoplasty are the preferred choices. Many of these patients require ICSC.

7. If the bladder cannot be made usable, transplantation in association with urinary diversion probably gives equivalent results, although there is an increased risk of complications.

8. Most experience has been gained with the ileal conduit. Continent urinary reservoirs may be an acceptable alternative if long-term follow-up supports the encouraging early reports.

9. Attention to the technical details of transplantation must be meticulous. No single operative procedure is best. Individual patients present individual problems.

10. Follow-up of patients must be obsessive. Urinary tract infections should be treated aggressively. Renal dysfunction must be investigated thoroughly, and every effort must be made to exclude minor degrees of urinary obstruction.

11. The cooperation of the urologist, transplant surgeon, nephrologist and radiologist is essential to offer patients with complex urological problems optimal treatment. Some of the unresolved issues could be approached more effectively if patients underwent transplantation in a limited number of centers in which the staff had a special interest and an expertise in these problems.

REFERENCES

Abbitt, P. L., Chevalier, R. L., Rodgers, B. M. and Howards, S. S. (1990). Acute torsion of a renal transplant: a course of organ loss. *Paediatr. Nephrol.* **4**, 174.

Alfrey, E. J., Salvatierra, O., Tanney, D. C., *et al.* (1997). Bladder augmentation can be problematic with renal failure and transplantation. *Paediatr. Nephrol.* **11**, 672.

Amin, M., Howerton, L. W. and Lich, R. (1977). Terminal loop cutaneous ureterostomy: a method of urinary drainage in kidney transplantation. *J. Urol.* **118**, 379.

Barnett, M., Bruskewitz, R., Glass, N., Sollinger, H., Uehling, D. and Belzer, F. O. (1985). Long-term clean intermittent self-catheterization in renal transplant recipients. *J. Urol.* **134**, 645.

Barnett, M. G., Bruskewitz, R. C., Belzer, F. O., Sollinger, H. W. and Uehling, D. T. (1987). Ileocecocystoplasty bladder augmentation and renal transplantation. *J. Urol.* **138**, 855.

Bricker, E. M. (1950). Bladder substitution after pelvic evisceration. *Surg. Clin. North Am.* **30**, 1511.

Bryant, J. E., Joseph, D. B., Kohaut, E. C. and Diethelm, A. G. (1991). Renal transplantation in children with posterior urethral valves. *J. Urol.* **146**, 1585.

Buerton, D., Vu, P., Terdjman, S., *et al.* (1987). Derivations urinaires et greffons intestinaux en transplantation renale chez l'enfant: rapport de huit cas. *Ann. Urol.* **21**, 49.

Cairns, H. S., Leaker, B., Woodhouse, C. R. J., Rudge, C. J. and Neild, G. H. (1991). Renal transplantation into the abnormal lower urinary tract. *Lancet* **338**, 1376.

Cairns, H. S., Spencer, S., Wilson, A. J., Rudge, C. J. and Nield, G. H. (1994). 99m Tc DMSA imaging with tomography in renal transplant recipients with abnormal lower urinary tracts. *Nephrol. Dial. Transplant.* **9**, 1157.

Casimir, F. and Merkel, F. K. (1977). The application of ileal conduits in pediatric renal transplantation. *J. Urol.* **118**, 647.

Castro, J. E., Mustapha, N., Mee, A. D. and Shackman, R. (1975). Ileal urinary diversion in patients with renal transplants. *Br. J. Urol.* **47**, 603.

Cendron, M. and Gearhart, J. B. (1991) The Mitrofanoff principle: technique and application in continent urinary diversion. *Urol. Clin. North Am.* **18**, 615.

Cerelli, J., Anderson, G. W., Evans, W. E. and Smith, J. P. (1976). Renal transplantation in patients with urinary tract abnormalities. *Surgery* **79**, 248.

Churchill, B. M., Sheldon, C. A., McLorie, C. A. and Arhus, G. S. (1988). Factors influencing patient and graft survival on 300 pediatric renal transplants. *J. Urol.* **140**, 1129.

Connolly, J. R., Miller, B. and Bretan, P. N. (1995). Renal transplantation in patients with posterior urethral valves: favourable long-term outcome. *J. Urol.* **154**, 1153.

Cornejo, F., Arango, O., Talbot-Wright, P., Carretero, P. and Gil-Vernet, J. M. (1988). Ileal conduit and orthotopic renal transplantation. *Eur. Urol.* **14**, 77.

Crowe, A., Cairns, H. S., Wood, S., *et al.* (1998). Renal transplantation following renal failure due to urological disorders. *Nephrol. Dial. Transplant.* **13**, 2065.

Dawahra, M., Martin, X., Tajra, L. C., *et al.* (1997). Renal transplantation using continent urinary diversion: long-term follow up. *Transplant. Proc.* **29**, 159.

Debruyne, F. M., Koene, R. A. P., Dam, V., Arendsen, H. J., Moonen, W. A. and Michiels, H. G. E. (1977). Renal transplantation into an ileal conduit. *Arch. Chir. Neerl.* **29**, 117.

Dunn, M., Roberts, J. B. M., Smith, P. J. B. and Slade, N. (1979). The long-term results of ileal conduit urinary diversion in children. *Br. J. Urol.* **51**, 458.

Ehrlich, O. and Brem, A. S. (1982). Urinary tract infections in patients treated with either intermittent clean self-catheterization or urinary diversion. *Pediatrics* **70**, 665.

Firlit, C. F. (1976). Use of defunctionalized bladders in paediatric renal transplantation. *J. Urol.* **116**, 634.

Firlit, C. F. and Merkel, F. K. (1977). The application of ileal conduits in pediatric renal transplantation. *J. Urol.* **118**, 647.

Flechner, S. M., Conley, B., Brewer, E. D., Benson, G. S. and Corriere, J. N., Jr. (1983). Intermittent clean catheterization: an alternative to diversion in continent transplant recipients with lower urinary tract dysfunction. *J. Urol.* **130**, 878.

Fontaine, E., Gagnadoux, M.-F., Niaudet, P., *et al.* (1998). Renal transplantation in children with augmentation cystoplasty: long-term results. *J. Urol.* **159**, 2110.

Fontaine, E., Salomon, L., Gagnadoux, M.-F., *et al.* (1997). Long-term results of renal transplantation in children with the prune-belly syndrome. *J. Urol.* **158**, 892.

Francis, D. M. and Millar, R. J. (1992). Renal transplantation using a continent ileocaecal urinary reservoir as a bladder substitute. *Transplantation* **53**, 937.

Garrison, R. N., Bentley, F. R. and Amin, M. (1989). Terminal loop cutaneous ureterostomy in cadaveric kidney transplantation. *Arch. Surg.* **124**, 467.

Gelet, A., Sanseverino, R., Salas, M., Martin, X., Marechal, J. M. and Dubernard, J. M. (1990). The AS800 urinary sphincter in renal transplantation. *Br. J. Urol.* **66**, 549.

Gill, I. S., Hayes, J. M., Hodge, E. E. and Novick, A. C. (1997). Clean intermittent catheterization and urinary diversion in the management of renal transplant recipients with lower urinary tract dysfunction. *J. Urol.* **148**, 1397.

Glass, N. R., Uehling, D., Sollinger, H. and Belzer, F. (1985). Renal transplantation using ileal conduits in 5 cases. *J. Urol.* **133**, 666.

Gleeson, M. J. and Griffith, D. P. (1990). Urinary diversion. *Br. J. Urol.* **66**, 113.

Gonzalez, R. (1997). Renal transplantation into the abnormal bladder. *J. Urol.* **158**, 895.

Griffin, P. J. A., Stephenson, T. P., Brough, S. and Salaman, J. R. (1994). Transplanting patients with abnormal lower urinary tracts. *Transpl. Int.* **7**, 288.

Groenewegen, A. A., Sukhai, R. N., Nauta, J., *et al.* (1993). Results of renal transplantation in boys treated for posterior urethral valves. *J. Urol.* **149**, 1517.

Hansson, S., Hjalmas, K., Sillen, V. and Friman, S. (1995). Clean intermittent catheterization in kidney transplant children with abnormal lower urinary tracts. *Transplant. Proc.* **27**, 3438.

Hatch, D. A. (1994). Kidney transplantation in patients with an abnormal lower urinary tract. *Urol. Clin. North Am.* **21**, 311.

Hatch, D. A., Belitsky, P., Barry, J. M., *et al.* (1993). Fate of renal allografts transplanted in patients with urinary diversions. *Transplantation* **56**, 838.

Heritier, P., Perraud, Y., Relave, M. H., *et al.* (1989). Renal transplantation and Kock pouch: a case report. *J. Urol.* **141**, 595.

Houle, A. M., Gilmour, R. F., Churchill, B. M., *et al.* (1993). What volume can a child normally store in the bladder at a safe pressure? *J. Urol.* **149**, 561.

Kashi, S. H., Wynne, K. S., Sadek, S. A. and Lodge, J. P. (1994). An evaluation of vesical urodynamics before renal transplantation and its effect on renal allograft function and survival. *Transplantation* **57**, 1455.

Kelly, W. D., Merkel, F. K. and Markland, C. (1966). Ileal urinary diversion in conjunction with renal homotransplantation. *Lancet* **1**, 222.

Kimbler, R. W., Zincke, H., Woods, J. E., Leary, F. J., Roses, J. and DeWeerd, J. H. (1977). Supravesical urinary diversion in renal transplantation. *Eur. Urol.* **3**, 193.

Kock, N. G., Nilsen, A. E. and Nilsson, L. O. (1982). Urinary diversion via a continent ileal reservoir: clinical results in 12 patients. *J. Urol.* **128**, 469.

Kogan, S. J., Weiss, R., Hanna, M. and Levitt, S. B. (1986). Successful renal transplantation in a patient with a neurogenic bladder managed by clean intermittent catheterization. *J. Urol.* **135**, 563.

Kreiger, J. N., Stubenbord, W. T. and Vaughan, E. D., Jr. (1980). Transplantation in children with end-stage renal disease of urologic origin. *J. Urol.* **124**, 508.

Landau, E. H., Jayanthi, V. R., Mclorie, G. A., *et al.* (1997). Renal transplantation in children following augmentation ureterocystoplasty. *Urology* **50**, 260.

Levey, R. H., Ingelfinger, J., Grupe, W. E., Toper, M. and Eraklis, A. J. (1978). Unique surgical and immunological features of renal transplantation in children. *J. Pediatr. Surg.* **13**, 576.

Levitt, S. B., Caberwal, D., Kogan, S. J., Romas, N. A. and Hardy, N. A. (1979). Use of preexisting ureterocutaneous anastomosis as a conduit in renal allotransplantation. *Urology* **13**, 377.

Lowe, B. S. and Woodside, J. B. (1990). Urodynamic evaluation of patients with continent urinary diversion using cecal reservoir and intussuscepted ileocecal valve. *Urology* **35**, 544.

Lucas, B. A., Munch, L. C., Wad, T. H., *et al.* (1992). Pull-through skin level allograft ureterostomy to isolate ileal stoma—report of 10 cases. *J. Urol.* **147**, 326A.

MacGregor, P., Novick, A. C., Cunningham, R., *et al.* (1986). Renal transplantation in end-stage renal disease patients with existing urinary diversion. *J. Urol.* **135**, 686.

Marchioro, T. L. and Tremann, J. A. (1974). Ureteroileostomy in renal transplant patients: a modified technique. *Urology* **3**, 171.

Marechal, J. M., Sanseverino, R., Gelet, A., Martin, X., Salas, M. and Dubernard, J. M. (1990). Continent cutaneous ileostomy (Kock pouch) prior to renal transplantation. *Br. J. Urol.* **65**, 317.

Markland, C., Kelly, W. O., Buselmeier, T., Kjellstrand, C., Simmons, R. and Najarian, J. S. (1972). Renal transplantation into ileal urinary conduits. *Transplant. Proc.* **4**, 629.

Marshall, F. F., Smolev, J. K., Spees, E. K., Jeffs, R. D. and Burdick, J. F. (1982). The urological evaluation and management of patients with congenital lower urinary tract anomalies prior to renal transplantation. *J. Urol.* **127**, 1078.

Marvin, R. G., Halff, G. A. and Elshihabi, I. (1995). Renal allograft torsion associated with prune-belly syndrome. *Paediatr. Nephrol.* **9**, 81.

McInerney, P. D., Picramenon, D., Koffman, C. G. and Munday, A. R. (1995). Is cystoplasty a safe alernative to urinary diversion in patients requiring renal transplantation? *Eur. Urol.* **27**, 117.

McLoughlin, M. B. (1976). Acute pyelonephritis in a transplant patient with an ileal loop mimicking rejection. *J. Urol.* **116**, 371.

Mitchell, M. E. and Piser, J. A. (1987). Intestinocystoplasty and total bladder replacement in children and young adults: a follow-up in 129 cases. *J. Urol.* **138**, 579.

Mitrofanoff, P. (1980). Cystostomie continte trans-appendiculaire dans le traitement des vessies neurologiques. *Chir. Pediatr.* **21**, 297.

Mundy, A. R. (1991). Artificial sphincters. *Br. J. Urol.* **67**, 225.

Neal, D. E., Hawkins, T., Gallagher, A. S., *et al.* (1985). The role of the ileal conduit in the development of upper tract dilatation. *Br. J. Urol.* **57**, 520.

Nguyen, D. H., Reinberg, Y., Gonzalez, R., Fryd, D. and Najarian, J. S. (1990). Outcome of renal transplantation after urinary diversion and enterocystoplasty: a retrospective, controlled study. *J. Urol.* **144**, 1349.

Pitts, W. R. and Muecke, E. C. (1979). A 20 year experience with ileal conduits: fate of kidneys. *J. Urol.* **122**, 154.

Popll, S., Davgirdas, J. T., Ing, T. S., Geis, W. P., Leehey, D. J. and Gandhi, V. C. (1985). Pyocystis in a renal transplant recipient with a defunctionalized bladder. *Am. J. Nephrol.* **5**, 431.

Rajagopalan, P. R., Hanevold, C. D., Orak, J. D., *et al.* (1994). Valve bladder does not affect the outcome of renal transplants in children with renal failure due to posterior urethral valves. *Transplant. Proc.* **26**, 115.

Rattazi, L. C., Simmons, R. L., Markland, C., Casali, R., Kjellstrand, C. M. and Najarian, J. S. (1975). Calculi complicating renal transplantation into ileal conduits. *Urology* **5**, 29.

Reinberg, Y., Bumgardner, G. L. and Aliabadi, H. (1990). Urologic aspects of renal transplantation. *J. Urol.* **143**, 1087.

Reinberg, Y., Gonzalez, R., Fryd, D., Mauer, S. M. and Najarian, J. S. (1988). The outcome of renal transplantation in children with posterior urethral valves. *J. Urol.* **140**, 1491.

Robards, V. L., Jr., Lubin, E. N. and Medlock, T. R. (1975). Renal transplantation and placement of ileal stoma. *Urology* **5**, 787.

Ross, J. H., Kay, R., Novick, A. C., *et al.* (1994). Long-term results of renal transplantation into the valve bladder. *J. Urol.* **151**, 1500.

Rudge, C. J. (1994). Transplantation into the abnormal bladder. In *Kidney Transplantation*, 4th ed., (P. J. Morris, ed.), W. B. Saunders, Philadelphia.

Sagalowsky, A. I., Kennedy, T. J., Davidson, I. and Peters, P. C. (1989). Pretransplant bladder rehabilitation in patients with abnormal lower urinary tracts. *Clin. Transplant.* **3**, 198.

Santiago-Delpin, E. A., Acosta-Otero, A. and Vazquez-Lugo, A. (1980). Ureteral implantation in kidney transplantation: the use of a mature end ureterostomy. *J. Urol.* **124**, 513.

Schick, E. and Tanagho, E. A. (1973). The effect of gravity on ureteric peristalsis. *J. Urol.* **109**, 187.

Schneidman, R. J., Pulliam, J. P. and Barry, J. M. (1984). CISC in renal transplant patients. *Transplantation* **38**, 312.

Schwarz, G. R. and Jeffs, R. D. (1975). Ileal conduit urinary diversion in children: computer analysis of follow-up from 2–16 years. *J. Urol.* **114**, 285.

Serrano, D. P., Flechner, S. T., Modlin, C. S., *et al.* (1996). Transplantation into the long-term defunctionalized bladder. *J. Urol.* **156**, 885.

Shandera, V. C., Rozanski, T. A. and Jaffers, G. (1996). The necessity of voiding cystourethrogram in the pre-transplant urologic evaluation. *Urology* **47**, 198.

Shapiro, S. R., Lebowitz, R. and Colodny, A. M. (1975). Fate of 90 children with ileal conduit urinary diversion a decade later: analysis of complications, pyelography, renal function and bacteriology. *J. Urol.* **114,** 289.

Sheldon, C. A., Gonzales, R., Burns, M. W., *et al.* (1994). Renal transplantation into the dysfunctional bladder: the role of adjunctive bladder reconstruction. *J. Urol.* **152,** 972.

Sheldon, C. A. and Welch, T. R. (1998). Total anatomic urinary tract replacement and renal transplantation: a surgical strategy to correct severe genitourinary anomalies. *J. Paediatr. Surg.* **33,** 635.

Shenasky, J. H., II. (1976). Renal transplantation in patients with urologic abnormalities. *J. Urol.* **115,** 490.

Shenasky, J. H. and Whelchel, J. D. (1976). Renal transplantation in the prune-belly syndrome. *J. Urol.* **115,** 112.

Skinner, D. G., Lieskovsky, G. and Boyd, S. D. (1984). Technique of creation of a continent internal ileal reservoir (Kock pouch) for urinary diversion. *Urol. Clin. North Am.* **11,** 741.

Stanley, O. H., Chambers, T. L. and Pentlow, B. D. (1983). Renal transplantation in children with occult neurogenic bladder drained by intermittent self-catheterisation. *B. M. J.* **286,** 1775.

Stenzel, K. H., Stubenbord, W. T., Whitsell, J. C., *et al.* (1974). Kidney transplantation: use of intestinal conduits. *J. A. M. A.* **229,** 534.

Thomalla, J. V., Mitchell, M. E., Leapman, S. B. and Filo, R. S. (1988). Renal transplantation in a patient with an artificial urinary sphincter device. *J. Urol.* **139,** 573.

Thomalla, J. V., Mitchell, M. E., Leapman, S. B. and Filo, R. S. (1989). Renal transplantation into the reconstructed bladder. *J. Urol.* **141,** 265.

Thuroff, J. W., Alken, P. and Riedmuller H., *et al* (1986). The Mainz pouch (mixed augmentation ileum and cecum) for bladder augmentation and continent diversion. *J. Urol.* **136,** 17.

Tunner, W. S., Whitsell, J. C., II, Rubin, A. L., *et al.* (1971). Renal transplantation in children with corrected abnormalities of the lower urinary tract. *J. Urol.* **106,** 133.

Warshaw, B. L., Edelbrock, H. H., Ettenger, R. B., *et al.* (1980). Renal transplantation in children with obstructive uropathy. *J. Urol.* **123,** 737.

Williams, J. L., Confer, D. J., DeLemos, R. A. and Montie, J. E. (1980). Colon conduit in pediatric renal transplantation. *J. Urol.* **124,** 515.

Woodhouse, C. R. and MacNeiley, A. E. (1994). The Mitrofanoff principle: expanding upon a versatile technique. *Br. J. Urol.* **74,** 447.

Zaragoza, M. R., Ritchey, M. L., Bloom, D. A., *et al.* (1993). Enterocystoplasty in renal transplantation candidates: urodynamic evaluation and outcome. *J. Urol.* **150,** 1463.

Anesthesia for Patients Undergoing Renal Transplantation

John W. Sear

Introduction

Patients with end-stage renal failure may receive replacement therapy by dialysis or by renal transplantation from a living related donor or a cadaver. Many of the factors that contribute to end-stage renal disease also increase the perioperative cardiovascular risk associated with anesthesia and surgery in these patients, including generalized atherosclerosis, uncontrolled hypertension and diabetes mellitus. Chronic renal failure increases the risks of ischemic heart disease and poor anesthetic outcome (Goldman, 1983).

In one of the first reports of the anesthetic problems associated with renal transplantation, Strunin (1966) described 36 patients who received a homograft renal transplant. Twenty of these patients died after surgery (4–143 days after the operation) from the sequelae of poor blood pressure control, hyperkalemia and hyperuremia. The formation of an arteriovenous fistula has been found to have a 30-day mortality of 2.8% (Solomonson et al., 1994)—the main adverse predictors are a myocardial infarction within the previous 6 months and increasing age. The patient with end-stage renal disease scheduled for renal transplantation presents with many clinical problems for the anesthesiologist:

Clinical problems of renal failure as related to anesthetic practice

Influence of renal failure on the pharmacokinetics and metabolism of anesthetic drugs

Intercurrent problems related to the underlying disease that caused the renal failure

Anesthetic management for renal transplantation

Clinical Problems Relevant to Anesthesia for Renal Transplantation

CARDIOVASCULAR DISEASE

There are three main cardiovascular effects of chronic renal failure: arterial hypertension, atherosclerosis and hyperlipidemia leading to ischemic heart disease and pericarditis. Hypertension and ischemic heart disease are common complications in patients presenting for renal transplantation. The incidence of preoperative hypertension is 68 to 94% in different reported series of patients undergoing renal transplantation (Heino et al., 1986; Marsland and Bradley, 1983; Morgan and Lumley, 1975). Similarly, the incidence of ischemic heart disease is high—about 1 in 20 of recipients aged younger than 55 years and higher in the elderly.

The cause of hypertension of chronic renal failure often is a consequence of volume expansion secondary to salt and water retention (Brown et al., 1971). It usually can be controlled with dialysis and appropriate antihypertensive therapy. In patients in whom the hypertension cannot be controlled by dialysis alone, it has been suggested that an abnormal relationship exists between plasma renin activity, intravascular fluid volume and blood pressure. There also may be an inappropriate level of sympathetic activity (Converse et al., 1992).

Improvements in dialysis technology have resulted in a significant reduction in the numbers of patients receiving antihypertensive therapy. Patients needing treatment often are refractory to single agents and require large doses of combinations of antihypertensive drugs (e.g., β-adrenoceptor blocking drugs, calcium channel blockers, vasodilators and angiotensin-converting enzyme inhibitors), which all may contribute to produce significant drug interactions with volatile and intravenous anesthetic agents (Sear et al., 1994).

In the posttransplant patient in whom there is correction of the uremia and fluid imbalance, persistence of hypertension may be due to acute or chronic rejection of the allograft, the presence of native diseased kidneys or transplant artery stenosis. Cyclosporine therapy also may produce hypertension; this often is accompanied by renal dysfunction. It appears to be a direct vasoconstrictor response and to be an action of cyclosporine on intracellular calcium homeostasis. Cyclosporine reduces renal tubular sensitivity to aldosterone. Other contributory factors include the presence of cyclosporine-induced hypomagnesemia and the renal production of thromboxane A_2.

Of patients receiving a renal transplant, 50 to 70% suffer marked swings in blood pressure during surgery ($\pm$ 30% shifts from the awake preinduction value) and show exaggerated vascular responses to induction of anesthesia, laryngoscopy and intubation and extubation. Induction of anesthesia is best achieved by combining a hypnotic agent supplemented with an opioid (fentanyl, alfentanil or sufentanil) or using a coinduction technique with midazolam. Patients on antihypertensive or antianginal treatment (especially those on β-adrenoceptor blocking drugs, angiotensin-converting enzyme inhibitors and calcium channel inhibitors) should receive appropriate therapy as part of their premedication. In patients not on therapy and presenting for surgery with elevated blood pressure, Stone and colleagues showed the efficacy of preoperative oral β-adrenoceptor blockade as an adjunct to premedication in reducing the hemodynamic lability in response to surgical stress and its associated incidence of myocardial ischemia (Stone et al., 1988; Fig. 13–1).

Patients with renal failure, especially those on dialysis, are prone to develop accelerated atherosclerosis. Left ventricular function may be compromised further by uremic cardiomyopathy and pericarditis. The cause of the pericarditis often is unknown but is seen late in the course of chronic renal disease and is commoner in undialyzed patients. If it is of the hemorrhagic type, the accompanying pericardial effusion may cause tamponade and further decreases in contractility and cardiac output. Treatment is by surgical pericardectomy.

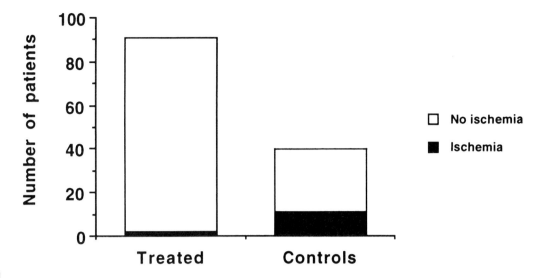

FIGURE 13-1

Reduction in the incidence of myocardial ischemia during surgery after pretreatment of untreated or poorly treated hypertensive patients with oral β-adrenoceptor antagonists. (Reproduced with permission from Stone *et al.*, 1988.)

ANEMIA

Anemia has been a major problem in the anesthetic management of patients with renal failure. Hemoglobin concentrations in patients on hemodialysis before transplantation often were 6 to 8 g 100 ml^{-1} with hematocrit values of 20 to 25%, although this is now uncommon with the more liberal use of erythropoietin in anemic renal failure patients, at least in the Western world. The normal picture is that of a normochromic, normocytic anemia of complex origin that usually is due to impaired erythropoiesis secondary to decreased erythropoietin synthesis and release. Other factors include a decreased red cell life span; increased hemolysis and bleeding; repeated blood loss during hemodialysis; aluminum toxicity; uremia-induced bone marrow suppression and iron, folate and vitamins B_6 and B_{12} deficiencies.

These problems can be reduced significantly by administration of biosynthetic erythropoietin, which increases hemoglobin concentrations toward normal (Winearls *et al.*, 1986). Important side effects have been observed when the hematocrit is increased greater than 35%, including hypertension, cerebrovascular accidents, thrombosis of fistulae and epileptiform activity (Eschbach *et al.*, 1987). Hemoglobin concentrations should be maintained at around 10 to 11 g dl^{-1}. The use of biosynthetic erythropoietin also is associated with reduction in the need for repeated blood transfusions (Eschbach *et al.*, 1989), which decreases the risk of sensitization.

In the absence of a correction of the anemia, there are compensatory mechanisms for the reduction in oxygen-carrying capacity. At a hemoglobin concentration of 6 to 8 g 100 ml^{-1}, the oxygen-carrying capacity of the blood is about 50% normal (i.e., about 10 ml oxygen per 100 ml blood). The normal tissue arteriovenous oxygen difference is 5 ml oxygen per 100 ml blood, although the heart extracts two to three times this amount. Various compensatory mechanisms exist to overcome the decrease in oxygen carrying capacity, including an increase in cardiac output and an increase in the red cell 2,3-diphosphoglycerate. The latter causes a shift of the oxygen dissociation curve to the right, improving tissue oxygenation. The shift appears to be greater in the uremic patient well managed by hemodialysis compared with the patient in renal failure poorly managed or not on dialysis. This difference may reflect the influence of acidosis on the position of the oxyhemoglobin dissociation curve.

Because of the need to maintain adequate tissue oxygenation, it is important to avoid sudden decreases in cardiac output or increase of pH during induction of anesthesia and the perioperative period. Although the policy of most transplantation units in the early 1970s was to avoid blood transfusion to correct existing anemia or acute operative blood loss because of the fear of sensitization of the recipient, the emphasis changed with the introduction of elective pregraft or perioperative transfusion to improve graft survival (see Chapter 39). Although the beneficial role of transfusion in graft survival is controversial in the cyclosporine era, there need be no hesitation in replacing volume losses with whole blood, keeping in mind that this may lead to an increase in plasma potassium levels. Severe anemia also affects the blood gas partition coefficient for the volatile anesthetic agents, with an increase in the rate of onset and recovery from anesthesia.

RESPIRATORY SYSTEM

Between dialyses, pulmonary congestion and edema often are seen with a resultant hypoxemia and hypocapnia. The use of peritoneal dialysis can aggravate the problem because the intraperitoneal fluid causes diaphragmatic splinting with basal pulmonary atelectasis and shunting. *Uremic lung* is a radiological entity characterized by perihilar pulmonary venous congestion secondary to fluid retention. Uremia can cause pleuritis. The immunosuppressed transplant patient is more susceptible to pulmonary infections, with preexisting disease often exacerbated by airway instrumentation and general anesthesia.

ACID-BASE STATUS AND ELECTROLYTE IMBALANCE

Patients with renal failure have an inability to excrete water, electrolytes and free acids. The presence of a metabolic acidosis with its associated electrolyte disturbances (hyponatremia, hyperchloremia and hyperkalemia) may cause problems with respect to the adequacy of reversal of residual neuromuscular blockade at the end of anesthesia. This possibility has become less important with the routine dialysis of all patients before transplantation. Intraoperative determination of plasma electrolytes is not routinely performed, unless there are specific indications, such as the administration of large quantities of blood or the diabetic patient.

With the introduction of routine dialysis in most patients before transplantation, preoperative electrolyte disturbances have largely disappeared. Of more importance is the blood potassium concentration. At serum concentrations greater than 7 mmol L^{-1}, abnormal electrocardiogram (ECG) changes are common, with the possibility of developing ventricular tachycardia and ventricular fibrillation. A high potassium level before anesthesia is potentially dangerous and must be avoided. Evidence exists, however, that uremic patients can tolerate mild to moderate degrees of hyperkalemia. It is probably safe to administer anesthesia in the presence of higher than normal potassium concentrations, unless there are ECG changes associated with hyperkalemia (high-peaked T waves, decreased amplitude of the R wave, widened QRS complexes and progressive diminution of P wave amplitude). Potassium values of greater than 5.5 mmol L^{-1} should be treated actively before anesthesia and surgery.

Methods available for the preoperative correction of hyperkalemia include glucose-insulin therapy, administration of bicarbonate, intravenous calcium gluconate or chloride, calcium resonium enema (30–60 g) and continuous hemofiltration or hemodialysis. Factors that may increase further the plasma potassium concentration (including infusions of stored blood, hypoventilation causing respiratory acidosis, and repeated doses of suxamethonium) are best avoided.

COAGULATION

Some patients show persistent heparinization after hemodialysis before transplantation (Hampers et al, 1966). A few uremic patients, normally those inadequately dialyzed or transplanted before requiring dialysis, exhibit a separate hemorrhagic diathesis.

Several abnormalities of the coagulation factors have been described (platelet dysfunction, decreased levels of platelet factor III resulting in poor adhesiveness and thrombocytopenia). Laboratory investigations show no alteration in prothrombin or partial thromboplastin time, but the bleeding time is prolonged. The decrease in platelet factor III occurs because of accumulation of toxic endogenous waste products, including guanininosuccinate, phenol and phenolic acid. These products are removed by adequate dialysis with a return to normal platelet function.

Other methods of treatment of uremic coagulopathy include platelet transfusion, cryoprecipitate, and subcutaneous boluses or continuous infusions (0.3 μg kg^{-1}) over 15 minutes of desmopressin acetate (DDAVP); DDAVP acts to increase the activity of coagulation factors VIII, XII, von Willebrand factor and high-molecular-weight kininogen (Mannucci, 1988; Mannucci *et al.*, 1983). Administration of DDAVP results in improved platelet function for about 4 hours.

Despite these theoretical problems, the blood loss during transplantation normally is less than 500 ml. If blood loss occurs, it may be rapid, and all replacement fluid should be administered through large venous catheters.

CENTRAL NERVOUS SYSTEM

The central nervous system features of uremia are initially malaise and reduced mental ability and an inability to concentrate but may proceed to myoclonus, seizures, coma and death. Patients complain of pruritus, which tends to be severe at night and at rest and is relieved by movement. Dialysis is associated with two neurological sequelae—the dysequilibrium syndrome and dementia. The former results from sudden changes in extracellular volume and electrolyte composition as well as cerebral edema. The dysequilibrium syndrome is characterized by dehydration, weakness, nausea and vomiting, hypotension and occasionally convulsions and coma. Treatment should be symptomatic and aggressive.

The dementia is a severe, life-threatening disorder that affects patients on long-term dialysis therapy and may be due to aluminum toxicity. The incidence of this complication has been reduced by using deionized fluids for dialyzing fluids and by avoiding excessive ingestion of aluminum in the form of antacids and dietary supplements. Peripheral neuropathies also may occur, especially in the lower limbs, and may involve the autonomic nervous system, leading to postural hypotension.

ENDOCRINE SYSTEM

Diabetic nephropathy is a common cause of end-stage renal disease and may be accompanied by accelerated atherosclerosis. Significant coronary artery disease may be a significant presenting feature of the triad of diabetes, hypertension and hyperlipidemia (the so-called syndrome X) (Williams, 1994). Diabetes may lead to an autonomic neuropathy that can cause gastroparesis and hemodynamic instability. Long-term problems in the diabetic patient include stiffening of the temporomandibular joints and difficulty with laryngoscopy and intubation (see later).

Uremic osteodystrophy encompasses many separate skeletal problems, including osteomalacia, osteosclerosis and osteitis fibrosa cystica—the last-mentioned developing as a result of secondary hyperparathyroidism. As renal function decreases, phosphate excretion falls, and the resulting hyperphosphatemia leads to a reduced absorption of calcium and hyperactivity of the parathyroid glands on an attempt to maintain the serum calcium concentration. The sequela is bone demineralization, making patients susceptible to spontaneous fracturing of long bones and vertebrae.

GASTROINTESTINAL TRACT

Common gastrointestinal symptoms in the uremic patient are anorexia, nausea and vomiting, gut bleeding, diarrhea and intractable hiccups. Most of these problems are attenuated by the introduction of dialysis before transplantation. Renal failure patients have delayed gastric emptying in addition to an increase in acidity and gastric volume. Patients benefit from administration of a histamine H_2-receptor antagonist as part of premedication. A rare but important complication of end-stage renal disease is ascites (accompanied by hypoalbuminemia), which may lead to splinting of the diaphragm and basal pulmonary atelectasis with resultant hypoxemia (Gluck and Nolph, 1987).

IMMUNE SYSTEM

Uremia impairs normal immune mechanisms, and these mechanisms may be obtunded further by administration of corticosteroids and immunosuppressant drugs for treatment of the underlying renal pathology (e.g., systemic lupus, scleroderma, nephrotic syndrome). As a result, sepsis remains a major cause of morbidity and mortality. Particular attention should be paid to strict aseptic techniques when inserting a urinary catheter, invasive monitoring devices or peripheral infusions.

PROBLEMS RESULTING FROM HEMODIALYSIS

The main sequelae resulting from hemodialysis are excessive or persistent heparinization after dialysis, abnormal fluid shifts and transmission of viral infections (e.g., hepatitis A, B and C; human immunodeficiency virus [HIV] and cytomegalovirus). Residual heparinization presents as a bleeding diathesis occurring 10 hours after hemodialysis. It is readily corrected by protamine.

Hepatitis is endemic in the dialysis population of some countries, and anesthesiologists should wear gloves to reduce the risk of transmission. Adequate screening and immunization for hepatitis A and B viruses should be conducted for medical and nursing personnel responsible for patients with chronic renal failure. The impact of HIV in the dialysis population is not of major significance to date in the United Kingdom, but there must be rigorous screening for the virus in all dialysis patients and in potential kidney donors (living related and cadaveric).

OTHER PREOPERATIVE COMPLICATIONS

Better preoperative selection and preparation of patients for renal transplantation have reduced the incidence of other complications of renal failure. Preoperative assessment should exclude the presence of congestive heart failure, pericardial or pleural effusions, ECG abnormalities resulting from myocardial ischemia and autonomic dysfunction in patients with diabetes mellitus.

With increasing numbers of elderly patients (>55 years old) and diabetic patients being accepted for renal transplantation, there is need for careful assessment of cardiorespiratory function before placement on the transplant list. This assessment should include referral, when appropriate, for an anesthetic consultant opinion and clear indication in the case notes of special problems relating to the individual patient at the time of surgery. The patient maintained on hemodialysis usually requires a dialysis session at some point during the 24- to 36-hour period before transplantation. Predialysis and postdialysis weight and electrolyte status should be recorded.

A common complication of dialysis in the preoperative transplant recipient is hypotension; this is predominantly due to ultrafiltration-induced hypovolemia, but it also may be due to the reduction in plasma osmolality; to reflex sympathetic inhibition or to the autonomic neuropathy associated with diabetes mellitus, systemic sepsis and electrolyte abnormalities (especially hypokalemia, hyperkalemia and hypocalcemia). Treatment is administered by infusing normal saline and reducing the rate of ultrafiltration if it occurs during preoperative dialysis.

PROTECTION OF VEINS, SHUNTS AND FISTULAE

Functional shunts or fistulae should be protected carefully during surgery, with the sphygmomanometer cuff placed on the other arm. Venous lines should be restricted when possible to peripheral veins on the dorsum of the hand, with the preservation of all forearm and antecubital fossa veins.

The monitoring of central venous pressure (CVP) is useful during transplantation because many patients come to surgery dehydrated after preoperative dialysis and may need extensive volume replacement to maintain a normal CVP. Although several previous reviews have stressed the problems of overhydration and electrolyte imbalance, this usually has been in poorly prepared or nondialyzed subjects. Central venous cannulation is best achieved using the subclavian or internal jugular approach. The current policy of fluid replacement is to load the circulating volume and raise the CVP during the period before completion of the vascular anastomoses.

NONANESTHETIC DRUGS GIVEN DURING RENAL TRANSPLANTATION

The policy relating to immunosuppressive therapy varies among units, but the anesthesiologist may be required to institute the appropriate therapy (hydrocortisone, prednisolone, azathioprine, cyclosporine, antilymphocytic globulin, OKT3 or other drugs) during the operation.

Influence of Renal Disease on Pharmacokinetics of Drugs Used During Anesthesia

PREMEDICATION DRUGS

Anticholinergic Drugs

Atropine and glycopyrrolate are eliminated by the kidney (20–50% of total) (Kirvela et al., 1993). Because they are administered only as single doses, however, accumulation with toxic side effects is unlikely to be a significant problem. The phenothiazine drugs (such as promethazine and chlorpromazine) are metabolized primarily by the liver, and their clearance is unaltered in patients with renal failure. One disadvantage of their use is their α-adrenoceptor blocking action, which may accentuate the cardiovascular instability commonly seen in the recently dialyzed patient undergoing transplantation.

Antacids and Prokinetic Drugs

The handling of the H_2-histamine receptor antagonists, such as cimetidine, ranitidine, famotidine and nizatidine, is largely unaltered by end-stage renal disease. Metoclopramide is eliminated by the kidney unchanged (<20%) and as N-4-sulfate (≦50%) and N-glucuronamide. Its kinetics are complex because the elimination half-life is dose dependent after intravenous and oral administration. When given to patients with end-stage renal disease, there is a significant reduction in clearance (16.7 L h^{-1} compared with 52.5 L h^{-1}) and prolongation of the terminal half-life (13.9 hours compared with 2.8 hours) (Bateman and Gokal, 1980). This change is not the result of reduced renal clearance but rather impaired metabolism and alteration in the amount of drug glucuronamide conjugates undergoing enterohepatic recirculation. In a further study in patients maintained on hemodialysis, Lehmann and colleagues confirmed the altered kinetics of metoclopramide and reported significant adverse side effects (drowsiness, restlessness and diarrhea) after single doses of 10 mg (Lehmann et al., 1985). Hemodialysis does not affect metoclopramide elimination from the body, however, and clearance of the drug subsequent to dialysis is unaltered (Wright et al., 1988).

Benzodiazepines

The handling of several drugs of the benzodiazepine group of sedative premedications is altered in patients with acute or chronic renal failure. Kangas et al. (1976) showed a decrease in the plasma protein binding of diazepam in patients with chronic renal failure; Andreasen (1974) found no correlation between the serum albumin concentration and protein binding of diazepam in patients in acute renal failure, however. In a further investigation of the disposition of diazepam in patients with chronic uremia, Ochs and associates found an increased volume of distribution and increased systemic clearance, both secondary to an increase in the free unbound drug fraction (from 1.4% to 7.9%) (Ochs et al., 1981).

There was no difference in free drug clearance in the uremic and healthy patients, although there was a smaller volume of distribution in the renal failure group.

Of greater interest to the anesthesiologist is the kinetics of the short-acting, water-soluble benzodiazepine midazolam (Vinik et al., 1983). There are significantly greater values for total drug clearance and volumes of distribution in patients with chronic renal failure when compared with healthy controls. These changes are secondary to an increased free drug fraction (6.5% compared with 3.9%). There were no differences in unbound drug kinetics, and the elimination half-life was similar in the two groups (4.6–4.9 hours). In an assessment of the dynamic properties of midazolam in patients with impaired renal function, no correlation was found between onset time of sedation and free drug fraction. This lack of correlation may have been due to inherent alterations in drug sensitivity in the uremic patient. Because the increased free fraction of unbound drug is distributed rapidly to the richly vascularized tissues, it is probably advisable to give intravenous midazolam at a slow rate, titrating dose to effect. In this way, the anesthesiologist can minimize any effects of relative overdosage of free drug to the heart, kidneys, liver and brain.

Odar-Cederlof and coworkers investigated the disposition of oxazepam in patients with renal failure (Odar-Cederlof et al., 1977). After an oral dose of 0.2 mg kg^{-1}, there was significant prolongation of the terminal half-life (5.9–25 hours in healthy subjects and 24–91 hours in uremic patients) and a decreased plasma protein binding in renal failure, coupled with an increased fecal excretion of the drug. Initial data analysis suggests unaltered systemic drug clearance; if correction is made for the decreased absorption of the oral drug in uremia, there is reduced clearance of oxazepam in renal failure. This reduced clearance has not been confirmed in a separate study by Murray et al. (1981).

Single-dose studies with lorazepam indicate no alterations in the terminal half-life in renal failure (Verbeeck et al., 1976); however, these same authors have described impaired drug elimination after long-term administration to two patients with uremia (Verbeeck et al., 1981). Although widely used as a premedication in this group of patients, there are no data on the kinetics or dynamics of temazepam in end-stage renal disease. The pharmacokinetic changes described for the benzodiazepines may account partly for the increased sensitivity to these drugs in patients with chronic renal failure and should serve as a caution to their injudicious use as sedation to supplement regional anesthesia in these patients. Our current practice in Oxford is to premedicate patients with temazepam (10–20 mg) 1 to 1.5 hours preoperatively, together with ranitidine and metoclopramide.

INDUCTION AGENTS

Barbiturates

Despite the increased sensitivity of patients in chronic renal failure to barbiturate drugs, thiopentone still is widely used for induction of anesthesia. Normal induction doses of thiopentone induced prolonged unconsciousness, the duration being related to the blood urea concentration (Dundee and Richards, 1954). Various suggestions have been made as to the cause of this effect. These include increased blood-brain barrier permeability (Freeman et al., 1962), increased unbound plasma barbiturate concentrations in uremic patients (Burch and Stanski, 1982; Christensen et al., 1983), qualitative plasma albumin abnormalities (Shoeman and Azarnoff, 1972) and abnormal cerebral uptake and metabolism of the barbiturate (Richet et al., 1970). If there is a

reduction in the serum albumin (as in the nephrotic syndrome), the bound fraction of drug is decreased. No change in dosing requirements could imply an increased potency in the presence of uremia; this also may relate to the effects of any acidosis causing an increased un-ionized (i.e., active) drug fraction.

Burch and Stanski (1982) investigated the disposition of thiopentone in patients with chronic renal failure. They found an unaltered total drug elimination half-life but an increased free drug fraction. There were, however, no differences compared with healthy patients in the unbound drug volumes of distribution and systemic clearance (Table 13–1). The increased free drug fraction results in higher brain concentrations of thiopentone. If there is assumed to be no alteration in brain or cardiovascular sensitivity to thiopentone in the patient with chronic renal failure, a decreased rate of administration rather than a decreased drug dosing should be used for induction of anesthesia. This hypothesis is supported by the studies of Christensen and colleagues, who found no differences in the dose of thiopentone required to induce anesthesia successfully in healthy and renal failure patients; there were no differences in arterial and venous drug concentrations at the point of hypnosis (Christensen and Andreasen, 1978; Christensen et al., 1983). This finding suggests that there is no alteration in brain sensitivity to the thiobarbiturate. There are presently no data on the disposition of methohexitone in patients with chronic renal failure. Pentobarbitone (an active metabolite of thiopentone) shows unaltered kinetics in patients with end-stage renal disease (Reidenberg et al., 1976).

Etomidate

No formal studies have been done on the disposition of the carboxylated imidazole etomidate in patients with renal failure, although several authors have shown a significant decrease in the plasma protein binding of etomidate in patients with uremia (Carlos et al., 1979; Meuldermans and Heykants, 1976). No available data suggest that this decrease may lead to altered dosage requirements.

The dynamic properties of etomidate in patients with impaired cardiovascular function may be useful, especially in the mildly hypovolemic patient. The well-documented adverse side effects of etomidate on the adrenal gland (to suppress steroidogenesis) are short-lived and are of little relevance in transplant patients concurrently receiving hydrocortisone for immunosuppression.

Ketamine

Ketamine is probably best avoided for induction of anesthesia for transplantation because it causes increases in heart rate and blood pressure, which may be deleterious in the patient with preexisting hypertension or coronary artery disease. In end-stage renal disease, elimination of the metabolites of ketamine (especially the active norketamine as well as the glucuronide conjugates) is reduced (Koppel et al., 1990).

Propofol

Kinetic studies after induction and maintenance of anesthesia with propofol indicate no alteration in terminal half-life or clearance in patients with renal failure (Ickx et al., 1998; Kirvela et al., 1992), although Ickx et al. (1998) reported a greater volume of distribution of propofol in end-stage renal disease. There is no significant effect of end-stage renal disease on plasma protein binding (Costela et al., 1996).

Morcos and Payne (1985) and Kirvela et al. (1992) reported the cardiovascular effects after propofol, 2 to 2.5 mg kg^{-1},

TABLE 13–1

INFLUENCE OF END-STAGE RENAL DISEASE ON THE DISPOSITION KINETICS OF COMMONLY USED INTRAVENOUS INDUCTION AGENTS

	Patients with Normal Renal Function				Patients with Impaired Renal Function			
	$T_{1/2}el$	Cl_p	V_{ss}	FF	$T_{1/2}el$	Cl_p	V_{ss}	FF
Thiopentone								
1	611	3.2	1.9	15.7	583	4.5*	3.0*	28.0*
2	588	2.7	1.4	11.0	1,069	3.9	3.2*	17.8*
Midazolam								
3	296	6.7	2.2	3.9	275	11.4*	3.8*	5.5*
Etomidate								
4	—	—	—	24.9	—	—	—	43.4*
Propofol								
5	1,714	11.8	19.8	—	1,638	12.9	22.6	—
6	—	—	—	0.98	—	—	—	1.11a
								0.87b
7	420†	33.5†	5.8†	—	513†	32.0†	11.3*†	—

Note. Mean values are given except where indicated.

$T_{1/2}el$, elimination half-life (min); Cl_p, systemic clearance (ml kg^{-1} min^{-1}); V_{ss}, apparent volume of distribution at steady-state (L kg^{-1}); FF, free or unbound fraction of drug (%). †: median values. *$P<0.05$ vs. healthy subjects. a. and b: before and after dialysis.

Sources of data: 1, Burch and Stanski, 1982; 2, Christensen *et al.*, 1983; 3, Vinik *et al.*, 1983; 4, Carlos *et al.*, 1979; 5, Kirvela *et al.*, 1992; 6, Costela *et al.*, 1996; and 7, Ickx *et al.*, 1998.

preceded by fentanyl, 3 to 5 μg kg^{-1}, in adequately volume-loaded end-stage renal failure patients and compared the data with those from healthy subjects. This induction sequence caused significant vasodilatation in all patients, with 24 to 30% decreases in systolic blood pressure and 22 to 32% decreases in diastolic blood pressure in the healthy subjects and 19 to 39% and 14 to 39% decreases in the renal disease patients. In the latter study, the maintenance of adequate antihypertensive therapy in these uremic patients up to the time of surgery may have contributed to the cardiovascular stability (Pouttu, 1989). Similar results have been reported in open studies by Nguyen *et al.* (1989) and Reiter *et al.* (1989). The induction agent of choice for patients undergoing renal transplantation is probably thiopentone, with the dose carefully titrated to clinical effect.

OPIOID DRUGS

In the healthy patient, most opioid drugs are metabolized to inactive compounds, which then are excreted in the urine or bile. For example, the metabolism of pethidine (meperidine), alfentanil, fentanyl, sufentanil and morphine may be 80 to 95%. Phenoperidine differs from these other opioids in that about 50% normally is eliminated in the urine in an unchanged form. In renal failure, the action of phenoperidine is likely to be prolonged.

Morphine

Morphine is still a widely used drug for the provision of perioperative and postoperative analgesia. Morphine is metabolized primarily in the liver, where it undergoes glucuronidation to the 3-glucuronide (M3G) (the main metabolite, ≤50%) and the 6-glucuronide (M6G) (about 10%). Other metabolites in humans include *N*-demethylation to normorphine. Although M6G is a more potent analgesic than the parent drug, M3G has been shown in animal models to antagonize the dynamic properties of morphine and M6G (Smith et al., 1990). Any change in the concentrations of these metabolites (or the parent drug) could have considerable dynamic sequelae.

Many authors have reported prolonged or exaggerated

clinical effects when intravenous morphine was given to patients with chronic renal failure (Don *et al.*, 1975; Mostert *et al.*, 1971; Stanley and Lathrop, 1977). Despite these important dynamic data, it is only more recently that substantive studies have been conducted on the disposition of analgesic drugs in patients with impaired renal function. The meaningful evaluation of the disposition of morphine by specific assays has allowed the clinician to examine critically the kinetics of single and multiple doses of the drug. Olsen and colleagues studied the plasma protein binding of morphine in healthy subjects and patients with renal failure; in uremia, they found an increased free drug fraction (from 65% to 70–75%) (Olsen *et al.*, 1975).

Several data sets examine the influence of end-stage renal disease on morphine disposition and metabolism in awake (Aitkenhead *et al.*, 1984; Sawe and Odar-Cederlof, 1987; Woolner *et al.*, 1986) and anesthetized patients (Chauvin *et al.*, 1987b; Sear *et al.*, 1989). All data sets show renal failure to have little effect on morphine clearance but to result in the accumulation of the various metabolites, M3G, M6G and normorphine (Fig. 13–2 and Table 13–2). The higher concentrations of M6G may account for the profound analgesia and sedation seen in the uremic patient who has received large doses of morphine or papaveretum (Omnopon) (Osborne *et al.*, 1986). In patients undergoing transplantation who received 10 mg of morphine intravenously as a supplement to nitrous oxide–oxygen anesthesia, we found the elimination half-lives of M3G and M6G to be 300 to 920 minutes and 220 to 900 minutes. These estimates are prolonged when compared with values of 100 to 200 minutes in the healthy anesthetized patient (Sear *et al.*, 1989) but are similar to the half-lives found when M6G was given by intravenous administration to patients with renal failure (Hanna *et al.*, 1993).

Although we would expect chronic renal impairment to result in larger areas under the concentration-time curve (AUC) 0 to 24 hours for both glucuronides, our data and those of Mazoit *et al.* (1990) and Sloan *et al.* (1991) also show greater AUC for morphine itself. These data all offer support to the notion that the kidney itself may play a role in morphine biotransformation as well as metabolite elimination. Although the papers of Mazoit and Sloan suggest that 30 to

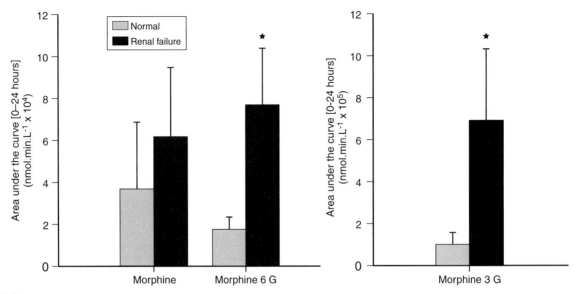

FIGURE 13–2

Areas under the concentration versus time curve for morphine and its two metabolites, morphine-6-glucuronide and morphine-3-glucuronide in five anesthetized healthy subjects with normal renal function (gray columns) and in 11 patients with renal failure receiving kidney grafts (solid columns)(*P<0.05). (Adapted with permission from Sear *et al.*, 1989.)

35% morphine elimination may be by nonurinary excretion, nonhepatic degradation (i.e., potentially by renal parenchymal metabolism), our data and those of Osborne *et al.* (1993) offer another explanation.

The increased plasma morphine concentrations (and larger AUC) could have occurred by hydrolysis of one or the other of the accumulating glucuronides (probably M3G) back to the parent compound. This would tend to reduce the

ratio AUC M3G/M6G. These represented a mean value in Osborne's study of around 5 in the healthy subjects and 3.9 and 4.5 in the groups of patients with end-stage renal disease (Osborne *et al.*, 1993). The same ratios in our patients were 8 in the healthy anesthetized subjects and 9 in patients undergoing transplantation (Sear *et al.*, 1989). We found no difference in the AUC M3G/M6G between the healthy subjects and patients with end-stage renal disease undergoing trans-

TABLE 13–2

INFLUENCE OF CHRONIC RENAL FAILURE ON THE DISPOSITION OF OPIOIDS IN THE ANESTHETIZED PATIENT

	Patients with Normal Renal Function				Patients with Impaired Renal Function			
	$T_{1/2}el$	Cl_p	V_{ss}	FF	$T_{1/2}el$	Cl_p	V_{ss}	FF
Morphine								
1	186	21.3	3.7	—	185	17.1	2.8*	—
2	307	11.4	3.8	—	302	9.6	2.4*	—
3	102	27.3	3.2	—	120	25.1	2.8*	—
Fentanyl								
4	405	14.8	7.7	—	594*	11.8	9.5	—
5	175†	17.1	2.7	—	229†	18.5	3.6	—
6	—	—	—	20.8	—	—	—	22.4
7	—	—	—	—	382	7.5	3.1	—
Alfentanil								
8	90	3.1	0.3	11.0	107	3.1	0.4*	19.0*
9	120	3.2	0.4	10.3	142	5.3*	0.6	12.4*
Sufentanil								
10	76	12.8	1.3	—	90	16.4	1.7	—
11	195	18.2	3.6	7.8	188	19.2	3.8	8.6
Remifentanil								
12	4.0	33.2	0.19	—	4.9	35.4	0.25	—
Oxycodone								
13	138	16.7	2.39	—	234	12.7	3.99	—

Note. Mean values are given throughout except for oxycodone, for which medians are given.

*$P<0.05$ versus healthy subjects.

†Mean residence time (rather than elimination half-life).

$T_{1/2}el$, elimination half-life (min); Cl_p, systemic clearance (ml kg^{-1} min^{-1}); V_{ss}, apparent volume of distribution at steady-state (L kg^{-1}); FF, free or unbound fraction of drug (%).

Sources of data: 1, Chauvin *et al.*, 1987b; 2, Sear *et al.*, 1989; 3, Osborne *et al.*, 1993, 4, Duthie, 1987; 5, Sear and Hand, 2000; 6, Bower, 1982; 7, Koehntop *et al.*, 1997; 8, Chauvin *et al.*, 1987a; 9, Bower and Sear, 1989; 10, Davis *et al.*, 1988; 11, Sear, 1989; 12, Hoke *et al.*, 1997; 13, Kirvela *et al.*, 1996.

plantation. The model of studying drug disposition during transplantation may be affected by the onset of renal drug elimination during the 24-hour study period.

The relationship between renal creatinine clearance and the renal clearances of morphine, M3G and M6G has been studied by Milne *et al.* (1992) in intensive care unit patients with variable degrees of renal impairment. For all three compounds, there was a linear relationship between free drug clearance and creatinine clearance. The unbound clearance of morphine exceeded that of creatinine, whereas the clearances of M3G and M6G were similar. The ratios of the plasma concentrations of M3G/morphine and M6G/morphine ranged from 4 to 170 and 0.79 to 51. Similar values have been reported by Petersen and colleagues in terminal cancer patients with impaired renal function receiving subcutaneous morphine (Petersen *et al.*, 1990). The mean plasma concentration ratio of M3G/M6G was 5.0 (similar to the ratios of AUC seen in the study of Osborne *et al.*, 1993). The unbound fractions for morphine, M3G and M6G were 74%, 85% and 89%, the first figure being significantly greater than that determined by Olsen *et al.* (1975).

Loetsch and coworkers have determined the half-lives of M3G and M6G in healthy volunteers to be on the order of 2.8 to 3.2 hours and 1.7 to 2.7 hours (Loetsch *et al.*, 1996). The longer half-lives of M3G and M6G (41–141 hours and 89–136 hours) reported by Osborne *et al.* (1986, 1993) and Sawe and Odar-Cederlof (1987) in patients with impaired renal function could be clinically important in the prolonged effect of the parent drug. In addition, Sawe and Odar-Cederlof (1987) showed a significant correlation between the M3G half-life and the plasma urea concentration. Although we did not find a significant correlation between the AUC of M3G and M6G and the immediate postoperative 24-hour creatinine clearance in the patients undergoing transplantation, there was an association between the creatinine clearance and the elimination half-life of the two glucuronide metabolites ($r = 0.87$ and $r = 0.63$; $P < 0.01$ and $P < 0.05$). There was no relationship between creatinine clearance and morphine clearance. Despite these data, we do not have sufficient information to derive a nomogram relating plasma creatinine, predicted or measured creatinine clearance and accumulation of the active M6G in the patient with renal impairment to determine the possibility of postoperative ventilatory depression.

If infusions of morphine are administered to patients with impaired renal function, accumulation of M6G may occur to give a clinical picture of a persistently narcotized patient (Hasselstrom *et al.*, 1989; Osborne *et al.*, 1986; Shelly *et al.*, 1986). The importance of M6G also can be seen in the case reported by Covington *et al.* (1989), in which severe respiratory depression was observed in a patient with end-stage renal disease receiving morphine patient-controlled analgesia for postcholecystectomy pain. The blood morphine concentration was 73 ng ml^{-1}, which is within the therapeutic range, but the M6G level was significantly elevated at 415 ng ml^{-1}. Similar data have been described by Carr and associates, in which the patient-controlled analgesia dose requirements after cadaveric renal transplantation were 3 to 4.7 mg h^{-1} compared with 4.6 to 23.6 mg h^{-1} in patients with normal renal function undergoing lower abdominal surgery (Carr *et al.*, 1998). As might be expected, the former group showed considerably greater AUC for M6G.

In a further study, D'Honneur and colleagues studied the transfer of morphine and its metabolites across the blood-brain barrier (D'Honneur *et al.*, 1994). Fourteen patients (6 with end-stage renal disease) received a single oral dose of morphine before the onset of continuous spinal anesthesia for peripheral vascular or orthopedic surgery. Plasma concen-

trations of morphine and both morphine glucuronides were greater in the renal failure patients; only the glucuronide concentrations (not the parent drug) were greater in the cerebrospinal fluid of the renal patients. This study did not address the key issue of whether the higher cerebrospinal fluid concentrations of M6G were associated with greater respiratory depression or sedation or prolonged analgesia, however.

The key question for the anesthesiologist providing analgesia during the perioperative period for surgery for renal transplantation is what the contribution is of the increased concentrations of M6G to the overall analgesia achieved with morphine. In patients with normal renal function, Portenoy and colleagues found that pain relief was greatest when the M6G/morphine molar ratio was greater than 0.7 with a significant correlation between the molar ratio and pain relief (Portenoy *et al.*, 1992).

There are data to suggest that increased concentrations of another morphine metabolite (normorphine) may be responsible for myoclonic activity, but this has not been confirmed by other researchers (Glare *et al.*, 1990). Similar alterations in the disposition of codeine, dihydrocodeine and propoxyphene (with active metabolite accumulation) have been observed in patients with renal failure (Barnes *et al.*, 1985; Gibson *et al.*, 1980; Guay *et al.*, 1988). Use of all of these drugs for postoperative pain relief is best avoided.

Whether the altered kinetics of morphine and its surrogates constitute the sole explanation for their prolonged dynamic effects is uncertain. Uremia is associated with central nervous system depression, and the increased sensitivity to central nervous system depressant drugs also may be due to increased receptor responsiveness or increased meningeal and/or cerebral permeability (Fishman, 1970; Lowenthal, 1974).

Fentanyl, Alfentanil and Sufentanil

Because of the exaggerated dynamic effects of morphine and its metabolite M6G, many anesthesiologists prefer to provide intraoperative analgesia with drugs of the phenylpiperidine type. Only a small fraction of each of the three main drugs (fentanyl, alfentanil and sufentanil) is excreted by the kidney unchanged.

The disposition of fentanyl in doses of 20 µg kg^{-1} intravenously was studied in awake patients with end-stage renal failure by Corall *et al.* (1980). They found an increased systemic clearance. Our data and those of other authors all show the wide interindividual variability in kinetic parameters in all subjects and no differences in the disposition of fentanyl in renal transplant patients compared with comparable patients undergoing lower abdominal surgery (Duthie, 1987; Koehntop and Rodman, 1997; Sear and Hand, 2000). Koehntop and Rodman (1997) found an inverse relationship between the degree of azotemia and fentanyl clearance, and two of their eight patients needed postoperative ventilation for prolonged respiratory depression after administration of fentanyl, 25 µg kg^{-1}. Bower (1982) showed no alteration in fentanyl binding in patients with uremia; we found no relationship between preoperative creatinine or urea and either the clearance or terminal elimination half-life when fentanyl, 5 to 10 µg kg^{-1}, was given as part of a balanced anesthetic technique for renal transplantation (Sear and Hand, 2000).

With alfentanil, there is an increased free drug fraction in patients with uremia, together with greater total drug clearance rates and volumes of distribution. There were no differences in the free drug volume of distribution or clearance, however. The metabolites of alfentanil are probably all inactive (Bower and Sear, 1989; Chauvin *et al.*, 1987a, 1987b).

Uremia has no effect on the plasma protein binding or disposition of sufentanil (Davis *et al.*, 1988; Fyman *et al.*, 1988; Sear, 1989). There are case reports of prolonged narcosis, however, after administration of sufentanil to patients with chronic renal failure, which probably is due to alterations in the dynamics of the opioid in the uremic patient (Fyman *et al.*, 1988; Wiggum *et al.*, 1985). Figure 13–3 summarizes data from our studies examining the perioperative disposition of morphine, the three phenylpiperidine drugs and buprenorphine and nalbuphine when given to provide analgesia during surgery for renal transplantation in patients receiving a balanced anesthetic technique with controlled ventilation to normocapnia.

Pethidine (Meperidine)

There are few kinetic data on the disposition of pethidine in patients with renal failure. The drug is metabolized mainly in the liver, with only 1 to 5% excreted unchanged in the urine. Chan and coworkers showed that the systemic clearance of pethidine depends on renal function, with accompanying reduced excretion of the metabolite norpethidine (Chan *et al.*, 1987). The dynamics of pethidine in patients with end-stage renal disease have been assessed by Burgess *et al.* (1994). They found that the renal failure group had a reduced ventilatory response to carbon dioxide, but administration of 1 mg kg^{-1} of pethidine subcutaneously did not

exaggerate the effect. Whether this observation is transferable from the laboratory to the clinical scenario is untested.

Similar to the effects with morphine, Szeto and colleagues found that when repeated doses of pethidine are given to patients in chronic renal failure, there is accumulation of the *N*-demethylated metabolite norpethidine (Szeto *et al.*, 1977). This compound has less analgesic but greater convulsant activity than the parent drug. Szeto *et al.* (1977) and Armstrong and Bersten (1986) reported patients in renal failure in which increased plasma ratios of norpethidine/pethidine were associated with excitatory signs. On these grounds, pethidine is best avoided as an analgesic drug in the patient undergoing renal transplantation.

Remifentanil

Although remifentanil is a piperidine derivative, its elimination does not depend on hepatic metabolism or renal elimination, but rather elimination occurs by plasma and tissue nonspecific esterase hydrolysis. The clearance of remifentanil is high (25–45 ml kg^{-1} min^{-1}), and its major metabolite has only minimal analgesic activity. The kinetics of remifentanil are unaltered in patients with end-stage renal disease (Hoke *et al.*, 1997). Because of its short half-life (4–9 minutes), the drug is best given by continuous infusion; it also has a short context-sensitive half-time (3 minutes) after prolonged periods of infusion—implying that a rapid offset of its analgesic and respiratory depressant effects would occur at the end of a surgical procedure. The main metabolite (GI 90291)

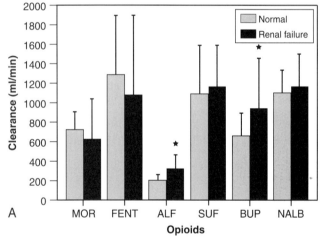

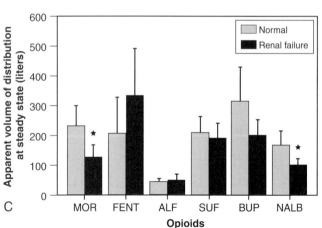

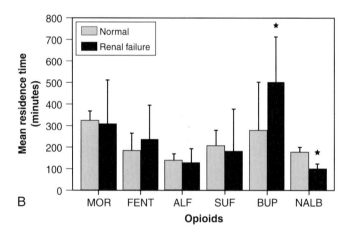

FIGURE 13–3

Perioperative disposition kinetics of six opioids used to provide analgesia as supplement to nitrous oxide–volatile anesthesia in renal failure patients undergoing kidney transplantation and age-matched anesthetized normal controls. Data shown for clearance (A), mean residence time (B) and apparent volume of distribution at steady state (C) (mean ± standard deviation; *P<0.05). AFL, alfentanil; MOR, morphine; SUF, sufentanil; BUP, buprenorphine; FENT, fentanil; NALB, nalbuphine. (Data from Bower and Sear, 1989 [alfentanil]; Sear *et al.*, 1989 [morphine]; Sear, 1989 [sufentanil]; Hand *et al.*, 1990 [buprenorphine]; Sear and Hand, 2000 [fentanil] and unpublished data for nalbuphine.)

has a longer terminal half-life and reduced clearance in patients with renal failure, but remifentanil's dynamics are unaffected, with no increased respiratory sensitivity. No reports have been published to date of the drug's use as a supplement to balanced anesthesia for renal transplantation.

Other Intraoperative Opioids

Two other drugs used to provide intraoperative analgesia for patients undergoing renal transplantation are buprenorphine and oxycodone. Buprenorphine is a partial opioid agonist about 30 times more potent than morphine. It is metabolized by dealkylation and glucuronidation to produce active (norbuprenorphine—40 times less potent than the parent drug) and inactive metabolites.

Hand and associates compared the disposition of buprenorphine after bolus dosing and continuous infusion in patients with impaired and normal renal function (Hand *et al.*, 1990). The renal group showed a nonsignificant prolongation of the terminal half-life; when given by continuous infusion, renal impairment was associated with increases in plasma concentrations of buprenorphine-3-glucuronide and norbuprenorphine—although the latter were thought unlikely to result in any prolongation of the drug's action.

When oxycodone disposition was compared in healthy anesthetized patients and patients undergoing cadaveric transplantation, Kirvela and associates found a prolonged elimination half-life resulting from a reduction in clearance and an increase in the volume of drug distribution (Kirvela *et al.*, 1996). There also were higher plasma concentrations of the metabolite noroxycodone. Kirvela and associates do not comment on any dynamic consequences of their findings, however. The drugs of choice for intraoperative analgesia in patients undergoing renal transplantation are presently fentanyl, alfentanil and sufentanil.

NEUROMUSCULAR RELAXANT DRUGS

The neuromuscular relaxant drugs are a group of ionized, water-soluble compounds that are filtered freely at the glomerulus. Most relaxants have low (<50%) plasma protein binding, and changes in plasma albumin concentrations (which may occur in patients with end-stage renal disease) are unlikely to affect the drugs' disposition. If the drug normally is excreted unchanged by the kidney, however, the kinetics and dynamics are altered in the patient with renal failure. Table 13–3 lists the extent of urinary excretion in the elimination of the various muscle relaxants.

Depolarizing Neuromuscular Relaxants

One of the main problems with neuromuscular blocking agents relates to the use of suxamethonium in chronic renal failure. Wyant (1967) reported a decrease in the activity of the enzyme pseudocholinesterase (and a decreased rate of degradation of suxamethonium) in patients being treated for renal failure by hemodialysis. This decrease does not seem to be a significant problem with current hemodialysis techniques, however. Prolongation of the action of suxamethonium is seen in some patients with chronic renal failure, but the exact incidence is unknown.

A second problem is suxamethonium-induced increases in serum potassium concentrations. Way *et al.* (1972) showed the increase in potassium in patients on hemodialysis to be comparable with that seen in normal healthy individuals, whereas Koide and Waud (1972) observed no difficulties with the use of the drug as long as the plasma potassium was less than 5.5 mmol L^{-1}. Pretreatment with nondepolarizing

TABLE 13–3

RENAL EXCRETION OF NEUROMUSCULAR BLOCKING DRUGS

Quaternary amines	
Suxamethonium	<10%
Gallamine	>95%
Benzylisoquinolinium compounds	
Tubocurarine	31–45%
Methyltubocurarine	42–52%
Atracurium	10%
Doxacurium	25–30%
Mivacurium	<10%
Cisatracurium	?
Aminosteroid compounds	
Pancuronium	35–50%
Vecuronium	15–20%
Pipercuronium	38%
Rocuronium	9%
Rapacuronium	30%

Note. Expressed as a mean percentage (or range) of total drug elimination.

neuromuscular blocking drugs prevents the onset of muscle fasciculations but not the increase in plasma potassium concentrations. For a rapid-sequence intubation in renal transplant recipients, suxamethonium remains the drug of choice, although large doses of some nondepolarizing drugs (especially atracurium, cisatracurium, mivacurium and rocuronium) offer an alternative in the patients with hyperkalemia.

Nondepolarizing or Competitive Neuromuscular Relaxants

Nondepolarizing or competitive neuromuscular relaxants can be divided broadly into agents showing significant alteration in the kinetics and duration of effect in the end-stage renal disease patient (and not useful in the anesthetic management of transplant recipients) and agents in which renal failure has little effect on drug dynamics.

Drugs Showing Significant Alterations in their Dynamics in Renal Disease

Tubocurarine. In healthy patients, about 70% of an intravenous dose of tubocurarine is recoverable from the urine. In renal failure, however, a compensatory increase occurs in the extent of biliary excretion. Prolonged paralysis in patients with chronic renal failure normally is seen only after administration of large or frequent doses of the relaxant (Gibaldi *et al.*, 1972). The duration of response to the drug primarily is determined by redistribution, with a terminal half-life in healthy patients of approximately 80 minutes (Table 13–4). Studies by Miller and coworkers have shown a decreased plasma clearance and a slower decline in the offset of paralysis in patients with renal failure (Miller *et al.*, 1977).

Dimethyltubocurarine. A significant decrease in the systemic clearance of dimethyltubocurarine in patients with chronic renal failure has been reported by Brotherton and Matteo (1981); this agent is best avoided in patients with renal failure.

Gallamine. Mushin *et al.* (1949) and Feldman *et al.* (1969) showed that 85 to 100% of gallamine was excreted by the kidney in humans; there are case reports of inadequate reversal or prolonged paralysis after its use in patients with renal insufficiency (Feldman and Levi, 1963; Lowenstein *et al.*, 1970). In a formal kinetic study, Ramzan and colleagues showed considerable prolongation of the elimination half-

TABLE 13–4

DISPOSITION OF NEUROMUSCULAR BLOCKING DRUGS IN PATIENTS WITH CHRONIC RENAL FAILURE

	Patients with Normal Renal Function			Patients with Impaired Renal Function		
	$T_{1/2}el$	Cl_p	V_{ss}	$T_{1/2}el$	Cl_p	V_{ss}
TUBOC 1	84	2.4	0.25	132*	1.5*	0.25
MTC 2	360	1.2	0.47	684*	0.4*	0.35
PANC 3	104	1.1	0.15	489*	0.3*	0.24
4	133	1.8	0.34	257	0.6*	0.33
ATRAC 5	21	6.1	0.19	24	6.7	0.26
6	17	5.9	0.14	21	6.9	0.21
VEC 7	53	5.3	0.2	83*	3.2*	0.24

Note. Mean values are given.

*$P<0.05$.

$T_{1/2}el$, elimination half-life (min); Cl_p; systemic clearance (ml kg^{-1} min^{-1}); V_{ss}, apparent volume of distribution at steady-state (L kg^{-1}); TUBOC, tubocurarine; MTC, methyltubocurarine; PANC, pancuronium; ATRAC, atracurium; VEC, vecuronium.

Sources of data: 1, Sheiner *et al.*, 1979; 2, Brotherton and Matteo, 1981; 3, McLeod *et al.*, 1976; 4, Somogyi *et al.*, 1977; 5, Fahey *et al.*, 1984; 6, De Bros *et al.*, 1986; 7, Lynam *et al.*, 1988.

life and reduction in clearance in patients with renal failure (Ramzan *et al.*, 1981).

Pancuronium. In healthy patients, about 40% of an intravenous dose of pancuronium is excreted in the urine, and another 10% is excreted in the bile. Augmentation of biliary excretion occurs in renal failure, but there still is a decrease in systemic clearance of pancuronium (Buzello and Agoston, 1978; McLeod *et al.*, 1976; Somogyi *et al.*, 1977) coupled with prolonged neuromuscular blockade (Geha *et al.*, 1976).

With other relaxants now widely available, there is no place for any of the aforementioned drugs as part of the anesthetic technique for renal transplantation.

Drugs Most Suited for Use in Patients Undergoing Renal Transplantation

Atracurium. Initial clinical studies by Hunter and colleagues showed no difference in the duration of neuromuscular blockade from an initial dose of atracurium or from repeated doses when the drug was administered to patients with normal function compared with patients who were anephric (Hunter *et al.*, 1982). This finding was confirmed by the dynamic-kinetic studies of Fahey *et al.* (1984) and De Bros *et al.* (1986), who showed that onset time, duration of action, recovery time (25–75% initial twitch height), and disposition kinetics were unaltered in patients with renal failure. A further study by Hunter and colleagues compared the properties of atracurium, vecuronium and tubocurarine in healthy subjects and patients with renal failure (Hunter *et al.*, 1984). After bolus dosing, atracurium and vecuronium were little affected by renal failure, but tubocurarine was longer acting, less predictable and not appropriate for use.

Atracurium may be administered by bolus dosing or continuous infusion to maintain neuromuscular blockade. After prolonged infusion, rapid recovery has been reported in the patient with renal failure (Russo *et al.*, 1986). Our studies confirm these findings, but we found considerable variability in recovery time (25–75% initial twitch height) in healthy subjects and in patients undergoing renal transplantation when infused during nitrous oxide in oxygen-narcotic anesthesia (Fig. 13–4). Nguyen and coworkers showed a pro-

longed recovery rate and longer time to 90% recovery of twitch height when administering atracurium by infusion to anephric patients anesthetized with nitrous oxide and increments of fentanyl (Nguyen *et al.*, 1985).

The degradation of atracurium is by Hofmann degradation and ester hydrolysis, although Fisher and colleagues showed that 50% of total systemic clearance cannot be accounted for by either of these mechanisms (Fisher *et al.*, 1985). An important metabolite of atracurium is laudanosine, which is eliminated in the urine and has been reported in animals to cause excitatory electroencephalogram (EEG) activity when administered in high doses. When given to nephrectomized cats, EEG changes of nonepileptiform spike activity were seen only at plasma concentrations 8 to 10 times those observed in patients during continuous infusions of atracurium (Ingram *et al.*, 1986). Ward and colleagues investigated the relationship between renal function and plasma concentrations of laudanosine (Ward *et al.*, 1987). After single doses of atracurium (0.3 mg kg^{-1}), there were no effects of renal failure on the disposition of atracurium or its two metabolites, laudanosine and the associated monoquaternary alcohol. Peak laudanosine concentrations were not significantly different in healthy subjects and patients with renal failure. Other studies by Fahey and coworkers have observed higher plasma laudanosine concentrations in cadaveric transplant recipients compared with healthy anesthetized subjects after larger doses of atracurium (Fahey *et al.*, 1985). In both of these articles and in the study by LePage *et al.* (1991), peak plasma laudanosine concentrations were considerably lower than those associated with EEG excitation in the anesthetized dog (Chapple *et al.*, 1987). Although elimination of laudanosine is by the kidney, and in the patient with a nonfunctioning allograft a prolongation of elimination half-life might be expected, some evidence exists *in humans* that other organs (such as the liver) may be involved in its elimination.

Vecuronium. The kinetics of 0.1 mg kg^{-1} of vecuronium in patients receiving cadaveric renal allografts and a control group of healthy subjects have been studied by Lynam *et al.* (1988). Anesthesia was maintained with nitrous oxide in oxygen and 1% end-tidal isoflurane. The duration of neuromuscular blockade and recovery from blockade were significantly

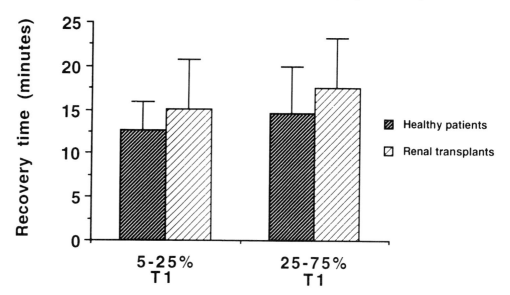

FIGURE 13–4

Times to recovery of normal neuromuscular transmission after infusions of atracurium to 10 patients undergoing renal transplantation and 9 healthy subjects. Anesthesia was provided by thiopentone, fentanyl and nitrous oxide. 5–25% T1, time for recovery of the first twitch of the *train-of-four* from 5 to 25% of initial twitch height; 25–75% T1, time for recovery from 25 to 75% of initial twitch height. Data shown are mean standard deviations.

prolonged in the renal failure group. No significant kinetic differences (i.e., clearance, elimination half-life) were seen. Many studies have produced data suggesting the accumulation of vecuronium in patients with renal failure, however (Bevan *et al.*, 1984; Cody and Dormon, 1987; LePage *et al.*, 1987; Starsnic *et al.*, 1989).

Because of the clinical importance of any dynamic interaction with renal failure, Beauvoir *et al.* (1993) conducted a metaanalysis of the available data. Based on six studies, they found renal failure to cause a significant increase in the duration of effect (measured as the time from injection to 25% recovery of twitch height) but no effect on the onset time or the 25 to 75% recovery time. Some of the explanation for these dynamic effects may lie in the biotransformation of vecuronium. It is metabolized by hepatic hydrolysis to yield three desacetyl metabolites—3 desacetyl, 17 desacetyl and 3.17 desacetyl ver*uronium*. The first of these is estimated to have the potency of about 80% of the parent drug, and there is good evidence that the 3 des metabolite accumulates in patients with renal failure (Segredo *et al.*, 1992).

Caution should be exercised to ensure complete return of neuromuscular function if multiple increments or infusions of the drug are used during prolonged surgery in anephric patients. Potentiation of neuromuscular blockade also may occur in patients with metabolic acidosis; the acidosis also opposes the reversal by neostigmine. In the uremic patient undergoing transplant surgery, potentiation of blockade may occur because of hypokalemia; hypocalcemia; hypermagnesemia or parenteral or topical use of some aminoglycoside antibiotics, such as gentamicin, furosemide, mannitol and methylprednisolone.

Newer Neuromuscular Blocking Drugs. Six new neuromuscular blocking agents show differing disposition profiles in renal failure (Table 13–5).

Pipecuronium. Pipecuronium is a bisquaternary aminosteroid, which is mainly eliminated unchanged by the kidney. Renal failure causes a prolonged elimination half-life and reduced clearance (Caldwell *et al.*, 1989).

Doxacurium. Doxacurium is a long-acting drug with an elimination half-life of 99 minutes and clearance of 2.7 ml kg^{-1} min^{-1}. It is mainly excreted unchanged by the kidney, although esterase hydrolysis may contribute, in part, to the termination of drug effect. Clearance is reduced in patients with renal failure, with accompanying prolongation of effect (Cashman *et al.*, 1992; Cook *et al.*, 1991).

Neither pipecuronium nor doxacurium should be used for neuromuscular blockade in the renal transplant recipient. The other four agents may be useful adjuncts to the anesthesiologist, however.

Mivacurium. Mivacurium is a short-acting benzyl-isoquinolinium compound that is metabolized by plasma esterases and presumably in the liver. In healthy subjects, de Bros and colleagues showed an elimination half-life of 17 minutes and a high clearance (54 ml kg^{-1} min^{-1}) (De Bros *et al.*, 1987). These kinetics and duration of effect are not prolonged in renal failure (Cook *et al.*, 1992).

Similar to atracurium, mivacurium has many stereoisomers (cis-trans, 37%; trans-trans, 57% and the less active cis-cis, 6%). Head-Rapson and colleagues examined the kinetics and dynamics of these three isomers in anesthetized patients with renal failure (Head-Rapson *et al.*, 1995). Although clearance of the cis-cis isomer was reduced significantly in renal failure, the disposition of the other two isomers was not. The clearance of each isomer correlated significantly with plasma cholinesterase activity. The median infusion rate required to achieve a common level of neuromuscular blockade (T1/T0, 10%) was similar in patients with renal failure compared with healthy subjects. Phillips and Hunter (1992) showed a prolonged duration of action in renal failure patients when compared with subjects with normal renal function—probably as a result of lowered plasma cholinesterase activity.

Cisatracurium. Cisatracurium is one of the 10 stereoisomers of atracurium and has the advantage of being three times more potent and releasing less histamine in animals. In contrast to the parent compound, its metabolism is mainly by Hofmann degradation with no ester hydrolysis. Studies by Kisor and associates confirm that the Hofmann pathway accounts for about 77% of total body clearance; organ clearance, 23% and renal clearance, 16% (Kisor *et al.*, 1996). The drug has an elimination half-life of 23 minutes and clearance in healthy subjects of about 5.2 ml kg^{-1} min^{-1}. The main metabolites are laudanosine and a monoquaternary acrylate.

Two studies have examined the dynamics and disposition of cisatracurium in renal failure. Boyd and colleagues found that at a dose of 2 × ED$_{95}$ (0.1 mg kg^{-1}), onset times were longer in the renal failure group, but recovery was not affected (Boyd *et al.*, 1995). In these patients, the clearance of cisatracurium was decreased by 13%, and the half-life was longer (34.2 minutes *vs.* 30 minutes). Although plasma con-

TABLE 13–5

DISPOSITION OF NEWER NEUROMUSCULAR BLOCKING DRUGS IN PATIENTS WITH CHRONIC RENAL FAILURE

	Patients with Normal Renal Function			Patients with Impaired Renal Function		
	$T_{1/2}el$	Cl_p	V_{ss}	$T_{1/2}el$	Cl_p	V_{ss}
CISATRAC						
1	30	4.2	—	34	3.8	—
MIVAC						
2						
cis-cis	68	3.8	0.23	80	2.4*	0.24
cis-trans	2.0	106	0.28	4.3	80	0.48
trans-trans	2.3	57	0.21	4.2	47	0.27
ROCUR						
3	71	2.9	0.26	97	2.9	0.21
4	104	3.7	0.21	97	2.5*	0.21
RAPACUR						
5	175	9.4	0.41	174	6.4	0.34
PIPERC						
6	137	2.4	0.31	263*	1.6*	0.44
DOXAC						
7	99	2.7	0.22	221*	1.2*	0.27

Note. Mean values are given.

*$P<0.05$.

$T_{1/2}el$, elimination half-life (min); Cl_p, systemic clearance (ml kg^{-1} min^{-1}); V_{ss}, apparent volume of distribution at steady-state (L kg^{-1}); CISATRAC, cisatracurium; MIVAC, mivacurium; ROCUR, rocuronium; RAPACUR, rapacuronium; PIPERC, pipercuronium; DOXAC, doxacurium.

Sources of data: 1, Eastwood et al., 1995; 2, Head-Rapson et al., 1995; 3, Szenohradszky et al., 1992; 4, Cooper et al., 1993; 5, Szenohradszky et al., 1999; 6, Caldwell et al., 1989; 7, Cook et al., 1991.

centrations of laudanosine were elevated in patients with renal failure, the values were about $\frac{1}{10}$ of those seen after atracurium (Eastwood et al., 1995). It also has been shown that cisatracurium causes no histamine release in humans at doses of eight times the ED_{95} dose—making the drug suitable for providing muscle relaxation in the atopic patient.

Rocuronium (ORG 9426). Rocuronium has a rapid onset of effect and intermediate duration of action and may be an alternative to suxamethonium for rapid-sequence intubation. Being a steroid molecule, it is metabolized primarily in the liver, with only 9% of the injected dose being recovered unchanged in the urine. In a comparison of its kinetics and dynamics in healthy anesthetized subjects and patients undergoing cadaveric renal transplantation, Szenohradszky and colleagues found renal failure to alter drug distribution but not systemic clearance (Szenohradszky et al., 1992). In a separate study, Cooper and associates found a decreased clearance of the relaxant in patients with renal failure during isoflurane anesthesia (Cooper et al., 1993).

Two studies have examined the dynamics of rocuronium in patients with chronic renal failure. Khuenl-Brady and colleagues found no differences in onset, duration of effect or recovery after doses of 0.6 mg kg^{-1} and three maintenance doses of 0.15 mg kg^{-1} (Khuenl-Brady et al., 1993). There were no significant differences in drug dynamics in the study by Cooper et al. (1993). Despite the chemical similarities of rocuronium to vecuronium, the former has a useful role in providing neuromuscular blockade to renally impaired patients without the problem of metabolite accumulation.

Rapacuronium (ORG 9487). Rapacuronium is another steroidal neuromuscular blocking agent presently undergoing clinical evaluation. It has two important properties—rapid onset of effect and short duration of action. It might be an appropriate drug to use when suxamethonium is contraindicated (i.e., in the presence of hyperkalemia). In doses of 1.5 to 2.5 mg kg^{-1}, complete blockade of the adductor pollicis muscle occurs in 60 to 90 seconds, with recovery to 25% of the first twitch of a *train-of-four* at 13 to 25 minutes. After prolonged administration (>60 minutes), there is likely to be a decreased recovery rate—probably as a result of the accumulation of an active metabolite, ORG 9488 (Schiere et al., 1999).

Szenohradszky and colleagues evaluated the kinetics and dynamics of rapacuronium in patients with renal dysfunction (Szenohradszky et al., 1999). They found small decreases in clearance and apparent volume of distribution in renal failure patients, but the dynamics of a single dose of 1.5 mg kg^{-1} were unaffected. Clearance of the metabolite was decreased by 85%, however, indicating that there is likely to be a longer duration of effect if repeated drug dosing is used in patients with renal failure.

Of the newer neuromuscular blocking drugs, cisatracurium and rocuronium offer suitable alternatives to atracurium in patients undergoing renal transplantation.

ANTICHOLINERGIC ESTERASES

All anticholinergic esterases are excreted through the kidney by glomerular filtration and tubular secretion. The pharmacokinetics of neostigmine, pyridostigmine and edrophonium were studied in patients with chronic renal failure by Cronnelly and Morris (1982). Significant decreases in the clearance of anticholinergic esterases are seen in the anephric patient, although pharmacokinetics parameters similar to those in patients with normal renal function can be shown in patients to whom the drugs are given approximately 1 hour after receiving a living related renal transplant (Table 13–6). The reduction in the plasma clearance of anticholinergic esterases in anephric patients exceeds that reported for relaxants such as pancuronium and tubocurarine, and residual neuromuscular blockade or recurarization in anephric patients is unlikely to be due to the muscle relaxant outlasting the antagonist. Because 75% of an intravenous dose undergoes renal elimination, the terminal half-life of pyridostigmine is more prolonged than that of neostigmine in patients with renal failure.

TABLE 13–6

INFLUENCE OF RENAL DISEASE ON THE DISPOSITION OF THE ANTICHOLINESTERASES

	Subjects with Normal Renal Function			Anephric Patients			Living Related Donor Renal Transplants			Renal Fraction of Total Clearance
	$T_{1/2}el$	Cl_p	V_{ss}	$T_{1/2}el$	Cl_p	V_{ss}	$T_{1/2}el$	Cl_p	V_{ss}	(%)
Neostigmine	80	9.0	0.7	183*	3.4*	0.8	104	9.4	1.0	54
Pyridostigmine	112	8.6	1.1	379*	2.1*	1.0	83	10.8	1.0	76
Edrophonium	110	9.6	1.1	206*	2.7*	0.7	87	9.9	0.9	66

*$P<0.05$ versus transplant patients and subjects with normal renal function.
$T_{1/2}el$, elimination half-life (min); Cl_p, systemic clearance (ml kg^{-1} min^{-1}); V_{ss}, apparent volume of distribution at steady-state (L kg^{-1}).
Adapted with permission from Cronnelly and Morris, 1982.

INHALATIONAL ANESTHETIC AGENTS

All volatile anesthetic agents are, to some extent, myocardial depressants and may reduce the cardiac output and blood flow to the transplanted kidney. Some agents (methoxyflurane, enflurane and sevoflurane) are biotransformed to a significant degree, leading to increased serum levels of inorganic fluoride. This biotransformation can lead to the development of high-output renal failure, and such agents would be inappropriate for anesthesia for renal transplantation.

Early studies with methoxyflurane established the nephrotoxic threshold in humans as a serum fluoride concentration of greater than 50 μmol L^{-1} (Cousins et al., 1974). In healthy patients, enflurane anesthesia does not produce renal damage, and inorganic fluoride concentrations in excess of 50 μmol L^{-1} are not likely to be achieved. After 2.4 hours of enflurane, Mazze et al. (1984) reported peak fluoride levels of about 19 μmol L^{-1}; this compares with increases of 3.5 μmol L^{-1} after 6 MAC-hours (MAC-hour = product of minimum alveolar concentration of a volatile anesthetic agent and time) of isoflurane and 1.2 μmol L^{-1} after 171 minutes of halothane anesthesia (Mazze et al., 1974, 1984).

When enflurane is used to provide anesthesia for patients undergoing living related donor renal transplantation, Wickstrom (1981) observed that administration of 2.4 MAC-hours of enflurane (mean duration, 189 minutes) caused a peak fluoride concentration of 21 μmol L^{-1}. In 1 of the 10 patients in this study, the serum fluoride concentration rose significantly to 40 μmol L^{-1}, which presents a risk of nephrotoxicity. There has been a case report of a deterioration in renal transplant function when enflurane was given to provide anesthesia for vascular access surgery (Loehning and Mazze, 1974). Enflurane should not be used as the sole anesthetic for renal transplantation.

Comparison of halothane, enflurane and isoflurane as volatile supplementation in patients undergoing living related donor renal transplantation has shown no influence of anesthesia on postoperative renal function (Cronnelly et al., 1984). When used to supplement nitrous oxide anesthesia, halothane, enflurane and isoflurane all cause a dose-related decrease in mean arterial pressure. Administration of a fluid challenge of 1,000 ml 0.154M sodium chloride results in similar increases of arterial pressure and CVP, regardless of the choice of anesthetic agent (Cronnelly et al., 1983a, 1983b).

The two newer volatile agents (desflurane and sevoflurane) differ in their molecular stability and biotransformation. Desflurane does not undergo breakdown by the liver or by contact with soda lime, and after 1 MAC-hour of anesthesia, the increase in inorganic fluoride is less than 1 μmol L^{-1}. Desflurane also has no deleterious effect on routine laboratory tests of renal function when given to patients with chronic renal disease (Zaleski et al., 1993).

In contrast, sevoflurane is less stable, with about 3% of the absorbed dose undergoing hepatic biotransformation. After prolonged anesthesia of an average of 13.4 hours to patients with normal renal function, peak serum fluoride concentrations of 42.5 μmol L^{-1} have been reported—with 5 of the 10 patients exceeding the nephrotoxic threshold of 50 μmol L^{-1} (Kobayashi et al., 1992). There were no cases of gross renal dysfunction, however. Similarly, Higuchi and colleagues found no evidence of any impairment in urinary concentrating ability to antidiuretic hormone administration after 10.6 MAC-hours of sevoflurane anesthesia despite a mean plasma fluoride concentration of 41.9 μmol L^{-1} and 1 of the 11 patients having a plasma fluoride concentration greater than 50 μmol L^{-1} (Higuchi et al., 1994).

When administered to patients with end-stage renal disease, sevoflurane (1–2.5%) supplementing nitrous oxide–oxygen anesthesia caused higher postoperative levels of blood urea, creatinine and serum and urinary β_2-microglobulins (Nishiyama et al., 1996). There were no differences, however, between these patients and controls in serum fluoride levels, the rate of elimination or AUC fluoride time. The renal failure patients had lower urinary fluoride concentrations than the healthy controls. In the only in vitro study examining the effects of fluorinated volatile anesthetics on proximal tubular function, Lochhead and colleagues found that all of the volatile agents potentially shared the tubulotoxic effects of methoxyflurane at clinically revelant concentrations (Lochhead et al., 1997). There also is controversy over the interaction between sevoflurane and carbon dioxide absorbents in closed or semiclosed breathing systems leading to the production of a vinyl derivative known as compound A. Although nephrotoxic in rats, there is no evidence to support this in humans.

Although some transplant units avoid its use, no absolute contraindication to nitrous oxide during transplant anesthesia exists; however, its use may result in increased bowel size because of gas diffusion. This increased bowel size may be relevant in young children undergoing transplantation, in whom intraabdominal space is limited for the placement of an adult-sized kidney. Patients with impaired renal function may develop cardiac arrhythmias secondary to alterations in plasma electrolyte concentrations. There is the additional risk of acute hemodynamic changes occurring during transplantation because of the release of catecholamines and renin from the revascularized kidney (Freilich et al., 1984). Halothane and to a lesser extent enflurane sensitize the myocardium to the effects of endogenous catecholamines with the resulting development of ventricular arrhythmias. These effects are not seen in patients receiving isoflurane, and this agent and desflurane presently are the volatile agents of choice as the supplement to nitrous oxide in oxygen anesthesia for renal transplantation.

Stimulus to Early Allograft Function

Loop diuretics and/or mannitol may be used to promote a diuresis from the grafted kidney. Use of mannitol (the reduced form of the 6-carbon sugar mannose) has been criticized (Salaman et al., 1969), but there is evidence to suggest that it may have a protective role as a free radical scavenger, preventing free radical–induced reperfusion injury. Mannitol reduces the incidence of impaired renal function immediately after transplantation from 55 to 14% (Weimar et al., 1983). It also has been shown to improve renal blood flow by a greater percentage than can be accounted for by plasma volume expansion alone (Johnston et al., 1979). It is a small molecule that equilibrates slowly with the extravascular and extracellular fluids and so causes an increased circulating blood volume. Mannitol is freely filtered by the renal glomerulus and not reabsorbed in the distal kidney tubules. Because of its osmotic effect, sodium and water also are excreted; this may lead to increases in the serum potassium by 0.7 mmol L^{-1}. Failure of adequate perfusion of the kidney and failure of glomerular excretion may lead to the development of intracellular dehydration.

Moote and Manninen (1987) examined the influence of mannitol on serum electrolytes in patients undergoing renal transplantation. A dose of 50 g of mannitol (four times the dose used in Oxford) increased the CVP and reduced serum concentrations of sodium, chloride and bicarbonate. The rise in potassium was small, but this may assume clinical importance in patients also receiving a blood transfusion. The thiazide diuretics and furosemide are not open to the same criticism, although their use should be coupled with preloading of the patient with isotonic (0.154M) saline. There is some evidence that furosemide has a direct protective effect against renal failure secondary to acute ischemia.

Besides use of mannitol and diuretics to establish a diuresis, it is important to maintain an adequate circulating volume. Dawidson and coworkers found that urine output is delayed after reperfusion in patients in whom the blood volume was less than 70 ml kg^{-1} (Dawidson et al., 1987). Rehydration requirements can be estimated from the CVP, using normal saline as the initial volume expander. If more than 40 to 90 ml kg^{-1} is required, colloid solutions should be added. The administration of this fluid load also acts as a physiological stimulus to urine production. This stimulus is important because most analgesic and inhalational anesthetic agents increase circulating antidiuretic hormone levels and decrease the glomerular filtration rate (Bastron and Deutsch, 1976).

When taken to the extreme, the use of loading with large volumes of fluid may lead to important adverse side effects. Carlier and colleagues examined the concept of *maximal hydration therapy* (infusing 100 ml kg^{-1} physiological saline during anesthesia) and its effect on early graft function (Carlier et al., 1982, 1986). Although the results are encouraging, fluid loads of this magnitude may precipitate pulmonary edema in patients with poor myocardial function or poor respiratory reserve. If this approach is used, it is mandatory to insert a pulmonary artery catheter before anesthesia and surgery.

Anesthesia for Renal Transplantation
RECOMMENDED PRACTICE

The following practices have been used in Oxford since the 1980s and are based on the physiological and pharmaco-

logical principles outlined previously. We use the same strategy for patients receiving either a cadaveric or a living related graft (the latter being about 10–20% of all grafts in the United Kingdom but 30–40% in the United States and Norway).

Premedication is important because many patients are anxious at the time of transplantation; suitable attenuation of this anxiety may be achieved with one of the orally administered benzodiazepines (usually temazepam, 10–20 mg). Intramuscular premedication is avoided because of the tendency of the uremic patient to have bleeding disorders. Vagolytic drugs (e.g., atropine) are given intravenously at time of induction of anesthesia if clinically indicated, for example, when suxamethonium is used to facilitate intubation or when the combination of an opioid and one of the hemodynamically neutral muscle relaxants is administered. The avoidance of pronounced bradycardias is particularly important in patients receiving long-term β-adrenoceptor blockade for the treatment of ischemic heart disease and hypertension. β-adrenoceptor blocking drugs, calcium channel inhibitors and other antihypertensive or antianginal therapy are continued up to the morning of surgery.

The routine prophylactic administration of antacids may be advocated for patients with symptoms of peptic ulceration; a single dose of sodium citrate (30 ml) in the anesthetic room is appropriate. Histamine H_2-receptor antagonists (such as rantidine, 150 mg orally) are given with the premedication to reduce gastric hyperacidity. Phenothiazine antiemetics or metoclopramide should be administered with care because they may cause prolonged sedation and extrapyramidal side effects in patients with renal failure (see earlier).

Anesthesia is best induced with a sleep dose of thiopentone coupled with a loading dose of fentanyl, 3 to 6 μg kg^{-1}. For patients with poor cardiac reserve, etomidate (0.3 mg kg^{-1}) may be preferred. Using the combination of a hypnotic and an opioid, the anesthesiologist can minimize the hemodynamic response to induction of anesthesia, laryngoscopy and intubation as well as to surgical incision. Neuromuscular blockade is provided by atracurium or cisatracurium in doses of 0.6 mg kg^{-1} or 0.15 to 0.4 mg kg^{-1}. To maintain neuromuscular blockade, increments of either drug are given when indicated clinically, with neuromuscular transmission monitored using a peripheral nerve stimulator. An alternative technique involves continuous infusion of either relaxant (atracurium, 6–8 μg kg^{-1} min^{-1} or cisatracurium, 1–2 μg kg^{-1} min^{-1}). For the patient in whom there is the added problem of a difficult airway or an inadequate period of starvation before surgery, suxamethonium (1.0–1.5 mg kg^{-1}) should be used to aid intubation.

Maintenance of anesthesia is achieved with isoflurane to supplement nitrous oxide; this has the advantage of nonrenal elimination and may be given with high inspired oxygen concentrations in the severely anemic patient. The arterial blood carbon dioxide tension should be kept at normocapnia or mild hypocapnia and monitored by end-tidal carbon dioxide sampling. Short periods of hypoventilation can lead to hemoglobin desaturation, whereas excess hyperventilation with low arterial carbon dioxide tension causes a shift of the oxyhemoglobin dissociation curve to the left. Intraoperative analgesia can be provided by morphine, 10 to 15 mg intravenously.

At the end of surgery, anesthesia is discontinued, and residual muscular paralysis is reversed with atropine or glycopyrrolate and neostigmine. Glycopyrrolate is preferred in patients with associated hypertensive or ischemic heart disease to avoid excessive tachycardias. An important interaction for the anesthesiologist to be aware of is that between cyclosporine and muscle relaxants. Sidi and associates found a greater incidence of postoperative respiratory failure in transplant patients receiving cyclosporine as the immunosuppressant drug (Sidi *et al.*, 1990). Once extubated, all transplant patients receive oxygen for 12 to 24 hours postoperatively.

Other approaches presently used for renal transplant anesthesia include total intravenous techniques, such as the combination of propofol and alfentanil (Kirvela *et al.*, 1994b), or neuroleptanesthesia (Lindahl-Nilsson *et al.*, 1980). The latter has no significant effect on peripheral hemodynamics and reduces solute, sodium and water clearance less than is seen with volatile anesthetic agents.

MONITORING DURING ANESTHESIA

The high incidence of ischemic and hypertensive heart disease in transplant patients makes it essential to monitor the ECG and blood pressure continuously during induction of anesthesia and the perioperative and immediate postoperative period. Blood pressure should be measured with the DINAMAP or similar automatic blood pressure apparatus placed on the nonfistula arm. Because of improvements in the preoperative preparation of kidney transplant recipients and because excessive blood loss is the exception rather than the rule, arterial cannulation is only rarely needed for the perioperative monitoring of blood pressure. The aim should be to maintain the systolic blood pressure greater than 110 mm Hg.

Measurement of the CVP is as important as measurement of blood pressure in patients undergoing renal transplantation. We use a triple-lumen catheter inserted into the internal jugular or subclavian vein. Intraoperative fluids are given generally as physiological saline and colloid, and blood generally is given only in the presence of excess blood loss, with the aim of increasing the CVP by 7 to 10 cm H_2O by the time of revascularization. In practice, we aim for a CVP of 15 to 20 cm H_2O in patients with good left ventricular function and 12 cm H_2O in patients whose function is impaired or elderly patients (>55–60 years of age). Sodium lactate (Ringer's) should be avoided because it contains potassium and because lactate metabolism is decreased in uremia. There is no contraindication to the administration of blood, which is always crossmatched and available in the operating room. Blood is given through a Sepacell filter.

The diabetic patient undergoing renal transplantation is given an infusion of glucose (5 g/h). The blood glucose level is titrated to normoglycemia with a separate infusion of a short-acting insulin (such as actrapid, Humulin S or Velosulin, 1–4 units/h).

Postoperative fluid requirements depend on early renal function but should be aimed at keeping the CVP at its intraoperative level. In our practice, this equates to a regimen of urine output plus 50 to 100 ml/h. Replacement fluids are given as crystalloid (equal volumes of 5% dextrose and normal saline), supplemented by colloid in cases of a fall in CVP accompanied by arterial hypotension. Persistent hypotension in the presence of an adequate CVP (5–10 cm H_2O) normally responds to dobutamine, 1 to 20 $\mu g\ kg^{-1}\ min^{-1}$. Some units routinely infuse dopamine, 2 to 3 $\mu g\ kg^{-1}\ min^{-1}$ from the time of renal revascularization to promote renal arteriolar vasodilatation. This infusion is continued until adequate urine is produced, then gradually tapered off. The accurate assessment of fluid balance postoperatively may be difficult in the predialysis patient who still has native urine production; after living-related transplantation, there may be a major response by the body to the high osmotic load of creatinine, urea and other solutes, with urine outputs of 40 L over the first 24 hours. This output tends to return to normal volumes by 24 to 48 hours. Because of this high fluid flux, the patient's

temperature should be carefully monitored intraoperatively, and heat balance should be maintained by warming all infused fluids and using a convection heater (such as the Bair Hugger). Other causes of a massive diuresis include the onset of the diuretic phase of acute tubular necrosis, which is characterized by large volumes of low osmolar urine.

Although we do not routinely measure perioperative electrolytes (particularly potassium), reports have appeared of sudden increases of plasma potassium levels leading to arrhythmias and cardiac arrest (Hirschmann and Edelstein, 1979). Several factors may be responsible, such as the administration of mannitol (Moreno *et al.*, 1969) or stored blood, severe metabolic acidosis and hyperkalemia or hyperglycemia (Goldfarb *et al.*, 1976). The cause of the latter mechanism is unknown. Prevention of this complication assumes greater significance in the diabetic patient undergoing renal transplantation (see later). If urine output is greater than 300 ml h^{-1}, the serum sodium and potassium levels should be checked every 4 to 6 hours. If output is greater than 1,000 ml h^{-1}, potassium supplements (10 mmol L^{-1}) may be needed. The excretion of large fluid volumes also may lead to intravascular and intracellular dehydration—presenting as tachycardia (ventricular tachycardia or atrial fibrillation) or seizures.

In patients with poor renal output in the absence of dehydration, electrolytes should be checked every 6 hours, checking of electrolytes, and accurate weighing should occur every 24 hours. Dialysis is to be avoided during the first 24 hours postoperatively but is indicated when there is massive weight gain, severe hypertension, fluid overload with pulmonary edema or a severe metabolic acidosis or hyperkalemia.

There are few indications for the use of dopamine in the transplant recipient. Two studies have failed to show any efficacy of dopamine by infusion for improving renal function. Brauser and Cronnelly (1987) found no increase in CVP or urinary volume after low-dose infusions of dopamine; they conclude that the newly transplanted kidney, which has been subjected to surgical denervation, trauma, ischemia, hypothermia and large doses of furosemide and mannitol, is less responsive to dopamine than the native kidney. In a more recent article, Kadieva and colleagues compared the hemodynamic effects of dopamine, 3 $\mu g\ kg^{-1}\ min^{-1}$, and a control group in 60 patients undergoing cadaveric renal transplantation (Kadieva *et al.*, 1993). They looked at two endpoints—initial graft function 1 week after transplantation and graft survival at 3 months. There were no differences in these two outcome measures; on that basis, these authors concluded that dopamine had no role in the patient without serious vascular disease or the absence of prolonged postrevascularization hypotension or prolonged preservation times.

POSTOPERATIVE CARE

Because of the multiple pathologies exhibited by transplant patients, they should be nursed postoperatively in either a high dependency or intensive care unit, where controlled oxygen therapy and full monitoring can be provided. The correct positioning of the triple-lumen catheter must be checked by a radiograph in the recovery area. If controlled ventilation is needed, admission to an intensive care unit is required. Strict monitoring of fluid input and output is essential; there should be regular monitoring of the ECG, blood pressure, heart rate, CVP and oxygen saturation by pulse oximetry.

Analgesia in the Postoperative Period

Analgesia should be titrated according to patient demand. The choice of drugs (opioids and oral nonnarcotic analgesics) must be carefully considered because accumulation of active metabolites of pethidine and morphine may occur in the patient with a nonfunctioning allograft. Excessive use of opioids may lead to delayed respiratory depression, sedation and convulsions (all related to both parent drug and active metabolite accumulation). Patient-controlled analgesia may aid the more efficient and safe titration of dosage to desired effect in the uremic patient, although there have been reports of excessive sedation and respiratory depression after use of patient-controlled analgesia in end-stage renal disease patients (Covington et al., 1989). We routinely prescribe a mixture of 60 mg of morphine and 5 mg of droperidol made up to 60 ml. Bolus doses of 1 to 2 mg are administered with a lockout of 5 to 10 minutes. We do not administer a background infusion of opioid as part of the patient-controlled analgesia.

Although only a small percentage of nonsteroidal anti-inflammatory drugs (NSAIDs) are eliminated unchanged by the kidney, there is evidence of reduced clearance of ketoprofen, fenoprofen, naproxen and carprofen in renal failure as a result of probable deconjugation of acyl glucuronide metabolites. More importantly, NSAIDs also can cause reversible kidney damage with reduction of renal blood flow and the glomerular filtration rate and edema, interstitial nephritis and papillary necrosis in the kidney. These effects probably are caused by the action of the NSAIDs on prostaglandin synthesis—the latter being integral for renal blood flow and glomerular filtration rate autoregulation. These drugs are avoided in all patients with renal impairment.

Anesthetic Outcomes After Renal Transplantation

The major postoperative anesthetic complications are vomiting and pulmonary inhalation; cardiac arrhythmias, which can lead to cardiac arrest; pulmonary edema; hypotension and hypertension and delayed respiratory depression. Cardiovascular complications in the transplant recipient are responsible for about 33% of all mortality (Divarkar et al., 1991), with about 50% of all patients showing arterial hypertension. Although usually a reflection of chronic rejection or excess renin release from the patient's native kidneys, rarer causes include the effects of the immunosuppressive drugs (particularly cyclosporine), recurrent glomerulonephritis and transplant renal artery stenosis. Transplant patients also appear to be at greater risk of developing left ventricular hypertrophy if the treatment of this hypertension requires two or more antihypertensive therapies (Harnett et al., 1987).

The posttransplant patient may manifest diabetes mellitus; this occurs in 3 to 16% of all recipients, with 4% of these patients requiring insulin. Usually the onset of hyperglycemia occurs within the first 3 months of transplantation or after the first bolus dose of steroid for the treatment of kidney graft rejection. Predisposing factors include preoperative glucose intolerance and the presence of HLA type B28.

With increasing awareness of the surgical risk factors present in the renal transplant patient, careful perioperative monitoring has led to low rates of perioperative mortality (0.03–0.06%). Factors that lead to increased risk in recipients include age greater than 60 years, coronary artery disease and diabetes mellitus (Tesi et al., 1994).

Alternative Methods of Anesthesia
REGIONAL ANESTHESIA FOR TRANSPLANTATION AND ASSOCIATED SURGERY

Although Vandam and colleagues described the use of regional anesthetic techniques for renal transplantation to avoid the potential interactions of general anesthesia with the uremic patient, this is no longer a significant problem with the development of modern dialysis techniques (Vandam et al., 1962). In a subsequent review by Linke and Merin (1976), they cite the advantages of regional anesthesia as the avoidance of neuromuscular blocking drugs and endotracheal intubation, the reduced likelihood of pulmonary regurgitation and pulmonary inhalation by the patient with a full stomach and the provision of pain-free conditions in the awake patient in the immediate postoperative period.

In chronic renal failure, onset of sensory analgesia occurs faster after subarachnoid blockade because of the combined effects of the metabolic acidosis causing a greater degree of ionization and a reduction in the volume of the epidural space secondary to distention of the epidural and spinal veins by a hyperdynamic circulation. The durations of sensory and motor blockades were shorter (20%) in the patients with renal failure, however, the increased cardiac output causing a faster washout of the local anesthetic from its site of action (Orko et al., 1986; Pitkanen et al., 1985).

There is concern over the possibility of extradural hematomata formation in patients with a disordered coagulatory system. Basta and Sloan (1999) have reported the first case of the development of an epidural hematoma in a chronic renal failure patient about 60 hours after catheter placement. Other possible complications include a difficulty in handling major blood loss in a vasodilated patient, an unpredictable response of the hypertensive renal patient on drug therapy to vasopressors, the maintenance of an awake patient's well-being during a long procedure and the medicolegal complexity of a postoperative peripheral neuropathy.

VASCULAR AND PERITONEAL ACCESS FOR DIALYSIS

Surgery for shunt insertion or fistula creation may be carried out under general or regional anesthesia. The anesthetic agent may be infiltrated locally, but for vascular access in the upper limb, anesthesia is best achieved by brachial plexus or axillary nerve blockade. The associated sympathetic nerve block abolishes vasospasm and ensures vasodilatation. The duration of brachial plexus anesthesia in patients suffering from end-stage renal disease is decreased by 39%, however (Bromage and Gertel, 1972). This decrease was thought to be the result of metabolic changes present in uremia (e.g., hyperkalemia) and the increase in cardiac output secondary to anemia. Two more recent articles fail to support these earlier data, however (Martin et al., 1988; McEllistrem et al., 1989). Bupivacaine disposition is unaltered after supraclavicular plexus blockade in uremic patients (Rice et al., 1991), and there is no direct correlation between the shortening of anesthetic action and the severity of anemia or uremia. Although bupivacaine is the agent of choice for local anesthetic procedures, a report by Gould and Aldrete (1981) described cardiotoxic effects after its use in normal doses in a patient with end-stage renal disease. Other drugs suitable for this group of patients include lignocaine, prilocaine and the two agents presently under evaluation, ropivacaine and bupivacaine. Compared with bupivacaine, lignocaine, mepivacaine and prilocaine have a faster onset of anesthesia but shorter in duration. As a general rule, the normal maximum doses for bupivacaine and other local anesthetic agents (Table 13–7) should be decreased by 25% in patients with end-stage renal disease because any accompanying acidosis would have the effect of decreasing the central nervous system threshold to the toxic effects of local anesthesia.

The use of regional anesthesia in the patient with uremic neuropathy generally is contraindicated. Similarly, use of

TABLE 13–7
MAXIMUM SAFE DOSES OF LOCAL ANESTHETIC AGENTS

	Plain Solution (mg)	With Added Epinephrine (1 : 200,000) (mg)	Relative Duration of Sensory Block
Lignocaine	300	500	1.5
Bupivacaine	175	250	8
Mepivacaine	300	500	1.5
Etidocaine	300	400	8
Prilocaine	400	600	1.5
Chloroprocaine	600	650	0.75
Procaine	500	600	1
Ropivacaine	250	—	1
L-Bupivacaine	175	—	1

*These doses are based on a 70-kg body weight. Doses should be decreased by 25% in the acidotic patient to avoid signs of central nervous system toxicity (e.g., lightheadedness, dizziness, disorientation, euphoria, dysarthria, slurring of speech, progressing to twitching and generalized convulsions).

vasoconstrictors such as epinephrine to prolong local anesthetic action is best avoided because of the risk of cardiac arrhythmias after systemic absorption in the acidotic, hyperkalemic patient. Other limitations of regional anesthesia are bleeding tendency, patient acceptance and a possible inadequate duration of analgesia. For more complex procedures (e.g., insertion of arteriovenous grafts, thigh shunts or continuous ambulatory peritoneal dialysis cannulation), general anesthesia usually is preferable.

Anesthetic Management of the Diabetic Patient Undergoing Renal Transplantation

The combined problems of diabetes and uremia are common because patients with juvenile-onset diabetes developing before the age of 30 years have a 1 in 5 chance of renal complications (Deckert et al., 1978). At present in the United Kingdom, about 10% of all renal transplants are in diabetic patients, the percentage in the United States being 20 to 25%. Although there has been some reluctance to offer a renal transplant, especially from a cadaver donor, to the diabetic patient because of the relatively poor results (see Chapter 36), an increasing number of units are faced with such patients for transplantation. There also is a move toward the combined transplantation of kidneys and pancreas in these patients. The problems presented by the diabetic patient for the anesthesiologist may be considered under the following headings:

Influence of uremia on carbohydrate metabolism
Preoperative assessment of patients
Anesthetic technique and postoperative management

INFLUENCE OF UREMIA ON CARBOHYDRATE METABOLISM

The influence of uremia on carbohydrate metabolism has been reviewed extensively by de Fronzo et al. (1973). The main defect appears to be a systemic insulin antagonism for which several factors may be implicated. Coupled with this hyperglycemic response, there is a glucose-induced hyperkalemia. Its exact cause is uncertain, although hypoaldosteronism and hyporeninism have been suggested.

PREOPERATIVE ASSESSMENT OF PATIENTS

Preoperative assessment does not differ from that of the nondiabetic patient undergoing renal transplantation, with the additional factor being that optimal glycemic control

should be achieved before surgery is begun. All patients with diabetes present an increased risk to the anesthesiologist, especially related to the complicating factors of hypertension and coronary artery disease (Burgos et al., 1989). This risk includes a greater need for intraoperative blood pressure support and aggressive treatment of any hypotension with vasoconstrictor drugs. In the diabetic patient with renal failure, there is a higher risk of perioperative myocardial ischemia and infarction, both of which may be silent because of the accompanying autonomic neuropathy. Another potential complication is the increased risk of wound infection.

Heino (1988) observed an increased perioperative morbidity and mortality in diabetic patients undergoing renal transplantation compared with nondiabetic transplant recipients. In a follow-up of 413 patients, Heino showed that diabetic patients with end-stage renal disease had a higher incidence of preoperative ST-T wave changes (62.2% vs. 39.8% in nondiabetic uremic patients) and a higher incidence of pulmonary congestion (14.5% vs. 5.2%) and pleural effusions (10.1% vs. 4.5%) on chest radiography. No differences were seen in the frequency of perioperative complications, although the diabetic patients had a greater mortality during the first postoperative month.

Many diabetics presenting for transplantation are poorly controlled and show blood glucose concentration lability. Concurrent administration of thiazine diuretics, diazoxide and β-adrenoceptor blocking drugs may complicate glucose homeostasis further. If the patients are normally maintained on continuous ambulatory peritoneal dialysis, this should be continued up to 1 hour before surgery. The dose of added insulin should be reduced in the final bag before operation, although the glucose in the dialysate does not always prevent the development of low intraoperative blood glucose levels. In general, the aim should be a blood glucose concentration of 4 to 8 mmol L^{-1}.

ANESTHETIC TECHNIQUE AND POSTOPERATIVE MANAGEMENT

After induction of anesthesia, uremic patients with diabetic neuropathy may show a greater systolic pressor response to intubation and other noxious stimuli (Kirvela et al., 1995). This response is due to an increased sensitivity to circulating catecholamines and a loss of baroreceptor control. The same authors have shown that diabetic patients exhibit greater QT$_c$ dispersion (Kirvela et al., 1994a), with an associated increased risk of sudden cardiorespiratory arrest (Reissell et al., 1994). The measurement of QT dispersion by 24-hour Holter ECG monitoring does not appear to be a sensitive method *per se* of detecting the cardiac autonomic neuropathy in these patients, however (Kirvela *et al.*, 1994a).

Because of the possible association of diabetes with gastroparesis and an increased gastric residual volume, all diabetic uremic patients should undergo a rapid-sequence intubation—with succinylcholine being used in the presence of normokalemia (Reissell *et al.*, 1992). Other suitable drugs may include rocuronium and rapacuronium in large doses. Studies on the handling of opiates during anesthesia in the diabetic patient with end-stage renal disease are limited. Koehntop *et al.* (1990) found an increased clearance of alfentanil (6.4 ml kg^{-1} min^{-1} *vs.* 4.1 ml kg^{-1} min^{-1}) in the diabetic compared with the nondiabetic uremic patient, in parallel with an enhanced clearance of theophylline in insulin-dependent diabetics (Korrapati *et al.*, 1995). Adithan and colleagues found no effect of diabetes on the biotransformation of paracetamol, however (Adithan *et al.*, 1988). Further studies of the effects of diabetes on anesthetic drug handling are needed.

Other potential anesthetic problems in these patients include temporomandibular joint rigidity and difficulties in intubation caused by tissue glycosylation (Hogan *et al.*, 1988; Salzarulo and Taylor, 1986). If there is any concern, the anesthetist should use suxamethonium as the relaxant of choice.

When transplantation of pancreas and kidney are carried out together, perioperative development of hypoglycemia may occur as a result of the production of endogenous insulin by the transplanted pancreatic tissue. This situation may be complicated further by residual effects of any preoperatively administered, long-duration insulin preparations. Diabetic control also is influenced by intraoperatively administered steroids given for immunosuppression as well as the use of mannitol. Perkins and coworkers found that reperfusion of the pancreatic graft can also lead to an *increase* in blood glucose levels as a result of the release into the circulation of graft preservation fluid, which contains high glucose concentrations (Perkins *et al.*, 1990).

Conclusions

Although Strunin (1966) reported an immediate perioperative mortality of 16% after renal transplantation, more recent series have recorded immediate mortality rates of 0.03% and 0.6% (Heino, 1988; Heino *et al.*, 1986; Marsland and Bradley, 1983). With present-day anesthetic techniques, the incidence of delayed extubation (owing to inadequate ventilatory performance) is low (<3% of patients).

From the discussion of drugs and techniques in this chapter, it is clear that there is no single correct technique for the anesthetic management of patients in end-stage renal failure. Effective and safe anesthesia for the renal transplantation patient depends on an understanding of the pathophysiology and biochemistry of uremia and its effect on the pharmacokinetics and metabolism of the drugs used. As the criteria for accepting patients into renal transplantation programs broaden, the anesthesiologist is likely to be faced with increasing problems of the interaction of other intercurrent diseases and multiple drug therapies.

REFERENCES

Adithan, C., Danda, D., Swaminathan, R. P., *et al.* (1988). Effect of diabetes on salivary paracetamol elimination. *Clin. Exp. Pharmacol. Physiol.* **15**, 465.

Aitkenhead, A. R., Vater, M., Achola, K., Cooper, C. M. S. and Smith, G. (1984). Pharmacokinetics of single-dose intravenous morphine in normal volunteers and patients with end-stage renal failure. *Br. J. Anaesth.* **56**, 813.

Andreasen, F. (1974). The effect of dialysis on the protein binding of drugs in the plasma of patients with acute renal failure. *Acta Pharmacol. Toxicol.* **34**, 284.

Armstrong, P. J. and Bersten, A. (1986). Normeperidine toxicity. *Anesth. Analg.* **65**, 536.

Barnes, J. N., Williams, A. J., Tomson, M. J. F., Toseland, P. A. and Goodwin, F. J. (1985). Dihydrocodeine in renal failure: further evidence for an important role of the kidney in the handling of opioid drugs. *B. M. J.* **290**, 740.

Basta, M. and Sloan, P. (1999). Epidural hematoma following epidural catheter placement in a patient with chronic renal failure. *Can. J. Anaesth.* **46**, 271.

Bastron, R. D. and Deutsch, S. (1976). *Anesthesia and the Kidney*, Grune & Stratton, Orlando.

Bateman, D. N. and Gokal, R. (1980). Metoclopramide in renal failure. *Lancet* **1**, 982.

Beauvoir, C., Peray, P., Daures, J. P., Peschaud, J. L. and D'Athis, F. (1993). Pharmacodynamics of vecuronium in patients with and without renal failure: a meta-analysis. *Can. J. Anaesth.* **40**, 696.

Bevan, D. R., Donati, F., Gyasi, H. and Williams, A. (1984). Vecuronium in renal failure. *Can. Anaesth. Soc. J.* **31**, 491.

Bower, S. (1982). Plasma protein binding of fentanyl: the effect of hyperlipidaemia and chronic renal failure. *J. Pharm. Pharmacol.* **34**, 102.

Bower, S. and Sear, J. W. (1989). Disposition of alfentanil in patients receiving a renal transplant. *J. Pharm. Pharmacol.* **41**, 654.

Boyd, A. H., Eastwood, N. B., Parker, C. J. H. and Hunter, J. M. (1995). Pharmacodynamics of the 1R-cis 1R'-cis isomer of atracurium (51W89) in health and chronic renal failure. *Br. J. Anaesth.* **74**, 400.

Brauser, S. D. and Cronnelly, R. (1987). Does dopamine improve function of the transplanted kidney? *Anesth. Analg.* **66**, s17.

Bromage, P. R. and Gertel, M. (1972). Brachial plexus anesthesia in chronic renal failure. *Anesthesiology* **36**, 488.

Brotherton, W. D. and Matteo, R. S. (1981). Pharmacokinetics and pharmacodynamics of metocurine in humans with and without renal failure. *Anesthesiology* **55**, 273.

Brown, J. J., Duesterdieck, G., Fraser, R., *et al.* (1971). Hypertension and chronic renal failure. *Br. Med. Bull.* **27**, 128.

Burch, P. G. and Stanski, D. R. (1982). Decreased protein binding and thiopental kinetics. *Clin. Pharmacol. Ther.* **32**, 212.

Burgess, K. R., Burgess, E. E. and Whitelaw, W. A. (1994). Impaired ventilatory response to carbon dioxide in patients in chronic renal failure: implications for the intensive care unit. *Crit. Care Med.* **22**, 413.

Burgos, L. G., Ebert, T. J., Asiddao, C., *et al.* (1989). Increased intraoperative cardiovascular morbidity in diabetics with autonomic neuropathy. *Anesthesiology* **70**, 591.

Buzello, W. and Agoston, S. (1978). Pharmacokinetics of pancuronium in patients with normal and impaired renal function. *Anaesthesist* **27**, 291.

Caldwell, J. E., Canfell, P. C., Castagnoli, K. P., *et al.* (1989). The influence of renal failure on the pharmacokinetics and duration of action of pipecuronium bromide in patients anesthetized with halothane and nitrous oxide. *Anesthesiology* **70**, 7.

Carlier, M., Squifflet, J. P., Pirson, Y., Alexandre, G. P. J., de Temmermann, P. and Gribomont, B. F. (1986). Anesthetic protocol in human renal transplantation: twenty two years of experience. *Acta Anaesthesiol. Belg.* **37**, 89.

Carlier, M., Squifflet, J. P., Pirson, Y., Gribomont, B. and Alexandre, G. P. J. (1982). Maximal hydration during anesthesia increases pulmonary arterial pressures and improves early function in human renal transplants. *Transplantation* **34**, 201.

Carlos, R., Calvo, R. and Erill, S. (1979). Plasma protein binding of etomidate in patients with renal failure or hepatic cirrhosis. *Clin. Pharmacokinet.* **4**, 144.

Carr, A. C., Stone, P. A., Serpell, M. G., Joel, S. P. and Tinker, L. (1998). Patient controlled morphine analgesia (PCA morphine) in cadaveric renal transplant recipients: does morphine-6-glucuronide accumulate? *Br. J. Anaesth.* **81**, 630.

Cashman, J. N., Luke, J. J. and Jones, R. M. (1992). Neuromuscular block with doxacurium (BW A938U) in patients with normal or absent renal function. *Br. J. Anaesth.* **64**, 186.

Chan, K., Tse, J., Jenning, F. and Orme, M. L. (1987). Pharmacokinetics of low-dose intravenous pethidine in patients with renal dysfunction. *J. Clin. Pharmacol.* **27**, 516.

Chapple, D. J., Miller, A. A., Ward, J. B. and Wheatley, P. L. (1987). Cardiovascular and neurological effects of laudanosine: studies in mice and rats, and in conscious and anaesthetized dogs. *Br. J. Anaesth.* **59**, 218.

Chauvin, M., Lebrault, C., Levron, J. C. and Duvaldestin, P. (1987a). Pharmacokinetics of alfentanil in chronic renal failure. *Anesth. Analg.* **66**, 53.

Chauvin, M., Sandouk, P., Scherrmann, J. M., Farinotti, R., Strumza, P. and Duvaldestin, P. (1987b). Morphine pharmacokinetics in renal failure. *Anesthesiology* **66**, 327.

Christensen, J. H. and Andreasen, F. (1978). Individual variation in response to thiopental. *Acta Anaesthesiol. Scand.* **22**, 303.

Christensen, J. H., Andreasen, F. and Jansen, J. (1983). Pharmacokinetics and pharmacodynamics of thiopental in patients undergoing renal transplantation. *Acta Anaesthesiol. Scand.* **27**, 513.

Cody, M. W. and Dormon, F. M. (1987). Recurarisation after vecuronium in a patient with renal failure. *Anaesthesia* **42**, 993.

Converse, R. L., Jacobsen, T. N., Toto, R. D., *et al.* (1992). Sympathetic overactivity in patients with chronic renal failure. *N. Engl. J. Med.* **327**, 1912.

Cook, D. R., Freeman, J. A., Lai, A. A., *et al.* (1991). Pharmacokinetics and pharmacodynamics of doxacurium in normal patients and in those with hepatic or renal failure. *Anesth. Analg.* **72**, 145.

Cook, D. R., Freeman, J. A., Lai, A. A., *et al.* (1992). Pharmacokinetics of mivacurium in normal patients and in those with hepatic or renal failure. *Br. J. Anaesth.* **69**, 580.

Cooper, R. A., Maddineni, V. R., Mirakhur, R. K., Wierda, J. M., Brady, M. and Fitzpatrick, K. T. (1993). Time course of neuromuscular effects and pharmacokinetics of rocuronium bromide (Org 9426) during isoflurane anaesthesia in patients with and without renal failure. *Br. J. Anaesth.* **71**, 222.

Corall, I. M., Moore, A. R. and Strunin, L. (1980). Plasma concentrations of fentanyl in normal surgical patients and those with severe renal and hepatic disease. *Br. J. Anaesth.* **52**, 101.

Costela, J. L., Jimenez, R., Calvo, R., Suarez, E. and Carlos, R. (1996). Serum protein binding of propofol in patients with renal failure or hepatic cirrhosis. *Acta Anaesthesiol. Scand.* **40**, 741.

Cousins, M. J., Mazze, R. I., Losek, J. C., Hitt, B. A. and Love, F. V. (1974). The etiology of methoxyflurane nephrotoxicity. *J. Pharmacol. Exp. Ther.* **190**, 530.

Covington, E. C., Gonsalves-Ebrahim, L., Currie, K. O., Shepard, K. V. and Pippenger, C. E. (1989). Severe respiratory depression from patient-controlled analgesia in renal failure. *Psychosomatics* **30**, 226.

Cronnelly, R., Kremer, P. F., Beaupre, P. N., Cahalan, M. K., Salvatierra, O. and Feduska, N. (1983a). Hemodynamic response to anesthesia in patients with end-stage renal disease. *Anesthesiology* **59**, A47.

Cronnelly, R., Kremer, P. F., Beaupre, P. N., Cahalan, M. K., Salvatierra, O. and Feduska, N. (1983b). Hemodynamic response to fluid challenge in anesthetized patients with end-stage renal disease. *Anesthesiology* **59**, A49.

Cronnelly, R. and Morris, R. B. (1982). Antagonism of neuromuscular blockade. *Br. J. Anaesth.* **54**, 183.

Cronnelly, R., Salvatierra, O. and Feduska, N. (1984). Renal allograft function following halothane, enflurane or isoflurane anesthesia. *Anesth. Analg.* **63**, 202.

Davis, P. J., Stiller, R. L., Cook, D. R., Brandom, B. W. and Davin-Robinson, K. A. (1988). Pharmacokinetics of sufentanil in adolescent patients with chronic renal failure. *Anesth. Analg.* **67**, 268.

Dawidson, I., Berglin, E., Brygner, H. and Reisch, J. (1987). Intravascular volumes and colloidal dynamics in relation to fluid management in living related kidney donors and recipients. *Crit. Care Med.* **15**, 631.

De Bros, F., Basta, S. J., Ali, H. H., Wargin, W. and Welch, R. (1987). Pharmacokinetics and pharmacodynamics of BW B1090U in healthy surgical patients receiving N_2O/O_2 isoflurane anaesthesia. *Anesthesiology* **67**, A609.

De Bros, F. M., Lai, A., Scott, R., *et al.* (1986). Pharmacokinetics and pharmacodynamics of atracurium during isoflurane anesthesia in normal and anephric patients. *Anesth. Analg.* **65**, 743.

Deckert, T., Poulsen, J. E. and Larsen, M. (1978). Prognosis of diabetics with diabetes onset before the age of thirty-one: I. survival, causes of death, and complications. *Diabetologica* **14**, 363.

de Fronzo, R. A., Andres, R., Edgar, P. and Gordon-Walker, W. (1973). Carbohydrate metabolism in uremia: a review. *Medicine (Baltimore)* **52**, 469.

D'Honneur, G., Gilton, A., Sandouk, P., Scherrmann, J. M. and Duvaldestin, P. (1994). Plasma and cerebrospinal fluid concentrations of morphine and morphine glucuronides after oral morphine: the influence of renal failure. *Anesthesiology* **81**, 87.

Divarkar, D., Bailey, R. R., Lynn, K. L. and Robson, R. A. (1991). Long-term complications following renal transplantation. *N. Z. J. Med.* **104**, 352.

Don, H. F., Dieppa, R. A. and Taylor, P. (1975). Narcotic analgesics in anuric patients. *Anesthesiology* **42**, 745.

Dundee, J. W. and Richards, R. K. (1954). Effect of azotemia upon the action of barbiturate anesthesia. *Anesthesiology* **13**, 333.

Duthie, D. J. R. (1987). Renal failure, surgery and fentanyl pharmacokinetics. Proceedings of VII European Congress of Anaesthesiology, volume II (main topics 7–12). *Beitr. Anaesthesiol. Intensivmed.* **20**, 374.

Eastwood, N. B., Boyd, A. H., Parker, C. J. H. and Hunter, J. M. (1995). Pharmacokinetics of 1R-cis 1R'-cis atracurium besylate (51W89) and plasma laudanosine concentrations in health and chronic renal failure. *Br. J. Anaesth.* **75**, 431.

Eschbach, J. W., Abdulladi, M. H., Browne, J. K., *et al.* (1989). Recombinant human erythropoietin (rHuEpo) in anemic patients with end-stage renal disease: results of a phase III multicenter trial. *Ann. Intern. Med.* **111**, 992.

Eschbach, J. W., Egrie, J. C., Downing, M. R., Browne, J. K. and Adamson, J. W. (1987). Correction of the anemia of end-stage renal disease with recombinant human erythropoietin: results of a combined phase I and II clinical trial. *N. Engl. J. Med.* **316**, 73.

Fahey, M. R., Rupp, S. M., Canfell, C., *et al.* (1985). Effect of renal failure on laudanosine excretion in man. *Br. J. Anaesth.* **57**, 1049.

Fahey, M. R., Rupp, S. M., Fisher, D. M., *et al.* (1984). The pharmacokinetics and pharmacodynamics of atracurium in patients with and without renal failure. *Anesthesiology* **61**, 699.

Feldman, S. A., Cohen, E. N. and Golling, R. C. (1969). The excretion of gallamine in the dog. *Anesthesiology* **30**, 593.

Feldman, S. A. and Levi, J. A. (1963). Prolonged paresis following gallamine: a case report. *Br. J. Anaesth.* **35**, 804.

Fisher, D. M., Canfell, C., Fahey, M. R., *et al.* (1985). Elimination of atracurium in humans: contribution of Hofmann elimination and ester hydrolysis versus organ-bound elimination. *Anesthesiology* **65**, 6.

Fishman, R. A. (1970). Permeability changes in experimental uremic encephalopathy. *Arch. Intern. Med.* **126**, 835.

Freeman, B. B., Sheff, M. F., Maher, J. F. and Schreiner, G. E. (1962). The blood-cerebrospinal fluid barrier in uremia. *Ann. Intern. Med.* **56**, 233.

Freilich, J. D., Waterman, P. M. and Rosenthal, J. T. (1984). Acute hemodynamic changes during renal transplantation. *Anesth. Analg.* **63**, 158.

Fyman, P., Reynolds, J., Moser, F., Avitable, M., Casthley, P. and Butt, K. (1988). Pharmacokinetics of sufentanil in patients undergoing renal transplantation. *Can. J. Anaesth.* **35**, 312.

Geha, D. G., Blitt, C. D. and Moon, B. J. (1976). Prolonged neuromuscular blockade with pancuronium in the presence of acute renal failure: a case report. *Anesth. Analg.* **55**, 343.

Gibaldi, M., Levy, G. and Hayton, E. L. (1972). Tubocurarine and renal failure. *Br. J. Anaesth.* **44**, 163.

Gibson, T. P., Giacomini, K. M., Briggs, W. A., Whitman, W. and Levy, G. (1980). Propoxyphene and norpropoxyphene plasma concentrations in the anephric patient. *Clin. Pharmacol. Ther.* **27**, 665.

Glare, P. A., Walsh, T. D. and Pippenger, C. E. (1990). Normorphine, a neurotoxic metabolite? *Lancet* **335**, 725.

Gluck, Z. and Nolph, K. D. (1987). Ascites associated with end-stage renal disease. *Am. J. Kidney Dis.* **10**, 9.

Goldfarb, S., Cox, M., Singer, I. and Goldberg, M. (1976). Acute hyperkalemia induced by hyperglycemia: hormonal mechanisms. *Ann. Intern. Med.* **84**, 426.

Goldman, L. (1983). Cardiac risk and complications of non-cardiac surgery. *Ann. Intern. Med.* **98**, 504.

Gould, D. B. and Aldrete, J. A. (1981). Bupivacaine cardiotoxicity in a patient with renal failure. *Acta Anaesthesiol. Scand.* **27**, 18.

Guay, D. R. P., Awni, W. M., Findlay, J. W. A., *et al.* (1988). Pharmacokinetics and pharmacodynamics of codeine in end-stage renal disease. *Clin. Pharmacol. Ther.* **43**, 63.

Hampers, C. L., Balufox, M. D. and Merrill, J. P. (1966). Anticoagulation rebound after hemodialysis. *N. Engl. J. Med.* **275**, 776.

Hand, C. W., Sear, J. W., Uppington, J., Ball, M. J., McQuay, H. J. and Moore, R. A. (1990). Buprenorphine disposition in patients with renal impairment: single and continuous dosing with especial reference to metabolites. *Br. J. Anaesth.* **64**, 276.

Hanna, M. H., D'Costa, F., Peat, S. J., *et al.* (1993). Morphine-6-glucuronide disposition in renal impairment. *Br. J. Anaesth.* **70**, 511.

Harnett, J. D., Parfrey, P. S., Griffith, S., Devlin, W. H. and Guttmann, R. D. (1987). Clinical and echocardiographic heart disease in renal transplant patients. *Transplant. Proc.* **19**, 3415.

Hasselstrom, J., Berg, U., Lofgren, A. and Sawe, J. (1989). Long lasting respiratory depression induced by morphine-6-glucuronide? *Br. J. Clin. Pharmacol.* **27**, 515.

Head-Rapson, A. G., Devlin, J. C., Parker, C. J. and Hunter, J. M. (1995). Pharmacokinetics and pharmacodynamics of the three isomers of mivacurium in health, in end-stage renal failure and in patients with impaired renal function. *Br. J. Anaesth.* **75**, 31.

Heino, A. (1988). Operative and postoperative non-surgical complications in diabetic patients undergoing renal transplantation. *Scand. J. Urol. Nephrol.* **22**, 53.

Heino, A., Orko, R. and Rosenberg, P. H. (1986). Anaesthesiological complications in renal transplantation: a retrospective study of 500 transplantations. *Acta Anaesthesiol. Scand.* **30**, 574.

Higuchi, H., Arimura, S., Sumikura, H., Satoh, T. and Kanno, M. (1994). Urine concentrating ability after prolonged sevoflurane anaesthesia. *Br. J. Anaesth.* **73**, 239.

Hirschmann, C. A. and Edelstein, G. (1979). Intraoperative hyperkalemia and cardiac arrest during renal transplantation in an insulin dependent diabetic patient. *Anesthesiology* **51**, 161.

Hogan, K., Rusy, D. and Springman, S. R. (1988). Difficult laryngoscopy and diabetes mellitus. *Anesth. Analg.* **67**, 1162.

Hoke, F. J., Shlugman, D., Dershwitz, M., *et al.* (1997). Pharmacokinetics and pharmacodynamics of remifentanil in persons with renal failure compared with healthy volunteers. *Anesthesiology* **87**, 533.

Hunter, J. M., Jones, R. S. and Utting, J. E. (1982). Use of atracurium in patients with no renal function. *Br. J. Anaesth.* **54**, 1251.

Hunter, J. M., Jones, R. S. and Utting, J. E. (1984). Comparison of vecuronium, atracurium and tubocurarine in normal patients and in patients with no renal function. *Br. J. Anaesth.* **56**, 941.

Ickx, B., Cockshott, I. D., Barvais, L., *et al.* (1998). Propofol infusion for induction and maintenance of anaesthesia in patients with end-stage renal disease. *Br. J. Anaesth.* **81**, 854.

Ingram, M. D., Sclabassi, R. J., Cook, D. R., Stiller, R. L. and Bennett, M. H. (1986). Cardiovascular and electroencephalographic effects of laudanosine in 'nephrectomized' cats. *Br. J. Anaesth.* **58(Suppl. 1)**, 14s.

Johnston, P. A., Bernard, D. B., Donohoe, J. F., Perrin, N. S. and Levinsky, N. G. (1979). Effect of volume expansion on hemodynamics of the hypoperfused rat kidney. *J. Clin. Invest.* **64**, 550.

Kadieva, V. S., Friedman, L., Margolius, L. P., Jackson, S. A. and Morrell, D. F. (1993). The effect of dopamine on graft function in patients undergoing renal transplantation. *Anesth. Analg.* **76**, 362.

Kangas, L., Kanto, J., Forsstrom, J. and Ilisalo, E. (1976). The protein binding of diazepam and M-dimethyldiazepam in patients with poor renal function. *Clin. Nephrol.* **5**, 114.

Khuenl-Brady, K. S., Pomaroli, A., Puhringer, F., Mitterschiffthaler, G. and Koller, J. (1993). The use of rocuronium (ORG 9426) in patients with chronic renal failure. *Anaesthesia* **48**, 873.

Kirvela, M., Ali-Melkkila, T., Kaila, T., Iisalo, E. and Lindgren, L. (1993). Pharmacokinetics of glycopyrronium in uraemic patients. *Br. J. Anaesth.* **71**, 437.

Kirvela, M., Lindgren, L., Seppala, T. and Olkkola, K. T. (1996). The pharmacokinetics of oxycodone in uremic patients undergoing renal transplantation. *J. Clin. Anesth.* **8**, 13.

Kirvela, M., Olkkola, K. T., Rosenberg, P. H., Yli-Hankala, A., Salmela, K. and Lindgren, L. (1992). Pharmacokinetics of propofol and haemodynamic changes during induction of anaesthesia in uraemic patients. *Br. J. Anaesth.* **68**, 178.

Kirvela, M., Scheinin, M. and Lindgren, L. (1995). Haemodynamic and catecholamine responses to induction of anaesthesia and tracheal intubation in diabetic and non-diabetic uraemic patients. *Br. J. Anaesth.* **74**, 60.

Kirvela, M., Yli-Hankala, A. and Lindgren, L. (1994a). QT dispersion and autonomic function in diabetic and non-diabetic patients with renal failure. *Br. J. Anaesth.* **73**, 801.

Kirvela, M., Yli-Hankala, A. and Lindgren, L. (1994b). Comparison of propofol/alfentanil anaesthesia with isoflurane/N$_2$O/fentanyl anaesthesia for renal transplantation. *Acta Anaesthesiol. Scand.* **38**, 662.

Kisor, D. F., Schmith, V. D., Wargin, W. A., Lien, C. A., Ornstein, E. and Cook, D. R. (1996). Importance of the organ-independent elimination of cisatracurium. *Anesth. Analg.* **83**, 901.

Kobayashi, Y., Ochiai, R., Takeda, J., Sekiguchi, H. and Fukushima, K. (1992). Serum and urinary inorganic fluoride levels after prolonged inhalation of sevoflurane in humans. *Anesth. Analg.* **74**, 753.

Koehntop, D. E., Noormoahmed, S. E. and Fletcher, C. V. (1990). Pharmacokinetics of alfentanil during renal transplantation in diabetic and non-diabetic patients. *Anesth. Analg.* **70**, s212.

Koehntop, D. E. and Rodman, J. H. (1997). Fentanyl pharmacokinetics in patients undergoing renal transplantation. *Pharmacotherapy* **17**, 746.

Koide, M. and Waud, B. E. (1972). Serum potassium concentrations after succinylcholine in patients with renal failure. *Anesthesiology* **36**, 142.

Koppel, C., Arndt, I. and Ibe, K. (1990). Effects of enzyme induction, renal and cardiac function on ketamine plasma kinetics in patients with ketamine long-term analgosedation. *Eur. J. Drug Metab. Pharmacokinet.* **15**, 259.

Korrapati, M. R., Vestal, R. E. and Loi, C.-M. (1995). Theophylline metabolism in healthy nonsmokers and in patients with insulin-dependent diabetes mellitus. *Clin. Pharmacol. Ther.* **57**, 413.

Lehmann, C. R., Heironius, J. D., Collins, C. B., *et al.* (1985). Metoclopramide kinetics in patients with impaired renal function, and clearance by hemodialysis. *Clin. Pharmacol. Ther.* **37**, 284.

LePage, J. Y., Athouel, A., Vecherini, M. F., Malinovsky, J. M. and Cozian, A. (1991). Evaluation of proconvulsant effect of laudanosine in renal transplant recipient. *Anesthesiology* **75**, A780.

LePage, J. Y., Malinge, M., Cozian, A., Pinaud, M., Blanloeil, Y. and Souron, R. (1987). Vecuronium and atracurium in patients with endstage renal failure. *Br. J. Anaesth.* **59**, 1004.

Lindahl-Nilsson, C., Lundh, R. and Groth, C.-G. (1980). Neurolept anaesthesia for the renal transplant operation. *Acta Anaesthesiol. Scand.* **24**, 451.

Linke, C. L. and Merin, R. G. (1976). A regional anesthetic approach for renal transplantation. *Anesth. Analg.* **55**, 69.

Lochhead, K. M., Kharasch, E. D. and Zager, R. A. (1997). Spectrum and subcellular determinants of fluorinated anesthetic-mediated proximal tubular injury. *Am. J. Pathol.* **150**, 2209.

Loehning, R. W. and Mazze, R. I. (1974). Possible nephrotoxicity from enflurane in a patient with severe renal disease. *Anesthesiology* **40**, 203.

Loetsch, J., Stockmann, A., Kobal, G., *et al.* (1996). Pharmacokinetics of morphine and its glucuronides after intravenous infusion of morphine and morphine-6-glucuronide in healthy volunteers. *Clin. Pharmacol. Ther.* **60**, 316.

Lowenstein, E., Goldfine, C. and Flacke, W. E. (1970). Administration of gallamine in the presence of renal failure—reversal of neuromuscular blockade by peritoneal dialysis. *Anesthesiology* **33**, 556.

Lowenthal, D. T. (1974). Tissue sensitivity to drugs in disease states. *Med. Clin. North Am.* **58**, 1111.

Lynam, D. P., Cronnelly, R., Castagnoli, K. P., *et al.* (1988). The pharmacodynamics and pharmacokinetics of vecuronium in patients anesthetized with isoflurane with normal renal function or with renal failure. *Anesthesiology* **69**, 227.

Mannucci, P. M. (1988). Desmopressin: a nontranfusional form of treatment for congenital and acquired bleeding disorders. *Blood* **72**, 1449.

Mannucci, P. M., Remuzzi, C. and Pusineri, F. (1983). Deamino-8-D-arginine vasopressin shortens the bleeding time in uremia. *N. Engl. J. Med.* **308**, 8.

Marsland, A. R. and Bradley, J. P. (1983). Anaesthesia for renal transplantation—5 years' experience. *Anaesth. Intensive Care* **11**, 337.

Martin, R., Beauregard, L. and Tetrault, J. P. (1988). Brachial plexus block and chronic renal failure. *Anesthesiology* **69**, 405.

Mazoit, J. X., Sandouk, P., Scherrmann, J.-M. and Roche, A. (1990). Extrahepatic metabolism of morphine occurs in humans. *Clin. Pharmacol. Ther.* **48**, 613.

Mazze, R., Sievenpiper, T. S. and Stevenson, J. (1984). Renal effects of enflurane and halothane in patients with abnormal renal function. *Anesthesiology* **60**, 161.

Mazze, R. I., Cousins, M. J. and Barr, G. A. (1974). Renal effects and metabolism of isoflurane in man. *Anesthesiology* **40**, 536.

McEllistrem, R. F., Schell, J., O'Malley, K., O'Toole, D. and Cunningham, A. J. (1989). Interscalene brachial plexus blockade with lidocaine in chronic renal failure—a pharmacokinetic study. *Can. J. Anaesth.* **36**, 59.

McLeod, K., Watson, M. J. and Rawlins, M. D. (1976). Pharmacokinetics of pancuronium in patients with normal and impaired renal function. *Br. J. Anaesth.* **48**, 341.

Meuldermans, W. E. G. and Heykants, J. J. P. (1976). The plasma protein binding and distribution of etomidate in dog, rat and human blood. *Arch. Int. Pharmacodyn. Ther.* **221**, 150.

Miller, R. D., Matteo, R. S., Benet, L. Z. and Sohn, T. I. (1977). The pharmacokinetics of d-tubocurarine in man with and without renal failure. *J. Pharmacol. Exp. Ther.* **202**, 1.

Milne, R. W., Nation, R. L., Somogyi, A. A., Bochner, F. and Griggs, W. M. (1992). The influence of renal function on the renal clearance of morphine and its glucuronide metabolites in intensive-care patients. *Br. J. Clin. Pharmacol.* **34**, 53.

Moote, C. A. and Manninen, P. H. (1987). Mannitol administered during renal transplantation produces profound changes in fluid and electrolyte balance. *Can. J. Anaesth.* **35**, s120.

Morcos, W. E. and Payne, J. P. (1985). The induction of anaesthesia with propofol (Diprivan) compared in normal and renal failure patients. *Postgrad. Med. J.* **61(Suppl. 3)**, S62.

Moreno, M., Murphy, C. and Goldsmith, C. (1969). Increase in serum potassium resulting from the administration of hypertonic mannitol and other solutions. *J. Lab. Clin. Med.* **73**, 291.

Morgan, M. and Lumley, J. (1975). Anaesthetic considerations in chronic renal failure. *Anaesth. Intensive Care* **3**, 218.

Mostert, J. W., Evers, J. L., Hobika, G. H., Moore, R. H. and Ambrus, J. L. (1971). Cardiorespiratory effects of anaesthesia with morphine or fentanyl in chronic renal failure and cerebral toxicity after morphine. *Br. J. Anaesth.* **43**, 1053.

Murray, T. G., Chiang, S. T., Koepke, H. H. and Walker, B. R. (1981). Renal disease, age and oxazepam kinetics. *Clin. Pharmacol. Ther.* **30**, 805.

Mushin, W. W., Wien, R., Mason, D. F. J. and Langston, G. T. (1949). Curare-like actions of tri-(diethylaminoethoxy)-benzene triethyliodide. *Lancet* **1**, 726.

Nguyen, H. D., Kaplan, R., Nagashima, H., Dunclaf, D. and Foldes, F. F. (1985). The neuromuscular effect of atracurium in anephric patients. *Anesthesiology* **63**, A335.

Nguyen, H. N., Delpech, Ph., Louville, Y., *et al.* (1989). Effets hemodynamiques de l'anesthesie au propofol, fentanyl, protoxyde d'azote, vecuronium pour la transplantation renale de l'adulte. *Cah. Anesthesiol.* **37**, 17.

Nishiyama, T., Aibiki, M. and Hanaoka, K. (1996). Inorganic fluoride kinetics and renal tubular function after sevoflurane anesthesia in chronic renal failure patients receiving hemodialysis. *Anesth. Analg.* **83**, 574.

Ochs, H. R., Greenblatt, D. J., Kaschel, H. J., Klehr, W., Divoll, M. and Abernethy, D. R. (1981). Diazepam kinetics in patients with renal insufficiency or hyperthyroidism. *Br. J. Clin. Pharmacol.* **12**, 829.

Odar-Cederlof, I., Vessman, J., Alvan, G. and Sjoqvist, F. (1977). Oxazepam disposition in uremic patients. *Acta Pharmacol. Toxicol.* **40(Suppl.)**, S52.

Olsen, G. D., Bennett, W. M. and Porter, G. A. (1975). Morphine and phenytoin binding to plasma proteins in renal and hepatic failure. *Clin. Pharmacol. Ther.* **17**, 677.

Orko, R., Pitkanen, M. and Rosenberg, P. H. (1986). Subarachnoid anaesthesia with 0.75% bupivacaine in patients with chronic renal failure. *Br. J. Anaesth.* **58**, 605.

Osborne, R., Joel, S., Grebenik, K., Trew, D. and Slevin, K. (1993). The pharmacokinetics of morphine and morphine glucuronides in kidney failure. *Clin. Pharmacol. Ther.* **54**, 158.

Osborne, R. J., Joel, S. P. and Slevin, M. L. (1986). Morphine intoxication in renal failure: the role of morphine-6-glucuronide. *B. M. J.* **292**, 1548.

Perkins, J. D., Fromme, G. A., Narr, B. J., *et al.* (1990). Pancreas transplantation at Mayo: II. operative and perioperative management. *Mayo Clin. Proc.* **65**, 483.

Petersen, G. M., Randall, C. T. C. and Paterson, J. (1990). Plasma levels of morphine and morphine glucuronides in the treatment of cancer pain: relationship to renal function and route of administration. *Eur. J. Clin. Pharmacol.* **38**, 121.

Phillips, B. J. and Hunter, J. M. (1992). Use of mivacurium chloride by constant infusion in the anephric patient. *Br. J. Anaesth.* **68**, 492.

Pitkanen, M., Tuominen, M. and Rosenberg, P. H. (1985). Bupivacaine spinal anesthesia compared with etidocaine epidural anesthesia in old and young patients. *Reg. Anesth.* **10**, 62.

Portenoy, R. K., Thaler, H. T., Inturrisi, C. E., Friedlanderklar, H. and Foley, K. M. (1992). The metabolite morphine-6-glucuronide contributes to the analgesia produced by morphine infusion in patients with pain and normal renal function. *Clin. Pharmacol. Ther.* **51**, 422.

Pouttu, J. (1989). Haemodynamic responses during general anaesthesia for renal transplantation in patients with and without hypertensive disease. *Acta Anaesthesiol. Scand.* **33**, 245.

Ramzan, M. I., Shanks, C. A. and Triggs, E. J. (1981). Gallamine disposition in surgical patients with chronic renal failure. *Br. J. Clin. Pharmacol.* **12**, 141.

Reidenberg, M. M., Lowenthal, D. T., Briggs, W. and Gasparo, M. (1976). Pentobarbital elimination in patients with poor renal function. *Clin. Pharmacol. Ther.* **20**, 67.

Reissell, E., Taskinen, M. R., Orko, R. and Lindgren, L. (1992). Increased volume of gastric contents in diabetic patients undergoing renal transplantation: lack of effect with cisapride. *Acta Anaesthesiol. Scand.* **36**, 736.

Reissell, E., Yli-Hankala, A., Orko, R. and Lindgren, L. (1994). Sudden cardiorespiratory arrest after renal transplantation in a patient with diabetic autonomic neuropathy and prolonged QT interval. *Acta Anaesthesiol. Scand.* **38**, 406.

Reiter, V., Fay, R., Pire, J. C., Lamiable, D. and Rendoing, J. (1989). Propofol a debit continu au cours des transplantations renales chez l'adulte. *Cah. Anesthesiol.* **37**, 23.

Rice, A. S. C., Pither, C. E. and Tucker, G. T. (1991). Plasma concentrations of bupivacaine after supraclavicular brachial plexus blockade in patients with chronic renal failure. *Anaesthesia* **46**, 354.

Richet, G., de Novales, E. L. and Verroust, P. (1970). Drug intoxication and neurological episodes in chronic renal failure. *B. M. J.* **2**, 394.

Russo, R., Ravagnan, R., Buzzetti, V. and Favini, P. (1986). Atracurium in patients with chronic renal failure. *Br. J. Anaesth.* **58(Suppl. 1)**, 63s.

Salaman, J. R., Calne, R. Y., Pera, J., Sells, R. A., White, H. J. O. and Yoffa, D. (1969). Surgical aspects of clinical renal transplantation. *Br. J. Surg.* **56**, 413.

Salzarulo, H. H. and Taylor, L. A. (1986). Diabetic 'stiff joint syndrome' as a cause of difficult endotracheal intubation. *Anesthesiology* **64**, 366.

Sawe, J. and Odar-Cederlof, I. (1987). Kinetics of morphine in patients with renal failure. *Eur. J. Clin. Pharmacol.* **32**, 337.

Schiere, S., Proost, J. H., Schuringa, M. and Wierda, J. M. K. H. (1999). Pharmacokinetics and pharmacokinetic-dynamic relationship between rapacuronium (Org 9487) and its 3-desacetyl metabolite (Org 9488). *Anesth. Analg.* **88**, 640.

Sear, J. W. (1989). Sufentanil disposition in patients undergoing renal transplantation: influence of choice of kinetic model. *Br. J. Anaesth.* **63**, 60.

Sear, J. W. and Hand, C. W. (2000). Fentanyl disposition in anaesthetized patient with renal failure using an iodine-labelled RIA. *Br. J. Anaesth.* **84**, 285.

Sear, J. W., Hand, C. W., Moore, R. A. and McQuay, H. J. (1989). Studies on morphine disposition: influence of renal failure on the kinetics of morphine and its metabolites. *Br. J. Anaesth.* **62**, 28.

Sear, J. W., Jewkes, C., Tellez, J.-C. and Foex, P. (1994). Does the choice of antihypertensive therapy influence haemodynamic responses to induction, laryngoscopy and intubation? *Br. J. Anaesth.* **73**, 303.

Segredo, V., Caldwell, J. E., Matthay, M. A., Sharma, M. L., Gruenke, L. D. and Miller, R. D. (1992). Persistent paralysis in critically ill patients after long-term administration of vecuronium. *N. Engl. J. Med.* **327**, 524.

Sheiner, L. B., Stanski, D. R., Vozeh, S., Miller, R. D. and Ham, J. (1979). Simultaneous modeling of pharmacokinetics and pharmacodynamics: applications to d-tubocurarine. *Clin. Pharmacol. Ther.* **25**, 358.

Shelly, M. P., Cory, E. P. and Park, G. R. (1986). Pharmacokinetics of morphine in two children before and after liver transplantation. *Br. J. Anaesth.* **58**, 1218.

Shoeman, D. W. and Azarnoff, D. L. (1972). The alterations of plasma proteins in uremia as reflected by their ability to bind digitoxin and diphenylhydratoin. *Pharmacology* **7**, 169.

Sidi, A., Kaplan, R. F. and Davis, R. F. (1990). Prolonged neuromuscular blockade and ventilatory failure after renal transplantation and cyclosporine. *Can. J. Anaesth.* **37**, 543.

Sloan, P. A., Mather, L. E., McLean, C. F., *et al.* (1991). Physiological disposition of intravenous morphine in sheep. *Br. J. Anaesth.* **67**, 378.

Smith, M. T., Watt, J. A. and Cramond, T. (1990). Morphine-3-glucuronide: a potent antagonist of morphine analgesia. *Life Sci.* **47**, 579.

Solomonson, M. D., Johnson, M. E. and Ilstrup, D. (1994). Risk factors in patients having surgery to create an arteriovenous fistula. *Anesth. Analg.* **79**, 694.

Somogyi, A. A., Shanks, C. A. and Triggs, E. J. (1977). The effect of renal failure on the disposition and neuromuscular blocking action of pancuronium bromide. *Eur. J. Clin. Pharmacol.* **12**, 23.

Stanley, T. H. and Lathrop, G. D. (1977). Urinary excretion of morphine during and after valvular and coronary-artery surgery. *Anesthesiology* **46**, 166.

Starsnic, M. A., Goldberg, M. E., Ritter, D. E., Marr, A. T., Sosis, M. and Larijani, G. E. (1989). Does vecuronium accumulate in the renal transplant patient? *Can. J. Anaesth.* **36**, 35.

Stone, J. G., Foex, P., Sear, J. W., Johnson, L. L., Khambatta, H. J. and Triner, L. (1988). Myocardial ischemia in untreated hypertensive patients: effect of a single small oral dose of a beta-adrenergic blocking agent. *Anesthesiology* **68**, 495.

Strunin, L. (1966). Some aspects of anaesthesia for renal homotransplantation. *Br. J. Anaesth.* **38**, 812.

Szenohradszky, J., Caldwell, J. E., Wright, P. M. C., *et al.* (1999). Influence of renal failure on the pharmacokinetics and neuromuscular blocking effects of a single dose of rapacuronium bromide. *Anesthesiology* **90**, 24.

Szenohradszky, J., Fisher, D. M., Segredo, V., *et al.* (1992). Pharmacokinetics of rocuronium bromide (ORG 9426) in patients with normal renal function or patients undergoing cadaver renal transplantation. *Anesthesiology* **77**, 899.

Szeto, H. H., Inturrisi, C. E., Houde, R., Saal, S., Cheigh, J. and Reidenberg, M. (1977). Accumulation of normeperidine, an active metabolite of meperidine in patients with renal failure or cancer. *Ann. Intern. Med.* **86**, 738.

Tesi, R. J., Elkhammas, E. A., Davies, E. A., Henry, M. L. and Ferguson, R. M. (1994). Renal transplantation in older people. *Lancet* **343**, 461.

Vandam, L. D., Harrison, J. H., Murray, J. E. and Merrill, J. P. (1962). Anesthetic aspects of renal homotransplantation in man. *Anesthesiology* **23**, 783.

Verbeeck, R., Tjandramanga, T. B., Verberckmoes, R. and de Schepper, P. J. (1976). Biotransformation and excretion of lorazepam in patients with chronic renal failure. *Br. J. Clin. Pharmacol.* **3**, 1033.

Verbeeck, R. V., Tjandramanga, T. B., Verberckmoes, R. and de Schepper, P. J. (1981). Impaired elimination of lorazepam following subchronic administration in two patients with renal failure. *Br. J. Clin. Pharmacol.* **12**, 749.

Vinik, H. R., Reves, J. G., Greenblatt, D. J., Abernethy, D. R. and Smith, L. R. (1983). The pharmacokinetics of midazolam in chronic renal failure patients. *Anesthesiology* **59**, 390.

Ward, S., Boheimer, N., Weatherley, B. C., Simmonds, R. J. and Dopson, T. A. (1987). Pharmacokinetics of atracurium and its metabolites in patients with normal renal function, and in patients in renal failure. *Br. J. Anaesth.* **59**, 697.

Way, W. L., Miller, R. D., Hamilton, W. K. and Layzer, R. B. (1972). Succinylcholine-induced hyperkalemia in patients with renal failure? *Anesthesiology* **36**, 138.

Weimar, W., Geerlings, S. W., Bijnen, A. B., *et al.* (1983). A controlled study on the effect of mannitol on immediate renal function after cadaver donor kidney transplantation. *Transplantation* **35**, 99.

Weir, P. H. C. and Chung, F. F. (1984). Anaesthesia for patients with chronic renal disease. *Can. Anaesth. Soc. J.* **31**, 468.

Wickstrom, I. (1981). Enflurane anaesthesia in living donor renal transplantation. *Acta Anaesthesiol. Scand.* **25**, 263.

Wiggum, D. C., Cork, R. C., Weldon, S. T., Gandolfi, A. J. and Perry, D. S. (1985). Postoperative respiratory depression and elevated sufentanil levels in a patient with chronic renal failure. *Anesthesiology* **63**, 708.

Williams, B. (1994). Insulin resistance: the shape of things to come. *Lancet* **344**, 521.

Winearls, C. G., Oliver, D. O., Pippard, M. J., Reid. C., Downing, M. R. and Cotes, P. M. (1986). Effect of human erythropoietin derived from recombinant DNA on the anaemia of patients maintained by chronic haemodialysis. *Lancet* **2**, 1175.

Woolner, D. F., Winter, D., Frendin, T. J., Begg, E. J., Lynn, K. L. and Wright, G. J. (1986). Renal failure does not impair the metabolism of morphine. *Br. J. Clin. Pharmacol.* **22**, 55.

Wright, M. R., Axelson, J. E., Rurak, D. W., *et al.* (1988). Effect of haemodialysis on metoclopramide kinetics in patients with severe renal failure. *Br. J. Clin. Pharmacol.* **26**, 474.

Wyant, G. M. (1967). The anaesthetist looks at tissue transplantation: three years' experience with kidney transplants. *Can. Anaesth. Soc. J.* **14**, 255.

Zaleski, L., Abello, D. and Gold, M. I. (1993). Desflurane versus isoflurane in patients with chronic hepatic and renal disease. *Anesth. Analg.* **76**, 353.

14

Early Course of the Patient with a Kidney Transplant

Stuart J. Knechtle • John D. Pirsch

Introduction

A successful long-term outcome for a new kidney transplant recipient depends on the early perioperative management and course after surgery. Important factors affecting long-term outcome include the occurrence of delayed graft function (Cecka, 1998; Troppmann et al., 1995), episodes of acute rejection (Cecka, 1998), early surgical complications (Aultman et al., 1999) such as obstruction, urine leak or vascular complications and sepsis (Almond et al., 1993). Toxicity from calcineurin inhibitors can lead to chronic transplant nephropathy later in the posttransplantation course. Donor and recipient factors affect long-term outcome, particularly the use of marginal donors (Cho, 1999) or highly sensitized recipients. The early management and amelioration of risk factors in the immediate postoperative period may lessen their long-term negative impact and improve outcome.

Overview

PERIOPERATIVE MANAGEMENT

Management of the transplant recipient begins in the immediate preoperative period. An initial assessment of the recipient includes a careful assessment of pretransplant fluid status to determine the need for dialysis and a careful physical examination to exclude potential contraindications to transplantation, such as significant cardiac disease or vascular insufficiency, which could preclude successful surgery. Knowledge of the donor status also is helpful in the early postoperative management of the transplant recipient. With an ideal donor or a living-related recipient, the expected outcome is an immediately functioning transplant that may preclude posttransplant dialysis. Marginal or older donors have a higher likelihood of delayed graft function, which can lead to volume overload and the need for urgent dialysis (Cho, 1999). Technical considerations include the need for vascular reconstruction, which may prolong surgery and contribute to postoperative delayed graft function. Recipient factors also affect the early postoperative course. Significant risk factors for early posttransplant dysfunction include pretransplant sensitization, obesity, younger or older age and patients with anatomic considerations that complicate the surgery.

In the early perioperative period, attention to fluid and electrolyte balance is crucial. Careful monitoring of urine output is essential, and any decrease in urine flow must be evaluated carefully. A decrease in urine volume may be due to acute tubular necrosis, hypovolemia, urinary leak, ureteric obstruction or, most significantly, vascular thrombosis. Assessment of the patient's volume status with the measurement of central venous pressure helps eliminate hypovolemia as a cause of decreasing urine output. Delayed graft function

(DGF) can be ascertained further with a nuclear scan or duplex ultrasonography to assess perfusion of the graft and to exclude renal artery or vein thrombosis. Duplex ultrasonography also allows the diagnosis of a urinary complication.

Measures to decrease the likelihood of DGF often are used during the operative procedure and in the perioperative period. Maintenance of adequate blood pressure and fluid status may be accomplished with intravenous albumin (Davidson et al., 1992) or crystalloid, the latter being preferable. Shorter cold ischemia or pulsatile perfusion of the donor organ also may decrease the likelihood of postoperative DGF. Some centers have used intraarterial calcium channel blockers, such as verapamil, to improve renal blood flow (Davidson et al., 1989). It is common practice to administer mannitol (12.5 g) around 10 minutes before the kidney is reperfused, which helps to trigger an osmotic diuresis and might be protective. Oral calcium channel blockers have been used to decrease the incidence of DGF (Dawidson et al., 1990). There is controversy about the early initiation of calcineurin inhibitors because of the potential for nephrotoxicity. Some centers delay the use of calcineurin inhibitors until there is established diuresis. If additional immunosuppression is desired, polyclonal or monoclonal anti–T cell antibodies may be used.

GRAFT DYSFUNCTION

Early complications of renal transplantation may be mechanical/surgical or medical. Early medical problems are commoner than posttransplant surgical problems (Table 14–1). The commonest early posttransplant medical problem is DGF. Delayed graft function occurs in 20% of patients from ideal cadaver donors and nearly 40% of patients with donors older than age 55 (Cecka, 1999). After or concomitant with DGF, acute rejection may become a significant clinical problem (Shoskes and Cecka, 1998; Troppmann et al., 1995; Woo et al., 1999). Other reasons for early medical complications

TABLE 14–1

EARLY SURGICAL AND MEDICAL COMPLICATIONS AFTER TRANSPLANTATION

Surgical/Mechanical	Medical
Obstruction	Acute rejection
Hematuria	Delayed graft function
Urinoma	Acute cyclosporine/tacrolimus nephrotoxicity
Arterial stenosis	Prerenal/volume contraction
Arterial thrombosis	Drug toxicity
Renal vein thrombosis	Infection
Postoperative hemorrhage	Recurrent disease
Lymphocele	

include acute cyclosporine or tacrolimus nephrotoxicity, prerenal azotemia, other drug toxicity, infection and early recurrent disease. A relatively uncommon but serious posttransplant medical problem is hemolytic uremic syndrome. This syndrome may be induced by rejection or as a secondary event from cyclosporine or tacrolimus therapy.

Mechanical problems usually are the result of complications of surgery or specific donor factors, such as multiple arteries, that lead to posttransplant dysfunction. Mechanical/surgical factors include obstruction of the transplant, hematuria, urine leak or urinoma and vascular problems, such as renal artery or vein stenosis or thrombosis. Postoperative bleeding is another potential complication that may cause compression of the transplant because the transplant usually is placed in the retroperitoneal space. Posttransplant lymphoceles are another common cause of early transplant dysfunction. Lymph drainage from transected lymph vessels accumulates in the perivascular and periureteral space and can cause ureteral obstruction or lower extremity swelling from iliac vein compression.

Surgical Complications

URINARY PROBLEMS

Urinary Obstruction

After implantation of a living donor kidney transplant, urine output begins immediately or within minutes. (See also Chapter 29 for a more complete discussion of urinary problems.) The same is not generally true of cadaveric kidneys, in which urine output may not be apparent for 1 hour or more after implantation and may be sluggish or nonexistent for days if the kidney has been injured (DGF) by donor factors or preservation. If a kidney that was formerly making urine slows down or stops and does not respond to

fluid administration, urinary obstruction has to be considered in the differential diagnosis. Initial evaluation is to check the patient's vital signs and central venous pressure to ensure adequate hydration and to check that the Foley catheter is functioning correctly. Obstruction of the Foley catheter by blood clots may occur easily and should be cleared by gentle irrigation. If these problems are not present, renal transplant ultrasound is the fastest, most accurate, and least expensive test to assess the renal pelvis for obstruction. Pelvicaliceal dilatation by ultrasound implies distal obstruction. If the bladder is collapsed rather than full, the problem is likely to be ureteral obstruction. Treatment should be immediate decompression of the renal transplant pelvis by percutaneous insertion of a nephrostomy tube. Subsequently (usually 1 or 2 days later to allow blood and edema to clear after nephrostomy tube placement), a nephrogram can be done to evaluate the ureter for stenosis or obstruction. The diagnosis is confirmed by a fall in the serum creatinine after decompression of the renal pelvis.

After the Foley catheter is removed, the commonest cause of urinary obstruction is not ureteral stenosis but rather bladder dysfunction. This cause is particularly common in diabetic patients with neurogenic bladders. Initial management is replacement of the Foley catheter and a trial of an α-blocker, such as doxazosin or terazosin. If bladder dysfunction persists after one or two such trials, it may be necessary to start intermittent self-catheterization. In rare instances in which bladder dysmotility is severe and urinary tract infections are common, it may be preferable to drain the transplant ureter into an ileal conduit to the anterior abdominal wall. Ideally the patient with a neurogenic bladder should have been evaluated before transplantation with urodynamic studies and a decision made about management at that time (see Chapters 4 and 12).

During the first 1 or 2 weeks posttransplant, obstruction usually is due to a technical problem related to surgery. If a

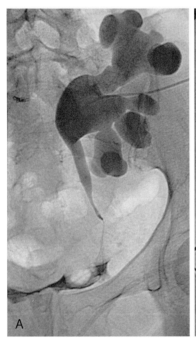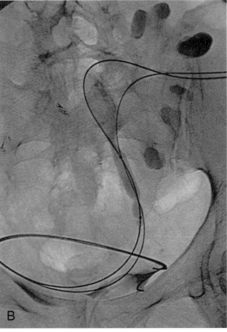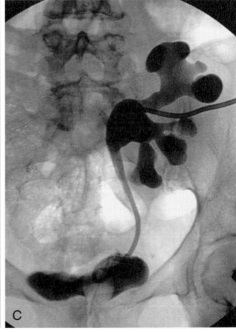

FIGURE 14–1

This patient presented with an elevated creatinine level. Ultrasound showed pelvicaliceal dilatation. A percutaneous nephrostomy tube was placed, and the following day a nephrostogram (A) was obtained. (B) The midureteral stenosis was crossed successfully with a guidewire, and the ureter was dilated with a balloon (the waist of the dilated balloon corresponds to the stricture). Subsequently a double-J stent was placed from the renal pelvis into the bladder across the dilated stricture (C).

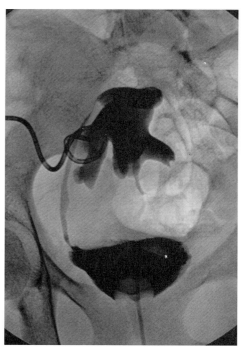

FIGURE 14–2

This intraabdominal kidney transplant was found by ultrasound to be obstructed. A nephrostomy tube was placed, and a nephrostogram was obtained the following day. The kidney had rotated medially and twisted the ureter proximally. The patient was managed operatively by placing the kidney laterally in a retroperitoneal pocket and performing a ureteroureterostomy using the ipsilateral native ureter.

ureteral stent was placed at the time of surgery, it is highly unusual to have obstruction. Possible explanations for obstruction are a twisted ureter or anastomotic narrowing. Generally, obstructions appear several weeks postoperatively, after the stent has been removed, and occur most frequently at the anastomosis between ureter and bladder (Ghasemian *et al.*, 1996). Usually, these can be crossed by a guidewire and dilated percutaneously by an interventional radiologist (Fig. 14–1). If the stenosis visualized by the nephrostogram shows a long (>2 cm) stricture, especially a proximal or midureteral stricture, it is likely that the problem is not amenable to balloon dilatation and that surgical repair is necessary (Fig. 14–2). The operation of choice for a long stricture or one that has failed balloon dilatation is ureteroureterostomy or ureteropyelostomy using the ipsilateral native ureter. The spatulated ends of the transplant and native ureters are anastomosed using running 5–0 absorbable suture. This anastomosis can be done over a 7F double-J stent, which is left in place for 4 to 6 weeks. If no ipsilateral ureter is available, it may be necessary to use contralateral ureter. If neither is available, alternatives include bringing the bladder closer to the kidney using a psoas hitch or fashioning a Boari flap (del Pizzo *et al.*, 1998), but these measures are rarely necessary. Another method is endoureterotomy (Erturk *et al.*, 1999), although experience with this method is limited.

Even if urinary obstruction is clinically silent (i.e., the patient is asymptomatic with a normal creatinine value), urinary obstruction manifested by dilatation of the pelvis and calyces on ultrasound should be treated because it ultimately leads to thinning of the renal cortex and loss of renal function. Urinary obstruction should be treated immediately to minimize damage to the transplanted kidney.

Bleeding into the Urinary System

Gross hematuria is common immediately postoperatively because of surgical manipulation of the bladder. The Leadbetter-Politano procedure for ureteroneocystostomy is associated with more hematuria compared with the extravesical approach typified by the Lich technique. The advantage of this technique is that it effectively prevents reflux and can be done with excellent long-term results. Occasionally, continuous bladder irrigation is necessary if gross hematuria is associated with clots, although intermittent manual irrigation usually is adequate. Obstruction of the bladder outlet by a blood clot is an emergency; vigilant nursing care is required to ensure that it does not occur. It is preferable not to distend the bladder in the immediate postoperative period to avoid disrupting the bladder sutures or causing a leak, and continuous bladder irrigation and cystoscopy ideally are avoided. Minor hematuria without clots is common in the first day or two regardless of the surgical method of ureteroneocystostomy and does not require treatment; it resolves over time without specific treatment.

Urine Leak

A leak of urine from the transplanted kidney in the early postoperative period may be clinically obvious if it presents with abdominal pain, a rising creatinine, and fall in urine output. Urine in the peritoneal cavity causes peritonitis and pain. More commonly, assuming that the kidney was placed in the retroperitoneal position, a urinoma collects around the kidney and bladder and causes a bulge in the wound and pain with direct displacement of adjacent viscera, including the bladder. The diagnosis should be suspected if the serum creatinine is rising (or not falling appropriately). Adjunctive tests to help make the diagnosis of urine leak, if it is not obvious clinically, include a renal scan, which would show urine in the retroperitoneal space surrounding the bladder or around loops of bowel, or an ultrasound, which would show a fluid collection outside the bladder and which aspirated has a high creatinine. Urine leak generally is due to a surgical problem with the ureteroneocytostomy or ischemic necrosis of the distal ureter. This leak should be repaired surgically immediately because the risk of wound infection increases with delay in treating this complication.

VASCULAR PROBLEMS
Arterial Stenosis

Transplant renal artery stenosis may present in the early postoperative period by (1) fluid retention, (2) elevated creatinine and (3) hypertension (Fervenza *et al.*, 1998; Wong *et al.*, 1996). (See also Chapters 28 and 30 for a more complete discussion of vascular problems.) Commonly the patient does not tolerate taking cyclosporine or FK506 because these drugs exacerbate the already existing ischemia at the glomerular arteriolar level. The aforementioned triad of clinical findings need not all be present, and the diagnosis should be suspected for any one of the three clinical reasons. If the creatinine is greater than 2 mg/dl, renal arteriography is best avoided because of the nephrotoxicity of the contrast dye. Magnetic resonance imaging angiography usually can give accurate delineation of the arterial anatomy. Ultrasound also is safe but not particularly discriminating and of help only if jetting of flow is seen.

As the population of renal transplant recipients has become increasingly older and included more diabetic patients and patients with vascular disease, transplant renal artery pseudostenosis has become increasingly common. Pseudostenosis refers to arterial stenosis in the iliac artery proximal to the implantation of the transplant renal artery. Although the anastomosis and renal artery may be completely normal, the problem is high renin output by the transplanted kidney resulting from its hypoperfusion.

Treatment of transplant renal artery stenosis and pseudostenosis includes balloon dilatation and surgery. In general, ostial stenosis, long areas of stenosis, and stenosis in tortuous arteries difficult to access radiographically are not treated as successfully with balloon dilatation as with surgery. Stenoses within smaller branches of the renal artery may be treatable only by angioplasty. Iliac artery disease causing pseudostenosis may be treated by angioplasty, but the risk is present of embolization or dissection causing thrombosis or further ischemia. Surgical options include bypass of the stenosis using autologous saphenous vein, a prosthetic graft, or an allogeneic arterial graft procured from a cadaveric donor. The risk of the procedure has to be weighed against the potential benefit of improving renal transplant blood flow. In addition to the serum creatinine, a biopsy may be useful to assess the quality of the renal parenchyma. In situations of advanced chronic rejection with a creatinine value greater than 2.5 mg/dl for more than a month, it may not be prudent to repair such arteries. Figure 14–3 shows a renal artery stenosis in the lower pole artery that was managed successfully by balloon angioplasty.

Arterial Thrombosis

Renal transplant arterial thrombosis usually occurs early (within 30 days) posttransplant (Penny et al., 1994) but should be a rare event because it is generally due to a technical error at the time of surgery. It usually is related to an intimal injury to the donor kidney during procurement or to anastomotic narrowing or iliac artery injury during implantation. Kidneys from donors less than 5 years of age have been associated with a higher risk of thrombosis (Singh et al., 1997). The kidney tolerates only 30 to 60 minutes of warm ischemia before it is irreversibly injured, making difficult the diagnosis and correction of this problem before it is too late to salvage the kidney. The diagnosis should be suspected in a patient who is hours to days posttransplant with a good urine output who has a sudden drop in urine output to zero. A high degree of suspicion has to be present, and the patient should be returned to the operating room promptly. If the patient

had urine output preoperatively from the native kidneys, the diagnosis is hard to make in a timely manner because urine output may continue after the renal transplant has thrombosed. The advantage of diagnostic ultrasound has to be weighed against the disadvantage of delaying a return to the operating room. Almost all kidney transplants with arterial thrombosis are lost because of ischemic injury.

In cases of more than one renal transplant artery in which arterial reconstruction is performed at implantation, there may be increased risk of thrombosis of one or more arteries. This increased risk is particularly a concern if there is a small accessory renal artery supplying the lower pole of the kidney and providing the ureteral blood supply. Thrombosis of a branch artery may present as a rise in serum creatinine associated with increased hypertension. Angiography shows partial thrombosis and loss of perfusion of a wedge-shaped section of renal parenchyma. The risk of this situation, in addition to potential long-term hypertension, is calyceal infarction and urine leak in the early postoperative period. Such kidneys, with partial infarction, generally can be salvaged. Urine leaks occurring through the outer cortex of the kidney after partial infarction may be managed by nephrostomy tube placement for urinary drainage and placement of another drain adjacent to the kidney to prevent a urinoma. In cases in which the transplant ureter necroses as a result of arterial ischemia, alternative urinary drainage needs to be provided surgically; this would be managed most often by ureteropyelostomy using the ipsilateral native ureter.

Renal Vein Thrombosis

Renal vein thrombosis may occur in cases in which the donor renal vein was narrowed by repair of an injury or in which the vein was twisted or compressed externally, but it may occur in the absence of a technical complication. The diagnosis is indicated by sudden onset of gross hematuria and fall in urine output, associated with pain and swelling over the graft. Ultrasound shows absence of flow in the renal vein, diastolic reversal of flow in the renal artery (Fig. 14–4) and an enlarged kidney often with surrounding blood. Ultrasound can point to this diagnosis definitively. Only if it is immediately recognized and repaired can this problem be reversible. Immediate surgical repair of the vein and control of bleeding are required, and it is generally necessary to remove the kidney and revise the venous anastomosis. Bleed-

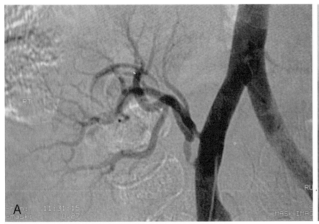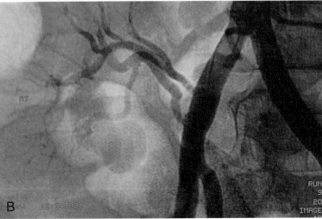

FIGURE 14–3

This patient presented with fluid retention, hypertension and an elevated creatinine level. (A) An arteriogram showed that the artery to the lower pole arising from a common aortic patch was stenotic proximally. This stenosis was successfully treated with balloon angioplasty (B) with resolution of the patient's symptoms.

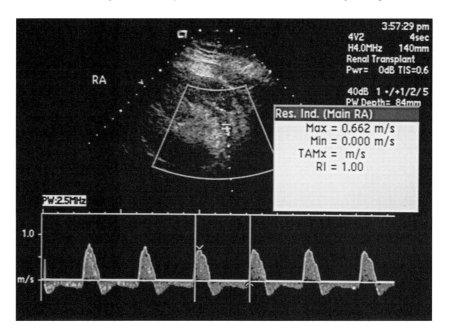

FIGURE 14–4

Ultrasound shows absence of flow in the renal vein and reversal of diastolic flow in the renal artery. This kidney was enlarged to 14 cm in length with a surrounding fluid collection that represented blood. These ultrasound findings were pathognomonic of transplant renal vein thrombosis. The condition was treated surgically with excision of the kidney, placement of a venous extension graft using donor iliac vein obtained from a third-party donor and reimplantation of the kidney. Three weeks later, the patient had a normally functioning kidney transplant.

ing from the swollen and cracked kidney surface usually can be controlled with hemostatic agents.

POSTOPERATIVE BLEEDING

As with all surgery, postoperative bleeding may complicate renal transplant outcomes. Bleeding generally occurs during the first 24 to 48 hours after the transplant and is diagnosed by a falling hematocrit, swelling over the graft with a bulging incision or significant blood seepage from the incision. Most often, this bleeding occurs in patients taking anticoagulation agents for other medical problems. If the hematoma is not clinically obvious, an ultrasound or computed tomography scan can define its size and help determine whether or not surgical evacuation is appropriate. Treatment includes immediate surgery and blood transfusions as necessary.

Rejection During the Early Postoperative Period

HYPERACUTE REJECTION

If a renal transplant is performed in the setting of ABO mismatch or a positive lymphocytotoxic crossmatch, the risk of hyperacute rejection is 85%. It is interesting that the incidence is not 100%; this presumably is due to some antibodies having lower affinity or not binding complement. There is no effective treatment for hyperacute rejection. It may be possible to prevent it by plasmapheresis to remove preformed antibodies, but variable results have been reported. Cases of blood type A2 donors being transplanted to O recipients have been reported because A2 expresses less of the putative antigen, but this strategy also has increased risk of graft loss (Hanto et al., 1993). In almost all transplant centers, a crossmatch-negative, ABO-compatible recipient can be identified or the kidney shipped to a center that has such a patient awaiting a kidney. A hyperacutely rejected kidney has no perfusion on renal scan (because of microvascular thrombosis) and needs to be removed.

ACCELERATED VASCULAR REJECTION

Despite a negative T-cell crossmatch test preoperatively, some patients may develop an early aggressive form of rejec-

tion, termed *accelerated vascular rejection*. This rejection is seen most often in sensitized patients with a panel-reactive antibody that is high and in patients with a previous transplant. The time course of this type of rejection is typically within 2 to 5 days of the transplant, and it tends to be poorly responsive to steroids and occasionally resistant to all forms of antirejection therapy. Histologically, such patients have fibrin deposition evident in the renal transplant biopsy and endothelialitis. Although successful prophylaxis of rejection has been described using OKT3 in highly sensitized patients, once this form of rejection has started there is no standard treatment. We use plasmapheresis in this setting because of the likely contribution of the humoral immune response.

ACUTE REJECTION

The commonest form of immunological rejection in the early posttransplant period is acute cellular rejection, mediated predominantly by host lymphocytes responding to the allogeneic donor kidney. Acute rejection typically occurs 5 to 7 days posttransplant, but it can occur at virtually any time after this. The highest incidence of acute rejection is within the first 3 months, and overall rates of rejection vary from 10 to 50% within the first 6 months depending on HLA matching and the immunosuppressive protocol. The clinical harbingers of acute rejection include a rising creatinine, weight gain, fever and graft tenderness. Since the introduction of cyclosporine and FK506, the latter two signs are seldom present. The diagnostic gold standard is kidney biopsy, which can be performed safely under local anesthesia with light sedation. An 18-gauge biopsy needle is introduced under ultrasound guidance and removes a core of tissue that can be evaluated immediately for histologic criteria of rejection (see Chapter 24). These criteria include tubulitis (invasion of tubules by lymphocytes) and arteritis (Racusen et al., 1999).

First-line treatment of acute cellular rejection is bolus steroid therapy with methylprednisolone sodium succinate (Solu-Medrol). Many regimens are used successfully, but a typical dose and duration are 500 mg intravenously, followed by 250 mg the following day, then a daily taper by 30-mg increments. Another commonly used regimen is three intravenous boluses of 0.5 g or 1.0 g of methylprednisolone

24 hours apart. About 85 to 90% of acute cellular rejection episodes are steroid responsive. If the patient's serum creatinine has not begun to decrease by day 4 of therapy, alternative treatment needs to be considered, such as ALG or OKT3 as lymphocytotoxic therapy. Rejection that does not respond to treatment with steroids, ALG or OKT3 occurs in less than 5% of patients, although more frequently in sensitized patients or retransplants.

Patients who experience acute cellular rejection while taking cyclosporine or FK506 should have their calcineurin phosphatase inhibitor held during treatment of rejection because the rise in creatinine makes them more susceptible to nephrotoxicity by these drugs, and there is generally no need for them to be taking cyclosporine while they are on high-dose steroids or antilymphocyte therapy. This measure eliminates the possibility that a further rise of creatinine is due to cyclosporine or FK506 nephrotoxicity.

The impact of acute cellular rejection on graft survival depends on the response to treatment. Whether or not an early rejection episode predisposes the kidney to chronic rejection remains controversial.

Graft Loss

During the early posttransplant period, if a renal transplant loses perfusion because of thrombosis or because of hyperacute, acute or accelerated vascular rejection, it must be removed. Otherwise, the systemic toxicity of a necrotic kidney may cause fever, graft swelling or tenderness and generalized malaise. Loss of perfusion can be assessed by nuclear scan or Doppler ultrasound. The technically easiest way to perform a transplant nephrectomy depends on how long the kidney has been in place. If nephrectomy is done within 2 weeks, there are minimal adhesions, and the vessels are exposed easily for ligation and transplant nephrectomy. At later times, it is usually easiest to reopen the transplant incision and enter the subcapsular plane around the kidney. The kidney is dissected free in the subcapsular space, and a large vascular clamp is placed across the hilum. The kidney is amputated above the clamp, and 3–0 Prolene is used to oversew the hilar vessels. The ureter also is oversewn.

Medical Complications
DELAYED GRAFT FUNCTION

Other than hyperacute rejection, DGF is the earliest and most frequent posttransplant complication that can occur. Delayed graft function is an extremely important posttransplant complication, particularly because its occurrence has early and long-term consequences for allograft survival. The mechanism and cellular events that may cause DGF include donor factors, such as age, cause of death of the donor, and postischemic reperfusion injury with subsequent injury and activation of the immune system leading to an increased incidence of acute rejection (Land, 1998).

Delayed graft function is one of the main predictors of poor graft survival in cadaveric renal transplantation. Delayed graft function typically is defined as the need for dialysis during the first week after transplantation. The incidence of DGF is significantly higher in cadaveric versus living donor transplants and is less common in first cadaveric grafts versus patients undergoing repeat transplantation. An analysis of 91,218 renal transplants reported to the United Network for Organ Sharing (UNOS) Scientific Renal Transplant Registry between October 1987 and 1997 showed an incidence of approximately 25% for first cadaver donors versus

5% for living donors (Shoskes and Cecka, 1998). An increase in DGF has been noted with advancing donor age. Young donors have a lower incidence of DGF (approximately 20%) compared with donors older than age 55 (38%). Prolonged cold ischemia time, at least 30 hours, does not appear to have a significant impact on the incidence of DGF, unless there is an episode of rejection.

The diagnosis of DGF usually is apparent during the first 24 hours posttransplant. Although some kidneys may make urine initially, a falloff in urine output unresponsive to fluid challenge is the commonest clinical scenario indicating DGF. The major differential diagnostic consideration in a patient with falling or absent urine output is an acute vascular or urological complication. This differential diagnosis can be determined easily with urgent ultrasound or radionuclide renal scanning. Typically a transplant with DGF shows good renal perfusion, good parenchymal uptake of orthoiodohippurate (^{123}I OIH) or mercaptoacetyltriglycine (^{99m}Tc MAG 3) with poor or no renal excretion. Once the diagnosis of DGF is established, careful attention to fluid status is paramount to decrease the frequency and necessity for dialysis. The usual time course of DGF is 10 to 14 days, and patients may require supportive dialysis therapy for management of fluid and electrolyte disturbances.

The major concern for transplant recipients for DGF is the potential for early acute rejection. Data are accumulating that the development of DGF may lead to up-regulation of the immune system with release of cytokine and adhesion molecules (Fuggle and Koo, 1998; Land, 1998; see Chapter 25). This situation may lead to an anti-MHC-directed alloimmune response, leading to an increased frequency of acute rejection. The diagnosis of rejection in patients with DGF may be hindered because the primary clinical monitoring tool is a fall in serum creatinine. For this reason, some centers use antilymphocyte therapy, such as Thymoglobulin or Atgam, to prevent early acute rejection in patients with DGF. Alternatively, frequent biopsies of patients with DGF have been proposed as a way to detect early acute rejection episodes. An early acute rejection episode after DGF significantly lowers short-term and long-term survival. Graft half-lives with DGF and no rejection average 6.7 years compared with 9.5 years for patients without DGF or rejection (Shoskes and Cecka, 1998). Patients with DGF and acute rejection have a graft half-life of 6.5 years. Prevention of DGF and early recognition of rejection are important goals to help improve early and long-term graft survival.

NEPHROTOXICITY FROM CALCINEURIN INHIBITORS

Early institution of calcineurin inhibitors (cyclosporine and tacrolimus) after transplantation is important in the prevention of acute rejection episodes. Because of the potential for additive nephrotoxicity, however, some centers avoid instituting calcineurin inhibitors until there is adequate function of the transplanted kidney. Most centers that delay the onset of calcineurin inhibitors use some form of sequential antibody induction therapy with humanized or chimeric interleukin-2 receptor inhibitors such as daclizumab or basiliximab, polyclonal antibodies such as Thymoglobulin or Atgam or a monoclonal antibody such as OKT3. Other centers begin administering calcineurin inhibitors early in the posttransplant course whether or not the allograft is functioning well or in DGF. Both of the calcineurin inhibitors, cyclosporine and tacrolimus, are effective in preventing acute rejection episodes but clearly can lead to nephrotoxicity primarily by decreasing renal blood flow in the afferent arteriole, leading to tubular injury (Mason, 1990; Perico et al., 1992). Because of variability of intestinal absorption in the early transplant period, underdosing and overdosing of these agents is common, which can lead to rejection episodes or cyclosporine nephrotoxicity or both events occurring in the same patient. Although there are many clinical parameters that have been advocated to differentiate calcineurin inhibitor nephrotoxicity from rejection, most clinical parameters are not of sufficient sensitivity to predict confidently the cause of the transplant dysfunction. In patients with DGF, it may be more difficult to diagnose acute rejection or calcineurin nephrotoxicity reliably. Monitoring cyclosporine and tacrolimus levels is of value in preventing significant increases in blood levels, which may lead to nephrotoxicity. Some centers routinely employ a high-dose calcineurin inhibitor protocol to prevent rejection and accept a certain level of nephrotoxicity as a consequence.

The most reliable way of differentiating calcineurin nephrotoxicity from rejection is percutaneous renal allograft biopsy. Generally, biopsies can be performed 3 to 5 days posttransplant using real-time ultrasonic imaging and automated biopsy needle devices. The histological hallmarks of calcineurin nephrotoxicity vary. Early functional nephrotoxicity is manifested most often by evidence of tubular injury. In patients with established calcineurin nephrotoxicity, lowering the dose or temporary discontinuation of cyclosporine or tacrolimus can lead to reversal of the renal injury.

The avoidance of subclinical or clinical episodes of nephrotoxicity may be important in terms of long-term allograft histology (Solez et al., 1998). A study that examined 2-year biopsy specimens of tacrolimus-treated and cyclosporine-treated recipients showed that chronic transplant nephropathy and fibrosis strongly correlate with episodes of early clinical nephrotoxicity from these agents. This study led to a reexamination of calcineurin-sparing protocols, and clinical studies are now in progress.

PRERENAL AND VOLUME CONTRACTION

Prerenal azotemia or volume contraction often may lead to allograft deterioration during the immediate postoperative period. Excessive use of diuretics and uncontrolled blood glucose are two of the commonest causes for the development of prerenal azotemia from volume contraction. Because most of these patients already are receiving calcineurin inhibitors, which decrease renal blood flow, the concomitant insult of volume contraction may lead to an elevated blood urea nitrogen and serum creatinine, which may be difficult to distinguish from an episode of acute rejection. Careful attention to daily weights, intake and output, and assessment of orthostatic blood pressure changes can diagnose reliably volume contraction as a contributing factor for renal allograft dysfunction. Volume repletion with intravenous or oral fluids is indicated.

OTHER DRUG TOXICITY

Transplant patients often have complex pharmacological regimens at the time of transplantation, which may include nephrotoxic medications or medications that may cause concomitant nephrotoxicity with calcineurin inhibitors (Lake and Canafax, 1995; Trotter, 1998). Examples of the former include nonsteroidal antiinflammatory drugs, nephrotoxic antibiotics such as amphotericin and aminoglycosides. Drugs that may interact with the metabolism of calcineurin inhibitors include calcium channel blockers such as diltiazem and verapamil, ketoconazole, erythromycin and fluconazole. Tacrolimus and cyclosporine are metabolized in the P450-3A4 system, and all of these agents may increase the blood levels of tacrolimus or cyclosporine. Grapefruit juice also has been shown to

increase the gastrointestinal absorption of cyclosporine. Routine drug level monitoring is paramount when drugs that are metabolized in the P450-3A4 system are used. Adjustment in the daily dose of cyclosporine and tacrolimus to attain therapeutic blood levels may help prevent episodes of nephrotoxicity from the concomitant use of these agents. Avoidance of concomitant medications that interfere with drug metabolism is desirable. Another class of pharmacological agents that need to be used with care include selective serotonin reuptake inhibitor antidepressants. In particular, Nefazodone and Fluvoxamine are metabolized in the P450-3A4 system and may increase calcineurin blood levels.

RECURRENT DISEASE

Most causes of renal failure do not recur in the transplant kidney; when they do, it is usually later in the posttransplant course. (See also Chapters 4 and 24 for further discussion of recurrent disease.) Two diseases may occur in the immediate posttransplant period and lead to significant graft dysfunction or graft loss if not treated aggressively. Focal glomerulosclerosis is the commonest glomerulonephritis that can recur in the immediate postoperative period (Artero et al., 1992, 1994). Presumably a *serum factor* is present that causes glomerular injury and massive early proteinuria (Savin et al., 1996). It is relatively uncommon but may occur immediately posttransplant. The diagnosis is established by the development of nephrotic range of proteinuria in a patient with a pretransplant diagnosis of focal segmental glomerulosclerosis (FSGS) and is confirmed on biopsy. Electron microscopy shows diffuse foot process effacement, which is diagnostic in this setting. Various strategies have been employed to treat recurrent FSGS, including high-dose calcineurin inhibitors, prednisone and plasmapheresis. Currently, plasmapheresis appears to be most effective in the treatment of recurrent FSGS; however, some patients may have only a partial remission or not respond to this modality (Artero et al., 1994). The usual course of therapy is 9 to 10 plasmapheresis treatments over several weeks. In some cases, plasma exchange may need to be repeated if there is an initial response and subsequent relapse. If patients do not have any response, it is unlikely that additional plasmapheresis therapy would be effective.

The other recurrent disease of concern in the immediate postoperative period is hemolytic uremic syndrome (Ducloux et al., 1998; Kaplan et al., 1998; Singh et al., 1996). Hemolytic uremic syndrome is multifactorial in origin. It is characterized clinically by a fall in hematocrit and/or platelet count with evidence of a microangiopathic process on peripheral blood smear, increased lactate dehydrogenase and transplant allograft dysfunction. Kidney biopsy specimens show fibrin clot in the small arterioles of the kidney. Hemolytic uremic syndrome has been noted to be induced by tacrolimus or cyclosporine. Discontinuation of the calcineurin inhibitor and plasmapheresis (Kaplan, 1999) have been beneficial in some series. The use of anticoagulants and aspirin is of uncertain benefit.

INFECTION

In the immediate postoperative period, most infections are related to the surgical procedure and usually involve wound infection, bacteremia from a central line, urinary tract infection or pneumonia (Rubin, 1998). (See also Chapter 31 for a complete discussion of infection.) Prevention of these infections involves meticulous surgical technique, careful line care and use, removal of the Foley catheter as soon as it is possible and early mobilization of the patient to prevent atelectasis or pneumonia. Most opportunistic infections do not occur until after the first 30 days. Of the opportunistic infections, cytomegalovirus is still common after transplant, particularly in recipients who are seronegative for cytomegalovirus and who receive seropositive organs. Epstein-Barr virus infection may occur early after transplantation and usually is related to heightened immunosuppression in a previously seronegative patient. In the past, *Pneumocystis carinii* pneumonia was a frequent complication of transplantation; however, most centers now employ routine prophylaxis with trimethoprim/sulfamethoxazole, which has nearly eliminated the occurrence of this infection in transplant patients. Other prophylactic strategies that have been employed include intravenous ganciclovir in the immediate postoperative period followed by high-dose oral acyclovir or oral ganciclovir for at least 3 months. The antiviral agents are effective at reducing the incidence and severity of cytomegalovirus infection (particularly oral ganciclovir); however, after stopping ganciclovir, cytomegalovirus may still occur. Other prophylactic agents include antifungal agents, such as fluconazole or clotrimazole troches, which can reduce the risk of mucosal *Candida* superinfection.

Highly resistant organisms have been detected with increasing frequency in transplant patients. Vancomycin-resistant *Enterococcus* (VREC) (Newell *et al.*, 1998; Orloff *et al.*, 1999; Papanicolaou *et al.*, 1996) and *Candida* (Nampoory *et al.*, 1996; Paya, 1993; Pirsch *et al.*, 1998) infections are becoming significant causes of morbidity in hospitalized transplant patients. Risk factors for VREC include prolonged hospitalization in the intensive care unit, extensive surgical procedures and intraabdominal infection. Treatment options for this infection are limited. Quinupristin/dalfopristin (Synercid), an investigational antibiotic, may be useful for control of serious VREC infections. The increase in *Candida* infection appears to be due to the routine use of clotrimazole or fluconazole to prevent *Candida* infection. Intravenous antibiotic pressure predisposes patients to fungal infection after transplantation.

Once an infection has occurred, aggressive management is indicated. This management may include removal of central venous catheters or Foley catheters. Any intraabdominal fluid collections should be aspirated and drained if found to be infected. Urinary tract infections should be treated promptly, preferably after the Foley catheter and ureteral stent have been removed.

HYPERTENSION

Hypertension develops in nearly 80% of renal transplant patients after transplantation (Curtis, 1993, 1994; First *et al.*, 1994; Pirsch and Friedman, 1994; Zeier *et al.*, 1998). (See also Chapter 30.) In kidney transplant recipients, hypertension may be due to intrinsic problems with the allograft (DGF, rejection, cyclosporine nephrotoxicity or donor allograft nephropathy) or due to extrinsic causes (hypertension from the native kidneys or familial hypertension). Because multiple causes may be present in the same patient, it often is difficult to ascertain the specific cause of hypertension after transplantation.

For some patients, hypertension is associated with immunosuppression. Cyclosporine, tacrolimus and corticosteroids all may contribute to the development of hypertension. Cyclosporine and tacrolimus cause afferent arteriole vasoconstriction, which may, in turn, stimulate the release of endothelin. Hypertension may ensue as a result of the activation of the renal angiotensin system. Patients with significant hypertension should be treated aggressively. Most centers prefer the use of calcium channel blockers and β-blockers as first-line agents, although angiotensin-converting enzyme inhibitors or angiotensin II receptor antagonists are being used more frequently. The major issue with the use of angiotensin-converting enzyme inhibitors or angiotensin II receptor inhibitors is anemia, which can be a problem in patients treated with calcineurin inhibitors. Patients who do not respond readily to antihypertensive therapy need to be evaluated further. Hypertension may be the result of renal artery or iliac artery stenosis, which may be compromising renal blood flow to the kidney and causing hypertension. A patient with a bruit over the transplant with poorly controlled hypertension and fluid retention needs to be evaluated carefully for renal artery or iliac artery stenosis. The advantages and potential side effects of antihypertensive agents in transplant recipients are shown in Table 14–2.

MANAGEMENT OF GRAFT DYSFUNCTION

The diagnosis and treatment of graft dysfunction are integral components of successful long-term management of the renal transplant recipient. Early diagnosis and directed therapy are crucial in the early posttransplant period to initiate

TABLE 14–2

ADVANTAGES AND POTENTIAL SIDE EFFECTS OF ANTIHYPERTENSIVE AGENTS IN TRANSPLANT RECIPIENTS

Class	Advantages/Indications	Side Effects
Diuretics	Salt-sensitive hypertension	Hyperuricemia Volume depletion
β-Blockers	Large selection Selective agents preferred	Adverse effect on lipids Relative contraindication with asthma, CHF, diabetes or peripheral vascular disease
α-Blockers	Useful with prostatic hypertrophy	Postural hypotension (first dose)
Central α-agonists	Clonidine useful in diabetic patients Clonidine available as transdermal patch	Dry mouth Rebound hypertension Fatigue
Calcium channel blockers	Improve renal blood flow May ameliorate cyclosporine nephrotoxicity	Drug interaction with cyclosporine (verapamil and diltiazem)
ACE inhibitors	Native kidney hypertension	May cause renal insufficiency Hyperkalemia
Angiotensin-receptor blockers	Proteinuria	Anemia

ACE = angiotensin-converting enzyme; CHF = congestive heart failure.

appropriate therapy and avoid potential overimmunosuppression. Evaluation of graft dysfunction should start with a careful history to see if there is a potential for nephrotoxicity from drugs or whether there is any likelihood of volume contraction contributing to the elevation of serum creatinine. A vigorous search for potential infection should follow, and if there is no obvious cause for deterioration in graft function, an ultrasound followed by a renal biopsy should be performed. If there is any clinical suspicion of renal artery or iliac artery stenosis, a magnetic resonance angiogram or arteriogram should be performed. The differentiation of calcineurin nephrotoxicity or rejection is ascertained most easily with percutaneous renal biopsy. Nephrotic range proteinuria in a patient whose original disease was FSGS or hemolytic uremic syndrome should prompt an immediate biopsy for diagnosis and potential treatment with plasmapheresis.

Summary

Optimization of outcomes after renal transplantation depends on rapid diagnosis and treatment of surgical and medical complications. In view of the invasiveness of the transplant procedure itself, the complexity of medical problems in this patient population and the side effects of nonspecific immunosuppressive therapy, close attention to the problems outlined in this chapter is crucial to avoid graft loss and patient death. Because the frequency of complications is greatest during the early posttransplant period, this is the time when vigilance should be highest.

REFERENCES

Almond, P. S., Matas, A., Gillingham, K., et al. (1993). Risk factors for chronic rejection in renal allograft recipients. *Transplantation* **55**, 752.

Artero, M., Biava, C., Amend, W., Tomlanovich, S. and Vincenti, F. (1992). Recurrent focal glomerulosclerosis: natural history and response to therapy. *Am. J. Med.* **92**, 375.

Artero, M. L., Sharma, R., Savin, V. J. and Vincenti, F. (1994). Plasmapheresis reduces proteinuria and serum capacity to injure glomeruli in patients with recurrent focal glomerulosclerosis. *Am. J. Kidney Dis.* **23**, 574.

Aultman, D. F., Sawaya, D. E., Zibari, G. B., et al. (1999). Are all successful renal transplants really successful? *Am. J. Kidney Dis.* **34**, 61.

Cecka, J. M. (1998). The UNOS Scientific Renal Transplant Registry—ten years of kidney transplants. *In Clinical Transplants 1997* (J. M. Cecka and P. I. Terasaki, eds.), p. 1, UCLA Tissue Typing Laboratory, Los Angeles.

Cecka, J. M. (1999). The UNOS Scientific Renal Transplant Registry. *In Clinical Transplants 1998* (J. M. Cecka and P. I. Terasaki, eds.), p. 1, UCLA Tissue Typing Laboratory, Los Angeles.

Cho, Y. W. (1999). Expanded criteria donors. *In Clinical Transplants 1998* (J. M. Cecka and P. I. Terasaki, eds.), p. 421, UCLA Tissue Typing Laboratory, Los Angeles.

Curtis, J. J. (1993). Management of hypertension after transplantation. *Kidney Int.* **43(Suppl.)**, S45.

Curtis, J. J. (1994). Hypertension following kidney transplantation. *Am. J. Kidney Dis.* **23**, 471.

Dawidson, I., Rooth, P., Alway, C., et al. (1990). Verapamil prevents posttransplant delayed function and cyclosporine A nephrotoxicity. *Transplant. Proc.* **22**, 1379.

Dawidson, I., Rooth, P., Fry, W. R., et al. (1989). Prevention of acute cyclosporine-induced renal blood flow inhibition and improved immunosuppression with verapamil. *Transplantation* **48**, 575.

Dawidson, I. J., Sandor, Z. F., Coorpender, L., et al. (1992). Intraoperative albumin administration affects the outcome of cadaver renal transplantation. *Transplantation* **53**, 774.

del Pizzo, J. J., Jacobs, S. C., Bartlett, S. T. and Sklar, G. N. (1998). The use of bladder for total transplant ureteral reconstruction. *J. Urol.* **159**, 750.

Ducloux, D., Rebibou, J. M., Semhoun-Ducloux, S., et al. (1998). Recurrence of hemolytic-uremic syndrome in renal transplant recipients: a meta-analysis. *Transplantation* **65**, 1405.

Erturk, E., Burzon, D. T. and Waldman, D. (1999). Treatment of transplant ureteral stenosis with endoureterotomy. *J. Urol.* **161**, 412.

Fervenza, F. C., Lafayette, R. A., Alfrey, E. J. and Petersen, J. (1998). Renal artery stenosis in kidney transplants. *Am. J. Kidney Dis.* **31**, 142.

First, M. R., Neylan, J. F., Rocher, L. L. and Tejani, A. (1994). Hypertension after renal transplantation. *J. Am. Soc. Nephrol.* **4(8 Suppl.)**, S30.

Fuggle, S. V. and Koo, D. D. (1998). Cell adhesion molecules in clinical renal transplantation. *Transplantation* **65**, 763.

Ghasemian, S. M. R., Guleria, A. S., Khawand, N. Y. and Light, J. A. (1996). Diagnosis and management of the urologic complications of renal transplantation. *Clin. Transplant.* **10**, 218.

Hanto, D. W., Brunt, E. M., Goss, J. A. and Cole, B. R. (1993). Accelerated acute rejection of an A2 renal allograft in an O recipient: association with an increase in anti-A2 antibodies. *Transplantation* **56**, 1580.

Kaplan, A. A. (1999). Therapeutic apheresis for renal disorders. *Ther. Apher.* **3**, 25.

Kaplan, B. S., Meyers, K. E. and Schulman, S. L. (1998). The pathogenesis and treatment of hemolytic uremic syndrome. *J. Am. Soc. Nephrol.* **9**, 1126.

Lake, K. D. and Canafax, D. M. (1995). Important interactions of drugs with immunosuppressive agents used in transplant recipients. *J. Antimicrob. Chemother.* **36(Suppl. B)**, 11.

Land, W. (1998). Postischemic reperfusion injury and kidney transplantation: prologue. *Transplant. Proc.* **30**, 4210.

Mason, J. (1990). Renal side-effects of cyclosporine. *Transplant. Proc.* **22**, 1280.

Nampoory, M. R., Khan, Z. U., Johny, K. V., et al. (1996). Invasive fungal infections in renal transplant recipients. *J. Infect.* **33**, 95.

Newell, K. A., Millis, J. M., Arnow, P. M., et al. (1998). Incidence and outcome of infection by vancomycin-resistant Enterococcus following orthotopic liver transplantation. *Transplantation* **65**, 439.

Orloff, S. L., Busch, A. M., Olyaei, A. J., et al. (1999). Vancomycin-resistant Enterococcus in liver transplant patients. *Am. J. Surg.* **177**, 418.

Papanicolaou, G. A., Meyers, B. R., Meyers, J., et al. (1996). Nosocomial infections with vancomycin-resistant Enterococcus faecium in liver transplant recipients: risk factors for acquisition and mortality. *Clin. Infect. Dis.* **23**, 760.

Paya, C. V. (1993). Fungal infections in solid-organ transplantation. *Clin. Infect. Dis.* **16**, 677.

Penny, M. J., Nankivell, B. J., Disney, A. P., Byth, K. and Chapman, J. R. (1994). Renal graft thrombosis: a survey of 134 consecutive cases. *Transplantation* **58**, 565.

Perico, N., Ruggenenti, P., Gaspari, F., et al. (1992). Daily renal hypoperfusion induced by cyclosporine in patients with renal transplantation. *Transplantation* **54**, 56.

Pirsch, J. D. and Friedman, R. (1994). Primary care of the renal transplant patient. *J. Gen. Intern. Med.* **9**, 29.

Pirsch, J. D., Odorico, J. S., D'Alessandro, A. M., et al. (1998). Posttransplant infection in enteric versus bladder-drained simultaneous pancreas-kidney transplant recipients. *Transplantation* **66**, 1746.

Racusen, L. C., Solez, K., Colvin, R. B., et al. (1999). The Banff 97 working classification of renal allograft pathology. *Kidney Int.* **55**, 713.

Rubin, R. H. (1998). Infectious diseases in transplantation/pre- and post-transplantation. *In Primer on Transplantation* (D. J. Norman and W. N. Suki, eds.), p. 141, American Society of Transplant Physicians, Thorofare, N.J.

Savin, V. J., Sharma, R., Sharma, M., et al. (1996). Circulating factor associated with increased glomerular permeability to albumin in recurrent focal segmental glomerulosclerosis. *N. Engl. J. Med.* **334**, 878.

Shoskes, D. A. and Cecka, J. M. (1998). Effect of delayed graft function on short- and long-term kidney graft survival. *In Clinical Transplants 1997* (J. M. Cecka and P. I. Terasaki, eds.), p. 297, UCLA Tissue Typing Laboratory, Los Angeles.

Singh, A., Stablein, D. and Tejani, A. (1997). Risk factors for vascular thrombosis in pediatric renal transplantation: a special report of the North American Pediatric Renal Transplant Cooperative Study. *Transplantation* **63**, 1263.

Singh, N., Gayowski, T. and Marino, I. R. (1996). Hemolytic uremic syndrome in solid-organ transplant recipients. *Transpl. Int.* **9**, 68.

Solez, K., Vincenti, F. and Filo, R. S. (1998). Histopathologic findings from 2-year protocol biopsies from a U.S. multicenter kidney transplant trial comparing tacrolimus versus cyclosporine: a report of the FK506 Kidney Transplant Study Group. *Transplantation* **66**, 1736.

Troppmann, C., Gillingham, K. J., Benedetti, E., *et al.* (1995). Delayed graft function, acute rejection, and outcome after cadaver renal transplantation: a multivariate analysis. *Transplantation* **59**, 962.

Trotter, J. F. (1998). Drugs that interact with immunosuppressive agents. *Semin. Gastrointest. Dis.* **9**, 147.

Wong, W., Fynn, S. P., Higgins, R. M., *et al.* (1996). Transplant renal artery stenosis in 77 patients—does it have an immunological cause? *Transplantation* **61**, 215.

Woo, Y. M., Jardine, A. G., Clark, A. F., *et al.* (1999). Early graft function and patient survival following cadaveric renal transplantation. *Kidney Int.* **55**, 692.

Zeier, M., Mandelbaum, A. and Ritz, E. (1998). Hypertension in the transplanted patient. *Nephron* **80**, 257.

Azathioprine and Steroids

Peter J. Morris

Introduction

Azathioprine and steroids were the backbone of immunosuppression in renal transplantation for many years and the only form of immunosuppression from the early 1960s to the early 1980s, when cyclosporine became available. After the introduction of cyclosporine, azathioprine and steroids were used in combination with cyclosporine or often after cessation of cyclosporine in so-called conversion protocols (see Chapter 16). One might wonder whether in the 5th edition of this book there still needs to be a chapter on azathioprine and steroids, bearing in mind the introduction of mycophenolate and the newer agent sirolimus, both of which are antiproliferative agents but with different mechanisms of action and which could replace azathioprine in immunosuppressive protocols (see Chapters 18 and 19). Azathioprine is an inexpensive agent, however, and it will continue to have a role in transplantation not only in the Western world in combination with cyclosporine but also, in particular, in developing countries where the cost of immunosuppression is a major factor in determining immunosuppressive protocols.

Steroids will continue to have a place in prevention of rejection and in the treatment of rejection. The introduction of more powerful immunosuppressive agents is allowing steroid-sparing protocols to be developed, however. As outlined later in this chapter, the complications of steroids are considerable, and a major aim of future immunosuppressive protocols will be to diminish the use of steroids.

6-Mercaptopurine was developed by Elion and Hitchings at Burroughs Wellcome as an anticancer agent in the 1950s (Elion et al., 1952, 1955). Subsequently, 6-mercaptopurine was shown to be an immunosuppressive agent by Schwartz and Dameshek (1959, 1960); it suppressed the humoral response to a foreign protein in rabbits and prolonged the survival of skin allografts in rabbits. The key paper by Schwartz and Dameshek on drug-induced immunological tolerance was noted by Calne (1960) in the United Kingdom and Zukoski et al. (1960) in the United States, and independently these investigators showed that 6-mercaptopurine could prevent rejection of renal allografts in dogs. In the original paper of Calne (1960), only two dogs survived the renal transplant operation for a short time, but when the dogs died from infection at a little more than a month posttransplantation, there was no histological evidence of rejection whatsoever, which was a unique finding. Similar results in a much larger series of experiments were published by Zukoski et al. (1960) from Richmond, Virginia. Soon after that, Elion et al. (1961, 1963) produced azathioprine, an imidazolyl derivative of 6-mercaptopurine, and this drug appeared to be somewhat less toxic than 6-mercaptopurine (Calne et al., 1962). Azathioprine first was used in the clinic at the Peter Bent Brigham Hospital, Boston, in 1961 (Murray et al., 1962, 1963). Soon thereafter, azathioprine was introduced into renal transplantation in a rapidly increasing number of renal transplant units throughout the world.

Steroids first were used to treat rejection (Goodwin et al., 1965) but then were added to azathioprine to prevent rejection from the time of transplantation because rejection seemed inevitable (Starzl et al., 1963). From the beginning of this so-called azathioprine era, arbitrarily large doses of steroids were given from the time of transplantation with a gradual reduction over 6 to 12 months to maintenance levels. The high doses of steroids used with azathioprine were responsible for most of the complications of transplantation (discussed later). It was not until the 1970s that a series of randomized trials as well as observational studies led slowly to the realization that low-dose steroids were as effective as high-dose steroids in preventing rejection and that there was a major reduction in steroid complications of transplantation with low-dose regimens. By the late 1970s, azathioprine and low-dose steroids, sometimes used together with an antilymphocyte serum or globulin for induction (particularly in North America), were the standard immunosuppressive therapy until the introduction of cyclosporine in the early 1980s.

Azathioprine
MECHANISM OF ACTION

Azathioprine and 6-mercaptopurine are thiopurines, and azathioprine is an imidazolyl derivative of 6-mercaptopurine. Azathioprine is metabolized in the liver before becoming active, and one metabolic pathway is through its conversion to 6-mercaptopurine, the active metabolite of 6-mercaptopurine being 6-thioinosinic acid. Azathioprine also is metabolized by other pathways independent of 6-mercaptopurine. Azathioprine inhibits DNA and RNA synthesis by preventing interconversion among the precursors of purine synthesis and suppressing de novo purine synthesis. Azathioprine and 6-mercaptopurine block proliferation in vitro and the production of interleukin-2, and this is probably an important aspect of its antiproliferative activity (Bach, 1975). Xanthine oxidase has an important role in the catabolism of 6-mercaptopurine, and if allopurinol is used with azathioprine, it is mandatory to reduce the dosage of azathioprine significantly because the allopurinol inhibits the xanthine oxidase pathway (Elion et al., 1963). This inhibition increases not only the immunosuppressive potency, but also the major side effect of azathioprine—marrow depression. Although the metabolites are excreted in the urine, these are inactive, and no reduction in dosage is required in the presence of a nonfunctioning kidney (Bach and Dardenne, 1971).

DOSAGE

Azathioprine is given as a single daily dose; if used with steroids alone, a suitable dose is 2.5 mg/kg/d. Careful monitoring of the leukocyte count is required, particularly in the early weeks posttransplantation, when the dosage is reduced only in the presence of leukopenia. Although the dose of azathioprine may be reduced somewhat with time, a maintenance dose of azathioprine, particularly in the presence of low-dose steroids, should not be lower than 2 mg/kg/d. An important multicenter randomized trial was carried out in Australia to test low-dose versus high-dose steroids used with azathioprine after transplantation. The trial failed to show that low-dose steroids were as effective as high-dose steroids (in contrast to earlier but smaller trials), until it was realized that the poorer outcome with low-dose steroids was associated with the use of low-dose azathioprine (i.e., <2 mg/kg/d) (D'Apice et al., 1984). A more recent analysis of data from the Collaborative Transplant Study suggested that long-term graft survival was related to the dose of azathioprine that patients were receiving for maintenance. Patients on azathioprine and steroids only, who were receiving greater than 1.5 mg/kg, had better graft survival than those receiving a lower maintenance dose of azathioprine (Opelz and Dohler, 2000).

When azathioprine is used with cyclosporine and steroids, lower doses are given. A fairly standard dose of azathioprine in a triple-therapy protocol is 1.5 mg/kg (see Chapter 16). At this level, hematological toxicity is common except in the presence of cytomegalovirus infection. There is some evidence in experimental models that azathioprine and cyclosporine are synergistic in terms of immunosuppression (Squiflet et al., 1982).

SIDE EFFECTS

The major complication of azathioprine therapy is bone marrow aplasia most commonly manifested as leukopenia, although in cases of more severe marrow depression, anemia and thrombocytopenia may be present. Regular monitoring of the leukocyte count is an important aspect of azathioprine therapy, and if the leukocyte count decreases to less than 3 $\times$ 10^9/L, the azathioprine dose should be reduced. Megaloblastic anemia has been described in association with the use of azathioprine. As already mentioned, if allopurinol is required for the prevention of gout, the azathioprine dose should be reduced to 25% of the previous dose.

Hepatotoxicity has been attributed to azathioprine for many years, and although undoubtedly azathioprine is associated with hepatic dysfunction, this is probably rare (see Chapter 32). Other causes of hepatic dysfunction in the presence of azathioprine need to be sought energetically before attributing this to azathioprine. Hair loss is a common side effect of azathioprine when used in therapeutic doses. Early observations of an increased incidence of squamous cell cancer in transplant patients was attributed to azathioprine. There does not seem to be any evidence, however, that squamous cell cancers have a greater incidence in patients treated with azathioprine and steroids compared with patients treated with cyclosporine and steroids. The increased incidence of squamous cell cancer in immunosuppressed patients probably relates to the overall immunosuppression rather than any specific drug activity (see Chapters 34 and 35).

Steroids
MECHANISMS OF ACTION

Steroids are administered as prednisone or prednisolone. These agents are absorbed rapidly from the gut, and peak plasma concentrations occur 1 to 3 hours after administration. The mechanism of action of steroids is extremely complex and is still not understood fully (Cupps and Fauci, 1982; Fauci, 1979). Steroids are antiinflammatory as well as being immunosuppressive. It was noted first by Billingham et al.

(1951) that cortisone would produce a modest prolongation of skin allografts in the rabbit. In the treatment of acute rejection, it is probably the antiinflammatory activity that produces the immediate response, whereas when used prophylactically it is the immunosuppressive activity that is predominant. A small randomized trial comparing prednisolone with a nonsteroidal antiinflammatory agent (ibuprofen) showed a higher rate of rejection in the patients receiving the nonsteroidal agent, confirming that the antiinflammatory effect of steroids is not its major role in renal transplantation (Kreis et al., 1984).

Steroids are metabolized in the liver, and prednisone is converted to prednisolone in the liver. Although it has been estimated that the bioavailability of prednisone is approximately 80% of that achieved by prednisolone, no evidence exists in practice that there is a difference in outcome between prednisone (used most commonly in the United States) or prednisolone (used most commonly in Europe) (Burleson et al., 1981; Gambertoglio et al., 1982). The half-life of steroids is short—about 60 minutes for prednisone and 200 minutes for prednisolone. These half-lives are increased substantially in the presence of hepatic dysfunction and are shorter in the presence of drugs such as phenytoin and rifampicin that induce hepatic enzymes. There is no evidence that these interactions have produced significant problems in clinical practice. It also has been shown that the clearance of prednisolone is slower in patients on cyclosporine compared with patients on azathioprine (Ost, 1987). A later study suggested, however, that cyclosporine did not influence the metabolism of methylprednisolone, but the authors noted a considerable variation of the metabolism of methylprednisolone among patients (Tornatore et al., 1993). More recently, the pharmacokinetics of prednisolone during sirolimus therapy has been studied with some evidence for a minor interaction between sirolimus and prednisolone in some patients (Jusko et al., 1996).

Steroids do have a significant effect in vitro on T-cell proliferation, blocking interleukin-2 production (Crabtree, 1989). A variety of other actions may augment their immunosuppressive activity (e.g., preventing the induction of interleukin-1 and interleukin-6 genes in macrophages) (Knudsen et al., 1987; Zanker et al., 1990). Its antiinflammatory activity perhaps is mediated by the inhibition of migration of monocytes to areas of inflammation (Fauci, 1979), and this same antiinflammatory activity has a marked deleterious effect on wound healing.

Dosage

Steroids have been used since the introduction of azathioprine to prevent rejection as well as to treat rejection. When used prophylactically, steroids were used initially in high doses (e.g., 100 mg/d), reducing to a maintenance dose of 10 mg/d over 6 to 9 months. As mentioned earlier, a maintenance dose of steroids in association with azathioprine requires a therapeutic dose of azathioprine in most instances—at least 2 mg/kg/d of azathioprine. McGeown and coworkers consistently reported excellent graft survival from Belfast with a low incidence of steroid-related complications using a dose of prednisolone of 20 mg/d given orally as a single morning dose, with a further reduction occurring at 6 months to a baseline maintenance dose of 10 mg/d (McGeown et al., 1977). Because many, if not most, of the Belfast patients had had bilateral nephrectomies and multiple transfusions, it was not clear whether the excellent results were related to the low dosage of steroids or to a transfusion effect, which was recognized widely as an important factor in improving graft outcome.

Initially, trials of low-dose steroids versus high-dose steroids were carried out at Oxford, then in many other centers, all of which showed not only that low-dose steroids were as effective as high-dose steroids in preventing rejection but also that there was a significant reduction in steroid-related complications in patients receiving low-dose steroids (Buckles et al., 1981; Chan et al., 1980, 1981; De Vecchi et al., 1985; Hricik et al., 1994; Isoniemi et al., 1990; Morris et al., 1982; Papadakis et al., 1983; Stabile et al., 1986). The results of these trials led quickly to the wide adoption of low-dose steroid regimens with azathioprine. In contrast, a study from Helsinki suggested that an initial high dose of methylprednisolone resulted in significantly better graft survival at 1 year (Hayry et al., 1984). The results of the large multicenter trial reported by D'Apice et al. (1984), already referred to, show that low-dose steroids are only equally effective as high-dose steroids in preventing rejection if therapeutic doses of azathioprine are used (i.e., >2 mg/kg/d).

With the introduction of cyclosporine, steroids still were used with or without azathioprine. In general, low-dose steroid protocols were continued, although there was a tendency, particularly in North America, to go back toward higher steroid dosage regimens in the first few weeks posttransplantation. Nevertheless, if steroids are used posttransplantation in association with cyclosporine or the newer immunosuppressive agents, low-dose protocols starting at 20 mg/d still are appropriate with a reduction to maintenance levels by 4 to 5 months posttransplantation. In the case of triple therapy, as discussed in Chapter 16 and later in this chapter, withdrawal of steroids may be appropriate about 1 year posttransplantation in the presence of stable function.

Whether steroids should be given as a single daily dose in the morning or in divided doses has not been resolved. Because of the short half-life of prednisone and prednisolone, divided doses may be more rational, but it could be argued that a single morning daily dose would be more appropriate taking into account the diurnal rhythm of glucocorticoid metabolism (Grant et al., 1985; Nichols et al., 1965). There is no clinical evidence that one or the other protocol is more effective or less likely to produce side effects.

For many years, maintenance doses of prednisone or prednisolone of 10 mg/d were standard therapy in association with azathioprine. In patients with long-surviving grafts with good function, steroid dosages have been reduced to 5 or 6 mg/d. It is unlikely, however, that many patients who are on long-term azathioprine and steroids would be able to have their steroid dosage reduced to less than 5 mg/d. Attempts in the past to withdraw steroids often have led to the onset of rejection when doses of less than 5 mg/d are reached. If patients have been on steroids for many years, their adrenals may not recover from the long-standing suppression, and this may produce clinical features of adrenocortical insufficiency (Naik et al., 1980). Patients receiving more potent immunosuppressive agents such as cyclosporine and tacrolimus may be weaned off steroids in the presence of stable function at approximately 1 year (as discussed later).

Alternate-day steroid therapy for maintenance also is used widely, especially in children in an attempt to reduce the side effects, particularly growth retardation (Breitenfield et al., 1980; Curtis, et al., 1982; De et al., 1980; Diethelm et al., 1976; Dumler, et al., 1982; Leb, 1979; McDonald et al., 1976; Potter et al., 1975). In children, alternate-day therapy may be associated with a greater incidence of rejection, but probably this is not the case in adults. A small randomized trial of alternate-day therapy failed to show any benefit over daily steroids, however (McDonald et al., 1976). Alternate-day therapy may lead to greater problems with respect to compliance, in contrast to a daily regimen of steroids. It had been common practice to administer a bolus of methylprednisolone prophylactically during the transplant operation with the aim of increasing immunosuppression and perhaps preventing delayed graft function, but a randomized prospective trial of bolus methylprednisolone versus placebo at the time of surgery did not show any benefit of the high perioperative intravenous dose of methylprednisolone (Kauffman et al., 1977).

TREATMENT OF ACUTE REJECTION

Steroids in high doses are the first approach to the treatment of an acute rejection episode. In some units in the early days of azathioprine, especially at the Necker Hospital in Paris, steroids were not administered prophylactically to prevent rejection but only if rejection occurred. In the case of HLA-identical sibling transplants, many patients never required steroids, but in cadaver transplantation, most had rejection and had to be treated with steroids (Kreis et al., 1978). Subsequently, as mentioned earlier, steroids were used prophylactically with azathioprine from the time of transplantation.

Early approaches to the treatment of an acute rejection episode involved either increasing the oral dosage of steroids to high levels (e.g., 200 mg/d for 3 days), with a rapid reduction over 10 days to the dosage levels of steroids being given before the acute rejection episode, or boluses of intravenous methylprednisolone (e.g., 0.5–1 g/d for 3–5 days). Probably both approaches are equally effective. In an early randomized prospective trial in Oxford, however, high intravenous doses were as effective as high oral doses in reversing rejection, but there was a definite suggestion that steroid-related complications were lower in those who received intravenous therapy (Gray et al., 1978). In a randomized study in children, a high intravenous dose of methylprednisolone (600 mg/m² daily for 3 days) was no more effective than low oral doses of prednisolone in reversing rejection—70% as opposed to 72% (Orta-Sibu et al., 1982).

The commonest form of high-dose intravenous therapy to treat acute rejection has been 1 g of methylprednisolone given intravenously as a single bolus daily for 3 days. The intravenous bolus should be administered slowly over 5 minutes because the sudden injection of the bolus can lead to cardiac arrhythmias (Thompson et al., 1983). It is probable that 1 g of methylprednisolone is a much greater dose than required; in Oxford for many years now we have used 0.5 g of methylprednisolone daily intravenously for 3 days, whereas the Stockholm unit has used 0.25 g daily intravenously for 3 days. The lower intravenous doses do not appear to be associated with any greater incidence of steroid-resistant rejection, as originally suggested by a prospective trial of high-dose versus low-dose intravenous steroids to treat rejection (Kauffman et al., 1979). Similarly in a small double-blind, randomized trial, Stromstrad et al. (1978) failed to show any therapeutic benefit of a 30 mg/kg bolus over a 3 mg/kg bolus, whereas Lui et al. (1989) failed to show any benefit of a bolus of 15 mg/kg of body weight over a bolus of 3 mg/kg.

SIDE EFFECTS

The side effects of continuous steroid therapy are numerous (Table 15–1). High-dose steroids were responsible for most complications of renal transplantation in the azathioprine era. With the widespread use of low-dose steroids, the incidence of serious side effects has been reduced markedly, but they still are a problem. Efforts to develop protocols that allow the withdrawal of steroids entirely or, ideally, avoid

TABLE 15–1

SIDE EFFECTS OF STEROIDS AFTER RENAL TRANSPLANTATION

Cushingoid facies	Hypertension
Wound healing	Psychiatric disturbance
Growth retardation	Cataracts
Diabetes	Pancreatitis
Hyperlipidemia	Skin changes
Bone disease	Peptic ulceration
Obesity	

their use at all are continuous. In a study of the cost of steroid side effects over 10 years in a cohort of 50 patients, the additional cost per patient attributable to a steroid complication was assessed at $5,300 (U.S. dollars) (Veenstra *et al.*, 1999).

Cushingoid Facies

Cushingoid facies used to be the hallmark of a renal transplant patient—a moon face, buffalo hump, acne, obese torso and thin, easily bruised skin, all representing the cumulative effect of high-dose steroids. With lower dose steroids, cushingoid facies is far less of a problem, although most patients show modest changes in their facies in the early months posttransplantation, particularly in association with the brutalization of the face associated with cyclosporine therapy. Most patients on low-dose steroids, which is the normal practice now with cyclosporine, have relatively minimal facial changes related to steroids.

Wound Healing

The antiinflammatory activity of steroids leads to poor wound healing. In the days of high-dose steroids, this was a major problem, influencing the healing not only of the incision, but also of the ureterovesical reconstruction. With low-dose steroids, poor wound healing is no longer a major problem, but nevertheless skin sutures are left *in situ* for at least 14 days.

Growth Retardation

Growth retardation is of particular concern in children after renal transplantation. One of the major advantages of cyclosporine is that it allows lower doses of steroids to be used in children, and growth retardation is less of a problem (Rizzoni *et al.*, 1986). As discussed in Chapter 37, however, growth retardation in children requiring a transplant is still a problem in that retardation resulting from renal failure already is present, and protocols for immunosuppression that might allow catchup growth are favored. Such a protocol requires the use of low-dose steroids or alternate-day steroids, or preferably no steroids. The use of growth hormone has had a significant impact on growth rates posttransplantation (Fine *et al.*, 1991).

Diabetes

Glycosuria and insulin-dependent and non–insulin-dependent diabetes are common after transplantation. The occurrence of diabetes is related, in part, to steroid usage (Isoniemi, 1991), but it has become commoner with the concomitant use of cyclosporine and tacrolimus, both of which can induce diabetes independently of steroids. In the presence of these two agents, the use of steroids augments

the potential for diabetes, and often patients who become diabetic on cyclosporine or tacrolimus have a regression of the diabetes when steroid therapy is discontinued.

Hyperlipidemia

Hypercholesterolemia and hypertriglyceridemia are associated with steroid use, as was evident in the azathioprine and steroid era. Hyperlipidemia has become a greater problem in the cyclosporine era because cyclosporine also leads to an increased incidence of hyperlipidemia (Drueke *et al.*, 1991; Kasiske and Umen, 1987; Markell and Friedman, 1989; see Chapter 30).

Bone Disease

Bone disease is a common and major problem posttransplantation, especially in the postmenopausal woman (Almond *et al.*, 1994; Grotz *et al.*, 1994, 1995; Horber *et al.*, 1994; Julian *et al.*, 1991; Wolpaw *et al.*, 1994). In the days of high-dose steroid therapy posttransplantation, avascular necrosis of bones, particularly of the head of the femur, was common, occurring with an incidence of approximately 10 to 15% within 2 years of transplantation (Fig. 15–1). All the evidence suggests that this incidence was due to a cumulative effect of steroid dosage. As low-dose steroid protocols were introduced, the incidence of avascular necrosis decreased dramatically. However, the cumulative dose of steroids received by a patient on a high-dose steroid regimen, as opposed to a low-dose regimen, is not that much higher after 6 months. Avascular necrosis of the hip should be treated by hip replacement relatively early to enable full rehabilitation to take place. In patients requiring hip replacement, every attempt should be made to withdraw steroids if that seems feasible.

Osteoporosis is associated with steroid therapy. In a randomized study, Hollander and colleagues showed that vertebral bone density was increased significantly in patients discontinuing steroids (Hollander *et al.*, 1997). Similar evidence was reported by Aroldi *et al.* (1997) in a randomized study of three different immunosuppressive protocols and vertebral bone density. These investigators showed that lumbar bone density decreased significantly in patients receiving cyclosporine and steroids but increased significantly in patients receiving cyclosporine alone without steroids. Many patients coming to renal transplantation have a degree of secondary hyperparathyroidism, and bone changes related to the hyperparathyroidism are enhanced by steroid therapy. Much more aggressive approaches to parathyroidectomy in patients with renal failure are being taken by most units now before transplantation. In patients after transplantation with raised parathormone levels, early parathyroidectomy also should be considered. Although there are no firm data in transplant patients, it is generally thought that women who are postmenopausal should receive hormone replacement therapy in an attempt to diminish the overall likelihood of significant bone disease, together with the use of protocols that would allow low-dose steroids to be used or steroids to be discontinued. A more recent study has suggested that deflazacort used instead of prednisone is associated with a decreased loss of total skeleton and lumbar spine density as well as improving the lipid profile (Lippuner *et al.*, 1998).

Obesity

Steroid therapy leads to a marked increase in appetite, and without any dietary restrictions after transplantation, all patients tend to gain weight, which is in addition to a weight increase resulting from salt and water retention. Many pa-

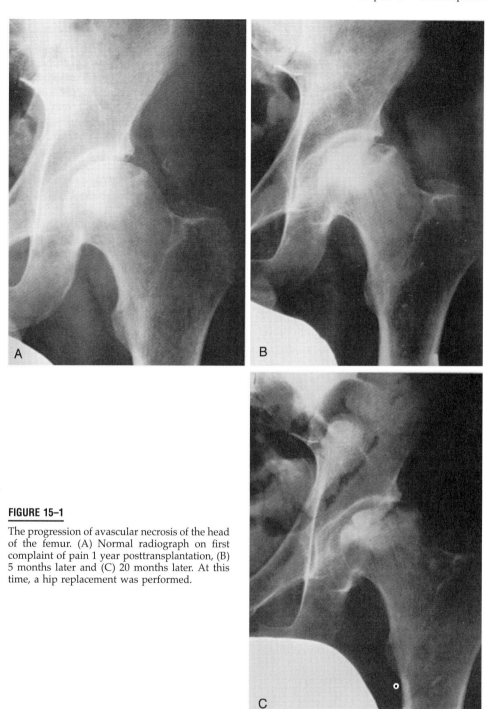

FIGURE 15–1

The progression of avascular necrosis of the head of the femur. (A) Normal radiograph on first complaint of pain 1 year posttransplantation, (B) 5 months later and (C) 20 months later. At this time, a hip replacement was performed.

tients become obese (body mass index >30), and this adds to the risks of poor survival. Every attempt should be made to advise patients from the time of transplantation to restrict calorie intake carefully because once patients have gained weight in the presence of steroid therapy, it is extremely difficult for them to reduce their weight.

Hypertension

Hypertension after transplantation is common and is related, in part, to steroids, but in the cyclosporine era, hypertension also is due to cyclosporine (see Chapter 30). In steroid withdrawal protocols, hypertension improves once steroids are discontinued (Ratcliffe *et al.*, 1996).

Psychiatric Disturbance

Psychiatric disturbance is evident in patients on steroids in two ways. In the early days posttransplantation, particularly with the need for high-dose steroids to treat rejection, significant psychiatric mood changes may be observed. Later, when steroids are being withdrawn or reduced to low doses, psychiatric mood changes, especially depression, also may occur.

Cataracts

Steroid-related cataracts are common after renal transplantation, occurring in approximately 25% of patients (Shun-Shin et al., 1990).

Pancreatitis

Acute pancreatitis occurs with a much greater incidence after renal transplantation than would be expected. Azathioprine and steroids have been associated with acute pancreatitis. The pancreatitis probably is related to overall immunosuppression and is often severe (Slakey et al., 1997). The clinical features of acute pancreatitis can be masked to some extent by steroids.

Skin Changes

Long-term steroids produced typical skin changes in renal transplant patients, the skin being thin, atrophic, easily bruised, and susceptible to knocks (see Chapter 34). A syndrome known as *transplant leg* is associated with long-term steroid usage; this occurs, for example, after bumping into a chair or a table, resulting in stripping a flap of skin from the lower leg.

Peptic Ulceration

Although it is debatable whether steroids do lead to development of peptic ulceration, most units use prophylactic H_2 antagonists in the early months posttransplantation, when steroid doses are at their highest. The advent of low-dose steroid therapy has been associated with a dramatic diminution in the incidence of peptic ulceration after transplantation.

Acute Abdomen

In all renal transplant patients who present with an acute abdomen, steroids may mask the symptoms noted by the patient. If this fact is not remembered, diagnosis of diverticulitis or a perforated peptic ulcer may be delayed with disastrous results.

Steroid Withdrawal

As a result of the significant number of complications associated with midterm and long-term steroid therapy in the renal transplant patient, many attempts have been made to reduce the cumulative dose of steroids posttransplantation as well as to withdraw steroids altogether. In the azathioprine era, reducing or withdrawing steroids was not possible, but with the advent of cyclosporine, there was renewed interest in reducing the dose of steroids as well as withdrawing steroids from immunosuppressive protocols. The availability of additional potent immunosuppressive agents, such as sirolimus, tacrolimus and mycophenolate mofetil, has allowed further steroid-sparing protocols to be developed.

STEROID WITHDRAWAL IN THE AZATHIOPRINE ERA

As discussed earlier, the side effects of steroids were improved somewhat by the use of alternate-day regimens. Attempts to withdraw steroids, mostly anecdotal, generally were associated with rejection, however. In patients on azathioprine and steroids, there appears to be a crucial dose level, below which there are likely to be problems with rejec-

tion (Naik et al., 1980). This crucial dose level is possibly around 5 to 6 mg of prednisolone per day. In one study from Edinburgh, patients with long-term surviving grafts were on azathioprine and 10 mg of prednisolone per day, a protocol that allowed for a slow reduction in the prednisolone dosage; many patients developed rejection when the daily steroid dose was reduced to less than 6 mg/d. As a result, the study directed at weaning patients with long- surviving transplants off steroids was abandoned (Anderton et al., 1977).

STEROID WITHDRAWAL IN THE CYCLOSPORINE ERA

Controversy still exists as to whether cyclosporine is best used with or without steroids (see Chapter 16). It would appear that if a high dose of cyclosporine is used, monotherapy may be satisfactory in many patients but with a greater risk of acute rejection often requiring the addition of steroids and perhaps with a greater risk of nephrotoxicity (De Sevaux et al., 1998; Hilbrands et al., 1996; Ponticelli et al., 1997; Schulak et al., 1990). The use of steroids perhaps allows the use of lower doses of cyclosporine, and steroids may decrease the incidence of nephrotoxicity in the early weeks posttransplantation, but there is no firm evidence for either of these suggestions (Griffin et al., 1987).

In a large retrospective analysis of data from the Collaborative Transplant Study, Opelz (1995) found that patients with a functioning graft at 1 year who had had steroids withdrawn had better graft and patient survival thereafter than patients remaining on steroids. The initial criticism of this study was that patients still on steroids at 1 year represented patients with poorer function as a result of rejection episodes or delayed graft function, but a subsequent analysis examining outcome only in patients with satisfactory renal function at 1 year found the same results. Opelz has mounted a prospective study to attempt to confirm these data.

The early withdrawal of steroids after transplantation in general is associated with a higher incidence of acute rejection, often requiring restarting steroids, in contrast to late withdrawal, which usually is successful (Hricik et al., 1992c). Hricik and colleagues performed a meta-analysis of seven randomized prospective trials of steroid avoidance or withdrawal in the first 3 months posttransplantation in patients receiving cyclosporine-based protocols (Hricik et al., 1993). In only one study, however, was follow-up of patients extended beyond 2 years. The results of this meta-analysis suggested that avoidance of steroids or early withdrawal increased the risk of acute rejection but did not affect patient or graft survival adversely. The meta-analysis could not address the question of long-term graft function. In children, the risk of acute rejection and graft loss after steroid withdrawal is much greater than in adults, and although steroid withdrawal is a worthy goal, especially in terms of growth, it is not recommended (Ingulli et al., 1993; Reisman et al., 1990; Roberti et al., 1994; Tejani et al., 1989).

More recent data from randomized prospective trials suggest that steroids may be withdrawn with a relative degree of safety and a low incidence of rejection in patients with stable graft function at around 1 year posttransplantation. Two such trials support this suggestion, one from Oxford and one from the Netherlands (Hollander et al., 1997; Ratcliffe et al., 1996). Some caution should be expressed, however, in view of the Canadian Multicentre Trial, in which prednisone withdrawal in patients on cyclosporine was compared with continuation of prednisone (Sinclair, 1992). Graft survival in the patients continuing on steroids was superior, and the conclusion was that steroids used with cyclosporine should not be withdrawn because of poorer graft outcome in the longer term (5 years).

In the Oxford trial (Ratcliffe *et al.*, 1996), patients who were receiving triple therapy (cyclosporine, azathioprine and steroids) and had stable function at least 1 year posttransplantation were randomized to have steroids withdrawn over a period of several months or continued at a maintenance level of 10 mg/d. Most patients had steroids withdrawn successfully, but there was a 10% deterioration in renal function at 1 year at the exit point of the trial, and this was accompanied by a further modest deterioration of renal function during the second year, but thereafter function appeared to be stable (Fig. 15–2). In the control group in which renal function was unchanged at 1 year, renal function deteriorated in the next year by the same 10% as the trial group primarily because most patients wished to discontinue steroids after seeing the beneficial effects in their trial cohorts who had had steroids withdrawn. This decrease in renal function, evidenced in serum creatinine and creatinine clearance, was of concern, but there is no evidence that further deterioration of function was occurring in a longer follow-up of patients in the trial (unpublished observations). The standard triple-therapy protocol at Oxford now includes cessation of steroids at around 1 year posttransplantation. Nevertheless, it was thought that caution concerning long-term renal function was appropriate in view of the Canadian Trial data referred to previously. There were significant benefits of steroid withdrawal in this trial, including a decline in blood pressure,

although not sustained in all patients; a significant drop in total cholesterol of 1 mmol/L and increases in plasma phosphate and alkaline phosphatase in the steroid withdrawal group.

In the Dutch study (Hollander *et al.*, 1997), which was similar to the Oxford study, patients with stable renal function at 1 year or longer posttransplantation were randomized to withdraw steroids or not. In two thirds of patients, steroids were withdrawn successfully, but acute rejection was the major cause of withdrawal failure. No grafts were lost from rejection. Benefits of withdrawal with respect to hypertension, hypercholesterolemia, hyperglycemia and appearance were noted. The authors concluded that steroids could be withdrawn safely after 1 year following kidney transplantation, provided that patients are followed carefully. Favorable changes associated with steroid withdrawal have been documented by other groups in studies of steroid withdrawal, including glucose tolerance and growth in children (Hricik *et al.*, 1991, 1992a, 1992b, 1994; Isoniemi, 1991).

STEROID WITHDRAWAL AND TACROLIMUS

A considerable amount of data, mostly from observational studies, suggest that tacrolimus is more steroid sparing than cyclosporine (see Chapter 17). In units using tacrolimus, many patients can have steroids withdrawn during the first year after transplantation. In one report from Pittsburgh, Shapiro and colleagues, who had noted previously that steroids could be discontinued in 70% of renal transplant patients receiving tacrolimus, reported a further longer term follow-up of approximately 289 patients not receiving steroids (Shapiro *et al.*, 1998). The patients in the steroid withdrawal group had an impressive 1- and 3-year graft survival of 98% and 94% compared with 90 patients in whom steroids had not been withdrawn, who had 1- and 3-year graft survival of 77% and 50%. Although the authors state that there was no difference between the two groups in terms of the proportion of living and cadaver donors, HLA matching, recipient sex, race or sensitization, the patients in whom steroids were not withdrawn were in general those who had delayed graft function or experienced acute rejection, both of which are factors having a significant deleterious impact on graft outcome (see Chapter 39). This type of observational study suggests that steroid withdrawal in renal transplant patients receiving tacrolimus-based immunosuppression is possible most of the time and is reasonably safe in short-term and medium-term follow-up after transplantation. Renal function remains stable in patients in whom steroids had been withdrawn, at least in the medium term. Another small prospective observational study of patients receiving tacrolimus, mycophenolate and steroids in whom steroids were withdrawn at 1 week showed an incidence of acute rejection of around 25%, but no grafts were lost (Grewal *et al.*, 1998).

STEROID WITHDRAWAL WITH MYCOPHENOLATE

There are no data in patients receiving mycophenolate and steroids only in whom steroids had been withdrawn, but there are data in patients receiving cyclosporine and mycophenolate in whom steroids were withdrawn. In one uncontrolled study in which steroids were withdrawn 4 to 30 months posttransplantation, no rejection episodes were noted after a mean follow-up of 10 months (Grinyo *et al.*, 1997). There has been a report of a multicenter, randomized prospective double-blind study of prednisone withdrawal from 3 months after transplantation in patients on cyclosporine, mycophenolate mofetil and prednisone. Patients were entered only if it was a primary graft and if no rejection

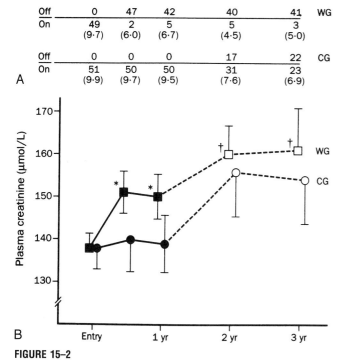

FIGURE 15–2

Changes in creatinine during the trial period and after 2 years of further follow-up. (A) Numbers at the top are number of patients in each of the original groups who were not taking (off) or taking (on) prednisolone, together with the mean daily dose of prednisolone in those taking steroids. (B) Mean plasma creatinine in each group at the trial endpoints (solid symbols) and subsequent follow-up (open symbols) for each group assigned by intention to treat (squares, withdrawal group; circles, control group). Bars indicate standard errors. Statistical comparison, with entry values by Student's two-tailed paired *t*-test. *$P < 0.001$. †$P < 0.05$. WG = withdrawal group; CG = control group. (Reproduced with permission of Ratcliffe *et al.*, 1996.)

episode had occurred in the first 3 months. The trial was stopped after 266 patients had been entered because of excess rejection in the prednisone withdrawal group (30.8% *vs.* 9.8% in the maintenance group). Risk was higher in black recipients. Patients in whom prednisone had been withdrawn successfully had lower cholesterol levels and required fewer antihypertensive drugs but had a higher creatinine (Steroid Withdrawal Study Group, 1999).

In a preliminary report in another study in patients receiving cyclosporine (Neoral) and sirolimus without steroids, only 1 of 28 patients in the protocol experienced an acute rejection episode (Pescovitz *et al.*, 1997). More information is required, and appropriate randomized trials of these newer immunosuppressive agents with or without steroids have to be done to assess whether it is possible to discontinue steroids, and it is important that long-term follow-up of renal function is available.

Conclusions

In the cyclosporine-based protocols, such as triple therapy, late steroid withdrawal is feasible in most patients with stable graft function, and the metabolic benefits of steroid withdrawal are considerable. Early withdrawal of steroids in cyclosporine-based protocols is far more likely to be associated with acute rejection. The advent of the newer immunosuppressive agents, tacrolimus, mycophenolate, and sirolimus, is likely to permit the development of further steroid-sparing protocols, but appropriately designed randomized studies are needed to clarify this issue. Bearing in mind the long-term results of the Canadian Multicentre Study, long-term follow-up for at least 5 years is required before a definite conclusion can be reached.

References

Almond, M. K., Kwan, J. T., Evans, K. and Cunningham, J. (1994). Loss of regional bone mineral density in the first 12 months following renal transplantation. *Nephron* **66**, 52.

Anderton, J. L., Fananapuzir, L., Eccleston, M. (1977). Minimum steroid requirements in renal transplant patients monitored by urinary fibrin degradation products and complement. *Proc. EDTA* **14**, 342.

Aroldi, A., Tarantino, A., Montagnino, G., *et al.* (1997). Effects of three immunosuppressive regimens on vertebral bone density in renal transplant recipients: a prospective study. *Transplantation* **63**, 380.

Bach, J. F. (1975). *The Mode of Action of Immunosuppressive Agents*, North Holland Publishing Company, Oxford.

Bach, J. F. and Dardenne, M. (1971). The metabolism of azathioprine in renal failure. *Transplantation* **12**, 253.

Billingham, R. E., Krohn, P. L. and Medawar, P. B. (1951). Effect of cortisone on survival of skin homografts in rabbits. *Br. M. J.* **1**, 1157.

Breitenfield, R. V., Herbert, L. A., Lemann, Jr., J., *et al.* (1980). Stability of renal transplant function with alternate-day corticosteroid therapy. *J. A. M. A.* **244**, 151.

Buckles, J. A. C., Mackintosh, P. and Barnes, A. D. (1981). Controlled trial of low- versus high-dose oral steroid therapy in 100 cadaveric renal transplants. *Proc. EDTA* **18**, 394.

Burleson, R. L., Marbarger, P. D., Jermanovich, N., Brennan, A. M. and Scruggs, B. F. (1981). A prospective study of methylprednisolone and prednisone as immunosuppressive agents in clinical renal transplantation. *Transplant. Proc.* **13**, 339.

Calne, R. Y. (1960). The rejection of renal homografts: inhibition in dogs by 6-mercaptopurine. *Lancet* **7**, 417.

Calne, R. Y., Alexandre, G. P. J. and Murray, J. E. (1962). A study of the effects of drugs in prolonging survival of homologous renal transplants in dogs. *Ann. N. Y. Acad. Sci.* **99**, 743.

Chan, L., French, M. E., Beare, J., *et al.* (1980). Prospective trial of high-dose versus low-dose prednisolone in renal transplant patients. *Transplant. Proc.* **12**, 323.

Chan, L., French, M. E., Oliver, D. O. and Morris, P. J. (1981). High- and low-dose prednisolone. *Transplant. Proc.* **13**, 336.

Crabtree, G. R. (1989). Corticosteroid-mediated immunoregulation in man. *Immunol. Rev.* **65**, 132.

Cupps, T. R. and Fauci, A. S. (1982). Corticosteroid-mediated immunoregulation in man. *Immunol. Rev.* **65**, 132.

Curtis, J. J., Galla, J. H., Woodford, S. Y., Lucas, B. A. and Luke, R. G. (1982). Effect of alternate-day prednisone on plasma lipids in renal transplant recipients. *Kidney Int.* **22**, 42.

D'Apice, A. J., Becker, G. J., Kincaid-Smith, P., *et al.* (1984). A prospective randomized trial of low-dose versus high-dose steroids in cadaveric renal transplantation. *Transplantation* **37**, 373.

De, V. A., Cantaluppi, A., Montagnino, G., *et al.* (1980). Long-term comparison between single-morning daily and alternate-day steroid treatment in cadaver kidney recipients. *Transplant. Proc.* **12**, 327.

De Sevaux, R. G., Hilbrands, L. B., Tiggeler, R. G., Koene, R. A. and Hoitsma, A. J. (1998). A randomized, prospective study on the conversion from cyclosporine-prednisone to cyclosporine-azathioprine at 6 months after renal transplantation. *Transpl. Int.* **11(Suppl. 1)**, S322.

De Vecchi, A., Rivolta, E., Tarantino, A., *et al.* (1985). Controlled trial of two different methylprednisolone doses in cadaveric renal transplantation. *Nephron* **41**, 262.

Diethelm, A. G., Sterline, W. A., Hartley, M. W. and Morgan, J. M. (1976). Alternate-day prednisone therapy in recipients of renal allografts: risk and benefits. *Arch. Surg.* **111**, 867.

Drueke, T. B., Abdulmassih, Z., Lacour, B., *et al.* (1991). Atherosclerosis and lipid disorders after renal transplantation. *Kidney Int.* **39**, S24.

Dumler, F., Levin, N. W., Szego, G., *et al.* (1982). Long-term alternate day steroid therapy in renal transplantation: a controlled study. *Transplantation* **34**, 78.

Elion, G. B., Bieber, S. and Hitchings, G. H. (1955). The fate of 6-mercaptopurine in mice. *Ann. N. Y. Acad. Sci.* **60**, 297.

Elion, G. B., Burgi, E. and Hitchings, G. H. (1952). Studies on condensed pyrimidine systems: IX. synthesis of some six-substituted purines. *J. Am. Chem. Soc.* **74**, 411.

Elion, G. B., Callahan, S., Bieber, S., Hitchings, G. H. and Rundles, R. W. (1961). A summary of investigations with 6-(1-methyl-4-nitro-r-imidazolyl)thio purine (BW 57-322). *Cancer Chemother. Rep.* **14**, 93.

Elion, G. B., Callahan, S., Nathan, H., Beiber, S., Rundles, R. W. and Hitchings, G. H. (1963). Potentiation by inhibition of drug degradation: 6-substituted purines and xanthine oxidase. *Biochem. Pharmacol.* **12**, 85.

Fauci, A. S. (1979). Mechanisms of the immunosuppressive and anti-inflammatory effects of gluco-corticosteroids. *J. Immunopharmacol.* **1**, 1.

Fine, R. N., Yadin, O., Nelson, P. A., *et al.* (1991). Recombinant human growth hormone treatment of children following renal transplantation. *Pediatr. Nephrol.* **5**, 147.

Gambertoglio, J. G., Frey, F. J., Holford, N. H., *et al.* (1982). Prednisone and prednisolone bioavailability in renal transplant patients. *Kidney Int.* **21**, 621.

Goodwin, W. E., Mims, M. M. and Kaufman, J. J. (1965). Human renal transplantation: III. technical problems encountered in 6 cases of homotransplantation. *Trans. Am. Assoc. Genitourin. Surg.* **54**, 116.

Grant, S. D., Forsham, P. H. and Di Raimondo, V. C. (1985). Suppression of 17-hydroxycorticosteroids in plasma and urine by single and divided doses of triamcinolone. *N. Engl. J. Med.* **273**, 1115.

Gray, D., Shepherd, H., Daar, A., Oliver, D. O. and Morris, P. J. (1978). Oral versus intravenous high-dose steroid treatment of renal allograft rejection: the big shot or not? *Lancet* **i**, 117.

Grewal, H. P., Thistlewaite, J. R., Loss, G. E., *et al.* (1998). Corticosteroid cessation one week following transplantation using tacrolimus/mycophenolate mofetil based immunosuppression. *Transplant. Proc.* **30**, 1378.

Griffin, P. J., Da Costa, C. A. and Salaman, J. R. (1987). A controlled trial of steroids in cyclosporine-treated renal transplant recipients. *Transplantation* **43**, 505.

Grinyo, J. M., Gil-Vernet, S., Seron, D., *et al.* (1997). Steroid withdrawal in mycophenolate mofetil-treated renal allograft recipients. *Transplantation* 63, 1688.

Grotz, W. H., Mundinger, F. A., Gugel, B., *et al.* (1994). Bone fracture and osteodensitometry with dual energy X-ray absorptiometry in kidney transplant recipients. *Transplantation* 58, 912.

Grotz, W. H., Mundinger, F. A., Gugel, B., *et al.* (1995). Bone mineral density after kidney transplantation: a cross-sectional study in 190 grafts recipients up to 20 years after transplantation. *Transplantation* 59, 982.

Hayry, P., Ahonen, J., Kock, B., *et al.* (1984). Glucocorticosteroids in renal transplantation: II. impact of high- versus low-dose postoperative methylprednisolone administration on graft survival and on the frequency and type of complications. *Scand. J. Immunol.* 19, 211.

Hilbrands, L. B., Hoitsma, A. J. and Koene, K. A. (1996). Randomized, prospective trial of cyclosporine monotherapy versus azathioprine-prednisone from three months after renal transplantation. *Transplantation* 61, 1038.

Hollander, A. A., Hene, R. J., Hermans, J., van Es L. A. and van der Woude, F. J. (1997). Late prednisone withdrawal in cyclosporine-treated kidney transplant patients: a randomized study. *J. Am. Soc. Nephrol.* 8, 294.

Horber, F. F., Casez, J. P., Steiger, U., *et al.* (1994). Changes in bone mass early after kidney transplantation. *J. Bone Miner. Res.* 9, 1.

Hricik, D. E., Almawi, W. Y. and Strom, T. B. (1994). Trends in the use of glucocorticoids in renal transplantation. *Transplantation* 57, 979.

Hricik, D. E., Bartucci, M. R., Moir, E. J., Mayes, J. T. and Schulak, J. A. (1991). Effects of steroid withdrawal on posttransplant diabetes mellitus in cyclosporine-treated renal transplant recipients. *Transplantation* 51, 374.

Hricik, D. E., Bartucci, M. R., Mayes, J. T. and Schulak, J. A. (1992a). The effects of steroid withdrawal on the lipoprotein profiles of cyclosporine-treated kidney and kidney-pancreas transplant recipients. *Transplantation* 54, 868.

Hricik, D. E., Lautman, J., Bartucci, M. R., *et al.* (1992b). Variable effects of steroid withdrawal on blood pressure reduction in cyclosporine-treated renal transplant recipients. *Transplantation* 53, 1232.

Hricik, D. E., O'Toole, M. A., Schulak, J. A. and Herson, J. (1993). Steroid-free immunosuppression in cyclosporine-treated renal transplant recipients: a meta-analysis. *J. Am. Soc. Nephrol.* 4, 1300.

Hricik, D. E., Whalen, C. C., Lautman, J., *et al.* (1992c). Withdrawal of steroids after renal transplantation—clinical predictors of outcome. *Transplantation* 53, 41.

Ingulli, E., Tejani, A. and Markell, M. (1993). The beneficial effects of steroid withdrawal on blood pressure and lipid profile in children posttransplantation in the cyclosporine era. *Transplantation* 55, 1029.

Isoniemi, H. (1991). Renal allograft immunosuppression: V. Glucose intolerance occurring in different immunosuppressive treatments. *Clin. Transplant.* 5, 268.

Isoniemi, H., Ahonen, J., Eklund, B., *et al.* (1990). Renal allograft immunosuppression: II. a randomized trial of withdrawal of one drug in triple drug immunosuppression. *Transpl. Int.* 3, 121.

Isoniemi, H. M., Ahonen, J., Tikkanen, M. J., *et al.* (1993). Long-term consequences of different immunosuppressive regimens for renal allografts. *Transplantation* 55, 494.

Julian, B. A., Laskow, D. A., Dubovsky, J., *et al.* (1991). Rapid loss of vertebral mineral density after renal transplantation. *N. Engl. J. Med.* 325, 544.

Jusko, W. J., Ferron, G. M., Mis, S. M., Kahan, B. D. and Zimmerman, J. J. (1996). Pharmacokinetics of prednisolone during administration of sirolimus in patients with renal transplants. *J. Clin. Pharm.* 36, 1100.

Kasiske, B. L. and Umen, A. J. (1987). Persistent hyperlipidaemia in renal transplant patients. *Medicine* 66, 309.

Kauffman, H. M., Sampson, D., Fox, P. S. and Stawicki, A. T. (1977). High dose (bolus) intravenous methylprednisolone at the time of kidney homotransplantation. *Ann. Surg.* 186, 631.

Kauffman, Jr., H. M., Stromstad, S. A., Sampson, D. and Stawicki, A. T. (1979). Randomized steroid therapy of human kidney transplant rejection. *Transplant. Proc.* 11, 36.

Knudsen, P. J., Dinarello, C. A. and Strom, T. B. (1987). Glucocorticoids inhibit transcription and post-transcriptional expression of interleukin-1. *J. Immunol.* 139, 4129.

Kreis, H., Chkoff, N., Droz, D., *et al.* (1984). Nonsteroid anti-inflammatory agents as a substitute treatment for steroids in ATGAM-treated cadaver kidney recipients. *Transplantation* 37, 139.

Kreis, H., Lacombe, M., Noel, L. H., *et al.* (1978). Kidney-graft rejection: has the need for steroids to be re-evaluated? *Lancet* 2, 1169.

Leb, D. E. (1979). Alternate-day prednisone treatment may increase kidney transplant rejection. *Proc. Dial. Transplant. Forum* 6, 136.

Lippuner, K., Casex, J. P., Horber, F. F. and Jaeger, P. (1998). Effects of deflazacort versus prednisone on bone mass, body composition, and lipid profile: a randomized, double blind study in kidney transplant patients. *J. Clin. Endocrinol. Metab.* 83, 3795.

Lui, S. F., Sweny, P., Scoble, J. E., Varghese, Z., Moorhead, J. F. and Fernando, O. N. (1989). Low-dose vs high-dose intravenous methylprednisolone therapy for acute renal allograft rejection in patients receiving cyclosporin therapy. *Nephrol. Dial. Transplant.* 4, 387.

Markell, M. S. and Friedman, E. A. (1989). Hyperlipidemia after organ transplantation. *Am. J. Med.* 87, 61N.

McDonald, F. D., Horensten, M. L., Mayor, G. B., *et al.* (1976). Effect of alternate-day steroids on renal transplant function: a controlled study. *Nephron* 17, 415.

McGeown, M. G., Kennedy, J. A., Loughridge, W. G., *et al.* (1977). One hundred kidney transplants in the Belfast City Hospital. *Lancet* 2, 648.

Morris, P. J., Chan, L., French, M. E. and Ting, A. (1982). Low dose oral prednisolone in renal transplantation. *Lancet* 1, 525.

Murray, J. E., Merrill, J. P., Damin, G. J., Dealy, J. B., Alexandre, G. P. J. and Harrison, J. H. (1962). Kidney transplantation in modified recipients. *Ann. Surg.* 156, 337.

Murray, J. E., Merrill, J. P., Harrison, J. H., Wilson, R. E. and Dammin, G. J. (1963). Prolonged survival of human-kidney homograft by immunosuppressive drug therapy. *N. Engl. J. Med.* 268, 1315.

Naik, R. B., Chakraborty, J., English, J., *et al.* (1980). Serious renal transplant rejection and adrenal hypofunction after gradual withdrawal of prednisolone two years after transplantation. *B. M. J.* 280, 1337.

Nichols, T., Nugent, C. A. and Tyler, F. H. (1965). Diurnal variation in suppression of adrenal function by glucocorticoids. *J. Clin. Endocrinol. Metab.* 25, 343.

Opelz, G. (1995). Influence of treatment with cyclosporine, azathioprine and steroids on chronic allograft failure. The Collaborative Transplant Study. *Kidney Int.* 52(Suppl.), S89.

Opelz, G. and Dohler, B. (2000). Critical threshold of azathioprine dosage for maintenance immunosuppression in kidney graft recipients. Collaborative Transplant Study. *Transplantation* 69, 818.

Orta-Sibu, N., Chantler, C., Bewick, M. and Haycock, G. (1982). Comparison of high-dose intravenous methylprednisolone with low-dose oral prednisolone in acute renal allograft rejection in children. *B. M. J. Clin. Res. Ed.* 285, 258.

Ost, L. (1987). Impairment of prednisolone metabolism by cyclosporine treatment in renal graft recipients. *Transplantation* 44, 533.

Papadakis, J., Brown, C. B., Cameron, J. S., *et al.* (1983). High versus 'low' dose corticosteroids in recipients of cadaveric kidneys: prospective controlled trial. *Br. M. J.* 286, 1097.

Pescovitz, M. D., Kahan, B. D., Julian, B., *et al.* (1997). ASTP abstracts. 16, 261.

Ponticelli, C., Tarantino, A., Segoloni, G. P., *et al.* (1997). A randomized study comparing three cyclosporine-based regimens in cadaveric renal transplantation. *J. Am. Soc. Nephrol.* 8, 638.

Potter, D. E., Holliday, M. A., Wilson, C. J., *et al.* (1975). Alternate-day steroids in children after renal transplantation. *Transplant. Proc.* 7, 79.

Ratcliffe, P. J., Dudley, C. R., Higgins, R. M., *et al.* (1996). Randomised controlled trial of steroid withdrawal in renal transplant recipients receiving triple immunosuppression. *Lancet* 348, 643.

Reisman, L., Lieberman, K. V., Burrows, L. and Schanzer, H. (1990). Follow-up of cyclosporine-treated pediatric renal allograft recipients after cessation of prednisone. *Transplantation* 49, 76.

Rizzoni, G., Broyer, M., Guest, G., *et al.* (1986). Growth retardation in children with chronic renal disease: scope of the problem. *Am. J. Kidney Dis.* 7, 256.

Roberti, I., Reisman, L., Lieberman, K. V. and Burrows, L. (1994). Risk of steroid withdrawal in pediatric renal allograft recipients (a 5-year follow-up). *Clin. Transplant.* 8, 405.

Schulak, J. A., Mayes, J. T., Moritz, C. E. and Hricik, D. E. (1990). A prospective randomized trial of prednisone versus no prednisone maintenance therapy in cyclosporine-treated and azathioprine-treated renal transplant patients. *Transplantation* **49**, 327.

Schwartz, R. S. and Dameshek, W. (1959). Drug-induced immunological tolerance. *Nature* **183**, 1682.

Schwartz, R. S. and Dameshek, W. (1960). The effects of 6-mercaptopurine on homograft reactions. *J. Clin. Invest.* **39**, 952.

Shapiro, R., Jordan, V. P., Scantlebury, G., *et al.* (1998). Outcome after steroid withdrawal in renal transplant patients receiving tacrolimus based immunosuppression. *Transplant. Proc.* **30**, 1375.

Shun-Shin, G. A., Ratcliffe, P., Bron, A. J., *et al.* (1990). The lens after renal transplantation. *Br. J. Ophthalmol.* **74**, 261.

Sinclair, N. R. (1992). Low-dose steroid therapy in cyclosporine-treated renal transplant recipients with well-functioning grafts. The Canadian Multicentre Transplant Study Group. *C. M. A. J.* **147**, 645.

Slakey, D. P., Johnson, C. P., Cziperle, D. J., *et al.* (1997). Management of severe pancreatitis in renal transplant recipients. *Ann. Surg.* **225**, 217.

Squiflet, J. P., Sutherland, D. E., Rynasiewicz, J. J., *et al.* (1982). Combined immunosuppressive therapy with cyclosporin A and azathioprine. A synergistic effect in three of four experimental models. *Transplantation* **34**, 315.

Stabile, C., Vincenti, F., Garoivoy, M., *et al.* (1986). Is a 'low' dose of prednisone better than a 'high' dose at the time of renal transplantation? *Braz. J. Med. Biol. Res.* **19**, 355.

Starzl, T. E., Marchioro, T. L. and Waddell, W. R. (1963). The reversal of rejection in human renal homografts with subsequent development of monograft. *Surg. Gynecol. Obstet.* **117**, 385.

Steroid Withdrawal Study Group. (1999). Prednisone withdrawal in kidney transplant recipients on cyclosporine and mycophenolate mofetil—a prospective randomised study. *Transplantation* **68**, 1865.

Stromstrad, S. A., Kauffman, H. M., Sampson, D. and Stawicki, A. T. (1978). Random steroid therapy of human kidney transplant rejection. *Surg. Forum* **29**, 376.

Tejani, A., Butt, K. M., Rajpoot, D., *et al.* (1989). Strategies for optimizing growth in children with kidney transplants. *Transplantation* **47**, 229.

Thompson, J. F., Chalmers, D. H., Wood, R. F., *et al.* (1983). Sudden death following high dose intravenous methylprednisolone. *Transplantation* **36**, 594.

Tornatore, K. M., Walshe, J. J., Reed, K. A., Holdsworth, M. T. and Venuto, R. C. (1993). Comparative methylprednisolone pharmacokinetics in renal transplant patients receiving double- or triple-drug immunosuppression. *Ann. Pharmacother.* **27**, 545.

Veenstra, D. L., Best, J. H., Hornberger, J., Sullivan, S. D. and Hricik, D. E. (1999). Incidence and long-term cost of steroid-related side effects after renal transplantation. *Am. J. Kidney Dis.* **33**, 829.

Wolpaw, T., Deal, C. L., Fleming-Brooks, S., *et al.* (1994). Factors influencing vertebral bone density after renal transplantation. *Transplantation* **58**, 1186.

Zanker, B., *et al.* (1990). Glucocorticoids block transcription of human interleukin-6 gene by accessory cells. *Transplantation* **49**, 183.

Zukoski, F. F., Lee, H. H. and Hume, D. M. (1960). The prolongation of functional survival of canine renal homografts by 6-mercaptopurine. *Surg. Forum* **11**, 470.

16

Cyclosporine
Peter J. Morris • Christine Russell

Introduction

Cyclosporine is a powerful immunosuppressive drug and has proved to be a potent agent in a wide variety of experimental models of tissue transplantation and in clinical organ transplantation. Cyclosporine was first isolated from two strains of imperfect fungus (*Cylindrocarpon lucidum* Booth and *Trichoderma polysporum* Rifai) from soil samples by the Department of Microbiology at Sandoz (Basel, Switzerland) as an antifungal agent of limited activity (Dreyfuss *et al.*, 1976). The latter, from which cyclosporine now is produced, is known more correctly as *Tolypocladium inflatum Gams* and was shown by Borel to have potent immunosuppressive activity in a variety of *in vitro* and *in vivo* experiments (Borel, 1982; Borel *et al.*, 1976, 1977). The drug has a molecular weight of 1200 kd and comprises 11 amino acids, one of which is unique and most of which are hydrophobic. Cyclosporine is soluble only in lipids or organic solvents.

After Borel's initial description of the immunosuppressive properties of cyclosporine, it was shown to suppress rejection of vascularized organ allografts in the rat, dog and rabbit (Calne and White, 1977; Green and Allison, 1978; Kostakis *et al.*, 1977). Similar observations in various models of vascularized organ allografts in many species followed quickly (Morris, 1981). Clinical trials of the drug in renal transplantation began in Cambridge in 1978 (Calne *et al.*, 1979); by the early 1980s, cyclosporine was licensed for use in renal transplantation, first in Europe and then in the United States.

Cyclosporine-based protocols rapidly became standard therapy in renal transplantation, unless restricted by cost, and now represent the conventional therapy against which new immunosuppressive agents are compared. Because cyclosporine was the first of the new immunosuppressive agents to enter the clinical arena, a relatively extensive review of the early experimental and clinical experience with the drug is justified; the advent of cyclosporine had an enormous impact not only on renal transplantation but also on liver and heart transplantation.

Experimental Transplantation of the Kidney

Many of the clinical applications of cyclosporine in kidney transplantation have arisen from experimental models of organ transplantation, especially kidney transplantation. A brief review of some of this work is relevant today. Much of the early work was performed with a kidney allograft model in rats. For example, rejection of a kidney allograft in rats was suppressed readily by a short course of cyclosporine given orally in olive oil with permanent survival of most animals at a dose of 10 mg/kg in this model across a strong major histocompatibility complex (MHC) barrier (Homan *et al.*, 1980d). This effect is dose dependent and time dependent, however (Tables 16–1 and 16–2). A short course of an appropriate dosage of cyclosporine given during the first few crucial days of exposure to the allograft resulted in prolonged

and indefinite survival of renal allografts. A large dosage of cyclosporine did not induce permanent graft survival, suggesting that at this dosage the generation of suppressor or regulatory T cells is inhibited (see later). After day 4, when the immune response to the graft was well established, cyclosporine had no effect on this reaction.

As might be expected from its known mechanism of action, cyclosporine was relatively ineffective in a specifically presensitized rat (Homan *et al.*, 1980b). The specificity of the tolerance to a renal allograft induced by cyclosporine in the rat was shown to be partially specific in that a third-party allograft was rejected when implanted 100 days after the induction of the tolerant state, but the cytotoxic antibody response to the third-party graft was suppressed (Homan *et al.*, 1979), probably representing an example of the phenomenon of *linked immunosuppression* (Wong *et al.*, 1997). The marked synergism seen in rats between cyclosporine and heterologous antilymphocyte serum is a finding that is relevant in clinical practice (Homan *et al.*, 1980c). Donor-specific transfusions in living related and living unrelated renal transplantation no longer are used, but tolerance to a renal allograft in rats can be produced by pretreatment with donor-specific antigen and cyclosporine (Foster *et al.*, 1988; Homan *et al.*, 1981b).

Similar to the reaction in rats, a short course of cyclosporine in rabbits produced prolonged survival of renal allografts (Dunne *et al.*, 1979; Green and Allison, 1978); the tolerance so induced appeared to be specific in some experiments but not in others (Dunne, 1981; Green and Allison, 1979). These differing results, together with those mentioned for rats, probably can be explained by the timing of the tests for specificity and the assays used. For example, in a rat cardiac allograft model, White and colleagues showed that the reactivity of the recipient depends on the time at which it is tested in relation to the cessation of cyclosporine administration, the immunodepression being nonspecific for 100 days, after which it is specific for the donor strain (White *et al.*, 1980).

In contrast to rats, renal allografts in dogs are rejected after cessation of cyclosporine administration even when given for 3 months. Provided that a therapeutic dose of cyclosporine is used, however, rejection is suppressed completely, the therapeutic dose being initially approximately 20 mg kg^{-1} d^{-1} (Homan *et al.*, 1980e, 1981a). Of relevance to clinical practice is that prednisolone with cyclosporine did not appear to increase the incidence of infectious complications and that conversion from cyclosporine to azathioprine and prednisolone in dogs at 3 months can be accomplished without loss of the graft (Homan *et al.*, 1981a). A combination of azathioprine and cyclosporine, in doses that were subtherapeutic, was effective in prolonging graft survival (Aeder *et al.*, 1983). Both these observations have been confirmed in clinical practice. Using a dog model, alternating daily doses of cyclosporine and azathioprine seemed to produce a significant degree of immunosuppression with fewer side effects (Collier *et al.*,

TABLE 16–1

EFFECT OF CYCLOSPORINE ON REJECTION OF DARK AGOUTI RENAL ALLOGRAFTS IN LEWIS RATS*

Dose of Cyclosporine (mg kg^{-1})	No. Rats	Survival (Days)	Median Survival (Days)
0	9	10×3, 11×6	11
2	5	10×2, 11×3	11
5	7	24, 66, 100×5	>100
10	5	77, 100×5	>100
20	10	26, 28×3, 29×2, 30, 35, 42, 61	29

*Cyclosporine was given orally for a maximum of 14 days or as long as the animal survived. An orthotopic renal transplant was performed with removal of the remaining kidney on day 7.
Adapted with permission of Homan *et al.*, 1980c.

1986), but this approach was not practical for widespread clinical application.

Delay in the administration of cyclosporine until day 4, at which time the rejection reaction should have been well under way, resulted in prolonged survival in some dogs (Homan *et al.*, 1980a), in contrast to similar experiments in rats (see Table 16–2). Gebhard and colleagues showed that the delayed administration of cyclosporine determined by evidence of rejection from fine-needle aspirates of dog renal allografts also could reverse rejection (Gebhard *et al.*, 1985). This demonstration suggests that it might be possible to use cyclosporine to treat a rejection reaction, although theoretically this would not be expected to be successful, as is evident later in the discussion on the mechanism of action of cyclosporine. Anecdotal data later became available in humans suggesting that cyclosporine may be effective in steroid-resistant acute rejection in patients immunosuppressed with azathioprine and steroids (MacDonald *et al.*, 1983; Margreiter *et al.*, 1983).

In primates, early studies in rhesus monkeys showed that cyclosporine in doses of 25 mg kg^{-1} d^{-1} suppressed rejection of renal allografts, although rejection occurred some 10 days after cessation of the drug (Cosimi *et al.*, 1978). Borleffs and colleagues confirmed these findings with a lower dose of cyclosporine, but more importantly they showed that continued administration of cyclosporine at a dose of 10 mg kg^{-1} d^{-1} led to prolonged survival of all renal allografts with continuing survival of three of five animals at 6 months (Borleffs *et al.*, 1982). The transfusion effect still was evident in these experiments. There was no evidence of nephrotoxicity, lymphomas or infections when cyclosporine was combined with azathioprine and prednisolone. In contrast to the

impressive results obtained in rhesus monkeys, which were similar to results obtained in dogs, cyclosporine proved less effective in prolonging renal allograft survival in chacma baboons. A dose of 20 mg kg^{-1} d^{-1}, given indefinitely, increased survival time only from a median of 11 to 22.5 days. A modest improvement in this survival was obtained by pretreatment with 30 mg d^{-1}, with indefinite administration of this dose afterward, despite the maintenance of what would be considered therapeutic levels of cyclosporine in the blood (Smit *et al.*, 1983). This appears to be the only model in which cyclosporine has proved to be relatively ineffective.

Mechanism of Action

It was apparent from many early *in vivo* experiments that cyclosporine exerts its effect at an early stage after exposure of the recipient to a tissue allograft. This situation was illustrated in the rat renal allograft model cited earlier (Homan *et al.*, 1980d; Morris *et al.*, 1983; see Table 16–2), showing that cyclosporine is relatively ineffective in this model if given after induction of the immune response has taken place or before the recipient animal has been exposed to the allogeneic histocompatibility antigens.

In vitro experiments correlated well with these *in vivo* observations. In several species, as well as in humans, cyclosporine has been shown to inhibit the proliferative response of lymphocytes to concanavalin A, phytohemagglutinin and pokeweed mitogen *in vitro* (Borel, 1981; Burckhardt and Guggenheim, 1979; Larsson, 1980; Leapman *et al.*, 1981; White *et al.*, 1979; Wiesinger and Borel, 1979). If cyclosporine is added 48 hours after the addition of mitogen to a culture, there is

TABLE 16–2

EFFECTS OF CYCLOSPORINE ON REJECTION OF DARK AGOUTI RENAL ALLOGRAFTS IN LEWIS RATS DEPENDING ON THE TIME OF ADMINISTRATION*

Treatment Period (Days)	Dose of Cyclosporine (mg kg^{-1})	No. Rats	Median Survival and Range (Days)
—	0	9	11 (10–11)
−14−−1	10	7	12 (10–13)
−2–0	10	6	12 (12–14)
0–2	10	5	22 (15–>100)
0–4	10	5	28 (20–>100)
0–14	10	7	>100 (all >100)
4–14	5	5	13 (11–14)
4–14	10	5	11 (10–11)
4–14	25	4	9 (9–10)

*Cyclosporine was given orally. An orthotopic renal transplant was performed on day 0 with removal of the remaining kidney on day 7.
Adapted with permission of Homan *et al.*, 1980c.

no inhibition of proliferation, and the effect is reversed by washing the lymphocytes and reexposing them to the mitogen (Wiesinger and Borel, 1979). Complete inhibition of the mixed lymphocyte reaction by cyclosporine has been shown in several species including humans (Hess and Tutschka, 1980; Horsburgh et al., 1980; Keown et al., 1981a, 1981b; Leapman et al., 1981; Tutschka et al., 1982). The generation of cytotoxic lymphocytes in the mixed lymphocyte reaction is prevented by cyclosporine, but once generated, cyclosporine has no effect on their cytotoxic activity (Bunjes et al., 1982; Hess and Tutschka, 1980; Hess et al., 1982a; Horsburgh et al., 1980; Keown et al., 1981b). Theoretically, cyclosporine might be expected to be less effective in preventing graft rejection in sensitized animals (Gratwohl et al., 1981; Homan et al., 1980b). Although it does not inhibit the secondary mixed lymphocyte reaction response or the generation of cytotoxic T lymphocytes in such a secondary reaction (Hess and Tutschka, 1980; Leapman et al., 1981), it does inhibit interleukin (IL)-2 production significantly (Andrus and Lafferty, 1981; Hess et al., 1982b), suggesting that cyclosporine could have some efficacy in sensitized recipients in the treatment of ongoing rejection.

Lymphocytes extracted from a rejecting renal allograft in the rat can be shown to exhibit specific cytotoxic activity and nonspecific cytotoxic activity in vitro because of macrophages and natural killer cells, but in animals treated with cyclosporine, the lymphocytes are not cytotoxic to specific target cells, although they display normal natural killer cell activity (Mason and Morris, 1984). The expression of the cytotoxic T-cell–associated serine protease granzyme A and perforin in the cellular infiltrate of heterotopic cardiac allografts was shown to be increased markedly in rejection of allografts in untreated mice but suppressed in animals treated with cyclosporine (Chen et al., 1993; Mueller et al., 1993). Cyclosporine also has been shown to reduce markedly the incidence of cytotoxic T lymphocytes in the blood of patients with a renal transplant compared with patients receiving azathioprine and prednisolone (Keown et al., 1985). This finding is compatible with the in vitro findings showing that cyclosporine inhibits the generation of cytotoxic T cells. In the same model, the induction of MHC class II antigen expression (resulting from release of interferon-γ) in the transplanted kidney is inhibited (Milton et al., 1986; see Chapter 2), and this is seen to a considerable extent in humans (Fuggle et al., 1986). Not only does cyclosporine inhibit the generation of cytotoxic T cells in this model but also it may reduce the antigenicity of the target organ.

The predominant action of cyclosporine is directed against CD4+ T (T-helper) lymphocytes (Borel, 1981; Borel et al., 1976; Burkhardt and Guggenheim, 1979; Cammisuli, 1982; Gordon and Singer, 1979; Kahan et al., 1982; Kunkle and Klaus, 1980). This effect on the CD4+ T cell prevents the production of lymphokines, especially IL-2 (Bunjes et al., 1982; Lafferty et al., 1983; Larsson, 1980; Palacios and Moller, 1981), which, in turn, inhibits the further proliferation of CD4+ T cells and the generation of the cytotoxic T cells from the cytotoxic T-cell precursor. This effect also may allow the uninhibited generation of nonspecific and specific suppressor or regulatory T lymphocytes, as suggested by the work of Leapman et al. (1981) and Hess et al. (1981, 1982b), which implied that T-suppressor cells are relatively resistant to cyclosporine. That the prolongation of renal allograft survival in the rat is due to the induction of T-suppressor cells has been shown in adoptive transfer assays (Barber et al., 1985; Chiu and Batchelor, 1986; Kupiec-Weglinski et al., 1985). The suppressor cells involved in the induction of tolerance in a renal allograft model (Hutchinson, 1986) all have been shown to be resistant

to cyclosporine in adoptive transfer assays (Rodriques et al., 1987).

Cyclosporine may inhibit the maturation of the cytotoxic T-cell precursor by preventing the development of receptors for IL-2 (Hess et al., 1983a) or by inhibiting another lymphokine produced by the T-helper cell that acts on the cytotoxic precursor cell and induces the production of IL-2 receptors (Bunjes et al., 1982). Conflicting data concerning the effect of cyclosporine on the expression of IL-2 receptors have been presented. No reduction of IL-2 receptor expression after mitogen stimulation of human lymphocytes was noted (Miyawaki et al., 1983; Ryffel et al., 1985), but IL-2 receptor expression was reduced in cyclosporine-treated human mixed lymphocyte reaction cultures (Hess et al., 1983b). Probably the effect of cyclosporine on IL-2 responsiveness and IL-2 receptor formation is more complex than originally believed.

Although, in general, cyclosporine has not been thought to inhibit the function of B lymphocytes (Borel et al., 1977; Burckhardt and Guggenheim, 1979; Gordon and Singer, 1979), there is some evidence to the contrary in humans (Paavonen and Hayry, 1980; Pisetsky and Haughton, 1986) and mice (Bouwer and Hinrichs, 1983; Klaus and Dongworth, 1982; Kunkle and Klaus, 1980). O'Garra and colleagues showed a cyclosporine-sensitive subpopulation of T-cell–independent B lymphocytes in mice and showed that cyclosporine can inhibit the production of murine B-cell–derived lymphokines (O'Garra et al., 1986).

Cyclosporine may have some inhibiting effect on the production of IL-1 by macrophages (Bunjes et al., 1982), although their response to lymphokines is not inhibited (Thomson et al., 1983). There is evidence that IL-3 production is inhibited by cyclosporine (Lafferty et al., 1983) and that the production of interferon-γ, but not interferon-α or interferon-β, is inhibited by cyclosporine (Kalman and Klimpel, 1983). Cyclosporine and FK506 (tacrolimus) have been shown to suppress markedly the steady-state level of IL-4 mRNA in a T-helper two-cell line but not to alter the level of IL-10 mRNA (Wang et al., 1991). Production of IL-10 in mice was inhibited by cyclosporine, however, if IL-10 production was stimulated by an anti-CD3 monoclonal antibody. It was augmented by cyclosporine if IL-10 production was stimulated by lipopolysaccharide (Durez et al., 1993). Cyclosporine does not appear to influence the inflammatory granulation response in vivo (Nemlander et al., 1983), which is consistent with the normal wound healing seen in clinical practice in patients receiving cyclosporine. Cyclosporine inhibits the in vitro immunological release of preformed (histamine) and de novo synthesized (leukotriene C_4 and prostaglandin D_2) mediators of inflammatory reactions from human basophils and mast cells (Marone et al., 1992).

Studies of the binding of cyclosporine to various cells suggest that although a large amount of the cell-associated drug is located in the cytosol, there may be a differential binding to different cells, with splenocytes and thymocytes showing particularly high activity (Merker et al., 1983). No evidence for a specific cyclosporine receptor has been found, and no evidence has been found for differential binding of cyclosporine to B cells, helper T cells or suppressor T cells (LeGrue et al., 1983). Within the cell, cyclosporine was shown to bind to calcium-dependent proteins and enzymes, such as calmodulin and cyclophilin (Handschumaker et al., 1984; Hess and Colambani, 1986). Initially, it was suggested that the blockade of these calcium-dependent intracellular proteins may block the calcium-dependent activation events, preventing the normal signals that initiate DNA and mRNA synthesis for the proinflammatory lymphokines, especially IL-2. LeGrue and coworkers had suggested first that the immunosuppressive activity of cyclosporine was not due to binding and inhibition of calmodulin-dependent processes (LeGrue et al., 1986). There was evidence in the 1980s that the transcription of mRNA for IL-2 and other lymphokines is inhibited but not that of other proteins (Elliot et al., 1984), but what happens between the intracellular localization of cyclosporine to calcium-dependent proteins and the blockade of the mRNA transcription for the lymphokines was not known until years later.

Several years later, there was a considerable increase in information about the mechanism of action of cyclosporine within the cell at a molecular level (Schreiber and Crabtree, 1992; Schreier et al., 1993; Sigal and Dumont, 1992). Cyclosporine binds within the cytosol to cyclophilin, a cis-trans-peptidyl-prolyl isomerase that has an important role in folding proteins and peptides into their native conformation (Fischer and Schmid, 1990). Cyclophilin has been found in a wide variety of cell types and organisms other than lymphocytes. It was the inhibition of this isomerase activity that was thought initially to be responsible for the immunosuppressive activity of cyclosporine (Fischer et al., 1989; Takahashi et al., 1989). There is a family of cyclophilins to which cyclosporine binds, although most of the drug binds to cyclophilin A, a 12-kd molecule. The cyclophilins belong to a larger family of immunophilins (proteins that bind immunosuppressive agents), FK-binding protein being another member of that family to which tacrolimus and rapamycin (sirolimus) bind. Tacrolimus and cyclosporine appear to have an identical mechanism of action that is quite different from that of rapamycin (see Chapters 17 and 19).

It is the complex of cyclosporine and cyclophilin that is the immunosuppressive molecule, cyclosporine being a prodrug and not of itself immunosuppressive. This complex of the drug and its immunophilin binds to a calcium-dependent and calmodulin-dependent phosphatase, calcineurin (Friedman and Weissman, 1991; Liu et al., 1991). Calcineurin appears to play a crucial role in the transduction of the calcium-dependent signal that leads to the activation of the enhancer region of the IL-2 gene (Clipstone and Crabtree, 1992; O'Keefe et al., 1992) because it dephosphorylates the cytosolic form of the nuclear factor of activated T cells (NFATc), which is necessary for its translocation into the nucleus as NFATn, which, in turn, activates the enhancer region of the IL-2 gene leading to its transcription (Granelli-Piperno et al., 1990). Undoubtedly, other transcription factors, such as NFIL-2 A and B, also are inhibited by cyclosporine (Mattila et al., 1990). The cyclosporine-immunophilin complex binds to calcineurin and blocks the dephosphorylation of NFATc and its translocation into the nucleus, preventing the transcription of the IL-2 gene (Flanagan et al., 1991; Granelli-Piperno, 1988). There is a second pathway of activation (the so-called second signal), however, mediated by CD28 with distinct signal pathways, including protein kinase C (Umlauf et al., 1993). Activation of this pathway also leads to IL-2 production and IL-2R expression, and this pathway is resistant to cyclosporine (Hess and Bright, 1991).

An additional action of cyclosporine has been shown: Cyclosporine enhances transforming growth factor (TGF)-β mRNA expression in normal human T cells and constrains new DNA synthesis through a TGF-β–dependent mechanism (Khanna et al., 1995; Liu et al., 1991). Because TGF-β may have an immunoregulatory role and be an immunosuppressive cytokine in its own right (Carel, 1990; Wallick et al., 1990), the immunosuppressive activity of cyclosporine not only might be due to suppression of expression of the proinflammatory cytokine IL-2, but also due to augmentation of the production of the immunosuppressive cytokine TGF-β (Khanna et al., 1995). As discussed later, the enhanced production of TGF-β by cyclosporine also may play a role in the development of fibrosis, a characteristic feature of chronic rejection.

Unraveling the molecular mechanism of action of these newer immunosuppressive agents such as cyclosporine and tacrolimus has led to a much more detailed understanding of the nature of signal transduction after the T-cell receptor has recognized alloantigen. This understanding, in turn, should allow drugs with specific actions to be designed, and this may be enhanced by the description of the three-dimensional structure of the cyclosporine-cyclophilin complex, which at a crystallographic level appears to be a pentamer with the two pentamers forming a sandwich with the cyclophilin pentamers on the outside and the cyclosporine molecules inside the sandwich (Pflugii et al., 1993; Theriault et al., 1993).

The major mechanism of action of cyclosporine is the inhibition of the transcription of the genes for IL-2 and other cytokines such as interferon in the CD4$^+$ T cell after recognition of alloantigen. This inhibition, in turn, leads to inhibition of many of the lymphokine-induced signals, such as the proliferation and generation of cytotoxic T-cell precursors.

Clinical Experience
EARLY EXPERIENCE

Cyclosporine first was used in renal transplantation by Calne and colleagues in Cambridge (Calne et al., 1979, 1981). Initially, it was used with other drugs, such as prednisolone or Asta 036.5122 (cytimum, an analogue of cyclophosphamide), but this proved a dangerous combination, with many patients dying of infection. For the first time, it became apparent that cyclosporine was nephrotoxic in humans, not a feature of the extensive experimental use of cyclosporine in animal models at that time, although becoming apparent later (Bennett, 1986; Whiting, 1982a, 1982b). Three lymphomas were seen in these early patients, which caused considerable alarm. A new policy was adopted at Cambridge whereby cyclosporine was used only in patients whose grafts were diuresing and was used alone, with high-dose methylprednisolone given to treat rejection. If more than 6 g of methylprednisolone was required, patients were converted to azathioprine and prednisolone. Following this policy, 60 cadaveric grafts were performed in 59 patients, all but one of whom had been transfused previously. Actuarial graft survival at 1 year was 82%. Six deaths occurred, five from infection, and 10 patients were converted to azathioprine and prednisolone because rejection was not controlled with cyclosporine (Calne and White, 1982). Many of these patients were not receiving steroids; many had never received any steroids.

This early experience in Cambridge prompted many controlled trials of cyclosporine—single-center trials in Minneapolis, Oxford, Pittsburgh and Sydney as well as multicenter trials in Europe and Canada and uncontrolled studies in Denver, Pittsburgh, Stockholm and Boston. In the European multicenter trial, only patients who were given grafts that were diuresing 6 hours after surgery were randomized to receive cyclosporine alone or conventional treatment with azathioprine and prednisolone, according to the custom of the unit. The trial was closed at the end of 1981 after 1 year, when slightly more than 200 patients had been entered. Actual survival at 1 year was 72% in the cyclosporine group and 52% in the control group (European Multicentre Trial, 1982, 1983), although many patients were converted to azathioprine and steroids because of apparent rejection on cyclosporine. At 5 years, there was a marked difference (but not as great) in graft survival in favor of cyclosporine—55%

versus 40% in the control group (Calne, 1987)—and at 10 years the difference was 35% versus 29%, with stable renal function in the cyclosporine group, although at a higher serum creatinine level than in the control group (European Multicentre Trial Group, 1993; Fig. 16–1). Undoubtedly, many of the grafts considered to be rejecting in this trial were suffering from nephrotoxicity in retrospect, an ever-present problem that is discussed later. Actual survival in the patients excluded from the trial and treated with conventional immunosuppression was similar to that of the control group within the trial.

An excellent multicenter trial was conducted in Canada, in which cyclosporine and prednisolone therapy was compared with standard therapy based on azathioprine and prednisolone in 209 cadaveric renal allograft recipients (Canadian Multicentre Transplant Study Group, 1983). In this first analysis, actuarial graft survival at 1 year was 84% in the cyclosporine group compared with 67% in those receiving standard therapy, with patient survivals of 97% and 90% in the two groups. At 3 years, graft survival was 69% in the cyclosporine-treated group and 58% in the control group, a less striking difference than in the initial analysis (Canadian Multicentre Transplant Study Group, 1986). Patient survival was 90% in the cyclosporine group and 82% in the control group. No transfusion effect was seen in the cyclosporine group, although this was evident in the control group (there were no nontransfused patients in the trial). A detrimental effect on graft survival was seen in cyclosporine-treated patients if they received kidneys that had been perfused for longer than 24 hours or if the surgical anastomosis time took longer than 45 minutes, suggesting that cyclosporine nephrotoxicity is more likely to occur in kidneys that have some ischemic damage.

In Minneapolis, all HLA-mismatched living or cadaveric donor transplants were eligible for the trial in which cyclosporine plus prednisolone was compared with conventional therapy of azathioprine, steroids and antilymphocyte globulin (Ferguson et al., 1982a; Najarian et al., 1983, 1985). All patients had had a splenectomy and at least 5 units of blood before transplantation. A total of 230 patients had been en-

tered into the trial, which included cadaver and living related transplants and diabetic and nondiabetic recipients. Overall graft survival rates at 2 years were 82% in the cyclosporine group and 77% in the control group, and patient survival was 88% and 91%. In the living related transplants, graft survival at 2 years was 87% in the cyclosporine group and 83% in the control group, whereas the 2-year graft survival figures in the cadaver transplants were 78% and 73%. These differences in survival were not significant, but the cumulative incidence of rejection episodes in the first year after transplantation in the cyclosporine group was half that in the control group, as was the incidence of infection.

Similarly, Starzl and colleagues, first at Denver (where treatment was not standardized) and then at Pittsburgh, reported impressive results with cyclosporine and prednisolone (at a maintenance dose of 20 mg d^{-1} after a burst of high-dose prednisolone) in primary and secondary cadaveric transplants (Starzl et al., 1982, 1983). Graft survival was about 90% at 1 year in primary cadaveric transplants. In 26 patients who received 27 cadaver retransplants, 1-year graft survival was 78%. After that initial experience, virtually all contraindications to the use of cyclosporine in renal transplantation were disregarded, and in 96 primary cadaveric grafts, patient survival at 1 year was predicted as 90% and graft survival as 80% (Starzl et al., 1983). Early anuria was not considered a contraindication to cyclosporine, which was sometimes considered to be the result of rejection and/or nephrotoxicity, although it did cause diagnostic problems in the management of their patients. In the controlled trial of cyclosporine versus azathioprine, prednisolone and antilymphocyte globulin in Sydney, 60 patients receiving first cadaveric grafts were entered, and graft survival of 70% at 1 year was similar in both groups. Persistent anuria after transplantation was a major problem in the cyclosporine group (Sheil et al., 1983).

In the Oxford trials, patients randomized to receive cyclosporine were converted at 3 months to azathioprine and prednisolone to reduce nephrotoxicity (Morris et al., 1982, 1987). This approach is discussed later in this chapter.

This early experience with cyclosporine in prospective controlled trials and in uncontrolled trials indicated that cy-

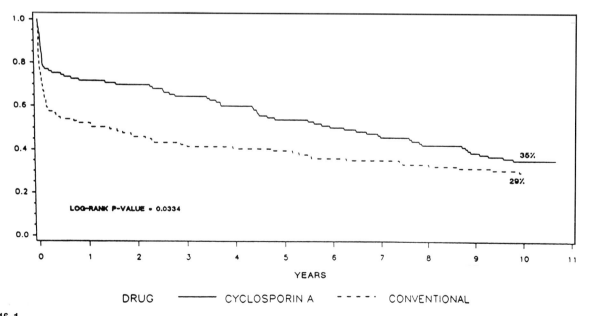

FIGURE 16–1

Cadaveric graft survival at 10 years in the European Multicentre Trial, in which 232 recipients were allocated randomly to receive either cyclosporine (n = 117) or azathioprine and steroids (n = 115). (Reproduced with permission of European Multicentre Trial Group, 1993.)

TABLE 16–3

CYCLOSPORINE-BASED PROTOCOLS THAT HAVE BEEN OR ARE USED IN RENAL TRANSPLANTATION

Cyclosporine (monotherapy)
Cyclosporine + prednisolone
Cyclosporine + azathioprine (dual therapy)
Cyclosporine + azathioprine + prednisolone (triple therapy)
ALG/OKT3 + azathioprine + prednisolone → cyclosporine + azathioprine + prednisolone (sequential therapy)
Cyclosporine + prednisolone → azathioprine + prednisolone (conversion therapy)
ALG/OKT3 + cyclosporine + azathioprine + prednisolone (quadruple therapy)

closporine was a major advance in immunosuppressive therapy, as was evident in the European Collaborative Study, which had data from more than 200 transplant centers and several thousand renal transplants (Opelz, 1986). Many side effects had become evident, the major one being nephrotoxicity, and so subsequent protocols were designed to obtain the same improved immunosuppression achieved with cyclosporine but with a reduction in side effects resulting from lower doses of cyclosporine (Table 16–3). There is no convincing evidence that one protocol is superior to another, at least for three protocols, as illustrated by an Australian multicenter trial (Hardie, 1993): Patient and graft survivals were identical for cyclosporine and prednisolone; cyclosporine and azathioprine and cyclosporine, azathioprine and prednisolone.

CYCLOSPORINE WITH OR WITHOUT STEROIDS

The initial use of cyclosporine in Europe was based on the experimental data and the early Cambridge experience, using a rather high dosage of cyclosporine alone, whereas in North America, cyclosporine was used with steroids. Gradu-

ally, most units added steroids to their cyclosporine protocols but not with any convincing evidence that steroids were necessary. In the United States, there had been a tendency to use high-dose steroids, at least in the early weeks after transplantation. Four prospective controlled trials comparing cyclosporine alone with cyclosporine and steroids were performed (De Vecchi et al., 1985; Griffin et al., 1986; Johnson et al., 1985; MacDonald et al., 1987; Stiller, 1983). None was able to confirm an additive effect of steroids in terms of immunosuppression. Two groups found an increased incidence of infection with steroids, although Griffin and co-workers suggested that steroids reduced the incidence of cyclosporine nephrotoxicity (Griffin et al., 1986). Schmidt and colleagues, in a morphological study of renal biopsy specimens 1 year after renal transplantation, found no difference in biopsy specimens from patients treated with cyclosporine with or without steroids, however (Schmidt et al., 1986). In these studies, steroids were used for the treatment of rejection, and in many patients with recurrent rejection steroids were added to cyclosporine.

Many patients can be managed without steroids or weaned off steroids relatively early, although the long-term outcome of the Canadian trial suggested that the withdrawal of steroids was associated with a poorer graft outcome (Sinclair, 1992). Patients who have not had steroids present an entirely different facies than what clinicians had become used to in the precyclosporine era (Fig. 16–2). Although the need for steroids in all patients treated with cyclosporine is unresolved, most patients are likely to need high-dose methylprednisolone for the treatment of acute rejection episodes. Most units have used steroids with cyclosporine from the time of transplantation. Two types of protocols were used. In North America, the tendency was to use high oral doses of prednisolone (e.g., 100 mg d^{-1}) from the time of transplantation, reducing rapidly to lower doses over the first 2 to 3 weeks, whereas in Europe, the trend was to use low doses from the time of transplantation (e.g., 20–30 mg d^{-1}), reduc-

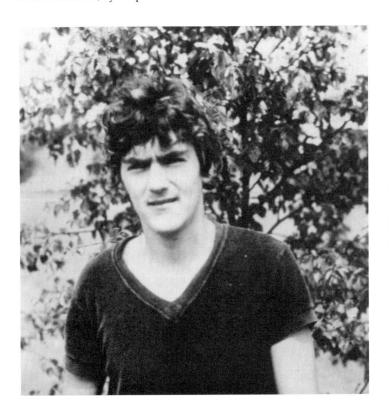

FIGURE 16–2

A young man 3 months after renal transplantation. He had received cyclosporine only (without steroids), and the absence of the usual cushingoid facies, which is most apparent in the early months after transplantation, is striking.

ing to maintenance doses over the first 3 to 6 months. There is no evidence that one approach is better than the other, and on general principles the low-dose steroid protocol should be favored if steroids are to be employed routinely with cyclosporine.

Cyclosporine alone has been used in the past at what would now be considered high doses (17.5 mg kg^{-1} d^{-1}), and many of the reported side effects of cyclosporine, most of which are dose related, can be attributed to these high doses. After the early years, cyclosporine doses gradually were reduced based on the maintenance of adequate trough blood levels (200–400 ng ml^{-1} in the early months), and this led to a reduction in nephrotoxicity and other side effects, but it has not led to the disappearance of nephrotoxicity. It is possible that the concurrent use of steroids with these lower doses of cyclosporine is important for adequate immunosuppression; that is the view held by most clinicians. The trials mentioned previously all used higher doses of cyclosporine. A randomized prospective trial comparing cyclosporine monotherapy with cyclosporine, azathioprine and prednisolone triple therapy did not show any difference in graft survival, but more severe rejections were seen in the monotherapy group, which required more high-dose steroid rejection treatments. Cyclosporine nephrotoxicity also was commoner in the monotherapy group, which was started on 15 mg kg^{-1} d^{-1} of cyclosporine, than in the triple therapy group, which received 8 mg kg^{-1} d^{-1} (Tarantino et al., 1991).

Cyclosporine is administered as a single daily dose or twice-daily dose with the older formulation (Sandimmune) or as two 12-hourly doses with the new microemulsion formulation (Neoral). After administration of Sandimmune, trough levels are reached at 12 to 18 hours, whereas with Neoral, which is much better absorbed and has an increased bioavailablity, trough levels are achieved at 10 to 12 hours. Sandimmune can be given as a single daily dose, whereas Neoral needs to be given twice daily (12 hourly). There is increasing concern that nephrotoxicity may be related more to high peak levels rather than high trough levels, and although there is no evidence that twice-daily doses of Sandimmune produced better immunosuppression, it was suggested that there was a greater incidence of nephrotoxicity (Savoldi et al., 1987). There is more recent evidence, however, to be discussed later, that low peak levels may predict rejection better than low trough levels.

CYCLOSPORINE WITH CONVERSION TO AZATHIOPRINE AND STEROIDS

The original development of a cyclosporine conversion protocol at Oxford was based on the recognition at Cambridge of nephrotoxicity and an apparent increase in the incidence of malignant lymphomas in patients receiving cyclosporine after renal transplantation. Conversion at 3 months after transplantation had proved effective in a dog renal transplant model (Homan et al., 1981a), and this protocol was used in a prospective controlled trial in which patients with nondiuresing kidneys and patients receiving HLA-DR–compatible kidneys were excluded (Morris et al., 1982). This small trial suggested that the conversion protocol appeared at least as satisfactory as conventional immunosuppression, and a second trial was begun in which all patients who were to receive a cadaver kidney were allocated randomly to receive cyclosporine alone with conversion to azathioprine and prednisolone at 90 days or continuous immunosuppression with azathioprine and low-dose steroids (Chapman and Morris, 1985; Chapman et al., 1985a; Morris et al., 1987). This trial was completed in 1984, and all patients had been followed for at least 5 years after transplantation. Patient and graft survivals (Fig. 16–3) in the conversion group were excellent (graft survival at 5 years was 67%) and significantly better than conventional therapy (graft survival at 5 years was 47%).

Five-year graft survival of the cyclosporine arm in the contemporaneous European Multicentre Trial (1982) was 55%. After conversion, there was a rapid improvement in renal function, which was maintained at 3 years, and other cyclosporine side effects, such as hypertension, gingival hypertrophy and hypercholesterolemia, were decreased. A similar improvement in cardiovascular risk factors was noted after conversion from cyclosporine to azathioprine by Sutherland et al. (1993). The main problem associated with conversion in the Oxford trial was that approximately one third of the patients had at least one acute rejection episode in the weeks after conversion, and one patient lost her graft as a result. In general, most patients responded readily to treatment with methylprednisolone, although some needed to be placed again on cyclosporine for recurrent rejection episodes.

Two other prospective controlled trials of cyclosporine conversion protocols (similar to the Oxford protocol) have

FIGURE 16–3

Actuarial patient and cadaveric graft survival in the Oxford Trial II of conversion from cyclosporine at 90 days to azathioprine and steroids versus azathioprine and steroids. The percentage actuarial graft survival rates at 1, 3 and 5 years (number of patients at entry) are given. Solid line = cyclosporine conversion group; broken line = azathioprine-prednisolone group. (From Morris et al., 1987; reproduced with permission from Lancet.)

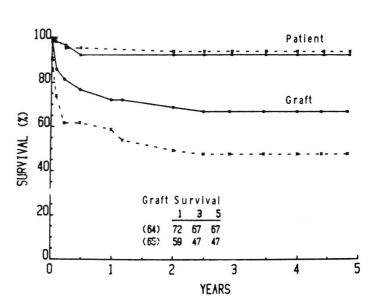

produced equally good results (Hall *et al.*, 1988; Hoitsma *et al.*, 1987). The Australian trial, in which only transfused recipients of first-cadaver grafts were entered, compared conversion not only with azathioprine plus prednisolone immunosuppression, but also with continuous cyclosporine therapy, and in both the cyclosporine groups graft survival at 1 year was approximately 80%.

Acute rejection after conversion was much less common in the Dutch and Australian trials, and it was suggested that this resulted from an overlap between discontinuation of cyclosporine and start of azathioprine and prednisolone in their trials, in contrast with the Oxford study, in which there was no such overlap. Stimulated by the early Oxford experience, other groups embarked on conversion protocols not only in the hope of decreasing the nephrotoxicity associated with cyclosporine, but also in some instances to reduce the cost of immunosuppression. In these uncontrolled trials of conversion protocols, there was considerable variation in experience (Chapman and Morris, 1987; Kasiske *et al.*, 1993). Mostly, there was a significant incidence of acute rejection after conversion that in some studies was considered unacceptable, whereas in others it was not considered a problem. Some authors suggested that there was a late loss of grafts after conversion that might have been avoided if cyclosporine had been continued, whereas other authors did not agree with this view. The results from the uncontrolled trials are confusing. The data of the three large prospective controlled trials of cyclosporine conversion at 3 months suggest that conversion is an acceptable protocol, at least in the short term and medium term, and leads to a significant improvement in renal function as well as regression of other cyclosporine side effects. As to the time of conversion, it is possible that delaying this for at least 6 months and perhaps longer after transplantation might be preferable, as suggested by Forwell *et al.* (1987) and confirmed in a study from Denmark by Pedersen *et al.* (1993). An overlap of immunosuppression around the time of conversion appears advisable.

The long-term follow-up of the Glasgow study, in which more than 200 patients with stable renal function at 1 year were randomized to convert from cyclosporine and steroids to azathioprine and steroids or remain on cyclosporine and steroids, showed no significant difference in patient or graft survival at 10 years (MacPhee *et al.*, 1998). Renal function was better in the conversion group, as was the need for treatment for hypertension.

Patients who have had a regraft possibly are more likely to reject after conversion, which always has been our impression in Oxford. Weimar and colleagues reported their results of conversion at 1 year in 23 cadaveric recipients in which 4 of 5 patients who had acute rejection after conversion were regrafts, whereas virtually no problems were encountered with conversion of patients with first grafts (Weimar *et al.*, 1987).

Conversion protocols are important because of the cost of cyclosporine compared with azathioprine and prednisolone. These protocols might allow cyclosporine to be used to achieve improved graft survival in transplantation programs for developing countries, although Sanders and coworkers advise caution in discontinuing cyclosporine in black patients in the United States (Sanders *et al.*, 1993). Although there has been a tendency to dismiss conversion protocols in favor of low-dose cyclosporine protocols, they are worthy of further attention, particularly in view of the excellent renal function obtained after conversion, which seems to persist for at least 3 years (Morris *et al.*, 1987). Meta-analysis of 10 randomized and 7 nonrandomized trials showed a greater combined rate of acute rejection among patients in whom cyclosporine was

withdrawn but a better graft survival rate in patients in whom cyclosporine was reduced (Kasiske *et al.*, 1993).

Conversion from cyclosporine to azathioprine and prednisolone was performed for nephrotoxicity and for acute rejection not responding to conventional treatment with methylprednisolone (Chapman and Morris, 1987). Conversion in steroid-resistant rejection rarely influenced the course of the rejection, and most grafts were lost. Morozumi and colleagues studied the histological outcome of grafts with cyclosporine-associated arteriolopathy in patients in whom cyclosporine was discontinued (Morozumi *et al.*, 1993). Although there was an improvement in the arteriolopathy after discontinuation of the drug in many patients, graft loss increased owing to vascular rejection and an increase in interstitial fibrosis. These investigators concluded that the only indication for the discontinuation of cyclosporine was the presence of a hemolytic uremic syndrome–like cyclosporine vasculopathy and that low-dose cyclosporine was preferable to cessation of the drug in the presence of this arteriolar lesion, which is an uncommon toxic association of cyclosporine.

TRIPLE THERAPY

In an attempt to maintain the improved immunosuppression provided by cyclosporine and to reduce the incidence of cyclosporine side effects, especially nephrotoxicity, triple therapy with low doses of cyclosporine, azathioprine and steroids was introduced by several groups (Fries *et al.*, 1985; Illner *et al.*, 1985; Simmons *et al.*, 1986; Slapak *et al.*, 1985). Data in experimental models suggested that azathioprine and cyclosporine might be synergistic in their immunosuppressive activity (Squifflet *et al.*, 1983).

The results of triple therapy were excellent (Fries *et al.*, 1987; Jones *et al.*, 1988a), with 1-year first cadaver graft survival rates of around 80% reported in most instances and with a substantial number of patients having no rejection. For example, 38% of patients with cadaver grafts in the Oxford experience had no clinical or histological rejection episodes in the first 3 months after transplantation (Jones *et al.*, 1988a). There does not appear to be an increase in the incidence of infection despite the possible enhancement of immunosuppression achieved with the triple therapy. This form of triple therapy soon became the most commonly used immunosuppressive therapy in renal transplantation, although today azathioprine is replaced by mycophenolate mofetil. Despite low doses of cyclosporine, renal function remained suboptimal and did not appear to be much improved over that seen in the Oxford Unit with the use of high doses of cyclosporine alone. Although triple therapy is a potent immunosuppressive regimen, it does not seem to be any more effective than some of the other cyclosporine protocols described in this section (Hardie, 1993). Its ease of use has made triple therapy an increasingly popular protocol in many units, with acceptable results that continue to improve (Fig. 16–4 and Table 16–4).

An attempt to resolve the problem of efficacy was reported first from Milan (Ponticelli *et al.*, 1988; Tarantino *et al.*, 1991) in a randomized controlled trial of triple therapy versus high-dose cyclosporine and steroids. Although patient and graft survival rates were similar in the two groups, there were more rejection episodes in the triple-therapy group and evidence of greater renal impairment and infection in the high-dose cyclosporine group. The second report was of a multicenter prospective trial from Australia comparing triple therapy with cyclosporine and prednisolone as well as cyclosporine and azathioprine (Hardie, 1993). Approximately 140 patients were entered into each arm of the trial, which in-

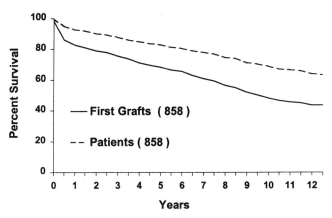

FIGURE 16–4

Actuarial survival of primary cadaveric grafts in 858 patients treated with triple therapy (cyclosporine, azathioprine and prednisolone) at the Oxford Transplant Centre.

cluded nondiabetic transfused recipients of first cadaver grafts. Patient and graft survival rates were excellent in all three groups—91% and 85% at 1 year. Of patients receiving cyclosporine and azathioprine, however, 36% required long-term prednisolone to control rejection. The investigators suggested that optimal therapy might involve the initial use of cyclosporine plus one other agent, with the possible addition of a third if required.

Many units have explored the possibility of dropping one of the three drugs, most commonly steroids, after several months of triple therapy. It appears that this can be done safely in most patients. In a trial from Finland, patients on triple therapy were randomized to drop one of the three drugs after 3 months (Hayry et al., 1988). The early experience of this trial suggested that any one of the three drugs can be discontinued safely with excellent graft survival being maintained in all three groups. More recently, a randomized prospective trial of steroid withdrawal in patients on triple therapy with stable renal function after 1 year was reported from Oxford (Ratcliffe et al., 1996). Complete steroid withdrawal was possible in most with significant improvement in cardiovascular risk factors (i.e., serum cholesterol and blood pressure) and in bone mineral metabolism. A modest reduction in graft function, of uncertain origin, was common but was not progressive, at least in the medium term. Withdrawal of steroids in patients on triple therapy has been shown

TABLE 16–4

TRIPLE-THERAPY PROTOCOL USED AT OXFORD TRANSPLANT CENTRE

Cyclosporine	8 mg/kg/d orally given as equally divided doses (first dose given before surgery) and reduced according to whole-blood trough levels (150–300 ng/ml in first 6 months, then maintained at 75–150 ng/ml)
Azathioprine	1.5 mg/kg/d orally; reduced if leukocyte count < 5,000
Prednisolone	20 mg/d given in divided doses orally and reduced to a maintenance dose of 10 mg/d by 6 months. The initial dose is reduced to 15 mg/d in patients < 60 kg body weight. In patients with stable renal function at 1 year, prednisolone is discontinued over a period of some months

to improve significantly the management of patients with posttransplant diabetes mellitus (Hricick et al., 1991). It seems reasonable to attempt withdrawal of steroids in all patients on triple therapy who have stable renal function. Whether this can be done earlier than 1 year after transplantation is uncertain.

As mentioned earlier, triple therapy can be undertaken with mycophenolate replacing azathioprine, resulting in a significant reduction in the incidence of acute rejection episodes in the first 6 months after transplantation, which, however, has not been reflected by better graft survival. This change has significant cost implications for immunosuppression.

QUADRUPLE THERAPY

The addition to triple therapy of a prophylactic course of heterologous antilymphocyte globulin or OKT3 or more recently a monoclonal antibody against the IL-2 receptor has been advocated by some groups, with delay of the administration of cyclosporine in patients with delayed primary function (Simmons et al., 1986). Although induction with an antilymphocyte agent is common practice in the United States, these are potent agents (antilymphocyte globulin or OKT3) associated with an increased risk of lymphoproliferative disease and infection and are not necessary in most patients receiving a renal transplant. Their use for induction in quadruple therapy protocols should be restricted to highly sensitized patients and patients with delayed graft function (see Chapters 20, 31 and 35 for further discussion). The use of humanized or chimeric monoclonal antibodies against the IL-2 receptor has resulted in less rejection without an apparent increase in infection or lymphoproliferative disease (Nashan et al., 1997; Vincenti et al., 1998; see Chapter 20), and these agents may prove to have a place in induction therapy.

SEQUENTIAL THERAPY

Sequential therapy has been used routinely by many units that previously gave antilymphocyte globulin or OKT3 with azathioprine and steroids (Benvenisty et al., 1990; Ferguson, 1988; Kreis et al., 1989; Sheild et al., 1988). Cyclosporine is not started until renal function has reached an acceptable level. The simplest approach used by the Basel group is to administer antilymphocyte globulin alone for the first 5 days before starting cyclosporine (Thiel et al., 1984). In general, the commoner approach is to give antilymphocyte globulin with low-dose azathioprine and prednisolone, starting cyclosporine after 7 or 14 days (Dierhoi et al., 1987; Somner et al., 1986). Although there is no firm evidence that this type of protocol is better than others, the graft survival figures from units employing this approach are impressive. In one prospective trial from Brussels, comparing sequential therapy using OKT3 with triple therapy, the graft survival rate was improved significantly—at 1 year in the OKT3-treated group, 83% versus 75% (Abramowicz et al., 1992). A subsequent report of a randomized prospective multicenter trial from the United States, in which sequential therapy using OKT3 for 14 days with the addition of cyclosporine on day 11 was compared with triple therapy, showed significantly fewer rejections in the OKT3 patients (51% vs. 66%), and 2-year patient and graft survival rates were 95% and 84% in the OKT3 group and 94% and 75% in the triple-therapy group (Norman et al., 1993). Although no increased morbidity was associated with the OKT3 in this trial, the routine use of antilymphocyte globulin or OKT3 induction therapy in low-risk renal transplant recipients seems to expose patients to

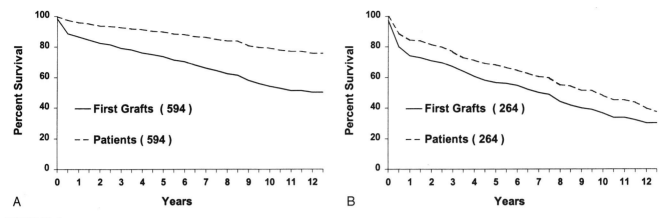

FIGURE 16–5

Actuarial survival of primary cadaveric grafts and patients, in recipients (A) younger than 55 years old and (B) 55 years old or older at the Oxford Transplant Centre using triple-therapy immunosuppression.

more potent immunosuppression than generally is required and is not justified in most patients.

CYCLOSPORINE IN HIGH-RISK PATIENTS

High-risk patients include a miscellaneous group of patients who may be at high risk for immunological or medical reasons, and these may be the ones who have benefited most from the use of cyclosporine.

1. *Elderly patients.* Cyclosporine has allowed transplantation to be offered to patients older than age 55 with end-stage renal failure, patients who would have been excluded from transplantation by most units in the azathioprine-prednisolone era because the risks of the procedure and immunosuppression were considered unacceptable. In that earlier era, however, the Stockholm group (Ost *et al.*, 1985) showed that transplantation represented the most satisfactory solution to end-stage renal failure in the elderly patient. Similar data were reported from Dallas using cyclosporine immunosuppression (Velez *et al.*, 1991). At Oxford, using triple-therapy immunosuppression, renal transplantation can be performed safely in most patients older than age 55 (Fig. 16–5). Although loss of grafts from rejection is rare in this group, graft survival is lower because of a greater death rate with a functioning graft, usually as a result of cardiovascular conditions. In patients younger than age 55, patient and graft survival are 96% and 87% at 1 year, compared with 84% and 74% in patients older than age 55. At 5 years, the corresponding figures are 90% and 74% in the younger cohort and 68% and 56% in the older cohort.

The pharmacokinetics of cyclosporine in the elderly do not appear to be different, the main problem being interaction with other medications that are eliminated by the same mechanisms, such as cytochrome P-450 and P-glycoprotein (Kovarik and Koelle, 1999). Because the elderly require less immunosuppression, attention should be paid to reducing cyclosporine levels to the lowest acceptable, and it is important in this group to withdraw steroids as early as possible—between 9 and 12 months after transplantation.

2. *Very young patients.* As described in detail in Chapter 37, cyclosporine has made transplantation an acceptable approach to renal failure in infants young children.

3. *Diabetic patients.* Patients with diabetes have done much better after renal transplantation with cyclosporine protocols than previously. Cadaver transplantation has become the

treatment of choice for diabetics with chronic renal failure (see Chapter 36).

4. *Sensitized patients.* Sensitized patients, particularly those having a regraft, show much improved graft survival rates with cyclosporine protocols than seen before with azathioprine and prednisolone (Bunzedahl *et al.*, 1986; Starzl *et al.*, 1983). This improvement has been particularly evident at Oxford (Fig. 16–6), most likely owing to the sophisticated analysis of the antibody status of sensitized recipients and the crossmatch between donor and recipient rather than cyclosporine (see Chapter 10).

CONVERSION TO CYCLOSPORINE

Conversion to cyclosporine from azathioprine and steroids may be considered for side effects of azathioprine and steroid therapy in an ever-decreasing cohort of patients or for steroid-resistant acute or chronic rejection (discussed later). In a phase I study at Oxford, nine patients with long-standing stable renal function were converted to cyclosporine because of steroid side effects. Although the early experience was encouraging (Thompson *et al.*, 1983a), the longer term follow-up was unsatisfactory: Only four patients remained on cyclosporine. Although the steroid side effects resolved,

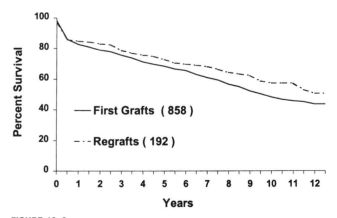

FIGURE 16–6

Actuarial survival of primary cadaveric grafts (n = 858) and regrafts (n = 192) at the Oxford Transplant Centre in patients receiving triple-therapy immunosuppression.

other problems arose: Two kidneys were lost, two patients died of sepsis, renal function declined in all grafts and one patient developed recurrent squamous cell carcinoma of the skin; hypertrichosis and gout were less serious problems. A more favorable experience was reported after conversion to cyclosporine for steroid side effects from Basel and Odense (Henriksen *et al.*, 1986; Thiel *et al.*, 1984), but follow-up in these patients was relatively short, which may be relevant, considering the initial favorable impression of conversion at Oxford. Although conversion to cyclosporine of long-term renal allograft recipients for steroid side effects does not place the graft at risk from rejection, problems may occur from cyclosporine nephrotoxicity and other side effects. Before adopting this approach in patients with severe steroid side effects, one should be aware of the potential problems, and only patients with excellent renal function should be considered as candidates for conversion. Otherwise, conversion to mycophenolate may be more satisfactory.

KETOCONAZOLE AND CYCLOSPORINE

Cyclosporine is metabolized by isoenzymes of the cytochrome P-450 system, whereas ketoconazole, a broad-spectrum antifungal agent, inhibits this enzyme system *in vitro* and *in vivo*. Cyclosporine toxicity has been reported in the presence of ketoconazole owing to high blood or serum levels of the drug (Daneshmend, 1982; Ferguson *et al.*, 1982b; Gluckman *et al.*, 1983). First and colleagues at Cincinnati first proposed that ketoconazole might be used to lower the dose of cyclosporine required for adequate blood levels, reducing the cost of the drug (First *et al.*, 1993). They have since reported the long-term follow-up data for patients given ketoconazole and cyclosporine for 3 years after renal transplantation. No adverse effects were apparent, and the reduction of cyclosporine dose at 1, 2 and 3 years was approximately 80% (First *et al.*, 1993). In the same report, these investigators presented a preliminary analysis of a prospective randomized trial in which patients received cyclosporine with or without ketoconazole. The cyclosporine dose in the ketoconazole group was less than 20% of that in the nonketoconazole group, and there was no difference in the incidence of rejection or graft loss. This approach to the use of cyclosporine could result in a dramatic reduction in the cost of immunosuppression and might be of particular relevance to the care of transplant patients in developing countries or the uninsured transplant patient in some areas of the Western world. Ketoconazole is used routinely for this purpose in the Cape Town unit in South Africa with acceptable results (D. Kahn, 1999, personal communication).

LIVING RELATED TRANSPLANTS

HLA-Identical Transplants

Although cyclosporine has had an impact on living related transplantation, its use for HLA-identical transplants is controversial because patient and graft survival are excellent with azathioprine and steroids, and most patients can be weaned off steroids after about 1 year. Fletchner and coworkers always had considered cyclosporine as the preferred therapy in these patients, however (Fletchner *et al.*, 1987). A thought-provoking analysis of renal transplantation between HLA-identical siblings treated with azathioprine and prednisone or cyclosporine and prednisone has been reported from New York (Sumrani *et al.*, 1990). Patient and graft survival rates were 100% and 97% in the cyclosporine group at 1 year compared with 91% and 85% in the azathioprine group. Although renal function remained stable in the azathioprine

group, there was a progressive deterioration in renal function in the cyclosporine group, a cause for considerable concern.

Further studies have looked at HLA-identical transplants. At the Cleveland Clinic, a group treated with azathioprine and prednisone was compared with a group treated with cyclosporine and prednisone. Five-year patient survival was 100% versus 96%, and graft survival was 92% versus 83%. A nonsignificant increase in serum creatinine level was noted in the cyclosporine patients (1.7 mg/dl) compared with azathioprine patients (1.3 mg/dl) (Gill *et al.*, 1994).

Non–HLA-Identical Transplants

The use of donor-specific transfusions in the early 1980s in patients with non–HLA-identical transplants led to a dramatic improvement in graft survival, approaching that of HLA-identical siblings (Salvatierra, 1986). Many patients become sensitized against the donor as a result of the transfusions, however, even with the concurrent administration of azathioprine (Anderson *et al.*, 1984). Kahan (1984) and Groth (1987) have advocated that donor-specific transfusions be abandoned because equally good results in this group can be obtained with cyclosporine (Flechner *et al.*, 1983a). The concurrent use of cyclosporine with donor-specific transfusions was explored by Hillis *et al.* (1987) and Cheigh *et al.* (1991): There were still some instances of sensitization, and it was not clear that results of the subsequent transplants were superior to those of transplants in patients given donor-specific transfusions alone. The use of cyclosporine without donor-specific transfusions before transplantation simplifies the whole procedure and is the protocol followed by the Oxford unit for non–HLA-identical living related transplants. The long-term outcome of the non–HLA-identical transplants pretreated with donor-specific blood under azathioprine cover remains impressive in the St. Louis experience (Anderson and Brennan, 1995). The role of prior donor-specific transfusion in this type of transplant is unresolved.

LIVING UNRELATED TRANSPLANTS

The improved results that have been obtained with cyclosporine have led many groups to embark on living unrelated transplants between highly motivated donors and recipients, usually spouses. The results of the Madison unit have been excellent. A protocol of donor-specific transfusions under azathioprine cover was followed by quadruple therapy with delayed start of cyclosporine after transplantation (Belzer *et al.*, 1987). A smaller study from Norway without donor-specific transfusions but using cyclosporine, either with prednisolone or azathioprine and prednisolone, also reported good early results for living unrelated transplantations (Sodal *et al.*, 1987).

These early results led to an increased number of living unrelated transplants throughout the world, mostly with spouse donors. Registry results from United Network for Organ Sharing (UNOS) and from the Collaborative Transplant Study (CTS) have confirmed the excellent outcome of these transplants being equivalent to that of one haplotype–disparate living related transplants (Terasaki *et al.*, 1995; Opelz *et al.*, 1999). With living unrelated transplants, outcome still is related to the degree of fortuitous matching between donor and recipient (Opelz *et al.*, 1999).

CYCLOSPORINE TO TREAT REJECTION

Cyclosporine has been reported by several groups to be effective in treating steroid-resistant acute rejection in patients on azathioprine and steroids (Hayry *et al.*, 1983; Margreiter *et al.,* 1984). This result is surprising in view of its proposed mechanism of action described earlier. Presumably the suppression of lymphokine production by activated T-helper lymphocytes can depress the clonal expansion of these cells and cytotoxic T-cell precursors, leading to reversal of an ongoing acute rejection episode. Conversion from azathioprine and steroids to cyclosporine in patients with chronic rejection not only is ineffective but also appears to hasten the deterioration of renal function (Henriksen *et al.,* 1986).

SIDE EFFECTS OF CYCLOSPORINE

Side effects of cyclosporine therapy are summarized in Table 16–5.

Renal Effects

Nephrotoxicity is unquestionably the most worrying side effect of cyclosporine and is of particular concern in renal transplantation, in which it has to be distinguished from rejection as a cause of deteriorating renal function. In the early rat and dog models of transplantation, nephrotoxicity was not noted. Nephrotoxicity became evident soon after initial clinical use (Calne *et al.,* 1979), however, and the investigators advocated the use of cyclosporine only in patients whose kidneys were diuresing after transplantation (Calne and White, 1982). Nephrotoxicity subsequently was shown in animal models using larger doses and more sophisticated evaluation of renal function, and some of the morphological changes attributed to nephrotoxicity in humans were observed (Whiting *et al.,* 1982a, 1982b).

Three clinical types of nephrotoxicity are observed with cyclosporine. The first occurs immediately after transplantation, usually in a kidney already damaged by ischemia and perhaps associated with use of intravenous cyclosporine. The nephrotoxic effect of cyclosporine in experimental models of ischemia of the kidney has been controversial in that one of the first attempts to show this interaction in the dog failed to do so (Homan *et al.,* 1980f). Since then, the susceptibility of the ischemic kidney to damage by cyclosporine has been well documented in rat models (Chow *et al.,* 1986; Jablonski *et al.,* 1986; Kanazi *et al.,* 1986). In humans, the incidence of delayed function after renal transplantation has tended to be higher in patients treated with cyclosporine than in those given azathioprine and steroids (Canadian Multicentre Transplant Study Group, 1983; Sheil *et al.,* 1983), although there is no general agreement about this (Flechner *et al.,* 1983b). The implications of the possible additive effects of cyclosporine

nephrotoxicity on an ischemic kidney are important because they suggest that protocols that delay the administration of cyclosporine until adequate renal function is established are more appropriate.

The second type of nephrotoxicity is seen any time after the first 2 or 3 weeks and is associated with deteriorating renal function, usually but not always associated with high blood levels of cyclosporine, and responds to a reduction in cyclosporine dosage. This type of nephrotoxicity has to be differentiated from an acute rejection episode. As pointed out in Chapter 14, this differentiation often is difficult because the florid signs of acute rejection previously seen in patients on azathioprine and prednisolone (i.e., fever, graft tenderness and swelling, oliguria and rapidly rising serum creatinine levels) are much less evident in patients treated with cyclosporine. Although high blood trough levels often are associated with nephrotoxicity and low levels with rejection, there are numerous exceptions to this (Holt *et al.,* 1986). If the serum creatinine level is greater than 300 μmol L^{-1}, it suggests rejection, and treatment for rejection should be started (e.g., 0.5 g of methylprednisolone intravenously daily for 3 days); this should be followed by an improvement in renal function (French *et al.,* 1983). At lower levels of serum creatinine, without any other clinical evidence of rejection, a significant reduction in the dose of cyclosporine (e.g., by 30%) should be implemented, and an improvement in renal function should follow rapidly if true nephrotoxicity is present.

Percutaneous biopsy or fine-needle aspiration of the kidney can be valuable in helping to make the correct diagnosis, and at Oxford, these two approaches are used in all cases of acute renal dysfunction in which the distinction between rejection and nephrotoxicity is unclear. The development of an automated percutaneous needle biopsy technique has made frequent biopsies quick, easy and safe. There are no morphological changes in biopsy specimens that implicate cyclosporine nephrotoxicity; the diagnosis still tends to be one of exclusion (d'Ardenne *et al.,* 1986; Neild *et al.,* 1986). A simple technique for measuring the intrarenal pressure has been described by Salaman and Griffin (1983); they claimed it distinguishes rejection (pressures > 40 mm Hg) from nephrotoxicity (pressures < 40 mm Hg) with a high degree of accuracy (Salaman and Griffin, 1985). This type of nephrotoxicity recovers rapidly with a cyclosporine dosage reduction or conversion to azathioprine and prednisolone (Chapman *et al.,* 1985a).

The mechanism of cyclosporine nephrotoxicity has not been clarified, but it would seem that a direct toxic action on proximal tubular cells is not a significant factor. A decrease in renal blood flow with an increased renal vascular resistance at the level of the afferent arteriole of the glomerulus and a decreased glomerular filtration rate is the primary cause of the nephrotoxicity (Perico and Remuzzi, 1991). The metabolites of cyclosporine also have a similar effect (Robey and Shaw, 1993). That acute cyclosporine nephrotoxicity is reversed so rapidly after cessation of the drug (within days) is compatible with the concept of renal vasoconstriction as the primary cause of the nephrotoxicity (Chapman *et al.,* 1985a; Curtis *et al.,* 1986). In rats, the sympathetic nervous system is important in the induction of nephrotoxicity because it can be prevented by denervating the kidney before administering cyclosporine (Paller and Murray, 1985). After renal transplantation in humans, however, the kidney is denervated, and nephrotoxicity occurs despite this so that sympathetic overactivity cannot be a significant feature of cyclosporine nephrotoxicity in renal transplantation in humans. Cyclosporine has been shown to stimulate the renin-angiotensin system in rats and dogs, but there is no evidence

TABLE 16–5

SIDE EFFECTS OF CYCLOSPORINE THERAPY

Renal	Nephrotoxicity, hemolytic-uremic syndrome
Hepatic	Hepatotoxicity
Neoplastic	Lymphomas, fibroadenoma of breast, squamous cell carcinoma
Dermatological	Thickening, rashes, hypertrichosis
Gastrointestinal	Anorexia, nausea, failure to gain weight
Metabolic	Hyperkalemia, hyperuricemia, hypomagnesemia, hyperglycemia
Neurological	Tremor, convulsions, burning sensation in limbs, malaise, depression
Cardiovascular	Fluid retention, hypertension, hypercholesterolemia, Raynaud's phenomenon, intravascular coagulation
Dental	Gingival hypertrophy
Hematological	Hemolytic anemia

suggesting that this system has a major involvement in cyclosporine nephrotoxicity.

Earlier work postulated that the effect of cyclosporine on the production of renal prostaglandins might be responsible for the vasoconstriction as well as the changes in intravascular coagulation that may occur in the presence of cyclosporine (Neild *et al.*, 1983). The kidney is a rich source of prostaglandin metabolites, and the main sites of prostaglandin synthesis are the arteries, arterioles and glomerular capillaries. The prostaglandins are potent renal vasodilators and are thought to play an important role in modulating the influence of various renal vasoconstrictor factors. There is some evidence that cyclosporine inhibits the production of the prostaglandin metabolites but may increase the production of thromboxane, which is a potent vasoconstrictor (Brown and Neild, 1987; Perico *et al.*, 1986). This effect of cyclosporine on the arachidonic acid metabolic pathway within the kidney could explain most of the observed functional and morphological changes of nephrotoxicity. There is some evidence for this explanation, at least in rats (Pasini *et al.*, 1990), whereas in humans, renal allograft function was improved by the administration of a thromboxane synthetase inhibitor in patients on cyclosporine (Coffman *et al.*, 1990). It is possible that the novel constrictor peptide, endothelin, also contributes to the hemodynamic alterations caused by cyclosporine (Perico and Remuzzi, 1991). Endothelin release was increased from smooth muscle cells in culture on exposure to cyclosporine, and in bone marrow–transplanted patients on cyclosporine, endothelin levels were increased significantly (Haug *et al.*, 1995). In a study of renal biopsy specimens, neither the mRNA of endothelin receptors A and B nor prepro-ER1 mRNA was increased (Asberg *et al.*, 1999).

Another possible uncommon manifestation of acute cyclosporine nephrotoxicity is a hemolytic-uremic syndrome-like condition that occurs in the first week after transplantation and a biopsy specimen shows striking arteriolopathy and thrombosis. Despite the striking nature of the histological findings, a return of renal function was noted with cessation of cyclosporine or the use of streptokinase and heparin (Keusch *et al.*, 1985; Remuzzi and Bertani, 1989; Somner *et al.*, 1986).

It has been reported that calcium channel blockers reduce the incidence of primary nonfunction in patients on cyclosporine (Hauser *et al.*, 1991; Neumayer *et al.*, 1989). Several calcium channel blockers have been studied in prospective trials. Diltiazem was associated with a marked reduction in cyclosporine dosage with fewer episodes of primary nonfunction and less severe rejection episodes (Chrysostomon *et al.*, 1993). Nifedipine was found to reduce the incidence of primary nonfunction (Donnelly *et al.*, 1993). Verapamil resulted in the need for lower cyclosporine doses but equivalent blood levels, but there was no reduction in nephrotoxicity or incidence of rejection (Pirsch *et al.*, 1993). A study by Ahmed *et al.* (1997) showed that isradipine, another calcium channel blocker, reduced blood pressure in hypertensive renal transplant recipients by decreasing renal vascular resistance. In rats, using single nephrons, lacidipine partially prevented the decrease in glomerular filtration rate and ultrafiltration coefficient caused by cyclosporine (Fassi *et al.*, 1999).

The third type of cyclosporine nephrotoxicity is a chronic condition in which there is a slow, steady deterioration in renal function, and the histology of the kidney may reveal severe interstitial fibrosis. This type of nephrotoxicity shows some improvement in renal function with a decrease in the cyclosporine dosage, but this improvement tends to be relatively short-lived. It is likely that many of the changes observed result from chronic immunological damage on which is superimposed some element of cyclosporine nephrotoxicity. That chronic changes of cyclosporine nephrotoxicity do occur is unquestioned in view of the striking morphological changes of interstitial fibrosis and tubular atrophy observed in the native kidneys of patients with uveitis treated with cyclosporine (Palestine *et al.*, 1986). After cardiac transplantation, this steady deterioration in renal function of patients on cyclosporine resulted in some patients requiring hemodialysis (Myers *et al.*, 1984), and this remains a problem in cardiac transplantation and is seen to a lesser extent in liver transplant patients. Chronic nephrotoxicity probably is a cumulative effect of initial ischemic damage to the kidney in association with high early doses of cyclosporine. A hypothesis has been put forward by Salomon (1991, 1992), however, in which he postulates that the deterioration of renal function in patients on cyclosporine is not due to cyclosporine nephrotoxicity but represents chronic rejection resulting from underimmunosuppression as doses of cyclosporine are reduced with time.

Transforming growth factor-β type 1 has been suggested to play a role in chronic cyclosporine nephrotoxicity. Transforming growth factor-β type 1 is a prosclerotic cytokine. Detectable levels have been found in the plasma of transplant recipients but not in healthy controls or those with membranous nephropathy. There was no difference in levels between patients with differing renal function, time since transplantation or cyclosporine trough levels (Coupes *et al.*, 1994). In isolated human renal proximal tubular cells, increasing concentrations of cyclosporine caused an increase in the production by the tubular cells of TGF-β and platelet-derived growth factor, both fibrogenic cytokines (Johnson *et al.*, 1999). In a study of renal biopsy specimens, TGF-β content correlated with cyclosporine toxicity, as opposed to acute tubular necrosis. Transforming growth factor-β also was expressed in biopsy specimens from patients with acute rejection, however, with more expression in patients with more severe rejection (Pankewycz *et al.*, 1996).

In rats receiving cyclosporine on a low-sodium diet, a model for cyclosporine toxicity that gives similar histological appearances to those of chronic cyclosporine toxicity in humans, mRNA expression of TGF-β was increased. Peripheral renin activity also was increased (Shihab *et al.*, 1997). Human mesangial cells and renal fibroblasts in culture also produced more collagen III on exposure to cyclosporine (Ghiggeri *et al.*, 1994).

Hepatic Effects

Hepatotoxicity has been observed in patients on cyclosporine after renal, cardiac and bone marrow transplantation (Hedley *et al.*, 1982; Klintmalm *et al.*, 1981; Oyer *et al.*, 1982; see Chapter 32). Generally, this hepatotoxicity has not been more than a temporary elevation of liver function tests that regressed on dosage reduction. These biochemical changes are uncommon with the lower doses used today. No histological changes have been described in association with these biochemical changes, but high doses of cyclosporine in rats produce ultrastructural changes and a deterioration in liver function (Thomson *et al.*, 1982). Cyclosporine is contraindicated in patients with abnormal liver function tests before renal transplantation because there is a risk of the development of frank cirrhosis in such patients (Hillebrand *et al.*, 1986). Because cyclosporine is metabolized in the liver, depressed liver function may alter blood levels of the drug, and careful attention must be paid to cyclosporine levels in such patients.

Neoplastic Effects

An apparent increased incidence of lymphomas in the early patients with a renal allograft and treated with cyclosporine caused considerable alarm (Bird, 1982; Bird et al., 1981; Thiru et al., 1981), but as time has passed, this increased incidence of lymphoma in renal and cardiac allograft recipients is no greater than that expected in recipients treated with conventional immunosuppressive therapy. Most of the patients who developed lymphomas received other drugs as well, such as prednisolone and antilymphocyte agents, suggesting that the occurrence of lymphoma is due to excessive immunosuppression rather than specifically to cyclosporine. The pathogenesis and incidence of lymphomas are described in detail in Chapter 35. Skin cancer, a major complication after transplantation in countries such as Australia with heavy sun exposure, appears just as commonly with cyclosporine immunosuppression, and this too is described in detail in Chapters 34 and 35. An observation has been made that cyclosporine produces striking morphological changes in vitro, including increased cell motility, and in vivo enhances tumor growth in immunodeficient SCID-beige mice. These effects appear to be mediated by TGF-β. It is possible that cyclosporine can promote tumor progression independent of its effect on the immune response (Hojo et al., 1999).

Dermatological Effects

Dermatological problems, of which hypertrichosis is the most worrisome, are discussed in detail in Chapter 34. In children, facial dysmorphism may be striking and was not seen in children receiving azathioprine and steroids (Crocker et al., 1993).

Gastrointestinal Effects

The development of a gelatin capsule for cyclosporine has been welcomed by most patients. The capsules are large and difficult to swallow, however, and some patients prefer to take the liquid form. Cyclosporine in the liquid form is unpleasant to take and is not disguised adequately even when taken with flavored drinks such as chocolate milk. The unpalatability of cyclosporine causes nausea and anorexia in some patients, particularly with large doses, but in general this is less of a problem with current low doses.

Metabolic Effects

Hyperkalemia is common in patients on cyclosporine (Adu et al., 1983; Foley et al., 1985) and is reversible with lowering of the dose or cessation of the drug (Chapman et al., 1985b). The mechanism is unclear, but the decreased potassium excretion may be due to decreased serum aldosterone levels (Adu et al., 1983; Bantle et al., 1985) or to a primary tubular defect (Bantle et al., 1985).

Renal handling of uric acid is affected by the use of cyclosporine, leading to higher serum urate levels in cyclosporine-treated patients after correction for elevated serum creatinine (Chapman et al., 1985a). The high urate levels return to normal slowly over several weeks on discontinuing the drug and probably reflect a tubular defect associated with cyclosporine nephrotoxicity. Gout occasionally occurs as a byproduct of the hyperuricemia, and urate levels may need to be lowered with allopurinol, remembering that the leukocyte count needs to be monitored carefully if the patient is on azathioprine as well as cyclosporine.

Hypomagnesemia is due to an increased magnesium clearance in patients on cyclosporine and usually is associated with high blood levels of cyclosporine (Allen et al., 1985a; June et al., 1985). Hypomagnesemia reflects another manifestation of cyclosporine nephrotoxicity. Convulsions, which may be another manifestation of cyclosporine toxicity (as discussed in the next section and in Chapter 33), have been attributed to hypomagnesemia.

Glycosuria may occur in patients on cyclosporine, often associated with an increased blood glucose level. Glycosuria is a manifestation of nephrotoxicity (Chan et al., 1987), but hyperglycemia may reflect a toxic effect of cyclosporine on β cells of the islets of Langerhans. This condition appears to be reversible. There is evidence in rats that cyclosporine produces glucose intolerance, probably through the inhibition of insulin secretion (Yale et al., 1985).

Neurological Effects

A variety of neurological complications have been reported with the use of cyclosporine, including tremor, convulsions, various paresthesias of the limbs, mania and depression (Atkinson et al., 1984; Beaman et al., 1985; Gross et al., 1982; Thompson et al., 1984; Wamboldt, 1984). These complications are discussed in detail in Chapter 33. Although not always clearly caused by cyclosporine, there is sufficient evidence that such neurological syndromes can be attributed to cyclosporine toxicity in many instances because they appear to be associated with high serum and blood levels. The syndrome is reversible on lowering the dose. These problems have become infrequent with current low doses of cyclosporine. Some evidence suggests that cyclosporine-induced hypomagnesemia may be the cause of these neurological complications, especially the convulsions, as already mentioned.

Cardiovascular Effects

Hypertension and hyperlipidemia are associated with the use of cyclosporine and are discussed in detail in Chapter 30. Cyclosporine appears to have complex effects on intravascular coagulation, and there have been reports of an increased incidence of renal artery and vein thrombosis (Canadian Multicentre Transplant Study Group, 1983; Jones et al., 1988b; Merion and Calne, 1985; Rigotti et al., 1986) and an increase in the incidence of deep venous thrombosis (Vanrentenghem et al., 1985), which was not confirmed at Oxford (Allen et al., 1987; see Chapter 28). Although it is attractive to attribute these complications, including the microangiopathy and hemolytic-uremic syndrome, to the effect of cyclosporine on the arachidonic acid metabolic pathway as discussed earlier, the evidence is too uncertain to draw any firm conclusions. Raynaud's phenomenon appears to be another uncommon complication of cyclosporine therapy (Deray et al., 1986), and one such case has occurred at Oxford.

Dental Effects

Gingival hypertrophy is associated with poor dental hygiene and high doses of cyclosporine (Seymour and Jacobs, 1992) and is discussed in detail in Chapter 34.

Hematological Effects

ABO autoimmune hemolytic anemia may occur after renal transplantation when a blood group O kidney is placed in a blood group A or B recipient. Several such cases have been reported (Bevan et al., 1985; Mangal et al., 1984; Nyberg et al., 1984b), although ABO autoimmune hemolytic anemia is commoner after liver transplantation (Ramsey et al., 1984).

The occurrence of this complication, a form of graft-versus-host reaction, reflects the better immunosuppression achieved with cyclosporine.

Genotoxicity and Breast-Feeding

Experimental animal and human data so far indicate that cyclosporine is unlikely to be genotoxic (Olshan et al., 1994). In studies so far, there has been no increase in congenital anomalies or genetic disease. Monitoring should be continued, however, to increase the sample size.

Cyclosporine concentrations in breast milk were similar to those in blood but below detection limits in breast-fed infants. No change in creatinine of the infants occurred over 12 months of continued breast-feeding (Nyberg et al., 1998).

MONITORING OF CYCLOSPORINE

Cyclosporine dosages are monitored by the measurement of whole-blood trough levels. The correlation between high trough levels and nephrotoxicity and low trough levels and rejection is not an exact one (Holt, 1986; Kahan, 1989). The differentiation between rejection and cyclosporine nephrotoxicity is difficult, and the cyclosporine levels provide additional information that help to make the distinction and allow appropriate action. Cyclosporine levels are particularly valuable in the first 2 weeks after transplantation in detecting patients who are not absorbing the drug adequately and later on in detecting lack of compliance. Many drugs may interact with cyclosporine (Table 16–6), and measuring cyclosporine levels is valuable in monitoring these interactions. The question that arises is whether trough levels are the most effective way of monitoring cyclosporine dosages or whether cyclosporine should be monitored by determining the area under the curve (AUC).

Area Under the Curve

Varying methods have been used to assess adequacy of cyclosporine exposure. One of the commonest is to measure a trough level, taken approximately 12 hours after the last dose (i.e. first thing in the morning, before the morning dose in a patient on a twice-daily cyclosporine (Neoral) dosage schedule). This level correlates poorly with total cyclosporine exposure as well as episodes of rejection. However, the Halifax group suggested that sparse sampling allows the AUC in the first 4 hours after dosage to be calculated and that a single sample at 3 hours not only correlates well with the AUC, but also is a better predictor of nephrotoxicity and rejection (Mahalati et al., 1999, 2000).

Total drug exposure or AUC is deemed to be the best way of monitoring cyclosporine dosage, and there is increasing pressure to change the long-standing methods of monitoring cyclosporine. Formal AUC testing involves many blood samples taken over a period of time and is too inconvenient and costly to perform routinely. This testing initially was performed using the old formulation of cyclosporine (Grevel et al., 1989), and trough levels were found to correlate poorly to dosage adjustments and AUC to correlate well to the dose in mg/kg. Using this method, fewer dosage adjustments were made per patient. This method involved blood measurements at 0, 2, 4, 6, 10, 14 and 24 hours, however.

Since the advent of the microemulsion formulation (Neoral), an AUC can be calculated from fewer blood tests because the microemulsion formulation is absorbed more rapidly, and an early sample at 2 or 3 hours usually is the maximum blood level. Gaspari and colleagues showed that best results were obtained with sampling at 1, 5, 8 and 11 hours, but 0, 1 and 3 hours gave excellent correlation (Gaspari et al., 1997). Vathsala (1999) showed that sampling at 2 and 6 hours provided an accurate picture of the AUC. Primmett and coworkers showed good correlation at 0 and 1 or 0 and 2 hours in 55 patients (Primmett et al., 1998). For patients on 8-hourly dosing strategies, such as children and some adults, levels at 2 and 4 hours gave accurate predictions of AUC (Meier-Kriesche et al., 1998). Trough levels never have correlated well with diagnosis of rejection. Area under the curve testing does correlate well, however, and it is possible that the whole basis on which cyclosporine is monitored is about to change as the evidence accumulates in favor

TABLE 16–6

WELL-ESTABLISHED DRUG INTERACTIONS WITH CYCLOSPORINE*

Drugs	Reference
Increase Cyclosporine Levels	
Ketoconazole	Daneshmend, 1982; Ferguson et al., 1982b; Gluckman et al., 1983
Erythromycin	Gino et al., 1986; Ptachcinski et al., 1985
Corticosteroids	Cockburn, 1986
Diltiazem	Neumayer and Wagner, 1986; Wagner et al., 1986
Decrease Cyclosporine Levels	
Isoniazid	Coward et al., 1985; Kahan, 1983
Phenobarbitone	Carstensen et al., 1986; Cunningham et al., 1983
Phenytoin	Freeman et al., 1984; Keown et al., 1984; Whiting et al., 1982b
Rifampicin	Allen et al., 1985b; Van Buren et al., 1984
Cause Additive Nephrotoxicity	
Aminoglycosides	Bennett, 1986; Whiting et al., 1982a, 1983
Amphotericin B	Kennedy et al., 1983
Melphalan	Dale et al., 1985
Sulfonamides/ cotrimoxazole	†
Trimethoprim	†

*For a listing of other reported interactions and a complete citation of all reports, contact Novartis Pharmaceuticals Medical Information Department, Basel, Switzerland.
†Kimmel et al., 1985; Nyberg et al., 1984a; Ringden et al., 1984; Thompson et al., 1983b.

of single sampling at 2 or 3 hours after dosage, especially in the first few weeks after transplantation (Cantarovich *et al.*, 1998; Charlebois *et al.*, 1997; Gaspari *et al.*, 1998; Kelles *et al.*, 1999; Lindholm and Kahan, 1993; Meyer *et al.*, 1993; Nankivell *et al.*, 1994; Primmett *et al.*, 1998; Warrens *et al.*, 1999). More intriguing is the possibility that cyclosporine has been used in a less effective way and that early dose monitoring using predicted AUC levels may lead to a significant reduction in the incidence of rejection and nephrotoxicity.

Neoral

Neoral, the microemulsion formulation of cyclosporine, was first approved for use in the United States in 1995. Many studies have looked at the absorption of Neoral and its effects on blood levels and total availability of the drug. The absorption appears to be more rapid, with peak levels occurring by 2 hours in most patients. Many trials have compared the old formulation with Neoral, one of the largest being from the Canadian Neoral study group. This group found that less drug was required in the Neoral group, with better absorption and a 40% greater exposure to the drug. Area under the curve could be calculated from measurements from 0 to 4 hours, and the maximum blood levels were reached by 2 hours in most patients. There was an initial transient increase in nephrotoxicity and in gastrointestinal and neurological side effects (Keown *et al.*, 1996). A second study from the International Sandimmune Neoral study group showed less rejection at 3 months, without an increase in nephrotoxicity (Keown and Niese, 1998).

An overview of the results from clinical trials has been performed by Frei (1999). It has been well established that Neoral is as safe and tolerable as Sandimmune. In randomized double-blind trials, there appeared to be no increase in side effects, although in contrast, in the open trials, there seemed to be more adverse effects (Frei, 1999). A meta-analysis of all published trials suggested that Neoral gave a lower rejection rate, but this was less clear when only randomized, prospective trials were assessed (Shah *et al.*, 1999).

In black patients, Neoral has better bioavailability than Sandimmune; this difference is more marked than in whites (Pollack *et al.*, 1999). The major metabolites of cyclosporine have similar AUC values for both preparations in the steady-state (Kovarik *et al.*, 1994).

A further microemulsion formulation of cyclosporine is now on the market; this formulation was developed by a company (Sangstat; Fremont, California) from 270 cyclosporine formulations. It appears bioequivalent to Neoral at the same dose (First *et al.*, 1998).

DRUG INTERACTIONS

Cyclosporine is metabolized almost entirely in the liver, probably through the cytochrome P-450 system. Most of the drug is excreted in the bile, with only trace amounts being excreted in the urine. Drugs that induce hepatic enzymes, such as rifampicin, increase the rate of metabolism of cyclosporine and lower blood levels of the parent compound. Other drugs that are potentially nephrotoxic, such as gentamicin, have an additive effect with cyclosporine on nephrotoxicity. It is important to be aware of known drug interactions and to remember the possibility of other, but as yet unconfirmed, interactions. The measurement of levels is important in detecting such interactions as well as in the monitoring of levels at which drugs with known interactions have to be used. The well-known interactions are listed in Table 16–6, and all known interactions are noted with the relevant

citations to the literature in the Sandimmune Drug Interactions, available from the Sandoz Medical Information Department (Basel, Switzerland); these are continually updated.

Conclusions

Cyclosporine represents a major advance in the immunosuppressive armamentarium, and all modern protocols of immunosuppression include cyclosporine. The development of a variety of protocols has been stimulated by the side effects of cyclosporine, the most serious of which is nephrotoxicity. All newer protocols are designed with the aim of using lower doses of cyclosporine and reducing the incidence of nephrotoxicity, while maintaining the enhanced immunosuppressive potency achieved with cyclosporine. Although all side effects, especially nephrotoxicity, have been reduced in severity and incidence, nephrotoxicity remains a problem. Whether this nephrotoxicity proves to be a long-term disadvantage of the drug is unclear, but at present, this possible long-term problem is outweighed by the significant improvement in graft survival achieved with cyclosporine in the short term and medium term after renal transplantation. The role of new drugs that might replace cyclosporine (e.g., tacrolimus and sirolimus) or might be used with cyclosporine, allowing a reduction or eventual withdrawal of cyclosporine (e.g., mycophenolate mofetil and sirolimus), is discussed in Chapters 17, 18 and 19, but at this time cyclosporine-based protocols remain the gold standard against which newer agents have to be evaluated.

REFERENCES

Abramowicz, D., Goldman, M., de Pauw, L., Vanherweghem, T. L., Kinnaert, P. and Vereerstraeten, P. (1992). The long-term effects of prophylactic OKT3 monoclonal antibody in cadaver transplantation—a single-center, prospective, randomized study. *Transplantation* **54**, 433.

Adu, D., Turney J., Michael, J. and McMaster, P. (1983). Hyperkalemia in cyclosporin treated renal allograft recipients. *Lancet* **2**, 370.

Aeder, M. I., Sutherland, D. E. R., Lewis, W. I. and Najarian, J. S. (1983). Combination immunotherapy with low-dose cyclosporin and azathioprine in splenectomized canine recipients of renal allografts. *Transplant. Proc.* **15**, 2933.

Ahmed, K., Michael, B. and Burke, J. F., Jr. (1997). Effects of isradipine on renal hemodynamics in renal transplant patients treated with cyclosporine. *Clin. Nephrol.* **48**, 307.

Allen, R. D., Hunnisett, A. G. and Morris, P. J. (1985a). Cyclosporin and magnesium. *Lancet* **1**, 980.

Allen, R. D., Hunnisett, A. G. and Morris, P. J. (1985b). Cyclosporin and rifampicin in renal transplantation. *Lancet* **1**, 1283.

Allen, R. D., Michie, C. A., Murie, J. A. and Morris, P. J. (1987). Deep venous thrombosis after renal transplantation. *Surg. Gynecol. Obstet.* **164**, 137.

Anderson, C. B. and Brennan, D. C. (1995). A sanguine outlook: the role of donor-specific transfusion in renal transplantation and tolerance. *Transplant. Rev.* **9**, 49.

Anderson, C. B., Tyler, J. D., Sicard, G. A., Anderman, C. K., Rodney, G. E. and Etheredge, E. E. (1984). Pretreatment of renal allograft recipient with immunosuppression and donor-specific blood. *Transplantation* **38**, 664.

Andrus, L. and Lafferty, K. J. (1981). Inhibition of T-cell activity by cyclosporin A. *Scand. J. Immunol.* **15**, 449.

Asberg, A., Attramadal, H., Midtvedt, K., *et al.* (1999). Gene expression of the renal endothelin system in renal transplant recipients on cyclosporine A based immunosuppression. *Transplantation* **67**, 1056.

Atkinson, K., Briggs, J. C., Darvenizia, P., Boland, J., Concannon, A. and Dodds, A. (1984). Cyclosporin associated central-nervous-system toxicity after allogenic bone marrow transplantation. *N. Engl. J. Med.* **310**, 527.

Bantle, J. P., Nath, K. A., Sutherland, D. E. R., Najarian, J. S. and

Ferrir, T. F. (1985). Effects of cyclosporin on the renin-angiotensin-aldosterone system and potassium excretion in renal transplant recipients. *Arch. Intern. Med.* **145**, 505.

Barber, W. H., Hutchinson, I. V. and Morris, P. J. (1985). The role of suppressor cells in maintaining passively enhanced rat kidney allografts. *Transplant. Proc.* **17**, 1391.

Beaman, M., Parvin, S., Veitch, P. S. and Walls, J. (1985). Convulsions associated with cyclosporin A in renal transplant recipients. *B. M. J.* **290**, 139.

Belzer, F. O., Kalayoghu, M. and Sollinger, H. W. (1987). Donor-specific transfusion in living-unrelated renal transplantation. *Transplant. Proc.* **19**, 1514.

Bennett, W. M. (1986). Comparison of cyclosporin nephrotoxicity with aminoglycoside nephrotoxicity. *Clin. Nephrol.* **25(Suppl. 1)**, S126.

Benvenisty, A. I., Cohen, D., Stegall, M. D. and Hardy, M. A. (1990). Improved results using OKT3 as induction immunosuppression in renal allograft recipients with delayed graft function. *Transplantation* **45**, 321.

Bevan, P. C., Seaman, M., Tolliday, B. and Chalmers, D. G. (1985). Interferon-induced parotitis and epididymitis. *Vox Sang.* **49**, 42.

Bird, A. B. (1982). Cyclosporin A, lymphomata and Epstein-Barr virus. *In Cyclosporin A,* (D. J. White, ed.), p. 307, Elsevier Biomedical, Amsterdam.

Bird, A. G., McGlachlan, S. M. and Britton, S. (1981). Cyclosporin A promotes spontaneous outgrowth in vitro of Epstein-Barr virus-induced B cell lines. *Nature* **289**, 300.

Borel, J. F. (1981). Cyclosporin A presents experimental status. *Transplant. Proc.* **13**, 344.

Borel, J. F. (1982). The history of cyclosporin A and its significance. *In Cyclosporin A,* (D. J. White, ed.), p. 5, Elsevier Biomedical, Amsterdam.

Borel, J. F., Feurer, C., Gubler, H. U. and Stahelin, H. (1976). Biological effects of cyclosporin A: a new antilymphocylic agent. *Agents Actions* **6**, 468.

Borel, J. F., Neuhaus, P., Marquet, C. and Stahelin, H. (1977). Effects of the new anti-lymphocytic peptide cyclosporin A in animals. *Immunology* **32**, 1017.

Borleffs, J. C., Neuhaus, P., Marquet, R. L., Zurcher, C. and Balner, H. (1982). Cyclosporin A and kidney transplantation in rhesus monkeys. *In Cyclosporin A,* (D. J. White, ed.), p. 329, Elsevier Biomedical, Amsterdam.

Bouwer, H. G. A. and Hinrichs, D. J. (1983). Cyclosporin effects on mitogen-induced T- and B-cell proliferation. *Transplant. Proc.* **15**, 2306.

Brown, Z. and Neild, G. H. (1987). Cyclosporine inhibits prostacyclin production by cultured human endothelial cells. *Transplant. Proc.* **19**, 1178.

Bunjes, D., Hardt, C., Solbach, W., Deusch, K., Rollinghoff, M. and Wagner, H. (1982). Studies on the mechanism of action of cyclosporin A in the murine and human T-cell response in vitro. *In Cyclosporin A,* (D. J. White, ed.), p. 261, Elsevier Biomedical, Amsterdam.

Bunzedahl, H., Bechstein, W., Wonigeit, K., *et al.* (1986). Effects of immunosuppression on renal allograft survival in immunized patients: a single center analysis. *Transplant. Proc.* **18**, 1067.

Burckhardt, J. J. and Guggenheim, B. (1979). Cyclosporin A: in vivo and in vitro suppression of rat T-lymphocytic function. *Immunology* **36**, 753.

Calne, R. Y. (1987). Cyclosporin in cadaveric renal transplantation: 5 year follow-up of a multicentre trial. *Lancet* **2**, 506.

Calne, R. Y., Rolles, K., White, D. J. G., *et al.* (1979). Cyclosporin A initially as the only immunosuppressant in 36 recipients of cadaveric organs: 32 kidney, 2 pancreas and 2 livers. *Lancet* **2**, 1033.

Calne, R. Y., Rolles, K., White, D. J. G., *et al.* (1981) Cyclosporin A in clinical organ grafting. *Transplant. Proc.* **13**, 349.

Calne, R. Y. and White, D. J. G. (1977). Cyclosporin A—a powerful immunosuppressant in dogs. *I. R. C. S. J. Med. Sci.* **5**, 595.

Calne, R. Y. and White, D. J. G. (1982). The use of cyclosporin A in clinical organ grafting. *Ann. Surg.* **196**, 330.

Cammisuli, S. (1982). The effect of cyclosporin A on cell interactions within the immune system. *In Cyclosporin A,* (D. J. White, ed.), p. 243, Elsevier Biomedical, Amsterdam.

Canadian Multicentre Transplant Study Group. (1983). A randomized clinical trial of cyclosporin in cadaveric renal transplantation. *N. Engl. J. Med.* **309**, 809.

Canadian Multicentre Transplant Study Group. (1986). A randomized clinical trial of cyclosporin in cadaveric renal transplantation. *N. Engl. J. Med.* **314**, 1219.

Cantarovich, M., Besner, J. G., Barkun, J. S., Elstein, E. and Loertscher, R. (1998). Two-hour cyclosporine level determination is the appropriate tool to monitor Neoral therapy. *Clin. Transplant.* **12**, 243.

Carel, J. C., Schreiber, R. D., Falgui, L. and Lacy, P. E. (1990). Transforming growth factor beta decreases the immunogenicity of rat islet xenografts (rat to mouse) and prevents rejection in association with treatment of the recipient with a monoclonal antibody to interferon-γ. *Proc. Natl. Acad. Sci.* **87**, 1591.

Carstensen, J. R., Jacobsen, W. and Dieperink, H. (1986). Interaction between cyclosporin A and phenobarbitone. *Br. J. Clin. Pharmacol.* **21**, 550.

Cecka, J. M. (1996). In sickness and health—high success rates of kidney transplants between spouses. *Transplant. Rev.* **10**, 216.

Chan, P., Chapman, J. R. and Morris, P. J. (1987). Glycosuria: an index of cyclosporine nephroxicity. *Transplant. Proc.* **19**, 1780.

Chapman, J. R., Griffiths, D., Harding, N. G. and Morris, P. J. (1985a). Reversibility of cyclosporin nephrotoxicity after three months treatment. *Lancet* **1**, 128.

Chapman, J. R. and Morris, P. J. (1985). Cyclosporin nephrotoxicity and the consequences of conversion to azathioprine. *Transplant. Proc.* **17(Suppl. 1)**, 254.

Chapman, J. R. and Morris, P. J. (1986). Long-term effects of short term cyclosporin. *Transplant. Proc.* **18(Suppl. 1)**, 186.

Chapman, J. R. and Morris, P. J. (1987). Cyclosporin conversion. *Transplant. Rev.* **1**, 197.

Chapman, J. R., Thompson, J. F., Wood, R. F. L. and Morris, P. J. (1985b). The problems associated with conversion to cyclosporin immunosuppression in long-term renal allograft recipients. *Transplant. Proc.* **17**, 1178.

Charlebois, J. E., Lum, B. L., Cooney, G. F., Mochon, M. and Kaiser, B. A. (1997). Comparison and validation of limited sampling equations for cyclosporine area under the curve monitoring calculations in pediatric renal transplant recipients. *Ther. Drug Monit.* **19**, 277.

Cheigh, J. S., Suthanthiran, M., Fotino, M., *et al.* (1991). Minimal sensitization and excellent renal allograft outcome following donor-specific blood transfusion with a short course of cyclosporin. *Transplantation* **51**, 378.

Chen, R. H., Ivens, K. W., Alpert, S., *et al.* (1993). The use of granzyme A as a marker of heart transplant rejection in cyclosporine or anti-CD4 monoclonal antibody-treated rats. *Transplantation* **55**, 146.

Chiu, Y.-L. and Batchelor, J. R. (1986). Mechanisms underlying continued survival of rat kidney allografts after a short period of chemical immunosuppression. *Transplantation* **40**, 150.

Chow, S. S., Thorner, P., Baumol, R. and Wilson, D. R. (1986). Cyclosporin and experimental renal ischemic injury. *Transplantation* **41**, 152.

Chrysostomon, A., Walker, R. G., Russ, G. R., d'Apice, A. J., Kincaid-Smith, P. and Mathew, T. H. (1993). Diltiazem in renal allograft recipients receiving cyclosporine. *Transplantation* **55**, 300.

Clipstone, N. A. and Crabtree, G. R. (1992). Identification of calcineamin as a key signalling enzyme in T-lymphocyte activation. *Nature* **357**, 695.

Cockburn, I. (1986). Cyclosporine A: clinical evaluation of drug interactions. *Transplant. Proc.* **18(Suppl. 5)**, 50.

Coffman, T. M., Smith, S. R., Creech, E. A., *et al.* (1990). The thromboxane (Tx) synthetase inhibitor CGS 13080 improves renal allograft function in patients taking cyclosporine (CSA). *Kidney Int.* **37**, 604.

Collier, S. J., Calne, R. Y., Thick, M., *et al.* (1986). Alternate day immunosuppression. *Lancet* **1**, 267.

Cosimi, A. B., Sheild, C. F., Peters, C., Burton, R. C., Scott, G. and Russell, P. S. (1978). Prolongation of allograft survival by cyclosporin A. *Surg. Forum* **30**, 287.

Coupes, B. M., Newstead, C. G., Short, C. D. and Brenchley, P. E. (1994). Transforming growth factor beta 1 in renal allograft recipients. *Transplantation* **57**, 1727.

Coward, R. A., Raftery, A. T., Brown, C. B., *et al.* (1985). Cyclosporin and antituberculous therapy. *Lancet* **1**, 1342.

Crocker, J. F., Dempsey, T., Schenk, M. E. and Renton, K. W. (1993). Cyclosporin A toxicity in children. *Transplantation Rev.* **7**, 72.

Cunningham, C., Whiting, P. H., Burke, M. D., Wheatley, D. M.

and Simpson, J. G. (1983). Increasing the hepatic metabolism of cyclosporine abolishes nephrotoxicity. *In Cyclosporine*, (B. D. Kahan, ed.) p. 496, Grune & Stratton, New York.

Curtis, J. J., Luke, R. G., Dubousky, E., Duthelm, G., Whelchel, J. D. and Jones, P. (1986). Benefits of removal of native kidneys in hypertension after renal transplantation. *Lancet* **2**, 477.

Dale, B. M., Sage, R. E., Norman, J. E., Barber, S. and Kotasek, D. (1985). Bone marrow transplantation following treatment with high dose melphalan. *Transplant. Proc.* **17**, 1711.

Daneshmend, T. K. (1982). Ketoconazole-cyclosporine interaction. *Lancet* **2**, 1342.

d'Ardenne, A. J., Dunnill, M. S., Thompson, J. F., McWhinnie, D. and Wood, R. F. M. (1986). Cyclosporin and renal graft histology. *J. Clin. Pathol.* **39**, 145.

Deray, G., Hoang, P., Achour, L., Hornych, A., Laudault, C. and Caraillon, A. (1986). Cyclosporin and Raynaud's phenomenon. *Lancet* **1**, 1092.

De Vecchi, A., Tarantino, A., Rivotta, E., Egidi, F. and Ponticelli, C. (1985). Need for steroid in cyclosporin (Cy) treated cadaveric renal transplant recipients (pts). *Kidney Int.* **28**, 394.

Dierhoi, M. H., Sollinger, H. W., Kulayoghu, M. and Belzer, F. O. (1987). Quadruple therapy for cadaveric renal transplantation. *Transplant. Proc.* **19**, 1917.

Donnelly, P. K., Feehally, J., Jurewicz, A., *et al.* (1993). Renal transplantation: nifedipine for the nonstarters? A prospective randomized study. *Transplant. Proc.* **25**, 600.

Dreyfuss, M., Harri, E., Hoftmann, H., Kobel, H., Pache, W. and Tscherter, H. (1976). Cyclosporin A and C: new metabolites from *Trichoderma polysporum* (Link ex Pers.) Rifai. *Eur. J. Appl. Microbiol.* **3**, 125.

Dunne, D. C. (1981). The specificity of post cyclosporin "tolerance." *Transplant. Proc.* **13**, 383.

Dunne, D. C., White, D. J. F., Herbertson, B. M. and Wade, J. (1979). Prolongation of kidney survival during and after cyclosporin A therapy. *Transplantation* **27**, 359.

Durez, P., Abramowicz, D., Gerard, C., *et al.* (1993). In vivo induction of interleukin 10 by anti-CD3 monoclonal antibody or bacterial lipoplysaccharide: differential modulation by cyclosporin A. *J. Exp. Med.* **177**, 551.

Elliot, J. F., Lin, Y., Mizel, S. B., Bleackley, R. C., Harnish, D. G. and Paetkam, V. (1984). Induction of interleukin 2 messenger RNA inhibited by cyclosporin. *Science* **226**, 1439.

European Multicentre Trial. (1982). Cyclosporin A as sole immunosuppressive agent in recipients of kidney allograft from cadaver donors. *Lancet* **2**, 57.

European Multicentre Trial. (1983). Cyclosporin in cadaveric renal transplantation: one-year follow-up of a multicentre trial. *Lancet* **2**, 986.

European Multicentre Trial Group. (1993). European Multicentre Trial of cyclosporine in renal transplantation: 10-year follow-up. *Transplant. Proc.* **25**, 527.

Fassi, A., Sangalli, F., Colombi, F., *et al.* (1999). Beneficial effects of calcium channel blockade on acute glomerular hemodynamic changes induced by cyclosporine. *Am. J. Kidney Dis.* **33**, 267.

Ferguson, R. M. (1988). A multicentre experience with sequential ALG/cyclosporine therapy in renal transplantation. *Clin. Transplant.* **2**, 285.

Ferguson, R. M., Rynasiewicz, J. J., Sutherland, D. E., Simmons, R. L. and Najarian, J. S. (1982a). Cyclosporin A in renal transplantation: a prospective randomized trial. *Surgery* **92**, 175.

Ferguson, R. M., Sutherland, D. E., Simmons, R. L. and Najarian, J. S. (1982b). Ketoconazole, cyclosporin metabolism and renal transplantation. *Lancet* **2**, 882.

First, M. R., Alloway, R. and Schroeder, T. J. (1998). Development of Sang-35: a cyclosporine formulation bioequivalent to neoral. *Clin. Transplant.* **12**, 518.

First, M. R., Schroeder, T. J., Michael, A., Hariharan, S., Weiskittel, P. and Alexander, J. W. (1993). Cyclosporine-ketonconazole interaction: long-term follow-up and preliminary results of a randomized trial. *Transplantation* **55**, 1000.

Fischer, G. and Schmid, F. X. (1990). The mechanism of protein folding: implications of in vitro refolding to de novo protein folding and traslocation in the cell. *Biochemistry* **29**, 2205.

Fischer, G., Wittmann-Liebold, B., Lang, K., Kiefhaben, T. and Schmid, F. X. (1989). Cyclophilin and peptidyl-prolyl cis-trans isomerase are probably identical proteins. *Nature* **337**, 476.

Flanagan, W. M., Corthesy, B., Bram, R. J. and Crabtree, G. R. (1991). Nuclear association of a T-cell transplantation factor blocked by FK506 and cyclosporin A. *Nature* **352**, 803.

Flechner, S. M., Kerman, R. H., van Burren, C. T., Lorber, M., Barker, C. J. and Kahan, B. D. (1987). Does cyclosporin improve results of HLA-identical renal transplantation? *Transplant. Proc.* **19**, 1485.

Flechner, S. M., Kerman, R. H., van Burren, C., Payne, W. D. and Kahan, B. D. (1983a). The using of cyclosporin and prednisolone for high MLC haploidentical living related renal transplantation. *Transplant. Proc.* **15**, 442.

Flechner, S. M., Payne, W. D., van Buren, C., Kerman, R. and Kahan, B. D., (1983b). The effect of cyclosporine on early graft function in human renal transplantation. *Transplantation* **36**, 268.

Foley, R. J., Hammer, R. W. and Weinmann, E. J. (1985). Serum potassium concentrations in cyclosporin- and azathioprine-treated renal patients. *Nephron* **40**, 280.

Forwell, M. H., Bradley, J. A., Briggs, J. D., *et al.* (1987). Low-dose cyclosporin or azathioprine one year after renal transplantation. *Transplant. Proc.* **19**, 1858.

Foster, S., Wood, K. J. and Morris, P. J. (1988). Production of indefinite renal allograft survival in the rat by pretreatment with viable and nonviable hepatocytes or liver membrane extracts. *Transplantation* **45**, 228.

Freeman, D. J., Laupacis, A., Keown, P. A., Stiller, C. R. and Carruthers, S. G. (1984). Evaluation of cyclosporin-phenytoin interaction with observations on cyclosporin metabolites. *Br. J. Pharmacol.* **18**, 887.

Frei, U. (1999). Overview of the clinical experience with Neoral in transplantation. *Transplant. Proc.* **31**, 1669.

French, M. E., Thompson, J. F., Hunniset, A. G., Wood, R. F. and Morris, P. J. (1983). Impaired function of renal allografts during treatment with cyclosporin A nephroxicity or rejection. *Transplant. Proc.* **15**, 485.

Friedman, J. and Weissman, I. (1991). Two cytoplasmic candidates for immunophilin action are revealed by affinity for a new cyclophilin: one in the presence and one in the absence of CSA. *Cell* **66**, 799.

Fries, D., Hiesse, C., Charpentier, B., *et al.* (1987). Triple combination of low dose cyclosporin, azathioprine and steroids in first cadaver donor renal allografts. *Transplant. Proc.* **19**, 1911.

Fries, D., Kechrid, C., Charpentier, B., Hammouche, M. and Moulin, B. (1985). A prospective study of a triple association: cyclosporin, corticosteroids and azathioprine in immunologically high risk renal transplantation. *Transplant. Proc.* **17**, 1213.

Fuggle, S. V., McWhinnie, D. L., Chapman, J. R., Taylor, H. M. and Morris, P. J. (1986). Sequential analysis of HLA-class II antigen expression in human renal allografts: induction of tubular class II antigens and correlation with clinical parameters. *Transplantation* **42**, 144.

Gaspari, F., Anedda, M. F., Signorini, O., *et al.* (1997). Prediction of cyclosporin area under the curve using a three-point sampling strategy after Neoral administration. *J. Am. Soc. Nephrol.* **8**, 647.

Gaspari, F., Perico, N., Signorini, O., Caruso, R. and Remuzzi, G. (1998). Abbreviated kinetic profiles in area under the curve monitoring of cyclosporine therapy: technical note. *Kidney Int.* **54**, 2146.

Gebhard, F., Hammer, C., Krombach, F., Bohn, D. and Brendel, W. (1985). Inflammatory cell during acute rejection in dog renal allografts under intermittent cyclosporin monotherapy. *Transplant. Proc.* **17**, 857.

Ghiggeri, G. M., Altieri, P., Oleggini, R., *et al.* (1994). Cyclosporine enhances the synthesis of selected extracellular matrix proteins by renal cells "in culture": different cell responses and phenotype characterization. *Transplantation* **57**, 1382.

Gill, E. S., Hodge, E. E., Novick, A. C., *et al.* (1994). Azathioprine vs cyclosporine in recipients of HLA-identical renal allografts. *Cleve. Clin. J. Med.* **61**, 206.

Gluckman, E., Devergie, A., Poirier, O. and Lokiec, F. (1983). Use of cyclosporin as prophylaxis of graft-vs.-host disease after human allogenic bone marrow transplantation: report of 38 patients. *Transplant. Proc.* **15(Suppl. 1–2)**, 2628.

Gordon, M. Y. and Singer, J. W. (1979). Selective effects of cyclosporin A on colony forming lymphoid and myeloid cells in man. *Nature* **279**, 433.

Granelli-Piperano, A. (1988). In situ hybridization for interleukin 2 and interleukin 2 receptor mRNA in T cells activated in the presence or absence of cyclosporin A. *J. Exp. Med.* **168**, 1649.

Granelli-Piperano, A., Nolan, P., Inabak, K. and Steinman, R. M. (1990). The effect of immunosuppressive agents on the induction of nuclear factors that bind to sites on the interleukin 2 promoter. *J. Exp. Med.* **172**, 1869.

Gratwohl, A., Forster, I. and Speck, B. (1981). Skin grafts in rabbits with cyclosporin A: absence of induction in tolerance and untoward side effects. *Transplantation* **31**, 136.

Green, C. T. and Allison, A. C. (1978). Kidney allograft survival after short term cyclosporin A treatment. *Lancet* **1**, 1182.

Green, C. T. and Allison, A. C. (1979). Induction of specific tolerance in rabbits by kidney allografting and short periods of cyclosporin A treatment. *Lancet* **2**, 1182.

Grevel, J., Welsh, M. S. and Kahan, B. D. (1989). Cyclosporine monitoring in renal transplantation: area under the curve monitoring is superior to trough-level monitoring. *Ther. Drug. Monit.* **11**, 246.

Griffin, P. J., Gomes da Costa, C. A. and Salaman, J. R. (1986). Renal transplantation without steroids: a controlled clinical trial. *Transplant. Proc.* **18**, 797.

Grino, J. M., Sabate, I., Castalao, A. M., Guardia, M., Seron, D. and Alsina, J. (1986). Erythromycin and cyclosporin. *Ann. Intern. Med.* **105**, 467.

Gross, M. L. P., Sewny, P., Pearson, R. M., Kennedy, J., Fernando, O. N. and Moorhead, J. F. (1982). Rejection encephalopathy: an acute neurological syndrome complicating renal transplantation. *J. Neurol. Sci.* **56**, 23.

Groth, C. G. (1987). There is no need to give blood transfusions as pretreatment for renal transplantation in the cyclosporine era. *Transplant. Proc.* **19**, 153.

Hall, B. M., Tiller, D. J., Hardie, I., *et al.* (1988). Comparison of three immuno-suppressive regimens in cadaver renal transplantation: long-term cyclosporine, short-term cyclosporine followed by azathioprine and prednisolone, and azathioprine and prednisolone without cyclosporine. *N. Engl. J. Med.* **318**, 1499.

Handschumaker, R. E., Harding, M. W., Rice, J. and Drugge, R. J. (1984). Cyclosporin A specific cytosolic binding protein for cyclosporin A. *Science* **226**, 544.

Hardie, I. R., for the Australian Collaborative Trials Committee. (1993). Optimal combination of immunosuppressive agents for renal transplantation: first report of a multicenter, randomized trial comparing cyclosporine + prednisolone with cyclosporin + azathioprine and with triple therapy in cadaver renal transplantation. *Transplant. Proc.* **25**, 583.

Haug, C., Duell, T., Voisard, R., *et al.* (1995). Cyclosporine A stimulates endothelin release. *J. Cardiovasc. Pharmacol.* **26**, S239.

Hauser, A. C., Derfler, K., Stockenhuber, F., Wamser, P., Marosi, L. and Balcke, P. (1991). Effect of calcium channel blockers on renal function in renal graft recipients treated with cyclosporine. *N. Engl. J. Med.* **324**, 1517.

Hayry, P., Ahonen, J., von Willebrand, E., *et al.* (1988). Discontinuation of one drug in triple drug immunosuppression with cyclosporin, azathioprine and steroids: an interim report. *Transplant. Proc.* **20**, 449.

Hayry, P., von Willebrand, E., Taskinen, E., *et al.* (1983). Cyclosporin in treatment of corticosteroid resistant episodes of rejection. *Arch. Surg.* **118**, 750.

Hedley, D., Powles, R. L. and Morgenstein, G. R. (1982). Toxicity of cyclosporin A in patients following bone marrow transplantation. *In Cyclosporin A,* (D. J. White, ed.), p. 545, Elsevier Biomedical, Amsterdam.

Henriksen, I., Hansen, B. L. and Birkeland, S. A. (1986). Conversion of long-term renal allograft recipients from prednisolone/azathioprine to cyclosporin. *Transplant. Proc.* **18**, 1002.

Hess, A. D. and Bright, E. C. (1991). Cyclosporin inhibits T-cell activation at two distinct levels: role of the CD 28 activation pathway. *Transplant. Proc.* **23**, 961.

Hess, A. D. and Colambani, P. M. (1986). Mechanism of action of cyclosporine: role of calmodulin, cyclosporin and other cyclosporine-binding proteins. *Transplant. Proc.* **18(Suppl. 5)**, 219.

Hess, A. D., Donnenburg, A. D., Tutschka, P. and Santos, G. W. (1983a). Effect of cyclosporin A on human lymphocyte response in vitro: V. analysis of responding T lymphocyte subpopulations in primary MLR with monoclonal antibodies. *J. Immunol.* **130**, 717.

Hess, A. D. and Tutschka, P. J. (1980). Effect of cyclosporin A on human lymphocyte responses in vitro: I. CsA allows for the expression of alloantigen-activated suppressor cells while prefer-

entially inhibiting the induction of cyclolytic effector lymphocytes in MLR. *J. Immunol.* **124**, 2601.

Hess, A. D., Tutschka, P. J. and Santos, G. W. (1981). Effect of cyclosporin A on human lymphocyte responses in vitro: II. induction of specific alloantigen unresponsiveness mediated by a nylon wool adherent suppressor cell. *J. Immunol.* **126**, 961.

Hess, A. D., Tutschka, P. J. and Santos, G. W. (1982a). The effect of cyclosporin A on T-lymphocyte subpopulations. *In Cyclosporin A,* (D. J. White, ed.), p. 209, Elsevier Biomedical, Amsterdam.

Hess, A. D., Tutschka, P. J. and Santos, G. W. (1982b). Effect of cyclosporin A on human lymphocyte responses in vitro: III. CsA inhibits the production of T lymphocyte growth factors in secondary mixed lymphocyte responses but does not inhibit the response of primed lymphocytes to TCGF. *J. Immunol.* **128**, 355.

Hess, A. D., Tutschka, P. J. and Santos, G. W. (1983b). Effect of cyclosporin on the induction of cytotoxic T lymphocytes: role of interleukin-1 and interleukin-2. *Transplant. Proc.* **15**, 2248.

Hillebrand, G., Castro, J. A., Habersetzer, R., *et al.* (1986). Chronic cyclosporin hepatotoxicity after renal transplantation. *Transplant. Proc.* **18**, 1020.

Hillis, A. N., Duguid, J., Evans, C. M., Bone, J. M. and Sells, R. A. (1987). Three year experience of donor specific transfusion and concomitant cyclosporin A. *Transplant. Proc.* **19**, 2248.

Hoitsma, A. J., Wetzels, J. F., van Lier, H. J., Berden, J. H. and Koene, R. A. (1987). Cyclosporin treatment with conversion after three months versus conventional immunosuppression in renal allograft recipients. *Lancet* **2**, 584.

Hojo, M., Morimoto, T., Maluccio, M. A., *et al.* (1999). Cyclosporine induces cancer progression by a cell autonomous mechanism. *Nature* **397**, 530.

Holt, D. W. (1986). Clinical interpretation of cyclosporin measurements. *Prog. Transplant.* **3**, 32.

Holt, D. W., Marsden, J. T., Johnston, A., Bewick, M. and Taube, D. H. (1986). Blood cyclosporin concentrations and renal allograft dysfunction. *B. M. J.* **293**, 1057.

Homan, W. P., Fabre, J. W., French, M. E., Millard, P. R., Denton, T. G. and Morris, P. J. (1980a). Reversal of acute rejection episodes by cyclosporin A in dogs receiving renal allografts. *Transplantation* **29**, 262.

Homan, W. P., Fabre, J. W., Millard, P. R. and Morris, P. J. (1980b). Effect of cyclosporin A upon second-set rejection of rat renal allografts. *Transplantation* **30**, 354.

Homan, W. P., Fabre, J. W., Millard, P. R. and Morris, P. J. (1980c). Interaction of cyclosporin A with anti lymphocyte serum and with enhancing serum for the suppression of renal allograft rejection in the rat. *Transplantation* **29**, 219.

Homan, W. P., Fabre, J. W. and Morris, P. J. (1979). Nature of the unresponsiveness induced by cyclosporin A in rats bearing renal allografts. *Transplantation* **28**, 439.

Homan, W. P., Fabre, J. W., Williams, K. A., Millard, P. R. and Morris, P. J. (1980d). Studies on the immunosuppressive properties of cyclosporin A in rats receiving renal allografts. *Transplantation* **29**, 361.

Homan, W. P., French, M. E., Millard, P. R., Denton, T. G., Fabre, J. W. and Morris, P. J. (1980e). Studies on the effects of cyclosporin A upon renal allograft rejection in the dog. *Surgery* **88**, 168.

Homan, W. P., French, M. E. and Morris, P. J. (1980f). Effects of cyclosporin A upon the function of ischemically damaged renal autografts in the dog. *Transplantation* **30**, 228.

Homan, W. P., French, M. E., Millard, P. R. and Morris, P. J. (1981a). A study of eleven drug regimens using cyclosporin A to suppress renal allograft rejection in the dog. *Transplant. Proc.* **13**, 397.

Homan, W. P., Williams, K. A., Millard, P. R. and Morris, P. J. (1981b). Prolongation of renal allograft survival in the rat by pretreatment with donor antigen and cyclosporin A. *Transplantation* **31**, 423.

Horsburgh, T., Wood, P. and Brent, L. (1980). Suppression of in vitro lymphocyte reactivity by cyclosporin A: existence of a population of drug-resistant cytotoxic lymphocytes. *Nature* **286**, 609.

Hows, J. M. and Smith, J. M. (1983). In vitro stability of cyclosporin A. *J. Clin. Pathol.* **36**, 720.

Hricik, D. E., Bartucci, M. R., Moir, E. J., Mayes, J. T. and Schulak, J. A. (1991). Effects of steroid withdrawal on post transplant diabetes mellitus in cyclosporin-treated renal transplant recipients. *Transplantation* **51**, 374.

Hutchinson, I. V. (1986). Suppressor T cells in allogenic models. *Transplantation* **41**, 547.

Illner, W. D., Land, W., Habersetzen, R., *et al.* (1985). Cyclosporine in combination with azathioprine and steroids in cadaveric renal transplantation. *Transplant. Proc.* **17**, 181.

Jablonski, P., Harrison, C., Howden, B., *et al.* (1986). Cyclosporin and the ischemic rat kidney. *Transplantation* **41**, 147.

Johnson, D. W., Saunders, H. J., Johnson, F. J., *et al.* (1999). Cyclosporin exerts a direct fibrogenic effect on human tubulointerstitial cells: roles of insulin-like growth factor I, transforming growth factor beta 1 and platelet-derived growth factor. *J. Pharmacol. Exp. Ther.* **289**, 535.

Johnson, R. W. G., Wise, M. H., Bukran, A., *et al.* (1985). A four-year prospective study of cyclosporin in cadaver renal transplantation. *Transplant. Proc.* **17**, 1197.

Jones, R. M., Murie, J. A. and Allen, R. D. (1988a). Triple therapy in cadaver renal transplantation. *Br. J. Surg.* **75**, 4.

Jones, R. M., Murie, J. A., Ting, A., Dunnill, M. S. and Morris, P. J. (1988b). Renal vascular thrombosis of cadaveric renal allografts in patients receiving cyclosporine, azathioprine and prednisolone triple therapy. *Clin. Transplant.* **2**, 122.

June, C. H., Thompson, C. B., Kennedy, M. S., Nims, J. and Thomas, E. D. (1985). Profound hypomagnesemia and renal magnesium wasting associated with the use of cyclosporin for marrow transplantation. *Transplantation* **39**, 620.

Kahan, B. D. (1983). The management of kidney recipients treated with cyclosporin. *Transplant. Proc.* **15(Suppl. 1–2)**, 2641.

Kahan, B. D. (1984). Donor specific transfusions—a balanced view. *Prog. Transplant.* **1**, 115.

Kahan, B. D. (1989). Cyclosporine. *N. Engl. J. Med.* **321**, 1725.

Kahan, B. D., Kerman, R. H., Agostino, G., Friedman, A. and LeGrue, S. J. (1982). The action of cyclosporin A on human lymphocytes. *In Cyclosporin A*, (D. J. White, ed.), p. 281, Elsevier Biomedical, Amsterdam.

Kalman, V. K. and Klimpel, G. R. (1983). Cyclosporin A inhibits the production of gamma interferon (IFN gamma), but does not inhibit production of virus-induced IFN alpha/beta. *Cell. Immunol.* **78**, 122.

Kanazi, G., Stowe, N., Steinmuller, D., Ho-Hsieg, H. and Novick, A. C. (1986). Effect of cyclosporine upon the function of ischemically damaged kidneys in the rat. *Transplantation* **41**, 782.

Kasiske, B. L., Heim-Duthoy, K. and Ma, J. Z. (1993). Elective cyclosporin withdrawal after renal transplantation: a meta analysis. *J. A. M. A.* **269**, 395.

Kelles, A., Herman, J., Tjandra-Maga, T. B. and Van Damme Lombaerts, R. (1999). Sandimmune to Neoral conversion and value of abbreviated AUC monitoring in stable pediatric kidney transplant recipients. *Pediatr. Transplant.* **3**, 282.

Kennedy, M. S., Deeg, H. J., Siegel, M., Growley, J. J., Storb, R. and Thomas, E. D. (1983). Acute renal toxicity with combined use of amphotericin B and cyclosporin after marrow transplantation. *Transplantation* **35**, 211.

Keown, P. A., Essery, G. L., Stiller, C. R., *et al.* (1981a). Mechanisms of immuno-suppression by cyclosporin. *Transplant. Proc.* **13**, 386.

Keown, P. A., Essery-Rice, G., Hellstrom, A., Sinclair, N. R. and Stiller, C. R. (1985). Inhibition of human in vitro cytotoxic T lymphocyte generation by cyclosporin following organ transplantation. *Transplantation* **40**, 45.

Keown, P. A., Landsberg, D., Halloran, P., *et al.* (1996). A randomized, prospective multicenter pharmacoepidemiologic study of cyclosporine emulsion in stable renal graft recipients. *Transplantation* **62**, 1744.

Keown, P. A., Laupacis, A., Carruthers, G., *et al.* (1984). Interaction between phenytoin and cyclosporin following organ transplantation. *Transplantation* **38**, 304.

Keown, P. A. and Niese, D. (1998). Cyclosporine microemulsion increases drug exposure and reduces acute rejection without incremental toxicity in de novo renal transplantation. *Kidney Int.* **54**, 938.

Keown, P. A., Stiller, C. R., Ulan, R. A., *et al.* (1981b). Immunological and pharmacological monitoring in the clinical use of cyclosporin A. *Lancet* **2**, 686.

Keusch, G., Baumgartner, D., Gmur, N. J., Burger, H. R., Larigiander, F. and Binswanger, V. (1985). Erythrocytosis (E) after kidney allotransplantation (KT): hematological characterization and complications. *Kidney Int.* **28**, 377.

Khanna, A., Li, B., Sehajpal, P. K., Sharma V. K. and Suthanthiran,

M. (1995). Mechanism of action of cyclosporine: a new hypothesis implicating transforming growth factor-β. *Transplant. Rev.* **9**, 41.

Kimmel, P. L., Philips, T. M., Kramer, N. C. and Thompson, A. M. (1985). In vitro and in vivo interaction of sulfamethoxazole (SNX) with cyclosporin A (CSA) measurements by high pressure liquid chromatography (HPLC). *Kidney Int.* **27**, 343.

Klaus, C. G. and Dongworth, D. W. (1982). Effects of cyclosporin A on B cell functions in the mouse. *In Cyclosporin A*, (D. J. White, ed.), p. 233, Elsevier Biomedical, Amsterdam.

Klintmalm, G. B., Iwatsuki, S. and Starzl, T. E. (1981). Cyclosporin A hepatotoxicity in 66 renal allograft recipients. *Transplantation* **32**, 488.

Kostakis, A. J., White, A. J. G. and Calne, R. Y. (1977). Prolongation of rat heart allograft survival by cyclosporin A. *I. C. R. S. J. Med. Sci.* **5**, 280.

Kovarik, J. M. and Koelle, E. U. (1999). Cyclosporin pharmacokinetics in the elderly. *Drugs Aging* **15**, 197.

Kovarik, J. M., Vernillet, L., Mueller, E. A., *et al.* (1994). Cyclosporine disposition and metabolite profiles in renal transplant patients receiving a microemulsion formulation. *Ther. Drug. Monit.* **16**, 519.

Kreis, H., Chkoff, N., Chatenoud, L., *et al.* (1989). A randomized trial comparing the efficacy of OKT3 used to prevent or to treat rejection. *Transplant. Proc.* **21**, 1741.

Kunkle, A. and Klaus, G. G. B. (1980). Selective effects of cyclosporin A on functional B cell subsets in the mouse. *J. Immunol.* **125**, 2526.

Kupiec-Weglinski, J. W., Araujo, J. L., Heidecke, C. D., Filho, M. A. and Tilney, N. L. (1985). Does cyclosporin inhibit T helper or spare T suppressor lymphocytes in the maintenance phase of allograft survival? *Transplant. Proc.* **17**, 1339.

Lafferty, K., Borel, J. F. and Hodgkin, P. (1983). Cyclosporine A (CSA): models for the mechanism of action. *Transplant. Proc.* **15**, 2242.

Larsson, E. L. (1980). Cyclosporin A and dexamethasone suppress T cell responses by selectively acting at distinct sites of the triggering process. *J. Immunol.* **124**, 2828.

Leapman, S. B., Filo, R. S., Smith, E. J. and Smith, P. G. (1981). Differential effects of cyclosporin A on lymphocyte subpopulations. *Transplant. Proc.* **13**, 405.

LeGrue, S., Freidman, A. and Kahan, B. D. (1983). Lack of evidence for a cyclosporin receptor on human lymphocyte membranes. *Transplant. Proc.* **15**, 2259.

LeGrue, S. J., Turner, R., Weisbrodt, N. and Dedman, J. R. (1986). Does the binding of cyclosporin to calmodulin result in immunosuppression? *Science* **234**, 68.

Lindholm, A. and Kahan, B. D. (1993). Influence of cyclosporine pharmacokinetics, trough concentrations, and AUC monitoring on outcome after kidney transplantation. *Clin. Pharmacol. Ther.* **54**, 205.

Liu, J., Farmer, J. D., Lane, W. S., Friedman, J., Weissman, I. and Schreiber, S. L. (1991). Calcineurin is a common target of cyclophilin-cyclosporine A and FKBP-FK506 complexes. *Cell* **66**, 807.

MacDonald, A. S., Belitsky, P., Cohen, A. D., White, J. and Lannon, S. G. (1983). Cyclosporin for steroid-resistant rejection in azathioprine-treated renal graft recipients. *Transplant. Proc.* **15**, 2535.

MacDonald, A. S., Daloze, P., Dandavino, R., *et al.* (1987). A randomized study of cyclosporin with and without prednisolone in renal allograft recipients. *Transplant. Proc.* **19**, 1865.

MacPhee, I. A., Bradley, J. A., Briggs, J. D., *et al.* (1998). Long-term outcome of a prospective randomized trial of conversion from cyclosporine to azathioprine treatment one year after renal transplantation. *Transplantation* **15**, 1186.

Mahalati, K., Belitsky, P., Sketris, I., West, K. and Panek, R. (1999). Neoral monitoring by simplified sparse sampling area under the concentration-time curve: its relation to acute rejection and cyclosporin nephrotoxicity early after kidney transplantation. *Transplantation* **68**, 55.

Mahalati, K., Lawen, J., Kiberd, B. and Belitsky, P. (2000). Is 3-hour cyclosporine blood level superior to trough level in early postrenal transplantation period? *J. Urol.* **163**, 37.

Mangal, A. K., Growe, G. H., Sinclair, M., Stillwell, G. F., Reeve, C. E. and Naiman, S. C. (1984). Acquired hemolytic anaemia due to "auto"-anti-A or "auto"-anti-B induced by group O homograft in renal transplant recipients. *Transfusion* **24**, 201.

Margreiter, R., Huber, C., Speilberger, M. and Konig, P. (1983). Cyclosporin in treatment of acute cadaveric kidney graft rejection refractory to high dose methylprednisolone. *Transplantation* **36**, 203.

Margreiter, R., Weimar, W., Heineman, E. and Jeekel, J. (1984). Inhibition of chronic kidney allograft rejection by cyclosporin. *Transplant. Proc.* **15(Suppl. 1)**, 2953.

Marone, G., Paulis, A., Casolaro, V., Ciccarelli, A., Spadaro, G. and Cirillo, R. (1992). In vitro and in vivo characterization of the anti-inflammatory effects of cyclosporin A. *Int. Arch. Allergy Immunol.* **99**, 279.

Mason, D. W. and Morris, P. J. (1984). Inhibition of the accumulation in rat kidney allografts of specific—but not nonspecific—cytotoxic cells by cyclosporin. *Transplantation* **37**, 46.

Mattila, P. S., Ullman, K. S., Fiering, S., *et al.* (1990). The actions of cyclosporin A and FK506 suggest a novel step in the activation of T lymphocytes. *EMBO J.* **9**, 4425.

Meier-Kriesche, H. U., Kaplan, B., Brannan, P., *et al.* (1998). A limited sampling strategy for the estimation of eight-hour Neoral areas under the curve in renal transplantation. *Ther. Drug Monit.* **20**, 401.

Merker, M., Rice, B., Schweitzer, B. and Handschumacher, R. E. (1983). Cyclosporin binding components in BW5147 lymphoblasts and normal lymphoid tissue. *Transplant. Proc.* **15**, 2265.

Merion, R. M. and Calne, R. Y. (1985). Allograft renal vein thrombosis. *Transplant. Proc.* **17**, 1746.

Meyer, M. M., Munar, M., Udeaja, J. and Bennett, W. (1993). Efficacy of area under the curve cyclosporine monitoring in renal transplantation. *J. Am. Soc. Nephrol.* **4**, 1306.

Milton, A. D., Spencer, S. C. and Fabre, J. W. (1986). The effect of cyclosporin on the induction of MHC antigens in heart and kidney allografts in the rat. *Transplantation* **42**, 338.

Miyawaki, T., Yachie, A., Ohzeki, S., Nagaoki, T. and Taniguchi, N. (1983). Cyclosporin A does not prevent expression of TAC antigen, a probable TCGF receptor molecule on mitogen-stimulated human T cells. *J. Immunol.* **130**, 2737.

Morozumi, K., Thiel, F., Gudat, F. and Mihatsch, M. J. (1993). Studies on morphological outcome of cyclosporine-associated arteriolopathy after discontinuation of cyclosporine inpatients with renal allografts. *Transplant. Proc.* **25**, 537.

Morris, P. J. (1981). Cyclosporin A. *Transplantation* **32**, 249.

Morris, P. J., Chapman, J. R., Allen, R. D., *et al.* (1987). Cyclosporin conversion versus conventional immunosuppression: long term follow-up and histological evaluation. *Lancet* **2**, 586.

Morris, P. J., French, M. E., Ting, A., Frostick, S. and Hunniset, A. (1982). A controlled trial of cyclosporin A in renal transplantation. *In Cyclosporin A*, (D. J. White, ed.), p. 355, Elsevier Biomedical, Amsterdam.

Morris, P. J., Mason, D. W. and Hutchinson, I. V. (1983). The effect of cyclosporin A on lymphocytes in animal models of tissue transplantation. *Transplant. Proc.* **15**, 2287.

Mueller, C., Shao, Y., Altermatt, H. J., Hess, M. W. and Shelby, J. (1993). The effects of cyclosporine treatment on the expression of genes encoding granzyme A and perforin in the infiltrate of mouse heart transplants. *Transplantation* **55**, 139.

Myers, B. D., Ross, J., Newton, L., Luetscher, J. and Pealroth, M. (1984). Cyclosporin-associated chronic nephropathy. *N. Engl. J. Med.* **311**, 699.

Najarian, J. S., Ferguson, R. M., Sutherland, D. E., Rynasiewicz, J. J. and Simmons, R. L. (1983). A prospective trial of the efficacy of cyclosporin in renal transplantation at the University of Minnesota. *Transplant. Proc.* **15**, 438.

Najarian, J. S., Fryd, D. S., Strand, M., *et al.* (1985). A single institution, randomized, prospective trial of cyclosporin immunosuppression in renal allograft recipients. *Ann. Surg.* **201**, 142.

Nankivell, B. J., Hibbins, M. and Chapman, J. R. (1994). Diagnostic utility of whole blood cyclosporine measurements in renal transplantation using triple therapy. *Transplantation* **58**, 989.

Nashan, B., Moore, R., Amlot, P. *et al.* (1997). Randomised trial of basiliximab versus placebo for control of acute cellular rejection in renal allograft recipients. CHIB 201 International Study Group. *Lancet* **350**, 1193.

Neild, G. H., Rocchi, G., Imberti, L., *et al.* (1983). Effects of cyclosporin A on prostacyclin synthesis by vascular tissue. *Thromb. Res.* **32**, 373.

Neild, G. H., Taube, D. H., Hartley, R. B., *et al.* (1986). Morphological differentiation between rejection and cyclosporin nephrotoxicity in renal allografts. *J. Clin. Pathol.* **39**, 152.

Nemlander, A., Ahonen, J., Wiktorowicz, K., *et al.* (1983). Effect of cyclosporin on wound healing. *Transplantation* **36**, 1.

Neumayer, H. H., Schreiber, M. and Wagner, K. (1989). Prevention of delayed graft function by diltiazem and iloprost. *Transplant. Proc.* **21**, 122.

Neumayer, H. H. and Wagner, K. (1986). Diltiazem and economic use of cyclosporin. *Lancet* **2**, 523.

Norman, D. J., Kahana, L., Stuart, F. P., *et al.* (1993). A randomized clinical trial of induction therapy with OKT3 in kidney transplantation. *Transplantation* **55**, 44.

Nyberg, G., Gabel, H., Althoff, P., Bjork, S., Herlitz, H. and Brynger, H. (1984a). Adverse effect of trimethoprim on kidney function in renal transplant patients. *Lancet* **1**, 394.

Nyberg, G., Haljamae, U., Frisenette-Fich, C., *et al.* (1998). Breast-feeding during treatment with cyclosporine. *Transplantation* **65**, 253.

Nyberg, G., Sandberg, L., Rydberg, L., *et al.* (1984b). ABO-autoimmune hemolytic anemia in renal transplant patient treated with cyclosporin: a case report. *Transplantation* **37**, 529.

O'Garra, A., Warren, D. J., Holman, M., Popham, A. M., Sanderson, C. J. and Klaus, C. G. (1986). Effects of cyclosporin in responses of murine B cells to T cell derived lymphokines. *J. Immunol.* **137**, 2220.

Ohlman, S., Lindholm, A., Hagglund, H., Sawe, J. and Kahan, B. D. (1993). On the intraindividual variability and chronobiology of cyclosporine pharmacokinetics in renal transplantation. *Eur. J. Clin. Pharmacol.* **44**, 265.

O'Keefe, S. J., Tamura, J., Kincaid, R. L., Tocci, M. J. and O'Neill, E. A. (1992). FK-506 and CSA-sensitive activation of the interleukin-2 promoter by calcineurin. *Nature* **357**, 692.

Olshan, A. F., Matison, D. R. and Zwanenburg, T. S. (1994). International Commission for Protection Against Environmental Mutagens and Carcinogens. Cyclosporine A: review of genotoxicity and potential for adverse human reproductive and developmental effects: report of a working group on the genotoxicity of cyclosporine A. August 18, 1993. *Mutat. Res.* **317**, 163.

Opelz, G. (1986). Multicenter impact of cyclosporin on kidney cadaver graft survival. *Prog. Allergy* **38**, 329.

Opelz, G., Wujciak, T., Dohler, B., Scherer, S. and Mytilineos, J. (1999). HLA compatibility and organ transplant survival. *Rev. Immunogenet.* **1**, 334.

Ost, L., Lundgren, G. and Groth, C. G. (1985). Renal transplants in the older patients. *Prog. Transplant.* **2**, 1.

Oyer, P. E., Stinson, E. B., Reitz, B. A., *et al.* (1982). Preliminary results with cyclosporin A in clinical cardiac transplantation. *In Cyclosporin A*, (D. J. White, ed.), p. 461, Elsevier Biomedical, Amsterdam.

Paavonen, T. and Hayry, P. (1980). Effects of cyclosporin A on T dependent and T independent immunoglobulin synthesis in vitro. *Nature* **287**, 542.

Palacios, R. and Moller, G. (1981). Cyclosporin A blocks receptors for HLA-DR antigens on T cells. *Nature* **290**, 792.

Palestine, A. G., Austin, H. A., Barlow, J. E., *et al.* (1986). Renal histopathologic alterations in patients treated with cyclosporin for uveitis. *N. Engl. J. Med.* **314**, 1293.

Paller, M. S. and Murray, B. M. (1985). Renal dysfunction in animal models of cyclosporin toxicity. *Transplant. Proc.* **17(Suppl. 1)**, 155.

Pankewycz, O. G., Miao, L., Isaacs, R., *et al.* (1996). Increased renal tubular expression of transforming growth factor beta in human allografts correlates with cyclosporine toxicity. *Kidney Int.* **50**, 1634.

Pasini, M., Perico, N. and Remuzzi, G. (1990). Roles for thromboxane (Tx) A_2 and sulfidopeptide leukotrienes (LT) in cyclosporine (CSA)-induced acute renal failure. *Kidney Int.* **37**, 350.

Pedersen, E. B., Hansen, H. E., Kornerups, H. J., Madsen, S. and Sorensen, A. W. S. (1993). Long-term graft survival after conversion from cyclosporin to azathioprine 1 year after renal transplantation: a prospective, randomized study from 1 to 6 years after transplantation. *Nephrol. Dial. Transplant.* **8**, 250.

Perico, N., Benigni, A., Zoja, C., Delani, F. and Remuzzi, G. (1986). Functional significance of exaggerated renal thromboxane A_2 synthesis induced by cyclosporin A. *Am. J. Physiol.* **251**, F581.

Perico, N. and Remuzzi, G. (1991). Cyclosporine-induced renal dysfunction in experimental animals and humans. *Transplant. Rev.* **5**, 63.

Pflugii, G., Kallen, J., Schirmer, T., Jansonius, J. N., Mauro, G. M. and Walkinshaw, M. D. (1993). X-ray structure of decameric cyclosporin-cyclosporin crystal complex. *Nature* **361**, 91.

Pirsch, J. D., D'Alessandro, A. M., Roecker, E. B., *et al.* (1993). A controlled, double-blind, randomized trial of verapamil and cyclosporine in cadaver renal transplant patients. *Am. J. Kidney Dis.* **21**, 189.

Pisetsky, D. S. and Haughton, G. (1986). Cyclosporin inhibition of a murine B cell lymphoma. *Clin. Exp. Immunol.* **63**, 549.

Pollack, R., Wong, R. L. and Chang, C. T. (1999). Cyclosporine bioavailability of Neoral and Sandimmune in white and black de novo renal transplant patients. Neoral study group. *Ther. Drug. Monit.* **21**, 661.

Ponticelli, C., Tarantinio, A., Montagnino, G., Aroldi, A., *et al.* (1988). The Milan clinical trial with cyclosporine in cadaveric renal transplantation. *Transplantation* **45**, 908.

Primmett, D. R., Levine, M., Kovarik, J. M., *et al.* (1998). Cyclosporine monitoring in patients with renal transplants: two- or three-point methods that estimate area under the curve are superior to trough levels in predicting drug exposure. *Ther. Drug Monit.* **20**, 276.

Ptachcinski, R. J., Carpenter, B. J., Burckart, G. J., Venkataramanan, R. and Rosenthal, J. T. (1985). Effect of erythromycin on cyclosporin levels. *N. Engl. J. Med.* **313**, 1416.

Ramsey, G., Nusbacher, J., Starzl, T. E. and Lindsey, G. D. (1984). Isohemagglutinins of graft origin after ABO-unmatched liver transplantation. *N. Engl. J. Med.* **311**, 1167.

Ratcliffe, P. J., Dudley, C. R., Higgins, R. M., Firth, J. D., Smith, B. and Morris, P. J. (1996). Randomised controlled trial of steroid withdrawal in renal transplant recipients receiving triple immunosuppression. *Lancet* **348**, 643.

Remuzzi, G. and Bertani, T. (1989). Renal vascular and thrombotic effects of cyclosporin. *Am. J. Kidney Dis.* **13**, 261.

Rigotti, P., Flechner, S. M., van Buren, C. T., Payne, W. T. and Kahan, B. P. (1986). Increased incidence of renal allograft thrombosis under cyclosporin immunosuppression. *Int. Surg.* **71**, 38.

Ringden, O., Myrenfors, P., Klintmalm, G., Tyden, G. and Ost, L. (1984). Nephrotoxicity by co-trimoxazole and cyclosporin in transplanted patients. *Lancet* **1**, 1016.

Robey, K. A. and Shaw, L. M. (1993). Effects of cyclosporine and its metabolites in the isolated perfused rat kidney. *J. Am. Soc. Nephrol.* **4**, 168.

Rodriques, M., Hutchinson, I. V. and Morris, P. J. (1987). Three phenotypically distinct populations of T suppressor cells resistant to cyclosporin A in the rat. *Transplant. Proc.* **19**, 4281.

Ryffel, B., Tammi, K., Greider, A. and Hess, A. D. (1985). Effects of cyclosporin on human T cell activation. *Transplant. Proc.* **17**, 1268.

Salaman, J. R. and Griffin, P. J. A. (1983). Fine needle intrarenal manometry: a new test for rejection in cyclosporin treated recipients of kidney transplants. *Lancet* **2**, 709.

Salaman, J. R. and Griffin, P. J. A. (1985). Fine needle intrarenal manometry in the management of renal transplant patients receiving cyclosporin. *Transplant. Proc.* **17**, 1275.

Salomon, D. R. (1991). An alternative view minimising the significance of cyclosporine nephrotoxicity and in favor of enhanced immunosuppression for long term kidney transplant recipients. *Transplant. Proc.* **23**, 2115.

Salomon, D. R. (1992). Cyclosporine nephrotoxicity and long-term renal transplantation. *Transplant. Rev.* **6**, 10.

Salvatierra, O., Jr. (1986). Donor-specific transfusions in living related transplantation. *World J. Surg.* **10**, 361.

Sanders, C. E., Curtis, J. J., Julian, B. A., *et al.* (1993). Tapering or discontinuing cyclosporine for financial reasons—a single-center experience. *Am. J. Kidney Dis.* **21**, 9.

Savoldi, S., Sandrini, S., Scolari, F., *et al.* (1987). Is cyclosporine administration in twice daily dose advantageous? *Transplant. Proc.* **19**, 1720.

Schreiber, S. L. and Crabtree, G. R. (1992). The mechanism of action of cyclosporin A and FK506. *Immunol. Today* **13**, 136.

Schreier, M. H., Baumann, G. and Zenke, G. (1993). Inhibition of T-cell signalling pathways by immunophilin drug complexes: are side effects inherent to immunosuppressive properties? *Transplant. Proc.* **25**, 501.

Schmidt, U., Mihatsch, M. J. and Albert, F. W. (1986). Morphologic findings of kidney transplants one year after treatment with cyclosporin A (CyA) alone or in combination with low dose steroids. *Transplant. Proc.* **18**, 1266.

Seymour, R. A. and Jacobs, D. J. (1992). Cyclosporin and the gingival tissues. *J. Clin. Periodontol.* **19**, 1.

Shah, M. B., Martin, J. E., Schroeder, T. J. and First, M. R. (1999). The evaluation of the safety and tolerability of two formulations of cyclosporine: Neoral and Sandimmune, a meta-analysis. *Transplantation* **67**, 1411.

Sheil, A. G. R., Hall, B. M., Tiller, D. J., *et al.* (1983). Australian trial of cyclosporin (Csa) in cadaveric donor renal transplantation. *Transplant. Proc.* **15**, 2485.

Sheild, C. F., Hughes, J. D. and Lemon, J. A. (1988). Prophylactic OKT3 and cadaveric renal transplantation at a single center. *Clin. Transplant.* **2**, 190.

Shihab, F. S., Andoh, T. F., Tanner, A. M. and Bennett, W. M. (1997). Sodium depletion enhances fibrosis and the expression of TGF-beta 1 and matrix proteins in experimental chronic cyclosporine nephropathy. *Am. J. Kidney Dis.* **30**, 71.

Sigal, N. H. and Dumont, F. J. (1992). Cyclosporin A, FK506 and rapamycin: pharmacologic probes of lymphocyte signal transduction. *Am. Rev. Immunol.* **10**, 519.

Simmons, R. I., Carafax, D. M., Fryd, D. S., *et al.* (1986). New immunosuppression drug combinations for mismatch related and cadaveric renal transplantation. *Transplant. Proc.* **18(Suppl. 1)**, 76.

Sinclair, N. R. (1992). Low dose steroid therapy in cyclosporine-treated renal transplant recipients with well-functioning grafts. The Canadian Multicentre Transplant Study Group. *C. M. A. J.* **147**, 645.

Slapak, M., Geoghegan, T., Digard, N., *et al.* (1985). The use of low dose cyclosporin in combination with azathioprine and steroids in renal transplantation. *Transplant. Proc.* **17**, 1222.

Smit, J. A., Drielsma, R. F., Myburgh, J. A., Laupacis, A. and Stiller, C. R. (1983). Renal allograft survival in the baboon using a pretreatment protocol with cyclosporine. *Transplantation* **36**, 121.

Sodal, G., Albrechtsen, D., Berg, K. J., *et al.* (1987). Renal transplantation from living donors mismatched for two HLA haplotypes. *Transplant. Proc.* **17**, 1509.

Somner, B. G., Henry, M. L. and Ferguson, R. M. (1986). Obliterative renal arteriopathy following cyclosporine therapy. *Transplant. Proc.* **18(Suppl. 1)**, 1285.

Squifflet, J. R., Sutherland, D. E. R., Field, J., *et al.* (1983). Synergistic immunosuppressive effect of cyclosporin A and azathioprine. *Transplant. Proc.* **15**, 520.

Starzl, T. E., Hakala, T. R., Iwatsuki, S., *et al.* (1982). Cyclosporin A and steroid treatment in 104 cadaveric renal transplantations. In *Cyclosporin A*, (D. J. White, ed.), p. 363, Elsevier Biomedical, Amsterdam.

Starzl, T. E., Hakala, T. R., Rosenthal, J. T., Iwatsuki, S. and Shaw, B. W. (1983). The Colorado-Pittsburgh cadaveric renal transplantation study with cyclosporin. *Transplant. Proc.* **15**, 2459.

Stiller, C. (1983). The requirements for maintenance steroids in cyclosporin-treated renal transplant recipients. *Transplant. Proc.* **15(Suppl. 1)**, 2490.

Sumrani, N., Delaney, V., Ding, Z., Butt, K. and Hong, J. (1990). HLA-identical renal transplants: impact of cyclosporine on intermediate-term survival and renal function. *Am. J. Kidney Dis.* **16**, 417.

Sutherland, E., Burgess, E., Klassen, J., Buckle, S. and Paul, L. C. (1993). Posttransplant conversion from cyclosporin to azathioprine: effect on cardiovascular risk profile. *Transplantation* **6**, 129.

Takahashi, N., Hayano, T. and Suzuki, M. (1989). Peptidyl-prolyl cistrans isomerase is the cyclosporin A-binding protein cyclophilin. *Nature* **337**, 473.

Tarantino, A., Aroldi, A., Stucchi, L., *et al.* (1991). A randomized prospective trial comparing cyclosporine monotherapy with triple-drug therapy in renal transplantation. *Transplantation* **52**, 53.

Terasaki, P. I., Cecka, J. M., Gjertson, D. W. and Takemoto, S. (1995). High survival rates of kidney transplants from spousal and living unrelated donors. *N. Engl. J. Med.* **333**, 333.

Theriault, Y., Logan, T. M., Meadows, R., *et al.* (1993). Solution structure of the cyclosporin A/cyclophilin complex by NMR. *Nature* **361**, 88.

Thiel, G., Loertscher, R., Brunner, F. B., *et al.* (1984). Conversion from conventional immunosuppression to cyclosporin A therapy in diabetic recipients of cadaveric kidney transplants. *Transplant. Proc.* **16**, 640.

Thiru, S., Calne, R. Y. and Nagington, J. (1981). Lymphoma in renal allograft patients treated with cyclosporin A as one of the immunosuppressive agents. *Transplant. Proc.* **13**, 359.

Thompson, C. B., June, C. H., Sullivan, K. M. and Thomas, E. D. (1984). Association between cyclosporin neurotoxicity and hypo-magnesaemia. *Lancet* **2**, 1116.

Thompson, J. F., Chalmers, D. H., Carter, N. P., Wood, R. F. and Morris, P. J. (1983a). Clinical and immunologic effects of conversion to cyclosporin-A therapy in long-term renal allograft recipients. *Transplant. Proc.* **15**, 1930.

Thompson, J. F., Chalmers, D. H., Hunnisett, A. G., Wood, R. F. and Morris, P. J. (1983b). Nephrotoxicity of trimethoprim and cortimoxazole in renal allograft recipients treated with cyclosporin. *Transplantation* **36**, 204.

Thomson, A. W., Moon, D. K., Geczy, C. L. and Nelson, D. S. (1983). Modification of delayed type hypersensitivity reaction to ovalbumin in cyclosporin A treated guinea pigs. *Immunology* **48**, 301.

Thomson, A. W., Whiting, P. H. and Simpson, J. G. (1982). Pathobiology of cyclosporin A in experimental animals. *In Cyclosporin A*, (D. J. White, ed.), p. 177, Elsevier Biomedical, Amsterdam.

Tutschka, P. J., Hess, A. D., Beschorner, W. E. and Santos, G. W. (1982). Cyclosporin A in allogeneic bone marrow transplantation: preclinical and clinical studies. *In Cyclosporin A*, (D. J. White, ed.), p. 519, Elsevier Biomedical, Amsterdam.

Umlauf, S. W., Beverly, B., Kang, S. M., Brorson, K., Tran, A. C. and Schwartz, R. H. (1993). Molecular regulation of the IL-2 gene: rheostatic control of the immune system. *Immunol. Rev.* **133**, 177.

Van Buren, D., Wideman, C. A., Ried, M., *et al.* (1984). The antagonistic effect of rifampin upon cyclosporin bioavailability. *Transplant. Proc.* **16**, 1642.

Vanrentenghem, Y., Roels, L., Lerut, J., *et al.* (1985). Thromboembolic complications and haemostatic changes in cyclosporin-treated cadaveric kidney allograft recipients. *Lancet* **1**, 1000.

Vathsala, A. (1999). Conversion from Sandimmune to Neoral in renal allograft recipients. *Transplant. Rev.* **13**, 1.

Velez, R. L., Brinker, P. J., Vergne-Marini, D. A., *et al.* (1991). Renal transplantation with cyclosporine in the elderly population. *Transplant. Proc.* **23**, 1749.

Vincenti, F., Kirkman, R., Light, S., *et al.* (1998). Interleukin-2-receptor blockade with daclizumab to prevent acute rejection in renal transplantation. *N. Engl. J. Med.* **338**, 161.

Wagner, K., Albrecht, S. and Neumayer, H. H. (1986). Prevention delayed graft function in cadaveric kidney transplantation by a calcium antagonist: preliminary result of two prospective randomized trials. *Transplant. Proc.* **18**, 510.

Wallick, S. C., Figari, I. S., Levinson, A. D. and Palladino, M. A.
(1990). Immunoregulatory role of transforming growth factor beta (TGF-beta) in development of killer cells: comparison of active and latent TGF-beta 1. *J. Exp. Med.* **172**, 1777.

Wamboldt, F. W., Weiler, S. J. and Kalin, N. H. (1984). Cyclosporin-associated mania. *Biol. Psychiatry* **19**, 1161.

Wang, S. C., Zeevi, A., Jordan, M. L., Simmons, R. L. and Tweardy, D. J. (1991). FK 506, rapamycin, and cyclosporin: effects on IL-4 and IL-10 mRNA levels in a T-helper 2 cell line. *Transplant. Proc.* **23**, 2920.

Warrens, A. N., Waters, J. B., Salama, A. D. and Lechler, R. I. (1999). Improving the therapeutic monitoring of cyclosporin A. *Clin. Transplant.* **13**, 193.

Weimar, W., Versluis, O. J., Wenting, G. J., Derkx, F. H., Schalekamp, M. A. and Jeekel, J. (1987). Prolonged cyclosporin therapy to induce solid engraftment after renal transplantation. *Transplant. Proc.* **19**, 1998.

White, D. J. G., Plumb, A. M., Pawelec, G. and Brons, G. (1979). Cyclosporin A: an immunosuppressive agent preferentially active against proliferating T cells. *Transplantation* **27**, 55.

White, D. J. G., Rolles, K. and Ottawa, T. (1980). Cyclosporin A induced long-term survival of incompatible skin and heart grafts in rats. *Transplant. Proc.* **12**, 261.

Whiting, P. H., Simpson, J. G., Davidson, R. J. and Thomson, A. W. (1982a). The toxic effects of combined administration of cyclosporin A and gentamicin. *Br. J. Exp. Pathol.* **63**, 554.

Whiting, P. H., Simpson, J. G., Davidson, R. J. and Thompson, A. W. (1983). Nephrotoxicity of cyclosporin in combination with aminoglycoside and cephalosporin antibiotics. *Transplant. Proc.* **15(Suppl. 1–2)**, 2702.

Whiting, P. H., Thomson, A. W., Blair, J. T. and Simpson, J. G. (1982b). Experimental cyclosporin A nephrotoxicity. *Br. J. Exp. Pathol.* **63**, 88.

Wiesinger, D. and Borel, J. F. (1979). Studies on the mechanism of action of cyclosporin A. *Immunobiology* **156**, 454.

Wong, W., Morris, P. J. and Wood, K. J. (1997). Pretransplant administration of a single donor class I major histocompatibility complex molecule is sufficient for the indefinite survival of fully allogeneic cardiac allografts: evidence for linked epitope suppression. *Transplantation* **63**, 1490.

Yale, J. F., Roy, R. D., Grose, M., Seemayer, T. A., Murphy, G. F. and Marliss, E. B. (1985). Effect of cyclosporin in glucose tolerance in the rat. *Diabetes* **34**, 1309.

Yatscoff, R. W., Rush, D. N. and Jefferey, J. R. (1984). Effects of sample preparation on concentrations of cyclosporin A measured in plasma. *Clin. Chem.* **30**, 1812.

Tacrolimus Therapy in Renal Transplantation

Sanjay Kulkarni • Adam Kopelan • E. Steve Woodle

Introduction

Tacrolimus (FK506, Prograf) is a macrolide antibiotic isolated from *Streptomyces tsukubaensis,* whose immunosuppressive properties were discovered in a large-scale screening process conducted by Fujisawa to identify new immunosuppressive agents. In contrast to all other U.S. Food and Drug Administration (FDA)–approved immunosuppressive agents developed to date, the clinical development of tacrolimus was conducted primarily in liver rather than kidney transplant recipients. After initial FDA approval of tacrolimus in liver transplantation in 1994, pivotal phase III studies were conducted in renal transplant recipients that led to an additional indication in renal transplantation in 1996. Although indications have not been achieved in other organs, tacrolimus has shown efficacy in rejection therapy and as a primary maintenance immunosuppressive agent in heart, lung, pancreas, and small bowel transplantation (Gruessner *et al.,* 1996; Jamieson, 1999; Kur *et al.,* 1999; Meiser *et al.,* 1999; Reddy *et al.,* 2000; Thompson, 1999). Clinical use of tacrolimus has increased markedly so that approximately three fourths of all new liver transplant recipients in the United States receive tacrolimus as their primary immunosuppressive agent, and one third of kidney transplant patients receive tacrolimus as their primary immunosuppressive agent. Tacrolimus is viewed widely as preferable to cyclosporine for maintenance immunosuppression in high–immunological risk renal allograft recipients (repeat renal transplant recipients, high–panel reactive antibody renal transplant recipients and combined kidney-pancreas transplant recipients). More recent experiences indicated that tacrolimus may have additional properties, including steroid-sparing properties, that may be superior to cyclosporine. The scientific foundation for the clinical application of tacrolimus in renal and pancreatic transplantation is based primarily on the studies outlined in this chapter.

Mechanism of Action

Tacrolimus and cyclosporine inhibit early T-cell calcium-dependent signaling events following T-cell receptor (TCR) triggering (see also Chapter 16). These inhibitory effects result in inhibition of expression of several cytokine genes, including interleukin (IL)-2, IL-3, IL-4, interferon-γ, and tumor necrosis factor-γ (Bierer *et al.,* 1993). Although cyclosporine and tacrolimus possess similar mechanisms of action, tacrolimus is 50 to 100 times more potent than cyclosporine in inhibiting T-cell activation *in vitro.* Tacrolimus and cyclosporine bind to intracellular receptors that are members of a family of intracytoplasmic proteins termed *immunophilins.* Cyclosporine binds intracellular receptors termed *cyclophilins,* whereas tacrolimus binds intracellular receptors termed *FK506 binding proteins* (FKBPs). Binding FKBPs by tacrolimus

results in formation of a drug-immunophilin complex that represents the active form of the drug. Immunophilins were first discovered to catalyze the cis-trans isomerization of Xaa-Pro amide bonds in oligopeptides (Braun *et al.,* 1995). Their *rotamase* activity was first thought to be linked to their immunosuppressant action but subsequently was found to be insufficient (Bierer *et al.,* 1993). Other analogues of tacrolimus and cyclosporine could inhibit rotomase activity without expressing immunosuppressive action (Bierer *et al.,* 1993).

The FK506/FKBP and cyclosporine/cyclophilin complexes have been shown to bind calcineurin, a serine/threonine phosphatase (Liu *et al.,* 1991). In initial studies with cyclosporine and tacrolimus, the level of calcineurin activity correlated with the amount of IL-2 produced after TCR ligation (Bierer *et al.,* 1993). Coupled with the finding that calcineurin phosphatase activity is a rate-limiting step in calcium-dependent T-cell activation (Mattila *et al.,* 1990), calcineurin was identified as the molecule responsible for the mechanism of action of tacrolimus and cyclosporine.

The binding of FK506/FKBP and cyclosporine/cyclophilin complexes to calcineurin causes a slight change in receptor structure that inactivates the phosphatase activity of calcineurin, an event now thought to be central to the inhibitory properties of these agents (Ho *et al.,* 1996). Calcineurin is normally activated following the intracellular rise in calcium after TCR ligation. Activation of calcineurin phosphatase activity results in dephosphorylation of the cytoplasmic component of nuclear factor of activated T cells (NF-AT$_c$), allowing its subsequent translocation to the nucleus (Clipstone and Crabtree, 1992). After translocation, NF-AT$_c$ combines with the nuclear component, and the resultant complex binds to the enhancer region of the IL-2 gene, leading to up-regulation of gene transcription (Schreiber and Crabtree, 1992). When FK506/FKBP or cyclosporine/cyclophilin complexes inactivate the phosphatase activity of calcineurin, NF-AT$_c$ no longer binds the enhancer region of the IL-2 gene and blocks its transcription (Schreiber and Crabtree, 1992; Sigal and Dumont, 1992). The primary mechanism by which cyclosporine and tacrolimus currently are thought to exert their immunosuppressive activity is by inhibition of calcineurin phosphatase activity (Braun *et al.,* 1995).

Clinical Experience in Renal Transplantation

Tacrolimus is unique among immunosuppressive drugs in that it was developed first in liver transplant recipients. The initial experiences with tacrolimus were in patients who were experiencing refractory hepatic allograft rejection (Demetris *et al.,* 1992; U.S. Multicenter FK506 Study Group, 1993). These experiences, combined with experiences from other centers (McDiarmid *et al.,* 1993; Woodle *et al.,* 1993a), showed the remarkable efficacy of tacrolimus in reversing refractory acute hepatic allograft rejection in patients receiving cyclo-

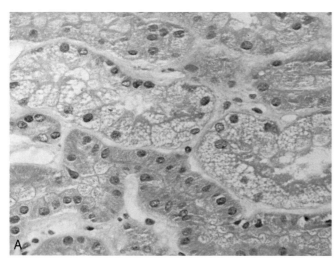
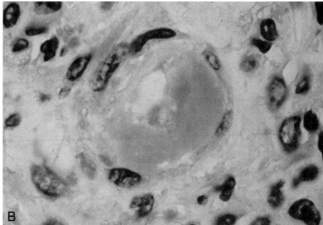

FIGURE 17-1

Histological manifestations of tacrolimus nephrotoxicity. (A) Tubular vacuolization. (B) Nodular arteriolar hyalinosis.

sporine as their primary immunosuppressive agent. The initial FDA-approved indication for tacrolimus was in the prevention of rejection after liver transplantation and was based on the results of two large-scale, randomized phase III pivotal trials conducted in liver transplant recipients (European FK 506 Multicenter Liver Study Group, 1994; U.S. Multicenter FK 506 Liver Study Group, 1994). These two open-label trials showed a statistically significant reduction in the incidence of acute rejection in patients treated with tacrolimus as compared with control patients who received cyclosporine. The trials also showed that tacrolimus therapy resulted in a reduction in the severity of rejection as compared with cyclosporine and showed salutary effects of tacrolimus on hypertension and serum lipid levels in comparison to cyclosporine. The incidence of nephrotoxicity was similar to that seen with cyclosporine (Fig. 17-1). These trials also showed that in contrast to cyclosporine, tacrolimus does not induce hirsutism or gingival hypertrophy, two major cosmetic side effects of cyclosporine.

REJECTION THERAPY

In a manner analogous to liver transplant recipients, the efficacy of tacrolimus was first shown in kidney transplant recipients as refractory rejection therapy. These observations are remarkable, in that refractory rejection patients represent the subset of patients who experience the most difficult rejection episodes to suppress. As outlined subsequently, tacrolimus therapy showed remarkable efficacy in therapy of refractory rejection. Even more impressive was the observation that refractory rejection episodes in cyclosporine-treated patients could be reversed simply by replacing cyclosporine with tacrolimus in their immunosuppressive regimens. A primary advantage of tacrolimus in the treatment of refractory rejection is that in contrast to antilymphocyte antibody preparations (e.g., OKT3 and polyclonal antibody preparations) that induce long-term suppression of T-cell responses, the immunosuppressive effects of tacrolimus could be titrated on a daily basis by adjusting dose because the immunosuppressive effects are readily reversible, in contrast to antilymphocyte antibodies.

The Pittsburgh group provided an early large experience with tacrolimus in treating refractory acute renal allograft rejection (Jordan *et al.*, 1991); 77 patients experiencing refractory acute renal allograft rejection under cyclosporine-based immunosuppressive therapy received tacrolimus as a substitute for cyclosporine in their immunosuppressive regimen. As in most studies of tacrolimus therapy for refractory acute renal allograft rejection, a significant majority (79%) of these patients had previously received antilymphocyte antibody therapy with OKT3 and/or antilymphocyte globulin (ALG) for acute rejection. Cessation of cyclosporine and conversion to tacrolimus resulted in salvage of 74% of kidney allografts with a mean serum creatinine of 2.35 ± 0.97 mg/dl (206 μmol/L) at 14 months after initiation of tacrolimus therapy. Patients with acute cellular rejection experienced graft salvage rates of 85%, whereas patients with acute cellular rejection and acute vascular rejection experienced a 65% salvage rate. Patients with acute cellular rejection in the presence of primary renal allograft nonfunction showed a 40% salvage rate. Of the 18 patients that were on hemodialysis at the time of tacrolimus conversion, half were rescued and did not require dialysis at 14 months posttreatment. One observation in this study was the ability to withdraw corticosteroids fully in 60% of rescued patients, although corticosteroid withdrawal was not performed under a predefined strict protocol. Several observations from this study have been confirmed by subsequent experiences and are now well accepted among transplant professionals, including (1) tacrolimus provides effective therapy for refractory acute renal allograft rejection, (2) tacrolimus often provides effective therapy for vascular rejection in kidney transplants and (3) the success of tacrolimus therapy for refractory acute renal allograft rejection is related to the severity and duration of rejection.

Subsequently, Jordan and colleagues presented 5-year follow-up of the Pittsburgh experience and showed good long-term renal allograft function in patients undergoing tacrolimus rescue therapy (Jordan *et al.*, 1997a, 1997b). A total of 169 patients were converted from cyclosporine to tacrolimus for steroid-resistant rejection, with a 74% success rate and a mean serum creatinine of 2.3 ± 1.1 mg/dl (202 μmol/L). Of the 17% of patients on dialysis at the time of tacrolimus initiation, 46% were salvaged with a mean serum creatinine of 2.15 ± 0.37 mg/dl (189 μmol/L). Improved response rates were noted in patients with acute cellular rejection plus acute vascular rejection compared with their initial experience because 75% of these patients were salvaged. As in their initial experience, corticosteroid withdrawal was accomplished while on tacrolimus because prednisone doses were reduced from 28 ± 1.1 mg/d to 8.5 ± 4.1 mg/d, with 22% of study patients off corticosteroids completely.

The first multicenter experience that evaluated the efficacy of tacrolimus in refractory acute renal allograft rejection was presented in 1996 (Woodle *et al.*, 1996d). This trial confirmed many of the observations from the initial Pittsburgh single-center experience. In this study, renal transplant patients with biopsy-proven rejection who had previously received antilymphocyte antibody for rejection therapy were entered into the trial (79% of all patients). Patients who were not candidates for antilymphocyte therapy also were eligible for study entry at the discretion of the investigator (21% of patients). A total of 73 patients with steroid-refractory rejection were converted from cyclosporine to tacrolimus therapy. Twelve-month actuarial patient and graft survival rates were 93% and 75%, with 1-year follow-up completed in 93% of patients. When renal function was analyzed, 78% of patients showed improvement, 18% were stable and 11% showed progressive deterioration. Improvement was defined as a repeat renal allograft biopsy showing reversal of rejection or at least a 10% decrease in serum creatinine; stabilization, as less than 10% reduction in serum creatinine during the first 6 months of therapy and progressive deterioration, as unrelenting deterioration in kidney function leading to allograft loss. The risk of experiencing progressive deterioration appeared to be related to pretacrolimus serum creatinine levels, with 39% of the study patients experiencing progressive deterioration with pretreatment serum creatinine of greater than 3.1 mg/dl (274 μmol/L). This important observation confirmed the same observations made by the single-center trials and suggested that early and aggressive initiation of tacrolimus therapy is paramount to the success of rescue therapy. Tacrolimus rescue therapy was associated with low rates of infection (4%) and posttransplant lymphoproliferative disease (PTLD) (1%), indicating that tacrolimus rescue therapy provided balanced immunosuppression.

Subsequently, many individual centers reported experiences with tacrolimus rescue therapy for refractory acute renal allograft rejection. In a single-center experience, Woodle and colleagues reported their experience with an aggressive approach that consisted of early initiation and aggressive dosing of tacrolimus (Woodle *et al.*, 1996a). This approach was based on the hypothesis that optimal results with tacrolimus therapy could be obtained by initiation of tacrolimus

therapy early in the rejection process and that aggressive dosing was more likely to provide prompt control of the rejection process. This approach was based on the observations from the early Pittsburgh experience, in which 24% of allografts were lost in the first year, and improvements in serum creatinine generally were not observed during the first 1 or 2 weeks of therapy. The failure of serum creatinine to show prompt improvement suggested that prompt control of the rejection process may not have been achieved by the dosing employed in the early series. Seventeen patients with steroid-resistant rejection were enrolled in the first report from this group, and a 100% rejection reversal rate was observed with a mean follow-up of 9 months. Patient and graft survival rates of 92% and 84% were observed. Good long-term renal function was observed (mean serum creatinine, 2.1 ± 0.6 mg/dl [186 μmol/L]). Six recurrent rejection episodes were observed in five patients, and each was successfully reversed. PTLD and posttransplant diabetes mellitus (PTDM) were not observed in this study.

Protocol biopsies were included so that the histological response to therapy could be assessed, providing a primary therapeutic gauge. The decision to include protocol biopsies was based on the early Pittsburgh experience, which showed minimal improvements in renal function in the first 2 weeks of tacrolimus rescue therapy. Protocol biopsies also provide a means to identify tacrolimus nephrotoxicity that resulted from the aggressive dosing and to distinguish between nephrotoxicity and ongoing rejection. In this study, protocol biopsies were performed at 48 hours, 1 week, 1 and 6 months and 1 year with additional biopsies performed until a histological reversal of rejection was observed. A subsequent analysis of 92 biopsy specimens in 23 patients provided a histological examination of the response to tacrolimus rescue therapy. This study revealed that histological changes did not correlate with serum creatinine changes during tacrolimus rejection therapy. At 1 week, 27% of patients did not show histological improvement, whereas 100% of patients showed improvement at 2 weeks on subsequent biopsy (Fig. 17–2). In the entire series, histological evidence of tacrolimus nephrotoxicity was observed in 21% of biopsy specimens, with most of the nephrotoxicity lesions being vascular rather than tubular in nature (Woodle *et al.*, 1996a). Finally, tacrolimus trough levels did not correlate with nephrotoxicity lesions,

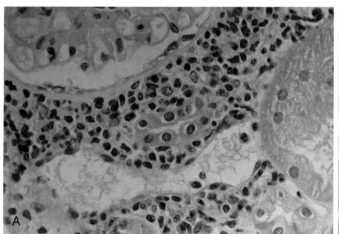
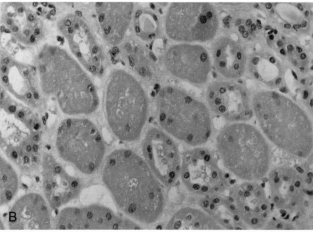

FIGURE 17–2

Serial renal allograft biopsy specimens during tacrolimus rejection therapy show histological reversal of rejection. (A) Hematoxylin and eosin stain of pretacrolimus biopsy specimen shows renal allograft rejection manifested by an intense interstitial infiltrate with tubulitis. (B) Repeat kidney biopsy specimen 1 week after initiation of tacrolimus therapy shows resolution of rejection.

regardless of whether they were associated with an elevated serum creatinine.

One important question regarding tacrolimus therapy is whether the results obtained in patients experiencing refractory acute renal allograft rejection are comparable to those previously reported with mycophenolate mofetil (MMF). To address this question, a metaanalysis of tacrolimus and MMF trials was conducted (Woodle *et al.*, 1998). This metaanalysis was distinct from other metaanalyses in that data from two of the three trials were reanalyzed so that the patient populations from all three trials were comparable. This metaanalysis revealed that tacrolimus and MMF provide effective therapy for refractory acute renal allograft rejection but that tacrolimus therapy allows reduced recurrent rejection rates, reduced requirements for repeat rejection therapy with antilymphocyte antibody, less cytomegalovirus infection and a lower incidence of serious adverse events. The results of this study showed that corticosteroid therapy is associated with lower efficacy and higher toxicities than MMF and tacrolimus. This metaanalysis indicated that tacrolimus provides advantages over MMF for treatment of refractory renal allograft rejection and that MMF and tacrolimus therapy are preferable to corticosteroid therapy. The authors of this study concluded that corticosteroids no longer should be used in patients experiencing refractory acute renal allograft rejection.

REJECTION THERAPY: ANTIBODY-MEDIATED REJECTION

Acute humoral rejection is a particularly virulent form of early rejection that has been associated with renal allograft loss rates that approximate 50% (Porter, 1991). Often occurring within the first 2 weeks after transplantation, acute humoral rejection frequently is associated with oliguria, graft tenderness, fever, leukocytosis and circulating antidonor antibodies. Pathological features of acute humoral rejection include polymorphonuclear or mixed polymorphonuclear and mononuclear cell infiltrates, tubulitis, endotheliitis and linear deposition of complement and IgG on immunohistological examination (Porter, 1991). Before the introduction of tacrolimus, combinations of bolus corticosteroids, plasmapheresis and antilymphocyte antibody preparations were used to treat acute humoral rejection with inconsistent and unsatisfactory response rates. Despite these aggressive regimens, graft losses remained high (Anderson and Newton, 1975; Berne *et al.*, 1976; Lucas *et al.*, 1970; Porter, 1991; Woodle *et al.*, 1998). Tacrolimus-based regimens for acute humoral rejection in renal transplant recipients were developed based on previous clinical experiences with tacrolimus therapy in liver and heart transplants experiencing acute humoral rejection (Phelan *et al.*, 1992; Woodle *et al.*, 1991, 1992, 1993c) as well as strong experimental evidence showing the potential of tacrolimus in limiting antibody responses (Inamura *et al.*, 1988; Stevens *et al.*, 1991; Walliser *et al.*, 1989; Wasik *et al.*, 1990).

Tacrolimus-based regimens for treating acute humoral rejection first were developed and reported in 1991 (Woodle *et al.*, 1991). These regimens were based on the removal of circulating antibody at the time of the rejection episode (by plasmapheresis), suppressing the formation of new antidonor antibody with high-dose tacrolimus and monitoring kidney allograft histology with frequent protocol biopsies. These regimens have provided graft salvage in patients with acute humoral rejection of renal, cardiac and liver allografts. The first use of tacrolimus for treatment of antibody-mediated rejection occurred in an ABO-incompatible hepatic allograft recipient who initially was treated with plasmapheresis and

OKT3 induction therapy (Woodle *et al.*, 1991). Tacrolimus therapy in this patient provided prompt rejection reversal without recurrence of rejection and provided long-term suppression of anti-A titers, indicating that tacrolimus provides effective long-term suppression of natural antibody levels. The decision to use tacrolimus in this patient was supported by considerable experimental evidence of antihumoral properties of tacrolimus (Inamura *et al.*, 1988; Stevens *et al.*, 1991; Walliser *et al.*, 1989; Wasik *et al.*, 1990; Woodle *et al.*, 1991). This experimental evidence included previous observations that tacrolimus is 2 to 3 logs more potent than cyclosporine in inhibiting B-cell activation *in vitro* and that tacrolimus inhibited antibody responses *in vivo* in experimental animals. Additional evidence of the ability of tacrolimus to treat antibody-mediated rejection effectively was reported subsequently in a cardiac allograft recipient who possessed antibodies against class I MHC antigens expressed by the donor (Phelan *et al.*, 1992; Woodle *et al.*, 1993c). A typical antibody-mediated rejection consisting predominantly of vasculitis rather than myocardial infiltrates was observed in this patient in the first postoperative week, despite induction therapy with plasmapheresis. Tacrolimus therapy in this patient was monitored by daily crossmatches performed against B cells from a third-party donor that expressed the same class I MHC antigen as the donor and by serial endomyocardial biopsies. As soon as antibody-mediated rejection was diagnosed, tacrolimus therapy was initiated and provided prompt control of the rejection process. The intensive monitoring of tacrolimus therapy showed the potent ability of tacrolimus to reverse humoral rejection mediated by antidonor MHC antibodies. Woodle and colleagues subsequently provided evidence of the ability of tacrolimus to reverse antibody-mediated rejection in renal allograft recipients (Woodle *et al.*, 1996c, 1997). These patients consisted of a highly sensitized patient experiencing acute accelerated renal allograft rejection, another patient with acute glomerular rejection, and two patients with delayed hyperacute rejection. Each of these patients showed aggressive rejection episodes that were confirmed by immunohistology (Fig. 17–3). All were successfully treated with an aggressive regimen consisting of daily plasmapheresis for 5 days and high-dose tacrolimus (initial target levels, 20–25 ng/ml) that provided prompt reversal and allowed long-term graft survival. To date, this regimen has not been associated with life-threatening opportunistic infections or PTDM, despite high target tacrolimus trough levels. An advantage of high-dose tacrolimus therapy is the ability to titrate tacrolimus doses on a daily basis, which allows daily titration of therapy and prompt increases or decreases in immunosuppression as necessary. In contrast, older methods that used OKT3 or polyclonal antibody therapy often resulted in profound, irreversible immunosuppression that provided variable control of the antibody-mediated rejection processes. The efficacy of tacrolimus in acute humoral rejection may have broad implications for tacrolimus regimens in highly sensitized patients.

After these early initial observations by Woodle and colleagues, another group reported success with a regimen remarkably similar to the tacrolimus-based regimen reported in the initial patients (Pascual *et al.*, 1998). In this later experience, MMF had become available and was used in combination with tacrolimus and plasmapheresis to treat patients experiencing acute humoral rejection in renal allografts. The availability of MMF allowed a reduction in the dose of tacrolimus in this regimen; however, the optimal dose of MMF in this setting remains to be established. This later experience confirmed the initial observations of Woodle and colleagues of the efficacy of tacrolimus in treating acute humoral rejection in renal allograft recipients. The ability of tacrolimus to

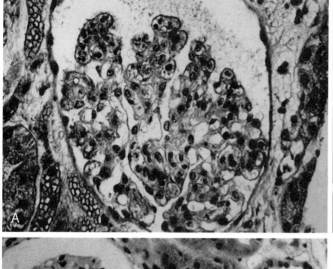

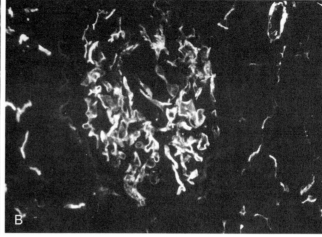

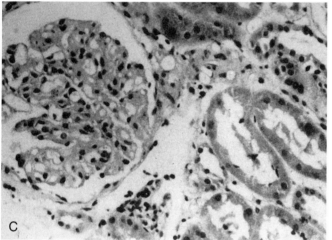

FIGURE 17–3

Serial renal allograft biopsy specimens during acute accelerated rejection of a renal allograft show evidence of the ability of tacrolimus rejection therapy to reverse antibody-mediated rejection. (A) Hematoxylin and eosin stain of pretacrolimus therapy renal allograft biopsy specimen in a patient experiencing acute accelerated rejection shows contracted glomerular capillary loops with marked polymorphonuclear infiltrates. (B) Immunohistological section shows IgG deposition in glomerular capillaries before tacrolimus therapy. (C) Biopsy specimen obtained 2 weeks after initiation of tacrolimus therapy shows resolution of glomerular infiltrates and improved glomerular perfusion.

reverse antibody-mediated rejection in cardiac and hepatic allograft recipients remains to be confirmed.

TACROLIMUS CONVERSION THERAPY FOR CYCLOSPORINE TOXICITY

Many studies have been published documenting the efficacy of tacrolimus conversion therapy for cyclosporine toxicities, including hemolytic uremic syndrome, hirsutism and gingival hyperplasia/gingivitis. Hemolytic uremic syndrome is a known complication of cyclosporine therapy, whose clinical severity may span a broad spectrum, from isolated mild nephrotoxicity (manifested by a modest increase in serum creatinine that results in renal allograft biopsy showing typical glomerular lesions) to a full-blown clinical syndrome including acute hemolytic anemia requiring transfusion and acute renal failure and graft loss. Cyclosporine and tacrolimus have been shown to be associated with hemolytic uremic syndrome (Abdalla et al., 1994; Ichihashi et al., 1992; McCauley et al., 1995; Schmidt et al., 1991), and clinical management of hemolytic uremic syndrome is similar for both agents. In mild cases manifested by moderate nephrotoxicity alone, reduction in cyclosporine or tacrolimus dose often is sufficient. More severe cases often require discontinuation of the calcineurin phosphatase inhibitor and a switch to the alternative agent. McCauley and associates reported four patients with cyclosporine-induced hemolytic uremic syndrome, in whom conversion to tacrolimus resulted in resolution of the hemolytic uremic syndrome in three. The fourth patient experienced graft loss but did not experience a recur-

rence of hemolytic uremic syndrome when a repeat transplant was performed under tacrolimus-based immunosuppression (McCauley et al., 1995). Abdalla and coworkers reported a case of cyclosporine-associated hemolytic uremic syndrome with microangiopathic hemolytic anemia and acute renal allograft failure in which tacrolimus conversion provided long-term function without hemolytic uremic syndrome recurrence (Abdalla et al., 1994).

MAINTENANCE IMMUNOSUPPRESSION

The indication for tacrolimus as a primary immunosuppressive agent in renal transplant recipients was based on the results of two large phase III registration trials that were analogous to the two pivotal phase III trials previously conducted in liver transplant recipients. The renal phase III trials provided results that were strikingly similar to those obtained in liver transplant recipients (Mayer et al., 1997; Pirsch et al., 1997), in that they showed that tacrolimus therapy results in approximately a one third reduction in the incidence of acute rejection.

The experience with tacrolimus in treating refractory renal allograft rejection provided a basis for assessing its efficacy as a primary immunosuppressive agent. Starzl and colleagues had previously noted in early experiences with tacrolimus that dual therapy with cyclosporine resulted in severe nephrotoxicity, obviating combined therapy with the two agents (Starzl et al., 1990). The early single-center and multicenter experiences with tacrolimus in patients experiencing refractory acute renal allograft rejection showed a low incidence of recurrent acute rejection, suggesting that tacrolimus may be effective in the prevention of acute rejection.

The first experience with tacrolimus as a primary immunosuppressive agent in renal transplant recipients was reported by Starzl et al. (1990). In this report, 36 patients had undergone kidney transplantation under tacrolimus therapy, many of whom were considered high-risk recipients. Overall graft survival in this group was 75%, and 39% experienced acute rejection, with 17% requiring OKT3 rejection therapy. Subsequently the Pittsburgh group reported a randomized trial of tacrolimus therapy in 57 low-risk renal transplant recipients (Shapiro et al., 1991). This study was the first in which tacrolimus was compared directly with cyclosporine as a primary immunosuppressive agent in renal transplant recipients. Patient and graft survival were similar in the two groups, although conversion from cyclosporine to tacrolimus was necessary in 31% of patients for rejection or toxicity. Mean serum creatinine was similar in both groups, but the tacrolimus group showed reduced serum cholesterol, a finding that has been reported many times in renal transplant recipients in subsequent studies. Corticosteroids were discontinued successfully in 54% of tacrolimus-treated patients but none of the cyclosporine-treated patients. No attempt was made to discontinue steroids in the cyclosporine arm. Toxicities, including diabetes mellitus, nephrotoxicity and neurotoxicity, were similar.

Subsequently the Pittsburgh group conducted a study comparing triple therapy with tacrolimus/azathioprine/corticosteroids versus double therapy with tacrolimus/corticosteroids in 395 patients (Shapiro et al., 1995b). Triple-therapy patients experienced a lower incidence of rejection (44% vs. 54%) with similar graft and patient survival. Prednisone was discontinued successfully in 49% of the successfully transplanted patients. The overall results in this study were balanced by higher infection rates in the triple-therapy patients.

A phase II multicenter, randomized, concentration-controlled trial was conducted at five U.S. centers that included 92 patients (Laskow et al., 1996). The purpose of this trial was to determine a target dose of tacrolimus that provided optimal balance between prevention of rejection and toxicity. This study examined three trough concentration ranges of tacrolimus (low, 5–14 ng/ml; medium, 15–25 ng/ml and high, 26–40 ng/ml) in combination with induction therapy, azathioprine and corticosteroids and compared them with a similar control group of cyclosporine-treated patients. The pooled tacrolimus patients experienced a lower rejection rate than the cyclosporine-treated patients (14% vs. 32%; $P < 0.05$). Rejection was observed in 21% of the low-dose tacrolimus group patients and 10% of the medium-dose and high-dose tacrolimus group patients. Toxicity was greatest in the high-dose tacrolimus group and lowest in the low-dose tacrolimus group. Tacrolimus was discontinued in only four patients, all of whom were in the high-dose tacrolimus group. This study indicated that the low-dose tacrolimus target level provided effective prevention of acute rejection while minimizing toxicity and provided a solid scientific foundation for the design and execution of pivotal phase III trials for the purpose of gaining regulatory agency approval in the United States and Europe.

The two phase III randomized, multicenter trials that led to FDA and European approval for tacrolimus in renal transplantation were conducted in the United States (Pirsch et al., 1997) and in Europe (Mayer et al., 1997). These trials were similar in scope and design. Both trials enrolled more than 400 patients into two limbs, one with tacrolimus-based immunosuppression and the other with cyclosporine-based immunosuppression. A primary difference between the two

trials was the inclusion of antibody induction therapy in the United States but not the European trial. The U.S. multicenter trial conducted by the FK506 Kidney Transplant Study Group (at 19 centers in the United States) compared the efficacy and safety of tacrolimus-based and cyclosporine-based immunosuppressive regimens. At the 1-year follow-up interval, no statistically significant difference was noted in patient or graft survival rates between the two regimens. A reduction in the incidence of acute rejection in the tacrolimus study arm of 30.7% compared with 46.4% in the cyclosporine study arm ($P = 0.001$) was observed, whereas moderate to severe rejection occurred 2.5 times more often in patients receiving cyclosporine. A significant reduction in antilymphocyte antibody therapy for rejection was observed in tacrolimus-treated patients compared with patients that received cyclosporine (10.7% vs. 25.1%; $P < 0.001$). The safety profile of tacrolimus was similar to that of cyclosporine, but patients on tacrolimus therapy tended to have higher incidences of neurological side effects (primarily tremors and paresthesias) as well as a higher incidence of PTDM. The risk for developing PTDM was higher in black Americans and Hispanics and in patients receiving higher doses of corticosteroids. Most tacrolimus-related toxicity responded to reductions in dose. In contrast, benefits of tacrolimus were evident in the reduced incidence of hyperlipidemia, hypercholesterolemia, gingival hyperplasia and hirsutism compared with patients that received cyclosporine.

Similar to the U.S. trial, the European Tacrolimus trial was conducted in a randomized, prospective fashion in 15 transplant centers across Europe (Mayer et al., 1997). Patients were recruited to receive tacrolimus (n = 303) or cyclosporine (n = 145) in conjunction with azathioprine and low-dose corticosteroids. No statistically significant difference was observed in 1-year actuarial patient and graft survival rates between both arms of the study. A reduction in the incidence of acute renal rejection was noted in tacrolimus study arm compared with the cyclosporine study arm (25.9% vs. 45.7%; $P < 0.001$). A primary difference between the United States and the European trials was the lower incidence of PTDM that was observed in the European trial, presumably as a result of omission of antibody induction and, in part, as a result of the lower rejection rates (i.e., reduced corticosteroid therapy) and the reduced number of blacks and Hispanics in the European trial as compared with the U.S. trial. Other than PTDM, the adverse events observed in this trial were comparable to those observed in the U.S. trial.

COMBINED THERAPY WITH MYCOPHENOLATE MOFETIL AND TACROLIMUS

Mycophenolate mofetil is an antiproliferative agent that was initially developed for use as an anticancer agent (see Chapter 18). Mycophenolate mofetil has been used and developed largely to replace azathioprine in modern immunosuppressive regimens because it has several theoretical advantages over azathioprine. In contrast to azathioprine, which acts by inducing permanent DNA mutations, MMF exerts its effect through a reversible inhibition of the enzyme inosine monophosphate dehydrogenase, a key enzyme in de novo purine synthesis. Mycophenolate mofetil was first approved for prophylaxis of acute rejection in kidney transplant recipients when used in combination with cyclosporine. Three large multicenter phase III pivotal trials showed that 2 to 3 g/d of MMF provided a one third reduction in the incidence of acute rejection compared with cyclosporine in combination with azathioprine or placebo (Matthew, 1998; Sollinger, 1995; Wiesel et al., 1998). These encouraging results with combined MMF and cyclosporine therapy raised the intriguing question as to whether combined therapy with MMF and tacrolimus could lead to greater reductions in acute rejection. Such potent combinations could lead to additional benefits for immunosuppressive therapy with tacrolimus, including allowing reduced dosages of tacrolimus (and/or corticosteroids), and provide reductions in PTDM. More potent immunosuppressive regimens may provide more potent means for reducing or eliminating corticosteroid therapy.

Three randomized, multicenter trials were conducted to evaluate tacrolimus/MMF combination therapy: the U.S. Dose-Ranging trial, the European Dose-Ranging trial and the U.S. Comparative trial (Miller *et al.*, 1997, 1999). These trials showed that tacrolimus and MMF combination therapy provide remarkably low rejection rates and that these rejection rates with 1 or 2 g/d of MMF were, in general, largely comparable to rejection rates observed with higher MMF doses (2–3 g/d) in cyclosporine-treated patients. More importantly, these studies showed reductions in PTDM rates to levels traditionally seen with cyclosporine therapy (e.g., 4–6%). These reductions in the incidence of PTDM likely were due to the reduced dose and target levels of tacrolimus and the marked reduction in corticosteroid use for treating acute rejection. These studies were an outstanding example of how careful analysis of phase III trial data and careful design of phase IV studies can reduce markedly the problems with newly approved drugs.

Pediatric Kidney Transplantation

The efficacy of tacrolimus immunosuppression in pediatric kidney transplantation has been shown in small single-center experiences. Shapiro and colleagues reported long-term follow-up data with primary tacrolimus therapy in pediatric kidney transplantation (Shapiro *et al.*, 1999). A total of 81 pediatric kidney recipients (mean age, 10.6 ± 5.2 years) underwent cadaveric or living related kidney transplantation under tacrolimus primary immunosuppression. Four-year actuarial patient and graft survival rates were 94% and 84%, with a mean serum creatinine of 1.1 ± 0.5 mg/dl (97 μmol/L) at follow-up. The incidence of acute rejection was 44%, but only 5% of these were resistant to steroid therapy and required administration of antilymphocyte antibody regimens.

The potential benefit of withdrawing corticosteroids under tacrolimus immunosuppression is of particular interest in pediatric patients. The effect of corticosteroids on the epiphyseal growth plates is well recognized and results in irreversible growth stunting. Experiences with steroid withdrawal in pediatric kidney transplant recipients receiving cyclosporine have yielded limited success. In a retrospective analysis, Roberti and associates reported late rejection episodes and graft dysfunction in 68.8% of pediatric kidney transplant recipients after steroid withdrawal under primary immunosuppression with cyclosporine (Roberti *et al.*, 1994). A predictor of poor outcome after steroid withdrawal was young age, which places the group most likely to benefit from steroid withdrawal at higher risk for graft loss.

Experience with corticosteroid withdrawal under tacrolimus therapy in pediatric patients has yielded promising results. Shapiro and coworkers reported that two thirds of the pediatric kidney transplant recipients were successfully withdrawn of corticosteroids with a low incidence of graft dysfunction or acute rejection (23%) (Shapiro *et al.*, 1999). Many of these patients showed a return to normal growth characteristics. Maintaining high tacrolimus levels during the first 2 weeks after transplantation appears to decrease the

rate of acute rejection, allowing early corticosteroid withdrawal.

Corticosteroid Withdrawal Under Tacrolimus Therapy

Corticosteroids have been a cornerstone of immunosuppressive therapy in kidney transplantation since the 1960s (see Chapter 15). Although the immunosuppressive efficacy of corticosteroids is well established, the morbidity associated with their use has prompted repeated attempts to reduce their use. Corticosteroid therapy has been shown to result in considerable morbidity, including glucose intolerance, weight gain, osteoporosis, hypertension, hyperlipidemia, growth retardation in pediatric patients, hirsutism and the development of cushingoid features.

Attempts have been made to withdraw corticosteroids from patients at varying times posttransplant or to avoid their use in maintenance therapy altogether (see Chapter 15). Failure of corticosteroid withdrawal or avoidance largely has been defined by the occurrence of an acute rejection episode during the absence of corticosteroid therapy. Success rates of 40 to 80% have been reported under cyclosporine-based immunosuppression (Hricik *et al.*, 1994). Most of the trials of corticosteroid withdrawal or avoidance under cyclosporine therapy were small and nonrandomized, however, and up to 1994, only two large randomized, double-blind trials of corticosteroid withdrawal have been conducted and reported in a peer-reviewed journal (Hricik *et al.*, 1994). The Canadian multicenter trial consisted of 500 patients who were randomized to long-term corticosteroid therapy or corticosteroid withdrawal. This trial has been quoted widely as providing evidence that corticosteroid withdrawal is associated with an increased risk of late renal allograft loss. In this trial, an 8% lower graft survival at 5 years was observed in patients in whom corticosteroids were withdrawn. This difference on multivariate analysis was not statistically significant, however, and pathological examination was not reported for the lost renal allografts. Additional studies are needed to assess the long-term effects of corticosteroid withdrawal on renal allograft survival (see Chapter 15).

Historically, rejection rates after corticosteroid withdrawal under cyclosporine and azathioprine or cyclosporine alone show an incidence of rejection of 3 to 75% (Hricik *et al.*, 1994). Hricik and colleagues performed a review of corticosteroid withdrawal and avoidance trials and found that most of these trials indicated an increased risk of acute rejection after corticosteroid withdrawal under cyclosporine therapy (Hricik *et al.*, 1994; see also discussion in Chapter 15).

The early experience with tacrolimus in treating refractory acute renal allograft rejection provided the initial observations of the potential steroid-sparing properties of tacrolimus (Cronin *et al.*, 1997; Jordan *et al.*, 1994, 1997b). The Pittsburgh group, in particular, was aggressive in the early stages of tacrolimus use and showed that many kidney transplant recipients could undergo late steroid withdrawal with acceptable levels of recurrent rejection episodes (Jordan *et al.*, 1994). Similarly, Woodle and colleagues withdrew corticosteroids after successful tacrolimus rescue therapy (Cronin *et al.*, 1997). Fourteen patients were enrolled in a trial of tacrolimus therapy for refractory renal rejection that included a prospective steroid withdrawal protocol. Corticosteroids were withdrawn successfully in 86% of patients, who had a 28% recurrent rejection rate at a mean follow-up of 38 months. One-year patient and graft survival rates were 100% and 92%. The ability of tacrolimus to allow steroid withdrawal is especially remarkable in this subset of patients, considering their high risk for recurrent rejection. Although these preliminary results are encouraging, larger additional studies are needed to assess the safety and efficacy of corticosteroid withdrawal after tacrolimus rescue therapy.

At the same time in which the three large randomized trials were being designed to evaluate the efficacy of combination therapy with tacrolimus and MMF, Woodle and colleagues initiated a single-center pilot trial of early corticosteroid cessation (at 1 week posttransplant) under tacrolimus and MMF maintenance immunosuppression without induction therapy (Grewal et al., 1998). The primary purpose in designing this trial was to maximize immunosuppressive therapy with a combination of high-dose tacrolimus and MMF therapy, allowing early discontinuation of corticosteroids at 7 days posttransplant. The aggressive tacrolimus and MMF dosing was expected to provide a low incidence of rejection, reducing the use of corticosteroids for rejection therapy. As a result of the reduced corticosteroid dosing, a low incidence of PTDM was expected. A total of 52 patients were enrolled, and 3-year follow-up has been analyzed. This analysis revealed an overall rejection rate of 25% with 96% graft survival and 100% patient survival. At 3 years, 81% of patients remained off corticosteroids. Patients also showed good renal function at 3 years with a mean serum creatinine of 1.9 mg/dl. An additional benefit of this study was the absence of weight gain, and mean weight did not increase from pretransplant up to 3 years posttransplant. A trend toward reduced systolic pressure was observed at 3 years. Of the 48 patients at risk to develop diabetes, only 6% developed PTDM. This observation is similar to those from the three randomized tacrolimus/MMF trials in renal transplantation. This experience with early corticosteroid withdrawal under tacrolimus and MMF immunosuppression indicates that it provides an effective regimen for early cessation of corticosteroids in renal transplant recipients.

Kidney-Pancreas Transplantation

Advances in surgical technique and immunosuppression have led to improved results in pancreas transplantation and have resulted in an increase in the number of pancreas transplants to more than 1,000 per year in the United States (Gruessner and Sutherland, 1999). As described earlier, combination therapy with tacrolimus and MMF has reduced the incidence of rejection after kidney transplantation and has been applied in pancreas transplantation. Tacrolimus therapy in pancreas after kidney (PAK) and pancreas transplant alone (PTA) and MMF in simultaneous pancreas-kidney (SPK) have prolonged graft survival rates, reduced acute rejection and decreased patient morbidity (Bartlett et al., 1996). This section reviews studies of tacrolimus immunosuppressive therapy in pancreas transplantation.

TACROLIMUS/AZATHIOPRINE/CORTICOSTEROIDS WITH INDUCTION THERAPY

The first large-scale experience with tacrolimus in SPK transplants was a multicenter study reported by Gruessner and colleagues in 1996 that included 154 pancreas allograft recipients (82 for induction and 61 for rescue) (Gruessner et al., 1996). In this trial, tacrolimus therapy was administered in conjunction with azathioprine, corticosteroids, and antilymphocyte antibody preparations. Of 82 patients in the induction group, 61 received a SPK transplant with or without simultaneous bone marrow transplant. The 6-month survival rate for SPK transplant recipients was 90%, with graft survival being 87% (vs. 70% for cyclosporine recipients in a

matched pair analysis), and the incidence of rejection was 35% within 6 months. In the rejection rescue group (cyclosporine to tacrolimus), patient and graft survival rates for SPK transplants at 6 months were 91% and 90% with a rejection rate of 44%. The authors concluded that tacrolimus was an efficacious agent associated with a low rate of graft loss and a high salvage rate for rescue therapy (Gruessner et al., 1996).

Several other groups have reported experiences with tacrolimus in pancreas transplants. Bartlett and colleagues reported on 27 PTA recipients who were prospectively treated with tacrolimus-based immunosuppression with percutaneous biopsy and compared them with 15 PTA recipients treated with cyclosporine and 113 SPK recipients (Bartlett et al., 1996). One-year pancreas graft survival was 90% in PTA recipients receiving tacrolimus versus 53% in cyclosporine-treated patients, whereas no differences in 1-year graft survival were noted in the SPK recipients receiving tacrolimus (87%). Jordan and coworkers evaluated 55 SPK recipients on an immunosuppression regimen of tacrolimus, corticosteroids and azathioprine or MMF without lymphocyte antibody induction therapy (Jordan et al., 1999). Even though 80% experienced rejection, 80% of those were corticosteroid-sensitive rejection episodes. Corticosteroids were tapered in patients with stable graft function (65%). The 3-year patient, kidney and pancreas survival were 96.5%, 91% and 80%. By contrast, Peddi and colleagues observed a 17% rejection incidence at 2 years in a series of 24 SPK transplants treated with tacrolimus, corticosteroids, azathioprine and antilymphocyte antibody induction (Peddi et al., 1998). Survival rates for patient, kidney and pancreas at 2 years were 100%, 100% and 78.4%, a finding consistent with other groups.

CYCLOSPORINE/MYCOPHENOLATE MOFETIL VERSUS TACROLIMUS/MYCOPHENOLATE MOFETIL THERAPY

Mycophenolate mofetil therapy in pancreas transplant recipients was first examined in combination with cyclosporine microemulsion. Merion and associates reported the results of a randomized multicenter trial of MMF versus azathioprine in combination with OKT3, cyclosporine (Neoral) and corticosteroids (Merion et al., 2000). The rejection incidences in the MMF and azathioprine groups were similar (22% and 30%), as were patient and graft survival rates. Odorico and colleagues studied 358 SPK transplant recipients receiving antilymphocyte antibody induction, cyclosporine, prednisone and either MMF or azathioprine (Odorico et al., 1998). They found a statistically significant reduction in acute renal and pancreas allograft rejection in the MMF versus the azathioprine groups, 75% versus 31% and 24% versus 7%. Although patient survival in the two groups was the same, kidney and pancreas survival rates favored the MMF group. Another series of 20 patients showed a lower rejection incidence in MMF/cyclosporine-treated patients versus azathioprine/cyclosporine-treated patients (45% vs. 65%) within 3 months after transplantation. No statistically significant differences in graft or patient survival were observed, however (Bruce et al., 1998).

Several studies have analyzed combined therapy with tacrolimus and MMF. Two multicenter studies evaluating the combination of tacrolimus and MMF in pancreas transplant recipients reported excellent patient and graft survival, low rates of acute rejection and rates of infection similar to cyclosporine/azathioprine-treated patients after 6 months (Gruessner et al., 1996; Stratta, 1999). The only randomized prospective trial evaluating MMF/tacrolimus versus MMF/cyclosporine in SPK transplants to date was reported by

Stegall *et al.* (1997). In this study, 36 patients were given OKT3 induction and prednisone and either MMF/tacrolimus (n = 18) or MMF/cyclosporine (n = 18). An 11% acute rejection rate was observed in the MMF/cyclosporine and MMF/tacrolimus groups after 3 months without statistically significant differences in graft or patient survival or in infection rates. The authors concluded that MMF could be used with tacrolimus or cyclosporine to achieve low acute rejection rates with similar graft function.

Kaufman and associates published a single-center experience using tacrolimus and MMF as primary maintenance immunosuppression in SPK transplantation (Kaufman *et al.*, 1999). Quadruple therapy with Atgam induction, prednisone, tacrolimus, and MMF was initiated in 50 consecutive SPK recipients. A 16% incidence of acute rejection at 6 months and a 27.8% incidence at 1 year was observed. There was a statistically significant increase of the rate of acute rejection in the nine patients converted to cyclosporine versus those who remained on tacrolimus (44.4% *vs.* 10.2%). The 2-year actuarial patient, kidney and pancreas survival rates were 97.7%, 93.3% and 90%. This group subsequently reported an additional 10 patients and showed that the overall incidence of acute rejection remained unchanged at 15.8% at 6 months. Two-year actuarial patient, kidney and pancreas survival rates remain relatively unchanged at 97.9%, 93.7% and 91.6%.

As described earlier, the common side effects of tacrolimus include nephrotoxicity, neurotoxicity, gastrointestinal toxicity, and glucose intolerance. Diabetogenicity has been one of the major concerns for using tacrolimus in the pancreas transplant population. Experimental models in animals have shown that tacrolimus causes reversible damage to islet cells, altering insulin secretion (Gruessner *et al.*, 1996). To date, the diabetogenic effect of tacrolimus has not been found to be of significance in pancreas transplant recipients.

In the multicenter analysis of tacrolimus and pancreas transplantation reported by Gruessner and colleagues, nephrotoxicity, neurotoxicity, gastrointestinal toxicity and glucose intolerance were reported at 13%, 16%, 9% and 0% in the induction group, whereas they were 25%, 23%, 21% and 5% in the rescue group (Gruessner *et al.*, 1996). They concluded that new-onset insulin-dependent diabetes was not noted in pancreas recipients who received tacrolimus for induction and maintenance therapy and that transient hyperglycemia, if present, is found frequently in recipients with concurrent rejection or infection episodes.

There are significant concerns regarding the combination of tacrolimus and MMF in SPK transplant recipients. Both agents have been associated with significant gastrointestinal toxicity in other solid organ transplant recipients. The gastrointestinal dysmotility present in many diabetic patients receiving SPK transplants could exacerbate the gastrointestinal toxicity of these agents. Stratta (1999) reported in the multicenter trial of tacrolimus and MMF that 50% of SPK transplant recipients experienced gastrointestinal toxicity with 6 of 30 requiring conversion to cyclosporine. Both Stegall and Kaufman reported less gastrointestinal toxicity in their SPK transplant recipients, which could be attributable to the lower doses of MMF (2 g/d *vs.* 3 g/d in the multicenter group). Tacrolimus has been shown to be an excellent immunosuppressive agent in SPK transplants, especially when used in conjunction with MMF for induction therapy.

Side Effects of Tacrolimus

In general, the side-effect profile of tacrolimus is similar to that of cyclosporine (Table 17–1). The physiological effects, including reduction in renal blood flow and glomerular fil-

TABLE 17–1
ADVERSE EFFECTS ASSOCIATED WITH TACROLIMUS THERAPY

Nephrotoxicity
  Reduced renal blood flow, glomerular perfusion
  Tubular and vascular toxicity
  Hemolytic uremic syndrome
Hepatotoxicity
Neurotoxicity
  Tremors
  Seizures
  Peripheral neuropathy
  Paresthesias
Metabolic disturbances
  Hyperkalemic, hyperchloremic acidosis
  Hypomagnesemia
  Diabetes mellitus
  Hyperuricemia
  Hypercholesterolemia
Hypertension
Gastrointestinal disturbances
  Diarrhea
  Anorexia, nausea and vomiting
  Epigastric cramping
Cosmetic
  Gingival hypertrophy and gingivitis
  Alopecia

tration, are similar between tacrolimus and cyclosporine. The pathological manifestations of tacrolimus and cyclosporine toxicity are similar because they induce tubular vacuolization and arteriolar nodular hyalinosis that are indistinguishable. In general, most studies have shown that the frequency of nephrotoxicity of tacrolimus and cyclosporine are similar.

The metabolic effects of cyclosporine and tacrolimus and their severities are similar, including hyperkalemic metabolic acidosis and hypomagnesemia. The U.S. Multicenter Phase III trial comparing tacrolimus and cyclosporine as primary immunosuppressive agents showed a higher incidence of PTDM with tacrolimus than with cyclosporine. Subsequent analyses of data from this trial indicated that the risk of PTDM in tacrolimus-treated patients was highly influenced by race, with blacks and Hispanics experiencing severalfold increases in risk compared with whites. Retrospective analyses indicated that the risk of PTDM was related to tacrolimus target levels and corticosteroid dose in the 30 days immediately preceding the development of PTDM. Development of tacrolimus/MMF and early corticosteroid withdrawal regimens under tacrolimus/MMF subsequently have allowed reduction in corticosteroid dosing (for maintenance and for rejection therapy owing to a reduction in the incidence of rejection) and tacrolimus dosing. These studies observed a reduced incidence of PTDM to ranges traditionally reported with cyclosporine (i.e., <10%). Posttransplant diabetes mellitus is no longer the Achilles' heel of tacrolimus therapy in renal transplant recipients.

Gastrointestinal disturbances (anorexia, nausea and abdominal cramping) are seen commonly with tacrolimus and are similar to those experienced with erythromycin therapy and are thought to be typical macrolide-antibiotic side effects. Tacrolimus neurotoxicity is similar to cyclosporine in manifestations, severity and frequency. Typical manifestations include sleep disturbance, tremor, nightmares, seizures and coma. Seizures when observed with tacrolimus should be treated in a manner similar to those that occur under cyclosporine therapy. Peripheral neuropathy may occur with tacrolimus and when observed requires immediate conversion to cyclosporine.

TABLE 17–2
DRUG INTERACTIONS ASSOCIATED WITH TACROLIMUS

Drugs that lower tacrolimus blood levels
  Carbamazepine
  Phenytoin (Dilantin)
  Isoniazid
  Phenobarbital
  Rifampin
Drugs that increase tacrolimus blood levels
  Cimetidine
  Ketoconazole, fluconazole, itraconazole
  Erythromycin, clarithromycin
  Sirolimus
  Diltiazem, verapamil, nicardipine
Drugs that exacerbate tacrolimus nephrotoxicity
  Aminoglycosides
  Amphotericin
  Nonsteroidal antiinflammatory drugs
  Sulfa derivatives

Cyclosporine induces serious cosmetic adverse effects consisting of gingival hyperplasia and gingivitis and hirsutism. Many studies have shown that both of these lesions respond almost uniformly and promptly to conversion to tacrolimus. There is no longer a need for gingival surgery for these lesions. Similarly, there is no reason for women and children to continue to suffer from disfiguring hirsutism associated with cyclosporine therapy.

Dosing and Therapeutic Monitoring

Tacrolimus therapy for rejection is commonly instituted at doses of 0.1 mg/kg given twice a day. Target trough concentrations should be in the range of 10 to 15 ng/ml or up to 20 ng/ml in patients experiencing more vigorous forms of rejection. Many investigators experienced with tacrolimus therapy have observed that short-term (a few days) exposure to higher levels of tacrolimus can provide control of rejection in the most refractory cases (Woodle et al., 1996b, d). Primary tacrolimus therapy is usually initiated at 0.05 to 0.1 mg/kg/d given twice daily with target concentration ranges between 8 and 20 ng/ml. Long-term tacrolimus therapy can be maintained at target concentration ranges between 4 and 8 ng/ml. The same drug interactions as seen with the use of cyclosporine apply to the use of tacrolimus (Table 17–2).

REFERENCES

Abdalla, A. H., Al-Sulaiman, M. H. and Al-Khader, A. A. (1994). FK506 as an alternative in cyclosporine-induced hemolytic uremic syndrome in a kidney transplant recipient. Transpl. Int. 7, 382.

Anderson, C. B. and Newton, W. T. (1975). Accelerated human renal allograft rejection. Arch. Surg. 110, 1230.

Bartlett, S. T., Schweitzer, E. J., Johnson, L. B., et al. (1996). Equivalent success of simultaneous pancreas kidney and solitary pancreas transplantation: a prospective trial of tacrolimus immunosuppression with percutaneous biopsy. Ann. Surg. 224, 440.

Becker, G., Witzke, O., Friedrich, J., et al. (1996). Tacrolimus (FK506) therapy in simultaneous pancreas and kidney transplantation. Transplant. Proc. 28, 3169.

Berne, T. V., Gustafson, L. A. and Chatterjee, S. N. (1976). Early severe renal allograft rejection. Arch. Surg. 111, 758.

Bierer, B. E., Hollander, G., Fruman, D., et al. (1993). Cyclosporin A and FK506: molecular mechanisms of immunosuppression and probes for transplantation biology. Curr. Opin. Immunol. 5, 763.

Braun, W., Kallen, J., Mikol, V., et al. (1995). Three dimensional structure and actions of immunosuppressants and their immunophilins. FASEB J. 9, 63.

Bruce, D. S., Woodle, E. S., Newell, K. A., et al. (1998). Effects of tacrolimus, mycophenolate mofetil, and cyclosporine microemulsion on rejection incidence in synchronous pancreas-kidney transplantation. Transplant. Proc. 30, 507.

Ciancio, G., Roth, D., Burke, G., et al. (1995). Renal transplantation in a new immunosuppressive era. Transplant. Proc. 27, 812.

Clipstone, N. A. and Crabtree, G. H. (1992). Identification of calcineurin as a key signaling enzyme in T-cell activation. Nature 357, 695.

Cronin, D. C., Bruce, D. S., Newell, K. A., et al. (1997). Tacrolimus therapy for refractory renal allograft rejection: experience with steroid withdrawal. Transplant. Proc. 29, 307.

D'Alessandro, A. M., Pirsch, J. D., Miller, C., et al. (1993). Use of FK 506 for the prevention of recurrent allograft rejection after successful conversion from cyclosporine for refractory rejection. Transplant. Proc. 25, 635.

Darras, F. S., Jordan, M. L., Shapiro, R., et al. (1991). Transplantation of pediatric en bloc kidneys under FK 506 immunosuppression. Transplant. Proc. 23, 3089.

Demetris, A. J., Fung, J. J., Todo, S., et al. (1992). Conversion of liver allograft recipients from cyclosporine to FK506 immunosuppressive therapy—a clinicopathologic study. Transplantation 53, 1056.

European FK 506 Multicenter Liver Study Group. (1994). Randomized trial comparing tacrolimus (FK 506) and cyclosporine in prevention of liver allograft rejection. Lancet 344, 423.

Felldin, M., Backman, L., Brattstrom, C., et al. (1995). Rescue therapy with tacrolimus (FK506) in renal transplant recipients—a multicenter analysis. Transplant. Proc. 27, 3425.

Fruman, D., Burakoff, S. and Bierer, B. (1994). Immunophilins in protein folding and immunosuppression. FASEB J. 8, 391.

Grewal, H. P., Thistlethwaite, J. R., Loss, G. E., et al. (1998). Corticosteroid cessation 1 week following renal transplantation using tacrolimus/mycophenolate mofetil-based immunosuppression. Transplant. Proc. 30, 1378.

Gruessner, R. W. G., Burke, G. W., Stratta, R., et al. (1996). A multicenter analysis of the first experience with FK 506 for induction and rescue therapy after pancreas transplantation. Transplantation 61, 261.

Gruessner, A. C. and Sutherland, D. E. (1999). Analysis of United States (U.S.) and non-US pancreas transplants as reported to the International Pancreas Transplant Registry (IPTR) and to the United Network for Organ Sharing (UNOS). In Clinical Transplants 1998 (J. M. Cecka and P. I. Terasaki, eds.), p. 53, UCLA Tissue Typing Laboratory, Los Angeles.

Ho, S., Clipstone, N., Timmermann, L., et al. (1996). The mechanism of action of cyclosporine A and FK 506. Clin. Immunol. Immunopathol. 80, S40.

Hricik, D. E., Kupin, W. L. and First, M. R. (1994). Steroid-free immunosuppression after renal transplantation. J. Am. Soc. Nephrol. 4(8 Suppl.), S10.

Ichihashi, T., Naoe, T., Yoshida, H., et al. (1992). Haemolytic uraemic syndrome during FK 506 therapy. Lancet 340, 60.

Inamura, N., Hashimoto, M., Nakahara, R., et al. (1988). Immunosuppressive effect of FK 506 on collagen-induced arthritis in rats. Clin. Immunol. Immunopathol. 46, 82.

Jamieson, N. V. (1999). Adult small intestinal transplantation in Europe. Acta Gastroenterol. Belg. 62, 239.

Jensen, C. W. B., Jordan, M. L., Schneck, F. X., et al. (1991). Pediatric renal transplantation under FK 506 immunosuppression. Transplant. Proc. 23, 3075.

Jordan, M. L., Naraghi, R., Shapiro, R., et al. (1997a). Tacrolimus rescue therapy for renal allograft rejection—five-year experience. Transplantation 63, 223.

Jordan, M. L., Naraghi, R. N., Shapiro, R., et al. (1997b). Five-year experience with tacrolimus rescue for renal allograft rejection. Transplant. Proc. 29, 306.

Jordan, M. L., Shapiro, R., Gritsch, H. A., et al. (1999). Long-term results of pancreas transplantation under tacrolimus immunosuppression. Transplantation 67, 266.

Jordan, M. L., Shapiro, R., Jensen, C. W. B., et al. (1991). FK 506 conversion of renal allografts failing cyclosporine immunosuppression. Transplant. Proc. 23, 3078.

Jordan, M. L., Shapiro, R., Naraghi, R., et al. (1996). Tacrolimus rescue therapy for renal transplant rejection. Transplant. Proc. 29, 2119.

Jordan, M. L., Shapiro, R., Vivas, C. A., et al. (1993). FK 506 salvage of renal allografts with ongoing rejection failing cyclosporine immunosuppression. *Transplant. Proc.* **25**, 638.

Jordan, M. L., Shapiro, R., Vivas, C., *et al.* (1994). FK506 "rescue" for resistant rejection of renal allografts under primary cyclosporine immunosuppression. *Transplantation* **57**, 860.

Kandaswamy, R., Humar, A., Gruessner, A. C., *et al.* (1999). Vascular graft thrombosis after pancreas transplantation: comparison of the FK 506 and cyclosporine eras. *Transplant. Proc.* **31**, 602.

Kaufman, D. B., Leventhal, J. R., Stuart, J., *et al.* (1999). Mycophenolate mofetil and tacrolimus as primary maintenance immunosuppression in simultaneous pancreas-kidney transplantation. *Transplantation* **67**, 586.

Kitamura, M., Hiraga, S., Kobayashi, D., *et al.* (1994). Clinical experience of FK 506 for renal allograft transplantation. *Transplant. Proc.* **26**, 1924.

Kur, F., Reichenspurner, H., Meiser, B. M., *et al.* (1999). Tacrolimus (FK506) as primary immunosuppressant after lung transplantation. *Thorac. Cardiovasc. Surg.* **47**, 174.

Laskow, D. A., Neylan, III, J. F., Shapiro, R. S., *et al.* (1998). The role of tacrolimus in adult kidney transplantation: a review. *Clin. Transplant.* **12**, 489.

Laskow, D. A., Vincenti, F., Neylan, J. F., Mendez, R. and Matas, A. (1996). An open-label, concentration-ranging trial of FK 506 in primary kidney transplantation. *Transplantation* **62**, 900.

Liu, J., Farmer, J. D., Lane, W. S., *et al.* (1991). Calcineurin is a common target of cyclophilin-cyclosporin A and FKBP-FK506 complexes. *Cell* **66**, 807.

Loss, G. E., Grewal, H., Siegel, C., *et al.* (1998). Reversal of delayed hyperacute renal allograft rejection with a tacrolimus-based therapeutic regimen. *Transplant. Proc.* **30**, 1249.

Lucas, Z. J., Coplon, N., Kempson, R. and Cohn, R. (1970). Early renal transplant failure associated with subliminal sensitization. *Transplantation* **10**, 522.

Mathew, A., Talbot, D., Minford, E. J., *et al.* (1995). Reversal of steroid-resistant rejection in renal allograft recipients using FK 506. *Transplantation* **60**, 1182.

Mathew, T. H. (1998). A blinded, long-term randomized multicenter study of mycophenolate mofetil in cadaveric renal transplantation: results at three years. Tricontinental Mycophenolate Mofetil Renal Transplantation Study Group. *Transplantation* **65**, 1450.

Mattila, P. S., Ullmann, K. S., Fiering, S., *et al.* (1990). The actions of cyclosporin A and FK506 suggest a novel step in the activation of T lymphocytes. *EMBO J.* **9**, 4425.

Mayer, A. D., Dmitrewski, J., Squifflet, J. P., *et al.* (1997). Multicenter randomized trial comparing tacrolimus (FK506) and cyclosporine in the prevention of renal allograft rejection. *Transplantation* **64**, 436.

McCauley, J., Shapiro, R., Scantlebury, V., *et al.* (1995). Hemolytic uremic syndrome and tacrolimus: the whole story. *American Society of Transplant Physicians Meeting*, May 14–17, Abstract P-53.

McDiarmid, S. V., Klintmalm, G. B. and Busuttil, R. W. (1993). FK506 conversion for intractable rejection of the liver allograft. *Transplant. Int.* **6**, 305.

Meiser, B. M., Pfeiffer, M., Schmidt, D., *et al.* (1999). Combination therapy with tacrolimus and mycophenolate mofetil following cardiac transplantation: importance of mycophenolic acid therapeutic drug monitoring. *J. Heart Lung Transplant.* **18**, 143.

Merion, R. M., Henry, M. L., Melzer, J. S., *et al.* (2000). Randomized prospective trial of mycophenolate mofetil versus azathioprine in prevention of acute renal allograft rejection after simultaneous kidney-pancreas transplantation. *Transplantation* **70**, 105.

Miller, J., Deierhoi, M. B., Filo, R. S., *et al.* (1999). Tacrolimus and mycophenolate mofetil in renal transplant recipients: one year results of a multicenter, randomized dose ranging trial. *Transplant. Proc.* **31**, 276.

Miller, J., Pirsch, J. D., Deierhoi, M., *et al.* (1997). FK 506 in kidney transplantation: Results of the U.S.A. randomized comparative phase III study. *Transplant. Proc.* **29**, 304.

Mycophenolate Mofetil Renal Refractory Rejection Study Group, Conti, D., Baker, J., Wynn, J., *et al.* (1996a). Mycophenolate mofetil for the treatment of refractory, acute, cellular renal transplant rejection. *Transplantation* **61**, 722.

Mycophenolate Mofetil Renal Refractory Rejection Study Group, Conti, D., Baker, J., Wynn, J., *et al.* (1996b). Rescue therapy with mycophenolate mofetil. *Clin. Transplant.* **10**, 131.

Ochiai, T., Fukao, K., Takahashi, K., *et al.* (1991). Japanese study of FK 506 on kidney transplantation: results of an early phase II study. *Transplant. Proc.* **23**, 3071.

Ochiai, T., Fukao, K., Takahashi, K., *et al.* (1993). Japanese study of FK 506 on kidney transplantation: results of late phase III study. *Transplant. Proc.* **25**, 649.

Ochiai, T., Fukao, K., Takahashi, K., *et al.* (1995a). FK 506: long-term study in kidney transplantation. *Transplant. Proc.* **27**, 818.

Ochiai, T., Fukao, K., Takahashi, K., *et al.* (1995b). Phase III study of FK 506 in kidney transplantation. *Transplant. Proc.* **27**, 829.

Odorico, J. S., Pirsch, J. D., Knechtle, S. J., D'Alessandro, A. M. and Sollinger, H. W. (1998). A study comparing mycophenolate mofetil to azathioprine in simultaneous pancreas-kidney transplantation. *Transplantation* **66**, 1751.

Pascual, M., Saidman, S., Tolkoff-Rubin, N., *et al.* (1998). Plasma exchange and tacrolimus-mycophenolate rescue for acute humoral rejection in kidney transplantation. *Transplantation* **66**, 1460.

Peddi, V. R., Kamath, S., Munda, R., *et al.* (1998). Use of tacrolimus eliminates acute rejection as a major complication following simultaneous kidney and pancreas transplantation. *Clin. Transplant.* **12**, 401.

Phelan, D. L., Thompson, C., Henschell, J., *et al.* (1992). Heart transplantation across preformed class I antibody using FK 506. *Hum. Immunol.* **34**, 70, 1992.

Pirsch, J. D., Miller, J., Deierhoi, M. H., *et al.* (1997). A comparison of tacrolimus (FK506) and cyclosporine for immunosuppression after cadaveric renal transplantation. *Transplantation* **63**, 977.

Porter, K. A. (1991). Renal transplantation. *In Pathology of the Kidney* (R. H. Heptinstall, ed.), p. 1861, Little, Brown, Boston.

Reddy, K. S., Stratta, R. J., Shokouh-Amiri, H., *et al.* (2000). Simultaneous kidney-pancreas transplantation without antilymphocyte induction. *Transplantation* **69**, 49.

Roberti, I., Resiman, L., Lieberman, K. V., *et al.* (1994). Risk of steroid withdrawal in pediatric renal allograft recipients (a 5-year follow-up). *Clin. Transplant.* **8**, 405.

Schmidt, R. J., Venkat, K. K. and Dumler, F. (1991). Hemolytic-uremic syndrome in a renal transplant recipient on FK 506 immunosuppression. *Transplant. Proc.* **23**, 3156.

Schreiber, S. L. and Crabtree, G. R. (1992). The mechanism of action of cyclosporin A and FK506. *Immunol. Today* **13**, 136.

Schulak, J. A. and Hricik, D. E. (1994). Steroid withdrawal after renal transplantation. *Clin. Transplant.* **8**, 211.

Shapiro, R., Jordan, M. L., Scantlebury, V. P., *et al.* (1991). FK 506 in clinical kidney transplantation. *Transplant. Proc.* **23**, 3065.

Shapiro, R., Jordan, M. L., Scantlebury, V. P., *et al.* (1995a). A prospective randomized trial of FK506-based immunosuppression after renal transplantation. *Transplant. Proc.* **59**, 485.

Shapiro, R., Jordan, M. L., Scantlebury, V. P., *et al.* (1995b). A prospective, randomized trial of FK 506/prednisone vs FK 506/azathioprine/prednisone in renal transplant patients. *Transplant. Proc.* **27**, 814.

Shapiro, R., Jordan, M. L., Scantlebury, V. P., *et al.* (1996). Tacrolimus in renal transplantation. *Transplant. Proc.* **28**, 2117.

Shapiro, R., Scantlebury, V. P., Jordan, M. L., *et al.* (1999). Pediatric renal transplantation under tacrolimus-based immunosuppression. *Transplantation* **67**, 299.

Sigal, N. H. and Dumont, F. J. (1992). Cyclosporin A, FK-506, and rapamycin: pharmacologic probes of lymphocyte signal transduction. *Ann. Rev. Immunol.* **10**, 519.

Sigal, N. H., Siekierka, J. J., Dumont, F. J., *et al.* (1990). Observations on the mechanism of action of FK-506—a pharmacologic probe of lymphocyte signal transduction. *Biochem. Pharmacol.* **40**, 2201.

Sollinger, H. W. (1995). Mycophenolate mofetil for the prevention of acute rejection in primary cadaveric renal allograft recipients. U.S. Renal Transplant Mycophenolate Mofetil Study Group. *Transplantation* **60**, 225.

Starzl, T. E., Fung, J., Jordan, M., *et al.* (1990). Kidney transplantation under FK 506. *J. A. M. A.* **264**, 63.

Stegall, M. D., Simon, M., Wachs, M. E., *et al.* (1997). Mycophenolate mofetil decreased rejection in simultaneous pancreas-kidney transplantation when combined with tacrolimus or cyclosporine. *Transplantation* **12**, 1695.

Stevens, C., Lempert, N. and Freed, B. M. (1991). The effects of immunosuppressive agent on in vitro production of human immunoglobulins. *Transplantation* **51**, 1240.

Stratta, R. J. (1999). Optimal immunosuppression in pancreas transplantation. *Transplant. Proc.* **31**, 619.

Sutherland, D. E. R., Cecka, M. and Gruessner, A. C. (1999). Report from the international pancreas transplant registry—1998. *Transplant. Proc.* **31**, 697.

Thompson, J. S. (1999). Intestinal transplantation: experience in the United States. *Eur. J. Paediatr. Surg.* **9**, 271.

Tolman, D. E., Frazier, O. H., Young, J. B. and Van Veldhuisen, P. (1999). A randomized, multicenter comparison of tacrolimus and cyclosporine immunosuppressive regimens in cardiac transplantation: decreased hyperlipidemia and hypertension with tacrolimus. *J. Heart Lung Transplant.* **18**, 336.

Turner, C., Bruce, D. S., Cronin, D. C., *et al.* (1998). Tacrolimus therapy for refractory acute renal allograft rejection: a four year experience with an aggressive approach. *Transplant. Proc.* **30**, 1234.

U.S. Multicenter FK 506 Liver Study Group. (1994). A comparison of tacrolimus (FK 506) cyclosporine for immunosuppression in liver transplantation. *N. Engl. J. Med.* **331**, 1110.

U.S. Multicenter FK 506 Liver Study Group, Klintmalm, G. B., Gonwa, T., Wiesner, R. H., *et al.* (1993). Prognostic factors for successful conversion from cyclosporine to FK 506-based immunosuppressive therapy for refractory rejection after liver transplantation. *Transplant. Proc.* **25**, 641.

Walliser, P., Berizie, C. R. and Kay, J. E. (1989). Inhibition of murine B lymphocyte proliferation by the novel immunosuppressant drug FK 506. *Immunology* **68**, 434.

Wasik, M., Stepien-Sopniewska, B., Lagodzinski, Z., *et al.* (1990). Effect of FK 506 and cyclosporine on human T and B lymphoproliferative responses. *Immunopharmacology* **20**, 57.

Wiesel, M., Carl, S., *et al.* (1998). A placebo-controlled study of mycophenolate mofetil used in combination with cyclosporine and corticosteroids for the prevention of acute rejection in renal allograft recipients: 1-year results. The European Mycophenolate Mofetil Cooperative Study Group. *J. Urol.* **159**, 28.

Woodle, E. S., Bruce, D. S., Josephson, M., *et al.* (1996a). FK 506 therapy for refractory renal allograft rejection: lessons from liver transplantation. *Clin. Transplant.* **10**, 323.

Woodle, E. S., Cronin, D., Newell, K. A., *et al.* (1996b). Tacrolimus therapy for refractory renal allograft rejection: definition of the histologic response by protocol biopsies. *Transplantation* **62**, 906.

Woodle, E. S., Jordan, M. L., Facklam, D. and Danovitch, G. A., for the Refractory Rejection Metaanalysis Study Group. (1998). Metaanalysis of FK 506 and mycophenolate mofetil refractory rejection trials in renal transplantation. *Transplant. Proc.* **30**, 1297.

Woodle, E. S., Marsh, J. W., Perdrizet, G. A., *et al.* (1993a). Recurrent rejection following FK 506 rescue therapy for acute hepatic allograft rejection. *Transplant. Proc.* **25**, 1988.

Woodle, E. S., Marsh, J. W., Perdrizet, G. A., *et al.* (1993b). FK 506 rescue therapy: early conversion improves efficacy. *Transplant. Proc.* **25**, 1990.

Woodle, E. S., Newell, K. A., Haas, M., *et al.* (1997). Reversal of accelerated renal allograft rejection with FK 506. *Clin. Transplant.* **11**, 2251.

Woodle, E. S., Perdrizet, G., Brunt, E. M., *et al.* (1991). FK-506: reversal of humorally-mediated rejection following ABO-incompatible liver transplantation. *Transplant. Proc.* **23**, 2992.

Woodle, E. S., Perdrizet, G., Brunt, E. M., *et al.* (1992). FK 506: inhibition of humoral mechanisms of hepatic allograft rejection. *Transplantation* **54**, 377.

Woodle, E. S., Perdrizet, G. A., So, S. K. S., White, H. M. and Marsh, J. W. (1995). FK506 rescue therapy for hepatic allograft rejection: experience with an aggressive approach. *Clin. Transplant.* **9**, 45.

Woodle, E. S., Phelan, D. L., Saffitz, J. E., *et al.* (1993c). FK 506: reversal of humorally-mediated cardiac allograft rejection in the presence of preformed anti-class I antibody. *Transplantation* **56**, 1271.

Woodle, E. S., Spargo, B., Ruebe, M. and Charette, J. (1996c). Treatment of acute glomerular rejection with FK 506. *Clin. Transplant.* **10**, 266.

Woodle, E. S., Thistlethwaite, J. R., Gordon, J. H., for the Tacrolimus Kidney Transplant Rescue Study Group. (1996d). A multicenter trial of FK 506 (tacrolimus) therapy in refractory acute renal allograft rejection. *Transplantation* **62**, 594.

Mycophenolate Mofetil

Timothy H. Mathew

Introduction

Mycophenolate mofetil (MMF) is an ester prodrug of the immunosuppressant mycophenolic acid (MPA). Mycophenolic acid is a selective and reversible uncompetitive inhibitor of inosine monophosphate dehydrogenase, an enzyme that is crucial for the proliferation of B and T lymphocytes but unimportant to other cell types that have access to alternative metabolic pathways.

Gozio (1896) initially derived MPA from several *Penicillium* species. Antibacterial and antifungal properties were identified in the 1940s, antiviral and antitumor activities were reported in 1968 (Williams *et al.*, 1968) and immunosuppressive properties were first studied in mice (Mitsui and Suzuki, 1969). These studies were confounded by the rapid metabolism of MPA in mice compared with other species. Studies in patients with psoriasis using MPA were performed in the 1970s but were discontinued because of concerns about immunosuppressive properties and carcinogenesis of MPA (Jones *et al.*, 1975). Further experience with this drug in the 1980s in 85 patients with psoriasis concluded that it was an effective treatment of moderate to severe psoriasis and that the long-term risks were acceptable. Gastrointestinal symptoms were prominent in the early years of the study but became infrequent (Epinette *et al.*, 1987).

Allison led a team at Syntex, Palo Alto Laboratories that rediscovered MPA in the early 1980s while searching for new ways to manipulate purine synthesis (Allison and Eugui, 1993). These investigators showed many of its *in vitro* effects (Allison and Eugui, 1996) and through allograft experiments in rats showed efficacy in transplantation (Morris *et al.*, 1989).

Allison recognized the need to improve the bioavailability and tolerability of MPA in patients and eventually his group found the answer in the morpholinoethyl ester of MPA, MMF. Sollinger (1996) conducted allograft experiments in many animal models with MMF and led the way with phase I and II clinical trials that showed safety and promising efficacy. Phase III clinical trials began in 1993 across three continents and represented the first rigorously conducted controlled trials in large numbers of transplant recipients. These trials established the safety and efficacy of MMF and showed superiority to azathioprine in preventing acute rejection episodes. These observations led to the registration of MMF for the prevention of rejection in kidney transplant recipients in the United States in 1995 and in many other countries soon after.

Other salts of MPA can be used as a prodrug to deliver MPA to the stomach and to the bloodstream. Clinical trials have begun using the sodium salt of MPA, which is believed to have less gastrointestinal toxicity than MMF. The efficacy and safety profile of these new salts, once absorbed, are likely to be similar if not identical to that established with MMF.

Chemistry

Mycophenolate mofetil is 2-morpholinoethyl(E)-6-(1,3-dihydro-4-hydroxy-6-methoxy-7-methyl-3-oxo-5-isobenzofuranyl)-4-methyl-4-hexanoate. The empirical formula is $C_{23}H_{31}NO_7$ with a molecular weight of 433.50. Mycophenolate mofetil is a white–to–off-white crystalline powder. The compound is stable with only a minor degree of sensitivity to intense light exposure.

Mechanism of Action

The active component of MMF is MPA, which inhibits inosine monophosphate dehydrogenase (IMPDH) (Allison and Eugui, 1993). This enzyme controls the rate of synthesis of guanosine monophosphate, an important nucleotide in the *de novo* purine pathway on which lymphocytes appear particularly dependent for normal function and proliferation because they cannot use a salvage purine pathway (Fig. 18–1). The net effect of the MMF-induced inhibition of IMPDH (down to about 50% of baseline activity) is to deplete levels of guanosine monophosphate and guanosine triphosphate as well as deoxyguanosine triphosphate. This depletion results in interruption of cell division of T and B lymphocytes, while allowing preservation of protein synthesis. There are two isoforms of IMPDH: Type I is predominantly found in leukocytes, whereas type II is present in many tissues. Mycophenolic acid inhibits the type II enzyme more than it does type I, and type II is expressed predominantly in activated lymphocytes. This characteristic along with the fact that cell types other than lymphocytes can use an alternative *salvage* pathway for the generation of nucleotides essential for DNA and RNA synthesis may explain the partially selective behavior of MPA.

Mycophenolic acid is rapidly glucuronidated to mycophenolic acid glucuronide (MPAG), which can be converted back to MPA by β-glucuronidase. Mycophenolic acid glucuronide is an inactive metabolite with little or no toxicity.

IN VITRO ACTIVITY

Human *in vitro* studies confirm the ability of MPA in clinically relevant concentrations to inhibit antigen-stimulated or mitogen-stimulated proliferation of B and T lymphocytes (Allison *et al.*, 1991; Weaver *et al.*, 1991; Zeevi *et al.*, 1991) more effectively than it inhibits proliferation of fibroblasts or endothelial cells (Eugui *et al.*, 1991a). Other effects include inhibition of antigen-induced B-lymphocyte antibody formation and a decrease in intracellular pools of guanosine triphosphate and deoxyguanosine triphosphate (by 40–80%). The antiproliferative effects can be reversed by the addition of guanosine triphosphate or deoxyguanosine triphosphate (Eugui *et al.*, 1991a). Human monocytes exposed to MMF showed inhibition of the transfer of fucose and mannose to

De Novo Pathway   Salvage Pathway

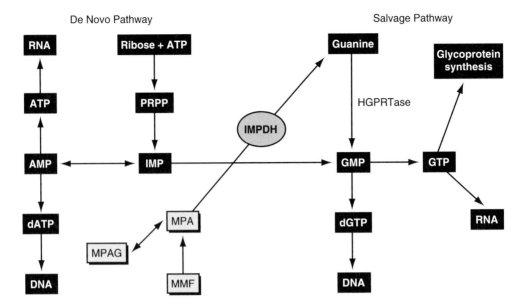

FIGURE 18–1

The effect of mycophenolate mofetil on the *de novo* and salvage metabolic pathways of purine synthesis. MPA inhibits inosine monophosphate dehydrogenase (IMPDH), preventing inosine monophosphate (IMP) converting to guanosine monophosphate (GMP). This promotes synthesis of the *de novo* pathway through increasing adenosine monophosphate (AMP), adenosine triphosphate (ATP) and deoxyadenosine triphosphate (dATP) and at the same time depletes GMP, guanosine triphosphate (GTP) and deoxyguanosine triphosphate (dGTP). These changes downregulate two rate-limiting enzymes, leading to diminished lymphocyte proliferation through a decrease in phosphoribosyl pyrophosphate (PRPP) and DNA polymerase activity. HGPRTase = hypoxanthine guanine phosphoribosyl transferase. (Adapted with permission from Simmons *et al.*, 1997.)

glycoproteins, some of which are adhesion molecules. This inhibition led to decreased adherence of leukocytes to endothelial cells, suggesting this might be an additional mechanism by which the rejection process could be influenced (Allison and Eugui, 1994; Laurent *et al.*, 1994).

IN VIVO ACTIVITY

In vivo studies have shown the ability of MPA to suppress antibody formation to sheep erythrocytes in mice (Eugui *et al.*, 1991b) and to inhibit the production of natural antibodies in a xenograft model in the rat using splenectomy and plasma exchange (Figueroa *et al.*, 1993; Soares *et al.*, 1993). Extensive testing in animals showed a beneficial effect on graft survival in rat cardiac allograft and various rat and baboon xenograft models, in dog hepatic allografts, in hamster to rat hepatic xenografts, in mouse and rat pancreatic allografts and in rat and dog renal allografts. Studies examined the prevention of acute and chronic rejection and rescue from acute rejection. The findings in these studies consistently showed benefit from MMF and were summarized by Sollinger (1996). In a rat aortic allograft model at 3 months, there was a striking lack of intimal hypertrophy compared with that seen in cyclosporine-treated controls (Steele *et al.*, 1993). Later observations indicated this change may not be sustained.

In humans, MMF at a standard dose was associated with a reduced incidence and lower titers of IgG anti-Atgam antibody formation in 47 patients receiving Atgam as part of induction therapy after renal transplantation (Kimball *et al.*, 1995). In a separate study, MMF was associated with a profound suppression of the humoral response to influenza vaccine. Of MMF-treated patients, 77% had no protective response to any antigen in the influenza vaccine compared with no response in 25% of the normal controls and in 36% of azathioprine-treated renal transplant recipients. Booster

vaccination did not alter the outcome (Smith *et al.*, 1998). These studies are significant for emphasizing the risks incurred by patients taking MMF and for the potential benefit this strong inhibitor of antibody formation may have in other antibody-mediated conditions.

These *in vitro* and *in vivo* studies were summarized by Fulton and Markham (1996). Overall the studies indicate that MMF has considerable potential for altering the acute rejection process through its selective antiproliferative and antiadhesion properties and for altering the chronic rejection process through its ability to suppress antibody production and intimal proliferation in vessels.

Toxicology

Single acute minimum lethal oral and subcutaneous doses were studied in the mouse (>4,000 mg/kg), rat (>250 mg/kg) and monkey (>1,000 mg/kg). Mortality occurred only in the rat, with deaths 3 to 6 days after dosing from gastrointestinal toxicity. In chronic dosing studies lasting 12 months, changes were present in the hematopoietic systems of the mouse (100 mg/kg/d) and rat (6 mg/kg/d) manifesting largely as anemia and were present in the lymphoid system of the dog (60 mg/kg/d) and monkey (45 mg/kg/d) manifesting as decreased lymphocyte counts and thymic atrophy. Immunosuppression in the rat and monkey was achieved at or below the dose levels for toxicity in the long-term studies, and recovery from hematopoietic and lymphoid toxicity occurred in the rat after a 1-month postdosing recovery period. An increased incidence of viral and parasitic infections occurred in monkeys (70 mg/kg/d) at 3 months, and gastrointestinal and renal toxicity were present in the dog and monkey at higher dose levels.

Mycophenolate mofetil failed to induce point mutations (Ames assay) or primary DNA damage in the presence or absence of metabolic activation. Mycophenolate mofetil was not mutagenic *in vivo* (mouse micronucleus assay) or *in vitro* with metabolic activation (CHO cell chromosomal aberration assay).

No effect on fertility of male rats in a 6-month toxicity study was seen in doses equivalent to clinical practice. In a female fertility and reproduction study in rats dosed at about one sixth of clinical levels, malformations (principally of the head and eyes) occurred in the first-generation pups in the absence of maternal toxicity. Similar malformations occurred at the highest dose levels in a rat teratology study using doses of 0.6 to 6 mg/kg/d. In a rabbit teratology study using doses of 10 to 90 mg/kg/d, malformations at the highest dose level affected head, eyes, cardiovascular, pulmonary and renal systems in the absence of maternal toxicity. The no-effect levels for teratological changes in rats and rabbits given MMF were 2 mg/kg/d and 30 mg/kg/d.

In a 2-year oral carcinogenicity study in mice, daily doses of MMF of 180 mg/kg/d were not tumorigenic. This dose level in the animal study equates with 6.3 times the recommended clinical dose (for a 70-kg person). In a 2-year rat study, MMF in a dose about half the equivalent clinical dose was not tumorigenic (Mycophenolate Mofetil, 1996).

Clinical Pharmacology and Blood Monitoring

The pharmacokinetic properties of MMF have been reviewed in detail (Bullingham *et al.*, 1996b; Fulton and Markham, 1996) and are only briefly summarized here with an emphasis on clinically relevant factors. The analytical methods for MMF have focused on its active metabolite MPA, given the almost complete first-pass conversion of MMF after oral dosing. Enzyme-multiplied immunoassay technique (EMIT) and high-performance liquid chromatography (HPLC) assays have been described, although neither EMIT nor HPLC has found a place in routine clinical practice. A comparison between the two assays identified that EMIT may overestimate MPA in plasma samples (by a mean of 1.9 times) perhaps by estimating metabolite. The HPLC method was favored on grounds of accuracy, reproducibility, speed and cost-effectiveness (Li and Yatscoff, 1995) and was shown to have a linear response from 0.1 to 50 mg/L with accuracy of about 98% (Beal *et al.*, 1998). Reference ranges for trough-level monitoring have not been published. The monitoring of MMF indirectly by its pharmacodynamic effect on IMPDH activity has been favored but not fully established (Yatscoff and Aspeslet, 1998).

Mycophenolate mofetil has been mainly used orally, although an intravenous preparation is available and approved for early postoperative use in liver transplantation. After oral administration, MMF is rapidly and essentially completely absorbed, then rapidly and completely hydrolyzed to MPA. Mycophenolate mofetil is not detectable in plasma after oral dosing, but radiolabeled intravenous dosing studies suggest the mean systemic clearance is about 6 L/min. The major metabolite of MPA in humans is the glucuronide conjugate, MPAG, which is found in higher concentrations than MPA in healthy subjects and renal transplant recipients. Mycophenolic acid glucuronide is a stable conjugate and pharmacologically inactive *in vitro*. The liver is the likely main site of conversion of MPA to MPAG, although extrahepatic glucuronidation probably occurs in the gut wall or kidney (Bullingham *et al.*, 1996b).

ABSORPTION

The absorption of MMF is believed to be complete because the same dose (1.5 g) by oral and intravenous routes results in similar MPA and MPAG total area under the concentration-time curves (AUC) and similar recovery of MPAG in the urine. The mean bioavailability of oral MMF based on MPA AUC was 94% compared with intravenous administration (Bullingham *et al.*, 1996a). The mean extent of absorption (as determined by the AUC) of MPA in repeat dosing studies increases in a dose-proportional fashion over a daily dosing range of 100 mg to 3 g (Sollinger *et al.*, 1992). The between-patient coefficient of variation of MPA AUC is 43% in steady-state renal transplant recipients.

After an oral dose to fasting healthy subjects, the plasma profile of MPA shows a rapid rise to peak values at about 1 hour. Food has no effect on the total MMF absorbed, although with food the Cmax for MPA was reduced by 40% and delayed to about 2 hours (Hoffmann La Roche, 1998). Following the peak, the decline of plasma MPA concentration is rapid, but secondary rises in plasma MPA concentration occur leading to an apparent mean terminal half-life of about 16 hours.

The secondary plasma peak MPA is characteristically seen at 6 to 12 hours after oral dosing of MMF, suggesting enterohepatic circulation (Wolfe *et al.*, 1997). Deconjugation of MPAG by colonic bacteria is believed to be important in this process, which allows uptake of MPA back into the circulation. Cholestyramine, presumably by binding MPAG directly in the bowel lumen, prevents this secondary peak of circulating MPA and reduces the total MPA AUC by a mean of 37%, adding further to the evidence for enterohepatic circulation. The presence of this large contribution of enterohepatic circulation to the plasma levels of MPA is considered to explain, in part, the interpatient variability of plasma MPA AUC values and underlines the need to consider dose adjustment if bile secretion is abnormal.

The plasma AUC of MPA has been shown to increase by about 50% at about 3 months posttransplant in renal allograft recipients relative to values found in the first few weeks posttransplant (Bullingham *et al.*, 1998). This increase with time restores the AUC values to those found in healthy subjects. The explanation may lie with the reduction in serum albumin levels consistently found for the first few weeks after transplantation and the plasma protein binding of MPA, which normally is approximately 97.5%. The plasma measurements of MPA include free and bound MPA, but it is only the free MPA that has pharmacological activity. These aspects of MMF pharmacokinetics need further elucidation. In an adult renal transplant recipient studied less than 40 days after transplant, a standard MMF dose of 1.0 g (being given regularly twice a day) results in a mean Tmax (time to peak concentration) of 1.31 hours (standard deviation, 0.76), Cmax of 8.16 mg/L (standard deviation, 4.5) and a 12-hour AUC of 27.3 mg/L/h (standard deviation, 10.9).

EXCRETION

The excretion of MMF is largely through the renal elimination of its major metabolite MPAG. Urinary excretion of MPA is negligible (Hoffmann La Roche, 1998). Only 6% of a radiolabeled oral dose was eliminated in the feces, whereas 93% was excreted in the urine (87% of which was in the form of MPAG). The renal route of excretion appears to involve the organic acid tubular pathway because concomitant probenecid increased the plasma MPAG AUC threefold in monkeys. Renal impairment, although predictably associated with increased plasma MPAG values (sixfold increase in severe renal impairment), has no consistent effect on plasma MPA AUC. Because MPAG has not been associated with any clinical toxicity, no dose adjustment is needed when MMF is used in patients with renal impairment. Hemodialysis is ineffective in removing MPA and MPAG because of the high degree of protein binding (MPAG is 82% protein bound). Limited data available on single dosing studies in cirrhotic patients showed no consistent change (Bullingham *et al.*, 1996).

TISSUE DISTRIBUTION

Tissue distribution has not been studied in humans. In rats, the highest concentrations of MMF were found in the stomach, intestine, liver and kidney, with lymphoid tissues also containing significant amounts. The brain had the lowest concentration of radioactivity, indicating the likelihood of poor transmission across the blood-brain barrier. Forty-eight hours after dosing, only the adrenals and bone marrow contained appreciable amounts of radioactivity. The volume of distribution of MPA in humans is approximately 4 L/kg (Lipsky, 1996).

No consistent variations were found in the pharmacokinetic studies in pediatric and elderly renal transplant recipients. Some reduction in plasma MPA AUC values were found in the pediatric group, but the studies were limited. The relatively small difference in clinical outcome seen between the adult groups receiving 2 g/d and 3 g/d in the pivotal trials suggests that the differences in measurable plasma MPA values resulting from pharmacokinetic factors are likely to be of little clinical significance.

CONCENTRATION-EFFECT RELATIONSHIP

Early clinical trials using doses of 1 g/d or less of MMF in combination with cyclosporine and steroids showed no benefit in reducing rejection episodes (Salaman *et al.*, 1993). Only a minor advantage (not statistically significant) was shown in the large pivotal trials by increasing the daily dose from 2 to 3 g (Halloran *et al.*, 1997). The effective dose range for reducing acute rejection episodes in renal transplantation is 1 to 3 g/d. The pivotal trials established an increased frequency of some adverse effects at the higher dose range (particularly involving the gastrointestinal tract).

An attempt to relate plasma concentrations of MMF to efficacy and safety in a 6-month period involved a study 150 renal transplant recipients. Dose adjustments were made on the basis of repeated AUC determinations and were aimed at maintaining one of three target AUC values of MPA. After each AUC analysis, a blind assessment led to a dose change recommendation. The results of this demanding study were that a low trough (predose) blood measurement and a low AUC of MPA were significantly related to the incidence of biopsy-proven rejection, whereas the higher doses of MMF were related to an increased occurrence of adverse events (largely gastrointestinal) (van Gelder *et al.*, 1999). About 10% of patients clustered at the lower end of plasma MPA AUC had increased rejection. Therapeutic monitoring to identify this at-risk group may be justified, but otherwise there is a consensus that MMF can be used safely and effectively without monitoring blood values.

METABOLISM

The administered dose of MMF can be accounted for fully as noted previously. Mycophenolic acid glucuronide is pharmacologically inactive being a phenolic glucuronide and is the major metabolite formed by glucuronyl transferases acting on MPA. The subconjugation of MPAG in the bowel and its reabsorption as active MPA accounts for more than one third of the plasma MPA AUC.

There is no evidence of genetic polymorphism in the metabolism of MMF, although there is substantial within-patient variation in MPA AUC (coefficient of variation, 17%) and between-patient variation (43%). Variables affecting these values include serum protein measurements, the degree of enterohepatic circulation and possibly age.

The plasma concentration and the AUC of MPAG increases twofold in renal transplant recipients compared with healthy subjects and may be threefold or fourfold higher in patients with delayed graft function. There is no evidence of increased toxicity or morbidity from MPAG even in these situations of greatly increased exposure to MPAG.

Drug Interactions

Mechanisms whereby drug interaction might occur with MMF include the following (Bullingham *et al.*, 1998):

Interference with enterohepatic recycling resulting in reduced MPA levels (noting that one third of the AUC of MPA depends on recycling)

Competition for glucuronidation, which might reduce the metabolism of the active component, resulting in increased exposure to MPA

Competition for renal tubular excretion by the organic acid pathway of the metabolite, MPAG, resulting in increased AUC for MPAG

The documented interactions were reviewed by Bardsley-Elliot *et al.* (1999).

ANTACIDS WITH MAGNESIUM AND ALUMINUM HYDROXIDES

A 33% reduction in AUC and 17% reduction in Cmax of MPA were observed when antacids containing magnesium and aluminum hydroxides were coadministered with MMF. It is recommended that MMF and antacids not be administered simultaneously (Hoffman La Roche, 1998).

ACYCLOVIR AND PROBENECID

Acyclovir and probenecid compete with MPAG for secretion by the renal tubules. The coadministration of MMF with each of these agents results in modest elevation of MPAG concentrations and elevation of acyclovir (22%) and probenecid concentrations. These changes are likely to be accentuated in the presence of renal impairment. Dose adjustment of these drugs does not appear necessary when MMF is coadministered with acyclovir or probenecid, but careful monitoring is recommended. Ganciclovir has not been shown to have a pharmacokinetic interaction with MMF. Probenecid given with MMF increases MPAG AUC threefold and MPA AUC twofold and is a reminder that any agent blocking the organic acid pathway may have the potential for an interaction with MMF (Hoffman La Roche, 1998).

CHOLESTYRAMINE

A 40% reduction of the AUC of MPA has been shown when cholestyramine is administered concomitantly with MMF because of predictable interference with the enterohepatic circulation of MPA and MPAG. Some degree of enterohepatic recycling is to be anticipated with the use of intravenous MMF. Cholestyramine should not be coadministered with MMF.

TACROLIMUS

A 156% increase was reported in the AUC of MPA when MMF was used with tacrolimus compared with cyclosporine.

This increase was associated with a 61% reduction in the AUC of MPAG, suggesting inhibition of the conversion of MPA to MPAG in the presence of tacrolimus (Zucker et al., 1997). This suggestion has led to trials of dose reduction of MMF in the presence of tacrolimus as well as the suggestion that more toxicity of MMF is seen in the group receiving the usual dose (2 g/d) of MMF (Mendez, 1998; Shapiro et al., 1998).

In vitro assays of uridine diphosphate–glucuronosyl-transferase using a substrate of MPA in the presence of clinically relevant amounts of tacrolimus and cyclosporine confirm the suggestion that tacrolimus affects the conversion of MPA to MPAG by this mechanism. The inhibition is dose dependent and present with cyclosporine and tacrolimus. Tacrolimus was 60 times more efficient at inhibition (Zucker et al., 1999).

Clinical evidence suggests there is a problem. One of the first reports on this combination was a retrospective assessment of 72 patients in whom there was a reduced rate of rejection but a higher incidence of diarrhea and leukopenia, often leading to discontinuation of MMF (Roth et al., 1998). The importance of monitoring MPA plasma levels was found in a trial combining tacrolimus and MMF in heart transplantation. On a fixed dose of MMF (2 g/d), rejection occurred in 10 of 15 patients and was associated with MPA less than 3.0 µg/ml. In a second phase of this experience, MMF dose adjustments were made to maintain MPA levels greater than 2.5 µg/ml, and only 3 of 30 cases had a rejection episode (Meiser et al., 1999). In clinical practice, an awareness of this issue and preparedness to reduce the dose of MMF in the face of adverse effects is necessary. As a working rule, it seems likely that a 2-g/d dose of MMF in combination with tacrolimus achieves plasma levels of MMF normally associated with the 3-g/d dose. Normal dosing probably should not exceed 2 g/d, and for most clinical situations an initial dose of 1.5 g/d is likely appropriate. Tacrolimus pharmacokinetics and dose requirements are not affected by the concomitant use of MMF in a steady-state.

OTHER AGENTS

Cyclosporine, oral contraceptives and cotrimoxazole have been examined in short-term studies without any significant interaction with MMF in either direction being observed. These findings do not exclude the possibility of interactions with long-term exposure.

Clinical Experience

Mycophenolate mofetil is approved for use in many countries for the prevention of rejection in renal and cardiac transplants. Some countries have approved the use of MMF for rescue from refractory renal allograft rejection. Trials in liver transplantation were delayed because of the need for an intravenous preparation to cover the early postoperative period. A satisfactory preparation has now been produced, and these trials are in progress.

MODE OF USE

Oral MMF is given as ongoing maintenance immunosuppression to patients receiving allogeneic transplants. The usual recommended dosage is 1 g twice daily taken with or without food. Anecdotal evidence suggests that gastrointestinal adverse effects may be reduced if MMF is taken with food or if the doses are divided further and spread throughout the day.

Mycophenolate mofetil has been used only in conjunction with additional immunosuppression, usually with both cyclosporine and steroids. It is generally believed that MMF on its own is not potent enough to prevent rejection satisfactorily. The ideal long-term immunosuppression regimen is not yet defined and may involve MMF in view of its low toxicity.

The maximum approved dose is 3 g/d. This dose was used in the pivotal trials and proved to have only a slight advantage in efficacy but to have increased adverse effects compared with the widely used 2-g/d dose. No reduction in dosage is needed for renal or hepatic impairment, although caution in not exceeding 2 g/d is advised when there is delayed graft function in the immediate posttransplant period.

Monitoring the complete blood count is recommended weekly for the first month of treatment, twice monthly for the second and third months, then monthly through the first year. If neutropenia (absolute neutrophil count $<1.3 \times 10^9$/L) appears, MMF should be suspended.

EFFICACY

Prevention of Rejection in Renal Allografts

The three simultaneously performed pivotal trials in renal transplant recipients were the first large, tightly controlled, randomly allocated and blinded clinical trials ever performed in the field of transplantation (European Mycophenolate Mofetil Cooperative Study Group, 1995; Tricontinental Mycophenolate Mofetil Renal Transplantation Study Group, 1996; U.S. Renal Transplant Mycophenolate Mofetil Study Group, 1995). These trials introduced a level of scientific critique new to the transplant community and set a standard against which future therapies in transplantation will be tested and judged.

The three trials have been subject to a pooled efficacy analysis (Halloran et al., 1997). This pooled analysis summarizes the outcome at 1 year of adding MMF to cyclosporine and corticosteroid treatment in renal allograft recipients. The three studies enrolled 1,493 patients. The first trial was placebo controlled and allowed no antilymphocyte globulin induction, the second was similar except it used azathioprine as a comparator to MMF and the third trial was similar to the second except the protocol allowed antilymphocyte globulin induction therapy. The three trials used identical assessment criteria.

In a pooled analysis of the three trials, MMF reduced significantly the incidence of biopsy-proven rejection episodes in the first year after transplantation from 40.8% for placebo/azathioprine patients to 19.8% for MMF 2 g/d and to 16.5% for MMF 3 g/d. The severity of rejection episodes was reduced in recipients on MMF (Table 18–1). The reduction in rejection was evident by the second month and was sustained to the end of the first year (Fig. 18–2) and was seen consistently across the three individual trials (Fig. 18–3). These data suggest that MMF did not simply delay acute rejection but prevented it while MMF treatment was continued. In the first year, the need for second courses of steroids was reduced, and the use of antilymphocyte therapy for severe rejection was decreased by 55% (Fig. 18–4). The incidence of graft loss from rejection in the first year was reduced by 60% in the MMF 2 g/d group (2.6%) compared with controls (6.3%) (Halloran et al., 1997).

Adverse events in the pooled analysis resulted in a greater proportion of patients withdrawing from the study (considered as treatment failures) in the MMF 3 g/d group (14.7%) compared with MMF 2 g/d (8.7%) and placebo/azathioprine groups (5.2%). An increased incidence of diarrhea, vomiting and leukopenia was observed (see later). The high number of

TABLE 18–1

POOLED EFFICACY ANALYSIS: ENDPOINTS (%) AT 1 YEAR*

	PLA/AZA (n = 498)	MMF2 g (n = 505)	MMF3 g (n = 490)
First biopsy-proven rejection	40.8	19.8†	16.5†
Grade I	16.9	9.9	8.4
Grade II	18.5	8.1	6.1
Grade III	5.4	1.8	2.0
Biopsy-proven rejection or treatment failure	53.8	36.8†	39.6†
Presumptive rejection	49.3	29.5	25.1

*Data from the pooled efficacy analysis of the three double-blind clinical studies in prevention of rejection (Halloran et al., 1997). The histopathological severity grading used was based on the Banff schema. The primary efficacy endpoint for the three trials was the combination of biopsy-proven rejection or treatment failure in the first 6 months after transplantation. Here the data relate to 1 year and can be seen to show statistically significant differences (adjusted for the Bonferroni correction) between mycophenolate mofetil at both dose levels and the control group.
†$P < 0.025$.
PLA/AZA = placebo/azathioprine; MMF2 g = mycophenolate mofetil, 2 g; MMF3 g = mycophenolate mofetil, 3 g.

withdrawals is not surprising in a complex clinical situation involving placebo controls.

Survival of grafts at 1 year was similar on MMF 2 g/d (90.4%) and MMF 3 g/d (89.2%) compared with placebo/azathioprine (87.6%), and this difference was not statistically significant. The data, displayed graphically as a cumulative incidence of graft failure, show that the small difference in outcome that was evident in early months is sustained through to 12 months (Fig. 18–5). Reports confirm that this difference continues out to 3 years in the three trials assessed separately (European Mycophenolate Mofetil Cooperative Study Group, 1999; Tricontinental Mycophenolate Mofetil Renal Transplantation Study Group, 1998; U.S. Renal Transplant Mycophenolate Mofetil Study Group, 1999). The individual trial 3-year graft survival figures show a consistent pattern favoring MMF with the mean (arithmetic mean of the individual trial results) showing a 4.9% difference between MMF 2 g/d and the comparator groups (Fig. 18–6). This difference in outcome has widened between 1 and 3 years (Fig. 18–7).

In these trials, MMF has shown an advantage of only about 4 to 5% in graft survival at the 3-year point after transplantation despite the marked reduction in the number and severity of early rejection episodes. The European trial showed a 7.6% reduction in the incidence of graft loss from rejection (excluding death) at 3 years, and all three trials showed a strong association between early rejection episodes

TABLE 18–2

CONTRIBUTION OF ACUTE REJECTION EPISODES TO GRAFT LOSS/DEATH AT 3 YEARS*

In First 6 Months	% Graft Loss/Death at 3 Years		
	US	TRI	EUR
Biopsy-proven rejection	40	26.1	31.5
No biopsy-proven rejection	6.6	9.8	5.7

*Data from the three pivotal trials (see text) show the percentage of graft loss or death at 3 years in each trial separately. The presence of biopsy-proven rejection in the first 6 months of each trial (regardless of drug allocation) shows a fourfold to fivefold increase in risk compared with those with no rejection.

and increased graft loss from all causes in the first 3 years (Table 18–2).

The initial trials were not powered to show this small survival difference to be statistically significant, and many observers have interpreted this lack of significance to be a negative outcome. Although the improvement is small, it is more difficult for any new therapy to show significance as 1-year graft survival improves to around 90%. The maximum potential graft survival is in reality probably near 95% (given the contribution of technical factors and death of patient to graft loss). Future trials seeking to establish efficacy of new agents will require larger numbers of patients to be enrolled to achieve sufficient power to show statistical significance.

The initial hope, based on experimental evidence, that MMF may decrease the incidence of chronic rejection appears unlikely to be realized. The analyses of mean serum creatinine levels and of proteinuria at 3 years failed to show any reduction in these markers of chronic allograft dysfunction in the groups receiving MMF (Tricontinental Mycophenolate Mofetil Renal Transplantation Study Group, 1998). Further follow-up of these groups to 5 years and a more detailed analysis of protocol biopsy specimens obtained at 3 years is required to resolve this question fully.

MMF-treated groups in these pivotal trials of efficacy and safety showed a marked reduction in the incidence and severity of early rejection episodes, a small improvement (not statistically significant) in graft survival at 3 years and no evidence of an impact on the incidence of chronic allograft dysfunction. The quality of this evidence is high given the blinded nature of the initial 12-month periods in each of the three trials and the continued blinding to 3 years in the Tricontinental trial. The trials were not powered to allow these modest changes in graft survival to be shown to be statistically significant, however. The reduction of rejection episodes to less than half of those seen in the control (placebo

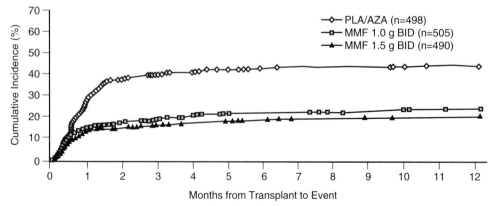

FIGURE 18–2

Cumulative incidence of first biopsy-proven rejection in first year (excludes 1-year protocol biopsies; Kaplan-Meier estimates). Data from the pooled efficacy analysis of the three double-blind clinical studies in prevention of rejection (Halloran et al., 1997). The separation between the curves occurs in the first 2 months and is sustained to the end of the observation period. PLA = placebo; AZA = azathioprine; MMF = mycophenolate mofetil.

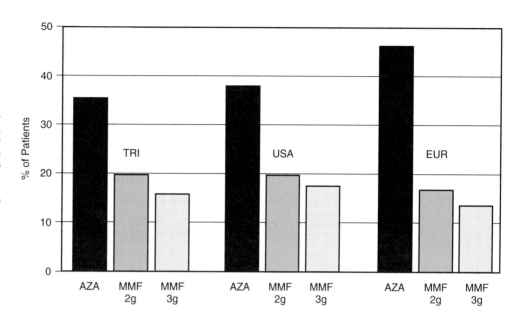

FIGURE 18–3

Incidence of biopsy-proven rejection in the three pivotal trials. The individual trial data show the incidence of biopsy-proven rejection in the first 6 months is consistent across the three trials. The mycophenolate mofetil 3 g/d dose was slightly superior to the 2 g/d dose in reducing rejection. AZA = azathioprine; MMF = mycophenolate mofetil.

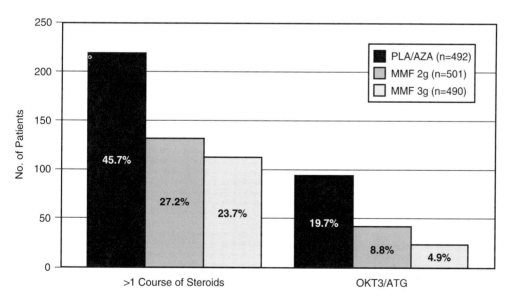

FIGURE 18–4

Course of treatment to reverse rejection. Data from the pooled efficacy analysis of the three double-blind clinical studies in prevention of rejection (Halloran et al., 1997). The reduction in number and severity of rejection episodes in the mycophenolate mofetil–treated groups is evident in the reduced number of second courses of steroids and the substantial reduction in the need for antilymphocyte therapy rescue. PLA = placebo; AZA = azathioprine; MMF = mycophenolate mofetil.

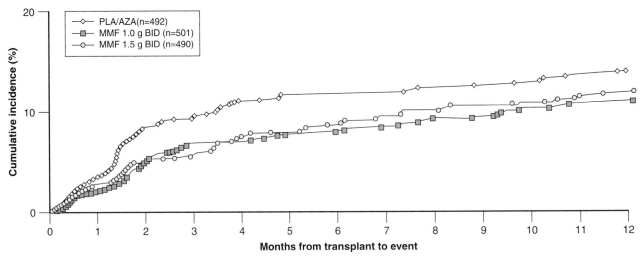

FIGURE 18–5

Cumulative incidence of graft loss or patient death (including on-study and posttermination events; Kaplan-Meier estimates). Data from the pooled efficacy analysis of the three double-blind clinical studies in prevention of rejection (Halloran *et al.*, 1997). The difference between the control group and mycophenolate mofetil groups is established in the first 2 months and is largely sustained to 12 months. PLA = placebo; AZA = azathioprine; MMF = mycophenolate mofetil.

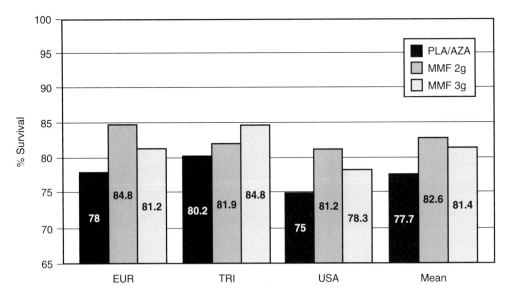

FIGURE 18–6

Graft survival (%) at 3 years in the pivotal trials. The individual trial results of graft survival (intent to treat) at 3 years show a consistent small benefit to the mycophenolate mofetil groups. The mean of the three individual trial results is shown on the right and indicates a 4.9% advantage at 3 years to the mycophenolate mofetil 2 g/d group compared with controls. PLA = placebo; AZA = azathioprine; MMF = mycophenolate mofetil.

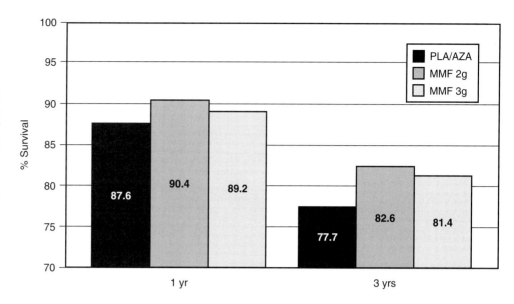

FIGURE 18-7

Graft survival at 1 and 3 years: mean result of three individual pivotal trials (EUR, TRI, USA; see text). The pooled analysis of the three trials at 1 year is compared with the mean of the individual results at 3 years (pooled analysis not available). The difference in outcome has increased with time emphasizing the need for longer term follow-up of these pivotal trials. PLA = placebo; AZA = azathioprine; MMF = mycophenolate mofetil.

or azathioprine) groups is clinically significant. The trials confirmed a strong association between the presence of acute rejection and future graft loss. The reduction in the use of antilymphocyte agents (a marker of the severity of rejection) from 20% in controls to 9% in the MMF 2 g/d group and to 5% in the MMF 3 g/d group was a particularly impressive result.

Comparative efficacy of MMF with the new anti-interleukin-2 receptor antagonists and with rapamycin and its analogues has not yet been established. It is generally believed that MMF is not a sufficiently potent immunosuppressive agent to replace calcineurin inhibition as initial therapy.

Prevention of Rejection in Other Organ Allografts

Heart

In the single multicenter double-blind, active controlled trial addressing the efficacy of MMF in preventing rejection in heart transplantation, 650 patients undergoing a first heart transplant were randomized to receive MMF (3 g/d) or azathioprine (1.5–3 mg/kg/d) in addition to cyclosporine and steroids. Follow-up was for 12 months, and primary endpoints were the proportion of patients who died or underwent retransplant and the proportion of patients with first biopsy-proven rejection with hemodynamic compromise or death. The study was confounded by 11% of patients withdrawing before receiving study drug. By chance, excess mortality occurred in those allocated but never receiving MMF. In the intention-to-treat analysis (which included 72 patients not receiving study medications and which included an imbalanced excess of deaths in the MMF allocated group), survival and rejection incidence were similar.

In the analysis of treated patients (i.e., actually receiving allocated study medications), the MMF group was associated with a significant reduction in mortality at 1 year (6.2% vs. 11.4%) and a significant reduction in requirement for rejection treatment (65.7% vs. 73.7%). Opportunistic infections, mostly herpes simplex, were increased in the MMF group (53.3% vs. 43.6%) (Kobashigawa et al., 1998).

The quality of the data here is modest given that there is only one trial and there is concern about cohorting. The trial has been sufficient to earn registration for MMF for this indication and is unlikely to be repeated. Other supporting evidence for the use of MMF in preventing cardiac rejection was reviewed by Bardsley-Elliot et al. (1999). Of particular

interest is the early report of secondary prevention in 30 patients, suggesting that MMF was more effective at maintaining coronary lumen size and graft perfusion than azathioprine (Pethig et al., 1999).

Other Organs

Mycophenolate mofetil has been reported to be useful in reducing rejection episodes, by allowing reduction or withdrawal of steroids and by allowing reduced doses of cyclosporine or tacrolimus in liver, lung and simultaneous pancreas/kidney transplantation. The experience has been small and often not well controlled but is generally favorable. The use of MMF in these organs was reviewed comprehensively by Bardsley-Elliot et al. (1999).

Treatment of Refractory Rejection in Renal Allografts

A single open study was conducted in 150 patients with biopsy-proven rejection, who were refractory to at least one course of an antilymphocyte agent. Patients were randomly allocated to ongoing treatment with MMF, 3 g/d, or a course of intravenous methylprednisolone, 5 mg/kg for 5 days tapered over the next 5 days to 20 mg/d. Graft loss and death were reduced by 45% in the MMF group, and subsequent rejection or treatment failure was reduced from 64% in the steroid group to 39% in the MMF group. The study was open and recruited modest numbers over an extended period. It addresses a complex clinical situation that is hard to categorize accurately. The evidence presented is suggestive of efficacy and has been sufficient to earn registration for this indication in some countries (Mycophenolate Mofetil Renal Refractory Rejection Study Group, 1996).

Initiation of Mycophenolate Mofetil at the Time of First Rejection Episode

Because about 50% of patients typically do not experience any rejection on a regimen of cyclosporine and steroids (with or without azathioprine), it seems unnecessary to submit this group to more intensive immunosuppression. To identify this cohort and focus on those most likely to benefit from the use of MMF, delaying the introduction of MMF until after the first rejection episode has occurred has been suggested.

This approach was studied in a double-blind, randomized trial of adding MMF or azathioprine to 221 renal transplant recipients experiencing a first rejection episode between 7 days and 6 months after transplantation. No patient received MMF before randomization, and all patients received cyclosporine and corticosteroids. Endpoints for the study were the use of antilymphocyte therapy, the number of courses of antirejection therapy in the first 6 months, and patient survival at 1 year (Pescovitz, for the Mycophenolate Mofetil Acute Renal Rejection Study Group, 1999).

By 6 months, the number of patients requiring full courses of antirejection therapy was 25% with MMF compared with 58% of controls. Additionally, 16.8% of MMF-treated patients and 41.7% of azathioprine-treated patients required at least one course of antilymphocyte therapy. By 1 year after enrollment, 8.9% of the MMF group had lost their graft or died compared with 14.8% in the controls. Of MMF-treated patients, 18% withdrew because of an adverse event compared with 10% of patients on azathioprine.

The results show that the delay in introducing MMF until the first rejection episode occurred was associated with a reduction in subsequent rejection episodes and still allowed a 91% 1-year graft survival to be achieved in the treated group. The 3-year results show 80.4% graft survival for patients on MMF and 75.9% for the azathioprine group, although the study was confounded by the premature termination of more than 50% of patients in both arms of the trial. Chronic renal allograft dysfunction was similar in each group at 3 years (Pescovitz, for the Mycophenolate Mofetil Acute Renal Rejection Study Group, 1999). The overall experience was promising, and this approach merits further trial.

Mycophenolate Mofetil as Dose-Sparing Agent for Steroids, Cyclosporine and Tacrolimus

The benign adverse effect profile for MMF, particularly its lack of nephrotoxicity, has led to the suggestion that it is an agent to be preferred to cyclosporine or tacrolimus in the long-term. Protocols to reduce, withdraw or avoid steroids have been published frequently over the last 15 years but have not gained widespread support because of the fear of breakthrough rejection (see Chapter 15). The increased immunosuppressive potency of MMF has led to many units testing this concept.

Cyclosporine-Sparing Studies

Promising results have been reported with MMF being used as an agent to allow cyclosporine dose reduction or withdrawal in the face of nephrotoxicity. In a pilot trial, 28 renal transplant recipients with progressive deterioration of renal function on cyclosporine and azathioprine at a mean of about 24 months after transplantation had azathioprine replaced by MMF and the cyclosporine dose halved. The mean serum creatinine at the point of change was 3.5 (± 1.2) mg/dl. Renal function improved in 21 of 28 patients, and only 1 patient continued to show deterioration of renal function over a mean observational period of 7 months. No acute rejection episodes occurred after the change in immunosuppression (Weir et al., 1997).

In 16 renal transplant recipients suspected of having cyclosporine nephrotoxicity, MMF, 2 g/d, was introduced and cyclosporine dose reduced to achieve a target of a subnormal whole blood trough level. The introduction of MMF allowed a 58% reduction in cyclosporine dose, which was associated with improved renal function, reduced transforming growth factor–β1 production and no episodes of acute rejection (Hueso et al., 1998).

Other small studies have been reported in which the dose of cyclosporine was reduced or the drug withdrawn in the face of proven or suspected nephrotoxicity (Ducloux et al., 1998; Wombolt et al., 1998), but none have been well controlled. The possibility that azathioprine might have allowed similar reduction in dosage without the addition of MMF has not been tested adequately. The safety and efficacy of this approach await to be resolved by further controlled evidence.

Other studies have examined the potential for a reduction in cyclosporine for all patients (usually stable at a fixed time point early in the posttransplant course). These randomized trials aimed to reduce prospectively cyclosporine complications and have tended to be larger trials and better controlled. Four such trials are illustrative:

1. In 159 stable renal transplant recipients at 12 months, patients were randomly submitted to cyclosporine withdrawal, tapered over 12 weeks (after the addition of MMF to a double-therapy regimen or its substitution for azathioprine in a triple-therapy regimen), or allocated to continuing on original therapy. There was improvement in renal function (creatinine clearance of 66 ml/min increasing to 73 ml/min vs. a slight decline in controls). Six patients had an acute rejection episode in the withdrawal group (compared with two in the controls) over a follow-up period of 183 days (median). This protocol was concluded to be safe and associated with improvement in renal function (Abramowicz et al., 1999).

2. In 110 patients allocated to low-dose or high-dose cyclosporine in addition to steroids and MMF, there was no difference in outcome (de Sevaux et al., 1998).

3. In 99 patients, high-dose monotherapy cyclosporine (targeted to blood levels) was compared with half-dose cyclosporine together with MMF. After 3 months, renal function was better and acute rejection was reduced in the MMF combination group (Sells et al., 1998).

4. In 94 stable renal transplant recipients, cyclosporine, MMF and steroid had been given. At 6 months, these patients were submitted to random allocation of prednisolone or cyclosporine withdrawal or continuation of triple therapy. Mycophenolate mofetil 2 g/d (which all patients had received initially) was continued in all patients. Six of 30 (20%) of the cyclosporine withdrawal patients had a rejection episode, and one third of these were steroid resistant, whereas there were no rejection episodes in the other two groups. There was no graft loss or patient death (de Sevaux et al., 1999).

This experience, although encouraging, is a reminder that the definitive study to assess the important question of safe cyclosporine withdrawal or dose reduction must be performed carefully with adequate numbers and controls and a long enough follow-up to be clinically meaningful.

Steroid-Sparing Studies

The case in favor of minimization of steroids after transplantation is persuasive and can be divided into steroid avoidance or steroid withdrawal (Mathew, 1992). Mycophenolate mofetil has been used for complete steroid avoidance with antilymphocyte induction therapy (Birkeland, 1998) and without induction (Elias et al., 1999). In both series, excellent long-term results were achieved, and almost half of all patients were managed with no steroid. The overall incidence of acute rejection episodes is higher with this approach, but most rejection episodes are mild and respond readily to steroids.

In a pilot study in 26 cadaveric renal transplant recipients on cyclosporine and MMF, steroids were withdrawn 4 to 30 months after transplantation. No rejection episodes occurred over a mean follow-up period of 10 months (Grinyo *et al.*, 1997). In a multicenter double-blinded study, 266 patients receiving cyclosporine, MMF and prednisone 3 months after transplantation were randomized to taper prednisone to zero over 8 weeks or to remain on the baseline dose (10–15 mg/ d). The incidence of rejection was found to be higher in the withdrawal group (19% *vs.* 5% at 1 year) (Matas *et al.*, 1999).

The penalty of this approach of steroid minimization appears to be an increase in the incidence of acute rejection, and MMF does not seem able to prevent this occurring. The risk-benefit equation of this approach is complex and will involve long-term, well-controlled studies to resolve.

Mycophenolate Mofetil in Combination with Tacrolimus

Mycophenolate mofetil in combination with tacrolimus displays pharmacological synergism (see earlier) and has been reported to produce results comparing favorably with cyclosporine with MMF. In a nonblinded trial randomizing 208 renal transplant recipients to tacrolimus/prednisone or tacrolimus/prednisone/MMF followed for a mean of 15 months, there was a significant reduction in rejection from 44% (without MMF) to 27% (with MMF). No difference in survival was shown (Shapiro *et al.*, 1999). In another study, 232 patients received tacrolimus/prednisolone, and MMF was randomly allocated in a dose of 1 g/d or 2 g/d or none. At 6 months, both MMF groups had a similar outcome with respect to rejection incidence (23% and 25%), being half the rate of that experienced in the double-therapy group (49%) but with no evidence of a significant difference in survival (Vanrenterghem *et al.*, 1998).

In a similar unblinded study using azathioprine as the comparator for two dose levels of MMF (1 g/d and 2 g/d) in combination with tacrolimus and steroids, 176 patients were followed for 1 year. The mean dose of MMF at 12 months in the MMF 1 g/d group was 1.0 g and in the MMF 2 g/d group was 1.5 g, indicating the difficulty in tolerating the 2-g/d dose in the presence of tacrolimus. Rejection (biopsy proven) occurred in 36%, 35% and 9% of the groups azathioprine, MMF 1 g/d and MMF 2 g/d. The mean time to first rejection was significantly longer and the use of antilymphocyte therapy was reduced in the MMF 2 g/d group. Overall survival was excellent, and the conclusion was that 2-g/d dose of MMF with adjustment was more efficacious than 1 g/d of MMF or azathioprine (Miller, for the FK506 Dose Ranging Kidney Transplant Study Group, 1999).

In another retrospective, nonrandomized study, 135 patients in various combinations of therapy were compared for rejection incidence and infection. The conclusion was that MMF in combination with tacrolimus provided potent immunosuppression resulting in less rejection, but that it also was associated with an increased rate of infection compared with MMF and cyclosporine (Daoud *et al.*, 1998).

More experience is needed with this combination, which appears at least as effective as cyclosporine and MMF and possibly is more effective. There are early indications that the price of increased efficacy may be more infections. The dose of MMF in the presence of tacrolimus should be adjusted carefully. A reduced dose (e.g., 1.5 g/d) may give the same MPA AUC as a higher dose (e.g., 2 g/d) on concomitant cyclosporine. The recommendation that when the combination of tacrolimus and MMF is used both drugs should have therapeutic monitoring of blood levels may prove appropriate (Meiser *et al.*, 1999).

SAFETY ISSUES
Overview

The adverse reaction profile for MMF is restricted largely to the gastrointestinal and hematopoietic systems. Some increase in infections and the rate of malignancy has been reported and is probably intrinsic to all effective immunosuppressive agents. There is no evidence of acute or chronic nephrotoxicity, hepatotoxicity or neurological toxicity and no effect on lipid metabolism. This benign adverse effect profile sets MMF apart from most other immunosuppressives used in organ transplantation.

The large well-conducted pivotal trials allowed a better definition of the adverse effects caused by MMF than previously introduced immunosuppressive agents. This account of the adverse effects of MMF accordingly draws mainly on this controlled experience, which allows a perspective to be placed on the reported side effects. Extension of the pivotal trials to 3 years of follow-up (European Mycophenolate Mofetil Cooperative Study Group, 1999; Tricontinental Mycophenolate Mofetil Renal Transplantation Study Group, 1998; U.S. Renal Transplant Mycophenolate Mofetil Study Group, 1999) and postmarketing experience for more than 3 years have not identified any additional areas of concern to those recorded in the first 12 months of treatment.

Withdrawals from Adverse Effects

In the first 6 months of the blinded pivotal trials, withdrawals attributed to drug-induced adverse effects occurred more frequently in the MMF groups than in placebo or azathioprine controls (Table 18–3). The larger dose of MMF (3 g/d) was associated with increased withdrawals. Gastrointestinal symptoms (diarrhea, abdominal pain and nausea) were the most frequent problems causing drug withdrawal followed by leukopenia and thrombocytopenia. In clinical practice, mainly using the 2-g/d dose, about 5% of renal transplant recipients prove unable to tolerate MMF. Most of these patients have persistent abdominal pain or diarrhea.

Potentially Life-Threatening or Other Serious Adverse Effects
Leukopenia and Anemia

Leukopenia and anemia occurred two to three times more frequently in MMF-treated patients (approximately 10%) than in those on placebo (2–4%). Pancytopenia and agranulocytosis were rare (<1%), and almost all hematological abnormalities resolved within 1 week (European Mycophenolate Mofetil Cooperative Study Group, 1995).

TABLE 18–3

PATIENTS (%) WITHDRAWN WITH DRUG-RELATED ADVERSE EFFECTS IN THE FIRST 6 MONTHS OF MYCOPHENOLATE MOFETIL PIVOTAL TRIALS*

	PLA (n = 166)	AZA (n = 326)	MMF2 g (n = 501)	MMF3 g (n = 490)
US		3.6	4.2	9.6
TRI		4.2	8	9.1
EUR	3.0		7.3	13.8

*The percentage of patients withdrawn because of adverse drug effects in the first 6 months of the three blinded pivotal trials (see text). In each trial, more withdrawals occurred in the higher dose mycophenolate mofetil group.

PLA = placebo; AZA = azathioprine; MMF2 g = mycophenolate mofetil, 2 g; MMF3 g = mycophenolate mofetil, 3 g.

The incidence of all hematological changes (leukopenia, anemia, thrombocytopenia and leukocytosis) in the azathioprine comparator trials was similar when MMF in a dose of 2 g/d was compared with azathioprine. With 3 g/d of MMF, leukopenia increased from 22 to 35%, but severe neutropenia (absolute neutrophil count, <500/ml) was infrequent and occurred in less than 2% of patients in these trials. These episodes of neutropenia reversed quickly with dose reduction and were not associated with more infective deaths.

Malignancy

Malignancy is a well-documented complication after transplantation that increases in incidence in a linear fashion with time at a rate of about 2.7% new cases per year. The most complete database is found in the ANZDATA registry. According to the ANZDATA registry, all renal transplant recipients have at least one cancer (including skin and non-skin cancers) by 35 years after transplantation (Disney et al., 1997).

The incidence of malignancy with MMF in the first 3 years after transplantation is similar to that seen in the control groups. There was a slight increase in the incidence of post-transplantation lymphoproliferative disease (PTLD) in the first 12 months in the MMF groups (0.6% for 2 g/d and 1% for 3 g/d) compared with placebo (0%) and azathioprine (0.3%). At 3 years, there had been little increase, with the incidence being azathioprine (0.6%), MMF 2 g/d (0.6%) and MMF 3 g/d (1.2%). These findings are well within the expected incidence of PTLD in protocols not including MMF.

Skin and nonskin cancers (excluding PTLD/lymphoma) occurred in 4.2% of azathioprine-treated patients and approximately 4% of MMF-treated patients. The overall pattern of malignancy with MMF in the early years does not raise particular concern (Fig. 18–8).

Infections

The pivotal trials did not indicate any increased overall risk of infection (including opportunistic infection) above that seen with azathioprine (Hoffman La Roche, 1998). Subgroup analysis showed an increase of tissue-invasive cytomegalovirus disease in MMF-treated patients (2 g/d, 8.3%, and 3 g/d, 11.5%) compared with azathioprine-treated patients (6.1%). Herpesvirus, *Candida* and other fungal infections were not increased. Of interest was the low incidence of *Pneumocystis carinii* infection in MMF-treated patients consistent with the observation that MMF has anti–*P. carinii* activity (Oz and Hughes, 1997). Fatal infection or sepsis occurred in less than 2% of MMF-treated patients in the pivotal trials.

Mycophenolate mofetil has been shown to potentiate the antiherpes activities of acyclovir, ganciclovir and penciclovir (Neytes et al., 1998). This effect may prove of clinical benefit not only in the treatment of herpes simplex, varicella zoster and cytomegalovirus infections in patients receiving mycophenolate, but also in those receiving any of these drugs for prophylaxis against these infections.

Symptomatic Adverse Effects

Gastrointestinal

The commonest and most significant adverse effects of MMF are abdominal pain, vomiting and diarrhea. The symptoms often do not appear until several weeks after transplantation and may subside spontaneously. These dose-related effects probably are due to direct gastric irritation (although evidence suggests that the same pattern is seen with the intravenous preparation) and can be reduced by dosing with food or dividing the same total daily dose into smaller increments. The incidence of diarrhea was 31% on 2 g/d of MMF and 36% on 3 g/d of MMF in the active comparator trials, although with azathioprine the incidence was 21%. In the pooled trial experience, about 2% of patients on MMF had to withdraw from the trial because of diarrhea or abdominal pain. Most gastrointestinal symptoms associated with MMF resolve when the dosage is reduced (Kobashigawa et al., 1998).

Other Effects

Multiple other adverse effects were recorded in the controlled trials, but none were in significant excess to the incidence in the controls. There were no biochemical abnormalities observed attributable to MMF, and in particular no adverse effect on liver function or lipid metabolism was noted.

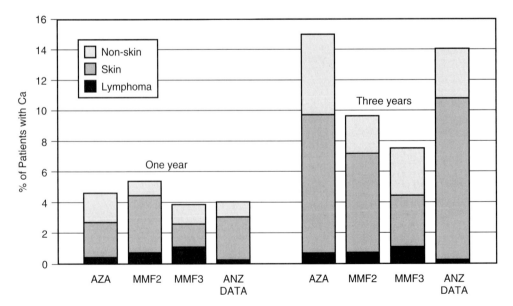

FIGURE 18–8

Mycophenolate mofetil and malignancy. The incidence of malignancy at 1 and 3 years after transplantation (data from the pivotal trials; see text) compared with that reported to ANZDATA registry. The data show that mycophenolate mofetil is not associated with an increased reporting rate of any type of malignancy in the early years after transplantation. MMF2 = mycophenolate mofetil, 2 g/d; MMF3 = mycophenolate mofetil, 3 g/d; AZA = azathioprine.

HIGH-RISK GROUPS
Neonates and Children

There is no recorded experience with neonates taking MMF. Animal studies have shown MMF to be excreted in breast milk, but no human experience is recorded, and breast-feeding is not advised.

In children, limited experience suggests that MMF is not as well tolerated as in adults and that gastrointestinal effects predominate. Generally, doses have been 600 mg/m² body surface area twice a day, and a study using this dose in pediatric renal transplant recipients examined in the first 3 weeks showed the concentration-time profile to be comparable to that of adults (Weber *et al.*, 1998). In pediatric renal transplant recipients in the presence of tacrolimus, reduction in the dose of MMF to 250 mg/m² twice a day has been recommended (Filler *et al.*, 1998).

Pregnant Women

Mycophenolate mofetil is relatively contraindicated in pregnancy. There is minimal clinical experience with MMF and pregnancy. This situation is a consequence of great caution because teratology studies showed fetal malformations to occur without maternal toxicity in two animal species at drug concentrations similar to those used clinically. Pregnancy categorizations have warned against pregnancy. The U.S. National Transplantation Pregnancy Registry has reported three pregnancies in women receiving MMF in the early stages of pregnancy. One patient had a miscarriage (relationship to MMF unclear), and the other two women had normal infants (Armenti *et al.*, 1999). Patients should be advised to avoid conception for 6 weeks after withdrawal of MMF.

No precaution exists about fathering children while taking MMF. There is no evidence that MMF has any effect on gonadal function or spermatogenesis.

Concurrent Disease

There is no evidence of any alteration of the pharmacokinetic profile of MMF in the presence of heart failure, hepatic disease or renal failure. No adjustment to dosage or any special monitoring is required when MMF is used in these patients.

Pharmacoeconomic Aspects of Mycophenolate Mofetil in Renal Transplantation

The costs of treating rejection and associated hospitalizations are reduced when the overall rejection incidence is low, and these savings can be put toward the higher acquisition costs of the treatment. This is the situation with MMF, in which the annual drug cost is approximately $4,000. In one Swiss study, the comparison of azathioprine and MMF in renal transplantation showed equal outcomes, but the cost for rejection treatment per patient was lowered eightfold and the number of transplant biopsies lowered threefold. This lowering more than balanced the increased cost of immunosuppression, which increased by 1.5 times (Wuthrich *et al.*, 1999).

Other studies in the first year have shown the use of MMF to be cost-effective with a savings of $1,300 (Sullivan, 1997) or $8,000 per patient (Khosla, 1998). Beyond the first year, when the clinical course of patients tends not to differ greatly despite a variety of treatment approaches, it is more difficult to show a financial advantage. One economic analysis based on a 10-year projection of graft survival claimed relatively poor cost-effectiveness over 10 years when MMF was given to all patients, but the cost-effectiveness improved when the drug was confined to patients at high risk of rejection (Schnitzler *et al.*, 1999).

The cost of new immunosuppressive therapies is going to form part of the overall equation determining their place in therapy. Apart from the direct savings mentioned, additional indirect savings come from a reduced expenditure on agents *spared* by the use of MMF. The cost of some of these agents is high and accounts for greater than 50% of ongoing cost of maintaining a transplant beyond the first year. Pharmacoeconomic assessment of these drug-sparing and dose-sparing protocols must follow the clinical demonstration of their efficacy.

Place of Mycophenolate Mofetil in Clinical Renal Transplantation

The clinical experience to date with MMF in renal transplantation has established it to be a well-tolerated adjunctive agent capable of reducing (not just delaying) acute rejection episodes to half the rate experienced when azathioprine or placebo is used. The reduction in acute rejection episodes in renal transplantation trials was associated strongly with reduction in late graft loss and resulted in a mean of 4.9% improvement in 3-year graft survival with MMF (2 g/d) across the three pivotal trials. This increase in graft survival does not achieve statistical significance for reasons discussed previously. An advantage in graft survival of 13% at 3 years is needed to establish statistical significance with cohorts of about 160 patients. To show statistical significance with a 5% difference requires cohort numbers three times this size. Future trials of new agents wishing to prove efficacy need to take heed of these facts.

This inability to show a significant difference in graft survival has led to considerable uncertainty about the place of MMF in therapy. The high ongoing cost of the medication is such that for many countries the small advantage of 4 to 5% increased survival at 3 years has not justified the increased expenditure required to fund MMF. Although one can show a pharmacoeconomic benefit in the first year of using MMF, the ongoing annual cost is increased, and the benefit not so evident.

The currently available immunosuppressive regimens control early rejection so effectively that acute rejection is no longer the prime cause of graft loss in the first year and contributes to late graft loss to an uncertain degree. The therapeutic issue has become reduction in short-term and long-term morbidity and premature mortality, which can be related in some part to the detrimental effects of long-term immunosuppression. This situation is most clearly evident in the increase in accelerated atherosclerosis well documented to complicate late outcome in renal transplant recipients. Cyclosporine in contributing to hypertension, lipid disturbance and nephrotoxicity; steroids in contributing to hypertension and glycemic and lipid disturbance; tacrolimus with its effect on glycemic control and rapamycin with its marked effect on lipid metabolism are all imperfect agents for long-term exposure. Mycophenolate mofetil stands out in having no obvious effect on the risk factors for cardiovascular disease and no nephrotoxicity. It appears to be an attractive candidate for long-term use in renal transplant recipients.

Apart from minimizing cardiovascular risk, the other therapeutic imperative is reduction in cancer risk. The early experience with MMF is reassuring in that it does not add to the early risk unacceptably, but in the longer term there is no experience. It must be assumed that because it is a more powerful agent than azathioprine at controlling rejection its effect on cancer risk would be similar or increased to that of azathioprine. These considerations add to the overall need to look urgently at protocols reducing the long-term immunosuppression burden on successfully treated renal transplant recipients. No longer is it appropriate to add another agent early, get good early results, but commit patients to lifelong treatment.

The first question is how long is it necessary to continue MMF? To date, all the large studies have continued MMF indefinitely, whereas the major clinical advantage appears to be gained in the first 3 months. Withdrawal of MMF at 3 to 6 months (perhaps accompanied by introduction of azathioprine) needs to be tested.

The next question is do all patients need to start on MMF? The trial, detailed earlier, initiating MMF at the time of the first rejection episode avoids its use in the approximately 50% of recipients destined not to have an early rejection episode, while achieving excellent outcome in those treated (Mycophenolate Mofetil Acute Renal Rejection Study Group, 1998). This cost-effective approach needs to be explored further.

The role of MMF in the rescue of renal allografts undergoing severe rejection is more problematic. The role of tacrolimus and antilymphocyte agents is likely to prove more impressive in this regard, although the evidence is that for patients not on MMF its introduction may be beneficial.

Can the ongoing use of MMF allow reduction or withdrawal of other agents such as cyclosporine and steroids and in the process minimize long-term toxicity? These studies are summarized in this chapter and conclude that the answer is yes, but probably at some cost of breakthrough rejection. The improvement in renal function seen with cyclosporine reduction (covered by the introduction of MMF) in the face of suspected nephrotoxicity has been particularly impressive.

The benefits of a reduction in the amount of long-term immunosuppression given to a patient must be balanced against the risk of losing control of the immune system. Patients and physicians often are most reluctant to risk losing the graft. The challenge in the management of immunosuppression is to address this issue. Programs need to allow for individualization of therapy and to be tailored to particular risk factors. Protocols will most likely use stronger immunosuppression in early months, weaning down to a less intense regimen for the long-term. Mycophenolate mofetil appears to have an important potential role in this process given its undoubted efficacy and benign adverse effect profile.

The role for MMF in renal transplantation awaits resolution of these issues. In particular to justify its continuing role in long-term therapy, it is essential to show some tradeoff or ability to spare other immunosuppressants, which would result in a lessening of long-term complications.

REFERENCES

Abramowicz, D., Manas, D., Lao, M., et al. (1999). Preliminary results of a randomised controlled study investigating the withdrawal of Neoral in stable renal transplant recipients receiving mycophenolate mofetil in addition to Neoral and steroids. *Transplantation* **67**, S240.

Allison, A. C., Almquist, S. J., Muller, C. D., et al. (1991). In vitro immunosuppressive effects of mycophenolic acid and an ester prodrug RS-61443. *Transplant. Proc.* **23(Suppl. 2)**, 10.

Allison, A. C. and Eugui, E. M. (1993). Mycophenolate mofetil a rationally designed immunosuppressive drug. *Clin. Transplant.* **7**, 96.

Allison, A. C. and Eugui, E. M. (1994). Preferential suppression of lymphocyte proliferation by mycophenolic acid and predicted long term effects of mycophenolate mofetil in transplantation. *Transplant. Proc.* **26**, 3205.

Allison, A. C. and Eugui, E. M. (1996). Purine metabolism and immunosuppressive effects of mycophenolate mofetil. *Clin. Transplant.* **10**, 77.

Armenti, V. T., Cosela, L. A., McGory, C. H., et al. (1999). Pregnancy outcomes in transplant recipients exposed to mycophenolate mofetil. *Transplantation* **67**, S623.

Bardsley-Elliot, A., Noble, S. and Foster, R. (1999). Mycophenolate mofetil: a review of its use in the management of solid organ transplantation. *Biodrugs* **12**, 363.

Beal, J. L., Jones, C. E., Taylor, P. J., et al. (1998). Evaluation of an immunoassay (EMIT) for mycophenolic acid in plasma from renal transplant recipients compared with high performance liquid chromatography assay. *Ther Drug Monit* **20**, 685.

Birkeland, S. A. (1998). Steroid free immunosuppression after kidney transplantation with antithymocyte globulin induction and cyclosporine and mycophenolate mofetil maintenance therapy. *Transplantation* **66**, 1207.

Bullingham, R. E. S., Monroe, S. and Nicholls, A. (1996a). Pharmacokinetics and bioavailability of mycophenolate mofetil in healthy subjects after single dose oral and intravenous administration. *J. Clin. Pharmacol.* **36**, 315.

Bullingham, R. E. S., Nicholls, A. and Hale, M. (1996b). Pharmacokinetics of mycophenolate mofetil: a short review. *Transplant. Proc.* **28**, 925.

Bullingham, R. E. S., Nicholls, A. and Kamm, B. R. (1998). Clinical pharmacokinetics of mycophenolate mofetil. *Clin. Pharmacokinet.* **34**, 429.

Daoud, A. J., Schroeder, T. J., Shah, M., et al. (1998). A comparison of the safety and efficacy of mycophenolate mofetil, prednisone and cyclosporine and mycophenolate mofetil, prednisone and tacrolimus. *Transplant. Proc.* **30**, 4079.

de Sevaux, R. G. L., Smak Gregoor, P. J. H., Hene, R. J., et al. (1998). A randomised study of conventional vs low dose cyclosporine in renal transplant recipients treated with cyclosporine, mycophenolate mofetil and prednisone. *Transplantation* **65**, S107.

de Sevaux, R. G. L., Smak Gregoor, P. J. H., Hene, R. J., et al. (1999). Withdrawal of cyclosporine or prednisone in renal transplant recipients treated with mycophenolate mofetil, cyclosporine and prednisone: a randomised trial. *Transplantation* **67**, S240.

Disney, A. P., Russ, G., Walker, R. and Shiel, A. G. (eds.) (1997). *ANZDATA Registry Report: Cancer Report in Australia and New Zealand Registry Report*, p. 145. Adelaide, South Australia.

Ducloux, D., Fournier, V., Bresson-Vautrin, C., et al. (1998). Mycophenolate mofetil in renal transplant recipients with cyclosporine associated nephrotoxicity. *Transplantation* **65**, 1504.

Elias, T. J., Bannister, K. M., Clarkson, A. R., et al. (2000). Excellent long term graft survival in low risk primary renal allografts treated with prednisolone avoidance immunosuppression. *Clin. Transplant.* **14**, 157.

Epinette, W. W., Parker, C. M., Jones, E. L., et al. (1987). Mycophenolic acid for psoriasis: a review of pharmacology, long term efficacy and safety. *J. Am. Acad. Dermatol.* **17**, 921.

Eugui, E. M., Almquist, S. J., Muller, C. D., et al. (1991a). Lymphocyte-selective cytostatic and immunosuppressive effects of mycophenolic acid in vitro: role of deoxyguanosine nucleotide depletion. *Scand. J. Immunol.* **33**, 161.

Eugui, E. M., Mirkovich, A. and Allison, A. C. (1991b). Lymphocyte selective antiproliferative and immunosuppressive effects of mycophenolic acid in mice. *Scand. J. Immunol.* **33**, 175.

European Mycophenolate Mofetil Cooperative Study Group. (1995). Placebo controlled study of mycophenolate mofetil combined with cyclosporin and corticosteroids for the prevention of acute rejection. *Lancet* **345**, 1321.

European Mycophenolate Mofetil Cooperative Study Group. (1999). Mycophenolate mofetil in renal transplantation: 3 year results from the placebo controlled trial. *Transplantation* **68**, 391.

Figueroa, J., Fuad, S. A. and Kunjunmen, B. D. (1993). Suppression of synthesis of natural antibodies by mycophenolate mofetil: its potential use in discordant xenografting. *Transplantation* **55**, 1371.

Filler, G., Lampe, D., Mai, I., et al. (1998). Dosing of mycophenolate mofetil in combination with tacrolimus for steroid-resistant vascular rejection in pediatric renal allografts. *Transpl. Int.* **11(Suppl. 1)**, S82.

Fulton, B. and Markham, A. (1996). Mycophenolate mofetil—a review of its pharmacodynamic and pharmacokinetic properties and clinical efficacy in renal transplantation. *Drugs* **51**, 278.

Gozio, B. (1896). Richerche Bacteriologiche e Chimiche sulle Alterazoni del Mais. *Riv. Igiene Sanita Publica Ann.* **7**, 825.

Grinyo, J. M., Gil-Vernet, S., Seron, D., *et al.* (1997). Steroid withdrawal in mycophenolate mofetil treated renal allograft recipients. *Transplantation* **63**, 1688.

Halloran, P., Mathew, T. H., Tomlanovich, S., *et al.* (1997). Mycophenolate mofetil in renal allograft recipients: a pooled efficacy analysis of three randomized, double blind clinical studies in the prevention of rejection. *Transplantation* **63**, 39.

Hoffmann La Roche. (1998). Mycophenolate mofetil: US prescribing information. Nutley, NJ.

Hueso, M., Bover, J., Seron, D., *et al.* (1998). Low dose cyclosporine and mycophenolate mofetil in renal allograft recipients with suboptimal renal function. *Transplantation* **66**, 1721.

Jones, E. L., Epinette, W. W., Hackney, V. C., *et al.* (1975). Treatment of psoriasis with oral mycophenolic acid. *J. Invest. Dermatol.* **65**, 537.

Khosla, U. M., Martin, J. E., Baker, G. M., *et al.* (1999). One year, single-center cost analysis of mycophenolate mofetil versus azathioprine following cadaveric renal transplantation. *Transplant. Proc.* **31**, 274.

Kimball, J. A., Pescovitz, M. D. and Book, B. K. (1995). Reduced human IgG anti-ATGAM antibody formation in renal transplant recipients receiving mycophenolate mofetil. *Transplantation* **60**, 1379.

Kobashigawa, J., Miller, L., Renlund, D., *et al.* (1998). A randomized active controlled trial of mycophenolate mofetil in heart transplant recipients. *Transplantation* **66**, 507.

Laurent, A. F., Dumont, S., Poindron, P., *et al.* (1994). Inhibition of mannosylation on human monocyte surface glycoprotein could explain some of the anti-inflammatory effects of mycophenolate mofetil. *Clin. Exp. Rheumatol.* **12(Suppl. 11)**, 110.

Li, S. G. and Yatscoff, R. W. (1995). Improved high performance liquid chromatographic assay for the measurement of mycophenolic acid in humans. *Proceedings International Congress on New Immunosuppressive Drugs*, Minnesota, p. 57.

Lipsky, J. J. (1996). Mycophenolate mofetil. *Lancet* **348**, 1357.

Matas, A. and Ewell, M., *et al.*, Cooperative Clinical Trials in Adult Transplantation Group. (1999). Prednisone withdrawal in kidney transplant recipients on Csa/Mmf—a prospective randomised study. *Transplantation* **67**, S269.

Mathew, T. H. (1992). Ideal immunosuppression after renal transplantation: are steroids needed? *International Yearbook of Nephrology* **4**, 299.

Meiser, B. M., Pfeiffer, M., Scmidt, D., *et al.* (1999). Combination therapy with tacrolimus and mycophenolate mofetil following cardiac transplantation: importance of MPA monitoring. *J. Heart Lung Transplant* **18**, 143.

Mendez, R. (1998). FK506 and mycophenolate mofetil in renal transplant recipients: six month results of a multicenter randomized dose ranging trial. *Transplant. Proc.* **30**, 1287.

Miller, J., for the FK506 Dose Ranging Kidney Transplant Study Group. (1999). Tacrolimus and mycophenolate mofetil in renal transplant recipients: one year results of multicenter randomized dose-ranging trial. *Transplant. Proc.* **31**, 276.

Mitsui, A. and Suzuki, S. (1969). Immunosuppressive effect of mycophenolic acid. *J. Antibiot. (Tokyo)* **22**, 363.

Morris, R. E., Hoyt, E. G., Eugui, E. M. and Allison, A. C. (1989). Prolongation of rat heart allograft survival by RS-61443. *Surg. Forum* **40**, 337.

Mycophenolate Mofetil. (1996). Investigational brochure, 11th ed., Syntex, San Francisco.

Mycophenolate Mofetil Acute Renal Rejection Study Group. (1998). Mycophenolate mofetil for the treatment of a first acute renal allograft rejection. *Transplantation* **65**, 235.

Mycophenolate Mofetil Renal Refractory Rejection Study Group. (1996). Mycophenolate mofetil for the treatment of refractory acute cellular renal transplant rejection. *Transplantation* **61**, 722.

Neytes, J., Andrei, G. and de Clercq, E. (1998). The novel immunosuppressive agent mycophenolate mofetil markedly potentiates the anti-herpes virus activities of acyclovir, ganciclovir and penciclovir in vitro and in vivo. *Antimicrob. Agents Chemother.* **42**, 216.

Oz, H. S. and Hughes, W. T. (1997). Novel anti pneumocystis carinii effects of the immunosuppressant mycophenolate mofetil in contrast to the provocative effects of tacrolimus, sirolimus and dexamethasone. *J. Infect. Dis.* **175**, 901.

Pescovitz, M. D., for the Mycophenolate Mofetil Acute Renal Rejection Study Group. (1999). Mycophenolate mofetil for the treatment of renal transplant rejection: three years of follow up. *Transplantation* **67**, S929.

Pethig, K., Wahlers, T., Heublein, B., *et al.* (1999). Mycophenolate mofetil for secondary prevention of allograft vasculopathy following heart transplantation: randomized, intravascular ultrasound controlled trial. *J. Heart Lung Transplant* **18**, 77.

Roth, D., Colona, J., Burke, G. W., *et al.* (1998). Primary immunosuppression with tacrolimus and mycophenolate mofetil for renal allograft recipients. *Transplantation* **65**, 248.

Salaman, J. R., Griffin, P. J. A. and Johnson, R. W. G. (1993). Controlled trial of RS-61443 in renal transplant patients receiving cyclosporine monotherapy. *Transplant. Proc.* **25**, 695.

Schnitzler, M. A., Woodard, R. S., Lowell, J. A., *et al.* (1999). Post marketing evaluation of mycophenolate mofetil based triple therapy immunosuppression compared with conventional azathioprine based regimen reveals enhanced efficacy and early pharmacoeconomic benefit. *3rd International Conference on New Trends in Clinical and Experimental Immunosuppression*, Geneva, Feb 12–15, p. 114.

Sells, R. A., Bakran, A., Brown, M. W., *et al.* (1998). A prospective randomised study of CSA monotherapy vs CSA plus mycophenolate mofetil in cadaveric renal transplant recipients. *Transplant. Proc.* **30**, 4098.

Shapiro, R., Jordan, M. L., Scantlebury, V. P., *et al.* (1998). A prospective, randomized trial to compare tacrolimus and prednisone with and without mycophenolate mofetil in patients undergoing renal transplantation: first report. *J. Urol.* **160**, 1982.

Shapiro, R., Jordan, M. L., Scantlebury, V. P., *et al.* (1999). A prospective, randomized trial of tacrolimus/prednisone vs tacrolimus/prednisone/mycophenolate mofetil in renal transplant recipients. *Transplantation* **67**, 411.

Simmons, W. D., Rayhill, S. C. and Sollinger, H. W. (1997). Preliminary risk benefit assessment of mycophenolate mofetil in transplant rejection. *Drug Saf.* **17**, 75.

Smith, K. G., Isbel, N. M., Catton, M. G., *et al.* (1998). Suppression of the humoral immune response by mycophenolate mofetil. *Nephrol. Dial. Transplant.* **13**, 160.

Soares, M. P., Latinne, D., Elsen, M., *et al.* (1993). In vivo depletion of the xenoreactive natural antibodies with an anti-u monoclonal antibody. *Transplantation* **56**, 1427.

Sollinger, H. W. (1996). From mice to man: the pre-clinical history of mycophenolate mofetil. *Clin. Transplant.* **10**, 85.

Sollinger, H. W., Deirerhoi, M. H., Belzer, F. O., *et al.* (1992). RS-61443—a phase 1 clinical trial and pilot rescue study. *Transplantation* **53**, 428.

Steele, D. M., Hullett, D. A., Bechstein, W. O., *et al.* (1993). Effects of immunosuppressive therapy on the rat aortic allograft model. *Transplant. Proc.* **25**, 754.

Sullivan, S. D., Garrison, L. P., Best, J. H. (1997). The cost effectiveness of mycophenolate mofetil in the first year after primary cadaveric transplant. U.S. Renal Transplant Mycophenolate Mofetil Study. *J. Am. Soc. Nephrol.* **8**, 1592.

Tricontinental Mycophenolate Mofetil Renal Transplantation Study Group. (1996). A blinded, randomized clinical trial of mycophenolate mofetil for the prevention of rejection in cadaveric renal transplantation. *Transplantation* **61**, 1029.

Tricontinental Mycophenolate Mofetil Renal Transplantation Study Group. (1998). A blinded long term randomized multicenter study of mycophenolate mofetil in cadaveric renal transplantation. *Transplantation* **65**, 1450.

U.S. Renal Transplant Mycophenolate Mofetil Study Group. (1995). Mycophenolate mofetil for the prevention of acute rejection in primary cadaveric renal allograft recipients. *Transplantation* **60**, 225.

U.S. Renal Transplant Mycophenolate Mofetil Study Group. (1999). Mycophenolate mofetil in cadaveric renal transplantation. *Am. J. Kidney Dis.* **34**, 296.

van Gelder, T., Hilbrands, L. B., Vanrenterghem, Y., *et al.* (1999). A randomized double-blind multicenter plasma concentration controlled study of the safety and efficacy of oral mycophenolate mofetil for the prevention of acute rejection after kidney transplantation. *Transplantation* **68**, 261.

Vanrenterghem, Y., Squifflet, J. P., Forsythe, J., *et al.* (1998). Coadministration of tacrolimus and mycophenolate mofetil in cadaveric renal transplant recipients. *Transplant. Proc.* **30**, 1290.

Weaver, J. L., Pine, P. S. and Aszalos, A. (1991). Comparison of the in vitro and biophysical effects of cyclosporine A, FK 506 and mycophenolic acid on human peripheral blood lymphocytes. *Immunopharmacol. Immunotoxicol.* **13**, 563.

Weber, L. T., Shipkova, M., Lamersdorf, T., *et al.* (1998). Pharmacokinetics of mycophenolic acid and the determinants of MPA free fraction in pediatric and adult renal transplant recipients. *J. Am. Soc. Nephrol.* **9**, 1511.

Weir, M. W., Anderson, L., Fink, J. C., *et al.* (1997). A novel approach to the treatment of chronic allograft nephropathy. *Transplantation* **64**, 1706.

Williams, R. H., Lively, D. H., DeLong, D. C., *et al.* (1968). Mycophenolic acid: antiviral and anti-tumour properties. *J. Antibiot. (Tokyo)* **21**, 463.

Wolfe, E. J., Mathur, V., Tomlanovich, S., *et al.* (1997). Pharmacokinetics of mycophenolate mofetil and intravenous ganciclovir alone and in combinatioon in renal transplant recipients. *Pharmacotherapy* **17**, 591.

Wombolt, D. G., McCune, T. R., Stewart, M., *et al.* (1998). Use of mycophenolate mofetil in patients with chronic cyclosporine nephrotoxicity. *Transplant. Proc.* **30**, 1194.

Wuthrich, R. P., Weinreich, T., Ambuhl, P. M., *et al.* (1999). Reduced kidney transplant rejection rate and pharmacoeconomic advantage of mycophenolate mofetil. *Nephrol. Dial. Transplant.* **14**, 394.

Yatscoff, R. W. and Aspeslet, L. J. (1998). The monitoring of immunosuppressive drugs: a pharmacodynamic approach. *Ther. Drug Monit.* **20**, 459.

Zeevi, A., Woan, M. and Yao, G. Z. (1991). Comparative in vitro studies on the immunosuppressive activities of mycophenolic acid, bredinin, FK 506, cyclosporine and rapamycin. *Transplant. Proc.* **23**, 2928.

Zucker, K., Rosen, A., Tsaroucha, A., *et al.* (1997). Unexpected augmentation of MPA pharmacokinetics in renal transplant patients receiving tacrolimus and mycophenolate mofetil in combination therapy and analogous in vitro findings. *Transpl. Immunol.* **5**, 225.

Zucker, K., Tsaroucha, A., Olson, L., *et al.* (1999). Evidence that tacrolimus augments the bioavailability of mycophenolate mofetil through the inhibition of MPA glucuronidation. *Ther. Drug Monit.* **21**, 35.

Sirolimus

Barry D. Kahan

Introduction

Sirolimus (SRL; Rapamune) is a macrocyclic lactone (Fig. 19–1) produced by *Streptomyces hygroscopicus*, an actinomycete discovered in the soil of the Vai Atari region of Rapa Nui (Easter Island). Macrocyclic lactones are lipophilic molecules bearing a 12-, 14- or 16-membered lactone ring substituted with hydroxyl, methyl and ethyl groups as well as carbonyl functions with one, two or three carbohydrate fragments.

Molecular and Cellular Mechanisms of Action

The emerging role of SRL relates to its unique mechanisms of action—its ability to inhibit the costimulatory pathways necessary for cytokine synthesis and the protein synthetic as well as DNA transcriptional processes mediating cell-cycle progression after cytokine stimulation (Kuo et al., 1992). On unimpeded entry into the cytoplasm, SRL complexes with FK-binding proteins (FKBP) to form the active inhibitor of cytosolic processes. In the co-stimulatory cascade necessary for the G_0-G_1 progression, SRL-FKBP complexes inhibit the activity of c-Rel, a crucial intermediate in the amplification of signal 1 activating the T-cell response (June et al., 1987). After autocrine or paracrine reception of the cytokine signal, a multifunctional kinase—mammalian target of rapamycin (mTOR)—exerts a variety of actions that regulate the phosphorylation of several sarcoma (src)-like, receptor-type, and cell cycle–dependent kinases (cdk). For example, the FKBP12-SRL-mTOR complex inhibits p70^{s6} $^{kinase\ kinase}$ but not the P85^{s6} enzyme, both of which lead to hyperphosphorylation of 40S ribosomal proteins (Brown et al., 1994, 1995). Inhibition of mTOR disrupts the dissociation of the elongation initiation factor (EIF$_4$), which is necessary for protein synthesis (Graves et al., 1995) and for hyperphosphorylation of retinoblastoma protein, a critical factor in cell-cycle progression. A fourth effect of SRL inhibition of mTOR is to prevent activation of the downstream serine-threonine protein kinases (Fig. 19–2), such as cyclin E and, more importantly, p34^{cdc2}, the latter effect facilitating the persistence of p27^{kip1} and the interruption of the formation of active p34^{cdc2}–cyclin D heterocomplexes that form a critical *maturation promotion factor*.

Sirolimus blocks Ca^{++}-dependent and Ca^{++}-independent activation pathways mediating transduction of proliferative and differentiation signals delivered by the lymphokines that act on T and B cells—interleukin (IL)-2, IL-3, IL-5, IL-6 and IL-15. The effects on T cells inhibit proliferation. On B cells, SRL blocks not only cytokine-dependent, but also *Staphylococcus aureus*–stimulated and soluble CD4 ligand–stimulated proliferative signals. SRL exerts a unique action to interrupt Ig class switching. In rodent models of tolerance induction, Ferraresso and colleagues observed that the state of allo-unresponsiveness induced by SRL was mediated by IgG$_{2c}$ antibodies, which are antigen specific and non–complement fixing (Ferraresso et al., 1994). These antibodies seem to down-regulate maturation of effector antidonor T cells. The drug apparently inhibited the action of interferon-γ to switch IgG$_1$ to IgG$_{2a}$ and IgG$_3$ antibody production and of transforming growth factor-β to switch subsequently to IgG$_{2b}$ and IgA production.

Not only *in vitro* but also apparently *in vivo* in humans, SRL inhibits, albeit less sensitively, signal transduction by a variety of other cytokines, including fibroblast growth factor, an effect that may explain problems with wound healing in SRL-treated patients; granulocyte colony-stimulating factor, leukopenia; IL-11, thrombocytopenia and insulin-like growth factor, hyperlipidemia. SRL disrupted other cytokine signals, such as the proliferation of nonstimulated vascular smooth muscle cells (Marx et al., 1995), cytokine-stimulated bovine or human endothelial cells (Akselband et al., 1991), rat aortic smooth muscle cell cultures (Graves et al., 1995), cardiac fibroblasts (Simm et al., 1997), bronchial smooth muscle cells (Scott et al., 1996) and rat smooth muscle cells (Obata et al., 1996). The effects on vascular endothelial and smooth muscle cell proliferation occur at SRL concentrations 10-fold to 100-fold greater than those required to inhibit the maturation of T and B cells and at concentrations about equal to the sensitivity of cytotoxic CD8$^+$ T, natural, lymphokine-activated and antibody-dependent killer cells. These actions may explain the beneficial effects of SRL to interrupt obliterative vascular lesions induced by balloon catheter injury and probably those associated with chronic rejection (Kahan, 1998b).

Prolongation of Transplants in Experimental Animals

Preliminary experiments documented that SRL prolongs the survival of heterotopic vascularized rat heart allografts (Calne et al., 1989). The immunosuppressive properties of the drug were confirmed using heterotopic vascularized grafts not only of heart in the mouse and rat, but also for rat kidney, heterotopic and orthotopic small bowel and pancreatic duodenal grafts (Stepkowski et al., 1991). Anecdotal experience supported a supraadditive interaction of SRL with cyclosporine (Neoral, Sandimmune) in mongrel dog (Knight et al., 1993) and subhuman primate models.

An extensive survey of available immunosuppressive agents using *in vitro* human lymphocyte proliferation assays and rat heart transplantations *in vivo* revealed that SRL acts in supraadditive (synergistic) fashion with cyclosporine but not with steroids or the antiproliferative agents azathioprine (Imuran), mycophenolic acid, or mizoribine (Kahan et al., 1991). The cyclosporine-SRL interaction included a pharmacokinetic component to increase drug concentrations mutually and a dynamic component (Stepkowski et al., 1996). The former interaction was attributed to competition between SRL and cyclosporine for metabolism by the cytochrome P450 (CYP) 3A4 system; the latter interaction, to the actions of SRL to disrupt the costimulation necessary for maximal transcription of cytokine genes during the G_0-G_1 transition as well as to interrupt the transduction of the humoral signals

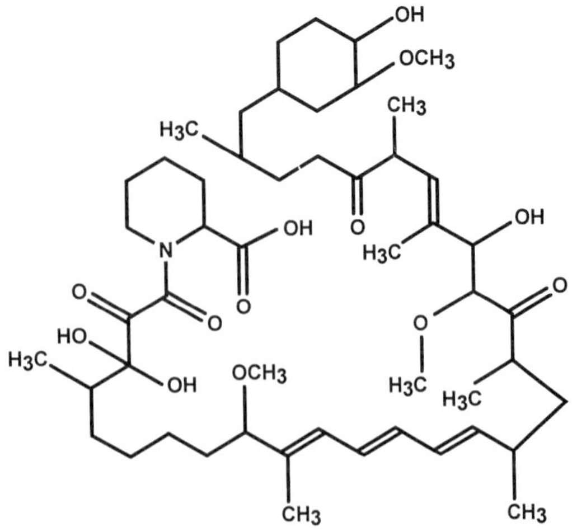

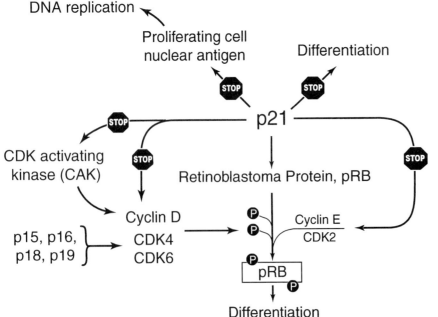

Sirolimus (RAPA, SRL)

FIGURE 19–1

Chemical structure of sirolimus.

necessary for the G_1 buildup for proliferative responses, both of which are complementary to the inhibition of calcineurin phosphatase activity by complexes of cyclosporine with its immunophilin cyclophilin.

Pharmacokinetic Properties

Macrocyclic lactones display four pharmacokinetic limitations, as follows:

1. Low and variable bioavailability has been attributed to sensitivity to gastric acid, incomplete intestinal absorption and first-pass hepatic metabolism.

2. Binding of the drug to plasma proteins varies from 10 to 93% at therapeutic concentrations.

3. There are widespread drug-drug pharmacokinetic interactions with coadministered pharmaceuticals at the level of CYP450 3A isozymes as a result of binding of macrocyclic lactone metabolite nitrosoalkanes to CYP450 iron (II), forming stable but inactive iron-metabolite complexes that prolong the half-lives of other drugs metabolized by this system.

4. Owing to marked differences in the activities of CYP 3A4 and the multidrug action efflux pump P-glycoprotein (P-gp), both of which are located in small intestinal enterocytes (Lown *et al.*, 1997), there is a large intersubject variability in the absorption and clearance of orally administered drug. For example, there is an 11-fold interindividual variation in the intestinal content of CYP 3A4 proteins (Hebert *et al.*, 1992; Wacher *et al.*, 1995). The prominent interactions when cyclosporine and SRL are delivered concomitantly to patients by the oral route may be reduced by spacing the drugs 4 hours apart (Kaplan *et al.*, 1998).

Sirolimus displays an oral bioavailability of about 15% and an average terminal half-life of 57 to 62 hours. After a single oral dose of 1 to 34 mg/m², whole blood peak concentrations usually occurred within 1 hour (range, 0.8–3 hours). Using a multiple-dose regimen, there was a good correlation ($r = 0.94$) between the trough (C_0) and the area under the concentration-time curve (AUC) concentrations, suggesting that C_0 values represent good indicators of total drug exposure (Napoli and Kahan, 1996; Zimmerman and Kahan, 1997), in contrast to cyclosporine, for which C_0 measurements are not representative of overall drug exposure (Kahan and Grevel, 1988). Although C_0 monitoring seems the most practical method, the problem with this strategy is the expensive and cumbersome nature of drug measurements by high-performance liquid chromatography (HPLC) with ultraviolet detection, an obstacle that may be addressed by an automated assay presently under development (IMx, Abbott Diagnostics, North Chicago, IL). Using the HPLC method in phase I/II trials, we observed that acute rejection prophylaxis was virtually guaranteed when the SRL C_0 were maintained between 10 and 15 ng/ml (Kahan *et al.*, 1998a) and cyclosporine exposure was set at average concentrations (C_{av}; the quotient of the AUC and the dosing interval) between 350 and 450 ng/ml; that is, cyclosporine concentrations that were

FIGURE 19–2

Actions of sirolimus on downstream activation events mediated by cycle-dependent kinases (cdk) and cyclins necessary for DNA replication and cellular differentiation.

40% lower than those used in cyclosporine/steroid regimens without SRL (Lindholm and Kahan, 1993). Concentration-controlled protocols that maintain SRL C_0 of less than 15 ng/ml have been associated with only modest drug toxicity.

Sirolimus shows extensive tissue distribution—a volume of distribution of 5.6 to 16.7 L/kg in stable renal transplant recipients (Yatscoff et al., 1995). Sirolimus whole blood concentrations are far higher than plasma concentrations because 94.5% of SRL is bound to red blood cells, 1% is bound to lymphocytes and granulocytes and 3.1% is free in plasma. The extensive partitioning of SRL in tissues results in a greater delay to steady-state concentrations and a relatively long terminal half-life that permits once-daily dosing (Zimmerman and Kahan, 1997). At least to expedite tissue loading partially, the first SRL dose generally is administered at three times the baseline amount. It also seems prudent to continue with twice the baseline amount for at least 3 days. For example, to achieve maximal rejection prophylaxis, the regimen is 15 mg on day 1 posttransplant; 10 mg on days 2, 3, and 4; and 5 mg daily thereafter.

The primary clinical trials of SRL used an oil-based liquid formulation that requires refrigeration for stabilization of the drug suspension; however, a solid SRL tablet was introduced (Kelly et al., 1999). A pharmacokinetic comparison of the liquid versus the pill formulation was performed in 12 renal transplant recipients who had been receiving liquid for more than 1 year. Concurrent 12-hour pharmacokinetic profiles of SRL and cyclosporine were conducted on the last dose of liquid and at 2, 4 and 8 weeks postconversion to the solid formulation. The only significant difference was a higher maximum concentration (Cmax) after administration of the liquid compared with the solid formulation. There were no significant differences among the pharmacokinetic parameters of cyclosporine AUC_{0-12}, dose-corrected SRL C_0, time to maximum SRL concentration (tmax) and relative oral bioavailability for the liquid versus the solid formulation.

Despite the promising results from initial clinical trials, exact recommendations for initial or maintenance dosing regimens, for therapeutic drug monitoring protocols and for patient management are unclear. To date, most clinical trials have sought to minimize SRL toxicities by combining modest doses of the drug with cyclosporine, exploiting the synergistic interactions of the two agents. Although phase III trials have confirmed that 2.0- or 5.0-mg SRL doses provide excellent prophylaxis of acute rejection episodes, some patients required dose reductions in response to toxic adverse events (see later). There may be a need to increase the long-term SRL dose to exploit its potential for chronic rejection prophylaxis (Kahan, 1998b).

Clinical Results with Sirolimus Therapy

ACUTE REJECTION PROPHYLAXIS

Phase I, II and III Studies in Combination with Cyclosporine

Based on the phase I results in quiescent renal transplant recipients (Murgia et al., 1996), an open-label, single-center, dose-escalation phase I/II trial was conducted to examine the safety and efficacy of de novo use of SRL to full therapeutic doses of cyclosporine in mismatched living donor renal transplants (Kahan et al., 1998a). The first cohort of 20 patients was divided into groups of 4 patients that were treated with ascending doses of SRL (0.5, 1.0, 2.0, 3.0 and 5.0 mg/m^2/d) in combination with cyclosporine and prednisone according to our usual steroid-tapering schedule. Because only one patient experienced an acute rejection episode (a black

recipient of a spousal transplant in the 0.5 mg/m^2/d dose group) and because we were concerned about the metabolic effects of long-term steroid treatment, we began to withdraw steroids (at a minimum of 5 months posttransplant) from the immunosuppressive regimen of this cohort. There were no rebound acute rejection episodes. To test the possibility of early withdrawal of patients from steroids, two additional cohorts of 10 patients each were treated with 7 mg/m^2/d of SRL in addition to cyclosporine and either 1-week or 1-month posttransplant courses of prednisone. Only one rejection episode occurred in each cohort. Among the 40 patients in this trial, there were three rejection episodes (two of which occurred among patients off steroids), yielding an overall 7.5% incidence of acute rejection episodes—a result that was significantly better than the 32% acute rejection rate in an historical cyclosporine/prednisone cohort (Kahan et al., 1998a).

A multicenter phase II trial showed that the addition of SRL allowed doses of cyclosporine (Sandimmune) to be reduced significantly among nonblack patients (Fig. 19–3); despite the reduced cyclosporine exposure, there was only a 12% incidence of acute rejection episodes (Kahan et al., 1999a). Based on these findings, we conducted a single-center de novo trial using markedly reduced doses of cyclosporine (a C_{av} target of 250 ng/ml rather than the usual target of 550 ng/ml) (Lindholm and Kahan, 1993), with excellent prophylaxis of acute rejection episodes among cadaveric kidney recipients of all races (unpublished data).

The pivotal multicenter, randomized, blinded, double dummy, clinical trial in 719 American renal transplant recipients compared the efficacy and safety of 2 mg/d (n = 284) or 5 mg/d (n = 274) doses of SRL with azathioprine (n = 161) in combination with a protocol-stipulated regimen of cyclosporine (Neoral) and prednisone (Kahan, for the Rapamune U.S. Study Group, 1998; 2000). Both doses of SRL resulted in a significant reduction in the overall rate of efficacy failure at 6 months compared with azathioprine—17.3% (P = 0.003), 17.9% (P = 0.009) and 29.2% (Fig. 19–4). Not only was there a reduced incidence, but also a milder severity of the acute rejection episodes as estimated by the Banff grade and by the number of patients who required antibody therapy to treat rejection episodes. Graft and patient survivals at 1 year were similar among all three treatment groups.

The pivotal global multicenter, randomized, blinded, single-dummy, clinical trial treated 576 recipients worldwide with 2 mg/d (n = 227) or 5 mg/d (n = 219) of SRL or with a placebo (n = 130). All groups received a baseline immunosuppressive regimen of cyclosporine and steroids (MacDonald, for the Rapamune Global Study Group, 1998). There was a reduction in the incidence of biopsy-proven rejection among the groups—19% (P = 0.076) and 11% (P = 0.001) compared with 37%. During the initial 6 months, there were no differences in patient (95–98%) or graft (88–93%) survival rates among the three treatment groups. The overall severity of acute rejection episodes was significantly lower among patients receiving 5 mg/d of SRL but not 2 mg/d of SRL compared with placebo. The need for antibody therapy to treat steroid-resistant episodes of acute rejection was reduced significantly in the 2 mg/d SRL group (2.2%) compared with placebo (7.7%; P = 0.025). These two pivotal studies show that SRL enhances the prophylactic effect of a cyclosporine/prednisone regimen in primary renal allograft recipients.

Phase II Trial of Sirolimus Therapy Without Calcineurin Inhibitors

Another phase II multicenter trial compared immunosuppressive regimens SRL/azathioprine/prednisone (41 pa-

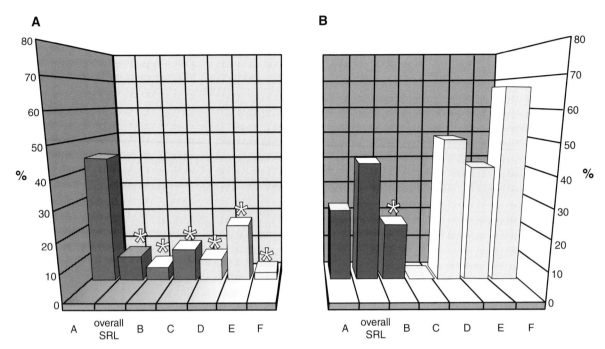

FIGURE 19-3

Incidence of acute rejection episodes among (A) nonblack and (B) black patients in the multicenter phase II trial. Asterisks indicate rejection rates that were significant ($P < 0.05$) compared with group A patients treated with full-dose cyclosporine/prednisone (CsA-Pred) only; group B received full-dose CsA-Pred plus sirolimus (SRL) 1 mg/m²; group C, full-dose CsA-Pred plus SRL, 3 mg/m²; group D, reduced-dose CsA full-dose Pred plus SRL, 1 mg/m²; group E, reduced-dose CsA full-dose Pred plus SRL, 3 mg/m²; group F, reduced-dose CsA full-dose Pred plus SRL, 5 mg/m².

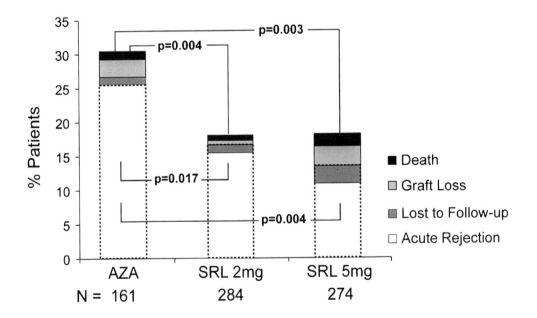

FIGURE 19-4

Results of pivotal U.S. multicenter trial. The full bar refers to the fraction of patients who displayed a composite endpoint of death, graft loss, loss to follow-up or acute rejection episodes within 6 months. *P* values above the bars refer to the composite endpoint. *P* values below the bars refer to comparisons of acute rejection episodes (*note*: loss to follow-up considered as experiencing a rejection episode for the sirolimus (SRL) but not the azathioprine (AZA) groups). *N* shows the number of patients in each treatment group. All comparisons were analyzed using log-rank tests.

tients) versus cyclosporine/azathioprine/prednisone (42 patients). The incidence of acute rejection episodes diagnosed clinically or on biopsy within 3 months of treatment was 49% versus 43% (Groth *et al.*, 1999). Three graft losses occurred in the cyclosporine group (one rejection and two thrombosis) and one in the SRL group (rejection plus sepsis). No deaths occurred in either group. The laboratory abnormalities that were observed more frequently in the SRL group included reduced leukocyte and platelet counts and increased triglyceride and cholesterol levels; however, renal function in the SRL cohort was at least transiently better than that among the cyclosporine patients. These results suggest that SRL may be as effective as cyclosporine in preventing acute rejection episodes in renal transplant patients receiving azathioprine and steroids. To select primary SRL over SRL/cyclosporine treatment, the clinician must decide whether the benefit on renal function is worth the increased risk of an acute rejection episode.

OTHER POSSIBLE INDICATIONS FOR SIROLIMUS

Refractory Renal Allograft Rejection

Renal allograft rejection refractory to treatment with antilymphocyte antibodies as evidenced by the persistence of vascular rejection (Banff grade IIB or III) on renal biopsy almost inevitably progresses to transplant loss. After an impressive result of SRL treatment in the first patient (Slaton and Kahan, 1996), we entered an additional 17 adult patients who had failed treatment with *at least one* 14-day course of OKT3, followed by a *second* 7-day course of OKT3 (n = 13) and/or a 14-day course of Atgam (n = 8) as well as treatment with mycophenolate mofetil in 5 patients. Sirolimus was initiated at 7 mg/m² for 5 days and continued thereafter at 5 mg/m². Cyclosporine doses were not changed; steroids were tapered or withdrawn as tolerated (Kahan *et al.*, 1998b). The actuarial 2-year patient survival was 85%; one patient succumbed to preexisting congestive cardiomyopathy and one patient to sudden death of unknown cause but with a functioning graft (creatinine, 1.5 mg/dl). Two other grafts were lost: one owing to persistent rejection and one owing to overwhelming, presumably infectious, diarrhea. Before inception of SRL therapy, the serum creatinine value at the end of the previous therapy and at the time of the confirmatory biopsy was 195% greater than the baseline value just before the acute episode. Among the nine patients (70%) with functioning grafts at 1 year, the mean serum creatinine value after inception of SRL was 2.15 mg/dl (range, 1.4–4.0 mg/dl). Five patients also were weaned from steroids. Sirolimus may represent a therapeutic alternative to treat allograft rejection episodes refractory to antilymphocyte antibodies and mycophenolate mofetil.

Steroid Withdrawal

Two cohorts of patients treated with *de novo* regimens of SRL/cyclosporine underwent steroid withdrawal: 40 recipients of HLA-mismatched living donors (phase IIA) and 35 recipients of cadaver (phase IIB) donor renal transplants. At the time of the reports, the minimum follow-up periods were 18 and 12 months. Among the 40 recipients in the phase IIA trial, 8 patients were ineligible for steroid withdrawal (Kahan *et al.*, 1998a). Among the other 32 recipients, 25 were withdrawn successfully from steroids (78%), with two episodes of acute rejection occurring thereafter (8%). After a 6-month period of SRL/cyclosporine/prednisone therapy, both of the patients who had experienced acute rejection episodes were withdrawn successfully the second time, such that all 25

patients were off steroids at 12 months and 24 were off steroids at 18 months. The patient who returned to steroid treatment had experienced a flare-up of preexisting lupus erythematosus. At 1 year, patients who had been withdrawn from steroids showed significant reductions in white blood cell count (presumably owing to lack of steroid stimulation of leukocytes) and, more importantly, in serum cholesterol and triglyceride values. The mean triglyceride value was 251 mg/dl for the SRL/cyclosporine group compared with 365 mg/dl for the SRL/cyclosporine/prednisone group (*P* = 0.02), and the mean values for the cholesterol were 244 mg/dl versus 278 mg/dl (*P* = 0.05). Among 35 cadaver recipients in a separate cohort within the phase IIB trial, 27 (77%) were entered into a steroid withdrawal protocol (Pescovitz *et al.*, 1997). Four episodes of acute rejection occurred after steroid withdrawal (15%), and four other patients required reinitiation of steroid treatment owing to medical reasons. The other 19 patients (54%) were rejection-free and steroid-free at 12 months, although they did not show any improvement in triglyceride or cholesterol levels. Of renal transplant recipients, 77% tolerated steroid withdrawal from a SRL/cyclosporine regimen, with success rates at 12 months of 96% among living and 54% among cadaver donor kidney recipients. Large multicenter trials of steroid withdrawal are planned during phase IV development of SRL.

Induction Immunosuppression

Because of its nonnephrotoxic properties (DiJoseph *et al.*, 1992), SRL offers a useful baseline drug for induction immunosuppression. Owing to the high 49% incidence of acute rejection episodes using a SRL/steroid regimen (Groth *et al.*, 1999), we added anti-IL-2R monoclonal antibodies (MAb) to an SRL-based regimen (Hong and Kahan, 1999) that is free of nephrotoxic calcineurin inhibitors. This regimen was used when there were adverse donor (or recipient) factors that placed the patient at high risk of delayed graft function, for example, donor age older than 10 years, cold ischemia time greater than 36 hours, adverse procurement conditions (hypotension, premature cardiac arrest), or perioperative complications (e.g., myocardial infarction). Five doses of daclizumab (Zenapax) were administered at doses of 1 mg/kg on alternate weeks, as had been documented to enhance the effects of cyclosporine (Vincenti *et al.*, 1998). Alternatively, two 20-mg doses of basiliximab (Simulect) were administered on days 0 and 4. SRL was begun at 15 mg on day 1; 10 mg on days 2, 3 and 4 and selected to achieve a C_0 value greater than 10 ng/ml. Once the serum creatinine value was less than 2.5 mg/dl, low doses of cyclosporine (50–100 mg twice a day) were instituted. None of the initial six patients experienced an acute rejection episode (Hong and Kahan, 1999). This is in contradistinction to the 50% rejection rate observed using induction therapy with daclizumab (Zenapax), and mycophenolate mofetil.

Prevention and/or Treatment of Chronic Rejection

Chronic rejection has become the major limitation to long-term renal allograft success. A review of the data reveals four observations that suggest SRL may be useful for the prevention of chronic rejection (Kahan, 1998b):

1. SRL inhibits growth factor–driven proliferation of endothelial and smooth muscle cells in six different *in vitro* models (see earlier) thought to reflect the processes producing the immunoobliterative vascular endothelial and smooth muscle as well as bronchial lesions that serve as histopathological hallmarks of chronic rejection in kidney, heart or lung transplant recipients.

2. Sirolimus exerts a beneficial effect to dampen vascular injury responses *in vivo*—the balloon catheter arterial injury (Gregory *et al.*, 1995) or restenosis response after angioplasty.

3. Sirolimus mitigates chronic rejection in rat (Calne *et al.*, 1989; Meiser *et al.*, 1991), pig (Calne *et al.*, 1989) and mouse (Morris *et al.*, 1995) models. Schmid and coworkers identified the degree of donor-recipient histoincompatibility and the SRL dose over the range of 0.5 to 2.0 mg/kg/d as determinants of the benefit of the drug on the development of transplant vasculopathy (Schmid *et al.*, 1997). The lowest SRL dose that was effective in rats (0.5 mg/kg/d)—a reduction in the incidence of vasculopathy from 62% ± 13% to 25% ± 15% ($P < 0.005$)—would translate to approximately 35 mg/d in humans, a dose that is more than double the largest amount used chronically in renal transplant trials (15 mg/d) (Kahan *et al.*, 1998a). Higher doses of SRL may be required to exploit its potency in chronic as opposed to acute rejection settings.

4. When used in combination with cyclosporine in humans, SRL reduces the incidence of acute rejection episodes, which are widely believed to forecast an increased risk of chronic rejection (Almond *et al.*, 1993; Kahan *et al.*, 1987). Administration of SRL at doses of 2 to 10 mg/d permits cyclosporine dose minimization during the early postoperative period, possibly mitigating the renal dysfunction, a disorder that may exacerbate other processes leading to chronic graft failure.

Toxic Side Effects

INFECTIONS

The initial impression from treatment of quiescent renal transplant recipients with a short course of ascending doses of SRL in the phase I study (Murgia *et al.*, 1996) was that the addition of the drug to a cyclosporine-based regimen increased only modestly the overall incidence of bacterial, viral or fungal infections. This impression was confirmed in the phase II study of *de novo* treatment of living-related kidney recipients (Kahan *et al.*, 1998a). In contrast, the adverse results with a high infection rate, particularly with *Pneumocystis carinii*, in the multicenter phase IIB trial on addition of SRL to a cyclosporine/prednisone regimen were observed owing to the policy of one center not to administer prophylactic agents (Kahan *et al.*, 1999a). This center reported six cases of the disease; prophylactic treatment with trimethoprim-sulfamethoxazole is now mandated for all patients receiving SRL. The only other process significantly increased in incidence by SRL is a oral aphthous ulcer, presumably owing to herpes simplex infections. Sirolimus treatment did not increase the rate of occurrence or the severity of cytomegalovirus disease compared with azathioprine-treated or placebo-treated controls despite the lack of routine antiviral prophylaxis in the phase II or III trials. The incidence of malignancies has not been increased by SRL. Only three cases of posttransplant lymphoproliferative disease have occurred among the 300 patients treated with SRL at our institution for periods of at least 1 and up to 5 years. All three cases occurred within 90 days posttransplant and were associated with excessive immunosuppression: one second transplant recipient treated by a physician parent with a regimen that produced extremely high concentrations of SRL and cyclosporine; one elderly man who received OKT3 to provide a cyclosporine holiday to permit renal allograft recovery from drug-induced nephrotoxicity and one woman with persistent renal allograft rejection refractory to murine OKT3, equine antihuman thymocyte globulin and rabbit thymoglobulin. These rates of malignancy are similar to those generally encountered among patients treated with cyclosporine/prednisone.

LACK OF NEPHROTOXICITY

Our phase I study of 40 stable renal transplant recipients documented that cyclosporine and SRL have few overlapping toxicities. In particular, SRL did not increase the degree of renal dysfunction or exacerbate hypertension during a 2-week treatment course (Murgia *et al.*, 1996). The observation of slightly worse renal function among SRL/cyclosporine/prednisone versus cyclosporine/azathioprine/prednisone or cyclosporine/prednisone patients in the pivotal trials probably relates to the pharmacokinetic interaction that increases renal tissue cyclosporine levels (Napoli *et al.*, 1998). In salt-deprived rat models, it was possible to account for the reduction in renal function solely based on the augmented cyclosporine kidney tissue concentration (Podder *et al.*, 1999).

CYTOPENIAS

The phase I study, including a 2-week treatment course in stable patients (Murgia *et al.*, 1996), and the phase I/II study in *de novo* transplant recipients (Kahan, 1998a) observed that SRL decreases the production of myeloid and erythroid elements as well as platelets. The changes usually occur during the first month, are modest in degree and resolve spontaneously. Drug dose reductions, which are rarely required, usually produce a reversal of the toxic effect beginning on day 5, with full recovery by 14 days. In the phase I/II trial, a greater incidence of adverse events appeared to be associated with SRL C_0 greater than 15 ng/ml. Overall the severity of the adverse events induced by SRL seemed mild compared with the potency of the immunosuppressive effects.

In the phase III trials, peripheral white blood cell counts less than 3,500/mm³ or platelet counts less than 100,000/mm³ pretransplant represented absolute contraindications to entry and posttransplant triggered more intense laboratory monitoring (Table 19–1). Patients who had white blood cell counts within the normal range pretransplant showed less myelosuppression than those in the blinded azathioprine-treated control arm (Fig. 19–5).

Sirolimus doses were decreased when platelet counts fell to less than 75,000/mm³ and were suspended when counts fell to less than 50,000/mm³. Although direct evidence is not available to clarify the issue, it appears that the presence of concomitant cytomegalovirus infection or pharmaceuticals that cause myelosuppression may exacerbate this toxicity of SRL. No patient required drug discontinuation for this reason. In cases of extreme low counts or the need to continue SRL therapy in the face of cytopenias, we have administered the nonimmunostimulatory cytokines—granulocyte colony-stimulating factor, erythropoietin or IL-11—to counter drug-induced effects on granulocytes, erythrocytes or platelets (see Table 19–1). This strategy is based on the hypothesis that the myelodepression is due to SRL-mediated inhibition of signal transduction through hematological growth factor receptors that use similar gp130 β chains with the lymphokine receptors that are the pharmacological target of drug action.

HYPERLIPIDEMIAS

Sirolimus seems to exacerbate cyclosporine-induced hypercholesterolemia and steroid-induced hypertriglyceridemia in dose-dependent fashion (Murgia *et al.*, 1996). Although the molecular mechanism is unclear, SRL appears to interfere with lipid clearance from low-density lipoproteins, possibly by inhibiting lipolysis and/or by disrupting signal transduc-

TABLE 19–1

CLINICAL MANAGEMENT OF THE ADVERSE EFFECTS OF SIROLIMUS THERAPY

Effect	Threshold for Action	Countermeasure Therapy
Thrombocytopenia	$<100,000/mm^3$	Dose reduction
	$<50,000/mm^3$	Drug suspension
	$<25,000/mm^3$	Oprelvekin (Neumega), 50 μg/kg/d
Absolute granulocytopenia	$<2,000/mm^3$	Dose reduction
	$<1,500/mm^3$	Drug suspension
	$<750/mm^3$	Filgrastim (Neupogen), 5 μg/kg/d (subcutaneous or intravenous)
Anemia	Hematocrit $<32\%$	Epoetin alfa (Epogen), 6,000 units, 3 times/wk
	Hematocrit $<25\%$	Epogen, 10,000 units, 3 times/wk
Hypertriglyceridemia	>300 ng/dl	Gemfibrozil, 600 mg daily
	>500 ng/dl	Gemfibrozil, 600 mg bid; fish oil, 2 tablets tid
	$>1,000$ ng/dl	Drug dose reduction
	$>1,500$ ng/dl	Drug suspension
Hypercholesterolemia	With hypertriglyceridemia	Pravastatin: dose proportionate to increase
	Without hypertriglyceridemia	Atorvastatin: dose proportionate to increase

tion by insulin or insulin-like growth factors necessary for fatty acid uptake by adipocytes.

Although the toxic effect occurs in a significant fraction of renal transplant recipients generally beginning in the second posttransplant month, most patients show spontaneous resolution of hyperlipidemia to only modest elevations that are well below the thresholds of 240 mg/dl cholesterol and 300 mg/dl triglycerides, which were proposed by the National Cholesterol Education Program to constitute a cardiovascular risk. The spontaneous resolution may be attributed to decreasing cyclosporine and steroid doses, improving dietary compliance or increasing exercise associated with recovery from end-stage renal disease. Patients with serum triglyceride values greater than 400 mg/dl and/or cholesterol values greater than 300 mg/dl should receive countermeasure therapy (see Table 19–1). Patients with isolated elevations of serum cholesterol (not triglyceride) levels are managed by administration of atorvastatin because it has less interaction with the cytochrome P450 3A4 system, produces only modest rhabdomyolysis as detected by increases in creatine phosphokinase levels and has a mild action to decrease serum triglyceride concentrations. Moderate to severe hypertriglyceridemia is more difficult to manage owing to the only modest activity of the combination of fibrates and fish oil. It is rare for SRL-treated patients to display serum triglyceride values greater than 1,000 mg/dl, the threshold associated with proclivity for the occurrence of pancreatitis, a complication that has not occurred in increased incidence among patients treated with SRL. Although hypercholesterolemia has been implicated as a cause for cardiovascular complications—now the leading cause of mortality for patients receiving dual-drug or triple-drug regimens—and possibly for an increased incidence of chronic rejection (Dimeny et al., 1993a, 1993b), the significance of SRL-induced hypertriglyceridemia to increase the incidence or severity of cardiovascular complications is less clear. Large phase III multicenter trials do not show an increased incidence of cardiovascular complications at 1 year among de novo treated transplant patients.

MISCELLANEOUS TOXICITIES

Among the side effects of macrocyclic lactones, gastrointestinal intolerance with diarrhea is the most prominent toxicity. Hepatotoxicity, pneumonitis, ototoxicity and dermatological effects represent less commonly reported reactions, and pancreatitis, hemolytic anemia and psychotic reactions are extremely unusual (Eichenwald, 1986). Of great interest are the apparently idiosyncratic, adverse cardiac toxicities that they may share with the somewhat related macrolides. Intravenous administration of tacrolimus (FK506, Prograf) (Hodak et al., 1998; Johnson et al., 1992) or erythromycin, particularly in women (Antzelevitch et al., 1996; Drici et al., 1998; Guelon et al., 1986), has been associated with the electrocardiographic sign of lengthening of the rate-correlated QT interval. This alteration may lead to the torsades de pointes ventricular arrhythmia in similar fashion as potassium channel blockers, such as quinidine and amiodarone. Coadministration of astemizole, cisapride, pimozide or terfenadine may increase the

FIGURE 19–5

Serial mean values (and standard deviations) of white blood cell counts (A) and platelet counts (B) over the first 12 months for patients in the U.S. pivotal trial of cyclosporine (CsA)/sirolimus (SRL)/prednisone (Pred) versus CsA/Aza/Pred. The CsA/SRL 5 mg/Pred group is indicated by □—□; CsA/SRL 2 mg/Pred group by △—△; CsA/Aza/Pred group by ○—○.

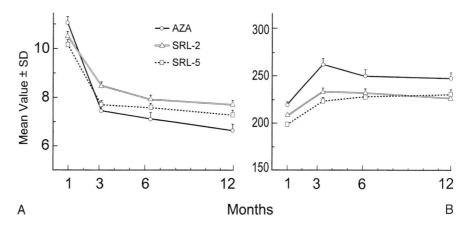

proclivity of macrocyclic lactones to produce cardiac effects.

Sirolimus displays little tendency to produce hepatotoxicity; only modest increases in serum glutamic-oxalic acid transaminase have been observed in randomized trials. There are anecdotal observations of an increased incidence of delayed wound healing, lymphocele formation, Achilles and plantar tendinitis and arthropathy, particularly in the heel. The incidence and significance of these side effects are expected to be clarified on further analysis of the phase III data comparing the clinical courses of SRL-treated versus azathioprine-treated (U.S. trial) and SRL-treated versus placebo-treated (global trial) patients.

SDZ-RAD

A rapamycin analogue (SDZ-RAD [RAD]) is an immunosuppressive macrolide bearing a stable 2-hydroxyethyl chain substitution at position 40 on the SRL structure. SDZ-RAD was developed in an attempt to improve the pharmacokinetic characteristics of SRL, particularly to increase the extent and reproducibility of its oral bioavailability and to reduce the extensive tissue distribution by virtue of its greater polarity.

A phase I, randomized, blinded, placebo-controlled study assessed the safety profile and pharmacokinetics of a 4-week course of once-daily, sequential ascending doses (0.75, 2.5 or 7.5 mg/d) of RAD capsules in renal transplant recipients on a stable regimen of cyclosporine and prednisone (Kahan *et al.*, 1999b). SDZ-RAD displayed a similar spectrum of side effects as that observed with SRL: an increased incidence of infections associated with the augmented immunosuppression and a dose-related occurrence of thrombocytopenia, hypercholesterolemia and hypertriglyceridemia, particularly at the 7.5-mg dose. The pharmacokinetic parameters of RAD showed dose proportionality, with a good correlation between C_0 and AUC concentrations but a moderate degree of drug accumulation (2.5-fold) at the 0.75-mg dose. The drug was absorbed rapidly, reaching a Cmax within 2 hours, and displayed a 16- to 19-hour half-life, which is significantly shorter than that of SRL, necessitating twice-daily dosing. SDZ-RAD concentrations reached a steady-state by 4 days. Preliminary kinetic-dynamic correlations indicate correlations between thrombocytopenia (but not hyperlipidemia) and AUC, Cmax and weight-adjusted dose. At the end of a 4-week course of simultaneous dosing, there was no evidence of a pharmacokinetic interaction between cyclosporine and RAD. Controlled, multicenter phase II/III pivotal trials are under way to assess the impact of the shorter half-life and increased hydrophilicity on the clinical outcomes of RAD compared with mycophenolate mofetil.

Macrocyclic Lactone Agents in the Matrix of New Immunosuppressives

INTERACTIONS WITH ANTI-INTERLEUKIN-2 RECEPTOR MONOCLONAL ANTIBODY

We have proposed a new immunosuppressive strategy—the cytokine paradigm—for induction immunosuppressive therapy (Hong and Kahan, 1998; Fig. 19–6). In addition to cyclosporine and SRL, the paradigm includes the administration of either the chimeric (basiliximab) or the humanized (daclizumab) anti-IL-2 receptor (IL-2R) MAbs. These reagents bind to the α (alpha) chain (CD25) of the IL-2R. Because CD25 does not bear an intracytoplasmic signaling mechanism, these MAbs do not elicit the cytokine release syndrome. They evoke the production of neutralizing antibodies only rarely. Administered in combination with cyclosporine and steroid therapy, they were shown in pivotal trials to reduce the incidence of acute rejection episodes by about 30% and to produce minimal side effects. The chimeric form is administered as two 20-mg doses (day 0 and day 4) because it is 10-fold more potent than the humanized form, which is prescribed as five 1-mg/kg doses of daclizumab at biweekly intervals. Induction immunosuppression with anti-IL-2R MAb and SRL has been used in six patients to permit extended periods of freedom from the administration of cyclosporine, which we subsequently introduced at low 50 to 100 mg twice-daily doses on resolution of the impaired function (Hong and Kahan, 1999). This beneficial effect might be explored further with longer courses of treatment with anti-IL-2R MAbs or by maintenance therapy with selective receptor antagonists possibly designed akin to the IL-1R antagonists presently in clinical use for treatment of rheumatoid conditions.

INTERACTIONS BETWEEN SIROLIMUS AND TACROLIMUS OR MYCOPHENOLATE MOFETIL

On introduction into clinical practice, SRL is likely to be applied widely in drug combinations. Because of the potency of its interaction with cyclosporine, it has been suggested that another calcineurin inhibitor, tacrolimus, might act synergistically with SRL (Mahalati *et al.*, 1999). This combination was not investigated extensively during the development of SRL because *in vitro* assays suggested that the drugs antagonize each other's effects when either one is used in molecular excess (Dumont *et al.*, 1990). *In vivo* studies claim that combinations of tacrolimus and SRL display more than additive interactions to prolong the survival of rat or mouse heart tissue allografts (Chen *et al.*, 1998; Vu *et al.*, 1997). These

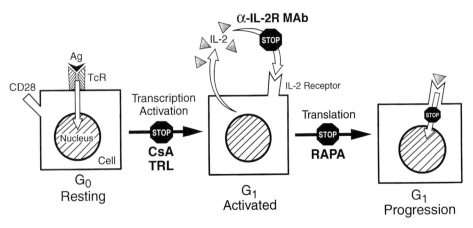

FIGURE 19–6

The cytokine paradigm: complementary sites of action of immunosuppressive drugs during lymphocyte activation. Cyclosporine (CsA) and tacrolimus (TRL) inhibit transcription of T-cell growth-promoting genes (e.g., interleukin [IL]-2). Anti-IL-2 (monoclonal antibodies MAs) block binding of IL-2 to its receptor. Sirolimus (SRL) blocks growth factor–initiated signal transduction. TcR = T-cell receptor; RAPA = rapamycin.

studies neither used rigorous methods to assess the drug interaction nor included simultaneous drug concentrations to assess the contribution of pharmacokinetic interactions to the apparent prolongation of graft survival. A final assessment must await clinical trials comparing tacrolimus/SRL with cyclosporine/SRL combination. Although these trials might be performed in concentration-controlled manner, it is difficult to imagine them being performed in blinded manner. Before embarking on such a trial, however, the physician should be aware that there may be a danger in conducting clinical trials based on results of experimental animal studies conducted in less than a rigorous manner. This danger is illustrated by the discrepancy between the claim of synergy between mycophenolate mofetil and SRL based on rat allograft survival (Vu et al., 1998) and the failure to observe a beneficial effect of SRL/mycophenolate mofetil/prednisone compared with SRL/azathioprine/prednisone combination in a European multicenter randomized trial.

Summary

Sirolimus is a promising new immunosuppressive agent with a unique mechanism of action to disrupt costimulatory and cytokine-stimulated T-cell activation through inhibition of a multifunctional kinase—mTOR. The drug has undergone development culminating in two large pivotal trials including more than 1,300 patients. These trials show that SRL reduces the incidence, time to onset and severity of acute rejection episodes. A parallel series of studies documented the capacity of SRL/azathioprine/prednisone or SRL/mycophenolate mofetil/prednisone to achieve similar 40% acute rejection rates as a cyclosporine/azathioprine/prednisone regimen but with somewhat improved renal function. Although the incidence and severity of infectious diseases was similar between SRL and control study groups, SRL displays myelodepressive and hyperlipidemic side effects. Although the former toxicities are generally reversible within 3 months posttransplant, hyperlipidemia, albeit at a level *below* the threshold definition of predisposition to arteriosclerotic complications (cholesterol, >240 mg/dl, and triglyceride, >400 mg/dl), may persist, leading to uncertainty concerning the long-term prognosis of patients. In the future, SRL is likely to be used in a variety of drug combination regimens, simultaneously and sequentially, to minimize early postretrieval renal injury, to avert acute rejection episodes and to forestall the chronic nephropathic process.

REFERENCES

Akselband, Y., Harding, M. W. and Nelson, P. A. (1991). Rapamycin inhibits spontaneous and fibroblast growth factor B-stimulated proliferation of endothelial cells and fibroblasts. *Transplant. Proc.* **23**, 2833.

Almond, P. S., Matas, A., Gillingham, K., et al. (1993). Risk factors for chronic rejection in renal allograft recipients. *Transplantation* **55**, 752.

Antzelevitch, C., Sun, Z. Q., Zhang, Z. Q., et al. (1996). Cellular and ionic mechanisms underlying erythromycin-induced long QT intervals and torsade de pointes. *J. Am. Coll. Cardiol.* **28**, 1836.

Brown, E. J., Albers, M. W., Shin, T. B., et al. (1994). A mammalian protein targeted by G1-arresting-rapamycin-receptor complex. *Nature* **369**, 756.

Brown, E. J., Beal, P. A., Keith, C. T., et al. (1995). Control of p70 s6 kinase by kinase activity of FRAP in vivo. *Nature* **377**, 441.

Calne, R. Y., Collier, D. S., Lim, S., et al. (1989). Rapamycin for immunosuppression in organ allografting. *Lancet* **2**, 227.

Chen, H., Qi, S., Xu, D., et al. (1998). Combined effect of rapamycin and FK506 in prolongation of small bowel graft survival in the mouse. *Transplant. Proc.* **30**, 2579.

DiJoseph, J. F., Sharma, R. N. and Chang, J. Y. (1992). The effect of rapamycin on kidney function in the Sprague-Dawley rat. *Transplantation* **53**, 507.

Dimeny, E., Fellstrom, B., Larsson, E., et al. (1993a). Hyperlipoproteinemia in renal transplant recipients: is there a linkage with chronic vascular rejection? *Transplant. Proc.* **25**, 2065.

Dimeny, E., Tufveson, G., Lithell, H., et al. (1993b). The influence of pretransplant lipoprotein abnormalities on the early results of renal transplantation. *Eur. J. Clin. Invest.* **23**, 572.

Drici, M. D., Knollmann, B. C., Wang, W. X., et al. (1998). Cardiac actions of erythromycin: influence of female sex. *J. A. M. A.* **280**, 1774.

Dumont, F. J., Melino, M. R., Staruch, M. J., et al. (1990). The immunosuppressive macrolides FK506 and rapamycin act as reciprocal antagonist in murine T cells. *J. Immunol.* **144**, 1418.

Eichenwald, H. F. (1986). Adverse reactions to erythromycin. *Pediatr. Infect. Dis.* **5**, 147.

Ferraresso, M., Tian, L., Ghobrial, R., et al. (1994). Rapamycin inhibits production of cytotoxic but not noncytotoxic antibodies and preferentially activates T helper 2 cells that mediate long-term survival of heart allografts in rats. *J. Immunol.* **153**, 3307.

Graves, L. M., Bornfeldt, K. E., Argast, G. M., et al. (1995). cAMP- and rapamycin-sensitive regulation of the association of eukaryotic initiation factor 4E and the translational regulator PHAS-I in aortic smooth muscle cells. *Proc. Natl. Acad. Sci. U. S. A.* **92**, 7222.

Gregory, C. R., Huang, X., Pratt, R. E., et al. (1995). Treatment with rapamycin and mycophenolic acid reduces arterial intimal thickening produced by mechanical injury and allows endothelial replacement. *Transplantation* **59**, 655.

Groth, C. G., Backman, L., Morales, J. M., et al. (1999). Sirolimus (rapamycin)-based therapy in human renal transplantation: similar efficacy and different toxicity compared with cyclosporine. *Transplantation* **67**, 1036.

Guelon, D., Bedock, B., Chartier, C., et al. (1986). QT prolongation and recurrent torsades de pointes during erythromycin lactobionate infusion. *Am. J. Cardiol.* **58**, 666.

Hebert, M. F., Roberts, J. P., Prueksaritanont, T., et al. (1992). Bioavailability of cyclosporine with concomitant rifampin administration is markedly less than predicted by hepatic enzyme induction. *Clin. Pharmacol. Ther.* **54**, 453.

Hodak, S. P., Moubarak, J. B., Rodriquez, I., et al. (1998). QT prolongation and near fatal cardiac arrhythmia after intravenous tacrolimus administration: a case report. *Transplantation* **66**, 535.

Hong, J. C. and Kahan, B. D. (1998). Two paradigms for new immunosuppressive strategies in organ transplantation. *Curr. Opin. Organ Transplant.* **3**, 175.

Hong, J. C. and Kahan, B. D. (1999). Use of anti-CD25 monoclonal antibody in combination with rapamycin to eliminate cyclosporine treatment during the induction phase of immunosuppression. *Transplantation* **68**, 701.

Johnson, M. C., So, S., Marsh, J. W., et al. (1992). QT prolongation and torsades de pointes after administration of FK506. *Transplantation* **53**, 929.

June, C. H., Ledbetter, J. A., Gilespie, M. M., et al. (1987). T-cell proliferation involving the CD28 pathway is associated with cyclosporine-resistant interleukin 2 gene expression. *Mol. Cell. Biol.* **7**, 4472.

Kahan, B. D. (1998a). Rapamycin: personal algorithms for use based on 250 treated renal allograft recipients. *Transplant. Proc.* **30**, 2185.

Kahan, B. D. (1998b). The role of rapamycin in chronic rejection prophylaxis: a theoretical consideration. *Graft* **1(Suppl. II)**, 93.

Kahan, B. D., for the Rapamune U.S. Study Group. (1998). A phase III comparative efficacy trial of Rapamune in renal allograft recipients. *Transplanation Society, XVII World Congress*, Montreal.

Kahan, B. D., for the Rapamune U.S. Study Group. (2000). Efficacy of sirolimus compared with azathioprine for reduction of acute renal allograft rejection: a randomized multicenter study. *Lancet* **356**, 194.

Kahan, B. D., Gibbons, S., Tejpal, N., et al. (1991). Synergistic interactions of cyclosporine and rapamycin to inhibit immune performances of normal human peripheral blood lymphocytes in vitro. *Transplantation* **51**, 232.

Kahan, B. D. and Grevel, J. (1988). Overview: optimization of cyclosporine therapy in renal transplantation by a pharmacokinetic strategy. *Transplantation* **46**, 631.

Kahan, B. D., Julian, B. A., Pescovitz, M. D., *et al.* (1999a). Sirolimus reduces the incidence of acute rejection episodes despite lower cyclosporine doses in Caucasian recipients of mismatched primary renal allografts: a phase II trial. *Transplantation* **68**, 1526.

Kahan, B. D., Mickey, R., Flechner, S. M., *et al.* (1987). Multivariate analysis of risk factors impacting on immediate and eventual cadaver allograft survival in cyclosporine-treated recipients. *Transplantation* **43**, 65.

Kahan, B. D., Podbielski, J., Napoli, K. L., *et al.* (1998a). Immunosuppressive effects and safety of a sirolimus/cyclosporine combination regimen for renal transplantation. *Transplantation* **66**, 1040.

Kahan, B. D., Podbielski, J. and Van Buren, C. T. (1998b). Rapamycin for refractory renal allograft rejection. *XVII Annual Meeting of the American Society of Transplant Physicians*, Chicago, Ill.

Kahan, B. D., Wong, R. L., Carter, C., *et al.* (1999b). A phase I study of a four-week course of the rapamycin analogue SDZ-RAD (RAD) in quiescent cyclosporine-prednisone-treated renal transplant recipients. *Transplantation* **68**, 1100.

Kaplan, B., Meier-Kriesche, H. U., Napoli, K. L., *et al.* (1998). The effects of relative timing of sirolimus and cyclosporine microemulsion formulation co-administration on the pharmacokinetics of each agent. *Clin. Pharmacol. Ther.* **63**, 48.

Kelly, P. A., Napoli, K. L., Dunne, C., *et al.* (1999). Conversion from liquid to solid sirolimus formulations in stable renal allograft transplant recipients. *Biopharm. Drug Dispos.* **20**, 249.

Knight, R., Ferraresso, M., Serino, F., *et al.* (1993). Low dose rapamycin potentiates the effects of subtherapeutic doses of cyclosporine to prolong renal allograft survival in the mongrel canine model. *Transplantation* **55**, 947.

Kuo, C. J., Chung, J., Fiorentino, D. F., *et al.* (1992). Rapamycin selectively inhibits interleukin-2 activation of p70 s6 kinase. *Nature* **358**, 70.

Lindholm, A. and Kahan, B. D. (1993). Influence of cyclosporine pharmacokinetics, trough concentrations, and AUC monitoring on outcome after kidney transplantation. *Clin. Pharmacol. Ther.* **54**, 205.

Lown, K. S., Mayo, R. R., Leichtman, A. B., *et al.* (1997). Role of intestinal P-glycoprotein (mdr1) in interpatient variation in the oral bioavailability of cyclosporine. *Clin. Pharmacol. Ther.* **62**, 248.

MacDonald, A. S., for the Rapamune Global Study Group (1998). A randomized, placebo-controlled trial of Rapamune in primary renal allograft recipients. *Transplantation Society XXVII World Congress*, Montreal.

Mahalati, K., McAlister, V., Peltikian, K., *et al.* (1999). A clinical pharmacokinetic study of tacrolimus and sirolimus combination immunosuppression. *18th Annual Scientific Meeting of the American Society of Transplantation*, Chicago, Ill.

Marx, S. O., Jayaraman, T., Go, L. O., *et al.* (1995). Rapamycin-FKBP inhibits cell cycle regulators of proliferation in vascular smooth muscle cells. *Circ. Res.* **76**, 412.

Meiser, B. M., Billingham, M. E. and Morris, R. E. (1991). Effects of cyclosporin, FK506, and rapamycin on graft-vessel disease. *Lancet* **338**, 1297.

Morris, R. E., Huang, X., Gregory, C. R., *et al.* (1995). Studies in experimental models of chronic rejection: use of rapamycin (sirolimus) and isoxazole derivatives (leflunomide and its analogue) for the suppression of graft vascular disease and obliterative bronchiolitis. *Transplant. Proc.* **27**, 2068.

Murgia, M. G., Jordan, S. and Kahan, B. D. (1996). The side effect profile of sirolimus: a phase I study in quiescent cyclosporine-prednisone-treated renal transplant patients. *Kidney Int.* **49**, 209.

Napoli, K. L. and Kahan, B. D. (1996). Routine clinical monitoring of sirolimus (rapamycin) whole-blood concentrations by HPLC with ultraviolet detection. *Clin. Chem.* **42**, 1943.

Napoli, K. L., Wang, M. E., Stepkowski, S. M., *et al.* (1998). Relative tissue distributions of cyclosporine and sirolimus after concomitant peroral administration to the rat: evidence for pharmacokinetic interactions. *Ther. Drug Monit.* **20**, 123.

Obata, T., Kashiwagi, A., Maegawa, H., *et al.* (1996). Insulin signaling and its regulation of system A amino acid uptake in cultured rat vascular smooth muscle cells. *Circ. Res.* **79**, 1167.

Pescovitz, M. D., Kahan, B. D., Julian, B., *et al.* (1997). Sirolimus (SRL) permits early steroid withdrawal from a triple therapy renal prophylaxis regimen. *XVI Annual Meeting of the American Society of Transplant Physicians*, Chicago, Ill.

Podder, H., Stepkowski, S. M., Napoli, K. L., *et al.* (1999). Sirolimus exacerbates cyclosporine-induced nephrotoxicity by raising cyclosporine blood trough levels, but does not impair renal function by a pharmacodynamic interaction. *XVIII Annual Scientific Meeting of the American Society of Transplantation*, Chicago, Ill.

Schmid, C., Heemann, U. and Tilney, N. L. (1997). Factors contributing to the development of chronic rejection in heterotopic rat heart transplantation. *Transplantation* **64**, 222.

Scott, P. H., Belham, C. M., Al-Hafidh, J., *et al.* (1996). Regulatory role for cAMP in phosphatidylinositol 3-kinase/p70 ribosomal S6 kinase-mediated DNA synthesis in platelet-derived-growth-factor-stimulated bovine airway smooth-muscle cells. *Biochem. J.* **318**, 965.

Simm, A., Nestler, M. and Hoppe, V. (1997). PDGF-AA: a potent mitogen for cardiac fibroblasts from adult rats. *J. Mol. Cell. Cardiol.* **29**, 357.

Slaton, J. W. and Kahan, B. D. (1996). Case report—sirolimus rescue therapy for refractory renal allograft rejection. *Transplantation* **61**, 977.

Stepkowski, S. M., Chen, H., Daloze, P., *et al.* (1991). Prolongation by rapamycin of heart, kidney, pancreas, and small bowel allograft survival in rats. *Transplant. Proc.* **23**, 507.

Stepkowski, S. M., Napoli, K. L., Wang, M. E., *et al.* (1996). Effects of the pharmacokinetic interaction between orally administered sirolimus and cyclosporine on the synergistic prolongation of heart allograft survival in rats. *Transplantation* **62**, 986.

Vincenti, F., Kirkman, R., Light, S., *et al.* (1998). Interleukin-2 receptor blockade with daclizumab to prevent acute rejection in renal transplantation. *N. Engl. J. Med.* **338**, 161.

Vu, M. D., Qi, S., Xu, D., *et al.* (1997). Tacrolimus (FK506) and sirolimus (rapamycin) in combination are not antagonistic but produce extended graft survival in cardiac transplantation in the rat. *Transplantation* **64**, 1853.

Vu, M. D., Qi, S., Xu, D., *et al.* (1998). Synergistic effects of mycophenolate mofetil and sirolimus in prevention of acute heart, pancreas, and kidney allograft rejection and in reversal of ongoing heart allograft rejection in the rat. *Transplantation* **66**, 1575.

Wacher, V. J., Wu, C. Y. and Benet, L. Z. (1995). Overlapping substrate specificities and tissue distribution of cytochrome P450 #A and P-glycoprotein: implications for drug delivery and activity in cancer chemotherapy. *Mol. Carcinog.* **13**, 129.

Yatscoff, R. W., Wang, P., Chan, K., *et al.* (1995). Rapamycin: distribution, pharmacokinetics, and therapeutic range investigations. *Ther. Drug Monit.* **17**, 666.

Zimmerman, J. and Kahan, B. D. (1997). Pharmacokinetics of sirolimus in stable renal transplant patients after multiple oral dose administration. *J. Clin. Pharmacol.* **37**, 405.

20

Antilymphocyte Globulin and Monoclonal Antibodies

Gregory A. Abrahamian • A. Benedict Cosimi

Introduction

Renal transplantation has become the treatment of choice for most patients with end-stage renal failure. Much of the success of kidney transplantation as well as liver, lung and heart transplantation has relied on the use of nonspecific immunosuppressive agents. However, the unpredictable control of the immune response provided by such nonspecific suppression and the consequences of lifelong administration continue to plague patients and practitioners.

Initial advances toward more selective control of the immune response occurred in 1967 with the introduction into clinical protocols of the polyclonal antilymphocyte preparations—antilymphocyte serum (ALS), antilymphoblast globulin (ALG) and antithymocyte globulin (ATG) (Starzl et al., 1967). The first trials using these preparations as part of induction or prophylactic immunosuppressive regimens were inconclusive. Subsequently, these agents were applied to the treatment of ongoing rejection in renal allograft recipients who were receiving conventional immunosuppression. This approach established the efficacy of antilymphocyte antibodies (Cosimi, 1981) and made available *triple-drug* therapeutic protocols, which could begin to provide acceptable survival rates for recipients of heart and liver allografts as well (Delmonico and Cosimi, 1988).

Despite the increased immunosuppressive specificity offered by the first antibody preparations, they continued to fall short of optimal selective suppression. Use of conventional techniques to immunize animals with T lymphocytes results in a polyclonal product containing a heterogeneous group of antibodies not only to most T-cell populations but also to B cells and nonlymphoid cells, together with many extraneous antibodies that reflect the individual animal's previous immunological activity. More specific antilymphocyte antibody preparations awaited the discovery of cell-hybridization techniques, which allowed the development of monoclonal antibodies (MAbs) to single-cell determinants (Kohler and Milstein, 1975). With MAb preparations directed at specific T-cell subsets, the therapeutic efficacy seen with polyclonal preparations could be maintained, while reducing greatly the administration of irrelevant proteins. The first agent applied clinically, OKT3, was a MAb reactive with a component of the antigen-recognition complex on T lymphocytes (T-cell receptor [TCR]). This MAb proved to be highly effective as treatment for steroid-resistant renal allograft rejection when it was introduced into clinical protocols in 1981 (Cosimi et al., 1981a). It was accepted quickly worldwide as the therapeutic agent of choice for severe renal, cardiac and hepatic allograft rejection (Cosimi et al., 1981a; Farges et al., 1992; Ortho Multicenter Transplant Study Group, 1985; Ponticelli et al., 1987; Robbins et al., 1992).

Despite the specificity of OKT3, it is a pan–T cell antibody and, similar to the polyclonal antilymphocyte preparations,

it affects all aspects of cell-mediated immunity. The ability to inhibit more selected cell populations in the effector pathway of rejection, while leaving the host's other immune pathways intact remained the goal of MAb development. Progress toward developing more selective suppression of the immune response has been slow, in part because of the complexity of the rejection reaction that must include alternate pathways that can mount an effective response successfully after known pathways have been selectively blocked (Baan et al., 1999).

Because the ideal MAb would affect only mechanisms involved in the rejection response, current agents are being designed to target molecules important for cytokine production or cell adhesion and costimulatory processes. As the complexities of the rejection response continue to unfold, further areas will be made available for exploration and potential targeting for MAbs. This chapter focuses on the preparation, mechanisms of action and clinical applications of the polyclonal and monoclonal antilymphocyte antibodies currently in clinical use and the newer agents under investigation.

Polyclonal Antilymphocyte Serum

PREPARATION

No tenets now exist dictating species selection for xenotypic antiserum production because the intensity of immune responses between different species is unpredictable. Within a species, the potency of antiserum obtained from individually immunized animals varies considerably. Pooling of preparations is recommended to achieve reasonable batch-to-batch consistency. On the basis of empirical considerations including cost, animal size and availability and efficacy of previously studied preparations, essentially all heterologous ALS used clinically is produced in horses or rabbits.

Cultured human lymphoblasts were the immunogen of choice for preparing ALG because these cells are free of contaminating blood cells or stromal elements that could induce unwanted antibodies and because they offer the advantages of reproducibility and ready availability; however, lymphoblasts have the disadvantage of being B cells rather than T cells. An immunogenic source of T cells, used for the preparation of ATG, may be obtained from human thymuses. Thymocytes obtained from cadaver donors or from patients undergoing cardiac surgery are reasonably free of contaminants. Lymphocyte membrane fractions also can be used to induce potent and relatively pure antiserum, requiring little absorption to remove antiplatelet and antierythrocyte antibodies.

After administration of the selected immunogen, serum is extracted from the animal (Fig. 20–1). The antiserum can be absorbed with platelets, erythrocytes and serum proteins to

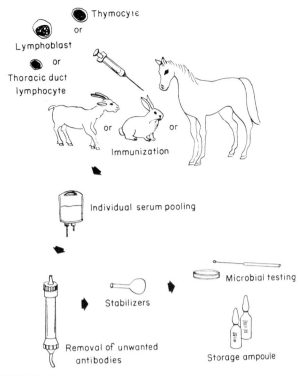

FIGURE 20-1

Basic method for preparing a polyclonal antiserum to human lymphocytes (ALS, ALG, ATG). The whole serum or the IgG fraction, containing multiple antibodies, is administered to patients.

remove contaminating antibodies. The resultant serum (ALS) can be administered without further purification (Niblack et al., 1987) or fractionated to obtain the immunosuppressive IgG component. Despite this extensive preparation process, greater than 95% of the final product consists of irrelevant horse or rabbit globulins, and it is estimated that only about 2% of the administered antibodies are specifically reactive with human T lymphocytes (Simpson and Monaco, 1995). Most clinically used preparations are prepared commercially, although some transplant centers prefer their own products (Hoitsma et al., 1985; Thomas et al., 1987). Generally the choice of the product to be used is based on local availability. Few controlled studies compared the different agents so that no standardized product has been defined as most efficacious. Antilymphocyte serum, ALG and ATG are described subsequently under the single rubric of ALS.

MECHANISM OF ACTION

The antigen specificity of various polyclonal preparations has been characterized (Bonnefoy-Berard et al., 1991; Bourdage and Hamlin, 1995; Rebellato et al., 1994). These studies reveal that antibodies in polyclonal ALS have varying specificities to common T-cell surface molecules. Most notably are antibodies directed against CD2, CD3, CD4, CD28 and TCR. Some preparations have significant reactivity against other leukocyte (CD20, CD40, CD16) and adhesion molecules (LFA-1, ICAM-1).

Considerable debate has persisted regarding the mechanism by which these preparations prolong graft survival. Absolute lymphopenia apparently is not necessary for immunosuppression, although prompt and sometimes profound lymphopenia usually follows the initial injections. Two possible mechanisms for this lymphopenia are complement-medi-

ated cell lysis and uptake by the reticuloendothelial system of opsonized T cells. Antilymphocyte serum apparently impairs the proliferative response of circulating T cells, and this impairment persists with cessation of treatment, when the number of circulating T cells gradually increases. This continued effect may result from the generation of nonspecific suppressor T cells; this has been shown in mouse (Maki et al., 1982) and monkey models (Thomas et al., 1982). Present evidence suggests that the initial interruption of cell-mediated graft destruction results from the elimination of T cells. Subsequent inhibition of proliferative responses may be maintained by nonspecific mechanisms, possibly including suppressor cells.

CLINICAL APPLICATIONS
Prophylactic Immunosuppression Using Antilymphocyte Serum

Before the introduction of cyclosporine, prospective controlled trials were conducted comparing azathioprine and steroids, with or without a 2- to 3-week ALS course beginning at the time of transplantation. This brief course of therapy typically delayed the onset of acute rejection and reduced the requirement for high-dosage steroids in the early postoperative period. Probably because of this lower steroid requirement, a significant decrease in the incidence of femoral avascular necrosis was noted in the ALS-treated group (Cosimi et al., 1976). A high incidence of rejection episodes occurred after ALS was stopped, however, and the improvement in long-term survival over that achieved in patients receiving azathioprine and prednisone without ALS often failed to reach statistical significance (Cosimi, 1981; Wechter et al., 1979). The multiple variables involved in such clinical trials and the difficulty in accruing enough patients to evaluate statistically differences in survival of only 10 to 15% were major factors leading to these inconclusive results (Howard et al., 1981; Streem et al., 1983). These variables continue to limit the usefulness of graft survival as a definitive endpoint for most trials of new immunosuppressive agents (Nashan et al., 1997; Vincenti et al., 1998).

The subsequent addition of cyclosporine to protocols based on azathioprine and steroids improved allograft survival in nearly all studies by an average of 17%, establishing cyclosporine as a key immunosuppressive agent (Stiller and Keown, 1984). Protocols combining ALS and subtherapeutic doses of cyclosporine greatly prolonged allograft survival, suggesting a synergistic interaction between the two agents (Homan et al., 1980). Initial clinical experience in patients receiving cyclosporine plus intensive conventional suppression revealed an unacceptably high incidence of lymphoproliferative disorders (Merion et al., 1984; Oyer et al., 1983), however, so that a general reluctance developed toward ALS administration to patients receiving cyclosporine.

Subsequent experience has indicated that prophylactic ALS in cyclosporine-based regimens may be efficacious, particularly for recipients of older donor kidneys, highly sensitized patients, retransplant recipients and patients with delayed graft function (Cecka et al., 1993; Cecka and Terasaki, 1991; Shield et al., 1997). The rationale is based on observations suggesting that irreversible allograft damage may develop if cyclosporine is administered when the allograft is recovering from preservation injury (Deierhoi et al., 1987; Sommer et al., 1987). These observations include reports of many of these allografts never functioning, in contrast to the typically temporary acute tubular necrosis observed in patients not treated with cyclosporine. Among cyclosporine-treated patients whose allografts do achieve function, the serum creatinine level usually remains higher in patients who had delayed graft function than in patients whose allografts never had acute tubular necrosis. Explanations for such irreversible renal damage include direct cyclosporine nephrotoxicity or unrecognized rejection that occurs during the sometimes prolonged period of initial nonfunction.

Because previous experience has emphasized that acute rejection seldom occurs while patients are receiving ALS, an approach in patients with delayed graft function is to use ALS without cyclosporine during the immediate posttransplant period. Such a strategy would eliminate the concerns regarding rejection and nephrotoxicity until baseline allograft function is established and cyclosporine can be added safely. Reports using such protocols have been encouraging, including significantly higher early posttransplant daily urine volumes, minimal increased risk of viral infections, rejection-free course in most patients and excellent long-term allograft survival (Stratta et al., 1989). The costs and potential risks of this approach have remained sources of concern to many centers, however, particularly because some studies failed to support the efficacy of such quadruple therapy (Michael et al., 1989; Slakey et al., 1993). The need for prophylactic ALS in cyclosporine-based regimens remains controversial, as it was during the azathioprine era (see also Chapter 16).

Particularly impressive results were reported from a trial comparing rabbit antithymocyte globulin (Thymoglobulin) with equine antithymocyte globulin (Atgam) for induction immunosuppression in renal allograft patients receiving cyclosporine maintenance therapy (Brennan et al., 1999). By 1 year after transplantation, 95% of the Thymoglobulin-treated patients and 75% of the Atgam-treated patients remained free of rejection.

Rejection Therapy Using Antilymphocyte Serum

The first randomized trial comparing ALS with high-dosage steroids for the treatment of established rejection was conducted in 1979 (Shield et al., 1979). All of the patients in that study were living related donor allograft recipients who had been treated with azathioprine and prednisone. Antilymphocyte serum proved to be as effective as high-dosage steroids with the added benefit of more rapid rejection reversal and fewer rerejection episodes. Further experience confirmed that a 1-year survival of greater than 90% could be achieved in recipients of haploidentical renal allografts treated for rejection with azathioprine, prednisone and ALS versus a survival of 74% in patients treated with steroids alone (Nelson et al., 1983).

In cyclosporine-treated renal allograft recipients, initial rejection therapy usually consists of high-dosage steroid boluses. If rejection persists, ALS therapy reverses 80% of the steroid-resistant rejection episodes (Benvenisty et al., 1987; Matas et al., 1986; Richardson et al., 1989), even in patients who had previously received ALS induction (Bock et al., 1995; Malinow et al., 1996). As discussed subsequently, the MAb OKT3 provides a possibly more reliable and clearly a more easily administered alternative therapy for steroid-resistant rejection. Nevertheless, ALS has remained since the 1960s a valuable option in rejection therapy, especially in patients who, because of previous MAb therapy, may not be candidates for a second course.

Thymoglobulin was compared with Atgam for the treatment of acute rejection after renal transplantation (Gaber et al., 1998). In a double-blind, randomized, multicenter clinical trial, Thymoglobulin had a significantly higher rejection reversal rate than Atgam (88% vs. 76%), and recurrent rejection occurred less frequently with Thymoglobulin (17%) compared with Atgam (36%) at 90 days after therapy. A similar

rate of 1-year patient and graft survival was observed, and there was no difference in adverse events in the two groups.

Tolerance Induction Using Antilymphocyte Serum

The feasibility of inducing allograft tolerance in adult recipients has been established in a number of experimental models, many of which have included ALS in the therapeutic protocol (Monaco and Wood, 1982). In an evolving series of murine models, highly specific unresponsiveness to donor antigens has been produced consistently using donor blood transfusions and ALS (Brent, 1981). Long-term renal allograft survival without the requirement for long-term immunosuppression has been extended to a nonhuman primate model (Thomas et al., 1983). With a brief course of posttransplant ALS therapy, donor bone marrow infusion and no further immunosuppression after day 5 posttransplant, these investigators achieved indefinite allograft survival in many recipients. On the basis of this extensive experience, a pilot trial in humans was undertaken in which 57 cadaveric renal allograft recipients received ALS followed by the transfusion of donor-specific bone marrow, and 54 similarly treated patients received the contralateral kidney without bone marrow transfusion (Barber et al., 1991). Both groups of patients received cyclosporine, azathioprine and prednisone. The allograft survival rates for the ALS-plus-bone marrow group were significantly improved at 12 months (90% vs. 71%). Although it was possible to withdraw steroids in many patients in the bone marrow group, no attempt was made to withdraw all immunosuppression as had been done in the nonhuman primate trial.

Data in fully major histocompatibility complex (MHC)–mismatched nonhuman primates showed that a state of multilineage hematologic mixed chimerism and donor-specific tolerance to renal allografts can be produced using a conditioning regimen that also includes ALS (Kawai et al., 1995; Kimikawa et al., 1997). In addition, a case was recently reported in which a patient with end-stage renal disease due to multiple myeloma underwent a nonmyeloablative preparative regimen, including ALS. A combined HLA matched bone marrow and renal transplant was then performed with the patient remaining clincally well and off all immunosuppression for over one year (Spitzer et al., 1999). These examples emphasize that tolerance induction in humans should be possible and that antilymphocyte antibodies probably would be a part of the initially applied conditioning regimens.

ADMINISTRATION

In general, the route of administration of polyclonal antilymphocyte preparations is relatively unimportant in determining the degree of suppression produced. Because local inflammatory reactions frequently result from subcutaneous or intramuscular injections, most clinicians prefer intravenous administration, which has the added advantages of allowing larger individual doses and presentation of the agent through a less immunogenic route. Because a painful chemical phlebitis may result from small peripheral vein administration, infusion of the agent into an arteriovenous fistula or a central venous catheter may be required but is not essential, depending on the source of the ALG.

Dilution of ALS in dextrose-containing or heparin-containing solutions may result in aggregation of the protein. It is usually administered in saline solution, at a concentration not exceeding 4 mg ml^{-1}. Rapid infusion may result in hypotension, whereas an unusually prolonged infusion at room temperature may be associated with antibody decomposition and aggregate formation. An in-line filter is recommended to prevent infusion of precipitates that may develop during storage. The dose depends on the source of the ALG and ranges from 1.5 mg kg^{-1} d^{-1} (Thymoglobulin) to 15 mg kg^{-1} d^{-1} (Atgam) infused over 4 to 6 hours. The duration of ALS therapy largely depends on center preference, generally ranging from 5 to 14 days.

MONITORING DURING ANTILYMPHOCYTE SERUM THERAPY

Because different ALS preparations as well as the same preparation in different patients have a varied immunosuppressive potency, attempts have been made to monitor the level of suppression that is being achieved (Cosimi et al., 1976). Monitoring T-cell numbers in peripheral blood with the use of MAbs is helpful in determining the appropriate dosage of ALS for individual patients and in predicting the likelihood of rejection resolution (Clark, 1996; Delmonico, 1984). Depression of CD3$^+$ cells (mature T lymphocytes) to less than 10% of pretreatment values generally has correlated with prompt clinical recovery. Some units repeat a dose of ALS only if the T-cell count rises above this level, which has significant cost implications. In contrast, persistent elevation of this cell population usually has been associated with unresolved rejection, requiring increased ALS doses or the addition of other immunosuppressants. Serial hematocrits and platelet counts should be monitored during therapy to avoid unacceptable anemia or thrombocytopenia resulting from antibodies to human erythrocytes and thrombocytes that contaminate most preparations. Dose adjustments of the administered ALS usually are effective in stabilizing any anemia or thrombocytopenia that may develop.

IMMUNOGENICITY OF POLYCLONAL ANTILYMPHOCYTE SERUM

After a course of therapy, serum antibodies to ALS can be detected in many patients (Niblack et al., 1987; Tatum et al., 1984). Such antibodies, if present in sufficient titer during therapy, could neutralize the beneficial effects of the agent and might explain why peripheral blood T cells are not depleted effectively in some patients. No consistent correlation has been shown between circulating levels of ALS and allograft survival, however.

Because one of the major concerns during therapy with a heterologous antiserum is the possibility of serum sickness, some units have recommended skin testing of patients who are to be treated or retreated with ALS to exclude the possibility of anaphylactic reactions (Bielory et al., 1988). Most clinicians have discontinued skin testing, however, because little correlation between skin reactivity and allergic reactions has been shown (Brooks et al., 1994). Anaphylactic reactions and serum sickness have been diagnosed infrequently. Many patients have been treated with ALS on repeated occasions without adverse effects. This lack of clinically relevant immune responses to the foreign protein presumably is due to multiple factors, including careful deaggregation of the products prepared for clinical infusion and the intravenous route of administration. Also important are the large doses employed, which should provide significant antigen excess and allow the development of only small, highly soluble complexes. Because these polyclonal antisera react with a variety of lymphocyte populations, the ALS presumably suppresses the immune response to itself as well.

TABLE 20–1

TABLE 20–1

SIDE EFFECTS OF ANTILYMPHOCYTE SERUM THERAPY IN RENAL ALLOGRAFT RECIPIENTS

Side Effect	Reported Incidence (%)
Chills, febrile reactions	75–80 with first infusion 5–10 with subsequent infusion
Erythema, pruritus	15–20
Thrombocytopenia	30–50
Local phlebitis	1–20
Serum sickness	0–20
Anaphylaxis	0–1

SIDE EFFECTS OF POLYCLONAL ANTILYMPHOCYTE SERUM

The incidence and severity of adverse clinical reactions after ALS administration varies with the preparation used. The most commonly reported side effects are listed in Table 20–1. Fever, often in association with significant chills, develops during the initial infusion in some patients. Because subsequent infusions usually are tolerated without incident, this reaction initially was presumed to result from pyrogen release during rapid lymphocytolysis and not from a hypersensitivity reaction to the foreign protein itself. More intensive evaluation of such *first-dose reactions* in recipients of polyclonal and monoclonal agents has indicated that increased serum cytokine levels, including tumor necrosis factor (TNF) and interleukin (IL)-6, as well as complement activation are correlated with side effects (Chatenoud et al., 1990; Debets et al., 1989; Vallhonrat et al., 1999). To limit the effects of this cytokine release, patients usually are premedicated with antipyretics, antihistamines and intravenous steroids before initiating ALS therapy. During ALS treatment, pruritic skin eruptions have been noted in 20% of recipients. Although this occurrence presumably represents some type of hypersensitivity to the agent, most patients can be continued successfully on the therapeutic protocol without development of more significant problems, particularly if antihistamines are administered for comfort.

Thrombocytopenia and/or anemia of varying severity has been reported in 50% of patients. This side effect generally is dose related, occurring in patients who require more than 12 to 15 mg kg^{-1} d^{-1} to depress adequately T-cell levels. A modest reduction in ALS dosage or further reduction in the concomitantly administered azathioprine or mycophenolate mofetil dose usually resolves this problem without the need for discontinuing ALS therapy. Although the thrombocytopenia presumably results from low levels of antiplatelet antibodies, reversible platelet aggregation within the pulmonary microcirculation in the absence of antiplatelet antibodies has been shown in dogs. These aggregates release vasoactive substances that could induce interstitial pooling and hypotensive reactions in the absence of hypersensitivity (Henricsson et al., 1977). Such a sequence of events could explain the hypotensive episodes sometimes seen after excessively rapid infusions of ALS.

Monoclonal Antibodies

As noted earlier, the production of polyclonal antilymphocyte preparations necessarily results in agents with lot-to-lot variation in potency and toxicity. These preparations react with many cell surface antigens and consequently preclude precise analysis and control of the immune response. In contrast, MAbs can be directed with exquisite selectivity against predetermined components of the immune system and can be produced uniformly in virtually unlimited quantity. They offer intriguing possibilities for the study and manipulation of immunological events occurring during rejection.

PREPARATION

The production of MAbs is based on two well-established observations. First, each B lymphocyte from an immunized animal produces a single specific antibody but has a short life span when cultured *ex vivo*; second, malignant myeloma cells can be grown permanently in culture but produce antibodies with no predefined specificity. The key breakthrough in MAb technology occurred when Kohler and Milstein (1975) succeeded in fusing both cell types, combining both essential properties: permanent growth and secretion of anti-

body with predefined specificity. Each fusion-derived hybridoma cell line secretes a MAb of known specificity plus the irrelevant myeloma protein.

The steps involved in producing antilymphocyte MAbs are depicted in Figure 20–2. Mice are primed and subsequently boosted with antigen in the form of T cells or membrane fragments. Isolated splenocytes from immunized animals are fused with mouse myeloma cells 4 to 6 weeks later. The hybridomas obtained are grown in media containing hypoxanthine, aminopterin and thymidine, which kill parental cells but allow hybrids to survive. The large numbers of growing hybrids are separated by random cloning. Only clones secreting the desired antibody are retained for *in vitro* or *in vivo* expansion. Typically the selected clones have been maintained by intraperitoneal passage in mice or by sequential tissue culture, from which large volumes of antibody-

FIGURE 20–2

Production of monoclonal antibodies. Fusion of a myeloma cell with a lymphocyte produces an immortal cell line that secretes a specific monoclonal antibody. This murine monoclonal antibody can be humanized with recombinant DNA technology.

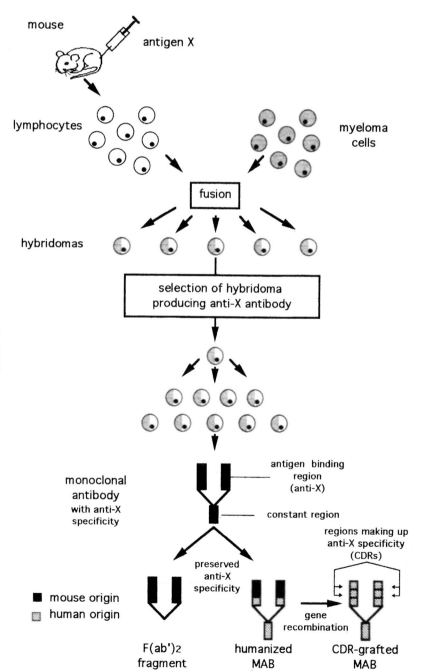

containing ascites or supernatant can be collected and puri-fied.

Human recipients of murine MAbs prepared by this tech-nique usually produce human antimouse antibodies (HAMA) (Chatenoud *et al.*, 1986). These HAMA cause rapid clearance of the murine antibody from the recipient's circula-tion, limiting the effectiveness of ongoing MAb treatment or precluding subsequent MAb administration (Schroeder *et al.*, 1990). One possible solution to this problem could be the use of F(ab')₂ fragments from MAbs (Hirsch *et al.*, 1990). Antilymphocyte antibody fragments generally have been found to be less immunosuppressive than the intact immuno-globulin. An alternative approach is to *humanize* the murine MAb. As a first step, the mouse variable region is joined to a human constant region. Then, using gene-recombinant techniques, this chimeric MAb is modified further so that only the essential antigen-combining sequences of mouse origin are retained (Boulianne *et al.*, 1984; Heinrich *et al.*, 1989). These segments, termed the *complementarity determin-ing regions* (CDRs), continue to confer antigenic specificity to the antibody. Because CDR-grafted antibodies differ from human immunoglobulins only at the epitope-combining site, however, the HAMA response to these agents seems to be reduced greatly and is predictably only antiidiotypic (Del-monico *et al.*, 1993). As a result, a therapeutic course of one humanized MAb should not prevent subsequent treatment with other MAbs bearing different idiotypes. Also, human-ized MAbs are less likely to induce the cytokine release syndrome described subsequently (Alegre *et al.*, 1994, 1995), and the effective half-life of the agent is greatly prolonged in the recipient's circulation (Vincenti *et al.*, 1997).

A further modification in the preparation of MAbs is the potential for constructing bispecific or trispecific MAbs. Such antibodies are secreted by fused hybridoma cells or are cre-ated by chemical cross-linking (Fanger *et al.*, 1991; Wong and Colvin, 1991). This technology creates MAbs that can bind several epitopes simultaneously and promote interactions be-tween the structures bearing these epitopes.

Through fusion technology, MAb immunoconjugates have been developed that exhibit potent immunosuppressive properties (Knechtle *et al.*, 1997; Mottram *et al.*, 1997). These conjugates allow precise delivery of drugs or toxins to target cells that have surface antigens reactive with the antibody portion of the therapeutic agent. Once antibody-antigen bind-ing occurs, internalization of the immunotoxin portion takes place by receptor-mediated endocytosis. The MAb immuno-conjugates tested in these studies have proved to be highly efficacious for inducing T-cell depletion.

MECHANISMS OF ACTION AND TARGET ANTIGENS OF MONOCLONAL ANTIBODIES

After being injected into the bloodstream, MAbs interact with the cell bearing the target antigen with several possible consequences, depending on the function of the antigen and the isotype of the MAb (Figs. 20–3 and 20–4). By a process termed *antigenic modulation* (see Fig. 20–3), some MAbs mod-ify the cell's antigenic characteristics or function without changing the total number of cells (Kerr and Atkins, 1989). Simple coating of the cell surface antigen also may occur, with no appreciable change in effector function (Jonker *et al.*, 1983). In other cases, the binding of a MAb may block interactions with other cells, cross-link different cells or trans-duce a signal to the cell, leading to its activation or inactiva-tion (Tite *et al.*, 1986; Wong *et al.*, 1990). Alternatively, cell death may result, particularly if a toxin has been conjugated to the MAb or if the Fc portion of a bound antibody triggers complement or effector leukocytes. Bispecific MAbs (Fanger *et al.*, 1991) can cross-link various cells, cytokines or toxins to redirect or amplify an immune response (see Fig. 20–4).

Target antigens for immunosuppressive MAbs typically are expressed on the surface of cells that are known to be involved in the immune response, particularly T cells. T cells are equipped with an array of cell surface molecules, some of which are illustrated in Figure 20–5, that mediate interactions between nonactivated T cells and antigen-presenting cells (APCs) or between cytotoxic T cells and their targets (e.g., allograft endothelium). These interactions, although incom-pletely understood, appear to be essential for sensitization and effector functions. Interference with the molecules medi-ating these interactions represents a logical approach to inter-rupting the immune response. Some of the molecules that

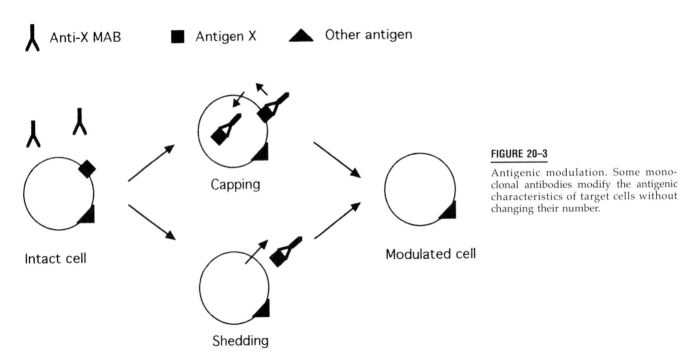

FIGURE 20–3

Antigenic modulation. Some mono-clonal antibodies modify the antigenic characteristics of target cells without changing their number.

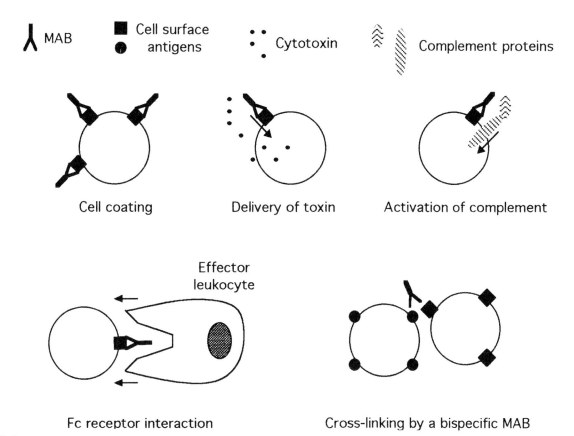

FIGURE 20–4

Mechanism of action of monoclonal antibodies. Depending on its isotype, a monoclonal antibody may coat the target cell, or it may activate complement or effector leukocytes, leading to cytolysis.

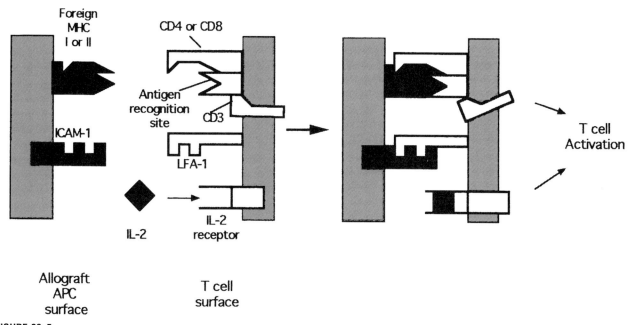

FIGURE 20–5

Some key surface antigens that are involved in interactions between T cells and antigen-presenting cells (APC) leading to T-cell activation.

TABLE 20–2

PROMISING TARGET ANTIGENS FOR MONOCLONAL ANTIBODY IMMUNOMODULATION

CD Antigen	Distribution	Ligand	Function
CD2	T and NK cells and thymocytes	CD58 (LFA-3)	Adhesion molecule, binding CD58
CD3	Mature T cells	MHC-peptide as part of TCR complex	Required for cell surface expression of and signal transduction by TCR
CD4	T cells (50–65%)	MHC class II	Coreceptor for MHC class II molecules
CD7	T cells, blasts	Unknown	T-cell proliferation
CD8	T cells (30–35%)	MHC class I	Coreceptor for MHC class I molecules
CD25	T, B and NK cells	IL-2	IL-2 ligation leading to T-cell proliferation
CD28/CTLA-4 (CD152)	T cells	CD80 (B7.1), CD86 (B7.2)	Activation of naive T cells, receptor for costimulatory signal
CD45	All leukocytes	CD22, galectin 1	Tyrosine phosphatase
CD52 (Campath-1)	Thymocytes, T cells, B cells, monocytes and granulocytes	Unknown	Unknown
CD54 (ICAM-1)	Endothelium, activated cells, B cells and dendritic cells	LFA-1, Mac-1	Leukocyte adhesion molecule, increased IL-12 production
CD154 (CD40L)	T and NK cells, basophils and monocytes	CD40	Costimulatory molecule
TCR	T cells	MHC class I or II	Antigen specificity

NK = natural killer; TCR = T-cell receptor; IL = interleukin.

already have been targeted effectively or appear to have significant clinical promise are listed in Table 20–2.

CD2

CD2, also known as the E-rosette receptor, T-11 or lymphocyte function antigen-2 (LFA-2), functions as an adhesion molecule to increase the sensitivity of antigen recognition by T cells. It is expressed on T cells, natural killer cells and thymocytes, and its ligand, CD58 (LFA-3), is expressed on APCs. Down-regulation of the CD2 receptor epitope has been shown to induce an anergic state (Boussiotis *et al.*, 1994), and CD2 inhibition has resulted in apoptosis of T cells (Rouleau *et al.*, 1994). Evaluation of the rat IgG2b anti-CD2 MAb, BTI-322 (formerly known as LO-CD2a), and its humanized IgG1 version, MEDI-507, revealed prolonged depletion of CD2 reactive cells when these agents were administered to chimpanzees. The antibodies are minimally mitogenic *in vitro*. Initial clinical evaluations of BTI-322 for induction therapy and treatment of acute rejection in cadaveric renal allografts or for graft-versus-host disease have been encouraging (Mourad *et al.*, 1997; Przepiorka *et al.*, 1998; Squifflet *et al.*, 1997). Clinical trials using MEDI-507 began in 1999.

CD3

A necessary step in the activation of T cells involves the recognition and binding of foreign antigen by the TCR. Closely linked to the antigenic recognition site of the TCR is a complex of three to seven subunits, designated *CD3*, that is present on essentially all mature T cells (Weiss, 1989a). Although the TCR engages its antigen outside the cell, the CD3 complex transduces an intracellular signal that is believed to be responsible for T-cell activation and up-regulation of IL-2 along with mitogenesis. OKT3, which has been the most widely used MAb in transplantation to date, targets this molecule (see later).

CD4

Other cell surface molecules define important subpopulations of T cells. CD4, in the past referred to as T4 or L3T4, is

a cell surface glycoprotein found on most mature thymocytes and about two thirds of peripheral T cells that bind MHC class II antigens. These cells were originally termed *helper* T cells. The molecule is believed to be necessary for alloactivation when MHC class II antigens are presented to CD4$^+$ T cells. As an accessory cell adhesion molecule, it stabilizes the interaction of the TCR-CD3 activation complex with the antigen–MHC class II complex. Many MAbs to CD4 have been tested; however, their clinical potential remains to be defined (see later).

CD5

Also known as Leu-1, T1 or Ly-1, CD5 is an adhesion molecule that binds to CD72 and apparently has a role in costimulatory signal transduction. It is expressed on thymocytes, T cells and a subset of B cells. Its importance remains unclear, however. XomaZyme-CD5 Plus (XomaZyme H65), a ricin-conjugated CD5 specific immunotoxin, has been evaluated in clinical trials to prevent graft-versus-host disease after bone marrow transplantation without any clear clinical benefit (Martin *et al.*, 1996).

CD6

The human CD6 is a cell surface glycoprotein expressed by thymocytes, mature T cells and a subset of B cells. CD6 has been shown to act as a costimulatory molecule that modulates TCR-mediated T-cell activation. Anti-CD6 MAbs inhibit the interaction of CD6 with a ligand named *activated leukocyte cell adhesion molecule* (ALCAM) (Starling *et al.*, 1996). Anti-T12, the only anti-CD6 MAb evaluated clinically, has not shown consistent efficacy (Kirkman *et al.*, 1983).

CD7

CD7 is a cell surface antigen present on pluripotential hematopoietic cells and T cells, whose expression is quantitatively increased on T-cell blasts such as those generated by alloactivation. CD7 has been thought to be an attractive target for MAb inhibition because of the possibility of removing donor-reactive T-cell blasts without removing resting cells from the circulation (see later).

CD8

Found on approximately one third of peripheral T cells, CD8 is a glycoprotein that binds MHC class I antigens. These lymphocytes also have been termed *cytotoxic* or *suppressor* T cells. CD8 is an important accessory molecule for antigen-dependent T-cell activation and probably functions to increase the affinity of T cells for their MHC class I–bearing target cells (Shevach, 1989). Anti-Leu2a, an MAb reactive with CD8, has been shown to deplete peripheral blood CD8$^+$ cells in humans; however, it had limited effects in reversing renal allograft rejection (Wee *et al.*, 1989). Another anti-CD8 MAb was shown to delay the onset of cardiac allograft vasculopathy in a large animal model (Allan *et al.*, 1997).

CD25

The significance of the cytokine IL-2 in rejection is highlighted by the potent effect of cyclosporine, which is thought to derive much of its immunosuppressive efficacy from the inhibition of IL-2 secretion. Interleukin-2, by reacting with its cell surface receptor, promotes T-cell differentiation and division, an early step in the rejection cascade. CD25, previously known as Tac or the IL-2 receptor, is found on activated T cells, B cells and monocytes. Three CD25 subunits are known: α (p45), β (p75), and γ (p64). The β and γ subunits have been given separate CD designations (CD122 and CD132); MAbs targeting the IL-2 receptor generally are referred to as anti-CD25 reagents. Many anti-CD25 MAbs have been developed, and two have been approved for clinical use (see later).

CD28

Present on T and B lymphocytes, CD28 is a receptor for costimulatory signals necessary for T-cell activation. It has two known ligands, CD80 (B7-1) and CD86 (B7-2), both of which are expressed on APCs. CTLA-4 (CD152) also is expressed on T cells and is structurally similar to CD28. It too binds CD80 and CD86; however, CTLA-4 transmits an inhibitory signal that acts to terminate the immune response (Walunas *et al.*, 1996). The recombinant fusion protein, CTLA-4-Ig, binds CD80 and CD86 and serves as a strong inhibitor of CD80/CD86:CD28-mediated T-cell costimulation (Linsley *et al.*, 1991). Rodent studies have shown that CTLA-4-Ig administration can prevent allograft rejection (Lenschow *et al.*, 1992; Turka *et al.*, 1992). Several trials using CTLA-4-Ig in primate models are currently under way.

CD52

The CD52 antigen (Campath-1) is a glycopeptide that is highly expressed on T and B lymphocytes and is coupled to the membrane by a glycosylphosphatidylinositol anchoring structure. The function of this antigen is unknown. Monoclonal antibodies to CD52 are efficient at mediating lymphocyte depletion *in vivo* through complement-mediated attack and antibody-dependent cellular cytotoxicity. In an unrandomized single-arm study, Campath-1H, a humanized anti-CD52 MAb, successfully reversed biopsy-proven rejection in renal transplant recipients (Friend *et al.*, 1995). The study was discontinued because of an unacceptable incidence of infection. In a small series of cadaveric renal transplant recipients receiving perioperative Campath-1H and low-dose cy-

closporine monotherapy, 12 of 13 patients were maintained successfully on only cyclosporine monotherapy for 11 months after surgery. Acute rejection occurred in only two patients and reversed with bolus steroid therapy (Calne *et al.*, 1998). A randomized trial is planned to compare this protocol with conventional therapy.

CD54

Another class of cell surface molecules, referred to as adhesion molecules, has a broad distribution among lymphocytes, granulocytes, monocytes and endothelium (Gahmberg *et al.*, 1990; Rothlein *et al.*, 1986; Springer *et al.*, 1987). These adhesion molecules promote optimal interactions between various cells. Included in this molecular class is LFA-1 (CD11a/CD18), expressed on all mature T cells. The major physiological ligand for LFA-1 is the intercellular adhesion molecule (ICAM-1 or CD54), present on APCs and endothelial cells.

The ICAM/LFA-1 system seems to recruit cells into areas of localized immune response. For instance, ICAM-1 appears in increased concentration on the endothelium of allografts undergoing rejection (Pober and Cotran, 1990; see Chapter 25). When this occurs, circulating leukocytes presumably adhere to allograft endothelium and migrate into the parenchyma, where they can amplify the rejection response. ICAM-1 also appears on the endothelium of organs during ischemia (Horgan *et al.*, 1991; Weiss, 1989b; see Chapter 25). The ICAM/LFA-1 system may play a role in the organ failure that sometimes follows ischemia secondary to shock or allograft preservation. Monoclonal antibodies targeting this interaction may be efficacious in limiting reperfusion injury as well as in prophylaxis and treatment of allograft rejection (see later).

CD154

Also known as CD40L (CD40 ligand), CD154 is the T-cell ligand for the CD40 complex on APCs. Two distinct signals are necessary for full T-cell activation (Janeway and Bottomly, 1994). The first signal is provided by the antigen itself and is responsible for the specificity of the immune response. The second signal, referred to as the *costimulatory signal*, is not antigen specific. In the absence of costimulatory signals, a T cell encountering an antigen undergoes abortive activation (Sayegh and Turka, 1998). The CD40/CD154 pathway has been defined as having a key role in T-cell activation (Durie *et al.*, 1994). Interaction of CD40 with its ligand leads to APC maturation, increased secretion of the inflammatory cytokine IL-2 and up-regulation of other costimulatory pathways including CD28/B7. The CD40/CD154 interaction also is important in B-cell activation, T cell–dependent macrophage activation and endothelial activation (Denton *et al.*, 1998). Short-term costimulatory blockade, using an anti-CD40L MAb, has been found to prolong heart and kidney allograft survival dramatically in nonhuman primates (Kirk *et al.*, 1997). A humanized MAb specific for CD154 (hu5C8), has provided longer renal allograft survival in nonhuman primates when administered intermittently over 5 months as the sole immunosuppressive therapy (Kirk *et al.*, 1999). Clinical trials have been suspended due to incidents involving thromboembolic events.

T-Cell Receptor

The TCR is a disulfide-bonded heterodimeric polypeptide that is part of a receptor complex on the cell membrane of T lymphocytes. The α and β heterodimers are expressed on most T cells (95%), and these cells respond to antigen in association with class I and class II MHC molecules. The remaining 5% of T cells express a γ/δ heterodimer whose function is unclear. The α and β chains are closely associated with the CD3 molecule, and given the dramatic immunosuppressive efficacy of the anti-CD3 MAb OKT3, anti-TCR MAbs could be useful clinically (see later).

Therapeutic Trials Using Monoclonal Antibodies

OKT3

The pan T-cell–reactive MAb OKT3 was selected for the first clinical trials because the efficacy of pan T-cell suppression for controlling rejection already had been shown in ALS trials, and the relative importance of various T-cell subpopulations was incompletely defined at the time (Cosimi et al., 1981b). In use since the 1980s, OKT3 remains the prototype MAb with proven efficacy, particularly for reversal of steroid-resistant rejection in every field of organ transplantation (Kreis et al., 1991), and remains the gold standard with which newer MAbs are compared for efficacy and toxicity.

Mechanism of Action

The OKT3 antibody is an IgG2a murine antibody that binds the epsilon portion of the human CD3 molecular complex on mature T lymphocytes. Cross-reactivity with other species is limited to chimpanzees. As a result, the in vivo evaluation of this MAb has been primarily in humans, in whom dramatic immunosuppressive effects have been observed (Cosimi et al., 1981a; Delmonico and Cosimi, 1988). Within minutes of the initial infusion, circulating T cells become essentially undetectable. This effect is exerted through opsonization with subsequent complement-mediated cytolysis or reticuloendothelial uptake and destruction of T cells. That this represents true T-cell depletion is confirmed by a fall in the total number of peripheral blood lymphocytes, a loss of reactivity with other T-cell markers and a lack of detectable cells coated with mouse immunoglobulin. After 3 to 5 days of therapy, T cells devoid of CD3 but expressing other cell surface markers (e.g., CD4, CD8) reappear in the circulation, indicating modulation of the CD3 antigen from the cell surface (see Fig. 20–3). Apparently the CD3-OKT3 complex is removed from the cell surface by endocytosis or by shedding (Chatenoud et al., 1990). Because the CD3 cell membrane site is a critical component of T cell–mediated cytotoxicity (Weiss, 1989a), cells denuded of CD3 are immunoincompetent.

The precise mechanism by which OKT3 produces rapid resolution of rejection is not entirely understood. Renal biopsy specimens after OKT3 treatment reveal varied depletion of CD3+ cells in allograft infiltrates, ranging from a few residual T cells to a substantial T-cell infiltrate despite the return of normal allograft function. Modulation of the CD3 antigen from these intragraft T cells is not as complete as that observed in the peripheral blood during OKT3 therapy (Kerr and Atkins, 1989). Persistence of allograft infiltrating T cells has not been found to correlate with an increased risk of recurrent rejection.

Clinical Applications

Rejection Therapy

The OKT3 antibody was evaluated first as treatment for established rejection at a time when azathioprine and steroids constituted the foundation of immunosuppressive induction

protocols (Cosimi et al., 1981a). The initial pilot trial showed that renal allograft rejection could be reversed with 1 to 2 mg of OKT3 administered daily. This observation led to the design of a multiinstitutional randomized study in which OKT3 was compared with conventional therapy for reversal of rejection. In this study, OKT3 reversed 94% of initial rejection episodes, in contrast to a reversal rate of approximately 70% in conventionally treated patients (Ortho Multicenter Transplant Study Group, 1985). This reversal rate resulted in significantly improved 1- and 2-year graft survival rates for the OKT3-treated population. Many subsequent reports confirmed the efficacy of OKT3 in reversing renal allograft rejection in patients on azathioprine and steroids (Goldstein, 1986; Thistlethwaite et al., 1984).

One limitation observed in these early trials was the frequent occurrence of subsequent rejection episodes (60–65% of patients), usually within the first 8 weeks after OKT3 had been discontinued. The introduction of cyclosporine partially addressed this limitation. In cyclosporine-based clinical protocols, 20 to 30% of renal allograft recipients required the addition of OKT3 if it was reserved for acute rejection unresponsive to two or three bolus doses of intravenous methylprednisolone (Delmonico and Cosimi, 1988; Thistlethwaite et al., 1987). The requirement for OKT3 has been further reduced to 10 to 20% of allograft recipients who receive induction therapy with mycophenolate mofetil and/or tacrolimus. In 80 to 85% of these patients, a 10-day course of OKT3 reverses the steroid-resistant rejection episode (Fig. 20–6). Recurrent rejection after OKT3 therapy is observed in 5 to 15% of these patients, compared with the greater than 60% incidence in patients that had been treated with azathioprine and steroids.

The dramatic efficacy of OKT3 when administered even later, as *rescue* therapy, has been confirmed in other studies. In a group of nearly 300 patients, treated by many different investigators, rejection that had failed to respond to cyclosporine, high-dose steroids and in many instances ALS was reversed in 65% of patients. Of these allografts, 56% that were at the point of abandonment under conventional therapy remained functional with a minimum of 6 months follow-up (Norman and Shield, 1986; Ponticelli et al., 1987). D'Alessan-

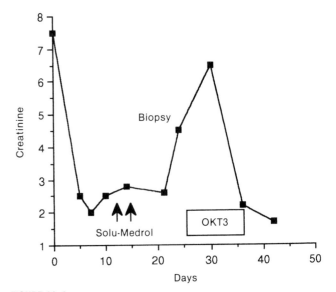

FIGURE 20–6

OKT3 treatment in a patient with acute rejection unresponsive to two high-dosage steroid boluses.

dro and colleagues extended the administration of OKT3 further to renal allograft recipients who experienced steroid-resistant or ALS-resistant rejection after a prophylactic regimen of prednisone, azathioprine, ALS and cyclosporine. Although OKT3 rescue was accomplished in nearly 83% of the recipients, recurrent rejection developed in more than 50% of these patients, and infectious complications were significant (D'Alessandro et al., 1989).

These observations document the potency of OKT3 therapy for reversing rejection; they also emphasize that excessive delay of OKT3 therapy is not advisable. The limitations of steroid treatment and the hazards of sequential courses of antilymphocyte antibody therapy are evident. Because of the well-established effectiveness of OKT3, most clinicians have advised limiting the administration of high-dose methylprednisolone to two or three doses. In patients with persistent rejection, OKT3 treatment is preferred to prolonged courses of steroid administration. Some centers advise earlier institution of OKT3 as a primary treatment approach for rejection (Tesi et al., 1993), especially in patients with evidence of more severe immunological injury on histopathological examination (Kamath et al., 1997).

Prophylactic Therapy

The dramatic success of OKT3 in treating already established rejection has prompted many prophylactic trials designed to prevent rejection. In an early randomized trial comparing OKT3 alone with azathioprine and steroids, the OKT3-treated patients were sensitized rapidly to the mouse antibody (Vigeral et al., 1986). Within 2 weeks of transplantation, all OKT3-treated patients developed acute rejection requiring the introduction of steroids. A subsequent randomized trial compared azathioprine and steroids with OKT3 administered in combination with these agents. This concomitant immunosuppression delayed the onset of HAMA production for 3 weeks (Debure et al., 1988). Fewer rejection episodes and a 2-year allograft survival of 89% were noted in the OKT3 group compared with only 70% in the control group. Because of the limited number of patients, this difference was not statistically significant. Others have evaluated the prophylactic use of OKT3 therapy (Norman et al., 1993). They similarly reported fewer episodes of acute rejection during the first month after transplantation. Nevertheless, acute rejection has been observed during or immediately after prophylactic OKT3 treatment (Haak et al., 1989). Because HAMA have usually developed in these patients, they are not candidates for OKT3 rescue, emphasizing a possible disadvantage of routine OKT3 prophylaxis.

For patients with acute tubular necrosis and delayed graft function, OKT3 prophylaxis may be indicated more clearly. This strategy can obviate the need for cyclosporine or tacrolimus administration at a time when the nephrotoxic effects of these agents may be synergistic with the ischemic damage. In a retrospective study of patients with acute tubular necrosis, OKT3 and cyclosporine induction were compared in combination with azathioprine and steroids (Benvenisty et al., 1990). OKT3 prophylaxis in these patients led to a significantly increased 1-year graft survival (80% vs. 55%), while markedly decreasing the incidence of rejection episodes (44% vs. 82%) and the duration of graft nonfunction (9.4 days vs. 14.9 days). In addition to avoiding cyclosporine nephrotoxicity, the benefit of OKT3 prophylaxis appeared to stem from the elimination of early rejection episodes that typically are difficult to diagnose in patients with an already poorly functioning allograft. Other investigators similarly have recommended the use of OKT3 rather than cyclosporine in patients with acute tubular necrosis (Kahana et al., 1990). Antilympho-

cyte serum prophylaxis, with OKT3 kept in reserve for severe rejection, is an alternative strategy in these patients.

Retreatment with OKT3

As noted earlier, approximately 5 to 15% of patients in whom rejection is reversed successfully by OKT3 experience subsequent allograft rejection episodes while being maintained on current cyclosporine-based or tacrolimus-based immunosuppressive protocols. The rerejection episode may be treated with methylprednisolone, another antilymphocyte preparation such as ALS or a second course of OKT3. The hazards of possibly fatal opportunistic infections or lymphoproliferative disorders greatly increase with sequential courses of antirejection therapy (Thistlethwaite et al., 1988). Dialysis, with possible subsequent retransplantation, often is the more prudent clinical plan for these renal allograft recipients.

Before retreatment with OKT3, the recipient's HAMA level should be assayed to rule out the presence of high titers of anti-OKT3 antibody (Legendre et al., 1992). Low levels of reactive endogenous antibodies to murine MAbs can be detected in a small proportion of individuals before initial therapy. Clinically evident reactions suggesting anaphylaxis have been unusual in these OKT3-treated allograft recipients, and the presence of these preexisting antibodies does not seem to alter the efficacy of therapy or predict the likelihood of subsequent rejection episodes (Jaffers et al., 1986).

Administration

A renal allograft biopsy is advisable before beginning OKT3 treatment to confirm the diagnosis of acute rejection and to exclude morphological changes associated with cyclosporine or tacrolimus toxicity (Stiller and Keown, 1984). OKT3 is administered by bolus intravenous infusion. Because a 1- to 5-mg dose generally is sufficient to saturate completely all the CD3 receptors of the targeted cell population, the typical adult dose is 5 mg d^{-1} (range, 1–15 mg d^{-1}). Once OKT3 therapy is begun, a 10- to 14-day course of daily intravenous injections usually is recommended. Initial response to therapy, indicated by stabilization of the serum creatinine level and a significant increase in urine output, commonly is observed within 4 days of starting OKT3 treatment. A return to the baseline serum creatinine level generally occurs within 7 days of the completion of OKT3 therapy, although patients have been reported to respond much later (Oh et al., 1988).

Just as cyclosporine nephrotoxicity may be synergistic with ischemic injury, it also may exacerbate the renal dysfunction associated with a rejection episode. In our initial OKT3 trials in cyclosporine-treated patients, the cyclosporine dose was maintained intentionally at the pre-OKT3 level. The mean creatinine level at completion of therapy in this group was 2.5 mg/dl, in contrast to our experience in azathioprine-treated recipients who routinely achieved a creatinine level of less than 2.0 mg/dl. This difference suggested that cyclosporine nephrotoxicity may have contributed to the allograft injury sustained during rejection (Delmonico et al., 1987). Consequently, we discontinued cyclosporine during OKT3 treatment in subsequent patients, an approach also adopted by other centers (Thistlethwaite et al., 1987). We concluded that low-dose cyclosporine (4–5 mg kg^{-1} d^{-1}) can be given safely during OKT3 therapy, and most groups now recommend that such low-dosage cyclosporine or tacrolimus be continued to limit the recipient's immune response to OKT3 and to reduce the incidence of recurrent rejection. Concomitantly administered azathioprine or mycophenolate mofetil dosages also should be reduced to limit the risks of viral infection and posttransplant lymphoproliferative disorder (PTLD).

Monitoring and Immune Response During OKT3 Therapy

Human antimouse antibodies frequently are detected in the recipient's serum after OKT3 treatment. In one large series, antibody formation after initial exposure to OKT3 occurred in 29% of patients (Schroeder et al., 1990). In the remaining patients, who were antibody negative after the first course of therapy, a similar fraction of patients (28%) made antibody after retreatment. Apparently the probability of HAMA response is relatively constant per exposure and is not influenced strongly by intrinsic differences in the patient's immune responsiveness (Colvin and Preffer, 1991). Concomitant immunosuppression does influence the likelihood of HAMA formation, which decreased from 36% in patients receiving double-drug immunosuppression to 21% in patients receiving triple-drug immunosuppression.

Two classes of anti-OKT3 antibodies have been identified (Chatenoud et al., 1986). The first type (antiisotypic) cross-reacts with all murine IgG2a immunoglobulins (Delmonico et al., 1989). These HAMA could interfere with subsequent therapy using OKT3 or any other IgG2a murine MAb. The second type (antiidiotypic) reacts specifically with the antigen-binding region of OKT3 and, if present in high titer, precludes another course of OKT3 but not of other murine MAbs (Legendre et al., 1992). As already mentioned, humanized MAbs may diminish the magnitude of the HAMA response.

In most patients, anti-OKT3 antibodies first become detectable 7 to 10 days after discontinuing therapy and do not interfere with the initial therapeutic effect. Occasionally the antibody response becomes detectable during the course of OKT3 therapy, resulting in prompt neutralization of the immunosuppressive effect and in resurgence of rejection activity. Because the development of HAMA is heralded by the reappearance of CD3$^+$ T cells in peripheral blood, flow cytometric monitoring is recommended every 3 to 4 days during OKT3 administration (Colvin and Preffer, 1991; Cosimi et al., 1981b; Hoffman and Hansen, 1981). A rise in detectable CD3$^+$ T cells may be overcome by increasing the OKT3 dose, reestablishing CD3 clearance and continued control of the rejection episode. It has been suggested that T-cell monitoring may be useful in predicting the likelihood of rejection after discontinuing OKT3 because correlation between early rejection and the rapidity of recovery of peripheral blood CD3$^+$ T-cell counts has been observed (Sheiner et al., 1997; Stephen et al., 1997). Because of the costs associated with sequential T-cell monitoring, some centers have adopted a routine escalating dose regimen to ensure adequate OKT3 serum levels without the need for frequent *in vitro* monitoring (Woodle et al., 1996).

Side Effects of OKT3

Nearly all patients develop an acute clinical syndrome after the first injection of OKT3 (Table 20–3). The reaction typically begins 45 to 60 minutes after the injection and lasts for several hours. It is manifested by chills, fever, diarrhea and occasionally chest tightness and wheezing. These symptoms are observed infrequently after subsequent doses, although diarrhea may persist for several days (Thistlethwaite et al., 1988). On rare occasions, a syndrome of aseptic meningitis has been noted in OKT3 recipients; the syndrome was

TABLE 20–3

SIDE EFFECTS OF OKT3 THERAPY IN RENAL ALLOGRAFT RECIPIENTS

Side Effect	Reported Incidence (%)
Chills, febrile reactions	70–75 (first infusion)
Nausea, vomiting	20 (first infusion)
Dyspnea, wheezing	15 (first infusion)
Diarrhea	20
Rash, pruritus	5

self-limited, whether OKT3 was discontinued or not (Martin et al., 1988).

Respiratory symptoms may be more severe for patients with nonfunctioning renal allografts and significant fluid retention. Pulmonary edema and cardiopulmonary arrests have been reported under these circumstances (Thistlethwaite et al., 1988). A chest radiograph and an accurate assessment of body weight and fluid status are recommended before instituting therapy.

As with ALS, these symptoms seldom occur with subsequent injections of OKT3. They were presumed to represent a physiological response to mediators released during the mitogenesis and lysis of T cells that occurs on initiation of therapy. Studies have confirmed that a massive and self-limited release of TNF, interferon-γ and other cytokines can be detected within hours of OKT3 administration. This mediator release coincides with the reversible acute clinical syndrome (Chatenoud et al., 1990; Gaston et al., 1991). Anti-TNF therapy with MAb or TNF-soluble receptors has been shown to decrease the severity of this syndrome (Charpentier et al., 1993; Eason et al., 1995). Corticosteroids, administered 15 to 60 minutes before OKT3 injection, also reduce the cytokine-release response (Chatenoud et al., 1991). It has been shown that complement activation fragments (C4d, Bb, iC3b and SC5b-9) also are rapidly produced *in vivo* after OKT3 administration, indicating that OKT3 activates the classic and alternative pathways of complement (Vallhonrat et al., 1999). These observations have led to the practice of routinely pretreating patients with steroids, antipyretic agents and antihistamines before the initial OKT3 infusion to limit the severity of the first-dose reactions (Shield et al., 1992).

The use of OKT3 has been reported to be associated with thrombosis in renal allografts during prophylactic therapy (Abramowicz et al., 1992). This complication could result from the procoagulant (endothelial activation) consequences of increased cytokine levels.

Antilymphocyte Serum Versus OKT3

Antilymphocyte serum and OKT3 are directed against T cells, admittedly with a differing degree of selectivity. Antilymphocyte serum products differ in terms of efficacy and side effects (Brennan et al., 1999; Gaber et al., 1998). Nevertheless, their uses overlap, and the preferred clinical indications for one versus the other remain controversial. Table 20–4 compares some of the important features that distinguish these two generations of antilymphocyte preparations. Generally, OKT3 administration is simpler and less expensive but has more pronounced side effects after the initial infusion. OKT3 appears to be more potent and reliable for treatment of acute rejection, as shown by its ability to rescue patients who failed to respond to ALS.

When used as prophylactic agents (Table 20–5), ALS and OKT3 have provided improved allograft survival in the subsets of recipients with increased risks of graft failure (Cecka

TABLE 20–4

COMPARISON OF ANTILYMPHOCYTE SERUM AND OKT3

	Antilymphocyte Serum	OKT3
Production	Cumbersome, small batches	Unlimited
Antibody content	Lot-to-lot variation of antibody classes, affinity and stability	Defined, homogeneous and reproducible
Cell target	T cells, B cells and platelets	Mature T cells
Reactivity	Multiple determinants (e.g., CD2, 3, 4, 8, 11), variable reactivity	CD3
Administration	Central (inpatient)	Peripheral (outpatient)
Typical dose/volume	1,000 mg/500 ml	5 mg/5 ml
Antibody formation	10–50% (second course frequently possible)	21–40% (second course frequently impossible)
Side effects	See Table 20–1	See Table 20–3

et al., 1993; Cecka and Terasaki, 1991). Antilymphocyte serum and OKT3 have virtually indistinguishable low rates of rejection and delayed graft function (Jonsson *et al.*, 1990). For example, a prospective randomized trial of ALS versus OKT3 prophylaxis resulted in comparable 1- and 2-year patient and graft survival rates (Frey *et al.*, 1992). In this study, ALS was associated with a significantly increased incidence of cytomegalovirus infections, whereas OKT3 was associated with more symptomatic side effects. Another prospective randomized trial comparing ALS and OKT3 in patients with acute tubular necrosis after cadaver donor renal transplantation revealed no statistically significant differences in graft survival, number of rejection episodes, time to first rejection or incidence of infections. OKT3 was associated with an increased incidence of side effects, such as hypotension and fever (Steinmuller *et al.*, 1991).

How does a clinician choose between ALS and OKT3? One approach is to use pharmacological therapy (cyclosporine or tacrolimus plus steroids) for baseline induction and maintenance immunosuppression. Only in renal recipients with delayed graft function is the introduction of cyclosporine or tacrolimus delayed in favor of ALS prophylaxis. This approach allows for subsequent rejection therapy with OKT3 if it is required. For initial acute rejection, two high-dose

steroid boluses are administered. If the rejection is not controlled, OKT3 therapy generally is begun. This approach takes into consideration the relative equivalence in prophylactic immunosuppression of pharmacological or antilymphocyte antibody induction therapy in patients with immediate allograft function, the apparent heightened susceptibility to cyclosporine or tacrolimus nephrotoxicity during periods of acute tubular necrosis and the greater reliability of OKT3 for treatment of acute rejection.

Infections and Malignancies with Antilymphocyte Preparations

Antilymphocyte preparations such as ALS and OKT3 as well as cyclosporine and tacrolimus, being T-cell reactive, tend to suppress cell-mediated immunity to viruses. The control of herpesvirus group infections, in particular, depends on cell-mediated immunity because these viruses spread only from cell to cell (Rubin and Tolkoff-Rubin, 1991). As a result, infections by these viruses frequently complicate pharmacological and antilymphocyte administration. Clinical presentation may range from annoying but usually controllable herpes simplex stomatitis to life-threatening leukopenia and pneumonitis of cytomegalovirus infections or Epstein-Barr virus–induced lymphoproliferative disorders.

Cytomegalovirus infections frequently complicated the early trials of ALS, until the importance of reducing concomitant immunosuppression was recognized (Rubin *et al.*, 1981). Important in determining the likelihood of this viral infection is the serological status of the donor and recipient. The risk is highest in a seronegative recipient of an allograft from a seropositive donor (58%), intermediate in a seropositive recipient (36%) and negligible when donor and recipient are seronegative (0%) (Hibberd *et al.*, 1992; see Chapter 31). Preemptive therapy using ganciclovir during the course of ALS treatment reduces the risk of disease in seropositive renal transplant recipients from 24% to 10% for induction and from 64% to 22% for antirejection therapy (Hibberd *et al.*, 1995). The risk of disease occurrence is reduced further when oral ganciclovir is administered for 3 to 4 months after preemptive intravenous therapy in seropositive patients (Turgeon *et al.*, 1998).

Latent Epstein-Barr virus is reactivated by antilymphocyte preparations, leading to the outgrowth of virally transformed

TABLE 20–5

PROPHYLACTIC ANTILYMPHOCYTE GLOBULIN OR OKT3 IN HIGH-RISK CADAVER RENAL ALLOGRAFT RECIPIENTS

	No ALS or OKT3		ALS or OKT3		
	% 1-Year Graft Survival	N	% 1-Year Graft Survival	N	*P* Value
First transplant	78	14,451	80	4,821	<0.001
DGF	64	3,694	70	1,185	<0.0001
Diabetic	76	2,831	80	1,026	<0.004
Donor age >55 years	68	922	76	357	0.006
CVA donor	74	4,056	78	1,406	<0.006
Retransplant	70	2,678	74	1,049	<0.006
DGF	53	965	60	386	<0.01
Diabetic	69	312	77	99	NS
Donor age >55 years	52	158	65	63	0.04
CVA donor	66	721	77	285	<0.001

ALS = antilymphocyte globulin; DGF = delayed graft function; CVA = cerebrovascular accident; NS = not significant.
Reproduced with permission of Cecka *et al.*, 1993.

B cells. These proliferating cells may then evolve from benign Epstein-Barr virus–dependent polyclonal B-cell lines to a malignant Epstein-Barr virus–independent monoclonal B-cell lymphoma (Malatack et al., 1991; Penn, 1994). The progression to lymphoma likely is related to the intensity of the immunosuppression, rather than specifically to the agent administered (Penn, 1990). For example, an increased incidence of lymphoproliferative disorders was noted retrospectively among 154 heart transplant patients after 2 weeks of OKT3 prophylaxis was introduced without reduction of concomitantly administered triple-drug therapy (Swinnen et al., 1990). In contrast, 1 month of OKT3 prophylaxis, in combination with azathioprine and steroids but without cyclosporine, did not result in any lymphomas in 150 renal transplant patients (Legendre, 1992).

These infectious complications emphasize the importance of decreasing the dosage of other immunosuppressive therapy administered during antilymphocyte therapy. We recommend at least a 50% reduction in the daily cyclosporine/tacrolimus and azathioprine/mycophenolate mofetil doses during the period of OKT3 or ALS administration.

ANTI-CD4 MONOCLONAL ANTIBODIES

A MAb targeting the CD4 T-cell subset should provide more selective immunosuppression than pan T-cell reactive MAbs (Wood et al., 1991; see Chapter 23). Because the activity of CD4-bearing T cells is most crucial during the initial stages of alloactivation when presentation of MHC class II alloantigen releases cytokines that amplify the rejection process (Delmonico and Cosimi, 1996), anti-CD4 MAbs should be predicted to be most effective if administered before or at the time of antigen presentation (Sablinski et al., 1992). These expectations have been confirmed by striking results obtained in experimental models. The anti-CD4 MAbs have provided not only significant prolongation, but also donor-specific tolerance of foreign tissues in rodents treated with antibody before transplantation (Madsen et al., 1987; Sablinski et al., 1991; Shizuru et al., 1990). These encouraging observations suggest that interference with the normal function of CD4+ T cells at the time of initial antigen processing could provide an approach to developing clinical protocols of donor-specific unresponsiveness.

Mechanism of Action

Monoclonal antibodies targeting CD4 may be classified as depleting or nondepleting based on their effect on peripheral blood CD4+ cell numbers. Depleting antibodies exert their effect by complement activation through the Fc portion of the molecule with resultant target cell lysis (Delmonico and Cosimi, 1996; Sablinski et al., 1991). The depletion of CD4+ cells in peripheral blood and graft infiltrates has correlated in most experimental models with the immunosuppressive activity of these antibodies. Rejection has been observed to occur promptly on the return of CD4+ cells to the circulation. A disadvantage of depleting antibodies can be the longevity of their effects. Peripheral blood CD4+ cell counts may remain depressed for 6 months after treatment in nonhuman primates (Powelson et al., 1994), and similar results have been reported in patients with depletion persisting for 2 years in one case (Horneff et al., 1991).

Nondepleting anti-CD4 MAbs may exert their effect through CD4 blockade or modulation. CD4 blockade may result from interference with interactions between CD4 and MHC or between CD4 and the TCR-CD3 complex. This interference might prevent the CD4 molecule from contributing to T-cell activation. It also is possible that CD4 bound by

MAb may transduce a negative signal to the T cell, suppressing its activation (Darby et al., 1994). Modulation presumably removes any contribution of the CD4 molecule to T-cell activation as an adhesion molecule or as a signal-transducing molecule. This modulation can lead to a significant delay of rejection in rats (Lehmann et al., 1992). Similarly, modulation of the CD4 molecule in monkeys was associated with prolonged renal allograft survival. In these animals, intragraft cells were found to be unresponsive to IL-2, suggesting that CD4 modulation prevents T-cell sensitization in the absence of depletion (Wee et al., 1992).

Preclinical Studies

Studies in nonhuman primate kidney allograft recipients have evaluated OKT4a, a murine IgG2a anti-CD4 MAb (Cosimi et al., 1990b). A single dose of 1 mg kg^{-1}, administered on the day of transplantation without any further immunosuppression, resulted in a mean allograft survival of 39 days versus 8 days in control animals. There was minimal depletion of peripheral blood CD4+ cells, suggesting that OKT4a, binding to the CD4 receptor, involved antigenic modulation with interference of signal transduction, blocking of the MHC class II–CD4 interaction, or suppressor cell induction.

Although no immune response to the administered anti-CD4 MAb was detected in rats, all monkey recipients of the murine OKT4a developed monkey antimouse antibodies (MAMA). In an attempt to limit this response, humanized versions of OKT4a were developed. Two CDR-grafted OKT4a MAbs were evaluated. A single intravenous injection of these humanized preparations extended renal allograft survival to 8 weeks, and the only MAMA response detected was idiotype specific (Powelson et al., 1994). This situation may explain why therapeutic serum levels of the humanized preparations were detectable for 24 days, in contrast to murine OKT4a serum levels, which routinely disappeared after 10 days. It is speculated that low-affinity antiidiotypic MAMA clear the MAb less efficiently than antiisotypic MAMA, resulting in prolonged therapeutic serum levels and immunosuppressive efficacy. The CDR-grafted MAb with the IgG1 isotype caused peripheral blood CD4+ cell depletion, a phenomenon not observed with the IgG4 isotype. This phenomenon presumably is related to the fact that human IgG1 antibodies activate complement, with resultant target cell lysis, whereas IgG4 antibodies do not (Greenwood et al., 1993).

Clinical Studies

Clinical trials using anti-CD4 MAbs have been conducted mostly in cadaveric renal allograft recipients. The murine preparation, OKT4a, has had variable efficacy as an induction immunosuppressive agent. Limited clinical trials revealed that this MAb was well tolerated, a HAMA response occurred in 82% of recipients and only 26% of patients suffered rejection episodes during the first 3 postoperative months (Delmonico and Cosimi, 1996). In a subsequent trial evaluating the CDR-grafted OKT4A (OKTcdr4a), biopsy-proven rejection episodes were observed in 18% of renal allograft recipients. No graft failures or antibody responses were observed in the recipients of this Mab; however, the dose used was insufficient to prevent rejection. Two other murine anti-CD4 MAbs of the IgG2a isotype, designated BL4 and MT151, have been evaluated in renal allograft recipients. These patients had a high incidence of early rejection (Land, 1991). A pilot study using B-F5, a murine IgG1 anti-CD4 MAb, reported a strong depleting effect on the CD4+ cell count with saturation of the remaining circulating CD4+ cells by the MAb. Of the patients, 50% had an acute rejection episode within the first 3 postoperative months, however (Dantal et al., 1996). The chimeric anti-CD4 MAb, cMT-412, has been evaluated in conjunction with cyclosporine-based triple-drug induction therapy in heart transplant recipients (Meisner et al., 1994). This antibody is a combination of the CD4-reactive murine hypervariable regions with human IgG1 constant region. The MAb-treated patients had less frequent and markedly delayed rejection episodes, fewer infectious complications despite long-lasting T-cell depletion and better overall survival than that observed in the ATG-treated control group. The HAMA response still occurred in 64% of patients despite the humanization of the MAb. These observations have stimulated continued clinical investigations of cMT-412.

There have been limited clinical trials using anti-CD4 MAbs for reversal of established renal allograft rejection. The anti-CD4 MAb, Max.16H5, initially was found to be effective in patients with rheumatoid arthritis (Horneff et al., 1991). In renal allograft recipients suffering late-onset rejection, Max.16H5 significantly depleted CD4$^+$ T cells (Reinke et al., 1995). Improved allograft function and clearing of the histopathological features of rejection were observed in most treated patients. Neither antiisotype nor antiidiotype antibodies to Max.16H5 were detected in any of the recipients. Despite these results, further trials using anti-CD4 MAbs for rejection have not yet been reported.

ANTI-CD7 MONOCLONAL ANTIBODY

CD7 MAbs inhibit T-cell proliferation in the allogeneic mixed lymphocyte reaction. The anti-CD7 MAb, SDZCHH380, produced through recombinant DNA techniques, is composed of human IgG1 and retains the parental murine hypervariable regions that determine the binding specificity (Lazarovits et al., 1993). A prospective randomized trial comparing SDZCHH380 with OKT3 induction in conjunction with cyclosporine-based immunosuppression was performed in renal allograft recipients. The SDZCHH380 was well tolerated, and the time to first rejection was comparable in both groups. No patients were sensitized to the SDZCHH380, in contrast to the 70% of OKT3 recipients with a HAMA response. Long-term analysis beyond 4 years has noted good allograft survival in the SDZCHH380-treated patients (Sharma et al., 1997). No further trials have yet been reported.

ANTI-CD25 (IL2-RECEPTOR) MONOCLONAL ANTIBODIES

Because the interaction between IL-2 and its receptor (CD25) is required for the generation of cytotoxic T cells and for T-cell proliferation, MAbs that interfere with this process should selectively suppress activated cells, such as those responding to an allograft (see Chapter 2). The validity of this hypothesis has been established in some mouse-strain combinations in which anti-CD25 MAb provides indefinite survival of vascularized heart transplants (Kupiec-Weglinski et al., 1988; Tellides et al., 1989).

ANTI-CD25 REJECTION PROPHYLAXIS

In human renal allograft recipients, the murine anti-Tac MAb in combination with cyclosporine, azathioprine and prednisone modestly delayed the onset of first rejection, but long-term functional results were similar to those in the control group (Kirkman et al., 1991). Two rat MAbs, 33B3.1 (Soulillou et al., 1990) and LO-Tact-1 (Hiesse et al., 1991), also have been studied in renal allograft recipients. These MAbs

are directed against the p55 chain, present on the low-affinity and the more important high-affinity forms of the IL-2 receptor (Gillis, 1989). In both trials, the investigators concluded that these anti-CD25 MAbs had comparable effects to ALS.

The murine anti-CD25 MAb, BT563, has been studied extensively and evaluated in randomized trials in kidney (van Gelder et al., 1995), liver (Langrehr et al., 1997; Nashan et al., 1996) and heart (van Gelder et al., 1996) allograft recipients. The incidence of rejection was reduced in the kidney and liver trials, although no significant improvement in allograft or patient survival was achieved. In the heart allograft trial, the frequency of rejection was similar in patients treated with BT563 or OKT3, but rejection occurred earlier in the BT563-treated group, suggesting that cytokines other than IL-2 may mediate early antidonor responses (Baan et al., 1999).

The varying results observed in these different trials may be due to two major limitations of rat MAbs. First, their immunogenicity and short circulating half-life may not induce adequate periods of immunosuppression. Second, because of their murine or rat structure, the MAbs are less effective than human antibodies in recruiting immune effector functions. Through genetic engineering, humanized and chimeric anti-CD25 MAbs have now been prepared. The chimeric anti-CD25 MAb, basiliximab, bears the murine variable region and human IgG1 constant region. The initial phase I/II trials in renal transplantation showed that basiliximab was well tolerated and had a prolonged serum half-life of 1 to 2 weeks with minimal immunogenicity (Amlot et al., 1995; Kovarik et al., 1997). A double-blind, placebo-controlled phase III trial (Kahan et al., 1999) reported that basiliximab in combination with cyclosporine and steroids reduced the proportion of patients who experienced biopsy-proven rejection by 28% (35.3% vs. 49.1%). Therapy was well tolerated, and adverse events were similar to the control group, who received only cyclosporine and steroids. These findings were similar to those observed in an earlier study by the CHIB201 International Study Group (Nashan et al., 1997). Similarly, daclizumab, a humanized anti-CD25 MAb, has a longer half-life and is less immunogenic than its murine parent antibody (anti-Tac) (Vincenti et al., 1997). The phase III clinical trial comparing five doses of daclizumab with placebo in a background of cyclosporine and steroid immunosuppression has been reported (Nashan et al., 1999). Biopsy-proven rejection occurred in 28% of the daclizumab-treated group compared with 47% in the placebo group. The need for subsequent treatment with antilymphocyte therapy was reduced, as was the development of infectious complications in the daclizumab group. In the setting of triple-drug therapy using cyclosporine, azathioprine and steroids, the addition of daclizumab reduced the incidence of biopsy-proven rejection from 35% to 22% (Vincenti et al., 1998). Both of these agents have received U.S. Food and Drug Administration approval for clinical use in renal transplant recipients.

ANTI-CD54 AND OTHER ADHESION MOLECULE MONOCLONAL ANTIBODIES

In addition to the specific interaction between foreign antigen and the TCR complex, several antigen-nonspecific accessory molecules promote attachment of T cells to their targets or APCs. LFA-1 (CD11a/CD18) and ICAM-1 (CD54) form one such critical adhesive receptor-ligand pair (see Fig. 20–5). As previously mentioned, these molecules may play a role in the progression of the reperfusion injury that sometimes follows an ischemic insult. As a barrier between blood and parenchyma, the endothelium is well positioned to regulate cellular migration from the circulation into tissues (Pober and Cotran, 1990).

Cell surface adhesion molecules have been grouped into three classes: selectins, integrins and immunoglobulins. Selectins are small glycoproteins expressed on activated endothelium, platelets or leukocytes and mediate the initial weak binding between endothelial cells and leukocytes. Selectin binding sets the stage for stronger binding by other adhesion molecules (Heeman et al., 1994). Integrins are larger molecules composed of two noncovalently linked polypeptide chains, each of which has a CD designation. Integrins span the cellular membrane and are well adapted to coordinate extracellular contacts with intracellular events (Heeman et al., 1994). The integrin LFA-1 (CD11a/CD18) is the ligand for CD54. The immunoglobulin supergene family includes the intercellular adhesion molecules (ICAM-1 or CD54, ICAM-2 and ICAM-3). Adhesion molecules in this family bind integrins or other members of the immunoglobulin family (TCR, MHC class I and II, CD3, CD4 and CD8). LFA-1 and CD54 have been of interest as possible targets for MAb therapy.

PRECLINICAL STUDIES

Antiadhesion molecule MAbs have been remarkably effective in some rat models targeting LFA-1 and CD54 (Isobe et al., 1992) or LFA-2 (CD2) and its ligand CD48 (Qin et al., 1994). BIRR1, an anti-CD54 murine MAb, was studied in monkey recipients of renal allografts (Cosimi et al., 1990a). A 12-day course of BIRR1 as the sole immunosuppressant administered to these monkeys led to significantly prolonged graft survival (24.2 vs. 9.2 days; P<0.001). Similar prolongation of skin allograft survival was observed in monkeys treated with anti-LFA-1 MAb (Berlin et al., 1992). An alternative approach to interruption of adhesion molecule interactions has been reported in which an entirely human fusion protein rather than the MAb was administered to monkey allograft recipients with encouraging prolongation of allograft survival (Kaplon et al., 1996). The mechanism of action involved in the anti-CD54-mediated immunosuppression appears to be through inhibition of ICAM-1-mediated functions, including antigen-independent interactions necessary for leukocyte adhesion and recruitment, as well as antigen-dependent functions, such as MHC peptide presentation and effector cytotoxicity (Adams, 1995).

Of potential relevance for recipients, particularly of cadaveric donor organs, has been the observation that reperfusion injury also is attenuated by therapies targeting these adhesion molecules (Byrne et al., 1992, 1993; DeMeester et al., 1996; Dragun et al., 1998; Kelly et al., 1994). Ischemia activates endothelium, resulting in adhesion molecule up-regulation. This up-regulation causes circulating neutrophils to adhere to vascular endothelium and infiltrate the reperfused ischemic tissue. There, they release toxic proteases and reactive oxygen metabolites resulting in damage to ischemic organs. Apparently this process can be inhibited by antiadhesion molecule therapy.

ANTI-CD54 REJECTION PROPHYLAXIS

A phase I clinical trial was undertaken using BIRR1 in cadaver donor renal allograft recipients (Haug et al., 1993). Because of the suggestive evidence that this MAb might be useful in limiting reperfusion injury, the initial trial selected recipients at high risk for delayed graft function. After 3 years' follow-up, 14 of 18 allografts (78%) continued with good-to-excellent function. The high-risk nature of the allograft donors in this trial was confirmed by the fate of the contralateral donor organs, which were transplanted into conventionally treated patients. Three of these were lost to primary nonfunction, and one was discarded because of con-

cern regarding the preservation history; overall contralateral allograft survival at 3 years was 50%. Subsequently a randomized multicenter trial in cadaveric renal transplantation was conducted in Europe. Enlimomab (BIRR1) or placebo was administered to 262 recipients for 6 days along with triple immunosuppressive therapy. No significant difference in the incidence of first acute rejection between the enlimomab-treated group (39%) and placebo group (45%) was found in this trial. Enlimomab did not reduce the incidence of delayed graft function, and both groups had equivalent patient and graft survival at 1 year (Salmela et al., 1999).

Clinical trials of MAbs targeting LFA-1, the ligand for the CD54 molecule, also have been undertaken. A randomized, multicenter trial compared an anti-LFA-1 MAb (odulimomab) with rabbit ATG as induction treatment in kidney transplant recipients. The incidence and severity of rejection as well as 1-year graft function were comparable between the two groups (Hourmant et al., 1996). A single report using an anti-LFA-1 MAb to treat established acute rejection in renal transplant recipients found this antibody to be ineffective in reversing rejection (Le Mauff et al., 1991).

ANTI–T CELL RECEPTOR MONOCLONAL ANTIBODY

The TCR, being essential for antigen recognition that, in conjunction with costimulatory signals, leads to T-cell activation, is an attractive target for immunomodulation. The MAb, T10B9.1A-31 (T10B9), is a murine IgM reactive with the α/β chain of the TCR. Approximately 99% of mature CD3+ cells are lysed in vitro by T10B9. This MAb is not mitogenic and does not induce the first-dose reactions associated with cytokine release (Brown et al., 1996). T10B9 has been evaluated in a prospective randomized trial of renal allograft recipients, comparing it with OKT3 for treatment of acute rejection (Waid et al., 1997a). Therapy with one of the MAbs was initiated after acute rejection occurred. Graft survival in both groups was excellent with a trend toward improved long-term survival in the T10B9-treated group. Recurrent rejection and the requirement for crossover to the other agent were similar in both groups. The incidence and severity of the first-dose symptoms were decreased in the T10B9-treated group, in association with lower TNF and interferon plasma levels in these patients. There was no significant difference in the incidence of infectious complications between the two treatment groups. The development of a HAMA response was similar in the two groups; however, there was no cross-reactivity of the HAMA of one MAb with those produced in response to treatment by the other MAb. An alternative therapy would be available should the first MAb fail or rerejection develop. A phase I study comparing T10B9 with OKT3 for induction immunosuppression in heart transplantation revealed no rejection during induction therapy with T10B9 (Waid et al., 1997b). One patient who developed rejection on OKT3 had the rejection reversed with T10B9 treatment. These results have been encouraging and have prompted further investigations.

Conclusion

New and more specific immunosuppressive agents have improved the 1-year survival of transplanted kidneys to the 85 to 95% range, depending on the selection of recipients. With the current availability of cyclosporine, tacrolimus, mycophenolate mofetil, ALS, OKT3, basiliximab and daclizumab, clinicians can devise multifaceted strategies, providing reliable prophylaxis and treatment of acute rejection, while limiting the nephrotoxicity of cyclosporine and tacrolimus in allografts with delayed function. A newer pan T-cell MAb, T10B9.1A-31, could provide more flexible immunosuppressive strategies because it could be used in patients who fail to respond to, or have been previously sensitized to, OKT3. It has not yet been approved for clinical use, however.

Despite these advances, it is evident that ALS, OKT3 and other pan T-cell MAbs do not lead to donor-specific tolerance, at least during the treatment of active rejection. These agents may result in prohibitive toxicity if indiscriminately combined with other immunosuppressive agents. The successful clinical application of OKT3 and more recently the anti-CD25 preparations has emphasized that MAbs are a potentially unique solution to many of the limitations of conventional immunosuppression. It is now possible to design rationally MAbs to components of the T-cell surface, rather than rely on serendipity for the discovery of new immunosuppressive agents.

There is much current interest in immunotoxin conjugates of MAbs (Ghetie and Vitetta 1994; Knechtle *et al.*, 1997; Thomas *et al.*, 1997) and in MAbs targeting costimulatory molecules, such as CD28 and CD154, because the accessory signals provided by these molecules are essential for immune activation (Eck *et al.*, 1997; Kirk *et al.*, 1999; Lenschow *et al.*, 1995). Based on the observation of graft survival after withdrawal of therapy with such agents in preclinical models, one anticipates that these MAbs may soon play an important role in clinical protocols.

One of the more promising additions to MAb technology is the recombinant DNA technology used to humanize murine or rat preparations. With these methods, novel antibody molecules that retain only short sequences from the rat variable region can now be constructed. Clinical trials suggest that these designer molecules are less immunogenic and that they can recruit more effectively, *in vivo*, the immune mechanisms necessary for lasting suppression. The development of these new molecular agents, more effectively directed to specific cellular targets, should play an increasingly important role in future clinical protocols and perhaps finally provide a means to achieve long-term tolerance in human transplant recipients.

References

Abramowicz, D., Pradier, O., Marchant, A., *et al.* (1992). Induction of thromboses within renal grafts by high-dose prophylactic OKT3. *Lancet* **339**, 777.

Adams, D. (1995). Therapeutic potential of inhibiting the ICAM-1/LFA-1 pathway of leukocyte adhesion. *In Recent Developments in Transplantation Medicine: Adhesion Molecules, Fusion Proteins, Novel Peptides and Monoclonal Antibodies*, (D. R. Salomon and H. Sollinger, eds.), p. 27, Physicians and Scientists, Glenview, Ill.

Alegre, M. L., Lenschow, D. J. and Bluestone, J. A. (1995). Immunomodulation of transplant rejection using monoclonal antibodies and soluble receptors. *Dig. Dis. Sci.* **40**, 58.

Alegre, M. L., Peterson, L. J., Xu, D., *et al.* (1994). A non-activating 'humanized' anti-CD3 monoclonal antibody retains immunosuppressive properties in vivo. *Transplantation* **57**, 1537.

Allan, J. S., Choo, J. K., Vesga, L., *et al.* (1997). Cardiac allograft vasculopathy is abrogated by anti-CD8 monoclonal antibody therapy. *Ann. Thorac. Surg.* **64**, 1019.

Amlot, P. L., Rawlings, E., Fernando, O. N., *et al.* (1995). Prolonged action of a chimeric interleukin-2 receptor (CD25) monoclonal antibody used in cadaveric renal transplantation. *Transplantation* **60**, 748.

Baan, D. C., Knoop, C. J., van Gelder, T., *et al.* (1999). Anti-CD25 therapy reveals the redundancy of the intragraft cytokine network after clinical heart transplantation. *Transplantation* **67**, 870.

Barber, W. H., Mankin, J. A., Laskow, D. A., *et al.* (1991). Long-term results of a controlled prospective study with transfusion of donor-specific bone marrow in 57 cadaveric renal allograft recipients. *Transplantation* **51**, 70.

Benveniraty, A. I., Cohen, D., Stegall, M. D. and Hardy, M. A. (1990). Improved results using OKT3 as induction immunosuppression in renal allograft recipients with delayed graft function. *Transplantation* **49**, 321.

Benveniraty, A. I., Tannenbaum, G. A., Cohen, D. I., *et al.* (1987). Use of antithymocyte globulin and cyclosporine to treat steroid-resistant episodes in renal transplant recipients. *Transplant. Proc.* **19**, 1889.

Berlin, P. J., Bacher, J. D., Sharrow, S. O., *et al.* (1992). Monoclonal antibodies against human T cell adhesion molecules—modulation of immune function in nonhuman primates. *Transplantation* **53**, 840.

Bielory, L., Wright, R., Niehuis, A. W., *et al.* (1988). Antithymocyte globulin hypersensitivity in bone marrow failure patients. *J. A. M. A.* **260**, 3164.

Bock, H. A., Gallati, H., Zurcher, R. M., *et al.* (1995). A randomized prospective trial of prophylactic immunosuppression with ATG-Fresenius versus OKT3 after renal transplantation. *Transplantation* **59**, 830.

Bonnefoy-Berard, N., Vincent, C. and Revillard, J. (1991). Antibodies against functional leukocyte surface molecules in polyclonal antilymphocyte and antithymocyte globulins. *Transplantation* **51**, 669.

Boulianne, G. L., Hozumi, N. and Shu!man, M. J. (1984). Production of functional chimeric mouse/human antibody. *Nature* **312**, 643.

Bourdage, J. S. and Hamlin, D. M. (1995). Comparative polyclonal antithymocyte globulin and antilymphocyte/antilymphoblast globulin anti-CD antigen analysis by flow cytometry. *Transplantation* **59**, 1194.

Boussiotis, V. A., Freeman, G. J., Griffin, J. D., *et al.* (1994). CD2 is involved in maintenance and reversal of human alloantigen-specific clonal anergy. *J. Exp. Med.* **180**, 1665.

Brennan, D. C., Flavin, K., Lowell, J. A., *et al.* (1999). A randomized, double-blinded comparison of thymoglobulin versus ATGAM for induction immunosuppressive therapy in adult renal transplant recipients. *Transplantation* **67**, 1011.

Brent, L. (1981). The continuing quest for specific unresponsiveness in tissue and organ transplantation. *Cell. Immunol.* **62**, 264.

Brooks, C. D., Karl, K. J. and Francom, S. F. (1994). ATGAM skin test standardization: comparison of skin testing techniques in horse-sensitive and unselected human volunteers. *Transplantation* **58**, 1135.

Brown, S. A., Lucas, B. A., Waid, T. H., *et al.* (1996). T10B9 (MEDI-500) mediated immunosuppression: studies on the mechanism of action. *Clin. Transplant.* **10**, 607.

Byrne, J. G., Murphy, M. P., Smith, W. J., *et al.* (1993). Prevention of CD18-mediated reperfusion injury enhances the efficacy of UW solution for 15-hr heart preservation. *J. Surg. Res.* **54**, 625.

Byrne, J. G., Smith, W. J., Murphy, M. P., *et al.* (1992). Complete prevention of myocardial stunning, contracture, low-reflow, and edema after heart transplantation by blocking neutrophil adhesion molecules during reperfusion. *J. Thorac. Cardiovasc. Surg.* **104**, 1589.

Calne, R., Friend, P., Moffatt, S., *et al.* (1998). Prope tolerance, perioperative campath 1H, and low-dose cyclosporin monotherapy in renal allograft recipients. *Lancet* **351**, 1701.

Cecka, J. M., Gjertson, D. and Terasaki, P. (1993). Do prophylactic antilymphocyte globulins (ALG and OKT3) improve renal transplant in recipient and donor high-risk groups? *Transplant. Proc.* **25**, 548.

Cecka, J. M. and Terasaki, P. I. (1991). The UNOS scientific renal transplant registry—1991. *In Clinical Transplants 1991*, (P. Terasaki, ed.), p. 1, UCLA Tissue Typing Laboratory, Los Angeles.

Charpentier, B., Hiesse, C., Lantz, O., *et al.* (1993). Evidence that antihuman tumor necrosis factor monoclonal antibody prevents OKT3-induced acute syndrome. *Transplantation* **54**, 997.

Chatenoud, L., Ferran, C., Legendre, C., *et al.* (1990). In vivo cell activation following OKT3 administration: systemic cytokine release and modulation by corticosteroids. *Transplantation* **49**, 697.

Chatenoud, L., Jonker, M., Villemain, F., *et al.* (1986). The human immune response to the OKT3 monoclonal antibody is oligoclonal. *Science* **232**, 1406.

Chatenoud, L., Legendre, C., Ferran, C., *et al.* (1991). Corticosteroid inhibition of the OKT3-induced cytokine-related syndrome-dosage and kinetics prerequisites. *Transplantation* **51**, 334.

Clark, K. (1996). Monitoring antilymphocyte globulin in renal transplantation. *Ann. R. Coll. Surg. Engl.* **78**, 536.

Colvin, R. B. and Preffer, F. I. (1991). Laboratory monitoring of therapy with OKT3 and other murine monoclonal antibodies. *Clin. Lab. Med.* **11**, 693.

Cosimi, A. B. (1981). The clinical value of antilymphocyte antibodies. *Transplant. Proc.* **13**, 462.

Cosimi, A. B., Burton, R. C., Colvin, R. B., *et al.* (1981a). Treatment of acute renal allograft rejection with OKT3 monoclonal antibody. *Transplantation* **32**, 535.

Cosimi, A. B., Colvin, R. B., Burton, R. C., *et al.* (1981b). Use of monoclonal antibodies to T-cell subsets for immunologic monitoring and treatment in recipients of renal allografts. *N. Engl. J. Med.* **305**, 308.

Cosimi, A. B., Conti, D., Delmonico, F. L., *et al.* (1990a). In vivo effects of monoclonal antibody to ICAM-1 (CD54) in nonhuman primates with renal allografts. *J. Immunol.* **144**, 4604.

Cosimi, A. B., Delmonico, F. L., Wright, J. K., *et al.* (1990b). Prolonged survival of nonhuman primate renal allograft recipients treated only with anti-CD4 monoclonal antibody. *Surgery* **108**, 406.

Cosimi, A. B., Wortis, H. H., Delmonico, F. L. and Russell, P. S. (1976). Randomized clinical trial of antithymocyte globulin in cadaver renal allograft recipients: importance of T cell monitoring. *Surgery* **80**, 155.

D'Alessandro, A. M., Pirsch, J. D., Stratta, R. J., *et al.* (1989). OKT3 salvage therapy in a quadruple immunosuppressive protocol in cadaveric renal transplantation. *Transplantation* **47**, 297.

Dantal, J., Ninin, E., Hourmant, M., *et al.* (1996). Anti-CD4 MoAb therapy in kidney transplantation—a pilot study in early prophylaxis of rejection. *Transplantation* **62**, 1502.

Darby, C. R., Bushell, A., Morris, P. J., *et al.* (1994). Nondepleting anti-CD4 antibodies in transplantation: evidence that modulation is far less effective than prolonged CD4 blockade. *Transplantation* **57**, 1419.

Debets, J. M. H., Leunissen, K. M. L., van Hooff, H. J., *et al.* (1989). Evidence of involvement of tumor necrosis factor in adverse reactions during treatment of kidney allograft rejection with antithymocyte globulin. *Transplantation* **47**, 487.

Debure, A., Chkoff, N., Chatenoud, L., *et al.* (1988). One-month prophylactic use of OKT3 in cadaver kidney transplant recipients. *Transplantation* **45**, 546.

Deierhoi, M. H., Sollinger, H. W., Kalayoglu, M. and Belzer, F. O. (1987). Quadruple therapy for cadaver renal transplantation. *Transplant. Proc.* **19**, 1917.

Delmonico, F. L. (1984). Antithymocyte globulin therapy after renal transplantation at the Massachusetts General Hospital. *Transplant. Proc.* **16**, 979.

Delmonico, F. L., Auchincloss, H. J., Rubin, R. H., *et al.* (1987). The selective use of antilymphocyte serum for cyclosporine treated patients with renal allograft dysfunction. *Ann. Surg.* **206**, 649.

Delmonico, F. L. and Cosimi, A. B. (1988). Monoclonal antibody treatment of human allograft recipients. *Surg. Gynecol. Obstet.* **166**, 89.

Delmonico, F. L. and Cosimi, A. B. (1996). Anti-CD4 monoclonal antibody therapy. *Clin. Transplant.* **10**, 397.

Delmonico, F. L., Cosimi, A. B., Kawai, T., *et al.* (1993). Non-human primate responses to murine and humanized OKT4A. *Transplantation* **55**, 722.

Delmonico, F. L., Fuller, T. C., Russell, P. S., *et al.* (1989). Variation in patient response associated with different preparations of murine monoclonal antibody therapy. *Transplantation* **47**, 92.

DeMeester, S. R., Molinari, M. A., Shiraishi, T., *et al.* (1996). Attenuation of rat lung isograft reperfusion injury with a combination of anti-ICAM-1 and anti-beta2 integrin monoclonal antibodies. *Transplantation* **62**, 1477.

Denton, M. D., Reul, R. M., Dharnidharka, V. R., *et al.* (1998). Central role for CD40/CD40 ligand (CD154) interaction in transplant rejection. *Pediatr. Transplant.* **2**, 6.

Dragun, D., Tullius, S. G., Park, J. K., *et al.* (1998). ICAM-1 antisense oligodesoxynucleotides prevent reperfusion injury and enhance immediate graft function in renal transplantation. *Kidney Int.* **54**, 590.

Durie, F. H., Foy, T. M., Masters, S. R., Laman, J. D. and Noelle, R. J. (1994). The role of CD40 in the regulation of humoral and cell-mediated immunity. *Immunol. Today* **15**, 40.

Eason, J. D., Wee, S. L., Kawai, T., *et al.* (1995). Inhibition of the effects of TNF in renal allograft recipients using recombinant human dimeric tumor necrosis factor receptors. *Transplantation* **59**, 300.

Eck, S. C., Chang, D., Wells, A. D. and Turka, L. A. (1997). Differential down-regulation of CD28 by B7-1 and B7-2 engagement. *Transplantation* **64**, 1497.

Fanger, M. W., Segal, D. M. and Romet-Lemonne, J. L. (1991). Bispecific antibodies and targeted cellular cytotoxicity. *Immunol. Today* **12**, 51.

Farges, C., Samuel, D. and Bismuth, H. (1992). Orthoclone OKT3 in liver transplantation. *Transplant. Sci.* **2**, 16.

Frey, D. J., Matas, A. J., Gillingham, K. L., *et al.* (1992). Sequential therapy—a prospective randomized trial of MALG versus OKT3 for prophylactic immunosuppression in cadaver renal allograft recipients. *Transplantation* **54**, 50.

Friend, P. J., Rebello, P., Oliveira, D., *et al.* (1995). Successful treatment of renal allograft rejection with a humanized antilymphocyte monoclonal antibody. *Transplant. Proc.* **27**, 869.

Gaber, A. O., First, M. R., Tesi, R. J., *et al.* (1998). Results of the double-blinded, randomized, multicenter, phase III clinical trial of Thymoglobulin versus ATGAM in the treatment of acute graft rejection episodes after renal transplantation. *Transplantation* **66**, 29.

Gahmberg, C. G., Nortamo, P., Kantor, C., *et al.* (1990). The pivotal role of the Leu-CAM and ICAM molecules in human leukocyte adhesion. *Cell Differ. Dev.* **32**, 239.

Gaston, R. S., Deierhoi, M. H., Patterson, T., *et al.* (1991). OKT3 first-dose reaction: association with T cell subsets and cytokine release. *Kidney Int.* **39**, 141.

Ghetie, M. A. and Vitetta, E. S. (1994). Recent developments in immunotoxin therapy. *Curr. Opin. Immunol.* **6**, 707.

Gillis, S. (1989). T-cell-derived lymphokines. In *Fundamental Immunology*, (W. E. Paul, ed.), p. 621, Raven Press, New York.

Goldstein, G. (1986). An overview of Orthoclone OKT3. *Transplant. Proc.* **18**, 927.

Greenwood, J., Clark, M. and Waldmann, H. (1993). Structural motifs involved in human IgG antibody effector functions. *Eur. J. Immunol.* **23**, 1098.

Haak, H. H., Weening, J. L., Rischen-Vos J., *et al.* (1989). Acute cellular rejection during effective early prophylactic OKT3 monoclonal antibody treatment after renal transplantation. *Transplantation* **48**, 352.

Haug, C. E., Colvin, R. B., Delmonico, F. L., *et al.* (1993). A phase I trial of immunosuppression with anti-ICAM-1 (CD54) mAb in renal allograft recipients. *Transplantation* **55**, 766.

Heeman, U. W., Tullius, S. G., Azuma, H., *et al.* (1994). Adhesion molecules and transplantation. *Ann. Surg.* **219**, 4.

Heinrich, G., Gram, H., Kocher, H. P., *et al.* (1989). Characterization of a human T cell-specific chimeric antibody (CD7) with human constant and mouse variable regions. *J. Immunol.* **143**, 3589.

Henricsson, A., Husberg, B. and Bergentz, S. E. (1977). The mechanism behind the effect of ALG on platelets in vivo. *Clin. Exp. Immunol.* **29**, 515.

Hibberd, P. L., Tolkoff-Rubin, N. E., Conti, D., *et al.* (1995). Preemptive ganciclovir therapy to prevent cytomegalovirus disease in cytomegalovirus antibody-positive renal transplant recipients. *Ann. Intern. Med.* **123**, 18.

Hibberd, P. L., Tolkoff-Rubin, N. E., Cosimi, A. B., *et al.* (1992). Symptomatic cytomegalovirus disease in the cytomegalovirus antibody seropositive renal transplant recipient treated with OKT3. *Transplantation* **53**, 68.

Hiesse, C., Lantz, O., Kriaa, F., *et al.* (1991). Treatment with Lo-Tact-1, a monoclonal antibody to the interleukin-2 receptor, in kidney transplantation. *Presse Med.* **20**, 2036.

Hirsch, R., Bluestone, J. A., DeNenno, L. and Gress, R. E. (1990). Anti-CD3 F(ab)2 fragments are immunosuppressive in vivo without evoking either the strong humoral response or morbidity associated with whole mAb. *Transplantation* **49**, 1117.

Hoffman, R. A. and Hansen, W. P. (1981). Immunofluorescent analysis of blood cells by flow cytometry. *Int. J. Immunopharmacol.* **3**, 249.

Hoitsma, A. J., van Lier, L. H., Reekers, P. and Koene, R. A. (1985). Improved patient and graft survival after treatment of acute rejections of cadaveric renal allografts with rabbit antithymocyte globulin. *Transplantation* **39**, 274.

Homan, W. P., Fabre, J. W., Millard, P. R. and Morris, P. J. (1980).

Interaction of cyclosporine A with antilymphocyte serum and with enhancing serum for the suppression of renal allograft rejection in the rat. *Transplantation* **29**, 274.

Horgan, M. J., Ge, M., Gu, J., *et al.* (1991). Role of ICAM-1 in neutrophil-mediated lung vascular injury after occlusion and reperfusion. *Am. J. Physiol.* **261**, H1578.

Horneff, G., Burmester, G. R., Emmrich, F. and Kalden, J. R. (1991). Treatment of rheumatoid arthritis with an anti-CD4 monoclonal antibody. *Arthritis Rheum.* **34**, 129.

Hourmant, M., Bedrossian, J., Durand, D., *et al.* (1996). A randomized multicenter trial comparing leukocyte function-associated antigen-1 monoclonal antibody with rabbit antithymocyte globulin as induction treatment in first kidney transplantations. *Transplantation* **62**, 1565.

Howard, R. J., Condie, R. M., Sutherland, D. E. R., *et al.* (1981). The use of antilymphoblast globulin in the treatment of renal allograft rejection. *Transplant. Proc.* **13**, 473.

Isobe, M., Yagita, H., Okumura, K. and Ihara, A. (1992). Specific acceptance of cardiac allograft after treatment with antibodies to ICAM-1 and LFA-1. *Science* **255**, 1125.

Jaffers, G. J., Fuller, T. C., Cosimi, A. B., *et al.* (1986). Monoclonal antibody therapy: anti-idiotype and non-anti-idiotype antibodies to OKT3 arising despite intense immunosuppression. *Transplantation* **41**, 572.

Janeway, C. A., Jr. and Bottomly, K. (1994). Signals and signs for lymphocyte responses. *Cell* **76**, 275.

Jonker, M., Malissen, B. and Mawas, C. (1983). The effect of in vivo application of monoclonal antibodies specific for human cytotoxic T cells in rhesus monkeys. *Transplantation* **35**, 374.

Jonsson, J., Light, J. A. and Korb, S. M. (1990). Renal transplantation at the Washington Hospital Center: experience with OKT3 and Minnesota antilymphoblast globulin for induction of immunosuppression. *Clin. Transplant.* **4**, 275.

Kahan, B. D., Rajagopalan, P. R., Hall, M., *et al.* (1999). Reduction of the occurrence of acute cellular rejection among renal allograft recipients treated with basiliximab, a chimeric anti-interleukin-2-receptor monoclonal antibody. *Transplantation* **67**, 276.

Kahana, L., Ackermann, J., Lefor, W., *et al.* (1990). Uses of orthoclone OKT3 for prophylaxis of rejection and induction in initial nonfunction in kidney transplantation. *Transplant. Proc.* **22**, 1755.

Kamath, S., Dean, D., Peddi, V. R., *et al.* (1997). Efficacy of OKT3 as primary therapy for histologically confirmed acute renal allograft rejection. *Transplantation* **51**, 1207.

Kaplon, R. J., Hochman, P. S., Michler, R. E., *et al.* (1996). Short course single agent therapy with an LFA-3-IgG fusion protein prolongs primate cardiac allograft survival. *Transplantation* **61**, 356.

Kawai, T., Cosimi, A. B., Colvin, R. B., *et al.* (1995). Mixed allogeneic chimerism and renal allograft tolerance in cynomolgus monkeys. *Transplantation* **59**, 256.

Kelly, K. J., Williams, W. W., Colvin, R. B., *et al.* (1994). Antibody to intercellular adhesion molecule 1 protects the kidney against ischemic injury. *Proc. Natl. Acad. Sci. U. S. A.* **91**, 812.

Kerr, P. G. and Atkins, R. C. (1989). The effects of OKT3 therapy on infiltrating lymphocytes in rejecting renal allografts. *Transplantation* **48**, 33.

Kimikawa, M., Sachs, D. H., Colvin, R. B., *et al.* (1997). Modification of the conditioning regimen for achieving mixed chimerism and donor-specific tolerance in cynomolgus monkeys. *Transplantation* **64**, 709.

Kirk, A. D., Burkly, L. C., Batty, D. S., *et al.* (1999). Treatment with humanized monoclonal antibody against CD154 prevents acute renal allograft rejection in nonhuman primates. *Nat. Med.* **6**, 686.

Kirk, A. D., Harlan, D. M., Davis, T. A., *et al.* (1997). CTLA 4 Ig and anti-CD40 ligand prevent renal allograft rejection in primates. *Proc. Natl. Acad. Sci. U. S. A.* **94**, 8789.

Kirkman, R. L., Araujo, J. L., Busch, G. J., *et al.* (1983). Treatment of acute renal allograft rejection with monoclonal anti-T12 antibody. *Transplantation* **36**, 620.

Kirkman, R. L., Shapiro, M. E., Carpenter, C. B., *et al.* (1991). A randomized prospective trial of anti-Tac monoclonal antibody in human renal transplantation. *Transplantation* **51**, 107.

Knechtle, S. J., Vargo, D., Fechner, J., *et al.* (1997). FN18-CRM9 immunotoxin promotes tolerance in primate renal allografts. *Transplantation* **63**, 1.

Kohler, G. and Milstein, C. (1975). Continuous cultures of fused cells secreting antibody of predefined specificity. *Nature* **256**, 495.

Kovarik, J., Wolf, P., Cisterne, J. M., *et al.* (1997). Disposition of basiliximab, an interleukin-2 receptor monoclonal antibody, in recipients of mismatched cadaveric renal allografts. *Transplantation* **64**, 1701.

Kreis, H., Legendre, C. and Chatenoud, L. (1991). OKT3 in organ transplantation. *Transplant. Rev.* **5**, 181.

Kupiec-Weglinski, J., Diamantstein, T. and Tilney, N. L. (1988). Interleukin 2 receptor-targeted therapy-rationale and applications in organ transplantation. *Transplantation* **46**, 785.

Land, W. (1991). Monoclonal antibodies in 1991: new potential options in clinical immunosuppressive therapy. *Clin. Transplant.* **5**, 493.

Langrehr, J. M., Nussler, N. C., Neumann, U., *et al.* (1997). A prospective randomized trial comparing interleukin-2 receptor antibody versus antithymocyte globulin as part of a quadruple immunosuppressive induction therapy following orthotopic liver transplantation. *Transplantation* **63**, 1772.

Lazarovits, A. I., Rochon, J., Banks, L., *et al.* (1993). Human mouse chimeric CD7 monoclonal antibody for the prophylaxis of kidney transplant rejection. *J. Clin. Invest.* **150**, 5163.

Legendre, C. M. (1992). Effect of immunosuppression on the incidence of lymphoma formation. *In Roundtable Report: Immunosuppression and Lymphoproliferative Disorders*, (I. Penn, ed.), p. 11, PRO/COM, Parsippany, N.J.

Legendre, C., Kreis, H., Bach, J. and Chatenoud, L. (1992). Prediction of successful allograft rejection retreatment with OKT3. *Transplantation* **53**, 87.

Lehmann, M., Sternkopf, F., Metz, F., *et al.* (1992). Induction of long-term survival of rat skin allografts by a novel, highly effective anti-CD4 monoclonal antibody. *Transplantation* **54**, 959.

Le Mauff, B., Hourmant, M., Rougier, J. P., *et al.* (1991). Effect of anti-LFA1 (CD11a) monoclonal antibodies in acute rejection in human kidney transplantation. *Transplantation* **52**, 291.

Lenschow, D. J., Zeng, Y., Hathcock, K. S., *et al.* (1995). Inhibition of transplant rejection following treatment with anti-B7-2 and anti-B7-1 antibodies. *Transplantation* **60**, 1171.

Lenschow, D. J., Zeng, Y., Thistlethwaite, J. R., *et al.* (1992). Long-term survival of xenogeneic pancreatic islet grafts induced by CTLA4Ig. *Science* **257**, 789.

Linsley, P. S., Brady, W., Urnes, M., *et al.* (1991). CTLA-4 is a second receptor for the B cell activation antigen B7. *J. Exp. Med.* **174**, 561.

Madsen, J. C., Peugh, W. N., Wood, K. J. and Morris, P. J. (1987). The effect of anti-L3T4 monoclonal antibody treatment on first set rejection of murine cardiac allografts. Transplantation **44**, 849.

Maki, T., Simpson, M. and Monaco, A. P. (1982). Development of suppressor T-cells by antilymphocyte serum treatment in mice. *Transplantation* **34**, 376.

Malatack, J. F., Gartner, J. C. J., Urbach, A. H. and Zitelli, B. J. (1991). Orthotopic liver transplantation, Epstein-Barr virus, cyclosporine, and lymphoproliferative disease: a growing concern. *J. Pediatr.* **118**, 667.

Malinow, L., Walker, J., Klassen, D. K., *et al.* (1996). Antilymphocyte induction immunosuppression in the post-Minnesota antilymphocyte globulin era: incidence of renal dysfunction and delayed graft function: a single center experience. *Clin. Transplant.* **10**, 237.

Martin, M. A., Massanari, M., Nghiem, D. D., *et al.* (1988). Nosocomial aseptic meningitis associated with administration of OKT3. *J. A. M. A.* **259**, 2002.

Martin, P. J., Nelson, B. J., Appelbaum, F. R., *et al.* (1996). Evaluation of a CD5-specific immunotoxin for treatment of acute graft-versus-host disease after allogeneic marrow transplantation. *Blood* **88**, 824.

Matas, A. J., Tellis, V. A., Quinn, T., *et al.* (1986). ALG treatment of steroid-resistant rejection in patients receiving cyclosporine. *Transplantation* **41**, 579.

Meisner, B. M., Reiter, C., Reichenspurner, H., *et al.* (1994). Chimeric monoclonal CD4 antibody—a novel immunosuppressant for clinical heart transplantation. *Transplantation* **58**, 419.

Merion, M., White, D. J. G., Thiru, S., *et al.* (1984). Cyclosporine: five years experience in cadaveric renal transplantation. *N. Engl. J. Med.* **310**, 148.

Michael, H. J., Francos, G. C., Burke, J. F., *et al.* (1989). A comparison of the effects of cyclosporine versus antilymphocyte globulin on delayed graft function in cadaver renal transplant recipients. *Transplantation* **48**, 805.

Monaco, A. P. and Wood, M. L. (1982). The potential for induction of specific unresponsiveness to organ allografts in clinical transplantation. *Heart Transplant.* **1**, 257.

Mottram, P. L., Han, W. R., Murray-Segal, L. J., *et al.* (1997). Idarubicin-anti-CD3: a new immunoconjugate that induces alloantigen-specific tolerance in mice. *Transplantation* **64**, 684.

Mourad, M., Besse, T., Malaise, J., *et al.* (1997). BTI-322 for acute rejection after renal transplantation. *Transplant. Proc.* **29**, 2353.

Nashan, B., Light, S., Hardie, I. R., *et al.* (1999). Reduction of acute renal allograft rejection by daclizumab. *Transplantation* **67**, 110.

Nashan, B., Moore, R., Amlot, P., *et al.* (1997). Randomized trial of basiliximab versus placebo for control of acute cellular rejection in renal allograft recipients. CHIB201 International Study Group. *Lancet* **350**, 1193.

Nashan, B., Schlitt, H. J., Schwinzer, R., *et al.* (1996). Immunoprophylaxis with a monoclonal anti-IL-2 receptor antibody in liver transplant patients. *Transplantation* **61**, 546.

Nelson, P. W., Cosimi, A. B., Delmonico, F. L., *et al.* (1983). Antithymocyte globulin as the primary treatment for renal allograft rejection. *Transplantation* **36**, 587.

Niblack, G., Johnson, K., Williams, T., *et al.* (1987). Antibody formation following administration of antilymphocyte serum. *Transplant. Proc.* **19**, 1896.

Norman, D. J., Kahana, L., Stuart, F. P., *et al.* (1993). A randomized clinical trial of induction therapy with OKT3 in kidney transplantations. *Transplantation* **55**, 44.

Norman, D. J. and Shield, C. F. (1986). Orthoclone OKT3: first-line therapy or last option? *Transplant. Proc.* **18**, 949.

Oh, C. S., Sollinger, H. W., Stratta, R. J., *et al.* (1988). Delayed response to orthoclone OKT3 treatment for renal allograft rejection resistant to steroid and antilymphocyte globulin. *Transplantation* **45**, 65.

Ortho Multicenter Transplant Study Group. (1985). A randomized clinical trial of OKT3 monoclonal antibody for acute rejection of cadaveric renal transplants. *N. Engl. J. Med.* **313**, 337.

Oyer, P. E., Stinson, E. B., Jamieson, S. W., *et al.* (1983). Cyclosporin-A in cardiac allografting: a preliminary experience. *Transplant. Proc.* **15**, 1247.

Penn, I. (1990). Cancers complicating organ transplantation. *N. Engl. J. Med.* **323**, 1767.

Penn, I. (1994). The problem of cancer in organ transplant recipients: an overview. *Transplant. Sci.* **4**, 23.

Pober, J. S. and Cotran, R. S. (1990). The role of endothelial cells in inflammation. *Transplantation* **50**, 537.

Ponticelli, C., Rivolta, E., Tarantino, A., *et al.* (1987). Treatment of severe rejection of kidney transplant with Orthoclone OKT3. *Clin. Transplant.* **1**, 99.

Powelson, J. A., Knowles, R. W., Delmonico F. L., *et al.* (1994). CDR-grafted OKT4A monoclonal antibody in cynomolgus renal allograft recipients. *Transplantation* **57**, 788.

Przepiorka, D., Phillips, G. L., Ratanatharathorn, V., et al. (1998). A phase II study of BTI-322, a monoclonal anti-CD2 antibody for treatment of steroid-resistant acute GVHD. *Blood* **92**, 4066.

Qin L, Chavin, K. D., Lin, J. and Yagita, H. (1994). Anti-CD2 receptor and anti-CD2 ligand (CD48) antibodies synergize to prolong allograft survival. *J. Exper. Med.* **179**, 341.

Rebellato, L. M., Gross, U., Verbanac, K. M. and Thomas, J. M. (1994). A comprehensive definition of the major antibody specificities in polyclonal rabbit antithymocyte globulin. *Transplantation* **57**, 685.

Reinke, P., Kern, F., Fietze, W., *et al.* (1995). Anti-CD4 monoclonal antibody therapy of late acute rejection in renal allograft recipients—CD4⁺ T cells play an essential role in the rejection process. *Transplant. Proc.* **27**, 859.

Richardson, A. J., Higgins, R. M., Liddington, M., Murie, J., Ting, A. and Morris, P. J. (1989). Antithymocyte globulin for steroid resistant rejection in renal transplant recipients immunosuppressed with triple therapy. *Transplant. Int.* **2**, 27.

Robbins, R. C., Oyer, P. E., Stinson, E. B. and Starnes, V. A. (1992). The use of monoclonal antibodies after heart transplantation. *Transplant. Sci.* **2**, 22.

Rothlein, R., Dustin, M. L., Marlin, S. D. and Springer, T. A. (1986). A human intercellular adhesion molecule (ICAM-1) distinct from LFA-1. *J. Immunol.* **137**, 1270.

Rouleau, M., Mollereau, B., Bernard, A., *et al.* (1994). Mitogenic CD2 monoclonal antibody pairs predispose peripheral T cells to undergo apoptosis on interaction with a third CD2 monoclonal antibody. *J. Immunol.* **152**, 4861.

Rubin, R. H., Cosimi, A. B., Hirsch, M. S., *et al.* (1981). Effects of antithymocyte globulin on cytomegalovirus infection in renal transplant recipients. *Transplantation* **31**, 143.

Rubin, R. H. and Tolkoff-Rubin, N. E. (1991). The impact of infection on the outcome of transplantation. *Transplant. Proc.* **23**, 2068.

Sablinski, T., Hancock, W. W., Tilney, N. L. and Kupiec-Weglinski, J. W. (1991). CD4 monoclonal antibodies in organ transplantation—a review of progress. *Transplantation* **52**, 579.

Sablinski, T., Sayegh, M. H., Kut, J. P., *et al.* (1992). The importance of targeting the CD4⁺ T cell subset at the time of antigenic challenge for induction of prolonged vascularized allograft survival. *Transplantation* **53**, 219.

Salmela, K., Wramner, L., Ekberg, H., *et al.* (1999). A randomized multicenter trial of the anti-ICAM-1 monoclonal antibody (Enlimomab), for the prevention of acute rejection and delayed onset of graft function in cadaveric renal transplantation. *Transplantation* **67**, 729.

Sayegh, M. H. and Turka, L. A. (1998). The role of T-cell costimulatory activation pathways in transplant rejection. *N. Engl. J. Med.* **338**, 1813.

Schroeder, T. J., First, M. R., Mansour, M. E., *et al.* (1990). Antimurine antibody formation following OKT3 therapy. *Transplantation* **49**, 48.

Sharma, L. C., Muirhead, N. and Lazarovits, A. I. (1997). Human mouse chimeric CD7 monoclonal antibody (SDZCHH380) for the prophylaxis of kidney transplant rejection: analysis beyond 4 years. *Transplant. Proc.* **29**, 323.

Sheiner, P. A., Guarrera, J. V., Grunstein, E., *et al.* (1997). Increased risk of early rejection correlates with recovery of CD3 cell count after liver transplant in patients receiving OKT3 induction. *Transplantation* **64**, 1212.

Shevach, E. M. (1989). Accessory molecules. *In Fundamental Immunology*, (W. E. Paul, ed.), p. 413, Raven Press, New York.

Shield, C. F., Cosimi, A. B., Tolkoff-Rubin, N. E., *et al.* (1979). Use of antithymocyte globulin for reversal of acute allograft rejection. *Transplantation* **28**, 461.

Shield, C. F., Edwards, E. B., Davies, D. B. and Daily, O. P. (1997). Antilymphocyte induction therapy in cadaver renal transplantation. *Transplantation* **63**, 1257.

Shield, C. F., Kahana, L., Pirsch, J., *et al.* (1992). Use of indomethacin to minimize the adverse reactions associated with orthoclone OKT3 treatment of kidney allograft rejection. *Transplantation* **54**, 164.

Shizuru, J. A., Seydel, K. B., Flavin, T. F., *et al.* (1990). Induction of donor-specific unresponsiveness to cardiac allografts in rats by pretransplant anti-CD4 monoclonal antibody therapy. *Transplantation* **50**, 366.

Simpson, M. A. and Monaco, A. P. (1995). Clinical uses of polyclonal and monoclonal antilymphoid sera. *In Monoclonal Antibodies in Transplantation*, (L. Chatenoud, ed.), p. 1, R. G. Landes, Austin.

Slakey, D. P., Johnson, C. P., Callaluce, R. D., *et al.* (1993). A prospective randomized comparison of quadruple versus triple therapy for first cadaver transplants with immediate function. *Transplantation* **56**, 827.

Sommer, B. G., Henry, M. L. and Ferguson, R. M. (1987). Sequential antilymphoblast globulin and cyclosporine for renal transplantation. *Transplant. Proc.* **19**, 1879.

Soulillou, J. P., Cantarovich, D., Le, M. B., *et al.* (1990). Randomized controlled trial of a monoclonal antibody against the interleukin-2 receptor (33B3.1) as compared with rabbit antithymocyte globulin for prophylaxis against rejection of renal allografts. *N. Engl. J. Med.* **322**, 1175.

Spitzer, T. R., Delmonico, F, Tolkoff-Rubin, N, *et al.* (1999). Combined histocompatibility leukocyte antigen-matched donor bone marrow and renal transplantation for multiple myeloma with end-stage renal disease: the induction of allograft tolerance through mixed lymphohaematopoietic chimerism. *Transplantation* **68**, 480.

Springer, T. A., Dustin, M. L., Kishimoto, T. K. and Marlin, S. D. (1987). The lymphocyte function associated LFA1, CD2 and LFA3 molecules: cell adhesion receptors of the immune system. *Ann. Rev. Immunol.* **5**, 223.

Squifflet, J. P., Besse, T., Malaise, J., *et al.* (1997). BTI-322 for induction therapy after renal transplantation: a randomized study. *Transplant. Proc.* **29**, 317.

Starling, G. C., Whitney, G. S., Siadak, A. W., *et al.* (1996). Characterization of mouse CD6 with novel monoclonal antibodies which enhance the allogeneic mixed leukocyte reaction. *Eur. J. Immunol.* **26**, 738.

Starzl, T. E., Porter, K. A., Iwasaki, Y., *et al.* (1967). The use of heterologous antilymphocyte globulins in human homotransplantation. *In Antilymphocyte Serum*, (G. E. W. Wolstenholme and M. O'Connor, eds.), p. 1, Little, Brown, Boston.

Steinmuller, D. R., Hayes, J. M., Novick, A. C., *et al.* (1991). Comparison of OKT3 with ALG for prophylaxis for patients with acute renal failure after cadaveric renal transplantation. *Transplantation* **52**, 67.

Stephen, R. N., Munschauer, C. E., Kohli, R. K., *et al.* (1997). Post-OKT3 induction therapy CD complex response predicts renal allograft rejection. *Transplantation* **63**, 1183.

Stiller, C. R. and Keown, P. A. (1984). Cyclosporine therapy in perspective. *Prog. Transplant.* **1**, 11.

Stratta, R. J., D'Alessandro, A. M., Armbrust, M. J., *et al.* (1989). Sequential antilymphocyte globulin/cyclosporine immunosuppression in cadaveric renal transplantation: effect of duration of ALG therapy. *Transplantation* **47**, 96.

Streem, S. B., Novick, A. C., Braun, W. E., *et al.* (1983). Low-dose maintenance prednisone and antilymphoblast globulin for the treatment of acute rejection. *Transplantation* **35**, 420.

Swinnen, L. J., Costanzo-Nordin, M. R., Fisher, S. G., *et al.* (1990). Increased incidence of lymphoproliferative disorder after immunosuppression with the monoclonal antibody OKT3 in cardiac-transplant recipients. *N. Engl. J. Med.* **323**, 1723.

Tatum, A. H., Bollinger, R. R. and Sanfilippo, F. (1984). Rapid serologic diagnosis of serum sickness from antilymphocyte globulin therapy using enzyme immunoassay. *Transplantation* **38**, 582.

Tellides, G., Dallman, M. J. and Morris, P. J. (1989) Mechanism of action of interleukin-2 receptor (IL2-R) monoclonal antibody (Mab) therapy: target cell depletion or inhibition of function? *Transplant. Proc.* **21**, 1022.

Tesi, R. J., Elkhammas, E. A., Henry, M. L. and Ferguson, R. M. (1993). OKT3 for primary therapy of the first rejection episode in kidney transplants. *Transplantation* **55**, 1023.

Thistlethwaite, J. R., Jr., Cosimi, A. B., Delmonico, F. L., *et al.* (1984). Evolving use of OKT3 monoclonal antibody for treatment of renal allograft rejection. *Transplantation* **38**, 695.

Thistlethwaite, J. R., Jr., Gaber, A. O., Haag, B. W., *et al.* (1987). OKT3 treatment of steroid-resistant renal allograft rejection. *Transplantation* **43**, 176.

Thistlethwaite, J. R., Jr., Stuart, J. K., Mayes, J. T., *et al.* (1988). Complications and monitoring of OKT3 therapy. *Am. J. Kidney Dis.* **11**, 112.

Thomas, F., Cunningham, P., Thomas, J., *et al.* (1987). Superior renal allograft survival and decreased rejection with early high-dose and sequential multi-species antilymphocyte globulin therapy. *Transplant. Proc.* **19**, 1874.

Thomas, J. M., Carver, F. M., Foil, M. B., *et al.* (1983). Renal allograft tolerance induced with ATG and donor bone marrow in outbred rhesus monkeys. *Transplantation* **36**, 104.

Thomas, J. M., Carver, F. M., Haisch, C. E., *et al.* (1982). Suppressor cells in Rhesus monkeys treated with antithymocyte globulin. *Transplantation* **34**, 83.

Thomas, J. M., Neville, D. M., Contreras, J. L., *et al.* (1997). Preclinical studies of allograft tolerance in rhesus monkeys. *Transplantation* **64**, 124.

Tite, J. P., Sloan, A. and Janeway, C. J. (1986). The role of L3T4 in T cell activation: L3T4 may be both an Ia-binding protein and a receptor that transduces a negative signal. *J. Mol. Cell. Immunol.* **2**, 179.

Turgeon, N., Fishman, J. A., Basgoz, N., *et al.* (1998). Effect of oral acyclovir or gangciclovir therapy after preemptive intravenous gangciclovir therapy to prevent cytomegalovirus disease in cytomegalovirus seropositive renal and liver transplant recipients receiving antilymphocyte antibody therapy. *Transplantation* **66**, 1780.

Turka, L. A., Linsley, P. S., Lin, H., *et al.* (1992). T-cell activation by the CD28 ligand B7 is required for cardiac allograft rejection in vivo. *Proc. Natl. Acad. Sci. U. S. A.* **89**, 11102.

Vallhonrat, H., Williams, W. W., Cosimi, A. B., *et al.* (1999). In vivo generation of C4b, Bb, iC3b, and SC5b-9 after OKT3 administration in kidney and lung transplant recipients. *Transplantation* **67**, 253.

van Gelder, T., Balk, A. H., Jonkman, F. A., *et al.* (1996). A randomized trial comparing safety and efficacy of OKT3 and monoclonal anti-interleukin-2 receptor antibody (BT563) in the prevention of acute rejection after heart transplantation. *Transplantation* **62**, 51.

van Gelder, T., Zietse, R., Mulder, A. H., *et al.* (1995). A double-blind, placebo-controlled study of monoclonal anti-interleukin-2 receptor antibody (BT563) administration to prevent acute rejection after kidney transplantation. *Transplantation* **60**, 248.

Vigeral, P., Chkoff, N., Chatenoud, L., *et al.* (1986). Prophylactic use of OKT3 monoclonal antibody in cadaver kidney recipients. *Transplantation* **41**, 730.

Vincenti, F., Kirkman, R., Light, S., *et al.* (1998). Interleukin-2-receptor blockade with daclizumab to prevent acute rejection in renal transplantation. Daclizumab Triple Therapy Study Group. *N. Engl. J. Med.* **338**, 161.

Vincenti, F., Lantz, M., Birnbaum, J., *et al.* (1997). A phase I trial of humanized anti-interleukin-2 receptor antibody in renal transplantation. *Transplantation* **63**, 33.

Waid, T. H., Lucas, B. A., Thompson, J. S., *et al.* (1997a). Treatment of renal allograft rejection with T10B9.1A31 or OKT3. *Transplantation* **64**, 224.

Waid, T. H., Thompson, J. S., McKeown, J. W., *et al.* (1997b). Induction immunotherapy in heart transplantation with T10B9.1A-31: a phase I study. *J. Heart Lung Transplant* **16**, 913.

Walunas, T. L., Bakker, C. Y. and Bluestone, J. A. (1996). CTLA-4 ligation blocks CD28-dependent T cell activation. *J. Exp. Med.* **183**, 2541.

Wechter, W. J., Morrell, R. M., Bergan, J., *et al.* (1979). Extended treatment with antilymphocyte globulin (ATGAM) in renal allograft recipients. *Transplantation* **28**, 365.

Wee, S. L., Colvin, R. B., Phelan, J. M., *et al.* (1989). Fc-receptor for mouse IgG1 (Fc gamma RII) and antibody-mediated cell clearance in patients treated with Leu2a antibody. *Transplantation* **48**, 1012.

Wee, S. L., Stroka, D. M., Preffer, F. L., *et al.* (1992). The effects of OKT4A monoclonal antibody on cellular immunity of nonhuman primate renal allograft recipients. *Transplantation* **53**, 501.

Weiss, A. (1989a). T lymphocyte activation. *In Fundamental Immunology*, (W. E. Paul, ed.), p. 359, Raven Press, New York.

Weiss, S. J. (1989b). Tissue destruction by neutrophils. *N. Engl. J. Med.* **320**, 365.

Wong, J. T. and Colvin, R. B. (1991). Selective reduction and proliferation of the CD4+ and CD8+ T cell subsets with bispecific monoclonal antibodies: evidence for inter-T cell-mediated cytolysis. *Clin. Immunol. Immunopathol.* **58**, 236.

Wong, J. T., Eylath, A. A., Ghobrial, I. and Colvin, R. B. (1990). The mechanism of anti-CD3 monoclonal antibodies: mediation of cytolysis by inter-T cell bridging. *Transplantation* **50**, 683.

Wood, K. J., Pearson, T. C., Darby, C. and Morris, P. J. (1991). CD4: a potential target molecule for immunosuppressive therapy and tolerance induction. *Transplant. Rev.* **5**, 150.

Woodle, E. S., Bruse, D. S., Josephson, M., *et al.* (1996). OKT3 escalating dose regimens provide effective therapy for renal allograft rejection. *Clin. Transplant.* **10**, 389.

Other Forms of Immunosuppression

Mark Waer • Jacques Pirenne • Chantal Mathieu

Inhibitors of Pyrimidine Biosynthesis

Two compounds, brequinar sodium and leflunomide, which were explored as immunosuppressants, were shown to inhibit the fourth enzyme, dihydroorotate dehydrogenase, in the *de novo* pyrimidine biosynthetic pathway. For both compounds, it is now believed that dihydroorotate dehydrogenase inhibition may not be the only mechanism of action and that they also may suppress tyrosine kinases that play key roles in activation pathways of T and B lymphocytes.

BREQUINAR SODIUM

Brequinar originally was developed as an antitumor drug and subsequently as an immunosuppressant for controlling transplant rejection. The interest in this drug in relation to transplantation was stimulated by the fact that there existed already an extensive safety database associated with its use as an antineoplastic drug and by the observation that it displayed a unique mechanism of action. The drug was shown to interfere with the *de novo* pyrimidine biosynthesis of lymphocytes. This different mechanism of action as compared with that of cyclosporine, for example, led to the expectation that brequinar might act synergistically with various other drugs.

Chemistry and Pharmacology

Brequinar is a substituted 4-quinoline carboxylic acid (6 fluoro-2-(2'-fluoro-1,1'-biphenyl-4-yl)-3 methyl-4-quinoline-carboxylic acid, sodium salt). It is a water-soluble compound that is absorbed readily after oral administration (Dexter *et al.*, 1985). Peak concentrations are obtained aproximately 2 hours after oral administration with a half-life in humans reported to be approximately 8 hours. Two thirds of the breakdown products are excreted in feces and one third in urine.

Mechanism of Action

As already mentioned, a first mechanism of action of brequinar is through its inhibition of the enzyme dihydroorotate dehydrogenase (Chen *et al.*, 1990). Dihydroorotate dehydrogenase is the fourth enzyme of the *de novo* pyrimidine biosynthetic pathway. Lymphocytes rely entirely on this *de novo* pathway for pyrimidine synthesis because they cannot use another, so-called pyrimidine salvage pathway. Consequently, nucleotide precursors uridine triphospate and cytidine triphosphate (UTP and CTP) necessary for the synthesis of RNA and DNA are depleted, and DNA and RNA synthesis are suppressed strongly by brequinar. This mode of action of brequinar explains its antiproliferative effect as well as its ability to decrease mRNA levels of interferon (IFN)-γ, interleukin (IL)-2 and IL-10 (Tian *et al.*, 1997). T and B lymphocytes are affected, explaining the effects of brequinar

on cell-mediated as well as humoral immunity. That the aforementioned mechanism of action is important is proved by the fact that *in vitro* as well as some *in vivo* effects of brequinar can be reversed by the administration of uridine (Xu *et al.*, 1997). Other immunosuppressive effects of brequinar are unaffected by similar administration of uridine, however, and pyrimidine levels are not decreased in the spleen of mice, suggesting that another mechanism of action may be involved. In this respect, it was shown that brequinar also was able to inhibit tyrosine phosphorylation in lymphocytes (Xu *et al.*, 1997).

It was found that brequinar inhibited protein tyrosine phosphorylation in anti-CD3-stimulated murine T lymphocytes and that it inhibited the activity of the protein tyrosine kinases p56lck and p59fyn. It was shown that lymphadenopathy and autoantibody production in MRL-lpr/lpr mice by brequinar depended on inhibition of pyrimidine nucleotide synthesis only partially and rather associated with *in vivo* inhibition of protein tyrosine phosphorylation (Xu *et al.*, 1997).

Experimental In Vitro and In Vivo Immunosuppressive Effects of Brequinar

Brequinar inhibits the mixed lymphocyte reaction in a dose-dependent manner. The concentration required to produce a 50% inhibition (IC50) is species dependent and varies from 0.025 μg/ml in humans to 40 μg/ml in monkeys. There is substantial interindividual variation in IC50 values in humans (Makowka and Cramer, 1992).

In rats, treatment three times weekly for 30 days was associated with permanent kidney and liver graft survival in most recipients. Heart graft survival prolongation was more difficult to achieve and required longer periods of administration (Cramer *et al.*, 1992a). Survival of small bowel allografts and hamster xenografts was prolonged in rats (Cramer *et al.*, 1992b).

There are at least three reasons why combination therapy with brequinar and cyclosporine was considered. First, a simultaneous use of cyclosporine might allow for lower doses of brequinar to be used and to provoke fewer side effects. Second, the cellular mechanism of action of cyclosporine and brequinar were different and complementary. Third, brequinar was shown to be active on B lymphocytes, whereas the main effect of cyclosporine is on T cells.

The humoral component of xenograft rejection is important and was inhibited successfully by combination therapy with brequinar and cyclosporine (Cramer *et al.*, 1992b). Treatment with brequinar before the transplantation of allogeneic hearts to sensitized recipients significantly delayed graft rejection in association with suppression of antibody responses to donor tissues (Yasunaga *et al.*, 1993). Although a synergistic effect of brequinar with cyclosporine was documented in various experimental models (Levy and Alexander, 1996), this synergism was complicated by enhanced toxicity of the two compounds (Pally *et al.*, 1998) as a result of drug accumulation.

Clinical Experience

After its approval for phase I studies in 1991, brequinar was tested in 32 patients within 48 hours after kidney transplantation. The patients received standard cyclosporine and steroid therapy and in addition brequinar on alternate days. The brequinar doses (50, 100 or 200 mg/kg) were adjusted to provide plasma levels of less than 2 mg/ml. There was evidence that the number of rejection episodes had been reduced significantly in this first series of patients (Cramer, 1996). These initial positive results were not confirmed in other centers, and enthusiasm for this drug was tempered because of its relatively narrow range of therapeutic effectiveness and an increased risk of thrombocytopenia at high dose levels.

Summary

Brequinar displays some characteristics that should make it an effective immunosuppressant. Its effect on pyrimidine metabolism means that it is exquisitely active in B cells, that it works synergistically with cyclosporine and that potential toxic effects should be reversed readily by uridine administration. It is relatively easy to monitor. The therapeutic window of brequinar seems to be relatively narrow, and its pharmacokinetic profile is subject to large interindividual variations. The future use of brequinar as a drug for transplantation patients is still uncertain. Because it was shown that the immunosuppressive effect of the drug is related more to peak plasma levels rather than to sustained levels, the future of this drug probably will depend on finding an analogue with a short plasma half-life limiting its toxicity.

LEFLUNOMIDE AND MALONITRILAMIDES

Leflunomide is an isoxazol derivative. These compounds initially were synthesized at Hoechst Research Laboratories (Germany) as potential agriculture herbicides. Subsequently it was found that leflunomide had immunosuppressive effects in models of adjuvent arthritis and graft-versus-host-disease (Bartlett *et al.*, 1989). Leflunomide has been shown to be effective and safe for the treatment of arthritis patients (Smolen *et al.*, 1999). The potential of leflunomide as an immunosuppressant for transplantation was shown extensively in various experimental studies. The long half-life (several days) of leflunomide could provide a problem of overimmunosuppression in transplant patients. Analogues from leflunomide's active metabolite (A771726) have been developed, which are called *malonitrilamides* (MNAs) and which have a much more acceptable pharmacokinetic profile. Most of the effects of leflunomide have been reproduced by the MNAs, making these compounds a potential new drug for transplantation purposes (Lin *et al.*, 1996a; Qi and Ekberg, 1998; Schorlemmer and Schleyerback, 1998).

Chemistry and Pharmacology

Leflunomide (N-(4))trifluoro-methylphenyl-5-methylisoxazol-4-carboxamide) is a prodrug easily converted to its open ring metabolite A771726. In almost all *in vitro* and *in vivo* assays described, A771726 has the activities described for leflunomide. As already mentioned, the MNAs are structurally similar to A771726. Leflunomide is insoluble in water and is suspended in 1% carboxymethylcellulose for oral adminstration.

Although rats tolerate leflunomide well after long-term administration, dogs readily develop anemia and gastrointestinal ulcerations. The commonest side effects in arthritis patients receiving long-term treatment are diarrhea (17%), nausea (10%), alopecia (8%) and rash (10%) (Smolen *et al.*, 1999), leading to a dropout rate of about 5% in arthritis trials. As already mentioned, the half-life of leflunomide is long in humans (>10 days), and the drug is metabolized predominantly by the liver.

Mechanism of Action

Leflunomide and its analogues have strong antiproliferative effects on T lymphocytes and especially on B lymphocytes. The production of IL-2 is not or only partially inhibited by leflunomide (Chong *et al.*, 1993).

Similar to brequinar, an effect on pyrimidine metabolism and on protein tyrosine kinase activity may explain the mechanism of action of leflunomide and the MNAs. Phosphorylation of the epidermal growth factor receptor of human fibroblasts has been shown to be inhibited by leflunomide (Mattar *et al.*, 1993). It was also shown that leflunomide directly inhibited the IL-2-stimulated protein tyrosine kinase activity of p56lck (Mattar *et al.*, 1993) and of p59fyn associated with the activation through the T-cell receptor/CD3 complex (Chong *et al.*, 1994). At higher concentrations, A771726 also inhibited IL-2-induced tyrosine phosphorylation of JAK1 and JAK3 protein tyrosine kinases, initiating signaling by the IL-2 receptor (Elder *et al.*, 1997). In a systematic effort to design inhibition of the antiapoptotic tyrosine kinase BTK (Bruton's tyrosine kinase), leflunomide analogues were shown to inhibit human BTK *in vitro* with IC50 values of about 15 nM (Mahajan *et al.*, 1999). Because BTK is a key factor for T cell–independent antibody formation, this effect of leflunomide may explain its potency in strongly suppressing T cell–independent IgM xenoantibodies (see later).

Kinetic studies involving activated lymphocytes showed that leflunomide retained its inhibitory activity when added 24 hours after stimulation and that addition of exogenous uridine reversed the proliferative effects of leflunomide (Siemaskao *et al.*, 1996). Inhibition of the pyrimidine synthesis was proposed to be an important mechanism of action. This proposal was confirmed on the molecular level by showing a direct inhibition of the enzyme dihydroorotate dehydrogenase by leflunomide (Williamson *et al.*, 1995).

Although in some reports it was mentioned that *in vivo* the immunosuppressive effect of A771726 was overcome by administering uridine (Stosic-Grujicic *et al.*, 1996), this was not confirmed in other models (Thoenes *et al.*, 1989). The *in vivo* mechanism of action of leflunomide may depend on factors such as drug levels, disposable uridine pools and immune-activation pathways involved. That more than one mechanism of action of leflunomide may occur *in vivo* was shown in mice, in which uridine restored proliferation and IgM production of lipopolysaccharide-stimulated B cells, whereas suppression of IgG production did not occur. The latter phenomenon correlated in a dose-dependent manner with tyrosine phosphorylation of JAK3 and STAT6 proteins, which are involved in IL-4-induced signal transduction pathways (Siemaskao *et al.*, 1998). The double *in vivo* mechanism of action was confirmed in rats, in which xenoreactivity was counteracted by the administration of uridine, whereas alloreactivity was not (Chong *et al.*, 1999). Some other effects of leflunomide and the MNAs were described. These drugs inhibited various macrophage functions, such as the production of oxygen radicals (Schorlemmer *et al.*, 1998), the inhibition of IgE-mediated hypersensitivity responses (Jarman *et al.*, 1999), the expression of IL-8 receptor type A (Mirmohammadsadegh *et al.*, 1998) and tumor necrosis factor–mediated NF-κB activation (Manna and Aggarwal, 1999).

In Vivo Transplantation Effects

In various transplantation experiments in rats, leflunomide was shown to be at least equally potent to cyclosporine (Bartlett *et al.*, 1991) and able to synergize with cyclosporine to induce tolerance (Lin *et al.*, 1996b). Some specific characteristics of leflunomide immunosuppression in rats were that it could interrupt ongoing acute rejections (Williams *et al.*, 1994) and that it was shown to be active in preventing and treating chronic vascular rejection (Xiao *et al.*, 1996).

One of the most attractive characteristics of leflunomide and the MNAs are their strong capacity to delay xenograft rejection (Lin *et al.*, 1998c) and to induce partial xenograft tolerance (Lin *et al.*, 1998a). This capacity may be related to the strong effects of leflunomide on T cell–independent xenoantibody formation as well as on the induction of natural killer cell nonresponsiveness (Lin *et al.*, 1998a) or xenoantigen expression (Lin *et al.*, 1998b).

Clinical Experience

Leflunomide has not been used yet in transplant patients because its pharmacokinetic profile is not considered optimal for this indication. The MNAs may be more suitable for transplantation, and clinical trials with these compounds are awaited with interest.

In arthritis patients, the efficacy and safety of leflunomide was evaluated carefully in a double-blind randomized multicenter trial (Smolen *et al.*, 1999). In this study, more than 350 patients were assigned randomly to leflunomide, placebo or sulfasalazine. Leflunomide and sulfasalazine were significantly superior to placebo. The commonest side effects in leflunomide-treated patients were diarrhea, nausea and rash. Three leflunomide patients showed abnormal liver function tests compared to five sulfasalazine patients. Overall, it was concluded that leflunomide was well tolerated and showed a similar efficacy to sulfasalazine.

Summary

Leflunomide and the MNAs are new immunosuppressants that deserve careful investigation in transplant patients, especially their effect on antibody formation and on chronic vascular lesions. Their synergism with cyclosporine or tacrolimus may be valuable. The major question that must be answered in the near future is whether MNA analogues may be developed for clinical transplantation use with an acceptable pharmacokinetic profile and a similar immunosuppressive effect as leflunomide.

15-Deoxyspergualin

In 1981, spergualin (a water-soluble peptide) was isolated from the culture filtrate of *Bacillus laterosporus* as a new anticancer or antibiotic substance (Takeuchi *et al.*, 1981). Spergualin was synthetically dehydroxylated to produce 15-deoxyspergualin (DSG), which subsequently became widely known as a promising new immunosuppressant. 15-Deoxyspergualin must be delivered parenterally because it has a poor oral bioavailability (Thomas *et al.*, 1993), and the drug is cleared rapidly, primarily through the kidney (Morris, 1991).

MECHANISMS OF ACTION

The precise mode of action of DSG is still unknown. 15-Deoxyspergualin specifically binds to Hsp 70, a heat-shock protein (Nadler *et al.*, 1992). It is believed that DSG may have its principal effect by inhibiting the activation of transcription factor NF-κB in antigen-presenting cells and monocytes (Halloran, 1996). This premise may explain why it inhibits monocyte and macrophage functions, such as antigen presentation, major histocompatibility class (MHC) II up-regulation, IL-1 release or superoxide production (Dickneite *et al.*, 1987; Waaga *et al.*, 1990). Specific T-cell functions, such as Con A blastogenesis, mixed lymphocyte reaction responsiveness or IL-2 production, are only poorly or not affected (Takahara *et al.*, 1992). In contrast, B lymphocyte maturation and antibody production are sensitive to DSG (Sterbenz and Tepper, 1993). Based on all of these characteristics, DSG has to be considered as a particular immunomodulatory agent with a unique mechanism of action that is totally different from other immunosuppressants.

EXPERIMENTAL ANIMAL MODELS

When used to prevent rejection, DSG did not seem to be effective in most animal experiments. When administered several days after transplantation, however, the drug was much more effective (Masuda *et al.*, 1987; Schorlemmer *et al.*, 1990). This finding suggested that DSG may be of use for the treatment of rejection crises, which was confirmed in dogs (Amemiya *et al.*, 1989), and subsequently this became the major indication for clinical use (see later). Because of its effects on monocytes, macrophages and B lymphocytes, DSG seems promising for xenotransplantation; this is illustrated by the fact that it is effective in stringent xenotransplant models such as that involving primary nonfunction of islet xenografts (Thomas *et al.*, 1995) and the induction of xenogeneic chimerism in the pig-into-baboon combination (Sablinski *et al.*, 1999).

CLINICAL USE

Based on the experimental studies showing that DSG was mainly effective as antirejection treatment, the major experience with DSG in clinical transplantation also was obtained in patients suffering from rejection. Between 1988 and 1991, many clinical trials were performed evaluating the effects of DSG for the treatment of kidney transplant rejections. The overall results indicated that as a 7- to 10-day monotherapy course, DSG reversed 70% of the acute rejections and 40% of the rejections that were already in a more chronic phase. When 3 days of high-dose methylprednisolone therapy was added, these results improved to 90% and 60% (Amemiya *et al.*, 1996).

In these clinical studies, the commonest subjective side effects were facial numbness and gastric discomfort. These symptoms disappeared as soon as the drip infusion was ended. Bone marrow suppression was the commonest serious side effect but responded effectively to a treatment with recombinant granulocyte colony–stimulating factor. Overall, further treatment of recurrent rejections was as effective as the first treatment.

Because of its effects on antibody formation, DSG also was explored in conjunction with cyclosporine, prednisolone and antilymphocyte globulin to inhibit secondary synthesis of preformed antibodies in ABO-incompatible or HLA-presensitized kidney transplant recipients as well as in pig islet xenograft recipients (Groth, 1993; Takahashi *et al.*, 1991). The experience in the latter studies is too limited to draw any firm conclusions, however.

FUTURE PROSPECTS

15-Deoxyspergualin has a particular mechanism of action that makes it an original immunomodulating agent that may broaden choices of immunosuppression. Until analogues are developed that allow for oral administration, the major clinical indication of DSG is limited to the treatment of rejection crises. 15-Deoxyspergualin may be an interesting alternative for steroids or antilymphocyte agents. The fact that it remains effective after recurrent administration is promising.

If in the future xenotransplantation becomes a reality, DSG may become important, especially for islet xenotransplantation. Because of its effects on macrophages and B lymphocytes, it may be essential to tackle the difficult problem of primary graft nonfunction in which these cells seem to be crucially involved. When new analogues are found that can be administered orally, the applications of DSG may be broadened (Lebreton et al., 1999).

FTY720

ORIGIN AND CHEMICAL STRUCTURE

FTY720 is a synthetic structural analogue of myriocin, a metabolite of the ascomycete *Isaria sinclairii* (Adachi et al., 1995). FTY720 has a molecular weight of 344 and is a 2-amino-2-[2-(4-octylphenyl)ethyl]-1,3-propanediol hydrochloride. This chemical structure is different from cyclosporine, tacrolimus and other current immunosuppressants.

ANTIREJECTION PROPERTIES IN SMALL AND LARGE ANIMALS

FTY720 given daily by oral gavage has marked antirejection properties in mice, rats, dogs and monkeys. FTY720 (0.1–10 mg/kg) prolongs survival of skin allografts in highly allogeneic rat models (Chiba et al., 1996). In a DA-to-LEW rat combination, a short course of peritransplant oral FTY720 (5 mg/kg; day −1 and 0) prolongs cardiac allograft survival and is as efficient as a 10-day posttransplant treatment with tacrolimus at 1 mg/kg (Xu et al., 1998a). Cardiac and liver allograft survival are prolonged in the ACI-to-Lew rat model by induction or maintenance treatment with FTY720 (Suzuki et al., 1996a). Delayed administration of FTY720 interrupts an ongoing allograft rejection, suggesting a role for FTY720 as a rescue agent (Suzuki et al., 1996b; Xu et al., 1998b). FTY720 blocks not only rejection, but also graft-versus-host disease after rat intestinal transplantation (Mitsusada et al., 1997). Peritransplant and posttransplant FTY720 (0.1–1 mg/kg/d) has profound immunosuppressive properties in dog and monkey kidney transplantation and in dog liver transplantation (Brinkmann et al., 1999b; Furukawa et al., 1999; Suzuki et al., 1999; Troncoso et al., 1999).

SYNERGY WITH OTHER IMMUNOSUPPRESSANTS

Small and large animal models provide evidence that FTY720 acts in synergy with calcineurin inhibitors, cyclosporine and tacrolimus and that this benefit does not result from pharmacokinetic interactions (Suzuki et al., 1996a). An induction course with FTY720 acts in synergy with posttransplant tacrolimus in prolonging cardiac allograft survival in rats (Xu et al., 1998a). A similar phenomenon is observed when FTY720 is used posttransplant in combination with cyclosporine in rat skin and heart allografts (Chiba et al., 1996; Hoshino et al., 1996; Kawaguchi et al., 1996; Suzuki et al., 1996b). FTY720 shows synergistic effect with tacrolimus and cyclosporine in heart and liver transplantation in the ACI-to-Lew rat model (Yamashita et al., 1999).

FTY720 shows synergy with cyclosporine in dog kidney (0.1–5 mg/kg/d) and monkey kidney (0.1–1 mg/kg/d) transplantation (Brinkmann et al., 1999b; Troncoso et al., 1999).

FTY720 (0.1 mg/kg) synergizes with cyclosporine and tacrolimus in dog liver transplantation (Furukawa et al., 1999). Synergy between FTY720 and rapamycin was observed in rat heart transplantation (Wang et al., 1998).

MECHANISMS OF ACTION

In contrast to cyclosporine and tacrolimus, FTY720 is a poor inhibitor of T-cell function *in vitro* (Brinkmann et al., 1999a; Troncoso et al., 1999). In particular, FTY720 does not influence antigen-induced IL-2 production. This lack of *in vitro* immunosuppressive activity contrasts with the marked antirejection properties of FTY720 seen *in vivo*.

Rats receiving one oral dose of 10 mg/kg of FTY720 show a rapid and profound decrease in peripheral lymphocyte counts. These counts remain significantly depressed but return to pretreatment levels within 14 days (Suzuki et al., 1996a). FACS analysis indicate a specific reduction in CD3 cells, with unchanged CD4/CD8 ratio (Xu et al., 1998a).

It was first suggested that FTY720-induced lymphocytopenia results from apoptotic lymphocyte death. *In vitro* exposure to high FTY720 concentrations (4×10^{-6}) induces chromatin condensation, typical DNA fragmentation and formation of apoptotic bodies (Suzuki et al., 1996a). Apoptosis after administration of FTY720 also has been documented *in vivo* (Chiba et al., 1996; Li et al., 1997b; Masubuchi et al., 1996; Suzuki et al., 1996a). FTY720 causes intragraft apoptotic lymphocytic death in animals with ongoing liver allograft rejection (Suzuki et al., 1998).

A second mechanism of action of FTY720 is through alteration of lymphocyte trafficking (Brinkmann et al., 1999a; Brunkhorst et al., 1999; Chiba et al., 1998). After FTY720 administration (4 or 8 mg/kg) in mice, labeled B and T cells immediately leave the peripheral blood and migrate to the peripheral lymph nodes, mesenteric lymph nodes and Peyer's patches. The labeled cells return to the peripheral blood after withdrawal of the drug and do not undergo apoptotic death. Migration is equivalent for T cells (CD4 and CD8 cells) and B cells (Yuzawa et al., 1999). This altered cell trafficking is accompanied by a reduction of lymphocyte infiltration into grafted organs (Yuzawa et al., 1999), a phenomenon that would contribute to the antirejection property of the drug.

Lymphocytes treated *ex vivo* with FTY720 and reintroduced *in vivo* similarly migrate to the peripheral lymphoid tissues, indicating that FTY720 acts directly on lymphocytes (Brinkmann et al., 1999a). The effect of FTY720 is abolished by previous exposure to pertussis toxin, suggesting that FTY720 modulates G protein–coupled chemokine receptors on the cell surface of the lymphocytes (Brinkmann et al., 1999a). The process of accelerated homing was blocked completely *in vivo* by coadministration of anti-CD62L, anti-CD49 and anti-CD11a monoclonal antibody, suggesting that FTY720 directly affects the homing receptors (Chiba et al., 1998).

FTY720, in presence of tumor necrosis factor-α, increases the expression of certain intercellular adhesion molecules on human umbilical vein endothelial cells *in vitro* (Li et al., 1997a). Alteration of cell trafficking by FTY720 may result not only from its direct action on lymphocytes, but also from an effect on endothelial cells.

TOXICITY

Pulmonary, cardiac and neurological toxicities have been reported but only in animals exposed to high doses of FTY720. The parent compound of FTY720 (myriocin) induces severe digestive toxicity, but not FTY720 itself (Adachi et al., 1995; Fujita et al., 1994, 1995). At therapeutic doses, FTY720 seems to be well tolerated. Doses of 5 mg/kg cause no clinical toxicity in rats. Studies in dogs indicate that doses of 5 mg/kg are equally well tolerated for periods of 90 days (Chiba *et al.*, 1996; Kawaguchi *et al.*, 1996). At 10 mg/kg, no toxicity was observed in heart grafted rats receiving posttransplant FTY720 (Chiba *et al.*, 1996; Hoshino *et al.*, 1996; Suzuki *et al.*, 1996a). A single dose of FTY720 at 10 mg/kg was lethal, however, when given pretransplant to liver rat recipients. Monkeys treated with FTY720 (0.1–1 mg/kg) showed no specific side effects (Troncoso *et al.*, 1999). Typical side effects of calcineurin inhibitors—nephrotoxicity, neurotoxicity and diabetogenicity—have not been observed with FTY720.

FTY720 IN HUMANS

Stable renal transplant patients maintained on cyclosporine tolerate well one oral dose of FTY720 (0.25–3.5 mg). In particular, no pulmonary toxicity was noted. Although clinically asymptomatic, a few episodes of bradycardia were observed. One episode of headache led to drug withdrawal.

Similar to its effect in animals, single doses of FTY720 cause a lymphocytopenia that is dose-dependent in intensity and duration and that equally affects CD4 cells, CD8 cells, memory T cells, naive T cells and B cells. Monocyte and granulocyte counts remain unchanged. Doses of 1 mg caused a rapidly reversible decrease in lymphocyte count with a nadir at about 6 to 12 hours. Higher doses of FTY720 result in more sustained and more profound lymphocytopenia.

Maximal concentration and area under the curve are proportional to the dose, indicating that the pharmacokinetic profile of FTY720 is linear. The volume of distribution is largely superior to the blood volume, indicating a widespread tissue penetration. FTY720 undergoes hepatic metabolism and has a long half-life (approximately 100 hours), indicating extended pharmacological action. Bioavailability is adequate, and intersubject variability is low (Brunkhorst *et al.*, 1999; Marino *et al.*, 1999; Neumayer *et al.*, 1999).

SUMMARY AND FUTURE PROSPECTS

FTY720 is a promising new type of immunosuppressive agent with unique structure and mechanism of action and a marked antirejection effect. FTY720 modifies lymphocyte trafficking through alteration of the expression or function of adhesion molecules. This alteration provokes a migration of lymphocytes from the peripheral blood to the secondary lymphoid tissues, a reduction in allograft lymphocyte infiltration and a peripheral lymphocytopenia. The effect is dose dependent and reversible on discontinuation of the drug. FTY720 also may cause lymphocyte apoptosis but probably only at higher doses. FTY720 can ameliorate or prevent rejection when used as induction or maintenance therapy. Ongoing acute rejection can be interrupted by posttransplant FTY720. FTY720 acts in synergy with calcineurin inhibitors cyclosporine and tacrolimus and with rapamycin. Further experimental work is needed to explore the detailed mechanisms of action of FTY720. Ongoing clinical trials will address the role of FTY720 in organ transplantation.

1,25-Dihydroxyvitamin D₃ and Its Analogues
MECHANISM OF ACTION

1,25-Dihydroxyvitamin D_3 (1,25(OH)$_2$D$_3$) and some of its new synthetic structural analogues are promising immunomodulators with effects in autoimmunity and transplantation immunology. The detection of the receptor for 1,25(OH)$_2$D$_3$ in almost all cells of the immune system, especially in antigen-

presenting cells (macrophages and dendritic cells) and in activated T lymphocytes, led to the investigation of a potential for 1,25(OH)$_2$D$_3$ as immunomodulator (Casteels *et al.*, 1995). Activated macrophages are able to synthesize and secrete 1,25(OH)$_2$D$_3$. After macrophage activation, the secretion of classic macrophage products such as cytokines (IL-1, tumor necrosis factor-α and IL-12) precedes the transcription of the vitamin D hydroxylase enzyme and as a consequence the production of 1,25(OH)$_2$D$_3$ (Overberg, L. *et al.*, 2000). The timing of its secretion is compatible with the concept of a suppressive, negative feedback signal.

1,25-Dihydroxyvitamin D₃ stimulates differentiation of monocytes and dendritic cells toward good phagocytosis and killing of bacteria, while suppressing the antigen-presenting capacity of these cells (Lemire, 1992). Essential for the latter is the suppression of expression of HLA class II molecules and of classic adhesion molecules necessary for full T-cell stimulation, such as B7.2 (Clavreul *et al.*, 1998). The crucial signals secreted by antigen-presenting cells for recruitment and activation of T cells are influenced directly by 1,25(OH)$_2$D$_3$. A key cytokine in the immune system, IL-12, is clearly inhibited by 1,25(OH)$_2$D$_3$ and analogues (Lemire *et al.*, 1994). This monocyte-produced cytokine is the major determinant of the direction in which the immune system is activated. By inhibiting IL-12 secretion, 1,25(OH)$_2$D$_3$ directly interferes with the heart of the immune cascade and shifts the reaction toward a Th2 profile (Casteels *et al.*, 1995).

1,25-Dihydroxyvitamin D₃ influences the secretion of other substances secreted by monocytes. Production of the suppressive factor prostaglandin E₃ is stimulated, whereas that of the monocyte-recruiter granulocyte-macrophage colony-stimulating factor is suppressed (Koren *et al.*, 1986; Towers and Freedman, 1998) by 1,25(OH)$_2$D$_3$.

Several T-cell cytokines, especially from the Th1 type, are direct targets for 1,25(OH)$_2$D$_3$ and its analogues. 1,25-Dihydroxyvitamin D₃-mediated inhibition of IL-2 secretion is due to impairment of NFAT complex formation, which normally binds to the distal NFAT binding site in the human IL-2 promoter (Takeuchi *et al.*, 1998). Interferon-γ is directly down-regulated by 1,25(OH)$_2$D$_3$ through a vitamin D–responsive element. Progressive deletion analysis of the IFN-γ promotor revealed that the negative regulation by 1,25(OH)$_2$D$_3$ may also be at the level of an upstream region containing an enhancer element (Cipitelli and Santoni, 1995).

PRECLINICAL MODELS

The fact that 1,25(OH)$_2$D$_3$ and its analogues influence the immune system by immunomodulation through induction of immune shifts and regulator cells makes these products appealing for clinical use, especially in the treatment and prevention of autoimmune diseases. In autoimmune diabetes in the NOD mouse, up-regulation of regulator cells and a shift from Th1 toward Th2 could be observed locally in the pancreas and islet grafts of treated mice. A restoration of the defective sensitivity to apoptosis seen in NOD lymphocytes was observed. This restoration led to better elimination of autoreactive effector cells (Casteels *et al.*, 1998a). This increased sensitivity to apoptosis by 1,25(OH)$_2$D$_3$ and its analogues has been described for different apoptosis-inducing signals. This mechanism may explain why an early and short-term treatment with these products before the clinical onset of autoimmunity can lead to long-term protection and restoration of self-tolerance (Casteels *et al.*, 1998b). A clear additive and synergistic effect was observed between 1,25(OH)$_2$D$_3$ or its analogues and other more classic immunomodulators, such as cyclosporine and sirolimus, *in vitro* and *in vivo* in an experimental encephalitis model (Branisteanu *et al.*, 1996).

1,25-Dihydroxyvitamin D_3 and its analogues were investigated in various transplantation models, such as in islet grafts in mice (Casteels *et al.*, 1998b; Mathieu *et al.*, 1998), murine cardiac allografts (Lemire *et al.*, 1992), mouse skin grafts (Jordan *et al.*, 1988; Veyron *et al.*, 1993), rat aortic allografts (Raisanen *et al.*, 1997) and rat heart allografts (Lewin *et al.*, 1994). The overall conclusion that can be drawn from these studies is that as a monotherapy for transplantation, $1,25(OH)_2D_3$ or its analogues are not potent. The latter is not surprising in view of its rather weak intrinsic effects on T cells. In conjunction with other immunosuppressants, there frequently is a strong synergistic effect, however. In view of its effect on antigen presentation and on directing the immune system in the Th2 direction, $1,25(OH)_2D_3$ may help to induce tolerance. A major concern remains the side effects of $1,25(OH)_2D_3$ on calcium and bone metabolism. To solve this problem, there is a great interest in finding $1,25(OH)_2D_3$ analogues with strong immune effects but lacking effects on bone metabolism.

Photopheresis

Extracorporeal photopheresis is an immunoregulatory technique in which lymphocytes are reinfused after exposure to a photoactive compound: 8-methoxypsoralen (8-MOP) and ultraviolet A light. The technique was developed for the treatment of erythrodermic cutaneous T-cell lymphoma (Edelson *et al.*, 1987). Subsequently the procedure was shown to be safe as an alternative treatment for various immune and autoimmune diseases (Perotti *et al.*, 1999). In rat (Perez *et al.*, 1989) and monkey experiments (Pepino *et al.*, 1989), the regimen was shown to result in extended skin or xenograft survival.

Photopheresis has been used to treat therapy-resistant rejection crises and as preventive therapy. Patients with refractory bronchiolitis obliterans complicating lung transplantation were treated successfully by phototherapy (O'Hagan *et al.*, 1999). In another study involving transplant patients with decreasing graft function and bronchiolitis obliterans, photopheresis resulted in a stabilization of graft function in five of eight patients and in some of these patients resulted in histological reversal of rejection (Salerno *et al.*, 1999).

The safety and efficacy of photopheresis in the prevention of acute rejection of cardiac allografts were evaluated in 60 primary cardiac allograft recipients, randomly assigned to standard triple-drug immunosuppressive therapy (cyclosporine, azathioprine and prednisone) alone or in conjunction with 24 photopheresis treatments administered during the first 6 months after transplantation. After 6 months of follow-up, phototherapy-treated patients developed significantly fewer rejection crises and significantly fewer multiple rejections. There were no significant differences in the rates or types of infection. Although there was no significant effect on graft survival rates at 6 or 12 months, this study indicates that phototherapy may be an effective new immunosuppressive regimen to be explored further in transplant recipients (Barr *et al.*, 1998).

Splenectomy

Splenectomy in the recipient before transplantation first was proposed by Starzl *et al.* in 1963 to improve graft survival. The role of splenectomy in enhancing graft survival has been controversial (Kauffman *et al.*, 1974; Opelz and Terasaki, 1973; Pierce and Hume, 1968; Renal Transplant Reg-

istry Advisory Committee, 1977; Starzl *et al.*, 1963; Stuart *et al.*, 1980), but a large prospective randomized trial of splenectomy in Minneapolis showed that splenectomy improved graft survival significantly (Fryd *et al.*, 1981). Longer term follow-up of patients in the trial showed that the early improvement in graft survival was lost because of an increased mortality from infection, however (Sutherland *et al.*, 1984). Several other single-center studies have shown an alarming risk of sepsis and death nullifying any early benefits of splenectomy on graft survival (Alexander *et al.*, 1984; Peters *et al.*, 1983), whereas a multicenter analysis from South Eastern Organ Procurement Foundation showed a modest improvement in graft survival after splenectomy but a relentless increase in patient mortality in the splenectomized patients (Lucas *et al.*, 1987). Splenectomy cannot be justified as a routine procedure, although it does have a place in patients who develop hypersplenism or who are being treated with azathioprine and who are consistently leukopenic, which is not generally a problem today with cyclosporine protocols.

Splenectomy may have a place in the preparation of a recipient who is to receive an ABO-incompatible graft, a practice that is likely to become more widely employed in living related donor transplantation in which an otherwise suitable ABO-incompatible donor is the only available donor. Alexandre's group reported a series of 38 such ABO-incompatible living donor transplants in which the recipient was prepared in general by plasmapheresis, donor-specific platelet transfusion and splenectomy. Although they believe that the need for plasmapheresis and donor-specific platelet transfusion should be reevaluated, they think that splenectomy may be important, in that 3 of the 38 recipients who did not have a splenectomy lost their grafts from acute vascular rejection, compared with 5 of 33 who had a splenectomy (Alexandre *et al.*, 1985, 1991; Reding *et al.*, 1987b). A small but successful experience of transplanting ABO-incompatible grafts that involved a splenectomy before transplantation also has been reported from Japan (Ishikawa *et al.*, 1998).

Plasmapheresis

Plasmapheresis has been used in three main situations. The first is in the treatment of an acute steroid-resistant rejection that morphologically is predominantly vascular and considered to be antibody mediated rather than cell mediated. Although some initial reports suggested a beneficial effect (Cardella *et al.*, 1978), controlled trials were unconvincing (Allen *et al.*, 1983; Kirubakaran *et al.*, 1981). The second situation is in the preparation of recipients of ABO-incompatible living donor kidneys, referred to earlier (Alexandre *et al.*, 1991; Reding *et al.*, 1987b), that may not be necessary because Brynger *et al.* (1982) reported some successful ABO-incompatible grafts without prior plasmapheresis of the recipient. Alexandre's group has not found a correlation between the posttransplant ABO isoagglutinin levels and the outcome of ABO-incompatible grafts (Reding *et al.*, 1987a).

The third situation is an attempt to reduce the titer and broad reactivity of HLA antibodies in highly sensitized patients on dialysis, combined with cyclophosphamide therapy to prevent reappearance of the antibodies so as to enable a negative crossmatch donor to be found and a transplant. Some encouraging early results of this approach have been reported but not without significant morbidity (Taube *et al.*, 1984). Immunoabsorption also has been used in place of plasmapheresis to remove antibody, and this is perhaps a more efficient method (Palmer *et al.*, 1989). Studies of this approach to transplantation of highly sensitized recipients are continuing with an emphasis on drugs that selectively may prevent synthesis of antibodies but perhaps may be associated with less toxicity than cyclophosphamide.

Cyclophosphamide

Cyclophosphamide in relatively high doses is an effective immunosuppressive agent in experimental allograft models (Winearls *et al.*, 1979) with perhaps some specificity for B lymphocytes (Turk *et al.*, 1972). Starzl *et al.* (1971) suggested that cyclophosphamide might be substituted for azathioprine in a report of a small series of patients followed only for several months because extremely good results were achieved with triple therapy using antilymphocyte globulin, cyclophosphamide and prednisolone with few complications. Previous experience with cyclophosphamide in small numbers of cases had not been good, probably because of the use of relatively large doses (Parsons *et al.*, 1966).

Cyclophosphamide has been combined with azathioprine and prednisolone (Berlyne and Danovitch, 1971) and has been used for the treatment of chronic steroid-resistant rejection allegedly with some benefit (Uldall *et al.*, 1971), although serious complications were noted in both reports. The administration of intermittent bolus doses of cyclophosphamide in the first few weeks after transplantation has been shown to be of no striking benefit in two small controlled trials (Jeffrey *et al.*, 1979; Wedgewood *et al.*, 1980). The complications of cyclophosphamide can be serious—leukopenia, thrombocytopenia, hemorrhagic cystitis, nausea and vomiting. These complications are rare with small doses and in cases in which cyclophosphamide has been used in a small number of patients at Oxford to replace azathioprine because of liver dysfunction at a dose of 1 mg kg^{-1}; there have been no side effects or any evidence of inadequate immunosuppression as judged by a subsequent deterioration in renal function. It is possible that cyclophosphamide has never been tested adequately at a sufficiently low dose to avoid most of the complications; this is suggested by the considerable experience of Yadav and colleagues at Chandigarh in India, in which cyclophosphamide has proved to be an apropriate alternative to azathioprine (Yadav *et al.*, 1988). In their unit, 29 living related transplant recipients were given cyclophosphamide instead of azathioprine (at a dose of 1.5–2.0 mg kg^{-1}) because of hepatic dysfunction or the cost and unavailability of azathioprine. Complications attributed directly to cyclophosphamide were minimal. The authors concluded that cyclophosphamide was a safe and effective alternative to azathioprine.

The only use of cyclophosphamide today is in attempts to desensitize highly sensitized recipients before renal transplantation (see Chapter 10). Most protocols involve repeated plasmaphereses, as described earlier, with cyclophosphamide, with or without steroids, being continued through the period of plasmapheresis until a kidney transplant can be performed (Alarabi *et al.*, 1997).

Bredinin (Mizoribine)

Bredinin, an imidazole nucleoside, has been used extensively in Japan in experimental renal transplantation in dogs (Amemiya *et al.*, 1988) and in place of azathioprine with seemingly a satisfactory outcome. Aso and colleagues reported the use of low-dose cyclosporine, prednisolone and bredinin in living related donor transplantation (Aso *et al.*, 1987; Tanabe *et al.*, 1999). In 23 haploidentical recipients treated with this triple therapy, no patient or graft was lost, but follow-up was quite short.

References

Adachi, K., Kohara, T., Nakano, N., *et al.* (1995). Design, synthesis, and structure-activity relationships of 2-substituted-2-amino-1,3-propanediols: discovery of a novel immunosuppressant, FTY720. *Bioorg. Med. Chem.* **5**, 853.

Alarabi, A., Backman, U., Wikstrom, B., Sjoberg, O. and Tufreson, G. (1997). Plasmapheresis in HLA-immunosensitized patients prior to kidney transplantation. *Int. J. Artif. Organs* **20**, 51.

Alexander, J. W., First, M. R., Majeski, J. A., *et al.* (1984). The late adverse effect of splenectomy on patient survival following cadaveric renal transplantation. *Transplantation* **37**, 467.

Alexandre, G. P., Latinne, D., Carlier, M., *et al.* (1991). ABO-incompatibility and organ transplantation. *Transplant. Rev.* **5**, 230.

Alexandre, G. P., Squifflet, J. P., De Bruyere, M., *et al.* (1985). Splenectomy as a prerequisite for successful human ABO-incompatible renal transplantation. *Transplant. Proc.* **17**, 138.

Allen, N. H., Dyer, P., Geoghegan, T., Harris, K, Lee, H. A. and Slapak, M. (1983). Plasma exchange in acute renal allograft rejection: a controlled trial. *Transplantation* **35**, 425.

Amemiya, H., Koyama, I., Kyo, M., *et al.* (1996). Outline and long-term prognosis in 15-deoxyspergualin-treated cases. *Transplant. Proc.* **28**, 1156.

Amemiya, H., Suzuki, S., Niya, S., *et al.* (1988). Synergistic effect of cyclosporine and mizoribine on survival of dog renal allografts. *Transplantation* **46**, 768.

Amemiya, H., Suzuki, S., Niya, S., *et al.* (1989). A new immunosuppressive agent, 15-deoxyspergualin in dog renal allorafting. *Transplant. Proc.* **21**, 3468.

Aso, K., Uchida, H., Sato, K., *et al.* (1987). Immunosuppression with low dose cyclosporine combined with bredinin and prednisolone. *Transplant. Proc.* **19**, 1955.

Barr, M. L., Meiser, B. M., Eisen, H. J., *et al.* (1998). Photopheresis for the prevention of rejection in cardiac transplantation. Photopheresis Transplantation Study Group. *N. Engl. J. Med.* **339**, 1744.

Bartlett, R. R., Dimitrijevic, M., Mattar, T., *et al.* (1991). Leflunomide (HWA 486), a novel immunomodulating compound for the treatment of autoimmune disorders and reactions leading to transplantation rejection. *Agents Actions* **32**, 10.

Bartlett, R. R., Mattar, T., Weithmann, U., *et al.* (1989). Leflunomide (HWA486): a novel immunorestoring drug. *In Therapeutic Approaches to Inflammatory Diseases*, (A. J. Lewis, N. S. Doherty and N. R. Ackerman, eds.), p. 215, Elsevier, New York.

Berlyne, G. M. and Danovitch, G. M. (1971). Cyclophosphamide for immunosuppression in renal transplantation. *Lancet* **2**, 924.

Branisteanu, D., Mathieu, C., Casteels, K., *et al.* (1996) Combination of vitamin D analogues and immunosuppressants: potential clinical use. *Clin. Immunother.* **6**, 465.

Brinkmann, V., Pinschewer, D. and Feng, L. (1999a). FTY720 suppresses immune responses by modulating G-protein coupled receptors on lymphocytes resulting in altered lymphocyte homing. *Proceedings of the AST Eighteenth Annual Meeting*, May 15–19, Chicago.

Brinkmann, V., Schuurman, H. J., Pinschewer, D., *et al.* (1999b). FTY720 efficiently prolongs allograft survival by suppressing T cell-dependent and T cell-independent immunity. *Proceedings of the AST Eighteenth Annual Meeting*, May 15–19, Chicago.

Brunkhorst, R., Neumayer, H.-H., Hiss, M., *et al.* (1999). Human safety and pharmacology of FTY720. *Proceedings of the AST Eighteenth Annual Meeting*, May 15–19, Chicago.

Brynger, H., Rydberg, I., Samuelsson, B., Blohme, I., Lindholm, A. and Sandberg, L. (1982). Renal transplantation across a blood group barrier—"A2" kidneys to "0" recipients. *Proc. Eur. Dial. Transplant. Assoc.* **19**, 427.

Cardella, C. J., Sutton, D. M., Falk, J. A., Kalz, A., Uldall, P. R. and de Vever, G. A. (1978). Effect of intensive plasma exchange on renal transplant rejection and serum cytotoxic antibody. *Transplant. Proc.* **10**, 617.

Casteels, K., Bouillon, R., Waer, M., *et al.* (1995). Immunomodulatory effects of 1,25-dihydroxyvitamin D$_3$. *Curr. Opin. Nephrol. Hypertens.* **4**, 313.

Casteels, K., Waer, M., Bouillon, R., *et al.* (1998a). 1,25-Dihydroxyvitamin D$_3$ restores sensitivity to cyclophosphamide-induced apoptosis in NOD mice and protects against diabetes. *Clin. Exp. Immunol.* **112**, 181.

Casteels, K., Waer, M., Laureys, J., *et al.* (1998b). Prevention of auto-immune destruction of syngeneic islet grafts in spontaneously diabetic nonobese diabetic mice by a combination of a vitamin₃ analog and cyclosporine. *Transplantation* **65**, 1225.

Chen, S.-F., Papp, L. M., Ardecky, R. J., *et al.* (1990). Structure activity relationship of quinoline carboxylic acids: a new class of inhibitors of DHODH. *Biochem. Pharmacol.* **40**, 709.

Chiba, K., Hoshino, Y., Suzuki, C., *et al.* (1996). FTY720, a novel immunosuppressant possessing unique mechanisms: I. prolongation of skin allograft survival and synergistic effect in combination with cyclosporine in rats. *Transplant. Proc.* **28**, 1056.

Chiba, K., Yanagawa, Y., Masubuchi, Y., *et al.* (1998). FTY720: a novel immunosuppressant, induces sequestration of circulating mature lymphocytes by acceleration of lymphocyte homing in rats: I. FTY720 selectively decreases the number of circulating mature lymphocytes by acceleration of lymphocyte homing. *J. Immunol.* **160**, 5037.

Chong, A. S., Xiao, F., Xu, X. L., *et al.* (1994). In vivo and in vitro immunosuppression with leflunomide. *In Recent Development in Transplantation Medicine,* (D. Przepiorka, ed.), p. 163, Physicians & Scientists, Glenview, Ill.

Chong, A. S. F., Gebel, H., Finnegan, A., *et al.* (1993). Leflunomide, a novel immunomodulatory agent: in vitro analyses of the mechanism of immunosuppression. *Transplant. Proc.* **25**, 747.

Chong, A. S. F., Huang, W., Liu, W., *et al.* (1999). In vivo activity of leflunomide. *Transplantation* **68**, 100.

Cipitelli, M. and Santoni, A. (1995). Vitamin D₃: a transcriptional modulator of the interferon-gamma gene. *Eur. J. Immunol.* **28**, 3017.

Clavreul, A., D'Hellencourt, C. L. M.-M. C., Potron, G., *et al.* (1998). Vitamin D differentially regulates B7.1 and B7.2 expression on human peripheral blood monocytes. *Immunology* **95**, 272.

Cramer, D. V. (1996). Brequinar sodium. *Transplant. Proc.* **28**, 960.

Cramer, D. V., Chapman, F. A., Jaffee, B. D., *et al.* (1992a). The effect of a new immunosuppressive drug, brequinar sodium, on heart, liver, and kidney allograft rejection in the rat. *Transplantation* **53**, 303.

Cramer, D. V., Chapman, F. A., Jaffee, B. D., *et al.* (1992b). The prolongation of concordant hamster-to-rat cardiac xenografts by brequinar sodium. *Transplantation* **54**, 701.

Dexter, D. L., Hesson, D. P., Ardecky, R. J., *et al.* (1985). Activity of a novel 4-quinolinecarboxylic acid, NSC368390, 6-fluoro-2-(2'-fluoro-1, 1'-biphenyl-4-yl)-3-methyl-4-quinoline carboxylic acid, sodium salt, against experimental tumors. *Cancer Res.* **45**, 5563.

Dickneite, G., Shorlemmer, H. U. and Sedlacek, H. H. (1987). Decrease of mononuclear phagocyte cell functions and prolongation of graft survival in experimental transplantation by 15-deoxyspergualin. *Int. J. Immunopharmacol.* **9**, 559.

Edelson, R., Berger, C., Gasparro, F., *et al.* (1987). Treatment of cutaneous T cell lymphoma by extracorporeal photochemotherapy: preliminary results. *N. Engl. J. Med.* **316**, 297.

Elder, R. T., Xu, X., Williams, J. W., *et al.* (1997). The immunosuppressive metabolite of leflunomide, A771726, affects murine T cells through two biochemical mechanisms. *J. Immunol.* **159**, 22.

Fryd, D. S., Sutherland, D. E. R., Simmons, R. L., Ferguson, R. M., Kjellstrand, C. M. and Najarian, J. S. (1981). Results of a prospective randomized study on the effect of splenectomy versus no splenectomy in renal transplant patients. *Transplant. Proc.* **13**, 48.

Fujita, T., Inoue, K., Yamamoto, S., *et al.* (1994). Fungal metabolites: Part II. a potent immunosuppressive activity found in *Isaria sinclairii* metabolite. *J. Antibiot. (Tokyo)* **47**, 208.

Fujita, T., Yoneta, M., Hirose, R., *et al.* (1995). Simple compounds, 2-alkyl-2-amino-1,3-propanediols, have potent immunosuppressive activity. *Bioorg. Med. Chem.* **5**, 847.

Furukawa, H., Suzuki, T., Jin, M. B., *et al.* (1999). Canine orthotopic liver transplantation treated with a novel immunosuppressant, FTY720, and subtherapeutic doses of conventional drugs. *Proceedings of the 25th Annual Scientific Meeting of the American Society of Transplant Surgeons,* May 19–21, Chicago.

Groth, C. G. (1993). Deoxyspergualin in allogeneic kidney and xenogeneic islet transplantation: early clinical trial. *Ann. N. Y. Acad. Sci.* **685**, 193.

Halloran, P. F. (1996). Molecular mechanisms of new immunosuppressants. *Clin. Transplant.* **10**, 118.

Hoshino, Y., Suzuki, C., Ohtsuki, M., *et al.* (1996). FTY720, a novel immunosuppressant possessing unique mechanisms: II. long-term graft survival induction in rat heterotopic cardiac allografts and synergistic effect in combination with cyclosporine A. *Transplant. Proc.* **28**, 1060.

Ishikawa, A., Itoh, M., Ushlyama, T., Suzuki, K. and Fujita, K. (1998). Experience of ABO-incompatible living kidney transplantation after double filtration plasmapheresis. *Clin. Transplant.* **12**, 80.

Jarman, E. R., Kuba, A., Montermann, E., *et al.* (1999). Inhibition of murine IgE and immediate cutaneous hypersensitivity responses to ovalbumin by the immunomodulatory agent leflunomide. *Clin. Exp. Immunol.* **115**, 221.

Jeffrey, J. R., Downs, A. R., Lye, C. and Ramsey, E. (1979). Immunosuppression with azathioprine, prednisolone and cyclophosphamide. *Transplantation* **28**, 10.

Jordan, S. C., Shibuka, R. and Mullen, Y. (1988). 1,25-Dihydroxyvitamin D₃ prolongs skin graft survival in mice. *In Vitamin D: Molecular, Cellular and Clinical Endocrinology,* (A. W. Norman, K. Schaefer, H.-G. Grigoleit, eds.), p. 346, Walter de Gruyter, Berlin.

Kauffman, H. M., Swanson, M. K. and McGregor, W. R. (1974). Splenectomy in renal transplantation. *Surg. Gynecol. Obstet.* **139**, 33.

Kawaguchi, T., Hoshino, Y., Rahman, F., *et al.* (1996). FTY720, a novel immunosuppressant possessing unique mechanisms: III. synergistic prolongation of canine renal allograft survival in combination with cyclosporine A. *Transplant. Proc.* **28**, 1062.

Kirubakaran, M. G., Disney, A. P., Norman, J., Pugsley, D. J. and Matthews, T. H. (1981). A controlled trial of plasmapheresis in the treatment of renal allograft rejection. *Transplantation* **32**, 164.

Koren, R., Ravid, A., Rotem, C., *et al.* (1986). 1,25-Dihydroxyvitamin D₃ enhances prostaglandin E₂ production by monocytes: a mechanism which partially accounts for the antiproliferative effect of 1,25(OH)₂D₃ on lymphocytes. *FEBS Lett.* **205**, 113.

Lebreton, L., Annat, J., Derrepas, P., *et al.* (1999). Structure-immunosuppressive activity relationships of new analogues of 15-deoxyspergualin: 1. structural modifications of the hydroxyglycine moiety. *J. Med. Chem.* **28**, 277.

Lemire, J. M. (1992). Immunomodulatory role of 1,25-dihydroxyvitamin D₃. *J. Cell. Biochem.* **49**, 26.

Lemire, J. M., Archer, D. C., Khulkarni, A., *et al.* (1992). Prolongation of the survival of murine cardiac allografts by the vitamin D₃ analogue 1,25-dihydroxy-delta¹⁶-cholecalciferol. *Transplantation* **54**, 762.

Lemire, J. M., Beck, L., Faherty, D., *et al.* (1994). 1,25-Dihydroxyvitamin D₃ inhibits the production of IL-12 by human monocytes and B cells. *In Vitamin D, A Pluripotent Steroid Hormone: Structural Studies, Molecular Endocrinology and Clinical Applications,* (A. W. Norman, R. Bouillon and M. Thomasset, eds.), p. 531, Walter de Gruyter, Berlin.

Levy, A. E. and Alexander, J. W. (1996). The significance of timing of additional short-term immunosuppression in the donor-specific transfusion/cyclosporine-treated rat. *Transplantation* **62**, 262.

Lewin, E. and Olgaard, K. (1994). The in vivo effect of a new, in vitro, extremely potent vitamin D₃ analog Kh1060 on the suppression of renal allograft rejection in the rat. *Calcif. Tissue Int.* **54**, 150.

Li, X. K., Enosawa, S., Kakefuda, T., *et al.* (1997a). FTY720, a novel immunosuppressive agent, enhances upregulation of the cell adhesion molecular ICAM-1 in TNF-α treated human umbilical vein endothelial cells. *Transplant. Proc.* **29**, 1265.

Li, X. K., Shinomiya, T., Kakefuda, T., *et al.* (1997b). Induction of lymphocyte apoptosis by a novel immunosuppressant, FTY720: relation with Fas, Bcl-2, and Bax expression. *Transplant. Proc.* **29**, 1267.

Lin, Y., Goebels, J., Xia, G., *et al.* (1998a). Induction of specific transplantation tolerance across xenogeneic barriers in the T-independent immune compartment. *Nat. Med.* **4**, 173.

Lin, Y., Ji, P., Xia, G., *et al.* (1998b). Blockade of induced xenoantigen expression prevents rejection after retransplantation of accommodated hamster-to-rat heart xenografts. *Transplantation* **65**, 340.

Lin, Y., Segers, C. and Waer, M. (1996a). Efficacy of the malononitrilamide X920715 as compared with leflunomide in cardiac allo- and xenotransplantation in rats. *Transplant. Proc.* **28**, 3036.

Lin, Y., Vandeputte, M. and Waer, M. (1996b). A short-term combination therapy with cyclosporine and rapamycin or leflunomide induces long-term heart allograft survival in a strongly immunogenic strain combination in rats. *Transpl. Int.* **9**, S328.

Lin, Y., Vandeputte, M. and Waer, M. (1998c). Accommodation and T-independent B cell tolerance in rats with long-term surviving hamster heart xenografts. *J. Immunol.* **160**, 369.

Lucas, B. A., Vaughan, W. K., Sanfilippo, F., Peters, T. G. and Alexander, J. W. (1987). Effects of pretransplant splenectomy: univariate and multi-centre analyses. *Transplant. Proc.* **19**, 1993.

Mahajan, S., Ghosh, S., Sudbeck, E. A., *et al.* (1999). Rational design and synthesis of a novel anti-leukemic agent targeting Bruton's tyrosine kinase (BTK), LFM-A13 [alpha-cyano-beta-hydroxy-beta-methyl-N-(2,5-dibromophenyl) propenamide]. *J. Biol. Chem.* **274**, 9587.

Makowka, L. and Cramer, D. V. (1992). Brequinar sodium: a new immunosuppressive drug for transplantation. *Transplant. Sci.* **2**, 50.

Manna, S. K. and Aggarwal, B. B. (1999). Immunosuppressive leflunomide metabolite (A77 1726) blocks TNF-dependent nuclear factor-kappa B activation and gene expression. *J. Immunol.* **162**, 2095.

Marino, M., Choudhury, S., Neumayer, H.-H., *et al.* (1999). Pharmacokinetic (PK)/pharmacodynamic (PD) model of FTY720 in humans. *Proceedings of the AST Eighteenth Annual Meeting*, May 15–19, Chicago.

Masubuchi, Y., Kawaguchi, T., Ohtsuki, M., *et al.* (1996). FTY720, a novel immunosuppressant possessing unique mechanisms: IV. prevention of graft-versus-host reactions in rats. *Transplant. Proc.* **28**, 1064.

Masuda, T., Mizutani, S., Lijima, M., *et al.* (1987). Immunosuppressive activity of 15-deoxyspergualin and its effect on skin allografts in rats. *J. Antibiot.* **49**, 1612.

Mathieu, C., Casteels, K., Waer, M., *et al.* (1998). Prevention of diabetes recurrence after islet transplantation in NOD mice by analogues of 1,25(OH)$_2$D$_3$ in combination with CyA. *Transplant. Proc.* **30(2)**, 541.

Mattar, T., Kochhar, K. and Bartlett, R. (1993). Inhibition of the epidermal growth factor receptor tyrosine kinase activity by leflunomide. *FEBS Lett.* **334**, 161.

Mirmohammadsadegh, A., Homey, B., Abts, H. F., *et al.* (1998). Differential modulation of pro- and anti-inflammatory cytokine receptors by N-(4-trifluoromethylphenyl-2-cyano-3-hydroxy-crotonic acid amide (A77 1726), the physiologically active metabolite of the novel immunomodulator leflunomide. *Biochem. Pharmacol.* **55**, 1523.

Mitsusada, M., Suzuki, S., Kobayashi, E., *et al.* (1997). Prevention of graft rejection and graft-versus-host reaction by a novel immunosuppressant, FTY720, in rat small bowel transplantation. *Transpl. Int.* **10**, 343.

Morris, R. E. (1991). 15-deoxyspergualin: a mystery wrapped within an emigma. *Clin. Transplant.* **5**, 530.

Nadler, S. G., Tepper, M., Schacter, B., *et al.* (1992). Interaction of the immunosuppressant deoxyspergualin with a member of the Hsp 70 family of heat shock proteins. *Science* **258**, 484.

Neumayer, H.-H., Brunkhorst, R., Budde, K., *et al.* (1999). Human pharmacokinetics of FTY720. *Proceedings of the AST Eighteenth Annual Meeting*, May 15–19, Chicago.

O'Hagan, A. R., Stillwell, P. C., Arroliga, A., *et al.* (1999). Photopheresis in the treatment of refractory bronchiolitis obliterans complicating lung transplantation. *Chest* **115**, 1459.

Opelz, G. and Terasaki, P. I. (1973). Effect of splenectomy on human renal transplants. *Transplantation* **15**, 605.

Overberg, L, Decallone, B., Valekx, D. *et al.* (2000). Identification and immune regulation of 25-hydroxyvitamin D-1-alpha-hydroxylase in murine macrophages. *Clin. Exp. Immunol.* **120**, 139.

Pally, C., Smith, D., Jaffee, B., *et al.* (1998). Side effects of brequinar and brequinar analogues, in combination with cyclosporine, in the rat. *Toxicology* **127**, 207.

Palmer, A., Taube, D., Welsh, K. I., Bewick, M. and Gjorstrop, P. (1989). Successful removal of anti-HLA antibodies by extracorporeal immunoabsorption to enable renal transplantation. *Lancet* **1**, 10.

Parsons, F. M., Fox, M., Anderson, C. R., Markland, C., Clark, P. B. and Raper, F. P. (1966). Cyclophosphamide in renal homotransplantation. *Br. J. Urol.* **38**, 673.

Pepino, P., Berger, C. L., Fuzesi, L., *et al.* (1989). Primate cardiac allo- and xenotransplantation: modulation of the immune response with photochemotherapy. *Eur. Surg. Res.* **21**, 105.

Perez, M., Edelson, R., Lori, J., *et al.* (1989). Inhibition of antiskin allograft immunity by infusions with syngeneic photoinactivated effector lymphocytes. *J. Invest. Dermatol.* **92**, 669.

Perotti, C., Torretta, L., Viarengo, G., *et al.* (1999). Feasibility and safety of a new technique of extracorporeal photochemotherapy: experience of 240 procedures. *Haematologica* **84**, 237.

Peters, T. G., Williams, J. W., Harmon, H. C. and Britt, L. G. (1983). Splenectomy and death in renal transplant patients. *Arch. Surg.* **118**, 795.

Pierce, J. C. and Hume, D. M. (1968). The effects of splenectomy on the survival of first and second renal homotransplants in man. *Surg. Gynecol. Obstet.* **127**, 1300.

Qi, Z. and Ekberg, H. (1998). Malononitrilamides 715 and 279 prolong rat cardiac allograft survival, reverse ongoing rejection, inhibit allospecific antibody production and interact positively with cyclosporin. *Scand. J. Immunol.* **48**, 379.

Raisanen-Sokolowski, A. K., Pakkala, I. S., Samila, S. P., *et al.* (1997). A vitamin D analog, MC1288, inhibits adventitial inflammation and suppresses intimal lesions in rat aortic allografts. *Transplantation* **63**, 936.

Reding, R., Squifflet, J. P., Latinne, D., De Bruyere, M., Pirson, Y. and Alexandre, G. P. (1987a). Early postoperative monitoring of natural-anti-A and anti-B isoantibodies in ABO-incompatible living donor relatted allografts. *Transplant. Proc.* **9**, 1989.

Reding, R., Squifflet, J. P., Prison, Y., *et al.* (1987b). Living related and unrelated donor kidney transplantation: comparison between ABO compatible and incompatible grafts. *Transplant. Proc.* **19**, 1511.

Renal Transplant Registry Advisory Committee. (1977). The 13th Report of the Human Renal Registry. *Transplant. Proc.* **9**, 9.

Sablinski, T., Emery, D. W., Monroy, R., *et al.* (1999). Long-term discordant xenogeneic (porcine-to-primate) bone marrow engraftment in a monkey treated with porcine-specific growth factors. *Transplantation* **67**, 972.

Salerno, C. T., Park, S. J., Krykes, N. S., *et al.* (1999). Adjuvant treatment of refractory lung transplant rejection with extracorporeal photopheresis. *J. Thorac. Cardiovasc. Surg.* **117**, 1063.

Schorlemmer, H., Dickneite, G. and Seiler, F. (1990). Treatment of acute rejection episodes and induction tolerance in rat skin allotransplantation by 15-deoxyspergualin. *Transplant. Proc.* **22**, 1626.

Schorlemmer, H. U., Kurrle, R. and Schleyerback, R. (1998). Leflunomide's active metabolite A77-1726 and its derivatives, the malononitrilamides, inhibit the generation of oxygen radicals in mononuclear phagocytes. *Int. J. Immunother.* **14**, 213.

Schorlemmer, H. U. and Schleyerback, R. (1998). Derivatives of leflunomide's active metabolite A77-1726, the malononitrilamides (MNAs), prevent the development of experimental arthritis. *Int. J. Immunother.* **14**, 177.

Siemaskao, K. F., Chong, A. S. F, Williams, J. W., *et al.* (1996). Regulation of B cell function by the immunosuppressive agent leflunomide. *Transplantation* **61**, 635.

Siemaskao, K., Chong, A. S.-F., Jäck, H.-M., *et al.* (1998). Inhibition of JAK3 and STAT6 tyrosine phosphorylation by the immunosuppressive drug leflunomide leads to a block in IgG1 production. *J. Immunol.* **160**, 1581.

Smolen, J. S., Kalden, J. R., Scott, D. L., *et al.* (1999). Efficacy and safety of leflunomide compared with placebo and sulphasalazine in active rheumatoid arthritis: a double-blind, randomised, multicentre trial. European Leflunomide Study Group. *Lancet* **253**, 259.

Starzl, T. E., Halgrimson, C. G., Penn, I., *et al.* (1971). Cyclophosphamide in human organ transplantation. *Lancet* **2**, 70.

Starzl, T. E., Marchioro, T. L. and Waddell, W. R. (1963). Human renal homotransplantation in the presence of blood group incompatibilities. *Proc. Exp. Biol. Med.* **113**, 471.

Sterbenz, K. G. and Tepper, M. A. (1993). Effects of 15-deoxyspergualin on the expression of surface immunoglobulin in 70Z/3.12 murine pre-B cell line. *Ann. N. Y. Acad. Sci.* **685**, 205.

Stosic-Grujicic, S., Dimitrijevic, M. and Bartlett, R. R. (1996). A novel immunomodulating agent, leflunomide, inhibits experimental autoimmune diabetes in mice. *Transplant. Proc.* **28**, 3072.

Stuart, F. P., Reckard, C. R., Ketel, B. L., *et al.* (1980). Effect of splenectomy on first cadaver kidney transplants. *Ann. Surg.* **192**, 553.

Sutherland, D. E. R., Fryd, D. S., Strand, M. H., *et al.* (1984). Results of the Minneosta randomized prospective trial of cyclosporin versus azathioprine-antilymphocyte globulin for immunosuppression in renal allograft recipients. *Am. J. Kidney Dis.* **5**, 318.

Suzuki, S., Enosawa, S., Kakefuda, T., *et al.* (1996a). A novel immunosuppressant, FTY720, with a unique mechanism of action, induces long-term graft acceptance in rat and dog allotransplantation. *Transplantation* **61**, 200.

Suzuki, S., Enosawa, S., Kakefuda, T., *et al.* (1996b). Long-term graft acceptance in allografted rats and dogs by treatment with a novel immunosuppressant, FTY720. *Transplant. Proc.* **28**, 1375.

Suzuki, S., Li, X., Tamura, A., *et al.* (1998). FTY720 induces lymphocyte apoptosis in vivo and reverses ongoing rejection in rat liver allografts. *Proceedings of New Dimensions in Transplantation*, February 16–19, Florence.

Suzuki, T., Shimamura, T., Jin, M. B., *et al.* (1999). Effect of a novel immunosuppressant, FTY720, on canine renal allograft. *Proceedings of the 25th Annual Scientific Meeting of the American Society of Transplant Surgeons*, May 19–21, Chicago.

Takahara, S., Jiang, H., Takano, Y., *et al.* (1992). The in vitro immunosuppressive effects of deoxyspergualin in man compared with FK 506 and cyclosporine. *Transplantation* **53**, 914.

Takahashi, K., Tanabe, K., Ooba, S., *et al.* (1991). Prophylactic use of a new immunosuppressive agent, deoxyspergualin, in patients with kidney transplantation from ABO incompatible or preformed antibody-positive donors. *Transplant. Proc.* **23**, 1078.

Takeuchi, T., Linuma, H., Kunimoto, S., *et al.* (1981). A new antitumor antibiotic, spergualin: isolation and antitumor activity. *Antibiotics* **34**, 1619.

Takeuchi, A., Redy, G. S., Kobayashi, T., *et al.* (1998). Nuclear factor of activated T cells (NFAT) as a molecular target for 1α,25-dihydroxyvitamin D₃-mediated effects. *J. Immunol.* **160**, 209.

Tanabe, K., Tokumoto, T., Ishikawa N., *et al.* (1999). Long-term results in mizoribine-treated renal transplant recipients: a prospective randomized trial of mizoribine and azathiaprine under cyclosporine-based immunosuppression. *Transplant. Proc.* **31**(7), 2877.

Taube, D., Williams, D. G., Cameron, J. S., *et al.* (1984). Renal transplantation after removal and prevention of resynthesis of HLA antibodies. *Lancet* **2**, 824.

Thoenes, G. H., Sitter, T., Langer, K. H., *et al.* (1989). Leflunomide (HWA 486) inhibits experimental autoimmune tubulointerstitial nephritis in rats. *Int. J. Immunopharmacol.* **11**, 921.

Thomas, F., Pittman, K., Ljung, T., *et al.* (1995). Deoxyspergualin is a unique immunosuppressive agent with selective utility in inducing tolerance to pancreas islet xenografts. *Transplant. Proc.* **27**, 417.

Thomas, F. T., Tepper, M. A., Thomas, J. M., *et al.* (1993). 15-Deoxyspergualin: a novel immunosuppressive drug with clinical potential. *Ann. N. Y. Acad. Sci.* **685**, 175.

Tian, L., Stepkowski, S. M., Qu, X. M., *et al.* (1997). Cytokine mRNA expression in tolerant heart allografts after immunosuppression with cyclosporine, sirolimus or brequinar. *Transpl. Immunol.* **5**, 189.

Towers, T. L. and Freedman, L. P. (1998). Granulocyte-macrophage colony-stimulating factor gene transcription is directly repressed by the vitamin D₃ receptor. *J. Biol. Chem.* **273**, 10338.

Troncoso, P., Stepkowski, S. M., Wang, M. E., *et al.* (1999). Prophylaxis of acute renal allograft rejection using FTY720 in combination with subtherapeutic doses of cyclosporine. *Transplantation* **67**, 145.

Turk, J. L., Parker, D. and Pulter, L. W. (1972). Functional aspects of the selective depletion of lymphoid tissue by cyclophosphamide. *Immunology* **23**, 493.

Uldall, R., Taylor, R. and Swiney, J. (1971). Cyclophosphamide in human organ transplantation. *Lancet* **2**, 258.

Veyron, P., Pamphile, R., Binderup, L., *et al.* (1993). Two novel vitamin D analogues, KH 1060 and CB 966, prolong skin allograft survival in mice. *Transpl. Immunol.* **1**, 72.

Waaga, A. M., Ulrichs, K., Krzymanski, M., *et al.* (1990). The immunosuppressive agent 15-deoxyspergualin induces tolerance and modulates MHC-antigen expression and interleukin-1 production in the early phase of rat allograft responses. *Transplant. Proc.* **22**, 1613.

Wang, M., Tejpal, N., Qu, X., *et al.* (1998). Immunosuppressive effect of FTY720 alone or in combination with cyclosporine and/or sirolimus. *Transplantation* **65**, 899.

Wedgewood, K. R., Guillan, P. J., Leveson, S. H., Davison, A. M. and Giles, G. T. (1980). A trial of intermittent intravenous cyclophosphamide in renal transplantation. *Br. J. Surg.* **67**, 835.

Williams, J. W., Xiao, F., Foster, P., *et al.* (1994). Leflunomide in experimental transplantation. *Transplantation* **57**, 1223.

Williamson, R. A., Yea, C. M., Robson, P. A., *et al.* (1995). Dihydroorotate dehydrogenase in a high affinity binding protein for A771726 and mediator of a range of biological effects of the immunomodulatory compound. *J. Biol. Chem.* **270**, 22467.

Winearls, C., Fabre, J. W., Millard, P. R. and Morris, P. J. (1979). Use of cyclophosphamide and enhancing serum to suppress renal allograft rejection in the rat. *Transplantation* **28**, 271.

Xiao, F., Shen, J., Chong, A., *et al.* (1996). Control and reversal of chronic xenograft rejection in hamster-to-rat cardiac transplantation. *Transplant. Proc.* **28**, 691.

Xu, M., Pirenne, J., Antoniou, E. A., *et al.* (1998a). Effect of peritransplant FTY720 alone or in combination with posttransplant FK 506 in a rat model of cardiac allotransplantation. *Transplant. Int.* **11**, 288.

Xu, M., Pirenne, J., Antoniou, S., *et al.* (1998b). FTY720 compares with FK506 as rescue therapy in rat heterotopic cardiac transplantation. *Transplant. Proc.* **30**, 2221.

Xu, X., Williams, J. W., Shen, J., *et al.* (1998). In vitro and in vivo mechanisms of action of the antiproliferative and immunosuppressive agent, brequinar sodium. *J. Immunol.* **160**, 846.

Xu, X. L., Gong, H. H., Blinder, L., *et al.* (1997). Control of lymphoproliferative and autoimmune disease in MRL-lpr/lpr mice by brequinar sodium: mechanisms of action. *J. Pharmacol. Exp. Ther.* **283**, 869.

Yadav, R. V., Indudhara, R., Kumar, P., Ghugh, K. S. and Gupta, K. L. (1988). Cyclophosphamide in renal transplantation. *Transplantation* **45**, 421.

Yamashita, K., Nomura, M., Takehara, M., *et al.* (1999). Effects of a novel immunosuppressant, FTY720, on heart and liver transplantations in rats. *Proceedings of the AST 18th Annual Meeting*, May 15–19, Chicago.

Yasunaga, C., Cramer, D. V., Chapman, F. A., *et al.* (1993). Cardiac graft rejection in hypersensitized recipients: prevention of antibody response and graft rejection using brequinar sodium. *Transplant. Proc.* **25(Suppl. 2)**, 65.

Yuzawa, K., Stepkowski, S., Wang, M., *et al.* (1999). FTY720 blocks allograft rejection by sequestration of T and B lymphocytes in peripheral lymphoid compartments. *Proceedings of the 25th Annual Scientific Meeting of the American Society of Transplant Surgeons*, May 19–21, Chicago.

Total Lymphoid Irradiation

Mark Waer

Introduction: Total Lymphoid Irradiation and Cellular Immunity in Hodgkin's Disease

For several decades, total lymphoid irradiation (TLI) has been used to treat Hodgkin's disease (Kaplan, 1980). Irradiation is delivered through two ports. A first so-called mantle port includes the lymph nodes of the neck, axilla and mediastinum. The other port is called the *inverted* Y and encompasses aortic, iliac and pelvic lymph nodes. In some patients, a splenectomy is performed as a standard procedure for the staging of the disease. If not, the spleen also is irradiated. Usually a total dose of 40 to 50 Gy (1 Gy = 100 rad) is administered in daily fractions of 1.5 to 2.5 Gy.

The possibility of using TLI as an immunosuppressant was discovered by investigators at Stanford University (Fuks *et al.*, 1976). In a study involving patients with Hodgkin's disease, these investigators found that various immunological tests of cellular immunity were strikingly depressed after TLI. The absolute number and the response of T lymphocytes to phytohemagglutinin and concanavalin A were decreased for 10 years after TLI. The mixed lymphocyte reaction, considered as the *in vitro* analogue of the rejection phenomenon, was paralyzed for about 2 years after TLI and recovered only 2 to 7 years later (Fuks *et al.*, 1976).

Despite the impairment of cellular immune functions, side effects most commonly encountered in patients with immune deficiency were not increased significantly. Secondary hematological tumors were observed rarely when patients were treated with TLI alone (Pedersen-Bjergaard and Olesen Larsen, 1982). The only infections that were commoner after TLI were localized herpes zoster infections (Goffinet *et al.*, 1972).

Total Lymphoid Irradiation in Transplantation Experiments in Animals

INDUCTION OF SPECIFIC TRANSPLANTATION TOLERANCE USING TOTAL LYMPHOID IRRADIATION IN MICE

Because efficient immunosuppression without clinically important side effects is a crucial goal in transplantation immunology, irradiation techniques were developed in mice to investigate TLI in transplantation experiments (Strober *et al.*, 1979). Mice were given 17 daily fractions of 2 Gy, delivered to upper and lower TLI fields concomitantly. Irradiated animals developed lymphopenia and a decrease of responses to phytohemagglutinin, concanavalin A and allogeneic lymphocytes to a similar extent for a relatively similar duration as that seen in Hodgkin's disease patients (Strober *et al.*, 1979).

The BALB/c mice receiving TLI and a fully allogeneic C57BL skin graft on the first day after TLI rejected the allograft after a mean of about 50 days compared with 10 days in control animals. When 30 × 10⁶ C57BL bone marrow cells

were injected on the day of skin grafting, the TLI-treated animals became stable hematopoietic chimeras without signs of graft-versus-host disease and developed permanent tolerance toward the skin allograft. This tolerance was specific because third-party C3H skin allografts, transplanted later, were rejected normally without any effect on the tolerated BALB/c skin graft (Strober *et al.*, 1979).

VARIABLES WITH CLINICAL RELEVANCE INFLUENCING ENGRAFTMENT AFTER TOTAL LYMPHOID IRRADIATION

For technical reasons and to allow a sufficient exposure of the infradiaphragmatic lymph nodes, the lower TLI field in mice has to be relatively wide, and consequently an almost panabdominal irradiation field is used (Strober *et al.*, 1979). That the width of the irradiation field is a vital factor was shown in the rat model, in which shielding of minor parts of the pelvic field prevented the induction of tolerance in all rats (Strober *et al.*, 1979). Widening of the TLI fields in the form of one or two total body irradiation (TBI) fractions impressively increased the efficacy of TLI in the mouse model (Waer *et al.*, 1984b).

The time of transplantation after TLI is crucial because skin grafts transplanted later than 1 week after the end of TLI were rejected rapidly (Strober *et al.*, 1979). The total TLI dose determines the engraftment after TLI (Strober *et al.*, 1979), and this is strain-specific: C57BL mice need higher radiation doses than BALB/c mice (Waer *et al.*, 1984b).

Presensitization, even to only minor transplantation antigens of the prospective bone marrow donor, prevented the induction of the stable chimerism after TLI (Strober *et al.*, 1979). Graft-versus-host disease cannot be prevented by TLI when a relatively high number of mature T lymphocytes are present in the bone marrow graft or when gut decontamination has not been performed (Waer *et al.*, 1984a).

MECHANISMS UNDERLYING THE IMMUNOLOGICAL TOLERANCE INDUCED BY TOTAL LYMPHOID IRRADIATION

Much of the experimental evidence collected with regard to the immunological mechanisms underlying the induction of tolerance after TLI point to the importance of suppressor cells (Strober, 1984). Strober (1984) found that spleen cells taken within the first days after TLI are able to block several mixed lymphocyte reaction combinations nonspecifically. That these suppressor cells are relevant to the *in vivo* action of TLI is suggested by the fact that a close correlation was found between the level of these cells after various TLI schedules and the capacity of the latter schedules to induce tolerance *in vivo* (Waer *et al.*, 1984a, 1984b).

It has become possible to clone the post-TLI suppressor cells, which express a surface phenotype similar to that reported for cloned natural killer (NK) cells (Thy I+, asialo-

GM +, Ig−, Lyt 1−, Lyt 2−, Ia−, MAC-1−), although they do not show NK activity (Schwadron and Strober, 1987). The cloned suppressor cells express full-length mRNA transcripts for the α, β and γ T-cell receptor cells, indicating they belong to the T-cell lineage (Hertel-Wulff et al., 1987a). The functional importance and activity of the cloned suppressor cells were proved by the demonstration that they could prevent graft-versus-host disease in vivo (Hertel-Wulff et al., 1987b). Because naturally occurring suppressor cells have been reported in the spleen of neonatal animals and because tolerance can be induced easily in the early neonatal period, it is now generally accepted that a situation is created after TLI that can be compared with early neonatal immunological immaturity (Strober, 1984).

The importance of regulatory asialo-GM1+ cells for the induction of transplantation tolerance after TLI was shown in bone marrow transplantation experiments peformed in mice. When BALB/c mice were injected after TLI with antibodies directed against the asialo-GM1 antigen, this resulted in the disappearance of suppressor cells after TLI and the occurrence of graft-versus-host disease when allogeneic bone marrow was infused (De Ruysscher et al., 1991).

Besides suppressor cells, changes in the intrinsic reactivity of T lymphocytes that occur after TLI also may be responsible for the post-TLI immunosuppression. The capacity of lymphocytes to proliferate and to secrete interleukin (IL)-2 but not to express IL-2 receptors seems impaired for several weeks after TLI (Bass and Strober, 1990; Field and Becker, 1989, 1992). This intrinsic T-cell defect depends on the irradiation of thymus and extrathymic tissues (Palathumpat et al., 1990).

After TLI, anergized T cells were shown to be incapable of proliferating in the presence of exogenous IL-2 (Field and Steinmuller, 1993). In other experiments, clonal deletion of donor-reactive or host-reactive lymphocytes was shown in the thymus of TLI-treated mice (Salam et al., 1994). Total lymphoid irradiation–treated mice also showed decreased antidonor cytotoxic T-cell precursor frequencies (Florence et al., 1990).

The recovery of the major T-helper lymphocyte subsets is different after TLI. Although so-called Th2 lymphocytes, which secrete IL-4, IL-5 and IL-10 and which mainly deliver help factors for B-cell lymphocytes, recover soon after TLI, this is not the case for Th1 lymphocytes. The latter subset, which secretes IL-2 and interferon and mediates delayed-type hypersensitivity and graft-versus-host reactions, is deficient for several months after TLI (Bass et al., 1989; Field and Rouse, 1995). This defect also can be prevented by shielding the thymus during irradiation (Bass and Strober, 1990). This Th2 dominance after TLI has been confirmed in large animals (Stark et al., 1994). It has been attempted to increase the tolerogenic effect of TLI by the injection of selected, mainly monocyte-dendritic donor type cells in conjunction with antithymocyte globulin (Hayamizu et al., 1998) or cyclophosphamide (Slavin et al., 1998).

TRANSPLANTATION EXPERIMENTS IN LARGE OUTBRED ANIMALS

After the promising results in mice, transplantation experiments were performed in dogs using TLI. Although bone marrow chimerism could be obtained easily, this did not guarantee the induction of tolerance to heart (Gottlieb et al., 1980) or kidney allografts (Howard et al., 1981), suggesting that bone marrow infusion and chimerism does not create tolerance toward organ-specific antigens. These observations, together with the uncertainty about the risk of graft-versus-host disease after TLI in humans, led to several experiments

designed to test synergy between TLI and various chemical immunosuppressants.

The combination of 18 fractions of 1 Gy of TLI together with postoperative azathioprine and antithymocyte globulin in the heart-allograft model in monkeys led to a high mortality and morbidity caused by leukopenia (Pennock et al., 1981). In the same model, the combination of TLI and continuous high-dose cyclosporine (17 mg/kg/d) was shown to be active but led to lethal lymphomas in 3 of 10 monkeys (Pennock et al., 1981). The same combination of TLI and cyclosporine, but given in low doses, was effective and clinically safe in rats (Rynasiewicz et al., 1981). Eighteen fractions of 1 Gy of TLI, followed by a 10-day course of postoperative antithymocyte globulin alone, induced permanent and specific transplantation tolerance toward heart allografts in about 40% of the transplanted dogs (Strober et al., 1983). These encouraging results led to a similar trial in clinical kidney transplantation (discussed later).

A different low-dose, wide-field TLI regimen was explored extensively at the University of Johannesburg in the baboon (Myburgh et al., 1987). These workers established the optimal schedule as 8 fractions of 1 Gy each delivered over 4 weeks. In two thirds of the baboons, specific and permanent tolerance toward solid grafts could be obtained. These models proved that tolerance can be achieved in larger animals without concomitant bone marrow transplantation, but they showed that immunosuppressive drugs have to be used, at least temporarily, to obtain clinically acceptable graft survival or that the TLI fields have to be expanded compared with those used in Hodgkin's disease.

POSTTRANSPLANTATION TOTAL LYMPHOID IRRADIATION

One major handicap for the clinical application of TLI is that it has to be completed within several weeks of transplantation, which poses serious problems for finding a suitable donor soon after finishing TLI. Some investigators explored the possibility of using TLI after transplantation. In mouse or rat heart allograft models, posttransplant TLI prolonged graft survival significantly when combined with anti-CD4 monoclonal antibody (Trager et al., 1989) or infusion of donor type dendritic cell precursors (Hayamizu et al., 1998). Posttransplantation TLI also seems clinically efficient as salvage therapy for heart transplant patients who are rejecting their grafts despite steroid and anti-T-cell antibody therapy (Hunt et al., 1991; Levin et al., 1989).

TOTAL LYMPHOID IRRADIATION IN EXPERIMENTAL MODELS OF XENOTRANSPLANTATION

Preoperative TLI combined with cyclosporine (Steinbrüchel et al., 1990), cyclosporine and pretransplant splenectomy (Yamaguchi et al., 1990), cyclosporine and anti-CD4 monoclonal antibody (Steinbrüchel et al., 1991) or deoxyspergualin (Marchman et al., 1991) resulted in significantly longer graft survival rates than any other combination had achieved to that point. In heart or heart-lung transplantation between xenogeneic primate species, preoperative TLI when administered in combination with cyclosporine and antithymocyte globulin (Sadeghi et al., 1991), cyclosporine and splenectomy (Bollinger et al., 1991) or cyclosporine and methylprednisolone (Panza et al., 1991) was more efficient than any other treatment regimen. In a pig islet-into-rat xenograft model, TLI in combination with deoxyspergualin was extremely effective (Thomas et al., 1995), and in a discordant lamb-into-pig model, TLI synergized with cyclosporine and azathioprine to provoke a 30-fold increase of the mean xenograft survival time (Tixier *et al.*, 1992). Pretransplant TLI combined with cyclosporine and methotrexate resulted in a more than 2-week-long graft survival time of pig heart-into-baboon. This regimen inhibited xenoreactive natural antibody production but not the xenoreactivity of macrophages (Xu *et al.*, 1998). In view of the growing interest in xenotransplantation in clinical practice, TLI in this particular area needs to be explored further.

Clinical Use of Total Lymphoid Irradiation

TOTAL LYMPHOID IRRADIATION COMBINED WITH POSTOPERATIVE AZATHIOPRINE AND PREDNISOLONE

The first clinical kidney transplants using TLI were performed at the University of Minnesota in patients who had previously rejected a first or second renal allograft (Najarian *et al.*, 1982). Historically, these patients had poor 2-year graft survival (<40%) with conventional immunosuppression. Doses of 10.5 to 40.5 Gy of TLI were administered in fractions of 1 or 1.25 Gy each two to five times weekly. In 9 of 20 patients, the interval between TLI and the time of transplantation exceeded 1 month because of problems of finding a crossmatch-negative kidney in these highly sensitized patients. As was shown in various animal experiments (Strober *et al.*, 1979), this factor could influence adversely the efficacy of TLI. All patients were given postoperative azathioprine and prednisolone, which was tapered after three different protocols. The graft survival was increased significantly in this group (70% at 2 years) and remained stable at 5 years (Kaufman *et al.*, 1989).

Four deaths occurred (two from Epstein-Barr virus–related lymphomas, one from sepsis and one from myocardial infarction). A total of 16 acute rejection episodes occurred in eight patients. Rejection episodes occurred only when the postoperative prednisolone dose was low (0.4 mg/kg/d) or when the time between TLI and transplantation was long (102 ± 32 days) A low number of T cell–depleted donor bone marrow cells (0.5×10^8 cells/kg) was given in five patients but did not result in chimerism, and it did not alter significantly the course of the kidney grafts. Because similar results (an increase of about 30% 1-year graft survival compared with historical control data) were achieved in this patient population using cyclosporine and because of ease of administration, the workers preferred cyclosporine over TLI (Sutherland *et al.*, 1983).

TOTAL LYMPHOID IRRADIATION WITH LOW-DOSE MAINTENANCE PREDNISOLONE

In the 1980s, 54 insulin-dependent patients with end-stage diabetic nephropathy received kidney cadaveric allografts at the University of Leuven. Half of the patients received pretransplant TLI followed by low-dose maintenance prednisone after transplantation. The other half were treated with cyclosporine and a similar low-dose prednisone protocol. Of these diabetic patients, 20 were enrolled in a controlled trial (Waer *et al.*, 1984c, 1987a, 1988). In the TLI patients, a minimal dose of 20 daily fractions of 1 Gy of TLI was administered, followed by one weekly extra TLI dose per week when a suitable donor was not found. In all patients, this was the case within 1 month after finishing the 20-Gy regimen. Total lymphoid irradiation was administered over the mantle and inverted-Y fields concomitantly, and splenectomy was performed before radiotherapy in eight patients to lower the risk of thrombocytopenia.

Although the 1-, 2- and 3-year posttransplant evaluation of the TLI-treated patients was considered satisfactory, a more long-term (8-year) follow-up revealed that patient and graft survival were significantly (P<0.05 and P<0.006) inferior in the TLI group. Total lymphoid irradiation patients developed more rejection crises, and in four patients azathioprine and in another five patients cyclosporine had to be introduced to prevent recurrent rejection crises. The excess mortality in the TLI-treated patients was due to sepsis, which was a consequence of high steroid administration needed to treat rejection crises in several TLI patients. The overall conclusion of this clinical study is that preoperative TLI in combination with low-dose postoperative prednisone is insufficient to guarantee good long-term kidney graft survival rates. Additional interventions, such as infusion of donor cells or administration of supplementary immunosuppressants, is needed to fulfill this aim in patients. This clinical experience confirms the animal data, which also showed that TLI by itself is insufficient to provoke long-term graft survival or tolerance and that extra manipulations are needed.

TOTAL LYMPHOID IRRADIATION WITH POSTOPERATIVE ANTITHYMOCYTE GLOBULIN AND LOW-DOSE PREDNISOLONE

Because of the encouraging results obtained with TLI combined with antithymocyte globulin in dogs, enabling specific tolerance to be induced in about 40% of the cases (Strober *et al.*, 1983), a similar treatment protocol was used for clinical kidney transplantation in a collaborative program between Stanford University in Palo Alto and Pacific Medical Center in San Francisco, California (Levin *et al.*, 1985). Between October 1982 and December 1986, 24 patients received a first and 1 patient received a second cadaveric renal allograft using TLI. Twenty fractions of 1 Gy each were administerd to the mantle and inverted-Y field consecutively. The mean duration of radiotherapy was 12 weeks, and a crossmatch-negative cadaveric donor was found at a mean interval of 9 days after the end of TLI. Six courses of 2 mg/kg of rabbit antithymocyte globulin were given intramuscularly every other day after transplantation. Low-dose prednisolone (0.2 mg/kg/d) was tapered to 0.15 mg/kg/d at 6 weeks and reduced further later in several patients. Six patients (of whom four could be considered as high risk—two diabetics and two >55 years old) died, four from cardiovascular complications in the second posttransplant year and two from viral infections occurring during treatment of a transplant rejection with another course of antithymocyte globulin and high doses of corticosteroids. The actuarial graft survival was 76% and 68% at 1 and 2 years. Ten of the 25 patients never had a rejection crisis despite an overall poor HLA matching between donor and recipient.

Immunological monitoring revealed data entirely comparable with those obtained at Leuven University. Further phenotyping of the suppressor/cytotoxic lymphocytes revealed that only 10% of the post-TLI suppressor/cytotoxic cells were cytotoxic (compared with about 50% in control subjects). The expansion within the suppressor/cytotoxic subpopulation observed after TLI was due to an increase of suppressor cells.

In 9 of the 11 patients who could be investigated during the second posttransplantation year, a specific mixed lymphocyte culture hyporesponsiveness or nonresponsiveness against donor-stimulator cells was shown (Chow *et al.*, 1987), and in three patients all immunosuppressive drugs could be withdrawn (Strober *et al.*, 1989). An evaluation (Levin *et al.*, 1989) in a larger group of 52 patients treated with the same protocol showed a 3-year graft survival of about 50%, which is less than in cyclosporine-treated patients (around 75%) at the same center. These results made the workers switch to add cyclosporine to a similar protocol. This switch yielded excellent short-term results (Levin *et al.*, 1989).

TOTAL LYMPHOID IRRADIATION WITH CYCLOSPORINE

The first team to explore the experimentally proven synergism between TLI and cyclosporine (Rynasiewicz *et al.*, 1981) was at the University of Rome (Cortesini *et al.*, 1985). In a study involving only high-risk patients, judged by the rapid rejection of a previous transplant or the finding of a high immune responder state, 10 patients were given 15 to 22 Gy of TLI followed by low-dose posttransplantation cyclosporine (12 mg/kg/d orally rapidly tapered to <5 mg/kg). These patients were compared with 10 patients treated with conventional immunosuppression (antilymphocyte globulin, prednisolone, azathioprine). Only one of the latter patients retained a functioning graft. Seven of the TLI patients had a functioning graft, among whom four never had a rejection crisis. Two diabetics and one nondiabetic patient died, two from pneumonia and one from myocardial infarction.

After obtaining promising results using a wide-field TLI regimen in baboons (Myburgh *et al.*, 1984), the transplantation team at the University of Johannesburg used a similar TLI schedule for clinical renal transplantation (Myburgh *et al.*, 1987, 1991). A wide TLI field involving the entire torso from the base of the skull down to and including the pelvis and proximal ends of the femora and humeri was used. Supradiaphragmatic ribs and the lungs were shielded. A cumulative dose of 8 Gy was given in fractions of 0.1 to 1.0 Gy administered twice weekly. Zero to two booster doses of 0.1 Gy at 4-week intervals were given if there were delays exceeding 1 month before transplantation.

This regimen was used in 73 patients receiving 56 cadaveric and 17 haploidentical living related renal allografts. Twenty-nine patients were children, 11 were retransplants and several were sensitized (showing panel-reactive antibodies of >30%). Actuarial graft survival at 1 and 5 years was 86% and 60% and significantly better for the unsensitized patients (80% at 5 years). Seven patients (9.6%) died from transplant-related causes, five with functioning grafts.

The fact that in two patients all immunosuppressive drugs could be stopped for several years and that in most of the others only low-dose maintenance immunosuppression (cyclosporine 3 mg/kg and prednisolone <10 mg/d orally) was used without any rejection crisis shows that this clinical feasibility study seems to confirm the results obtained in the baboon model, in which more than 50% of the animals became specifically tolerant (Myburgh *et al.*, 1984). About one third of the patients in this study were children, however. It is possible that children are more likely to develop tolerance after TLI than adults.

POSTTRANSPLANT TOTAL LYMPHOID IRRADIATION IN HEART TRANSPLANT PATIENTS

Posttransplant TLI in combination with anti-CD3 monoclonal antibodies or with antithymocyte globulin together with donor-specific blood transfusions seemed effective in a rat heart allograft model (Woodley *et al.*, 1993). Based on these results, the efficacy of 10 fractions of 0.8 Gy of TLI was evaluated in heart transplant patients with therapy-resistant or early vascular rejection at the University of Alabama (Salter *et al.*, 1993). This regimen resulted in a significant reduction of rejection recurrences, an effect that was maintained for at least 2 years. These favorable results have been confirmed by two other groups (Trachiotis *et al.*, 1998; Valentine *et al.*, 1996).

CONCLUSIONS

A first conclusion that can be drawn from the clinical TLI studies is that it is a safe immunosuppressive regimen. In all studies, the mortality of TLI-treated patients did not exceed that of the control groups. Only in our own study in diabetics was mortality significantly increased in the TLI group. As already mentioned, however, this was mainly due to the administration of high doses of steroids causing sepsis in several of these diabetic recipients. Because these steroids were needed to treat rejection crises, this increased mortality was more an indirect indication of the lack of efficacy of the TLI regimen as used rather than a sign of toxicity of TLI itself.

A concern when using radiotherapy is the risk for tumors. In more than 200 transplant patients treated, the incidence and the nature of cancers were not different from what may be expected in transplant patients. In view of a report showing a high incidence of solid tumors starting from 15 years after radiotherapy in children treated with TLI for Hodgkin's disease, however, a close follow-up of the TLI-treated transplant patients is warranted (Bhatia *et al.*, 1996).

Future Perspectives

At the end of the 1970s, before the cyclosporine era, the discovery of the immunosuppressive effects of TLI raised much enthusiasm and hope among transplantation immunologists and physicians. This hope has not been entirely fulfilled: With a few exceptions, operational tolerance has not been achieved in TLI-treated transplant recipients. Several aspects of TLI still make it a possible immunomodulatory regimen. First, despite profound effects on the number of lymphoid cells and on T-cell reactivity, TLI still can be considered as a safe procedure in the clinical setting. The experience in the several hundreds of TLI-treated transplant recipients shows that it is at least as safe as the commonly used immunosuppressive schedules. In view of more recent studies revealing an increased incidence of tumors more than 10 years after radiotherapy in young TLI-treated Hodgkin's disease patients (Bhatia *et al.*, 1996), the former claim still must be made with caution.

Second, in view of the increasing interest in xenotransplantation, the potential of TLI to interfere with xenoreactivity must be explored further. The fact that TLI may influence concomitantly T cell–dependent and T cell–independent immunity may be important because both immune arms now are known to be equally important for the rejection of xenografts.

Third, based on the animal experiments, it was clear that by itself TLI was insufficient to induce tolerance and that the most effective way to achieve this was to combine TLI with the infusion of donor type hematopoietic cells. This hypothesis has been confirmed in the patient studies: Without bone marrow infusion, transplantation tolerance was not achieved—not even in conjunction with the administration of other immunosuppressive drugs. If in the future the donor type cells can be identified that have the strongest capacity to induce tolerance without the risk of graft-versus-host disease, infusing these cells after TLI should be explored as a means to induce clinical tolerance.

Finally, in more recent studies, it became clear that posttransplantation TLI may be a safe and efficient approach to treat therapy-resistant rejection crises, especially in heart or heart-lung transplant recipients in whom the loss of a transplant in most cases must be considered as a lethal event. If these results can be confirmed, even if it is only for the latter indication, TLI deserves its place as an immunomodulatory regimen in clinical transplantation.

REFERENCES

Bass, H., Mosmann, T. and Strober, S. (1989). Evidence for mouse TH1 and TH2-like helper T cells in vivo. *J. Exp. Med.* **170**, 1495.

Bass, H. and Strober, S. (1990). Deficits in T helper cells after total lymphoid irradiation (TLI): reduced IL-2 secretion and normal IL-2 receptor expression in the mixed leucocyte reaction MLR. *Cell. Immunol.* **126**, 129.

Bhatia, S., Robison, L., Oberlin, O., *et al.* (1996). Breast cancer and other second neoplasms after childhood Hodgkin's disease. *N. Engl. J. Med.* **334**, 745.

Bollinger, R. R., Fabian, M. A., Harland, R. C., *et al.* (1991). Total lymphoid irradiation for cardiac xenotransplantation in nonhuman primates. *Transplant. Proc.* **23**, 587.

Chow, B., Saper, V. and Strober, S. (1987). Renal transplant patients treated with total lymphoid irradiation show specific unresponsiveness to donor antigens in MLR. *J. Immunol.* **130**, 3746.

Cortesini, R., Renna Molajoni, E., Monari, C., *et al.* (1985). Total lymphoid irradiation in clinical transplantation: experience in 30 high-risk patients. *Transplant. Proc.* **17**, 1291.

De Ruysscher, D., Sobis, H. and Vandeputte, M. (1991). A subset of asialo GM1+ cells play a protective role in the occurrence of graft versus host disease in mice. *J. Immunol.* **146**, 4065.

Field, E. and Becker, G. (1989). The immunosuppressive mechanism of total lymphoid irradiation. *Transplantation* **48**, 499.

Field, E. and Becker, G. (1992). Blocking of mixed lymphocyte reaction by spleen cells from total lymphoid irradiated mice involves interruption of the IL2-pathway. *J. Immunol.* **148**, 354.

Field, E. H. and Rouse T. M. (1995). Alloantigen priming after total lymphoid irradiation alters alloimmune cytokine responses. *Transplantation* **60**, 695.

Field, E. H. and Steinmuller, D. (1993). Nondeletional mechanisms of tolerance in total-lymphoid irradiation-induced bone marrow chimeras. *Transplantation* **56**, 250.

Florence, L. S., Ito, T., Ang, K. U., *et al.* (1989). The synergistic effect of total lymphoid irradiation with extracted donor alloantigen in inducing transplantation unresponsiveness. *Transplantation* **47**, 156.

Florence, L. S., Jiang, G. L., Ang, K. K., *et al.* (1990). In vitro analysis of T cell-mediated cytotoxicity displayed by rat heart allograft recipients rendered unresponsive by total-lymphoid irradiation and extracted donor antigen. *Transplantation* **49**, 436.

Fuks, Z., Strober, S., Bobrove, A. M., *et al.* (1976). Long term effects of radiation on T and B lymphocytes in peripheral blood of patients with Hodgkin's disease. *J. Clin. Invest.* **58**, 803.

Goffinet, D. R., Glatstein, E. and Merigan, R. D. (1972). Herpes zoster-varicella infections and lymphoma. *Ann. Intern. Med.* **76**, 235.

Gottlieb, M., Strober, S., Hoppe, R. T., *et al.* (1980). Engraftment of allogeneic bone marrow without graft-versus-host disease in mongrel dogs using total lymphoid irradiation. *Transplantation* **29**, 487.

Hayamizu, K., Huie, P., Sibley, R. K., *et al.* (1998). Monocyte-derived dendritic cell precursors facilitate tolerance to heart allografts after total lymphoid irradiation. *Transplantation* **66**, 1285.

Hertel-Wulff, B., Lindsten, T., Schwadron, R., *et al.* (1987a). Rearrangement and expression of T cell receptor genes in cloned murine natural suppressor cell lines. *J. Exp. Med.* **166**, 1168.

Hertel-Wulff, B., Palathumpat, V., Schwadron, R. B., *et al.* (1987b). Prevention of GVHD by natural suppressor cells. *Transplant. Proc.* **19**, 536.

Howard, R. J., Sutherland, D. E. R., Lum, C. T., *et al.* (1981). Kidney allograft survival in dogs treated with total lymphoid irradiation. *Ann. Surg.* **193**, 196.

Hunt, S. A., Strober, S., Hoppe, R. T., *et al.* (1991). Total lymphoid irradiation for treatment of intractable cardiac allograft rejection. *J. Heart Lung Transplant* **10**, 211.

Kaplan, H. S. (1980). *Hodgkin's Disease*, 2nd ed., p. 1, Harvard University Press, Cambridge, Mass.

Kaufman, D. B., Kim, T. H., Slavin, S., *et al.* (1989). Long term clinical studies of high-risk renal retransplant recipients given total lymphoid irradiation. *Transplant. Proc.* **21**, 1798.

Levin, B., Bohanson, V., Warvariv, V., *et al.* (1989). Total lymphoid irradiation (TLI) in the cyclospoprine era: use of TLI in resistant cardiac allograft rejection. *Transplant. Proc.* **21**, 1793.

Levin, B., Collins, G., Waer, M., *et al.* (1985). Treatment of cadaveric renal transplant recipients with total lymphoid irradiation, antithymocyte globulin, and low-dose prednisone. *Lancet* **2**, 1321.

Marchman, W., Araneda, D., De Masi, R., *et al.* (1991). Therapy with 15-deoxyspergualin and total lymphoid irradiation blocks xenograft rejection and antibody formation after xenografting. *Transplant. Proc.* **23**, 210.

Myburgh, J. A., Meyers, A. M., Botha, J. R., *et al.* (1987). Wide field low-dose total lymphoid irradiation in clinical kidney transplantation. *Transplant. Proc.* **19**, 1974.

Myburgh, J. A., Meyers, A. M., Margolius, L., *et al.* (1991). Total lymphoid irradiation in clinical renal transplantation: results in 73 patients. *Transplant. Proc.* **23**, 2033.

Myburgh, J. A., Smit, J. A., Stark, J. H., *et al.* (1984). Total lymphoid irradiation in kidney and liver transplantation in the baboon: prolonged graft survival and alterations in T cell subsets with low cumulative dose regimens. *J. Immunol.* **132**, 1019.

Najarian, J. S., Ferguson, R. M., Sutherland, D. E. R., *et al.* (1982). Fractionated total lymphoid irradiation as preparative immunosuppression in high risk renal transplantation. *Ann. Surg.* **196**, 442.

Palathumpat, V., Vandeputte, M. and Waer, M. (1990). Effects of thymus irradiation on the immune competence of T cells after total lymphoid irradiation. *Transplantation* **50**, 95.

Panza, A., Roslin, M. S., Coons, M., *et al.* (1991). One year survival of heterotopic heart primate xenografts treated with total lymphoid irradiation and cyclosporine. *Transplant. Proc.* **23**, 483.

Pedersen-Bjergaard, J. and Olesen Larsen, S. (1982). Incidence of acute nonlymphocytic leukemia, preleukemia, and acute myeloproliferative syndrome up to 10 years after treatment of Hodgkin's disease. *N. Engl. J. Med.* **207**, 965.

Pennock, J. L., Reitz, B. A., Bieber, C. P., *et al.* (1981). Survival of primates following orthotopic cardiac transplantation treated with total lymphoid irradiation and chemical immune suppression. *Transplantation* **32**, 467.

Rynasiewicz, J. J., Sutherland, D. E. R., Kawahara, K., *et al.* (1981). Total lymphoid irradiation: critical timing and combination with cyclosporin A for imunosuppression in a rat heart allograft model. *J. Surg. Res.* **30**, 365.

Sadeghi, A. M., Laks, H., Drinkwater, D. L., *et al.* (1991). Heart-lung xenotransplantation in primates. *J. Heart Lung Tranplant* **10**, 442.

Salam, A., Vandeputte, M. and Waer, M. (1994). Clonal deletion and clonal anergy in allogeneic bone marrow chimeras prepared with TBI or TLI. *Transpl. Int.* **7**, S457.

Salter, S. P., Slater, M. M., Kirklin, J. K., *et al.* (1995). Total lymphoid irradiation in the treatment of early or recurrent heart transplant rejection. *Int. J. Radiat. Oncol. Biol. Phys.* **33**, 83.

Schwadron, R. B. and Strober, S. (1987). Cloned natural suppressor cells derived from the neonatal spleen: in vitro action and lineage. *Transplant. Proc.* **19**, 533.

Slavin, S., Gurevitch, O. and Prighozina, T. (1998). Induction of bilateral transplantation tolerance to cellular and perfused allografts and xenografts with donor hematopoietic cells. *Ann. N. Y. Acad. Sci.* **863**, 37.

Stark, J. H., Smit, J. A. and Myburgh, J. A. (1994). Nonspecific mixed lymphocyte culture inhibitory antibodies in sera of tolerant transplanted baboons conditioned with total lymphoid irradiation. *Transplantation* **57**, 1103.

Steinbrüchel, D. A., Madsen, H., Nielsen, B., *et al.* (1990). Treatment with total lymphoid irradiation, cyclosporin A and a monoclonal anti-T-cell antibody in a hamster-to-rat heart transplantation model: graft survival and morphological analysis. *Transpl. Int.* **3**, 36.

Steinbrüchel, D. A., Madsen, H., Nielsen, B., *et al.* (1991). The effect of combined treatment with total lymphoid irradiation: cyclosporin A and anti-CD4 monoclonal antibodies in a hamster-to-rat heart transplantation model. *Transplant. Proc.* **23**, 579.

Strober, S. (1984). Natural suppressor (NS) cells, neonatal tolerance, and total lymphoid irradiation: exploring obscure relationships. *Ann. Rev. Immunol.* **2**, 97.

Strober, S., Dhillon, M., Schubert, M., *et al.* (1989). Acquired immune tolerance to cadaveric renal allografts: a study of three patients treated with total lymphoid irradiation. *N. Engl. J. Med.* **321**, 28.

Strober, S., Modry, D. L., Hoppe, R. T., *et al.* (1983). Induction of specific unresponsiveness to heart allografts in mongrel dogs treated with total lymphoid irradiation and anti-thymocyte globulin. *J. Immunol.* **132**, 1013.

Strober, S., Slavin, S., Gottlieb, M., *et al.* (1979). Allograft tolerance after total lymphoid irradiation (TLI). *Immunol. Rev.* **46**, 87.

Sutherland, D. E. R., Ferguson, R. M., Aeder, M. I., *et al.* (1983). Total lymphoid irradiation and cyclosprine. *Transplant. Proc.* **15**, 2881.

Thomas, F., Pittman, K., Ljung, T., *et al.* (1995). Deoxyspergualin is a unique immunosuppressive agent with selective utility inducing tolerance to pancreas islet xenografts. *Transplant. Proc.* **27**, 417.

Tixier, D., Levy, C., Le Bourgeois, J. P., *et al.* (1992). Discordant heart xenografts: experimental study in pigs conditioned by total lymphoid irradiation and cyclosporine A. *Presse Med.* **21**, 1941.

Trachiotis, G. D., Johnston, T. S., Vega, J. D., *et al.* (1998). Single-field total lymphoid irradiation in the treatment of refractory rejection after heart transplantation. *J. Heart Lung Transplant* **17**, 1045.

Trager, D. K., Banks, B. A., Rosenbaum, G., *et al.* (1989). Cardiac allograft prolongation in mice treated with combined posttransplantation total-lymphoid irradiation and anti-L3T4 antibody therapy. *Transplantation* **47**, 587.

Valentine, V. G., Robbins, R. C., Wehner, H. H., *et al.* (1996). Total lymphoid irradiation for refractory acute rejection in heart-lung and lung allografts. *Chest* **109**, 1184.

Waer, M., Ang, K. K., van der Schueren, E., *et al.* (1984a). Allogeneic bone marrow transplantation in mice after total lymphoid irradiation: influence of breeding conditions and strain of recipient mice. *J. Immunol.* **132**, 991.

Waer, M., Ang, K. K., van der Schueren, E., *et al.* (1984b). Influence of radiation field and fractionation schedule of total lymphoid irradiation (TLI) on the induction of suppressor cells and stable chimerism after bone marrow transplantation in mice. *J. Immunol.* **132**, 985.

Waer, M., Ceuppens, J. L., Vanrenterthem, Y., *et al.* (1986). Identification of a major Leu 7/Okt 8 positive T-lymphocyte subpopulation in renal transplant patients pre-treated with total lymphoid irradiation. *Leuk. Res.* **10**, 883.

Waer, M., Palathumpat, V., Sobis, H., *et al.* (1990). Induction of transplantation tolerance in mice across major histocompatibility barrier using allogeneic thymus transplantation and total lymphoid irradiation (TLI). *J. Immunol.* **145**, 499.

Waer, M., Vanrenterghem, Y., Ang, K. K., *et al.* (1984c). Comparison of the immunosuppressive effect of fractionated total lymphoid irradiation (TLI) vs. conventional immunosuppression (CI) in renal cadaveric allotransplantation. *J. Immunol.* **132**, 1041.

Waer, M., Vanrenterghem, Y., Roels, L., *et al.* (1987a). Immunological and clinical observations in diabetic kidney graft recipients pre-treated with total lymphoid irradiation. *Transplantation* **43**, 271.

Waer, M., Vanrenterghem, Y., Roels, L., *et al.* (1988). Renal cadaveric transplantation in diabetics using lethal lymphoid irradiation or cyclosporin A: a controlled randomized study. *Transpl. Int.* **1**, 64.

Waer, M., Vanrenterghem, Y., van der Schueren, E., *et al.* (1987b). Identification and function of a major OKT3, OKT8, Leu-7, positive lyymphocyte subpopulation in renal transplant recipients treated with total lymphoid irradiation. *Transplant. Proc.* **14**, 1570.

Woodley, S. L., Gurley, K. E., Hoffmann, S. L., *et al.* (1993). Induction of tolerance to heart allografts in rats using posttransplant total lymphoid irradiation and anti-T cell antibodies. *Transplantation* **56**, 1443.

Xu, H., Gundry, S. R., Hancock, W. W., *et al.* (1998). Prolonged discordant xenograft survival and delayed xenograft rejection in a pig-to-baboon orthotopic cardiac xenograft model. *J. Thorac. Cardiovasc. Surg.* **115**, 1342.

Yamaguchi, Y., Halperin, E. C., Harland, R. C., *et al.* (1990). Significant prolongation of hamster liver transplant survival in Lewis rats by total lymphoid irradiation, cyclosporin and splenectomy. *Transplantation* **49**, 13.

23

Approaches to the Induction of Tolerance

Kathryn J. Wood

Introduction

NEED FOR TOLERANCE IN CLINICAL TRANSPLANTATION

When the immune system encounters an antigen, it has to decide which type of response to make. Many factors are taken into account as the decision is made, including where the contact with the antigen took place and the environmental conditions that prevailed at the time the antigen was encountered. Components of the innate and the adaptive immune systems participate in the decision-making process (Fearon and Locksley, 1996).

The molecular mechanisms that influence the decision and the way the outcome develops, either activation or unresponsiveness, hold the key to the ability to manipulate the immune system effectively for therapeutic purposes. Insights into the nature of these processes at a molecular level enable the identification of novel approaches for inhibiting immune responses in patients after cell or organ transplantation as well as in patients who have autoimmune disease or allergy.

At present, immunosuppressive drugs are used to control unwanted immune responses. The improvements in short-term (1 year) graft survival seen since the 1970s in large part are due to the introduction of new immunosuppressive drugs into clinical practice as well as improvements in patient management (Cecka and Terasaki, 1998; Morris *et al.*, 1999 and data provided by UNOS [United Network for Organ Sharing] at www.unos.org). In the context of solid-organ transplantation, the drugs that currently are available for clinical use, including azathioprine, cyclosporine, tacrolimus, mycophenolate mofetil, antithymocyte globulin, anti-CD25 monoclonal antibodies and steroids (see Chapters 15–20), are effective at suppressing the processes that lead to early activation of the immune system. The drugs can be used with good success to prevent or control acute allograft rejection. These drugs are less effective at controlling the response to injury and chronic activation of the immune system. They also appear to be unable to promote the development of unresponsiveness or tolerance to the donor antigens consistently in the way they are used clinically at present. Experimental studies suggest that some of these agents may block the development of unresponsiveness under certain circumstances (Larsen *et al.*, 1996b). For most transplant patients, the continued survival of the allograft depends on the lifelong administration of one or more immunosuppressive drugs.

The inability of current immunosuppressive drug regimens to induce tolerance to donor antigens may be due, in part, to the nonspecific nature of the immunosuppression achieved by using drug therapy. Drugs, such as those listed previously, are unable to distinguish between the potentially harmful immune response mounted against the organ graft and responses that could be beneficial, protecting the recipient from infectious pathogens as well as providing mechanisms to control the development of malignant cells. In general, the drugs act by interfering with lymphocyte activation or proliferation regardless of the antigen specificity of the lymphocyte targeted (see Chapters 15–19). This lack of immunological specificity means that the immune system of patients treated with these immunosuppressive drugs is compromised not only in its ability to respond to the transplant but also in its ability to respond to any other antigenic stimuli that may be encountered after transplantation. The patient is more susceptible to infection and at a higher risk of developing cancer (Penn, 1998; Sheil, 1998; see Chapters 34 and 35). It has been suggested that some of the drugs used to treat transplant patients, in particular cyclosporine, may have additional properties that play a role in enhancing tumor growth in a manner that is unrelated to the drugs' effects on the immune system (Hojo *et al.*, 1999).

The full potential of organ transplantation may not be realized until alternative approaches to nonspecific immunosuppression are identified. Novel strategies that lead to the targeting of only the immune response directed against the transplant in the short-term or the long-term are needed. If tolerance to donor antigens of the graft could be achieved reliably, it would ensure that only lymphocytes in the patient's immune repertoire responding to donor antigens were suppressed, leaving most lymphocytes immunocompetent and able to perform their normal function of protecting the body from infection and cancer after transplantation. The development of transplantation tolerance in the short-term or the long-term after transplantation appears to offer the best possibility of achieving effectiveness and specificity in the control of the immune system after transplantation.

WORKING DEFINITION OF TOLERANCE

To define *tolerance* in the context of transplantation is challenging. In simple terms, transplantation tolerance is the continued survival and function of a graft in the absence of continuing immunosuppression. Although this is only a functional definition that does not define any one particular mechanism as being responsible for the tolerant state, this definition may not be inappropriate because it is becoming increasingly clear that multiple mechanisms can be used to promote the development and maintenance of tolerance to a defined set of antigens *in vivo*. What is most important is that the tolerant state in operation is effective and that it can allow the survival and function of a graft in the absence of a destructive immune response against the transplanted tissue. This chapter reviews the mechanisms of tolerance and highlights some of the novel strategies that are being explored to switch off immune responses to induce antigen-specific tolerance after transplantation.

OVERVIEW OF T-CELL ACTIVATION

Understanding of the mechanisms of activation and regulation of the immune system is important in the development of novel approaches for tolerance induction in the context of transplantation. Although it is easy to feel overwhelmed by the wealth of data on immune activation coming constantly into the literature, these findings are crucial if strategies for targeting the immune system are to be developed in the future. T-cell activation is covered in depth in Chapter 2. Following is a brief outline of events that sets the scene for discussing the different approaches to tolerance induction being explored most actively at present.

Antigen-presenting cells and T lymphocytes are pivotal to the adaptive arm of the immune response. They can act as helper and effector cells and play a major role in the destructive immune response that occurs after transplantation of a mismatched graft (Mason *et al.*, 1984). T cells also can act as regulator cells and have been shown to participate in the regulation or control of ongoing immune responses as well as in the suppression of unwanted immune responses (see later).

After transplantation, donor-derived passenger leukocytes are triggered to migrate out of the graft, in part by the proinflammatory environment created as a result of the transplantation procedure itself (Larsen *et al.*, 1990). The release of chemokines and cytokines, complement and endothelial cell activation influence the events leading to the initiation of the immune response. As the dendritic cells migrate from the graft to the T-cell areas of the draining lymphoid tissue, they *mature*. The maturation process results in the increased expression of major histocompatibility complex (MHC)–peptide complexes at the cell surface as well as up-regulation of other accessory and costimulatory molecules that are essential for triggering the response of naive T cells (Banchereau and Steinman, 1998; Fig. 23–1). In this way, immunostimulatory antigen-presenting cells expressing donor-type MHC-peptide complexes are brought into close proximity to naive T cells that may have T-cell receptors (TCRs) capable of recognizing the donor antigens through the direct pathway of allorecognition.

Damage to the graft as a result of removal from the donor and implantation into the recipient causes the release of donor antigen from the graft. The proinflammatory environment within the graft attracts recipient-derived antigen-presenting cells to the graft site. In this situation, donor alloantigens are taken up by recipient antigen-presenting cells. Immature forms of these cells are well designed to capture antigen because they are phagocytic and have the ability to take up material by micropinocytosis (Reis e Sousa *et al.*, 1993). Antigens taken up by one of these routes enter the endocytic pathway and are processed into peptides that can be expressed at the cell surface bound to recipient MHC class II molecules. In addition, recipient dendritic cells can take up apoptotic cells (Albert *et al.*, 1999) that may be generated as a result of ischemia-reperfusion injury after transplantation, and this can lead to antigen presentation in the context of recipient MHC class I molecules. Presentation of donor-derived allopeptides by recipient antigen-presenting cells triggers recipient T cells to respond to donor alloantigen through the indirect pathway (Shoskes and Wood, 1994). T cells responding through the direct and the indirect pathway of allorecognition contribute to allograft rejection (Gould and Auchincloss, 1999).

When a T cell recognizes the MHC-peptide complexes expressed by an antigen-presenting cell, through its TCR, the molecules present in the membrane contact area between the T cell and the antigen-presenting cell are reorganized (van

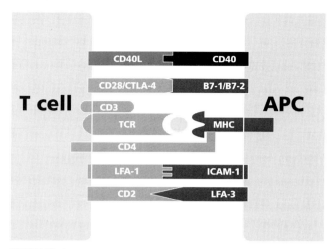

FIGURE 23–1

Cell surface molecules when antigen-presenting cells (APC) interact with naive CD4+ T cells. T-cell activation requires at least two signals. Signal 1 is delivered to the T cell when major histocompatibility complex (MHC) class II–peptide complexes (APC) are recognized specifically by the T-cell receptor/CD3 complex expressed by the T cell. CD4 (T cell) interacts with the MHC class II molecule, fulfilling an adhesion and a signaling function. Second signals or costimulation is provided by additional cell surface interactions. CD28 (T cell) can bind to B7.2 (CD86) and B7.1 (CD80) expressed by the APC. This interaction delivers a signal to the T cell that lowers the threshold for T-cell activation. CD40 on the APC can bind to its ligand, CD40L (CD154) (T cell). This interaction provides additional signals to the T cell but, in contrast to the CD28 pathway, also delivers signals to the APC resulting in an increase in expression of B7.1 and B7.2. To ensure that the T cell engages the APC for sufficient time for the signaling events to occur, adhesion molecules, including ICAM-1 (intracellular adhesion molecule 1) and LFA-1 (lymphocyte function antigen 1), also engage each other.

der Merwe *et al.*, 2000). This highly orchestrated series of events results in the formation of the immunological synapse, which has been visualized in many studies (Grakoui *et al.*, 1999). These events ensure that all of the cell surface structures, TCR, costimulation and adhesion molecules, required to initiate effective T-cell activation are brought into the correct spatial orientation (Lanzavecchia *et al.*, 1999; see Fig. 23–1).

For a T cell to become activated fully, a threshold number of TCRs need to be engaged (Valitutti and Lanzavecchia, 1997). T-cell receptor recognition of a donor MHC-peptide complex present on an antigen-presenting cell results in signal transduction through the CD3 proteins that associate with the TCR at the cell surface. This signal transduction initiates a cascade of biochemical signaling pathways that are contributed to by interactions between accessory, costimulatory and adhesion molecules and culminate ultimately in cytokine production, proliferation of the triggered T cell and its differentiation into an effector cell.

Accessory and costimulatory molecules that have been shown to be important in triggering T-cell activation on the T-cell side include CD4, CD11b/CD18 (LFA-1), CD28 and CD154 (CD40 ligand) (see Fig. 23–1). These molecules must engage their ligands on antigen-presenting cells, MHC class II, ICAM, CD86/CD80 (B7-1/B7-2) and CD40 to ensure that the threshold for activation of a naive T cell is overcome once antigen recognition has occurred.

The cytokine and chemokine milieu present at the time these molecular engagements occur affects the differentiation pathway a T cell takes and the course of the response

(O'Garra, 1998). Cytokines and chemokines can modulate the expression of the cell surface molecules mentioned previously as well as the expression of cytokine and chemokine receptors themselves. This modulation can result in differential signaling in the T cell and antigen-presenting cell, tipping the balance of the response from full to partial activation or, in some circumstances, inactivation of the cells involved, modifying dramatically the downstream events (i.e., cell migration patterns and the generation of effector cells).

Mechanisms of Tolerance to Donor Antigens

The immune system is constantly in a state of balance to ensure that its response to any challenge is effective but not excessive. Natural mechanisms already exist to ensure that the immune system does not respond in an uncontrolled way. It may be possible to take advantage or harness these mechanisms to induce or maintain tolerance to donor antigens.

The mechanisms identified as responsible for inducing or maintaining tolerance to donor antigens include the following:

Deletion of donor reactive cells centrally in the thymus as well as in the periphery

Active regulation of the immune response to donor antigens by suppressor or immunoregulatory T cells

Immune deviation by alteration of the cytokine microenvironment in the recipient, particularly in the graft itself

T-cell ignorance or helplessness, a state of unresponsiveness that might be particularly relevant to grafts placed at sites such as the brain

Exhaustion, in which the ability of donor reactive cells simply is eliminated as a result of overstimulation

Anergy, a state of unresponsiveness that is refractory to further stimulation

Each of these mechanisms is not unique to the deliberate induction of tolerance in the context of transplantation. All of them also have been described as responsible for tolerance to self-antigens and are used by the body as mechanisms for the prevention of autoimmune disease (Mason and Powrie, 1998).

The induction and maintenance of tolerance is a dynamic process, and often it is not possible to assign a single mechanism as responsible for the tolerant state. More likely, multiple mechanisms operate in concert with one another, with each taking a more or less significant role as the process develops. The same situation applies to the development and maintenance of tolerance to self-antigens and the prevention of autoimmune disease. An overriding feature that is essential for the successful operation of each of these mechanisms is the persistent presence of donor antigen throughout the period of tolerance *in vivo*.

PERSISTENCE OF DONOR ANTIGEN

One of the key requirements for maintaining tolerance before or after transplantation, regardless of the precise nature of the mechanism that is operating, is the persistence of donor antigen; this has been shown in many experimental models (Bushell *et al.*, 1994; Hamano *et al.*, 1996; Khan *et al.*, 1996; Scully *et al.*, 1994). The source of the antigen can be donor-derived cells introduced before transplantation, as is the case in models of mixed chimerism (Khan *et al.*, 1996), or the graft itself after transplantation (Hamano *et al.*, 1996). In the absence of antigen, tolerance is lost gradually because the mechanisms responsible for maintaining tolerance are

no longer stimulated. During the induction phase and the maintenance phase of tolerance, the presence of alloantigen is the key factor driving the outcome. As is often the case with the immune system, the same element can influence the response positively and negatively. In the case of donor antigen, presentation in the wrong context could lead to activation with the potential of destroying the tolerant state and triggering graft rejection.

DELETION OF DONOR REACTIVE LEUKOCYTES

Deletion is a mechanism that can be used to eliminate donor reactive T cells and B cells from the recipient repertoire (Goodnow *et al.*, 1990; Kappler *et al.*, 1987). This discussion focuses on T cells and T-cell deletion, which can occur centrally in the thymus or in the periphery.

Clonal deletion of T cells in the thymus is the major mechanism by which tolerance to self-antigens is induced (Kappler *et al.*, 1987; Stockinger, 1999). Thymocytes expressing a functional αβ TCR develop into mature T cells in the thymus only if the constraints for positive and negative selection are met. The interaction between the TCR and the self-MHC–peptide complexes in the thymus is crucial for this process to enable T cells with some reactivity for self-MHC to be positively selected, while those with high affinity and avidity for self-MHC-self peptides are deleted or negatively selected (Goldrath and Bevan, 1999; Sebzda *et al.*, 1999). This process is essential to ensure that a diverse T-cell repertoire is produced and maintained.

Clonal deletion in the thymus depends on the affinity and avidity of the TCR for the selecting ligand (Jameson *et al.*, 1995). This dependence implies that there is a spectrum of responses depending on the *strength of interaction* between the T cell and the MHC-peptide complex. T cells with high affinity and avidity for the ligand are deleted, whereas T cells with lower affinity and avidity are not. The process of deletion of T cells in the thymus may be incomplete. Although residual T cells have a TCR only with a lower affinity and avidity for the selecting ligand, they still are present and have the potential to react with the selecting antigen or by cross-reactivity with another antigen at a later stage (Kawai and Ohashi, 1995).

Central deletion of T cells in the thymus can be exploited as a mechanism for inducing tolerance to donor antigens. This mechanism has been particularly successful in the context of therapeutic strategies using donor bone marrow in combination with nonmyeloablative therapy, such as T-cell depletion or costimulation blockade, for the induction of tolerance (Wekerle and Sykes, 1999). In mixed allogeneic chimeras in the mouse, donor-derived dendritic cells have been shown to be resident and persist in the recipient thymus (Manilay *et al.*, 1998; Tomita *et al.*, 1994). As a result, there is continuous deletion of donor reactive thymocytes, leading to the absence of donor reactive T cells in the periphery and tolerance.

Intrathymic injection of donor antigen or allopeptides directly into the thymus results in the deletion of donor reactive cells (Jones *et al.*, 1997, 1998; Markmann *et al.*, 1993). If this injection of antigen is combined with leukocyte or T-cell depletion in the periphery, it can lead to the successful induction of operational donor-specific tolerance in rodents (Jones *et al.*, 1997; Posselt *et al.*, 1990; Remuzzi *et al.*, 1991). In contrast to the situation that occurs in stable mixed chimeras, after intrathymic delivery of donor antigen, the antigen persists in the thymus only for a defined period after injection. Intrathymic delivery of donor antigen provides a window of opportunity in which to transplant a solid-organ graft rather than producing persistent deletion of thymocytes in the long-term (Jones *et al.*, 1998; Fig. 23–2).

Antigen-reactive T cells can be deleted in the periphery (Webb *et al.*, 1990). The introduction of high doses of defined antigens intravenously or orally has been shown to result in deletion of mature T cells in peripheral lymphoid organs (Kearney *et al.*, 1994). CD4[+] and CD8[+] T cells can be eliminated by peripheral deletion, but in many cases deletion was incomplete even when high doses of antigen were used. When analyzed, the residual antigen-reactive cells remaining in the periphery were shown to be hyperresponsive to further stimulation by the same antigen, showing that additional mechanisms of tolerance were in operation (Pape *et al.*, 1998; see later).

The mechanisms by which T cells are deleted in the thymus and periphery has been an area of active investigation. The Fas pathway has been shown to play an essential role in the homeostasis of the peripheral lymphocyte compartment as well as in the effector mechanisms used by cytotoxic T lymphocytes and natural killer cells to destroy target cells (Nagata, 1997; see Chapter 2). The Fas pathway has been implicated as one of the mechanisms operating to delete antigen-reactive cells centrally and in the periphery.

The Fas receptor (CD95, APO-1) is a type I membrane protein of the tumor necrosis factor (TNF) receptor superfamily (Nagata, 1997). When it finds its natural ligand (CD95L, Fas-ligand), a complex signaling cascade is initiated, which can result in death of the Fas-expressing cell by apoptosis (Krammer, 1999). Although there are conflicting data about the role of the Fas pathway in the thymus, the overall impression from many analyses suggests that the Fas pathway can play a role in antigen-specific deletion of thymocytes but only at high concentrations of antigen. When antigen is present in low doses, deletion in the thymus appears to be Fas independent (Theofilopoulos, 1995).

The Fas pathway has been shown to play a greater role in deletion of T cells at particular sites in the periphery, so-called immune privileged sites (Bellgrau and Duke, 1999). At these sites, transplantation of allogeneic tissues results in the prolonged survival of the transplanted tissue relative to the survival obtained after transplantation of the same tissue at other sites. These sites include the anterior chamber of the eye and the testis. Fas-ligand expression has been shown to be important for these sites to maintain their immune privilege status (Bellgrau and Duke, 1999; Griffith *et al.*, 1995). Fas-ligand–mediated apoptosis has been shown to be the mechanism by which inflammatory cells entering these sites are eliminated. The Fas pathway also has been implicated in

deletional tolerance after administration of allogeneic bone marrow (George *et al.*, 1998). In the periphery, the Fas pathway may be important in deletion of antigen-reactive cells, when antigen is present at high concentration or at particular sites of the body where Fas-ligand is expressed endogenously.

To try to harness the potential of immune privileged sites, attempts have been made to engineer the expression of Fas-ligand on tissue at the site of transplantation. These attempts have met with varying degrees of success (Kang *et al.*, 1997; Lau *et al.*, 1996; Turvey *et al.*, 2000). In certain settings, expression of Fas-ligand on the transplanted allogeneic tissue itself or on tissue transplanted alongside the graft has been reported to prolong graft survival (Lau *et al.*, 1996).

Deletion of antigen-reactive cells can occur as a result of T-cell activation in the periphery. This process is incomplete in the absence of a functional Fas pathway, suggesting that Fas is involved at least in part (van Parijs *et al.*, 1996). Activation-induced cell death is a natural mechanism that is used to reduce the size of the population of T cells responding to a particular antigen challenge (clonal downsizing) (Bluestone, 1998; Lenardo, 1996). In this way, homeostasis in the lymphocyte compartment is maintained, preventing the accumulation of any one particular clone of lymphocytes. In addition to the Fas pathway, many other mechanisms have been implicated in clonal downsizing after the elimination of antigen, including up-regulation of expression of CD152 (CTLA4) on T cells, a molecule that is thought to prevent further costimulation by competing for binding to CD80 and CD86 (B7-1 and B7-2) on the antigen-presenting cell and by delivering negative signals to the responding cells, shutting down further clonal expansion (Bluestone, 1998; van Parijs and Abbas, 1998).

Loss of antigen-reactive cells through activation-induced cell death rapidly eliminates reactivity toward the stimulating antigen. In normal circumstances (i.e., during responses to nominal antigens), this process is used to balance the response. Antigen-reactive T cells no longer are activated once the antigen has been eliminated. After transplantation, antigen stimulation potentially continues as long as the organ continues to function. Expansion of donor reactive T cells could occur indefinitely, unless the response were actively controlled. Activation-induced cell death may be one of the mechanisms that is used to ensure that the size of the population of leukocytes responding to donor antigen is kept at a manageable level. Certain immunosuppressive drugs, such as rapamycin, may be able to facilitate this process (Li *et al.*, 1999b; Wells *et al.*, 1999).

FIGURE 23–2

Hypothesis to explain the role of the allograft in the maintenance of tolerance after T-cell depletion. Depletion of T cells below a certain threshold level in the thymus and the periphery can lead to long-term graft acceptance. T-cell depletion can be achieved by the use of monoclonal antibody therapy alone or in combination with the injection of donor antigen directly into the thymus. New T cells with specificity for donor alloantigens emerge from the thymus (recent thymic emigrants) once the antibody therapy decays. If the graft expressing high levels of donor antigen is present as the T cells repopulate, rejection of the graft does not occur. One possibility is that donor reactive T cells are deleted as they contact donor antigen in the graft.

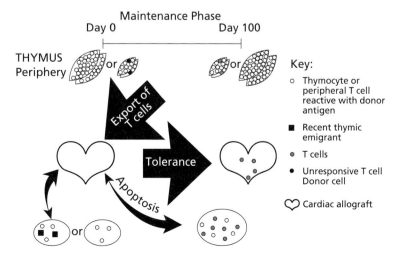

The reappearance of donor reactive cells at a functional level can be controlled or prevented by the continuing presence of donor antigen in the form of the organ graft or active immunoregulation. This process results in the long-term survival of the graft, provided that the rate of deletion is maintained or that additional mechanisms that can promote tolerance to the graft are induced. In some situations, this process is described as *exhaustion* because the response to a particular antigen can be effectively exhausted by chronic stimulation of the responding populations. Such a situation occurs most commonly in chronic viral infection (Zinkernagel *et al.*, 1999).

ACTIVE SUPPRESSION AND REGULATION

Suppression was described first in the 1970s after the demonstration that antigen-specific unresponsiveness could be transferred from one recipient to another (Gershon and Kondo, 1971). In this situation, mechanisms other than deletion of antigen-reactive cells are in operation, and populations of cells present among those transferred adoptively must be capable of regulating the response of naive cells to the same antigen.

Active regulation and suppression of immune responses has been described as a mechanism for inducing and maintaining tolerance to donor antigens in the context of transplantation as well as to self-antigens, preventing the onset of autoimmune disease (Hutchinson, 1986; Waldmann and Cobbold, 1998). It has been suggested that for the maintenance of tolerance to self-antigens, active regulation of self-reactive leukocytes in the periphery is essential for the prevention of autoimmune disease (Mason and Powrie, 1998). Two of the lines of evidence in support of this hypothesis are as follows. The deletion of self-reactive T cells in the thymus is incomplete. Cells with the potential to cause destruction of those tissues can be isolated from the T cells present in normal individuals. Alongside these potentially destructive self-reactive leukocytes, other leukocyte populations capable of controlling their activity exist (Sakaguchi *et al.*, 1996). These cells have been isolated and are in the process of being characterized.

To exploit suppression and regulation of the immune response to an organ graft for therapeutic purposes, a clearer understanding of the mechanisms by which the phenomenon operates is required. Although regulation could be operating exclusively through deletional mechanisms, at present there is little evidence to support this as the dominant mechanism for active immunoregulation or suppression. The demonstration that immunoregulatory cells can be used to transfer unresponsiveness adoptively from a transplant recipient with a long-term surviving graft to a fresh naive recipient through many generations of cells, the process known as *infectious tolerance*, suggests that this population of regulatory or suppressor cells can generate further cohorts by influencing the differentiation patterns of naive cells *in vivo* (Qin *et al.*, 1993; Waldmann and Cobbold, 1998). These cells appear to function not by eliminating donor reactive aggressive leukocytes, but by silencing their functional activity *in vivo*.

In most experimental systems in rodents, the regulatory or suppressor cells reside in the CD4[+] T-cell compartment (Bushell *et al.*, 1995; Hall *et al.*, 1985; Quigley *et al.*, 1989). CD8[+] regulatory T cells also are described but are less common except in humans (Hutchinson, 1986; Li *et al.*, 1999a). Many groups have been trying to identify molecular markers that allow these specialized populations of regulatory and suppressor cells to be identified more precisely. To date, many candidate cell surface markers have been reported to be expressed by cells with immunoregulatory properties to self-antigens or alloantigens, including particular isoforms of

CD45 (CD45RB[low] [mouse], CD45RC[low] [rat]) (Hara *et al.*, 2000; Josien *et al.*, 1995; Powrie and Mason, 1990; Yang *et al.*, 1995), CD25 (Gao *et al.*, 1999; Sakaguchi *et al.*, 1995) and CD152 (CTLA4) (Read and Powrie, unpublished data).

When these immunoregulatory leukocytes are present *in vivo*, they could suppress the reactivity of aggressive cells in many ways. One hypothesis attracting particular interest at present is the possibility that these cells represent a third subset of T cells with a specialized cytokine and functional profile. Roles for transforming growth factor (TGF)-β and interleukin (IL)-10 alone or in combination have been proposed in many different models of immunoregulation and anergy, including the anterior chamber of the eye, after oral or nasal delivery of antigen and in models of tolerance to self-antigen or alloantigen (Asseman *et al.*, 1999; Josien *et al.*, 1998; Powrie *et al.*, 1996; Wilbanks *et al.*, 1992). Transforming growth factor-β has been reported to modulate the function of the antigen-presenting cell promoting TH2 responses (Bridoux *et al.*, 1997; King *et al.*, 1998; see later). The relationship between TGF-β and IL-10 in the development of tolerance still is being characterized as different models show differential requirements for one or both of these mediators at particular stages in the response (Miller *et al.*, 1999). From these data, it seems reasonable to propose that there are certain soluble mediators that can promote the development of unresponsiveness when present in the correct microenvironment, TGF-β and IL-10 being two examples. Similar to many immunological mediators, the presence of TGF-β and IL-10 in the right place at a certain concentration is key to the way in which they function. When present in the wrong place at the wrong time with respect to tolerance induction, TGF-β can cause fibrosis, and IL-10 can trigger acute graft rejection (Blazar *et al.*, 1998; Moore *et al.*, 1993; Moses *et al.*, 1990; Qian *et al.*, 1996; Qin *et al.*, 1996; Wahl, 1994). These and other soluble mediators not yet identified likely act in combination with cell surface structures to promote the development of tolerance.

A CD4[+] T-cell clone secreting a unique pattern of cytokines (IL-10 and TGF-β) has been generated in tissue culture by growing naive cells in IL-10 (Groux *et al.*, 1997). This population has been termed *T-regulatory 1*. These cells appear similar to the cells described previously after oral delivery of a defined antigen that produced large amounts of TGF-β on restimulation with antigen (TH3 cells) (Weiner, 1997). Whether T-regulatory 1 cells are the same as the cells responsible for inducing or maintaining tolerance to alloantigens remains to be shown. In the future, however, if it were possible to differentiate and expand cells with immunoregulatory function to a defined antigen reliably *in vitro*, this would offer great opportunities for using cellular therapy to control immune responses.

An alternative but complementary hypothesis to explain the action of regulatory T cells suggests that regulatory T cells control the ability of antigen-presenting cells to trigger T-cell activation (Li *et al.*, 1999a; Taams *et al.*, 1998). Antigen-presenting cells have been shown to become *licensed* to trigger effector cell activation once they have encountered an activated T helper (CD4) cell (Bennett *et al.*, 1998; Lanzavecchia, 1998; Ridge *et al.*, 1998). This hypothesis eliminates the need for clusters of helper and cytotoxic T cells to be brought together in the vicinity of the antigen-presenting cell at the same time to ensure that only effector cells with the appropriate antigen specificity are activated. Rather the hypothesis suggests that once an antigen-presenting cell has presented antigen and activated a T helper cell, the T helper cell changes the functional activity of the antigen-presenting cell to enable activation of an effector T cell to be triggered in its absence.

A similar scenario has been envisaged for regulatory T cells. When regulatory cells are mixed into cultures of antigen-presenting cells and helper T cells, they can inhibit proliferation of the responding T cells. It has been shown that regulatory T cells can inhibit the up-regulation of costimulatory molecules on antigen-presenting cells when they are present in these cultures (Li et al., 1999a; Taams et al., 1998). These and other data suggest that regulatory cells can change the function of antigen-presenting cells, preventing them from triggering T-cell activation.

One potentially powerful effect of regulatory and suppressor cells is their ability to link the unresponsive state to more than one antigen, the phenomenon known as *linked unresponsiveness* (Davies et al., 1996a, b; Madsen et al., 1988; Wong et al., 1996). This phenomenon has been described in transplantation and autoimmune models, and the data show that it is possible to manipulate the immune response to a variety of different antigens by initially targeting just one. For example, if the recipient's immune system is exposed to a defined alloantigen before transplantation, alone or in combination with a T cell–modulating agent, the response to that antigen can be switched off *in vivo* (Madsen et al., 1988; Saitovitch et al., 1996; Wong et al., 1997a, 1997b). As the unresponsive state to this defined antigen develops, it can be linked to other molecules present on the graft, provided that the initiating antigen is present (Table 23–1; Fig. 23–3). Linked unresponsiveness has been shown in many different systems. In our studies using a mouse model of transplantation, we have shown that when recipients are pretreated with cells expressing a single donor class I molecule, such as H-2K^b, alone (Madsen et al., 1988) or in combination with anti-CD4 monoclonal antibody (Saitovitch et al., 1996; Wong et al., 1997a, 1997b), specific unresponsiveness to H-2K^b is induced before transplantation (Table 23–1). After transplantation, this state of unresponsiveness to H-2K^b can be linked to MHC and minor histocompatibility complex antigens expressed by the graft (Table 23–1). In other words, if one transplants an organ graft expressing the initial antigen and other alloantigens, unresponsiveness to the triggering antigen as well as the alloantigens expressed by the transplant develops in the long-term after transplantation.

The mechanisms underlying linked unresponsiveness are under active investigation. Data from the analysis of anergized T-cell clones *in vitro* and regulatory cells *in vivo* show that the process is active and requires cell-cell contact (Hara et al., 2000; Lombardi et al., 1994). In many systems, the initiating antigen is seen indirectly by the recipients' immune system (Hara et al., 2000), after processing of the donor molecule by recipient antigen-presenting cells. The cells have been described as possessing the phenotype of regulatory cells because they can function in adoptive transfer systems.

This phenomenon has important clinical implications, particularly when alloantigen is administered before transplantation in the form of blood transfusions. The mechanism implies that tolerance established to one set of antigens can spread to others if they are presented on the same graft or the same antigen-presenting cells. It might be possible to expose a recipient to one or more defined HLA antigens that they themselves do not express. When an organ donor became available, the graft might express at least one of the antigens to which unresponsiveness has been induced before transplantation. In this way, the presentation of this same donor molecule on allograft would allow linked unresponsiveness to develop to the mismatched antigens expressed by the organ donor.

In many studies in which lymphocytes have been shown to have regulatory properties *in vivo*, the same functional attributes have not been replicated when the cells have been analyzed *in vitro* (Batchelor and Welsh, 1976; Pearce et al., 1993; Young et al., 1997). Assays designed to investigate the functional activity of donor reactive cells present in tolerant recipients (e.g., mixed leukocyte cultures or by the generation of cytotoxic responses), have failed to reveal the tolerant state. Under the conditions used routinely for these assays, the cells appear to respond as if they were naive. This response suggests that the conditions in the *in vitro* assays do not reflect accurately the microenvironment that exists within the organ graft or within the periphery of tolerant recipients that enables the cells responsible for maintaining tolerance to operate efficiently in this setting.

IMMUNE DEVIATION FROM A TH1 TO A TH2 RESPONSE

T cells exhibit distinct cytokine profiles after chronic stimulation with antigen (Mosmann et al., 1986). TH1 CD4$^+$ T-cell clones secrete the inflammatory signature cytokines interferon (IFN)-γ, TNF-α and IL-2, which are linked to cell-mediated immune responses. In contrast, CD4$^+$ T-cell clones with a TH2 cytokine profile produce the signatory cytokines IL-4, IL-5, IL-6, IL-10 and IL-13, which are associated with a humoral immune response (Mosmann et al., 1991; O'Garra, 1998). Clones with similar cytokine profiles have been found after chronic antigen stimulation of CD8$^+$ T cells, referred to as *TC1* and *TC2* cells.

When naive T cells first encounter antigen, they are considered to be unpolarized (TH0) and capable of secreting low levels of TH1 and TH2 cytokines. The signals that the cells receive when they recognize antigen and the microenvironment in which the encounter takes place determine which pathway the response adopts. Once the choice is made, the

TABLE 23–1

Experiments Showing Linked Unresponsiveness in a Cardiac Allograft Mouse Model*

Source of Antigen Used to Pretreat CBA (H-2^k) Recipients in Combination with Anti-CD4	Strain and MHC Haplotype of Heart Donor	Initiating Antigens	Graft Survival (Median Survival Time) (d)
B10 − H-2^b	B10 − H-2^b	B10 − H-2^b	100
B10 − H-2^b	BALB − H-2^d	None	25
CBK − H-2K^b + H-2^d	B10 − H-2^b	H-2K^b	100
CBK − H-2K^b + H-2^k	(CBK × BALB)F1 H-2K^b + H-2^d	H-2K^b	100
CBK − H-2K^b + H-2^k	(CBA × BALB)F1 H-2^k + H-2^d	None	25

*The recipient is pretreated with antigen in the form of blood under an umbrella of anti-CD4 monoclonal antibody.
MHC = major histocompatibility complex.

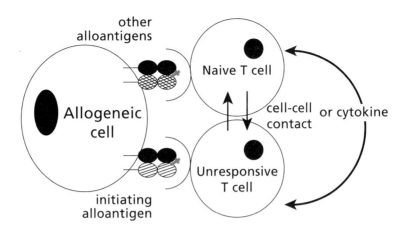

FIGURE 23–3

Linked unresponsiveness. After T cells encounter alloantigen, they can be rendered unresponsive to a subsequent encounter with the same antigen. Unresponsive T cells can develop regulatory or suppressor properties that can be transferred or linked to other alloantigens expressed by the antigen-presenting cell. In a mouse model, we have shown that recipient T cells that recognize donor MHC class I antigen after intravenous delivery by the indirect pathway can regulate the response to other alloantigens expressed by the allograft, preventing graft rejection and promoting the induction of operational tolerance. The mechanism of action of the regulatory cells is under active investigation at present. Several possibilities have been proposed, including the production of cytokines, such as interleukin-10 or transforming growth factor-β, by the unresponsive T cell and the interaction between cell surface molecules expressed by the three interacting cell populations or the unresponsive T cell and the antigen-presenting cell.

differentiation toward a TH1 or a TH2 phenotype is reinforced by positive feedback by cytokines and signaling pathways on the selected self type, whereas additional mechanisms suppress the development of cells of the opposite cytokine's phenotype (O'Garra, 1998).

It has been proposed that inhibition of graft rejection and the onset of autoimmune diseases is a consequence of preferential blockade of potentially destructive TH1 immune responses in favor of less aggressive TH2 responses (Rocken and Shevach, 1996). In the context of organ transplantation, much of the supporting evidence for this hypothesis came from reports of an absence of TH1 cytokines in animals with long-term graft survival (Mottram et al., 1995; Onodera et al., 1997; Sayegh et al., 1995). The presence of TH2 cells in tolerant recipients is not a uniform finding, however (Hall et al., 1998). Studies have failed to show that TH2 cytokines actively promote the development of tolerance or that TH1 cytokines can promote only graft rejection (Bushell et al., 1999; Qian et al., 1996). The absence of the TH1 cytokines IFN-γ and IL-2 has been shown to prevent the induction of tolerance (Dai et al., 1998; Konieczny et al., 1998).

It is still a matter of some debate as to the relative significance of TH2 cytokine profiles in transplantation tolerance. There are many reports that the presence of TH2 cytokines within the microenvironment of the graft actively promote the development of chronic changes (Russell et al., 1994). Studies in which some of the signature cytokines of TH2 cells, particularly IL-4, have been neutralized have failed to show convincingly that this cytokine, and by inference TH2 immune deviation, is key for promoting long-term graft survival and tolerance (Bushell et al., 1999; Davies et al., 1996a, b). These and other data suggest that immune deviation alone cannot account for peripheral tolerance, although it cannot be ruled out that deviation of cytokine production toward a TH2 phenotype promotes the recruitment and activation of other mechanisms that all contribute to the tolerance state. Taken together, the available data suggest that interplay within the cytokine network is crucial for controlled unresponsiveness and that immune deviation as a mechanism to explain tolerance *in vivo* is overly simple.

LESSONS THAT CAN BE LEARNED FROM SITUATIONS IN WHICH TOLERANCE DEVELOPS WITHOUT INTERVENTION

Transplantation tolerance has been reported to develop spontaneously after transplantation of liver grafts across a full MHC mismatch and of kidney and heart grafts that are mismatched for one or more major or minor antigens in some donor-recipient combinations (Gallico et al., 1979; Kamada, 1985; Peugh et al., 1986; Qian et al., 1994). In these situations, the grafts are accepted without any immunosuppression being administered. In many situations in rodents and large animals, notably the pig, liver and kidney allografts are accepted after administration of only a short course of immunosuppression (Calne et al., 1969; Gianello et al., 1995). It generally is accepted that there is a hierarchy with respect to the ease of inhibition of immune response directed against different organ grafts, with liver allografts and skin grafts being at the two opposite ends of the spectrum. In clinical transplantation, it often is noted that the liver appears to protect other organs that are transplanted alongside it from the full force of the rejection response—the *liver effect*.

The mechanisms of spontaneous acceptance of liver allografts have been investigated actively to try to understand why the liver appears to promote the development of unresponsiveness. The initial posttransplant phase after liver grafting is associated with the activation of donor-specific helper and cytotoxic T cells as well as infiltration of the graft by T cells and macrophages (Kamada, 1985). The level of infiltration subsides after a few months, however, and the grafts survive long-term. When the characteristics of the cellular infiltrates and the cytokines that the infiltrating leukocytes produce have been examined in the early posttransplant period in tolerant and rejecting liver allografts, they have been found to be essentially the same with some changes in the B-cell compartment (Farges et al., 1994a; Sun et al., 1994). An early down-regulation of IL-4 expression also has been reported, but the relationship between this and the tolerant state has not been clarified (Farges et al., 1994b).

Analysis of rejecting and nonrejecting kidney allografts in

the early posttransplant period have failed to identify one key parameter that distinguishes rejecting from nonrejecting grafts (Dallman *et al.*, 1987; Wood *et al.*, 1987). This lack of success may reflect the fact that only previously identified molecules were explored in these studies. Many groups are searching for new genes that are expressed in tolerant T cells. Some genes are beginning to be identified (Korthauer *et al.*, 2000), and these might hold the key to tolerance. Alternatively the liver effect might result from a combination of parameters that were not easy to identify in the analyses carried out to date. New techniques, including gene array technology, may facilitate these investigations in the future.

It has been proposed that the ability of a liver allograft to protect itself from acute rejection and in the long-term reverse the rejection response to itself and to a second organ graft may be due to the large antigen load delivered by the liver graft itself (Sun *et al.*, 1996). This hypothesis is supported, in some sense, by the finding that simultaneous transplantation of multiple hearts or kidneys into the same host also can promote acceptance of all of the grafts in the absence of immunosuppression, whereas in the same situation transplantation of a single graft would result in rapid rejection. Transplantation of multiple heart or kidney grafts on its own does not induce transplantation tolerance even though graft survival is prolonged. If donor leukocytes also are infused, however, tolerance is induced. This observation may offer more clues as to why the liver is particularly potent in inducing unresponsiveness on its own (Sun *et al.*, 1996).

The liver contains large numbers of passenger leukocytes. It has been suggested that these hold the key to the liver effect (Starzl *et al.*, 1992). The migration of these cells from the graft in the early posttransplant phase might contribute to the deletion and inactivation of donor reactive cells through activation-induced cell death (see earlier) as well as providing a long-term source of donor antigen in the recipient, microchimerism. It has been shown that elimination of these cells before transplantation prevents tolerance induction, and, as mentioned earlier, tolerance can be restored by infusing extra donor leukocytes (Sun *et al.*, 1996). It has been postulated that the persistence of donor-derived passenger cells from the liver allograft is key to the development of the unresponsive state in the long-term. Data suggest, however, that the presence of the donor leukocytes is required only in the relatively short-term after transplantation and that thereafter the passenger leukocytes play no significant role (Ko *et al.*, 1999). These data imply that in the long-term other mechanisms are responsible for maintaining the survival of the liver graft. Other mechanisms that have been proposed to explain the spontaneous acceptance of liver grafts include the production of large quantities of soluble donor class I molecules that may block the functional activity or induce apoptosis of CD8$^+$ T cells as well as setting up regulatory populations of T cells that can control the downstream response made by the host against the graft (Zavazava and Kronke, 1996) and the production of immunoregulatory molecules such as IL-10 by the liver posttransplantation (Le Moine *et al.*, 1994).

Approaches to the Induction of Tolerance

The strategies for tolerance induction being explored most actively at present invoke one or more of the mechanisms of tolerance described previously. These mechanisms include the continuous deletion of donor reactive leukocytes by establishing the presence of high levels of donor cells in the recipient (mixed chimerism), short-term depletion and/or deletion of donor reactive leukocytes combined with the

establishment of immunoregulation and suppression of responses to donor alloantigens in the longer term after transplantation and costimulation blockade leading to the induction of T-cell unresponsiveness in the presence of the organ graft.

Most of the approaches being explored, with the exception of mixed chimerism, do not aim to induce tolerance to donor antigens before transplantation. Instead, they attempt to use novel strategies that are nonspecific in their mode of action at the time of transplantation to create an environment that promotes the development of operational tolerance to the graft in the long-term. Although in an ideal world it would be preferable to switch off the response to donor antigens before the graft is transplanted, in the short term, this may not be realistic with the tools currently available. The development of tolerance to the graft in the long-term would have major benefits for patients because it would enable the total amount of immunosuppressive drug therapy to be reduced over the transplant course and might enable drug therapy to be eliminated from the treatment regimen at some point. Many of these approaches being developed rely on the use of biological molecules, monoclonal antibodies or soluble recombinant ligands in the form of fusion proteins, alone or in combination with donor antigen to enable targeting of specific components of the immune system.

STRATEGIES BASED ON CENTRAL DELETION OF ANTIGEN-REACTIVE CELLS

Deletion of donor reactive cells is an effective way of eliminating donor reactivity in the recipient's immune system if deletion can be maintained throughout the posttransplant course. It has been shown elegantly that the development of macrochimerism as a result of bone marrow infusion under the appropriate conditions can be used to achieve this goal (Sykes and Sachs, 1988). A few bone marrow transplant recipients who subsequently required a renal transplant were transplanted with a kidney from their bone marrow donor (Jacobsen *et al.*, 1994; Sayegh *et al.*, 1991; Sorof *et al.*, 1995). In these cases, long-term immunosuppression was unnecessary because the recipient already was unresponsive to the donor alloantigens as a result of the allogeneic chimerism that developed after the successful bone marrow transplant. Bone marrow transplantation is not an appropriate approach to consider for most recipients on transplant waiting lists. Fully allogeneic chimerism has the drawback of reducing the immunocompetence of the recipient's immune system in some situations. Nevertheless, from these cases, it is clear that if it were possible to introduce donor bone marrow cells into the recipient under conditions that would allow macrochimerism to develop and be maintained, this would be an effective approach for inducing tolerance *in vivo* (Wood and Sachs, 1996).

Many different approaches have been used to try to achieve this goal. Total lymphoid irradiation alone or in combination with bone marrow infusion has been shown to be effective at inducing tolerance in some recipients in rodents, primates and human patients (Myburgh *et al.*, 1984; Slavin *et al.*, 1977; Strober *et al.*, 1989). The requirement for irradiation in these systems has inhibited their development and clinical application to the fullest extent.

An alternative system has been developed and refined by Sykes and Sachs (1988) and others (Wekerle and Sykes, 1999). In a mouse model, they showed that it is possible to use nonmyeloablation in combination with high-dose bone marrow infusion to promote deletion of donor reactive cells in the thymus (Manilay *et al.*, 1998; Tomita *et al.*, 1994). Use of costimulation blockade has been shown to eliminate the need for cytoreduction (Wekerle *et al.*, 1998, 2000). In a large animal model, T-cell depletion has been shown to be effective in producing stable mixed chimerism (Huang *et al.*, 2000). Persistent macrochimersim after bone marrow infusion means that the unresponsive state persists long-term in the absence of a solid-organ graft. Once macrochimerism has been established, grafts from the bone marrow donor can be transplanted at any time thereafter because deletion of the donor reactive cells continues indefinitely.

This type of protocol has been translated successfully to a primate model of transplantation (Kawai *et al.*, 1995) and more recently to a clinical study in which mixed chimerism was used to treat a patient with multiple myeloma who required a renal transplant (Spitzer *et al.*, 1999). In primates in which fully mismatched allografts were transplanted, it has proved difficult to eliminate some of the more toxic elements of the pretransplant protocol (Kimikawa *et al.*, 1997). The pretransplant workup includes thymic irradiation, whole-body irradiation, splenectomy and donor marrow infusion, then relies on the administration of a short course of cyclosporine posttransplantation. To reduce or eliminate the toxicity of the protocol, alternative approaches for achieving reliable, stable mixed chimerism in large animals are required. The finding that T-cell depletion or costimulation blockade is effective in small animals is encouraging, and both of these strategies require careful evaluation in large animal models. Although in the short-term the state of chimerism established by bone marrow infusion is important in inducing tolerance to the graft, in large animals it may not be the only mechanism that operates in the long-term after transplantation, when immunoregulation may become an important contributor to the unresponsive state that persists. The maintenance of the macrochimeric state up to the time of transplantation may be sufficient to enable the graft to be transplanted without long-term immunosuppressive drug therapy (see later).

STRATEGIES BASED ON DEPLETION OF LEUKOCYTES AT THE TIME OF TRANSPLANTATION

The elimination of recipient leukocytes at the time of transplantation may be a successful approach to the development of tolerance. Many strategies that result in the depletion of leukocytes (antithymocyte globulin, anti-CD52) or T cells (anti-CD3 with or without immunotoxin, CD2, CD4 and CD8) have been investigated in small and large animal studies (Waldmann, 1989). In small animals, the short-term depletion of T cells appears to be sufficient in some situations for tolerance to develop and be maintained in the long-term. The success rate can be enhanced by removing the thymus before transplantation to prevent repopulation of the periphery with T cells after transplantation (Monaco *et al.*, 1966). Data from primates using an anti-CD3 immunotoxin conjugated alone before transplantation or in combination with deoxyspergualin at the time of transplantation suggest that T-cell depletion can be used to induce tolerance to donor alloantigens (Fechner *et al.*, 1997; Knechtle *et al.*, 1997; Thomas *et al.*, 1999).

Depletion of leukocytes at the time of transplantation creates a transient immunodeficiency in the recipient, compromising the recipient's ability to reject the transplant. The degree and duration of leukocyte depletion achieved determine how effective and for how long the graft is protected from immune attack. The downstream events that occur once leukocytes begin to reappear in the recipient's circulation are not understood clearly. Using TCR transgenic recipients, we have shown that when leukocytes are depleted, the maintenance of tolerance depends on transplantation of the graft

within a window of depletion of donor reactive cells in the thymus and the periphery (Jones *et al.*, 1998). If the organ graft is transplanted at the appropriate time, donor reactive cells fail to repopulate from the thymus in an antigen-selective manner. Although donor reactive cells do not reappear in the periphery, cells with reactivity to other antigens are present in the periphery of recipients with long-term surviving organ grafts. These data can be used to suggest a mechanism for the long-term allograft survival observed in primates treated with a anti-CD3 immunotoxin complex. In this case, one can argue that the CD3$^+$ T cells are depleted by the immunotoxin before transplantation. A window of opportunity is created such that when renal allograft is transplanted, no donor reactive cells are present in the periphery. As cells repopulate the periphery with time after transplantation, all of the donor reactive cells are deleted or eliminated as a result of the presence of the surviving graft.

This approach has been taken one step further and translated into a pilot clinical study using the monoclonal antibody Campath 1H, which reacts with the lymphocyte cell surface molecule CD52 and targets T cells and B cells for depletion. In a series of patients transplanted in Cambridge, Campath was administered in the early posttransplant course in the absence of any other immunosuppression. The patients then were given low-dose cyclosporine as monotherapy beginning on day 5. The interim analysis of this cohort of patients is encouraging and has prompted a larger randomized study to be initiated (Calne *et al.*, 1998). The effects of T-cell depletion can be enhanced by combining this approach with the administration of donor antigen to try to achieve some level of chimerism at least in the short-term (Cobbold *et al.*, 1986; Thomas *et al.*, 1983, 1987; Wood and Monaco, 1980).

STRATEGIES BASED ON TARGETING ACCESSORY MOLECULES

Initially, administration of depleting anti-CD4 and anti-CD8 monoclonal antibodies was shown to result in prolonged graft survival (Cobbold and Walmann, 1986; Cobbold *et al.*, 1986; Madsen *et al.*, 1987; Shizuru *et al.*, 1987). That this treatment strategy resulted in antigen-specific tolerance was shown first most clearly when a protein antigen was administered in conjunction with a depleting anti-CD4 monoclonal antibody (Benjamin and Waldmann, 1986; Benjamin *et al.*, 1988; Gutstein and Wofsy, 1986). Refinements of these types of protocols have resulted in the ability to achieve long-term T-cell unresponsiveness to protein and alloantigens in the absence of T-cell depletion in experimental models (Benjamin *et al.*, 1988; Cobbold *et al.*, 1996; Darby *et al.*, 1992; Qin *et al.*, 1987).

CD4 and CD8 are not the only accessory molecules that can be targeted to block immune activation. Monoclonal antibodies reacting with other accessory and adhesion molecules, including CD3, CD2, LFA1 and I-CAM, have been shown to prolong the survival of MHC-mismatched grafts when administered in rodents (Benjamin *et al.*, 1988; Isobe *et al.*, 1992; Krieger *et al.*, 1996; Nicolls *et al.*, 1993; Punch *et al.*, 1999). Tolerance to allogeneic bone marrow using these approaches has been shown when combined with antibody therapy (Qin *et al.*, 1989).

Operational tolerance induced by these strategies has been shown to develop over several weeks after the initial antigen encounter (Pearson *et al.*, 1993; Scully *et al.*, 1994). When a combination of donor antigen and monoclonal antibody therapy targeting accessory molecules is used, the precise mechanism of tolerance induction in part depends on the amount of antigen infused (Pearson *et al.*, 1992). With high doses of donor bone marrow, deletion also may be used as one of the mechanisms of tolerance initially (Bemelman *et al.*, 1998). With lower doses of antigen, immunoregulation is the mechanism in operation (Bemelman *et al.*, 1998; Bushell *et al.*, 1995, 1999). When antibodies targeting accessory molecules are used as therapeutic agents at the time of transplantation, immunoregulation is the dominant mechanism that comes into play to maintain tolerance in the longer term (Waldmann and Cobbold, 1998).

In these systems, tolerance to donor antigens is induced and/or maintained as a result of the development of a population of regulatory and suppressor T cells that can mediate unresponsiveness to the initiating donor antigen as well as other antigens present on the graft, the phenomenon of linked unresponsiveness (Wong *et al.*, 1996; see Table 23–1). In mice and rats, this type of tolerance has been shown to be infectious (Qin *et al.*, 1993); it can be transferred from one generation of cells to another, provided that there is a sufficient period of contact between the two populations.

The maintenance of tolerance in these systems requires the persistent presence of antigen in the form of the organ when the thymus is still functional (Hamano *et al.*, 1996). In the absence of donor antigen, tolerance eventually is lost, presumably as a result of the export of naive T cells from the thymus into the periphery. Quantitatively, if these cells fail to encounter antigen, they eventually outnumber the unresponsive T cells induced by the monoclonal antibody therapy.

STRATEGIES BASED ON BLOCKADE OF COSTIMULATION

Monoclonal antibodies and recombinant fusion proteins targeting costimulatory molecules are capable of inducing tolerance to donor antigens *in vivo*. CD86 and CD80 are expressed as cell surface molecules by antigen-presenting cells and are responsible for delivering additional signals to T cells when they interact with CD28 (Greenfield *et al.*, 1998; Schwartz, 1992). CD86 appears to interact preferentially with CD28 and may be the most important ligand for T-cell activation. CD86 and CD80 can interact with a second molecule, CD152 (CTLA4), which is expressed by T cells later in the activation process. CD80 may bind preferentially to CD152 (Thompson, 1995). In contrast to CD28, CTLA4 negatively regulates T-cell activation when it engages its ligand on the antigen-presenting cell and, as described previously, is implicated in the control of clone size to maintain normal homeostasis in the immune system (Bluestone, 1998; Thompson and Allison, 1997). The role of each of these pathways in alloimmune responses is being investigated with a battery of reagents, including monoclonal antibodies, fusion proteins and knock-out mice (Judge *et al.*, 1999). Additional molecules expressed by antigen-presenting cells or T cells that also can participate in T-cell costimulation are being described (Abbas and Sharpe, 1999; Dong *et al.*, 1999; Hutloff *et al.*, 1999; Yoshinago *et al.*, 1999). The significance of these new pathways in the rejection process is not determined.

When an immunoglobulin fusion protein of CTLA4 (CTLA4Ig) was produced, it was shown to inhibit graft rejection in xenogeneic and allogeneic systems (Larsen *et al.*, 1996b; Lenschow *et al.*, 1992). In rodent models, CTLA4Ig therapy alone has been shown to induce tolerance to the graft (Lenschow *et al.*, 1992; Pearson *et al.*, 1994), an effect that was enhanced when donor antigen is included in the treatment protocol (Lin *et al.*, 1993; Pearson *et al.*, 1996; Sayegh *et al.*, 1997). This effect has not been found in every experimental model examined, however. For example, the use of CTLA4Ig monotherapy in primates has not been re-

ported to be capable of inducing long-term graft survival (Kirk *et al.*, 1997).

The mechanism by which CTLA4Ig promotes long-term graft survival has been investigated in a mouse model. Blockade of CD86 and CD80 at the time of alloantigen recognition triggers deletion of antigen-reactive cells in the early phase after transplantation (Li *et al.*, 1999b; Wells *et al.*, 1999). When an antiapoptotic gene, *bcl-x*, was expressed in the responding lymphocytes, deletion did not occur, and graft prolongation was prevented. This finding suggests that an early reduction in clone size facilitates the development of long-term graft function promoted by treatment with CTLA4Ig by reducing the number of donor reactive cells that have to be controlled downstream in the posttransplant course.

The precise relationship between peripheral tolerance and CTLA4 engagement of its ligands requires further clarification. Some studies suggest that CTLA engagement is essential to promote T-cell tolerance (Perez *et al.*, 1997). Differential blockade of CD80 and CD86 has been shown to have different effects in the treatment of autoimmune diabetes and transplant rejection (Lenschow *et al.*, 1995a, 1995b). The finding that immunoregulatory T cells use CTLA4 to control immune responsiveness would confirm that this molecule is likely to be important. CTLA4Ig therapy may need to be used at doses below saturation *in vivo* to ensure that the interaction with CD80 and CD86 is not blocked completely.

CD40-CD154 PATHWAY

A second pathway that has been shown to be important in the initiation of T-cell responses, the CD40-CD154 pathway, has been targeted using monoclonal antibody therapy to inhibit graft rejection (Larsen *et al.*, 1996a, 1996b). CD154 (CD40-ligand) is a type 2 membrane protein of the TNF family (Armitage *et al.*, 1992; Hollenbaugh *et al.*, 1992). It is expressed predominantly by activated CD4$^+$ T cells and a small proportion of CD8$^+$ T cells (Noelle, 1996). Structural models predict that CD154 forms a homotrimer that binds to CD40 on the surface of antigen-presenting cells.

The CD40-CD154 interaction is pivotal for the induction of humoral and cellular responses. The importance of CD154 for B-cell activation first was shown by *in vitro* studies. A CD40-Ig fusion protein and a blocking monoclonal antibody to CD154 were shown to inhibit B-cell cycling, proliferation and differentiation into plasma cells in response to T cell–dependent antigens (Noelle *et al.*, 1992). *In vivo* studies using the anti-CD154 monoclonal antibody, CD40 or CD154 knockout mice (Kawabe *et al.*, 1994; Xu *et al.*, 1994) all showed a crucial role for this interaction in the generation of primary and secondary humoral responses to T cell–dependent antigens, class switching to antigen switching RGG1 responses and development of germinal centers. The lack of humoral response in the absence of the CD40-CD40L interaction is due to not only lack of signaling through CD40 on the B-cell surface, but also the inhibition of priming of CD4$^+$ T cells through CD40L (Grewal *et al.*, 1996).

The CD40-CD154 pathway is bidirectional. Not only does CD154 engagement on T cells augment T-cell activation, but also CD40 triggering on the antigen-presenting cell primes the antigen-presenting cell for stimulation. Signals through CD40 have been shown to up-regulate expression of CD80 and CD86 as well as induce IL-12 (Gurunathan *et al.*, 1998). Activation of dendritic cells through CD40 promotes their ability to present antigen to T cells; this may explain why targeting CD154 and blocking its ability to interact with CD40 has a profound effect on T cell–dependent immune responses *in vivo*. If modification of antigen-presenting cell function is a route to tolerance, this pathway also may be involved when the behavior of antigen-presenting cells is modified after interaction with immunoregulatory and suppressor T cells (Liu et al., 1999).

Treatment with anti-CD154 monoclonal antibody alone administered at the time of transplantation has been shown to induce prolonged survival of fully MHC-mismatched cardiac, renal and islet allografts in mice and primates (Larsen et al., 1996a, 1996b; Markees et al., 1997; Niimi et al., 1998; Parker et al., 1995). In rodents, anti-CD154 therapy has been shown to induce operational tolerance in a proportion of recipients. The tolerant state induced appears to be more robust in rodents when anti-CD154 has been combined with donor antigen before transplantation tolerance has been induced (Markees et al., 1997; Niimi et al., 1998; Parker et al., 1995). There appear to be fewer long-term changes in graft architecture when donor antigen is included in the treatment protocol (Ensminger et al., 2000a).

Interest in this approach was stimulated further with the report that a humanized monoclonal antibody specific for CD154 (HU5C8) was capable of prolonging the survival of renal and islet allografts in rhesus monkeys (Kenyon et al., 1999; Kirk et al., 1997, 1999). The initial data from these primate studies looked encouraging with rejection-free survival of the kidney grafts obtained, provided that antibody therapy at a relatively high dose (25 mg/kg) was continued in the first 6 months posttransplant. When anti-CD154 therapy was discontinued after the first month posttransplant, rejection episodes did occur. Analysis of the status of recipients with long-term surviving grafts carried out to date show that peripheral lymphocytes from the monkeys do not respond in vitro to donor antigen. The recipients do develop antidonor antibody, however, and when biopsy samples were taken from some of the long-term surviving grafts, a T-cell infiltrate was present. As documented in many experimental studies, the presence of a T-cell infiltrate does not mean that grafts will experience rejection. It is essential that these studies are continued and that the long-term follow-up data are reported. Together, these observations were sufficiently encouraging to initiate a pilot clinical study using this antibody in renal transplant patients. How to use these novel reagents in the clinical arena—in other words how to combine them with conventional immunosuppression—is not clear (see later).

Further exploration of CD154 monoclonal antibody therapy in rodent models has been undertaken as a result of the data produced in primates. These data have proved interesting and informative and may enable further improvements in this as well as other novel therapeutic approaches to be made. Exploration of the efficacy of CD154 blockade in different donor recipient combinations in mouse models has revealed that only when rejection is dependent on CD4$^+$ T cells is CD154 blockade on its own effective. In donor-recipient combinations in which CD8$^+$ T cells also play a role in rejection, many studies have shown that the CD8$^+$ T-cell subset is unaffected by CD154 monoclonal antibody therapy (Ensminger et al., 2000b; Honey et al., 1999; Jones et al., 2000; Trambley et al., 1999). In some cases, this situation can lead to the rejection of grafts despite CD154 blockade. CD8$^+$ T cells are refractory to inhibition by anti-CD154 in response to antigen stimulation. Data from our laboratory in a transplantation model have shown that CD8$^+$ T cells become activated, proliferate and home to the graft in the presence of high-dose continued anti-CD154 monoclonal antibody therapy in vivo (Jones et al., 2000). These data together with other data from transplant models and virus infection (Whitmire et al., 1999) studies raise questions as to the potential ability of anti-CD154 monotherapy to control rejection in every situation. At this stage, it is unclear why anti-CD154

was so successful in primates if the CD8 compartment was functional.

Anti-CD154 monoclonal antibody therapy alone, although capable of promoting graft prolongation in some situations, may not be able to prevent transplant vasculopathy. This observation was reported first by Larsen and colleagues, and analysis of data from our own studies has confirmed this observation (Ensminger et al., 2000b; Larsen et al., 1996a, b). When we investigated this observation in more detail in a vascular allograft model, we found that blockade of CD154 alone does not have a significant effect on the development of transplant arteriosclerosis. Only when CD8$^+$ T cells were removed from the recipient was the disease state inhibited. Long-term follow-up of these recipients has revealed that the disease process in the absence of CD8$^+$ T cells is delayed rather than inhibited completely. These observations have important implications for the use of monoclonal antibody in the clinical setting. None of the experimental data showing the role of CD8$^+$ T cells and the development of transplant arteriosclerosis has combined the anti-CD154 monoclonal antibody therapy with other immunosuppressive agents, however.

In the mouse models used by Larsen and colleagues, anti-CD154 always was more effective in prolonging graft survival as well as preventing the development of transplant arteriosclerosis when it was combined with CTLA-Ig (Larsen et al., 1996b). Blocking the CD28 costimulatory pathway and the CD40-CD154 pathway appeared to be more efficacious than manipulation of either pathway alone. In the primate studies reported by Kirk and colleagues, CTLA-Ig appeared to have little effect on the rejection process (Kirk et al., 1997). It remains to be seen whether this finding is replicated in other experimental models. It is worth considering further the possibility of blocking both of these pathways and analyzing the potential of this approach in more depth in the future.

Effect of Immunosuppressive Drugs on Tolerance Induction

The introduction of any novel strategy for tolerance induction into clinical practice at present necessitates combining the approach with one or more immunosuppressive drugs at the time of transplantation. How successful this approach would be is unclear. Data from many experimental studies in which a biological agent has been combined with one of the calcineurin inhibitors given simultaneously at the time of transplantation suggest that calcineurin inhibitors might block or inhibit the development of unresponsiveness (Kirk et al., 1999; Larsen et al., 1996b). This inhibition could be linked to the inhibition of IL-2 gene transcription in the presence of calcineurin inhibitors. Studies in IL-2 knock-out mice have shown that operational tolerance to alloantigens is not induced in this setting (Dai et al., 1998). Apoptosis triggered by costimulation blockade is blocked in the presence of calcineurin inhibitors (Wells et al., 1999). If deletion of alloantigen reactive cells is an essential part of the mechanism that operates during the induction of unresponsiveness as a consequence of costimulation blockade at the time of antigen recognition, it may not be surprising that inclusion of calcineurin inhibitors in the treatment protocol blocks graft prolongation.

Examination of data from clinical studies in which biological agents have been used as part of the therapeutic strategy supports the experimental findings outlined previously. When OKT3 was given simultaneously with cyclosporine at the time of transplantation, the long-term graft survival rate was poorer than when cyclosporine was introduced in a delayed fashion. The protocol adopted for the Campath 1H study has been designed to take these observations into account (Calne *et al.*, 1998).

Whether all immunosuppressive drugs have a similar effect on the development of unresponsiveness when used in combination with biological agents requires further careful evaluation. Preliminary data from primate studies using anti-CD154 suggest that there are differential effects (Kirk *et al.*, 1999). In mice, data have been reported showing that sirolimus may promote apoptosis in combination with costimulation blockade, having a beneficial effect on graft outcome (Li *et al.*, 1999b). Further work is essential to enable an acceptable treatment regimen for use in combination with novel agents to be identified if the translation to the clinic of strategies designed to promote the development of tolerance is going to be successful.

REFERENCES

Abbas, A. and Sharpe, A. (1999). T cell costimulation: an abundance of B7s. *Nat. Med.* **5**, 1345.

Albert, M., Sauter, B. and Bhardwaj, N. (1999). Dendritic cells acquire antigen from apoptotic cells and induce class-1 restricted CTLs. *Nature* **392**, 86.

Armitage, R., Fanslow, W., Strockbine, L., *et al.* (1992). Molecular and biological characterisation of a murine ligand for CD40. *Nature* **357**, 80.

Asseman, C., Mauze, S., Leach, M. W., *et al.* (1999). An essential role for interleukin-10 in the function of regulatory T cells that inhibit intestinal inflammation. *J. Exp. Med.* **190**, 995.

Banchereau, J. and Steinman, R. (1998). Dendritic cells and the control of immunity. *Nature* **392**, 245.

Batchelor, J. and Welsh, K. (1976). Mechanisms of enhancement of kidney allograft survival: a form of operational tolerance. *Br. Med. Bull.* **32**, 113.

Bellgrau, D. and Duke, R. (1999). Apoptosis and CD95 ligand in immune privileged sites. *Int. Rev. Immunol.* **18**, 547.

Bellgrau, D., Gold, D., Selawry, H., *et al.* (1995). A role for CD95 ligand in preventing graft rejection. *Nature* **377**, 630.

Bemelman, F., Honey, K., Adams, E., *et al.* (1998). Bone marrow transplantation induces either clonal deletion or infectious tolerance depending on the dose. *J. Immunol.* **160**, 2645.

Benjamin, R. J., Qin, S., Wise, M .P., *et al.* (1988). Mechanisms of monoclonal antibody-facilitated tolerance induction: a possible role for the CD4 (L3T4) and CD11a (LFA-1) molecules in self-non-self discrimination. *Eur. J. Immunol.* **18**, 1079.

Benjamin, R. J. and Waldmann, H. (1986). Induction of tolerance by monoclonal antibody therapy. *Nature* **320**, 449.

Bennett, S., Carbone, F., Karamalis, F., *et al.* (1998). Help for cytotoxic T-cell responses is mediated by CD40 signalling. *Nature* **332**, 161.

Blazar, B. R., Taylor, P. A., Panoskaltsis-Mortara, A., *et al.* (1998). Interleukin-10 dose-dependent regulation of CD4+ and CD8+ T cell-mediated graft-versus-host disease. *Transplantation* **66**, 1220.

Bluestone, J. (1998). Is CTLA-4 a master switch for peripheral T cell tolerance? *J. Immunol.* **158**, 1989.

Bridoux, F., Badou, A., Saoudi, A., *et al.* (1997). Transforming growth factor β (TGF-β)-dependent inhibition of T helper cell (Th2)-induced autoimmunity by self-major histocompatibility complex (MHC) class II-specific, regulatory CD4+ T cell lines. *J. Exp. Med.* **185**, 1769.

Bushell, A., Morris, P. and Wood, K. (1994). Anti-CD4 antibody combined with random blood transfusion leads to authentic transplantation tolerance in the mouse: a protocol with significant clinical potential. *Transplantation* **58**, 133.

Bushell, A., Morris, P. and Wood, K. (1995). Transplantation tolerance induced by antigen pretreatment and depleting anti-CD4 antibody depends on CD4+ T cell regulation during the induction phase of the response. *Eur. J. Immunol.* **25**, 2643.

Bushell, A., Niimi, M., Morris, P. J., *et al.* (1999). Evidence for immune regulation in the induction of transplantation tolerance: a conditional but limited role for IL-4. *J. Immunol.* **162**, 1359.

Calne, R. Y., Friend, P., Morratt, S., *et al.* (1998). Prope tolerance,

perioperative campath 1H, and low dose cyclosporine monotherapy in renal allograft recipients. *Lancet* **351**, 1701.

Calne, R. Y., Sells, R. A., Pena, J. R., *et al.* (1969). Induction of immunological tolerance by porcine liver allografts. *Nature* **223**, 472.

Cecka, J. and Terasaki, P. (1998). *Clinical Transplants 1998*, p. 80, UCLA Tissue Typing Laboratory, Los Angeles.

Cobbold, S. and Waldmann, H. (1986). Skin allograft rejection by L3T4+ and LYT-2+ T cell subsets. *Transplantation* **41**, 634.

Cobbold, S. P., Adams, E., Marshall, S. E., *et al.* (1996). Mechanisms of peripheral tolerance and suppression induced by monoclonal antibodies to CD4 and CD8. *Immunol. Rev.* **149**, 5.

Cobbold, S. P., Martin, G., Qin, S., *et al.* (1986). Monoclonal antibodies to promote marrow engraftment and tissue graft tolerance. *Nature* **323**, 164.

Dai, Z., Konieczny, B., Baddoura, F., *et al.* (1998). Impaired alloantigen-mediated T cell apoptosis and failure to induce long-term allograft survival in IL-2 deficient mice. *J. Immunol.* **161**, 1659.

Dallman, M. J., Wood, K. J. and Morris, P. J. (1987). Specific cytotoxic T cells are found in the non-rejected kidneys of blood transfused rats. *J. Exp. Med.* **165**, 566.

Darby, C. R., Morris, P. J. and Wood, K. J. (1992). Evidence that long-term cardiac allograft survival induced by anti-CD4 monoclonal does not require depletion of CD4+ T cells. *Transplantation* **54**, 483.

Davies, D. D., Leong, L. Y., Mellor, A., *et al.* (1996a). T cell suppression in transplantation tolerance through linked recognition. *J. Immunol.* **156**, 3602.

Davies, J. D., Martin, G., Phillips, J., *et al.* (1996b). T cell regulation in adult transplantation tolerance. *J. Immunol.* **157**, 529.

Dong, H., Zhu, G., Tamada, K., *et al.* (1999). B7-H1, a third member of the B7 family, costimulates T cell proliferation and IL-10 secretion. *Nat. Med.* **5**, 1365.

Ensminger, S., Billing, S., Spriewald, B., *et al.* (2000a). Reduction in transplant vasculopathy when donor alloantigen is administered with anti-CD154 at the time of transplantation. (submitted).

Ensminger, S., Witzke, O., Spriewald, B., *et al.* (2000b). Vascular rejection despite CD154 blockade is mediated by CD8+ T cells. *Transplantation* **69**, 2609.

Farges, O., Morris, P. and Dallman, M. (1994a). Spontaneous acceptance of liver graft: analysis of the immune response. *Transplantation* **57**, 171.

Farges, O., Morris, P. and Dallman, M. (1994b). Spontaneous acceptance of rat liver allografts is associated with an early down regulation of intragraft interleukin-4 messenger RNA expression. *Hepatology* **21**, 767.

Fearon, D. and Locksley, R. (1996). The instructive role of innate immunity in the acquired immune response. *Science* **272**, 50.

Fechner, J., Vargo, D., Geissler, E., *et al.* (1997). Split tolerance induced by immunotoxin in a rhesus kidney allograft model. *Transplantation* **63**, 1339.

Foy, T., Laman, J., Ledbetter, J., *et al.* (1994). gp39-CD40 interactions are essential for germinal centre formation and the development of B cell memory. *J. Exp. Med.* **180**, 157.

Foy, T., Shepherd, D., Durie, F., *et al.* (1993). In vivo CD40-gp39 interactions are essential for thymus-dependent humoral immunity: II. prolonged suppression of the humoral immune response by an antibody to the ligand for CD40, gp39. *J. Exp. Med.* **178**, 1567.

Gallico, G., Butcher, G. and Howard J. (1979). The role of subregions of the rat histocompatibility complex in the rejection and passive enhancement of renal allografts. *J. Exp. Med.* **149**, 244.

Gao, O., Rouse, T., Kazmerzak, K., *et al.* (1999). CD4+ CD25+ cells regulate CD8 cell anergy in neonatal tolerance. *Transplantation* **68**, 1891.

George, J., Sweeney, S., Kirklin, J., *et al.* (1998). An essential role for Fas ligand in transplantation tolerance induced by donor bone marrow. *Nat. Med.* **4**, 333.

Gershon, R. and Kondo, K. (1971). Infectious immunological tolerance. *Immunology* **21**, 903.

Gianello, P., Fishbein, J., Rosengard, B., *et al.* (1995). Tolerance to class I-disparate renal allografts in miniature swine. *Transplantation* **59**, 772.

Goldrath, A. and Bevan, M. (1999) Selecting and maintaining a diverse T cell repertoire. *Nature* **402**, 255.

Goodnow, C., Adelstein, S. and Basten, A. (1990). The need for central and peripheral tolerance in the B cell repertoire. *Science* **248**, 1373.

Gould, D. and Auchincloss, H. (1999). Direct and indirect recognition: the role of MHC antigens in graft rejection. *Immunol. Today* **20**, 77.

Grakoui, A., Bromley, S., Sumen, C., *et al.* (1999). The immunological synapse: a molecular machine controlling T cell activation. *Science* **285**, 221.

Greenfield, E., Nguyen, K. and Kuchroo, V. (1998). CD28/B7 costimulation: a review. *Crit. Rev. Immunol.* **18**, 389.

Grewal, I., Feollmer, H., Grewal, K., *et al.* (1996). Requirement for CD40 ligand in costimulation induction, T cell activation, and experimental allergic encephalomyelitis. *Science* **274**, 1864.

Griffith, T., Brunner, T., Fletcher, S., *et al.* (1995). Fas ligand-induced apoptosis as a mechanism of immune privilege. *Science* **270**, 1189.

Groux, H., O'Garra, A., Bigler, M., *et al.* (1997). A CD4+ T-cell subset inhibits antigen-specific T-cell responses and prevents colitis. *Nature* **389**, 737.

Gurunathan, S., Irvine, K., Wu, C., *et al.* (1998). CD40 ligand/trimer DNA enhances both humoral and cellular immune responses and induces protective immunity to infectious and tumor challenge. *J. Immunol.* **161**, 4563.

Gutstein, N. L. and Wofsy, D. (1986). Administration of F(ab')₂ fragments of monoclonal antibody to L3T4 inhibits humoral immunity in mice without depleting L3T4+ cells. *J. Immunol.* **137**, 3414.

Hall, B., Jelbart, M., Gurley, K., *et al.* (1985). Specific unresponsiveness in rats with prolonged cardiac allograft survival after treatment with cyclosporine: mediation of specific suppression by T helper/inducer cells. *J. Exp. Med.* **162**, 1683.

Hall, B. M., Fava, L., Chen, J., *et al.* (1998). Anti-CD4 monoclonal antibody-induced tolerance to MHC-incompatible cardiac allografts maintained by CD4+ suppressor T cells that are not dependent upon IL-4. *J. Immunol.* **161**, 5147.

Hamano, K., Rawsthorne, M., Bushell, A., *et al.* (1996). Evidence that the continued presence of the organ graft and not peripheral donor microchimerism is essential for the maintenance of tolerance to alloantigen in anti-CD4 treated recipients. *Transplantation* **62**, 856.

Hara, M., Niimi, M., Read, S., *et al.* (2000). IL-10 dependent regulatory T cells mediate tolerance to alloantigens in vivo. (submitted).

Hojo, M., Morimoto, T., Maluccio, M., *et al.* (1999). Cyclosporine induces cancer progression by a cell-autonomous mechanism. *Nature* **397**, 530.

Hollenbaugh, D., Grosmaire, L., Kullas, C., *et al.* (1992). The human T cell antigen gp39, a member of the TNF gene family, is a ligand for the CD40 receptor: expression of a soluble form of gp39 with B cell costimulatory activity. *EMBO J.* **11**, 4313.

Honey, K., Cobbold, S. and Waldmann, H. (1999). CD40 ligand blockade induces CD4+ T cell tolerance and linked suppression. *J. Immunol.* **163**, 4805.

Huang, C., Fuchimoto, Y., Scheier-Dolberg, R., *et al.* (2000). Stable mixed chimerism and tolerance using a non-myeloablative preparative regimen in a large animal model. *J. Clin. Invest.* **105**, 173.

Hutchinson, I. V. (1986). Suppressor T cells in allogeneic models. *Transplantation* **41**, 547.

Hutloff, A., Dittrich, A., Beler, K., *et al.* (1999). ICOS is an inducible T-cell costimulator structurally and functionally related to CD28. *Nature* **397**, 263.

Isobe, M., Yagita, H., Omumura, K., *et al.* (1992). Specific acceptance of cardiac allografts after treatment with antibodies to ICAM-1 and LFA-1. *Science* **255**, 1125.

Jacobsen, N., Taaning, E., Ladefoged, J., *et al.* (1994). Tolerance to an HLA-B, DR disparate kidney allograft after bone marrow transplantation from the same donor. *Lancet* **343**, 800.

Jameson, S., Hogquist, K. and Bevan, M. (1995). Positive selection of thymocytes. *Ann. Rev. Immunol.* **13**, 93.

Jones, N., Fluck, N., Mellor, A., *et al.* (1997). Deletion of alloantigen-reactive thymocytes as a mechanism of adult transplantation tolerance induction following intrathymic antigen administration. *Eur. J. Immunol.* **27**, 1591.

Jones, N., Fluck, N., Mellor, A., *et al.* (1998). The induction of transplantation tolerance by intrathymic delivery of alloantigen: a critical relationship between intrathymic deletion, export of new T cells and the timing of transplantation. *Inter. Immunol.* **10**, 1637.

Jones, N., van Maurik, A., Hara, M., *et al.* (2000). CD40-CD40L

independent activation of CD8+ T cells can trigger allograft rejection. *J. Immunol.* **165**, 1111.

Josien, R., Douillard, P., Guillot, C., *et al.* (1998). A critical role for transforming growth factor beta in donor transfusion induced allograft tolerance. *J. Clin. Invest.* **102**, 1920.

Josien, R., Pannetier, C., Douillard, P., *et al.* (1995). Graft-infiltrating T helper cells, CD45RC phenotype, and TH1/TH2-related cytokines in donor-specific transfusion induced in adult rats. *Transplantation* **60**, 1131.

Judge, T., Wu, Z., Zheng, X., *et al.* (1999). The role of CD80, CD86, and CTLA4 in alloimmune responses. *J. Immunol.* **162**, 1947.

Kamada, N. (1985). The immunology of experimental liver transplantation in the rat. *Immunology* **55**, 369.

Kang, S.-M., Hofamann, A., Le, D., *et al.* (1997). Immune response and myoblast that express Fas ligand. *Science* **278**, 1322.

Kappler, J. W., Roehm, N. and Marrack, P. (1987). T cell tolerance by clonal elimination in the thymus. *Cell* **49**, 273.

Kawabe, T., Naka, T., Yoshida, K., *et al.* (1994). The immune responses in CD40-deficient mice: impaired immunoglobulin class switching and germinal centre formation. *Immunity* **1**, 167.

Kawai, K. and Ohashi, P. (1995). Immunological function of a defined T-cell population tolerized to low-affinity self antigens *Nature* **374**, 68.

Kawai, T., Cosimi, A., Colvin, R., *et al.* (1995). Mixed allogeneic chimerism and renal allograft tolerance in cynomolgus monkeys. *Transplantation* **59**, 256.

Kearney, E., Pape, K., Loh, D., *et al.* (1994). Visualisation of peptide-specific T cell immunity and peripheral tolerance induction in vivo. *Immunity* **1**, 327.

Kenyon, N., Chatzipetrou, M., Masetti, M., *et al.* (1999). Long-term survival and function of intrahepatic islet allografts in rhesus monkeys treated with humanized anti-CD154. *Proc. Natl. Acad. Sci. U. S. A.* **96**, 8132.

Khan, A., Tomita, Y. and Sykes, M. (1996). Thymic dependence of loss of tolerance in mixed allogeneic bone marrow chimeras after depletion of donor antigen. *Transplantation* **62**, 380.

Khoury, S. J., Hancock, W. W. and Weiner, H. L. K. (1992). Oral tolerance to myelin basic protein and natural recovery from experimental autoimmune encephalomyelitis are associated with downregulation of inflammatory cytokines and differential upregulation of transforming growth factor beta, interleukin 4, and prostaglandin E expression in the brain. *J. Exp. Med.* **17**, 1355.

Kimikawa, M., Sachs, D., Colvin, R., *et al.* (1997). Modifications of the conditioning regimen for achieving mixed chimerism and donor-specific tolerance in cynomolgus monkeys. *Transplantation* **64**, 709.

King, C., Davies, J., Mueller, R., *et al.* (1998). TGF-β1 alters APC preference, polarizing islet antigen responses toward a Th2 phenotype. *Immunity* **8**, 601.

Kirk, A., Burkly, L., Batty, D., *et al.* (1999). Treatment with humanised monoclonal antibodies against CD154 prevents acute renal allograft rejection in nonhuman primates. *Nat. Med.* **5**, 686.

Kirk, A., Harlan, D., Armstrong, N., *et al.* (1997). CTLA4-Ig and anti-CD40 ligand prevent renal allograft rejection in primates. *Proc. Natl. Acad. Sci. U. S. A.* **94**, 8789.

Knechtle, S., Vargo, D., Fechner, J., *et al.* (1997). FN18-CRM9 immunotaxin promotes tolerance in primal renal allografts. *Transplantation* **63**, 1.

Ko, S., Dewick, A., Jager, M., *et al.* (1999). The functional relevance of passenger leukocytes and microchimerism for heart allograft acceptance in the rat. *Nat. Med.* **5**, 1292.

Konieczny, B., Dai, Z., Elwood, E., *et al.* (1998). IFN-γ is critical for long-term allograft survival induced by blocking the CD28 and CD40 ligand T cell costimulation pathways. *J. Immunol.* **160**, 2059.

Korthauer, U., Nagel, W., Davis, E., *et al.* (2000). Anergic T lymphocytes selectively express an integrin regulatory protein of the cytohesin family. *J. Immunol.* **164**, 308.

Krammer, P. (1999). CD95 (AP)/Fas mediated apoptosis: live and let die. *Adv. Immunol.* **71**, 163.

Krieger, N., Most, D., Bromberg, J., *et al.* (1996). Coexistence of TH1 and TH2-type cytokine profiles in anti-CD2 monoclonal antibody induced tolerance. *Transplantation* **62**, 1285.

Lanzavecchia, A. (1998). Licence to kill. *Nature* **398**, 413.

Lanzavecchia, A., Lezzie, G. and Viola, A. (1999). From TCR engagement to T cell activation: a kinetic view of T cell behaviour. *Cell* **96**, 1.

Larsen, C., Alexander, D., Hollenbaugh, D., *et al.* (1996a). CD40-gp39 interactions play a critical role during allograft rejection. *Transplantation* **61**, 4.

Larsen, C., Morris, P. and Austyn, J. (1990). Migration of dendritic leukocytes from cardiac allografts into host spleens: a novel pathway for initiation of rejection. *J. Exp. Med.* **171**, 307.

Larsen, P., Elwood, E., Alexander, D., *et al.* (1996b). Long-term acceptance of skin and cardiac allografts after blocking CD40 and CD28 pathways. *Nature* **381**, 434.

Lau, H., Yu, M., Fontana, A., *et al.* (1996). Prevention of islet allograft rejection with engineered myoblasts expressing FasL in mice. *Science* **273**, 109.

Le Moine, S., Marchant, A., Durand, F., *et al.* (1994). Systemic release of interleukin-10 during orthotopic liver transplantation. *Hepatology* **20**, 889.

Lenardo, M. (1996). Fas and the art of lymphocyte maintenance. *J. Exp. Med.* **183**, 721.

Lenschow, D., Ho, S., Sattar, H., *et al.* (1995a). Differential effects of anti-B7-1 and anti-B7-2 monoclonal antibody treatment on the development of diabetes in the non-obese diabetic mouse. *J. Exp. Med.* **181**, 1145.

Lenschow, D., Zeng, Y., Hathcock, K., *et al.* (1995b). Inhibition of transplant rejection following treatment with anti-B7-2 and anti-B7-1 antibodies. *Transplantation* **60**, 1171.

Lenschow, D. J., Zeng, Y., Thistlethwaite, J. R., *et al.* (1992). Long-term survival of xenogeneic pancreatic islet grafts induced by CTLA4Ig. *Science* **257**, 789.

Li, J., Liu, Z., Jiang, S., *et al.* (1999a). T suppressor lymphocytes inhibit NF-kappa B mediated transcription of CD86 gene in APC. *J. Immunol.* **163**, 6386.

Li, Y., Li, X., Zheng, X., *et al.* (1999b). Blocking both signal 1 and signal 2 of T cell activation prevents apoptosis of alloreactive T cells and induction of peripheral allograft tolerance. *Nat. Med.* **5**, 1298.

Lin, H., Bolling, S. F., Linsley, P. S., *et al.* (1993). Long-term acceptance of major histocompatibility complex mismatched cardiac allografts induced by CTLA4Ig plus donor-specific transfusion. *J. Exp. Med.* **178**, 1801.

Liu, Z., Tugulea, S., Cortesini, R., *et al.* (1999). Inhibition of CD40 signaling pathway in antigen presenting cells by T suppressor cells. *Hum. Immunol.* **60**, 568.

Lombardi, G., Sidhu, S., Batchelor, R., *et al.* (1994). Anergic T cells as suppressor cells in vitro. *Science* **264**, 1587.

Madsen, J. C., Peugh, W. N., Wood, K. J., *et al.* (1987). The effect of anti-L3T4 monoclonal antibody on first-set rejection of murine cardiac allografts. *Transplantation* **44**, 849.

Madsen, J. C., Superina, R. A., Wood, K. J., *et al.* (1988). Immunological unresponsiveness induced by recipient cells transfected with donor MHC genes. *Nature* **332**, 161.

Manilay, J., Pearson, D., Sergio, J., *et al.* (1998). Intrathymic deletion of alloreactive T cells in mixed bone marrow chimeras prepared with a nonmyeloablative conditioning regime. *Transplantation* **66**, 96.

Markees, T., Phillips, N., Noelle, R., *et al.* (1997). Prolonged survival of mouse skin allografts in recipients treated with donor splenocytes and antibody to CD40 ligand. *Transplantation* **64**, 329.

Markmann, J., Odorico, J., Bassiri, H., *et al.* (1993). Deletion of donor-reactive T lymphocytes in adult mice after intrathymic inoculation with lymphoid cells. *Transplantation* **55**, 871.

Mason, D. and Powrie, F. (1998). Control of immune pathology by regulatory T cells. *Curr. Opin. Immunol.* **10**, 649.

Mason, D. W., Dallman, M. J., Arthur, R. P., *et al.* (1984). Mechanisms of allograft rejection: the roles of cytotoxic T cells and delayed type hypersensitivity. *Immunol. Rev.* **77**, 167.

Miller, C., Ragheb, J., and Schwartz, R. (1999). Anergy and cytokine-mediated suppression as distinct superantigen-induced tolerance mechanisms in vivo. *J. Exp. Med.* **190**, 53.

Monaco, A. P., Wood, M. L., and Russel, P. S. (1966). Studies on heterologous anti-lymphocyte serum in mice: III. immunologic tolerance and chimerism produced across the H-2 locus with adult thymectomy and anti-lymphocyte serum. *Ann. N. Y. Acad. Sci.* **129**, 190.

Moore, K., O'Garra, A., de Waal, M. R., *et al.* (1993). Interleukin-10. *Ann. Rev. Immunol.* **11**, 165.

Morris, P., Johnson, R., Fuggle, S., *et al.* (1999). Analysis of factors that affect the outcome of primary cadaveric renal transplantation in the UK. HLA task force of the kidney advisory group of the United Kingdom Transplant Support Service Authority (UKTSSA). *Lancet* **354**, 1147.

Moses, H. L., Yang, E. Y. and Pietenpol, J. A. (1990). TGF-β stimulation and inhibition of cell proliferation: new mechanistic insights. *Cell* **63**, 245.

Mosmann, T. R., Cherwinski, H., Bond, M. W., *et al.* (1986). Two types of murine helper T cell clone: I. definition according to profiles of lymphokine activities and secreted proteins. *J. Immunol.* **136**, 2348.

Mosmann, T. R., Schumacher, J. H., Street, N. F., *et al.* (1991). Diversity of cytokine synthesis and function of mouse CD4+ T cells. *Immunol. Rev.* **123**, 209.

Mottram, P. L., Han, W.-R., Purcell, L. J., *et al.* (1995). Increased expression of IL-4 and IL-10 and decreased expression of IL-2 and interferon-γ in long-surviving mouse heart allografts after brief CD4-monoclonal antibody therapy. *Transplantation* **59**, 559.

Myburgh, J. A., Smit, J. A., Stark, J. H., *et al.* (1984). Total lymphoid irradiation in kidney and liver transplantation in the baboon: prolonged graft survival and alteration in cell subsets with low cumulative dose regimens. *J. Immunol.* **132**, 1019.

Nagata, S. (1997). Apoptosis by death factor. *Cell* **88**, 355.

Nicolls, M. R., Aversa, G. G., Pearce, N. W., *et al.* (1993). Induction of long-term specific tolerance to allografts in rats by therapy with an anti-CD3-like monoclonal antibody. *Transplantation* **55**, 459.

Niimi, M., Pearson, T., Larsen, C., *et al.* (1998). The role of the CD40 pathway in alloantigen induced hyporesponsiveness in vivo. *J. Immunol.* **161**, 5331.

Noelle, R. (1996). CD40 and its ligand in host defence. *Immunity* **4**, 415.

Noelle, R., Roy, M., Shepherd, D., *et al.* (1992). A 39-kDa protein on activated helper T cells binds CD40 and transduces the signal for cognant activation of B cells. *Proc. Natl. Acad. Sci. U. S. A.* **89**, 6550.

O'Garra, A. (1998). Cytokines induce the development of functionally heterogenous T helper cell subsets. *Immunity* **8**, 275.

Onodera, K., Hancockm, W. W., Graserm, E., *et al.* (1997). Type 2 helper T cell-type cytokines and the development of "infectious" tolerance in rat cardiac allograft recipients. *J. Immunol.* **158**, 1572.

Pape, K., Merica, R., Mondino, A., *et al.* (1998). Direct evidence that functionally impaired CD4+ T cells persist in vivo following the induction of peripheral tolerance. *J. Immunol.* **160**, 4719.

Parker, D., Greiner, D., Phillips, N., *et al.* (1995). Survival of mouse pancreatic islet allografts in recipients treated with allogeneic small lymphocytes and antibody to CD40 ligand. *Proc. Natl. Acad. Sci. U. S. A.* **92**, 9560.

Pearce, N., Berger, M., Gurley, K., *et al.* (1993). Specific unresponsiveness in rats with prolonged cardiac allograft survival after treatment with cyclosporinee: VI. in vitro alloreactivity of T cell subsets from rats with long-surviving allografts. *Transplantation* **55**, 380.

Pearson, T., Alexander, D., Hendrix, R., *et al.* (1996). CTLA4-Ig plus bone marrow induces long-term allograft survival and donor-specific unresponsiveness in the murine model. *Transplantation* **61**, 997.

Pearson, T. C., Darby, C., Bushell, A. R, *et al.* (1993). The assessment of transplantation tolerance induced by anti-CD4 monoclonal antibody in the murine model. *Transplantation* **55**, 361.

Pearson, T. C., Madsen, J. C., Larsen, C., *et al.* (1992). Induction of transplantation tolerance in the adult using donor antigen and anti-CD4 monoclonal antibody. *Transplantation* **54**, 475.

Penn, I. (1998). Occurrence of cancers in immunosuppressed organ transplant recipients. *Clin. Transplant.* **12**, 147.

Perez, V. L., Van Parijs, L., Biuckians, A., *et al.* (1997). Induction of peripheral T cell tolerance in vivo requires CTLA-4 engagement. *Immunity* **6**, 411.

Peugh, W. N., Superina, R. A., Wood, K. J., *et al.* (1986). The role of H2 and non-H2 antigens and genes in the rejection of murine cardiac allografts. *Immunogenetics* **23**, 30.

Posselt, A. M., Barker, C. F., Tomaszewski, J. E., *et al.* (1990). Induction of donor-specific unresponsiveness by intrathymic islet transplantation. *Science* **249**, 1293.

Powrie, F., Carlino, J., Leach, M. W., Mauze, S. and Coffman, R. L. (1996). A critical role for transforming growth factor-β but not interleukin-4 in the suppression of T helper type 1-mediated colitis by CD45RB^low CD4+ T cells. *J. Exp. Med.* **183**, 2669.

Powrie, F. and Mason, D. (1990). Ox-22[high] CD4[+] T cells induce wasting disease with multiple organ pathology: prevention by the Ox-22[low] subset. *J. Exp. Med.* **172**, 1701.

Punch, J., Lin, J., Bluestone, J., *et al.* (1999). CD2 and CD3 receptor-mediated tolerance: constraints on T cell activation. *Transplantation* **67**, 741.

Qian, S., Demetris, A., Murase, N., *et al.* (1994). Murine liver allograft transplantation: tolerance and donor cell chimerism. *Hepatology* **19**, 916.

Qian, S., Li, W., Li, Y., *et al.* (1996). Systemic administration of cellular interleukin-10 can exacerbate cardiac allograft rejection in mice. *Transplantation* **62**, 1709.

Qin, L., Chavin, K., Ding, Y., *et al.* (1996). Retrovirus mediated gene transfer of viral IL-10 gene prolongs murine cardiac allograft survival. *J. Immunol.* **156**, 2316.

Qin, S., Cobbold, S., Benjamin, R., *et al.* (1989). Induction of classical transplantation tolerance in the adult. *J. Exp. Med.* **169**, 779.

Qin, S., Cobbold, S., Pope, H., *et al.* (1993). "Infectious" transplantation tolerance. *Science* **259,** 974.

Qin, S., Cobbold, S., Tighe, H., *et al.* (1987). CD4 monoclonal antibody pairs for immunosuppression and tolerance induction. *Eur. J. Immunol.* **17**, 1159.

Quigley, R. L., Wood, K. J. and Morris, P. J. (1989). Mediation of antigen-induced suppression of renal allograft rejection by a CD4 (W3/25[+]) T cell. *Transplantation* **47**, 684.

Reis e Sousa, C., Stahl, P. and Austyn, J. (1993). Phagocytosis of antigens by Langerhans cells in vitro. *J. Exp. Med.* **178**, 509.

Remuzzi, G., Rossini, M., Imberti, O., *et al.* (1991). Kidney graft survival in rats without immunosuppressants after intrathymic glomerular transplantation. *Lancet* **337**, 750.

Ridge, J., Di Rosa, F. and Matzinger, P. (1998). A conditional dendritic cell can be a temporal bridge between a CD4[+] T-helper and a T-killer cell. *Nature* **393**, 474.

Rocken, M. and Shevach, E. (1996). Immune deviation—the third dimension of nondeletional T cell tolerance. *Immunol. Rev.* **149**, 175.

Russell, P., Chase, C., Winn, H., *et al.* (1994). Coronary atherosclerosis in transplanted mouse hearts: I. time course, immunogenetic and immunopathological considerations. *Am. J. Pathol.* **144,** 260.

Saitovitch, D., Morris, P. and Wood, K. (1996). Recipient cells expressing single donor MHC locus products can substitute for donor specific transfusions in the induction of transplantation tolerance when pretreatment is combined with anti-Cd4 monoclonal antibody: evidence for a vital role of Cd4[+] T cells in the induction of tolerance to class I molecules. *Transplantation* **61**, 1532.

Sakaguchi, S., Sakaguchi, N., Asano, M., *et al.* (1995). Immunologic self tolerance maintained by activated T cells expressing IL-2 receptor alpha chains (CD25): breakdown of a single mechanism of self tolerance causes various autoimmune diseases. *J. Immunol.* **155**, 1151.

Sakaguchi, S., Toda, M., Asano, M., *et al.* (1996). T cell mediated maintenance of natural self tolerance: its breakdown as a possible cause of various autoimmune diseases. *J. Autoimmun.* **9**, 211.

Sayegh, M., Akalin, E., Hancocok, W., *et al.* (1995). CD28-B7 blockade after alloantigenic challenge in vivo inhibits Th1 cytokines but spares Th2. *J. Exp. Med.* **181**, 1869.

Sayegh, M., Fine, N., Smith, J., *et al.* (1991). Immunologic tolerance to renal allografts after bone marrow transplants from the same donors. *Ann. Intern. Med.* **114**, 954.

Sayegh, M., Zheng, X., Magee, C., *et al.* (1997). Donor antigen is necessary for the prevention of chronic rejection in CTLA4 Ig-treated murine cardiac allograft recipients. *Transplantation* **64**, 1646.

Schwartz, R. H. (1992). Costimulation of T lymphocytes: the role of CD28, CTLA-4, and B7/BB1 in interleukin-2 production and immunotherapy. *Cell* **71**, 1065.

Scully, R., Qin, S., Cobbold, S., *et al.* (1994). Mechanisms in CD4 antibody-mediated transplantation tolerance: kinetics of induction, antigen dependency and role of regulatory T cells. *Eur. J. Immunol.* **24**, 2383.

Sebzda, E., Mariathasan, S., Ohteki, T., *et al.* (1999). Selection of the T cell repertoire. *Ann. Rev. Immunol.* **17**, 829.

Sheil, A. (1998). Cancer in immune suppressed organ transplant recipients: aetiology and evolution. *Transplant. Proc.* **30**, 2055.

Shizuru, J. A., Gregory, A. K., Chao, C.T.-B., *et al.* (1987). Islet allograft survival after a single course of treatment of recipient with antibody to L3T4. *Science* **237,** 278.

Shoskes, D. and Wood, K. (1994). Indirect presentation of MHC antigens in transplantation. *Immunol. Today* **15**, 1.

Slavin, S., Strober, S., Fuks, Z., *et al.* (1977). Induction of specific tissue transplantation tolerance using fractionated total lymphoid irradiation in adult mice: long-term survival of allogeneic bone marrow and skin grafts. *J. Exp. Med.* **146**, 34.

Sorof, J., Koerper, M., Portale, A., *et al.* (1995). Renal transplantation without chronic immunosuppression after T cell depleted HLA-mismatched bone marrow transplantation. *Transplantation* **59**, 1633.

Spitzer, T., Delmonico, F., Tolkoff-Rubin, N., *et al.* (1999). Combined histocompatibility leukocyte antigen-matched donor bone marrow and renal transplantation for multiple myeloma with end stage renal disease: the induction of allograft tolerance through mixed lymphohematopoietic chimerism. *Transplantation* **68**, 480.

Starzl, T. E., Demetris, A. J., Murase, N., *et al.* (1992). Cell migration, chimerism and graft acceptance. *Lancet* **339**, 1579.

Stockinger, B. (1999). T lymphocyte tolerance: from thymic deletion to peripheral control mechanisms. *Adv. Immunol.* **71**, 229.

Strober, S., Dhillon, M., Schubert, M., *et al.* (1989). Acquired immune tolerance to cadaveric renal allografts: a study of three patients treated with total lymphoid irradiation. *N. Engl. J. Med.* **321**, 28.

Sun, J., McCaughan, G., Matsumoto, Y., *et al.* (1994). Tolerance to rat liver allograft: I. differences between tolerance and rejection are more marked in the B cell compared to the T cell or cytokine response. *Transplantation* **57**, 1349.

Sun, J., Sheil, A., Wang, C., *et al.* (1996). Tolerance to rat liver allograft: IV. tolerance depends on the quantity of donor tissue and donor leukocytes. *Transplantation* **62**, 1725.

Sykes, M. and Sachs, D. H. (1988). Mixed allogeneic chimerism as an approach to transplantation tolerance. *Immunol. Today* **9**, 23.

Taams, L., van Rensen, A., Poelen, M., *et al.* (1998). Anergic T cells actively suppress T cell responses via the antigen presenting cell. *Eur. J. Immunol.* **28**, 2901.

Theofilopoulos, A. (1995). The basis of autoimmunity: Part I. mechanisms of aberrant self recognition. *Immunol. Today* **16**, 90.

Thomas, F. T., Carver, F. M. and Foil, M. B. (1983). Long-term incompatible kidney survival in outbred higher primates without chronic immunosuppression. *Ann. Surg.* **198**, 370.

Thomas, J., Contreras, J., Jiang, X., *et al.* (1999). Peritransplant tolerance induction in macaques: early events reflecting the unique synergy between immunotoxin and deoxyspergualin. *Transplantation* **68**, 660.

Thomas, J. M., Carver, M. and Cunningham, P. (1987). Promotion of incompatible allograft acceptance in rhesus monkeys given posttransplant anti-thymocyte globulin and donor bone marrow: I. in vivo parameters and immunohistologic evidence suggesting microchimerism. *Transplantation* **43**, 332.

Thompson, C. (1995). Distinct roles for the costimulatory ligands B7-1 and B7-2 in T helper cell differentiation? *Cell* **81**, 879.

Thompson, C. and Allison, J. (1997). The emerging role of CTLA-4 as an immune attenuator. *Immunity* **7**, 445.

Tomita, Y., Khan, A. and Sykes, M. (1994). Role of intrathymic clonal deletion and peripheral anergy in transplantation tolerance induced by bone marrow transplantation in mice conditioned with a non-myeloablative regimen. *J. Immunol.* **153**, 1087.

Trambley, J., Bingaman, A., Lin, A., *et al.* (1999). Asialo GM1[+] CD8[+] T cells play a critical role in costimulation blockade resistant allograft rejection. *J. Clin. Invest.* **104**, 1715.

Turvey, S., Gonzalez-Nicolini, V., Kingsley, C., *et al.* (2000). Fas ligand transfected myoblasts and islet cell transplantation. *Transplantation* **69**, 1972.

Valitutti, S. and Lanzavecchia, A. (1997). Serial triggering of TCRs: a basis for the sensitivity and specificity of antigen recognition. *Immunol. Today* **18**, 299.

van der Merwe, A., Davis, S., Shaw, A., *et al.* (2000). Cytoskeletal polarization and redistribution of cell surface molecules during T cell antigen recognition. *Semin. Immunol.* **12**, 5.

van Parijs, L. and Abbas, A. (1998). Homeostasis and self-tolerance in the immune system: turning lymphocytes off. *Science* **280**, 243.

van Parijs, L., Ibraghimov, A. and Abbas, A. (1996). The roles of costimulation and Fas in T cell apoptosis and peripheral tolerance. *Immunity* **4**, 321.

Wahl, S. (1994). Transforming growth factor β: the good, the bad, and the ugly. *J. Exp. Med.* **180**, 1587.

Waldmann, H. (1989). Manipulation of T-cell responses with monoclonal antibodies. *Ann. Rev. Immunol.* **7**, 407.

Waldmann, H. and Cobbold, S. (1998). How do monoclonal antibodies induce tolerance? A role for infectious tolerance? *Ann. Rev. Immunol.* **16**, 619.

Webb, S., Morris, C., and Sprent, J. (1990). Extrathymic tolerance of mature T cells: clonal elimination as a consequence of immunity. *Cell* **63**, 1249.

Weiner, H. (1997). Oral tolerance: immune mechanisms and treatment of autoimmune diseases. *Immunol. Today* **18**, 335.

Wells, A., Li, X., Li, Y., *et al.* (1999). Requirement for T cell apoptosis in the induction of peripheral transplantation tolerance. *Nat. Med.* **5**, 1303.

Wekerle, T., Sayegh, M. H., Hill, J., *et al.* (1998). Extrathymic T cell deletion and allogeneic stem cell engraftment induced with costimulatory blockade is followed by central T cell tolerance. *J. Exp. Med.* **187**, 2037.

Wekerle, T. and Sykes, M. H. (1999). Mixed chimerism as an approach for the induction of transplantation tolerance. *Transplantation* **68**, 459.

Wekerle, T., Kurtz, J., Ito, H., *et al.* (2000). Allogeneic bone marrow transplantation with co-stimulatory blockade induces macrochimerism and tolerance without cytoreductive host treatment. *Nat. Med.* **6**, 464.

Whitmire, J., Flavell, R., Grewal, I., *et al.* (1999). CD40-CD40 ligand costimulation is required for generating antiviral CD4 T cell responses but is dispensable for CD8 T cell responses. *J. Immunol.* **163**, 3194.

Wilbanks, G. A., Mammolenti, M. and Streilein, J. W. (1992). Studies on the induction of anterior chamber-associated immune deviation (ACAID): III. induction of ACAID depends upon intraocular transforming growth factor-beta. *Eur. J. Immunol.* **22**, 165.

Wong, W., Morris, P. and Wood, K. (1996). Syngeneic bone marrow expressing a single donor class I MHC molecule permits acceptance of a fully allogeneic cardiac allograft. *Transplantation* **62**, 1462.

Wong, W., Morris, P. and Wood, K. (1997a). Pretransplant administration of a single donor class I MHC molecule is sufficient for the indefinite survival of fully allogeneic cardiac allografts: evidence for linked epitope suppression. *Transplantation* **63**, 1490.

Wong, W., Stranford, S., Morris, P., *et al.* (1997b). Retroviral gene transfer of a donor class I MHC gene to recipient bone marrow cells induces tolerances to alloantigens in vivo. *Transplant. Proc.* **29**, 1130.

Wood, K. J., Hopley, A., Dallman, M. J., *et al.* (1987). Donor major histocompatibility antigens are induced on non-rejected renal allografts in transfused rats. *Transplantation* **42**, 759.

Wood, K. J. and Sachs, D. (1996). Chimerism and transplantation tolerance: cause and effect. *Immunol. Today* **12**, 584.

Wood, M. L. and Monaco, A. P. (1980). Suppressor cells in specific unresponsiveness to skin allografts in ALS-treated, marrow-injected mice. *Transplantation* **29**, 196.

Xu, J., Foy, T., Laman, J., *et al.* (1994). Mice deficient for the CD40 ligand. *Immunity* **1**, 423.

Yang, C.-P., McDonagh, M., and Bell, E. (1995). CD45RC⁺ CD4 T cell subsets are maintained in an unresponsive state by the persistence of transfusion-derived alloantigen. *Transplantation* **60**, 192.

Yoshinaga, S., Whoriskey, J., Khare, S., *et al.* (1999). T cell costimulation through B7RP-1 and ICOS. *Nature* **402**, 827.

Young, N., Roelen, D., Iggo, N., *et al.* (1997). Effect of one-HLA-haplotype-matched and HLA-mismatched blood transfusions on recipient T lymphocyte allorepertoires. *Transplantation* **63**, 1160.

Zavazava, N. and Kronke, M. (1996). Soluble HLA class I molecule induce apoptosis in alloreactive cytotoxic T lymphocytes. *Nat. Med.* **2**, 1005.

Zinkernagel, R., Planz, O., Ehl, S., *et al.* (1999). General and specific immunosuppression caused by anti-viral responses. *Immunol. Rev.* **168**, 301.

Pathology of Kidney Transplantation
Shamila Mauiyyedi • Robert B. Colvin

Renal Allograft Biopsy

Renal biopsy remains the gold standard for the diagnosis of episodes of graft dysfunction, which occur in 30 to 50% of patients after transplantation. All large studies have confirmed the practical value of the renal allograft biopsy: Pathological diagnosis changed the clinical diagnosis in 30 to 42% and therapy in 38 to 83% of patients (Kiss *et al.*, 1992; Kon *et al.*, 1997; Pascual *et al.*, 1999). In a prospective trial at Massachusetts General Hospital, the biopsy diagnosis changed patient management in 42% of graft dysfunction episodes (39% in the first month, 56% in the first year and 39% after 1 year), and unnecessary immunosuppression was avoided in 19% of patients (Pascual *et al.*, 1999). The biopsy also is a good source of information on pathogenetic mechanisms and a generator of hypotheses that can be tested in experimental animal studies and clinical trials. The biopsy serves, in turn, to validate the hypotheses tested in such trials.

This chapter describes the relevant light, immunofluorescence and electron microscopy findings of the commonest lesions that affect the renal allograft, then discusses their differential diagnoses. We have updated and excerpted previous reviews that should be consulted for further citations and illustrations (Colvin, 1995, 1998). Here references are limited largely to human pathological studies after 1980.

OPTIMAL TISSUE

At least seven nonsclerotic glomeruli and two arteries (bigger than arterioles) must be present in a renal allograft biopsy specimen for adequate evaluation (Colvin *et al.*, 1997; Solez *et al.*, 1993a). Using these criteria, the sensitivity of a single core is approximately 90%, and the predicted sensitivity of two cores is about 99% (Colvin *et al.*, 1997). The adequacy of the biopsy sample depends entirely on the lesions seen, however. One artery with endothelialitis is sufficient for the diagnosis of acute rejection if no glomerulus is present; similarly, immunofluorescence or electron microscopy of one glomerulus is adequate to diagnose *de novo* membranous glomerulonephritis. In contrast, a large portion of cortex with a minimal infiltrate does not exclude rejection. Subcapsular biopsy specimens often show inflammation and fibrosis and are not representative samples. Conversely, normal medulla is not sufficient to rule out rejection because rejection is less common in the medulla than in the cortex (Wang *et al.*, 1995). Frozen sections for light microscopy are of limited value because freeze artifacts preclude accurate evaluation. The diagnostic accuracy of frozen sections was 89% when compared with paraffin sections (Cohen *et al.*, 1991). Rapid (2-hour) processing for paraffin sections is used at Massachusetts General Hospital and provides satisfactory preparations.

MICROSCOPY

The biopsy specimen is examined for glomerular, tubular, vascular and interstitial pathology, including (1) acute or chronic allograft glomerulopathy and *de novo* or recurrent glomerulonephritis; (2) tubular injury and inflammation (e.g., isometric vacuolization and tubulitis); (3) vascular lesions (e.g., endarteritis, fibrinoid necrosis, thrombi, myocyte necrosis, nodular medial hyalinosis and chronic allograft arteriopathy); (4) nature and degree of the interstitial cellular infiltrate (e.g., activated mononuclear cells, edema and neutrophils) and (5) degree of fibrosis and scarring (interstitial fibrosis, tubular atrophy and glomerulosclerosis). Arteries and arterioles are particularly scrutinized because the diagnostic lesion often lies there.

Our standard immunofluorescence panel detects IgG, IgA, IgM, C3, C4d, albumin and fibrin. C4d complement fragment identifies antibody-mediated rejection and is the most important reason for staining biopsy specimens with possible acute rejection (Collins *et al.*, 1999). Immunoperoxidase studies are included when lymphoproliferative or viral diseases are in the differential diagnosis. Electron microscopy is valuable when *de novo* or recurrent glomerular disease is suspected.

CLASSIFICATION OF PATHOLOGICAL DIAGNOSES IN THE RENAL ALLOGRAFT

The ideal diagnostic classification of renal allograft pathology should be based on pathogenesis, have therapeutic relevance and be reproducible; the classification in Table 24–1 meets these criteria (Colvin, 1998). This discussion is divided broadly into allograft rejection and nonrejection pathology, with an emphasis on differential diagnosis of acute and chronic allograft dysfunction. Grading systems of acute and chronic rejection are discussed further in those sections.

Donor Kidney

Biopsy of the cadaveric donor kidney sometimes is used to determine the suitability of the kidney for transplantation. Objective pathological criteria based on outcome that could be applied to the renal biopsy as a screening test have not been established because donor biopsies are not performed routinely, and controlled trials have not been done. In one large study, only 38% were normal: 29% had arteriolar hyalinosis, 8% had interstitial fibrosis, 3% had glomerulosclerosis, 5% had glomerular IgA deposits and 7% had intravascular coagulation (Curschellas *et al.*, 1991). The initial and late renal functions were independent of these morphological findings, however. In another series, tubular cell degeneration did not correlate with delayed graft function, but the presence of arteriosclerotic lesions was associated with a small but significant difference in 2-year graft survival (66% *vs.* 72%) (Taub *et al.*, 1999). Glomerulosclerosis greater than 20% has been correlated with poor graft outcome (Gaber *et al.*, 1995). Of donor kidneys with greater than 20% glomerulosclerosis, 87% developed delayed graft function, and 38% were lost. In contrast, grafts with less than 20% glomerulosclerosis had

PATHOLOGICAL CLASSIFICATION OF RENAL ALLOGRAFT LESIONS

I. Immunological rejection
  A. Hyperacute rejection
  B. Acute allograft rejection
    1. T cell–mediated (acute cellular rejection)
      a. Tubulointerstitial (CCTT/Banff type I)
      b. Endarteritis (CCTT/Banff type II)
      c. Glomerular (acute allograft glomerulopathy)
    2. Antibody mediated (acute humoral rejection)
      a. Capillary (peritubular ± glomerular)
      b. Arterial (fibrinoid necrosis; CCTT/Banff type III)
  C. Chronic allograft rejection (humoral or unknown pathogenesis)
    1. Tubulointerstitial
    2. Vascular (chronic allograft arteriopathy)
    3. Glomerular (chronic allograft glomerulopathy)
  D. Other alloantibody-mediated renal diseases
    1. *De novo* membranous glomerulonephritis
    2. Anti-GBM disease (in Alport's syndrome)
    3. Anti-TBM disease
II. Nonrejection injury
  A. Acute ischemic injury (acute tubular necrosis)
  B. Perfusion injury
  C. Calcineurin inhibitor nephrotoxicity (cyclosporine/ tacrolimus)
    1. Acute toxicity
    2. Thrombotic microangiopathy
    3. Chronic toxicity
  D. OKT3 toxicity (thrombotic angiopathy)
  E. Major artery or vein thrombosis (e.g., renal vein thrombosis)
  F. Renal artery stenosis
  G. Obstruction, lymphocele, reflux
  H. Infection (viral, bacterial, fungal)
  I. Acute tubulointerstitial nephritis (drug allergy)
III. *De novo* glomerular disease
  A. FSGS (hyperfiltration/collapsing)
  B. Diabetic nephropathy
  C. Other specific types
  D. Posttransplant lymphoproliferative disease
IV. Recurrent primary disease
  A. Immunological (e.g., IgA nephropathy, lupus, anti-GBM disease)
  B. Metabolic (e.g., amyloidosis, diabetes, oxalosis)
  C. Unknown (e.g., dense deposit disease, FSGS)

CCTT = Cooperative Clinical Trials in Transplantation; GBM = glomerular basement membrane; TBM = tubular basement membrane; FSGS = focal segmental glomerular sclerosis.
Modified with permission of Colvin, 1998.

delayed graft function in less than 33% of recipients, and only 7% were lost. Measurements of serum creatinine in the donors did not distinguish the different degrees of glomerulosclerosis found on biopsy. These data suggest that donor glomerulosclerosis greater than 20% increases the risk of delayed graft function and poor outcome of transplanted kidneys. If confirmed in a larger series, routine biopsy of high-risk kidneys before transplantation could be useful. No kidney is perfect histologically, however, and the criteria must be standardized to avoid a high rate of unused kidneys.

Other lesions may cause the transplant surgeon or pathologist to argue against use of the graft. Thrombotic microangiopathy with widespread glomerular thrombi, with or without vascular thromboses, is a contraindication to transplant in our opinion. This scenario is especially common in victims of head injury, in whom increased levels of released thromboplastin mediate severe coagulopathy. Reversal of diabetic glomerulosclerosis in a donor kidney transplanted into a nondiabetic recipient was documented by loss of proteinuria and mesangial hypercellularity at 7 months; cadaver kidneys

with mild diabetic lesions are potentially usable (Abouna *et al.*, 1983). Thin glomerular basement membrane (GBM) disease (a common cause of benign recurrent hematuria) requires electron microscopy and is not detected readily at the time of transplant; the suitability of such kidneys has not been established. We observed a case of donor-derived thin GBM disease in which the graft developed hypertrophy and secondary focal segmental sclerosis over 2 years, probably from increased susceptibility to hyperfiltration injury given the original GBM abnormality.

Hyperacute Rejection

Hyperacute rejection refers to immediate rejection (typically within 10 minutes to 1 hour) of the kidney on perfusion with recipient blood, in which the recipient is presensitized to alloantigens on the surface of the graft endothelium. During surgery, the graft kidney becomes soft, flabby and livid, mottled and purple or cyanotic in color; urine output ceases (Gaber *et al.*, 1992b; Kissmeyer-Nielsen *et al.*, 1966; Myburgh *et al.*, 1969; Starzl *et al.*, 1968). The kidney subsequently swells, and widespread hemorrhagic cortical necrosis and medullary congestion occur. The large vessels sometimes are thrombosed. Some cases may be delayed and become evident 8 hours to 2 days posttransplant (Gaber *et al.*, 1992b) because circulating antibody titer may be insufficient at the time of grafting.

Early lesions show marked accumulation of platelets in glomerular capillary lumina that appear as amorphous pale pink, finely granular masses in hematoxylin and eosin–stained slides (negative on periodic acid–Schiff [PAS] stains). Neutrophil and platelet margination occurs over the next hour or so along damaged endothelium of small arteries, arterioles, glomeruli and peritubular capillaries, and the capillaries fill with sludged (compacted) red cells and fibrin (Williams *et al.*, 1968). The larger arteries usually are spared. The neutrophils do not infiltrate initially but form chainlike figures in the peritubular capillaries without obvious thrombi (Williams *et al.*, 1968). The endothelium is stripped off the underlying basal lamina, and the interstitium becomes edematous and hemorrhagic. Intravascular coagulation occurs, and cortical necrosis ensues over 12 to 24 hours. The medulla is relatively spared but ultimately is affected as the whole kidney becomes necrotic (Kissmeyer-Nielsen *et al.*, 1966). Widespread microthrombi usually are found in the arterioles and glomeruli and can be detected in totally necrotic samples. The small arteries may show fibrinoid necrosis. Mononuclear infiltrates typically are sparse.

By immunofluorescence, fibrin, immunoglobulin (especially IgM) and complement (e.g., C3 and C4d) staining may be seen in vessels and glomeruli (Busch *et al.*, 1971b; Collins *et al.*, 1999; Matas *et al.*, 1976; Williams *et al.*, 1968). Mesangial deposition of IgG, IgM, C3 and properdin has been reported (Gaber *et al.*, 1992b; Matas *et al.*, 1976; Williams *et al.*, 1968). The site of antibody and complement deposition is determined by the site of the target alloantigen. Antibody-mediated hyperacute rejection caused by preexisting anti-HLA class I antibodies may show C3 and fibrin throughout the microvasculature (Halloran *et al.*, 1990). ABO antibodies (primarily IgM) also deposit in all vascular endothelium. Cases with anti-class II antibodies may have IgG and/or IgM primarily in glomerular and peritubular capillaries, where class II antigens normally are conspicuous (Ahern *et al.*, 1982). In antiendothelial-monocyte antigen cases, IgG primarily is in peritubular capillaries, rather than glomeruli or arteries (Paul *et al.*, 1979). Often, antibody cannot be detected in the vessels (Sibley and Payne, 1985), however, which may be due to endothelial loss and degradation or washing away of the membrane-bound antibody. In these cases, staining for C4d should be positive in peritubular capillaries (Collins *et al.*, 1999).

Acute Renal Allograft Rejection

Acute rejection typically develops in the first 2 to 6 weeks after transplantation but can arise in a normally functioning kidney 3 days to 10 years or more later or in a graft affected by other conditions, such as acute tubular necrosis (ATN), cyclosporine toxicity or chronic rejection. Acute rejection may be cell mediated and/or humoral (see Table 24–1). *Acute cellular rejection* is mediated primarily by T cells reacting to donor histocompatibility antigens in the kidney and is much commoner than *acute humoral rejection* resulting from donor-specific antibodies, although the latter now is recognized with greater frequency.

ACUTE CELLULAR REJECTION

Tubulointerstitial Rejection (Type I)

The prominent microscopic feature of acute cellular rejection is a pleiomorphic interstitial infiltrate of mononuclear cells, accompanied by interstitial edema and sometimes hemorrhage (Fig. 24–1A). The infiltrating cells primarily are T cells and macrophages. The T cells typically are activated (lymphoblasts), with increased basophilic cytoplasm, nucleoli and occasional mitotic figures, indicative of increased synthetic and proliferative activity. Interstitial neutrophils can be focally prominent in severe rejection. When they are conspicuous, the possibility of humoral rejection should be considered. Eosinophils are present in about 30% of biopsy specimens with rejection (Nickeleit *et al.*, 1998) and can be abundant but rarely are more than 2 to 3% of the infiltrate (Kormendi and Amend, 1988; Weir *et al.*, 1986). Basophils comprise a minor component of the infiltrate and invade tubules and can be the predominant granulocyte (5% of the infiltrate) (Colvin and Dvorak, 1974). Acute rejection with abundant plasma cells has been described in the first month

and is associated with poor graft survival (Charney *et al.*, 1999).

Mononuclear cells invade tubules and insinuate between tubular epithelial cells, a process termed *tubulitis* (Fig. 24–1B), best shown on a PAS-stained section that outlines the tubular basement membrane (TBM). All cortical tubules (proximal and distal) as well as the medullary tubules and the collecting ducts may be affected. Disruption of the TBM and leakage of Tamm-Horsfall protein into the interstitium has been described in 64% of biopsy specimens, especially evident on PAS stains (Cohen *et al.*, 1984).

CD8[+] and CD4[+] cells invade tubules (Tuazon *et al.*, 1987). Intratubular T cells with cytotoxic granules accumulate selectively in the tubules, compared with the interstitial infiltrate (Meehan *et al.*, 1997). T cells proliferate once inside the tubule, as judged by the marker Ki67 (MIB-1), which labels 15% of the intratubular lymphocytes (Robertson *et al.*, 1995). This proliferation probably contributes to their concentration within tubules, in addition to selective invasion (Meehan *et al.*, 1997). Increased tubular HLA-DR (Bishop *et al.*, 1986; Fuggle *et al.*, 1987), tumor necrosis factor-α (Morel *et al.*, 1993), interferon-γ receptor (Noronha *et al.*, 1993), interleukin (IL)-2 receptor (Kooijmans-Coutinho *et al.*, 1995) and IL-8 are detectable by immunoperoxidase study of acute cellular rejection. Several adhesion molecules are increased on tubular cells during rejection, including ICAM-1 (CD54) and VCAM-1 that correlate with the degree of T-cell infiltration (Briscoe *et al.*, 1992).

Signs of tubular cell injury can be detected by the terminal deoxynucleotide transferase-uridine-nick end label assay (TUNEL) for apoptosis. Increased numbers of TUNEL-positive tubular cells are present in acute rejection, compared with normal kidneys (Ito *et al.*, 1995; Meehan *et al.*, 1997). The frequency was significantly lower in cyclosporine toxicity or ATN (Meehan *et al.*, 1997). The degree of apoptosis correlates with the cytotoxic cells in the infiltrate, consistent with a pathogenetic relationship (Meehan *et al.*, 1997). Prominent apoptosis of the infiltrating T cells also has been detected at a frequency comparable to that in the normal thymus (1.8% of cells) (Meehan *et al.*, 1997). Others have described occasional TUNEL-positive lymphocytes (Ito *et al.*, 1995).

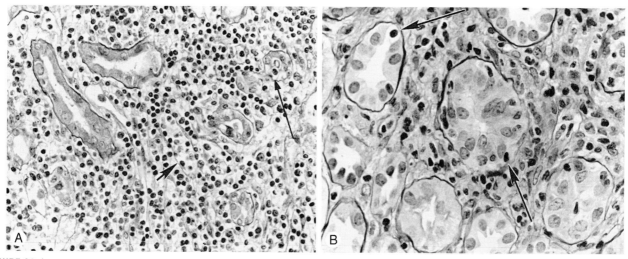

FIGURE 24–1

Acute cellular rejection, type I. (A) Mononuclear cell infiltrate in the interstitium composed of activated lymphocytes and macrophages. The peritubular capillaries (short arrow) are dilated containing abundant mononuclear cells. Tubulitis is prominent (long arrow). (B) Tubulitis affecting proximal tubules, where mononuclear cells are interposed between the tubular epithelial cells. The invading mononuclear cells (arrows) appear dark, with scant cytoplasm and often are surrounded by a clear halo, which helps distinguish them from the adjacent tubular epithelial cells. (A, PAS × 400; B, PAS × 500.)

Apoptosis probably occurs in infiltrating T cells as a result of activation-induced cell death and would serve to limit the immune reaction (Meehan *et al.*, 1997). Little, if any, immunoglobulin deposition is found by immunofluorescence in acute cellular rejection, which is characterized primarily by accumulation of extravascular fibrin and/or fibrinogen in the interstitium and not uncommonly increased C3 along the TBM.

By electron microscopy, lymphocytes in the tubules accumulate between the epithelium and the TBM, frequently surrounded by a clear zone (Shimamura *et al.*, 1966). The tubular epithelial cells remain in contact with the TBM, but the lymphocytes are separated from the TBM by a thin layer of epithelial cytoplasm; the TBM rarely shows breaks (Nadasdy *et al.*, 1988). The tubular epithelial cells in the vicinity of mononuclear cells often show signs of injury, including vacuolization (Shimamura *et al.*, 1966), necrosis and apoptosis (Nadasdy *et al.*, 1988). In contrast, the tubular epithelium in drug-induced interstitial nephritis is reported not to be injured in the vicinity of the lymphocytes (Ivanyi *et al.*, 1992). Occasional leakage of Tamm-Horsfall protein into the interstitium through fractured TBM has been described. The peritubular capillaries show mononuclear cells in the lumen, mostly lymphocytes, which sometimes are flattened in contact with the endothelium or when emigrating through the wall (Ivanyi *et al.*, 1992). The endothelium becomes activated, as judged by cytoplasmic and nuclear enlargement, increased ribosomes, endoplasmic reticulum, mitochondria and Golgi complex; the fenestrations may disappear completely (Ivanyi *et al.*, 1992).

Several studies reported provocative results with polymerase chain reaction to amplify mRNA from biopsy specimens or fine-needle aspirates. These studies attempted to define the pathogenetically or diagnostically relevant cytokines synthesized in the tissue but generally had scanty pathological correlations. Among the most specific and sensitive measures of rejection by polymerase chain reaction seem to be the mRNA for certain proteins of cytotoxic cells, granzyme B, perforin, Fas and Fas ligand (Pavlakis *et al.*, 1996; Sharma *et al.*, 1996; Strehlau *et al.*, 1997). A combination of two of the three markers is highly predictive of acute rejection, more so than the cytokines (Strehlau *et al.*, 1997). This finding may argue that the cytolytic pathway is more active than the cytokine delayed hypersensitivity mechanisms, but that ap-

plies only to the time of the biopsy, which is relatively late in the inflammatory process. Acute rejection arising late after transplantation has a cytokine profile similar to delayed hypersensitivity reactions with little evidence of cytotoxic mechanisms (Ode-Hakim *et al.*, 1996).

Endarteritis (Type II Rejection)

Infiltration of mononuclear cells under arterial and arteriolar endothelium is the pathognomonic lesion of acute cellular rejection (Fig. 24–2). Many terms have been used for this process, including *endothelialitis, endovasculitis, intimal arteritis* and *endarteritis*. We prefer the last term, which emphasizes the type of vessel (artery *vs.* vein) involved and the site of inflammation. Endarteritis in acute cellular rejection must not be confused with fibrinoid necrosis of arteries. The latter is characteristic of acute humoral rejection and can be seen in thrombotic vasculopathy. Some workers, regrettably, still do not separate these lesions, regarding all vascular rejection as predominantly humoral.

Endarteritis has been reported in 35 to 56% of renal biopsy specimens with acute cellular rejection (Bates *et al.*, 1999; Colvin *et al.*, 1997; Kooijmans-Coutinho *et al.*, 1996; Nickeleit *et al.*, 1998; Schroeder *et al.*, 1991; Sibley *et al.*, 1983). Many workers do not find the lesion as often, which may be ascribed to inadequate sampling, overdiagnosis of rejection (increasing the denominator), or timing of the biopsy with respect to antirejection therapy. Endarteritis lesions affect arteries of all sizes including the arteriole, although lesions affect larger vessels preferentially. For example, in a detailed analysis, 27% of the artery cross-sections were affected versus 13% of the arterioles (Nickeleit *et al.*, 1998). A sample of four arteries would have an estimated sensitivity of about 75% in the detection of type II rejection (Nickeleit *et al.*, 1998). A sample may not be considered adequate to rule out endarteritis unless several arteries are included.

Endothelial cells typically are reactive with increased cytoplasmic volume and basophilia. The endothelium shows disruption and lifting from supporting stroma by infiltrating inflammatory cells (Alpers *et al.*, 1990). Occasionally, endothelial cells are necrotic or absent. Mononuclear cells that sometimes are attached to the endothelial surface are insufficient for the diagnosis of endarteritis; however, they probably represent the early phase of this lesion. The medium usually

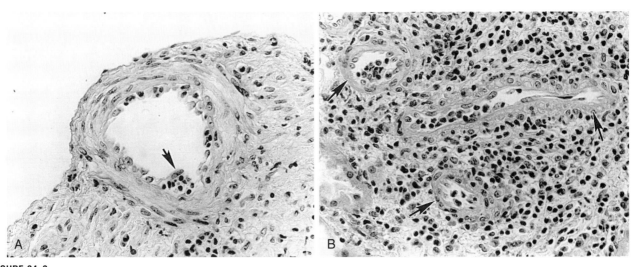

FIGURE 24–2

Acute cellular rejection, type II. (A) Endarteritis in a small-sized artery. The endothelium (arrow) is lifted by undermining mononuclear cells, without involvement of the media. (B) Endothelitis affecting three arterioles (arrows). (A, H&E × 400; B, H&E × 400.)

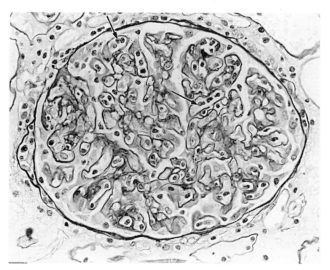

FIGURE 24–3

Glomerulitis. Scattered mononuclear cells (arrows) in glomerular capillary loops. (PAS × 400.)

During acute rejection, the endothelium of arteries expresses increased HLA-DR (Fuggle *et al.*, 1985; Tuazon *et al.*, 1987) and ICAM-1 and VCAM-1 (Brockmeyer *et al.*, 1993; Faull and Russ, 1989). The up-regulation of the adhesion molecules occurs in association with CD3+ (Briscoe *et al.*, 1992) and CD25+ (Fuggle *et al.*, 1993) infiltrating mononuclear cells. Endothelial cells also have decreased endothelin expression in rejection with endarteritis but not in tubulointerstitial rejection (Watschinger *et al.*, 1994).

Glomerular Lesions

In most cases of acute cellular rejection, the glomeruli are spared or show minor changes, typically a few scattered mononuclear cells (T cells and monocytes) and occasionally segmental endothelial damage, termed *glomerulitis* (Bishop *et al.*, 1986; Harry *et al.*, 1984; Tuazon *et al.*, 1987; Fig. 24–3). In a few cases, a severe, diffuse form of glomerular injury is evident and dominates the histological pattern (Fig. 24–4). In 1981, Richardson *et al.* drew attention to a distinctive, acute allograft glomerulopathy, characterized by hypercellularity, injury and enlargement of endothelial cells, infiltration of glomeruli by mononuclear cells and webs of PAS-positive material. The glomeruli contain numerous CD3+ and CD8+ T cells and monocytes (Hiki *et al.*, 1986; Tuazon *et al.*, 1987). The lymphocytes have an activated phenotype, as judged by the presence of IL-2 receptor and HLA-DR. The glomeruli have increased staining for HLA class I antigens (Tuazon *et al.*, 1987). By immunofluorescence, fibrin and scant immunoglobulin and complement deposits are found in glomeruli. This severe form of glomerulopathy has been observed in 4 to 7% of biopsy specimens taken for allograft dysfunction, typically 1 to 4 months after transplantation (Axelsen *et al.*, 1985; Herrera *et al.*, 1986; Maryniak *et al.*, 1985a; Richardson *et al.*, 1981). Acute allograft glomerulopathy is believed to be an unusual variant of cellular rejection, sometimes promoted by cytomegalovirus infection; hepatitis C virus also has been associated with acute glomerulopathy (Cosio *et al.*, 1996b). T cells, not antibodies, are detected regularly in glomeruli immunohistochemically (Hiki *et al.*, 1986; Tuazon *et al.*, 1987), and OKT3 can reverse the lesion (Hibberd *et al.*, 1991). For

shows little change. In severe cases, a transmural mononuclear infiltrate may be seen. The cells infiltrating the endothelium and intima are T cells and monocytes but not B cells (Alpers *et al.*, 1990; Tuazon *et al.*, 1987). CD8+ and CD4+ cells invade the intima in early grafts, but later CD8+ cells predominate (Tuazon *et al.*, 1987), suggesting that class I antigens are the primary target. Some of the T cells express a cytotoxic phenotype (Meehan *et al.*, 1997). Tumor necrosis factor receptors are detectable in the endothelium of arteries (Noronha *et al.*, 1993). Apoptosis of vascular endothelial cells can be detected in sites of endarteritis (Ito *et al.*, 1995; Meehan *et al.*, 1997). The endarteritis lesions have been little studied ultrastructurally, presumably because of the difficulty in sampling.

Normal arterial endothelial cells express class I antigens, weak ICAM-1, and little or no class II antigens, or VCAM-1.

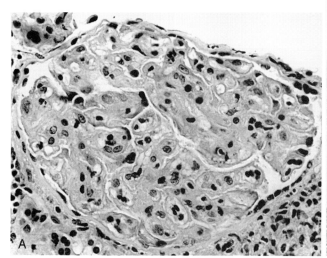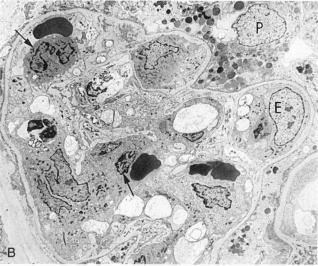

FIGURE 24–4

Acute allograft glomerulopathy. (A) Light microscopy shows glomerular capillary loops occluded by swollen endothelium and scattered mononuclear inflammatory cells. (B) Electron microscopy shows reactive glomerular capillary endothelium, (E), with increased cytoplasm, organelles, enlarged nucleus, prominent nucleolus and loss of fenestrae. Mononuclear cells, including lymphocytes, are in capillary lumina (arrows). Red blood cells are trapped in the obliterated capillary lumina. (A, H&E × 400; B, EM × 2,200.)

unknown reasons, rejection becomes focused on glomerular components; florid glomerulopathy may occur with little interstitial inflammation, although cellular endarteritis is common.

Electron microscopy of acute allograft glomerulopathy reveals that many endothelial cells are enlarged and reactive, with marked increase in cytoplasmic organelles (ribosomes, mitochondria and endoplasmic reticulum), an enlarged nucleus with open chromatin, prominent nucleoli and loss of fenestrae (Fig. 24–4B). The endothelial swelling may obliterate the lumen. Some GBM may be bare of endothelium or wrinkled and collapsed. The glomerular capillary lumina contain monocytes and activated lymphocytes, with occasional neutrophils, platelets and fibrin. The mesangium has loose matrix and sometimes monocytes. Amorphous electron dense deposits are sparse and limited to subendothelial spaces and the mesangium (Richardson *et al.*, 1981).

ACUTE HUMORAL REJECTION

Acute humoral rejection is a form of renal allograft rejection caused by the posttransplant production of circulating antibodies to donor alloantigens on endothelium, including HLA class I (Halloran *et al.*, 1992), class II (Collins *et al.*, 1999; Scornik *et al.*, 1992) or non–major histocompatibility complex (MHC) antigens (Kooijmans-Coutinho *et al.*, 1996; Miltenburg *et al.*, 1989; Yard *et al.*, 1993). The antibodies arise *after* transplant, in contrast to hyperacute rejection (low titers may sometimes be detected before transplant, insufficient to trigger an immediate rejection). Other terms used historically for acute humoral rejection are *accelerated acute rejection, necrotizing arteritis* and *fibrinoid necrosis*. Acute humoral rejection coexists with T cell–mediated injury in most cases (62%) and probably contributes to graft injury more often than generally is appreciated (Collins *et al.*, 1999). Cytotoxic antidonor class I antibodies are found in the circulation at the time of acute rejection in 20 to 25% of patients (Halloran *et al.*, 1992; Lobo *et al.*, 1995). Such antibodies correlate with an increased risk of clinically severe acute rejection and graft loss (Halloran *et al.*, 1992; Lobo *et al.*, 1995). These results fit with old data that showed 15% of eluates from acutely rejected kidneys had anti–T cell cytotoxic antibodies and 21% had anti–B cell

antibodies (Soulillou *et al.*, 1981). In our experience, about 29% of acute rejection episodes have a humoral component (Crespo *et al.*, 2000).

Identification of acute humoral rejection in biopsy specimens is difficult because none of the histological features is diagnostic (Collins *et al.*, 1999; Halloran *et al.*, 1992; Lobo *et al.*, 1995; Salmela *et al.*, 1992; Trpkov *et al.*, 1996). The diagnosis of acute humoral rejection previously was made by identification of suspicious morphological features on biopsy with subsequent serological confirmation of circulating antidonor antibodies.

Typical histological findings are a scant-to-moderate infiltrate in the interstitium, which usually contains mononuclear cells and prominent neutrophils. The interstitial infiltrate probably is actually focused on the peritubular capillaries (Fig. 24–5A). Peritubular capillaries have neutrophils in 46% of cases with circulating anti–HLA class I antibody; neutrophils also are detected in 5% of cases without such antibodies (Trpkov *et al.*, 1996). Interstitial edema and hemorrhage can be prominent. Neutrophils are common in glomerular capillaries (Halloran *et al.*, 1992; Fig. 24–6A). Glomerulitis with mononuclear cells in glomerular capillaries and endothelial swelling is commoner in the presence of anti–class I antibody (46% *vs.* 10%) (Trpkov *et al.*, 1996). The glomeruli may show necrosis and thrombosis (Salmela *et al.*, 1992). Similar lesions occur in pig–to–nonhuman primate xenografts, in which the peritubular capillaries are the principal target, and show apoptosis before an infiltrate is detectable (Shimizu *et al.*, 2000). Acute tubular injury, sometimes severe, can be identified in many cases and may be the first manifestation of acute humoral rejection. Focal necrosis of whole tubular cross-sections, similar to cortical necrosis, has been reported; 38 to 70% of acute humoral rejection cases may have patchy infarction (Lobo *et al.*, 1995; Trpkov *et al.*, 1996). Little mononuclear cell tubulitis is found, although a neutrophilic tubulitis (Fig. 24–6B) with or without neutrophil casts may be prominent (Trpkov *et al.*, 1996).

Fibrinoid arterial necrosis (type III rejection) is found in 3 to 5% of cases with acute rejection (Bates *et al.*, 1999; Nickeleit *et al.*, 1998). Fibrinoid necrosis is more characteristic of humoral than cellular rejection, detected in biopsy specimens in 20 to 25% of patients with anti-HLA antibodies versus 5

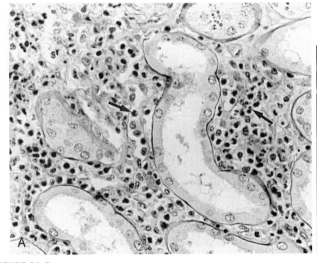
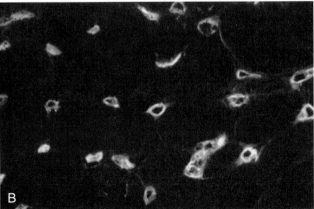

FIGURE 24–5

Acute humoral rejection. (A) Dilated peritubular capillaries contain numerous neutrophils (arrows). The endothelium is prominent and reactive. (B) Immunofluorescence microscopy shows widespread bright staining of peritubular capillaries with C4d (monoclonal antibody), a marker of acute humoral rejection, which strongly correlates with the presence of circulating donor-specific antibody. (A, PAS × 400; B, streptavidin-FITC × 400.) (See color plate.)

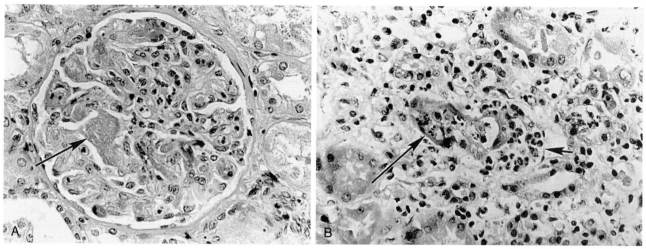

FIGURE 24–6

Acute humoral rejection. (A) Glomerulus with scattered neutrophils in capillary loops and fibrinoid necrosis (arrow). (B) Neutrophilic tubulitis with neutrophils invading tubules (long arrow); an adjacent peritubular capillary is engorged with neutrophils (short arrow). (A, H&E × 400; B, H&E × 400.)

to 7% of patients without such antibodies (Trpkov *et al.*, 1996). Another study noted 53% of 17 patients had fibrinoid necrosis (24%) or transmural arterial inflammation (18%) or both (12%) (Lobo *et al.*, 1995). In affected arteries, the media show myocyte necrosis and fragmentation of elastica with accumulation of brightly eosinophilic material called *fibrinoid necrosis* with little mononuclear infiltrate in the intima or adventitia (Fig. 24–7). A scant infiltrate of neutrophils, eosinophils and thrombosis may be present in the walls. Eosinophil cationic protein deposits have been shown in the necrotic vascular walls (Hallgren *et al.*, 1991). The presence of endarteritis in cases of acute humoral rejection indicates an added component of T cell–mediated rejection. Arterial thrombosis can be found in 10%, and a pattern resembling thrombotic microangiopathy has been reported (Lobo *et al.*, 1995). Normal arteries in a biopsy specimen do not exclude acute humoral rejection. Of biopsy specimens from patients with cir-

culating anti–class I antibody, 25% had no arterial lesions at all (Trpkov *et al.*, 1996).

Immunofluorescence for IgG, IgM, C3 or fibrin is not as helpful as one might expect, revealing no statistically significant difference between those with and without circulating antibody (Collins *et al.*, 1999; Trpkov *et al.*, 1996). It was discovered, however, that the peritubular capillaries show bright staining for C4d (see Fig. 24–5B) in acute humoral rejection (Collins *et al.*, 1999). Feucht and colleagues first drew attention to C4d as a marker of severe rejection, although without clinicopathological correlation with the features of acute humoral rejection (Feucht *et al.*, 1991). C4d, a fragment of complement component C4, is released during activation of the classic complement pathway by antigen-antibody interaction. Because C4d contains a thioester bond, it binds covalently to tissues at the local site of activation. C4d staining rarely is seen in pure acute cellular rejection or acute cyclosporine toxicity. However, cellular and humoral rejection coexist in about 45% of cases with C4d (Crespo *et al.*, 2000). In our experience, 100% of cases with acute humoral rejection (circulating anti-HLA antibody) had C4d versus 0% of cases with acute cellular rejection (Collins *et al.*, 1999). Lesions of fibrinoid necrosis contain IgG and/or IgM, C3 and fibrin (Busch *et al.*, 1971b; McKenzie and Whittingham, 1968).

By electron microscopy, the peritubular capillaries are dilated and contain neutrophils. The endothelium is reactive and shows loss of fenestrations. The glomerular endothelium is separated from the GBM by a widened lucent space with swelling of endothelial cells (Trpkov *et al.*, 1996) and loss of endothelial fenestrations, indicative of injury. Platelets, fibrin and neutrophils are found in glomerular and peritubular capillaries. The small arteries with fibrinoid necrosis show marked endothelial injury and loss, smooth muscle necrosis and deposition of fibrin tactoids.

To explain why peritubular capillaries are the major target of circulating HLA antibodies, sometimes in the absence of obvious glomerular inflammation, we hypothesized that peritubular capillaries may have less anticomplement protective pathways than glomeruli (Collins *et al.*, 1999). Four major cell-surface inhibitors of complement activation are abundant in normal human glomeruli: decay accelerating factor (DAF, CD55); membrane cofactor protein (MCP, CD46) and CR1 (CD35), which inactivate C3 and/or C5 convertases of the

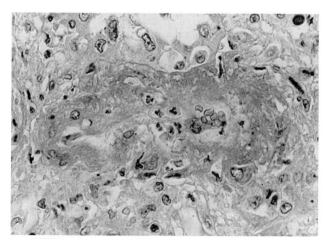

FIGURE 24–7

Fibrinoid arterial necrosis. An arteriole with destruction of the medial wall smooth muscle cells by fibrinoid necrosis. Some neutrophils are present underneath the reactive and swollen endothelium. This vascular change is distinct from that of endarteritis (compare with Fig. 24–2) and can be seen in acute humoral rejection and type III acute rejection. (H&E × 800.)

classic and alternative pathways, and protectin (CD59), which inhibits the formation of the membrane attack complex (Cosio et al., 1989; Ichida et al., 1994; Nakanishi et al., 1994). In contrast, only CD59 is prominent in normal cortical peritubular capillaries by immunofluorescence.[121] At the peritubular capillary surface, classic pathway activation of C4 is relatively unopposed. The importance of these regulators of complement activation in resistance to humoral rejection has been proved by the prevention of pig xenograft hyperacute rejection using organs from pigs transgenic for human CD55 and CD59 (Byrne et al., 1997).

The prognosis of acute humoral rejection is uniformly worse than that of acute cellular rejection (Collins et al., 1999; Halloran et al., 1992; Kooijmans-Coutinho et al., 1996; Lobo et al., 1995; Trpkov et al., 1996; Yard et al., 1993). Patients that recover from the acute episode of acute humoral rejection have a similar long-term outcome (Trpkov et al., 1996), however, suggesting that the pathogenetic humoral response can be transient if treated effectively. Plasmapheresis combined with mycophenolate mofetil and tacrolimus can be successful in reversing acute humoral rejection and restoring graft function (Pascual et al., 1998). These important clinical implications as well as interest in xenotransplantation have stimulated efforts to improve the diagnosis and therapy of acute humoral rejection. The optimal treatment has not been determined. Standard current immunosuppressive therapies are directed at the T cell and only indirectly affect B-cell responses (through inhibition of T cells). It would be of interest to determine whether plasmapheresis or some of the newer drugs that affect humoral antibody (e.g., anti-CD20) can improve the survival rate.

CLASSIFICATION SYSTEMS

Several classification systems have been proposed for renal allograft rejection. The early schema had more gradations at the severest end of the spectrum and emphasized thrombotic features, and endarteritis was not recognized as a distinct lesion (Colvin et al., 1997). The Banff working schema (Banff 93–95) attempted to promote uniform allograft biopsy grading for drug trials and routine diagnostic use (Sulez et al., 1993). The Banff schema had a beneficial effect in the standardization of definitions. The complexities, subjectivity and lack of reproducibility have limited use of Banff, however. Banff 93–95 had five categories for acute rejection: borderline, Grade I, IIa, IIb and III. These grades were based on mild, moderate or severe scores for each of the following: degree of interstitial infiltrate, tubulitis and vascular lesions. The threshold between *borderline* category and *grade I* rejection was the presence of tubulitis with greater than four mononuclear cells/tubular cross-section or group of 10 tubular cells and greater than 25% interstitial infiltration. Published data do not support prognostic significance of the extent of the infiltrate or tubulitis, even if it could be graded accurately (Banfi et al., 1981; Bates et al., 1999; Matas et al., 1983; Visscher et al., 1991). Grade II rejection was divided into IIa and IIb based on the absence or presence of *mild or moderate intimal arteritis*. Grade III was *severe intimal arteritis*, including arterial fibrinoid necrosis as well as focal infarction and interstitial hemorrhage in the definition. These grades separate lesions that should be together and combine those that should be separate.

A simple, rational scoring system for acute rejection was developed by a panel of renal pathologists participating in the National Institutes of Health Cooperative Clinical Trials in Transplantation (CCTT) (Colvin et al., 1997). The panel defined three types of acute rejection—tubulointerstitial, endarteritis and fibrinoid necrosis—and added criteria that re-

flect ongoing parenchymal injury (edema, tubular injury) or immunological activity (activated lymphocytes) to help separate out active rejection from inactive infiltrates (Table 24–2). The CCTT system excludes the subcapsular area for scoring (which often shows mild inflammation and fibrosis) and does not score tubulitis in areas of tubular atrophy (where it often is seen nonspecifically). The CCTT classification regards the presence or absence of endarteritis as potentially more fundamental, and it is the basis of separating type I from type II. The interobserver reproducibility of the CCTT classification was satisfactory, with 91% agreement on the presence or absence of rejection (κ, 0.80) (Colvin et al., 1997). The agreement was almost as good for the type of rejection (κ, 0.72) and the presence or absence of endarteritis (κ, 0.65). Banff 93–95 compares unfavorably with the CCTT in κ values (Marcussen et al., 1995). Banff has a higher threshold for the degree of interstitial infiltrate in grade I rejection than CCTT (25% vs. 5%). The CCTT study results indicated that 31% of type I rejection cases had an interstitial infiltrate involving less than 25% of the cortex. The CCTT system would classify many of the Banff borderlines as a type I rejection.

The CCTT classification types correlate with clinical severity: Type I rejection (tubulointerstitial type) more often is completely steroid responsive (Nickeleit et al., 1998). Type II rejection (endarteritis) was six times more likely to be clinically severe than type I (Colvin et al., 1997), confirming several studies suggesting that endarteritis has adverse prognostic significance (Bates et al., 1999; Magil et al., 1980; Schroeder et al., 1991; Visscher et al., 1991). Type III rejection (fibrinoid necrosis of the arterial wall) has a well-known adverse prognostic significance in all series (Banfi et al., 1981; Bates et al., 1999; Burke et al., 1995b; Matas et al., 1983; Visscher et al., 1991). A definitive study by Bates et al. (1999) at Oxford independently showed that CCTT categories fit well with prognosis. In biopsy specimens from 293 patients 2 to 35 days posttransplant, the 3-month graft survival was about 95% for type I (including the Banff borderline, I and IIa, which behaved the same), 85% for type II and 10% for type III; the graft survival at 5 years was 78%, 60% and 0%. The CCTT system has certain objective and major advantages, notably simplicity and reproducibility, while retaining sensitivity, specificity and clinically relevant prognostic implications.

Driven by the limitations of the initial Banff formulation, a fundamental revision was achieved by consensus in 1997 (Racusen, 1999; Table 24–3). The changes recognized the strengths of the CCTT system (simplicity and clear and clini-

TABLE 24–2

COOPERATIVE CLINICAL TRIALS IN TRANSPLANTATION CRITERIA FOR ACUTE RENAL ALLOGRAFT REJECTION

Type I	At least 5% of the cortex must have interstitial mononuclear infiltration with at least 2 of the following 3 features present: edema, tubular degeneration and/or injury or reactive lymphoblasts. Tubulitis must be present, with at least 3 tubules affected in 10 serial high-power fields (× 40) from the areas with the most infiltrate
Type II	Arterial mononuclear endothelial inflammation (endarteritis or endotheliitis) is present (with or without features of type I)
Type III	Arterial fibrinoid necrosis or transmural inflammation. May be accompanied by thrombosis, parenchymal necrosis and/or recent infarction or hemorrhage

Reproduced with permission of Colvin et al., 1997.

TABLE 24–3

COMPARISON OF CLASSIFICATION SYSTEMS FOR ACUTE RENAL ALLOGRAFT REJECTION

Common Name	Banff 93–95*	Revised Banff Classification†	CCTT‡
Tubulointerstitial Rejection			
	Borderline[1]	Suspicious[1, 2]	Type I
	Grade I[1]	Type I (a,b)[1, 3]	
	Grade IIa[1]		
Endarteritis (intimal arteritis)			
	Grade IIb	Type II (a,b)[5]	Type II
	Grade III[4]		
Fibrinoid necrosis/transmural inflammation			
	Grade III[6]	Type III[7]	Type III

*Solez *et al.,* 1993a.
†Racusen *et al.,* 1999.
‡Colvin *et al.,* 1997.
[1]Differ in the degree of tubulitis and infiltration. Does not require tubular injury, lymphoblasts or edema *vs.* CCTT type I.
[2]Same as previous borderline, but with the lower limit of infiltrate defined as 10% (instead of *trivial*).
[3]Type Ia and Ib differ in the extent of infiltrate and tubulitis (Ia is the old I; Ib is the old IIa). The combination of suspicious and category I is equivalent to CCTT type I (except for the edema, activated lymphocytes and tubular injury).
[4]Subset of grade III with severe endarteritis.
[5]Endarteritis required; no longer includes severe tubulointerstitial rejection (old IIa); mild-to-moderate endarteritis is now IIa (formerly IIb); severe endarteritis is now IIb (formerly part of grade III). Identical to CCTT type II.
[6]Subset of grade III with fibrinoid necrosis or transmural inflammation.
[7]Type III no longer includes severe endarteritis (moved to IIb) or hemorrhage or infarction as the only abnormality. Identical to CCTT type III.
CCTT = Cooperative Clinical Trials in Transplantation. Reproduced with permission of Colvin, 1998.

cally meaningful categories), while retaining the opportunity to *Banff score* individual features. The grades were changed to the CCTT types, with one exception: The Banff *borderline* category was retained and renamed *suspicious for rejection.* The rationale for the term *suspicious* is that many but not all of these cases are rejection; if the clinician has any other evidence that favors rejection (e.g., a rise in creatinine), these are scored as type I rejection in the CCTT, provided that the criteria of edema and activated lymphocytes and/or tubular injury are met. Banff still does not require evidence of injury and/or activation for the diagnosis of active rejection, in contrast to CCTT. Hemorrhage and infarction were removed as criteria for Banff type III rejection because they may have other causes.

At present, for practical clinical use, we can see little added value in the microscoring of the Banff system and prefer the basic categories of CCTT, as in the revised Banff/CCTT system. The *suspicious* category warrants further study because, in our opinion, most of the cases are probably active rejection, either clinical or subclinical (see the discussion of protocol biopsies later). The suspicious category particularly would be a classification problem for drug trials that have *histologically confirmed* rejection as a primary endpoint. The CCTT system has no ambiguity, and if any trend were evident in our studies, cases with the least infiltrate tended to have a worse prognosis (Nickeleit *et al.,* 1999). We now propose an additional category for acute humoral rejection, with separation of cases with capillary involvement (peritubular and/or glomerular capillaries) from cases with fibrinoid necrosis (see Table 24–1).

Chronic Rejection

Although slow, progressive loss of renal function occurs in about 25% of patients, when all renal allografts functioning and nonfunctioning at death are considered, the nature of the lesion is debated (Hostetter, 1994). Many workers use the term *chronic rejection* to encompass the myriad of structural and functional alterations that develop slowly (months) and generally lead to graft loss in a period of years. We prefer to reserve the term *chronic rejection* for chronic injury primarily mediated by an immune reaction to donor alloantigens. When the cause is unknown, *chronic allograft nephropathy* can be used, but its lack of specificity is a testimony to an inability to make a more definitive diagnosis. Although some have argued that the renal biopsy is not useful in analyzing graft dysfunction after 1 year, the data show that in 8 (Kon *et al.,* 1997) to 39% (Pascual *et al.,* 1999) of patients, the biopsy led to a change in management that improved renal function.

The chronically rejected kidney is pale and fibrotic with a dense, thick, adherent capsule. The weight may be normal or increased because of previous compensatory hypertrophy. If the patient returns to dialysis (or receives another graft), the remaining original graft usually becomes progressively smaller and fibrotic and may undergo calcification. The cortical surface typically is smooth, indicating uniform atrophy, and the cortex and medulla are proportionately affected. The thickened, obliterated arcuate arteries often can be appreciated at the corticomedullary junction. The larger arteries also are commonly affected by the rejection process and show fibrous intimal thickening up to the point of anastomosis with the recipient artery (Porter *et al.,* 1963).

CHRONIC GLOMERULAR LESIONS

Glomerular abnormalities first were recognized in long-term grafts and related to rejection by Porter *et al.* (1967). The morphological definition of chronic allograft glomerulopathy may be taken as duplication of the GBM with modest mesangial expansion, in the absence of specific *de novo* or recurrent glomerular disease. The glomeruli show an increase in mesangial cells and matrix with various degrees of scarring and adhesions. In some cases, mesangiolysis or webbing of the mesangium may be prominent. Most cases show the classic duplication of the GBM, segmentally or globally, on PAS or silver stains, with associated cellular (mononuclear or mesangial cell) interposition (Fig. 24–8A). The nonduplicated GBM may become slightly thickened, attributable to compensatory hypertrophy. Variable global or segmental glomerulosclerosis is seen. Focal adhesion of the tip of the glomerular

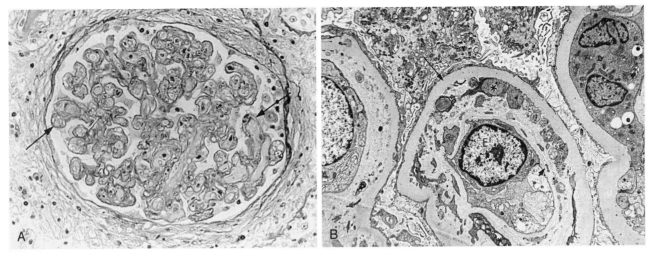

FIGURE 24–8

Chronic allograft glomerulopathy. (A) Widespread duplication of the glomerular basement membrane (GBM) and cellular interposition (arrows). The mesangium is slightly prominent, but cellularity and matrix are not increased; rather, mesangiolysis or webbing is observed in areas. (B) High-power electron microscopy of a glomerular capillary shows duplication of the GBM; the new or second layer of GBM (short arrowhead) forms underneath the endothelium (E) and is separated from the old GBM layer (long arrow) by the cellular (mononuclear or mesangial cell) interposition. (A, PAS × 250; EM × 7,700.)

tuft to the origin of the tubule, the so-called glomerular tip lesion, is common after 1 year (Lee and Howie, 1988). In serial sections, 18% of glomeruli were found to be *atubular* (without a proximal tubular orifice) in recipients with chronic rejection, compared with 1 to 2% in normal donors (Pagtalunan *et al.*, 1996). Atubular glomeruli were about 30% smaller in volume but could not be distinguished otherwise from open glomeruli by their appearance on single sections. Immunofluorescence microscopy typically shows scant segmental granular deposits of immunoglobulin (typically IgM and IgG, rarely IgA), C3 and sometimes fibrin in the capillary wall and in the mesangium (Busch *et al.*, 1971a; McKenzie and Whittingham, 1968; Porter *et al.*, 1968).

Electron microscopy reveals duplication of the GBM (Fig. 24–8B), often accompanied by cellular (mononuclear or mesangial cell) interposition, widening or lucency of the subendothelial space and a moderate increase in mesangial matrix and cells (Habib and Broyer, 1993). The GBM typically has rarefactions, microfibrils and cellular debris but little deposits (Busch *et al.*, 1971a; Hsu *et al.*, 1980; Porter *et al.*, 1967). These changes have been categorized into five ultrastructural types by Olsen *et al.* (1974). Type I is categorized by the presence of electron-lucent subendothelial flocculent material, which is common and may be seen in acute rejection as well. In one study, subendothelial lucency was present in 74% of the routine biopsy specimens taken at about 2 years (Porter *et al.*, 1967). This glomerular change may be seen in the absence of other features of chronic rejection (Porter *et al.*, 1967). Type II is categorized by the presence of granular electron dense deposits, similar to immune complexes in other diseases, and may be subendothelial or mesangial (Olsen *et al.*, 1974; Petersen *et al.*, 1975). Type III and IV deposits are small (III) and large (IV) vesicles scattered about along the GBM (and may be seen in mesangium as well) and probably represent cellular debris. These were once thought to be viruses. The type V deposits in the GBM are membranous ribbons that may be remnants of the slit diaphragms or other membranous debris. Endothelial cells may appear reactive with loss of fenestrae, probably undergoing *dedifferentiation* (Colvin, 1998; Hsu *et al.*, 1980; Porter *et al.*, 1967). Podocyte foot process effacement ranges from minimal to quite extensive (Hsu *et al.*, 1980), corresponding to the degree of proteinuria.

TUBULES AND INTERSTITIUM

Tubular atrophy and interstitial fibrosis are regular but nonspecific features of chronic rejection and do not serve to distinguish rejection from other causes, such as cyclosporine toxicity or ischemic injury. Tubular atrophy may be focal or widespread accompanied by the interstitial fibrosis. The TBMs of atrophied tubules are thickened and duplicated. Atrophic tubules typically have thickened, duplicated TBMs and intratubular mononuclear cells and mast cells (Colvin *et al.*, 1974). This appearance should not be confused with the tubulitis of acute rejection. The interstitium typically has a sparse mononuclear infiltrate, with small lymphocytes, plasma cells and mast cells (Colvin and Dvorak, 1974). Nodular collections of quiescent-appearing lymphoid cells sometimes are found around small arcuate arteries. Abundant plasma cells may be present; some of these patients respond to antiviral drugs. The presence of monomorphic immature lymphoid cells or necrosis should raise the possibility of posttransplant lymphoproliferative disease (PTLD).

The TBM commonly has deposition of C3 in a broad segmental pattern. This deposition is an exaggeration of similar changes found in normal kidneys and probably represents residue from prior episodes of tubular injury or possibly a persistent chronic injury. Linear IgG TBM deposits and associated circulating anti-TBM antibodies may be detected in about 3% of cases (Rotellar *et al.*, 1986). Of the biopsy specimens, 48% with linear TBM deposits were from stable patients, and 32% had only minimal histological changes. Linear IgG did not correlate with prior rejection episodes or graft survival, although those with circulating antibodies were not analyzed separately. The TBM shows pronounced thickening and duplication of the basement membrane in chronic rejection (Nadasdy *et al.*, 1995; Reinholt *et al.*, 1990). These changes probably are nonspecific and related to tubular atrophy that can be seen in other conditions of chronic renal failure. These changes do not correlate with deposition of immune reactants by immunofluorescence (Reinholt *et al.*, 1990).

PERITUBULAR CAPILLARIES

Peritubular capillaries may be dilated and prominent, with thick basement membranes, or may disappear alto-

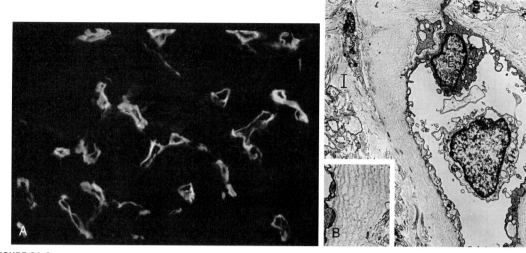

FIGURE 24–9

Chronic humoral rejection. (A) Immunofluorescence microscopy shows peritubular capillaries with bright and diffuse staining for C4d (monoclonal antibody), indicating activation of the classic complement pathway, triggered by humoral antidonor antibodies (See color plate). (B) Electron microscopy shows high magnification of a peritubular capillary with multilamination (arrow) of the basement membrane. Inset is a higher magnification of the area marked by the arrow. E-endothelium; I-interstitium. (A, streptavidin-FITC, × 400; B, EM × 5,200; inset, × 11,200.)

gether, leaving only occasional traces of the original basement membrane behind (Bishop *et al.*, 1989). Peritubular capillaries generally are negative for immunoglobulin staining, and only focal C3 and fibrin staining may be identified. Most cases of chronic renal allograft rejection (60%) have prominent C4d deposition (Mauiyyedi *et al.*, 2000; Fig. 24–9A), however. Cases with C4d deposition typically had circulating antidonor HLA class I or II reactive antibodies by *in vitro* cytotoxicity (82% *vs.* 0% of controls, P<.003). Cases without C4d did not have circulating antidonor antibody. Most, but not necessarily all, of the antibodies are reactive to donor HLA antigens expressed on lymphocytes.

Electron microscopy often reveals splitting and multilayering of the peritubular capillary basement membrane (Mazzucco *et al.*, 1994; Monga *et al.*, 1992; Fig. 24–9B). These lesions were described in 75% of transplant specimens (the sampling was skewed to the more chronic lesions because 60% had chronic transplant glomerulopathy). The severity of the lesions, but not the prevalence, is associated with the presence of glomerulopathy. The pattern of the ultrastructural changes in the glomeruli and capillaries was similar, which suggested that they share the same pathogenetic mechanisms, probably resulting from immunological endothelial cell damage. Basement membrane lamination and C4d deposition in peritubular capillaries in chronic rejection are highly correlated, arguing that the lamination may be the result of repair after antibody-mediated damage (Mauiyyedi *et al.*, 2000b).

CHRONIC ARTERIAL LESIONS

Small and large arteries 1 month after transplantation can begin to develop severe intimal proliferation and luminal narrowing (Burke *et al.*, 1995a; Colvin *et al.*, 1995). The intimal change is most prominent in the larger arteries but can be seen at all levels, from interlobular arteries to the main renal artery. The intima shows pronounced, concentric fibrous thickening with invasion and proliferation of spindle-shaped myofibroblasts. This vascular change has been termed *chronic allograft arteriopathy*. A variable infiltrate of mononuclear cells may be present in the intima, which is characteristic of chronic rejection (Fig. 24–10). The subendothelial mononu-

clear cells remain one of the most distinctive features of chronic allograft arteriopathy and argue that the endothelium itself is a target.

The intimal matrix generally is loose, somewhat pale in hematoxylin and eosin–stained sections, containing acid mucopolysaccharides with increased hyaluronic acid (Wells *et al.*, 1990), collagen and sometimes elastic fibers. The internal elastica may be disrupted and duplicated. Fibrin sometimes is deposited in a bandlike subendothelial location or mural thrombus. Foamy macrophages containing lipid droplets characteristically are seen along the internal elastica and can be found 4 weeks after transplantation. Focal myocyte loss from the media occurs in association with a sparse T-cell infiltrate, as shown in mouse and rat studies (Russell *et al.*, 1994a). Immunofluorescence often shows IgM, C3 and fibrin

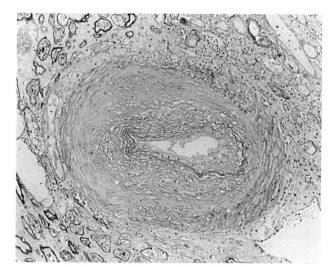

FIGURE 24–10

Chronic allograft arteriopathy. An interlobular artery with prominent intimal fibroplasia and reduplication of the internal elastic lamina. The presence of scattered mononuclear cells in the intima is characteristic of chronic rejection. (PAS × 200.)

and/or fibrinogen staining along the endothelium, in the intima or in the media, as a diffuse blush or focal granular deposits (Andres et al., 1970; Busch et al., 1971a; Jeannet et al., 1970; McKenzie and Whittingham, 1968; Petersen et al., 1975). Sometimes these deposits may be accompanied by IgG deposition.

The intima of affected arteries shows accumulation of myointimal cells (α-smooth muscle actin positive), a mononuclear infiltrate of T cells (CD4$^+$, CD8$^+$ and CD45RO$^+$), macrophages (HLA-DR positive) and dendritic cells (S100 positive) (Gouldesbrough and Axelsen, 1994; Oguma et al., 1988; Salomon et al., 1991). The T cells express cytotoxic markers, including perforin (Fox et al., 1993) and GMP-17 (Meehan et al., 1997). No B cells (CD20) were detected (Gouldesbrough and Axelsen, 1994). Proliferation of mononuclear cells, spindle cells and endothelium was detected with proliferating cell nuclear antigen which stained a few of the cells (Gouldesbrough and Axelsen, 1994). The endothelium expresses increased adhesion molecules, notably ICAM-1 and VCAM-1. Antagonism of ICAM-1 binding and/or expression inhibits chronic rejection (Russell et al., 1995), and in humans certain ICAM-1 genetic polymorphisms (e.g., exon 4, the Mac-1 binding site) appear to confer higher risk for chronic rejection (McLaren et al., 1999). The endothelium generally remains of donor origin (Hruban et al., 1993; Sedmak et al., 1988); however, some of the spindle-shaped cells that contribute to the intimal thickening are of recipient origin (Kennedy and Weissman, 1971; Oguma et al., 1988).

The myointimal cells stain prominently for α-smooth muscle actin, sometimes so strikingly that a *double media* seems to be formed (Sacchi et al., 1993). This phenomenon also has been described as the development of a new artery inside and concentric with the old (Howie et al., 1992), with elastic laminae and a muscular media, separated poorly from the old internal elastic lamina by cellular tissue. The extracellular matrix in the thickened intima consists of collagen, fibronectin, tenascin, proteoglycans and acid mucopolysaccharides (Colvin, 1995; Gould et al., 1992; McManus et al., 1995). The fibronectin has the extra domain A of cellular fibronectin, typical of embryonic or wound healing fibronectin (Gould et al., 1992). The vessels synthesize the proteoglycans biglycan and decorin, and proteoglycan proteins are increased in the intima (McManus et al., 1995). Several growth factors and cytokines have been detected. Platelet-derived growth factor A chain protein is primarily in endothelial cells, whereas the B chain is in macrophages and smooth muscle cells (Alpers et al., 1996). Enhanced platelet-derived growth factor B-type receptor protein was found on intimal cells and on smooth muscle cells of the proliferating vessels (Fellstrom et al., 1989). Fibroblast growth factor-1 and its receptor are present in the thickened intima (Kerby et al., 1996). Tumor necrosis factor-α is in the smooth muscle of vessels with chronic rejection in contrast to normal kidneys (Noronha et al., 1992).

By electron microscopy, the thickened arterial intima consists of myofibroblasts, collagen fibrils, basement membrane material and a loose amorphous electron lucent ground substance (Porter, 1990). Scattered lymphocytes and macrophages usually are present, the latter sometimes filled with fine lipid droplets corresponding to the foam cells by light microscopy. With time, the cellularity diminishes, and the amount of collagen increases (Busch et al., 1971b). Scanning electron microscopy shows endothelial cell injury, disorganization of the endothelium and gaps between endothelial cells, often with leukocytes and platelets (Young-Ramsaran et al., 1993).

The vascular lesions of renal allografts can be divided into three stages, which probably differ in mechanism and reversibility (Colvin, 1998). The stage 1 lesion is endarteritis, characteristic of type II acute cellular rejection. This lesion lacks matrix formation. This acute stage is believed to be T cell mediated, primarily directed at the endothelium. Stage 2 lesions have intimal matrix production and accumulation of myofibroblasts forming a neointima. This lesion may contain mononuclear cells (T cells and macrophages) that are believed to be active. This stage clearly arises as a result of an immunological rejection reaction, as proposed by Porter et al. (1963), and can be distinguished from other causes of intimal fibrosis by virtue of the infiltrate. Humoral antibody is believed to promote transition to the fibrous stage (see later in discussion of pathogenesis). Secondary factors probably become increasingly important as the lesion progresses to stage 3, where the intima is fibrous and inflammatory cells are scant. This stage is largely irreversible. Stage 2 and 3 arterial lesions have been termed *graft atherosclerosis, accelerated atherosclerosis, chronic allograft arteriosclerosis, graft vascular disease, allograft vascular sclerosis* and *chronic allograft arteriopathy*, among other terms. The authors prefer the last term because it specifies a chronic process of allograft arteries, in which *arteriopathy* reflects the uncertain pathogenesis and may totally lack lipid. A fourth category resembling natural atherosclerosis with cholesterol clefts and calcification has been proposed (Gouldesbrough and Axelsen, 1994).

Arterioles generally do not show the intimal changes but may have subendothelial hyaline deposits (hyalin or hyalinosis). Such lesions may not be due to rejection and may represent donor disease, recipient diabetes, hypertension, aging or chronic cyclosporine toxicity. It has been observed in the precyclosporine era, however, that afferent and efferent hyalinization is commonest when there is also chronic transplant glomerulopathy (Porter et al., 1966).

The pathogenesis of chronic rejection has been investigated actively, and there is now direct proof in animals that the prototypical process that affects arteries (chronic allograft arteriopathy) is immunologically mediated (Colvin, 1998). The vast experimental data can be summarized as follows:

1. The lesions do not routinely arise in isografts.
2. The target antigens can be major or minor histocompatibility antigens (Adams et al., 1992; Cramer et al., 1989; Russell et al., 1994a).
3. The specific initiator is probably T cells followed by antibody (antibody is necessary and sufficient for the fibrous lesion in mice).
4. The target cell is probably the endothelium, but the smooth muscle also may be affected.
5. Secondary nonimmunologic mechanisms analogous to those in atherosclerosis are important in the progression of the lesion.
6. Ultimately the process may be independent of specific antidonor immunological activity.

Studies in inbred genetically altered mice have provided further arguments in favor of an important, if not crucial, role for antibodies. Antibodies were able to initiate florid graft intimal fibrosis without participation of T cells in immunodeficient *scid* mice given repeated doses of anti–class I alloantibody. Under these conditions, the allografts develop fibrous intimal thickening of coronary arteries over 1 to 2 months (Russell et al., 1994b). Conversely, although T cells are sufficient to initiate cellular vascular lesions in B cell–deficient mice, the lesions do not progress to fibrosis in the absence of antibody (Russell et al., 1997). Fibrous lesions also are reduced markedly in strain combinations that fail to elicit a humoral antibody response.

The evidence in humans for a role of antibodies has been largely circumstantial. Alloantibodies to graft class I antigens are a specific risk factor for chronic transplant arteriopathy in human renal allografts (Davenport et al., 1994; Jeannet et al., 1970). There are several interpretations of the correlation between chronic transplant arteriopathy and circulating antibody: (1) The antibodies are a consequence of rejection, not a cause; (2) the antibodies are secondary to another immune reactivity, the latter causing the arteriopathy (e.g., Th2) and (3) the antibodies cause the arteriopathy. We have obtained direct pathological evidence (C4d deposition) that a substantial subset of chronic rejection in humans has a detectable humoral component, as described earlier (Mauiyyedi et al., 1999, 2000c). This evidence argues that a major subset of chronic rejection is mediated by antibodies, usually to HLA antigens, that fix complement at the level of the peritubular capillaries.

CLASSIFICATION SYSTEMS FOR CHRONIC REJECTION

The classification systems for chronic rejection are still primitive, largely as a result of ignorance of pathogenesis. The systems for grading chronic rejection generally are based on adding the scores of three component parts—tubulo-interstitial, vascular and glomerular (Isoniemi et al., 1994; Kasiske et al., 1991; Racusen et al., 1999). The primary assumption is that these components are part of the same process (i.e., the consequence of chronic endothelial damage); however, many workers would argue that different pathogenetic factors contribute to each lesion. The Banff system grades the different elements into three categories, as various degrees of *chronic transplant nephropathy* (Solez, 1994).

The chronic allograft damage index system (Isoniemi et al., 1994) has been used and shown to correlate with long-term outcome. The components scored are interstitial fibrosis, tubular atrophy, arterial intimal thickening, glomerular sclerosis, mesangial expansion and GBM duplication (Kasiske et al., 1991). The sum score in biopsy specimens taken at 2 years correlated with graft function at 6 years, but there was a fair amount of scatter (Isoniemi et al., 1994). Similarly a chronic graft damage score calculated at 6 months is associated strongly with graft loss 2 to 3 years after transplantation (Dimeny et al., 1995). It is hoped that a new system will be developed in the future with pathogenetically based diagnostic categories, such as chronic humoral rejection, and indicators of ongoing activity, such as apoptosis or proliferative markers.

Protocol Biopsies

Protocol biopsies are, by definition, performed at specific times for evaluation of the status of the renal allograft, independent of renal function, usually as part of a clinical research trial. Subclinical processes can be detected, such as immunological rejection, calcineurin inhibitor toxicity or recurrent disease, which may warrant treatment. That an infiltrate occurs in stable grafts, especially in the first 2 months, has been known since the 1980s (Burdick et al., 1984; McWhinnie et al., 1986). This knowledge implied that an allograft infiltrate is not sufficient to diagnose rejection. Interest has been raised by the systematic studies of Rush and colleagues, however, who made the surprising observation that 30% of biopsy specimens from stable patients 1 to 3 months posttransplant showed histological rejection (Rush et al., 1994), and grafts with these lesions show later loss of renal function (Rush et al., 1995, 1998). A study by Legendre and colleagues made the equally surprising observation that 25% of recipients of cadaveric kidneys who had no clinically overt rejection episodes had chronic allograft nephropathy evident histologically in protocol biopsy specimens at 3

months, and 50% had such lesions at 6 months (Legendre et al., 1998).

The first question is whether the inflammation detected is truly subclinical rejection and, if so, whether any structural or molecular features distinguish subclinical active rejection from innocent inflammation. In one of the early clinicopathological correlative studies, Rush and colleagues found that patients with the least inflammation in the protocol biopsy specimens at 1 to 6 months (as judged by the cumulative *Banff Score for Inflammatory Changes*) had the most normal histology and the lowest serum creatinine value at 12 months (Rush et al., 1995). Similar data were reported by Legendre and colleagues, who found that subclinical type I rejection in a 3-month protocol was associated with progression of histological lesions at 6 months (Legendre et al., 1998). This experience argues that inflammation in the renal allograft, even if subclinical, is pathogenic. By polymerase chain reaction analysis, protocol biopsy specimens with an infiltrate that meet the criteria of rejection have an enhanced expression of proinflammatory gene transcripts (e.g., cytotoxic T-cell effector molecules and interferon-γ), arguing that the process is pathogenetic, despite the stable renal function at the time (Lipman et al., 1998).

Are there features that correlate with aggressive infiltrates (i.e., rejection)? Published data in human biopsy specimens suggest that the following features are more typical of active than subclinical rejection: an increased number of CD8$^+$ cells (Hammer et al., 1983), especially diffuse infiltrates (Ibrahim et al., 1995); a denser infiltrate of T memory and/or activated cells (CD45RO$^+$) (Ibrahim et al., 1995); invasion of tubules by CD57$^+$ cells (Beschorner et al., 1985; Marcussen et al., 1996) and apoptosis (Ito et al., 1995). One exceptional patient from Rush's first study had endothelialitis (CCTT/Banff type II rejection) and developed clinically overt rejection a few days after the biopsy (Rush et al., 1994). Few if any of the protocol biopsy specimens in other studies (including our own in experimental animals) show type II rejection, suggesting that this type of rejection is rarely subclinical.

Investigation in animals, which can be done with greater experimental control, has revealed that not all infiltrates are aggressive. Grafts in animals that are developing tolerance typically have graft infiltrates, which we have termed the *acceptance reaction* (Shimizu et al., 1997). The acceptance infiltrate differed from that in rejecting grafts, in certain features, including less infiltration by CD3$^+$ T cells and macrophages, less T-cell activation (CD25, proliferating cell nuclear antigen), absent endarteritis and less apoptosis of graft cells. The grafts also expressed less interferon-γ and more IL-10 than rejecting grafts by Northern blotting (Blancho et al., 1997). In certain class I disparate murine and pig renal allografts, the intense infiltrate disappears spontaneously and is followed by indefinite graft survival (Blancho et al., 1997; Russell et al., 1978). The fascinating question raised by these studies is whether the infiltrate contains immunoregulatory cells important in the adaptation of the host to the graft.

A second question to be answered by protocol biopsies is whether any features predict the later development of chronic rejection. A study by Nickerson et al. (1998) addressed this question—to identify early clinical and pathological variables that predict independently diminished renal allograft function at 24 months posttransplant. Seventy-one patients in whom protocol renal biopsies were performed at 1, 2, 3, 6 and 12 months posttransplant were studied, and the findings were correlated with the 24-month serum creatinine. The best histological predictor of the 24-month serum creatinine or the rise from 6 to 24 months was the protocol biopsy score at 3 and 6 months. In an effort to identify early predictors of chronic rejection, Furness and colleagues studied a consecutive series of 52 renal transplant recipients with protocol biopsies at 1, 3, and 6 months. They found that the morphometric extent of immunostained collagen III at 6 months (using 40% of the area as a threshold) correlated with a significantly lower glomerular filtration rate at 24 months and a progressive deterioration in graft function (Nicholson et al., 1999).

Another reason for interest in protocol biopsies is the possibility that newer immunosuppressive drugs may reduce the frequency of clinically overt rejection but not prevent subclinical injury (Sollinger, 1995). Nickerson and colleagues showed that 17 patients taking mycophenolate mofetil and cyclosporine had a decreased incidence of clinical overt rejection episodes in the first 3 months but had the same prevalence of early subclinical rejection on biopsy specimens as patients taking azathioprine and cyclosporine in the past (Nickerson et al., 1999).

The most important question is whether treatment of subclinical rejection is beneficial (and then what therapy is optimal). The definitive answer depends on randomized treatment of patients who undergo protocol biopsies. To date, no trial has been done in which treatment was randomized according to the biopsy results. The closest trial, done by Rush's group, randomized patients to undergo biopsies or not at 1, 2, and 3 months; those whose biopsy specimens showed rejection were treated with increased corticosteroids, and the outcome (including biopsies at 6 and 12 months) was compared with the control group who did not undergo early biopsies (Rush et al., 1998). Compared with controls, patients in the biopsy arm had a significant decrease in acute rejection episodes 9 months posttransplant, reduced tubular atrophy and interstitial fibrosis at 6 months (all underwent biopsy then) and a lower serum creatinine at 24 months. This study supports the hypothesis that the treatment of early subclinical rejection with corticosteroids leads to better long-term outcomes (Rush et al., 1998). The correct answer must be obtained in rigorous clinical trials because every treatment with immunosuppression carries a risk. In some animal tolerance regimens, treatment of subclinical infiltrates with steroids triggers rejection (Yamada et al., 1999).

Acute Tubular Necrosis

The morphological basis of delayed graft function is usually acute ischemic injury, commonly called *acute tubular necrosis* (ATN). The term is a misnomer in human pathology because necrosis of the tubular cells is not generally conspicuous. The term *acute tubular injury* or *ischemia* is preferred. Necrotic and apoptotic tubular cells are found by electron microscopy in transplant ATN more frequently than in native kidney ATN, however (Olsen et al., 1989; Solez et al., 1993). Broad zones of actual tubular necrosis are due to vascular thrombosis and/or occlusion, surgical trauma or severe rejection.

The commonest feature histologically of ATN in our experience is loss of the brush borders of proximal tubular cells, best shown on PAS stain. The tubular lumen appears larger than normal and lacks the usual artifactual sloughing of the apical cytoplasm in human renal biopsy specimens (this sloughing has occurred *in vivo* and was washed downstream) (Fig. 24–11). The other features of ATN include flattening of the cytoplasm and loss of cell nuclei as a result of apoptosis and/or death of individual tubular epithelial cells and covering of the TBM by the remaining cells. The lumina contain individual apoptotic detached cells (*anoikis*) and inflammatory cells. Reactive changes in the tubular epithelium are seen after 24 to 48 hours, including large basophilic nuclei

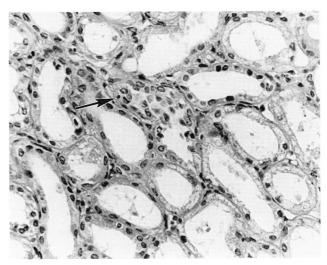

FIGURE 24–11

Acute tubular necrosis. Dilated rigid-appearing tubular lumina with loss of brush borders, cytoplasmic flattening and nuclear apoptoses (arrow). (H&E × 400.)

with prominent nucleoli, increased cytoplasmic basophilia and occasionally mitoses. In our experience, mitoses rarely are found in patients taking cyclosporine. In confirmation of this impression, nuclear staining of tubules for proliferating cell nuclear antigen, principally in proximal tubules, was lower in patients taking cyclosporine, suggesting that cyclosporine may have an inhibitory effect on cell regeneration (Nadasdy et al., 1995). Some interstitial infiltrates of mononuclear cells or neutrophils may be present, but usually these are not prominent.

Immediate graft failure can result from machine or manual perfusion injury, a problem that was commoner in the past (Spector et al., 1976). Biopsy specimens show loss of endothelial cells and plugs of platelet aggregates and fibrin in the microvasculature, especially in glomeruli with sparse neutrophils (Evan et al., 1983; Spector et al., 1976). Mechanical flushing of cadaveric kidneys with organ preservation fluid immediately before transplantation, which has been advocated by some workers, was associated with abnormal cellular debris within the tubules, eosinophilic proteinaceous material within Bowman's capsule and increased frequency of delayed graft function (Roake et al., 1996).

Cyclosporine and Tacrolimus Nephrotoxicity

Cyclosporine nephrotoxicity has been divided into three categories—acute nephrotoxicity, chronic nephrotoxicity, and thrombotic microangiopathy (hemolytic-uremic syndrome) (Mihatsch et al., 1983, 1995b). Cyclosporine binds to the *cyclophilins*, a family of peptidyl-prolyl cis-trans isomerases, also known as *immunophilins*, which includes the FK binding proteins (Borel and Kis, 1991). The cyclosporine-cyclophilin and the tacrolimus-FKBP complexes inhibit calcineurin, a phosphatase involved in signal trafficking to the nucleus, necessary to trigger T-cell cytokine synthesis. Nephrotoxicity also seems to be related to calcineurin inhibition because all cyclosporine congeners that lack nephrotoxicity also lack immunosuppressive potency (Sigal et al., 1991). Cyclosporine and tacrolimus induce the same spectrum of renal lesions, and perhaps the term *calcineurin inhibitor nephrotoxicity* is more apt. Pathological diagnosis of cyclosporine toxicity was made in 61% of renal allograft biopsy specimens in an early series (Sibley *et al.*, 1983) and in 38% almost a decade later (Kiss *et al.*, 1992). The only patients in whom cyclosporine toxicity can be excluded are those not receiving the drug (Colvin, 1998).

ACUTE CYCLOSPORINE TOXICITY

The biopsy features of acute toxicity are variable—from no morphological abnormality to acute tubular injury, marked tubular vacuolization and vascular smooth muscle apoptosis. A normal biopsy specimen is found in *functional cyclosporine toxicity*, which is due to reversible vasospasm (Remuzzi and Perico, 1995).

The proximal tubules show the most conspicuous morphological changes of acute cyclosporine toxicity with loss of brush borders and isometric (uniformly sized), clear, fine vacuolization (or microvacuoles) in the epithelial cells (Fig. 24–12). The microvacuoles contain clear aqueous fluid rather than lipid and are indistinguishable from those caused by osmotic diuretics or ischemia. Electron microscopy shows that the vacuoles in cyclosporine toxicity are due to dilatation of the endoplasmic reticulum and appear empty (Mihatsch *et al.*, 1988). Isometric vacuolization is said to predominate in the straight portion of the proximal tubule (Mihatsch *et al.*, 1988), although in our experience, it also occurs in the convoluted portion. The degree of vacuolization does not correlate with blood cyclosporine levels; some patients with cyclosporine toxicity lack the vacuolar change (Nast *et al.*, 1989), and isometric vacuoles can be found in a few patients with stable renal function (Solez *et al.*, 1993). Repeat renal biopsy specimens after reduction of the cyclosporine dose have shown disappearance of tubular vacuolization (Versluis *et al.*, 1988).

Arterioles are a significant target of cyclosporine toxicity. The most characteristic acute changes include individual medial smooth muscle cell degeneration, necrosis and/or apoptosis and loss of smooth muscle cells (Mihatsch *et al.*, 1988). The apoptotic smooth muscle cells are later replaced by rounded, lumpy protein deposits or hyalinosis, which is the beginning of the chronic arteriolopathy (Mihatsch *et al.*, 1988). Accumulation of glycogen (PAS positive, diastase sensitive) in smooth muscle cells has been described in patients on high-dose cyclosporine (Larsen *et al.*, 1989). Endothelial

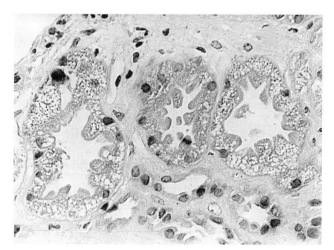

FIGURE 24–12

Acute cyclosporine nephrotoxicity. Isometric vacuolization of tubular epithelium. This change is commonly associated with acute cyclosporine toxicity but can be seen in other conditions, such as ischemia, acute tubular necrosis and secondary to osmotic diuretics. (H&E × 400.)

cells can have prominent vacuolization and some swelling. Immunofluorescence microscopy of the vessels often shows deposits of IgM, C3 and sometimes fibrin and/or fibrinogen, but these changes are nonspecific (Bergstrand *et al.*, 1985). A tendency of mononuclear cells to remain in the peritubular capillaries, rather than infiltrate the interstitium, was once regarded as characteristic of cyclosporine toxicity (Sibley *et al.*, 1983). This idea has not been confirmed in later studies because this tendency can be seen as an early feature of acute cellular rejection in patients who have not received cyclosporine (Alpers *et al.*, 1991).

THROMBOTIC MICROANGIOPATHY

Thrombotic microangiopathy (hemolytic-uremic syndrome) resulting from cyclosporine was first reported in bone marrow transplant recipients (Shulman *et al.*, 1981) and occurs in about 1 to 4% of renal allograft recipients even with careful attention to blood cyclosporine levels, suggesting that it is dose independent and probably idiosyncratic (Candinas *et al.*, 1994; Hochstetler *et al.*, 1994). Patients typically present with acute renal failure, thrombocytopenia, microangiopathic hemolytic anemia, elevated lactic dehydrogenase and hyperbilirubinemia. Encephalopathy may be present. Despite these characteristic features, the clinical syndrome often is not recognized before biopsy (Hochstetler *et al.*, 1994). The full syndrome does not always occur, and the thrombotic microangiopathy may be limited to the kidney without systemic signs. Most cases present with a delayed onset and a slower loss of function 1 to 5 months posttransplant (Sommer *et al.*, 1985).

The pathological changes are the same as in thrombotic microangiopathy from other causes. The glomeruli typically have swollen bloodless capillaries with scattered fibrin-platelet thrombi, particularly in the hilum (Shulman *et al.*, 1981), the so-called pouch lesion (Mihatsch *et al.*, 1994). The endothelial cells are swollen and may obliterate the capillary lumina completely (Fig. 24–13A). The GBM is segmentally duplicated with cellular (mononuclear or mesangial cell) interposition best seen by electron microscopy, which also shows the loss of fenestrae and swelling of the endothelial cytoplasm. Variable mesangial expansion, sclerosis and mesangiolysis (Mihatsch *et al.*, 1994) may be seen. Marked congestion and focal, global or segmental necrosis can be present (Van den Berg-Wolf *et al.*, 1988). Mihatsch and colleagues commented that the affected glomeruli usually are supplied by an arteriole with cyclosporine arteriolopathy (Mihatsch *et al.*, 1994).

The small arteries and arterioles have mucoid intimal thickening with acid mucopolysaccharides and extravasated red cells and fragments; necrosis and thrombi may be prominent (Fig. 24–13B). Apoptosis of endothelial and smooth muscle cells is seen. The medial smooth muscle can develop a mucoid appearance with loss of a clear definition of the cells (Neild *et al.*, 1986). The arterioles may show hypertrophy of the endothelial cells and have a constricted appearance (Neild *et al.*, 1986). The vascular lumina may be obliterated partially or completely by intimal proliferation and endothelial swelling. The vascular lesions are severest in the interlobular and arcuate-sized arteries and can lead to cortical infarction (Sommer *et al.*, 1985). By immunofluorescence microscopy, the vessels stain with IgM, C3 and fibrin.

CHRONIC CYCLOSPORINE TOXICITY

Irreversible chronic renal failure resulting from cyclosporine toxicity first was shown in native kidneys of heart transplant patients who received cyclosporine for more than 1 year (Myers *et al.*, 1984). Biopsy specimens showed intersti-

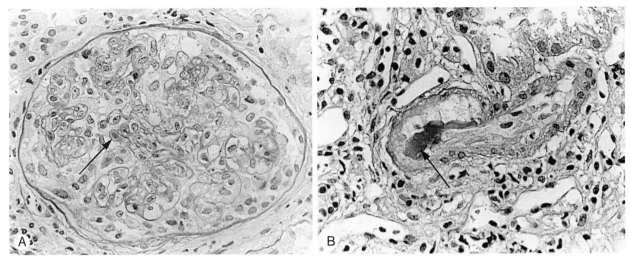

FIGURE 24–13

Thrombotic microangiopathy associated with cyclosporine. (A) Glomerulus with widespread endothelial swelling, segmental glomerular basement membrane duplication and focal fibrin thrombus in a capillary loop (arrow). (B) Small artery with endothelial swelling and fibrin thrombus (arrow). (A, PAS × 400; B, PAS × 500.)

tial fibrosis, tubular atrophy, arteriolar hyalinosis and sometimes focal glomerular scarring. These findings have been confirmed and extended in numerous other studies (Bergstrand et al., 1985). The current consensus is that cyclosporine can cause irreversible renal failure, but the risk is low with the lower doses now employed. Overall, renal allografts have better survival with cyclosporine than without. Because many features resemble chronic rejection in the kidney, the most convincing pathological data come from non–renal transplant patients taking cyclosporine (Dische et al., 1988; Nizze et al., 1988). Predisposing factors for chronic cyclosporine toxicity lesions are renal ischemia and a history of acute nephrotoxicity.

Glomerular Lesions

After 1 year on cyclosporine, glomeruli show increased numbers with global or segmental sclerosis (Dische et al., 1988; Nizze et al., 1988). Focal, segmental sclerosis was commoner in cyclosporine-treated bone marrow (13%) and heart transplant (27%) recipients at autopsy than their respective noncyclosporine controls (0% and 14%) (Nizze et al., 1988). Heart transplant recipients have an increase in the heterogeneity of glomerular volume and size, with more small and large glomeruli (compensatory hypertrophy), compared with controls (living kidney donors) (Myers et al., 1988b). The shift to smaller glomeruli becomes more extreme with chronic renal failure, and the hypertrophied glomeruli disappear (Myers et al., 1988a). Hyperfiltration injury probably causes the progressive glomerular proteinuria and sclerosis. Bone marrow and heart transplant patients at autopsy show glomerular collapse in 59% of patients on cyclosporine versus 8% of patients not on cyclosporine (Nizze et al., 1988). Immunofluorescence findings are nonspecific (IgM and C3). Electron microscopy in cardiac transplant recipients showed diffuse expansion of the mesangial matrix, with little hypercellularity (Myers et al., 1988a). No significant GBM or podocyte abnormality was appreciated. Mild GBM thickening and wrinkling with normal podocytes were described in liver transplant patients with chronic cyclosporine toxicity (Dische et al., 1988). The endothelium may show loss of its normal fenestrae.

Tubules and Interstitium

Tubular atrophy was recognized as a feature of chronic cyclosporine toxicity in early studies, affecting 30% of the cortex by 6 to 8 months (Thiru et al., 1983). This feature was more prominent than increased interstitial fibrosis, perhaps a reflection of direct tubular toxicity. The interstitium has prominent patchy fibrosis, with a scanty infiltrate. Bandlike (striped) narrow zones of fibrosis and tubular atrophy are regarded as characteristic of cyclosporine (Farnsworth et al., 1984; Rosen et al., 1990; Sibley et al., 1983), suggesting a vascular mechanism or damage to the medullary rays. After 1 year, interstitial fibrosis was unchanged or mildly increased compared with 1-month biopsy specimens (Bignardi et al., 1987). In biopsy specimens, it is not easy to appreciate the striped pattern, which appears as nondescript patchy fibrosis with intervening spared cortex. Interstitial fibrosis also develops in nontransplant patients (e.g., therapy for psoriasis, uveitis, type I diabetes) taking cyclosporine (Mihatsch et al., 1991; Palestine et al., 1986; Young et al., 1994; Zachariae et al., 1992) and has been identified in biopsy specimens taken about 1 month after discontinuing cyclosporine (Messana et al., 1995). Low doses of cyclosporine can cause significant and presumably permanent loss of renal function by inducing chronic tubulointerstitial nephritis.

Arteriolopathy

The chronic phase of cyclosporine-associated arteriolopathy is characterized by replacement of the degenerated medial smooth muscle cells with hyalinlike deposits in a beaded pattern along the peripheral, outer media (Fig. 24–14A). This condition has been referred to as *nodular protein (hyalin) deposits* (Mihatsch et al., 1995), in a *pearllike pattern* (Bergstrand et al., 1985) and *peripheral medial nodular hyalinosis*. The current evidence supports the view that this type of arteriolopathy is specific for cyclosporine. In heart and bone marrow transplant recipient autopsy studies, 55% of cases on cyclosporine had this type of arteriolopathy in the native kidneys compared with 0% in cases not on cyclosporine (Nizze et al., 1988). Evidence of apoptosis sometimes is found in the form of karyorrhectic debris in the media but fibrinoid necrosis is

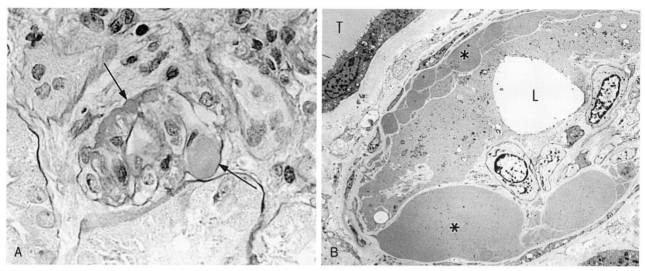

FIGURE 24–14

Chronic cyclosporine arteriolopathy. (A) An arteriole with peripheral nodular hyalinosis, in which hyalin deposits (arrows) replace necrotic and/or apoptotic smooth muscle cells in the outermost media. (B) Electron microscopy shows an artery that has beads of hyalin (*) along the outer media. L-arteriolar lumen; T-tubule. (A, PAS × 800; B, EM × 2,700.)

not observed (Myers *et al.*, 1988b). In severe cases, the media is nearly devoid of smooth muscle cells (Myers *et al.*, 1988b).

Electron microscopy reveals a distinctive replacement of individual smooth muscle cells of afferent arterioles with amorphous electron dense material that contains cell debris and protrudes into the adventitia (Bergstrand *et al.*, 1985; Rossmann *et al.*, 1991; Yamaguchi *et al.*, 1989; Fig. 24–14B). This replacement gives rise to the beaded hyalinosis distribution in the outer media noted by light microscopy. The myocyte nuclei are condensed (apoptotic), and the residual cytoplasm sometimes is vacuolated. In severe cases, the myocytes are depleted. Edema and hypergranulation, dilated endoplasmic reticulum, degenerated mitochondria, lipofuscin granules, multivesicular bodies and a disarray of microfibrils have been noted. The matrix between the myocytes is expanded and filled with similar granular and vesicular material and collagen. Intercellular junctions are decreased, and myocytes with two nuclei and mitotic figures can be observed (Yamaguchi *et al.*, 1989). The endothelium sometimes appears swollen, protruding into and narrowing the lumen and having reduced cell junctions; aggregates of platelets are rare (Antonovych *et al.*, 1988; Yamaguchi *et al.*, 1989). These findings support the view that the smooth muscle myocyte of the afferent arteriole is a primary target of cyclosporine injury. Immunofluorescence microscopy shows IgM and C3 in a relatively nonspecific but conspicuous sheathing of the arterioles (Bergstrand *et al.*, 1985).

The lesion begins and predominates in the afferent arterioles but may progress to the small arteries and efferent arterioles (Bergstrand *et al.*, 1985; Yamaguchi *et al.*, 1989). In severe cyclosporine arteriopathy, there is a decrease in renin immunostaining in the juxtaglomerular apparatus, suggesting a loss of renin-containing arteriolar cells (Strom *et al.*, 1995). This observation led to the hypothesis that the prime target of cyclosporine is the renin-producing smooth muscle cell in the afferent arteriole, also the primary site of the nodular hyalinosis. The frequency of arterioles affected with cyclosporine-associated arteriolopathy is typically small (<15%), and the lesions can be overlooked easily (Strom *et al.*, 1994). In renal transplant patients taking cyclosporine, 15% of protocol biopsy specimens at 6 months showed cyclosporine hyalinosis arteriolopathy, which increased to 45% in

18-month protocol biopsy specimens (Savoldi *et al.*, 1988). In contrast, the *nonspecific* hyalinosis shows no such progressive increase. The arteriolar lesions also develop in native kidneys of patients who receive lower doses of cyclosporine (<5 mg/kg/d) for 2 years (Pei *et al.*, 1994; Young *et al.*, 1994).

TACROLIMUS TOXICITY

Tacrolimus so far has shown a nephrotoxicity in humans that is similar in frequency and identical in pathology to cyclosporine, including reversible acute renal failure (Japanese FK Study Group, 1993; Randhawa *et al.*, 1993), hemolytic-uremic syndrome (Randhawa *et al.*, 1993; Schmidt *et al.*, 1991) and chronic lesions of arteriolar hyalinosis and striped fibrosis (Randhawa *et al.*, 1993). Neurotoxicity and insulin-dependent diabetes are commoner adverse effects with tacrolimus than with cyclosporine. Diabetes developed in 12% on tacrolimus (Vincenti *et al.*, 1996) and it also occurs in children (Furth *et al.*, 1996).

Drug-Induced Acute Tubulointerstitial Nephritis

Drug-induced interstitial nephritis in the allograft is similar to that in the native kidney and resembles tubulointerstitial rejection. Both conditions are characterized by an intense mononuclear interstitial infiltrate and tubulitis and have variable numbers of eosinophils. Acute rejection occasionally has a prominent eosinophilic infiltrate (Almirall *et al.*, 1993; Hallgren *et al.*, 1991; Hongwei *et al.*, 1994; Kormendi and Amend, 1988; Ten *et al.*, 1989; Weir *et al.*, 1986); conversely, drug-induced interstitial nephritis may have no eosinophils, especially that caused by nonsteroidal antiinflammatory drugs (Colvin and Fang, 1994). Endarteritis, if present, is unequivocal evidence for rejection. Strong (but perhaps not so absolute) evidence for a drug cause is the invasion of multiple tubules by eosinophils and eosinophils in tubular casts (Colvin, unpublished observation), usually attributed to prophylactic trimethoprim-sulfamethoxazole (Bactrim). We have also seen one case of severe acute interstitial nephritis and serum sickness–like syndrome secondary to the horse antithymocyte globulin.

Infections

CYTOMEGALOVIRUS

Cytomegalovirus, a herpesvirus, is one of the commonest pathogens in renal transplant recipients, typically causing symptomatic infection in the first 2 to 3 months after transplantation, manifested by fever, leukopenia, viremia and hepatitis or pneumonitis (Rubin and Colvin, 1998). The renal allograft is affected directly by the cytomegalovirus infection or indirectly by a modification or intensification of the allograft rejection reaction.

A few allografts have shown prominent cytomegalovirus cytopathic changes (nuclear and cytoplasmic inclusions) and an acute tubulointerstitial nephritis (Cameron et al., 1982; Herrera et al., 1986; Payton et al., 1987). In these cases, graft failure was attributed to cytomegalovirus infection rather than rejection. Cytopathic changes were reported in glomerular and peritubular endothelial cells in addition to the usual tubular sites (Payton et al., 1987). In contrast to latent and/or asymptomatic infections, the viral genome was detected primarily in focal clusters of infiltrating mononuclear cells (Gnann et al., 1988). Cytomegalovirus interstitial nephritis and rejection have an infiltrate primarily of CD8[+] cells (Platt et al., 1985; Sanfilippo et al., 1985; Tuazon et al., 1987). Rarely, cytomegalovirus infects glomerular cells and causes an acute glomerulonephritis (Beneck et al., 1986).

Lopez and colleagues suggested that cytomegalovirus infection was associated with an increased risk of allograft dysfunction and loss (Lopez et al., 1974). Subsequent studies showed that cytomegalovirus appears to exert most of its effects through activation of the rejection process, which commonly becomes focused on glomeruli or vessels (Rubin and Colvin, 1998). The frequency of late rejection was fivefold higher in patients with proven cytomegalovirus disease (86%) compared with patients without cytomegalovirus disease (17%) (von Willebrand et al., 1986).

Acute glomerulopathy sometimes has been related to cytomegalovirus infection (Richardson et al., Tuazon et al., 1987) as well as chronic allograft glomerulopathy (Cosio et al., 1996a). Further studies have shown that cytomegalovirus is neither necessary nor sufficient for acute glomerulopathy. A metaanalysis of the 175 reported cases of acute allograft glomerulopathy reveals that 67% had cytomegalovirus infection, compared with a 47% frequency of cytomegalovirus in the 146 cases in the same reports without glomerulopathy ($P<.001$ by chi-square analysis) (Colvin, 1998). Two studies have shown the essential requirement for the renal allograft itself (rather than native kidney) (Battegay et al., 1988; Herrera et al., 1986). Any glomerular effect of the cytomegalovirus must be through an alteration of the rejection process, perhaps through systemic cytokine effects, and the acute glomerulopathy should be considered a rare feature of acute rejection (see earlier). Hepatitis C virus also has been associated with acute glomerulopathy (see later).

POLYOMAVIRUS

A new polyomavirus was originally isolated from B.K., a Sudanese patient who had distal donor ureteral stenosis, 3 months after a living related transplant (Gardner et al., 1971). BK virus is related to JC virus (which also inhabits the human urinary tract) and to simian kidney virus SV40. These viruses are members of the papavirus group, which includes the papillomaviruses. The BK virus commonly infects urothelium but rarely causes morbidity in immunocompetent individuals. In renal transplant recipients, three lesions have been attributed to BK virus: hemorrhagic cystitis, ureteral stenosis

(Coleman et al., 1978; Gardner et al., 1984; Hogan et al., 1980a) and interstitial nephritis. Many cases have been reported, particularly in patients taking tacrolimus (Drachenberg et al., 1999; Mathur et al., 1997; Nickeleit et al., 1999; Pappo et al., 1996).

BK virus infection causes tubulointerstitial nephritis in allografts (Pappo et al., 1996). Concurrent acute cellular rejection may be present. Animal studies indicate that the native kidney also may be infected (van Gorder et al., 1999). Urine cytology may show *decoy cells* with inclusions (Gardner et al., 1984; Hogan et al., 1980b). The recognition of viral nuclear inclusions is the key step in diagnosis. The affected nuclei usually are enlarged, atypical with smudgy, basophilic chromatin. These nuclear inclusions tend to be grouped in tubules, particularly collecting ducts in the cortex and outer medulla, and often can be spotted at low power. The mononuclear interstitial infiltrate is associated with the infected tubular cells and can be patchy. The infiltrate often contains plasma cells, which sometimes invade the tubules (Fig. 24–15A). Immunohistochemistry and electron microscopy confirm the diagnosis. The polyomaviruses are characteristically 40 to 50 nm in diameter, smaller than papillomaviruses (52–55 nm). Monoclonal antibodies are commercially available that react with BK-specific determinants and with the large T antigen of several polyomavirus species (Fig. 24–15B). We have obtained good results with paraffin/microwave techniques. Electron microscopy reveals the characteristic intranuclear paracrystalline arrays of viral particles (Fig. 24–15C). The treatment is decreased immunosuppression, and some patients respond by complete recovery.

HEPATITIS C VIRUS

Approximately 10% of candidates for renal transplantation in the United States have serum antibodies to hepatitis C virus (Cosio et al., 1996b). Hepatitis C virus has been associated with an increased risk of acute allograft glomerulopathy (Cosio et al., 1996b; Gallay et al., 1995). Hepatitis C virus–positive recipients had a ninefold increase in frequency of acute allograft glomerulopathy in biopsy specimens obtained for graft dysfunction in the first 6 months compared with hepatitis C virus–negative controls who received hepatitis C virus–negative kidneys (55% vs. 6%) (Cosio et al., 1996b). Hepatitis C virus–negative recipients who received hepatitis C virus–positive kidneys also had a higher frequency of glomerulopathy (40%). The glomerulopathy resembled membranoproliferative glomerulonephritis (MPGN) or chronic allograft glomerulopathy in two cases (Dussol et al., 1995; Gallay et al., 1995) and acute allograft glomerulopathy, with variable occlusion of glomerular capillaries by hypertrophic endothelial cells, lymphocytes and monocytes in about 20 patients (Cosio et al., 1996a, 1996b). Electron microscopy and immunofluorescence studies were not performed. Acute endarteritis was twice as common (60%) than in controls (28%), as was chronic vascular rejection (60% vs. 31%), which tended to occur early (within 1 month in 64%). Posttransplant hepatitis C virus infection of renal allografts may be a factor in the development of chronic allograft dysfunction, morphologically appearing as *de novo* MPGN or chronic allograft glomerulopathy (Fig. 24–16A), usually with glomerular immune complex deposits (Mauiyyedi et al., 2000a; Fig. 24–16B). Thrombotic microangiopathy (Fig. 24–17) also occurs in hepatitis C virus–positive recipients with a relatively high frequency (30%), associated with high titers of antiphospholipid antibodies (Baid et al., 1999).

OTHER INFECTIONS

Herpesvirus type 1 and 2 has caused interstitial nephritis in renal allografts but only rarely. In the one reported case,

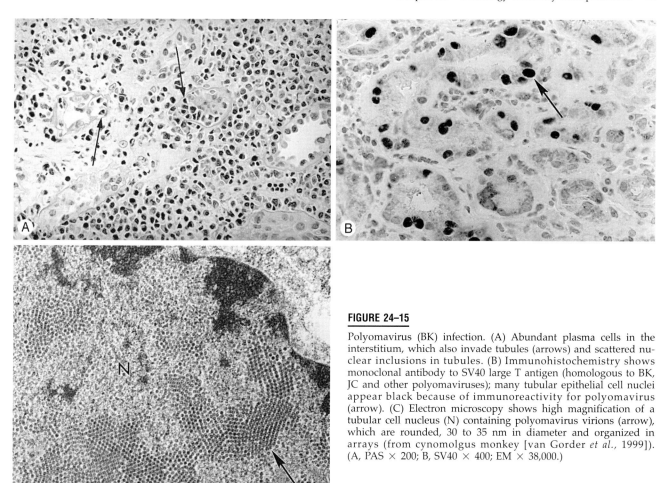

FIGURE 24–15

Polyomavirus (BK) infection. (A) Abundant plasma cells in the interstitium, which also invade tubules (arrows) and scattered nuclear inclusions in tubules. (B) Immunohistochemistry shows monoclonal antibody to SV40 large T antigen (homologous to BK, JC and other polyomaviruses); many tubular epithelial cell nuclei appear black because of immunoreactivity for polyomavirus (arrow). (C) Electron microscopy shows high magnification of a tubular cell nucleus (N) containing polyomavirus virions (arrow), which are rounded, 30 to 35 nm in diameter and organized in arrays (from cynomolgus monkey [van Gorder *et al.*, 1999]). (A, PAS × 200; B, SV40 × 400; EM × 38,000.)

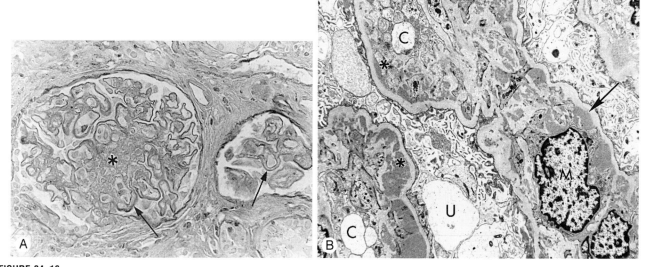

FIGURE 24–16

Hepatitis C virus infection and chronic allograft glomerulopathy. (A) Two glomeruli with glomerular basement membrane duplication (arrows) and an increase in mesangial matrix and cells (*). (B) Electron microscopy shows high magnification of glomerular capillary loops with electron dense deposits in the subendothelial region (*) and mesangium (arrow). M-mesangial cell; C-capillary lumen; U-urinary space. (A, PAS × 160; B, EM × 5,900.)

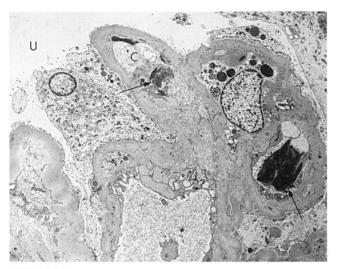

FIGURE 24–17

Hepatitis C virus infection–associated thrombotic microangiopathy with presence of anticardiolipin antibodies. Electron microscopy shows a portion of glomerular tuft with aggregated fibrin tactoids in capillary lumina (arrows), subendothelial lucency and loss of endothelial fenestrae. C-capillary lumen; U-urinary space. (EM × 4,300.)

the diagnosis was made in an allograft removed 3 weeks posttransplant (Silbert *et al.*, 1990). Nuclear clearing, necrosis and inclusions in tubular cells, with occasional multinucleated cells suggested a viral infection by light microscopy. The infiltrate was rich in neutrophils with a mild mononuclear component. Immunoperoxidase stains for herpesvirus type 1 and 2 antigens were strongly positive. A few other cases are presumably in pathology files misclassified as rejection.

Adenovirus can cause necrotizing hemorrhagic tubulointerstitial nephritis, hemorrhagic cystitis and renal failure in immunocompromised patients (Ito *et al.*, 1991). Tubular cells had intranuclear inclusions with a distinct halo surrounded by a ring of marginated chromatin and glassy smudged nuclei. The clues that lead to the diagnosis are the glassy-appearing nuclear smudging, with more extensive tubular necrosis and less extensive interstitial infiltrate than typical graft rejection. The diagnosis is established by immunoperoxidase stains for viral antigen. Adenovirus antigens were in tubular cells, which contain intranuclear crystalline arrays of 75- to 80-nm viral particles. Immune complexes also may contribute to the injury.

Acute pyelonephritis is an uncommon but potentially devastating complication of transplantation. Pyelonephritis can present as acute renal failure (Gillum and Kelleher, 1985; Yang *et al.*, 1994) and cause graft loss (Hansen *et al.*, 1988; Kalra *et al.*, 1993). Pyelonephritis arises most often 1 year or more posttransplantation (80% of episodes) (Pearson *et al.*, 1980). *Escherichia coli* is the commonest organism (80%). Acute pyelonephritis can often be detected on renal biopsy, despite the expectation that the process is patchy (Yang *et al.*, 1994). The pathology is similar to that in native kidneys.

Rare cases of fatal emphysematous pyelonephritis resulting from gas-producing organisms have developed in nondiabetic recipients (Kalra *et al.*, 1993). Perinephric abscesses resulting from anaerobic bacteria also have been described (Brook, 1994). Xanthogranulomatous pyelonephritis has developed rarely *de novo* in allografts (Elkhammas *et al.*, 1994; Jones *et al.*, 1989). On the biopsy specimen, the sheets of lipid-filled macrophages (Elkhammas *et al.*, 1994) are char-

acteristic. Malakoplakia may spread from the recipient urinary tract and require withdrawal of immunosuppressive therapy (Barker, 1984; Biggar *et al.*, 1985; Stern *et al.*, 1994). The diagnosis is made by detection of pathognomonic PAS-positive Michaelis-Gutmann bodies that are basophilic, laminated, intracellular inclusions that contain calcium and glycolipids.

Arterial or Venous Thrombosis

Most arterial thromboses develop in the early posttransplant period, presenting as delayed graft function with anuria (Bakir *et al.*, 1996). The pathological features in the kidney are those of acute infarction with microthrombi and scant inflammation. Evidence for underlying rejection should be sought by careful examination of the larger arteries for endarteritis. Some workers have reported a high frequency of arterial thrombosis in patients receiving high-dose prophylactic OKT3 (Pradier *et al.*, 1992), but this was not detected by others (Bakir *et al.*, 1996).

Acute renal vein thrombosis usually presents as sudden pain at the transplant site, graft swelling, hematuria and proteinuria (Merion and Calne, 1985). In a series of 557 consecutive renal transplants, the prevalence of renal vein thrombosis was 0.4%. Morphologically the kidneys are swollen and purple with thrombosis of the veins (Fig. 24–18A). The cortex shows severe hemorrhagic congestion (Fig. 24–18B) and extensive infarction and necrosis (Merion and Calne, 1985), sometimes with diffuse microcapillary thrombi. Intracapillary leukocytes can be a clue as in native kidneys. Graft rupture may occur (Said *et al.*, 1994).

Late renal vein thrombosis is associated with proteinuria resulting from membranous glomerulonephritis or transplant glomerulopathy (First *et al.*, 1984a, 1984b; Liano *et al.*, 1988), sometimes with graft loss (Schwarz *et al.*, 1994). Lupus anticoagulant has been detected in a few patients (Liano *et al.*, 1988; Marcen *et al.*, 1990).

De Novo Glomerular Disease

Patients without previous glomerular disease occasionally develop lesions in the allograft that resemble a primary glomerular disease, rather than the usual chronic allograft glomerulopathy. Although some are coincidental, at least two are related to an alloimmune response to the allograft: membranous glomerulonephritis and anti-GBM disease in Alport's syndrome. A third glomerular disease, focal segmental glomerular sclerosis (FSGS), is believed to be related to hyperfiltration injury of the allograft.

MEMBRANOUS GLOMERULONEPHRITIS

De novo membranous glomerulonephritis is typically a late complication, with a prevalence of about 1 to 2% (Schwarz *et al.*, 1994). Children may have a higher risk, with a frequency of 9% in biopsy specimens and/or nephrectomies (Antignac *et al.*, 1988; Heidel *et al.*, 1994). The risk of *de novo* membranous glomerulonephritis increases with time after transplant, reaching 5.3% at 8 years. The presence of *de novo* membranous glomerulonephritis in a first graft increases the risk in a second graft (Heidel *et al.*, 1994). No other risk factors have been identified. Patients often present with proteinuria in the nephrotic range (Antignac *et al.*, 1988; Schwarz *et al.*, 1994), although about 20 to 30% of patients never have proteinuria (Antignac *et al.*, 1988). The presence of the nephrotic syndrome is correlated with an adverse prognosis (Truong *et al.*, 1989). Three grafts that were lost from *de novo* membranous

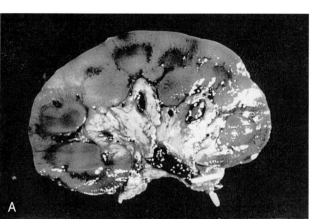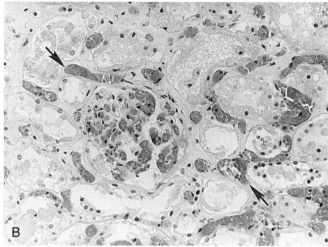

FIGURE 24–18

Renal vein thrombosis. (A) Gross specimen of a renal allograft nephrectomy with thrombi in renal veins, hemorrhage and infarction of the renal parenchyma, including cortex and medulla. (B) Light microscopy shows cortex, congested peritubular capillaries (arrows), necrotic tubules and congested glomerular capillary loops. (B, H&E × 250.)

glomerulonephritis had renal vein thrombosis (First *et al.*, 1984a; Schwarz *et al.*, 1994), occasionally associated with anti-phospholipid antibody (Liano *et al.*, 1988).

Light microscopy usually shows rather mild GBM changes. Mesangial hypercellularity is found in about 33%. Mononuclear cells can be abundant in glomerular capillaries, raising the possibility of acute rejection or renal vein thrombosis (Monga *et al.*, 1993). Changes of chronic rejection also may be present. Immunofluorescence shows granular deposits along the GBM that stain for IgG, C3, C3d and factor H (Cosyns *et al.*, 1986); about 35% are more irregular and segmental in distribution than typical primary (idiopathic) membranous glomerulonephritis (Monga *et al.*, 1993; Truong *et al.*, 1989). By electron microscopy, subepithelial electron dense deposits are present (Fig. 24–19), which are smaller and more irregular in distribution than primary membranous glomerulonephritis; the basement membrane spikes are also smaller (Truong *et al.*, 1989). In contrast to primary membranous glomerulonephritis, the deposits often are in different stages (I–III) in the same biopsy specimen (Monga *et al.*, 1993; Truong *et al.*, 1989). Repeat biopsy specimens have shown persistence or progression of the deposits in most cases, with resolution in occasional cases (Antignac *et al.*, 1988; Monga *et al.*, 1993). The pathogenesis of *de novo* membranous glomerulonephritis has not been established. The literature supports the hypothesis that *de novo* membranous glomerulonephritis may be a form of antibody-mediated rejection or directed at minor histocompatibility antigens in the glomerulus, presumably on the podocyte, or a special type of chronic rejection (Colvin, 1998; Thoenes *et al.*, 1979; Truong *et al.*, 1989).

ANTI–GLOMERULAR BASEMENT MEMBRANE NEPHRITIS

Although the overall experience with transplantation in Alport's syndrome or hereditary nephritis is good, crescentic glomerulonephritis caused by *de novo* anti-GBM antibodies has been reported (Diaz *et al.*, 1994; McCoy *et al.*, 1982) in these patients who lack the normal GBM component, α5 chain of type IV collagen. The α5 chain is necessary for the phenotypic expression of the α3 chain of type IV collagen in the GBM, whose NC1 terminal domain is the usual autoantigen of anti-GBM nephritis. The time of occurrence varies

from a few days to several months posttransplant. Among several large series, anti-GBM antibodies developed in only about 10% of Alport's patients, and none developed nephritis (Gobel *et al.*, 1992; Nyberg *et al.*, 1995; Querin *et al.*, 1986). Linear glomerular IgG deposits without overt glomerular injury or circulating antibodies also is reported (Querin *et al.*, 1986), suggesting that another factor may be necessary, as in recurrent anti-GBM disease. Successful second transplantation and recurring anti-GBM nephritis in successive allografts have occurred (Diaz *et al.*, 1994; Milliner *et al.*, 1982; personal experience). The 5-year graft survival may be equal to that of non-Alport's recipients (Gobel *et al.*, 1992).

NEPHROTIC SYNDROME IN CONGENITAL NEPHROSIS

Two children who had congenital nephrotic syndrome developed nephrotic syndrome shortly after transplantation

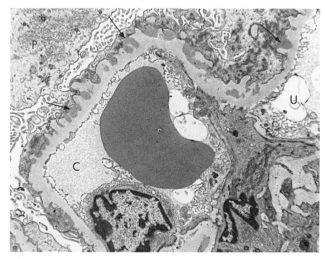

FIGURE 24–19

De novo membranous glomerulonephritis. Subepithelial electron dense deposits (arrows) along the glomerular basement membrane with intervening basement membrane spikes. Podocyte (P) foot processes are effaced. C-capillary lumen; U-urinary space. (EM × 10,300.)

that responded to steroids or cyclophosphamide; this was believed to be *de novo* minimal change disease rather than recurrence (Flynn *et al.*, 1992; Lane *et al.*, 1991). The genetic defect in this autosomal recessive disease was shown to be in the gene encoding nephrin, a component of the filtration slit membrane between podocytes (Tryggvason, 1999). We suspect that the recurrence is due to an autoantibody to nephrin, analogous to the anti-GBM disease of hereditary nephritis.

FOCAL SEGMENTAL GLOMERULAR SCLEROSIS

De novo focal segmental glomerular sclerosis (FSGS) has been described in adult recipients of pediatric kidneys (Neumayer *et al.*, 1994; Woolley *et al.*, 1988), in which the presumed pathogenesis is hyperfiltration injury; in long-standing grafts, in which parenchymal loss resulting from cyclosporine toxicity and/or chronic rejection leads to hyperfiltration injury of residual glomeruli (see cyclosporine section), and as the collapsing variant of FSGS, with an unknown pathophysiology (Meehan *et al.*, 1998).

The collapsing variant of FSGS (Fig. 24–20) can arise *de novo* in renal transplants (Detwiler *et al.*, 1994; Meehan *et al.*, 1998). Five cases of the collapsing variant of FSGS have been reported to arise *de novo* in renal allografts (Meehan *et al.*, 1998); patients presented 6 to 25 months posttransplant with marked proteinuria (2–12 g/d). Diffuse or focal, global or segmental collapse of glomeruli was evident with prominent hyperreactive podocytes. Arteriolar hyalinosis, arteriosclerosis and interstitial fibrosis were present. A rapid progression to renal failure occurred in 80% of the patients (2–12 months). The cause is unknown; all patients were human immunodeficiency virus negative. Two cases arose at the same time in kidneys obtained from a single donor that were transplanted into different recipients, consistent with a transmittable agent. We have seen the disease only after 1992.

The donor and the recipient of an adult kidney are not expected to develop FSGS owing to hyperfiltration because the frequency of FSGS after adult unilateral nephrectomy is extremely low (Kiprov *et al.*, 1982). Focal segmental glomerular sclerosis has been reported in occasional living related donors, sometimes with a rapidly progressive course (Ismail-

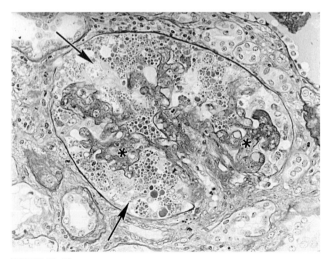

FIGURE 24–20

De novo collapsing glomerulopathy. Collapsed glomerular capillaries (*) and prominent podocyte proliferation, hypertrophy and abundant reabsorption droplets (arrows). (PAS × 250.)

Allouch *et al.*, 1993). In one case, the donor, but not the recipient, developed FSGS 11 years posttransplantation (Said and Soyannwo, 1996). One *tolerant* patient developed FSGS after 32 years while on no immunosuppression for 7 years (Trimarchi *et al.*, 1999).

Recurrent Renal Disease

Recurrent disease is a small but significant cause of allograft failure, estimated to occur in 1 to 5% of recipients (Cameron, 1991; Ramos and Tisher, 1994). Isografts (identical twins), in contrast, have a higher recurrence rate attributed to the total lack of immunosuppression (Glassock *et al.*, 1968). Recurrence may become a greater problem in the future with longer graft survival and development of tolerance protocols that require no immunosuppression. The reader is referred to a comprehensive review for detailed information regarding specific diseases (Colvin, 1998). The frequency and clinical significance of recurrence vary with the disease. The diagnosis of recurrence requires accurate classification of the original disease and lesions that differ from chronic allograft glomerulopathy. Diseases may be grouped into four categories by frequency of recurrence, then by whether there is an adverse effect on graft outcome or risk of unique complications (Colvin, 1998; Table 24–4). A few general observations are made here.

Recurrent disease in renal allografts provides unique opportunities for insight into the basic disease mechanisms. Recurrence may be taken as strong evidence for a blood-borne causative agent. Two idiopathic glomerular diseases were first shown to be caused by blood-borne factors by recurrence in the graft (FSGS and dense deposit disease). The evidence that FSGS is due to a circulating factor led to the use of plasmapheresis to treat recurrence and to partial characterization of a putative serum factor (Savin *et al.*, 1996). Recurrence of anti-GBM disease can be avoided by postponing transplantation for 6 to 12 months after the serum becomes negative by a sensitive test for anti-GBM antibody (Collins and Colvin, 1997). Series have recurrence rates of 5% or less (Daly *et al.*, 1996). In IgA nephropathy, some apparent recurrences, particularly in HLA-identical sibling grafts, are probably asymptomatic IgA deposits in the donor (Brensilver *et al.*, 1988; Tolkoff *et al.*, 1978). The IgA deposits disappear within a few months (Sanfilippo *et al.*, 1982; Silva *et al.*, 1982).

Conversely, failure to recur proves that the disease is intrinsic to the kidney (e.g., hereditary nephritis, autosomal dominant polycystic kidney disease, congenital nephrotic syndrome) or that the pathogenetic mechanisms have ceased (anti-GBM antibody nephritis, lupus nephritis). In patients with hemolytic-uremic syndrome, the prime risk factor in recurrence is the cause of the original hemolytic-uremic syndrome. Cases without an infectious cause are at highest risk (Bassani *et al.*, 1991; Hebert *et al.*, 1991).

Transplantation can illuminate uniquely the early pathological events that precede clinical signs and determine the reversibility of preexisting lesions in the donor kidney (e.g., diabetes, IgA nephropathy). For example, in dense deposit disease (Fig. 24–21), the glomerular electron dense deposits can recur 3 weeks after transplantation, preceding C3 accumulation (Droz *et al.*, 1979), and are not necessarily symptomatic. The development of diabetic nephropathy begins with an increase in allograft glomerular volume at 6 months (Osterby *et al.*, 1992), followed by increases in mesangial volume (Wilczek *et al.*, 1995). Thickening of the GBM appears later, with a progressive increase that is first evident after 2 to 3 years (Bohman *et al.*, 1985; Wilczek *et al.*, 1995). Arteriolar hyalinosis may precede glomerular changes and can be de-

TABLE 24–4

CLASSIFICATION OF RECURRENT RENAL DISEASE

Usually recur (>50% patients)	
Adverse effect*	Primary HUS
	Primary oxalosis
	Dense deposit disease
	Collapsing FSGS†
Little or no adverse effect	Immunotactoid/fibrillary glomerulopathy†
	Systemic light chain disease†
	Diabetes mellitus‡
Commonly recur (5–50%)	
Adverse effect	FSGS
	Membranoproliferative GN, type I
	Membranous GN
	ANCA-related diseases
	Wegener's granulomatosis
	Pauciimmune GN
	Microscopic polyarteritis
	Progressive systemic sclerosis
	Sickle cell nephropathy†
Little or no adverse effect	IgA nephropathy
	Henoch-Schönlein purpura
	Amyloidosis
Rarely recur (<5%)	
Adverse effect	Anti-GBM disease
Little or no adverse effect	Systemic lupus erythematosus
	Fabry's disease
	Cystinosis
Never recur (0%)	
Unique complications	Hereditary nephritis/Alport's syndrome (anti-GBM disease)
	Congenital nephrosis (nephrotic syndrome; nephrin autoantibody?)
No unique complications	Polycystic disease (all genetic types)
	Osteo-onychodysplasia (nail-patella)†
	Acquired cystic disease
	Secondary HUS (infection)
	Secondary FSGS
	Familial FSGS†
	Postinfectious acute glomerulonephritis†
Unclassified, recurrence reported§	Thrombotic thrombocytopenic purpura
	Adenosine phosphoribosyl transferase deficiency
	Familial fibronectin glomerulopathy
	Lipoprotein glomerulopathy
	Malacoplakia

*Adverse effect defined as graft loss of >5% (when disease recurs)
†Limited experience: few cases reported (n <10).
‡Arteriolar and glomerular lesions recur to some degree in most if not all cases, but severe form (nodular) delayed until >5 years.
§Recurrence occurs, but too few cases reported to classify frequency or consequences.
HUS = hemolytic uremic syndrome; FSGS = focal segmental glomerulosclerosis; GN = glomerulonephritis; ANCA = antineutrophil cytoplasmic antibody; GBM = glomerular basement membrane.

tectable in early biopsy specimens (Mauer *et al.*, 1976). Nodular diabetic glomerulosclerosis (Fig. 24–22) has been reported as a late complication, 5 to 15 years posttransplant (Hariharan *et al.*, 1996; Maryniak *et al.*, 1985; Mauer *et al.*, 1976). Nodular diabetic glomerulosclerosis in native kidneys has a latency of 8 to 10 years and will become more prevalent in long surviving allografts.

Differential Diagnosis of Biopsy Specimens
LESIONS WITH SCANT INFLAMMATION

Hyperacute Rejection Versus Acute Tubular Necrosis and Major Vessel Thrombosis

Hyperacute rejection typically has more hemorrhage, necrosis and neutrophil accumulation in glomeruli and peritubular capillaries than perfusion injury; glomerular neutrophils alone were associated with ischemic perfusion injury in one series (Gaber *et al.*, 1992a). Major arterial thrombosis has

predominant necrosis with little hemorrhage or microthrombi, and peritubular capillary neutrophils are not prominent. Renal vein thrombosis shows marked congestion and relatively little neutrophil response. The presence of antiphospholipid antibodies should be sought in cases of major vessel thromboses. Although the finding of antibody and C3 deposition in small vessels is helpful, negative immunofluorescence stains for IgG, IgM and C3 do not exclude hyperacute rejection. C4d should be positive in peritubular capillaries. The pretransplant serum should be retested against donor T and B cells, monocytes and erythrocytes. If no antibodies are revealed, antiendothelial antibodies should be sought by antibody-dependent cytotoxicity or indirect immunofluorescence.

Acute Cyclosporine Toxicity Versus Acute Tubular Necrosis

The differential diagnosis of acute cyclosporine toxicity versus ATN can be impossible. The acute tubular toxicity

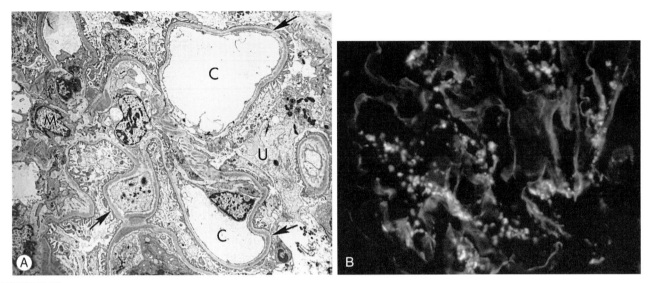

FIGURE 24–21

Recurrent dense deposit disease. (A) Electron microscopy shows widespread electron dense deposits that are continuous, linear and embedded in the glomerular basement membrane proper (i.e., intramembranous [arrows]). Similar deposits are also seen in the mesangium (M). C-capillary lumen; U-urinary space. (B) On immunofluorescence microscopy, staining for C3 shows broad linear, ribbonlike deposits along the glomerular basement membrane and bloblike deposits in the mesangium (mesangial rings). (A, EM × 3,300; B, IF, C3-FITC × 400.) (See color plate.)

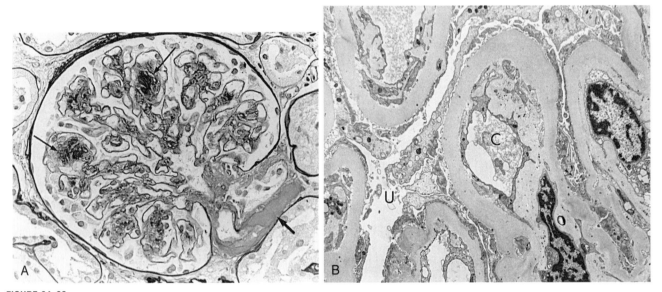

FIGURE 24–22

Recurrent diabetic nephropathy. (A) Glomerulus with prominent Kimmelstiel-Wilson mesangial nodules (thin arrows) and arteriolar hyalinosis (thick arrow). (B) Electron microscopy shows homogeneous thickening of the glomerular basement membrane to 1,100 nm. C-capillary lumen; U-urinary space. (A, PAS × 400; B, EM × 5,400.)

of cyclosporine may be indistinguishable from ischemia or osmotic diuretics (e.g., mannitol), and vacuoles may be seen by light microscopy in all three. By electron microscopy, a coarser and varied vacuolization is typical of ATN and the periphery of infarcts (Mihatsch *et al.*, 1988) compared with the isometric (uniform) vacuoles of cyclosporine toxicity. The vacuoles of osmotic diuretic injury do not involve the endoplasmic reticulum, as do those of cyclosporine toxicity (Mihatsch *et al.*, 1994). A tubular lesion that may discriminate reliably between ATN and acute cyclosporine toxicity is necrosis of tubular cells, which is significantly commoner in ATN (0.5% of tubules), characteristically involving whole tubular cross-sections (Solez *et al.*, 1993b). Acute medial apoptosis and/or degeneration in arterioles is the only definitive finding favoring cyclosporine toxicity.

Acute Humoral Rejection Versus Acute Tubular Necrosis

In ATN, focal interstitial, peritubular capillary and glomerular neutrophils may be present, although not as prominently as in acute humoral rejection. Severe acute tubular injury may be seen in acute humoral rejection and ATN. C4d deposition in peritubular capillaries (immunofluorescence microscopy) is typically present only in acute humoral rejection but not in ATN.

Thrombotic Microangiopathy

Morphology alone cannot distinguish the various causes of thrombotic microangiopathy, whether cyclosporine or other causes (Loomis *et al.*, 1989). In renal transplants, the key conditions to distinguish from cyclosporine-associated thrombotic microangiopathy are recurrent thrombotic microangiopathy, acute humoral rejection and hepatitis C virus–associated thrombotic microangiopathy. Recurrence always should be the first choice when the recipient's original disease was thrombotic microangiopathy in the native kidney (unless associated with a diarrheal illness). If acute humoral rejection is suspected, C4d staining (immunofluorescence) of the renal allograft biopsy specimen helps distinguish between them; C4d deposition in peritubular capillaries is present in acute humoral rejection but absent in cyclosporine-associated thrombotic microangiopathy (see section on acute humoral rejection). Serum should be tested for anti-HLA class I, class II and antiendothelial antibodies. Hepatitis C virus–positive renal allograft recipients may develop thrombotic microangiopathy with associated elevation of circulating anticardiolipin antibody (Baid *et al.*, 1999); hepatitis serology and anticardiolipin antibody determination could help distinguish between hepatitis C virus versus cyclosporine in the cause of thrombotic microangiopathy.

LESIONS WITH ACUTE INFLAMMATION

Acute Cellular Rejection Versus Acute Humoral Rejection

Acute cellular rejection and acute humoral rejection are two major forms of acute rejection that can coexist (Table 24–5). In acute humoral rejection, neutrophils are the predominant inflammatory cells in peritubular capillaries, glomeruli, tubules and interstitium, with or without accompanying fibrinoid necrosis. The vascular lesion of acute humoral rejection is fibrinoid necrosis of the wall, whereas in acute cellular rejection endarteritis is the usual lesion. C4d deposition in peritubular capillaries (immunofluorescence microscopy) is typically present only in acute humoral rejection but

TABLE 24–5

DIFFERENTIATION BETWEEN ACUTE HUMORAL REJECTION AND ACUTE CELLULAR REJECTION

	Acute Humoral Rejection	Acute Cellular Rejection
Interstitium		
Infiltrate	Variable	Moderate–severe
Edema	Present	Present
Peritubular capillaries	Neutrophils	Mononuclear cells
C4d*	Positive	Negative
Tubules		
Acute tubular necrosis	Can be present	Usually absent
Tubulitis	Can be neutrophilic	Mononuclear cell
Vessels		
Endarteritis	Can be present	Present in type II
Fibrinoid necrosis	Typically present	Present in type III
Glomeruli		
Inflammatory cells	Neutrophils	Mononuclear cells
Fibrinoid necrosis	Can be present	Typically absent

*C4d staining in peritubular capillaries indicates activation of the classic complement pathway by humoral antibody (monoclonal antibody, immunofluorescence microscopy).

not in acute cellular rejection. Testing for circulating antidonor antibody is useful to confirm the diagnosis of acute humoral rejection, although some cases are probably due to non-HLA antibodies.

Acute Cellular Rejection Versus Cyclosporine Toxicity

The criteria for morphological distinction of cyclosporine toxicity and acute rejection have received much attention (Table 24–6). Patients with rejection typically have a diffuse, interstitial mononuclear cell infiltrate, whereas patients with

TABLE 24–6

DIFFERENTIATION BETWEEN ACUTE REJECTION AND ACUTE CYCLOSPORINE TOXICITY

	Acute Rejection	Cyclosporine Toxicity
Interstitium		
Infiltrate	Moderate–marked	Absent–mild
Edema	Usual	Can be present
Tubules		
Tubular injury	Usual	Usual
Vacuoles	Occasional	Common
Tubulitis	Prominent	Minimal–Absent
Arterioles		
Endotheliitis	Can be present	Absent
Smooth muscle degeneration	Absent	Sometimes present
Mucoid intimal thickening with red cells	Absent	Sometimes present (TMA)
Arteries		
Endotheliitis	Common	Absent
Glomeruli		
Mononuclear cells	Often	Rare
Thrombi	Occasional	Occasionally prominent (TMA)

TMA = thrombotic microangiopathy.
Reproduced with permission of Colvin, 1998.

cyclosporine toxicity and patients with stable function have only focal mononuclear cell infiltrates. Scattered eosinophils may be seen in either condition. Most cases of acute cyclosporine toxicity do not have an associated eosinophilic interstitial infiltrate. Endarteritis is found extremely rarely, if ever, in cyclosporine toxicity (0–1%) and is the most discriminating feature between acute rejection and cyclosporine toxicity (Neild *et al.*, 1986; Sibley *et al.*, 1983; Taube *et al.*, 1985) in the differential diagnosis of acute allograft dysfunction. Endothelial and medial smooth muscle cell vacuolization has been noted in cyclosporine toxicity, best appreciated by electron microscopy. The frequency of vacuolization probably does not distinguish between cyclosporine toxicity and rejection or stable grafts (Neild *et al.*, 1986).

Acute Cellular Rejection Versus Acute Tubular Necrosis and Obstruction

Tubulitis is less prominent in ATN, particularly in the proximal tubules (Marcussen *et al.*, 1996). Tubulitis has been documented in renal transplants with dysfunction resulting from lymphoceles (obstruction) and in urine leaks, possibilities that need to be considered and excluded by other techniques (Curtis *et al.*, 1996). Acute obstruction typically has some dilatation of the collecting tubules, especially in the outer cortex. Edema and a mild mononuclear infiltrate are common. Endarteritis is absent.

Acute Cellular Rejection Versus Other Interstitial Nephritis

Interstitial mononuclear inflammation and tubulitis occur in a variety of diseases other than acute rejection, such as drug-induced (allergic) or infectious tubulointerstitial nephritis. When eosinophils are more abundant than usual for rejection and eosinophils invading tubules are identified, drug allergy may be favored over rejection. The presence of endarteritis permits a definitive diagnosis of active rejection (Nickeleit *et al.*, 1998). Lymphocytes commonly surround vessels (without medial involvement), a nonspecific feature, and must not be confused with endarteritis. Tubulitis often is present in atrophic tubules and does not indicate acute rejec-

tion. The diagnosis of acute pyelonephritis should be considered when active inflammation and abundant intratubular neutrophils are present. In acute humoral rejection, neutrophilic tubulitis with neutrophil casts can be seen; a C4d stain helps in distinguishing between these. A positive urine and blood culture also separates infection from rejection.

Acute Cellular Rejection Versus Polyomavirus

The usual diagnostic feature of polyoma interstitial nephritis (BK virus) is the enlarged, hyperchromatic tubular nuclei with lavender viral nuclear inclusions, often in collecting ducts. These nuclei may be inconspicuous, however, and diligent study of multiple sections may be required. Other clues are prominent apoptosis of tubular cells and abundant plasma cells, which invade tubules (a pathognomonic finding in our experience). Immunohistochemistry for polyomavirus large T antigen and electron microscopy (even of paraffin) confirm the diagnosis. Sometimes BK virus infection, with its exuberant plasmacytic infiltration and activated immunoblasts, may be confused with the plasmacytic hyperplasia form of PTLD.

Acute Cellular Rejection Versus Posttransplant Lymphoproliferative Disease

The most helpful feature that raises the suspicion of PTLD in our experience is the presence of a dense sheet of monomorphic lymphoblasts without edema or granulocytes (Fig. 24–23A). Serpiginous necrosis of the lymphoid cells (irregular patches) is distinctive but not always present (Randhawa *et al.*, 1996). The other features found to be helpful include nodular and expansile aggregates of immature lymphoid cells; the nuclei are enlarged and vesicular with prominent nucleoli that may be multiple. Immunohistochemistry is helpful in identifying the predominance of B cells in the infiltrate, which is not seen in rejection alone. If the cells have a monoclonal κ or λ phenotype, the diagnosis is confirmed. The definitive diagnosis of PTLD is *in situ* hybridization for Epstein-Barr virus–encoded RNA (Fig. 24–23B).

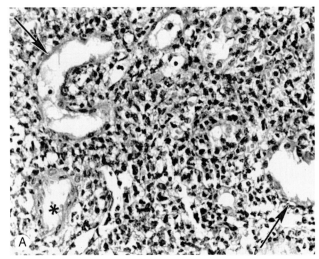
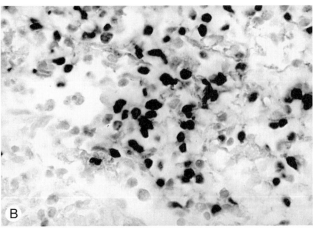

FIGURE 24–23

Posttransplant lymphoproliferative disease. (A) Dense mononuclear cell infiltrate centered predominantly in the interstitium that obliterates the normal renal architecture. Occasional surviving tubules (arrows) and vessels (*) may be identified. (B) On *in situ* hybridization, nuclei of mononuclear cells stain dark, brown-black for Epstein-Barr virus–encoded RNA, which is the definitive test for the diagnosis of posttransplant lymphoproliferative disease. (A, H&E, × 400; B, EBER × 630.)

LESIONS WITH CHRONIC INFLAMMATION OR FIBROSIS

The differential diagnosis of chronic allograft dysfunction includes chronic rejection; chronic cyclosporine toxicity; recurrent and *de novo* glomerulonephritis and other conditions such as hypertension, scarring from prior acute rejection episodes, viral infections (notably hepatitis C virus) and unknown causes.

Chronic Rejection Versus Chronic Cyclosporine Toxicity

The most difficult differential diagnosis in the renal transplant recipient is between chronic rejection and chronic cyclosporine toxicity (Table 24–7). The finding that favors cyclosporine toxicity most decisively is the arteriolopathy, provided that it is distinctive (isolated smooth muscle cell degeneration and string-of-pearls replacement by hyalinosis in the outer media). The arterioles are relatively spared in chronic rejection compared with chronic cyclosporine toxicity. Peripheral hyalinosis replacing smooth muscle cells in the arterioles strongly favors cyclosporine toxicity (Mihatsch *et al.*, 1995b). Features that favor chronic rejection over chronic cyclosporine toxicity are duplication of the GBM and marked intimal fibrosis of the small arteries (Mihatsch *et al.*, 1995b). The pattern of tubular atrophy and interstitial fibrosis is not discriminating. In cases of chronic allograft dysfunction in which neither cyclosporine-associated arteriolopathy nor chronic rejection lesions are identified, the nonspecific interstitial fibrosis, tubular atrophy and glomerular scarring changes still may be attributable to chronic cyclosporine toxicity but without certainty. Other causes must be excluded. Numerous plasma cells in the infiltrate are more typical of chronic rejection; plasma cells were an average of 21% of the infiltrate in chronic rejection versus 3% in cyclosporine toxicity (Nadasdy *et al.*, 1991). C4d deposits in peritubular capillaries is helpful in distinguishing most chronic rejection cases from other causes of chronic allograft dysfunction.

Chronic Rejection Versus Hypertensive Vascular Disease

Arterial lesions are the cardinal features of chronic rejection (Sibley, 1994). The proliferative endarteritis is characteristic, but the fully developed active lesion may not be present in all cases. Findings more specific for rejection are a mononuclear infiltrate in the intima or media, intimal foam cells against the internal elastica, and a moth-eaten, thin media resulting from loss of smooth muscle cells. Marked duplication of the internal elastica, a normal or thickened media and relative sparing of the larger arteries (arcuate and larger) are more typical of hypertension (Porter, 1990). The healing phase of thrombotic microangiopathy may leave intimal fibrosis that resembles chronic rejection, but without the intimal mononuclear cells.

Cyclosporine Arteriolopathy Versus Diabetic or Hypertensive Hyalinosis

The usual hyalinosis deposits in hypertension or diabetes are subendothelial and concentric. Although some overlap of these patterns occurs, when the hyalinosis has multiple, discrete nodules similar to the size and location of the medial smooth muscle cells, chronic cyclosporine toxicity should be the first choice. Intimal fibrosis and elastic duplication, as commonly found in hypertension and aging, are not regarded as related to cyclosporine administration, and the

TABLE 24–7

DIFFERENTIATION BETWEEN CHRONIC REJECTION AND CHRONIC CYCLOSPORINE TOXICITY

	Chronic Rejection	Cyclosporine Toxicity
Interstitium		
Infiltrate	Plasma cells	Mild
Fibrosis	Patchy	Patchy, striped
Peritubular capillaries	Often C4d$^+$	C4d$^-$
Tubules		
Tubular atrophy	Usual	Usual
Vacuoles	Occasional	Occasional
Arterioles		
Smooth muscle degeneration	Absent	Usual
External nodular hyalinosis	Absent	Present
Arteries		
Intimal fibrosis	Usual	Can be present
Mononuclear cells intima	Often present	Absent
Glomeruli		
Duplication GBM	Usual	Absent
Mesangial expansion	Can be present	Can be present

GBM = glomerular basement membrane.

intimal proliferative lesions commonly seen in chronic rejection are not regarded as related to cyclosporine (Falkenhain *et al.*, 1996; Mihatsch *et al.*, 1988, 1994; Myers *et al.*, 1988b). In the study of protocol biopsies of renal transplants noted previously, fibrous intimal thickening did not progress and was correlated with the donor age (Savoldi *et al.*, 1988).

Chronic Allograft Glomerulopathy Versus Primary or Recurrent Glomerular Disease

Chronic allograft glomerulopathy, although typically seen in chronic rejection, is not specific and can be seen in other diseases in which the endothelium is the target of injury, such as thrombotic microangiopathy, scleroderma and eclampsia. If immune complex deposits are found more than occasionally, especially when in a subepithelial or subendothelial location, recurrent or *de novo* glomerulonephritis should be suspected. Chronic hepatitis C virus infection should be considered when MPGN is found in the allograft (either *de novo* or recurrent) (Dussol *et al.*, 1995; Gallay *et al.*, 1995). Schistosomiasis can also cause recurrent MPGN in allografts, as shown in one of the two patients from Brazil who developed nephrotic syndrome and recurrence 3 years posttransplant (Azevedo *et al.*, 1987). Biopsy specimens taken for this differential diagnosis should include immunofluorescence and electron microscopy.

References

Abouna, G. M., Al Adnani, M. S., Kremer, G. D., *et al.* (1983). Reversal of diabetic nephropathy in human cadaveric kidneys after transplantation into non-diabetic recipients. *Lancet* **2**, 1274.

Adams, D. H., Tilney, N. L., Collins, J. J., *et al.* (1992). Experimental graft arteriosclerosis: I. the Lewis-to-F-344 allograft model. *Transplantation* **53**, 1115.

Ahern, A. T., Artruc, S. B., DellaPelle, P., *et al.* (1982). Hyperacute rejection of HLA-AB-identical renal allografts associated with B lymphocyte and endothelial reactive antibodies. *Transplantation* **33**, 103.

Almirall, J., Campistol, J. M., Sole, M., *et al.* (1993). Blood and graft eosinophilia as a rejection index in kidney transplant. *Nephron* **65**, 304.

Alpers, C., Graham-Christopher, T. and Mallea, M. (1991). Peritubular capillary congestion in renal allograft biopsies may be an unreliable marker for cyclosporine nephrotoxicity. *Am. J. Kidney Dis.* **18**, 413.

Alpers, C. E., Davis, C. L., Barr, D., *et al.* (1996). Identification of platelet-derived growth factor A and B chains in human renal vascular rejection. *Am. J. Pathol.* **148**, 439.

Alpers, C. E., Gordon, D. and Gown, A. M. (1990). Immunophenotype of vascular rejection in renal transplants. *Mod. Pathol.* **3**, 198.

Andres, G. A., Accinni, L., Hsu, K. C., *et al.* (1970). Human renal transplants: III. immunopathologic studies. *Lab. Invest.* **22**, 588.

Antignac, C., Hinglais, N., Gubler, M. C., *et al.* (1988). De novo membranous glomerulonephritis in renal allografts in children. *Clin. Nephrol.* **30**, 1.

Antonovych, T. T., Sabnis, S. G., Austin, H. A., *et al.* (1988). Cyclosporine A-induced arteriolopathy. *Transplant. Proc.* **20**, 951.

Axelsen, R. A., Seymour, A. E., Mathew, T. H., *et al.* (1985). Glomerular transplant rejection: a distinctive pattern of early graft damage. *Clin. Nephrol.* **23**, 1.

Azevedo, L. S., de Paula, F. J., Ianhez, L. E., *et al.* (1987). Renal transplantation and schistosomiasis mansoni. *Transplantation* **44**, 795.

Baid, S., Pascual, M., Williams, W. W., Jr., *et al.* (1999). Renal thrombotic microangiopathy associated with anticardiolipin antibodies in hepatitis C-positive renal allograft recipients. *J. Am. Soc. Nephrol.* **10**, 146.

Bakir, N., Sluiter, W. J., Ploeg, R. J., *et al.* (1996). Primary renal graft thrombosis. *Nephrol. Dial. Transplant.* **11**, 140.

Banfi, G., Imbasciati, E., Tarantino, A., *et al.* (1981). Prognostic value of renal biopsy in acute rejection of kidney transplantation. *Nephron* **28**, 222.

Barker, T. H. (1984). Malakoplakia in a renal allograft. *Br. J. Urol.* **56**, 549.

Bassani, C. E., Ferraris, J., Gianantonio, C. A., *et al.* (1991). Renal transplantation in patients with classical haemolytic-uraemic syndrome. *Pediatr. Nephrol.* **5**, 607.

Bates, W. D., Davies, D. R., Welsh, K., *et al.* (1999). An evaluation of the Banff classification of eary renal allograft biopsies and correlation with outcome. *Nephrol. Dial. Transplant.* **14**, 2364.

Battegay, E. J., Mihatsch, M. J., Mazzucchelli, L., *et al.* (1988). Cytomegalovirus and kidney. *Clin. Nephrol.* **30**, 239.

Beneck, D., Greco, M. A. and Feiner, H. D. (1986). Glomerulonephritis in congenital cytomegalic inclusion disease. *Hum. Pathol.* **17**, 1054.

Bergstrand, A., Bohmann, S. O., Farnsworth, A., *et al.* (1985). Renal histopathology in kidney transplant recipients immunosuppressed with cyclosporin A: results of an international workshop. *Clin. Nephrol.* **24**, 107.

Beschorner, W. E., Burdick, J. F., Williams, G. M., *et al.* (1985). Phenotypic identification of intraepithelial lymphocytes (IEL) in acute renal allograft rejection. *Kidney Int.* **27**, 206.

Biggar, W. D., Crawford, L., Cardella, C., *et al.* (1985). Malakoplakia and immunosuppressive therapy: reversal of clinical and leukocyte abnormalities after withdrawal of prednisone and azathioprine. *Am. J. Pathol.* **119**, 5.

Bignardi, L., Neild, G. H., Hartley, R. B., *et al.* (1987). Histopathological changes in cyclosporin-treated renal allografts biopsied at one and twelve months. *Nephrol. Dial. Transplant.* **2**, 366.

Bishop, G. A., Hall, B. M., Duggin, G. G., *et al.* (1986). Immunopathology of renal allograft rejection analyzed with monoclonal antibodies to mononuclear cell markers. *Kidney Int.* **29**, 708.

Bishop, G. A., Waugh, J. A., Landers, D. V., *et al.* (1989). Microvascular destruction in renal transplant rejection. *Transplantation* **48**, 408.

Blancho, G., Gianello, P. R., Lorf, T., *et al.* (1997). Molecular and cellular events implicated in local tolerance to kidney allografts in miniature swine. *Transplantation* **63**, 26.

Bohman, S. O., Tyden, G., Wilczek, H., *et al.* (1985). Prevention of kidney graft diabetic nephropathy by pancreas transplantation in man. *Diabetes* **34**, 306.

Borel, J. F. and Kis, Z. L. (1991). The discovery and development of cyclosporine (Sandimmune). *Transplant. Proc.* **23**, 1867.

Brensilver, J. M., Mallat, S., Scholes, J., *et al.* (1988). Recurrent IgA nephropathy in living-related donor transplantation: recurrence or transmission of familial disease? *Am. J. Kidney Dis.* **12**, 147.

Briscoe, D. M., Pober, J. S., Harmon, W. E., *et al.* (1992). Expression of vascular cell adhesion molecule-1 in human renal allografts. *J. Am. Soc. Nephrol.* **3**, 1180.

Brockmeyer, C., Ulbrecht, M., Schendel, D. J., *et al.* (1993). Distribution of cell adhesion molecules (ICAM-1, VCAM-1, ELAM-1) in renal tissue during allograft rejection. *Transplantation* **55**, 610.

Brook, I. (1994). The role of anaerobic bacteria in perinephric and renal abscesses in children. *Pediatrics* **93**, 261.

Burdick, J. F., Beschorner, W. E., Smith, W. J., *et al.* (1984). Characteristics of early routine renal allograft biopsies. *Transplantation* **38**, 679.

Burke, B. A., Chavers, B. M., Gillingham, K. J., *et al.* (1995a). Chronic renal allograft rejection in the first 6 months posttransplant. *Transplantation* **60**, 1413.

Burke, G. W., Cirocco, R., Markou, M., *et al.* (1995b). Acute graft loss secondary to necrotizing vasculitis: evidence for cytokine-mediated Shwartzman reaction in clinical kidney transplantation. *Transplantation* **59**, 1100.

Busch, G. J., Galvanek, E. G. and Reynolds, E. S. (1971a). Human renal allografts: analysis of lesions in long-term survivors. *Hum. Pathol.* **2**, 253.

Busch, G. J., Reynolds, E. S., Galvanek, E. G., *et al.* (1971b). Human renal allografts: the role of vascular injury in early graft failure. *Medicine* **50**, 29.

Byrne, G. W., McCurry, K. R., Martin, M. J., *et al.* (1997). Transgenic pigs expressing human CD59 and decay-accelerating factor produce an intrinsic barrier to complement-mediated damage. *Transplantation* **63**, 149.

Cameron, J., Rigby, R. J., van Deth, A. G., *et al.* (1982). Severe tubulo-interstitial disease in a renal allograft due to cytomegalovirus infection. *Clin. Nephrol.* **18**, 321.

Cameron, J. S. (1991). Recurrent primary disease and de novo nephritis following renal transplantation. *Pediatr. Nephrol.* **5**, 412.

Candinas, D., Keusch, G., Schlumpf, R., *et al.* (1994). Hemolytic-uremic syndrome following kidney transplantation: prognostic factors. *Schweiz. Med. Wochenschr.* **124**, 1789.

Charney, D. A., Nadasdy, T., Lo, A. W., *et al.* (1999). Plasma cell-rich acute renal allograft rejection. *Transplantation* **68**, 791.

Cohen, A. H., Border, W. A., Rajfer, J., *et al.* (1984). Interstitial Tamm-Horsfall protein in rejecting renal allografts. *Lab. Invest.* **50**, 519.

Cohen, A. H., Gonzalez, S., Nast, C. C., *et al.* (1991). Frozen-section analysis of allograft renal biopsy specimens: reliable histopathologic data for rapid decision making. *Arch. Pathol. Lab. Med.* **115**, 386.

Coleman, D. V., MacKenzie, E. F. D., Gardner, S. D., *et al.* (1978). Human polyoma virus (BK) infection and ureteric stenosis in renal allograft recipients. *J. Clin. Pathol.* **31**, 338.

Collins, A. B. and Colvin, R. B. (1997). Kidney and lung disease mediated by glomerular basement membrane antibodies: detection by western blot analysis. In *Manual of Clinical Laboratory Methods*, (N. R. Rose, E. C. de Macario, J. D. Folds, H. C. Lane and R. M. Nakmura, eds.), p. 1008, ASM Press, Washington, D.C.

Collins, A. B., Schneeberger, E. E., Pascual, M., *et al.* (1999). Deposition of C4d in peritubular capillaries is a marker of acute humoral renal allograft rejection. *J. Am. Soc. Nephrol.* **10**, 2208.

Colvin, R., Chase, C., Winn, H., *et al.* (1995). Chronic allograft arteriopathy: insights from experimental models. In *Transplant Vascular Sclerosis*, (C. Orosz, ed.), p. 7, R.G. Landes Biomedical Publishers, Austin, Tx.

Colvin, R. B. (1995). Pathology of renal allografts. In *Diagnostic Immunopathology*, (R. B. Colvin, A. K. Bhan and R. T. McCluskey, eds.), p. 329, Raven Press, New York.

Colvin, R. B. (1998). Renal transplant pathology. In *Heptinstall's Pathology of the Kidney*, (J. C. Jennette, J. L. Olson, M. L. Schwartz and F. G. Silva, eds.), p. 1409, Lippincott-Raven, Philadelphia.

Colvin, R. B., Cohen, A. H., Saiontz, C., *et al.* (1997). Evaluation of pathologic criteria for acute renal allograft rejection: reproducibility, sensitivity, and clinical correlation. *J. Am. Soc. Nephrol.* **8**, 1930.

Colvin, R. B., Dvorak, A. M. and Dvorak, H. F. (1974). Mast cells in the cortical tubular epithelium and interstitium in human renal disease. *Hum. Pathol.* **5**, 315.

Colvin, R. B. and Dvorak, H. F. (1974). Basophils and mast cells in renal allograft rejection. *Lancet* **1**, 212.

Colvin, R. B. and Fang, L. S.-T. (1994). Interstitial nephritis. In *Renal Pathology*, (C. C. Tisher and B. M. Brenner, eds.), p. 723, J.B. Lippincott, Philadelphia.

Cosio, F. G., Roche, Z., Agarwal, A., *et al.* (1996a). Prevalence of hepatitis C in patients with idiopathic glomerulonephritis in native and transplant kidneys. *Am. J. Kidney Dis.* **28**, 752.

Cosio, F. G., Sedmak, D. D., Henry, M. L., *et al.* (1996b). The high prevalence of severe early posttransplant renal allograft pathology in hepatitis C positive recipients. *Transplantation* **62**, 1054.

Cosio, F. G., Sedmak, D. D., Mahan, J. D., *et al.* (1989). Localization of decay accelerating factor in normal and diseased kidneys. *Kidney Int.* **36**, 100.

Cosyns, J. P., Kazatchkine, M. D., Bhakdi, S., *et al.* (1986). Immunohistochemical analysis of C3 cleavage fragments, factor H, and the C5b-9 terminal complex of complement in de novo membranous glomerulonephritis occurring in patients with renal transplant. *Clin. Nephrol.* **26**, 203.

Cramer, D. V., Qian, S. Q., Harnaha, J., *et al.* (1989). Cardiac transplantation in the rat: I. the effect of histocompatibility differences on graft arteriosclerosis. *Transplantation* **47**, 414.

Crespo, M., Pascual, M., Tolkoff-Rubin, N, *et al.* (2000). Acute humoral rejection in renal allograft recipients. I. Incidence, serology and clinical characteristics. *Transplantation* (in press).

Curschellas, E., Landmann, J., Durig, M., *et al.* (1991). Morphologic findings in "zero-hour" biopsies of renal transplants. *Clin. Nephrol.* **36**, 215.

Curtis, J. J., Julian, B. A., Sanders, C. E., *et al.* (1996). Dilemmas in renal transplantation: when the clinical course and histological findings differ. *Am. J. Kidney Dis.* **27**, 435.

Daly, C., Conlon, P. J., Medwar, W., *et al.* (1996). Characteristics and outcome of anti-glomerular basement membrane disease: a single-center experience. *Ren. Fail.* **18**, 105.

Davenport, A., Younie, M. E., Parsons, J. E., *et al.* (1994). Development of cytotoxic antibodies following renal allograft transplantation is associated with reduced graft survival due to chronic vascular rejection. *Nephrol. Dial. Transplant.* **9**, 1315.

Detwiler, R. K., Falk, R. J., Hogan, S. L., *et al.* (1994). Collapsing glomerulopathy: a clinically and pathologically distinct variant of focal segmental glomerulosclerosis. *Kidney Int.* **45**, 1416.

Diaz, J. I., Valenzuela, R., Gephardt, G., *et al.* (1994). Anti-glomerular and anti-tubular basement membrane nephritis in a renal allograft recipient with Alport's syndrome. *Arch. Pathol. Lab. Med.* **118**, 728.

Dimeny, E., Wahlberg, J., Larsson, E., *et al.* (1995). Can histopathological findings in early renal allograft biopsies identify patients at risk for chronic vascular rejection? *Clin. Transplant.* **9**, 79.

Dische, F. E., Neuberger, J., Keating, J., *et al.* (1988). Kidney pathology in liver allograft recipients after long-term treatment with cyclosporin A. *Lab. Invest.* **58**, 395.

Drachenberg, C. B., Beskow, C. O., Cangro, C. B., *et al.* (1999). Human polyoma virus in renal allograft biopsies: morphological findings and correlation with urine cytology. *Hum. Pathol.* **30**, 970.

Droz, D., Nabarra, B., Noel, L. H., *et al.* (1979). Recurrence of dense deposits in transplanted kidneys: I. sequential survey of the lesions. *Kidney Int.* **15**, 386.

Dussol, B., Tsimaratos, M., Lerda, D., *et al.* (1995). Viral hepatitis C and membranoproliferative glomerulonephritis in a renal transplant patient. *Nephrologie* **16**, 223.

Elkhammas, E. A., Mutabagani, K. H., Sedmak, D. D., *et al.* (1994). Xanthogranulomatous pyelonephritis in renal allografts: report of 2 cases. *J. Urol.* **151**, 127.

Evan, A. P., Gattone, V. H., 2d., *et al.* (1983). Glomerular endothelial injury related to renal perfusion: a scanning electron microscopic study. *Transplantation* **35**, 436.

Falkenhain, M. E., Cosio, F. G. and Sedmak, D. D. (1996). Progressive histologic injury in kidneys from heart and liver transplant recipients receiving cyclosporine. *Transplantation* **62**, 364.

Farnsworth, A., Hall, B. M., Ng, A., *et al.* (1984). Renal biopsy morphology in renal transplantation. *Am. J. Surg. Pathol.* **8**, 243.

Faull, R. J. and Russ, G. R. (1989). Tubular expression of intercellular adhesion molecule-1 during renal allograft rejection. *Transplantation* **48**, 226.

Fellström, B., Klareskog, L., Heldin, C. H., *et al.* (1989). Platelet-derived growth factor receptors in the kidney—upregulated expression in inflammation. *Kidney Int.* **36**, 1099.

Feucht, H. E., Felber, E., Gokel, M. J., *et al.* (1991). Vascular deposition of complement-split products in kidney allografts with cell-mediated rejection. *Clin. Exp. Immunol.* **86**, 464.

First, M. R., Mendoza, N., Maryniak, R. K., *et al.* (1984a). Membranous glomerulopathy following kidney transplantation: association with renal vein thrombosis in two of nine cases. *Transplantation* **38**, 603.

First, M. R., Vaidya, P. N., Maryniak, R. K., *et al.* (1984b). Proteinuria following transplantation: correlation with histopathology and outcome. *Transplantation* **38**, 607.

Flynn, J. T., Schulman, S. L., deChadarevian, J. P., *et al.* (1992). Treatment of steroid-resistant post-transplant nephrotic syndrome with cyclophosphamide in a child with congenital nephrotic syndrome. *Pediatr. Nephrol.* **6**, 553.

Fox, W. M., Hameed, A., Hutchins, G. M., *et al.* (1993). Perforin expression localizing cytotoxic lymphocytes in the intimas of coronary arteries with transplant-related accelerated arteriosclerosis. *Hum. Pathol.* **24**, 477.

Fuggle, S. V., McWhinnie, D. L., Chapman, J. R., *et al.* (1985). Sequential analysis of HLA class II antigen expression in human renal allografts: induction of tubular class II antigens and correlation with clinical parameters. *Transplantation* **42**, 144.

Fuggle, S. V., McWhinnie, D. L. and Morris, P. J. (1987). Precise specificity of induced tubular HLA-class II antigens in renal allografts. *Transplantation* **44**, 214.

Fuggle, S. V., Sanderson, J. B., Gray, D. W., *et al.* (1993). Variation in expression of endothelial adhesion molecules in pretransplant and transplanted kidneys—correlation with intragraft events. *Transplantation* **55**, 117.

Furth, S., Neu, A., Colombani, P., *et al.* (1996). Diabetes as a complication of tacrolimus (FK506) in pediatric renal transplant patients. *Pediatr. Nephrol.* **10**, 64.

Gaber, L. W., Gaber, A. O., Tolley, E. A., *et al.* (1992a). Prediction by postrevascularization biopsies of cadaveric kidney allografts of rejection, graft loss, and preservation nephropathy. *Transplantation* **53**, 1219.

Gaber, L. W., Gaber, A. O., Vera, S. R., *et al.* (1992b). Successful reversal of hyperacute renal allograft rejection with the anti-CD3 monoclonal OKT3. *Transplantation* **54**, 930.

Gaber, L. W., Moore, L. W., Alloway, R. R., *et al.* (1995). Glomerulosclerosis as a determinant of posttransplant function of older donor renal allografts. *Transplantation* **60**, 334.

Gallay, B. J., Alpers, C. E., Davis, C. L., *et al.* (1995). Glomerulonephritis in renal allografts associated with hepatitis C infection: a possible relationship with transplant glomerulopathy in two cases. *Am. J. Kidney Dis.* **26**, 662.

Gardner, S. D., Field, A. M., Coleman, D. V., *et al.* (1971). New human papovavirus (B.K.) isolated from urine after renal transplantation. *Lancet* **1**, 1253.

Gardner, S. D., MacKenzie, E. F., Smith, C., *et al.* (1984). Prospective study of the human polyomaviruses BK and JC and cytomegalovirus in renal transplant recipients. *J. Clin. Pathol.* **37**, 578.

Gillum, D. M. and Kelleher, S. P. (1985). Acute pyelonephritis as a cause of late transplant dysfunction. *Am. J. Med.* **78**, 156.

Glassock, R. J., Feldman, D., Reynolds, E. S., *et al.* (1968). Human renal isografts: a clinical and pathologic analysis. *Medicine* **47**, 411.

Gnann, J. W., Jr., Ahlmen, J., Svalander, C., *et al.* (1988). Inflammatory cells in transplanted kidneys are infected by human cytomegalovirus. *Am. J. Pathol.* **132**, 239.

Gobel, J., Olbricht, C. J., Offner, G., *et al.* (1992). Kidney transplantation in Alport's syndrome: long-term outcome and allograft anti-GBM nephritis. *Clin. Nephrol.* **38**, 299.

Gould, V. E., Martinez, L. V., Virtanen, I., *et al.* (1992). Differential distribution of tenascin and cellular fibronectins in acute and chronic renal allograft rejection. *Lab. Invest.* **67**, 71.

Gouldesbrough, D. R. and Axelsen, R. A. (1994). Arterial endothelialitis in chronic renal allograft rejection: a histopathological and immunocytochemical study. *Nephrol. Dial. Transplant.* **9**, 35.

Habib, R. and Broyer, M. (1993). Clinical significance of allograft glomerulopathy. *Kidney Int.* **43(Suppl.)**, S95.

Hallgren, R., Bohman, S. O. and Fredens, K. (1991). Activated eosinophil infiltration and deposits of eosinophil cationic protein in renal allograft rejection. *Nephron* **59**, 266.

Halloran, P. F., Schlaut, J., Solez, K., *et al.* (1992). The significance of the anti-class I antibody response: II. clinical and pathologic features of renal transplants with anti-class I-like antibody. *Transplantation* **53**, 550.

Halloran, P. F., Wadgymar, A., Ritchie, S., *et al.* (1990). The significance of the anti-class I antibody response: I. clinical and pathologic features of anti-class I-mediated rejection. *Transplantation* **49**, 85.

Hammer, C., Land, W., Stadler, J., *et al.* (1983). Lymphocyte subclasses in rejecting kidney grafts detected by monoclonal antibodies. *Transplantation* **5**, 870.

Hansen, B. L., Rohr, N., Svendsen, V., *et al.* (1988). Bacterial urinary tract infection in cyclosporine-A immunosuppressed renal transplant recipients. *Scand. J. Infect. Dis.* **20**, 425.

Hariharan, S., Smith, R. D., Viero, R., *et al.* (1996). Diabetic nephropathy after renal transplantation: clinical and pathologic features. *Transplantation* **62**, 632.

Harry, T. R., Coles, G. A., Davies, M., *et al.* (1984). The significance of monocytes in glomeruli of human renal transplants. *Transplantation* **37**, 70.

Hebert, D., Kim, E. M., Sibley, R. K., *et al.* (1991). Post-transplantation outcome of patients with hemolytic-uremic syndrome: update. *Pediatr. Nephrol.* **5**, 162.

Heidet, L., Gagnadoux, M. E., Beziau, A., *et al.* (1994). Recurrence of de novo membranous glomerulonephritis on renal grafts. *Clin. Nephrol.* **41**, 314.

Herrera, G. A., Alexander, R. W., Cooley, C. F., *et al.* (1986). Cytomegalovirus glomerulopathy: a controversial lesion. *Kidney Int.* **29**, 725.

Hibberd, A. D., Nanra, R. S., White, K. H., *et al.* (1991). Reversal of acute glomerular renal allograft rejection: a possible effect of OKT3. *Transpl. Int.* **4**, 246.

Hiki, Y., Leong, A. Y., Mathew, T. H., *et al.* (1986). Typing of intraglomerular mononuclear cells associated with transplant glomerular rejection. *Clin. Nephrol.* **26**, 244.

Hochstetler, L. A., Flanigan, M. J. and Lager, D. J. (1994). Transplant-associated thrombotic microangiopathy: the role of IgG administration as initial therapy. *Am. J. Kidney Dis.* **23**, 444.

Hogan, T. F., Borden, E. C., McBain, J. A., *et al.* (1980a). Human polyomavirus infections with JC virus and BK virus in renal transplant patients. *Ann. Intern. Med.* **92**, 373.

Hogan, T. F., Padgett, B. L., Walker, D. L., *et al.* (1980b). Rapid detection and identification of JC virus and BK virus in human urine by using immunofluorescence microscopy. *J. Clin. Microbiol.* **11**, 178.

Hongwei, W., Nanra, R. S., Stein, A., *et al.* (1994). Eosinophils in acute renal allograft rejection. *Transpl. Immunol.* **2**, 41.

Hostetter, T. H. (1994). Chronic transplant rejection. *Kidney Int.* **46**, 266.

Howie, A. J., Bryan, R. L. and Gunson, B. K. (1992). Arteries and veins formed within renal vessels: a previously neglected observation. *Virchows Arch.* **420**, 301.

Hruban, R. H., Long, P. P., Perlman, E. J., *et al.* (1993). Fluorescence in situ hybridization for the Y-chromosome can be used to detect cells of recipient origin in allografted hearts following cardiac transplantation. *Am. J. Pathol.* **142**, 975.

Hsu, H. C., Suzuki, Y., Churg, J., *et al.* (1980). Ultrastructure of transplant glomerulopathy. *Histopathology* **4**, 351.

Ibrahim, S., Dawson, D. V. and Sanfilippo, F. (1995). Predominant infiltration of rejecting human renal allografts with T cells expressing CD8 and CD45RO. *Transplantation* **59**, 724.

Ichida, S., Yuzawa, Y., Okada, H., *et al.* (1994). Localization of the complement regulatory proteins in the normal human kidney. *Kidney Int.* **46**, 89.

Ismail-Allouch, M., Burke, G., Nery, J., *et al.* (1993). Rapidly progressive focal segmental glomerulosclerosis occurring in a living related kidney transplant donor: case report and review of 21 cases of kidney transplants for primary FSGS. *Transplant. Proc.* **25**, 2176.

Isoniemi, H., Taskinen, E. and Hayry, P. (1994). Histological chronic allograft damage index accurately predicts chronic renal allograft rejection. *Transplantation* **58**, 1195.

Ito, H., Kasagi, N., Shomori, K., *et al.* (1995). Apoptosis in the human allografted kidney: analysis by terminal deoxynucleotidyl transferase–mediated DUTP-botin nick end labeling. *Transplantation* **60**, 794.

Ito, M., Hirabayash, N., Uno, Y., *et al.* (1991). Necrotizing tubulointerstitial nephritis associated with adenovirus infection. *Hum. Pathol.* **22**, 1225.

Ivanyi, B., Hamilton-Dutoit, S. J., Hansen, H. E., et al. (1996). Acute tubulointerstitial nephritis: phenotype of infiltrating cells and prognostic impact of tubulitis. *Virchows Arch.* **428**, 5.

Ivanyi, B., Hansen, H. E. and Olsen, T. S. (1992). Postcapillary venule-like transformation of peritubular capillaries in acute renal allograft rejection: an ultrastructural study. *Arch. Pathol. Lab. Med.* **116**, 1062.

Japanese FK Study Group. (1993). Morphological characteristics of renal allografts showing renal dysfunction under FK 506 therapy: is graft biopsy available to reveal the morphological findings corresponding with FK 506 nephropathy? *Transplant. Proc.* **25**, 624.

Jeannet, M., Pinn, V. W., Flax, M. H., *et al.* (1970). Humoral antibodies in renal allotransplantation in man. *N. Engl. J. Med.* **282**, 111.

Jones, B. F., Nanra, R. S., Grant, A. B., *et al.* (1989). Xanthogranulomatous pyelonephritis in a renal allograft: a case report. *J. Urol.* **141**, 926.

Kalra, O. P., Malik, N., Minz, M., *et al.* (1993). Emphysematous pyelonephritis and cystitis in a renal transplant recipient—computed tomographic appearance. *Int. J. Artif. Organs* **16**, 41.

Kasiske, B. L., Kalil, R. S., Lee, H. S., *et al.* (1991). Histopathologic findings associated with a chronic, progressive decline in renal allograft function. *Kidney Int.* **40**, 514.

Kennedy, L. J. and Weissman, I. L. (1971). Dual origin of intimal cells in cardiac allograft arteriosclerosis. *N. Engl. J. Med.* **285**, 884.

Kerby, J. D., Verran, D. J., Luo, K. L., *et al.* (1996). Immunolocalization of FGF and FGF receptors in the vascular lesions of chronic renal allograft vasculopathy. *Transplantation* **62**, 467.

Kiprov, D. D., Colvin, R. B. and McCluskey, R. T. (1982). Focal and segmental glomerulosclerosis and proteinuria associated with unilateral renal agenesis. *Lab. Invest.* **46**, 275.

Kiss, D., Landman, J., Mihatsch, M., *et al.* (1992). Risks and benefits of graft biopsy in renal transplantation under cyclosporin-A. *Clin. Nephrol.* **38**, 132.

Kissmeyer-Nielsen, F., Olsen, S., Peterson, V. P., *et al.* (1966). Hyperacute rejection of kidney allografts, associated with pre-existing humoral antibodies against donor cells. *Lancet* **2**, 662.

Kon, S. P., Templar, J., Dodd, S. M., *et al.* (1997). Diagnostic contribution of renal allograft biopsies at various intervals after transplantation. *Transplantation* **63**, 547.

Kooijmans-Coutinho, M. F., Bruijn, J. A., Hermans, J., *et al.* (1995). Evaluation by histology, immunohistology and PCR of protocollized renal biopsies 1 week post-transplant in relation to subsequent rejection episodes. *Nephrol. Dial. Transplant.* **10**, 847.

Kooijmans-Coutinho, M. F., Hermans, J., Schrama, E., *et al.* (1996). Interstitial rejection, vascular rejection, and diffuse thrombosis of renal allografts: predisposing factors, histology, immunohistochemistry, and relation to outcome. *Transplantation* **61**, 1338.

Kormendi, F. and Amend, W. (1988). The importance of eosinophil cells in kidney allograft rejection. *Transplantation* **45**, 537.

Lane, P. H., Schnaper, H. W., Vernier, R. L., *et al.* (1991). Steroid-dependent nephrotic syndrome following renal transplantation for congenital nephrotic syndrome. *Pediatr. Nephrol.* **5**, 300.

Larsen, S., Brun, C., Duun, S., *et al.* (1988). Early arteriolopathy following "high-dose" cyclosporine in kidney transplantation. *A. P. M. I. S.* **4(Suppl.)**, 66.

Lee, S. J. and Howie, A. J. (1988). Changes at the glomerulo-tubular junction in renal transplants. *J. Pathol.* **156**, 311.

Legendre, C., Thervet, E., Skhiri, H., *et al.* (1998). Histologic features of chronic allograft nephropathy revealed by protocol biopsies in kidney transplant recipients. *Transplantation* **65**, 1506.

Liano, F., Mampaso, F., Garcia-Martin, F., *et al.* (1988). Allograft membranous glomerulonephritis and renal-vein thrombosis in a patient with a lupus anticoagulant factor. *Nephrol. Dial. Transplant.* **3**, 684.

Lipman, M. L., Shen, Y., Jeffery, J. R., *et al.* (1998). Immune-activation gene expression in clinically stable renal allograft biopsies: molecular evidence for subclinical rejection. *Transplantation* **66**, 1673.

Lobo, P. I., Spencer, C. E., Stevenson, W. C., *et al.* (1995). Evidence demonstrating poor kidney graft survival when acute rejections are associated with IgG donor-specific lymphocytotoxin. *Transplantation* **59**, 357.

Loomis, L. J., Aronson, A. J., Rudinsky, R., *et al.* (1989). Hemolytic uremic syndrome following bone marrow transplantation: a case report and review of the literature. *Am. J. Kidney Dis.* **14**, 324.

Lopez, C., Simmons, R. L., Mauer, S. M., *et al.* (1974). Association of renal allograft rejection with virus infections. *Am. J. Med.* **56**, 280.

Magil, A., Rubin, J., Ladewig, L., *et al.* (1980). Renal biopsy in acute allograft rejection: significance of moderate vascular lesions in long-term graft survival. *Nephron* **26**, 180.

Marcen, R., Pascual, J., Quereda, C., *et al.* (1990). Lupus anticoagulant and thrombosis of kidney allograft vessels. *Transplant. Proc.* **22**, 1396.

Marcussen, N., Lai, R., Olsen, T. S., *et al.* (1996). Morphometric and immunohistochemical investigation of renal biopsies from patients with transplant ATN, native ATN, or acute graft rejection. *Transplant. Proc.* **28**, 470.

Marcussen, N., Olsen, T. S., Benediktsson, H., *et al.* (1995). Reproducibility of the Banff classification of renal allograft pathology: inter- and intraobserver variation. *Transplantation* **60**, 1083.

Maryniak, R., First, R. M. and Weiss, M. A. (1985a). Transplant glomerulopathy: evolution of morphologically distinct changes. *Kidney Int.* **27**, 799.

Maryniak, R. K., Mendoza, N., Clyne, D., *et al.* (1985b). Recurrence of diabetic nodular glomerulosclerosis in a renal transplant. *Kidney Int.* **27**, 799.

Matas, A. J., Scheinman, J. I., Rattazzi, L. C., *et al.* (1976). Immunopathological studies of the ruptured human renal allograft. *Transplantation* **22**, 420.

Matas, A. J., Sibley, R., Mauer, M., *et al.* (1983). The value of needle renal allograft biopsy: I. a retrospective study of biopsies performed during putative rejection episodes. *Ann. Surg.* **197**, 226.

Mathur, V. S., Olson, J. L., Darragh, T. M., *et al.* (1997). Polyomavirus induced interstitial nephritis in two renal transplant recipients: case reports and review of the literature. *Am. J. Kidney Dis.* **29**, 754.

Mauer, S. M., Barbosa, J., Vernier, R. L., *et al.* (1976). Development of diabetic vascular lesions in normal kidneys transplanted into patients with diabetes mellitus. *N. Engl. J. Med.* **295**, 916.

Mauiyyedi, S., Baid, S., Pascual, M., *et al.* (2000a). Chronic allograft glomerulopathy related to hepatitis C virus infection. *Mod. Pathol.* **13**, 176A.

Mauiyyedi, S., Della Pelle, P., Saidman, S., *et al.* (2000c). C4d deposits in peritubular capillaries in chronic renal allograft rejection. *J. Am. Soc. Nephrol.*, in press.

Mauiyyedi, S., Nelson, C., Tolkoff-Rubin, N., *et al.* (2000b). Peritubular capillary lamination: a marker of antibody mediated chronic rejection of renal allografts. *Mod. Pathol.* **13**, 176A.

Mazzucco, G., Motta, M., Segoloni, G., *et al.* (1994). Intertubular capillary changes in the cortex and medulla of transplanted kidneys and their relationship with transplant glomerulopathy: an ultrastructural study of 12 transplantectomies. *Ultrastruct. Pathol.* **18**, 533.

McCoy, R. C., Johnson, H. K., Stone, W. J., *et al.* (1982). Absence of nephritogenic GBM antigen(s) in some patients with hereditary nephritis. *Kidney Int.* **21**, 642.

McKenzie, I. and Whittingham, S. (1968). Deposits of immunoglobulin and fibrin in human renal allografted kidneys. *Lancet* **2**, 1313.

McLaren, A. J., Marshall, S. E., Haldar, N. A., *et al.* (1999). Adhesion molecule polymorphisms in chronic renal allograft failure. *Kidney Int.* **55**, 1977.

McManus, B. M., Malcom, G., Kendall, T. J., *et al.* (1995). Prominence of coronary arterial wall lipids in human heart allografts: implications for pathogenesis of allograft arteriopathy. *Am. J. Pathol.* **147**, 293.

McWhinnie, D. L., Thompson, J. F., Taylor, H. M., *et al.* (1986). Morphometric analysis of cellular infiltration assessed by monoclonal antibody labeling in sequential human renal allograft biopsies. *Transplantation* **2**, 352.

Meehan, S., McCluskey, R., Pascual, M., *et al.* (1997). Cytotoxicity and apoptosis in human renal allografts: identification, distribution, and quantitation of cells with a cytotoxic granule protein GMP-17 (TIA-1) and cells with fragmented nuclear DNA. *Lab. Invest.* **76**, 639.

Meehan, S. M., Pascual, M., Williams, W. W., *et al.* (1988). De novo collapsing glomerulopathy in renal allografts. *Transplantation* **65**, 1192.

Merion, R. M. and Calne, R. Y. (1985). Allograft renal vein thrombosis. *Transplant. Proc.* **17**, 1746.

Messana, J. M., Johnson, K. J. and Mihatsch, M. J. (1995). Renal structure and function effects after low dose cyclosporine in psoriasis patients: a preliminary report. *Clin. Nephrol.* **43**, 150.

Mihatsch, M., Thiel, G. and Ryffel, B. (1988). Cyclosporine nephrotoxicity. *Adv. Nephrol.* **17**, 303.

Mihatsch, M. J., Gudat, F., Ryffel, B., *et al.* (1994). Cyclosporine nephropathy. *In Renal Pathology: With Clinical and Functional Correlations*, (C. C. Tisher and B. M. Brenner, eds.), p. 1641, J.B. Lippincott, Philadelphia.

Mihatsch, M. J., Helmchen, U., Casanova, P., *et al.* (1991). Kidney biopsy findings in cyclosporine-treated patients with insulin-dependent diabetes mellitus. *Klin. Wochenschr.* **69**, 354.

Mihatsch, M. J., Morozumi, K., Strom, E. H., *et al.* (1995a). Renal transplant morphology after long-term therapy with cyclosporine. *Transplant. Proc.* **27**, 39.

Mihatsch, M. J., Ryffel, B. and Gudat, F. (1995b). The differential diagnosis between rejection and cyclosporine toxicity. *Kidney Int.* **52(Suppl.)**, S63.

Mihatsch, M. J., Theil, G., Spichtin, H. P., *et al.* (1983). Morphological findings in kidney transplants after treatment with cyclosporine. *Transplant. Proc.* **15(Suppl. 1)**, 2821.

Milliner, D. S., Pierdes, A. M. and Holley, K. E. (1982). Renal transplantation in Alport's syndrome: anti-glomerular basement membrane glomerulonephritis in the allograft. *Mayo Clin. Proc.* **57**, 35.

Miltenburg, A. M., Meijer Paape, M. E., Weening, J. J., *et al.* (1989). Induction of antibody-dependent cellular cytotoxicity against endothelial cells by renal transplantation. *Transplantation* **48**, 681.

Monga, G., Mazzucco, G., Basolo, B., *et al.* (1993). Membranous glomerulonephritis (MGN) in transplanted kidneys: investigation on 256 renal allografts. *Mod. Pathol.* **6**, 249.

Monga, G., Mazzucco, G., Messina, M., *et al.* (1992). Intertubular capillary changes in kidney allografts: a morphologic investigation on 61 renal specimens. *Mod. Pathol.* **5**, 125.

Morel, D., Normand, E., Lemoine, C., *et al.* (1993). Tumor necrosis factor alpha in human kidney transplant rejection—analysis by in situ hybridization. *Transplantation* **55**, 773.

Myburgh, J. A., Cohen, I., Gecelter, L., *et al.* (1969). Hyperacute rejection in human-kidney allografts: Shwartzman or Arthus reaction? *N. Engl. J. Med.* **281**, 131.

Myers, B. D., Newton, L., Boshkos, C., *et al.* (1988a). Chronic injury of human renal microvessels with low-dose cyclosporine therapy. *Transplantation* **46**, 694.

Myers, B. D., Ross, J., Newton, L., *et al.* (1984). Cyclosporine-associated chronic nephropathy. *N. Engl. J. Med.* **311**, 699.

Myers, B. D., Sibley, R., Newton, L., *et al.* (1988b). The long-term course of cyclosporine-associated chronic nephropathy. *Kidney Int.* **33**, 590.

Nadasdy, T., Krenacs, T., Kalmar, K. N., *et al.* (1991). Importance of plasma cells in the infiltrate of renal allografts: an immunohistochemical study. *Pathol. Res. Pract.* **187**, 178.

Nadasdy, T., Laszik, Z., Blick, K. E., *et al.* (1995). Human acute tubular necrosis: a lectin and immunohistochemical study. *Hum. Pathol.* **26**, 230.

Nadasdy, T., Ormos, J., Stiller, D., *et al.* (1988). Tubular ultrastructure in rejected human renal allografts. *Ultrastruct. Pathol.* **12**, 195.

Nakanishi, I., Moutabarrik, A., Hara, T., *et al.* (1994). Identification and characterization of membrane cofactor protein (CD46) in the human kidneys. *Eur. J. Immunol.* **24**, 1529.

Nast, C. C., Blifeld, C., Danovitch, G. M., *et al.* (1989). Evaluation of cyclosporine nephrotoxicity by renal transplant fine needle aspiration. *Mod. Pathol.* **2**, 577.

Neild, G. H., Taube, D. H., Hartley, R. B., *et al.* (1986). Morphological differentiation between rejection and cyclosporin nephrotoxicity in renal allografts. *J. Clin. Pathol.* **39**, 152.

Neumayer, H. H., Huls, S., Schreiber, M., *et al.* (1994). Kidneys from pediatric donors: risk versus benefit. *Clin. Nephrol.* **41**, 94.

Nicholson, M. L., Bailey, E., Williams, S., *et al.* (1999). Computerized histomorphometric assessment of protocol renal transplant biopsy specimens for surrogate markers of chronic rejection. *Transplantation* **68**, 236.

Nickeleit, V., Hirsch, H. H., Binet, I. F., *et al.* (1999). Polyomavirus infection of renal allograft recipients: from latent infection to manifest disease. *J. Am. Soc. Nephrol.* **10**, 1080.

Nickeleit, V., Vamvakas, E. C., Pascual, M., *et al.* (1998). The prognostic significance of specific arterial lesions in acute renal allograft rejection. *J. Am. Soc. Nephrol.* **9**, 1301.

Nickerson, P., Jeffery, J., Gough, J., *et al.* (1998). Identification of clinical and histopathologic risk factors for diminished renal function 2 years posttransplant. *J. Am. Soc. Nephrol.* **9**, 482.

Nickerson, P., Jeffery, J., Gough, J., *et al.* (1999). Effect of increasing baseline immunosuppression on the prevalence of clinical and subclinical rejection: a pilot study. *J. Am. Soc. Nephrol.* **10**, 1801.

Nizze, H., Mihatsch, M. J., Zollinger, H. U., *et al.* (1988). Cyclosporine-associated nephropathy in patients with heart and bone marrow transplants. *Clin. Nephrol.* **30**, 248.

Noronha, I. L., Eberlein-Gonska, M., Hartley, B., *et al.* (1992). In situ expression of tumor necrosis factor-alpha, interferon-gamma, and interleukin-2 receptors in renal allograft biopsies. *Transplantation* **54**, 1017.

Noronha, I. L., Hartley, B., Cameron, J. S., *et al.* (1993). Detection of IL-1 beta and TNF-alpha message and protein in renal allograft biopsies. *Transplantation* **56**, 1026.

Nyberg, G., Friman, S., Svalander, C., *et al.* (1995). Spectrum of hereditary renal disease in a kidney transplant population. *Nephrol. Dial. Transplant.* **10**, 859.

Ode-Hakim, S., Docke, W. D., Kern, F., *et al.* (1996). Delayed-type hypersensitivity-like mechanisms dominate late acute rejection episodes in renal allograft recipients. *Transplantation* **61**, 1233.

Oguma, S., Banner, B., Zerbe, T., *et al.* (1988). Participation of dendritic cells in vascular lesions of chronic rejection of human allografts. *Lancet* **2**, 933.

Olsen, S., Bohman, S. O. and Petersen, V. P. (1974). Ultrastructure of the glomerular basement membrane in long term renal allografts with transplant glomerular disease. *Lab. Invest.* **30**, 176.

Olsen, S., Burdick, J. F., Keown, P. A., *et al.* (1989). Primary acute renal failure ("acute tubular necrosis") in the transplanted kidney: morphology and pathogenesis. *Medicine* **68**, 173.

Osterby, R., Nyberg, G., Karlberg, I., *et al.* (1992). Glomerular volume in kidneys transplanted into diabetic and non-diabetic patients. *Diabet. Med.* **9**, 144.

Pagtalunan, M. E., Oberbauer, R., Haas, M., *et al.* (1996). Atubular glomeruli in patients with chronic allograft rejection. *Transplantation* **61**, 1166.

Palestine, A. G., Austin, H. A., III, Balow, J. E., *et al.* (1986). Renal histopathologic alterations in patients treated with cyclosporine for uveitis. *N. Engl. J. Med.* **314**, 1293.

Pappo, O., Demetris, A. J., Raikow, R. B., *et al.* (1996). Human polyoma virus infection of renal allografts: histopathologic diagnosis, clinical significance, and literature review. *Mod. Pathol.* **9**, 105.

Pascual, M., Saidman, S., Tolkoff-Rubin, N., *et al.* (1998). Plasma exchange and tacrolimus-mycophenolate rescue for acute humoral rejection in kidney transplantation [published erratum appears in *Transplantation* 1999 Feb 15;67(3):495]. *Transplantation* **66**, 1460.

Pascual, M., Vallhonrat, H., Cosimi, A. B., *et al.* (1999). The clinical usefulness of the renal allograft biopsy in the cyclosporine era: a prospective study. *Transplantation* **67**, 737.

Paul, L., Class, F., van Es, L., *et al.* (1979). Accelerated rejection of a renal allograft associated with pretransplantation antibodies directed against donor antigens on endothelium and monocytes. *N. Engl. J. Med.* **300**, 1258.

Pavlakis, M., Strehlau, J., Lipman, M., *et al.* (1996). Use of intragraft gene expression in the diagnosis of kidney allograft rejection. *Transplant. Proc.* **28**, 2019.

Payton, D., Thorner, P., Eddy, A., *et al.* (1987). Demonstration by light microscopy of cytomegalovirus on a renal biopsy of a renal allograft recipient: confirmation by immunohistochemistry and in situ hybridization. *Nephron* **47**, 205.

Pearson, J. C., Amend, W. J., Jr., Vincenti, F. G., *et al.* (1980). Post-transplantation pyelonephritis: factors producing low patient and transplant morbidity. *J. Urol.* **123**, 153.

Pei, Y., Scholey, J. W., Katz, A., *et al.* (1994). Chronic nephrotoxicity in psoriatic patients treated with low-dose cyclosporine. *Am. J. Kidney Dis.* **23**, 528.

Petersen, V. P., Olsen, T. S., Kissmeyer, N. F., *et al.* (1975). Late failure of human renal transplants: an analysis of transplant disease and graft failure among 125 recipients surviving for one to eight years. *Medicine* **54**, 45.

Platt, J. L., Sibley, R. K. and Michael, A. F. (1985). Interstitial nephritis associated with cytomegalovirus infection. *Kidney Int.* **28**, 550.

Porter, K. A. (1990). Renal transplantation. *In The Pathology of the Kidney*, (R. H. Heptinstall, ed.), p. 1799, Little, Brown, Boston.

Porter, K. A., Andres, G. A., Calder, M. W., *et al.* (1968). Human renal transplants: II. immunofluorescence and immunoferritin studies. *Lab. Invest.* **18**, 159.

Porter, K. A., Dossetor, J. B., Marchioro, T. L., *et al.* (1967). Human renal transplants: I. glomerular changes. *Lab. Invest.* **16**, 153.

Porter, K. A., Owen, K., Mowbray, J. F., *et al.* (1963). Obliterative vascular changes in four human kidney homotransplants. *B. M. J.* **2**, 639.

Porter, K. A., Rendall, J. M., Stolinski, C., *et al.* (1966). Light and electron microscopic study of biopsies from 33 human renal allografts and an isograft 1 3/4 to 2 1/2 years after transplantation. *Ann. N. Y. Acad. Sci.* **129**, 615.

Pradier, O., Marchant, A., Abramowicz, D., *et al.* (1992). Procoagulant effect of the OKT3 monoclonal antibody: involvement of tumor necrosis factor. *Kidney Int.* **42**, 1124.

Querin, S., Noel, L. H., Grunfeld, J. P., *et al.* (1986). Linear glomerular IgG fixation in renal allografts: incidence and significance in Alport's syndrome. *Clin. Nephrol.* **25**, 134.

Racusen, L. C., Solez, K., Colvin, R. B., *et al.* (1999). The Banff 97 working classification of renal allograft pathology. *Kidney Int.* **55**, 713.

Ramos, E. L. and Tisher, C. C. (1994). Recurrent diseases in the kidney transplant. *Am. J. Kidney Dis.* **24**, 142.

Randhawa, P. S., Magnone, M., Jordan, M., *et al.* (1996). Renal allograft involvement by Epstein-Barr virus associated post-transplant lymphoproliferative disease. *Am. J. Surg. Pathol.* **20**, 563.

Randhawa, P. S., Shapiro, R., Jordan, M. L., *et al.* (1993). The histopathological changes associated with allograft rejection and drug toxicity in renal transplant recipients maintained on FK506: clinical significance and comparison with cyclosporine. *Am. J. Surg. Pathol.* **17**, 60.

Reinholt, F. P., Bohman, S. O., Wilczek, H., *et al.* (1990). Ultrastructural changes of tubular basement membranes in immunologic renal tubular lesions in humans. *Ultrastruct. Pathol.* **14**, 121.

Remuzzi, G. and Perico, N. (1995). Cyclosporine-induced renal dysfunction in experimental animals and humans. *Kidney Int.* **52(Suppl.)**, S70.

Richardson, W. P., Colvin, R. B., Cheeseman, S. H., *et al.* (1981). Glomerulopathy associated with cytomegalovirus viremia in renal allografts. *N. Engl. J. Med.* **305**, 57.

Roake, J. A., Fawcett, J., Koo, D. D., *et al.* (1996). Late reflush in clinical renal transplantation: protection against delayed graft function not observed. *Transplantation* **62**, 114.

Robertson, H., Wheeler, J., Thompson, V., *et al.* (1995). In situ lymphoproliferation in renal transplant biopsies. *Histochem. Cell. Biol.* **104**, 331.

Rosen, S., Greenfeld, Z. and Brezis, M. (1990). Chronic cyclosporine-induced nephropathy in the rat. *Transplantation* **49**, 445.

Rossmann, P., Jirka, J., Chadimova, M., *et al.* (1991). Arteriolosclerosis of the human renal allograft: morphology, origin, life history and relationship to cyclosporine therapy. *Virchow Arch.*, **418**, 129.

Rotellar, C., Noel, L. H., Droz, D., *et al.* (1986). Role of antibodies directed against tubular basement membranes in human renal transplants. *Am. J. Kidney* **7**, 157.

Rubin, R. H. and Colvin, R. B. (1998). Impact of cytomegalovirus infection on renal transplantation. *In Kidney Transplant Rejection: Diagnosis and Treatment*, (L. C. Racusen, K. Solez and J. F. Burdick, eds.), p. 605, Marcel Dekker, New York.

Rush, D., Nickerson, P., Gough, J., *et al.* (1998). Beneficial effects of treatment of early subclinical rejection: a randomized study. *J. Am. Soc. Nephrol.* **9**, 2129.

Rush, D. N., Henry, S. F., Jeffery, J. R., *et al.* (1994). Histological findings in early routine biopsies of stable renal allograft recipients. *Transplantation* **57**, 208.

Rush, D. N., Jeffery, J. R. and Gough, J. (1995). Sequential protocol biopsies in renal transplant patients: clinico-pathological correlations using the Banff schema. *Transplantation* **59**, 511.

Russell, P. S., Chase, C. M. and Colvin, R. B. (1995). Coronary atherosclerosis in transplanted mouse hearts: IV. effects of treatment with monoclonal antibodies to intercellular adhesion molecule-1 and leukocyte function-associated antigen-1. *Transplantation* **60**, 724.

Russell, P. S., Chase, C. M. and Colvin, R. B. (1997). Alloantibody- and T cell-mediated immunity in the pathogenesis of transplant arteriosclerosis: lack of progression to sclerotic lesions in B cell-deficient mice. *Transplantation* **64**, 1531.

Russell, P. S., Chase, C. M., Colvin, R. B., *et al.* (1978). Kidney transplants in mice: an analysis of the immune status of mice bearing long-term, H-2 incompatible transplants. *J. Exp. Med.* **147**, 1449.

Russell, P. S., Chase, C. M., Winn, H. J., *et al.* (1994a). Coronary atherosclerosis in transplanted mouse hearts: I. time course and immunogenetic and immunopathological considerations. *Am. J. Pathol.* **144**, 260.

Russell, P. S., Chase, C. M., Winn, H. J., *et al.* (1994b). Coronary atherosclerosis in transplanted mouse hearts: II. importance of humoral immunity. *J. Immunol.* **152**, 5135.

Sacchi, G., Bertalot, G., Cancarini, C., *et al.* (1993). Atheromatosis and double media: uncommon vascular lesions of renal allografts. *Pathologica* **85**, 183.

Said, R., Duarte, R., Chaballout, A., *et al.* (1994). Spontaneous rupture of renal allograft. *Urology* **43**, 554.

Said, R. and Soyannwo, M. (1996). Renal failure in a living-related kidney donor: case report and review of the literature. *Am. J. Nephrol.* **16**, 334.

Salmela, K. T., von Willebrand, E. O., Kyllonen, L. E., *et al.* (1992). Acute vascular rejection in renal transplantation—diagnosis and outcome. *Transplantation* **54**, 858.

Salomon, R. N., Hughes, C. C., Schoen, F. J., *et al.* (1991). Human coronary transplantation-associated arteriosclerosis: evidence for a chronic immune reaction to activated graft endothelial cells. *Am. J. Pathol.* **138**, 791.

Sanfilippo, F., Croker, B. P. and Bollinger, R. R. (1982). Fate of four cadaveric donor renal allografts with mesangial IgA deposits. *Transplantation* **33**, 370.

Sanfilippo, F., Kolbeck, P. C., Vaughn, W. K., *et al.* (1985). Renal allograft cell infiltrates associated with irreversible rejection. *Transplantation* **40**, 679.

Savin, V. J., Sharma, R., Sharma, M., *et al.* (1996). Circulating factor associated with increased glomerular permeability to albumin in recurrent focal segmental glomerulosclerosis. *N. Engl. J. Med.* **334**, 878.

Savoldi, S., Scolari, F., Sandrini, S., *et al.* (1988). Cyclosporine chronic nephrotoxicity: histologic follow up at 6 and 18 months after renal transplant. *Transplant. Proc.* **20**, 777.

Schmidt, R. J., Venkat, K. K. and Dumler, F. (1991). Hemolytic-uremic syndrome in a renal transplant recipient on FK 506 immunosuppression. *Transplant. Proc.* **23**, 3156.

Schroeder, T. J., Weiss, M. A., Smith, R. D., *et al.* (1991). The efficacy of OKT3 in vascular rejection. *Transplantation* **51**, 312.

Schwarz, A., Krause, P. H., Offermann, G., *et al.* (1991). Recurrent and de novo renal disease after kidney transplantation with or without cyclosporine A. *Am. J. Kidney Dis.* **17**, 524.

Schwarz, A., Krause, P. H., Offermann, G., *et al.* (1994). Impact of de novo membranous glomerulonephritis on the clinical course after kidney transplantation. *Transplantation* **58**, 650.

Scornik, J. C., LeFor, W. M., Cicciarelli, J. C., *et al.* (1992). Hyperacute and acute kidney graft rejection due to antibodies against B cells. *Transplantation* **54**, 61.

Sedmak, D., Sharma, H., Czajka, C., *et al.* (1988). Recipient endothelialization of renal allografts: an immunohistochemical study utilizing blood group antigens. *Transplantation* **46**, 907.

Sharma, V. K., Bologa, R. M., Li, B., *et al.* (1996). Molecular executors of cell death—differential intrarenal expression of Fas ligand, Fas, granzyme B, and perforin during acute and/or chronic rejection of human renal allografts. *Transplantation* **62**, 1860.

Shimamura, T., Gyorkey, F., Morgen, R. O., *et al.* (1966). Fine structural observations in human kidney homografts. *Invest. Urol.* **3**, 590.

Shimizu, A., Cooper, D. K. C., Meehan, S. M., *et al.* (2000). Acute humoral xenograft rejection: Destruction of the microvascular capillary endothelium in pig-to-nonhuman primate renal grafts. *Lab. Invest.* **80**, 815

Shimizu, A., Yamada, K., Meehan, S. M., *et al.* (1997). Intragraft cellular events associated with tolerance in pig allografts: the "acceptance reaction." *Transplant. Proc.* **29**, 1155.

Shulman, H., Striker, G., Deeg, H. J., *et al.* (1981). Nephrotoxicity of cyclosporin A after allogeneic marrow transplantation: glomerular thromboses and tubular injury. *N. Engl. J. Med.* **305**, 1392.

Sibley, R. K. (1994). Morphologic features of chronic rejection in kidney and less commonly transplanted organs. *Clin. Transplant.* **8**, 293.

Sibley, R. K. and Payne, W. (1985). Morphologic findings in the renal allograft biopsy. *Semin. Nephrol.* **5**, 294.

Sibley, R. K., Rynasiewicz, J., Ferguson, R. M., *et al.* (1983). Morphology of cyclosporine nephrotoxicity and acute rejection in patients immunosuppressed with cyclosporine and prednisone. *Surgery* **94**, 225.

Sigal, N. H., Dumont, F., Durette, P., *et al.* (1991). Is cyclophilin involved in the immunosuppressive and nephrotoxic mechanism of action of cyclosporin A? *J. Exp. Med.* **173**, 619.

Silbert, P. L., Matz, L. R., Christiansen, K., *et al.* (1990). Herpes simplex virus interstitial nephritis in a renal allograft. *Clin. Nephrol.* **33**, 264.

Silva, F. G., Chandler, P., Pirani, C. L., *et al.* (1982). Disappearance of glomerular mesangial IgA deposits after renal allograft transplantation. *Transplantation* **33**, 214.

Solez, K. (1994). International standardization of criteria for histologic diagnosis of chronic rejection in renal allografts. *Clin. Transplant.* **8**, 345.

Solez, K., Axelsen, R. A., Benediktsson, H., *et al.* (1993a). International standardization of criteria for the histologic diagnosis of renal allograft rejection: the Banff working classification of kidney transplant pathology. *Kidney Int.* **44**, 411.

Solez, K., Racusen, L. C., Marcussen, N., *et al.* (1993b). Morphology of ischemic acute renal failure, normal function, and cyclosporine toxicity in cyclosporine-treated renal allograft recipients. *Kidney Int.* **43**, 1058.

Sollinger, H. W. (1995). Mycophenolate mofetil for the prevention of acute rejection in primary cadaveric renal allograft recipients. U.S. Renal Transplant Mycophenolate Mofetil Study Group. *Transplantation* **60**, 225.

Sommer, B. G., Innes, J. T., Whitehurst, R. M., *et al.* (1985). Cyclosporine-associated renal arteriopathy resulting in loss of allograft function. *Am. J. Surg.* **149**, 756.

Soulillou, J. P., DeMougon-Cambon, A., Duboid, C., *et al.* (1981). Immunological studies of eluates of 83 rejected kidneys. *Transplantation* **32**, 368.

Spector, D., Limas, C., Frost, J. L., *et al.* (1976). Perfusion nephropathy in human transplants. *N. Engl. J. Med.* **295**, 1217.

Starzl, T. E., Lerner, R. A., Dixon, F. J., *et al.* (1968). Shwartzman reaction after human renal homotransplantation. *N. Engl. J. Med.* **278**, 642.

Stern, S. C., Lakhani, S. and Morgan, S. H. (1994). Renal allograft dysfunction due to vesicoureteric obstruction by nodular malakoplakia. *Nephrol. Dial. Transplant.* **9**, 1188.

Strehlau, J., Pavlakis, M., Lipman, M., *et al.* (1997). Quantitative detection of immune activation transcripts as a diagnostic tool in kidney transplantation. *Proc. Natl. Acad. Sci. U. S. A.* **94**, 695.

Strom, E. H., Epper, R. and Mihatsch, M. J. (1995). Ciclosporin-associated arteriolopathy: the renin producing vascular smooth muscle cells are more sensitive to ciclosporin toxicity. *Clin. Nephrol.* **43**, 226.

Strom, E. H., Thiel, G. and Mihatsch, M. J. (1994). Prevalence of cyclosporine-associated arteriolopathy in renal transplant biopsies from 1981 to 1992. *Transplant. Proc.* **26**, 2585.

Taub, H. C., Greenstein, S. M., Lerner, S. E., *et al.* (1994). Reassessment of the value of post-vascularization biopsy performed at renal transplantation: the effects of arteriosclerosis. *J. Urol.* **151**, 575.

Taube, D. H., Neild, G. H., Williams, D. G., *et al.* (1985). Differentiation between allograft rejection and cyclosporin nephrotoxicity in renal transplant recipients. *Lancet* **2**, 171.

Ten, R. M., Gleich, G. J., Holley, K. E., *et al.* (1989). Eosinophil granule major basic protein in acute renal allograft rejection. *Transplantation* **47**, 959.

Thiru, S., Maher, E. R., Hamilton, D. V., *et al.* (1983). Tubular changes in renal transplant recipients on cyclosporine. *Transplant. Proc.* **15**, 2846.

Thoenes, G. H., Pielsticker, K. and Schubert, G. (1979). Transplantation-induced immune complex kidney disease in rats with unilateral manifestations in the allografted kidney. *Lab. Invest.* **41**, 321.

Tolkoff-Rubin, N. E., Cosimi, A. B., Fuller, T., *et al.* (1978). IgA nephropathy in HLA-identical siblings. *Transplantation* **26**, 430.

Trimarchi, H. M., Gonzalez, J. M., Truong, L. D., *et al.* (1999). Focal segmental glomerulosclerosis in a 32-year-old kidney allograft after 7 years without immunosuppression. *Nephron* **82**, 270.

Trpkov, K., Campbell, P., Pazderka, F., *et al.* (1996). Pathologic features of acute renal allograft rejection associated with donor-specific antibody: analysis using the Banff grading schema. *Transplantation* **61**, 1586.

Truong, L., Gelfand, J., D'Agati, V., *et al.* (1989). De novo membranous glomerulonephropathy in renal allografts: a report of ten cases and review of the literature. *Am. J. Kidney Dis.* **14**, 131.

Tryggvason, K. (1999). Unraveling the mechanisms of glomerular ultrafiltration: nephrin, a key component of the slit diaphragm. *J. Am. Soc. Nephrol.* **10**, 2440.

Tuazon, T. V., Schneeberger, E. E., Bhan, A. K., *et al.* (1987). Mononuclear cells in acute allograft glomerulopathy. *Am. J. Pathol.* **129**, 119.

Van den Berg-Wolf, M. G., Kootte, A. M., Weening, J. J., *et al.* (1988). Recurrent hemolytic uremic syndrome in a renal transplant recipient and review of the Leiden experience. *Transplantation* **45**, 248.

van Gorder, M. A., Della Pelle P., Henson, J. W., *et al.* (1999). Cynomolgus polyoma virus infection: a new member of the polyoma virus family causes interstitial nephritis, ureteritis, and enteritis in immunosuppressed cynomolgus monkeys. *Am. J. Pathol.* **154**, 1273.

Versluis, D. J., Ten, K. F. J., Wenting, G. J., *et al.* (1988). Histological lesions associated with cyclosporin: incidence and reversibility in one year old kidney transplants. *J. Clin. Pathol.* **41**, 498.

Vincenti, F., Laskow, D. A., Neylan, J. F., *et al.* (1996). One-year follow-up of an open-label trial of FK506 for primary kidney transplantation: a report of the U.S. Multicenter FK506 Kidney Transplant Group. *Transplantation* **61**, 1576.

Visscher, D., Carey, J., Oh, H., *et al.* (1991). Histologic and immunophenotypic evaluation of pretreatment renal biopsies in OKT3-treated allograft rejections. *Transplantation* **51**, 1023.

von Willebrand, E., Pettersson, E., Ahonen, J., Hayry, P. (1986). CMV infection, class II antigen expression, and human kidney allograft rejection. *Transplantation* **42**, 364.

Wang, H., Nanra, R. S., Carney, S. L., *et al.* (1995). The renal medulla in acute renal allograft rejection: comparison with renal cortex. *Nephrol. Dial. Transplant.* **10**, 1428.

Watschinger, B., Vychytil, A., Attar, M., *et al.* (1994). Pattern of endothelin immunostaining during rejection episodes after kidney transplantation. *Clin. Nephol.* **41**, 86.

Weir, M. R., Hall, C. M., Shen, S. Y., *et al.* (1986). The prognostic value of the eosinophil in acute renal allograft rejection. *Transplantation* **41**, 709.

Wells, A. F., Larsson, E., Tengblad, A., *et al.* (1990). The location of hyaluronan in normal and rejected human kidneys. *Transplantation* **50**, 240.

Wilczek, H. E., Jaremko, G., Tyden, G., *et al.* (1995). Evolution of diabetic nephropathy in kidney grafts: evidence that a simultaneously transplanted kidney exerts a protective effect. *Transplantation* **59**, 51.

Williams, G. M., Hume, D. M., Huson, R. P., Jr., *et al.* (1968). "Hyperacute" renal-homograft rejection in man. *N. Engl. J. Med.* **279**, 611.

Woolley, A. C., Rosenberg, M. E., Burke, B. A., *et al.* (1988). De novo focal glomerulosclerosis after kidney transplantation. *Am. J. Med.* **84**, 310.

Yamada, K., Gianello, P. R., Ierino, F. L., *et al.* (1999). Role of the thymus in transplantation tolerance in miniature swine: II. effect of steroids and age on the induction of tolerance to class I mismatched renal allografts. *Transplantation* **67**, 458.

Yamaguchi, Y., Teraoka, S., Yagisawa, T., *et al.* (1989). Ultrastructural study of cyclosporine-associated arteriolopathy in renal allografts. *Transplant. Proc.* **21**, 1517.

Yang, C. W., Kim, Y. S., Yang, K. H., *et al.* (1994). Acute focal bacterial nephritis presented as acute renal failure and hepatic dysfunction in a renal transplant recipient. *Am. J. Nephrol.* **14**, 72.

Yard, B. A., Spruyt-Gerritse, M., Class, F., *et al.* (1993). The clinical significance of allospecific antibodies against endothelial cells detected with an antibody-dependent cellular cytotoxicity assay for vascular rejection and graft loss after renal transplantation. *Transplantation* **55**, 1287.

Young, E. W., Ellis, C. N., Messana, J. M., *et al.* (1994). A prospective study of renal structure and function in psoriasis patients treated with cyclosporin. *Kidney Int.* **46**, 1216.

Young-Ramsaran, J. O., Hruban, R. H., Hutchins, G. M., *et al.* (1993). Ultrastructural evidence of cell-mediated endothelial cell injury in cardiac transplant–related accelerated arteriosclerosis. *Ultrastruct. Pathol.* **17**, 125.

Zachariae, H., Hansen, H. E., Kragballe, K., *et al.* (1992). Morphologic renal changes during cyclosporine treatment of psoriasis: studies on pretreatment and posttreatment kidney biopsy specimens. *J. Am. Acad. Dermatol.* **26**, 415.

Immunohistology of the Transplanted Kidney

Susan V. Fuggle • Dicken D. H. Koo

Introduction

Immunohistochemical analysis of transplant biopsy material has contributed significantly to understanding of the immunological processes involved after transplantation and has added to knowledge of the rejection reaction in the transplanted kidney as seen on routine histology. Many investigations have been performed to examine the role of molecules that may be involved in the generation of a host alloimmune response against the graft. The expression of major histocompatibility complex (MHC) antigens has been of particular interest, especially in mismatched grafts, in which a host alloimmune response may be initiated. Expression of cytokine-inducible molecules, such as endothelial adhesion molecules and chemokines, may be of additional interest because these molecules are involved in the recruitment of specific leukocyte subsets into the graft. Phenotypic characterization and analysis for the expression of effector molecules may indicate the functional capacity of the cellular infiltrate. The focus of many immunohistological studies has been to examine whether expression of any of these markers may act as a diagnostic tool for events that may influence renal allograft outcome.

We first review information obtained from immunohistochemical analyses of donor kidney biopsy specimens obtained before transplantation with particular reference to donor factors that may be associated with causing differing levels of antigen expression. Next, data from postreperfusion transplant biopsy specimens are reviewed with reference to ischemia/reperfusion injury, concentrating on analysis of leukocyte infiltration and expression of MHC antigens and adhesion molecules. In the final section, we discuss information from transplant biopsy specimens obtained routinely after transplantation or during periods of allograft dysfunction.

Pre-Transplant Kidneys

Immunohistochemical analyses of donor kidney biopsy specimens obtained before transplantation provide a useful baseline for determining changes that may result once the kidney is transplanted. The localization of the MHC antigens in the kidney is important because of their pivotal role in stimulating an alloimmune response. Once the expression of these molecules was found to be up-regulated by cytokines during an inflammatory response, there was interest in the possibility that the presence of up-regulated levels of MHC antigens within a transplanted organ may be indicative of allograft rejection and provide a diagnostic tool. The induced class II antigen is of potential importance within transplanted tissue because cells expressing donor class II antigens may be able to augment the immune response and themselves become targets for alloreactive T cells.

The MHC class I antigens, in humans termed *human leukocyte antigen (HLA) class I antigens,* are expressed on all structures within a kidney. Glomeruli, intertubular structures and large vessel endothelium all stain intensely positive, whereas the renal tubules are more weakly stained (Fleming *et al.,* 1981; Fuggle *et al.,* 1983). The HLA class II antigens are detected consistently on glomerular endothelium, mesangium, intertubular capillaries and interstitial dendritic cells (Fuggle *et al.,* 1983). Although distal tubules do not express class II antigens, cytoplasmic class II antigens have been detected in the proximal tubules by some investigators (Barrett *et al.,* 1987; Evans *et al.,* 1985; Hancock *et al.,* 1982; Raftery *et al.,* 1989) but not others (Koyama *et al.,* 1979; Natali *et al.,* 1981; Scott *et al.,* 1981). Analysis using reagents specific for the individual HLA-DR, HLA-DQ and HLA-DP products showed that HLA-DR antigen distribution is identical to the class II antigen expression described earlier (Fig. 25–1A) but that HLA-DP (Fig. 25–1B) and HLA-DQ antigens are not detected normally on the renal tubules and are expressed more weakly on glomeruli and intertubular structures (Evans *et al.,* 1986; Fuggle *et al.,* 1987).

Donor kidneys contain few interstitial leukocytes before transplantation, provided that the organ is free of preexisting disease and has not been damaged before or during procurement. The predominant resident leukocyte population comprises cells with a dendritic morphology (McWhinnie *et al.,* 1986).

Other molecules that have been studied in some detail are the cytokine-inducible adhesion molecules, which by interaction with their respective ligands on the leukocyte surface mediate the recruitment of leukocytes at the site of an inflammatory response. Two such markers are the selectin molecules, P-selectin and E-selectin, which mediate the initial events of tethering and rolling. P-selectin and E-selectin are markers of activated endothelium, P-selectin being expressed rapidly on the endothelial surface within minutes of stimulation without a requirement for *de novo* protein synthesis and E-selectin being expressed maximally within hours of stimulation because of the requirement for mRNA and protein synthesis. Once tethered at the endothelial surface, leukocytes require activation by chemoattractants and chemokines, which are synthesized and retained at an inflammatory site introducing specificity into the type of leukocyte recruited. The presence of these molecules has been studied in transplant biopsy specimens and is discussed later. Firm adhesion is mediated by interaction of integrins with molecules such as the cytokine-inducible molecules, intercellular adhesion molecule-1 (ICAM-1) and vascular cell adhesion molecule-1 (VCAM-1), on the endothelial surface. Leukocytes migrate to the interstitium by means of a haptotactic gradient at the endothelial cell junctions, mediated in part by platelet/endothelial cell adhesion molecule-1 (PECAM-1 [CD31]). This molecule is constitutively expressed on endothelium and as

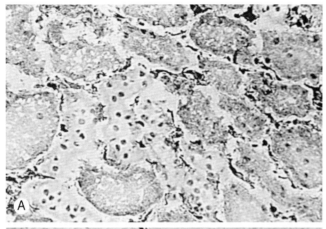

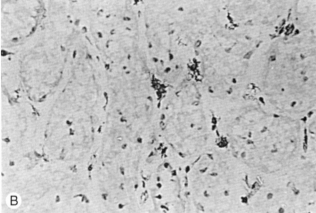

FIGURE 25–1

Comparison of the distribution of HLA-DR and HLA-DP antigens in pretransplant renal biopsy specimens. (A) HLA-DR is strongly expressed on the intertubular structures, proximal tubules are weakly positive and distal tubules are negative. (B) HLA-DP is expressed on intertubular structures, but all of the renal tubules are negative. Cryostat sections of biopsy tissue were stained by an indirect immunoperoxidase technique and counterstained with hematoxylin. (Original magnification × 350.)

such provides a useful indicator of endothelial destruction in transplant biopsy specimens (Fuggle *et al.*, 1993; Gibbs *et al.*, 1993; Table 25–1).

The level of expression of ICAM-1, VCAM-1 and E-selectin and P-selectin varies among preanastomosis renal biopsy specimens in a manner analogous to that reported for the class II antigens (Fuggle *et al.*, 1983, 1993). Intercellular adhesion molecule-1 (ICAM-1) is constitutively expressed on all of the vascular endothelium, distal tubules are negative, but proximal tubular expression has been detected variably and where present appears most intensely expressed apically at the brush borders (Anderson *et al.*, 1992; Bishop and Hall, 1989; Brockmeyer *et al.*, 1993; Dustin *et al.*, 1986; Faull and Russ, 1989; Fuggle *et al.*, 1993; Gibbs *et al.*, 1993; Hill *et al.*, 1995; Nickeleit *et al.*, 1993). Vascular cell adhesion molecule-1 (VCAM-1) has a more restricted distribution in the kidney, being constitutively strongly expressed on parietal epithelial cells of the Bowman's capsule, weakly expressed on the glomerular mesangium and possibly detected on an occasional intertubular structure (capillary endothelium or leukocyte). Distal tubules are negative, but there is considerable variation in proximal tubular staining, ranging from an isolated focus of basolateral staining (usually surrounding a

nucleus) in a small proportion of proximal tubules to a much more widespread staining (Alpers *et al.*, 1993; Anderson *et al.*, 1994; Brockmeyer *et al.*, 1993; Fuggle *et al.*, 1993; Gibbs *et al.*, 1993; Hill *et al.*, 1995; Lin *et al.*, 1993; Rice *et al.*, 1990; Seron *et al.*, 1991). VCAM-1 also may be expressed weakly on occasional intertubular structures and veins. There is considerable variation in the level of E-selectin expression in the pretransplant biopsy specimens, ranging from specimens being entirely negative to having multiple foci of positively stained intertubular capillaries, veins and venules. Glomerular capillaries do not appear to express E-selectin (Anderson *et al.*, 1994; Brockmeyer *et al.*, 1993; Fuggle *et al.*, 1993; Gibbs *et al.*, 1993). P-selectin is expressed at a low level in pretransplant biopsy specimens, in which it is localized to arterial or less frequently venous endothelium and occasional intertubular capillaries (Fuggle *et al.*, 1995; Koo *et al.*, 1998, 1999).

CADAVER VERSUS LIVING RELATED DONOR KIDNEYS

To investigate the possibility that pathophysiologically harmful events within the donor may be the cause of the variation in levels of expression of these cytokine-inducible antigens, we compared biopsy specimens obtained from cadaver and living related donor kidneys. There were no significant differences in the level of T lymphocytes, neutrophils or resident macrophages between biopsy specimens from living related donor and cadaver donor kidneys, but clear differences were detected in adhesion molecule and HLA-DR antigen expression between the two groups of specimens (Fig. 25–2). Although in accordance with previous findings, high levels of tubular HLA-DR, ICAM-1 and VCAM-1 were detected in 66%, 62% and 46% of cadaver kidneys respectively and endothelial E-selectin in 54%; all living related donor kidneys were negative for tubular ICAM-1, VCAM-1 and endothelial E-selectin and only 7% of living related donor kidneys were positive for tubular HLA-DR antigens. In the analysis, there was a highly significant association between elevated expression of the three tubular markers studied. This finding is not surprising because *in vitro* analyses on cytokine-stimulated cultured tubular cells have shown the kinetics of induction of HLA-DR, ICAM-1 and VCAM-1 to be similar, with peak levels being detected 1 to 2 days after stimulation (Kirby *et al.*, 1993; Lin *et al.*, 1992, 1993; Wilson *et al.*, 1995). This timing is later than the peak of endothelial E-selectin expression that occurs 4 to 6 hours after cytokine stimulation, with the expression returning to basal levels by 24 hours (Bevilacqua *et al.*, 1987). This situation may explain the absence of a correlation between up-regulated expression of the tubular markers and E-selectin in the pretransplant biopsy specimens.

Consistent with the theory that antigen induction in the kidney may be caused by systemic cytokine release in the donor, elevated levels of tubular antigens were found to be associated with traumatic death, prolonged ventilator support in the donor and infection in the donor (Koo *et al.*, 1999). High levels of endothelial E-selectin in the cadaver donor biopsy specimens were found to be associated with administration of the antidiuretic ʟ-arginine vasopressin analogue, DDAVP (1-desamino-8-ᴅ-arginine vasopressin), to the donor before retrieval. DDAVP also is used in the treatment of bleeding disorders (Manucci, 1988), and it has been shown that DDAVP stimulates platelet and endothelial P-selectin expression and increased platelet-activating factor expression on monocytes (Hashemi *et al.*, 1993; Kanwar *et al.*, 1995; Wun *et al.*, 1995). It is possible that DDAVP administration has secondary effects on hemostasis and endothelial activation.

A further factor that may contribute to the differences in

TABLE 25–1

NOMENCLATURE FOR ANTIGENS

Antigen	Main Cellular Expression	Comments and Function
CD3	T lymphocytes	CD3 is associated with the T-cell receptor and is involved in signal transduction after antigen recognition
CD4	Helper T-lymphocyte subpopulation (MHC class II restricted) monocytes, macrophages, thymocytes	CD4 binds to MHC class II molecules on antigen-presenting cells; involved in signal transduction
CD8	Cytotoxic T-lymphocyte subpopulation (MHC class I restricted), thymocytes	CD8 binds to MHC class I molecules on antigen-presenting cells; involved in signal transduction
CD14	Monocytes, macrophages, some granulocytes	Receptor for lipopolysaccharide complexed to its binding protein
CD25	Activated T and B lymphocytes, macrophages	CD25 (α-chain (55 kd) of interleukin-2 receptor); functions as a low-affinity receptor for interleukin-2 and in combination with β-chain (75 kd) forms a high-affinity receptor
CD31	Platelets, monocytes, macrophages, granulocytes, endothelial cells	Alternative names: platelet endothelial cell adhesion molecule-1 (PECAM-1); adhesion molecule
CD45	Leukocytes	Leukocyte common antigen, 5 isoforms result from differential splicing; CD45 plays a role in signal transduction
CD57	Natural killer cells, some T and B lymphocytes	Also known as HNK-1, CD57 is a 110-kd glycoprotein
CD69	Activated T and B lymphocytes, activated macrophages, natural killer cells	Also known as the activator-inducer molecule; involved in early events after cellular activation
Perforin	Cytotoxic lymphocytes, natural killer cells	Pore-forming protein that acts in concert with granzyme proteases for cytolytic activity
Granzymes A/B	Cytotoxic lymphocytes, natural killer cells	Serine proteases that contribute to DNA fragmentation and cell death
Fas-ligand	Activated T lymphocytes, natural killer cells	Interaction of Fas-ligand with target cells expressing Fas antigen may result in apoptotic cell death
ICAM-1	Broad reactivity, many activated cells	Also referred to as CD54, cytokine inducible adhesion molecule; ligands include lymphocyte function antigen-1 (LFA-1, CD11a/CD18) and Mac-1 (CD11b/CD18) expressed on leukocytes
VCAM-1	Activated endothelium, follicular dendritic cells	Also referred to as CD106, a cytokine-inducible adhesion molecule; ligand VLA-4 (CD49d/CD29)
E-selectin	Activated endothelium	Endothelial leukocyte adhesion molecule-1 (CD62E); cytokine-inducible adhesion molecule primarily involved in neutrophil adherence to endothelium; carbohydrate ligands include sialyl-Lewis x
P-selectin	Stimulated endothelium and platelets	Adhesion molecule (CD62P), also referred to as GMP-140; mobilized from intracellular storage granules to cell surface on activation to mediate adhesion to leukocyte ligands (e.g., PSGL-1)

levels of expression of these molecules between cadaver and living donor kidneys is that the patients requiring ventilator support are close to brain death. The physiological effects of brain death on neurological and hormonal functions are well defined (Pratschke *et al.*, 1999). Dramatically increased levels of interleukin (IL-6) and severe hormonal imbalances have been detected in blood samples from patients after the diagnosis of brain death (Amado *et al.*, 1995). There is evidence from a rat model of acutely induced brain death showing increased levels of inflammatory cytokines, up-regulated levels of MHC antigens, adhesion molecules and the costimulatory molecule B7 present in peripheral organs 6 hours after brain death (Takada *et al.*, 1998).

There are potentially significant consequences of the presence of up-regulated levels of proinflammatory molecules in donor organs. E-selectin on the endothelium of donor kidneys may mediate a more immediate infiltration of leukocytes after transplantation. Expression of higher levels of tubular MHC antigens may increase the immunogenicity of the transplant and together with up-regulated adhesion molecules increase the susceptibility to immune attack. Convincing *in vitro* data show that renal tubular epithelial cells with induced ICAM-1 and VCAM-1 are capable of binding leukocytes (Jevnikar *et al.*, 1990; Kirby *et al.*, 1993; Lin *et al.*, 1992, 1993). The localization of VCAM-1 to the basolateral surface of the proximal tubules provides a mechanism for leukocyte migration into the tubular cytoplasm after extravasation. The

variation in expression of these molecules in cadaver kidneys before transplantation indicates that they are not "normal", but they are essential in providing a baseline against which to compare subsequent posttransplant biopsy specimens.

Postreperfusion Biopsies

In the early experience in clinical renal transplantation, biopsy specimens frequently were obtained 1 hour after revascularization of the kidney, and a neutrophil infiltration in the glomeruli was considered indicative of antibody-mediated damage to the kidney (Kincaid-Smith *et al.*, 1968; Williams *et al.*, 1968). Subsequent studies did not show a direct correlation between neutrophil infiltration and hyperacute or acute rejection (McDicken *et al.*, 1975; Perloff *et al.*, 1973; Valenzuela *et al.*, 1980). The introduction of sensitive crossmatching and refined antibody screening procedures virtually has eliminated hyperacute rejection in modern clinical practice, and thus there have been relatively few studies of postreperfusion biopsy specimens. Nevertheless in one such study, polymorphonuclear leukocytes were detected in postreperfusion biopsy specimens from cadaver renal allografts. The interpretation of the findings was confounded by the presence of hyperacute rejection in 4 of the 57 transplants, but the results showed there to be a significant association between the presence of neutrophil infiltration and longer

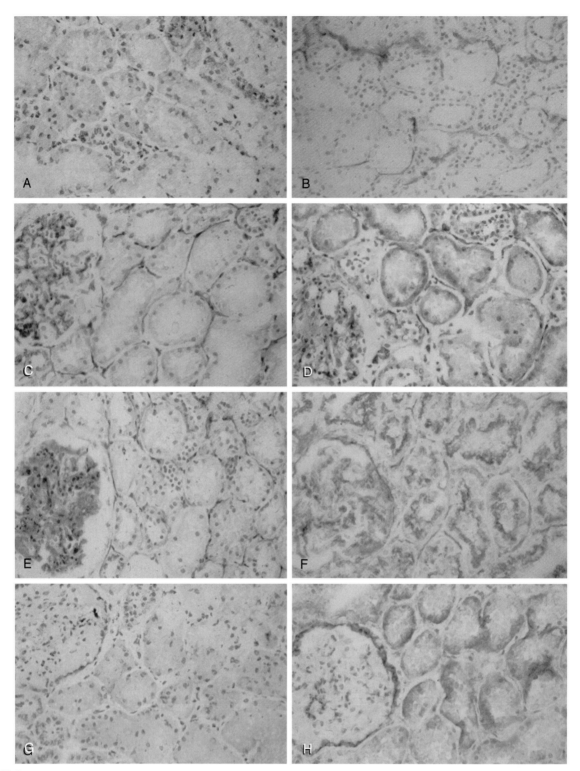

FIGURE 25–2

Differences in adhesion molecule and HLA-DR antigen expression between cadaveric and living related donor (LRD) kidneys. All biopsy specimens were stained with monoclonal antibodies using an indirect immunoperoxidase technique. (A) LRD kidney stained for E-selectin shows negative expression and (B) a cadaveric kidney with high levels of E-selectin on the intertubular capillaries. (C) LRD kidney with no tubular expression of HLA-DR antigens and (D) a cadaveric kidney with strong expression of HLA-DR antigens on the proximal tubules. (E) Intercellular adhesion molecule-1 (ICAM-1) was absent on the tubules of all LRD kidneys, whereas (F) tubular ICAM-1 was detected at high levels in a proportion of the cadaver kidneys. (G) None of the LRD kidneys expressed tubular vascular cell adhesion molecule-1 (VCAM-1), whereas (H) a proportion of the cadaveric kidneys expressed high levels of proximal tubular VCAM-1. (Original magnification × 250.)

(See color plate.)

(Reproduced with permission from the International Society of Nephrology [Koo *et al.*, 1999].)

periods of cold ischemia (Gaber *et al.*, 1992). This study suggests that the infiltration may be a manifestation of ischemia/reperfusion injury, but prereperfusion biopsy specimens were not available to provide a baseline. Therefore it was not certain whether the cells entered on reperfusion and were not already present within the donor kidney.

To investigate changes that may be attributable to ischemia/reperfusion injury, we compared biopsy specimens obtained from cadaver and living related renal transplants obtained before and approximately 30 to 45 minutes after reperfusion of the transplanted kidney. In this study, the preanastomosis biopsy specimen in each case provided a control for preexisting donor leukocytes and the level of antigen expression within the organ. There was no detectable infiltration of macrophages or T lymphocytes after reperfusion, but an increased neutrophil infiltration, as determined by staining for CD15s and neutrophil elastase, was detected in 29 of 55 (53%) cadaver allografts (Koo *et al.*, 1998; Fig. 25-3A and B). The neutrophil infiltration was localized to the glomeruli in 16 of 29 (55%) and to the interstitium in 25 of 29 (86%) postreperfusion biopsy specimens from cadaver allografts. Staining performed with antibodies specific for recipient MHC class I antigens confirmed that these infiltrating cells were of recipient origin. Analysis of adhesion molecule expression showed staining patterns of VCAM-1, ICAM-

1 and E-selectin to be consistent between preanastomosis and postanastomosis biopsy specimens (as may be anticipated because these molecules require protein synthesis for upregulation of expression). In contrast, there was a noticeable increase in expression of P-selectin after reperfusion in 24 of 55 (44%) cadaver renal allografts (Fig. 25-3C and D). P-selectin is stored in the α granules of platelets and in the Weibel-Palade bodies of endothelial cells and on activation is expressed within minutes of stimulation on the cell surface. In the postreperfusion biopsy specimens, double staining showed that the P-selectin was expressed by platelets adhering to the endothelium. The analysis of the biopsy specimens from the living donors showed a different picture, with none of the postreperfusion biopsy specimens being infiltrated by neutrophils, and only 1 of 11 had an increase in P-selectin expression (Koo *et al.*, 1998).

The infiltration of neutrophils into the glomeruli of cadaver renal allografts was significantly associated with prolonged cold ischemia times. This finding provides evidence that cold ischemia and reperfusion may be, in part, responsible for initiating an early inflammatory response within the graft. The infiltration was associated with an increased incidence of delayed graft function and poor graft function 6 months after transplantation. These results suggest that the inflammatory response generated as a result of cold ische-

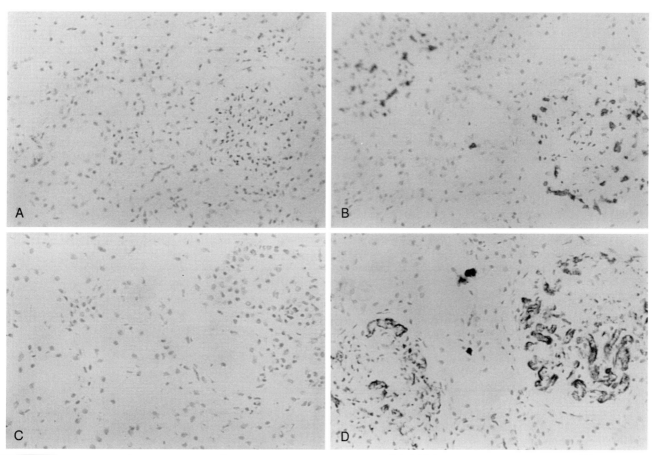

FIGURE 25–3

Changes observed after reperfusion of cadaver renal allografts. (A) Prereperfusion biopsy specimen stained with an antineutrophil elastase antibody shows the absence of neutrophils, and (B) a postreperfusion biopsy specimen from the same kidney stained with the antineutrophil elastase antibody shows neutrophil infiltration into the glomerulus. (C) Prereperfusion biopsy specimen shows negative staining for P-selectin and (D) postreperfusion biopsy specimen from the same kidney shows deposition of P-selectin on the glomerular capillaries. (Original magnification × 250.)

(A and B reproduced with permission from the American Society for Investigative Pathology [Koo *et al.*, 1998].)

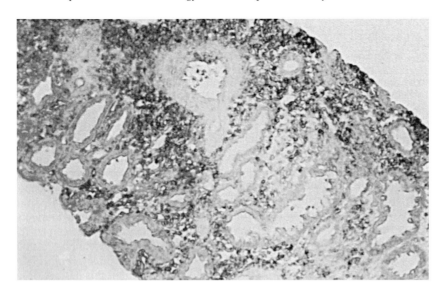

FIGURE 25–4

Paraffin section of a renal transplant biopsy specimen stained for CD45 (leukocyte common antigen) to show leukocyte infiltration during rejection. APAAP technique counterstained with hematoxylin. (Original magnification × 115.)

mia/reperfusion injury may contribute to the association observed between cold ischemia and delayed graft function in many single-center and multicenter studies (Chertow et al., 1996; Najarian et al., 1994; Peters et al., 1995; Pfaff et al., 1998; Shoskes and Halloran, 1996). Immunohistochemical analysis of prereperfusion and postreperfusion biopsy specimens may provide a simple means of assessing the level of ischemia/reperfusion injury in cadaver renal allografts.

Post-transplant Kidneys

Leukocyte migration into the transplant kidney begins immediately after vascularization of the graft, and significant numbers of cells can be detected in the interstitium within hours (Perloff et al., 1973). Leukocyte infiltration is one of the hallmarks of acute rejection (Fig. 25–4), but the realization that leukocyte infiltration also may be present in well-functioning renal allografts, albeit at a lower level, occurred only after the analysis of routine transplant biopsy specimens (Burdick et al., 1984; McWhinnie et al., 1986). Leukocyte infiltration also was found to be present when acute tubular necrosis was apparent (Burdick et al., 1984). In grafts with clinically stable function, peak levels of infiltration are seen within 3 weeks after transplantation, then decrease thereafter, but leukocyte infiltration still may be present in successful renal allografts several years after transplantation (McWhinnie et al., 1986; Fig. 25–5). Similar observations were reported in rat renal allograft models in which mononuclear cells were detected in the graft despite the effective suppression of rejection by treatment with donor-specific antibody (Bradley et al., 1985; French and Batchelor, 1969) or whole blood (Armstrong et al., 1987; Dallman et al., 1987).

At the Oxford Transplant Centre, a prospective randomized trial was performed to compare the utility of different biopsy techniques for monitoring recipients of renal allografts (Gray et al., 1992). The techniques used were conventional histology, immunohistological analysis based on quantitation of the leukocyte infiltration (Foot et al., 1989; McWhinnie et al., 1986, 1987, 1989) and fine-needle aspiration cytology. Conventional histology and immunohistology yielded similar results for the detection of clinical rejection, with a sensitivity of 75% and 79% and specificity of 87% and 80%. The presence of infiltration preceding or following clinical rejection accounted for most of the inaccuracy of the immunohistological results.

COMPOSITION OF THE LEUKOCYTE INFILTRATION

The early immunohistological studies exploited the potential of monoclonal antibodies to determine the cellular composition and the CD4 and CD8 phenotypes of the infiltrating leukocytes (Table 25–2). As anticipated, macrophages and T lymphocytes constitute the major cell types, with B lymphocytes and natural killer cells being in the minority. An example of the leukocyte and T-lymphocyte infiltration is shown in Figure 25–6. CD4+ and CD8+ cells are found in transplant biopsy specimens, but because CD4 is expressed on macrophages in humans (Wood et al., 1983), it is difficult to determine the precise proportions of each T-lymphocyte subset by immunohistochemistry; the reports of the relative contribution of these cellular subsets to the overall infiltration varied in the early literature (Hall et al., 1984a; Hancock et al., 1983; McWhinnie et al., 1986; Platt et al., 1982; Tufveson et al., 1983; van Es et al., 1984). The goal of these immunohistological studies was to identify differences in the cellular composition

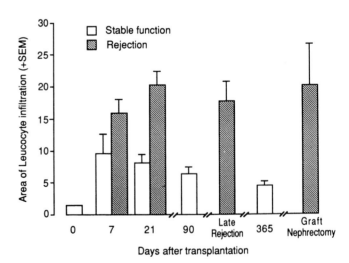

FIGURE 25–5

Leukocyte infiltration into renal allograft biopsy specimens from cyclosporine-treated recipients during rejection or stable graft function. Late rejection biopsy specimens were obtained from grafts rejecting after the first month following transplantation and graft nephrectomy specimens from renal allografts with irreversible acute rejection.

TABLE 25–2

LEUKOCYTE INFILTRATION AND CD25 EXPRESSION IN RENAL ALLOGRAFT BIOPSY SPECIMENS*

Clinical Circumstances	Total Leukocyte Infiltration % CD45 staining ± SEM	CD25+ Infiltration % CD25 staining ± SEM
No rejection (n = 32)	9.4 ± 1.0	0.9 ± 0.2
<7 days before rejection (n = 6)	27.9 ± 3.5	7.1 ± 1.4
During rejection (n = 12)	30.9 ± 2.3	9.5 ± 2.5
Postrejection (n = 12)	11.4 ± 2.0	1.4 ± 0.5

*Biopsy sections were stained for CD45 (leukocyte common antigen, total leukocytes) and CD25 (interleukin-2 receptor) using indirect immunoperoxidase techniques and the percentage area positively stained quantitated by morphometric point counting. For analysis, biopsy specimens were grouped according to the recipient's clinical circumstances.

and/or distribution that may be of diagnostic value, in particular in the CD4 or CD8 phenotype of the infiltrating cells. With this objective in view, several studies were performed with discrepant findings, and the approach has not proved to have clinical value (Beschorner *et al.*, 1985; Bishop *et al.*, 1986a; Hancock *et al.*, 1983; McWhinnie *et al.*, 1986; Sako *et al.*, 1987; Sanfilippo *et al.*, 1985; van Es *et al.*, 1984; Waltzer *et al.*, 1987).

MARKERS ASSOCIATED WITH IMMUNE ACTIVATION

The phenotype of a cell is not necessarily related to its functional capacity, and many studies have been performed in an attempt to define infiltration actively involved in graft rejection and destruction. One approach is to examine biopsy specimens for leukocyte surface markers expressed *de novo* or that become up-regulated during cellular proliferation and activation (e.g., CD25, α chain of the IL-2 receptor [Schwarting and Stein, 1989], and CD69, activator inducer molecule [Schwarting *et al.*, 1989]). The results from initial comparative studies of biopsy specimens showed a significant increase in CD25+ cells in biopsy specimens from rejecting renal allografts (Hancock *et al.*, 1985; Seron *et al.*, 1989). Our analysis of activation markers in routine clinical material produced more heterogeneous results. The grouped data showed a significant increase in the proportion of CD25+ leukocytes in the infiltration before and during rejection (see Table 25–2), but the results were sufficiently diverse to preclude the application of this type of analysis as a routine diagnostic tool.

Another approach is to examine biopsy specimens for the presence of molecules involved in the effector mechanisms of cell-mediated rejection. Cytolytic effector molecules, such as Fas-ligand, perforin and the serine proteases or granzymes, are ideal candidates being found preferentially in cells with cytolytic capacity, particularly cytotoxic T lymphocytes and natural killer cells (Berke, 1995; Henkart, 1994). Initial immunohistochemical analyses of human renal transplant biopsy specimens were performed with antibodies to human perforin and granzymes. Significantly increased levels of perforin-positive cells were found in a small study of rejecting renal allografts (Kataoka *et al.*, 1992), and granzyme A–expressing cells and granzyme B–expressing cells have been detected in biopsy specimens obtained during allograft rejection (Kummer *et al.*, 1995). The advent of reverse-transcriptase polymerase chain reaction technology has enabled the detection of low-abundance mRNA transcripts

within clinical material. The technology enables the study of many combinations of gene transcripts related to cellular activation.

Elevated levels of granzymes, perforin and Fas-ligand have been shown to be associated with acute renal allograft rejection (Lipman *et al.*, 1992, 1994; Strehlau *et al.*, 1996, 1997; Suthanthiran, 1997; Vasconcellos *et al.*, 1998). The potential of these markers as a diagnostic tool has been shown by Strehlau and coworkers, who achieved 100% sensitivity and 100% specificity for the diagnosis of acute rejection in a combined analysis of Fas ligand, perforin or granzyme B expression (Strehlau *et al.*, 1997). Concomitant gene expression of these molecules has been detected in peripheral blood in acutely rejecting allograft biopsy specimens, suggesting that less invasive allograft monitoring may be possible (Vasconcellos *et al.*, 1998).

Differences in the profiles of immunoregulatory cytokines in clinical material may be useful in determining the activity of the leukocyte infiltration. This whole area has been the subject of extensive study at the protein and mRNA level. One of the first reports was of the detection of IL-6 mRNA by *in situ* hybridization in biopsy specimens from patients

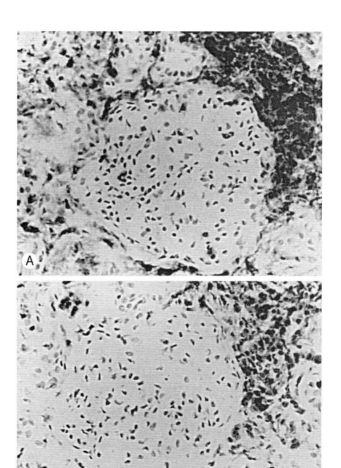

FIGURE 25–6

Cellular infiltration in a rejecting allograft shows periglomerular distribution of (A) leukocytes (CD45 staining) and (B) T lymphocytes (CD3 staining). Cryostat sections of biopsy tissue were stained using an indirect immunoperoxidase technique and counterstained with hematoxylin. (Original magnification × 350.)

with acute renal allograft rejection (Vandenbroecke *et al.*, 1991). Many studies have shown the presence of cytokines such as IL-2, IL-7, IL-8, IL-10, IL-12, IL-15, IL-17 and interferon-γ to be associated significantly with acute rejection, although variation in the cytokine profiles was reported in the different studies (Budde *et al.*, 1997; de Mattos *et al.*, 1997; Kirk *et al.*, 1995; Strehlau *et al.*, 1996, 1997; Suthanthiran, 1997; van Kooten *et al.*, 1998; Xu *et al.*, 1995).

The variation in the level of cytokine expression detected in these different studies and in the associations between different cytokines and acute rejection reflects the complexity of this type of study. The discrepancies probably arise from differences in the timing of the biopsies relative to the onset of rejection and rejection therapy. Data from studies performed in our center, where fine-needle aspiration biopsy specimens were analyzed on a daily basis, showed that the expression of cytokines may be transient or dynamic, confounding such analyses of core biopsy material obtained at specific time points (Dallman *et al.*, 1992; McLean *et al.*, 1997). The observation that immune activation, cytokine and cytolytic gene transcripts can be detected in protocol biopsy specimens from stable grafts with subclinical rejection also may contribute to these discrepant conclusions. The presence of these transcripts also raises the possibility that an ongoing subclinical rejection response may have a detrimental effect on long-term graft function and survival (Lipman *et al.*, 1998).

HUMAN LEUKOCYTE ANTIGEN EXPRESSION

The expression of HLA antigens in transplanted organs became an area of intense interest in the mid-1980s, and many studies in clinical biopsy specimens and material from animal models were performed. It was shown that as in normal tissue the glomerular and intertubular capillaries still express high levels of class II antigens, but increased levels of tubular class II antigen expression may occur within the transplanted kidney (Armstrong *et al.*, 1987; Barrett *et al.*, 1987; Benson *et al.*, 1985; Copin *et al.*, 1995; Fuggle *et al.*, 1986; Hall *et al.*, 1984b; Hayry and von Willebrand, 1986; Henny *et al.*, 1986; Milton *et al.*, 1986a; Raftery *et al.*, 1989; von Willebrand *et al.*, 1986; Wood *et al.*, 1988). In our study of a series of human renal allograft biopsy specimens, the expression of class II antigens could be classified as normal, focal or generalized, characterized by intense positive staining within the tubular cytoplasm and on the cell membranes. Focal induction usually was perivascular or associated with focal leukocyte infiltration that also contained class II–positive cells. In biopsy specimens with generalized induction of class II antigens, the large vessel endothelium also was intensely positive (Fuggle *et al.*, 1986).

Analyses of the specificity of the induced class II antigens using locus-specific and polymorphic antibodies showed that the induced antigen has HLA-DR (Fig. 25–7A), HLA-DQ and HLA-DP (Fig. 25–7B; compare Fig. 25–1A and B) components and is of donor origin (Evans *et al.*, 1986; Fuggle *et al.*, 1987). In biopsy specimens with generalized induction of HLA-DR antigens on all renal tubules, however, induced HLA-DQ and HLA-DP antigens sometimes were detected only on the proximal and not on the distal tubules. The renal tubules may have a differential susceptibility to induction. In a rat model, intravenous administration of interferon-γ caused induction of class II antigens in proximal but not distal renal tubules (Skoskiewicz *et al.*, 1985).

It is clear from *in vitro* studies that cellular expression of class I antigens is up-regulated after stimulation by cytokines, and an up-regulation after transplantation has been shown by quantitative analysis of tissue from animal models of transplantation (Milton *et al.*, 1986a). The high constitutive

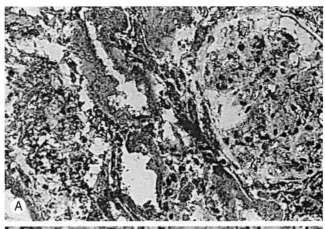
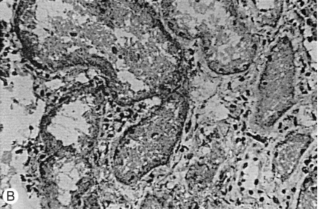

FIGURE 25–7

Distribution of HLA-DR and HLA-DP antigens in a renal allograft with up-regulated class II antigen expression. HLA-DR (A) and HLA-DP (B) are strongly expressed on the renal tubules. Cryostat sections of biopsy tissue were stained by an indirect immunoperoxidase technique and counterstained with hematoxylin. (Original magnification × 350.)

level of expression in normal human kidney largely has precluded immunohistochemical analysis of clinical material for HLA class I antigens.

There is a close correlation between class II induction and increased levels of interstitial leukocyte infiltration within the graft (Fuggle *et al.*, 1986; Fig. 25–8). These observations are consistent with the hypothesis that tubular class II antigens are induced by cytokines released from activated T lymphocytes. Hayry and von Willebrand (1986) showed that induced class II antigen expression was found in association with an infiltration that included a blastogenic component. The kinetics of antigen induction and decay are difficult to study clinically. *In vitro*, HLA-ABC induction precedes that of HLA-DR, and persistent exposure to cytokines is required to maintain the high levels of expression (Bishop *et al.*, 1986b).

It was thought that the presence of up-regulated class II antigens might prove to be a useful tool in the diagnosis of allograft rejection, but the expectations have not been fulfilled. A correlation between HLA class II antigen induction and renal allograft rejection first was described by Hall *et al.* (1984b), and although this finding has been reported by others (Hayry and von Willebrand, 1986; Henny *et al.*, 1986), our data from sequential biopsy specimens suggest a more indirect association between clinical rejection and class II induction (Fuggle, 1989; Fuggle *et al.*, 1986; Fig. 25–9); induced class II antigen expression may be detected in the absence

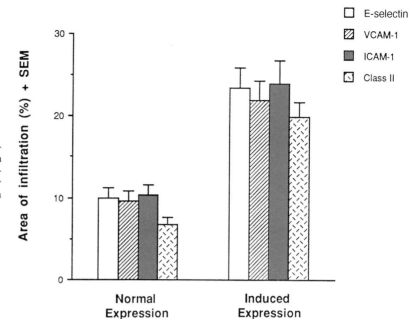

FIGURE 25–8

Leukocyte infiltration in biopsy specimens with normal or increased levels of expression of adhesion molecules and class II antigens. There is a significantly higher level of leukocyte infiltration in biopsy specimens with induced levels of antigen expression when compared with those with normal expression.

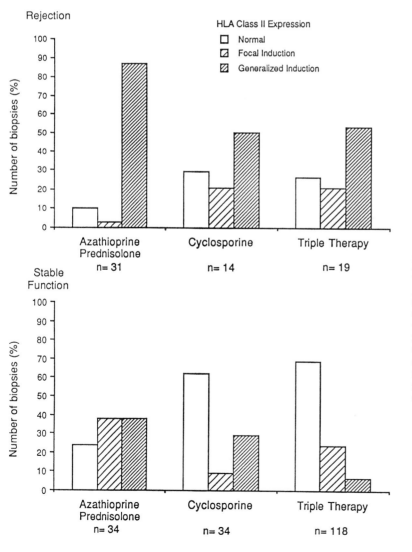

FIGURE 25–9

Comparison of HLA class II expression in renal allograft biopsy specimens taken during clinical rejection or stable function from recipients receiving azathioprine/prednisolone, cyclosporine or triple-therapy immunosuppression. Class II antigens are induced more frequently and intensely in rejecting kidneys from patients treated with azathioprine and prednisolone than in patients receiving cyclosporine or triple-therapy immunosuppression. Similarly, there is a greater incidence of induced class II antigen expression in stable function biopsy specimens from azathioprine and prednisolone–treated patients than in patients receiving cyclosporine or triple-therapy immunosuppression. Generalized class II antigen induction rarely occurs in stable function biopsy specimens from recipients immunosuppressed with triple therapy, suggesting a decreased level of subliminal rejection with this powerful immunosuppressive regimen.

of clinical rejection and vice versa. Consistent with these observations, induced class II antigens have been detected in nonrejecting grafts early after transplantation (Raftery et al., 1989) and in biopsy specimens from patients with cyclosporine nephrotoxicity (Fuggle et al., 1989) and chronic vascular rejection (Bogman et al., 1989). It has been shown in rat models that up-regulation of parenchymal class II antigens may result from ischemic injury (Shackleton et al., 1990; Shoskes et al., 1990) and occur in nonrejected renal allografts in which rejection is prevented by pretransplant donor-specific transfusion (Armstrong et al., 1987; Wood et al., 1988).

The influence of immunosuppression on class II antigen expression has been shown in dog (Groenewegen et al., 1985a) and rat models (Autenreid and Halloran, 1985; Milton et al., 1986a), in which cyclosporine inhibits the induction of class II antigens, probably as a result of the suppression of interferon-γ release (Bishop and Hall, 1988; Groenewegen et al., 1985b; Halloran et al., 1988; Reem et al., 1983). In the clinical situation, cyclosporine monotherapy and triple therapy result in a decreased incidence of class II induction in clinical rejection and stable function when compared with immunosuppression with azathioprine and low-dose prednisolone (Fuggle, 1989; see Fig. 25–9).

Despite the fact that presence of induced class II antigens has not provided information applicable to the diagnosis of acute rejection, it is possible that persistent high levels of expression may be indicative of subliminal rejection and of a poorer overall long-term prognosis. Induced class II antigen is of potential importance within transplanted tissue because cells that express donor class II antigens may be able to stimulate the alloimmune response, a rejection response, and themselves become targets for alloreactive T cells.

EXPRESSION OF CHEMOKINES AND ADHESION MOLECULES

The coordinated expression of particular chemoattractants and adhesion molecules at specific time points after initiation of an inflammatory response results in the recruitment of specific leukocyte subsets to the area (Baggiolini et al., 1997; Fuggle and Koo, 1998; Springer, 1994, 1995). Leukocytes are recruited to inflammatory sites by the production of chemokines (Baggiolini et al., 1997; Melter et al., 1999; Rollins, 1997). Chemokines bind to G-protein receptors on leukocytes, resulting in leukocyte activation, expression of high-affinity integrin molecules and binding of leukocytes to endothelium. Chemokines have been classified into subfamilies according to the amino acid sequence at the N-terminus. CC chemokines have adjacent cysteine residues, whereas CXC chemokines have cysteine residues separated by a single amino acid. Functionally, CC chemokines act primarily on T lymphocytes, monocytes and macrophages, whereas CXC chemokines act on granulocytes. Additional families of chemokines have been identified, the C chemokine, lymphotactin, and the CX_3C chemokine family, which has three amino acids between the two cysteine residues. To date, more than 40 chemokines have been described that interact with the chemokine receptors. Although particular leukocyte subsets express specific chemokine receptors, there is considerable redundancy because each chemokine receptor may recognize more than one chemokine. The recruitment of particular leukocyte subsets into the transplant during allograft rejection depends on the presence of particular chemokines within the transplanted organ.

Studies in animal models have shown that the CC chemokines, RANTES (regulated on activation, normal T cell expressed and secreted) and MCP-1 (monocyte chemoattractant protein-1) which are chemoattractants for monocytes and T lymphocytes, are up-regulated in the kidney after allogeneic renal transplantation (Nadeau et al., 1995; Nagano et al., 1997). In clinical renal transplantation, RANTES mRNA and protein have been detected on the tubules, intertubular capillaries and infiltrating mononuclear cells in 17 of 20 biopsy specimens from kidneys with cellular rejection (Pattison et al., 1994). Similarly, expression of MCP-1 has been detected in biopsy specimens from acutely rejecting renal allografts showing a direct correlation with the level of monocyte infiltration. Urinary levels of MCP-1 correlated significantly with renal MCP-1 gene expression and acute rejection, suggesting its potential application as an early diagnostic marker of acute rejection (Grandaliano et al., 1997).

Renal tubular epithelial cells may play a role in amplifying the inflammatory response within a rejecting allograft by the production of chemokines. Gene expression of the CXC chemokine ENA-78 has been detected in acutely rejecting renal allograft biopsy specimens and in cultured renal tubular epithelial cells stimulated with IL-1β (Schmouder et al., 1995). Further evidence for the direct involvement of tubules has been provided from an analysis of rejecting renal allograft biopsy specimens by scanning laser confocal microscopy showing expression of RANTES, MCP-1, MIP 1α (macrophage inflammatory protein-1α) and MIP -1β (macrophage inflammatory protein-1β) on the basolateral surfaces of tubular epithelial cells (Robertson et al., 1998).

The particular leukocyte subsets that are recruited within a rejecting renal allograft partly depend on the particular chemokine receptors they express. In 13 of 14 rejecting renal allograft biopsy specimens, mononuclear leukocytes expressing chemokine receptors CCR5 and CXCR4 were identified by in situ hybridization. These receptors were absent from other renal structures (Eitner et al., 1998a, 1998b). Concurrent analysis for chemokine gene expression was not performed on these biopsy specimens to identify the chemokines involved in the recruitment of leukocytes expressing these chemokine receptors. A comprehensive range of monoclonal antibodies is available commercially, and it should be possible to determine the interrelationship between the expression of chemokines and their receptors in transplantation.

In transplanted kidneys, significant levels of up-regulated P-selectin and E-selectin may be detected on intertubular capillaries and larger vessels, often associated with areas of leukocyte infiltration (Anderson et al., 1994; Brockmeyer et al., 1993; Fuggle et al., 1993, 1995; Gibbs et al., 1993; von Willebrand et al., 1995; Fig. 25–10A). Because ICAM-1 is expressed constitutively on endothelium in the kidney and the basal expression is so high, it is difficult to detect up-regulated levels using conventional histochemical methods, but up-regulated levels of ICAM-1 are evident after cytokine stimulation of endothelium in vitro. Nevertheless, up-regulation of ICAM-1 may be detected on proximal tubules after transplantation, where it is expressed most strongly at the brush border (Anderson et al., 1992; Bishop and Hall, 1989; Brockmeyer et al., 1993; Faull and Russ, 1989; Fuggle et al., 1993; Gibbs et al., 1993; Hill et al., 1995; Moolenaar et al., 1991; Nickeleit et al., 1993; von Willebrand et al., 1995). Up-regulated levels of VCAM-1 are found on proximal tubules after transplantation, but in this case the expression usually is localized to the basolateral surface and on the intertubular capillaries and large vessel endothelium (Alpers et al., 1993; Briscoe et al., 1992; Brockmeyer et al., 1993; Fuggle et al., 1993; Gibbs et al., 1993; Hill et al., 1995; Lin et al., 1993; Nickeleit et al., 1993; Fig. 25–10B and C).

Up-regulation of ICAM-1, VCAM-1 and E-selectin in transplant biopsy specimens occurs on the same cell types as the variation in expression in the pretransplant biopsy specimen (Fuggle et al., 1993) and frequently is focal and associ-

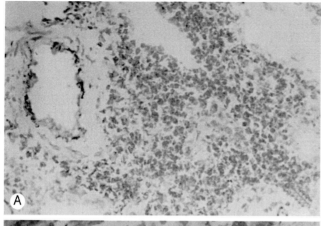

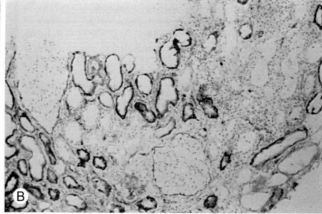

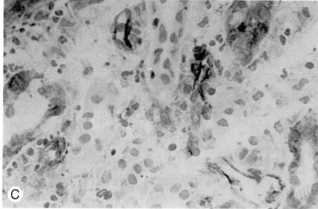

FIGURE 25–10

Up-regulated levels of adhesion molecules in transplanted kidneys. (A) Transplant kidney biopsy specimen shows periarterial leukocyte infiltration and up-regulated expression of E-selectin on the vessel endothelium. (B) Up-regulated tubular and (C) endothelial VCAM-1 expression in a transplanted kidney. Indirect immunoperoxidase staining. (Original magnifications A, × 400; B, × 250; C, × 400.)

ated with mononuclear cell infiltration. In our study of transplant biopsy specimens in which the level of infiltration was quantitated, there was a significantly higher level of infiltration in biopsy specimens with induced adhesion molecule expression (Fuggle *et al.*, 1993; see Fig. 25–8). In this biopsy material, there was generally concomitant expression of induced ICAM-1, VCAM-1 and E-selectin. Increased levels of adhesion molecules may amplify the damage caused by alloreactive cells because results from *in vitro* analyses have shown that increased levels of adhesion molecules on the renal tubular epithelial cells can enhance the binding of alloreactive lymphocytes and augment cell-mediated damage (Lin *et al.*, 1993; Suranyi *et al.*, 1991).

It was postulated that changes in the expression of endothelial adhesion molecules may be of value in transplant monitoring, but the results of the studies show that similar caveats to those discussed in relation to class II antigen expression apply. Cytomegalovirus infection is a confounding factor when assessing the diagnostic value of up-regulated antigen expression. Cytokines released during the response to cytomegalovirus-infected cells can increase the level of expression of MHC antigens, ICAM-1 and VCAM-1 on endothelial cells (Waldman and Knight, 1996). Cytomegalovirus infection does not appear to up-regulate endothelial HLA class II, VCAM-1 or E-selectin expression directly, but ICAM-1 is markedly up-regulated, leading to sustained, extensive expression after an infection with cytomegalovirus (Sedmak *et al.*, 1994a, 1994b). In a similar manner to HLA class II antigens, immunosuppressive agents, in particular cyclosporine, can modulate adhesion molecule expression (De Caterina *et al.*, 1995; Frishberg *et al.*, 1996).

Adhesion molecules are important at many stages in the alloimmune response, in particular in the initial transmigra-

tion of leukocytes into the transplanted organ, then in the effector phase of the response. The presence of induced MHC class II antigens together with adhesion molecules may make the transplant more susceptible to damage from alloreactive effector lymphocytes.

Conclusion

Immunohistochemical studies of transplant biopsy material can provide important information about the donor kidney itself and the changes that may occur in the allograft immediately after transplantation as a result of ischemia/reperfusion injury. In biopsy specimens obtained in the longer term, immunohistochemical analysis complements the information derived from routine pathology, providing invaluable insights into the immunological events that occur in the transplanted kidney not only during episodes of allograft rejection, but also during periods of stable graft function.

References

Alpers, C. E., Hudkins, K. L., Davis, C. L., *et al.* (1993). Expression of vascular cell adhesion molecule-1 in kidney allograft rejection. *Kidney Int.* **44**, 805.

Amado, J. A., Lopez-Espadas, F., Vazquez-Barquero, A., *et al.* (1995). Blood levels of cytokines in brain-dead patients: relationship with circulating hormones and acute-phase reactants. *Metabolism* **44**, 812.

Anderson, C. B., Blaehr, H., Ladefoged, S. and Larsen S. (1992). Expression of the intercellular adhesion molecule-1 (ICAM-1) in human renal allografts and cultured human tubular cells. *Nephrol. Dial. Transplant.* **7**, 147.

Anderson, C. B., Ladefoged, S. D. and Larsen, S. (1994). Acute kidney graft rejection: a morphological and immunohistochemical study on 'zero-hour' and follow-up biopsies wiht special emphasis on cellular infiltrates and adhesion molecules. *A. P. M. I. S.* **102**, 23.

Armstrong, H. E., Bolton, E. M., McMillan, I., Spencer, S. C. and Bradley, J. A. (1987). Prolonged survival of actively enhanced rat renal allografts despite accelerated cellular infiltration and rapid induction of both Class I and Class II MHC antigens. *J. Exp. Med.* **165**, 891.

Autenreid, P. and Halloran, P. (1985). Cyclosporine blocks the induction of class I and class II molecules in mouse kidney by graft-vs.-host disease. *J. Immunol.* **135**, 3922.

Baggiolini, M., Dewald, B. and Moser, B. (1997). Human chemokines: an update. *Ann. Rev. Immunol.* **15**, 675.

Barrett, M., Milton, A. D., Barrett, J., *et al.* (1987). Needle biopsy evaluation of class II major histocompatibility complex antigen expression for the differential diagnosis of cyclosporine nephrotoxicity from kidney graft rejection. *Transplantation* **44**, 223.

Benson, E. M., Colvin, R. and Russell, P. S. (1985). Induction of Ia antigens in murine renal transplants. *J. Immunol.* **134**, 7.

Berke, G. (1995). Unlocking the secrets of CTL and NK cells. *Immunol. Today* **16**, 343.

Beschorner, W. E., Burdick, J. F., Williams, G. F. and Solez, K. (1985). The presence of Leu-7 reactive lymphocytes in renal allografts undergoing acute rejection. *Transplant. Proc.* **17**, 618.

Bevilacqua, M. P., Pober, J. S., Mendrick, D. L., Cotran, R. S. and Gimbrone, M. A., Jr. (1987). Identification of an inducible endothelial-leukocyte adhesion molecule. *Proc. Natl. Acad. Sci. U. S. A.* **84**, 9238.

Bishop, G. A. and Hall, B. M. (1988). Effects of immunosuppressive drugs on functions of activated T lymphocytes: cyclosporine inhibition of gamma interferon production in the presence of interleukin 2. *Transplantation* **45**, 967.

Bishop, G. A. and Hall, B. M. (1989). Expression of leucocyte and lymphocyte adhesion molecules in the human kidney. *Kidney Int.* **36**, 1078.

Bishop, G. A., Hall, B. M., Duggin, G. G., Horvath, J. S., Sheil, A. G. and Tiller, D. J. (1986a). Immunopathology of renal allograft rejection analyzed with monoclonal antibodies to mononuclear cell markers. *Kidney Int.* **29**, 708.

Bishop, G. A., Hall, B. M., Suranyi, M. G., Tiller, D. J., Horvath, J. S. and Duggin, G. G. (1986b). Expression of HLA antigens on renal tubular cells in culture: I. evidence that mixed lymphocyte culture supernatants and gamma interferon increase both class I and class II HLA antigens. *Transplantation* **42**, 671.

Bogman, M. J. J. T., Dooper, I. M. M. and van de Winkel, J. G. J. (1989). Diagnosis of renal allograft rejection by macrophage immunostaining with a CD14 monoclonal antibody, WT14. *Lancet* **2**, 235.

Bradley, J. A., Mason, D. W. and Morris, P. J. (1985). Evidence that rat renal allografts are rejected by cytotoxic T cells and not by nonspecific effectors. *Transplantation* **39**, 169.

Briscoe, D. M., Pober, J. S., Harmon, W. E. and Cotran, R. S. (1992). Expression of vascular cell adhesion molecule-1 in human renal allografts. *J. Am. Soc. Nephrol.* **3**, 1180.

Brockmeyer, C., Ulbrecht, M., Schendel, D. J., *et al.* (1993). Distribution of cell adhesion molecules (ICAM-1, VCAM-1, ELAM-1) in renal tissue during allograft rejection. *Transplantation* **55**, 610.

Budde, K., Waiser, J., Ceska, M., Katalinic, A., Kurzdorfer, M. and Neumayer, H. H. (1997). Interleukin-8 expression in patients after renal transplantation. *Am. J. Kidney Dis.* **29**, 871.

Burdick, J. F., Beschorner, W. E., Smith, W. J., *et al.* (1984). Characteristics of early routine renal allograft biopsies. *Transplantation* **38**, 679.

Chen, R. H., Ivens, K. W., Alpert, S., *et al.* (1993). The use of granzyme A as a marker of heart transplant rejection in cyclosporine or anti-CD4 monoclonal antibody-treated rats. *Transplantation* **55**, 146.

Chertow, G. M., Milford, E. L., Mackenzie, H. S. and Brenner, B.M. (1996). Antigen-independent determinants of cadaveric kidney transplant failure. *J. A. M. A.* **276**, 1732.

Copin, M. C., Noel, C., Hazzan, M., *et al.* (1995). Diagnostic and predictive value of an immunohistochemical profile in asymptomatic acute rejection of renal allografts. *Transpl. Immunol.* **3**, 229.

Dallman, M. J., Roake, J., Hughes, D., Toogood, G. and Morris, P. J. (1992). Sequential analysis of IL-2 gene transcription in renal transplants. *Transplantation* **53**, 683.

Dallman, M. J., Wood, K. J. and Morris, P. J. (1987). Specific cytotoxic T cells are found in the nonrejected kidneys of blood-transfused rats. *J. Exp. Med.* **165**, 566.

De Caterina, R., Tanaka, H., Nakagawa, T., Hauptman, P. J. and Libby, P. (1995). The direct effect of injectable cyclosporine and its vehicle, cremophor, on endothelial vascular cell adhesion molecule-1 expression: ricinoleic acid inhibits coronary artery endothelial activation. *Transplantation* **60**, 270.

de Mattos, A. M., Meyer, M. M., Norman, D. J., Bennett, W. M., Sprague, J. and Bakke, A. C. (1997). Interleukin-12 p40 mRNA expression in human kidney allograft biopsies. *Transpl. Immunol.* **5**, 199.

Dustin, M. L., Rothlein, R., Bhan, A. K., Dinarello, C. A. and Springer, T. A. (1986). Induction by IL 1 and interferon-gamma: tissue distribution, biochemistry, and function of a natural adherence molecule (ICAM-1). *J. Immunol.* **137**, 245.

Eitner, F., Cui, Y., Hudkins, K. L. and Alpers, C. E. (1998a). Chemokine receptor (CXCR4) mRNA-expressing leukocytes are increased in human renal allograft rejection. *Transplantation* **66**, 1551.

Eitner, F., Cui, Y., Hudkins, K. L., *et al.* (1998b). Chemokine receptor (CCR5) expression in human kidneys and in the HIV infected macaque. *Kidney Int.* **54**, 1945.

Evans, P. R., Trickett, L. P., MacIver, A. G. and Smith, J. L. (1986). Heterogeneity of expresssion of HLA-Class II antigens DR, DQ and DP on the normal renal endothelium. *Dis. Markers* **3**, 185.

Evans, P. R., Trickett, L. P., Smith, J. L., MacIver, A. G., Tate, D. and Slapak, M. (1985). Varying expression of major histocompatibility complex antigens on human renal endothelium and epithelium. *Br. J. Exp. Pathol.* **66**, 79.

Faull, R. J. and Russ, G. R. (1989). Tubular expression of intercellular adhesion molecule-1 during renal allograft rejection. *Transplantation* **48**, 226.

Fleming, K. A., McMichael, A. J., Morton, J. A., Woods, J. and McGee, J. O. D. (1981). Distribution of HLA class I antigens in normal human tissue and in mammary cancer. *J. Clin. Pathol.* **34**, 779.

Foot, R. A., Fuggle, S. V., McWhinnie, D. L., Carter, N. P. and Morris, P. J. (1989). The diagnosis of renal allograft rejection: an improved assessment of graft infiltration using image analysis. *Transplant. Proc.* **21**, 1905.

French, M. E. and Batchelor, J. R. (1969). Immunological enhancement of rat kidney grafts. *Lancet* **2**, 1103.

Frishberg, Y., Meyers, C. and Kelly, C. J. (1996). Cyclosporine A regulates T cell-epithelial adhesion by altering LFA-1 and ICAM-1 expression. *Kidney Int.* **50**, 45.

Fuggle, S. V. (1989). MHC antigen induction in vascularised organ allografts: clinical correlations and significance. *Transplant. Rev.* **3**, 81.

Fuggle, S. V., Carter, A. S., Gray, D. W. and Morris, P. J. (1995). Endothelial cell panel mAb with normal tissue and pre-transplant and transplanted kidneys. In *Leucocyte Typing V: White Cell Differentiation Antigens*, vol. 2, (S. F. Schlossman, L. Boumsell, W. Gilks, *et al.*, eds.), p. 1790, Oxford University Press, Oxford.

Fuggle, S. V., Errasti, P., Daar, A. S., Fabre, J. W., Ting, A. and Morris, P. J. (1983). Localization of major histocompatibility complex (HLA-ABC and DR) antigens in 46 kidneys: differences in HLA-DR staining of tubules among kidneys. *Transplantation* **35**, 385.

Fuggle, S. V. and Koo, D. D. H. (1998). Cell adhesion molecules in clinical renal transplantation. *Transplantation* **65**, 763.

Fuggle, S. V., McWhinnie, D. L., Chapman, J. R., Taylor, H. M. and Morris, P. J. (1986). Sequential analysis of HLA-class II antigen expression in human renal allografts: induction of tubular class II antigens and correlation with clinical parameters. *Transplantation* **42**, 144.

Fuggle, S. V., McWhinnie, D. L. and Morris, P. J. (1987). Precise specificity of induced tubular HLA-class II antigens in renal allografts. *Transplantation* **44**, 214.

Fuggle, S. V., McWhinnie, D. L. and Morris, P. J. (1989). Immunohistological analysis of renal allograft biopsies from cyclosporin treated patients: correlation with intragraft events. *Transpl. Int.* **2**, 123.

Fuggle, S. V., Sanderson, J. B., Gray, D. W., Richardson, A. and Morris, P. J. (1993). Variation in expression of endothelial adhesion molecules in pretransplant and transplanted kidneys—correlation with intragraft events. *Transplantation* **55**, 117.

Gaber, L. W., Gaber, A. O., Tolley, E. A. and Hathaway, D. K. (1992). Prediction by postrevascularization biopsies of cadaveric kidney allografts of rejection, graft loss, and preservation nephropathy. *Transplantation* **53,** 1219.

Gibbs, P., Berkley, L. M., Bolton, E. M., Briggs, J. D. and Braley, J. A. (1993). Adhesion molecule expression (ICAM-1, VCAM-1, E-selectin and PECAM) in human kidney allografts. *Transpl. Immunol.* **1,** 109.

Grandaliano, G., Gesualdo, L., Ranieri, E., Monno, R., Stallone, G. and Shena, F. P. (1997). Monocyte chemotactic peptide-1 expression and monocyte infiltration in acute renal transplant rejection. *Transplantation* **63,** 414.

Gray, D. W. R., Richardson, A., Hughes, D., *et al.* (1992). A prospective, randomised, blind comparison of three biopsy techniques in the management of patients after renal transplantation. *Transplantation* **53,** 1226.

Groenewegen, G., Buurman, W. A., Jeunhomme, G. M. A. A. and van der Linden, C. J. (1985b). Effect of cyclosporine on MHC Class II antigen expression on arterial and venous endothelium in vitro. *Transplantation* **40,** 21.

Groenewegen, G., Buurman, W. A. and van der Linden, C. J. (1985a). Lymphokine dependence of in vivo expression of MHC class II antigens by endothelium. *Nature* **316,** 361.

Hall, B. M., Bishop, G. A., Farnsworth, A., *et al.* (1984a). Identification of the cellular subpopulations infiltrating rejecting cadaver renal allografts: preponderance of the T4 subset of T cells. *Transplantation* **37,** 564.

Hall, B. M., Duggin, C. G., Phillips, J., Bishop, G. A., Horvath, J. S. and Tiller, D. J. (1984b). Increased expression of HLA-DR antigen on renal tubular cells in renal transplants: relevance to the rejection response. *Lancet* **2,** 246.

Halloran, P. F., Urmson, J., Farkas, S., *et al.* (1988). Effects of cyclosporine on systemic MHC expression: evidence that non T-cells produce interferon-gamma in vivo and are inhibitable by cyclosporine. *Transplantation* **46,** 68.

Hancock, W. W., Gee, D., De Moerloose, P., Rickles, F. R., Ewan, V. A. and Atkins, R. C. (1985). Immunohistological analysis of serial biopsies taken during human allograft rejection. *Transplantation* **39,** 430.

Hancock, W. W., Kraft, N. and Atkins, R. C. (1982). The immunohistochemical demonstration of major histocompatibility antigens in the human kidney using monoclonal antibodies. *Pathology* **14,** 409.

Hancock, W. W., Thomson, N. M. and Atkins, R. C. (1983). Composition of interstitial cellular infiltrate identified by monoclonal antibodies in renal biopsies of rejecting human renal allografts. *Transplantation* **35,** 458.

Hashemi, S., Palmer, D. S., Aye, M. T. and Ganz, P. R. (1993). Platelet-activating factor secreted by DDAVP-treated monocytes mediates von Willebrand factor release from endothelial cells. *J. Cell. Physiol.* **154,** 496.

Hayry, P. and von Willebrand, E. (1986). The influence of the pattern of inflammation and administration of steroids on Class II MHC antigen expression in renal transplants. *Transplantation* **42,** 358.

Henkart, P. A. (1994). Lymphocyte-mediated cytotoxicity: two pathways and multiple effector molecules. *Immunity* **1,** 343.

Henny, F. C., Weening, J. J., Baldwin, W. M., *et al.* (1986). Expression of HLA-DR antigens on peripheral blood T lymphocytes and renal graft tubular epithelial cells in association with rejection. *Transplantation* **42,** 479.

Hill, P. A., Main, I. W. and Atkins, R. C. (1995). ICAM-1 and VCAM-1 in human renal allograft rejection. *Kidney Int.* **47,** 1383.

Jevnikar, A. M., Wuthrich, R. P., Takei, F., *et al.* (1990). Differing regulation and function of ICAM-1 and class II antigens on renal tubular cells. *Kidney Int.* **38,** 417.

Kanwar, S., Woodman, R. C., Poon, M. C., *et al.* (1995). Desmopressin induces endothelial P-selectin expression and leukocyte rolling in postcapillary venules. *Blood* **86,** 2760.

Kataoka, K., Naomoto, Y., Shiozaki, S., *et al.* (1992). Infiltration of perforin-positive mononuclear cells into the rejected kidney allograft. *Transplantation* **53,** 240.

Kincaid-Smith, P., Morris, P. J., Saker, B. M., Ting, A. and Marshall, V. C. (1968). Immediate renal-graft biopsy and subsequent rejection. *Lancet* **2,** 748.

Kirby, J. A., Rajasekar, M. R., Lin, Y., Proud, G. and Taylor, R. M. R. (1993). Interaction between T lymphocytes and kidney epithelial cells during renal allograft rejection. *Kidney Int.* **43(Suppl. 39),** S124.

Kirk, A. D., Bollinger, R. R. and Finn, O. J. (1995). Rapid, comprehensive analysis of human cytokine mRNA and its application to the study of acute renal allograft rejection. *Hum. Immunol.* **43,** 113.

Koo, D. D. H., Welsh, K. I., McLaren, A. J., Roake, J. A., Morris, P. J. and Fuggle, S. V. (1999). Cadaver versus living donor kidneys: impact of donor factors on antigen induction before transplantation. *Kidney Int.* **56,** 1551.

Koo, D. D. H., Welsh, K. I., Roake, J. A., Morris, P. J. and Fuggle S. V. (1998). Ischemia/reperfusion injury in human kidney transplantation: an immunohistochemical analysis of changes after reperfusion. *Am. J. Pathol.* **153,** 557.

Koyama, K., Fukunishi, T., Barcos, M., Tanigaki, N. and Pressman, D. (1979). Human Ia-like antigens in non-lymphoid organs. *Immunology* **38,** 333.

Kummer, J. A., Wever, P. C., Kamp, A. M., ten Berge, I. J., Hack, C. E. and Weening, J. J. (1995). Expression of granzyme A and B proteins by cytotoxic lymphocytes involved in acute renal allograft rejection. *Kidney Int.* **47,** 70.

Lin, Y., Kirby, J. A., Browell, D. A., *et al.* (1993). Renal allograft rejection: expression and function of VCAM-1 on tubular epithelial cells. *Clin. Exp. Immunol.* **92,** 145.

Lin, Y., Kirby, J. A., Clark, K., *et al.* (1992). Renal allograft rejection: induction and function of adhesion molecules on cultured epithelial cells. *Clin. Exp. Immunol.* **90,** 111.

Lipman, M. L., Shen, Y., Jeffery, J. R., *et al.* (1998). Immune-activation gene expression in clinically stable renal allograft biopsies: molecular evidence for subclinical rejection. *Transplantation* **66,** 1673.

Lipman, M. L., Stevens, C., Bleackley, C., *et al.* (1992). The strong correlation of cytotoxic T lymphocyte specific serine protease gene transcripts with renal allograft rejection. *Transplantation* **53,** 73.

Lipman, M. L., Stevens, A. C. and Strom, T. B. (1994). Heightened intragraft CTL gene expression in acutely rejecting renal allografts. *J. Immunol.* **152,** 5120.

Manucci, P. M. (1988). Desmopressin: a nontransfusional form of treatment for congenital and acquired bleeding disorders. *Blood* **72,** 1449.

McDicken, I. W., Hawking, K. M., Lameyer, L. D., Blok, A. P. R. and Westbroek, D. L. (1975). Prognostic value for immediate function of one-hour renal allograft biopsy. *B. M. J.* **4,** 559.

McLean, A. G., Hughes, D., Welsh, K. I., *et al.* (1997). Patterns of graft infiltration and cytokine gene expression during the first 10 days of kidney transplantation. *Transplantation* **63,** 374.

McWhinnie, D. L., Fuggle, S. V., Azevedo, L. S., Carter, N. P. and Morris, P. J. (1989). Correlation of HLA Class II antigen induction and cellular infiltration in renal allograft rejection. *Transplant. Proc.* **21,** 320.

McWhinnie, D. L., Fuggle, S. V., Azevedo, L. S., Jones, R. M. and Morris, P. J. (1987). HLA class II induction and cellular infiltration are effectively suppressed by triple therapy in renal allografts. *Transplant. Proc.* **19,** 3628.

McWhinnie, D. L., Thompson, J. F., Taylor, H. M., *et al.* (1986). Morphometric analysis of cellular infiltration assessed by monoclonal antibody labeling in sequential human renal allograft biopsies. *Transplantation* **42,** 352.

Melter, M., McMahon, G., Fang, J., Ganz, P. and Briscoe, D. M. (1999). Current understanding of chemokine involvement in allograft transplantation. *Pediatr. Transplant.* **3,** 10.

Milton, A. D., Spencer, S. C. and Fabre, J. W. (1986a). Detailed analysis and demonstration of the differences in the kinetics of induction of Class I and Class II major histocompatibility antigens in rejecting cardiac and kidney allografts in the rat. *Transplantation* **41,** 499.

Milton, A. D., Spencer S. C. and Fabre J. W. (1986b). The effects of cyclosporine on the induction of donor class I and class II MHC antigens in heart and kidney allografts in the rat. *Transplantation* **42,** 337.

Moolenaar, W., Bruijn, J. A., Schrama, E., *et al.* (1991). T-cell receptors and ICAM-1 expression in renal allografts during rejection. *Transpl. Int.* **4,** 140.

Mueller, C., Shelby, J., Weissman, I. L., Perinat-Frey, T. and Eichwald, E. J. (1991). Expression of the protease gene HF as a marker in rejecting allogeneic murine heart transplants. *Transplantation* **51,** 514.

Nadeau, K. C., Azuma, H. and Tilney, N. L. (1995). Sequential cytokine dynamics in chronic rejection of rat renal allografts: roles for cytokines RANTES and MCP-1. *Proc. Natl. Acad. Sci. U. S. A.* **92,** 8729.

Nagano, H., Nadeau, K. C., Takada, M., Kusaka, M. and Tilney, N. L. (1997). Sequential cellular and molecular kinetics in acutely rejecting renal allografts in rats. *Transplantation* **63,** 1101.

Najarian, J. S., Gillingham, K. J., Sutherland, D. E., Reinsmoen, N. L., Payne, W. D. and Matas, A. J. (1994). The impact of the quality of initial graft function on cadaver kidney transplants. *Transplantation* **57,** 812.

Natali, P. G., De Martino, C., Quaranta, V., *et al.* (1981). Expression of Ia-like antigens in normal human nonlymphoid tissues. *Transplantation* **31,** 75.

Nickeleit, V., Miller, M., Cosimi, B. A., *et al.* (1993). Adhesion molecules in human renal allograft rejection: immunohistochemical analysis of ICAM-1, ICAM-2, ICAM-3, VCAM-1 and ELAM-1. In *Structure, Function, and Regulation of Molecules Involved in Leukocyte Adhesion,* (P. E. Lipsky, R. Rothlein, T. K. Kishimoto, R. B. Faanes and C. W. Smith, eds.), p. 380, Springer-Verlag, New York.

Pattison, J., Nelson, P. J., Huie, P., *et al.* (1994). RANTES chemokine expression in cell-mediated transplant rejection of the kidney. *Lancet* **343,** 209.

Perloff, L. J., Goodloe, S. J., Jenis, E. H., Light, J. A. and Spees, E. K. (1973). Value of one-hour renal-allograft biopsy. *Lancet* **2,** 1294.

Peters, T. G., Shaver, T. R., Ames, J. E., Santiago-Delpin, E. A., Jones, K. W. and Blanton, J. W. (1995). Cold ischemia and outcome in 17,937 cadaveric kidney transplants. *Transplantation* **59,** 191.

Pfaff, W. W., Howard, R. J., Patton, P. R., Adams, V. R., Rosen, C. B. and Reed, A. I. (1998). Delayed graft function after renal transplantation. *Transplantation* **65,** 219.

Platt, J. L., LeBien, T. W. and Michael, A. F. J. (1982). Interstitial mononuclear cell populations in renal graft rejection: identification by monoclonal antibodies in tissue sections. *J. Exp. Med.* **155,** 17.

Pratschke, J., Wilhelm, M. J., Kusaka, M., *et al.* (1999). Brain death and its influence on donor organ quality and outcome after transplantation. *Transplantation* **67,** 343.

Raftery, M. J., Seron, D., Koffman, G., Hartley, B., Janossy, G. and Cameron, J. S. (1989). The relevance of induced class II HLA antigens and macrophage infiltration in early renal allograft biopsies. *Transplantation* **48,** 238.

Reem, G. M., Cook, L. A. and Vilcek, J. (1983). Gamma interferon synthesis by human thymocytes and T lymphocytes inhibited by Cyclosporine A. *Science* **221,** 63.

Rice, G. E., Munro, J. M. and Bevilacqua, M. P. (1990). Inducible cell adhesion molecule 110 (INCAM-110) is an endothelial receptor for lymphocytes: a CD11/CD18-independent adhesion mechanism. *J. Exp. Med.* **171,** 1369.

Robertson, H., Wheeler, J., Morley, A. R., Booth, T. A., Talbot, D. and Kirby, J. A. (1998). Beta-chemokine expression and distribution in paraffin-embedded transplant renal biopsy sections: analysis by scanning laser confocal microscopy. *Histochem. Cell. Biol.* **110,** 207.

Rollins, B. J. (1997). Chemokines. *Blood* **90,** 909.

Sako, H., Nakane, Y., Okino, K., *et al.* (1987). Immunohistochemical study of the cells infiltrating human renal allografts by the ABC and IGSS method using monoclonal antibodies. *Transplantation* **44,** 43.

Sanfilippo, F., Kolbeck, P. C., Vaughan, W. K. and Bollinger, R. R. (1985). Renal allograft cell infiltrates associated with irreversible rejection. *Transplantation* **40,** 679.

Schmouder, R. L., Strieter, R. M., Walz, A. and Kunkel, S. L. (1995). Epithelial-derived neutrophil-activating factor-78 production in human renal tubule epithelial cells and in renal allograft rejection. *Transplantation* **59,** 118.

Schwarting, R., Niedobitek, G. and Stein, H. (1989). Cluster report: CD69. In *Leucocyte Typing IV: White Cell Differentiation Antigens,* (W. Knapp, ed.), p. 428, Oxford University Press, Oxford.

Schwarting, R. and Stein, H. (1989). Cluster report: CD25. In *Leucocyte Typing IV: White Cell Differentiation Antigens,* (W. Knapp, ed.), p. 399, Oxford University Press, Oxford.

Scott, H., Brandtzaeg, P., Hirschberg, H., Solheim, B. G. and Thorsby, E. (1981). Vascular and renal distribution of HLA-DR-like antigens. *Tissue Antigens* **18,** 195.

Sedmak, D. D., Guglielmo, A. M., Knight, D. A., Birmingham, D. J., Huang, E. H. and Waldman, W. J. (1994a). Cytomegalovirus inhib-

its major histocompatibility class II expression on infected endothelial cells. *Am. J. Pathol.* **144,** 683.

Sedmak, D. D., Knight, D. A., Vook, N. C. and Waldman, J. W. (1994b). Divergent patterns of ELAM-1, ICAM-1, and VCAM-1 expression on cytomegalovirus-infected endothelial cells. *Transplantation* **58,** 1379.

Seron, D., Alexopoulos, E., Raftery, M. J., Hartley, R. B. and Cameron, J. S. (1989). Diagnosis of rejection in renal allograft biopsies using the presence of activated and proliferating cells. *Transplantation* **47,** 811.

Seron, D., Cameron, J. S. and Haskard, D. O. (1991). Expression of VCAM-1 in the normal and diseased kidney. *Nephrol. Dial. Transplant.* **6,** 917.

Shackleton, C. R., Ettinger, S. L., McLoughlin, M. G., Scudamore, C. H., Miller, R. R. and Keown, P. A. (1990). Effect of recovery from ischemic injury on class I and class II MHC antigen expression. *Transplantation* **49,** 641.

Shoskes, D. A. and Halloran, P. F. (1996). Delayed graft function: etiology, management and long-term significance. *J. Urol.* **155,** 1831.

Shoskes, D. A., Partrey, N. A. and Halloran, P. F. (1990). Increased major histocompatibility complex antigen expression in unilateral ischemic acute tubular necrosis in the mouse. *Transplantation* **49,** 201.

Skoskiewicz, M. J., Colvin, R. B., Schneeberger, E. E. and Russell, P. S. (1985). Widespread and selective induction of major histocompatibility complex-determined antigens in vivo by gamma-interferon. *J. Exp. Med.* **162,** 1645.

Springer, T. A. (1994). Traffic signals for lymphocyte recirculation and leukocyte emigration: the multistep paradigm. *Cell* **76,** 301.

Springer, T. A. (1995). Traffic signals on endothelium for lymphocyte recirculation and leukocyte emigration. *Annu. Rev. Physiol.* **57,** 827.

Strehlau, J., Pavlakis, M., Lipman, M., Maslinski, W., Shapiro, M. and Strom, T. B. (1996). The intragraft gene activation of markers reflecting T cell activation and cytotoxicity analyzed by quantitative RT-PCR in renal transplantation. *Clin. Nephrol.* **46,** 30.

Strehlau, J., Pavlakis, M., Lipman, M., *et al.* (1997). Quantitative detection of immune activation transcripts as a diagnostic tool in kidney transplantation. *Proc. Natl. Acad. Sci. U. S. A.* **94,** 695.

Suranyi, M. G., Bishop, G. A., Clayberger, C., *et al.* (1991). Lymphocyte adhesion molecules in T cell-mediated lysis of human kidney cells. *Kidney Int.* **39,** 312.

Suthanthiran, M. (1997). Molecular analyses of human renal allografts: differential intragraft gene expression during rejection. *Kidney Int.* **51(Suppl. 58),** S15.

Takada, M., Nadeau, K. C., Hancock, W. W., *et al.* (1998). Effects of explosive brain death on cytokine activation of peripheral organs in the rat. *Transplantation* **65,** 1533.

Tufveson, G., Forsum, V., Claesson, K., *et al.* (1983). T-lymphocyte subsets and HLA-DR-expressing cells in rejected human kidney grafts. *Scand. J. Immunol.* **18,** 37.

Valenzuela, R., Hamway, S. A., Deodhar, S. D., *et al.* (1980). Histologic, ultrastructural, and immunomicroscopic findings in 96 one hour human renal allograft biopsy specimens. *Hum. Pathol.* **11,** 187.

Vandenbroecke, C., Caillat-Zucman, S., Legendre, C., *et al.* (1991). Differential in situ expression of cytokines in renal allograft rejection. *Transplantation* **51,** 602.

van Es, A., Baldwin, W. M., Oljans, P. J., Tanke, H. J., Ploem, J. S. and van Es, L. A. (1984). Expression of HLA-DR on T lymphocytes following renal transplantation, and association with graft-rejection episodes and cytomegalovirus infection. *Transplantation* **37,** 65.

van Kooten, C., Boonstra, J. G., Paape, M. E., *et al.* (1998). Interleukin-17 activates human renal epithelial cells in vitro and is expressed during renal allograft rejection. *J. Am. Soc. Nephrol.* **9,** 1526.

Vasconcellos, L. M., Asher, F., Schachter, D., *et al.* (1998). Cytotoxic lymphocyte gene expression in peripheral blood leukocytes correlates with rejecting renal allografts. *Transplantation* **66,** 562.

von Willebrand, E., Krogerus, L., Salmela, K., *et al.* (1995). Expression of adhesion molecules and their ligands in acute rejection of human kidney allografts. *Transplant. Proc.* **27,** 917.

von Willebrand, E., Petterson, E., Ahonen, J. and Hayry, P. (1986). CMV infection, class II antigen expression, and human kidney allograft rejection. *Transplantation* **42,** 364.

Waldman, W. J. and Knight, D. A. (1996). Cytokine-mediated induction of endothelial adhesion molecule and histocompatibility leukocyte antigen expression by cytomegalovirus-activated T cells. *Am. J. Pathol.* **148,** 105.

Waltzer, W. C., Miller, F., Arnold, A., Anaise, D. and Rapaport, F. (1987). Immunohistologic analysis of human renal allograft dysfunction. *Transplantation* **43,** 100.

Williams, G. M., Hume, D. M., Hudson, R. P., Morris, P. J., Kano, K. and Milgrom F. (1968). "Hyperacute" renal-homograft rejection in man. *N. Engl. J. Med.* **279,** 611.

Wilson, J. L., Proud, G., Forsythe, J. L. R., Taylor, R. M. R. and Kirby, J. A. (1995). Renal allograft rejection: tubular epithelial cells present alloantigen in the presence of costimulatory CD28 antibody. *Transplantation* **59,** 91.

Wood, G. S., Warner, N. L. and Warnke, R. A. (1983). Anti-Leu-3/T4 antibodies react with cells of monocyte/macrophage and Langerhans lineage. *J. Immunol.* **131,** 212.

Wood, K. J., Hopley, A., Dallman, M. J. and Morris, P. J. (1988). Lack of correlation between the induction of donor class I and class II major histocompatibility complex antigens and graft rejection. *Transplantation* **45,** 759.

Wun, T., Paglieroni, T. G. and Lachant, N. A. (1995). Desmopressin stimulates the expression of P-selectin on human platelets in vitro. *J. Lab. Clin. Med.* **125,** 401.

Xu, G.-P., Sharma, V. K., Li, B., *et al.* (1995). Intragraft expression of IL-10 messenger RNA: a novel correlate of renal allograft rejection. *Kidney Int.* **48,** 1504.

Fine-Needle Aspiration Cytology of the Transplanted Kidney

David Hughes

Introduction

Fine-needle aspiration biopsy (FNAB), together with the cytological evaluation of the specimens (fine-needle aspiration cytology [FNAC]), has become an established practical method for monitoring kidney transplant patients (Kreis, 1984; Leone *et al.*, 1995; von Willebrand, 1989). The aspiration biopsy technique was developed for clinical practice by Franzen *et al.* in 1960 and applied to human renal transplants for the first time in 1968 by Pasternack in Helsinki. In the 1970s, based on experimental work in rat and human allografts (Hayry *et al.*, 1979; von Willebrand and Hayry, 1978; von Willebrand *et al.*, 1979), the cytoimmunological sequence of events in renal allograft rejection became better understood. It was obvious from experimental models that the inflammation (i.e., immunoactivation) associated with rejection is seen earlier and more specifically in the kidney transplant than in the peripheral blood of the recipient. In the 1980s and 1990s, immunocytology and molecular biology techniques were applied extensively to FNAB samples to study various aspects of immune activity within renal allografts (Bolton *et al.*, 1984; Dallman *et al.*, 1992; McLean *et al.*, 1997).

The advantage of FNAB is that it can be performed daily, if necessary, to monitor human renal allografts without risk to the graft or the patient (Hayry and von Willebrand, 1981a; von Willebrand, 1989). With experience of 13,000 FNABs in the Helsinki center alone, the method has proved to be safe, quick and well suited to close monitoring of the transplant patient during the early postoperative period, when the risk of acute rejection is greatest (Hayry *et al.*, 1981b). Many reports in the literature have evaluated the clinical usefulness (Almirall *et al.*, 1992a; Birkeland *et al.*, 1994; Gouldesborough *et al.*, 1992; Leone *et al.*, 1995; Surachno *et al.*, 1987; Ubhi *et al.*, 1988) and cost-effectiveness (Burdick and Kittur, 1991; Delaney *et al.*, 1993) of transplant aspiration cytology.

Performance of Fine-Needle Aspiration Biopsy

The FNAB technique is not difficult and requires only simple equipment. To ensure that representative samples with sufficient cell yield and minimal blood contamination are obtained, the following technical details are recommended (Hayry and von Willebrand, 1981b; von Willebrand, 1980). The biopsy is performed at the bedside under aseptic conditions and without local anesthesia. A 23- or 25-gauge spinal needle is inserted percutaneously into the kidney cortex, preferably using ultrasound guidance. The stylet is removed, and a 20-ml syringe is connected to the needle. The needle is moved up and down three to four times through a distance of 0.5 to 1.5 cm while exerting constant suction by hand or with a "pistol grip." In this way, the needle traverses

through a more representative area of cortex, sampling scantily dispersed inflammatory foci. The needle is withdrawn rapidly from the kidney, and 10 to 50 μl of cell suspension is recovered. The needle is flushed immediately with FNAB transport medium composed of 5 ml of RPMI-1640 tissue culture medium containing 5% human serum albumin, 50 IU ml^{-1} heparin and 1% HEPES buffer. Although the cells survive well in this medium and can be kept in a refrigerator overnight, samples ideally are processed immediately. If polymerase chain reaction (PCR) studies are planned, ethylenediaminetetraacetic acid (EDTA) should be used as an anticoagulant (0.1 mM in RPMI-1640) because heparin interferes with PCR. Also, the monocyte component of an aspirated cell population is less likely to adhere to the plastic container in the presence of EDTA. To assess the level of blood contamination of the aspiration specimen, either a blood sample of similar size is drawn from the fingertip into another syringe and diluted in the same medium or 1 ml of anticoagulated peripheral venous blood should be taken to accompany the biopsy specimen.

Duplicate FNAB specimens are processed similarly. Samples are diluted further in medium to give 5×10^5 nucleated cells/ml. Cytocentrifuge preparations are made by spinning 100-μl aliquots onto microscope slides at 800 rpm for 8 minutes. The slides are air-dried and for routine cytological diagnostic purposes are stained using a conventional May-Grunwald-Giemsa procedure or one of the commercially available rapid Romanowsky staining kits. Using the latter approach, it is possible to produce a cytomorphological diagnosis within 30 minutes of the FNAB specimen being taken. Extra cytospin slides may be prepared for immunocytological analysis using monoclonal antibodies for the identification of the different inflammatory cell types or demonstration of activation markers, such as the interleukin-2 (IL-2) receptors and HLA class II antigens. Such slides may be immunolabeled immediately or wrapped in aluminum foil and stored between −20°C and −40°C for future studies.

Representative Aspects of Fine-Needle Aspiration Cytology Samples

For adequate evaluation, the aspiration biopsy specimen must be representative. The cellular infiltrate of acute rejection is always most pronounced in the kidney cortex, and samples should contain enough proximal or distal tubule epithelial cells to be representative. Samples can be assessed by evaluating the proportion of tubule cells to white blood cells. Cytological criteria defining the representative and reproducible basis to FNAC have been established by analyzing duplicate aspirates (von Willebrand and Hayry, 1984) in which a correlation coefficient of 0.95 was obtained in human renal allografts if both specimens contained at least 7 tubule cells/100 leukocytes. When the ratio of tubule cells to leukocytes in either specimen fell below this, the correlation coefficient fell remarkably. Other groups reported similar results for double biopsy analysis (Belitsky et al., 1985; Vereerstraeten et al., 1985b). Too much blood contamination in the biopsy specimen affects markedly the reliability of the results and is the main reason for false-negative findings and day-to-day variations. Using representative samples, FNAB has been shown to have good intraobserver and interobserver reproducibility (Manfro et al., 1995).

Cytomorphological Interpretation of Fine-Needle Aspiration Cytology Preparations

PARENCHYMAL CELLS

In contrast to histological specimens, aspiration biopsy specimens consist mostly of single cells, although clumps of renal tubule cells and whole glomeruli are encountered regularly. The following parenchymal cells can be identified in routine, May-Grünwald-Giemsa–stained, cytological specimens: small (proximal) tubule cells, large (distal) tubule cells, endothelial cells and whole glomeruli or parts of glomeruli (Figs. 26–1A and 26–2). These cells are quite distinct from the erroneously sampled small, deep-staining cuboidal cells of the medullary lower nephron and columnar palisades of the calices. Immunocytological analysis of parenchymal cells is especially useful when there are morphological changes, vacuolation and degeneration in the tubule and endothelial cells. Using relevant monoclonal antibodies, these cells can be identified precisely. Cytokeratin antibodies stain tubule cells and do not stain endothelial cells or macrophages. The URO range of monoclonal reagents permits the precise identification of cells from different regions of the nephron (Cordon-Carlo et al., 1984). Endothelial cells can be stained with antibodies to factor VIII–related antigen, CD62E (E-selectin, ELAM), CD105 (endoglin), CD144 (VE-cadherin) or vimentin antibodies, which do not stain tubule cells.

MORPHOLOGICAL CHANGES IN RENAL PARENCHYMAL CELLS

Characteristic cytological findings in acute tubule necrosis of the kidney transplant are swollen tubule cells with irregular vacuolation and cytoplasmic degeneration (see Figs. 26–1B and 26–2). These changes usually are due to prolonged cold ischemia and become normal as graft function improves. Uncomplicated cases of acute tubular necrosis do not have signs of immunoactivation. Acute tubular necrosis is common in cadaver grafts (Sanfilippo et al., 1984), with approximately 30 to 40% of the grafts showing signs of delayed onset of function during the first week or so after transplantation.

Similar but more pronounced changes appear in the tubule cells in acute cyclosporine nephrotoxicity. Tubule cells are swollen, with prominent isometric or "shotgun" vacuolation of the cell cytoplasm (Egidi et al., 1985a; Hayry and von Willebrand, 1981a, 1981b; Santelli et al., 1985). Typically the isometric vacuolation is perinuclear and seen most often in proximal tubule cells, but distal tubule cells and endothelial cells also may be affected. Cytoplasmic vacuolation as such is a feature of cell degeneration and nonspecific. The prominent isometric vacuolation in cyclosporine toxicity appears to be characteristic of the condition, however, and has been reported in experimental kidney transplantation models (Whiting et al., 1982). Intracellular deposits of cyclosporine and its metabolites can be shown by specific monoclonal antibodies and immunofluorescence techniques (von Willebrand and

Hayry, 1983). After reduction of the cyclosporine dose, the deposits disappear, and the graft function improves. The morphological changes take a longer time to normalize, however. With triple-drug immunosuppression and lower cyclosporine doses, this complication is uncommon.

During acute cellular rejection, without any signs of acute tubular necrosis or cyclosporine toxicity, the graft tubule and endothelial cells usually appear normal in the beginning, but with prolonged rejection, their morphology gradually deteriorates until in irreversible rejection necrotic parenchymal cells appear in the aspirates. In transient, easily reversible rejections, tubule cells retain their normal morphology.

Necrotic changes in the graft parenchymal cells also are seen in graft infarction (e.g., consequent to renal vein thrombosis) when kidney parenchymal cells become degenerate, stain pale and acquire pyknotic nuclei. The only other cells present are macrophages and neutrophils. Frequent monitoring may show a progressive increase in the proportion of necrotic to viable cells as more of the graft becomes necrotic. Occasionally, graft infarction may be only local or polar, and FNAC samples from different regions of the kidney are most useful in providing a clearer picture (Hughes et al., 1992). The information derived from graft parenchymal cell morphology is useful in the differential diagnosis of graft complications, but the interpretation of these changes requires concomitant evaluation of the inflammatory infiltrate and knowledge of the clinical data of the patient (Ahonen, 1984).

INFLAMMATORY CELLS

The following lymphoid inflammatory cell types can be identified adequately (Hayry and von Willebrand, 1981b; von Willebrand, 1980) in the routine May-Grunwald-Giemsa–stained smears: small lymphocytes and activated lymphocytes with increased cytoplasmic basophilia. Lymphoid blast cells (Figs. 26–1C and 26–3A, B) also can be identified by their large size (15–25 μm in diameter), intense cytoplasmic basophilia and pale perinuclear halo. Of the lymphoid blast cells, approximately 50% are B blasts containing intracytoplasmic immunoglobulins as visualized in immunofluorescence staining. T-blast cells are identified more easily with surface markers and immunolabeling. Mature plasma cells are seen occasionally in aspirates during immunoactivation. Large granular lymphocytes (Fig. 26–3C), which are the morphological form of natural killer cells, also may be present (Saksela et al., 1979).

Granulocytes are not recorded in excess over the blood background until late in irreversible rejection when necrotic changes appear in the graft. Basophils are seen rarely. Eosinophils (Fig. 26–3D) are more frequent during the early stages of the immune response to a graft in the aspirates and in the patient's blood, especially when the steroid dose is low (Almirall et al., 1993; Lautenschlager et al., 1985). In the aspirates, eosinophils are often vacuolated, and degranulating forms are seen, which could explain why higher numbers often are seen in the patient's blood. Monocytic cells (Fig. 26–3E) may appear in different forms and sizes—small monocytes with a morphology of normal blood monocytes, large monocytes that often have irregular multilobulated nuclei, early monoblasts and tissue macrophages at different points of maturation. Macrophages (see Figs. 26–1D and 26–3F) are large cells 60 μm in diameter, and the typical forms have prominently vacuolated cytoplasm and a pyknotic elongated nucleus in the cell periphery. Some macrophages may be encountered in the aspirates shortly after transplantation, especially during acute tubular necrosis, when they may contain engulfed cell debris in varying stages of digestion.

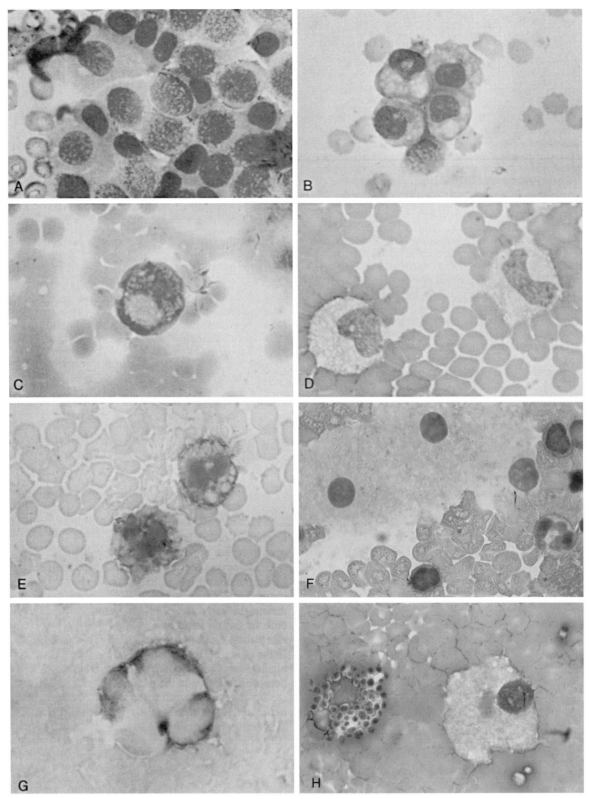

FIGURE 26–1

Cells sampled from human renal allografts using fine-needle aspiration biopsy may include (A) well-preserved tubule epithelial cells associated with good graft function or (B) tubule cells with swollen, vacuolated cytoplasm that are more characteristic of acute tubular necrosis. Typical of cells seen during acute cellular rejection are (C) a lymphoblast with deeply basophilic cytoplasm and a prominent perinuclear halo, (D) macrophages, (E) CD14-labeled macrophages, (F) Fas-ligand–labeled lymphocytes with faintly labeled tubule cells, (G) ICAM-1–labeled tubule cells and (H) kidney tubule cells in a fine-needle aspiration biopsy sample taken in a case of early fungal pyelonephritis at 7 days posttransplantation; one cell is laden with *Candida glabrata*. (A–D and H, May-Grünwald-Giemsa stain; E–G, alkaline phosphatase anti–alkaline phosphatase monoclonal antibody labeling. Magnification × 800.) (See color plate.)

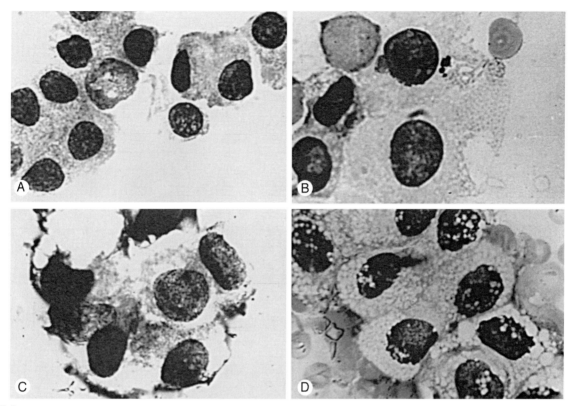

FIGURE 26–2

Parenchymal cells in fine-needle aspirates. (A) A group of normal tubule cells. (B) Endothelial cells (in the middle) with normal morphology and tubule cells (to the left). (C) Swelling and vacuolization in tubule cells in acute tubular necrosis. (D) Tubule cells with swelling and strong isometric vacuolization in the cytoplasm.

Usually, numerous macrophages are seen in severe, prolonged and irreversible rejections.

Thrombocytes may be part of the allograft rejection picture (Leithner et al., 1980; Smith et al., 1979). Small solitary thrombocytes are difficult to visualize in ordinary May-Grünwald-Giemsa staining, but aggregates are seen easily. Thrombocytes can be identified more accurately by specific immunolabeling (von Willebrand et al., 1985). The thrombocyte aggregates seen in FNAB specimens during rejection are mostly loose aggregates, often with granulocytes, and they disappear from the graft during successful rejection treatment. Aggregation of thrombocytes on graft endothelial cells occurs primarily in severe, irreversible rejections.

Quantitation of Inflammation

Fine-needle aspirates of renal transplants are always contaminated with various amounts of blood. Evaluation of inflammation is done by comparing the aspirate cell differential with the blood leukocyte differential using an incremental scoring method: White blood cell differential counts are performed on FNAC and blood specimens, and the blood values are subtracted from biopsy values to obtain the increment of inflammatory cells (Fig. 26–4). The number of parenchymal cells/100 leukocytes is recorded in the same microscopic fields with a separate counter to ensure sample adequacy.

All inflammatory cells in allograft rejection do not have equal diagnostic significance. When comparing experimental rat renal allografts with autografts, the cell types most characteristic of the allograft inflammatory infiltrate are the different types of blast cells and tissue macrophages (von Willebrand et al., 1979). The lymphoid blast cells are most

prominent in the early stages of acute cellular rejection (ACR), whereas macrophages are commoner in advanced and irreversible rejection. Consequently, in calculating a corrected increment, these cells have been assigned a full correction factor of ×1.0 (Hayry and von Willebrand, 1981a, 1981b). The correction factors for all inflammatory cells are given in Figure 26–4. The sum of the corrected increment values (i.e., the total corrected increment) describes the intensity of inflammation in the graft. The total number of blast cells/cytopreparation also is counted, which gives a good picture of overall inflammatory reaction. In a stable graft, no blast cells are seen, but during immunoactivation, the number of blast cells may rise to 50 cells/cytopreparation. The total corrected incremental scoring (TCIS) method makes it possible to describe the fine-needle aspirate cell findings by single numerical values instead of using detailed morphological description, although such a description is important, too. Despite the arbitrary element to the TCIS method, the system performs well in routine use and has become generally accepted, although it is probable that the increment structure will be refined in time (Jorgensen et al., 1989). The range of incremental scores encountered in practice may be grouped into a more easily interpreted set of grades: grade 5, high probability of no rejection (TCIS 0–0.5); grade 4, moderate probability of no rejection (TCIS 0.5–2.5); grade 3, borderline zone (TCIS 2.5–3.5); grade 2, moderate probability of rejection (TCIS >3.5 with no lymphoblasts) and grade 1, high probability of rejection (TCIS >3.5 with lymphoblasts) (Hughes, 1993). Such a grading system not only simplifies diagnostic reporting (see Fig. 26–4) but also facilitates the comparison of FNAC results with other graded modalities, such as the needle core biopsy (NCB), and clinical indications of rejection (Gray et al., 1992).

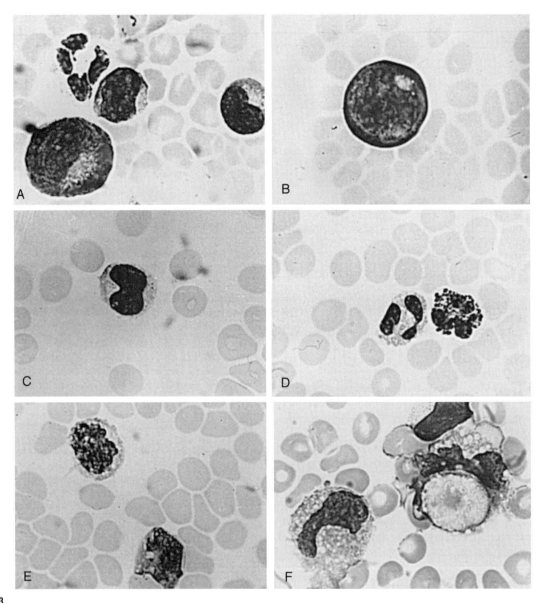

FIGURE 26–3

Inflammatory cells in fine-needle aspirates during rejection. (A) A blast cell with intense cytoplasmic basophilia and perinuclear halo; two activated lymphocytes. (B) A blast cell with less prominent perinuclear halo. (C) A large granular lymphocyte with azurophilic granulation in the cytoplasm. (D) An eosinophil and a basophil. (E) Monocytes with normal morphology. (F) Macrophages with vacuolization and inclusions in the cytoplasm.

FINE-NEEDLE ASPIRATION CYTOLOGY SCORE SHEET

OXFORD TRANSPLANT CENTRE

<u>Patient: xx</u>   <u>Date:</u>   <u>x/x/99</u>   <u>Days Post-Tx: 8</u>

<u>Case: yy[1] / 99</u>   <u>Clinical Details:</u>   <u>Tenderness over graft; rise in serum creatinine</u>

	FNAB	Blood	FNAB-Blood	Correction Factor	TOTAL
Lymphoblasts	5	0	5	x 1.0	5.0
Activated lymphocytes	6	0	6	x 0.5	3.0
Large granular lymphocyte	1	0	1	x 0.2	0.2
Small, inactive lymphocytes	28	11	17	x 0.1	1.7
Metamyelocytes	3	3	0	x 0.1	0
Neutrophils	25	72	-	x 0.1	-
Eosinophils	8	4	4	x 0.1	0.4
Basophils	0	0	0	x 0.1	0
Monocytes	18	10	8	x 0.2	1.6
Macrophages/Monoblasts	6	0	6	x 1.0	6.0
Parenchymal cells per 100 FNAB leucocytes	64			Total Corrected Incremental Score (TCIS):	17.9
				GRADE:	1

COMMENTS: Poorly preserved renal tubule cells. Blastogenic rejection picture.

FIGURE 26–4

Fine-needle aspiration cytology (FNAC) report. Example from a patient with strong acute rejection. For details, see text.

When the rejection grades for 1,270 FNAB samples taken during routine graft monitoring at the Oxford Transplant Centre were compared with corresponding similarly graded clinical indications of rejection, greater than 50% of adequate samples were in complete agreement with the clinical grading (Fig. 26–5). A further 31% of samples disagreed with the clinical diagnosis by only one grade, half of these overdiagnosing and half underdiagnosing rejection. A disagreement between the FNAC and clinical diagnoses of two or more grades was seen in 17% of samples, with a tendency for the cytology to overdiagnose rejection; only three samples disagreed totally with the clinical grading. Fine-needle aspiration biopsy samples were inadequate in 16% of the cases. When a likelihood ratio analysis is performed to examine the power of different TCIS grades to revise the pretest probability of rejection (Fig. 26–6), incremental scores less than 3.0 showed a strong ability to predict the absence of rejection; conversely, scores greater than 3.5 strongly predicted rejection. This finding supports the use of a TCIS cutoff for rejection of approximately 3.0. When the likelihood ratio is plotted against a range of TCIS cutoff points, values less than 5.0 are more powerful for diagnosing rejection than higher values, which reflects a false-positive effect exerted by the nonspecific presence of monocytes and macrophages in high scores (Fig. 26–7).

Monitoring the Graft Using Fine-Needle Aspiration Cytology

CYTOLOGICAL FINDINGS IN ACUTE CELLULAR REJECTION

Sequential follow-up of a renal transplant with frequent aspiration biopsies enables the monitoring of the onset, type, size and duration of the inflammatory episodes of rejection and analysis of the impact of inflammation on graft parenchymal cells. The effect of immunosuppressive treatment on these parameters can be monitored.

Lymphocytes and monocytes are the first inflammatory cells seen in the transplant in most early acute episodes of inflammation. This type of lymphocyte-dominated mild inflammation often disappears without additional rejection treatment and does not cause clinical signs of rejection. The typical cytological hallmark of early acute rejection in the graft is the lymphoid blast response (Table 26–1), which also usually is associated with deteriorating graft function. As

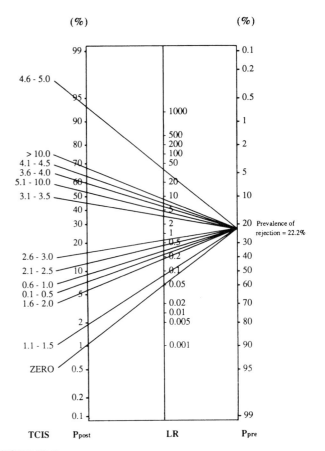

FIGURE 26–6

A bayesian nomogram showing how the likelihood ratio (LR) method of data analysis may be used to investigate the power of different total corrected incremental scoring (TCIS) cutoff levels to confirm the presence or absence of cellular rejection. The nomogram is derived from the results of 1,270 fine-needle aspiration biopsy samples taken during the routine monitoring of 368 cadaveric renal transplants maintained on conventional triple-therapy immunosuppression at the Oxford Transplant Centre. The pretest probability (P_Pre) of rejection, based on clinical evidence available at the time of sampling, was 22.2%. Following an established procedure (Radack et al., 1986), the likelihood ratios for each TCIS cutoff group were calculated from the levels of agreement between the TCIS scores and the subsequent retrospective clinical diagnosis and are plotted against the nomogram to give the posttest (P_Post) probability of rejection. Total corrected incremental scoring values less than 3.0 showed a strong ability to revise correctly the pretest probability of rejection to a diagnosis of no rejection. Samples containing lymphoblasts, particularly those within the TCIS range 4.5 to 5.0, were the most powerful predictors of rejection. The power of TCIS values greater than 5.0 to predict rejection was weakened in general by a high nonspecific macrophage presence. Such a nomogram may be used to great effect in clinical practice for interpreting the significance of different TCIS results.

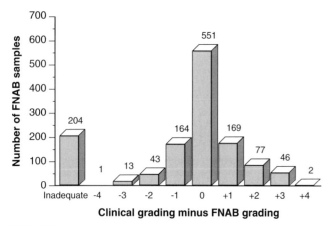

FIGURE 26–5

Graph shows the measure of agreement between fine-needle aspiration biopsy and clinical gradings of acute rejection for 1,270 samples.

immunosuppressive medication is increased, the inflammatory cells disappear from the graft, and the graft function improves. In advanced severe rejections, mononuclear phagocytes dominate the cell infiltrate, macrophage accumulation usually being the hallmark of irreversible rejection (see Table 26–1). In most cases of early ACR, the inflammation follows the cytological pattern just described. In individual patients, however, different inflammatory profiles can be seen (Fig. 26–8. Occasionally, only a short peak is observed with minimal clinical signs; occasionally, inflammation may persist for days or weeks. Sometimes multiple peaks with fre-

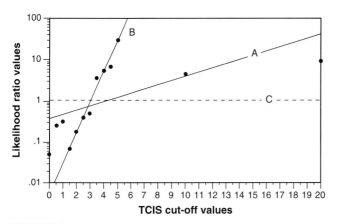

FIGURE 26–7

Graphic comparison of total corrected incremental scoring (TCIS) values and their corresponding likelihood ratios (data taken from Fig. 26–6). (A) A plot of the entire TCIS range of 0 to 20. (B) A more restricted TCIS range of 1.5 to 5.0, in which the graph is much steeper, showing a stronger ability within this region to revise the probability of rejection. (C) The likelihood ratio of 1.0, the level below which rejection is indicated by fine-needle aspiration biopsy to be less probable (TCIS = 3.0) and above which rejection is more probable (TCIS = 3.5).

quent exacerbations and remissions are observed. In some cases, the) inflammation mounts slowly and precedes the appearance of clinical signs by 1 to 2 days, whereas in others, an intense inflammatory response appears rapidly.

The immunosuppressive protocol influences the cytological pattern of rejection. With older immunosuppressive protocols consisting of azathioprine and low-dose steroids, acute rejections were early and intense with strong blast response (Hayry and von Willebrand, 1984; Hayry et al., 1982). With the advent of cyclosporine in immunosuppression, rejection profiles changed remarkably: The onset of rejection was delayed, and the intensity was reduced (Egidi et al., 1985b; Hayry et al., 1983). The institution of triple-drug treatment with cyclosporine, azathioprine and steroids delayed and reduced the inflammatory episodes of rejection more. In Helsinki, with this combined treatment, only approximately 30% of cadaver kidney grafts displayed any immunoactivation during the first postoperative month compared with 70% under older treatment modalities (Hayry et al., 1988; Isoniemi et al., 1990).

CYTOLOGICAL FINDINGS IN ACUTE VASCULAR REJECTION

Diagnosis of acute vascular rejection (AVR) always is based on histology. Earlier studies suggested that mononu-

TABLE 26–1

TYPICAL INFLAMMATORY CELL PICTURES IN FINE-NEEDLE ASPIRATION BIOPSY SPECIMENS DURING DIFFERENT STAGES OF AN ACUTE CELLULAR REJECTION EPISODE

Cell Type	Early Rejection (%)	Late Rejection (%)
Blast cells	5	0
Activated lymphocytes	7	1
Lymphocytes	57	17
Monocytes	9	21
Macrophages	0	6
Granulocytes	22	55

clear phagocyte–dominated inflammation is seen more often in cytological specimens in AVR than in ACR (Cooksey et al., 1985; Reeve et al., 1986; von Willebrand et al., 1983).

In analyses of 30 consecutive kidney transplants, with histologically verified AVR, cytological findings characteristic of AVR in FNAC specimens were evaluated (Salmela et al., 1992; von Willebrand et al., 1992a, 1992b). In transplants with a combination of AVR and ACR, the inflammatory infiltrate consisted of lymphocytes, mononuclear phagocytes and lymphoid blast cells. In reversible AVR, the intensified immunosuppressive treatment cleared away the inflammation, but in irreversible AVR, the inflammation continued with a macrophage-dominated pattern along with a continuing blast response. When histological evidence in acute rejection showed only a vascular component, the inflammation consisted of lymphocytes and especially mononuclear phagocytes, and no blast response could be detected. In irreversible AVR, the inflammation continued with a macrophage-dominated pattern despite the intensified treatment. These findings suggest a central role for mononuclear phagocytes in AVR in which lymphoid blast cells and lymphocytic infiltrates are not a prominent feature.

Immunocytological Analysis of Fine-Needle Aspiration Cytology Preparations

Further information on the intragraft events may be obtained by using monoclonal antibodies and immunocytological methods on the specimens. The immunoperoxidase technique allows differentiation of the infiltrating cells in the graft, different T-lymphocyte subsets, B lymphocytes, mononuclear phagocytes and parenchymal cells (Bolton et al., 1984; Wood et al., 1982). Immunogold-silver staining with Romanowsky counterstaining enables the simultaneous immunocytological and morphological study of aspirated cells (Hughes et al., 1988a). The alkaline phosphatase anti–alkaline phosphatase method, initially introduced for working with hematological preparations, is highly reliable with FNAC cytopreparations. Immunolabeling and flow cytometry have been applied to FNAB samples to study lymphocyte phenotype and activation status (Oliveira et al., 1997a).

In most episodes of ACR, the CD8 T cells dominate the CD4 cells in the graft (Table 26–2), although at the beginning of the rejection episode the CD4 T cells seem to be frequent (Vereerstraeten et al., 1985a; von Willebrand, 1983; Waugh et al., 1985). A persistence of CD4 dominance in the graft has been connected with severe or irreversible rejection (Lautenschlager et al., 1986). The amount of CD2$^+$ or CD3$^+$ T lymphocytes in the graft usually is smaller than the sum of the CD8 and CD4 cells. A few lymphocytes express CD8 and CD4 antigens. B lymphocytes expressing surface immunoglobulins usually are not numerous during rejection (around 5–20% of the lymphocytes), but of the lymphoid blast cells the proportion of B-blast cells usually is approximately 50%, the rest being T-blast cells. B-blast cells can be identified by immunofluorescence staining of the intracytoplasmic immunoglobulins (von Willebrand, 1985). Different forms of mononuclear phagocytes can be stained and identified with CD14 monoclonal antibodies (see Fig. 26–1E). CD14 immunolabeling has been used to show the ubiquitous macrophage activity occurring in early renal allografts in relation to IL-10 gene expression (McLean et al., 1997) and IL-1 receptor antagonist (IL-1ra) up-regulation (Oliveira et al., 1997b). The CD68 antibodies also may be useful, although some reactivity with tubule cells occurs as well. T-lymphocyte phenotypic subpopulations in the graft vary, however, during different phases of rejection and during viral infections and

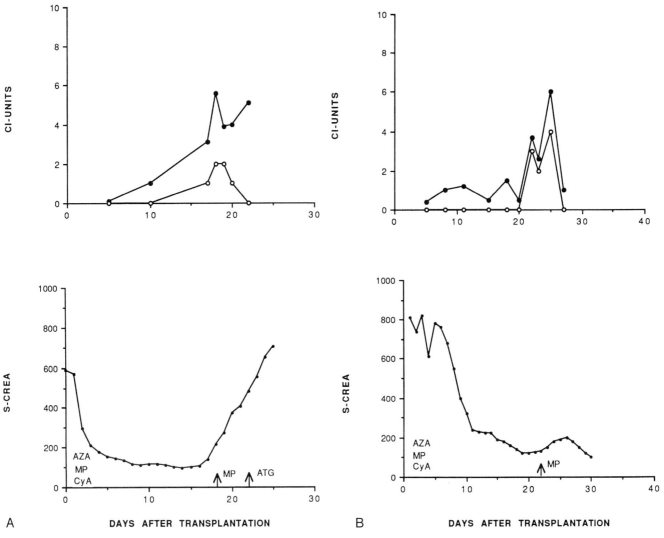

FIGURE 26–8

Correlation of fine-needle aspiration findings (CI = units) with patient's clinical course after transplantation. (S-Creat = serum creatinine level). Closed circles = total corrected increment; open circles = blast cells in corrected increment (CI) units; arrows = rejection treatment. (A) Strong irreversible rejection in a patient receiving triple-drug treatment, azathioprine (AZA), methylprednisolone (MP) and cyclosporine (CyA). Rejection was treated first with MP, then with antithymocyte globulin (ATG) with no response. A necrotic graft was removed 25 days after transplantation. (B) A reversible moderate rejection in a graft with delayed function. Rejection was treated with MP with good response. Basic immunosuppression was achieved with triple-drug treatment.

TABLE 26–2

IMMUNOLABELING CHARACTERISTICS OF LYMPHOID CELLS DURING ACUTE REJECTION AS SEEN USING FINE-NEEDLE ASPIRATION CYTOLOGY

Predominant Reactivity	Cluster Designation	%
T lymphocytes	CD3	40–60
T-helper inducer	CD4	10–30
T-suppressor killer	CD8	30–50
Natural killer cells	CD57	up to 30
B lymphocytes	CD19	5–20
HLA-DR–positive lymphocytes		10–30
Interleukin-2 receptor–positive lymphocytes	α-chain—CD25; β-chain—CD122	5–25
Activation inducer molecule–positive lymphocytes	CD69	up to 15
Perforin-positive lymphocytes		up to 70
Granzyme B–positive lymphocytes		up to 40
Fas-ligand–positive lymphocytes	CD95L	up to 40

as such cannot be used as diagnostic findings. Quantitative analysis of the different inflammatory subsets gives important additional information about the graft.

ACTIVATION MARKERS IN ACUTE CELLULAR REJECTION

Analysis of activation markers of the graft inflammatory cells and parenchymal cells gives important additional information of the graft state, whether there is immunoactivation in the graft or not (Ribeiro *et al.*, 1998). Because of the transitory nature of activation molecule expression, the facility to perform frequent regular biopsies in following these markers is a powerful aspect of the FNAC procedure. The association between tubule cell class II induction and renal allograft rejection has been confirmed in several studies (Almirall *et*

al., 1992b; Fuggle *et al.*, 1986; Hall *et al.*, 1984; Hayry *et al.*, 1981a, 1981b; see Chapter 25). After steroid treatment for rejection, class II expression may diminish rapidly in reversible rejections (Hayry and von Willebrand, 1986), but this is not always observed (Fuggle *et al.*, 1986). The induction of IL-2 receptors (CD25) on activated lymphoid cells in the graft inflammatory infiltrate has been shown during ACR, when it closely followed the pattern of blastogenic inflammation (Hancock *et al.*, 1985; von Willebrand and Hayry, 1987; Fig. 26–9A, B). Cell proliferation markers such as Ki-67 also may be used to identify lymphocyte activation (Almirall *et al.*, 1992c). The expression of CD25 on lymphocytes may be preceded by the more transient appearance of the activation-inducer molecule (CD69) (McLean *et al.*, 1997). With successful rejection treatment, the blast cells and the IL-2-receptor–positive cells disappear rapidly. Studies have shown that

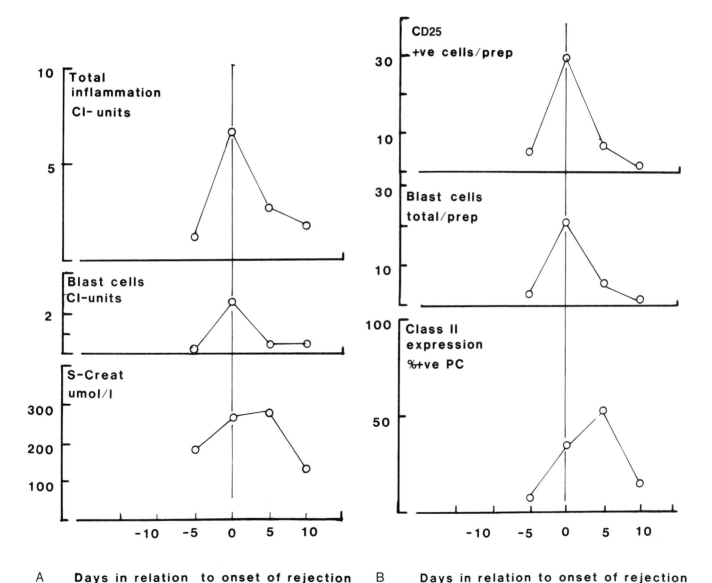

A   **Days in relation to onset of rejection**   B   **Days in relation to onset of rejection**

FIGURE 26–9

Correlation of (A) total inflammation and blast response in the graft with expression of (B) activation markers (class II expression on parenchymal cells and interleukin-2 receptors on lymphoid cells) during rejection. The total inflammation and blast cells are expressed in corrected increment (CI) units in (A). S-Creat = serum creatinine. (B) Interleukin-2 receptor (CD25)–expressing lymphoid cells (blast cells and activated lymphocytes) and blast cells are expressed as the total number of positive cells in the preparation, and the parenchymal cells expressing HLA class II antigens are expressed as the percentage of positive parenchymal cells in the preparation.

combined immunolabeling of aspirated cell populations using monoclonal antibodies to the cytotoxic T-lymphocyte activation markers perforin, granzyme B and Fas-ligand increases significantly the accuracy of FNAB reporting compared with TCIS scoring alone (Pascoe et al., 2000; see Fig. 26–1F).

ACTIVATION MARKERS IN ACUTE VASCULAR REJECTION

The induction of the activation markers, class II expression on the tubule cells and IL-2-receptor expression on activated lymphoid cells, is well established in ACR, but little is known about induction of activation markers in AVR. To elucidate, the expression of class II antigens on the graft tubule cells and the IL-2-receptor expression on the lymphoid cells were analyzed in a study in which serial aspiration biopsy specimens were taken from 30 consecutive transplants with AVR (von Willebrand et al., 1992a, 1992b). Based on histology, two main groups were seen: Eleven grafts had features of AVR only, and 19 grafts had a combination of AVR and ACR. In this latter group of grafts, the AVR findings were predominant. In the grafts with a combination of AVR and ACR, clear induction of class II antigens and IL-2 receptors was seen, similar to that in ACR. The induction continued along with the ongoing inflammation in the irreversible rejections but returned to normal in the reversible rejections. Instead, no class II and IL-2-receptor induction could be observed in the grafts with pure AVR and irreversible rejection, and there were no blast cells in the rejection infiltrate. This pattern, shown by immunocytology, suggests that AVR is a heterogeneous group of rejection patterns. Humoral mechanisms might be involved in AVR.

EXPRESSION OF ADHESION MOLECULES IN ACUTE CELLULAR REJECTION

The expression of different adhesion molecules on the graft endothelial and tubule cells can be assessed from FNAC cytopreparations with immunoperoxidase staining and monoclonal antibodies. Normal kidneys and stable grafts express constitutively several adhesion molecules on the endothelial cells of intertubular capillaries, arteries and veins, for instance, intercellular adhesion molecule (ICAM-1) and vascular cell adhesion molecule (VCAM-1) as described in Chapter 25. Normally, tubule cells do not express these molecules or only in small amounts on the luminal surfaces, but during rejection, induction of ICAM-1 has been shown on tubule cells in histological biopsy specimens (Bishop and Hall, 1989). In a study with serial aspiration biopsy specimens (von Willebrand et al., 1992a, 1992b), induction of ICAM-1 on the graft tubule cells was shown in all of 10 grafts with reversible ACR episodes (see Fig. 26–1G). The ICAM-1 induction occurred early during rejection and disappeared rapidly when rejection subsided. The 10 control grafts with no rejection displayed no ICAM-1 induction on tubule cells. A relationship also has been shown between ICAM-1 and class II expression in ACR of human kidney allografts (von Willebrand et al., 1993). The role of different adhesion molecules in kidney graft rejection currently is being studied extensively. A combined cytochemical and immunocytochemical study of daily, sequential FNAB preparations has shown that there is an early increase in oxygen free radical activity in kidney tubule and endothelial cells that is apparent in postrevascularization samples but peaks by day 1. This increase is accompanied by an increase in the number of cells expressing P-selectin (peaking by day 5) and is followed by increases in free radical scavenging enzyme activation

(identified using monoclonal antibodies to superoxide dismutase and glutathione peroxidase) and a monocyte influx into the graft (identified using a monoclonal antibody to CD14) (Hughes et al., 1995).

Correlations with Renal Transplant Histology

The best way to evaluate events in a transplanted kidney is to sample the graft itself, and the most frequently used method is the classic NCB. The NCB gives an excellent "snapshot" of the situation at the biopsy site and usually is representative of the whole transplant. It is not used often for repeated monitoring of the events in the graft because of possible bleeding complications. In early studies, the diagnostic value of FNAC was evaluated by correlating FNAC findings with the clinical course of rejection and with the response to treatment (Hayry and von Willebrand, 1981a, 1981b; von Willebrand, 1980). The cytological findings also were correlated with the histology of the rejected grafts and with the cytological composition of the inflammatory infiltrate after enzymatic disaggregation of the rejected transplants (Hayry and von Willebrand, 1981b). Since then, several groups of investigators have reported a high concordance of simultaneous FNAC and NCB findings in different clinical situations but particularly in acute cellular blastogenic rejection, acute tubular necrosis and acute cyclosporine toxicity and especially when the graft situation was stable (Dendorfer et al., 1985; De Vecchi et al., 1984; Droz et al., 1984; Egidi et al., 1985a, 1985b; Koller et al., 1984; Sobh et al., 1987). A relationship exists between the severity (mild, moderate or severe) of acute rejection in NCB and the level of inflammation in FNAC (Hughes et al., 1988c). There was no difference in the FNAC scores, however, when NCB showed mild acute or chronic rejection.

The FNAC and histology findings have been compared in the monitoring of ACR in a study with dog renal allografts (Belitsky et al., 1985; Gupta et al., 1985) in which a high concordance was shown between serial FNAC and NCB specimens over the entire course of rejection. Later, diagnostic sensitivity and specificity of greater than 90% were reported (Helderman et al., 1988) in a prospective study that included serial FNAC and NCB specimens from 21 patients. A blind study was performed, comparing 200 consecutive NCB and FNAC specimens taken from 200 kidney transplants (Reinholt et al., 1990) in which high sensitivity and specificity were found in ACR (81% and 92%) and in stable kidney grafts (78% and 82%). A prospective, randomized, blind comparison of FNAC and NCB employing a clinical and biochemical diagnosis of rejection as the gold standard was performed at Oxford (Gray et al., 1992). A total of 219 FNAC and NCB specimens (processed for conventional histology and for immunohistology) were taken from 50 patients. The FNAC, conventional NCB and immuno-NCB showed sensitivities of 59%, 75% and 77% and specificities of 96%, 87% and 80%. In this analysis, the FNAC had an increased tendency to miss clinically important rejection but, especially with its significantly superior adequacy rate, proved most reliable for routine monitoring of stable or nonfunctioning grafts. Immunocytological analysis of FNAC and simultaneous NCB also revealed a close correlation in the phenotypic frequency of different inflammatory cell subsets (Bolton et al., 1983). Reports comparing cytology with histology (Cooksey et al., 1984; Reeve et al., 1986; von Willebrand et al., 1983, 1992a, 1992b) have shown that the cytological pattern of AVR in aspiration cytology is lymphocyte-dominated and mononuclear phagocyte–dominated inflammation without a clear blastogenic response. For a diagnosis of AVR, histology always is needed.

TABLE 26-3

CORRELATION BETWEEN FINE-NEEDLE ASPIRATION BIOPSY CYTOLOGY AND HISTOLOGY

Histology	Fine-Needle Aspirate Cytology (%)								
	BL	ActL	LGL	SL	Mo	MØ	TCIS	Total Blasts	RTMS
Normal graft	0	0.3	1	11	7	0	1.2	0	1.3
Acute cellular rejection	1.5	1.7	2.3	21	11	0	6.3	13	1.8
Acute vascular rejection	0.4	1	2	18	12	2.1	5.5	3	2.1
Chronic rejection	0.1	1	3.1	20	9	1.1	4.3	1	2.3
Acute cyclosporine toxicity	0	0.3	3.1	19	9	0	2	0.3	2.2
Graft infarction	0	0	0	0	8	3	3.8	0	4.0

BL = blast cells; ActL = activated lymphocytes; LGL = large granular lymphocytes; SL = small lymphocytes; Mo = monocytes; MØ = macrophages; TCIS = total corrected increment score; Total Blasts = total number of blast cells/cytopreparation; RTMS = graft renal tubule cell morphology score (1 = normal, 4 = necrosis).

The correlation between histological diagnosis and cytological findings is presented in Table 26–3 (von Willebrand, 1989). In normal grafts with good function, the cytological findings also were normal, the TCIS values were low (0–3) with no blast cells and the tubule cell morphology score (RTMS) was normal. In ACR, total corrected increment was high (4–15) with blast cells and lymphocytic infiltration and activation. In AVR, the cell infiltrate was dominated by mononuclear phagocytes with only a few blast cells and tubule cells showing degeneration. In chronic rejection, there was a lymphocytic-monocytic–dominated inflammation with no blast cells and degenerative changes in the parenchymal cells. Typical of cytology in acute cyclosporine toxicity was morphological alterations in the tubule cells, mostly swelling, degeneration and isometric vacuolation but no inflammation in the graft and no blast cells.

Aspiration Cytology in the Differential Diagnosis of Early Renal Transplant Failure

In the differential diagnosis of early renal transplant failure, the following intragraft disorders may be diagnosed by the FNAC: immunoactivation (ACR), acute tubular necrosis and acute cyclosporine nephrotoxicity. On most occasions, acute rejection is diagnosed easily when the renal transplant has good initial function. If the transplant is not functioning initially because of acute tubular necrosis, the clinical diagnosis of rejection is more difficult. In these cases, frequent aspiration biopsies make it possible to evaluate the onset of rejection and to treat it according to FNAC findings. Distinct tubule cell changes with isometric vacuolation and deposits of cyclosporine are compatible with acute cyclosporine nephrotoxicity. Such alterations are sometimes seen together with blastogenic inflammation, indicating combined rejection and cyclosporine nephrotoxicity. The diagnostic value of FNAC in early and late transplant complications is presented in Table 26–4.

Cytological Detection of Bacterial, Fungal and Viral Infections

Although FNAC has found primary importance in monitoring for rejection, useful applications also have been described in the identification of the bacterial infection of the graft, which sometimes complicates the diagnosis of rejection (Surachno et al., 1986). Fine-needle aspiration cytology has been used to provide direct evidence of previously unsus-

pected renal allograft infection with *Candida albicans* at day 19 posttransplant (Palmer et al., 1989) and with a fluconazole-resistant *Candida glabrata* at day 4 (Hughes et al., 1999). In addition to extracellular organisms, macrophages and tubule cells (see Fig. 26–1H) may be seen laden with fungal bodies.

Viral infections, especially cytomegalovirus infection, often cause differential diagnostic problems in transplant patients. Clinical cytomegalovirus infection seems to induce a general immunoactivation in the patient; lymphoid blast cells, activated lymphocytes and large granular lymphocytes are found in blood and in the fine-needle aspirate (Nast et al., 1991; Nguyen et al., 1985; Tufveson et al., 1985; von Willebrand et al., 1989). Some patients also develop acute rejection during cytomegalovirus infection (Ouziala et al., 1985; von Willebrand et al., 1986). Induction of class II antigens on graft tubule cells has been shown during cytomegalovirus infection (von Willebrand et al., 1989), but the interrelationship between virus infection, up-regulation of graft class II antigens and rejection remains unclear. Patients with frequent rejections have more cytomegalovirus infections, which undoubtedly is related, in part, to increased immunosuppression. Developments in cytomegalovirus diagnostic procedures, especially the new rapid immunocytological staining methods (Ho et al., 1998; Van der Bij et al., 1988), hybridization and PCR techniques, have been helpful in this differential diagnostic problem.

TABLE 26-4

DIAGNOSTIC ABILITY OF FINE-NEEDLE ASPIRATION BIOPSY IN RENAL TRANSPLANTATION

Good
Acute cellular rejection
Acute tubular necrosis
Acute cyclosporine toxicity
Infarction of the graft
Normal graft

Possible
Acute vascular rejection
Lymphocele, hematoma
Bacterial or fungal infection in the graft
Viral infection, cytomegalovirus (immunocytochemistry)

Not Satisfactory
Chronic rejection
Chronic cyclosporine toxicity
Recurrence of the original disease

Value of Functional Studies and Sequential Monitoring Using Fine-Needle Aspiration Cytology

In the past, NCB has been used to obtain tissue from the graft to study cellular and molecular activity. It is inadvisable on safety grounds alone, however, to obtain NCB specimens on a regular basis. Immune activity within the renal allograft is a dynamic process, and changes in the molecular activity are best followed on at least a daily basis. Applications have already been mentioned for FNAC in immunocytochemical studies. Functional studies also have been made of aspirated cells in culture (Horsburgh *et al.*, 1988). A pilot study at Oxford (Dallman *et al.*, 1992) showed that, using PCR, it is possible to detect and monitor changes in IL-2 gene expression in daily FNAC samples. Such expression often precedes clinical, biochemical and sometimes cytomorphological evidence of rejection. Interleukin-2 gene expression may fluctuate during antirejection therapy even though cytological examination suggests continuing rejection. γ-Interferon gene expression in FNAB samples also has been shown to be predictive of cellular rejection (Nast, 1995; Nast *et al.*, 1994).

A PCR study of daily FNAB samples taken for the first 10 days after transplantation showed that, during the first 4 days, all grafts developed a low-grade, monocyte-rich mononuclear cell infiltrate, accompanied by IL-10 expression (McLean *et al.*, 1997). Rejecting and nonrejecting dense infiltrates were associated with a biphasic pattern of IL-2 and γ-interferon gene expression, preceding and accompanying graft infiltration. Grafts that did not develop dense infiltrates had no detectable IL-2 or γ-interferon gene expression and did not develop cellular rejection during the study period. The appearance of rejecting and nonrejecting infiltrates was associated strongly with DR mismatches between donor and recipient. Interleukin-2 and γ-interferon gene expression are necessary but not sufficient for the development of ACR and are related most closely to the period leading up to rejection rather than with the period of graft dysfunction.

Cell culture studies using FNAB samples have shown that graft-infiltrating cells have greater IL-2-driven proliferative capacity during rejection (Oliveira *et al.*, 1997c) and that IL-2 synthesis identified from culture supernatants could predict impending acute rejection (Oliveira *et al.*, 1998). Cytokine patterns suggest that acute rejection is associated with Th1 cytokine profiles, stable function with Th0/Th2 and chronic rejection with Th2 patterns rejection (Oliveira *et al.*, 1998).

Conclusions

Fine-needle aspiration cytology is a diagnostic and investigative method developed for continuous monitoring of intragraft events in clinical transplantation. The advantage of FNAC is that it can be performed daily, if necessary, on human renal transplants without risk to the graft or to the patient. Repeated aspiration biopsy specimens give a dynamic picture of the process in the graft and make it possible to assess the onset, type and intensity of inflammatory episodes of rejection; to monitor the concomitant morphological changes in transplant parenchymal cells and to evaluate the effect of changes in patient treatment on these parameters. By applying new immunocytological and molecular biology techniques, the nature of cellular infiltrates and the stage of activation and specificity of different cell types can be characterized in more detail.

The main drawback of the aspiration cytology method is that the information derived from FNAC is in certain respects limited when compared with architectural information provided by NCB. This limitation in many ways is compensated for by the detailed cytomorphological information obtained, particularly in relation to the types of leukocytes present and their levels of activation. Episodes of ACR can be diagnosed with certainty, but AVR and chronic rejections are more difficult to diagnose. Vascular changes in a kidney graft cannot be evaluated without a needle biopsy. In routine practice, the two procedures ideally should be used in combination, with FNAC providing most of the routine monitoring, particularly during initial poor graft function. Needle core biopsy then may be used to confirm positive cytological findings, to clarify equivocal cytological cases and to provide baseline architectural information on graft status. The interpretation of cytological and immunological preparations requires special expertise and preferably should be performed by experienced clinicians, which is analogous to the interpretation of renal transplant histology specimens.

As knowledge of allograft immunity expands, FNAC will continue to provide an important means of studying intragraft events. The most convincing argument for FNAB becoming widely accepted in clinical practice, however, would come from a large prospective randomized trial showing that graft survival is improved by using aspiration biopsy monitoring, but it is unlikely that such data will become available soon (Bogman, 1995). In addition to aspiration biopsy, the examination of cells washed from NCB samples (Hughes *et al.*, 1988b) has been shown to provide useful information on cellular rejection, and urine cytology, although not a substitute for biopsy, has been an underused method for studying intragraft events, particularly in children, in whom a noninvasive, easily repeated indicator of rejection may be helpful (Corey, 1997).

References

Ahonen, J. (1984). Clinical use of FNAC in renal transplantation. In *Renal Transplant Cytology*, (H. Kreis and D. Droz, eds.), p. 31, Wichtig Editore, Milan.

Almirall, J., Campistol, J. M., Sole, M., Andreu, J. and Revert, L. (1993). Blood and graft eosinophilia as a rejection index in kidney transplantation. *Nephron* **65**, 304.

Almirall, J., Sole, M., Campistol, J. M., *et al.* (1992a). Clinical usefulness of conventional fine-needle aspiration cytology in kidney transplantation—influence of different immunosuppressive protocols. *Transplant. Proc.* **1**, 71.

Almirall, J., Sole, M., Campistol, J. M., *et al.* (1992b). HLA-DR expression on tubular cells in kidney transplantation. *Transplant. Proc.* **24**, 69.

Almirall, J., Sole, M., Campistol, J. M., *et al.* (1992c). Lymphocyte activation and proliferation markers in the material obtained by fine-needle aspiration cytology. *Transplant. Proc.* **24**, 67.

Belitsky, P., Campbell, J. and Gupta, R. (1985). Serial biopsy controlled evaluation of fine needle aspiration in renal allograft rejection. *Lab. Invest.* **53**, 580.

Birkeland, S. A., Elbirk, A., Rohr, N. and Jorgensen, K. A. (1994). Analysis of the inflammatory leucocyte mobilization in 838 fine needle aspiration biopsies in non-rejecting (day 1–90) kidney grafts and 465 biopsies in grafts before, during and after acute cellular rejection. *Transpl. Immunol.* **2**, 308.

Bishop, G. A. and Hall, B. M. (1989). Expression of leucocyte and lymphocyte adhesion molecules in the human kidney. *Kidney Int.* **36**, 1078.

Bogman, M. J. J. T. (1995). Fine-needle aspiration biopsy of the renal transplant—is it worthwhile or a waste of time? *Nephrol. Dial. Transplant.* **10**, 2182.

Bolton, E. M., Thompson, J. F., Wood, R. F. and Morris, P. J. (1983). Immunoperoxidase staining of fine needle aspiration biopsies and needle core biopsies from renal allografts. *Transplantation* **36**, 728.

Bolton, E. M., Thompson, J. F., Wood, R. F. M. and Morris, P. J. (1984). Lymphocyte sub-populations in fine needle aspiration biopsies determined by immunoperoxidase staining. In *Renal Transplant*

Cytology, (H. Kreis and D. Droz, eds.), p. 207, Wichtig Editore, Milan.

Burdick, J. F. and Kittur, D. S. (1991). Factors affecting early diagnosis of organ allograft rejection. *Transplant. Proc.* **23**, 2047.

Cooksey, G., Reeve, R. S., Paterson, A. D., Cotton, R. E. and Blamey, R. W. (1985). Lymphocyte sub-populations in cytologic aspirates from human renal allografts. *Transplant. Proc.* **17**, 630.

Cooksey, G., Reeve, R. S., Wenham, P. W., Cotton, R. E. and Blamey, R. W. (1984). Comparison of fine needle aspiration cytology with histology in the diagnosis of renal allograft rejection. *In Renal Transplant Cytology*, (H. Kreis and D. Droz, eds.), p. 73, Wichtig Editore, Milan.

Cordon-Carlo, C., Bander, N. H. and Fradet, Y. (1984). Immunoanatomic dissection of the human urinary tract by monoclonal antibodies. *J. Histochem. Cytochem.* **32**, 1035.

Corey, H. E. (1997). Urine cytology: an underused method to diagnose acute renal allograft rejection. *Pediatr. Nephrol.* **11**, 226.

Dallman, M. J., Roake, J., Hughes, D., Toogood, G. and Morris, P. J. (1992). Sequential analysis of IL-2 gene transcription in renal transplants. *Transplantation* **53**, 683.

Delaney, V., Ling, B. N., Campbell, W. G., et al. (1993). Comparison of fine-needle aspiration biopsy, Doppler ultrasound, and radionuclide scintigraphy in the diagnosis of acute renal allograft dysfunction in renal transplant recipients: sensitivity, specificity, and cost analysis. *Nephron* **63**, 263.

Dendorfer, U., Hammer, C., Schleibner, S., et al. (1985). Comparison of renal transplant cytology with histological findings. *Transplant. Proc.* **17**, 2583.

De Vecchi, A., Egidi, F., Banfi, G., Imabsciati, E., Tarantino, A. and Ponticelli, C. (1984). Comparison of fine needle aspiration biopsy and needle biopsy in renal transplantation. *In Renal Transplant Cytology*, (H. Kreis and D. Droz, eds.), p. 67, Wichtig Editore, Milan.

Droz, D., Campos, H., Noel, L. H., Adafer, E. and Kreis, H. (1984). Renal transplant fine needle aspiration cytology: correlations to renal histology. *In Renal Transplant Cytology*, (H. Kreis and D. Droz, eds.), p. 59, Wichtig Editore, Milan.

Egidi, F., De Vecchi, A., Banfi, G., Tarantino, A., Imbasciati, E. and Ponticelli, C. (1985a). Comparison of renal biopsy and fine needle aspiration biopsy in renal transplantation. *Transplant. Proc.* **17**, 61.

Egidi, F., De Vecchi, A., Pagliari, B., Moriggi, M. and Ponticelli, C. (1985b). Lack of relationship between blood cyclosporine levels and nephrotoxicity as assessed by fine needle aspiration biopsy of renal allografts. *Transplant. Proc.* **17**, 2096.

Franzen, S., Giertz, G. and Zaijcek, J. (1960). Cytological diagnosis of prostatic tumors by transrectal aspiration biopsy. *Br. J. Urol.* **32**, 193.

Fuggle, S. V., McWhinnie, D. L., Chapman, J. R., Taylor, H. M. and Morris, P. J. (1986). Sequential analysis of HLA-Class II antigen expression in human renal allografts: induction of tubule Class II antigens and correlation with clinical parameters. *Transplantation* **42**, 144.

Gouldesborough, D. R., McLigeyo, S. O. and Anderton, J. L. (1992). Renal transplant aspiration cytology: role for simple morphological criteria. *Cytopathology* **3**, 119.

Gray, D. W. R., Richardson, A., Hughes, D., et al. (1992). A prospective, randomized, blind comparison of three biopsy techniques in the management of patients after renal transplantation. *Transplantation* **53**, 1226.

Gupta, R., Campbell, J., Om, A. and Belitsky, P. (1985). Serial monitoring of cellular rejection by simultaneous histology and fine needle aspiration cytology. *Transplant. Proc.* **17**, 2123.

Hall, B. M., Duggin, G. G., Philips, J., Bishop, G. A., Horvarth, J. S. and Tiller, D. J. (1984). Increased expression of HLA-DR antigens on renal tubular cells in renal transplants: relevance to the rejection response. *Lancet* **2**, 247.

Hancock, W. W., Gee, D., De Moerloose, P., Rickles, F. R., Ewan, V. A. and Atkins, R. C. (1985). Immunohistological analysis of serial biopsies taken during human renal allograft rejection: changing profile of infiltrating cells and activation of the coagulation system. *Transplantation* **39**, 430.

Hayry, P., Ahonen, J. and von Willebrand, E. (1983). Effect of cyclosporin A on the in situ inflammatory response of human renal allograft rejection: a preliminary report. *Scand. J. Immunol.* **16**, 135.

Hayry, P. and von Willebrand, E. (1981a). Monitoring of human renal allograft rejection with fine-needle aspiration cytology. *Scand. J. Immunol.* **13**, 87.

Hayry, P. and von Willebrand, E. (1981b). Practical guidelines for fine needle aspiration biopsy of human renal allografts. *Ann. Clin. Res.* **13**, 288.

Hayry, P. and von Willebrand, E. (1984). Transplant aspiration cytology. *Transplantation* **38**, 7.

Hayry, P. and von Willebrand, E. (1986). The influence of the pattern of inflammation and administration of steroids on Class II MHC antigen expression in renal transplants. *Transplantation* **42**, 358.

Hayry, P., von Willebrand, E., Ahonen, J., Eklund, B. and Lautenschlager, I. (1981a). Monitoring of organ allograft rejection by transplant aspiration cytology. *Ann. Clin. Res.* **13**, 264.

Hayry, P., von Willebrand, E., Ahonen, J. and Eklund, B. (1981b). Do well-to-do and repeatedly rejecting renal allografts express the transplantation antigens similarly on their surface? *Scand. J. Urol. Nephrol.* **64(Suppl.)**, 52.

Hayry, P., von Willebrand, E., Ahonen, J. and Eklund, B. (1982). Glucocorticosteroids in renal transplantation: I. impact of high vs. low dose postoperative methyl-prednisolone administration on the first episode(s) of rejection. *Scand. J. Immunol.* **16**, 39.

Hayry, P., von Willebrand, E. and Ahonen, J. (1988). Effects of cyclosporine, azathioprine and steroids on the renal transplant, on the cytological patterns of intra-graft inflammation and on concomitant rejection-associated changes in the recipient blood. *Transplant. Proc.* **20**, 153.

Hayry, P., von Willebrand, E. and Soots, A. (1979). In situ effector mechanisms in rat kidney allograft rejection: III. kinetics of the inflammatory response and generation of donor-directed killer cells. *Scand. J. Immunol.* **10**, 95.

Helderman, J. H., Hernandez, J., Sagalowsky, A., et al. (1988). Confirmation of the utility of fine needle aspiration biopsy of the renal allograft. *Kidney Int.* **34**, 376.

Ho, S. K. N., Lo, C.-Y., Cheng, I. K. P. and Chan, T.-M. (1998). Rapid cytomegalovirus pp65 antigenaemia assay by direct erythrocyte lysis and immunofluorescence staining. *J. Clin. Microbiol.* **36**, 638.

Horsburgh, T., Brown, S., Veitch, P. S. and Bell, P. R. F. (1988). Cell culture of fine-needle aspirates and Tru-Cut biopsies. *Transplant. Proc.* **20**, 679.

Hughes, D. (1993). Fine-needle aspiration biopsy in rejection diagnosis. *In The HLA System in Clinical Transplantation*, (B. G. Solhein, S. Ferrone, and E. Moller, eds.), p. 339, Springer Verlag, Heidelberg.

Hughes, D. A., Davies, D. R., Young, R., et al. (1999). Fine-needle aspiration cytology (FNAC) detection of early renal allograft infection with *Candida glabrata*—a case report. *Cytopathology* **10**, 349.

Hughes, D. A., Kempson, M. G., Carter, N. P. and Morris, P. J. (1988a). Immunogold-silver/Romanowsky staining: simultaneous immunocytochemical and morphologic analysis of fine-needle aspirate biopsies. *Transplant. Proc.* **20**, 575.

Hughes, D. A., McLean, A., Roake, J. A., Gray, D. W. R. and Morris, P. J. (1995). Free oxygen species (FOS), FOS-scavenging enzyme, P-selectin and monocyte activity in cell populations aspirated from early human renal allografts. *Transplant. Proc.* **27**, 2879.

Hughes, D. A., McWhinnie, D. L., Jones, R., et al. (1988b). Evaluation of needle-core biopsy washings for monitoring rejection in human renal allografts. *Transplant. Proc.* **20**, 579.

Hughes, D. A., McWhinnie, D. L., Sutton, R., et al. (1988c). Can incremental scoring of fine-needle aspirates predict histopathologic renal allograft rejection? *Transplant. Proc.* **20**, 690.

Hughes, D. A., Rapoport, J., Roake, J. A., Toogood, G. J., Gray, D. W. R. and Morris, P. J. (1992). Confirmation of renal allograft infarction using fine-needle aspiration cytology. *In Contributions to Transplantation Medicine: Transplant Monitoring*, (A. Yussim and C. Hammer, eds.), Wolfgang Pabst Verlag, Lengerich, Germany.

Isoniemi, H., Ahonen, J. and Eklund, B. (1990). Renal allograft immunosuppression: early inflammatory and rejection episodes in triple drug treatment compared to double drug combinations or cyclosporin monotherapy. *Transpl. Int.* **3**, 92.

Jorgensen, K. A., Strate, M., Svendsen, V., Rohr, N., Elbirk, A. and Birkeland, S. A. (1989). Are FNAB correction factors correct? *Transplant. Proc.* **21**, 3603.

Koller, C., Hammer, C., Gokel, J. M., et al. (1984). Correlation between core biopsy and aspiration cytology. *Transplant. Proc.* **16**, 1298.

Kreis, H. A. (1984). Use of fine needle aspiration cytology to diagnose rejection. *Transplant. Proc.* **16**, 1569.

Lautenschlager, I., von Willebrand, E. and Hayry, P. (1985). Blood eosinophilia, steroids and rejection. *Transplantation* **40**, 354.

Lautenschlager, I., von Willebrand, E. and Hayry, P. (1986). Does T4 predominance in the graft signify severe rejection? *Transplant. Proc.* **18**, 1311.

Leithner, O. H., Sinzinger, H., Angelberger, P. and Syre, P. (1980). Indium-111 labeled platelets in chronic kidney transplant rejection. *Lancet* **2**, 213.

Leone, G., Puliatti, C., Morale, W., Alo, P. L., Di Tondon, U. and Leone, F. (1995). Fine-needle aspiration biopsy (FNAB) in immediate post-operative period of transplant: a valid support to discriminate acute rejection vs acute tubule necrosis. *Clin. Nephrol.* **44**, 139.

Manfro, R. C., Goncalves, L. F. S. and Ribeiro de Moura, L. A. (1995). Reproducibility of fine-needle aspiration biopsy in the diagnosis of acute rejection of renal allografts. *Nephrol. Dial. Transplant.* **10**, 2306.

McLean, A. G., Hughes, D., Welsh, K. I., et al. (1997). Patterns of graft infiltration and cytokine gene expression in the first ten days of kidney transplantation. *Transplantation* **63**, 374.

Nast, C. C. (1995). Renal transplant fine needle aspiration and cytokine gene expression. *Pediatr. Nephrol.* **9(Suppl.)**, S56.

Nast, C. C., Wilkinson, A., Rosenthal, J. T., et al. (1991). Diagnosis of cytomegalovirus infection in renal allografts using fine needle aspiration biopsy. *Transplant. Proc.* **23**, 1354.

Nast, C. C., Zuo, X.-J., Prehn, J., Danovitch, G. M., Wilkinson, A. and Jordan, S. C. (1994). Gamma-interferon gene expression in human renal allograft fine-needle aspirates. *Transplantation* **57**, 498.

Nguyen, L., Hammer, C., Dendorfer, U., Castro, L., Schleibner, C. and Land, W. (1985). Changes in large granular lymphocyte size and number in kidney transplant patients during rejection and viral infection. *Transplant. Proc.* **17**, 2110.

Oliveira, J. G. G., Ramos, J. P., Xavier, P., et al. (1997a). Analysis of fine-needle aspiration biopsies by flow cytometry in kidney transplant patients. *Transplantation* **64**, 97.

Oliveira, J. G. G., Xavier, P., Neto, S., et al. (1997b). Monocytes-macrophages and cytokines/chemokines in fine-needle aspiration biopsy cultures. *Transplantation* **63**, 1751.

Oliveira, G., Xavier, P., Mendes, A. and Guerra, L. E. (1997c). Cultures of aspiration biopsy specimens in the immunological monitoring of renal transplants. *Nephron* **76**, 310.

Oliveira, G., Xavier, P., Murphy, B., et al. (1998). Cytokine analysis of human renal allograft aspiration biopsy cultures supernatants predicts acute rejection. *Nephrol. Dial. Transplant.* **13**, 417.

Ouziala, M., Santelli, G., Charpentier, B. and Fries, D. (1985). Diagnostic value of fine needle aspiration biopsy during viral infections in renal transplant recipients. *Transplant. Proc.* **17**, 2098.

Palmer, B. F., Hernandez, J., Segalowsky, A., Dawidson, I. and Helderman, J. (1989). Documentation of fungal pyelonephritis of the renal allograft by fine-needle aspiration cytology. *Transplant. Proc.* **21**, 3598.

Pascoe, M. D., Marshall, S. E., Welsh, K. I., Fulton, L. M. and Hughes, D. A. (2000). Increased accuracy of renal allograft rejection diagnosis using combined perforin, granzyme B and Fas-ligand fine-needle aspiration immunocytology. *Transplantation* **69**, 2547.

Pasternack, A. (1968). Fine-needle aspiration biopsy of human renal homografts. *Lancet* **2**, 82.

Radack, K. L., Rouan, G. and Hedges, J. (1986). The likelihood ratio: an improved measure for reporting and evaluating diagnostic test results. *Arch. Pathol. Lab. Med.* **110**, 689.

Reeve, R. S., Cooksey, G., Wenham, P. W., et al. (1986). A comparison of fine needle aspiration cytology and Tru-cut tissue biopsy in the diagnosis of acute renal allograft rejection. *Nephron* **42**, 68.

Reinholt, F. P., Bohman, S.-O., Wilczek, H., von Willebrand, E. and Hayry, P. (1990). Fine needle aspiration cytology and conventional histology in 200 renal allografts. *Transplantation* **49**, 910.

Ribeiro, D. D. S., David, N. E., Castro, M. C., et al. (1998). Contribution of the expression of ICAM-1, HLA-DR and IL-2R to the diagnosis of acute rejection in renal allograft aspirative cytology. *Transpl. Int.* **1(Suppl.)**, S19.

Saksela, E., Timonen, T., Ranki, A. and Hayry, P. (1979). Morphological and functional characterization of isolated effector cells responsible for human natural killer cell activity to fetal fibroblasts and to cultured cell line targets. *Immunol. Rev.* **44**, 71.

Salmela, K., von Willebrand, E., Kyllonen, L., et al. (1992). Acute

vascular rejection in renal transplantation: diagnosis and outcome. *Transplantation* **54**, 858.

Sanfilippo, F., Vaughn, W. K., Spees, E. K. and Lucas, B. A. (1984). The detrimental effects of delayed graft function in cadaver donor renal transplantation. *Transplantation* **38**, 643.

Santelli, G., Ouziala, M., Charpentier, B. and Fries, D. (1985). Predictive value of fine needle aspiration biopsy for cyclosporine nephrotoxicity. *Transplant. Proc.* **17**, 2094.

Smith, N., Chandler, S., Hawker, R. J., Hawker, L. M. and Barnes, A. D. (1979). Indium-labelled autologous platelets as diagnostic aid after renal transplantation. *Lancet* **2**, 1241.

Sobh, M. A., Moustaffa, F. E. and Ghonheim, M. A. (1987). Fine-needle aspiration biopsy: a reproducibility study and a correlation with the Tru-cut biopsy evaluation of renal allotransplants. *Nephrol. Dial. Transplant.* **2**, 562.

Surachno, S., van Oers, M. H. J., Kox, C. and Wilmink, J. M. (1987). The relevance of transplant aspiration cytology (TAC) for the clinical management of renal allograft recipients. *Clin. Transplant.* **1**, 290.

Surachno, S., van Oers, M. H. J. and Wilmink, J. M. (1986). Early diagnosis of bacterial infection of renal allografts using fine-needle aspiration biopsy. *Lancet* **1**, 686.

Tufveson, G., Backman, U., Claesson, K., Frodin, L., Stenquist, B. and Wahlberg, J. (1985). Renal transplant cytology: impact of different immunosuppressive protocols and biopsy techniques. *Transplant. Proc.* **17**, 2087.

Ubhi, C. S., Baker, J. M., Guillou, P. J. and Giles, G. R. (1988). Use of fine needle aspirates to monitor the treatment of acute renal allograft rejection. *Clin. Transplant.* **2**, 216.

Van der Bij, W., Toresma, R., van Son, W. J., et al. (1988). Rapid immunodiagnosis of active cytomegalovirus infection by monoclonal antibody staining of blood leucocytes. *J. Med. Virol.* **25**, 179.

Vereerstraeten, P., Romasco, F., Kinnaert, P., Dupont, E., Wybran, J. and Toussaint, C. (1985a). T cell subset patterns in peripheral blood and in fine needle aspiration lymphocytes after kidney transplantation. *Transplant. Proc.* **17**, 2115.

Vereerstraeten, P., Romasco, F. and Monsieur, R. (1985b). Representativeness and reproducibility of WBC counts in fine needle aspiration specimens from kidney transplants. *Transplant. Proc.* **17**, 2106.

von Willebrand, E. (1980). Fine needle aspiration cytology of human renal transplants. *Clin. Immunol. Immunopathol.* **17**, 309.

von Willebrand, E. (1983). OKT 4/8 ratio in the blood and in the graft during episodes of human allograft rejection. *Cell. Immunol.* **77**, 196.

von Willebrand, E. (1985). Fine needle aspiration cytology of renal transplants: background and present applications. *Transplant. Proc.* **17**, 2071.

von Willebrand, E. (1989). Long-term experience with fine needle aspiration in kidney transplant patients. *Transplant. Proc.* **21**, 3568.

von Willebrand, E. and Hayry, P. (1978). Composition and in vitro cytotoxicity of cellular infiltrates in rejecting human kidney allografts. *Cell. Immunol.* **41**, 358.

von Willebrand, E. and Hayry, P. (1983). Cyclosporin A deposits in renal allografts. *Lancet* **2**, 189.

von Willebrand, E. and Hayry, P. (1984). Reproducibility of the fine needle aspiration biopsy: analysis of 93 double biopsies. *Transplantation* **38**, 314.

von Willebrand, E. and Hayry, P. (1987). Relationship between cellular and molecular markers of inflammation in human kidney allograft rejection. *Transplant. Proc.* **19**, 1644.

von Willebrand, E., Lautenschlager, I. and Ahonen J. (1989). Cellular activation in the graft and in the blood during cytomegalovirus disease. *Transplant. Proc.* **21**, 2080.

von Willebrand, E., Loginov, R., Salmela, K., Isoniemi, H. and Hayry, P. (1993). The relationship between ICAM-1 and Class II expression in acute cellular rejection of human kidney allografts. *Transplant. Proc.* **25**, 870.

von Willebrand, E., Pettersson, E., Ahonen, J. and Hayry, P. (1986). CMV infection, Class II antigen expression, and human kidney allograft rejection. *Transplantation* **42**, 364.

von Willebrand, E., Salmela, K., Isoniemi, H., Krogerus, L., Taskinen, E. and Hayry, P. (1992a). Induction of HLA Class II antigen and interleukin 2 receptor expression in acute vascular rejection of human kidney allografts. *Transplantation* **53**, 1077.

von Willebrand, E., Salmela, K., Isoniemi, H., Taskinen, E., Krogerus,

L. and Hayry, P. (1992b). Expression of activation markers, HLA Class II and IL-2R in AVR of human renal allografts. *Transpl. Int.* **5(Suppl. 1)**, 690.

von Willebrand, E., Soots, A. and Hayry, P. (1979). In situ effector mechanisms in rat kidney allograft rejection: I. characterization of the host cellular infiltrate in rejecting allograft parenchyma. *Cell. Immunol.* **46**, 309.

von Willebrand, E., Taskinen, E., Ahonen, J. and Hayry, P. (1983). Recent modifications in the fine needle aspiration biopsy of human renal allografts. *Transplant. Proc.* **15**, 1195.

von Willebrand, E., Zola, H. and Hayry, P. (1985). Thrombocyte aggregates in renal allografts: analysis by the fine needle aspiration biopsy and monoclonal anti-thrombocyte antibodies. *Transplantation* **39**, 258.

Waugh, J., Bishop, G. A., Hall, B., *et al.* (1985). T cell subsets in fine needle aspiration biopsies from renal transplant recipients. *Transplant. Proc.* **17**, 1701.

Whiting, P. H., Thomson, A. W., Blair, J. T. and Simpson, J. G. (1982). Experimental cyclosporin A nephrotoxicity. *Br. J. Pathol.* **63**, 88.

Wood, R. F. M., Bolton, E. M., Thompson, J. F. and Morris, P. J. (1982). Monoclonal antibodies and fine needle aspiration cytology in detecting renal allograft rejection. *Lancet* **2**, 278.

Chronic Renal Transplant Rejection

Leendert C. Paul • Johan W. de Fijter • Yvo W. J. Sijpkens

Introduction

After the early posttransplant months, up to 40% of renal transplants develop slow but progressive graft dysfunction and ultimately fail within a decade, despite the use of immunosuppressive drugs in doses sufficient to prevent acute rejection. This form of graft failure was described first by Porter *et al.* in 1963 and was called *chronic rejection*. Today it is one of the most prevalent causes of end-stage renal disease, accounting for 25 to 30% of patients on renal transplant waiting lists. Because immune and nonimmune factors seem involved in its pathogenesis (Paul, 1995), the term *chronic allograft dysfunction* has been proposed to describe the condition clinically and the term *chronic allograft nephropathy* to describe the histopathology. These terms are used interchangeably with chronic rejection, however.

Magnitude of the Problem

Chronic rejection is the most prevalent cause of graft failure in the initial 10 posttransplant years and occurs in 25% of patients (Schweitzer *et al.*, 1991). In an analysis of 654 renal transplants performed at our center between 1983 and 1996, chronic rejection accounted for 37% of graft losses after the first 6 months (Sijpkens *et al.*, 1999), which is similar to the 25 to 50% graft loss reported in other studies (Cole *et al.*, 1995). It is often stated that the graft half-life, the time period in which 50% of grafts that survived the first year are lost, has remained unchanged since the 1960s. An analysis of the United States Renal Data System material has shown, however, that the median cadaveric graft survival improved from 64.5 months in 1986–1987 to 101.8 months in 1992–1993 (USRDS, 1999), an improvement of 50%.

Manifestations and Differential Diagnosis

Clinically, chronic rejection is characterized by a relatively slow but variable rate of decline in glomerular filtration rate after the initial 3 posttransplant months, often in combination with proteinuria and hypertension (Paul *et al.*, 1993). In more than 80% of patients, there is progressive loss of function as determined by the plot of the reciprocal of the serum creatinine concentration over time (Kasiske *et al.*, 1991; Riggio *et al.*, 1985). The prevalence of proteinuria is variable; 20 to 28% of patients have greater than 0.5 g proteinuria/24 hours compared with 6 to 8% of patients free of chronic rejection (Massy *et al.*, 1996). The diagnostic significance of posttransplant hypertension is limited because of its high prevalence in renal patients (Raine, 1995). None of the clinical manifestations of chronic rejection is specific, and other causes of graft dysfunction, such as acute rejection, chronic drug toxicity, or recurrent glomerulonephritis have to be excluded.

The histopathology of chronic rejection is not specific and consists of atherosclerosis, transplant glomerulopathy and glomerulosclerosis, multilayering of the peritubular capillary basement membranes, interstitial fibrosis and tubular atrophy (Fig. 27–1). These findings often are accompanied by variable degrees of infiltration with macrophages and lymphocytes. Graft atherosclerosis consists of mostly concentric intimal thickening of large parts of the arteries and arterioles. The intimal thickening is thought to result from the migration of myofibroblasts from the media into the intima, their local proliferation and the deposition of extracellular matrix proteins. The intimal thickening, as assessed by histopathology, does not predict the luminal area available for blood flow *in vivo*, however (Wehr *et al.*, 1997).

The glomerular lesions of chronic rejection are variable and include wrinkling and collapse of the glomerular tuft, glomerular hypertrophy, mesangial matrix expansion and focal glomerulosclerosis (Barrientos *et al.*, 1994; Cheigh *et al.*, 1983). In 1964, Hamburger *et al.* described transplant glomerulopathy, a lesion characterized by enlargement of the glomeruli with swelling of the endothelial and mesangial cells, mesangiolysis, infiltration with mononuclear cells, mesangial matrix expansion and widening of the subendothelial zone with interposition of mesangial cells and matrix (Olsen, 1992; Fig. 27–2).

Since 1991, there has been an ongoing effort to standardize renal transplant pathology interpretations (Racusen *et al.*, 1999; Solez *et al.*, 1993). Although most of the work focused on the classification of acute rejection, chronic rejection has received more attention recently. Recognizing that tubulointerstitial changes are sampled most accurately, the grading of severity of chronic allograft nephropathy focused initially on interstitial fibrosis and tubular atrophy, but chronic glomerular and vascular changes are graded now also (Racusen *et al.*, 1999).

On electron microscopic examination, circumferential multilamellation of the peritubular capillary basement membranes is found in 80% of grafts (Monga *et al.*, 1992), but the lesion is not specific. Subsequent studies have suggested that the presence of more than seven layers of basement membrane is specific and is found in 40% of chronic allograft nephropathy specimens (Ivanyi *et al.*, 2000).

Immunohistochemical studies of chronic rejection have shown deposits of extracellular matrix proteins in the glomeruli and interstitium that are qualitatively not different from the matrix proteins observed in other renal diseases (Gould *et al.*, 1992; Habib *et al.*, 1993; Vleming *et al.*, 1995). A study by Abrass and colleagues shows *de novo* expression of collagen type IV α chain 3 and laminin-β2 in cortical tubular basement membranes and its adjacent interstitium in acute or chronic rejection, whereas in cyclosporine nephrotoxicity there is generalized accumulation of collagens I and III (Abrass *et al.*, 1999).

The vascular, glomerular and interstitial lesions may emerge as a result of immune-mediated damage and scarring of the various compartments of the kidney. Alternatively, some of the lesions emerge in response to loss of renal mass, as described in the section tissue response to injury. Based

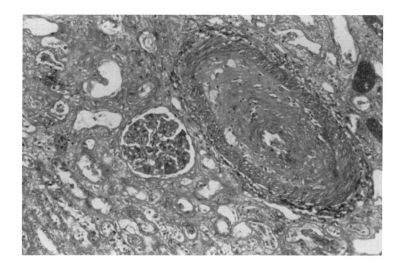

FIGURE 27–1

Photomicrograph of a renal transplant removed because of chronic rejection. There is extensive intimal thickening with narrowing of the vascular lumen, glomerulosclerosis with expansion of the mesangial matrix, interstitial fibrosis and tubular atrophy. (Trichrome staining.) (See color plate.)

on histopathological studies in rats, Demetris and colleagues proposed that chronic rejection emerges as a result of disruption of the graft microvascular lymphatic drainage secondary to foci of tissue inflammation within the parenchyma (Demetris *et al.*, 1997). Lymphatics from a renal transplant reconnect to recipient lymph vessels within 10 to 14 days (Malek *et al.*, 1969). During acute rejection, there is an increased production of lymph fluid and a disruption of the lymphatic microvascular endothelial junctions, which retards lymphatic flow (Eliska *et al.*, 1986). Obstruction of the lymphatics that drain the vessel wall can cause vessel wall lesions as observed in chronic rejection (Solti *et al.*, 1991).

The differential diagnosis of chronic allograft nephropathy includes membranoproliferative and membranous glomerulonephritis (Habib *et al.*, 1987), hepatitis C–associated glomerulopathy (Morales *et al.*, 1997) and chronic cyclosporine or tacrolimus nephrotoxicity. Immunofluorescent studies are indispensable to exclude the C3 deposits characteristic of membranoproliferative glomerulonephritis. Immunofluorescent studies of glomeruli with chronic allograft nephropathy show in most cases a nondiagnostic pattern of immunoglobulin deposits, often IgM, although some cases display linear IgG deposits along the glomerular basement membrane or granular deposits of IgG or IgA in peripheral capillary loops (Habib *et al.*, 1987). Electron microscopy shows an electron-lucent zone of finely flocculent material in the subendothelial space in chronic allograft nephropathy, whereas type I mem-

branoproliferative glomerulonephritis is characterized by subendothelial electron dense deposits (Andresdottir *et al.*, 1998).

Risk Factors

Analysis of risk factors of chronic allograft nephropathy mostly has focused on posttransplantation events, but several risk factors at the time of transplantation correlate with late graft loss. In a multivariate analysis of the Leiden transplant database of grafts that failed more than 6 months after transplantation because of chronic rejection, recipient age, original renal disease, degree of sharing of cross-reactive groups of class I antigens, donor age, baseline immunosuppression and cigarette smoking were all independently correlated with late graft loss (Sijpkens *et al.*, 1999; Table 27–1 and Table 27–2). Donor age seems to have a particularly strong effect on long-term outcome because it explains about 30% of the variance in graft outcome beyond 1 year (Gjertson, 1997).

After transplantation, several other factors influence long-term outcome. Transplants with prolonged ischemic exposure and delayed graft function experience more often inferior long-term outcome (McLaren *et al.*, 1999; Shoskes and Cecka, 1998) as do grafts that have undergone acute rejection episodes (Almond *et al.*, 1993). In our own material, we found a significant correlation of late graft loss and the serum creati-

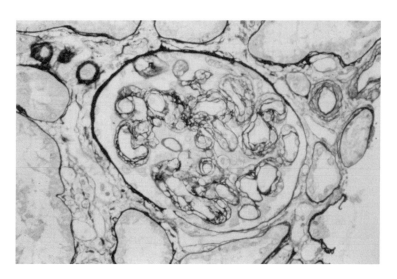

FIGURE 27–2

Photomicrograph of a renal transplant with transplant glomerulopathy. There is splitting of the glomerular basement membrane. (Silver-methenamine staining.) (See color plate.)

TABLE 27–1

INDEPENDENT RISK FACTORS, KNOWN AT TIME OF TRANSPLANTATION, ASSOCIATED WITH GRAFT LOSS FROM CHRONIC REJECTION

Characteristic	RR	95% CI	P Value
Recipient age (<50 y)	2.04	1.13–3.68	0.0175
Original disease:* systemic versus inherited	3.90	1.63–9.34	0.0022
Cigarette smoking	1.67	1.05–2.62	0.0286
Donor age (>50 y)	2.18	1.35–3.53	0.0015
CREG† (1–3 vs. 4–8 shares)	2.12	1.31–3.43	0.0022
Azathioprine vs. cyclosporine	1.94	1.06–3.55	0.0319

*The original diseases were grouped into inherited (polycystic disease, Alport's disease), glomerular and systemic (nephrosclerosis, diabetes, lupus) diseases.
†MHC I antigens were assigned to one or more cross-reactive groups (CREG) based on the amino acid residue system proposed for United Network for Organ Sharing (UNOS) allocation (see Table 27–3). The term *shares* is used for the number of corresponding HLA antigens between donor and recipient.
RR = relative risk; CI = confidence interval.

nine concentration, degree of proteinuria and rejection episodes at 6 months (Sijpkens et al., 1999). Repeated, severe and prolonged acute rejection episodes (Matas et al., 1994) as well as rejection episodes that occur months or years after transplantation are at high risk to evolve into chronic rejection (Massy et al., 1996). Acute vascular rejection and endarteritis is a highly statistically significant adverse prognostic feature compared with tubulointerstitial rejection (Nickeleit et al., 1998; Van Saase et al., 1995; Table 27–2). Other biopsy features that correlate with chronic rejection are tissue infiltration with large numbers of monocytes or macrophages and large numbers of class II–positive tubular and interstitial cells (Alexopoulos et al., 1998).

Graft biopsy specimens from patients with elevated cholesterol levels display often more severe chronic damage than biopsy specimens from patients with lower cholesterol levels, although not all studies find this association (Brazy et al., 1992; Dimeny et al., 1995). In multivariate analysis, hypertriglyceridemia is an independent risk factor of late graft loss (Massy et al., 1996). Recipient hypertension also portends a poorer outcome with a faster decline in function and a greater likelihood of return to dialysis compared with patients with a normal blood pressure (Opelz et al., 1998). Impaired graft function at 6 or 12 months also is a risk factor for late graft loss (Opelz, 1997; Sijpkens et al., 1999). Cytomegalovirus infections enhance chronic vascular rejection in cardiac transplant patients and experimental animals, but such a correlation has not been found in renal transplant patients (Massy et al., 1996). Studies of transplants with chronic rejection have failed to show cytomegalovirus mRNA or protein in such grafts. The role of maintenance immuno-suppressive drugs in relation to the long-term prognosis has been reviewed extensively (Paul, 1998).

A study analyzed the risk factors of tubulointerstitial fibrosis and transplant glomerulopathy separately (Kupin et al., 1997). Significantly more black recipients, female donors and preceding steroid-sensitive rejection episodes were found in the transplant glomerulopathy group, whereas the donor/recipient surface area ratio, a surrogate marker for donor/recipient size matching, was significantly lower compared with the patients with interstitial fibrosis, suggesting that glomerular hyperfiltration or hypertension plays a role in transplant glomerulopathy (Kupin et al., 1997). The degree of HLA mismatching was higher in patients with tubulointerstitial fibrosis, supporting the hypothesis that immune mechanisms play a dominant role in tubulointerstitial fibrosis of chronic allograft nephropathy.

More recent studies have focused on the definition of risk factors at the genetic level. McLaren and coworkers studied the genotypes for five polymorphisms in intercellular adhesion molecule-1 (ICAM-1), E-selectin, and L-selectin. Frequency data for the polymorphisms in the chronic allograft failure group and their matched controls were compared with a group of recipients with graft survival for more than 10 years and a group of controls (McLaren et al., 2000). A variant allele in exon 4 of ICAM-1 (R241) was commoner in the chronic allograft failure recipients compared with long-term survivors and controls. Stratification by time to graft failure caused by chronic allograft failure revealed more rapid failure in the presence of another ICAM-1 variant in the recipient (E469) in exon 6.

The level of transforming growth factor (TGF)-β synthesis

TABLE 27–2

INDEPENDENT RISK FACTORS, KNOWN AT 6 MONTHS POSTTRANSPLANT, ASSOCIATED WITH GRAFT LOSS FROM CHRONIC REJECTION

Characteristic	RR	95% CI	P Value
Recipient age (<50 y)	1.95	1.02–3.71	0.04
Original disease:* systemic versus inherited	4.99	1.91–13.1	0.001
Donor age† (>50 y)	1.68	1.01–2.80	0.04
CREG‡ (1–3 vs. 4–8 shares)	2.20	1.29–3.75	0.004
Azathioprine vs. cyclosporine	2.13	1.06–4.28	0.03
Acute rejection: interstitial vs. no rejection	2.04	1.04–3.97	0.04
Acute rejection: vascular vs. no rejection	3.52	1.72–7.18	0.001
Proteinuria at 6 mo (>1 positive dipstick vs. negative)	2.86	1.29–6.35	0.01
Serum creatinine at 6 mo (>150 μmol/L)	3.41	1.96–5.94	<0.001

*The original diseases were grouped into inherited (polycystic disease, Alport's disease), glomerular and systemic (nephrosclerosis, diabetes, lupus) diseases.
†Donor age is an independent risk factor after removal of serum creatinine from the model.
‡MHC I antigens were assigned to one or more cross-reactive groups (CREG) based on the amino acid residue system proposed for United Network for Organ Sharing (UNOS) allocation (see Table 27–3). The term *shares* is used for the number of corresponding HLA antigens between donor and recipient.
RR = relative risk; CI = confidence interval.

varies among individuals and depends on inheritable differences in the gene encoding TGF-β. Of particular interest are two polymorphisms in the region of the gene encoding the leader sequence of the protein, resulting in variations in the amino acid sequences at codon 10 and codon 25. In the allelic variation of codon 10, proline is exchanged for leucine, which results in a modification of the charge and distortion of an α helix structure. In the allelic variation at codon 25, arginine is replaced by proline, which results in an alteration of the charge and structure of an enzyme cleavage site. The highest TGF-β production is associated with the presence of leucine at codon 10 and arginine at codon 25 (Hutchinson, 1999). Genotypically high TGF-β producers may be at an increased risk to develop chronic allograft nephropathy (Inigo et al., 1999).

Immunology of Chronic Rejection
INVOLVEMENT OF IMMUNE REACTIONS

Because chronic rejection develops in an allograft within a relatively short time compared with lesions that may emerge in syngeneic or autologous grafts, it may result from classic immunological reactions in response to allogeneic incompatibilities between donor and recipient. Immunohistochemistry of grafts with chronic rejection supports this view because it shows in various stages of the process variable amounts of macrophages and T cells, enhanced expression of cell adhesion molecules and deposits of immunoglobulins and complement. Because of the protracted time course, however, it has been difficult to show convincingly the participation of various immunological mechanisms. Tangible evidence came from experiments that showed that pretransplant immunizations with donor splenocytes accelerates chronic rejection (Cramer et al., 1990), whereas manipulations aimed at induction of tolerance inhibit the process (Azuma et al., 1996). Retransplantation of allogeneic kidney grafts back into the original donor strain of rats prevents chronic rejection if the retransplant is done within the first 3 months, suggesting that at least the initial stage depends on allogeneic immune reactivity (Tullius et al., 1994). Several immunosuppressive drugs inhibit chronic rejection in well-controlled experimental conditions.

IMMUNE MEDIATORS OF CHRONIC REJECTION

The role of various immune mediators in the pathogenesis of chronic rejection is unresolved. Heterotopic carotid transplants in B cell–deficient mice do not develop graft vasculopathy (Shi et al., 1996), whereas serum transferred from mice immunized with isolated class I alloantigens or major histocompatibility complex (MHC) class I, class II and minor alloantigens induces proliferative vascular lesions of the donor-type heart graft (Russell et al., 1994a). It was shown that fully allogeneic hearts transplanted into B cell–deficient mice develop endothelialitis, but intimal proliferation or vessel fibrosis does not emerge (Russell et al., 1997). B cell–deficient mice grafted with aortic vessels mismatched for MHC class I and II alloantigens undergo intimal thickening indistinguishable from that of normal immunocompetent recipients (Chow et al., 1996). In some other models, neither antibodies nor cytotoxic T-lymphocyte activity seems involved (Le Moine et al., 1998).

INDUCTION OF THE IMMUNE RESPONSE IN CHRONIC REJECTION

If classic immunological mechanisms are involved in chronic rejection, how is the immune response initiated? Two

pathways of antigen recognition have been described, and each of these pathways generates different sets of T-cell clones. In the *direct* pathway, recipient T cells recognize allo-MHC molecules on the surface of allogeneic donor cells in conjunction with various other peptides, including donor MHC peptides bound in the MHC groove. In the *indirect* pathway, T cells recognize antigens that have been shed from the graft and processed and presented by self–antigen presenting cells. Although both activation routes are activated in acute rejection, the loss of donor antigen-presenting cells from the graft in the weeks or months after transplantation suggests that the direct antigen presentation route is not involved in the induction of chronic rejection. Studies of T lymphocytes from renal transplant patients with chronic rejection have shown that these cells have been primed *in vivo* to react to incompatible donor class II peptides presented by recipient but not donor antigen-presenting cells (Vella et al., 1997).

SPECIFICITY OF THE RESPONSE

Although clinical data show a beneficial effect of HLA matching on long-term graft survival (Opelz, 1992), experimental studies have shown that chronic rejection may occur when recipients and donors differ at minor histocompatibility antigens or at isolated MHC class I or class II antigens (Le Moine et al., 1998; Russell et al., 1994c; Shi et al., 1996). The absence of class I or class II antigens does not prevent the emergence of chronic rejection (Mannon et al., 1999), suggesting that other antigens may be involved.

The correlation of peripheral blood lymphocyte reactivity with donor MHC peptides and chronic rejection has been alluded to (Vella et al., 1997). Many studies have documented a correlation between de novo appearance of posttransplant antibodies and chronic rejection (Buchler et al., 1995; Costa et al., 1997). Older studies using an antibody-dependent cell-mediated cytotoxicity assay or the mixed antiglobulin reaction showed a correlation between antidonor lymphocyte antibodies and chronic rejection (Pierce et al., 1975; Thomas et al., 1976). Suciu-Foca and colleagues reported impaired long-term graft survival in patients who develop posttransplant anti-HLA antibodies (Suciu-Foca et al., 1991). Patients with long-surviving grafts who had antibodies against one of their mismatched HLA antigens had specific antiidiotypic antibodies, whereas such antibodies were not found in patients with chronic rejection (Suciu-Foca et al., 1991). Other studies found predominantly anti–B cell antibodies in patients with chronic rejection (Abe et al., 1997; Davenport et al., 1994). In addition to circulating antibodies, several groups have shown the binding of such antibodies to graft parenchymal cells.

In addition to lymphocytotoxic antibodies, serum antibodies against kidney parenchymal cells have been reported (Kirby et al., 1990; Mohanakumar et al., 1981; Paul et al., 1985). We found that rats with chronic kidney graft rejection produce antibodies against cryptic basement membrane antigens, glomerular mesangial cell focal adhesion plaque proteins and the small proteoglycan molecules biglycan and decorin, molecules synthesized and secreted by activated mesangial cells (De Heer et al., 1994; Paul et al., 1998). Other groups have reported immune reactivity against heat-shock proteins (Liu et al., 1996), proteins identified in cells exposed to inflammation, ischemia, infection and acute rejection episodes (Liu et al., 1996).

Tissue Response to Injury and Fibrogenesis

From the review of risk factors, it is clear that chronic rejection is associated closely with previous tissue injury.

Injury results in structural damage and tissue activation, followed by a stereotypic inflammatory response characterized by an influx of mononuclear cells, proliferation of tissue fibroblasts and deposition of extracellular matrix material. A myriad of cytokines, enzymes and growth factors, such as TGF-β, platelet-derived growth factor (PDGF), interleukin (IL-1β), tumor necrosis factor-α, IL-6 (Gaweco et al., 1999), vascular endothelial growth factor (VEGF) (Pilmore et al., 1999), angiotensin II and endothelin (Simonson et al., 1998), seem involved in various stages of the tissue reaction after injury. These mediators are synthesized and secreted by tissue invading inflammatory cells and activated graft parenchymal cells. Inflammation may produce obliteration of small vessels and ischemia in distal areas (Bohle et al., 1981), which, in turn, may induce further inflammation (Shoskes et al., 1990). Although such processes often result in extensive fibrosis, several animal models have shown that scarring may be reversible, depending on, at least in part, up-regulation of matrix degrading enzymes.

In addition to antigen-driven chronic inflammation directed by allogeneic incompatibilities between donor and recipient, the situation in kidney transplants with chronic rejection is complicated further by other mechanisms. Reduction in renal mass causes an increase in glomerular capillary blood flow and pressure in the remaining nephrons (Hostetter et al., 1981), increased glomerular permeability for macromolecules (Remuzzi and Bertani, 1990), glomerular hypertrophy (Yoshida et al., 1989), changes in renal metabolism (Alfrey, 1994; Nath et al., 1985) and the emergence of lipoprotein disorders secondary to uremia and proteinuria (Keane et al., 1988). Micropuncture studies have shown glomerular hypertension in rat kidney grafts with chronic rejection (Junaid et al., 1995; Kingma et al., 1993; Mackenzie et al., 1995), whereas lowering of the pressure results in improved graft survival, decreased proteinuria and preservation of structure (Benediktsson et al., 1996; Mackenzie et al., 1994). Glomerular hypertension is not sufficient to explain chronic rejection, however, because glomerular hypertension in syngeneic grafts does not result in chronic rejection lesions within the same period (Kingma et al., 1993). Glomerular hypertension seems to be a progression factor. Consistent with this hypothesis are the clinical correlations suggesting that an imbalance between recipient metabolic demands and graft renal mass is associated with more late graft loss. The 3-year graft survival rates of transplants from female, black, very young or very old donors is less compared with grafts from donors who are supposedly endowed with a larger nephron mass (Brenner et al., 1992). Studies that examined more directly the relationship of nephron mass, recipient metabolic needs and long-term outcome have been inconsistent, in part, because of difficulties in measuring nephron mass. There is consensus that high recipient weights are associated with shortened graft survival (Feldman et al., 1996; Pirsch et al., 1995; Terasaki et al., 1994), but it is not clear whether this results from glomerular hyperfiltration and hypertension, inadequacies of immunosuppressive medication or some other as yet undefined mechanism. It has been argued that focal glomerulosclerosis, the histopathological hallmark of glomerular hyperfiltration and hypertension, is not a prominent feature of human chronic rejection (Halloran et al., 1999). No data are available regarding glomerular hypertension in humans, but glomerular hyperfiltration does occur in human kidney transplants with chronic rejection (Rosenberg et al., 1995; Salahudeen et al., 1992). These observations, together with experimental data (Amuchastegui et al., 1998; Benediktsson et al., 1996; Mackenzie et al., 1994; Remuzzi and Perico, 1998), strongly suggest that glomerular hypertension plays a modulating role in chronic allograft nephropathy, at least in the

group of patients with transplant glomerulopathy (Kupin et al., 1997).

Besides hemodynamics, when the glomerular permselective property is lost, increased glomerular filtration of macromolecules results in the delivery of abnormal amounts of protein in the tubular filtrate. Filtered plasma proteins are endocytosed by proximal tubular epithelial cells, followed by degradation in the lysosomes (Wall and Maack, 1985). Increasing the protein load beyond the tubular capacity for this process results in lysosomal rupture and exposure of the tubular interstitium to the injurious effects of lysosomal enzymes (Maack, 1967). Oxidant-mediated injury to tubular cells could result from the reabsorption of iron, which is released from transferrin at the acidic pH of the proximal tubular fluid (Zager et al., 1993). Filtered complement components can be activated nonimmunologically at the surface of damaged tubules and mediate further local interstitial injury (Nath et al., 1985). Protein overload in tubular epithelial cells results in an up-regulation of proinflammatory and vasoactive mediators, such as monocyte chemoattract protein (MCP-1), osteopontin and endothelin (Remuzzi et al., 1997).

As discussed previously, an increase in myofibroblasts and extracellular matrix material in an architecturally disrupted tissue is the hallmark of chronic rejection in which interstitial fibroblasts and dedifferentiated smooth muscle cells are key players. Interstitial fibroblasts cultured from diseased human kidneys show hyperproliferative responses, an increased mitotic life span and an increased collagen synthesis compared with normal renal fibroblasts (Rodeman and Muller, 1990). Excessive matrix production also may result from increased synthesis by renal tubular epithelial cells and interstitial macrophages (Nath, 1992). Tubular epithelial cells in culture produce a variety of collagens including interstitial collagen type I and III (Wolf et al., 1990), whereas interstitial tissue macrophages synthesize collagen I and fibronectin (Vaage and Lindblad, 1990). The amount of extracellular matrix produced likely is determined by the genetic programming of the cells involved as well as several exogenous influences, such as growth factors, cytokines, vitamins, hormones, cell-cell contacts and contacts of the cells with extracellular matrix proteins. Similar processes influence the myofibroblast behavior in the vessel wall (Ross, 1995).

In addition to increased synthesis of extracellular matrix material, matrix degradation is another important factor that determines the net amount of scar tissue. Metalloproteases such as collagenases, gelatinases and stromelysins degrade virtually all matrix components (Stetler-Stevenson, 1996). They are regulated by inhibitors of metalloproteases such as tissue inhibitor of metalloproteinases (TIMP-1, TIMP-2 and TIMP-3). In several models of interstitial fibrosis, TIMP-1 is increased, as are plasminogen activator inhibitors (Eddy, 1996). Overexpression of such enzyme inhibitors and decreased expression of proteases may contribute to fibrogenesis and atherosclerosis, but this has not been examined in renal transplants with chronic rejection.

Hypothesis to Explain Chronic Allograft Nephropathy
CHRONIC REJECTION

Kidney grafts undergoing chronic rejection show at various stages features of immune-mediated inflammation, which raises the possibility that chronic rejection results from a chronic, smoldering, low-grade immune reaction against transplantation antigens. The distinction between acute and chronic rejection could be in the intensity of the immune reaction, its specificity or differences in the tissue resistance to injury. As discussed previously, antibodies and T cells specific for various antigens have been described in chronic rejection. Conceivably the response is directed against MHC gene products that are up-regulated during tissue activation, or the response is against cryptic antigens. Cryptic antigens are not detectable in noninjured tissues but become readily accessible after tissue injury (De Heer et al., 1994).

After tissue activation, many genes are up-regulated that suppress the proinflammatory response and protect the cells from apoptosis. A20 is an example of a tissue-protective gene that inhibits activation of NF-κB, a transcription factor that plays a key role in the induction of proinflammatory events (Bach et al., 1997). Bcl-2 and Bcl-x are antiapoptotic genes, and hemoxygenase-1 prevents oxidant-stressed endothelial induction of adhesion molecules (Habib et al., 1993). Hemoxygenase-1 also can ameliorate tissue damage through the generation of heme breakdown products, such as bilirubin, which exerts anticomplement or antioxidant effects, and carbon monoxide, which has vasodilatory and antiplatelet effects (Bach et al., 1997). In chronic rejection, such tissue-protective genes may protect the graft from acute rejection, but they may be unable to prevent chronic rejection.

Because of the correlation between acute rejection and long-term graft prognosis, it is conceivable that the degree of tissue inflammation correlates with the extent of tissue scarring and fibrosis. If there is a direct correlation between tissue inflammation and chronic rejection, however, it is expected that drugs that decrease the incidence and extent of acute rejection will result in a decrease in chronic rejection. The introduction of cyclosporine in the 1980s and the introduction of mycophenolate mofetil in the 1990s decreased the incidence and severity of acute rejection episodes substantially, but there has been no discernible effect on the rate of late graft loss (Gjertson, 1991; Mathew, 1998).

CYTOKINE EXCESS THEORY

It has been proposed that repetitive injury over a short time results in excessive production of fibrogenic cytokines, including but not restricted to TGF-β. These cytokines promote deposition of extracellular matrix proteins with or without concomitant impaired breakdown. As discussed previously, genotypically high TGF-β producers seem at increased risk of losing their graft late after transplantation (Inigo et al., 1999). Transforming growth factor-β mRNA and protein expression are enhanced in kidney grafts with chronic rejection (Paul et al., 1996; Shihab et al., 1995). Transforming growth factor-β is a multifunctional cytokine that plays a central role in extracellular matrix production and degradation, and its net effect, in general, is to promote the accumulation of extracellular matrix. The regulation of the amount of biologically active TGF-β is complex and is a function of its production rate, its rate of enzymatic release from a complex of active TGF-β and an N-terminal latency associated protein, the availability of a signal-transducing TGF-β receptor and the presence of soluble or cellular TGF-β binding molecules (Border et al., 1992; Roy-Chaudhury et al., 1997). Kidney transplants with chronic allograft nephropathy have enhanced expression of urokinase plasminogen activator, its receptor and plasminogen activator inhibitor type 1 (Tang et al., 1998), and it is believed that urokinase plasminogen activator activates TGF-β.

We showed that rats with chronic rejection produce antibodies against mesangial cell focal adhesion plaque proteins (Paul et al., 1998) and various as yet only partly characterized molecules such as biglycan and decorin. The latter compounds are small proteoglycan molecules produced by activated mesangial cells that bind and inactivate TGF-β and

stimulate the release of matrix metalloproteinase collagenases by fibroblasts (Huttenlocher et al., 1996). It is conceivable that antibodies against biglycan and decorin bind to and inactivate these molecules in vivo, resulting in less active TGF-β binding molecules, decreased production of collagenases, and impaired fibrillogenesis. A role of decorin in limiting glomerular sclerosis has been illustrated in a rat model of mesangial glomerulonephritis (Border et al., 1992).

Experiments using neutralizing anti-interferon (IFN)-γ monoclonal antibodies or IFN-γ knock-out mice have shown the pivotal role played by this cytokine in graft vasculopathy (Nagano et al., 1997; Russell et al., 1994b).

INTERFERENCE IN TISSUE REPAIR AFTER INJURY

Animals with chronic rejection often produce antibodies against various molecules involved in tissue repair. As discussed previously, animals with chronic rejection mount an antibody response to heat-shock proteins, proteins identified in cells exposed to inflammation, ischemia, infection and acute rejection episodes (Liu et al., 1996). Heat-shock proteins mediate the assembly, folding and translocation of intracellular polypeptides and protect against their degradation and interaction with receptors (Ellis and Vies, 1991; Gething and Sambrook, 1992). It is conceivable that an immune response to such molecules interferes with their function in tissue repair, resulting in chronic fibrous organ disease. We found antibodies to mesangial cell focal adhesion plaques, and conceivably such antibodies disrupt important signaling molecules associated with focal adhesion complexes (Simonson and Herman, 1993) and result in increased cell proliferation or matrix formation. Similarly the antibodies against biglycan and decorin found in chronic kidney graft rejection in rats (Paul et al., 1985) could interfere in the function of these molecules as enhancing proteolytic enzyme activity. It is also conceivable that kidneys from older donors are less efficient in tissue repair processes.

LOSS OF SUPPORTING EXTRACELLULAR MATRIX ARCHITECTURE

The importance of a disruption of the three-dimensional extracellular matrix has not received much attention in the pathogenesis of chronic rejection. Anatomical structures such as blood vessels can regenerate after tissue damage, but other structures such as renal tubules are dependent on an intact extracellular matrix framework that determines and maintains the tissue organization. Tubular epithelial cells must find an intact tubular basement membrane on which to attach, to proliferate and to organize their polarity; if they do not find this structure, they undergo integrin-dependent apoptosis (Frisch and Francis, 1994) or perhaps transdifferentiate to fibroblasts (Strutz et al., 1995). When the tubular basement membrane is disrupted, tubular epithelial cells that have been lost through cytotoxic (Wever et al., 1998) or apoptotic mechanisms are not able to regenerate, and fibrosis ensues. The role of antibodies against basement membrane antigens as found in chronic rejection presently is unknown (De Heer et al., 1994; Paul et al., 1979).

PREMATURE SENESCENCE THEORY

It has been proposed that chronic rejection represents the senescent state of graft endothelial or tubular cells (Halloran, 1998; Halloran et al., 1999). Somatic cells in culture are limited in the number of cell divisions they can undergo, a phenomenon referred to as the Hayflick limit (Hayflick and Moorhead, 1961). After this finite number of divisions, cells become senescent and shut down irreversibly many processes, such as replication and energy generation. Histologically, senescence is characterized by atrophy. The multitude of stresses that act on graft cells may lead to their premature senescence and consequent failure to exert their regulatory influence over a variety of functions, such as tissue repair after injury. Fibrosis arises, according to this hypothesis, from an exhaustion of graft cells after multiple stresses.

Chronic rejection may result from diverse processes: the induction and the persistence of alloimmune or autoimmune responses against cryptic graft antigens exposed to the recipient immune system in a proinflammatory milieu, an excessive scarring response as a result of a dysregulation of normal tissue repair mechanisms, apoptosis as a result of lack of survival signals or the accelerated senescence of graft parenchymal cells after multiple stresses. Whatever the ultimate mechanism turns out to be, tissue damage and activation seem to play a key role, and measures to prevent chronic rejection should aim primarily to minimize graft damage and activation.

Prevention and Treatment of Chronic Rejection: the Future

Although none of the recommendations proposed to avoid chronic rejection clinically have been tested formally, it would seem prudent to recommend the following strategies. The most important principle to avoid chronic rejection is likely the prevention of graft activation at any stage of the harvesting and transplant process. With emerging knowledge on the pathophysiology of brain death, it is conceivable that interventions are explored that prevent the induction of a proinflammatory state of the organs to be transplanted (Takada et al., 1998). Although the administration of superoxide dismutase at the time of surgery may be effective to prevent chronic renal transplant rejection (Land, 1994), it does not prevent chronic rejection universally (Myllarniemi et al., 1996), and the drug is not available commercially. Optimal donor management and short ischemic exposure seem presently the only ways to deal with this issue. Although acute rejection episodes are correlated strongly with late graft loss, they should be treated aggressively to ensure complete restoration of function (Opelz, 1997). The use of high intravenous doses of methylprednisolone is the treatment most commonly used for acute rejection episodes, but such doses do not reverse the acute rejection lesions histologically in 25% of cases (Mazzucchi et al., 1999). Surveillance biopsies perhaps are useful to diagnose subclinical rejections, which, if treated, could result in better long-term outcome (Nickerson et al., 1998).

The role of matching for HLA antigens or the broadly reactive cross-reactive groups (Table 27–3; Sijpkens et al., 1999) is unknown, but protocol biopsy specimens from HLA-identical living donor kidneys at 2 years showed no chronic allograft nephropathy versus 50% in grafts from cadaveric donors (Legendre et al., 1998). It is expected that effective maintenance immunosuppression will be the cornerstone to prevent chronic rejection (Chandraker et al., 1998). Experimental studies have shown that immune tolerance in animals prevents chronic allograft failure (Azuma et al., 1996; Larsen et al., 1996), but there is no evidence in humans that such protocols are clinically feasible. Some of the newer immunosuppressive drugs, especially those that also inhibit smooth muscle cell proliferation, seem effective in animal models when given prophylactically (Azuma et al., 1995; Schmid et al., 1995), but their efficacy to improve long-term outcome clinically is unknown.

TABLE 27–3

HLA-A AND B ANTIGENS ASSIGNED TO CROSS-REACTIVE GROUPS

CREG	Antigens Included
A01C	A1, 3, 11, 29, 30, 31, 36
A02C	A2, 23, 24, 28, B57, 58
A10C	A25, 26, 32, 33, 34, 66
B05C	B18, 35, 51, 52, 53
B07C	B7, 8, 13, 27, 41, 47, 55, 56, 60, 61
B08C	B8, 14, 18, 38, 39
B12C	B13, 37, 41, 44, 45, 47, 49, 50, 60, 61
B21C	B35, 49, 50, 51, 52, 53, 57, 58, 62, 63, 70
BW4	A23, 24, 25, 32, B13, 27, 37, 38, 44, 47, 49, 51, 52, 53, 57, 58, 63
BW6	B7, 8, 14, 18, 35, 39, 41, 45, 50, 55, 56, 60, 61, 62, 70

CREG = cross-reactive group.

The impact of antiviral therapy on chronic rejection in humans is unknown. Data are available on the beneficial effect of the lipid-lowering agent pravastatin in heart transplant patients (Kobashigawa et al., 1995), but there are no clinical data on pravastatin's efficacy to prevent chronic renal graft nephropathy. There now is some evidence that hyperlipidemia is associated with chronic renal allograft failure, and so there is no justification to ignore posttransplant hyperlipidemia because it is also likely to have an impact on patient cardiovascular morbidity and mortality (Arend et al., 1997; Kasiske et al., 1996; McLaren et al., 2000).

Limited data are available on the effect of antihypertensive drugs on late graft loss. Based on animal data, the use of antihypertensive drugs, especially angiotensin-converting enzyme inhibitors or angiotensin receptor blockers, prolongs graft survival in chronic rejection, although calcium channel blockers seem ineffective (Amuchastegui et al., 1998; Benediktsson et al., 1996). A retrospective clinical study supports the hypothesis that angiotensin-converting enzyme inhibitors are beneficial in chronic allograft nephropathy (Barnas et al., 1996), but controlled clinical trials are needed to provide proof.

Several other nonimmunosuppressive drugs have been tested in experimental models, including eicosanoid and platelet-activating factor antagonists (Hayry et al., 1993a), heparinoids (Aziz et al., 1993), somatostatin analogues (Hayry et al., 1993b), insulin-like growth factor (IGF) antagonists (Hayry et al., 1995), estrogens (Lou et al., 1996b), nitric oxide donors (Lou et al., 1996a) and protein thyrosine kinase inhibitors (Sihvola et al., 1999). Hayry's group blocked the binding of IGF-1 to its receptor using stable D-peptide analogues of IGF-1 and observed a diminished replication rate of smooth muscle cells in association with 30% inhibition of intimal thickening in a rat aortic allograft model (Myllarniemi et al., 1997). Blocking the signaling pathway of PDGF receptors using PDGF-receptor tyrosine kinase inhibitors also reduces migration and proliferation of smooth muscle cells and inhibits vascular intimal thickening by 50% (Myllarniemi et al., 1997; Sihvola et al., 1999).

The use of somatostatin analogues in various models of vascular injury has yielded inconsistent results. It is now known, however, that there are two subfamilies of somatostatin receptors that are differentially expressed at different time intervals after injury and that the wrong set of receptors has been targeted (Patel, 1997).

Estrogens inhibit heart graft coronary vessel disease significantly (Lou et al., 1996b). It was shown in a rat renal allograft model that testosterone treatment of ovariectomized female rats results in increased urinary protein excretion and extended glomerulosclerosis, interstitial fibrosis and severe vascular lesions, whereas estradiol treatment resulted in improved graft function, reduction in glomerular sclerosis and diminished cellular infiltration. This beneficial effect of estradiol is independent of donor gender (Muller *et al.*, 1999). The discovery that disruption of the classic estrogen receptor α does not interfere with the vasculoprotective properties of estrogens together with the definition of the estrogen receptor β makes it feasible to provide vascular or tissue protection without the pleiotropic effect on a variety of other tissues (Kuiper *et al.*, 1996, 1997).

Conclusion

Chronic rejection is the main problem facing long-term survival of allogeneic organ grafts. Its pathophysiology is complex and involves immunological and nonimmunological factors. The nonimmunological factors are likely progression factors. Several mechanisms have been described that may result in excessive fibrosis as observed in chronic rejection. Experimentally, various interventions seem successful to prevent chronic rejection, but these have not yet been implemented clinically. Efficacy studies in chronic rejection would be difficult to conduct because of difficulties in trial design and entry criteria, the need to enroll large numbers of patients and the need to follow patients for long periods. For the short term, appropriate surrogate biomarkers for late graft loss should be tested and defined to guide future studies with hard outcomes (Kasiske *et al.*, 1995; Paul, 1999).

References

Abe, M., Kawai, T., Futatsuyama, K., *et al.* (1997). Postoperative production of anti-donor antibody and chronic rejection in renal transplantation. *Transplantation* **63**, 1616.

Abrass, C. K., Berfield, A. K., Stehman-Breen, C., Alpers, C. E. and Davis, C. L. (1999). Unique changes in interstitial extracellular matrix composition are associated with rejection and cyclosporine toxicity in human renal allograft biopsies. *Am. J. Kidney Dis.* **33**, 11.

Alexopoulos, E., Leontsini, M. and Papadimitriou, M. (1998). Macrophages and HLA-DR (+) cells in acutely rejecting kidney transplants predict subsequent graft survival, even after reversal of the acute episode. *Nephrology* **4**, 113.

Alfrey, A. C. (1994). Role of iron and oxygen radicals in the progression of chronic renal failure. *Am. J. Kidney Dis.* **23**, 183.

Almond, P. S., Matas, A., Gillingham, K. J., *et al.* (1993). Risk factors for chronic rejection in renal allograft recipients. *Transplantation* **55**, 752.

Amuchastegui, S. C., Azzollini, N., Mister, M., Pezzotta, A., Perico, N. and Remuzzi, G. (1998). Chronic allograft nephropathy in the rat is improved by angiotensin II receptor blockade but not by calcium channel antagonism. *J. Am. Soc. Nephrol.* **9**, 1948.

Andresdottir, M. B., Assmann, K. J., Koene, R. A. and Wetzels, J. F. (1998). Immunohistological and ultrastructural differences between recurrent type I membranoproliferative glomerulonephritis and chronic transplant glomerulopathy. *Am. J. Kidney Dis.* **32**, 582.

Arend, S. M., Mallat, M. J. K., Westendorp, R. J. W., Van der Woude, F. J. and Van Es, L. A. (1997). Patient survival after renal transplantation: more than 25 years follow up. *Nephrol. Dial. Transplant.* **12**, 1672.

Aziz, S., Tada, Y., Gordon, D., McDonald, T. O., Fareed, J. and Verrier, E. D. (1993). A reduction in accelerated graft coronary disease and an improvement in cardiac allograft survival using low molecular weight heparin in combination with cyclosporine. *J. Heart Lung Transplant.* **12**, 634.

Azuma, H., Binder, J., Heemann, U., Tullius, S. G. and Tilney, N. L. (1995). Effect of RS61443 on chronic rejection of rat kidney allografts. *Transplant. Proc.* **27**, 436.

Azuma, H., Chandraker, A., Nadeau, K., *et al.* (1996). Blockade of T-

cell costimulation prevents development of experimental chronic renal allograft rejection. *Proc. Natl. Acad. Sci. U. S. A.* **93**, 12439.

Bach, F. H., Hancock, W. W. and Ferran, C. (1997). Protective genes expressed in endothelial cells: a regulatory response to injury. *Immunol. Today* **18**, 483.

Barnas, U., Schmidt, A., Haas, M., Oberbauer, R. and Mayer, G. (1996). The effects of prolonged angiotensin-converting enzyme inhibition on excretory kidney function and proteinuria in renal allograft recipients with chronic progressive transplant failure. *Nephrol. Dial. Transplant.* **11**, 1822.

Barrientos, A., Portoles, J., Herrero, J. A., *et al.* (1994). Glomerular hyperfiltration as a nonimmunologic mechanism of progression of chronic renal rejection. *Transplantation* **57**, 753.

Benediktsson, H., Chea, R., Davidoff, A. and Paul, L. C. (1996). Antihypertensive drug treatment in chronic renal allograft rejection in the rat: effect on structure and function. *Transplantation* **62**, 1634.

Bohle, A., Von Gise, H., Mackensen-Haen, S. and Stark-Jakob, B. (1981). The obliteration of the postglomerular capillaries and its influence upon the function of both glomeruli and tubuli: functional interpretation of morphologic findings. *Klin. Wochenschr.* **59**, 1043.

Border, W. A., Noble, N. A., Yamamoto, T., *et al.* (1992). Natural inhibitor of transforming growth factor-β protects against scarring in experimental kidney disease. *Nature* **360**, 361.

Brazy, P. C., Pirsch, J. D. and Belzer, F. O. (1992). Factors affecting renal allograft function in long-term recipients. *Am. J. Kidney Dis.* **19**, 558.

Brenner, B. M., Cohen, R. A. and Milford, E. L. (1992). In renal transplantation, one size may not fit all. *J. Am. Soc. Nephrol.* **3**, 162.

Buchler, M., Al Najjar, A., Guerraoui, A., *et al.* (1995). Posttransplant anti-HLA antibodies: risk factor for chronic rejection? *Transplant. Proc.* **27**, 2478.

Chandraker, A., Azuma, H., Nadeau, K., *et al.* (1998). Late blockade of T cell costimulation interrupts progression of experimental chronic allograft rejection. *J. Clin. Invest.* **101**, 2309.

Cheigh, J. S., Mouradian, J., Soliman, M., *et al.* (1983). Focal segmental glomerulosclerosis in renal transplants. *Am. J. Kidney Dis.* **2**, 449.

Chow, L. H., Huh, S., Jiang, J., Zhong, R. and Pickering, J. G. (1996). Intimal thickening develops without humoral immunity in a mouse aortic allograft model of chronic vascular rejection. *Circulation* **94**, 3079.

Cole, E., Naimark, D., Aprile, M., *et al.* (1995). An analysis of predictors of long term cadaveric renal allograft survival. *Clin. Transplant.* **9**, 282.

Costa, A. N., Scolari, M. P., Iannelli, S., *et al.* (1997). The presence of posttransplant HLA-specific IgG antibodies detected by enzyme-linked immunosorbent assay correlates with specific rejection pathclogies. *Transplantation* **63**, 167.

Cramer, D. V., Chapman, F. A., Wu, G. D., Harnaha, J. B., Qian, S. Q. and Makowka, L. (1990). Cardiac transplantation in the rat: II. alteration of the severity of donor graft arteriosclerosis by modulation of the host immune response. *Transplantation* **50**, 554.

Davenport, A., Younie, M. E., Parsons, J. E. M. and Klouda, P. T. (1994). Development of cytotoxic antibodies following renal allograft transplantation is associated with reduced graft survival due to chronic vascular rejection. *Nephrol. Dial. Transplant.* **9**, 1315.

De Heer, E., Davidoff, A., Van der Wal, A., Van Geest, M. and Paul, L. C. (1994). Chronic renal allograft rejection in the rat: transplantation-induced antibodies against basement membrane antigens. *Lab. Invest.* **70**, 494.

Demetris, A. J., Murase, N., Ye, Q., *et al.* (1997). Analysis of chronic rejection and obliterative arteriopathy—possible contributions of donor antigen-presenting cells and lymphatic disruption. *Am. J. Pathol.* **150**, 563.

Dimeny, E., Wahlberg, J., Lithell, H. and Fellstrom, B. (1995). Hyperlipidaemia in renal transplantation—risk factor for long-term graft outcome. *Eur. J. Clin. Invest.* **25**, 574.

Eddy, A. A. (1996). Molecular insights into renal interstitial fibrosis. *J. Am. Soc. Nephrol.* **7**, 2495.

Eliska, O., Eliskova, P. and Mirejovsky, M. (1986). Lymph vessels of the transplanted kidney. *Nephron* **44**, 136.

Ellis, R. J. and Vies, S. M. V. (1991). Molecular chaperones. *Ann. Rev. Biochem.* **60**, 321.

Feldman, H. I., Fazio, I., Roth, D., *et al.* (1996). Recipient body size and cadaveric renal allograft survival. *J. Am. Soc. Nephrol.* **7**, 151.

Frisch, S. M. and Francis, H. (1994). Disruption of epithelial cell-matrix interactions induces apoptosis. *J. Cell. Biol.* **124**, 619.

Gaweco, A. S., Mitchell, B., Lucas, B., McClatchey, K. D. and Van Thiel, D. H. (1999). Concerted induction of NF-κB activation and expression of NF-κB-inducible IL-6 in human chronic renal allograft rejection. *Transplantation* **67**, S11.

Gething, J. R. and Sambrook, J. F. (1992). Protein folding in the cell. *Nature* **355**, 33.

Gjertson, D. W. (1991). Survival trends in long-term first cadaver-donor kidney transplants. In *Clinical Transplants 1991*, (P. I. Terasaki, J. M. Cecka, eds.), p. 225, UCLA Tissue Typing Laboratory, Los Angeles.

Gjertson, D. W. (1997). A multi-factor analysis of kidney graft outcomes at one and five years posttransplantation: 1996 UNOS update. In *Clinical Transplants 1996*, (J. M. Cecka, P. I. Terasaki, eds.), p. 343, UCLA Tissue Typing Laboratory, Los Angeles.

Gould, V. E., Martinez-Lacabe, V., Virtanen, I., Sahlin, K. M. and Schwartz, M. M. (1992). Differential distribution of tenascin and cellular fibronectins in acute and chronic renal allograft rejection. *Lab. Invest.* **67**, 71.

Habib, R., Antigua, C., Hinglais, N., Gagnadoux, M. F. and Broyer, M. (1987). Glomerular lesions in the transplanted kidney in children. *Am. J. Kidney Dis.* **10**, 198.

Habib, R., Zurowska, A., Hinglais, N., et al. (1993). A specific glomerular lesion of the graft: allograft glomerulopathy. *Kidney Int.* **44(Suppl. 42)**, S104.

Halloran, P. F. (1998). Non-immunologic tissue injury and stress in chronic allograft dysfunction. *Graft* **1**, 23.

Halloran, P. F., Melk, A. and Barth, C. (1999). Rethinking chronic allograft nephropathy—the concept of accelerated senescence. *J. Am. Soc. Nephrol.* **10**, 167.

Hamburger, J., Crosnier, J. and Dormont, J. A. (1964). Observations in patients with a well tolerated homotransplanted kidney. *Ann. N. Y. Acad. Sci.* **120**, 558.

Hayflick, L. and Moorhead, P. S. (1961) The serial cultivation of human diploid cell strains. *Exp. Cell. Res.* **25**, 585.

Hayry, P., Isoniemi, H., Yilmaz, S., et al. (1993a). Chronic allograft rejection. *Immunol. Rev.* **134**, 33.

Hayry, P., Myllarniemi, M., Aavik, E., et al. (1995). Stable D-peptide analogue of insulin-like growth factor-1 inhibits smooth muscle proliferation after carotid ballooning injury in the rat. *FASEB J.* **9**, 1336.

Hayry, P., Raisanen, A., Ustinov, J., Mennander, A. and Paavonen, T. (1993b). Somatostatin analog Lanreotide inhibits myocyte replication and several growth factors in allograft arteriosclerosis. *FASEB J.* **7**, 1055.

Hostetter, T. H., Olson, J. L., Rennke, H. G., Venkatachalam, M. A. and Brenner, B. M. (1981). Hyperfiltration in remnant nephrons: a potentially adverse response to renal ablation. *Am. J. Physiol.* **241**, F85.

Hutchinson, I. V. (1999). The role of transforming growth factor-β in transplant rejection. *Transplant. Proc.* **31 (suppl 7A)**, 95.

Huttenlocher, A., Werb, Z., Tremble, P., Huhtala, P., Rosenberg, L. and Damsky, C. H. (1996). Decorin regulates collagenase gene expression in fibroblasts adhering to vitronectin. *Matrix Biol.* **15**, 239.

Inigo, P., Lario, S., Campistol, J. M., Oppenheimer, F. and Rivera, F. (1999). Relation between transforming growth factor β1 (TGFβ) gene polymorphisms and the development of chronic allograft nephropathy in renal transplant recipients. *9th Congress of the European Society for Organ Transplantation*, Oslo, Norway.

Ivanyi, B., Fahmy, H., Brown, H., et al. (2000). Peritubular capillaries in chronic renal allograft rejection: a quantitative ultrastructural study. *Hum. Pathol.* **31**, 1129.

Junaid, A., Kren, S. M., Rosenberg, M. E., Nath, K. A. and Hostetter, T. H. (1995). Physiological and structural responses to chronic experimental renal allograft injury. *Am. J. Physiol.* **267**, F1102.

Kasiske, B. L., Guijarro, C., Massy, Z. A., Wiederkehr, M. R. and Ma, J. Z. (1996). Cardiovascular disease after renal transplantation. *J. Am. Soc. Nephrol.* **7**, 158.

Kasiske, B. L., Heim-Duthoy, K. L., Tortorice, K. L. and Rao, K. V. (1991). The variable nature of chronic declines in renal allograft function. *Transplantation* **51**, 330.

Kasiske, B. L., Massy, Z. A., Guijarro, C. and Ma, J. Z. (1995). Chronic renal allograft rejection and clinical trial design. *Kidney Int.* **48(Suppl. 52)**, S116.

Keane, W. F., Kasiske, B. L. and O'Donnell, M. P. (1988). Lipids and progressive glomerulosclerosis. *Am. J. Nephrol.* **8**, 261.

Kingma, I., Chea, R., Davidoff, A., Benediktsson, H. and Paul, L. C. (1993). Glomerular capillary pressures in long-surviving rat renal allografts. *Transplantation* **56**, 53.

Kirby, J. A., Givan, A. L., Shenton, B. K., et al. (1990). Renal allograft rejection: possible involvement of antibody-dependent cell-mediated cytotoxicity. *Transplantation* **50**, 225.

Kobashigawa, J. A., Katznelson, S., Laks, H., et al. (1995). Effect of pravastatin on outcomes after cardiac transplantation. *N. Engl. J. Med.* **333**, 621.

Kuiper, G. G., Carlsson, B., Grandien, K., et al. (1997). Comparison of the ligand binding specificity and transcript tissue distribution of estrogen receptors alpha and beta. *Endocrinology* **138**, 863.

Kuiper, G. G., Enmark, E., Pelto, H. M., Nilsson, S. and Gustafsson, J. A. (1996). Cloning of a novel receptor expressed in rat prostate and ovary. *Proc. Natl. Acad. Sci. U. S. A.* **93**, 5925.

Kupin, W., Nakhleh, R., Lee, M., et al. (1997). Separate risk factors for the development of transplant glomerulopathy vs chronic tubulointerstitial rejection. *Transplant. Proc.* **29**, 245.

Land, W. (1994). The potential impact of the reperfusion injury on acute and chronic rejection events following organ transplantation. *Transplant. Proc.* **26**, 3169.

Larsen, C. P., Elwood, E. T., Alexander, D. Z., et al. (1996). Long-term acceptance of skin and cardiac allografts after blocking CD40 and CD28 pathways. *Nature* **381**, 434.

Legendre, C., Thervet, E., Skhiri, H., et al. (1998). Histologic features of chronic allograft nephropathy revealed by protocol biopsies in kidney transplant recipients. *Transplantation* **65**, 1506.

Le Moine, A., Flamand, V., Noel, J. C., Fayt, I., Goldman, M. and Abramowicz, D. (1998). Chronic rejection of major histocompatibility complex class II-disparate skin grafts after anti-CD3 therapy. *Transplantation* **66**, 1537.

Liu, K., Moliterno, R., Qian, J., et al. (1996). Role of heat shock proteins in heart transplant rejection. *J. Heart Lung Transplant.* **15**, 222.

Lou, H., Kodama, T., Wang, Y. N., Katz, N., Ramwell, P. and Foegh, M. L. (1996a). L-Arginine prevents heart transplant arteriosclerosis by modulating the vascular cell proliferative response to insulin-like growth factor-1 and interleukin-6. *J. Heart Lung Transplant.* **15**, 1248.

Lou, H., Kodama, T., Zhao, Y. J., et al. (1996b). Inhibition of transplant coronary arteriosclerosis in rabbits by chronic estradiol treatment is associated with abolition of MHC class II antigen expression. *Circulation* **94**, 3355.

Maack, T. (1967). Changes in the activity of acid hydrolases during renal reabsorption of lysozyme. *J. Cell. Biol.* **35**, 268.

Mackenzie, H. S., Azuma, H., Rennke, H. G., Tilney, N. L. and Brenner, B. M. (1995). Renal mass as a determinant of late allograft outcome: insights from experimental studies in rats. *Kidney Int.* **48(Suppl. 52)**, S38.

Mackenzie, H. S., Tullius, S. G., Heemann, U. W., et al. (1994). Nephron supply is a major determinant of long-term renal allograft outcome in rats. *J. Clin. Invest.* **94**, 2148.

Malek, P., Vrubel, J. and Kolc, J. (1969). Lymphatic aspects of experimental and clinical transplantation. *Bull. Soc. Int. Chir.* **28**, 110.

Mannon, R. B., Kopp, J. B., Ruiz, P., et al. (1999). Chronic rejection of mouse kidney allografts. *Kidney Int.* **55**, 1935.

Massy, Z. A., Guijarro, C., Wiederkehr, M. R., Ma, J. Z. and Kasiske, B. L. (1996). Chronic renal allograft rejection: immunologic and nonimmunologic risk factors. *Kidney Int.* **49**, 518.

Matas, A. J., Gillingham, K. J., Payne, W. D. and Najarian, J. S. (1994). The impact of an acute rejection episode on long-term renal allograft survival (t1/2). *Transplantation* **57**, 857.

Mathew, T. H., for the Tricontinental Mycophenolate Mofetil Renal Transplantation Study Group. (1998). A blinded, long-term, randomized multicenter study of mycophenolate mofetil in cadaveric renal transplantation—results at three years. *Transplantation* **65**, 1450.

Mazzucchi, E., Lucon, A. M., Nahas, W. C., et al. (1999). Histological outcome of acute cellular rejection in kidney transplantation after treatment with methylprednisolone. *Transplantation* **67**, 430.

McLaren, A. J., Fuggle, S. V., Welsh, K. I., Gray, D. W. R. and Morris, P. J. (2000). Chronic allograft failure in human renal transplantation: a multivariate analysis. *Ann. Surg.* **232**, 98.

McLaren, A. J., Jassem, W., Gray, D. W., Fuggle, S. V., Welsh, K. I. and Morris, P. J. (1999a). Delayed graft function: risk factors and the relative effects of early function and acute rejection on long-term survival in cadaveric renal transplantation. *Clin. Transplant.* **13**, 266.

McLaren, A. J., Marshall, S. E., Haldar, N. A., *et al.* (1999b). Adhesion molecule polymorphisms in chronic allograft failure. *Kidney Int.* **55**, 1977.

Mohanakumar, T., Waldrep, J. C., Phibbs, M., Mendez-Picon, G., Kaplan, A. M. and Lee, H. M. (1981). Serological characterization of antibodies eluted from chronically rejected human renal allografts. *Transplantation* **32**, 61.

Monga, G., Mazzucco, G., Messina, M., Motta, M., Quaranta, S. and Novara, R. (1992). Intertubular capillary changes in kidney allografts: a morphologic investigation on 61 renal specimens. *Mod. Pathol.* **5**, 125.

Morales, J. M., Campistol, J. M., Andres, A. and Rodicio, J. L. (1997). Glomerular diseases in patients with hepatitis C virus infection after renal transplantation. *Curr. Opin. Nephrol. Hypertens.* **6**, 511.

Muller, V., Szabo, A., Viklicky, O. *et al.* (1999). Sex hormones and gender-related differences: their influence on chronic renal allograft rejection. *Kidney Int.* **55**, 2011.

Myllarniemi, M., Calderon, L., Lemstrom, K., Buchdunger, E. and Hayry, P. (1997). Inhibition of platelet-derived growth factor receptor tyrosine kinase inhibits vascular smooth muscle cell migration and proliferation. *FASEB J.* **11**, 1119.

Myllarniemi, M., Raisanen-Sokolowski, A., Vuoristo, P., Kallio, E., Land, W. and Hayry, P. (1996). Lack of effect of recombinant human superoxide dismutase on cold ischemia-induced arteriosclerosis in syngeneic rat aortic transplants. *Transplantation* **61**, 1018.

Nagano, H., Mitchell, R. N., Taylor, M. K., Hasegawa, S., Tilney, N. L. and Libby, P. (1997). Interferon-gamma deficiency prevents coronary arteriosclerosis but not myocardial rejection in transplanted mouse hearts. *J. Clin. Invest.* **100**, 550.

Nath, K. A. (1992). Tubulointerstitial changes as a major determinant in the progression of renal damage. *Am. J. Kidney Dis.* **20**, 1.

Nath, K. A., Hostetter, M. K. and Hostetter, T. H. (1985). Pathophysiology of chronic tubulo-interstitial disease in rats: interactions of dietary acid load, ammonia and complement component C3. *J. Clin. Invest.* **76**, 667.

Nickeleit, V., Vamvakas, E. C., Pascual, M., Poletti, B. J. and Colvin, R. B. (1998). The prognostic significance of specific arterial lesions in acute renal allograft rejection. *J. Am. Soc. Nephrol.* **9**, 1301.

Nickerson, P., Jeffery, J., Gough, J., *et al.* (1998). Identification of clinical and histopathologic risk factors for diminished renal function 2 years posttransplant. *J. Am. Soc. Nephrol.* **9**, 482.

Olsen, T. S. (1992). Pathology of allograft rejection. In *Kidney Transplant Rejection: Diagnosis and Treatment*, (J. F. Burdick, L. C. Racusen, K. Solez, and G. M. Williams, eds.), p. 333, Marcel Dekker, New York.

Opelz, G. (1997). Critical evaluation of the association of acute with chronic graft rejection in kidney and heart transplant recipients. *Transplant. Proc.* **29**, 73.

Opelz, G., for the Collaborative Transplant Study. (1992). Collaborative transplant study—10-year report. *Transplant. Proc.* **24**, 2342.

Opelz, G., Wujciak, T., Ritz, E. and Collaborative Transplant Study. (1998). Association of chronic kidney graft failure with recipient blood pressure. *Kidney Int.* **53**, 217.

Patel, Y. C. (1997). Molecular pharmacology of somatostatin receptor subtypes. *J. Endocrinol. Invest.* **20**, 348.

Paul, L. C. (1995). Chronic renal transplant loss. *Kidney Int.* **47**, 1491.

Paul, L. C. (1998). Immunosuppressive drug-induced toxicities compromising the half-life of renal allografts. *Transplant. Proc.* **30(Suppl. 8A)**, 7S.

Paul, L. C. (1999). Surrogate end points in chronic kidney graft rejection studies. *Transplant. Proc.* **31**, 1293.

Paul, L. C., Baldwin, W. M. and Van Es, L. A. (1985). Vascular endothelial alloantigens in renal transplantation. *Transplantation* **40**, 117.

Paul, L. C., Hayry, P., Foegh, M., *et al.* (1993). Diagnostic criteria for chronic rejection/accelerated graft atherosclerosis in heart and kidney transplants: joint proposal from the Fourth Alexis Carrel Conference on Chronic Rejection and Accelerated Arteriosclerosis in Transplanted Organs. *Transplant. Proc.* **25**, 2022.

Paul, L. C., Muralidharan, J., Muzaffar, S. A., *et al.* (1998). Antibodies against mesangial cells and their secretory products in chronic renal allograft rejection in the rat. *Am. J. Pathol.* **152**, 1209.

Paul, L. C., Saito, K., Davidoff, A. and Benediktsson, H. (1996). Growth factor transcripts in rat renal transplants. *Am. J. Kidney Dis.* **28**, 441.

Paul, L. C., Van Es, L. A., Stuffers-Heiman, M., De la Riviere, G. B. and Kalff, M. W. (1979). Antibodies directed against tubular basement membranes in human renal allograft recipients. *Clin. Immunol. Immunopathol.* **14**, 231.

Pierce, J. C., Kay, S. and Lee, H. M. (1975). Donor-specific IgG antibody and the chronic rejection of human renal allografts. *Surgery* **78**, 14.

Pilmore, H. L., Eris, J. M., Painter, D. M., Bishop, G. A. and McCaughan, G. W. (1999). Vascular endothelial growth factor expression in human chronic renal allograft rejection. *Transplantation* **67**, 929.

Pirsch, J. D., Armbrust, M. J., Knechtle, S. J., *et al.* (1995). Obesity as a risk factor following renal transplantation. *Transplantation* **59**, 631.

Porter, K. A., Owen, K., Mowbray, J. F., Thomson, W. B., Kenyon, J. R. and Peart, W. S. (1963). Obliterative vascular changes in four human kidney homotransplants. *B. M. J.* **14**, 639.

Racusen, L. C., Solez, K., Colvin, R. B., *et al.* (1999). The Banff 97 working classification of renal allograft pathology. *Kidney Int.* **55**, 713.

Raine, A. E. G. (1995). Does antihypertensive therapy modify chronic allograft failure? *Kidney Int.* **48(Suppl. 52)**, S107.

Remuzzi, G. and Bertani, T. (1990). Is glomerulosclerosis a consequence of altered glomerular permeability to macromolecules? *Kidney Int.* **38**, 384.

Remuzzi, G. and Perico, N. (1998). Protecting single-kidney allografts from long-term functional deterioration. *J. Am. Soc. Nephrol.* **9**, 1321.

Remuzzi, G., Ruggenenti, P. and Benigni, A. (1997). Understanding the nature of renal disease progression. *Kidney Int.* **51**, 2.

Riggio, R. R., Haschemeyer, R., Suthanthiran, M., *et al.* (1985). Predictability of renal allograft failure time in long-term survivors: a hypothesis. *Transplant. Proc.* **17**, 2311.

Rodeman, H. P. and Muller, G. A. (1990). Abnormal growth and clonal proliferation of fibroblasts derived from kidneys with interstitial fibrosis. *Proc. Soc. Exp. Biol. Med.* **195**, 57.

Rosenberg, M. E., Salahudeen, A. K. and Hostetter, T. H. (1995). Dietary protein and the renin-angiotensin system in chronic renal allograft rejection. *Kidney Int.* **48(Suppl. 52)**, S102.

Ross, R. (1995). Cell biology of atherosclerosis. *Annu. Rev. Physiol.* **57**, 791.

Roy-Chaudhury, P., Simpson, J. G. and Power, D. A. (1997). Endoglin, a transforming growth factor-beta-binding protein, is upregulated in chronic progressive renal disease. *Exp. Nephrol.* **5**, 55.

Russell, P. S., Chase, C. M. and Colvin, R. B. (1997). Alloantibody- and T cell-mediated immunity in the pathogenesis of transplant arteriosclerosis: lack of progression to sclerotic lesions in B cell-deficient mice. *Transplantation* **64**, 1531.

Russell, P. S., Chase, C. M., Winn, H. J. and Colvin, R. B. (1994a). Coronary atherosclerosis in transplanted mouse hearts: II. importance of humoral immunity. *J. Immunol.* **152**, 5135.

Russell, P. S., Chase, C. M., Winn, H. J. and Colvin, R. B. (1994b). Coronary atherosclerosis in transplanted mouse hearts: III. effects of recipient treatment with a monoclonal antibody to interferon-gamma. *Transplantation* **57**, 1367.

Russell, P. S., Chase, C. M., Winn, H. J. and Colvin, R. B. (1994c). Coronary atherosclerosis in transplanted mouse hearts: I. time course and immunogenetic and immunopathological considerations. *Am. J. Pathol.* **144**, 260.

Salahudeen, A. K., Hostetter, T. H., Raatz, S. K. and Rosenberg, M. E. (1992). Effects of dietary protein in patients with chronic renal transplant rejection. *Kidney Int.* **41**, 183.

Schmid, C., Heemann, U., Azuma, H. and Tilney, N. L. (1995). Rapamycin inhibits transplant vasculopathy in long-surviving rat heart allografts. *Transplantation* **60**, 729.

Schweitzer, E. J., Matas, A. J., Gillingham, K. J., *et al.* (1991). Causes of renal allograft loss: progress in the 1980s, challenges for the 1990s. *Ann. Surg.* **214**, 679.

Shi, C., Lee, W. S., He, Q., *et al.* (1996). Immunologic basis of transplant-associated arteriosclerosis. *Proc. Natl. Acad. Sci. U. S. A.* **93**, 4051.

Shihab, F. S., Yamamoto, T., Nast, C. C., et al. (1995). Transforming growth factor-β and matrix protein expression in acute and chronic rejection of human renal allografts. *J. Am. Soc. Nephrol.* **6**, 286.

Shoskes, D. A. and Cecka, J. M. (1998). Deleterious effects of delayed graft function in cadaveric renal transplant recipients independent of acute rejection. *Transplantation* **66**, 1697.

Shoskes, D. A., Parfrey, N. A. and Halloran, P. F. (1990). Increased major histocompatibility complex antigen expression in unilateral ischemic acute tubular necrosis in the mouse. *Transplantation* **49**, 201.

Sihvola, R., Koskinen, P., Myllärniemi, M., et al. (1999). Prevention of cardiac allograft arteriosclerosis by protein-tyrosine kinase inhibitor selective for platelet-derived growth factor receptor. *Circulation* **99**, 2295.

Sijpkens, Y. W. J., Doxiadis, I. I. N., De Fijter, J. W., et al. (1999). Sharing crossreactive groups (CREG) of MHC class I antigens improves long-term graft survival. *Kidney Int.* **56**, 1920.

Simonson, M. S., Emancipator, S. N., Knauss, T. and Hricik, D. E. (1998). Elevated neointimal endothelin-1 in transplantation-associated arteriosclerosis of renal allograft recipients. *Kidney Int.* **54**, 960.

Simonson, M. S. and Herman, W. H. (1993). Protein kinase C and protein tyrosine kinase activity contribute to mitogenic signalling by endothelin-1: cross-talk between G protein-coupled receptors and pp60c-src. *J. Biol. Chem.* **268**, 9347.

Solez, K., Axelsen, R. A., Benediktsson, H., et al. (1993). International standardization of criteria for the histologic diagnosis of renal allograft rejection: the Banff working classification of kidney transplant pathology. *Kidney Int.* **44**, 411.

Solti, F., Jellinek, H., Schneider, F., Lengyel, E., Berczi, V. and Kekesi, V. (1991). Lymphatic arteriopathy: damage to the wall of the canine femoral artery after lymphatic blockade. *Lymphology* **24**, 54.

Stetler-Stevenson, W. G. (1996). Dynamics of matrix turnover during pathologic remodeling of the extra-cellular matrix. *Am. J. Pathol.* **148**, 1345.

Strutz, F., Okada, H., Lo, C. W., et al. (1995). Identification and characterization of a fibroblast marker: FSP1. *J. Cell. Biol.* **130**, 393.

Suciu-Foca, N., Reed, E., D'Agati, V. D., et al. (1991). Soluble HLA antigens, anti-HLA antibodies, and antidiotypic antibodies in the circulation of renal transplant recipients. *Transplantation* **51**, 593.

Takada, M., Nadeau, K. C., Hancock, W. W., et al. (1998). Effects of explosive brain death on cytokine activation of peripheral organs in the rat. *Transplantation* **12**, 1533.

Tang, W. H., Friess, H., Di Mola, F. F., et al. (1998). Activation of the serine proteinase system in chronic kidney rejection. *Transplantation* **65**, 1628.

Terasaki, P. I., Koyama, H., Cecka, J. M. and Gjertson, D. W. (1994). The hyperfiltration hypothesis in human renal transplantation. *Transplantation* **57**, 1450.

Thomas, J. M., Thomas, F. T., Kaplan, A. M. and Lee, H. M. (1976). Antibody-dependent cellular cytotoxicity and chronic renal allograft rejection. *Transplantation* **22**, 94.

Tullius, S. G., Hancock, W. W., Heemann, U., Azuma, H. and Tilney, N. L. (1994). Reversibility of chronic renal allograft rejection: critical effect of time after transplantation suggests both host immune dependent and independent phases of progressive injury. *Transplantation* **58**, 93.

United States Renal Data System (USRDS) (1999). Renal transplantation: access and outcomes. *In Annual Data Report 1998,* http://www.med.umich.edu/usrds.

Vaage, J. and Lindblad, W. J. (1990). Production of collagen type I by mouse peritoneal macrophages. *J. Leukoc. Biol.* **48**, 274.

Van Saase, J. L. C. M., Van der Woude, F. J., Thorogood, J., et al. (1995). The relation between acute vascular and interstitial renal allograft rejection and subsequent chronic rejection. *Transplantation* **59**, 1280.

Vella, J. P., Spadafora-Ferreira, M., Murphy, B., et al. (1997). Indirect allorecognition of major histocompatibility complex allopeptides in human renal transplant recipients with chronic graft dysfunction. *Transplantation* **64**, 795.

Vleming, L. J., Baelde, J. J., Westendorp, R. G. J., Daha, M. R., Van Es, L. A. and Bruijn, J. A. (1995). Progression of chronic renal disease in humans is associated with the deposition of basement membrane components and decorin in the interstitial extracellular matrix. *Clin. Nephrol.* **44**, 211.

Wall, D. A. and Maack, T. (1985). Endocytic uptake, transport, and catabolism of proteins by epithelial cells. *Am. J. Physiol.* **248**, C12.

Wehr, S., Rudin, M., Joergensen, J., Hof, A. and Hof, R. P. (1997). Allo- and autotransplantation of carotid artery—a new model of chronic graft vessel disease—evaluation by magnetic resonance imaging and histology. *Transplantation* **64**, 20.

Wever, P. C., Boonstra, J. G., Laterveer, J. C., et al. (1998). Mechanisms of lymphocyte-mediated cytotoxicity in acute renal allograft rejection. *Transplantation* **66**, 259.

Wolf, G., Killen, P. D. and Neilson, E. G. (1990). Cyclosporin A stimulates transcription and procollagen secretion in tubulointerstitial fibroblasts and proximal tubular cells. *J. Am. Soc. Nephrol.* **1**, 918.

Yoshida, Y., Fogo, A. and Ichikawa, I. (1989). Glomerular hemodynamic changes vs. hypertrophy in experimental glomerular sclerosis. *Kidney Int.* **35**, 654.

Zager, R. A., Schimpf, B. A., Bredl, C. R. and Gmur, D. J. (1993). Inorganic iron effects on in vitro hypoxic proximal renal tubular cell injury. *J. Clin. Invest.* **91**, 702.

28

Vascular and Lymphatic Complications After Renal Transplantation

Derek W. R. Gray

Introduction

The initial description of vascular anastomoses for renal transplantation was by Carrel in the early part of the 20th century, for which he received the Nobel Prize in 1912 (see Chapter 1). Ensuring the vascular supply of the kidney transplant is a basic principle for management of the transplant patient at all stages. In the early years of kidney transplantation, the techniques for vascular anastomosis were rapidly refined (see Chapter 11), and although safe, reliable techniques and sutures are standard, vascular complications and their management are an important aspect of renal transplantation.

Vascular Anastomoses

The techniques for suturing the transplant renal artery and vein to the iliac vessels are described in Chapter 11, but it is worthwhile to emphasize several points that may help to avoid complications. If the external iliac vessels are used for end-to-side anastomoses, it is important to place the anastomoses as high as possible on the external iliac artery and vein so that the kidney can be placed comfortably in the parapsoas gutter. If this advice is unheeded and the anastomoses are made just above the inguinal ligament (a tempting site for the venous anastomosis because access is easier), the kidney is jammed against the abdominal wall and the inguinal ligament. The pressure and tension on the vessels is a recipe for subsequent thrombosis. It is important before selecting the sites for the anastomosis to visualize the placement of the kidney and the course the vessels will run from the proposed anastomoses. The kidney commonly is placed in the opposite iliac fossa to the side of origin because this position usually gives satisfactory placement of the vessels and places the renal pelvis and ureter anterior to the vessels.

To allow safe anastomosis of a short renal vein (usually of the right kidney) without tension, it may be necessary to bring up the iliac vein by dividing the internal iliac vein and one or two adjacent tributaries. This can be a difficult maneuver, not to be undertaken by an inexperienced surgeon without supervision. The major disaster is losing control of the distal cut vein as a result of the ligature slipping, and as a precaution, the use of suture ligation may be advisable when a short length of vein is available. Sometimes, it may be necessary also to divide the internal iliac artery to free the underlying vein, which can be done safely, provided that the other internal iliac artery is patent. Consideration then can be given to using the divided internal iliac artery for the arterial anastomosis, this being the normal choice for live donor transplantation because a Carrel patch is not available. In most cases in which a Carrel patch is available, however, end-to-side arterial anastomosis to the external or common

iliac is preferable because there is less risk of anastomotic stenosis in less experienced hands. In cases of repeat transplantation, ligation of both internal iliac arteries should be avoided, especially in young men because subsequent vasculogenic impotence can occur (Billet *et al.*, 1982).

The technique used for arterial anastomosis varies among surgeons, but some general points include the need for judicious placement of the arteriotomy for end-to-side anastomosis: It often may be placed to the lateral or medial side of the vessel to give an advantageous curve of the renal artery, depending on its length. Sometimes the aortic patch or the recipient vessel is heavily diseased with atheroma and may require a *large bite* anastomosis using heavier suture. It may be necessary to reverse the anastomosis suture bite to ensure that an intimal flap is not lifted in the worst-affected vessel.

When the graft has multiple vessels, in general it is best to undertake bench surgery to convert the situation to a single venous and arterial anastomosis, and some of the techniques for multiple arteries are outlined in Chapter 11. Provided that one of the renal veins is at least 1.5-cm caliber, it is safe to ligate the smaller veins because there is good cross-anastomosis, but ligation of larger dominant veins has produced venous infarction. For the renal arteries, all vessels to the parenchyma must be preserved when technically possible. It is particularly important to preserve lower polar vessels because these may be the sole blood supply for the transplant ureter.

The venous anastomosis usually is made between the renal vein and the external or common iliac veins (noting the points made on mobilization of the internal iliac veins above), and the renal vein is prepared by excising the attached vena cava with a 3- to 4-mm rim of vena cava, sufficient to insert the anastomosis sutures. Leaving any more of the vena cava makes the anastomosis longer, to no advantage. Left kidneys sometimes have a remarkably long renal vein, and it is the practice of some surgeons routinely to shorten the vein back to the gonadal tributary, using the junction of the vessels to widen the anastomosis. This shortening is not mandatory, and a correctly placed long renal vein may allow placement with a gentle curve to the vein and an advantageous inflow angle at the anastomosis. Although anastomosis to the external iliac vein commonly is made medial to the arterial anastomosis, the more proximal external iliac and common iliac veins may lie directly posterior or lateral to the artery, especially on the right side, and the vein mobilization and anastomosis may be made more conveniently on the lateral side of the iliac arteries in some patients.

Although individual surgeons have their own style of venous anastomosis technique, some points should be standard, including the placement of tied sutures at each end of the anastomosis, which should be to a venotomy that is large enough to stretch open the renal vein. The use of at least one stay suture is recommended to prevent inadvertent picking up of the opposite wall. A common finding that should be sought is the presence of a valve in the renal or iliac vein. In either site, the valve presents a danger for inadvertent tethering by sutures and should be excised carefully.

Complications at Time of Surgery

The placement of venous and arterial clamps is a matter of personal preference, but the accidental loosening of a clamp during anastomosis is more significant than during a routine vascular operation because the kidney is perfused with warm blood. Care should be taken to avoid such an event by careful support of clamps that may be subject to leverage, covering the clamp handles with damp towels. An extra click on the ratchet of the clamps above that used for normal vessel control in arterial surgery probably is justified. If inadvertent perfusion of the kidney occurs before the anastomosis is completed, preventing full release of the clamps, the kidney should be kept cold, and intravascular clotting should be prevented by local injection of heparinized saline. Once the kidney has been perfused fully, the latter option is no longer appropriate if the blood supply needs to be clamped off again.

If the kidney vasculature has to be controlled for a large venous bleed after letting off the clamps, and if it looks likely that the repair will take some time, it is better to release the arterial clamp every 2 minutes and let oxygenated blood through the kidney for about 20 seconds, venting the blood to waste (about 50 ml) if the venous clamps cannot be released. This practice is preferable to leaving the kidney clamped off with warm ischemia or attempting to reperfuse and cool the kidney *in situ*. This practice maintains kidney viability and has been used by the author for a 20-minute period, after which primary function of the kidney was still obtained. Gentle clamping of the renal vessels must used (fingers are best if a careful assistant is available), and the anesthesiologist must be informed and keep up with blood lost during this period.

Routine intravenous administration of heparin is not used for most patients because often patients on dialysis have a reduced hematocrit and defective platelet function as a result of uremia. If there is extensive recipient arterial atheroma and if the hemoglobin is greater than 11.0 g/dl, it is the author's practice to administer heparin before clamping, but caution in the dosage should be used. If available, thromboelastography is useful for controlling the heparin dosage, but in the absence of such aids 3,000 U of sodium heparin is appropriate for the average patient. If these measures are not undertaken, thrombosis of the iliac artery may occur while the vessel is occluded by clamps. This complication must be detected before release of blood to the artery or vein of the kidney, and this is best detected by soft clamping both of the renal vessels (which can be done with the fingers), while releasing both of the venous and then the arterial iliac clamps, in that order. When pulsatile flow is confirmed in the iliac artery (with no excessive bleeding from either anastomosis), it is safe to release blood into the kidney. If no pulse is seen or blood loss is excessive, the renal vessels can be clamped directly and the kidney kept cold and nonperfused (see earlier).

The most obvious technical error, which may first become apparent on releasing the clamps, is the presence of a partial or complete twist on the artery or vein. This is a particularly easy mistake to make, and time taken to confirm that the vein is placed correctly before tying down the initial sutures, taking into account the likely final positioning of the kidney,

is time well spent. As mentioned earlier, by routinely placing the right kidney in the left side and vice versa, the normal lie of the aortic patch is such that the angulated takeoff of the renal artery is in the correct orientation, which is helpful in detecting partial twists of the artery. If a twist or partial twist of a vessel is detected after completing the anastomosis, the surgeon *never* should be tempted to *place* the kidney and accept the position. It is always better to repeat the anastomosis before perfusing the kidney rather than risk later thrombosis.

A less obvious but equally dangerous threat to the arterial flow is the presence of an intimal flap within the renal artery. This flap may arise as a consequence of excessive traction on the artery during retrieval (one should be wary of the presence of bruising in the arterial adventitia on first examination of a donated kidney) or injudicious perfusion of the renal artery using a hard cannula after removal of the kidney. Careful inspection of the artery and its ostium from within while preparing the kidney on the bench should detect this problem, which can be corrected by placing an intimal tacking stitch or by shortening the renal artery to a point distal to the damage.

Rapid bleeding from undetected venous tears (or unligated major tributaries of vein or artery) can cause hasty reapplication of clamps, which may be prevented by avoiding excessive hilar dissection and testing the vein while preparing the kidney on the bench using gentle installation of cold saline. Occasionally the renal vein is extremely thin and fragile, and tears may develop during the anastomosis. Excised excess aortic and vena caval tissue always should be kept available because this can act as a useful patch, for example, to repair tears of the renal vein, which should be sought and repaired before releasing the venous clamps.

Postoperative Thrombosis
INCIDENCE AND ETIOLOGY

Several centers have reported an increase in graft vessel thromboses, affecting chiefly the renal vein, but also the artery. With the reduction in rejection as a cause of graft loss using modern immunosuppression, some centers now report thrombosis to be the commonest cause of graft loss. Early reports of vascular complications after renal transplantation quoted a 1% incidence of graft arterial thrombosis, all ascribed to technical causes (Lacombe, 1975), but some early reports described renal venous thrombosis and cited an incidence of 4% (Nerstrom et al., 1972). A study from Oxford in 1978 noted one renal vein thrombosis in 158 patients who received azathioprine and steroid immunosuppression after renal transplantation. A subsequent report from Oxford in 1988 described six venous thromboses in 110 patients on cyclosporine-based triple-drug therapy (5%) (Jones et al., 1988), and an incidence of 4% was noted in patients taking cyclosporine and prednisolone in Glasgow (Akyol et al., 1991). An incidence of 6% was reported by a single center using a predominantly cyclosporine-based regimen (Bakir et al., 1996). Children receiving pediatric kidney transplants have a well-recognized tendency to thrombose, with the risk being highest in the youngest patients (2–5 years old, 9%) (Singh et al., 1997).

None of the aforementioned reports was prospective, and one must question whether these reports represent a true increase in incidence or simply are the result of more accurate diagnosis. Graft loss resulting from rejection used to be common, and a few thromboses could have been ascribed to rejection in the absence of biopsy evidence. Many centers have routinely subjected all graft nephrectomy specimens to histological examination, and the finding of diffuse infarction with clot in the main vessels is so distinctive that it is hard to believe the problem was missed previously.

The cause of the apparent rise in thrombosis is unproven, and a study of cases reported to the Australian and New Zealand Transplant Registry failed to identify any factor apart from a slight association with increased donor age, female sex of donor and prolonged cold ischemia (Penny et al., 1994); however, the data available to registries may be inadequate to answer the question. Detailed single-center studies, all retrospective, have resulted in many suggestions being made, with moderately good supportive evidence in some cases. A prothrombotic tendency in some renal transplant patients has been documented (Fischereder et al., 1998), especially in diabetic patients (Reissell et al., 1994), and the role of diabetes has been suggested by other studies (Bergentz et al., 1985), including the author's experience in Oxford. Other suggested factors include a raised platelet count with (Higgins et al., 1995; Reissell et al., 1994) or without (Higgins et al., 1995) diabetes, plasminogen activator inhibitor-1 (Wang et al., 1994) and gene polymorphisms for prothrombin (Oh et al., 1999) and factor V Leiden (Irish et al., 1997).

Other specific suggested factors, supported by limited evidence, include continuous ambulatory peritoneal dialysis (Murphy et al., 1994; Ojo et al., 1999) and certain graft perfusion fluids (Benoit et al., 1994). Antiphospholipid antibodies have been suggested to play a role, not only in lupus patients, in whom they are well recognized, but also in other patients across a broad diagnostic range of end-stage renal disease (Knight et al., 1995; Vaidya et al., 1999; Wagenknecht et al., 1999). In some of these patients, the causes of the original renal failure are unlikely to have been missed lupus (Knight et al., 1995). The fact that 28% (Ducloux et al., 1999) of transplant patients appear to develop antiphospholipid antibodies and presumably have evidence of autoimmunity despite (or perhaps because of?) immunosuppression is fascinating and potentially important.

The advent of cyclosporine was associated with a significant rise in graft survival and was an undoubted advance in transplantation, but several groups also have timed the increase in graft thromboses to coincide with the introduction of this immunosuppressant. Other drugs introduced over the same period also have been implicated, for example, OKT3 (Abramowicz et al., 1992). As mentioned previously, early changes in procoagulation may be attributed more to surgical trauma than either agent individually (Deira et al., 1998). In 1985, Merion and Calne reported a 7.6% incidence of renal vein thrombosis in 79 patients treated with cyclosporine versus 1.1% incidence in 89 patients treated with azathioprine and steroid and suggested that the increase might be attributable directly to cyclosporine.

An investigation of the effects of cyclosporine on blood flow and coagulation provides several rational reasons for why cyclosporine may promote thrombosis, including a well-proven reduction in renal blood flow (McKenzie et al., 1985) with increased concentration of thrombosis promoters such as thromboxane (Petric et al., 1988), reduced production of prostacyclin by endothelial cells (Brown and Neild, 1987; Neild et al., 1983), evidence for endothelial cell damage by high levels of cyclosporine (Brown et al., 1986) and enhanced adenosine diphosphate–induced platelet aggregation in the presence of cyclosporine (Vanrenterghem et al., 1985), with in vitro evidence of enhanced hemostasis and reduced thrombolysis (Baker et al., 1990; Thomson et al., 1985) and varied alterations in clotting factors and thrombosis inhibitors such as antithrombin III (Watzke et al., 1986). Transplant patients taking cyclosporine have been shown to be hypercoagulable

compared with general surgical patients in the early postoperative period and to have sustained enhancement of in vitro hemostasis and reduced thrombolysis (Baker et al., 1990). Cyclosporine has a proven association with intraglomerular thrombosis (Neild et al., 1984, 1985) and microangiopathy, including hemolytic-uremic syndrome (Dowling et al., 1986; Van Buren et al., 1985), although the relationship to large-vessel thrombosis is not clear.

Not all investigators have linked cyclosporine therapy to increased incidence of thromboses (Bergentz et al., 1985; Gruber et al., 1989; Zazgornik et al., 1985). A prospective randomized study looked at early prothrombotic changes in clotting indices and compared patients who underwent kidney transplantation with cyclosporine versus OKT3 as induction agents. The prothrombotic changes seen in the first 6 hours were marked but similar in both groups, suggesting the real culprit was surgical trauma (Deira et al., 1998). A later role for cyclosporine is not excluded by this study, however. One large single-center study noted no increase in thrombosis in the cyclosporine era (Gruber et al., 1989). The center in question frequently used antilymphocyte globulin induction, however, and delayed cyclosporine introduction in these patients. Because the peak incidence of thrombosis is in the first 7 days posttransplantation (see later), the absence of thromboses in the latter study may reflect the absence of cyclosporine during the high-risk period, conversely providing support for the hypothesis.

If it is accepted that thrombosis is commoner in patients receiving cyclosporine, should routine thrombosis prophylaxis be given to all patients? The major defect caused by cyclosporine is of platelet function, and presumably platelet adhesion is a major initiating factor. Agents such as heparin have little rationale and have been found to be ineffective clinically in a retrospective study (Mohan et al., 1999). The author found that thromboses still occurred in the presence of full anticoagulation with heparin.

A more logical alternative is low-dose aspirin therapy, which was introduced for all renal transplant recipients in Oxford in 1991. The dosage used is 75 mg/d, given orally preoperatively and continued for 1 month. The experience has been a dramatic drop in the incidence of renal vein thromboses. In the 6-year period from July 1985 to June 1991, there were 27 cases of renal vein thrombosis in 475 transplants (5.6%). In the subsequent 6-year period, there were 6 cases of renal vein thrombosis in 480 transplants (1.2%) ($P<0.01$) (Robertson, 2000; Fig. 28–1). The author noted 13 cases of major bleeding after the introduction of aspirin (2.7%). These cases included 8 bleeds after core biopsy of the graft (1.6%) and 3 bleeds early posttransplant. Three patients required exploration and evacuation of hematoma. It is difficult to be sure of the role of aspirin in these cases, although it is likely to be at least a contributing factor. The incidence of clinically relevant bleeding after transplant biopsy has been reported to be 0.3 to 12.6% (Hanas et al., 1992; Riehl et al., 1994). Gastrointestinal bleeding has not been a problem, probably because most patients receive aspirin only for 1 month and receive peptic ulcer prophylaxis. The results are in keeping with reports of lack of detrimental effect of low-dose aspirin on surgery in transplant recipients (Werner and Schubert, 1997).

RENAL ARTERY THROMBOSIS

The failure of a kidney transplant to produce urine in the immediate postoperative period is a relatively common event. Many transplants fail to produce urine at all for several weeks and are labeled as suffering from acute tubular necrosis. This relatively benign condition is not always the

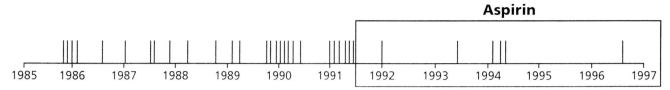

FIGURE 28–1

Time plot to show kidney graft renal vein thromboses from July 1985 to June 1997. Aspirin started preoperatively was introduced midway through 1991. A total of 475 transplants was performed in the 6 years before aspirin, and 490 transplants were performed after aspirin introduction (all patients were on cyclosporine-based immunosuppression regimens). (Reproduced with permission of Robertson *et al.*, 2000.)

reason for anuria, and sometimes the absence of function is caused by thrombosis of the graft artery. The index of suspicion of such an event is high if the kidney ordinarily would be expected to function immediately, as in transplantation of a kidney from a living donor, but in any case urgent diagnosis is unnecessary because it is never possible to salvage a kidney from such an event. In general, this disaster should be a rarity: Some large series quote figures of 1% (Nerstrom *et al.*, 1972).

The cause of acute arterial thrombosis probably is multifactorial, although most authors blame technical errors (Nerstrom *et al.*, 1972), which undoubtedly do occur. Other possible contributory factors include persistent hypotension (from any cause), dehydration (usually owing to excessive preoperative dialysis) and procoagulant conditions such as lupus anticoagulant and diabetes. The problem seems to be more frequent in highly sensitized recipients, especially when transplanted across an *acceptable* positive crossmatch, suggesting that antibody-mediated endothelial damage may have a role, despite the absence of hyperacute rejection on subsequent histological examination. The presence of antiendothelial antibodies has been suggested to be contributory, at least in pediatric transplants (Harmer *et al.*, 1990). At Oxford, it has been noted that highly sensitized patients tend to have a high incidence of *vascular spasm* with poor perfusion at the end of the operation, even in crossmatch-negative patients.

Apart from anuria of the transplanted kidney (often masked by residual function from the patient's own kidneys), there are no diagnostic features of early graft artery thrombosis. Any patient that fails to show satisfactory graft function within the first 2 days posttransplantation should undergo an isotope perfusion scan or color duplex scanning (Reuther *et al.*, 1989; Taylor *et al.*, 1987), preferably the latter because isotopic scanning has a low but definite diagnostic error rate. Graft necrosis also can be confirmed by biopsy using core needle or fine-needle technique before to graft nephrectomy.

Spontaneous late thrombosis of the renal artery is a rare but well-documented event (Nerstrom *et al.*, 1972), and renal artery stenosis is an obvious risk factor (Fig. 28–2). Similarly, thrombosis of a diseased iliac artery on the side of the transplant may result in sudden loss of renal function, but there often is no clearly identifiable cause. Thrombosis of long-term grafts after intervention such as angiography (Nerstrom *et al.*, 1972) or attempted angioplasty is commoner than spontaneous renal artery thrombosis. The diagnosis is relatively simple using isotopic scanning, duplex scanning and biopsy. Occasionally, renal tissue viability may be preserved by a polar artery (Fig. 28–2) and may be confirmed by a biopsy directed to the affected part of the kidney; if biopsy confirms infarction, nephrectomy is advisable.

RENAL VEIN THROMBOSIS

Venous thrombosis has been noted to occur in the early phase after transplantation in 4 (Nerstrom *et al.*, 1972) to 6%

(Jones *et al.*, 1988) of cases. The possible link with cyclosporine therapy already has been described, and technical factors, such as twists on the vein and placing the vein too low such that the graft and vein are compressed, are discussed at the beginning of this section. Occasionally a perfectly functioning graft undergoes sudden torsion, with occlusion of the vein and subsequent thrombosis. The clinical features vary, with the effect on urine output ranging from primary nonfunction similar to that seen with arterial thrombosis to sudden loss of urine output and rising creatinine in an otherwise perfectly functioning graft. The peak incidence is at 3 to 9 days (Nerstrom *et al.*, 1972). The clinical signs are striking, with often severe pain resulting from rapid local graft swelling: Presumably the pain arises from the stretching of surrounding tissues rather than the graft itself. The leg on the side of the graft anastomosis also may swell rapidly. The diagnosis is confirmed by a finding of nonperfusion on an isotope renogram or a color duplex examination, and the ultrasound scan shows a swollen graft, with often considerable perigraft hemorrhage.

If graft vein thrombosis is diagnosed early enough, there are well-documented cases of successful evacuation of venous clot with subsequent long-term function (Nerstrom *et al.*, 1972). The window of opportunity for this approach is probably within 1 hour of the thrombotic event, however, and by the time the diagnosis becomes clear the graft often is not salvageable. Whenever the diagnosis is made, surgery always should be undertaken as an emergency because apart from the necessity to relieve the pain, delay is associated with an increasing risk of graft rupture, which may result in catastrophic graft hemorrhage (Kootstra *et al.*, 1974; Lord *et al.*, 1973). Renal vein thrombosis was not recognized previously as a cause of allograft rupture, which usually was ascribed to acute irreversible rejection with patent vessels (Lord *et al.*, 1973), but since the advent of cyclosporine, renal vein thrombosis has become the commonest cause of rupture (Richardson *et al.*, 1990a, 1990b).

At operation, the graft usually is grossly swollen, purple and clearly nonviable with clot palpable in the renal vein and often in the iliac vein. Early capsular tears, harbingers of full rupture, are common (Fig. 28–3). Vascular clamps should be reapplied to the iliac vein, and clot should be removed from the renal vein and adjacent iliac vein through a venotomy in the renal vein above the anastomosis. It may be worth closing the venotomy and allowing the kidney time to reperfuse, but if the appearance does not improve, the graft should be removed.

Late thrombosis of the graft renal vein is a rare but well-recognized cause of deteriorating function. In some cases, there is swelling of the graft, which occasionally grows slowly to a dramatic size, but in most cases, the graft is confined by the tough fibrous false capsule that develops around most kidney transplants, and there are no other symptoms. A relatively constant finding is the sudden development of severe proteinuria. The diagnosis is confirmed by

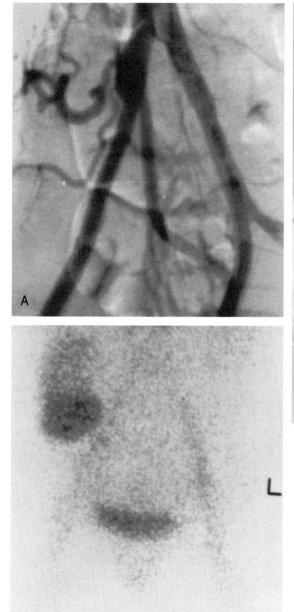

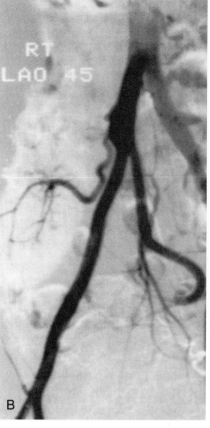

FIGURE 28–2

(A) Angiogram of a right renal transplant shows tight renal artery stenosis of a large upper polar vessel arising from an aortic patch with a smaller lower polar artery arising from the same patch. (B) Later angiogram of the same patient as in A shows thrombosis of upper polar vessel but continued perfusion of the lower polar artery. (C) Isotope perfusion scan of the same patient as in A and B shows continued perfusion of the upper lobe of the transplant kidney. The kidney was salvaged successfully by saphenous vein bypass to the distal upper pole vessel.

findings of severe edema on biopsy, and venography with selective venous catheterization may be diagnostic as well as allow therapeutic thrombolysis therapy after pushing the catheter into the clot. Surgical intervention has little to offer in terms of restoration of graft function, although eventual nephrectomy may become necessary.

OTHER VENOUS THROMBOEMBOLISM

Femoroiliac segment venous thrombosis can occur alone without affecting renal function and has been described in one series as being present in 10% of cases (Nerstrom et al., 1972), when usually the side ipsilateral to the kidney was affected, with contralateral thrombosis being less common and bilateral thrombosis being rare. Venous thrombosis at sites other than the graft and iliac vessels is not unusual in renal transplant recipients. A study from Oxford found an overall incidence of 8% (Allen et al., 1987). There were two

peaks of incidence (Fig. 28–4). The first peak was during the perioperative period and first month and presumably was related to the usual operative and bed rest factors. The second peak occurred in the fourth month, perhaps related to the rising hematocrit that is usual in patients with a functioning graft at that time. From 4 months onward, sporadic thromboembolic events were seen with an even distribution. Overall, 60% of patients manifested a predisposing factor, such as the development of a lymphocele or infection. Although spontaneous deep vein thrombosis can occur in ambulatory patients, the risk is insufficient to justify routine anticoagulation in all patients. Any kidney transplant patient admitted to the hospital has a high risk of deep vein thrombosis and thromboembolism, however, and the use of routine subcutaneous heparin therapy and antiembolism stockings is recommended in all patients admitted to the hospital 3 months after successful transplantation. Any patient developing signs of deep vein thrombosis or pulmonary embolism

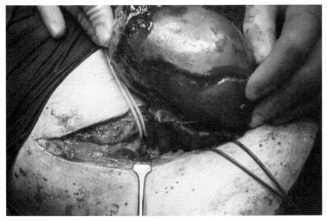

FIGURE 28–3

Photograph taken at operation for acute renal vein thrombosis. An early capsule rupture is present. (See color plate.)

should have this confirmed by either ultrasound or venography and either ventilation-perfusion scans or pulmonary angiography and be treated by anticoagulation with heparin, and then with warfarin anticoagulation in the standard manner.

ACCESS THROMBOSIS

The maintenance of a functioning dialysis access site is important after transplantation because many grafts fail to function initially and may fail altogether later, necessitating a return to dialysis. The thrombotic tendency noted in the discussion on renal graft artery thrombosis probably extends to vascular access sites, and thrombosis of dialysis shunts and fistulae is a common event after transplantation. These problems are preventable to some extent by careful attention to hydration during the operative procedure, avoidance of direct pressure to fistulae by wrapping the limb in cotton wool during anesthesia and not using the fistula limb for blood pressure measurement or intravenous infusion. Postoperatively the access site should be checked regularly to confirm it is still patent, and if thrombosis occurs, urgent thromboembolectomy, if necessary under local anesthetic, often restores flow.

Lymphocele

INCIDENCE

The lymphatic drainage of the leg follows closely the course of the iliac vessels, and some lymphatics inevitably are divided when the vessels are mobilized for arterial anastomosis. Considering the frequency with which the iliac vessels are exposed in routine vascular operations and the rarity of lymphatic complications, it came as a surprise when the severity of lymphatic leakage after renal transplantation first was appreciated (Diethelm, 1972; Inocencio et al., 1969; Madura et al., 1970; Zinke et al., 1975). Although the occurrence of lymphocele was well recognized after operations such as lymphadenectomy (Byron et al., 1966), early reports after kidney transplantation, based on clinical presentation, variously estimated the incidence in large series to be around 2% (Schweizer et al., 1972; Zinke et al., 1975), with occasional reports of incidence of 18% (Braun et al., 1974). The advent of ultrasound for routine examination of the graft caused the average figure to be revised to 10% of grafts (Morris et al., 1978) and led to the realization that many lymphatic collections remain subclinical; 50% of patients may show a small (<50 ml) collection on ultrasound scanning after renal transplantation (Pollak et al., 1988), and most resolve spontaneously. The lymphatic origin was confirmed in early studies by biochemical analysis showing the electrolyte content to be similar to that of serum with a low protein content and microscopy showing lymphocytes in the fluid (Inocencio et al., 1969; Madura et al., 1970).

ETIOLOGY

The obvious suspected source of lymphatic leakage after kidney transplantation is the graft itself. The normal kidney has a well-developed lymphatic drainage, and lymphatics are divided and usually left unligated when the organ is transplanted. Studies of lymphatic drainage from the transplanted kidney of animals such as the sheep suggested that 10 L a day of lymphatic drainage pass through the lymphatics of a single kidney during allograft rejection (Pedersen and Morris, 1970). Similarly, large amounts of lymph have been shown to be produced from the human renal transplant (Hamburger et al., 1971). It came as a surprise when studies of injected radiopaque dyes and radiolabeled substances suggested that most lymphoceles originated from leakage of

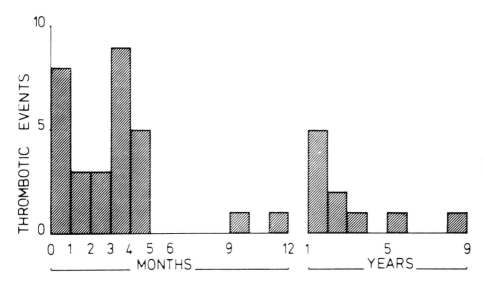

FIGURE 28–4

Time of diagnosis of thrombotic events after renal transplantation. (Reproduced with permission of Allen et al., 1987.)

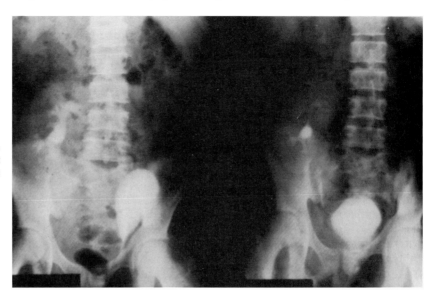

FIGURE 28–5

A lymphocele before (left) and after (right) internal drainage (fenestration). Note the displacement of the bladder and caliceal dilatation, which were corrected after surgery.

lymph from unligated iliac vessel lymphatics of the recipient (Madura *et al.*, 1970; Ward *et al.*, 1978). This finding has led to the recommendation that all lymphatics seen during the iliac dissection should be clipped or tied (not subjected to diathermy—lymph has no clotting factors) (Griffiths *et al.*, 1979), which is the best approach to prevention (Howard *et al.*, 1976).

Why the transplant kidney lymph contributes so little remains unexplained. Presumably the presence of the kidney in some way exacerbates the lymphatic leakage from the iliac vessels: Probably the inflammatory processes associated with the presence of an allograft increase the flow of lymph (Pedersen and Morris, 1970), preventing normal sealing of the vessels or absorption of the fluid, as must occur after other retroperitoneal operations on the iliac vessels. The immunosuppression also may have a role in preventing the normal healing processes from sealing the lymphatic vessels (Greenberg *et al.*, 1985). There is some evidence that the incidence of lymphocele has decreased since the introduction of low-dose steroid regimens. The pressure inside a lymphocele does not appear to have been recorded in the literature but is easily sufficient to produce compression of the ureter and iliac veins if these are located adjacent to the wall of the collection (Braun *et al.*, 1974). The occurrence of lymphocele after trauma has been described (Pernthaler *et al.*, 1991; Roney and Wellington, 1985).

PRESENTATION

As noted earlier (Pollak *et al.*, 1988), routine ultrasound examination of grafts has shown that most lymphoceles are less than 3 cm in diameter, contain less than 100 ml of lymph and are clinically silent, resolving spontaneously with time. Larger collections may present clinically and usually do so at 2 weeks to 6 months after transplantation, the peak incidence being at 6 weeks (Pollak *et al.*, 1988). The commonest presentation is of deteriorating renal function in the presence of perigraft swelling and ipsilateral painless leg edema. Many presentations have been recognized, including hypertension, pain, fever, urinary frequency (Braun *et al.*, 1974; Schweizer *et al.*, 1972), infection (Greenberg *et al.*, 1985) and ipsilateral thrombophlebitis (Braun *et al.*, 1974). Presentation after trauma (Roney and Wellington, 1985) and late presentation 8 years posttransplantation also has been described (DeCamp and Tilney, 1988; Thompson and Neale, 1989).

DIAGNOSIS

Although renal scintigraphy has been shown to be capable of detecting large lymphoceles (Bingham *et al.*, 1978), ultrasound examination is the key to diagnosis (Pollak *et al.*, 1988) and usually can distinguish a lymphocele from blood clot collections by the characteristic homogeneity and distinctive shape and position (van Sonnenberg *et al.*, 1986; Fig. 28–5). The distinction of an infected lymphocele from a noninfected lymphocele is important clinically because the treatment of infection should be by external drainage rather than internal fenestration. Infection is detectable by the presence of a complex echo pattern within the cavity (Ridge *et al.*, 1987). Most lymphoceles occur inferior to the lower pole of the transplant kidney but are clearly separate from the bladder, which can be confirmed easily, if necessary, by passage of a urinary catheter and repeat ultrasound. The examination also may show whether the lymphocele is producing obstruction of the ureter with dilated calices. The diagnosis can be confirmed by ultrasound-guided drainage, allowing biochemical and cytological analysis of the fluid consistent with the presence of lymph. Adjunctive radiological procedures, such as computed tomography, nuclear magnetic resonance scanning and intravenous urography, are unnecessary except in complicated or unclear cases.

TREATMENT

As mentioned earlier, prevention by careful ligation of lymphatics during the iliac dissection is better than cure (Griffiths *et al.*, 1979; Howard *et al.*, 1976). Ultrasound-guided drainage provides not only diagnosis, but also initial treatment, which allows relief of urinary obstruction and restoration of renal function, in effect taking the urgency out of the situation. Small symptomless collections are common, as noted earlier, and usually resolve if left alone (Pollak *et al.*, 1988). Although simple aspiration is sometimes curative (Greenberg *et al.*, 1985; Pollak *et al.*, 1988) and may be repeated on several occasions, the likelihood of spontaneous resolution becomes small after three aspirations followed by recurrence (Pollak *et al.*, 1988); every aspiration brings a small risk of infection (Pollak *et al.*, 1988).

Prolonged external drainage, open (Zaontz and Firlit, 1988) or through a percutaneously inserted catheter (Burgos *et al.*, 1988; Cohan *et al.*, 1987), has been advocated by some but involves a long hospital stay and an increased infection risk. Injection of sclerosants has been described. Tetracycline did not appear to be effective (Pollak *et al.*, 1988), but the injection of povidone-iodine in association with external drainage has been claimed to be effective (Burgos *et al.*, 1988; Gilliland *et al.*, 1989; Teruel *et al.*, 1983). The failure rate of povidone-iodine injection has been reported to be less than 11%, but the technique has the drawback of taking 20 to 30 days before drainage ceases (Teruel *et al.*, 1983), which may not be significantly less than the effect of simple drainage alone, and there has been no randomized comparison of the two approaches. The risk of infection also remains.

The operation of choice has been called incorrectly *marsupialization* by some (Greenberg *et al.*, 1985; Howard *et al.*, 1976) but is known correctly as *unroofing* (Byron *et al.*, 1966) or as *fenestration*. This operation can be achieved by reopening the transplant wound or preferably through a lower midline abdominal incision and a transperitoneal approach to the lymphocele. The lymphocele is seen at operation to bulge into the peritoneal cavity, and it is normally an easy matter to create a 5-cm opening between the two, taking care to avoid damage to any structures that may be running between the wall of the collection and the peritoneum, bearing in mind the inconstant anatomy of the transplanted structures. Simple incision of the wall between the cavities is followed by a small but significant recurrence rate. To avoid recurrence, various authors have recommended maneuvers such as excision of a 5-cm disk of the wall of the lymphocele, oversewing the edges and mobilizing the omentum, which then is stitched down into the graft (Bry *et al.*, 1990). A novel suggestion is to use the peritoneal dialysis catheter, if still in place, as a stent into the cyst cavity (Nicholson and Veitch, 1990). Routine fenestration at the end of the transplant operation has been suggested as a prophylactic measure in children (Zaontz *et al.*, 1988).

There has been considerable interest in the use of laparoscopic surgery to excise a disk from the lymphocele wall, fenestrating the lymphocele into the peritoneal cavity. First described in 1991 by McCullough *et al.*, many case reports followed. Sufficient numbers have accumulated in larger centers to justify publication of results of reasonably large series (Lledo Garcia *et al.*, 1996; Melvin *et al.*, 1997).

As in other fields in which laparoscopy has been introduced, perhaps a little too enthusiastically, there have been descriptions of disaster, the most at-risk structure being the transplant ureter (Shokeir *et al.*, 1994). It is sometimes easy to confuse the swelling made by the extraperitoneal kidney with that made by the lymphocele, and the useful role of intraoperative ultrasound in avoiding that problem has been stressed (Melvin *et al.*, 1997), allowing a perfect outcome record. If intraoperative ultrasound is not available, however, it is the author's opinion that a deeply placed lower pole lymphocele is treated more safely by an open operative approach.

COMPLICATIONS

Most lymphoceles are treated without complications, but infection can be a difficult problem, especially with organisms such as yeast in severely immunosuppressed patients. Prolonged surgical drainage and antimicrobial therapy are likely to be necessary. Lymphoceles that compress the renal or iliac veins may predispose to venous thrombosis, with the features noted earlier.

Graft Renal Arterial Disease
RENAL ARTERY STENOSIS

In the early days of transplantation, the kidneys used for transplantation, whether from live or cadaveric donors, were

always free of significant arterial disease, and the first descriptions of graft arterial stenosis after transplantation caused some surprise (Hume, 1968; Morris *et al.*, 1971; Newton *et al.*, 1967; Smellie *et al.*, 1969). Subsequently, all transplant centers began to recognize the problem. Early series variously suggested an incidence of 1% (Margules *et al.*, 1973), 3% (Smellie *et al.*, 1969), 10% (Munda *et al.*, 1977) and 12% (Lacombe, 1975). Series in the late 1980s quoted incidences of 1.5% (Roberts *et al.*, 1989), 4% (Hohnke *et al.*, 1987) and 7% (Benoit *et al.*, 1987; Greenstein *et al.*, 1987). The reason for the varied incidence is uncertain but may relate to the problems of retrospective surveys, and there is some difficulty in comparing reports because some units have a more liberal policy for angiography to determine renal artery stenosis than others (Kincaid-Smith *et al.*, 1969; Morris *et al.*, 1971), and the exact definition of what constitutes stenosis varies. Some studies that have described the results of arteriography on all functioning grafts have shown renal artery stenosis in 23% of patients examined (Lacombe, 1975), confirming that radiological stenoses often do not represent a functional stenosis.

Etiology

The fact that the early reports of graft arterial stenosis were in kidneys from young donors without vascular disease excluded the possibility of preexisting disease progressing more rapidly because of the transplantation process (Smellie *et al.*, 1969), although today, with older donors, this may be a factor in some cases. Damage to the renal artery during retrieval, usually as a result of undue traction on the kidney, may result in an intimal fracture, which subsequently may present as a renal artery stenosis, or similarly intimal damage may be produced by cannulation during perfusion. Sometimes the problem arises because of the propensity for the excessively long renal artery (usually on a right kidney) to kink if the kidney has to be placed too close to the anastomosis (Morris *et al.*, 1971). This situation is particularly likely if the renal vein is short and is another reason for dividing the internal iliac vein to allow more mobility of the implanted kidney.

Other technical errors include poor anastomotic technique, particularly in the case of end-to-end anastomoses of the internal iliac artery to the renal artery or if an atheromatous plaque is present in the recipient vessel at the origin (Munda *et al.*, 1977). Another possible causative factor is clamp damage to the renal artery, although this must be rare because most surgeons are aware of the possibility and have no need to clamp the renal artery directly in most transplant operations.

Severe acute rejection can affect the renal artery (Morris *et al.*, 1971), but most cases of renal artery stenosis arise many months after transplantation in grafts with previously good function, and the process is acquired after the initial phase of transplantation. Histological examination of most excised lesions reveals extensive fibrous endarteritis and intimal thickening (Lacombe, 1975). Although the cause of these changes has been suggested to be subintimal dissection or perfusion cannula damage (Smellie *et al.*, 1969), the most likely explanation is that the graft artery is subject to chronic immune attack, possibly antibody mediated, with subsequent fibrosis and atheroma formation. In support of this idea, the incidence of renal artery stenosis in live donor kidney recipients is lower, approximately half that seen in cadaveric cases (Lacombe, 1975). This theory fails to explain why the lesions often are localized to one area of the artery, and an alternative explanation, that of disturbed hemodynamics, is possible (Morris *et al.*, 1971), perhaps combined with the effects of rejection (Kincaid-Smith *et al.*, 1969). One study

(Morris *et al.*, 1971) found that renal artery stenosis was particularly common after end-to-side compared with end-to-end anastomosis and suggested this was due to turbulent flow adjacent to the end-to-side anatomosis. A subsequent study found renal artery stenosis to be commoner after end-to-end anastomosis, however (Munda *et al.*, 1977).

Presentation

The usual time of presentation is 3 months to 2 years after transplantation, with a peak incidence at 6 months (Lacombe, 1975), and the usual mode of presentation is increasingly severe hypertension with or without a rising creatinine level. Polycythemia has been claimed to be associated with graft renal artery stenosis (Schramek *et al.*, 1975), but this has been disputed by others (Ulrych and Langford, 1975). The mechanism for production of hypertension is thought to be similar to the mechanism that operates in the native kidney with renal artery stenosis—involvement of the renin-angiotensin axis. The advent of angiotensin-converting enzyme (ACE) inhibitors such as captopril and enalapril as treatment for hypertension has introduced a new presentation, with sudden, often dramatic deterioration in renal function after introduction of ACE inhibitors (Curtis *et al.*, 1983; see Chapter 30). Some patients may become profoundly hypotensive with complete anuria, especially if full doses of the drugs are used. For this reason, ACE inhibitor treatment for hypertension always must be introduced at a low dose, preferably in the hospital or under constant close supervision, and the patient must have renal function checked within the following 3 days and regularly during the subsequent weeks. A second classic presentation is the development of sudden left ventricular failure for no obvious reason. The electrocardiogram often shows no abnormality other than left ventricular strain pattern.

Clinical examination may reveal the presence of a bruit, a sign that originally was claimed to be present in 100% of cases (Smellie *et al.*, 1969), although it is now recognized that the sensitivity and specificity of this sign are poor, and renal artery stenosis can be present with no audible bruit (Lacombe, 1975). Normal femoral pulses always should be sought because occlusive aortoiliac disease may mimic graft arterial stenosis (see later). The graft may be somewhat small on palpation, but this usually is not clinically evident.

Diagnosis

The key to diagnosis is to consider the possibility of renal artery stenosis in all patients with deteriorating function and/or sudden onset of hypertension or hypertension requiring more drug therapy to control. This diagnosis is not difficult in patients who were previously normotensive with good graft function, but many patients remain hypertensive after transplantation, and many have suboptimal function as a result of rejection episodes. The progression of hypertension to the requirement of four drugs to control blood pressure in conjunction with gradually deteriorating graft function may happen slowly and be ascribed to continuing chronic rejection, when renal artery stenosis is the cause. All patients with deteriorating graft function should undergo ultrasound examination to exclude urinary obstruction, and a biopsy is then advisable. In the presence of renal artery stenosis, signs of rejection are likely to be absent, and the renal structure likely is to be preserved better than the degree of functional deterioration would suggest. The classic features of glomerular crowding are seen rarely (M. Dunnill, 1993, personal communication).

The deleterious effect of ACE inhibitor administration for hypertension, mentioned previously, can be used judiciously as a diagnostic test for the presence of renal artery stenosis (Hricik, 1987). Sudden deterioration in renal function with improved blood pressure control is highly suggestive of renal artery stenosis. Some cases are less dramatic, and the deterioration in renal function may become obvious only after 2 to 3 weeks. The absence of any deterioration in graft function on full-dose ACE inhibitor therapy is good evidence that significant graft arterial stenosis is not present, particularly if the hypertension has been well controlled by ACE inhibitor therapy.

Despite some early enthusiastic reports (Lindsey *et al.*, 1975), in general the measurement of renal vein renin values has not been of assistance in making the diagnosis (Gupta *et al.*, 1976; Lacombe, 1975). The addition of an ACE inhibitor challenge was reported to improve the diagnostic value of plasma renin measurements (Holdaas *et al.*, 1988), but a prospective study failed to confirm this view; the specificity of the test was 75% and the sensitivity 67%, too low to recommend this as a useful test (Erley *et al.*, 1992). The reason why renin measurement is inaccurate may be that most patients are on multiple antihypertensive drugs when the possible diagnosis is raised, and the frequent presence of the patient's own kidneys complicates the situation further. Isotope renography with the addition of ACE inhibitor therapy has been recommended as a diagnostic test (Miach *et al.*, 1989), but a prospective study showed the test has a sensitivity of 75% and specificity of 67% and cannot be recommended as a diagnostic test (Erley *et al.*, 1992).

Radiological Diagnosis

Angiography or, more accurately, digital subtraction angiography, remains the gold standard for diagnosis of transplant renal artery stenosis, being diagnostic in 93% of cases (Arlart, 1985). It is invasive, however, and there has been a considerable effort to replace angiography with a noninvasive or relatively noninvasive test.

Duplex ultrasound scanning, particularly with the addition of color flow display, has been investigated by several groups for diagnosis of graft renal artery stenosis (Murphy *et al.*, 1987; Taylor *et al.*, 1987). One study examined 88 transplants by duplex scanning and diagnosed renal artery stenosis in seven patients, six of whom (85%) turned out to have stenotic lesions (Taylor *et al.*, 1987). A prospective comparison with other noninvasive tests for transplant renal artery stenosis reported a sensitivity for color duplex scanning of 100% and a specificity of 75%, suggesting the test has value for screening (bearing in mind the operator dependency), but arteriographic confirmation still is required because the positive predictive value was only 56% (Erley *et al.*, 1992). Many centers use this test as a noninvasive screen for less clear-cut cases.

The advent of sophisticated tests such as computed tomography, spiral computed tomography and magnetic resonance imaging with gadolinium enhancement has improved the accuracy of assessment of vasculature such that native renal arteries can be imaged as accurately as with angiography, for example, in potential live kidney donors (Bakker *et al.*, 1999; Dachman *et al.*, 1998; Tello *et al.*, 1998). The variable anatomy of the transplant kidney presents a more formidable challenge and until recently neither computed tomography nor magnetic resonance imaging gave sufficiently reliable results to replace angiography (Loubeyre *et al.*, 1996). Technical improvements in imaging combined with the addition of gadolinium enhancement to magnetic resonance imaging has improved vascular imaging, however, and it has been suggested that a degree of accuracy now can be obtained to

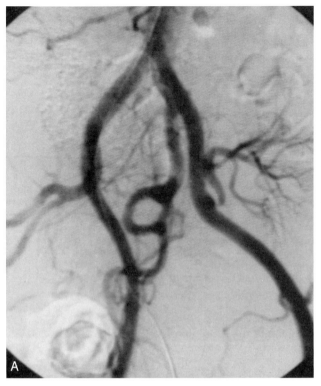

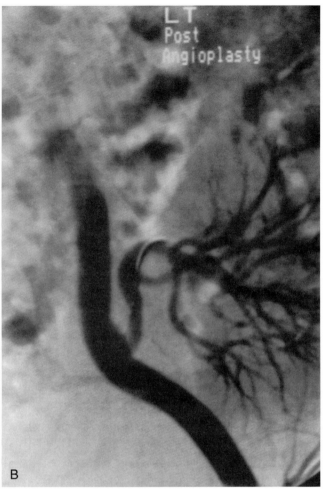

FIGURE 28–6

(A) Angiogram shows tight renal artery stenosis at the origin of the renal artery to a left-sided renal transplant. Oblique views were needed to show the stenosis. (B) Successful angioplasty of same stenosis as in A.

replace angiography for diagnosis of transplant renal artery stenosis (Bakker *et al.*, 1998; Johnson *et al.*, 1997). A multicenter prospective randomized trial is not available, however, and such evidence may be required before most centers change to magnetic resonance imaging as the gold standard.

The diagnostic investigation of choice remains selective graft arterial catheterization and angiography (Erley *et al.*, 1992), although 50% of hypertensive transplant patients show abnormalities of the renal artery if subjected to angiography (Morris *et al.*, 1971; Smellie *et al.*, 1969). For this reason, apart from the invasive nature of the investigation, angiography should be reserved for patients with features that are compatible with graft artery stenosis, such as poorly controlled hypertension and/or deteriorating renal function with or without a bruit (Morris *et al.*, 1971). Because of the variable anatomy of the transplant vasculature, the catheterization and interpretation are often difficult, and the procedure should be performed by the femoral route by an experienced radiologist, preferably using digital subtraction angiography. Multiple angled views should be taken before a lesion can be excluded (Fig. 28–6). The injection of contrast material directly into the graft renal artery has been associated with sudden deterioration in graft function in the past, and it has been recommended that as little contrast material as possible be used, although this risk is slight if the newer nonionic contrast media are used (Barrett *et al.*, 1992). Injection of contrast material should not be used as an excuse for performing a less than adequate examination.

The major problem in diagnosis is establishing that a

radiological stenosis is truly a functional stenosis. The presence of hypertension, deteriorating renal function, perhaps a positive response to ACE inhibitors, and a biopsy specimen relatively free of the changes of chronic rejection all support the diagnosis of a functional stenosis requiring treatment. Final proof when there is doubt can be obtained by measuring the pressure gradient across the stenosis: A drop of greater than 20 mm is significant (Nahman *et al.*, 1994)

Treatment

Three options are available: conservative treatment, transluminal angioplasty with or without stenting and surgery. If the stenosis is relatively minor and the blood pressure controllable with reasonable levels of medication yet the creatinine remains stable at a level of less than 200 μmol/L, it is reasonable to continue with conservative management: Deterioration is not inevitable, and some patients appear to improve. The conservative option becomes particularly attractive if the lesion is unsuitable for angioplasty or angioplasty is tried and fails.

The success of transluminal angioplasty for lesions in the coronary and peripheral circulation led to hopes that the technique would provide the answer for graft arterial stenosis. Early reports of success were encouraging (Greenstein *et al.*, 1987; Grossman *et al.*, 1982; Sniderman *et al.*, 1980), but more recent studies have modified this enthusiasm (Roberts *et al.*, 1989). Follow-up series have reported that transluminal angioplasty of graft renal artery stenosis is successful initially in 60 to 80% of those attempted (Benoit *et al.*, 1987; Clements *et al.*, 1987; Greenstein *et al.*, 1987; Hohnke *et al.*, 1987; Roberts *et al.*, 1989). Earlier reports were the most optimistic; one study described a 76% initial success rate with few complications and no recurrence of the stenosis at 30 months (Greenstein *et al.*, 1987). Other series have agreed with this finding (Clements *et al.*, 1987; Greenstein *et al.*, 1987; Hohnke *et al.*, 1987; Sniderman *et al.*, 1980; Thomas *et al.*, 1992), although some noted a higher recurrence rate of 33% at 2 years (Benoit *et al.*, 1987). A further study from a large center described an entirely different experience, with initial success in only 58% of cases and a recurrence rate of 16% (Roberts *et al.*, 1989). Technical complications of angioplasty were 21% with graft loss and/or mortality in 9%. This latter study has introduced a note of caution into the use of angioplasty for graft renal artery stenosis.

In part, the difference in the success rates quoted may reflect a differing definition of *success* in terms of improvement versus cure of hypertension and improved graft function. Another explanation may be the type of lesion treated in different series. Most authors agree that the most suitable lesions for angioplasty are localized stenoses of the main renal artery distal to the anastomosis (Fig. 28–7); these are the majority of lesions treated in the most successful series. The poor results come from a series in which almost all the stenoses appeared to occur at the anastomosis itself, in which dilatation was associated with a poor success rate and high risk of complication (Roberts *et al.*, 1989). Although one report described successful angioplasty of perianastomotic graft artery strictures (Greenstein *et al.*, 1987), a poor outcome corresponds with the experience of most vascular centers in dilating perianastomotic strictures at other sites, although there are exceptions (Fig. 28–7).

Because of the aforementioned findings, the recommendation now is that the lesions most suitable for graft arterial angioplasty are localized lesions more than 1 cm from the anastomosis. Lesions close to or at the anastomosis are not as easy to dilate successfully and are associated with a high risk of rupture. Such lesions should be considered for angioplasty only in circumstances in which a surgical alternative is difficult or graft loss would be an acceptable risk. Other lesions thought to be unsuitable are long diffuse stenoses, particularly those that extend into the branches of the renal artery. Even in centers that have fairly successful angioplasty programs, complications such as rupture or thrombosis occur in 10% (Benoit *et al.*, 1987), and the patient always should be aware of the possibility of graft loss. It is wise not to undertake graft angioplasty unless operating facilities are available for immediate reconstruction in the event of complications.

Coronary angioplasty has been enhanced significantly by the use of expandable intraluminal stents, and the use of stents for transplant renal artery stenosis, especially recurrent stenosis, is becoming common. The results reported are still anecdotal (Chan *et al.*, 1995; Newman-Sanders *et al.*, 1995; Nicita *et al.*, 1998; Sierre *et al.*, 1998) but are sufficiently encouraging to allow recommendation of a stent as treatment for stenoses that have recurred more than once.

The final alternative is surgical correction. This surgery should not be undertaken lightly because the procedure can be one of the most difficult operations in vascular surgery (Osborn *et al.*, 1976), owing to the variable anatomy and extensive fibrosis that occurs around the allograft kidney.

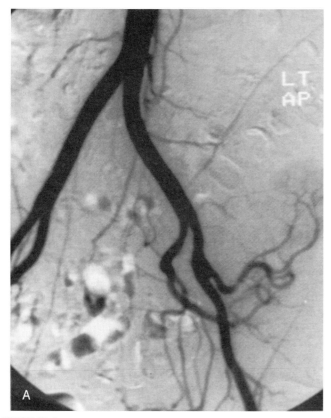
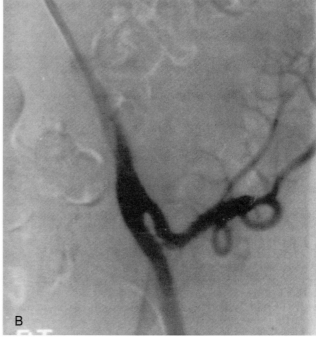

FIGURE 28–7

(A) Stenosis at the midpoint of the renal artery of a left-sided renal transplant. This lesion is eminently suitable for angioplasty. (B) Successful angioplasty of same stenosis as in A.

Surgical alternatives include local resection of the stenosed area, vein patch angioplasty or vein graft interposition (Lacombe, 1975; Margules et al., 1973). A difficult problem is maintenance of kidney viability while the vessel is nonperfused because in contrast to surgery for renal artery stenosis in the native kidney, there are few capsular vessels to maintain viability during arterial clamping. Cooling the kidney in situ is not a practical option, and most surgeons rely on a speedy anastomosis.

Retransplantation of the same graft is a theoretical possibility, although none of the reported series have used this technique. Surgery should be undertaken only for graft arterial stenosis if the other alternatives of angioplasty or conservative treatment are not appropriate. The earliest reports of surgery for graft arterial stenosis claimed a near 100% success rate (Lacombe, 1975; Margules et al., 1973) with no subsequent recurrence of the lesion. Later series described initial success rates of 66% (Smith et al., 1976), 72% (Roberts et al., 1989) and 75% (Hohnke et al., 1987), although a cautionary note came from one center where only 33% of operative corrections were successful. Long-term follow-up indicates that lesions can recur after surgery in 12% of cases (Benoit et al., 1987), and some patients may require repeat procedures that may be more difficult.

Despite the enthusiasm with which some surgeons have recommended surgical treatment (rather than angioplasty) for graft arterial stenosis (Roberts et al., 1989), most centers agree that angioplasty is the procedure of first choice for most patients, if the lesion appears suitable on angiography. Surgery can be successful and probably gives better results than angioplasty (Benoit et al., 1987), but it is a difficult operation with a risk of graft loss. Occasionally, retransplantation may be a simpler alternative, and hypertension may resolve completely, making it not always necessary to remove the first graft.

RENAL ARTERY ANEURYSM

Most aneurysms that occur after renal transplantation are false aneurysms resulting from anastomotic dehiscence (Fig. 28–8). In some cases, subsequent evidence of local infection is found, and these are truly mycotic, but infection may not always be present. A well-recognized risk factor for aneurysm rupture in other sites is pregnancy, and such cases have been recognized in transplant patients (Richardson et al., 1990c). Any transplant patient who is pregnant should undergo regular ultrasound scanning of the fetus with the radiologist aware of the possibility of graft arterial aneurysm. Presentation may be as an asymptomatic lesion found on ultrasound examination, local pain and pressure symptoms resulting from expansion or rupture. In the case of rupture, urgent repair is necessary to save the patient's life, and the graft is rarely salvaged. If the aneurysm is recognized before rupture, elective repair using a vein graft may be possible, but if mycotic aneurysm is present, graft nephrectomy with ligation of the recipient vessels and replacement with an autogenous vein graft is the most prudent course to avoid repeated anastomotic dehiscence from infection. Ligation is particularly appropriate if the presentation is with massive hemorrhage from the anastomosis owing to infection (Kyriakides et al., 1976; Owens et al., 1979) and is usually tolerated without limb ischemia.

Aneurysms resulting from traumatic arteriovenous fistula formation within the kidney substance are common because of repeated needle core biopsy and are shown easily with the advent of color duplex ultrasonography (Hubsch et al., 1990). Occasionally, duplex scanning may detect a fistula between the main vessels (Taylor et al., 1987). The widespread

introduction of smaller needle core biopsy systems using spring-loaded biopsy machines probably has lowered the incidence of this complication. Arteriovenous fistulae within the kidney usually are asymptomatic, although an impressive bruit may be present on auscultation. Expansion is unusual, perhaps because of the constricting fibrotic capsule that surrounds most transplant kidneys. In most cases, conservative management is advocated. Occasionally, heavy hematuria may require intervention with selective arterial catheterization and embolization.

Other Arterial Surgery in the Renal Transplant Patient
GENERAL ASPECTS

Several factors conspire to increase the likelihood of coexistent vascular disease in the renal transplant recipient (Ibels et al., 1977). Patients with functioning grafts performed two or more decades ago are becoming elderly, and an increasing number of candidates for transplantation are elderly. Vascular disease is more frequent with increasing age; an increasingly common cause of kidney failure requiring dialysis and transplantation in the elderly is renovascular occlusion secondary to atheroma. An increasing proportion of patients is receiving grafts for renal failure secondary to diabetes, and the progression of microvascular and macrovascular disease is not halted by transplantation. The severity of peripheral vascular disease has been shown to vary with coronary vascular lesions in this group (Manske et al., 1997). As is discussed in Chapter 30, transplant patients in general have considerably increased risk factors for vascular disease, including hyperlipidemia and hypertension (Ibels et al., 1977). The high incidence of atherosclerosis may not be attributable only to traditional risk factors such as hyperlipidemia, however (Barbagallo et al., 1999). All transplant patients should be encouraged to give up smoking, but some continue despite advice, adding to the already considerable danger of vascular disease. The result of these multiple risk factors is an incidence of vascular disease that is eight times higher than an age-matched population (Ibels et al., 1977), and cardiovascular mortality is the major cause of premature death in the renal transplant population.

In general, the management of vascular disease follows established practice: however, there are some general points to remember regarding investigation and treatment of vascular disease in the transplant patient. There is an impression, unsubstantiated by hard evidence to date, that vascular disease in the transplant (and renal) patient tends to be severe, with more distal disease and extensive calcification reducing the likelihood of success from maneuvers such as transluminal angioplasty. Angiography often is more difficult because of vascular calcification and usually should be performed from the opposite side to avoid the transplant renal artery. The dangers of contrast infusion already have been alluded to. Transplant patients with dry gangrene—for example, in the toes—are less likely to demarcate and autoamputate than nontransplant patients, and the likelihood of spreading infection is higher. An expectant policy should be undertaken only with a high degree of supervision, particularly in the diabetic.

Patients submitted to surgery may be more prone to infection and poor wound healing, especially if they have been taking steroids for many years (Gouny et al., 1991). Prophylactic antibiotic use is mandatory for all procedures. The danger of infection tends to preclude use of synthetic grafts in situations such as femoropopliteal bypass, and the use of a contralateral leg vein or arm vein may be justified.

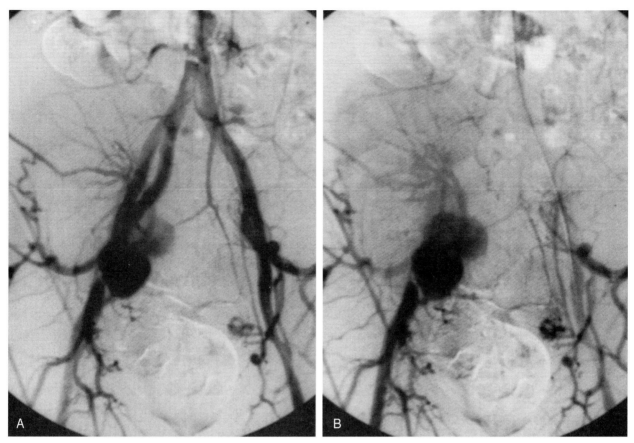

FIGURE 28–8

(A and B) Consecutive films from an angiogram in a patient with deteriorating graft function show a false anastomotic aneurysm, which was found to be due to infection at operation. The graft was removed at surgery.

Consideration should be given to staging of procedures (Gouny, *et al.*, 1991). Lastly, the transplant kidney is exquisitely sensitive to dehydration and hypotension. Great care must be taken during anesthesia for any surgery to ensure that these pitfalls are avoided. Mannitol should be given for all but the more minor procedures and the renal function monitored daily after the procedure.

ILIAC AND AORTIC OCCLUSIVE VASCULAR DISEASE

Occlusive disease of the great vessels proximal to the likely anastomosis site of a kidney transplant must be excluded pretransplantation by palpating the femoral pulse, and if in any doubt angiography should be performed. Significant lesions found should be corrected before transplantation (Gouny *et al.*, 1991). Stenotic lesions of the aorta or iliac vessels after kidney transplantation may affect renal function and cause hypertension, mimicking renal artery stenosis. Presumably the mechanism is the same. For this reason, the femoral pulses always should be sought in patients with deteriorating renal function in whom the possibility of renal artery stenosis is being raised. Any doubt about the femoral pulse strength can be resolved by measuring femoral pressures and the response to papaverine injection (Parvin *et al.*, 1985). The results of bypass grafting or endarterectomy in this situation are generally good (Gouny *et al.*, 1991), as are those of transluminal angioplasty (Weigele, 1991).

AORTIC AND ILIAC ARTERY ANEURYSM

Patients presented for transplantation may have preexisting aortoiliac aneurysmal disease, and particularly in the older male population the aorta should be palpated carefully before acceptance on the transplant waiting list. If an aneurysm is found, it should be repaired before transplantation: Successful repair does not preclude a subsequent transplant. The importance of repairing aortic aneurysms before transplantation was shown in Oxford when a patient ruptured a small and unsuspected abdominal aortic aneurysm within days of receiving a renal transplant.

After transplantation, patients have a greater risk of aneurysm formation than the average population. Screening by ultrasound scanning of all patients aged 55 in the Oxford transplant population revealed a prevalence of 3%, which is similar to the results of screening for aneurysm in men older than age 70 in the normal population. The prevalence is high enough to suggest that all transplant patients (men and women) older than age 50 should be screened every 5 years for aortic aneurysm formation. The indications for surgery seem to be similar to those in the ordinary population, with possibly more emphasis on elective repair because the kidney transplant is unlikely to survive the aortic cross-clamping necessary to control a ruptured aortic aneurysm, even if the patient does so. Elective repair is advised for any aneurysm that is larger than 5 cm, growing rapidly or locally tender.

The absence of functioning native kidneys simplifies the procedure to some extent because the aortic cross-clamp can be applied above the renal vessels if necessary, but the functioning transplanted kidney below the aneurysm presents a problem for preserving graft function. Many approaches have been tried to preserve blood flow to the kidney during aortic cross-clamping, including bypass from the aorta above the clamp to the iliac or femoral vessels below, axillofemoral bypass, femorofemoral bypass, hypothermic shunts and a variety of other shunts with or without oxygenators (Lacombe, 1991). One large series has reported the results of simply cross-clamping the aorta and performing rapid graft insertion in 15 cases without permanent loss of graft function, although temporary deterioration was frequent (Lacombe, 1991). The investigators questioned the need for bypass during aortic cross-clamping, showing that there was still continued perfusion of the kidney, although at low pressure, from iliac and lumbar collaterals. The advocates of bypass insertion point out, however, that the no-bypass technique leaves no leeway for error during the graft insertion, and grafts with suboptimal function before the procedure may be damaged more severely or permanently if a shunt is not used.

Patients who have diseased or ligated internal iliac vessels may have little collateral perfusion. In an emergency or when the vascular anatomy is unknown, it may be best to set up bypass if possible. For elective surgery, the choice remains a matter for the personal preference of the surgeon; aorta-to-iliac artery bypass has been the procedure used in Oxford.

Many patients present with an aortic or iliac aneurysm before transplantation, and the usual advice has been for the patient to undergo elective aneurysm repair before renal transplantation. Although this approach is relatively safe, it also is relatively safe to performed a combined aneurysm repair and renal transplant procedure if the patient is to be the recipient of a live donor graft, and this results in reduced time in the hospital and reduced costs (Wright *et al.*, 1991).

REFERENCES

Abramowicz, D., Pradier, O., Marchant, A., *et al.* (1992). Induction of thromboses within renal grafts by high-dose prophylactic OKT3. *Lancet* **339**, 777.

Akyol, A. M., Briggs, J. D., Junor, B. J. R., Rodger, R. S. C., MacPherson, S. G. and Bradley, J. A. (1991). Renal vein thrombosis after cadaveric renal transplantation. Presented to the *Association of Surgeons of Great Britain and Ireland*, Oxford, U.K.

Allen, R. D., Michie, C. A., Murie, J. A. and Morris, P. J. (1987). Deep venous thrombosis after renal transplantation. *Surg. Gynecol. Obstet.* **164**, 137.

Arlart, I. P. (1985). Digital subtraction angiography (DSA) in renal and renovascular hypertension: diagnostic value and application in follow-up studies after PTA. *Uremia Invest.* **9**, 217.

Baker, L. R., Tucker, B. and Kovacs, I. B. (1990). Enhanced in vitro haemostasis and reduced thrombolysis in cyclosporine-treated renal transplant recipients. *Transplantation* **49**, 905.

Bakir, N., Sluiter, W. J., Ploeg, R. J., van Son, W. J. and Tegzess, A. M. (1996). Primary renal graft thrombosis. *Nephrol. Dial. Transplant.* **11**, 140.

Bakker, J., Beek, F. J., Beutler, J. J., *et al.* (1998). Renal artery stenosis and accessory renal arteries: accuracy of detection and visualization with gadolinium-enhanced breath-hold MR angiography. *Radiology* **207**, 497.

Bakker, J., Ligtenberg, G., Beek, F. J., van Reedt Dortland, R. W. and Hene, R. J. (1999). Preoperative evaluation of living renal donors with gadolinium-enhanced magnetic resonance angiography. *Transplantation* **67**, 1167.

Barbagallo, C. M., Pinto, A., Gallo, S., *et al.* (1999). Carotid atherosclerosis in renal transplant recipients: relationships with cardiovascular risk factors and plasma lipoproteins. *Transplantation* **67**, 366.

Barrett, B. J., Parfrey, P. S., Vavasour, H. M., O'Dea, F., Kent, G. and Stone, E. (1992). A comparison of nonionic, low-osmolality radiocontrast agents with ionic, high-osmolality agents during cardiac catheterization. *N. Engl. J. Med.* **326**, 431.

Benoit, G., Hiesse, C., Icard, P., *et al.* (1987). Treatment of renal artery stenosis after renal transplantation. *Transplant. Proc.* **19**, 3600.

Benoit, G., Jaber, N., Moukarzel, M., *et al.* (1994). Incidence of vascular complications in kidney transplantation: is there any interference with the nature of the perfusion solution? *Clin. Transplant.* **8**, 485.

Bergentz, S. E., Bergvist, D., Bornmyr, S., Brunkwall, J. and Husberg, B. (1985). Venous thrombosis and cyclosporin. *Lancet* **2**, 101.

Billet, A., Dagher, F. J. and Queral, L. A. (1982). Surgical correction of vasculogenic impotence in a patient after bilateral renal transplantation. *Surgery* **91**, 108.

Bingham, J. B., Hilson, A. J. and Maisey, M. N. (1978). The appearances of renal transplant lumphoceles during dynamic renal scintigraphy. *Br. J. Radiol.* **5**, 342.

Braun, W. E., Banowsky, L. H., Straffon, R. A., *et al.* (1974). Lymphoceles associated with renal transplantation. *Am. J. Med.* **57**, 714.

Brown, Z. and Neild, G. H. (1987). Cyclosporin inhibits prostacyclin production by cultured human endothelial cells. *Transplant. Proc.* **19**, 1178.

Brown, Z., Neild, G. H., Willoughby, J. J., Somia, N. V. and Cameron, S. J. (1986). Increased Factor VIII as an index of vascular injury in cyclosporin nephrotoxicity. *Transplantation* **42**, 150.

Bry, J., Hull, D., Bartus, S. A. and Schweizer, R. T. (1990). Treatment of recurrent lymphoceles following renal transplantation: remarsupialization with omentoplasty. *Transplantation* **49**, 477.

Burgos, F. J., Teruel, J. L., Mayayo, T. *et al.* (1988). Diagnosis and management of lymphoceles after renal transplantation. *Br. J. Urol.* **61**, 289.

Byron, R. L., Yonemoto, R. H., Davajan, V., *et al.* (1966). Lymphocysts: surgical correction and prevention. *Am. J. Obstet. Gynecol.* **94**, 203.

Chan, H. W., Ho, Y. W., Chan, C. M., Yiu, T. F., Tong, M. K. and Wong, P. H. (1995). Treatment of anastomotic ostial allograft and renal artery stenosis with the Palmaz stent. *Transplantation* **59**, 436.

Clements, R., Evans, C. and Salaman, J. R. (1987). Percutaneous transluminal angioplasty of renal transplant artery stenosis. *Clin. Radiol.* **38**, 235.

Cohan, R. H., Saeed, M., Sussman, S. K., *et al.* (1987). Percutaneous drainage of pelvic lymphatic fluid collections in the renal transplant patient. *Invest. Radiol.* **22**, 864.

Curtis, J. J., Luke, R. G., Whelchel, J. D., Diethelm, A. G., Jones, P. and Dustan, H. P. (1983). Inhibition of angiotensin-converting enzyme in renal-transplant recipients with hypertension. *N. Engl. J. Med.* **308**, 377.

Dachman, A. H., Newmark, G. M., Mitchell, M. T. and Woodle, E. S. (1998). Helical CT examination of potential kidney donors. *A.J.R. Am. J. Roentgenol.* **171**, 193.

DeCamp, M. M. and Tilney, N. L. (1988). Late development of intractable lymphocele after renal transplantation. *Transplant. Proc.* **20**, 105.

Deira, J., Alberca, I., Lerma, J. L., Martin, B. and Tabernero, J. M. (1998). Changes in coagulation and fibrinolysis in the postoperative period immediately after kidney transplantation in patients receiving OKT3 or cyclosporine A as induction therapy. *Am. J. Kidney Dis.* **32**, 575.

Diethelm, A. G. (1972). Anuria secondary to perirenal lymphocele: a complication of renal transplantation. *South. Med. J.* **65**, 350.

Dowling, J. P., D'Apice, A. F. and Kincaid-Smith, P. S. (1986). De novo microangiopathy: occurrence and diagnosis in three transplant patients. *Kidney Int.* **30**, 614.

Ducloux, D., Pellet, E., Fournier, V., *et al.* (1999). Prevalence and clinical significance of antiphospholipid antibodies in renal transplant recipients. *Transplantation* **67**, 90.

Erley, C. M., Duda, S. H., Wakat, J.-P., *et al.* (1992). Noninvasive procedures for diagnosis of renovascular hypertension in renal transplant recipients—a prospective analysis. *Transplantation* **54**, 863.

Fischereder, M., Gohring, P., Schneeberger, H., *et al.* (1998). Early loss of renal transplants in patients with thrombophilia. *Transplantation* **65**, 936.

Gilliland, J. D., Spies, J. B., Brown, S. B., Yrizarry, J. M. and Greenwood, L. H. (1989). Lymphoceles: percutaneous treatment with povidone-iodine sclerosis. *Radiology* **171**, 227.

Gouny, P., Lenot, B., Decaix, B., *et al.* (1991). Aortoiliac surgery and kidney transplantation. *Ann. Vasc. Surg.* **5**, 26.

Greenberg, B. M., Perloff, L. J., Grossman, R. A., Naji, A. and Barker, C. F. (1985). Treatment of lymphocele in renal allograft recipients. *Arch. Surg.* **120**, 501.

Greenstein, S. M., Verstandig, A., McLean, G. K., *et al.* (1987). Percutaneous transluminal angioplasty, the procedure of choice in the hypertensive renal allograft recipient with renal artery stenosis. *Transplantation* **43**, 29.

Griffiths, A. B., Fletcher, E. W. and Morris, P. J. (1979). Lymphocele after renal transplantation. *Aust. N. Z. J. Surg.* **49**, 626.

Grossman, R. A., Dafoe, D. C., Shoenfeld, R. B., *et al.* (1982). Percutaneous transluminal angioplasty treatment of renal transplant artery stenosis. *Transplantation* **34**, 339.

Gruber, S. A., Chavers, B., Payne, W. D., *et al.* (1989). Allograft renal vascular thrombosis: lack of increase with cyclosporine immunosuppression. *Transplantation* **47**, 475.

Gupta, S. K., Rao, T. K., Butt, K. M., Kountz, S. L. and Friedman, E. A. (1976). Renal artery stenosis in renal transplant recipients. *Proc. Clin. Dial. Transplant. Forum* **226**, 162.

Hamburger, J., Dimitrin, A., Bunkir, L., Debray-Sachs, M. and Aurent, J. (1971). Collection of lymph from kidneys homotransplanted in man: all transformation in vivo. *Nature* **232**, 633.

Hanas, E., Larsson, E., Fellstrom, B., *et al.* (1992). Safety aspects and diagnostic findings of serial renal allograft biopsies, obtained by an automatic technique with a midsize needle. *Scand. J. Urol. Nephrol.* **26**, 413.

Harmer, A. W., Kaskard, D., Koffman, C. G. and Welsh, K. I. (1990). Novel antibodies associated with unexplained loss of renal allografts. *Transpl. Int.* **3**, 66.

Higgins, R. M., Gray, D. W. and Morris, P. J. (1995). Association of thrombosis after renal transplantation with elevation of the platelet count. *Transplantation* **59**, 1353.

Hohnke, C., Abendroth, D., Schleibner, S. and Land, W. (1987). Vascular complications in 1,200 kidney transplantations. *Transplant. Proc.* **19**, 3691.

Holdaas, H., Talseth, T., Berg, K. G., Fauchald, P., Nordal, K. P. and Hartmann, A. (1988). Diagnostic value of peripheral plasma renin response to a single dose of captopril in suspected renal transplant arter stenosis. *Transplant. Proc.* **20**, 423.

Howard, R. J., Simmons, R. L. and Najarian, J. S. (1976). Prevention of lymphoceles following renal transplantation. *Ann. Surg.* **184**, 166.

Hricik, D. E. (1987). Antihypertensive and renal effects of enalapril in post-transplant hypertension. *Clin. Nephrol.* **27**, 250.

Hubsch, P. J., Mostbeck, G., Barton, P. P., *et al.* (1990). Evaluation of arteriovenous fistulas and pseudoaneurysms in renal allografts following percutaneous needle biopsy. *J. Ultrasound Med.* **9**, 95.

Hume, D. M. (1968). *In Human Transplantation*, (D. M. Hume, ed.), p. 110, Grune & Stratton, New York.

Ibels, L. S., Stewart, J. H, Mahony, J. F., Neale, F. C. and Sheil A. R. (1977). Occlusive arterial disease in uraemic and haemodialysis patients and renal transplant recipients. *Q. J. M.* **46**, 197.

Inocencio, N. F., Pierce, J. M., Rosenberg, J. C., *et al.* (1969). Renal allograft with massive perirenal accumulation of lymph. *B. M. J.* **3**, 452.

Irish, A. B., Green, F. R., Gray, D. W. and Morris, P. J. (1997). The factor V Leiden (R506Q) mutation and risk of thrombosis in renal transplant recipients. *Transplantation* **64**, 604.

Johnson, D. B., Lerner, C. A., Prince, M. R., *et al.* (1997). Gadolinium-enhanced magnetic resonance angiography of renal transplants. *Magn. Reson. Imaging* **15**, 13.

Jones, R. M., Murie, J. A., Ting, A., Dunnill, M. S. and Morris, P. J. (1988). Renal vascular thrombosis of cadaveric renal allografts in patients recieving cyclosporine, azathioprine and prednisolone triple therapy. *Clin. Transplant.* **2**, 122.

Kincaid-Smith, P., Hare, W. S., Morris, P. J. and Marshall, V. C. (1969). Renal artery stenosis due to the vascular lesions of rejection in cadaveric allografts. *Proc. Eur. Dial. Transpl. Assoc.* **6**, 235.

Knight, R. J., Schanzer, H., Rand, J. H. and Burrows, L. (1995). Renal allograft thrombosis associated with the antiphospholipid antibody syndrome. *Transplantation* **60**, 614.

Kootstra, G., Meijer, S. and Elema, J. D. (1974). "Spontaneous" rupture of homografted kidneys. *Arch. Surg.* **108**, 107.

Kyriakides, G. K., Simmons, R. L. and Najarian, J. S. (1976). Mycotic aneurysms in transplant patients. *Arch. Surg.* **111**, 472.

Lacombe, M. (1975). Arterial stenosis complicationg renal allotransplantation in man. *Ann. Surg.* **181**, 293.

Lacombe, M. (1991). Aortoiliac surgery in renal transplant patients. *J. Vasc. Surg.* **13**, 712.

Lindsey, E. S., Garbus, S. B., Golladay, E. S. and McDonald, J. C. (1975). Hypertension due to renal artery stenosis in transplanted kidneys. *Ann. Surg.* **181**, 604.

Lledo Garcia, E., Hernandez Fernandez, C., Escribano Patino, G., *et al.* (1996). Lymphocele after renal transplantation: therapeutic controversies in the age of laparoscopy. *Actas Urol. Esp.* **20**, 648.

Lord, R. S., Effeney, D. J., Hayes, J. M. and Tracey, G. D. (1973). Renal allograft rupture: cause, clinical features and management. *Ann. Surg.* **177**, 268.

Loubeyre, P., Cahen, R., Grozel, F., *et al.* (1996). Transplant renal artery stenosis: evaluation of diagnosis with magnetic resonance angiography compared with color duplex sonography and arteriography. *Transplantation* **62**, 446.

Madura, J. A., Dunbar, J. D. and Cerelli, G. J. (1970). Perirenal lymphocele as a complication of renal homotransplantation. *Surgery* **68**, 310.

Manske, C. L., Wilson, R. F., Wang, Y. and Thomas, W. (1997). Atherosclerotic vascular complications in diabetic transplant candidates. *Am. J. Kidney Dis.* **29**, 601.

Margules, R. M., Belzer, R. F. and Kountz, S. L. (1973). Surgical correction of renovascular hypertension following renal allotransplantation. *Arch. Surg.* **106**, 13.

McCullough, C. S., Soper, N. J., Clayman, R. V., So, S. S., Jendrisak, M. D. and Hanto, D. W. (1991). Laparoscopic drainage of a posttransplant lymphocele. *Transplantation* **51**, 725.

McKenzie, N., Deviveni, R., Vezina, W., Keown, P. and Stiller, C. (1985). The effect of cyclosporin on organ blood flow. *Transplant. Proc.* **17**, 1973.

Melvin, W. S., Bumgardner, G. L., Davies, E. A., Elkhammas, E. A., Henry, M. L. and Ferguson, R. M. (1997). The laparoscopic management of post-transplant lymphocele: a critical review. *Surg. Endosc.* **11**, 245.

Merion, R. M. and Calne, R. Y. (1985). Allograft renal vein thrombosis. *Transplant. Proc.* **17**, 1746.

Miach, P. J., Ernest, D., McKay, J. and Dawborn, J. K. (1989). Renography with captopril in renal transplant recipients. *Transplant. Proc.* **21**, 1953.

Mohan, P., Murphy, D. M., Counihan, A., Cunningham, P. and Hickey, D. P. (1999). The role of intraoperative heparin in cyclosporine treated cadaveric renal transplant recipients. *J. Urol.* **162**, 682.

Morris, P. J., Oliver, D., Bishop, M., *et al.* (1978). Results from a new renal transplantation unit. *Lancet* **2**, 1353.

Morris, P. J., Yadar, R. V., Kincaid-Smith, P., *et al.* (1971). Renal artery stenosis in renal transplantation. *Med. J. Aust.* **1**, 1255.

Munda, R., Alexander, J. W., Miller, S., First, M. R. and Fidler, J. P. (1977). Renal allograft artery stenosis. *Am. J. Surg.* **134**, 400.

Murphy, A. M., Robertson, R. J. and Dubbins, P. A. (1987). Duplex ultrasound in the assessment of renal transplant complications. *Clin. Radiol.* **38**, 229.

Murphy, B. G., Hill, C. M., Middleton, D., *et al.* (1994). Increased renal allograft thrombosis in CAPD patients. *Nephrol. Dial. Transplant.* **9**, 1166.

Nahman, N. S., Jr., Maniam, P., Hernandez, R. A., Jr., *et al.* (1994). Renal artery pressure gradients in patients with angiographic evidence of atherosclerotic renal artery stenosis. *Am. J. Kidney Dis.* **24**, 695.

Neild, G. H., Ivory, K. and Williams, D. G. (1984). Glomerular thrombosis and cortical infarction in cyclosporin-treated rabbits with acute serum sickness. *Br. J. Exp. Pathol.* **65**, 133.

Neild, G. H., Reuben, R., Hartley, R. B. and Cameron, J. S. (1985). Glomerular thrombi in renal allografts associated with cyclosporin treatment. *J. Clin. Pathol.* **38**, 253.

Neild, G. H., Rocchi, G., Imberti, L., *et al.* (1983). Effect of cyclosporin A on prostacyclin sythesis by vascular tissue. *Thromb. Res.* **32**, 377.

Nerstrom, B., Ladefoged, J. and Lund, F. (1972). Vascular complications in 155 consecutive kidney transplantations. *Scand. J. Urol. Nephrol.* **6(Suppl. 15)**, 64.

Newman-Sanders, A. P., Gedroyc, W. G., al-Kutoubi, M. A., Koo, C., and Taube, D. (1995). The use of expandable metal stents in transplant renal artery stenosis. *Clin. Radiol.* **50**, 245.

Newton, W. T, Keltner, R. M., Jr. and Shankel, S. W. (1967). Acquired renovascular hypertension in a patient with renal allotransplantation. *Am. J. Surg.* **113**, 292.

Nicholson, M. L. and Veitch, P. S. (1990). Treatment of lymphocele associated with renal transplant. *Br. J. Urol.* **65**, 240.

Nicita, G., Villari, D., Marzocco, M., Li Marzi, V., Trippitelli, A. and Santoro, G. (1998). Endoluminal stent placement after percutaneous transluminal angioplasty in the treatment of post-transplant renal artery stenosis. *J. Urol.* **159**, 34.

Oh, J., Schaefer, F., Veldmann, A., *et al.* (1999). Heterozygous prothrombin gene mutation: a new risk factor for early renal allograft thrombosis. *Transplantation* **68**, 575.

Ojo, A. O., Hanson, J. A., Wolfe, R. A., *et al.* (1999). Dialysis modality and the risk of allograft thrombosis in adult renal transplant recipients. *Kidney Int.* **55**, 1952.

Osborn, D. E., Castro, J. E. and Shackman, R. (1976). Surgical correction of arterial stenosis in renal allografts. *Br. J. Urol.* **48**, 221.

Owens, M. L., Wilson, S. E., Maxwell, J. G., Bordner, A., Smith, R. and Ehrlich, R. (1979). Major hemorrhage after renal transplantation. *Transplantation* **27**, 285.

Parvin, S. D., Evans, D. H. and Bell, P. R. F. (1985). Peripheral resistance measurements in the assessment of severe peripheral vascular disease. *Br. J. Surg.* **72**, 751.

Pedersen, N. C. and Morris, B. (1970). The role of the lymphatic system in the rejection of homografts: a study of the lymph from renal transplants. *J. Exp. Med.* **131**, 936.

Pernthaler, H., Schmid, T., Sandbichler, P. and Margreiter, R. (1991). Lymphocele following renal graft trauma. *Br. J. Urol.* **67**, 659.

Penny, M. J., Nankivell, B. J., Disney, A. P., Byth, K. and Chapman, J. R. (1994). Renal graft thrombosis: a survey of 134 consecutive cases. *Transplantation* **58**, 565.

Petric, R., Freeman, D., Wallace, C., McDonald, J., Stiller, C. and Keown, P. (1988). Effect of cyclosporine on urinary prostinoid excretion, renal blood flow and glomerulotubular function. *Transplantation* **45**, 883.

Pollak, R., Veremis, S. A., Maddux, M. S. and Mozes, M. F. (1988). The natural history of and therapy for perirenal fluid collections following renal transplantation. *J. Urol.* **140**, 716.

Reissell, E., Lalla, M., Hockerstedt, K. and Lindgren, L. (1994). Coagulation abnormalities in diabetic patients undergoing renal transplantation. *Ann. Chir. Gynaecol.* **83**, 251.

Reuther, G., Wanjura, D. and Bauer, H. (1989). Acute renal vein thrombosis in renal allografts: detection with duplex doppler US. *Radiology* **170**, 557.

Richardson, A. J., Higgins, R. M., Jaskowski, A. J., Murie, M., Dunnill, M. S. and Morris, P. J. (1990a). Renal allograft rupture and renal vein thrombosis. *Transplant. Proc.* **22**, 1419.

Richardson, A. J., Higgins, R. M., Jaskowski, A. J., *et al.* (1990b). Spontaneous rupture of renal allografts: the importance of renal vein thrombosis in the cyclosporin era. *Br. J. Surg.* **77**, 558.

Richardson, A. J., Liddington, M., Jaskowski, A., Murie, J. A., Gillmer, M. and Morris, P. J. (1990c). Pregnancy in a renal transplant recipient complicated by rupture of a transplant renal artery aneurysm. *Br. J. Surg.* **77**, 228.

Ridge, J. A., Manco Johnson, M. L. and Weil, R. (1987). Ultrasonographic diagnosis of infected lymphocele after kidney transplantation. *Eur. Urol.* **13**, 31.

Riehl, J., Maigatter, S., Kierdorf, H., Schmitt, H., Maurin, N. and Sieberth, H. G. (1994). Percutaneous renal biopsy: comparison of manual and automated puncture techniques with native and transplanted kidneys. *Nephrol. Dial. Transplant.* **9**, 1568.

Roberts, J. P., Ascher, N. L., Fry, D. S., *et al.* (1989). Transplant renal artery stenosis. *Transplantation* **48**, 580.

Robertson, A. J., Nargund, V., Gray, D. W., and Morris, P. J. (2000). Low dose aspirin as prophylaxis against renal vein thrombosis in renal transplant recipients. *Nephrol. Dial. Transplant.* **15**, 1865.

Roney, P. D. and Wellington, J. L. (1985). Traumatic lymphocele following renal transplantation. *J. Urol.* **134**, 322.

Schramek, A., Better, O. S., Adler, O., *et al.* (1975). Hypertensive crisis, erythrocytosis, and uraemia due to renal artery stenosis of kidney transplants. *Lancet* **1**, 70.

Schweizer, R. T., Cho, S, Kountz, S. L. and Belzer, F. O. (1972). Lymphoceles following renal transplantation. *Arch. Surg.* **104**, 42.

Shokeir, A. A., Eraky, I., el-Kappany, H. and Ghoneim, M. A. (1994). Accidental division of the transplanted ureter during laparoscopic drainage of lymphocele. *J. Urol.* **151**, 1623.

Sierre, S. D., Raynaud, A. C., Carreres, T., Sapoval, M. R., Beyssen, B. M. and Gaux, J. C. (1998). Treatment of recurrent transplant renal artery stenosis with metallic stents. *J. Vasc. Interv. Radiol.* **9**, 639.

Singh, A., Stablein, D. and Tejani, A. (1997). Risk factors for vascular thrombosis in pediatric renal transplantation: a special report of the North American Pediatric Renal Transplant Cooperative Study. *Transplantation* **63**, 1263.

Smellie, W. A., Vinik, M. and Hume, D. M. (1969). Angiographic investigation of hypertension complicating human renal transplantation. *Surg. Gynecol. Obstet.* **128**, 963.

Smith, R. B., Cosimi, A. B., Lordon, R., Thompson, A. L. and Ehrlich, R. M. (1976). Diagnosis and management of arterial stenosis causing hypertension after successful renal transplantation. *J. Urol.* **115**, 639.

Sniderman, K. W., Sprayregen, S., Sos, T. A., *et al.* (1980). Percutaneous transluminal dilatation in renal transplant arterial stenosis. *Transplantation* **30**, 440.

Taylor, K. J., Morse, S. S., Rigsby, C. M., Bia, M. and Schiff, M. (1987). Vascular complications in renal allografts: detection with duplex Doppler US. *Radiology* **162**, 31.

Tello, R., Mitchell, P. J., Witte, D. J. and Thomson, K. R. (1998). Detection of renal arteries with fast spin-echo magnetic resonance imaging. *Australas. Radiol.* **42**, 179.

Teruel, J. L., Escobar, E. M., Quereda, C., Mayayo, T. and Ortuno, J. (1983). A simple and safe method for management of lymphocele after renal transplantation. *J. Urol.* **130**, 1058.

Thomas, C. P., Riad, H., Johnson, B. F. and Cumberland, D. C. (1992). Percutaneous transluminal angioplasty in transplant renal arterial stenoses: a long-term follow-up. *Transpl. Int.* **5**, 129.

Thompson, T. J. and Neale, T. J. (1989). Acute perirenal lymphocele formation 8 years after renal transplantation. *Aust. N. Z. J. Surg.* **59**, 583.

Thomson, A. W., Webster, L. M., Aldridge, R. D. and Morrice, L. N. (1985). Cyclosporin and leucocyte procoagulant activity. *Lancet* **1**, 1396.

Ulrych, M. and Langford, H. G. (1975). Erythrocytosis and renal artery stenosis in transplants. *Lancet* **1**, 867.

Vaidya, S., Wang, C., Gugliuzza, K. and Fish, J. C. (1999). Antiphospholipid antibody syndrome and posttransplant renal thrombosis. *Transplant. Proc.* **31**, 230.

Van Buren, D., Van Buren, C. T., Flechner, S. M., Maddox, A. M., Verani, R. and Kahan, B. D. (1985). De novo hemolytic syndrome in renal transplant recipients immunosuppressed with cyclosporin. *Surgery* **98**, 54.

Vanrenterghem, Y., Roels, L., Lerut, J., *et al.* (1985). Thromboembolic complications and haemostatic changes in cyclosporine-treated cadaveric kidney allograft recipients. *Lancet* **1**, 999.

van Sonnenberg, E., Witlich, G. R., Casola, G., *et al.* (1986). Lymphoceles: imaging characteristics and percutaneous management. *Radiology* **161**, 593.

Wagenknecht, D. R., Fastenau, D. R., Torry, R. J., Carter, C. B., Haag, B. W. and McIntyre, J. A. (1999). Antiphospholipid antibodies are a risk factor for early renal allograft failure: isolation of antiphospholipid antibodies from a thrombosed renal allograft. *Transplant. Proc.* **31**, 285.

Wang, Y., Turner, N., An, S. F., Fleming, K. A. and Thompson, E. M. (1994). Gene expression of plasminogen activator inhibitor 1 in transplant kidneys complicated by renal vein thrombosis: a combined study by in-situ hybridization and immunohistochemistry. *Nephrol. Dial. Transplant.* **9**, 296.

Ward, K., Klingensmith, W. C., Sterioff, S. and Wagner, H. N. (1978). The origin of lymphoceles following renal transplantation. *Transplantation* **25**, 346.

Watzke, H., Spielberger, C., Steiner, E., *et al.* (1986). Hemostasis after renal transplantation: comparison of three different immunosuppressive regimens. *Transplant. Proc.* **18**, 1025.

Weigele, J. B. (1991). Iliac artery stenosis causing renal allograft-mediated hypertension: angiographic diagnosis and treatment. *A. J. R. Am. J. Roentgenol.* **157**, 513.

Werner, W. and Schubert, J. (1997). Preoperative aspirin therapy—a contraindication for kidney transplantation? *Zentralbl. Chir.* **122**, 374.

Wright, J. G., Tesi, R. J, Massop, D. W., *et al.* (1991). Safety of simultaneous aortic reconstruction and renal transplantation. *Am. J. Surg.* **162**, 126.

Zaontz, M. R. and Firlit, C. F. (1988). Pelvic lymphocele after pediatric renal transplantation: a successful technique for prevention. *J. Urol.* **139**, 557.

Zazgornik, J., Kopsa, H., Balcke, P., Minar E. and Shaheen, F. (1985). Untitled letter. *Lancet* **2**, 102.

Zinke, H., Woods, J. E., Aguilo, J. J., *et al.* (1975). Experience with lymphoceles after renal transplantation. *Surgery* **77**, 444.

Urological Complications After Renal Transplantation

D. Cranston • D. Little

Introduction

The urological complications of renal transplantation are relatively uncommon although the incidence differs between centers. The quoted incidence of urological complications ranges from 5 to 14% (Loughlin et al., 1984; Mundy et al., 1981). Although rarely life-threatening, urological complications are associated with significant morbidity in the immunosuppressed patient and ultimately may be associated with long-term allograft dysfunction and loss. Early diagnosis and treatment are important. Prevention is better than cure and is best achieved by careful attention to detail in every stage of the transplant operation, which begins with the donor nephrectomy, includes the bench dissection of the kidney and concludes with the recipient operation. Meticulous attention to detail is mandatory in transplanting a kidney into an immunosuppressed patient in renal failure who may have impaired healing and increased risk of developing infections. The three relevant stages of the transplant operation are discussed in more detail, then the specific early and late urological complications are discussed together with their management.

Prevention of Complications
DONOR OPERATION

Cadaveric donor surgery is a difficult procedure to do well. Living related donor surgery often is technically demanding and always emotionally taxing. The technical aspects of removal of donor kidneys are described in Chapter 7, but an understanding of the anatomy of the kidney and ureter, and in particular, the blood supply, is important in prevention of urological complications. The normal blood supply to the ureter arises from the ureteral branches of the renal artery, branches from the gonadal artery, the common iliac or internal iliac artery and the superior or inferior vesical artery. Branches of all these arteries have free anastomoses in the ureteral adventitia (Daniel and Shackman, 1952). Although most kidneys derive their blood supply from one renal artery, in 25% of the population there are multiple arteries to one kidney, and in 10 to 15% multiple arteries supply both kidneys (Grant, 1962). When a lower polar artery is present, the ureteral blood supply may arise from this lower polar vessel, damage to which compromises the ureter.

The transplant ureter depends entirely on the renal artery for its blood supply, and it is important to avoid two errors in removal of the kidney and ureter. The first error is excessive stripping of the connective and adventitial tissue surrounding the ureter, which may lead to necrosis of the distal ureter. The second error is dissecting too far proximally into the renal hilum, which may compromise the ureteral branch of the renal artery resulting in ischemic necrosis of the ureter.

The surgeon should avoid dissection in the "golden triangle" (Fig. 29–1) between the lower pole of the kidney and the gonadal vessels on the left-hand side and the lower pole of the kidney and the lower border of the junction between the renal vein and the inferior vena cava on the right-hand side (Salvatierra et al., 1974). Loughlin and associates found the urological complication rate higher in recipients of kidneys from living related donors and considered that this may be due to more limited exposure at the time of the removal of the kidney and more extensive hilar dissection of the kidney after removal (Loughlin et al., 1984). The same was found to be the case by Cimic and colleagues, but they do not describe which approach they used to remove the kidneys (Cimic et al., 1997). Trauma to the renal artery during donor nephrectomy can lead to ischemia and consequent ureteral necrosis, and for that reason some centers use an anterior transperitoneal approach for removing the kidney from a living related donor, which gives excellent exposure to the hilum. Disruption of the intima of the renal artery by excessive traction on the renal vessels during removal or damage with a cannula during perfusion can result in ischemia, and care must be exercised in both of these areas. The en-bloc removal of cadaveric kidneys (described in Chapter 7) reduces the risk of damage to aberrant lower polar vessels and compromise to the ureteral blood supply.

The upper age limit of cadaveric donors has been steadily rising over the years. For example, the Nottingham group reported that 22% of the adult transplant recipients between 1983 and 1986 in their series received kidneys from donors older than 50 years of age (Foster et al., 1988), and now approximately 20% of donors are older than age 60. The Nottingham group believed that the results using older donors were inferior to those achieved with younger donors. Their incidence of technical complications was higher mainly because of anastomoses involving diseased vessels. These investigators did not comment on the urological complication rate, although given the close relationship between urological complications and ischemia, kidneys from marginal donors at the extremes of age might be associated with more urological complications.

CONGENITAL ABNORMALITIES IN RENAL DONORS

Bauer and associates reported an overall incidence of 0.6% of ureteral duplication in a series of 51,880 autopsies (Bauer et al., 1992). If there is ureteric duplication, it is important not to separate the ureters but to dissect them en bloc with their common adventitial sheath and periureteral fat to protect the ureteral blood supply. The technique of uretereoneocystostomy is the same as that for a single ureter except the distal ends of the ureters are spatulated and anastomosed together before implantation in the bladder (see also Chapter 11). If the Leadbetter-Politano method of implantation is em-

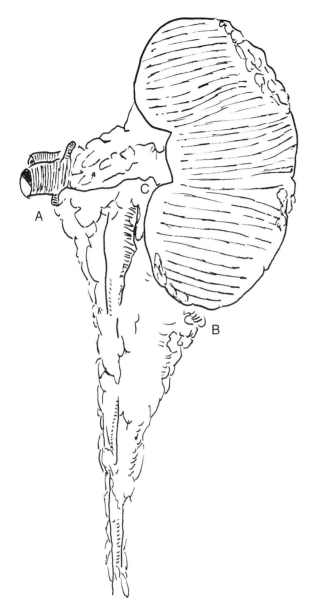

FIGURE 29–1

The golden triangle (as outlined by A, B and C). Dissection in this area should be avoided during removal and preparation of the kidney for transplantation.

ployed, a generous submucosal tunnel is made for the ureters, which are then brought intravesically side by side.

Occasionally, complications arise from a preexisting pathology in the donor kidney: Preexisting pelviureteral obstruction in a transplanted kidney, which was present in the donor kidney beforehand but not recognized, has been described. Stones may be present in the donor kidney that subsequently cause obstruction after the kidney has been transplanted. Congenital renal abnormalities do not necessarily exclude the use of the kidneys for transplantation. Successful transplantation of horseshoe kidneys, separated at the isthmus or transplanted as a single unit, has been reported (Lowell et al., 1994; Menezes de Goes et al., 1981). The two kidneys from a donor with crossed, nonfused renal ectopia also have been transplanted successfully into two recipients (Barry and Fincher, 1984; Rosenthal and Khetan, 1989).

BENCH DISSECTION

After removal of the kidneys and perfusion with or without storage, some further dissection usually is done on the bench before transplantation into the recipient. This dissection is a further source of potential complications, and particular care must be taken of small aberrant lower polar vessels, which may be difficult to see when the circulation is absent. Division of the vessels to the lower pole may impair seriously the ureteral blood supply, as already indicated.

In a cadaveric donor, double arteries often can be taken together on a Carrel patch. Occasionally in a living related donor, it is necessary to remove a kidney with a double renal artery, and a Carrel patch cannot be used. In this situation, preservation of the lower polar vessel is essential. This preservation can be achieved by anastomosing the lower polar vessel in an end-to-side manner to the main renal artery, or if it is a reasonably large artery, it may be spatulated and anastomosed to the spatulated main renal artery to form a single conduit (see Chapter 11). Particular care needs to be taken during bench dissection of horseshoe kidneys and from donors with cross-renal ectopia that may or may not be fused and usually have multiple abnormal renal vessels. Bench surgery is performed with the kidney in ice so that careful, meticulous reconstruction can be performed without any sense of urgency. This approach is of particular use with multiple arteries or congenital abnormal kidneys, and care at this point minimizes subsequent complications (Chinn, 1989).

RECIPIENT OPERATION

The vesicoureteric anastomosis is performed after revascularization of the kidney. Several techniques for performing this anastomosis have been described (see Chapter 11). The two most commonly employed techniques involve either an extravesical ureteroneocystostomy anastomosis of the distal ureter to the bladder mucosa or implantation of the ureter into the bladder through a submucosal tunnel. In the former, closure of the detrusor layer over this anastomosis provides an antireflux mechanism. Alternatively the ureter is tunneled submucosally and sutured to the bladder mucosa by a separate anterior cystotomy in a technique referred to as the *Leadbetter-Politano technique* (see Chapter 11). Each technique has its proponents and antagonists. Proponents of the extravesical ureteroneocystostomy technique argue that it allows for use of a shorter length of ureter with improved blood supply and a minimal cystotomy. The separate anterior cystotomy of the Leadbetter-Politano technique has been reported to be the site of urinary leak and of significant hematuria postoperatively (Thrasher et al., 1990). A further established disadvantage of the Leadbetter-Politano technique is the risk of ureterovesical junction obstruction as a result of kinking of the ureter in the new submucosal tunnel. Excessive handling of the ureter in placing it in the submucosal tunnel has been reported to compromise further the already precarious blood supply of the distal ureter, increasing the risk of ischemic stenosis. An early report showed that there was a relatively high incidence of reflux after the extravesical procedure compared with the Leadbetter-Politano technique (Yadav et al., 1972). The significance of posttransplant vesicoureteral reflux remains controversial, however. Some investigators have found that patients with reflux have a higher incidence of urinary infection and early graft failure (Mathew et al., 1977). Others have shown no association with infection or impaired allograft function (Nghiem et al., 1981; Ohl et al., 1988; Whittier et al., 1974). Well-designed, prospective studies directly comparing the long-term results obtained with the two techniques have not been reported.

A retrospective study by Butterworth *et al.* (1997) directly comparing the two techniques, in which the Leadbetter-Politano technique was performed in 140 consecutive transplant patients and an extravesical anastomosis was performed in 108 patients, showed a significantly lower complication rate with the extravesical technique. Similar conclusions were noted in a review of 320 patients by Thrasher and coworkers, who quote a urological complication rate of 9.4% in patients undergoing Leadbetter-Politano implantation versus 3.7% using the extravesical technique (Thrascher *et al.*, 1990). The duration of follow-up for these patients was not indicated, however. Shah and colleagues found no significant difference in urological complications with a rate of 4% in both groups (Shah *et al.*, 1988). Gibbons and colleagues described a 2.1% incidence of ureteral complications using an extravesical technique (Gibbons *et al.*, 1992). No data regarding long-term follow-up were included in this study, however, in which urological complications occurring only in the first 6 weeks posttransplantation were reported. Obstruction at the anastomotic site may occur months or years after transplantation (Gibbons *et al.*, 1992).

Further controversy arises as to the appropriate use of stents in the extravesical ureteroneocystostomy. Benoit and coworkers prospectively randomized a series of 194 kidney transplant recipients (97 with and 97 without a double-J stent) and reported a reduced incidence of urinary leak in the stented group (1% *vs.* 6%) (Benoit *et al.*, 1996). There was a 35% urinary tract infection rate in both groups, and no significant difference in 1-year patient and allograft survival was shown. There was no significant difference in serum creatinine at 1 year in the stented and unstented groups. In 1993, Nicol *et al.* reviewed the routine placement of a stent in 358 renal transplants performed in 355 patients and concluded that urinary leak rate was reduced in the stented ureters. These investigators outlined unique problems relating to stent placement, however, including stent migration, breakage, ureteric obstruction, calculus and infection. Koo and associates confirmed the finding that primary insertion of double-J stents abolished the complications of ureteric leak and obstruction, and they described no complications attributable to the placement of a stent in 100 patients evaluated (Koo *et al.*, 1993).

Whichever technique is chosen, care must be taken to avoid twisting the ureter or leaving an excess length of ureter. Preferably the kidney should not be put in upside down, although this does not seem to affect urine drainage adversely and may facilitate drainage of a transplant ureter into an ileal conduit (see Chapter 12).

Diagnosis and Management of Complications

Urological complications are a source of frequent morbidity and occasional mortality after renal transplantation. The incidence of urological complications in the early days of renal transplantation ranged from 10 to 25% (Loughlin *et al.*, 1984; Starzl *et al.*, 1970) with an associated 20 to 30% mortality (Colfry *et al.*, 1974; Mundy *et al.*, 1981). The incidence of complications has fallen dramatically since the 1970s, however. Current rates of urological complications vary but are approximately 5 to 10% with minimal morbidity; graft loss should be avoided in virtually all cases (Loughlin *et al.*, 1984; Nicholson *et al.*, 1991).

At Oxford, the urological complication rate at any time after transplantation in our first 1,535 transplants was 8.5%. In the first 207 transplants up to 1979, it was 16%. The major factor in this reduction was the change from high-dose to low-dose steroids in the immunosuppressive regimens

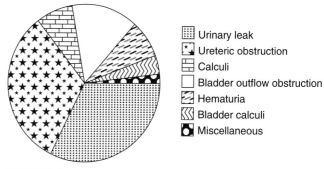

FIGURE 29–2

The composition of 132 urological complications in 1,535 consecutive kidney transplant patients at Oxford.

(Jaskowski *et al.*, 1987; Shoskes *et al.*, 1995). Thereafter the complication rate fell to less than 5% but has been rising in more recent years, possibly as a result of an increased use of marginal donors. Many complications are technical in nature, and the contribution of rejection to ureteral damage has yet to be clarified (Katz *et al.*, 1988). Urological complications can be divided into early and late categories. Early complications are defined as those that occur within 3 months of the transplant, and late complications are those that occur after this time. The relative proportions of common urological complications encountered in Oxford are shown in Figure 29–2. Complications consist of urinary fistulae or leaks, ureteral obstruction, vesicoureteral reflux, stones, bladder outflow obstruction (including the problem of prostatic enlargement in an increasingly elderly male recipient population) and problems related to posttransplant renal biopsies. Leaks tend to occur early, although obstruction may occur at any stage posttransplant.

URINARY LEAKS

Principles of Management

As already stated, urinary fistulae or leaks usually occur early in the postoperative course. The most frequent site of leakage is from the ureteroneocystostomy or the bladder closure (in the case of the Leadbetter-Politano technique). Other sites of urine leakage include a ureterocutaneous fistula or more rarely a caliceal-cutaneous fistula. Depending on the site and extent of the leak, the patient may present clinically with pain over the allograft, local edema extending to the thigh and perineum of the affected side and fever. These symptoms and signs usually are associated with deterioration in renal function. Intestinal ileus may develop in the presence of a large retroperitoneal collection. In our experience of 45 cases of urinary fistula (3%), median time to onset was 29 days (range 0–275), with all but 2 cases within the first 120 days (Table 29–1). Of the predisposing factors identified, damage during retrieval and an ischemic, necrotic lower ureter were the most important.

Ultrasound and nuclear renal scans (technetium 99m–mercaptoacetyltriglycine, technetium 99m–diethylenetriaminepentaacetic acid) are sensitive screening techniques for the detection of urinary extravasation. Additional information may be obtained from contrast-enhanced computed tomography or cystography. If a collection of fluid consistent with a urinoma is identified, the fluid can be aspirated percutaneously under ultrasonic guidance and analyzed for creatinine to distinguish it from a lymphocele. If the fluid is urine, the creatinine concentration is high relative to serum,

TABLE 29–1

URINARY LEAK (n = 45) IN 1,535 OXFORD TRANSPLANT RECIPIENTS

Location (n)	Onset in Weeks (Median)	Treatment (n)
Upper (5)	0–7 (3.5)	Conservative (from nephrostomy site) (1)
		Retrograde stent (1)
		Suture defect in renal pelvis (1) and stent (1)
		Ureteroureterostomy (1)
Lower (14)	0–38 (3)	Nephrostomy (1)
		Open drainage (1)
		Open stent insertion (3)
		Reimplantation (3)
		Native ureteropyelostomy (2)
		Ureteroureterostomy (3)
		Boari flap (1)
Bladder (6)	0–51 (6.5)	Prolonged catheter drainage (3)
		Percutaneous drainage (1)
		Repair of vesical defect (2)
Ureteric necrosis (19)	1–10 (5)	Reimplantation (5)
		Native ureteropyelostomy (13)
		Boari flap (1)
No site identified (1)	2	Death from cardiac arrest (1)

whereas lymph has the same creatinine concentration as serum. Alternatively, if the peritoneum was opened at the time of surgery and the patient was dialyzed through a Tenckhoff catheter, fluid from the catheter, if still in place, may be analyzed for creatinine concentration.

Early detection and appropriate treatment are important in reducing the morbidity and mortality arising from urinary leaks. Treatment depends on the site and cause of the leak and whether urine is escaping through a drain externally or is leaking internally and forming a urinoma or an intraperitoneal leak. In the past, early exploration of the transplanted kidney with identification and reconstruction of the leak was advised in all cases (Palmer and Chatterjee, 1978). Applying the urological principle that an adequately drained urinary extravasation will resolve if there is no distal obstruction of the ureter, however, many endoscopic procedures can be applied in the management of urinary leaks, including antegrade and retrograde stenting of the ureter with or without percutaneous drainage of the collection. If these methods are employed, the fact that these patients are immunosuppressed must be borne in mind, and early open surgical reconstruction should be considered if the urinary leakage persists.

Leaks from the bladder usually close spontaneously with drainage through a urinary catheter in the current era of low-dose steroids. With adequate drainage and stenting and no urinary collection, one often can afford to be patient and allow a fistula to heal spontaneously. After reexploration for leakage and reconstruction of the urinary tract, stenting and drainage are prudent measures even if not used in the initial transplant operation.

Endoscopic Surgical Management

Double-J stents have been available since 1978 (Finney, 1978) and have had a considerable impact on urological practice (Fig. 29–3). In transplantation, these stents are useful in obstruction, leakage and any urinary injury at the time of organ removal (Nicholson *et al.*, 1991). Double-J stents can be inserted percutaneously in an antegrade manner or from the bladder in a retrograde manner with a rigid or flexible cystoscope. Retrograde pyelography and double-J stent insertion through a cystoscope often are difficult because of the angle at which the transplanted ureter enters the bladder. In the early postoperative period, edema at the transplant ureteral opening can make instrumentation difficult. The flexible cystoscope may make placement of a guidewire and double-J stent easier than is the case with the rigid cystoscope, especially in a male, because it allows the transplant ureteral orifice to be seen end-on rather than at an acute angle.

Open Surgical Management

Open surgery to the transplant ureter poses different problems from surgery on a native ureter. A transplant ureter cannot be divided and reanastomosed as is the case with a normal ureter because this leaves no blood supply to the distal ureter. Transplantation patients are on steroids and have impaired healing, and the choice of suture material is important. Catgut should not be used; a longer lasting, absorbable material, such as Vicryl, Maxon or Dexon, is preferred. Nonabsorbable suture generally should be avoided in the urinary tract because it may act as a nidus for calculus formation and infection. Open surgical techniques to repair a urinary leak include anastomosis of the transplant pelvis to the adjacent native ureter and anastomosis of the transplant ureter to the adjacent native ureter. Debate exists in the literature as to which method should be best employed (Baquero *et al.*, 1985). A significant disadvantage of employing pyeloureterostomy instead of ureteroureterostomy as a first line of treatment is that it limits the options for further reconstruction if necessary. Whichever method of reconstruction is employed, the recipient ureter normally can be tied off proximally without any complications and does not require an ipsilateral native nephrectomy (Lord *et al.*, 1991).

OBSTRUCTION

Principles of Management

Urinary obstruction can occur early or late after transplantation. Early obstruction usually is diagnosed by a rising serum creatinine level and is confirmed by ultrasound examination of the transplanted kidney. The common causes of ureteral obstruction are listed in Table 29–2. Because the transplant kidney is denervated, the pain and renal colic usually associated with ureteric obstruction are normally absent. An antegrade pyelogram shows the site of obstruction; usually, strictures present at the distal end of the ureter, presumably as a result of ischemia (Fig. 29–4). Rarely, obstruction can occur without hydronephrosis. When this obstruction occurs, it often is due to the ureter and renal pelvis being surrounded by fibrosis, which may be secondary to

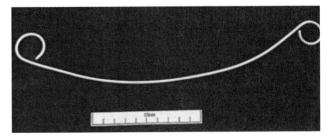

FIGURE 29–3

A double-J stent.

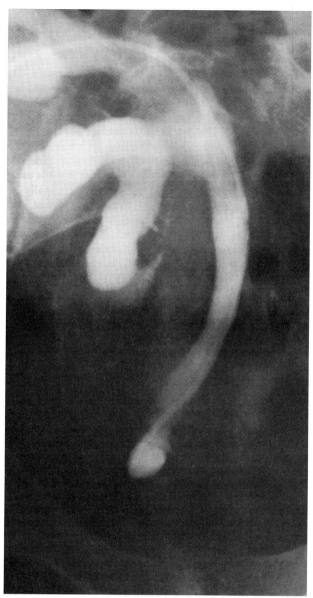

FIGURE 29–4

Antegrade study in a transplanted kidney showing an obstructed lower ureter.

urine leakage or infection. Occasionally the situation arises when there is a modest degree of hydronephrosis with some ureteral stenosis, and it is unclear whether there is true obstruction or not. A diuresis renogram often provides the answer to this question, although equivocal results still occur in 17% of cases. The F-15 renogram also can be definitive:

TABLE 29–3

URINARY OBSTRUCTION (n = 53) IN 1,535 OXFORD TRANSPLANT RECIPIENTS

Location (n)	Treatment (n)
Upper/PUJ (10)	Antegrade stent (4)
	Ureteral dilatation (1)
	Pyeloplasty (1)
	Division of obstructing vessel (1)
	Native ureteropyelostomy (3)
Middle (10)	Antegrade stent (3)
	Retrograde stent (1)
	Open exploration (1) and stent (1)
	Native ureteropyelostomy (2)
	Ureteroureterostomy (2)
Lower/VUJ (33)	Nephrostomy (2)
	Antegrade stent (6)
	Balloon dilatation (2)
	Endoscopic removal of suture (1)
	Native ureteropyelostomy (2)
	Reimplantation (20)

PUJ = pelviureteric junction; VUJ = vesicoureteric junction.

Furosemide is administered 15 minutes before the injection of isotope and results in maximal urinary flow rates at the start of the renogram, decreasing the percentage of false-positive results in dilated or poorly functioning systems. The increase in the urinary flow rate also can clarify systems that obstruct at high flow rates (Upsdell et al., 1992). With modern imaging techniques, the Whitaker test, once popular for the diagnosis of ureteral obstruction, almost never is required.

Treatment in mild cases of obstruction depends on deterioration of renal function and other complicating factors such as urinary tract infections. More harm can be done by treating mild cases of obstruction aggressively rather than by leaving them alone and monitoring the patient carefully—with a low threshold for intervention if the obstruction gets worse.

Endoscopic Surgical Management

Our experience of 1,535 transplants involved 46 cases of primary obstruction, with a further 7 cases due to extrinsic compression from a lymphocele (6) or obstructing blood vessels (1). Many were cured by a single procedure (Table 29–3). Before 1985, all cases required open surgery, but with increasing expertise, endoscopic surgery has become more effective. In the presence of hydronephrosis, a nephrostomy tube, an antegrade pyelogram and a subsequent J stent placement constitute the most appropriate approach (Goldstein et al., 1981; Hunter et al., 1983; Lieberman et al., 1981). A retrograde examination and the insertion of a J stent also can be attempted, but these often are technically more difficult, especially if the Leadbetter-Politano method of ureteric implantation has been employed. Balloon dilatation of a stenotic

TABLE 29–2

CAUSES OF URETERAL OBSTRUCTION

Early Obstruction	Late Obstruction	Obstruction Occurring at Any Stage
Badly placed suture	Ureteral stricture from ischemia	Donor abnormality: pelviureteric junction, renal calculi
Twisted ureter	Periureteral fibrosis	Lymphocele
Edema at vesicoureteric junction	Fungus ball	Blood clot in ureter following biopsy
Ureteral compression by hematoma	Renal calculi	

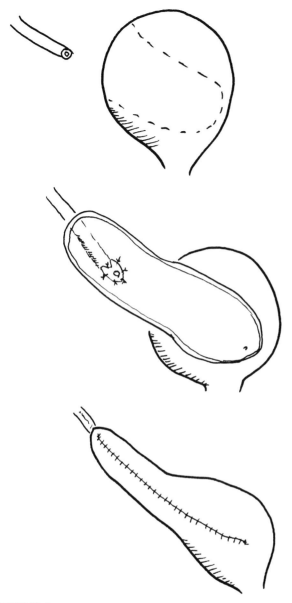

FIGURE 29–5

The creation of a Boari flap to enable implantation of a short transplant ureter.

ureter may be useful (Lieberman et al., 1982). A 50% success rate at 1 year has been reported (Streem et al., 1988). Reports in the literature indicate that advances in minimally invasive procedures practiced in general urology can be applied to the transplant ureter. Erturk et al. (1999) and Youssef et al. (1994) report the safe and successful treatment of two small independent series of patients with distal transplant ureteric stenosis treated with Acucise endoureterotomy.

Obstruction can still occur with a J stent in place, especially if the stent is a tight fit in the ureter and becomes kinked, blocking the internal lumen (Gedroyc et al., 1988). Open surgery is reserved for failed endoscopic procedures, recurrent problems that cannot be cured by endoscopic means and the occasional major problem in which it is evident from the outset that reexploration is necessary.

Open Surgical Management

If there is sufficient length of donor ureter and the obstruction is distal, it usually is possible to remove the strictured

portion of the ureter and redo the ureteroneocystostomy. If there is insufficient length or the stricture is higher, ipsilateral native ureterotransplant ureterostomy or native ureterotransplant pyelostomy may be the reconstructive method of choice. This procedure normally can be done safely by tying off the proximal native ureter without complications (Glass et al., 1982; Lord et al., 1991). An extraperitoneal or intraperitoneal approach may be taken. If there has been infection in the vicinity of the ureter with a lot of fibrosis, an intraperitoneal route may provide the best approach, and the insertion of a ureteral catheter in the native ureter cystoscopically at the start of the procedure helps to localize the native ureter.

A Boari flap and psoas hitch (Figs. 29–5 and 29–6) performed in the standard fashion are useful treatments for obstructed lower ureters when there is insufficient length after removing the obstructing segment to allow the ureter to be reimplanted in the bladder. Vesicopyelostomy and ureterocalicostomy have been described (Jarowenko and Flechner, 1985), and vesicocalicostomy has been used for a difficult case of recurrent hydronephrosis and neurogenic bladder when other reconstructive surgery had failed.

URINARY TRACT INFECTION

Urinary tract infections are one of the commonest sources of infection posttransplantation and are discussed in more detail in Chapter 31. The clinical entity of encrusted cystitis and pyelitis deserves mention, however, because of the predilection of immunosuppressed patients to become infected with urea-splitting microorganisms, in the presence of alkaline urine (Aguado et al., 1993; Meria et al., 1998; Morales et al., 1992). Many bacteria have been shown in this infection,

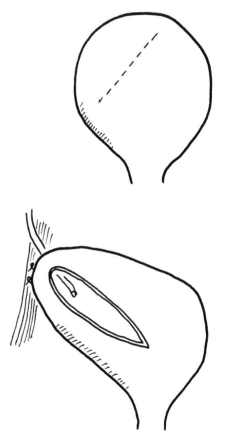

FIGURE 29–6

The psoas hitch, enabling implantation of a short transplant ureter.

but *Corynebacterium* group D2 is implicated most frequently. The result of this infection is chronic inflammation of the bladder mucosa or pelvicaliceal system associated with encrustations. Endoscopic visualization of encrusted cystitis reveals a marked inflammatory appearance of all or part of the bladder with ulcerations and whitish plaques. The zones of predilection for these encrustations are the trigone, bladder neck and sites of previous endoscopic resections surrounded by a vivid red, edematous and hemorrhagic mucosa. These lesions may be impossible to distinguish from carcinoma *in situ* or malacoplakia. Treatment of encrusted cystitis and encrusted pyelitis consists of treatment of the infection, acidification of the urine and elimination of calcified plaques that contain microorganisms.

The issue of transplanting patients who perform clean intermittent self-catheterization has been well described. Inevitably, these patients develop bacteriuria. As in the nontransplanted, immunocompetent patient, antibiotic treatment of these patients should be reserved until they manifest signs of systemic infection. The use of prophylactic antibiotics in a patient who is correctly performing clean intermittent self-catherization promotes development of resistant organisms.

VESICOURETERIC REFLUX

Preexisting vesicoureteric reflux as the cause of end-stage renal failure has a negative impact on the long-term survival of the transplanted kidney (Fontana *et al.*, 1998; Park *et al.*, 1994). This impact probably reflects a functional defect of the bladder, predisposing the patient to recurrent urinary tract infections and graft pyelonephritis. A micturating cystogram shows reflux up the transplant ureter (Fig. 29–7). There is no strong evidence that sterile reflux of urine into the transplant results in increased graft loss, and conservative management may be adopted. Persistent infections with no demonstrable pathology other than reflux should lead to consideration of surgery, however. Submucosal injection of polytetrafluoroethylene (Teflon) close to the transplant ureteric orifice has been described in a few case reports. Alternatively, anastomosis of the transplant ureter to native ureter can be performed if there is no reflux up the native ureter, or the transplant ureter can be reimplanted in the bladder using a Leadbetter-Politano antireflux procedure.

CALCULI

Urinary calculi are a relatively uncommon complication of renal transplantation. Calculi may have been present in the donor kidney or may develop after transplantation. Transplantation patients are at an increased risk for calculi compared with the general population, with an incidence of 1 to 2% (Cho *et al.*, 1988; Jain *et al.*, 1986). This increased risk is due to hypercalcemia, recurrent urinary tract infection, decreased fluid intake and increased incidence of urinary tract obstruction. Because of the denervation of the transplant kidney, renal colic frequently is not experienced by the patient.

Cho and coworkers identified nine stones in 544 transplant patients, an incidence of 1.7% (Cho *et al.*, 1988). Four of these were bladder calculi, and two stones passed spontaneously; three stones were present in the transplant kidney. At Oxford, two patients presented with stones in the first 1,000 transplants, an incidence of 0.2%. Predisposing factors include obstructive uropathy, recurrent urinary tract infection, hypercalciuria, hyperoxaluria, alkaluria, aciduria, internal stents and nonabsorbable suture material. Motayne and associates reported an instance of 6.3% of calculi when a

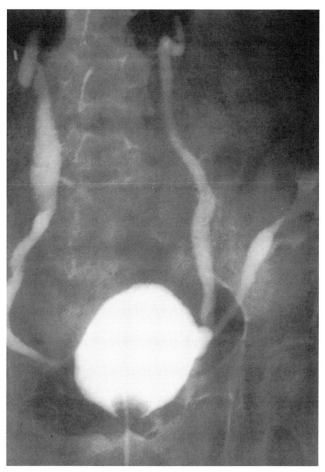

FIGURE 29–7

Voiding cystogram shows reflux up both native ureters (a bilateral nephrectomy had been performed previously) as well as up the ureter of the transplanted kidney.

stapled ureteroureterostomy was used, and in all cases the calculus formed on the staple line (Motayne *et al.*, 1984).

Open stone removal is rarely necessary. Complete stone removal usually is possible by standard endourological techniques, although extracorporeal shock-wave lithotripsy may be difficult to employ because of the position of the transplanted kidney in the iliac fossa. Radiological localization of the stone is impossible owing to the bones of the pelvis, and a lithotripsy machine using ultrasonic localization of the stone is preferable. Lithotripsy has been practiced successfully in children who have had renal transplants (Ellis *et al.*, 1989). After lithotripsy treatments of transplant kidneys, one must watch carefully for signs of obstruction in what is effectively a solitary kidney. Use of J stents before lithotripsy is debatable. Percutaneous removal of the calculi normally is straightforward because access to the transplanted kidney is much easier than to a native kidney (Fig. 29–8). Ureteral stones may be extracted through an antegrade percutaneous approach, via a nephrostomy.

LYMPHOCELES

Lymphoceles sometimes may cause ureteral obstruction (Braun *et al.*, 1974). Most cases occur within 6 months of transplantation (see Chapter 28). The classic triad at presentation is decreased urine output, hydronephrosis and ipsilateral leg edema. Treatment in the first instance involves aspiration,

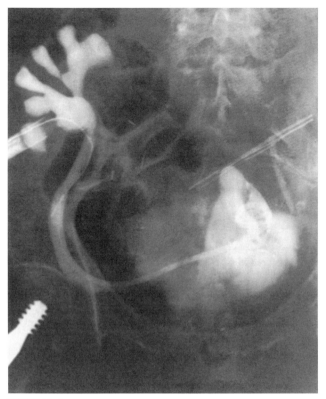

FIGURE 29–8

Percutaneous removal of stones in ureter and pelvis (not seen) of a transplanted kidney, in which a double-J stent had been inserted previously for relief of obstruction.

but if recurring, fenestration into the peritoneal cavity is performed at open operation or by endoscopic techniques.

BLADDER OUTFLOW OBSTRUCTION

Prostatic outflow obstruction can occur after surgery. This obstruction is likely to become an increasing problem in the transplantation population as more older men are undergoing transplantation. Transurethral resection can be carried out safely according to standard surgical principles, although in our experience it is important to avoid overdistention of the bladder and high-pressure reflux of irrigation fluid and potentially infected urine into the transplant kidney. It also is important to avoid inadvertent damage to the transplant ureter, which has been mistaken for a bladder tumor by clinicians who are inexperienced in cystoscopy of transplant patients.

Men older than age 50 should be evaluated carefully before transplantation with respect to prostatic outflow obstruction by obtaining a thorough history and examination, together with appropriate investigations as indicated. These investigations may include ultrasound scanning of the bladder, measurement of the residual urine, determination of urinary flow rate and cystoscopy. Significant obstruction is best dealt with before transplantation. Transurethral resection of the prostate should be avoided in a patient with little or no native urine output pretransplant, however, because of the high urethral stricture rate. Medical treatment in transplant patients with prostatic outflow obstruction with selective androgen ablation or α blockade is an option. Prostatic stents may be feasible, but they introduce a foreign body into the

urethra of an immunosuppressed patient. For this reason, stents should be considered only when there is no alternative.

Urethral strictures can occur posttransplant as a result of catheterization, especially if it has been traumatic. The strictures are managed by the standard urological techniques of dilatation, optical urethrotomy, stenting or occasionally urethroplasty. Clean intermittent self-catheterization has been shown to be safe for transplant patients with abnormal bladders and safe for patients with recurrent urethral strictures (Flechner *et al.*, 1983; Kogan *et al.*, 1986).

ERECTILE DYSFUNCTION

Disturbances in male sexual and reproductive function occur frequently in chronic renal failure. The pathophysiology has been related to multiple factors, including psychological, biochemical, endocrinological, hematological, neurological, pharmacological and vasculogenic elements. Patients undergoing successful renal transplantation appear to experience improvement in erectile function compared with patients treated with dialysis or patients having a failed renal transplant. Sperm count, motility and plasma testosterone also have been observed to return to normal after transplantation (Wayne, 1981). Vasculogenic impotence may result from iatrogenic occlusion of the internal iliac artery after renal transplantation. Gittes and Waters (1979) found the incidence of sexual impotence to be 10% after the first transplant compared with 65% after two transplants, when bilateral internal iliac arteries were employed. In 1998, Taylor reported the views of transplant surgeons in Great Britain and Ireland regarding the sequential use of the internal iliac artery for renal transplantation. They concluded that the sequential use of the contralateral internal iliac artery for vascularization of a second renal allograft confers a risk of impotence in more than 25% of cases.

Treatment of erectile dysfunction posttransplant is similar to that in nontransplant patients. Successful use of penile prosthetic devices in men after transplant has been described (Kabalin and Kessler, 1989; Rowe *et al.*, 1993). Intracorporeal injections of agents such as papaverine and prostaglandins should be performed with caution because frequently renal transplant patients have occult cardiovascular disease, and systemic absorption of these agents may be deleterious. Similar to in nontransplant patients, priapism may occur. Likewise, use of newer pharmacological agents, such as sildenafil, a selective inhibitor of phosphodiesterase type 5, should be prescribed with caution in these patients, but as yet no interactions with immunosuppressive drugs have been reported.

TRANSPLANT BIOPSY

Transplant biopsy has complications (Rao, 1986). Hematuria and clot retention are the commonest urological complications and may cause anuria. Normally the bleeding resolves spontaneously, but occasionally it may be necessary to pass an irrigating catheter into the bladder to evacuate blood clots.

MALIGNANCY

The incidence of neoplasia of the genitourinary tract varies from 0.64 to 1.67% in patients after renal transplantation (Schmidt *et al.*, 1995; see also Chapter 35). Data from the Cincinnati Tumor Registry confirm genitourinary malignancy as occurring in approximately 2% of renal transplant recipients. As indicated in Chapter 35, risk factors such as immunosuppression, oncogenic viruses, loss of T-cell suppressor function and intensification of the normal age-related incidence of cancer are implicated in carcinogenesis. Increased recipient age at the time of transplantation has implications for the development of genitourinary malignancy because older patients have a higher prevalence of prostate and bladder cancers. The use of older donors also probably increases the risk of transmitted disease, particularly occult renal cell carcinomas.

De novo tumors of the genitourinary tract posttransplant frequently affect the native kidneys and bladder. Patients on prolonged dialysis before transplantation are at increased risk of developing acquired cystic disease of the kidney. The development of acquired cystic disease of the kidney has been estimated to increase the prevalence of renal cell carcinoma to a rate approximately four to six times greater than in the general population. Reports suggest a role for ultrasound screening of native kidneys before transplantation (Gulanikar *et al.*, 1998). Similar to in nontransplant patients, most bladder cancers are transitional cell in origin (>90%), although 10% are squamous cell carcinomas, commonly occurring in association with infection, stones or chronic irritation. Patients with abnormal lower urinary tracts, such as bladder exstrophy, are at increased risk of developing adenocarcinoma. Nephrogenic adenoma, which is an unusual form of metaplastic transformation of urothelial cells, also is reported to be commoner in renal transplant recipients (Banyai-Falger *et al.*, 1998; Tse *et al.*, 1997). Review of data provided by the Australia and New Zealand Dialysis and Transplant Cancer Registry shows a risk ratio of 4.9 for bladder cancer (observed *vs.* expected) and a 168-fold increased risk for ureteral cancer (particularly associated with end-stage renal failure secondary to analgesia abuse) (see Chapter 35). Penn (1993) confirmed this increased risk and highlighted the aggressive nature of these urothelial tumors. A report from Swindle and colleagues recommends routine screening for *de novo* transitional cell carcinoma of the genitourinary tract in patients transplanted for analgesic nephropathy (Swindle *et al.*, 1998). Treatment of urothelial tumors usually involves surgical resection as well as posing the difficult clinical dilemma as to the feasibility of continuing immunosuppression in the presence of malignancy.

Conclusion

Transplant patients who present with urological complications can be challenging, but the potential for intervention and graft salvage is excellent. An understanding of basic urological principles, together with their modification in the transplant patient, is essential for safe surgery and satisfactory outcome.

REFERENCES

Aguado, J. M., Morales, J. M., Salto, E., *et al.* (1993). Encrusted pyelitis and cystitis by *Corynebacterium urealyticum* (CDC group D2): a new and threatening complication following renal transplant. *J. Urol.* **56**, 617.

Banyai-Falger, S., Maier, U., Susani, M., *et al.* (1998). High incidence of nephrogenic adenoma of the bladder after renal transplantation. *Transplantation* **65**, 511.

Baquero, A., Ginsberg, P. C., Kaschak, D., *et al.* (1985). Experience with pyeloureterostomy associated with simple ligation of native ureter without ipsilateral nephrectomy in renal transplantation. *J. Urol.* **133**, 386.

Barry, J. M. (1983). Unstented extravesical ureteroneocystostomy in kidney transplantation. *J. Urol.* **129**, 918.

Barry, J. M. and Fincher, R. D. (1984). Transplantation of a horseshoe kidney into two recipients. *J. Urol.* **131**, 1162.

Barry, J. M., Hefty, T. R., Nelson, K. A. and Johnston, T. (1990). Ten years of training community urologists and general surgeons to do cadaver kidney retrievals. *J. Urol.* **143**, 897.

Barry, J. M., Lawson, R. K., Strong, D. and Hodges, C. V. (1974). Urologic complications in 173 kidney transplants. *J. Urol.* **112**, 567.

Bauer, S. B., Permutter, A. D. and Retik, A. B. (1992). Anomalies of the upper urinary tract. *In Campbell's Urology*, (P. C. Walsh, A. B. Retik, T. A. Stamey and E. D. Vaughan, eds.), 6th ed., p. 1406, W.B. Saunders, Philadelphia.

Benoit, G., Blanchet, P., Eschwege, P., Alexander, L., Bensadoun, H. and Charpentier, B. (1996). Insertion of a double pigtail ureteral stent for the prevention of urological complications in renal transplantation: a prospective randomized study. *J. Urol.* **156**, 881.

Braun, W. E., Banowsky, L. H., Straffon, R. A., *et al.* (1974). Lymphoceles associated with renal transplantation: report of 15 cases and review of the literature. *Am. J. Med.* **57**, 714.

Butterworth, P. C., Horsburgh, P. S., Veitch, P. S., Bell, P. R. F. and Nicholson, M. L. (1997). Urological complications in renal transplantation: impact of a change of technique. *Br. J. Urol.* **79**, 499.

Chinn, J. L. (1989). Microvascular reconstruction "bench" surgery for donor kidneys before transplantation. *J. Urol.* **142**, 23.

Cho, D. K., Zackson, D. A., Cheigh, J., Stubenbord, W. T. and Stenzel, K. H. (1988). Urinary calculi in renal transplant recipients. *Transplantation* **45**, 899.

Cimic, J., Meuleman, E. J. H., Oosterhof, G. O. N. and Hoitsma, A. J. (1997). Urological complications in renal transplantation: a comparison between living related and cadaveric grafts. *Eur. Urol.* **31**, 433.

Colfry, A. J., Schlegel, J. U., Lindsey, E. S. and McDonald, J. C. (1974). Urological complications in renal transplantation. *J. Urol.* **112**, 564.

Daniel, O. and Shackman, R. (1952). The blood supply of the human ureter in relation to ureterocolic anastomosis. *Br. J. Urol.* **24**, 334.

Dunn, S. P., Vinocur, C. A., Hanevold, C., *et al.* (1987). Pyelonephritis following pediatric renal transplant: increased incidence with vesicoureteral reflux. *J. Pediatr. Surg.* **22**, 1095.

Ellis, E., Wagner, C., Arnold, W., Hulbert, W. and Barnett, T. (1989). Extracorporeal shock wave lithotripsy in a renal transplant patient. *J. Urol.* **141**, 98.

Erturk, E., Burzon, D. T. and Waldman, D. (1999). Treatment of transplant ureteral stenosis with endoureterotomy. *J. Urol.* **161**, 412.

Finney, R. P. (1978). Experience with new double J ureteral catheter stent. *J. Urol.* **120**, 678.

Flechner, S. M., Conley, S. B., Brewer, E. D., *et al.* (1983). Intermittent clean catheterisation: An alternative to diversion in continent transplant recipients with lower urinary tract dysfunction. *J. Urol.* **130**, 878.

Fontana, I., Ginevri, F., Arcuri, V., *et al.* (1998). Impact of vesicoureteral reflux on graft survival in paediatric kidney transplants. *Transplant. Proc.* **30**, 2000.

Foster, M. C., Wenham, P. W., Rowe, P. A., *et al.* (1988). The use of older patients as cadaveric kidney donors. *Br. J. Surg.* **75**, 767.

Gedroyc, W. M. W., Koffman, G. and Saunders, A. J. S. (1988). Ureteric obstruction in stented renal transplants. *Br. J. Urol.* **62**, 123.

Gibbons, W. S., Barry, J. M. and Hefty, T. R. (1992). Complications following unstented parallel incision extra vesical ureteroneocystostomy in 1,000 kidney transplants. *J. Urol.* **148**, 38.

Gittes, R.F. and Waters, W.B. (1979) Sexual impotence: the overlooked complication of a second renal transplant. *J. Urol.* 121:719.

Glass, N. R., Fisher, D. T., Lieberman, R., Crummy, A. B., Uehling, D. T. and Belzer, F. O. (1982). Management of ureteral obstruction after transplantation by percutaneous antegrade pyelography and pyeloureterostomy. *Urology* **20**, 15.

Goldstein, I., Cho, S. I. and Olsson, C. A. (1981). Nephrostomy drainage for renal transplant complications. *J. Urol.* **126**, 159.

Grant, J. C. B. (1962). *An Atlas of Anatomy*, 5th ed., Williams & Wilkins, Baltimore.

Gulanikar, A. C., Daily, P. P., Kilambi, N. K., Hamrick-Turner, J. E. and Butkus, D. E. (1998). Prospective pretransplant ultrasound screening in 206 patients for acquired renal cysts and renal cell carcinoma. *Transplantation* **66**, 1669.

Hefty, T. R. (1985). Experience with parallel incision extravesical ureteroneocystostomy in renal transplantation. *J. Urol.* **134**, 455.

Hunter, D. W., Castaneda-Zuniga, W. R., Coleman, C. C., Herrera, M. and Amplatz, K. (1983). Percutaneous techniques in the management of urological complications in renal transplant patients. *Radiology* **148**, 407.

Jain, A. B., Angrisani, L. and McMaster, P. (1986). Staghorn calculous in a renal allograft. *Transplant. Proc.* **18**, 959.

Jarowenko, M. V. and Flechner, S. M. (1985). Recipient ureterocalycostomy in a renal allograft: case report of a transplant salvage. *J. Urol.* **133**, 844.

Jaskowski, A., Jones, R. M., Murie, J. A. and Morris, P. J. (1987). Urological complications in 600 consecutive renal transplants. *Br. J. Surg.* **74**, 922.

Kabalin, J. N. and Kessler, R. (1989). Successful implantation of penile prosthesis in organ transplant patients. *Urology* **33**, 282.

Katz, J. P., Greenstein, S. M., Hakki, A., Miller, A., Katz, S. M. and Simonian, S. (1988). Transitional epithelial lesions of the ureter in renal transplant rejection. *Transplantation* **45**, 710.

Khauli, R. B. (1994). Genitourinary malignancies in organ transplant recipients. *Semin. Urol.* **12**, 224.

Kogan, S. J., Weiss, M. H. and Levitt, S. B. (1986). Successful renal transplantation in a patient with a neurogenic bladder managed by clean intermittent catherization. *J. Urol.* **135**, 563.

Koo Seen Lin, L. C., Bewick, M. and Koffman, C. G. (1993). Primary use of a double J silicone ureteric stent in renal transplantation. *Br. J. Urol.* **72**, 697.

Lieberman, R. P., Crummy, A. B., Glass, N. R. and Belzer, F. O. (1981). Fine-needle antegrade pyelography in the renal transplant. *J. Urol.* **126**, 155.

Lieberman, S. F., Keller, F. S., Barry, J. M. and Rosch, J. (1982). Percutaneous antegrade transluminal ureteroplasty for renal allograft ureteral stenosis. *J. Urol.* **128**, 122.

Lord, R. H., Pepera, T. and Williams, G. (1991). Ureteroureterostomy and pyeloureterostomy without native nephrectomy in renal transplantation. *Br. J. Urol.* **67**, 349.

Loughlin, K. R., Tilney, N. L. and Richie, J. P. (1984). Urologic complications in 718 renal transplant patients. *Surgery* **95**, 297.

Lowell, J. A., Taylor, R. J., Cattral, M., Stevenson Bynon, J., Brennan, D. C. and Stratta, R. J. (1994). En bloc transplantation of a horseshoe kidney from a high risk multi-organ donor: case report and review of the literature. *J. Urol.* **152**, 468.

Mathew, T. H., Kincaid-Smith, P. and Vikraman, P. (1977). Risks of vesicoureteric reflux in the transplanted kidney. *N. Engl. J. Med.* **297**, 414.

McDougall, M. L., Welling, L. W. and Wiegman, T. B. (1984). Acquired renal cystic kidney disease: occurrence, prevalence and renal adenocarcinoma in patients on long-term hemodialysis. *N. Engl. J. Med.* **310**, 390.

Menezes de Goes, G., De Campos Freire, G., Borelli, M., Pompeo, A. C. L. and Wrociawski, E. R. (1981). Transplantation of a horseshoe kidney. *J. Urol.* **126**, 537.

Meria, P., Desgrippes, A., Arfi, C. and Le Duc, A. (1998). Encrusted cystitis and pyelitis. *J. Urol.* **160**, 3.

Morales, J. M., Aguado, R., Diaz-Gonzalez, R., *et al.* (1992). Alkaline-encrusted pyelitis/cystitis and urinary tract infection due to *Corynebacterium urealyticum*: a new severe complication after renal transplantation. *Transplant. Proc.* **24**, 81.

Motayne, G. G., Jindal, S. L., Irvine, A. H. and Abele, R. P. (1984). Calculus formation in renal transplant patients. *J. Urol.* **132**, 448.

Mundy, A. R., Podesta, M. L., Bewick, M., Rudge, C. J. and Ellis, F. G. (1981). The urological complications of 1,000 renal transplants. *Br. J. Urol.* **53**, 397.

Nghiem, D. D., Goldman, M. H., Mendez, G. P. and Lee, P. (1981). Significance of vesicoureteral reflux in renal transplantation. *Urology* **18**, 542.

Nicholson, M. L., Donnelly, P. K., Veitch, P. S. and Bell, P. R. F. (1991). Urological complications of renal transplantation: the impact of double J ureteric stents. *Ann. R. Coll. Surg. Engl.* **73**, 316.

Nicol, D. L., P'Ng, K., Hardie, D. R., Wall, D. R. and Hardie, I. R. (1993). Routine use of indwelling ureteral stents in renal transplantation. *J. Urol.* **150**, 1375.

Ohl, D. A., Konnak, J. W., Campbell, D. A., Dafoe, D. C., Merion, R. M. and Turcotte, J. G. (1988). Extravesical ureteroneocystostomy in renal transplantation. *J. Urol.* **139**, 499.

Palmer, J. M. and Chatterjee, S. N. (1978). Urologic complications in renal transplantation. *Surg. Clin. North Am.* **58**, 305.

Park, C. H., Ryu, D. S., Kim, K. S., Cho, W. H., Park, S. B. and Kim, H. C. (1994). Vesicoureteric reflux following renal transplantation: significance and risks. *Transplant. Proc.* **26**, 2191.

Penn, I. (1993). Effect of immunosuppression on pre-existing cancers. *Transplant. Proc.* **25**, 1380.

Rao, K. V. (1986). Urological complications associated with a kidney transplant biopsy: report of 3 cases and review of the literature. *J. Urol.* **135**, 768.

Rosenthal, J. T. and Khetan, U. (1989). Transplantation of cadaver kidneys from a donor with crossed non-fused renal ectopia. *J. Urol.* **141**, 1184.

Rowe, S. J., Montague, D. K., Steinmuller, D. R., Lakin, M. M. and Novick, A. C. (1993). Treatment of organic impotence with penile prosthesis in renal transplant patients. *Urology* **41**, 16.

Salvatierra, O., Kountz, S. L. and Belzer, F. O. (1974). Prevention of ureteral fistula after renal transplantation. *J. Urol.* **112**, 445.

Schmid, T., Spielberger, M., Sandbichler, P. and Margreiter, R. (1988). Modified ureterocystostomy: a low rate of urological complication in kidney transplantation. *Dtsch. Med. Wochenschr.* **113**, 1134.

Schmidt, R., Stippel, D., Krings, F. and Pollok, M. (1995). Malignancies of the genito-urinary system following renal transplantation. *Br. J. Urol.* **75**, 572.

Shah, S., Nath, V., Gopalkrishnan, G., Pandey, A. P. and Shastri, J. C. M. (1988). Evaluation of extravesical and Leadbetter-Politano ureteroneocystostomy in renal transplantation. *Br. J. Urol.* **62**, 412.

Sheil, A. G. R. (1992). Development of malignancy following renal transplantation in Australia and New Zeland. *Transplant. Proc.* **24**, 1275.

Shoskes, D. A., Hanbury, D., Cranston, D. and Morris, P. J. (1995). Urological complications in 1000 consecutive renal transplant recipients. *J. Urol.* **153**, 18.

Starzl, T. E., Groth, C. G., Putnam, C. W., *et al.* (1970). Urological complications in 216 human recipients of renal transplants. *Ann. Surg.* **172**, 1.

Streem, S. B., Novick, A. C., Steinmuller, D. R., and Another, A. N. (1988). Long-term efficacy of ureteral dilation for transplant ureteral stenosis. *J. Urol.* **140**, 32.

Swindle, P., Falk, M., Rigby, R., Petrie, J., Hawley, C. and Nicol, D. (1998). Transitional cell carcinoma in renal transplant recipients: the influence of compound analgesics. *Br. J. Urol.* **81**, 229.

Taylor, R. M. R. (1998). Impotence and the use of the internal iliac artery in renal transplantation. *Transplantation* **65**, 745.

Thrasher, J. B., Temple, D. R. and Spees, E. K. (1990). Extravesical versus Leadbetter-Politano ureteroneocystostomy: a comparison of urological complications in 320 renal transplants. *J. Urol.* **144**, 1105.

Tse, V., Khadra, M., Eisinger, D., Mitterdorfer, A., Boulas, J. and Rogers, J. (1997). Nephrogenic adenoma of bladder in renal transplant and non-renal transplant patients—a review of 22 cases. *Urology* **50**, 690.

Upsdell, S. M., Testa, H. J. and Lawson, R. S. (1992). The F-15 diuresis renogram in suspected obstruction of the upper urinary tract. *Br. J. Urol.* **69**, 126.

Van Son, W. J., Hooykaas, J. A., Slooff, M. J. and Tegzess, A. M. (1986). Vesicocalicostomy as ultimate solution for recurrent urological complications after cadaveric renal transplantation in a patient with poor bladder function. *J. Urol.* **136**, 889.

Wayne, W. C. (1981). Sexual and reproductive function in men treated with hemodialysis and renal transplantation. *J. Urol.* **126**, 713.

Whittier, F., Staab, E., Rhamy, R., Elliott, R. and Ginn, P. (1974). Vesicoureteral reflux after renal transplantation. *J. Urol.* **747**, 1097.

Yadav, R. V., Johnson, W., Morris, P. J., Sprague, P., Yoffa, D. and Marshall, V. C. (1972). Vesico-ureteric reflux following renal transplantation. *Br. J. Surg.* **59**, 33.

Youssef, N. I., Jindal, R., Babayan, R. J., *et al.* (1994). The Acucise catheter: a new endourological method for correcting transplant ureteric stenosis. *Transplantation* **57**, 1398.

Cardiovascular Complications After Renal Transplantation

C. R. V. Tomson

Introduction

As graft survival rates have increased, owing to advances in histocompatibility testing and better immunosuppression, the leading cause of graft loss has become death with a functioning graft; cardiovascular disease now is the leading cause of death with a functioning graft. Cardiovascular disease would be less of a problem if life expectancy after transplantation were normal, but life expectancy remains much poorer in transplant recipients than in the general population (Arend *et al.*, 1997). Premature cardiovascular disease is a major target for intervention in patients undergoing renal transplantation.

Numerous distinct cardiovascular diseases contribute to premature cardiovascular morbidity and mortality in renal transplant recipients, including classic atherosclerosis, arteriosclerosis, hypertensive vascular and cardiac disease and cardiac valvular diseases. These abnormalities may be present before the onset of renal disease, may evolve with the progression of renal disease to end-stage renal failure or may occur *de novo* as a direct result of renal replacement therapy—all of which have different implications for attempts at prevention of premature cardiovascular morbidity and mortality. Selection of transplant candidates should include assessment of the presence and extent of preexisting cardiovascular disease, the consequent risk of death during anesthesia and the effect of transplantation on the subsequent progression of cardiovascular disease. In a patient free of overt atherosclerotic disease at transplantation, however, impaired graft function and drug treatment may cause hypertension, dyslipidemia, diabetes and proteinuria, resulting in myocardial infarction, stroke or amputation for peripheral vascular disease. An increased risk of cardiovascular disease is not seen to the same extent in liver transplant recipients. This difference suggests strongly that the roots of the problem lie in the damage to the vasculature caused by chronic renal failure, rather than by transplantation itself.

Cardiovascular Disease in End-Stage Renal Failure

Despite improvements in dialysis therapy, life expectancy among dialysis patients remains as poor as for many forms of cancer (Port, 1994). Cardiovascular disease is one of the major causes of premature death in patients on dialysis treatment, with mortality rates at least 10-fold higher among nondiabetic dialysis patients than in the general population and 44-fold higher among diabetic dialysis patients (Brown *et al.*, 1994; Raine *et al.*, 1992). The increased risk conferred by end-stage renal failure is greatest among younger patients, to the extent that a 25- to 35-year-old dialysis patient has the same risk of cardiovascular disease as an 80-year-old in the

general population (Levey *et al.*, 1998; Fig. 30–1). Early series suggested that this increased risk was due to *accelerated atherosclerosis* as a result of dialysis or the accompanying dietary modifications (Lindner *et al.*, 1974), but larger series of more representative patients have not supported this suggestion (Burke *et al.*, 1978; Nicholls *et al.*, 1980). Prospective studies have not confirmed a high rate of development of *de novo* ischemic heart disease in dialysis patients (Parfrey *et al.*, 1996; Rostand *et al.*, 1979, 1984), with the exception of patients with diabetes. The concept of accelerated atherosclerosis also is refuted by observations that death rate from myocardial infarction is highest in the first year of hemodialysis and falls subsequently (Mailloux *et al.*, 1991; Raine, 1994b), that the risk of acute myocardial infarction is highest early after initiation of dialysis (Herzog, 1999) and that the duration of dialysis before transplantation is not a predictor of cardiovascular mortality after transplantation (Arend *et al.*, 1997), findings that are consistent with the suggestion that the initiation of dialysis causes the clinical expression of hitherto silent coronary disease acquired in the predialysis period. The presence of clinically diagnosed atherosclerotic disease before end-stage renal failure is a potent risk marker for poor survival (Churchill *et al.*, 1992; Farias *et al.*, 1994), as exemplified by the dismal survival in dialysis patients with atherosclerotic renal vascular disease (Conlon *et al.*, 1998; Mailloux *et al.*, 1994b).

Several angiographic studies have shown a high incidence among dialysis patients of angina with normal or near-normal coronary arteries (Koch *et al.*, 1997a; Kremastinos *et al.*, 1992; Roig *et al.*, 1981; Rostand *et al.*, 1984, 1986), probably as a result of increased oxygen demand from left ventricular hypertrophy, anemia and arteriovenous fistulae, and of increased susceptibility to ischemia as a result of metabolic abnormalities (Raine *et al.*, 1993b)—emphasizing the multifactorial nature of cardiovascular disease in renal failure. Data from the United States Renal Data System suggest that approximately 22% of deaths from cardiac causes among patients on dialysis are due to acute myocardial infarction. A study using this database of 34,189 patients on dialysis in the United States between 1977 and 1995 showed an extraordinarily high mortality after myocardial infarction of 59% at 1 year, 73% at 2 years and 90% at 5 years, with higher mortality in older patients and patients with diabetes (Herzog *et al.*, 1998). The same authors reported a low use of thrombolytic therapy in dialysis patients with acute myocardial infarction, possibly because of atypical clinical presentation (Herzog, 1999).

Although most commentators have focused on coronary disease, carotid disease also is an important cause of morbidity and mortality in renal failure. Stroke is associated closely with hypertension in Japanese hemodialysis patients (Iseki and Fukiyama, 1996); associations with apolipoprotein (a) phenotypes (Kronenberg *et al.*, 1994) and apolipoprotein E

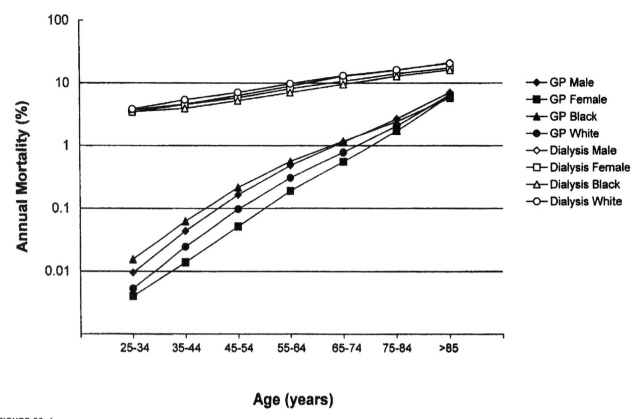

FIGURE 30–1

Cardiovascular mortality by age, race and sex in the general U.S. population (GP) compared with dialysis patients. (Reproduced with permission of Levey *et al.*, 1998.)

genotypes (Lim *et al.*, 1997) have been described. Peripheral vascular disease is common in dialysis patients, although how frequently it develops *de novo* in patients free of vascular disease at the start of renal replacement therapy is uncertain (Fishbane *et al.*, 1995; Webb *et al.*, 1993).

Much of the available data on cardiovascular deaths comes from epidemiological studies based on national registries. Although valuable, data collection for these registries requires categorization of the cause of death in broad categories—*cardiovascular, infective, malignancy*—in a way that makes it difficult to identify accurately possible contributors to the increased death rate (e.g., to distinguish the contributions of atherosclerotic coronary heart disease and hypertensive heart disease). Data from the European Dialysis and Transplantation Registry suggested that the risk of cardiovascular death was higher in Northern than in Southern Europe and that this geographical difference in risk applied to the general population and, amplified 17-fold, to patients with renal failure (Raine *et al.*, 1992). Prospective studies in Manchester and Milan with precise guidelines for classification of the causes of death showed no difference in cardiovascular morbidity or mortality between the two centers, however, suggesting that the difference in the registry data might be due to systematic underrecording of cardiovascular deaths in countries where such deaths are much rarer in the general population (Brown *et al.*, 1998).

Cardiovascular Disease After Transplantation

Early surveys from individual units stressed that nonfatal occlusive vascular disease was common in transplant recipients. A series from Sydney reported a cumulative incidence

of occlusive disease (coronary heart disease, peripheral arterial disease and cerebral thrombosis) of 42% at 6 years in patients free of clinical evidence of vascular disease before transplantation (Ibels *et al.*, 1977). Much of this excess risk may have been attributable to the high prevalence of smoking, hypertension and dyslipidemia in these patients, however.

Cardiovascular disease is the dominant cause of death after transplantation in modern series (Lindholm *et al.*, 1995; Raine, 1995). Deaths from ischemic heart disease accounted for 53% of deaths with a functioning graft in a Scandinavian study of 1,347 grafts over 5 years; the risk of death from ischemic heart disease in patients aged 55 to 64 years compared with that in the general population was 6.4 in nondiabetic transplant recipients, 20.8 in diabetic transplant recipients and 8.6 in patients remaining on dialysis (Lindholm *et al.*, 1995). Similarly, in a study from the Netherlands, the standardized mortality ratio (age-adjusted and sex-adjusted mortality compared with the general population) was 14.7 for recipients of first renal transplants in the first year after transplantation and 4.4 in subsequent years; the cardiovascular standardized mortality ratio was 12.1 (95% confidence interval, 4.9–19.2) in the first year and 9.1 (95% confidence interval, 6.7–11.5) in subsequent years (Arend *et al.*, 1997).

The question of whether renal transplantation *per se* increases the risk of death compared with continued dialysis treatment is important. After controlling for other risk factors, two early studies concluded that life expectancy was similar in dialysis patients and transplant recipients (Burton and Walls, 1987; Hutchinson *et al.*, 1984). Port and colleagues showed that the relative risk of death after transplantation compared with remaining on the waiting list was increased initially, after adjustment for age, sex, race and primary renal disease, but fell to a relative risk of 0.36 in individuals surviving for at least 1 year after transplantation (Port et al., 1993). The improvement in life expectancy conferred by successful transplantation was greatest among diabetics and was not significant in patients with renal failure resulting from glomerulonephritis, suggesting that, similar to other interventions that reduce cardiovascular mortality (e.g., statins, antihypertensive treatment), the greatest benefit is seen among patients at highest risk (Port et al., 1993). Similarly, successful transplantation increases life expectancy among older patients (age > 60 years) (Schaubel et al., 1995). A small study from Poland showed a decrease in cardiovascular mortality after adjustment for the presence of cardiovascular disease at the start of renal replacement therapy (Surdacki et al., 1995). The likelihood of death with a functioning graft increases with age and diabetes (Hirata et al., 1996), however, and these observations do not imply that scarce cadaveric organs should be allocated preferentially to high-risk recipients; the number of quality-adjusted life years gained by allocation to fit, younger patients is likely to be considerably higher.

Few studies have addressed the relative contribution of risk factors to atherosclerosis in renal transplant recipients. In an extension of a previous study of 403 patients transplanted in one center (Kasiske, 1988), risk factors for the development of definite ischemic heart disease, peripheral vascular disease and cerebral vascular disease were analyzed by multiple regression analysis, using time-averaged values for variables such as cholesterol and blood pressure. Many of the earlier patients in the series underwent pretransplant splenectomy. Of patients, 35% were transplanted in the cyclosporine era, the remainder receiving azathioprine and prednisolone; most received induction treatment with antilymphocyte globulin. By 15 years, 23% of surviving patients had developed ischemic heart disease; 15%, cerebral vascular disease and 15%, peripheral vascular disease (Fig. 30–2). In all analyses, pretransplant vascular disease was a strong predictor of posttransplant vascular disease, and ischemic heart disease, peripheral vascular disease and cerebral vascular disease all were predictive of each other. Independent risk factors for ischemic heart disease were age, diabetes, male sex, splenectomy, number of acute rejection episodes and low high-density lipoprotein (HDL) cholesterol. In the earlier series from the same center, total cholesterol, blood pressure and smoking all were significant risk factors (Kasiske, 1988); their absence in the later series may be explained partly by aggressive treatment of hypertension and the introduction of lipid-lowering treatment. For cerebral vascular disease, risk factors were diabetes, smoking, splenectomy, number of acute rejection episodes and hypoalbuminemia. For peripheral vascular disease, diabetes was an extremely powerful risk factor (unadjusted relative risk, 25.7), with male sex, smoking and hypoalbuminemia all independently associated (Kasiske et al., 1996).

A retrospective longitudinal study from the Netherlands found age greater than 40 years, hypertension, male sex, smoking and diabetes to be associated significantly with posttransplant mortality, although the impact of these individual factors on mortality was small. Standardized mortality was 14 times the population average in the first year and remained 4 times the population average in subsequent years posttransplant (Arend et al., 1997). An earlier study from the same center found increased cardiovascular morbidity and mortality in patients with polycystic kidney disease compared with other nondiabetic transplant recipients (Florijn et al., 1994). A smaller longitudinal study in Poland confirmed that cardiovascular disease at the time of transplantation was highly predictive of posttransplant cardiovascular mortality,

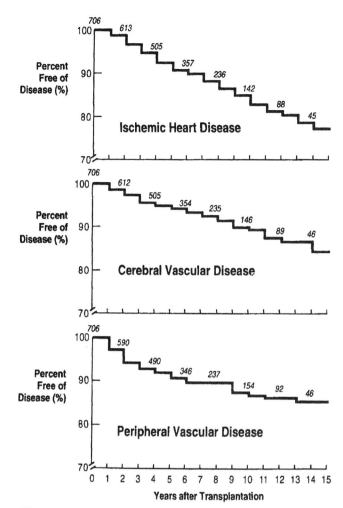

FIGURE 30–2

Actuarial incidences of ischemic heart disease, cerebral vascular disease and peripheral vascular disease in renal transplant patients free of disease at the time of transplantation, Minnesota, 1976–1991. (Reproduced with permission of Kasiske et al., 1996.)

although it also was found that patients receiving successful transplants had a reduced risk of death compared with patients remaining on dialysis after adjustment for preexisting cardiovascular disease (Surdacki et al., 1995).

In a cross-sectional multicenter study of 406 stable transplant recipients from Norway, where cardiovascular mortality after transplantation is particularly high, ischemic heart disease was commoner in men and in diabetics and was associated with age and total cholesterol but not with blood pressure. Cerebrovascular disease was associated only with age, and peripheral vascular disease was associated with age, male sex and systolic blood pressure (Aakhus et al., 1999). The association between diabetes (present in 17%) and ischemic heart disease was lost on multiple regression analysis. In this study, in contrast to the longitudinal study described earlier, symptomatic angina was accepted as evidence of ischemic heart disease. Only a single blood pressure measurement was used in the analysis, and a significant number of patients with electrocardiographic evidence of left ventricular hypertrophy were classified as normotensive—illustrating the difficulties of assessing risk factors from a single cross-sectional analysis.

As noted earlier, dialysis patients have a high cumulative

mortality in the 5 years after myocardial infarction. The same study showed much lower mortality rates in transplant patients after myocardial infarction, with mortality of 24% at 1 year, 30% at 2 years and 47% at 5 years: The difference between dialysis and transplant patients remained after statistical adjustment for demographic characteristics, cause of renal failure, duration of pretransplant dialysis, calendar year and coexisting illnesses, with an adjusted relative risk of all-cause death of 2.72 for dialysis patients compared with transplant patients. It remains highly likely, however, that part of this difference was due to selection of fitter patients for transplantation (Herzog et al., 1998).

Arterial Pathology in Renal Disease

Patients with renal disease are at risk not only of atherosclerosis, as a result of well-recognized risk factors such as dyslipidemia, hypertension and smoking, but also of vascular calcification (Budisavljevic et al., 1996) and of accelerated aging or degenerative arterial disease, often termed *arteriosclerosis* (London and Druecke, 1997). As mentioned earlier, angina often can occur despite normal coronary arteries in renal patients, as a result of increased demand and metabolic abnormalities. This combination of numerous pathologies may explain why many small series in transplanted patients have failed to show a relationship between a risk factor (e.g., hypercholesterolemia) and cardiovascular events.

Only a few systematic studies of arterial histopathology in renal disease have been reported. Vincenti and coworkers examined the iliac arteries histologically in 50 nondiabetic dialysis patients at the time of transplantation (Vincenti et al., 1980). Arterial disease was present in 62%, and its severity was related to age and especially to previous hypertension, although not to serum cholesterol or to duration of dialysis. Although the authors used the term *atherosclerosis* to describe the abnormalities, they commented on the prominence of fragmentation of the internal elastic lamellae, smooth muscle proliferation and intimal fibrosis and the rarity of mucopolysaccharide deposition, calcification and lipid deposition (Vincenti et al., 1980). A similar absence of lipid deposition, with intimal fibrosis and damage to elastic lamellae, was reported in three other clinical series (Ejerblad et al., 1979; Ibels et al., 1979; Tomson et al., 1988).

Vascular calcification is extremely common in patients with renal disease. Although vascular calcification in patients without renal disease nearly always is associated with atherosclerosis, this is not the case in uremic patients, in whom calcification frequently is confined to the arterial media and is associated with hyperparathyroidism, hypertension and chronic elevation of the calcium phosphate product (Goldsmith et al., 1997). Although usually asymptomatic, vascular calcification occasionally can result in calciphylaxis, a syndrome of skin necrosis associated with small vessel occlusion as a result of thrombosis and severe vascular calcification that frequently is fatal (Budisavljevic et al., 1996; Wilkinson et al., 1988). Parathyroidectomy is of probable benefit (Hafner et al., 1995); hyperbaric oxygen therapy has been reported to be helpful in accelerating healing.

One clinical counterpart to these pathological findings is decreased conduit artery compliance, reflecting decreased elasticity (London et al., 1996). Decreased conduit artery compliance, as measured by pulse wave velocity, has been shown to be a strong independent predictor of death among dialysis patients (Blacher et al., 1999). Coronary artery calcification can be detected by fluorography, standard computed tomography (CT), and electron-beam CT, but whether this finding carries the same prognostic value in renal patients as in those without renal disease (Dixon and Coulden, 1997) is uncertain. One study in renal transplant candidates showed that digital subtraction fluorography had a sensitivity of 78% and a specificity of 66% for the prediction of angiographic coronary stenoses (Marwick et al., 1989); newer techniques have not been evaluated extensively.

These findings emphasize the high rate of vascular disease and its relation to hypertension in patients *coming* to renal transplantation, and it is relevant that the strongest predictor of posttransplant vascular disease in Kasiske's study was the presence of pretransplant vascular disease (Kasiske, 1993). An understanding of the risk factors known to contribute to cardiovascular disease in the general population as well as the extra risk factors thought to operate in uremia is essential for all clinicians who manage patients at any stage of renal disease.

Hypertension in Renal Disease
EFFECT OF HYPERTENSION ON PATIENT AND GRAFT SURVIVAL

Numerous studies have shown associations between hypertension and chronic renal allograft dysfunction and, as in other populations with established renal dysfunction, an association between the severity of hypertension and the rate of decline of renal function (Cheigh et al., 1989; Kokado et al., 1996; Modena et al., 1991; Warholm et al., 1995). Cosio and associates reported that the presence of poorly controlled posttransplant hypertension was associated with poor graft survival in black American but not in white American transplant recipients (Cosio et al., 1995) and that posttransplant hypertension in black Americans was associated with higher body weight and with pretransplant hypertension (Cosio et al., 1997). A study from Germany showed a stronger association between hypertension at the time of transplantation and subsequent chronic renal allograft dysfunction than with the degree of HLA matching (Frei et al., 1995), suggesting that hypertension may be part of the cause, rather than simply the result, of graft dysfunction (Bock, 1995).

Cheigh and colleagues found that graft survival was impaired similarly in patients with well-controlled hypertension and poorly controlled hypertension compared with normotensive patients (Cheigh et al., 1989), suggesting that hypertension simply is a manifestation of impaired graft function. Similarly, Massy and coworkers found that although hypertension was a risk factor for chronic renal allograft dysfunction on univariate analysis, it was not independent of other nonimmunological risk factors, including hypoalbuminemia, proteinuria and hypertriglyceridemia (Massy et al., 1996a). Controlled trials comparing two target levels of blood pressure control in patients at risk of chronic renal allograft dysfunction have not been performed. The evidence from other populations with proteinuric progressive renal disease that tight blood pressure control reduces progression of renal dysfunction is strong, however (Giatras et al., 1997; Gruppo Italiano di Studi Epidemiologici in Nefrologia, 1997; Kasiske et al., 1993; Klahr et al., 1994; Maschio et al., 1996), suggesting that similar blood pressure targets should be adopted in patients with renal transplants (Levey et al., 1998). There are no data proving that posttransplant hypertension is associated with increased cardiovascular morbidity or mortality, although a trend toward higher cardiovascular mortality in patients with hypertension (six events among 32 hypertensives compared with one event among 23 normotensives over 7 years' follow-up) was noted in one study (van Ypersele de Strihou et al., 1983).

MECHANISMS OF HYPERTENSION IN RENAL DISEASE

A progressively greater incidence of hypertension is found as renal function declines (Buckalew et al., 1996), in keeping with the central role of the kidneys in the maintenance of normal blood pressure (Cowley and Roman, 1996; Guyton, 1987; Guyton et al., 1972; Raine, 1994a). Numerous factors contribute to the maintenance of high arterial blood pressure in renal patients (Preston et al., 1996; Raine, 1994a). Classically, hypertension in the presence of renal impairment has been attributed to the interplay of two major factors: (1) salt and water retention as a result of a reset relationship between arterial pressure and sodium excretion and (2) renin overproduction by diseased kidneys (Raine, 1994b). Logically, hypertension resulting from salt and water retention should respond to dietary salt restriction together with diuretics in patients with pre–end-stage renal impairment and to adequate removal of salt and water by ultrafiltration combined with dietary salt restriction in dialysis-dependent patients. Hypertension resulting from renin overproduction is less common and responds to bilateral nephrectomy and to a greater or lesser extent to β-blockers, angiotensin-converting enzyme (ACE) inhibitors or angiotensin II receptor blockade.

A major role for overactivity of the sympathetic nervous system in the hypertension of chronic renal failure has been supported by observations that postganglionic sympathetic nerve discharge to skeletal muscle blood vessels, recorded directly by microelectrodes in the peroneal nerve, was more than twice as high in hypertensive dialysis patients than in normal subjects or in dialysis patients who had undergone bilateral nephrectomy and were normotensive (Converse et al., 1992). These results suggest that in renal failure there may be reversible sympathetic activation, mediated by an afferent signal originating in the failing kidneys. It was shown that ACE inhibition decreases sympathetic overactivity in chronic renal failure (Ligtenberg et al., 1999).

Impaired vasorelaxation as a result of decreased release or activity of the endogenous vasodilator nitric oxide may contribute to hypertension in renal disease. Accumulation of asymmetrical dimethylarginine (ADMA), an endogenous inhibitor of nitric oxide synthesis, has been reported in chronic renal failure (Vallance et al., 1992). A study showed higher levels of ADMA in hemodialysis patients than in healthy controls, with higher levels among hemodialysis patients with clinically manifest atherosclerotic disease than in patients without (Kielstein et al., 1999), but no study has yet shown a relationship between ADMA levels and blood pressure, and the relevance of the increased ADMA levels remains uncertain (Anderstam et al., 1997). Other mechanisms that may contribute to hypertension in renal disease include hyperparathyroidism (Raine et al., 1993a) and increased endothelin release (Takahashi et al., 1994), although the clinical relevance of raised endothelin levels in renal patients is uncertain (Hand et al., 1999).

MECHANISMS OF HYPERTENSION AFTER RENAL TRANSPLANTATION

Impaired Graft Function

As noted earlier, hypertension is a nearly uniform feature of chronic renal allograft dysfunction as well as of chronic renal impairment caused by disease of native kidneys; the development of hypertension in a previously normotensive transplant patient is correlated closely with morphological evidence of chronic rejection or recurrent disease if other causes such as graft artery stenosis have been ruled out (Olmer et al., 1988). Decreased nephron number is thought to cause sodium-sensitive hypertension, and this may be one mechanism by which *nephron underdosing* or early loss of nephrons because of rejection contributes to the later development of chronic renal allograft dysfunction (Brenner and Mackenzie, 1997). This hypothesis has not been tested by systematic studies of salt intake and blood pressure at various levels of transplant function or by studies of the effect of dietary sodium restriction on blood pressure and progression.

Native Kidneys

Cross-sectional studies of the prevalence of hypertension after transplantation in relation to the presence of native kidneys show that hypertension is more frequent when native kidneys are *in situ* in most cases (Huysmans et al., 1987; Pollini et al., 1979). This situation is not seen in all cases (Kirkman et al., 1982), and the cause of renal failure may be important. In dialysis patients whose disease was chronic pyelonephritis, there was no difference in blood pressure after transplantation in patients who had undergone pretransplant bilateral nephrectomy and in a control group with the same diagnosis matched for age and sex who had not had this procedure (Darby et al., 1993).

The influence of native kidneys on posttransplant hypertension usually is attributed to hypersecretion of renin by the native kidneys. Renal vein catheterization of host and transplanted kidneys has shown hyperreninemia arising from native kidneys (Grunfeld et al., 1975), although measurement of plasma renin activity does not predict reliably blood pressure or the response to nephrectomy in transplant patients (Zeier et al., 1998). Increased sympathetic activity as a result of an afferent signal arising in diseased native kidneys is an additional possible explanation (Converse et al., 1992) and would account for the observation (Huysmans et al., 1988) that β-blockade produced no changes in blood pressure in renal transplant patients who had undergone bilateral nephrectomy, in contrast to patients with host kidneys *in situ*, in whom β-blockade reduced mean blood pressure by 15 mmHg.

Transplanted Kidneys

There is increasing evidence that alterations in renal sodium handling are primarily responsible for the genesis of many forms of hypertension and that these abnormalities may be transmitted with the kidney by transplantation, indicating that they are intrinsic to the kidney itself (Cowley and Roman, 1996; Jelakovic and Mayer, 1995; Koomans et al., 1996). In experimental rats, transplantation of kidneys from hypertensive strains into normotensive recipients results in hypertension, even if the donor rats were rendered normotensive from birth by drug treatment (Rettig, 1993). The development of hypertension after cross-transplantation from a hypertensive to a normotensive strain is preceded by sodium retention (Rettig et al., 1996).

In humans, there is evidence from the precyclosporine era that preexisting essential hypertension in renal transplant recipients could be reversed by receipt of a kidney from a normotensive donor (Curtis et al., 1983a). Conversely, recipients of kidneys retrieved from cadaveric donors who had died of subarachnoid hemorrhage were more likely to develop hypertension than those receiving kidneys from donors who had died of head injury or cerebral tumor; heart weights in the donors with subarachnoid hemorrhage were significantly higher, consistent with a higher blood pressure in this group (Strandgaard and Hansen, 1986). Retrospective (Guidi et al., 1985) and prospective (Guidi et al., 1996) studies in patients not receiving calcineurin inhibitors have shown that kidneys from donors with a family history of hypertension increase the risk of posttransplant hypertension only in recipients who do not have a family history of hypertension. This group of recipients (normotensive family, hypertensive kidney) were more at risk of hypertension and suffered a greater degree of renal damage during acute rejections than all other recipients (Guidi *et al.*, 1998). Beyond their theoretical interest, these findings are relevant to the cause of hypertension after transplantation.

Immunosuppressive Treatment

Cyclosporine, tacrolimus and corticosteroids all contribute to hypertension after renal transplantation, an effect shown clearly in numerous case-control and conversion studies, whereas neither azathioprine nor mycophenolate has any effect on blood pressure (Curtis, 1994; Zeier *et al.*, 1998). The mechanism by which cyclosporine causes hypertension is complex (Haas and Mayer, 1997). It stimulates the renin-angiotensin system in laboratory rodents, but in humans the major mechanism by which cyclosporine causes hypertension is sodium retention and volume expansion, with relative suppression of the renin-angiotensin axis (Curtis *et al.*, 1988). Studies in heart transplant recipients show that cyclosporine induces increased sympathetic activity (Scherrer *et al.*, 1990), possibly through an effect on central nervous system immunophilins (Sander *et al.*, 1996), an effect that may be responsible for sodium retention (Mark, 1990). In all species, cyclosporine causes intrarenal vasoconstriction, acting predominantly at the afferent glomerular arteriole, an effect that can be antagonized by calcium channel blockers (Curtis, 1994). Enhanced release of the powerful endogenous vasoconstrictor endothelin may play an important role (Meyer-Lehnert *et al.*, 1997). Cyclosporine also up-regulates angiotensin II receptors in human vascular smooth muscle cells, enhancing calcium entry on stimulation (Avdonin *et al.*, 1999). These mechanisms provide a rationale for the use of sodium restriction, diuretics, α-blockers and β-blockers, calcium channel blockers and ACE inhibitors or angiotensin II receptor blockers in cyclosporine-associated hypertension.

Tacrolimus therapy causes hypertension, probably by similar mechanisms. Hypertension has been reported to improve in many reports of conversion from cyclosporine to tacrolimus (Copley *et al.*, 1998; Friemann *et al.*, 1998), although interpretation of these studies is complicated by the fact that renal excretory function often improved as a result of rescue therapy. In the large randomized studies of cyclosporine versus tacrolimus in kidney transplantation, the incidence of hypertension at 12 months' follow-up was only marginally lower with tacrolimus (Jensik, 1998; Shapiro *et al.*, 1991) or no different (Mayer *et al.*, 1997; Pirsch *et al.*, 1997), although two short-term studies have shown a lower incidence of hypertension in patients randomized to tacrolimus (Radermacher *et al.*, 1998; Schleiber *et al.*, 1995).

Although hypertension is a well-recognized feature of Cushing's syndrome, the impact of corticosteroid treatment on blood pressure after renal transplantation is variable. Numerous observations of the effect of different steroid regimens and of the effects on blood pressure of steroid withdrawal support the concept that corticosteroids predispose patients to hypertension after renal transplantation (Hricik *et al.*, 1992b; Morris *et al.*, 1982; Raine, 1994b). Two randomized studies of late steroid withdrawal confirmed a beneficial effect on blood pressure of steroid withdrawal (Hollander *et al.*, 1997; Ratcliffe *et al.*, 1996), although the apparent improvement in blood pressure appeared to be transient, being

no longer evident 1 year after steroid withdrawal (Ratcliffe *et al.*, 1996).

Transplant Renal Artery Stenosis

Graft artery stenosis should be suspected whenever hypertension develops or worsens relatively rapidly in a transplant recipient, especially in association with a decline in graft function or a bruit audible over the allograft. Other presentations include recurrent hypertensive heart failure (so-called flash pulmonary edema), particularly in the presence of well-preserved left ventricular function (Lye *et al.*, 1996), and a rise in serum creatinine after introduction or increase in the dose of an ACE inhibitor or addition of diuretic therapy (Curtis *et al.*, 1983b; Hricik, 1987; Mourad *et al.*, 1989; van der Woude *et al.*, 1985). The incidence of this complication has been estimated to be 1 to 25%, reflecting the various definitions used and the fact that the gold standard test, direct renal angiography, is an invasive procedure that cannot be used indiscriminately (Fervenza *et al.*, 1998). Stenosis may occur at the anastomosis, proximal to the anastomosis or distal to it. Possible contributing factors include trauma to the artery during retrieval or reimplantation, by excessive traction, intimal damage during cannulation or clamping; poor suture technique; need for endarterectomy in the internal iliac artery before end-to-end anastomosis (Sutherland *et al.*, 1993b); preexisting atheromatous disease or fibromuscular dysplasia; turbulence distal to the anastomosis; acute rejection (Wong *et al.*, 1996) and cytomegalovirus infection (Pouria *et al.*, 1998).

There is no consensus on how best to select patients suspected of having transplant renal artery stenosis for angiography. Measurement of peripheral plasma renin levels are not helpful because of renin production from native kidneys and of salt and water retention as a result of underperfusion of the transplant (Fervenza *et al.*, 1998). Isotope renography before and after administration of an ACE inhibitor (usually captopril) relies on the fact that in the presence of impaired renal perfusion, maintenance of glomerular filtration rate depends on increased local production of angiotensin II, which results in vasoconstriction of the efferent arteriole. Prevention of the formation of angiotensin II results in an acute decline in glomerular filtration rate. Performance of this test is too poor for it to be relied on to exclude transplant renal artery stenosis (Erley *et al.*, 1992), although some evidence suggests that this functional test is a better predictor of the response to revascularization than the angiographic appearances (Shamlou *et al.*, 1994). Duplex ultrasound is highly observer dependent and time-consuming but appears reliable in some centers. Alternative noninvasive techniques include helical CT angiography and magnetic resonance angiography (Gedroyc *et al.*, 1992), although a high false-positive rate has been reported with the latter (Loubeyre *et al.*, 1996). The choice of investigation depends on local expertise.

Because of early concerns over graft loss and mortality associated with operative repair of graft artery stenosis, percutaneous transluminal angioplasty has been widely employed in the 1990s and is now the procedure of first choice, unless evidence exists that the transplant artery is excessively long with kinking, in which case primary surgical repair should be undertaken (Benoit *et al.*, 1990; Fauchald *et al.*, 1992). The initial results are good for blood pressure control and renal excretory function, but several series have reported a high restenosis rate after angioplasty (Benoit *et al.*, 1990; Fervenza *et al.*, 1998), and a high index of suspicion must be maintained. Although stent insertion may prevent restenosis, this has yet to be proved. The options in a patient with restenosis are repeat angioplasty with or without stent insertion and surgical revascularization. This is an individual decision that should be based on an assessment of surgical risk and local expertise.

Extrinsic compression of the transplant by lymphocele is a rare reversible cause of hypertension (Vanwalleghem *et al.*, 1997). This phenomenon of hypertension caused by extrinsic compression is well recognized in native kidneys (the *Page kidney*), usually after blunt trauma, and in animal models (*cellophane wrap hypertension*). Whether other cases of transplant compression by a dense pseudocapsule are being missed is a matter for speculation.

Correction of Anemia

Successful transplantation induces a rapid rise in hemoglobin concentration and hematocrit. In patients maintained on dialysis, rapid correction of anemia frequently is associated with exacerbation of preexisting hypertension, the mechanism for which is complex but involves a failure of cardiac output to normalize after correction of anemia and may be related, at least in part, to persisting extracellular volume expansion, which helps to maintain oxygen delivery to the tissues in anemia (Anastassiades *et al.*, 1993; Raine and Roger, 1991). Whether or not similar mechanisms apply after transplantation, when volume homeostasis is controlled by the transplanted kidney rather than by adjustment of the dialysis prescription, is uncertain. One nonrandomized study in 12 patients with posttransplant erythrocytosis, using ambulatory blood pressure measurements, showed a fall of mean 24-hour blood pressure from 153/95 to 139/85 mmHg after reduction of hemoglobin concentration from 18.7 to 14.6 g/dl by phlebotomy (Barenbrock *et al.*, 1993).

MANAGEMENT OF HYPERTENSION AFTER RENAL TRANSPLANTATION
Measurement

Accurate and repeated measurement of blood pressure is essential for rational decisions about treatment of hypertension after transplantation; casual, single measurements of blood pressure to the nearest 10 mmHg with equipment that is not regularly calibrated as soon as the patient has sat down in the clinic are inadequate and introduce levels of imprecision that never would be tolerated in a biochemical measurement of kidney function. Accurate measurement requires a cuff of at least 80% of the arm circumference; with the arm supported at heart level; measured in a patient who has not ingested caffeine or smoked within 30 minutes; after 5 minutes' rest; with a mercury sphygmomanometer, a recently calibrated aneroid sphygmomanometer or a validated electronic device. At least two measurements should be taken, 2 minutes apart, and the results averaged; additional readings should be taken if the first two readings differ by more than 5 mmHg (Joint National Committee, 1997; World Health Organization, 1999). The more measurements that are taken, the more reliance can be placed on them. Ambulatory and home blood pressure measurements increase the amount of information available but give systematically lower measurements than clinic-based measurements, usually being 7 to 10 mmHg lower. The daytime mean blood pressure is the most clinically relevant summary measurement from ambulatory blood pressure recordings, although transplant patients often may show lack of a nocturnal dip in blood pressure, which may be an adverse prognostic indicator.

Diagnosis of Hypertension

The threshold for introduction of antihypertensive treatment in an individual patient not only should depend on

repeated careful measurements of blood pressure but also on the cardiovascular risk profile for that patient. Because transplant recipients are at such high risk of cardiovascular disease, they should be considered to be in the highest risk category, on a par with elderly patients with severe hypertension, hyperlipidemia and a positive personal and family history of ischemic heart disease (Levey *et al.*, 1998); treatment should be initiated if blood pressure is greater than 140 mmHg systolic or 90 mmHg diastolic, or both. Because several studies have shown a beneficial effect of lower blood pressure targets in renal patients with significant proteinuria, the aim of treatment should be to reduce blood pressure to less than 125/75 mmHg in transplant recipients with proteinuria and to less than 130/85 mmHg in transplant patients without proteinuria (Levey *et al.*, 1998). Proteinuria is defined, for these purposes, as greater than 1 g/24 h or a protein/creatinine ratio of greater than 100 mg/mmol on an early morning urine sample.

Nondrug Treatment

Given that posttransplant hypertension often results from impaired excretion of dietary salt, it seems rational to advise dietary salt restriction as part of treatment—doubly so because the effectiveness of some drug treatments is amplified by dietary salt restriction. This policy has not been tested formally, however. Additional measures that may improve blood pressure control are weight reduction in obese patients, regular aerobic exercise and avoidance of excess alcohol intake.

Drug Treatment

Given the myriad mechanisms of posttransplant hypertension, it is not surprising that it is impossible to state with certainty which drug or drug class is most appropriate for an individual patient. Dihydropyridine calcium channel blockers ameliorate the nephrotoxicity of calcineurin inhibitors (Harper *et al.*, 1996) and probably are the drugs of first choice in patients receiving this type of immunosuppression, although they may exacerbate gingival hyperplasia in patients receiving cyclosporine and are a frequent cause of lower limb edema. Many calcium channel blockers (including verapamil, diltiazem, nicardipine and amlodipine but not nifedipine) interact with the cytochrome P-450 system and increase cyclosporine levels; this interaction has been used to generate cost savings, although the effect of diltiazem wanes with time (Patton *et al.*, 1994).

Angiotensin-converting enzyme inhibitors may be particularly beneficial in proteinuric patients, in whom the risk of progressive renal dysfunction is high, because of the extra protection these agents appear to offer against progression, particularly if attainment of the target blood pressure of 125/75 mmHg is difficult (Levey *et al.*, 1998). Angiotensin-converting enzyme inhibitors also are useful in the treatment of posttransplant erythrocytosis (Beckingham *et al.*, 1995), but ACE inhibitors can exacerbate anemia in the presence of renal impairment (Gossmann *et al.*, 1996), in both instances probably by interfering with erythropoietin release. Use of ACE inhibitors mandates regular measurement of serum creatinine, in view of the potential for these drugs to cause deterioration in renal function in the presence of renal artery stenosis (Curtis *et al.*, 1983b; Mourad *et al.*, 1989; van der Woude *et al.*, 1985), particularly after addition of loop diuretic treatment (Hricik, 1987). A similar phenomenon has been reported with small-vessel disease (Davin and Mahieu, 1985). As add-on treatment, α-blockers and β-blockers frequently are useful, as are loop diuretics, which potentiate the antihypertensive and antiproteinuric effects of ACE inhibitors. An assocation between loop diuretic use and posttransplant hyperparathyroidism (Bittar et al., 1989) has not been confirmed or refuted by other studies. Centrally acting sympatholytic agents are a rational choice, given the evidence of sympathetic overactivity, but the older agents (e.g, clonidine) are difficult to use, and experience with moxonidine in transplant recipients is limited. Optimal adjustment of immunosuppressive medication is an essential part of the therapeutic management of posttransplant hypertension, given the evidence that steroids and calcineurin inhibitors contribute to the pathogenesis of hypertension in these patients.

Native Nephrectomy

Presence of native kidneys is associated strongly with hypertension after transplantation (Huysmans et al., 1987; Kasiske, 1987). The likely reasons for this link include renin release from the native kidneys (Grunfeld et al., 1975) and sympathetic activation through reflexes arising in the failed kidneys (Converse et al., 1992). The latter phenomenon may explain commonly observed cases in which fluid volume control and use of ACE inhibitors fail to control blood pressure.

Bilateral native kidney nephrectomy may cure resistant hypertension in transplant patients, while improving renal allograft renal plasma flow, probably as a result of reduction of renin-angiotensin system activity (Curtis et al., 1985). It is a less hazardous procedure than in the past, in particular with use of the translumbar approach (Darby et al., 1991), although similar improvements in blood pressure have been reported after bilateral radiological embolization of the native kidneys (Thompson et al., 1984). Laparoscopic nephrectomy has become an important option. An improvement in graft survival has been reported, although this advantage was lost by 10 years (Yasamura et al., 1981); a note of caution is sounded by one report suggesting that the procedure may increase the risk of recurrent glomerulonephritis in recipients of cadaveric grafts (Odorico et al., 1996). Bilateral nephrectomy before transplantation may worsen anemia or increase erythropoietin requirements but has no impact on the restoration of normal hemoglobin levels after successful transplantation (Darby et al., 1993), although it may be associated with a lower risk of posttransplant polycythemia (Frei et al., 1982).

Cardiac Structure and Function After Renal Transplantation
ABNORMALITIES BEFORE TRANSPLANTATION

Abnormalities on echocardiography are extremely common in dialysis patients: Left ventricular dilatation, left ventricular hypertrophy and systolic dysfunction are all predictive of premature death (with a threefold increase in risk) compared with dialysis patients without these abnormalities (Foley et al., 1995b; Parfrey and Foley, 1999; Silberberg et al., 1989a). The roots of these disorders are complex and lie in the early predialysis phase of chronic renal failure.

Left Venticular Hypertrophy

Left ventricular hypertrophy is a powerful predictor of poor prognosis in patients with essential hypertension, and there is convincing evidence that regression of left ventricular hypertrophy may be induced by antihypertensive therapy, particularly with ACE inhibitors and calcium channel antagonists (Schmeider et al., 1998), and that regression is associated with an improved prognosis (Muiesan et al., 1995). Left ventricular hypertrophy is common in predialysis patients (Johnstone et al., 1996; Saggar-Malik et al., 1994; Tucker et al., 1997) and in dialysis patients (Foley et al., 1995b; Harnett et al., 1994; Savage et al., 1998). It is associated with hypertension and anemia (Levin et al., 1996; Silberberg et al., 1989b); a role for increased endothelin release also has been suggested (Demuth et al., 1998). Partial regression after correction of anemia by erythropoietin (Macdougall et al., 1990; Silberberg et al., 1990) has been reported, and there is plentiful evidence that antihypertensive treatment also causes regression in dialysis patients (Dyadyk et al., 1997; Rockstroth et al., 1997). As in the general population, left ventricular hypertrophy is a powerful predictor of premature death in patients with renal disease (Foley et al., 1995a, 1995b; Parfrey et al., 1990; Silberberg et al., 1989a), but it is not yet known whether treatments that cause its regression improve the prognosis in this group. The priority must be to prevent its development by control of hypertension and anemia early in the course in chronic renal failure.

Left Ventricular Dilatation and Systolic Dysfunction

The pathogenesis of left ventricular dilatation is related to anemia, salt and water overload and the presence of high-flow arteriovenous fistulae and may represent the late stage of hypertensive heart disease (London et al., 1987). Systolic dysfunction may result from end-stage hypertensive heart disease, from ischemic heart disease or from a number of other conditions including hyperparathyroidism. Both abnormalities carry a poor prognosis (Foley et al., 1995a; Parfrey et al., 1990), as does a clinical diagnosis of heart failure in dialysis patients (Harnett et al., 1995), notwithstanding the difficulty in distinguishing between the effects of cardiac dysfunction and fluid overload with a normal heart (Parfrey and Foley, 1999).

Whether or not uremia itself impairs cardiac contraction remains uncertain. Few studies have separated adequately the effects of changes in loading conditions as a result of fluid removal, changes in electrolyte concentrations and changes in the concentration of uremic metabolites. In one elegant study of changes in cardiac performance during dialysis, it was shown that the apparent improvement in systolic function during isovolemic hemodialysis solely was due to an increase in plasma ionized calcium and was not seen if a low calcium dialysate was used (Henrich et al., 1984).

Diastolic Dysfunction

There is plentiful evidence of impaired cardiac relaxation (diastolic dysfunction) in uremic patients, resulting in increased susceptibility to hypotension during fluid removal on dialysis (Rozich et al., 1991; Ruffmann et al., 1990). Diastolic dysfunction may result partly from increased left ventricular stiffness as a result of muscular hypertrophy and can result from dialysis-induced increases in serum ionized calcium concentration (Nappi et al., 1999), but one study in hemodialysis patients suggests that this abnormality is independent of left ventricular mass and is a specific uremic defect (Facchin et al., 1995).

Histological Abnormalities

In uremic animals and in human studies, there is evidence of a diffuse intermyocardiocytic fibrosis (Amann et al., 1994), which appears to be due to a specific failure of capillary supply to match myocyte hypertrophy, resulting in a decreased density of capillaries in the uremic myocardium, an alteration highly likely to increase susceptibility to ischemia

(Amann *et al.*, 1998). Factors contributing to this failure of capillary development may include increased angiotensin II, sympathetic overactivity, endothelin, erythropoietin deficiency and secondary hyperparathyroidism.

CHANGES IN CARDIAC STRUCTURE AND FUNCTION AFTER TRANSPLANTATION

Left Ventricular Hypertrophy

Successful renal transplantation results in partial regression of left ventricular hypertrophy (Himelman *et al.*, 1988; Ikaheimo *et al.*, 1982; Teruel *et al.*, 1987), and this observation remains true in the cyclosporine era if transplantation is associated with a reduction in blood pressure (Parfrey *et al.*, 1995; Peteiro *et al.*, 1994), although it is likely that correction of anemia also contributes. Left ventricular hypertrophy remains common in patients with functioning transplants, however. Studies using 24-hour ambulatory blood pressure monitoring and echocardiographic determination of left ventricular mass in apparently normotensive renal transplant recipients have shown a close correlation between 24-hour blood pressure, but not clinic blood pressure, and left ventricular mass. Of patients in this study, 25% had left ventricular hypertrophy despite absence of hypertension as assessed in the clinic. Ventricular hypertrophy was commoner in cyclosporine-treated (38%) than non–cyclosporine-treated patients (8%). An attenuated nocturnal fall in blood pressure also was observed in cyclosporine-treated patients (Lipkin *et al.*, 1993). The particular association of hypertension and left ventricular hypertrophy with cyclosporine may have relevance to the significant increase in cardiovascular mortality observed in long-term follow-up of cyclosporine-treated patients in the Minnesota randomized trial, compared with patients receiving prednisolone and azathioprine (Canafax *et al.*, 1986).

Development of left ventricular hypertrophy after transplantation is commoner in recipients with the DD genotype of the ACE gene, which confers higher angiotensin II levels—an unsurprising finding in view of the fact that angiotensin II has trophic actions on cardiac myocytes (Hernandez *et al.*, 1997). A study in dialysis patients suggested that regression of left ventricular hypertrophy was related solely to the degree to which blood pressure was reduced and that the less pronounced regression in patients with the DD genotype was due to poorer control of hypertension (Cannella *et al.*, 1998).

The effect of immunosuppressive drugs on left ventricular structure is uncertain. One case report has been published in which five pediatric recipients of bowel and/or liver transplants treated with tacrolimus, with high trough levels, developed hypertrophic cardiomyopathy, which resolved after reduction of the dose or conversion to cyclosporine (Atkison *et al.*, 1995), but this has not been reported from other centers or in the context of kidney transplantation. Some animal studies suggest that calcineurin inhibitors might prevent the development of cardiac hypertrophy through an action on one major target of calcineurin, NFAT-3, which appears to mediate the hypertrophic response (Force *et al.*, 1999), although in patients any such action is likely to be offset by drug-induced systemic hypertension.

Left Ventricular Volume and Function

Successful transplantation results in normalization of cavity size, possibly owing to better control of fluid balance and anemia and to improvement in systolic function (Himelman *et al.*, 1988; Ikaheimo *et al.*, 1982), but no improvement in diastolic function despite regression of hypertrophy (Himel-

man *et al.*, 1988). Dramatic improvements in systolic contraction in patients who were thought to have severe cardiomyopathy before transplantation and might have been considered poor operative candidates have been reported (Burt *et al.*, 1989; Fleming *et al.*, 1985). Similarly, in the Canadian cohort study, systolic dysfunction and left ventricular dilatation normalized after transplantation (Parfrey *et al.*, 1995). These improvements are most likely to be due to correction of previously unrecognized fluid overload, as has been reported in dialysis patients (Toz *et al.*, 1998). These abnormalities should not automatically be considered contraindications to transplantation.

Dyslipidemia

Abnormalities of lipid metabolism are, with hypertension and smoking, the most important treatable risk factors for atherosclerotic disease in the general population (Berenson *et al.*, 1998; Tunstall-Pedoe *et al.*, 1997), and there is no doubt that drug treatment to lower total serum cholesterol results in reduction in cardiovascular morbidity and mortality, the greatest benefit being seen in the populations at highest risk (Pitt *et al.*, 1999; Sacks *et al.*, 1996; 4S Study Group, 1994; Shepherd *et al.*, 1995).

The question of whether hypertriglyceridemia is an independent risk factor for cardiovascular disease is important, given the high prevalence of this abnormality in chronic renal failure and dialysis patients. Hypertriglyceridemia usually is associated closely with low HDL cholesterol (Castelli, 1986; Criqui *et al.*, 1993) (as well as with other atherogenic alterations, such as an increase in small dense low-density lipoprotein [LDL]). Within groups with low HDL cholesterol, who already are at high risk, hypertriglyceridemia is associated with greater risk, although as yet there is little evidence that drug treatment that corrects hypertriglyceridemia improves outcome (Sattar *et al.*, 1998).

Lipoprotein (a), a lipoprotein-containing apoprotein (a) linked to apoprotein B100 by a disulfide bridge and bearing a close homology to plasminogen, is recognized to be a strong independent risk factor for coronary heart disease (Rader and Brewer, 1992). At present, its concentration cannot be normalized by drug treatment.

DYSLIPIDEMIA IN CHRONIC RENAL DISEASE

Proteinuria and the Nephrotic Syndrome

Minor degrees of albuminuria are associated with an atherogenic lipid profile. Nephrotic syndrome is associated with marked elevations of total and LDL cholesterol resulting from enhanced hepatic synthesis of lipoprotein lipids (Appel *et al.*, 1984; Joven *et al.*, 1990) and with increased lipoprotein (a) (Steinvinkel *et al.*, 1993; Wanner and Bartens, 1994). There is a more variable increase in very-low-density lipoprotein cholesterol and serum triglycerides. Probably as a result, patients with nephrotic syndrome have a markedly increased risk of developing ischemic heart disease (Ordonez *et al.*, 1993).

Chronic Renal Failure and Hemodialysis

The classic abnormalities seen are hypertriglyceridemia and decreased HDL cholesterol, with a normal serum total cholesterol (Attman *et al.*, 1988, 1996). In addition to these abnormalities, numerous alterations in lipoprotein composition have been reported, most of which would be expected to be atherogenic, including low apolipoprotein A1 and high apolipoprotein B levels and increased lipoprotein (a), together with increased concentrations of remnant particles (Cheung et al., 1993). Low-density lipoprotein from hemodialysis patients is taken up more readily than normal by the macrophage scavenger pathway, which is implicated in early atherogenesis (Ambrosch et al., 1998). These changes result from delayed catabolism of triglyceride-rich particles owing to inhibition of the lipolytic enzymes lipoprotein lipase, triglyceride lipase and lecithin:cholesterol acyltransferase by insulin resistance, hyperparathyroidism and inflammatory cytokines (Nishizawa et al., 1997; Wanner et al., 1997).

In addition to these changes in the activity of the enzymes regulating lipid turnover, there is evidence of nonenzymatic modification of lipid particles in uremia, as a result of peroxidation owing to decreased antioxidant activity, formation and decreased clearance of advanced glycation end products and carbamylation (chemical modification by urea) (Becker et al., 1997; Galle and Wanner, 1997; Miyata et al., 1999; Roxborough and Young, 1995). All of these changes enhance the atherogenicity of LDL particles.

Peritoneal Dialysis

Peritoneal dialysis is characterized by peritoneal protein losses of similar magnitude to those seen in nephrotic syndrome, together with lipoprotein losses and glucose absorption from the dialysate and the impaired lipolysis seen in chronic renal failure. Hypercholesterolemia, hypertriglyceridemia and low HDL cholesterol concentrations result. Elevated lipoprotein (a) concentrations have been reported and may be caused by hypoalbuminemia (Yang et al., 1997). A longitudinal study showed that raised triglycerides or raised total cholesterol/HDL cholesterol ratio was associated significantly with reduced survival in patients with and without clinically overt cardiovascular disease at inception (Little et al., 1998).

Dyslipidemia as a Risk Factor for Vascular Disease in Uremia

Not surprisingly in view of the complex alterations in lipid chemistry seen in uremia, many studies have failed to show the expected association between hypercholesterolemia and vascular disease in uremic patients. Large-scale registry studies have shown an inverse relationship, survival being poorest in patients with the lowest serum cholesterol (Degoulet et al., 1982; Goldwasser et al., 1993; Lowrie and Lew, 1990, 1992), likely to be due to the association of malnutrition, underdialysis and chronic inflammation with hypocholesterolemia. Numerous smaller studies in renal failure patients have failed to find an association between hypercholesterolemia and cardiovascular morbidity or mortality. Many studies have found associations between vascular morbidity or mortality and dyslipidemia, including associations with hypercholesterolemia, hypertriglyceridemia and raised concentrations of the apolipoproteins B, CII and E (Attman and Alaupovic, 1991; Attman et al., 1987); apolipoprotein B, the low-molecular-weight apolipoprotein (a) phenotype, male sex, age, high plasma fibrinogen and low HDL cholesterol (Koch et al., 1997c); hypertriglyceridemia and low HDL cholesterol (Hahn et al., 1983); hypertriglyceridemia, at least when combined with hypertension or smoking (Haire et al., 1978; Kates et al., 1995); hypercholesterolemia in continuous ambulatory peritoneal dialysis patients (Gamba et al., 1993) and increased concentration or altered composition of lipoprotein (a) (Cressman et al., 1992; Kronenberg et al., 1999; Webb et al., 1994). A prospective study in diabetic patients on hemodialysis reported higher cholesterol, LDL cholesterol and apolipoprotein B in patients dying of myocardial in-

farction than in survivors (Tschope et al., 1993); however, a later expanded study from the same group showed that death was predicted by apolipoprotein A, fibrinogen, age and history of stroke but not by serum lipid concentrations (Koch et al., 1997b). Selenium deficiency, a cause of impaired antioxidant activity, also has been found to be associated with a history of vascular disease among dialysis patients (Girelli et al., 1993).

The relationship between atherosclerotic vascular disease and hypercholesterolemia is not as convincing in renal failure as in the general population. Although this situation partly may be due to the small sample size of many studies, it also may reflect the fact that altered lipoprotein composition, in particular atherogenic modifications such as peroxidation, glycation, carbamylation and accumulation of remnant particles owing to impaired lipolysis, is responsible for atherogenesis in these patients.

DYSLIPIDEMIA AFTER RENAL TRANSPLANTATION

The lipid abnormalities seen after renal transplantation are a complex mix, attributable partly to drug treatment with steroids, cyclosporine and antihypertensives, partly to impaired renal function and proteinuria and partly to other factors such as persistent hyperparathyroidism (Massy and Kasiske, 1996). The typical pattern includes marked hypercholesterolemia and moderate hypertriglyceridemia with increased apolipoprotein B (Kasiske and Umen, 1987; Vathsala et al., 1989). Factors related to dyslipidemia after transplantation include age, body weight, pretransplant lipid abnormalities and impaired graft function. A comparison of lipid abnormalities in 275 renal transplant recipients in Oxford with a large age-matched and sex-matched cohort (n = 4,055) from the local general population found that total cholesterol and triglycerides were higher in all age groups of transplanted patients, and these differences were particularly striking in women. For example, in 50-year-old female transplant recipients, triglycerides were increased by 70% and cholesterol by 33% compared with the general population (Bittar et al., 1990). Diuretic therapy is associated with hypercholesterolemia and hypertriglyceridemia and β-blocker therapy with hypertriglyceridemia (Bittar et al., 1990; Wheeler et al., 1996). In cyclosporine-treated patients, increased lipoprotein (a) and increased susceptibility of LDL to oxidation have been reported (Massy and Kasiske, 1996).

Effect of Immunosuppression

There is convincing evidence that corticosteroid therapy causes hypertriglyceridemia, by causing insulin resistance resulting in impaired lipolysis and by increasing hepatic triglyceride production. Although numerous studies have found an association between steroid usage, particularly with high-dosage regimens, and hypercholesterolemia, the mechanisms underlying this association remain unclear (Massy and Kasiske, 1996; Raine, 1994b; Vathsala et al., 1989). Steroid therapy also is associated with raised HDL cholesterol compared with cyclosporine monotherapy (Wheeler et al., 1996), which would be expected to ameliorate any increased cardiovascular risk conferred by steroid treatment. No differences in cholesterol or triglyceride levels were seen in patients randomized to receive low-dose alternate-day prednisolone in addition to cyclosporine in a Canadian multicenter trial in 523 patients (Sinclair, 1992). Elective withdrawal of steroids has been reported to cause not only a reduction of total cholesterol, but also of HDL cholesterol (Hricik et al., 1992a). In patients randomized after 3 months of cyclosporine and prednisolone either to cyclosporine monotherapy or to azathioprine and prednisolone, withdrawal of prednisolone resulted in a large decrease in HDL cholesterol and an increase in triglycerides; apolipoprotein (a) levels were higher in the cyclosporine monotherapy group; all these changes were associated with increased risk. These data do not support the idea that withdrawal of steroids improves the risk of vascular disease (Hilbrands et al., 1995). In one randomized study of steroid withdrawal, total cholesterol decreased, but HDL cholesterol was not reported (Ratcliffe et al., 1996); in another, no change was seen in lipid levels but lipid-lowering treatment was initiated more commonly in patients continuing on steroids (Hollander et al., 1997).

Cyclosporine treatment contributes to increases in total cholesterol and LDL cholesterol after transplantation, as shown by cyclosporine withdrawal (Harris et al., 1986; Sutherland et al., 1993a) and by prospective comparison of cyclosporine-based and cyclosporine-free treatment (Raine et al., 1988). Kasiske and colleagues analyzed serum lipid changes in 573 patients 3 to 52 weeks after transplantation and observed a 15 to 20% increase in total cholesterol and LDL cholesterol concentrations in association with cyclosporine use (Kasiske et al., 1991). The mechanism underlying this change is uncertain. Cyclosporine is highly lipophilic, binding to cell membranes and lipoprotein particles, and may enter the cell through the LDL receptor (Kahan, 1989). Possibly, binding of cyclosporine to LDL cholesterol may lead to impaired clearance of LDL from the circulation through cell-surface LDL receptors. Severe hypercholesterolemia has been reported to impair the efficacy of cyclosporine, possibly by competitive reduction of cellular uptake of LDL-bearing particles (Ingulli and Tejani, 1992). Cyclosporine also increases the susceptibility of LDL particles to lipid peroxidation (Apanay et al., 1994; van den Dorpel et al., 1997), resulting in alterations in LDL composition and an increased frequency of autoantibodies to oxidized LDL in transplanted patients (Ghanem et al., 1996). Lipid peroxidation can be ameliorated by antioxidant therapy (Wang and Salahudeen, 1995).

Tacrolimus appears to have less impact on cholesterol, LDL cholesterol and triglyceride levels than cyclosporine, seen in the randomized trials (Jensik, 1998; Shapiro et al., 1991) and in conversion studies (Copley et al., 1998; Friemann et al., 1998; McCune et al., 1998). Compared with cyclosporine containing an antioxidant, α-tocopherol (Neoral), tacrolimus enhances the susceptibility of LDL to peroxidation unless given with vitamins C and E as antioxidants (Varghese et al., 1999). Preliminary data indicate that sirolimus treatment is associated with marked increases in serum cholesterol and triglyceride levels (Rajagopalan and Rapamune Global Study Group, 1999).

Prognostic Importance of Posttransplant Dyslipidemia

Given the close association between hypercholesterolemia and cardiovascular disease in the general population, it appears likely that the lipid abnormalities present after renal transplantation may exert an adverse effect on cardiovascular morbidity and mortality. In the longitudinal studies from Minnesota, an association was found between total serum cholesterol and cardiovascular events in the first report (Kasiske, 1988) but not in the later, extended report from the same group, possibly because of the introduction of aggressive lipid-lowering therapy (Kasiske, 1993). Cardiovascular complications also were commoner in transplant patients with hyperlipidemia within the first year of transplantation in a survey of 500 transplant recipients on cyclosporine and prednisolone therapy (Vathsala et al., 1989). Similarly, in a study from Paris, total cholesterol and triglycerides as well

as associated apolipoproteins were higher in patients with posttransplant vascular events than in those without (Druecke et al., 1991). In a study from Trondheim, posttransplant ischemic heart disease was associated with hypercholesterolemia and peripheral vascular disease with systolic hypertension (Aakhus et al., 1999). In one study that found no association between posttransplant hyperlipidemia and graft or patient survival, lipid values were available only in 182 of 665 consecutive patients (Bumgardner et al., 2000). In contrast, other studies have found an association between hyperlipidemia and chronic renal allograft dysfunction (Isoniemi et al., 1994; Massy et al., 1996a; McLaren et al., 2000). One small case-control study has shown an association between hypercholesterolemia and stroke in transplant patients (Massy et al., 1998).

Treatment of Hyperlipidemia

There are no randomized controlled trial data on the impact of lipid-lowering therapy in renal failure or after transplantation (Yukawa et al., 1999), although several trials are now being planned or performed. For now, the clinician must balance the possible benefits of lipid-lowering therapy, based on observations in the general population and the associations of hyperlipidemia with posttransplant disease discussed previously, with the possible harm and cost of adding to the dietary or drug treatment of transplant patients.

In addition to the associations with drug treatment described earlier, hyperlipidemia after transplantation is associated with obesity. Attempts at weight reduction by restriction of calorie-rich foods, in particular fat intake, together with exercise are an important first step in treatment. A meta-analysis, which included 40 studies in transplant patients, showed that dietary intervention was of proven benefit (Massy et al., 1995). The choice of drug treatment lies, at present, between a fibrate derivative and a hydroxymethylglutaryl-coenzyme A reductase inhibitor (statin). Fibrates in general are more effective at correcting hypertriglyceridemia, but many of the drugs in this class are nephrotoxic and should be avoided in transplant recipients. Statins are more effective at correcting hypercholesterolemia and reducing LDL cholesterol, but these agents also have some triglyceride-lowering effects (Arnadottir and Berg, 1997; Massy and Kasiske, 1996; Massy et al., 1995).

The effect of lipid-lowering therapy on the effectiveness of cyclosporine is uncertain, but the fact that cyclosporine binds to LDL particles and may enter the cell through the LDL receptor raises the possibility of an interaction. A study in nephrotic syndrome suggested that cholesterol-lowering treatment resulted in response in previously cyclosporine-resistant children (Ingulli and Tejani, 1992), but this possibility has not been studied systematically in transplant recipients. Similar to in cardiac transplant recipients (Kobashigawa et al., 1995), one study has reported a significant reduction in rejection in renal transplant recipients randomized to pravastatin, 20 mg daily on day 7 posttransplant (Katznelson et al., 1996). Whether this reduction is due to enhanced immunosuppression or to effects of statins on the production of compounds other than cholesterol from its precursor, mevalonate, is uncertain (Massy et al., 1996b).

The major concern surrounding the use of statins after transplantation centers on the possibility of an enhanced risk of myopathy in patients also taking cyclosporine. Myopathy is a rare side effect of statin therapy, characterized by a spectrum of illness ranging from asymptomatic elevation of creatine kinase levels through muscle pain and tenderness with a characteristic histological pattern of muscle fiber necrosis to acute rhabdomyolysis with acute renal failure, all eventually reversible on withdrawal of therapy. Most reports have been in patients taking high doses or in patients in whom a preexisting muscle disorder (e.g., mitochondrial myopathy, hypothyroidism) was unmasked by treatment. Myopathy is commoner in patients receiving combination therapy with other lipid-lowering agents (fibrates, niacin) and those treated with erythromycin and cyclosporine, which cause delayed metabolism or hepatic clearance of the statin. The probable mechanism is reduced production within the muscle cell of coenzyme Q and heme, both derived from mevalonate; this results in mitochondrial damage (Alejandro and Petersen, 1994). Water-soluble statins (e.g., pravastatin, fluvastatin) may be less likely to enter muscle cells than lipid-soluble agents; although this apparent advantage may be offset by reduced binding to plasma proteins, few cases of myopathy have been reported in patients receiving pravastatin, and no myopathy was reported in three reports involving a total of 100 transplant patients on cyclosporine and pravastatin, 10 to 40 mg/d (Hsu et al., 1995). Another reason for the low incidence of myopathy with pravastatin and cyclosporine therapy may be the lack of accumulation after multiple doses compared with lovastatin (Olbricht et al., 1997). Fluvastatin levels are increased only minimally in cyclosporine-treated patients (Goldberg and Roth, 1996). Most studies of lipid-lowering therapy after transplantation are far too small to give any useful data on the risk of myopathy, however. There are no published data on the use of atorvastatin in combination with cyclosporine. Whichever drug is used, it should be used in the lowest effective dose, and the patient and physician should remain aware of the possibility of myopathy.

Diabetes as a Risk Factor for Vascular Disease

The increased risk of macrovascular disease in patients with diabetes is well recognized (Kannel and McGee, 1979; see also Chapter 36), and this results in many patients starting renal replacement therapy with already well-established vascular disease, with the result that diabetes is a potent predictor of poor survival in such patients (Braun, 1990; Braun et al., 1981; Brown et al., 1994; Herzog et al., 1998; Kasiske, 1988; Kasiske et al., 1996; Lindholm et al., 1995; Mailloux et al., 1994a; Najarian et al., 1977; Port, 1994; Port et al., 1993). In one large series of type I diabetics undergoing transplantation, 30% died within a mean follow-up of 47

months; 57% of these deaths were cardiovascular. The incidence of stroke, myocardial infarction and amputation was 14%, 28% and 36% (Lemmers and Barry, 1991). Series employing coronary angiography in diabetic transplant candidates have shown rates of clinically significant coronary artery stenoses (variously defined) of 25 to 43% (Table 30–1). The severity of coronary artery disease is a potent predictor of outcome; for instance, over a mean follow-up of 12 months, the mortality of patients without coronary disease (defined as any stenosis > 50%) was 5.4% compared with 43.5% in those with disease and 62.5% in the subgroup with severe disease (Philipson et al., 1986). In a more recent series, 55% of patients with at least one coronary stenosis of greater than 75% had experienced a cardiovascular event, most frequently amputation, within 36 months: Patients with any significant coronary disease had a sevenfold increased risk of amputation, and six of seven strokes in this series of 198 patients were in patients with coronary disease (Manske et al., 1997). As in other high-risk groups, transplantation may improve survival compared with continued dialysis (Khauli et al., 1986), but it is difficult to exclude selection bias in such comparisons, and overall prognosis is poor with either modality.

In all of the published series, symptoms of angina were absent in a high proportion of patients with significant coronary disease (and angina present in a significant number with minor disease), and few patients had had documented myocardial infarction at the time of assessment. The only way to be certain about the presence or absence of significant coronary disease is to perform angiography. The Minneapolis group has developed an algorithm allowing identification of a low-risk subgroup: Coronary disease was unlikely in type I diabetic patients younger than age 45 with no smoking history, no ST-T wave changes on the electrocardiogram and a duration of diabetes of less than 25 years (Manske et al., 1993).

Which patients should be offered revascularization is controversial. In the only randomized study, the Minneapolis group randomized 26 of 31 patients with asymptomatic coronary artery disease and well-preserved left ventricular function to revascularization (8 angioplasty, 5 bypass grafting) or medical treatment with aspirin and an unspecified calcium channel blocker. The study was stopped prematurely because of a highly significant reduction in cardiovascular events in the patients undergoing revascularization (Manske et al., 1992a; Fig. 30–3). Four of 13 medically managed patients had a fatal myocardial infarction within 16 months. Medical

TABLE 30–1

REPORTED SERIES OF CORONARY ANGIOGRAPHY IN DIABETIC PATIENTS UNDERGOING ASSESSMENT FOR TRANSPLANTATION*

Center (Reference)	n	% with Significant CAD	Comments
Portland (Bennett et al., 1978)	11	36 (>50% stenosis)	None had angina; 8/11 died within 20 months
Boston (Weinrauch et al., 1978)	21	43 (>50% stenosis)	24-month survival; 87% no CAD, 22% CAD
Cleveland (Braun et al., 1984)	100	25 (>70% stenosis)	Higher mortality in CAD group; 4 MIs within 51 months in patients without >70% stenosis; 2 with CAD survived transplantation after CABG
Pittsburgh (Philipson et al., 1986)	60	38 (>50% stenosis)	7 with normal thallium stress tests not subjected to angiography; mortality 5.4% with no CAD, 43.5% with CAD
Yale (Lorber et al., 1987)	77	32 (not defined)	Includes 13 with past history of myocardial infarction
Minneapolis (Manske et al., 1992b)	110	28 (>75% stenosis) 47 (>50% stenosis)	Associated with age, smoking, hemoglobin$_{A1c}$ No patient > 45 years old had normal coronaries
Dusseldorf (Koch et al., 1997a)	105	36 (>50% stenosis)	Poor correlation between angina and coronary disease; no correlation with dyslipidemia

*All but the series from Dusseldorf were limited to type I diabetics.
CAD = coronary artery disease; CABG = coronary artery bypass graft.

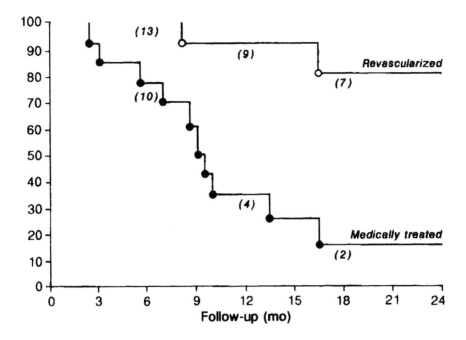

FIGURE 30–3

Cardiovascular events in type I diabetics with asymptomatic, angiographically proven coronary artery disease and end-stage renal failure, randomized to revascularization or to medical treatment with aspirin and a calcium channel blocker. (Modified with permission of Manske *et al.*, 1992a.)

management of such patients now would involve aggressive lipid-lowering treatment, β-blockade and (possibly) avoidance of dihydropyridine calcium channel blockers (Estacio *et al.*, 1998; Tatti *et al.*, 1998).

Hyperhomocysteinemia

Moderate elevations of plasma homocysteine are associated, probably causally, with an increased risk of coronary heart disease (Nygard *et al.*, 1997) and cerebrovascular disease (Perry *et al.*, 1995) in the general population (Hankey and Wikelboom, 1999; Welch and Loscalzo, 1988). Mild hyperhomocysteinemia is multifactorial, with contributions from polymorphisms in methylene tetrahydrofolate reductase, homozygosity for cystathione β-synthase deficiency (homozygosity for which causes classic homocystinuria), dietary folate and dietary pyridoxine deficiency. Moderate degrees of renal impairment are associated with marked hyperhomocysteinemia (Bostom and Culleton, 1999; Wilcken *et al.*, 1981). In populations with renal disease, prospective studies have confirmed the findings in the nonrenal population of increased risk of vascular disease (Bostom and Culleton, 1999; Moustapha *et al.*, 1998) and of access thrombosis (Shemin *et al.*, 1999). Hyperhomocysteinemia in renal disease can be ameliorated but seldom corrected fully by folate and/or pyridoxine supplementation (Arnadottir *et al.*, 1993; Bostom *et al.*, 1996; Perna *et al.*, 1997; van Guldener *et al.*, 1998b, 1998c; Wilcken *et al.*, 1981, 1988); partial correction does not improve endothelial function as measured by postischemic brachial artery vasodilatation (van Guldener *et al.*, 1998b, 1998c). Decreased clearance of homocysteine from plasma can be shown in renal impairment (Guttormsen *et al.*, 1997), but there is no evidence that the normal kidney clears homocysteine by excretion or extraction (van Guldener *et al.*, 1998a), suggesting that the mechanism is impaired metabolism as a result of accumulation of an unknown metabolite.

HYPERHOMOCYSTEINEMIA AFTER RENAL TRANSPLANTATION

Case-control studies in renal transplant recipients have confirmed the association between hyperhomocysteinemia and cardiovascular disease (Arnadottir *et al.*, 1996; Massy *et al.*, 1994). It has been suggested that cyclosporine causes hyperhomocysteinemia independent of the level of renal function (Arnadottir *et al.*, 1998). Other authors have claimed that this apparent association is due to failure to correct for the effect of minor degrees of renal impairment on plasma total homocysteine levels, however (Bostom and Culleton, 1999). There is no evidence to support a policy of screening for hyperhomocysteinemia in renal transplant recipients with a view to folate supplementation, but this is an area of active research.

Abnormalities of Coagulation in Renal Disease

Disorders of the coagulation cascade, including inherited deficiency of antithrombin III, protein S and protein C; factor V Leiden, causing resistance to activated protein C; antibodies to phospholipids (anticardiolipin) causing the lupus anticoagulant phenomenon and polymorphisms in the factor VII and fibrinogen genes, are well recognized as important risk factors for venous thrombosis. The role of these abnormalities in the genesis of arterial disease is less clear-cut, although there is epidemiological evidence implicating polymorphisms associated with high factor VII levels in coronary disease (Iacovello *et al.*, 1998). A study from Oxford showed that renal transplant recipients have a chronic hypercoagulable state, with higher factor VII coagulation activity in patients with cardiovascular disease or metabolic complications than in the remainder (Irish and Green, 1997). In chronic renal failure patients, including those on dialysis, there is evidence that high factor VII activity is associated with a persistent inflammatory response, including an inverse association between factor VII coagulant activity and serum albumin (Irish and Green, 1998). Several studies have found an increased risk of renal vein thrombosis and/or acute rejection in renal transplant recipients with thrombophilia (Fischereder et al., 1998, 1999; Heidenreich et al., 1998; Irish et al., 1997; see Chapter 28); one of these studies reported an increased risk of vascular events (including venous thromboembolism, coronary artery disease and ischemic stroke) among renal transplant recipients with thrombophilia (Heidenreich et al., 1998). Controlled studies of anticoagulant strategies in patients with thrombophilia have not been reported, although there is anecdotal evidence from Oxford that the regular use of low-dose aspirin (75 mg/d) has markedly reduced the incidence of renal vein thrombosis (see Chapter 28). The incidence of anticardiolipin antibodies and lupus anticoagulant appears to be increased in renal failure, but their significance is uncertain (Brunet et al., 1995).

Polycythemia is common after transplantation, particularly in patients with good graft function treated with cyclosporine, and is a risk factor for thromboembolic events (Wickre et al., 1983). The need for regular phlebotomy can be avoided with ACE inhibitors (see earlier) or theophylline (Bakris et al., 1990; Grekas et al., 1995).

Renal Dysfunction as a Risk Factor for Cardiovascular Disease

The extremely high prevalence of cardiovascular disease among patients starting renal replacement therapy (Furth et al., 1998; Joki et al., 1997; Jungers et al., 1997, 1999; Luke, 1998), the observation that cardiovascular mortality in dialysis patients falls relative to other causes over time (Mailloux et al., 1991) and the fact that one of the strongest risk markers for cardiovascular mortality among transplant patients is a history of cardiovascular disease before the onset of end-stage renal failure (Kasiske et al., 1996) focus attention on the predialysis phase of chronic renal failure as the period in which the vastly increased risk of cardiovascular disease is acquired. This topic is particularly relevant to renal transplantation, which returns many patients to a state of moderate renal insufficiency, often with proteinuria, rather than restoring renal function completely to normal. Proteinuria (Grimm et al., 1997; Yudkin et al., 1988) is a potent risk marker for cardiovascular disease, although this may be because proteinuria acts as a sensitive marker of the presence of generalized vascular dysfunction. A raised serum creatinine also is a potent predictor of cardiovascular disease (Fried et al., 1998; Shulman et al., 1989; Wannamethee et al., 1997).

Chronic Inflammation and Hypoalbuminemia

Atherosclerosis is an inflammatory disease, with active involvement by cytokines and adhesion molecules at sites of endothelial damage in the process of adhesion of monocytes and subsequent cellular infiltration and lipid deposition in the arterial wall (Ross, 1999). As in the general population, moderately raised concentrations of C-reactive peptide are associated strongly with early death in dialysis patients (Ikizler et al., 1999; Owen and Lowrie, 1998; Steinvinkel et al., 1999b; Wanner et al., 1997; Zimmermann et al., 1999). The fact that serum albumin falls during an acute-phase response may be the explanation for the strong association between hypoalbuminemia and death in dialysis patients (Foley et al., 1996; Goldwasser et al., 1993; Iseki et al., 1997; Lowrie and Lew, 1990, 1992; Owen et al., 1993). The cause as well as the most appropriate treatment of a persistent acute-phase

response in a hemodialysis patient in the absence of clinically evident infection is often hard to determine: One study suggests an association with chronic chlamydial infection (Steinvinkel et al., 1999a). Repeated exposure to dialysis membranes with poor *biocompatibility* also is a possible contributor; use of more biocompatible membranes is associated with higher serum albumin levels (Parker et al., 1996) and lower risk of death from coronary artery disease (Bloembergen et al., 1999). In addition to being a marker for inflammation and possibly for malnutrition, hypoalbuminemia also may be a direct cause of increased lipoprotein (a) (Yang et al., 1997) and increased factor VII and fibrinogen levels (Kim et al., 1998).

Hypoalbuminemia after renal transplantation is associated with age, diabetes, proteinuria and cytomegalovirus infection and is a strong independent predictor of poor outcome (Guijarro et al., 1996). Although there is no hard evidence to support the suggestion, it is highly likely that chronic immunological stimulation by the presence of an allograft increases the risk not only of progressive arterial damage within the graft, as seen in chronic renal allograft dysfunction, but also elsewhere in the recipient.

Insulin Resistance and Posttransplant Diabetes

In the general population, insulin resistance—an impaired ability of insulin to stimulate glucose uptake in peripheral tissues, mainly muscle—is part of a metabolic syndrome also involving dyslipidemia, endothelial dysfunction and hypertension and is an independent risk factor for ischemic heart disease (Despres et al., 1996). This syndrome frequently is present in essential hypertension and central obesity as well as in type 2 diabetes mellitus. Insulin resistance frequently is present in patients with renal disease (Alvestrand, 1997). Increased sympathetic activity may be a contributing cause (Krentz and Evans, 1998), which would explain the finding of insulin resistance in patients with normal glomerular filtration rate (Fliser et al., 1998). Other causes include uremic acidosis (Mak, 1998), anemia (Alvestrand, 1997), and hyperparathyroidism or decreased activity of 1,25-dihydroxycholecalciferol (Gunal et al., 1997; Rostand and Druecke, 1999). After transplantation, corticosteroid therapy is a major cause of insulin resistance.

Posttransplant diabetes is associated with increased risk of cardiovascular disease (Kasiske et al., 1996) and of graft failure (Miles et al., 1998; Sumrani et al., 1991), but this is attributable largely to the presence of other cardiovascular risk markers in these patients. Corticosteroid therapy causes insulin resistance; however, the mechanism by which calcineurin inhibitors cause diabetes is more complex and is related mainly to impaired insulin secretion as a result of direct effects on β cells (Jindal et al., 1997). The risk of posttransplant diabetes is higher with tacrolimus than with cyclosporine (Knoll and Bell, 1999).

Assessment of the Potential Transplant Recipient

HISTORY AND INVESTIGATION: IDENTIFICATION OF THE HIGH-RISK PATIENT

Recognition of the high risk of cardiovascular morbidity after renal transplantation has resulted in increasing awareness of the need to screen potential renal transplant recipients for coronary artery disease. Patients with a history of coronary artery disease, stroke or peripheral vascular disease and patients with type 1 diabetes are at high risk and require careful evaluation with a view to revascularization. In patients without symptoms or diabetes, conventional exercise tests have proved difficult because of a high incidence of false-positive and false-negative results. An exhaustive review of the literature on pretransplant assessment for cardiovascular disease concluded that there were insufficient data to allow strong recommendations on which noninvasive tests, such as thallium redistribution scanning and dobutamine echocardiography, are useful in identifying renal transplant candidates at high risk; the choice of screening strategy depends on local resources (Kasiske *et al.*, 1995).

MANAGEMENT
Coronary Revascularization

Several nonrandomized studies have reported a remarkably high restenosis rate after percutaneous transluminal coronary angioplasty (PTCA) in dialysis patients compared with the outcome of coronary artery bypass grafting (CABG) (Ahmed *et al.*, 1994; Collins *et al.*, 1996; Ivens *et al.*, 1996; Kahn *et al.*, 1990; Koyanagi *et al.*, 1996; Rinehart *et al.*, 1995), despite higher initial morbidity after CABG (Herzog *et al.*, 1999). No randomized trials are likely to occur, but these observations cast doubt on the utility of PTCA in dialysis patients other than for short-term relief of symptomatic angina. Numerous series attest to the feasibility of CABG in patients on dialysis and in transplant recipients (Batiuk *et al.*, 1991). A case-control series suggested that CABG in dialysis patients improved outcome, with remarkably good long-term survival (Opsahl *et al.*, 1988). There is little doubt, however, that morbidity is increased in dialysis patients compared with patients without renal disease, as illustrated by a case-control series from Pennsylvania (Deutsch *et al.*, 1989); adverse outcomes are associated with age, heart failure and diabetes (Ashraf *et al.*, 1995; Garrido *et al.*, 1995; Kaul *et al.*, 1994).

Medical Management

Many patients, particularly in countries where access to angiography and revascularization are limited, come to transplantation with silent coronary artery disease, and others are listed for transplantation with known coronary artery disease not sufficiently severe to justify revascularization. For these patients, several strategies may minimize the risk of perioperative complications, including perioperative β-blockade or centrally acting sympatholytic agents, aspirin and correction of anemia (Sonksen *et al.*, 1998; Wizemann *et al.*, 1992). After the initial postoperative phase, attention should turn to control of the risk factors discussed earlier.

Conclusions

Cardiovascular disease after renal transplantation often is the expression of a disease process that first started with the onset of renal dysfunction many years before, and its prevention starts with the early predialysis phase of chronic renal failure, with aggressive treatment of hypertension and dyslipidemia. The evidence that dialysis treatment itself accelerates arterial damage is poor. After transplantation, however, many patients are restored to a state not of normal renal function but of chronic renal impairment and have drug-induced hypertension and dyslipidemia, resulting in a vastly increased risk of atherosclerosis. Further research is required on the optimal strategies to prevent or ameliorate cardiovascular disease and in particular to establish the roles of lipid-lowering therapy in chronic renal failure and after transplantation.

REFERENCES

Aakhus, S., Dahl, K. and Wideroe, T. E. (1999). Cardiovascular morbidity and risk factors in renal transplant patients. *Nephrol. Dial. Transplant.* **14**, 648.

Ahmed, W. H., Shubrooks, S. J., Gibson, M., Baim, D. S. and Bittl, J. A. (1994). Complications and long-term outcome after percutaneous coronary angioplasty in chronic hemodialysis patients. *Am. Heart J.* **128**, 252.

Alejandro, D. S. J. and Petersen, J. (1994). Myoglobinuric acute renal failure in a cardiac transplant patient taking lovastatin and cyclosporine. *J. Am. Soc. Nephrol.* **5**, 153.

Alvestrand, A. (1997). Carbohydrate and insulin metabolism in renal failure. *Kidney Int.* **52(Suppl. 62)**, S48.

Amann, K., Breitbach, M., Ritz, E. and Mall, G. (1998). Myocyte/capillary mismatch in the heart of uremic patients. *J. Am. Soc. Nephrol.* **9**, 1018.

Amann, K., Mall, G. and Ritz, E. (1994). Myocardial interstitial fibrosis in uraemia: is it relevant? *Nephrol. Dial. Transplant.* **9**, 127.

Ambrosch, A., Domroese, U., Westphal, S., *et al.* (1998). Compositional and functional changes of low-density lipoprotein during hemodialysis in patients with ESRD. *Kidney Int.* **54**, 608.

Anastassiades, E. E., Howarth, D., Howarth, J., *et al.* (1993). Influence of blood volume on the blood pressure of predialysis and peritoneal dialysis patients treated with erythropoietin. *Nephrol. Dial. Transplant.* **8**, 621.

Anderstam, B., Katzarski, K. and Bergstrom, J. (1997). Serum levels of NG, NG-dimethyl-L-arginine, a potential endogenous nitric oxide inhibitor in dialysis patients. *J. Am. Soc. Nephrol.* **8**, 1437.

Apanay, D. C., Neylan, J. F., Ragab, M. S. and Sgoutas, D. S. (1994). Cyclosporine increases the oxidizability of low-density lipoproteins in renal transplant recipients. *Transplantation* **58**, 663.

Appel, G. B., Blum, C. B., Chien, S., Kunis, C. L. and Appel, A. S. (1984). The hyperlipidemia of the nephrotic syndrome: relationship to plasma albumin concentration and viscosity. *N. Engl. J. Med.* **312**, 1544.

Arend, S. M., Mallat, M. J., Westendorp, R. J., van der Woude, F. J. and van Es, L. A. (1997). Patient survival after renal transplantation: more than 25 years follow-up. *Nephrol. Dial. Transplant.* **12**, 1672.

Arnadottir, M. and Berg, A. L. (1997). Treatment of hyperlipidemia in renal transplant recipients. *Transplantation* **63**, 339.

Arnadottir, M., Brattstrom, L., Simonsen, O., *et al.* (1993). The effect of high-dose pyridoxine and folic acid supplementation on serum lipid and plasma homocysteine concentrations in dialysis patients. *Clin. Nephrol.* **40**, 236.

Arnadottir, M., Hultberg, B., Vladov, V., Nilsson-Ehle, P. and Thysell, H. (1996). Hyperhomocysteinemia in cyclosporine-treated renal transplant recipients. *Transplantation* **61**, 509.

Arnadottir, M., Hultberg, B., Wahlberg, J., Fellstrom, B. and Dimeny, E. (1998). Serum total homocysteine concentration before and after renal transplantation. *Kidney Int.* **54**, 1380.

Ashraf, S. S., Shaukat, N., Kamaly, I. D., *et al.* (1995). Determinants of early and late mortality in patients with end-stage renal disease undergoing cardiac surgery. *Scand. J. Thorac. Cardiovasc. Surg.* **29**, 187.

Atkison, P., Joubert, G., Barron, A., *et al.* (1995). Hypertrophic cardiomyopathy associated with tacrolimus in paediatric transplant patients. *Lancet* **345**, 894.

Attman, P. O. and Alaupovic, P. (1991). Lipid and apolipoprotein profiles of uremic dyslipoproteinemia—relation to renal function and dialysis. *Nephron* **57**, 401.

Attman, P. O., Alaupovic, P. and Gustafson, A. (1987). Serum apolipoprotein profile of patients with chronic renal failure. *Kidney Int* **32**, 368.

Attman, P. O., Alaupovic, P., Tavella, M. and Knight Gibson, C. (1996). Abnormal lipid and apolipoprotein composition of major lipoprotein density classes in patients with chronic renal failure. *Nephrol. Dial. Transplant.* **11**, 63.

Attman, P. O., Gustafson, A., Alaupovic, P. and Wang, C. S. (1988). Lipid metabolism in patients with chronic renal failure in the predialytic phase. *Contrib. Nephrol.* **65**, 24.

Avdonin, P. V., Cottet-Maire, F., Afanesjeva, G. V., Loktionova, S. A., Lhote, P. and Ruegg, U. T. (1999). Cyclosporine A up-regulates angiotensin II receptors and calcium responses in human vascular smooth muscle cells. *Kidney Int.* **55**, 2407.

Bakris, G. L., Sauter, E. R., Hussey, J. L., Fisher, J. W., Gaber, A. O. and Winsett, R. (1990). Effects of theophylline on erythropoietin production in normal subjects and in patients with erythrocytosis after renal transplantation. *N. Engl. J. Med.* **323**, 86.

Barenbrock, M., Spieker, C., Rahn, K. H. and Zidek, W. (1993). Therapeutic efficiency of phlebotomy in posttransplant hypertension associated with erythrocytosis. *Clin. Nephrol.* **40**, 241.

Batiuk, T. D., Kurtz, S. B., Oh, J. K. and Orszulak, T. A. (1991). Coronary artery bypass operation in dialysis patients. *Mayo Clin. Proc.* **66**, 45.

Becker, B. N., Himmelfarb, J., Henrich, W. L. and Hakim, R. M. (1997). Reassessing the cardiac risk profile in chronic hemodialysis patients: a hypothesis on the role of oxidant stress and other non-traditional cardiac risk factors. *J. Am. Soc. Nephrol.* **8**, 475.

Beckingham, I. J., Woodrow, G., Hinwood, M., *et al.* (1995). A randomized placebo-controlled study of enalapril in the treatment of erythrocytosis after renal transplantation. *Nephrol. Dial. Transplant.* **10**, 2316.

Bennett, W. M., Kloster, F., Rosch, J., Barry, J. and Porter, G. A. (1978). Natural history of asymptomatic coronary arteriographic lesions in diabetic patients with end-stage renal disease. *Am. J. Med.* **65**, 779.

Benoit, G., Moukarzel, M., Hiesse, C., Verdelli, G., Charpentier, B. and Fries, D. (1990). Transplant renal artery stenosis: experience and comparative results between surgery and angioplasty. *Transpl. Int.* **3**, 137.

Berenson, G. S., Srinivasan, S. S., Bao, W., Newman, W. P., Tracy, R. E. and Wattigney, W. A. (1998). Association between multiple cardiovascular risk factors and atherosclerosis in children and young adults. *N. Engl. J. Med.* **338**, 1650.

Bittar, A. E., Ratcliffe, P. J., Richardson, A. J., Brown, R. C., Woodhead, J. S. and Morris, P. J. (1989). Hyperparathyroidism, hypertension, and loop diuretic medication in renal transplant recipients. *Nephrol. Dial. Transplant.* **4**, 740.

Bittar, A. E., Ratcliffe, P. J., Richardson, A. J., *et al.* (1990). The prevalence of hyperlipidemia in renal transplant recipients: associations with immunosuppressive and antihypertensive therapy. *Transplantation* **50**, 987.

Bloembergen, W. E., Hakim, R. M., Stannard, D. C., *et al.* (1999). Relationship of dialysis membrane and cause-specific mortality. *Am. J. Kidney Dis.* **33**, 1.

Bock, H. A. (1995). Chronic rejection and hypertension: a chicken-and-egg problem. *Nephrol. Dial. Transplant.* **10**, 1126.

Bostom, A. G. and Culleton, B. F. (1999). Hyperhomocysteinemia in chronic renal disease. *J. Am. Soc. Nephrol.* **10**, 891.

Bostom, A. G., Shemin, D., Lapane, K. L., *et al.* (1996). High-dose B-vitamin treatment of hyperhomocysteinemia in dialysis patients. *Kidney Int.* **49**, 147.

Braun, W. E. (1990). Long-term complications of renal transplantation. *Kidney Int.* **37**, 1363.

Braun, W. E., Phillips, D., Vidt, D. G., *et al.* (1981). Coronary arteriography and coronary artery disease in 99 diabetic and nondiabetic patients on chronic hemodialysis or renal transplantation programs. *Transplant. Proc.* **13**, 128.

Braun, W. E., Phillips, D. F., Vidt, D. G., *et al.* (1984). Coronary artery disease in 100 diabetics with end-stage renal failure. *Transplant. Proc.* **16**, 603.

Brenner, B. M. and Mackenzie, H. S. (1997). Nephron mass as a risk factor for progression of renal disease. *Kidney Int.* **52(Suppl. 63)**, S124.

Brown, J. H., Fellin, G., Hunt, L. P., Vites, N. P., D'Amico, G. and Mallick, N. P. (1998). Comparison between two prospective studies of cardiovascular disease carried out amongst renal replacement patients in UK and Italy. *Nephrol. Dial. Transplant.* **13**, 449.

Brown, J. H., Hunt, L. P., Vites, N. P., Short, C. D., Gokal, R. and Mallick, N. P. (1994). Comparative mortality from cardiovascular disease in patients with chronic renal failure. *Nephrol. Dial. Transplant.* **9**, 1136.

Brunet, P., Aillaud, M. F., San Marco, M., *et al.* (1995). Antiphospholipids in hemodialysis patients: relationship between lupus anticoagulant and thrombosis. *Kidney Int.* **48**, 794.

Buckalew, V. M., Jr., Berg, R. L., Wang, S. R., Porush, J. G., Rauch, S. and Schulman, G. (1996). Prevalence of hypertension in 1,795 subjects with chronic renal disease: the modification of diet in renal disease study baseline cohort. Modification of Diet in Renal Disease Study Group. *Am. J. Kidney Dis.* **28**, 811.

Budisavljevic, M. N., Cheek, D. and Plot, D. W. (1996). Calciphylaxis in chronic renal failure. *J. Am. Soc. Nephrol.* **7**, 978.

Bumgardner, G. L., Wilson, G. A., Tso, P. L., *et al.* (1995). Impact of serum lipids on long-term graft and patient survival after renal transplantation. *Transplantation* **60**, 1418.

Burke, J. F., Francos, G. C., Moore, L. L., Cho, S. Y. and Lasker, N. (1978). Accelerated atherosclerosis in chronic-dialysis patients—another look. *Nephron* **21**, 181.

Burt, R. K., Gupta Burt, S., Suki, W. N., Barcenas, C. G., Ferguson, J. J. and Van Buren, C. T. (1989). Reversal of left ventricular dysfunction after renal transplantation. *Ann. Intern. Med.* **111**, 635.

Burton, P. R. and Walls, J. (1987). Selection-adjusted comparison of life-expectancy of patients on continuous ambulatory peritoneal dialysis, haemodialysis, and renal transplantation [published erratum appears in *Lancet* 1987 Jun 6;1(8545),1330]. *Lancet* **1**, 1115.

Canafax, D. M., Simmons, R. L., Sutherland, D. E., **et al.** (1986). Early and late effects of two immunosuppressive drug protocols on recipients of renal allografts: results of the Minnesota randomized trial comparing cyclosporine versus antilymphocyte globulin-azathioprine. *Transplant. Proc.* **18**, 192.

Cannella, G., Paoletti, E., Barocci, S., *et al.* (1998). Angiotensin-converting enzyme gene polymorphism and reversibility of uremic left ventricular hypertrophy following long-term antihypertensive therapy. *Kidney Int.* **54**, 618.

Castelli, W. P. (1986). The triglyceride issue: a view from Framingham. *Am. Heart J.* **112**, 432.

Cheigh, J. S., Haschemeyer, R. H., Wang, J. C. L., *et al.* (1989). Hypertension in kidney transplant recipients: effects on long-term renal allograft survival. *Am. J. Hypertens.* **2**, 341.

Cheung, A. K., Wu, L. L., Kablitz, C. and Leypoldt, J. K. (1993). Atherogenic lipids and lipoproteins in hemodialysis patients. *Am. J. Kidney Dis.* **22**, 271.

Churchill, D. N., Taylor, D. W., Cook, R. J., *et al.* (1992). Canadian Hemodialysis Morbidity Study. *Am. J. Kidney Dis.* **19**, 214.

Collins, A., Ma, J. and Herzog, C. (1996). A national comparison of PTCA vs. CAB in chronic dialysis patients. *J. Am. Soc. Nephrol.* **7**, 1443.

Conlon, P. J., Athirakul, K., Kovalik, E., *et al.* (1998). Survival in renal vascular disease. *J. Am. Soc. Nephrol.* **9**, 252.

Converse, R. L., Jr., Jacobsen, T. N., Toto, R. D., *et al.* (1992). Sympathetic overactivity in patients with chronic renal failure. *N. Engl. J. Med.* **327**, 1912.

Copley, J. B., Staffeld, C., Lindberg, J., *et al.* (1998). Cyclosporine to tacrolimus: effect on hypertension and lipid profiles in renal allografts. *Transplant. Proc.* **30**, 1254.

Cosio, F. G., Dillon, J. J., Falkenhain, M. E., *et al.* (1995). Racial differences in renal allograft survival: the role of systemic hypertension. *Kidney Int.* **47**, 1136.

Cosio, F. G., Falkenhain, M. E., Pesavento, T. E., *et al.* (1997). Relationships between arterial hypertension and renal allograft survival in African-American patients. *Am. J. Kidney Dis.* **29**, 419.

Cowley, A. W., Jr. and Roman, R. J. (1996). The role of the kidney in hypertension. *J. A. M. A.* **275**, 1581.

Cressman, M. D., Heyka, R. J., Paganini, E. P., O'Neil, J., Skibinski, I. and Hoff, H. F. (1992). Lipoprotein (a) is an independent risk factor for cardiovascular disease in hemodialysis patients. *Circulation* **86**, 475.

Criqui, M. H., Heiss, G., Cohn, R., *et al.* (1993). Plasma triglyceride level and mortality from coronary heart disease. *N. Engl. J. Med.* **328**, 1220.

Curtis, J. J. (1994). Hypertension following kidney transplantation. *Am. J. Kidney Dis.* **23**, 471.

Curtis, J. J., Luke, R. G., Diethelm, A. G., Whelchel, J. D. and Jones, P. (1985). Benefits of removal of native kidneys in hypertension after renal transplantation. *Lancet* **2**, 739.

Curtis, J. J., Luke, R. G., Dustan, H. P., *et al.* (1983a). Remission of essential hypertension after renal transplantation. *N. Engl. J. Med.* **309**, 1009.

Curtis, J. J., Luke, R. G., Jones, P. and Diethelm, A. G. (1988). Hypertension in cyclosporine-treated renal transplant recipients is sodium-dependent. *Am. J. Med.* **85**, 134.

Curtis, J. J., Luke, R. G., Whelchel, J. D., Diethelm, A. G., Jones, P. and Distan, H. P. (1983b). Inhibition of angiotensin converting enzyme in renal-transplant recipients with hypertension. *N. Engl. J. Med.* **308**, 377.

Darby, C., Raine, A. E., Cranston, D. and Morris, P. J. (1993). Effect of prior bilateral nephrectomy on haemoglobin and blood pressure outcome after transplantation. *Nephrol. Dial. Transplant.* **8**, 1151.

Darby, C. R., Cranston, D., Raine, A. E. G. and Morris, P. J. (1991). Bilateral nephrectomy before transplantation: indications, surgical approach, morbidity and mortality. *Br. J. Surg.* **78**, 305.

Davin, J. C. and Mahieu, P. R. (1985). Captopril-associated renal failure with endarteritis but not renal-artery stenosis in transplant recipient. *Lancet* **1**, 820.

Degoulet, P., Legrain, M., Reach, I., *et al.* (1982). Mortality risk factors in patients treated by chronic hemodialysis: report of the Diaphane collaborative study. *Nephron* **31**, 103.

Demuth, K., Blacher, J., Guerin, A. P., *et al.* (1998). Endothelin and cardiovascular remodelling in end-stage renal disease. *Nephrol. Dial. Transplant.* **13**, 375.

Despres, J. P., Lamarche, B., Mauriege, P., *et al.* (1996). Hyperinsulinemia as an independent risk factor for ischemic heart disease. *N. Engl. J. Med.* **334**, 952.

Deutsch, E., Bernstein, R. C., Addonizio, P. and Kussmaul, W. G. I. (1989). Coronary artery bypass surgery in patients on chronic hemodialysis: a case-control study. *Ann. Intern. Med.* **110**, 369.

Dixon, A. K. and Coulden, R. A. (1997). Coronary artery calcification on computed tomography. *Lancet* **350**, 1265.

Druecke, T. B., Abdulmassih, Z., Lacour, B., Bader, C., Chevalier, A. and Kreis, H. (1991). Atherosclerosis and lipid disorders after renal transplantation. *Kidney Int.* **39(Suppl. 31)**, S24.

Dyadyk, A. I., Bagriy, A. E., Lebed, I. A., Yarovaya, N. F., Schukina, E. V. and Taradin, G. G. (1997). ACE inhibitors captopril and enalapril induce regression of left ventricular hypertrophy in hypertensive patients with chronic renal failure. *Nephrol. Dial. Transplant.* **12**, 945.

Ejerblad, S., Ericsson, J. L. E. and Eriksson, I. (1979). Arterial lesions of the radial artery in uraemic patients. *Acta Chir. Scand.* **145**, 415.

Erley, C. M., Duda, S. H., Wakat, J. P., *et al.* (1992). Noninvasive procedures for diagnosis of renovascular hypertension in renal transplant recipients—a prospective analysis. *Transplantation* **54**, 863.

Estacio, R. O., Jeffers, B. W., Hiatt, W. R., Biggerstaff, S. L., Gifford, N. and Schrier, R. W. (1998). The effect of nisoldipine as compared with enalapril on cardiovascular outcomes in patients with non-insulin dependent diabetes and hypertension. *N. Engl. J. Med.* **338**, 546.

Facchin, L., Vescovo, G., Levedianos, G., *et al.* (1995). Left ventricular morphology and diastolic function in uraemia: echocardiographic evidence of a specific cardiomyopathy. *Br. Heart J.* **74**, 174.

Farias, M. A. G., McClellan, W., Soucie, J. M. and Mitch, W. E. (1994). A prospective comparison of methods for determining if cardiovascular disease is a predictor of mortality in dialysis patients. *Am. J. Kidney Dis.* **23**, 382.

Fauchald, P., Vatne, K., Paulsen, D., *et al.* (1992). Long-term clinical results of percutaneous transluminal angioplasty in transplant renal artery stenosis. *Nephrol. Dial. Transplant.* **7**, 256.

Fervenza, F. C., Lafayette, R. A., Alfrey, E. J. and Petersen, J. (1998). Renal artery stenosis in kidney transplants. *Am. J. Kidney Dis.* **31**, 142.

Fischereder, M., Gohring, P., Schneeberger, H., et al. (1998). Early loss of renal transplants in patients with thrombophilia. *Transplantation* **65**, 936.

Fischereder, M., Schneeberger, H., Gohring, P., Hillebrand, G., Schlondorff, D. and Land, W. (1999). Early graft failure with thrombophilia and effects of anticoagulation. *Transplant. Proc.* **31**, 360.

Fishbane, S., Youn, S., Kowalski, E. J. and Frei, G. L. (1995). Ankle-arm blood pressure index as a marker for atherosclerotic vascular diseases in hemodialysis patients. *Am. J. Kidney Dis.* **25**, 34.

Fleming, S. J., Caplin, J. L., Banim, S. O. and Bakder, L. R. I. (1985). Improved cardiac function after renal transplantation. *Postgrad. Med. J.* **61**, 525.

Fliser, D., Pacini, G., Engelleiter, R., *et al.* (1998). Insulin resistance and hyperinsulinemia are already present in patients with incipient renal disease. *Kidney Int.* **53**, 1343.

Florijn, K. W., Chang, P. C., van der Woude, F. J., van Bockel, J. H. and van Saase, J. L. (1994). Long-term cardiovascular morbidity and mortality in autosomal dominant polycystic kidney disease patients after renal transplantation. *Transplantation* **57**, 73.

Foley, R. N., Parfrey, P. S., Harnett, J. D., *et al.* (1995a). Clinical and echocardiographic disease in patients starting end-stage renal disease therapy. *Kidney Int.* **47**, 186.

Foley, R. N., Parfrey, P. S., Harnett, J. D., Kent, G. M., Murray, D. C. and Barre, P. E. (1995b). The prognostic signficance of left ventricular geometry in uremic cardiomyopathy. *J. Am. Soc. Nephrol.* **5**, 2024.

Foley, R. N., Parfrey, P. S., Harnett, J. D., Kent, G. M., Murray, D. C. and Barre, P. E. (1996). Hypoalbuminemia, cardiac morbidity, and mortality in end-stage renal disease. *J. Am. Soc. Nephrol.* **7**, 728.

Force, T., Rosenzweig, A., Choukroun, G. and Hajjar, R. (1999). Calcineurin inhibitors and cardiac hypertrophy. *Lancet* **353**, 1290.

Frei, D., Guttmann, R. D. and Gorman, P. (1982). A matched-pair control study of postrenal transplant polycythaemia. *Transplant. Proc.* **11**, 36.

Frei, U., Schindler, R., Wieters, D., Grouven, U., Brunkhorst, R. and Koch, K. M. (1995). Pre-transplant hypertension: a major risk factor for chronic progressive renal allograft dysfunction? *Nephrol. Dial. Transplant.* **10**, 1206.

Fried, L. P., Kronmal, R. A., Newman, A. B. A., *et al.* (1998). Risk factors for 5-year mortality in older adults: the cardiovascular health study. *J. A. M. A.* **279**, 585.

Friemann, S., Feuring, E., Padberg, W. and Ernst, W. (1998). Improvement of nephrotoxicity, hypertension and lipid metabolism after conversion of kidney transplant recipients from cyclosporine to tacrolimus. *Transplant. Proc.* **30**, 1240.

Furth, S., Herman, J. A. and Powe, N. R. (1998). Cardiovascular risk factors, comorbidity, and survival outcomes in black and white dialysis patients. *Semin. Dial.* **11**, 102.

Galle, J. and Wanner, C. (1997). Oxidative stress and vascular injury—relevant for atherogenesis in uraemic patients? *Nephrol. Dial. Transplant.* **12**, 2480.

Gamba, G., Mekia, J. L., Saldivar, S., Pena, J. C. and Correa-Rotter, R. (1993). Death risk on CAPD patients. *Nephron* **65**, 23.

Garrido, P., Bobadilla, J. F., Albertos, J., *et al.* (1995). Cardiac surgery in patients under chronic hemodialysis. *Eur. J. Cardiothorac. Surg.* **9**, 36.

Gedroyc, W. M. W., Negus, R., Al-Kutoubi, A., Palmer, A., Taube, D. and Hulme, B. (1992). Magnetic resonance angiography of renal transplants. *Lancet* **339**, 789.

Ghanem, H., van den Dorpel, M. A., Weimar, W., Manin, T. V. A. J., El-Kannishy, M. H. and Jansen, H. (1996). Increased low density lipoprotein oxidation in stable kidney transplant recipients. *Kidney Int.* **49**, 488.

Giatras, I., Lau, J. and Levey, A. S. (1997). Effect of angiotensin-converting enzyme inhibitors on the progression of nondiabetic renal disease: a meta-analysis of randomized trials. Angiotensin-Converting-Enzyme Inhibition and Progressive Renal Disease Study Group. *Ann. Intern. Med.* **127**, 337.

Girelli, D., Olivieri, O., Stanzial, A. M., *et al.* (1993). Low platelet glutathione peroxidase activity and selenium concentration in patients with chronic renal failure: relations to dialysis treatments, diet and cardiovascular complications. *Clin. Sci.* **84**, 611.

Goldberg, R. and Roth, D. (1996). Evaluation of fluvastatin in the treatment of hypercholesterolemia in renal transplant patients taking cyclosporine. *Transplantation* **62**, 1559.

Goldsmith, D. J. A., Covic, A., Sambrook, P. A. and Ackrill, P. (1997). Vascular calcification in long-term haemodialysis patients in a single unit: a retrospective analysis. *Nephron* **77**, 37.

Goldwasser, P., Mittman, N., Antignani, A., *et al.* (1993). Predictors of mortality in hemodialysis patients. *J. Am. Soc. Nephrol.* **3**, 1613.

Gossmann, J., Thurmann, P., Bachmann, T., *et al.* (1996). Mechanism of angiotensin converting enzyme inhibitor-related anemia in renal transplant recipients. *Kidney Int.* **50**, 973.

Grekas, D., Dioudis, C., Valkouma, D., Papoulidou, F. and Tourkantonis, A. (1995). Theophylline modulates erythrocytosis after renal transplantatoin. *Nephron* **70**, 25.

Grimm, R. H., Svendsen, K. H., Kasiske, B., Keane, W. F. and Sahi, M. M. (1997). Proteinuria is a risk factor for mortality over 10 years of follow-up. *Kidney Int.* **52(Suppl. 63)**, S10.

Grunfeld, J. P., Kleinknecht, D., Moreau, J. F., *et al.* (1975). Permanent hypertension after renal homotransplantation in man. *Clin. Sci. Mol. Med.* **48**, 391.

Gruppo Italiano di Studi Epidemiologici in Nefrologia. (1997). Randomised placebo-controlled trial of effect of ramipril on decline in glomerular filtration rate and risk of terminal renal failure in proteinuric, non-diabetic nephropathy. The GISEN Group (Gruppo Italiano di Studi Epidemiologici in Nefrologia). *Lancet* **349**, 1857.

Guidi, E., Bianchi, G., Rivolta, E., *et al.* (1985). Hypertension in man with a kidney transplant: role of familial versus other factors. *Nephron* **41**, 14.

Guidi, E., Cozzi, M. G., Minetti, E. and Bianchi, G. (1998). Donor and recipient family histories of hypertension influence renal impairment and blood pressure during acute rejections. *J. Am. Soc. Nephrol.* **9**, 2102.

Guidi, E., Menghetti, D., Milani, S., Montagnino, G., Palazzi, P. and Bianchi, G. (1996). Hypertension may be transplanted with the kidney in humans: a long-term historical prospective follow-up of recipients grafted with kidneys coming from donors with or without hypertension in their families. *J. Am. Soc. Nephrol.* **7**, 1131.

Guijarro C., Massy, Z. A., Wiederkehr, M. R., Ma, J. Z. and Kasiske, B. L. (1996). Serum albumin and mortality after renal transplantation. *Am. J. Kidney Dis.* **27**, 117.

Gunal, A. I., Celiker, H., Celebi, H., Ustundag, B. and Gunal, S. Y. (1997). Intravenous alfacalcidol improves insulin resistance in hemodialysis patients. *Clin. Nephrol.* **48**, 109.

Guttormsen, A. B., Ueland, P. M., Svarstad, E. and Refsum, H. (1997). Kinetic basis of hyperhomocysteinemia in patients with chronic renal failure. *Kidney Int.* **52**, 495.

Guyton, A. C. (1987). Renal function curve—a key to understanding the pathogenesis of hypertension. *Hypertension* **10**, 1.

Guyton, A. C., Coleman, T. G., Cowley, A. V., Jr., Scheel, K. W., Manning, R. D., Jr. and Norman, R. A., Jr. (1972). Arterial pressure regulation: overriding dominance of the kidneys in long-term regulation and in hypertension. *Am. J. Med.* **52**, 584.

Haas, M. and Mayer, G. (1997). Cyclosporin A-associated hypertension—pathomechanisms and clinical consequences. *Nephrol. Dial. Transplant.* **12**, 395.

Hafner, J., Keusch, G., Wahl, C., *et al.* (1995). Uremic small-artery disease with medial calcification and intimal hyperplasia (so-called calciphylaxis): a complication of chronic renal failure and benefit from parathyroidectomy. *J. Am. Acad. Dermatol.* **33**, 954.

Hahn, R., Oette, K., Mondorf, H., Finke, K. and Sieberth, H. G. (1983). Analysis of cardiovascular risk factors in chronic hemodialysis patients with special attention to the hyperlipoproteinemias. *Atherosclerosis* **48**, 279.

Haire, H. M., Sherrard, D. J., Scardapane, R. N., Curtis, F. K. and Brunzell, J. D. (1978). Smoking, hypertension, and mortality in a maintenance dialysis population. *Cardiovasc. Med.* **3**, 1163.

Hand, M. F., Haynes, W. G. and Webb, D. J. (1999). Reduced endogenous endothelin-1-mediated vascular tone in chronic renal failure. *Kidney Int.* **55**, 613.

Hankey, G. J. and Wikelboom, J. W. (1999). Homocysteine and vascular disease. *Lancet* **354**, 407.

Harnett, J. D., Foley, R. N., Kent, G. M., Barre, P. E., Murray, D. and Parfrey, P. S. (1995). Congestive heart failure in dialysis patients: prevalence, incidence, prognosis, and risk factors. *Kidney Int.* **47**, 884.

Harnett, J. D., Kent, G. M., Barre, P. E., Taylor, R. and Parfrey, P. S. (1994). Risk factors for the development of left ventricular hypertrophy in a prospectively followed cohort of dialysis patients. *J. Am. Soc. Nephrol.* **4**, 1486.

Harper, S. J., Moorhouse, J., Abrams, K., *et al.* (1996). The beneficial effects of oral nifedipine on cyclosporin-treated renal transplant recipients—a randomised prospective study. *Transpl. Int.* **9**, 115.

Harris, K. P. G., Russell, G. I., Parvin, S. D., Veitch, P. S. and Walls, J. (1986). Alterations in lipid and carbohydrate metabolism attributable to cyclosporin A in renal transplant recipients. *B. M. J.* **292**, 16.

Heidenreich, S., Dercken, C., August, C., Koch, H. G. and Nowak-Gottl, U. (1998). High rate of acute rejections in renal allograft recipients with thrombophilic risk factors. *J. Am. Soc. Nephrol.* **9**, 1309.

Henrich, W. L., Hunt, J. M. and Nixon, J. V. (1984). Increased ionized calcium and left ventricular contractility during hemodialysis. *N. Engl. J. Med.* **310**, 19.

Hernandez, D., Lacalzada, J., M. R., *et al.* (1997). Prediction of left ventricular mass changes after renal transplantation by polymorphism of the angiotensin converting enzyme gene. *Kidney Int.* **51**, 1205.

Herzog, C. A. (1999). Acute myocardial infarction in patients with end-stage renal disease. *Kidney Int.* **56(Suppl. 71)**, S130.

Herzog, C. A., Ma, J. Z. and Collins, A. J. (1998). Poor long-term survival after acute myocardial infarction among patients on long-term dialysis. *N. Engl. J. Med.* **339**, 799.

Herzog, C. A., Ma, J. Z. and Collins, A. J. (1999). Long-term outcome of dialysis patients in the United States with coronary revascularization procedures. *Kidney Int.* **56**, 324.

Hilbrands, L. B., Demacker, P. N., Hoitsma, A. J., Stalenhoef, A. F. and Koene, R. A. (1995). The effects of cyclosporine and prednisone on serum lipid and (apo)lipoprotein levels in renal transplant recipients. *J. Am. Soc. Nephrol.* **5**, 2073.

Himelman, R. B., Landzberg, J. S., Simonson, J. S., *et al.* (1988). Cardiac consequences of renal transplantation: changes in left ventricular morphology and function. *J. Am. Coll. Cardiol.* **12**, 915.

Hirata, M., Cho, Y. W., Cecka, J. M. and Terasaki, P. I. (1996). Patient death after renal transplantation—an analysis of its role in graft outcome. *Transplantation* **61**, 1479.

Hollander, A. A., Hene, R. J., Hermans, J., van Es, L. A. and van der Woude, F. J. (1997). Late prednisone withdrawal in cyclosporine-treated kidney transplant patients: a randomized study. *J. Am. Soc. Nephrol.* **8**, 294.

Hricik, D. E. (1987). Antihypertensive and renal effects of enalapril in post-transplant hypertension. *Clin. Nephrol.* **27**, 250.

Hricik, D. E., Bartucci, M. R., Mayes, J. T. and Schulak, J. A. (1992a). The effects of steroid withdrawal on the lipoprotein profiles of cyclosporine-treated kidney and kidney-pancreas transplant recipients. *Transplantation* **54**, 868.

Hricik, D. E., Lautman, J., Bartucci, M. R., Moir, E. J., Mayes, J. T. and Schulak, J. A. (1992b). Variable effects of steroid withdrawal on blood pressure reduction in cyclosporine-treated renal transplant recipients. *Transplantation* **53**, 1232.

Hsu, I., Spinler, S. A. and Johnson, N. E. (1995). Comparative evaluation of the safety and efficacy of HMG-CoA reductase inhibitor monotherapy in the treatment of primary hypercholesterolemia. *Ann. Pharmacother.* **29**, 743.

Hutchinson, T. A., Thomas, D. C., Lemieux, J. C. and Harvey, C. E. (1984). Prognostically controlled comparison of dialysis and renal transplantation. *Kidney Int.* **26**, 44.

Huysmans, F. T., Hoitsma, A. J. and Koene, R. A. (1987). Factors determining the prevalence of hypertension after renal transplantation. *Nephrol. Dial. Transplant.* **2**, 34.

Huysmans, F. T., van Heusden, F. H., Wetzels, J. F., Hoitsma, A. J. and Koene, R. A. (1988). Antihypertensive effect of beta blockade in renal transplant recipients with or without host kidneys. *Transplantation* **46**, 234.

Iacovello, L., Di Castelnuovo, A., De Knijff, P., *et al.* (1998). Polymorphisms in the coagulation factor VII gene and the risk of myocardial infarction. *N. Engl. J. Med.* **338**, 79.

Ibels, L. S., Alfrey, A. C., Huffer, W. E., Craswell, P. W., Anderson, J. T. and Weil, R. (1979). Arterial calcification and pathology in uremic patients undergoing dialysis. *Am. J. Med.* **66**, 790.

Ibels, L. S., Stewart, J. H., Mahony, J. F., Neale, F. C. and Sheli, A. G. R. (1977). Occlusive arterial disease in uraemic and haemodialysis patients and renal transplant recipients. *Q. J. M.* **46**, 197.

Ikaheimo, M., Linnaluoto, M., Huttunen, K. and Takkunen, J. (1982). Effects of renal transplantation on left ventricular size and function. *Br. Heart J.* **47**, 155.

Ikizler, T. A., Wingard, R. L., Harvell, J., Shyr, Y. and Hakim, R. M. (1999). Association of morbidity with markers of nutrition and inflammation in chronic hemodialysis patients: a prospective study. *Kidney Int.* **55**, 1945.

Ingulli, E. and Tejani, A. (1992). Severe hypercholesterolemia inhibits cyclosporine A efficacy in a dose-dependent manner in children with nephrotic syndrome. *J. Am. Soc. Nephrol.* **3**, 254.

Irish, A. B. and Green, F. R. (1997). Environmental and genetic determinants of the hypercoagulable state and cardiovascular disease in renal transplant recipients. *Nephrol. Dial. Transplant.* **12**, 167.

Irish, A. B. and Green, F. R. (1998). Factor VII coagulant activity (VIIc) and hypercoagulability in chronic renal disease and dialysis: relationship with dyslipidaemia, inflammation, and factor VII genotype. *Nephrol. Dial. Transplant.* **13**, 679.

Irish, A. B., Green, F. R., Gray, D. W. R. and Morris, P. J. (1997). The factor V Leiden (R506Q) mutation and risk of thrombosis in renal transplant recipients. *Transplantation* **64**, 604.

Iseki, K. and Fukiyama, K. (1996). Predictors of stroke in patients receiving chronic hemodialysis. *Kidney Int.* **50**, 1672.

Iseki, K., Miyasato, F., Tokuyama, K., *et al.* (1997). Low diastolic blood pressure, hypoalbuminemia, and risk of death in a cohort of chronic hemodialysis patients. *Kidney Int.* **51**, 1212.

Isoniemi, H., Nurminen, M., Tikkanen, M. J., *et al.* (1994). Risk factors predicting chronic rejection of renal allografts. *Transplantation* **57**, 68.

Ivens, K., Heering, P., Leschke, M. and Grabensee, B. (1996). Percutaneous coronary angioplasty (PTCA) or coronary artery bypass grafting (CABG)—which is the appropriate therapy of coronary artery disease in uraemic patients? *Nephrol. Dial. Transplant.* **11**, 1949.

Jelakovic, B. and Mayer, G. (1995). A renocentric view of essential hypertension: lessons to be learnt from kidney transplantation. *Nephrol. Dial. Transplant.* **10**, 1510.

Jensik, S. C. (1998). Tacrolimus (FK506) in kidney transplantation: three-year survival results of the US multicenter, randomized, comparative trial. The FK506 Kidney Transplant Study Group. *Transplant. Proc.* **30**, 1216.

Jindal, R. M., Sidner, R. A. and Milgrom, M. L. (1997). Post-transplant diabetes mellitus: the role of immunosuppression. *Drug Saf.* **16**, 242.

Johnstone, L. M., Jones, C. L., Grigg, L. E., Wilkinson, J. L., Walker, R. G. and Powell, H. R. (1996). Left ventricular abnormalities in children, adolescents and young adults with renal disease. *Kidney Int.* **50**, 998.

Joint National Committee. (1997). The sixth report of the Joint National Committee on prevention, detection, evaluation, and treatment of high blood pressure [published erratum appears in *Arch. Intern. Med.* 1998 Mar 23;158(6),573]. *Arch. Intern. Med.* **157**, 2413.

Joki, N., Hase, H., Nakamura, R. and Yamaguchi, T. (1997). Onset of coronary artery disease prior to initiation of haemodialysis in patients with end-stage renal disease. *Nephrol. Dial. Transplant.* **12**, 718.

Joven, J., Villabona, C., Vilella, E., Masana, L., Alberti, R. and Valles, M. (1990). Abnormalities of lipoprotein metabolism in patients with the nephrotic syndrome. *N. Engl. J. Med.* **323**, 579.

Jungers, P., Khoa, T. N., Massy, Z. A., *et al.* (1999). Incidence of atherosclerotic arterial occlusive accidents in predialysis and dialysis patients: a multicentric study in the Ile de France district. *Nephrol. Dial. Transplant.* **14**, 898.

Jungers, P., Massy, Z. A., Nguyen Khoa, T., *et al.* (1997). Incidence and risk factors of atherosclerotic cardiovascular accidents in predialysis chronic renal failure patients: a prospective study. *Nephrol. Dial. Transplant.* **12**, 2597.

Kahan, B. D. (1989). Cyclosporine. *N. Engl. J. Med.* **321**, 1725.

Kahn, J. K., Rutherford, B. D., McConahay, D. R., Johnson, W. L., Giorgi, L. V. and Hartzler, G. O. (1990). Short- and long-term outcome of percutaneous transluminal coronary angioplasty in chronic dialysis patients. *Am. Heart J.* **119**, 484.

Kannel, W. B. and McGee, D. L. (1979). Diabetes and cardiovascular disease. *J. A. M. A.* **241**, 2035.

Kasiske, B. L. (1987). Possible causes and consequences of hypertension in stable renal transplant patients. *Transplantation* **44**, 639.

Kasiske, B. L. (1988). Risk factors for accelerated atherosclerosis in renal transplant recipients. *Am. J. Med.* **84**, 985.

Kasiske, B. L. (1993). Risk factors for cardiovascular disease after renal transplantation. *Miner. Electrolyte Metab.* **19**, 186.

Kasiske, B. L., Guijarro, C., Massy, Z. A., Wiederkehr, M. R. and Ma, J. Z. (1996). Cardiovascular disease after renal transplantation. *J. Am. Soc. Nephrol.* **7**, 158.

Kasiske, B. L., Kalil, R. S. N., Bain, R. P. and Rohde, R. D. (1993). Effect of antihypertensive therapy in the kidney in patients with diabetes: a meta-analysis. *Ann. Intern. Med.* **118**, 129.

Kasiske, B. L., Ramos, E. L., Gaston, R. S., *et al.* (1995). The evaluation of renal transplant candidates: clinical practice guidelines. Patient Care and Education Committee of the American Society of Transplant Physicians. *J. Am. Soc. Nephrol.* **6**, 1.

Kasiske, B. L., Tortorice, K. L., Heim-Duthoy, K. L., Awni, W. M. and

Rao, K. V. (1991). The adverse impact of cyclosporine on serum lipids in renal transplant recipients. *Am. J. Kidney Dis.* **17**, 700.

Kasiske, B. L. and Umen, A. J. (1987). Persistent hyperlipidemia in renal transplant patients. *Medicine* **66**, 309.

Kates, D. M., Haas, L., Brunzell, J. and Sherrard, D. J. (1995). Risk factors for cardiovascular disease in end-stage renal failure patients: a 21 year study. *J. Am. Soc. Nephrol.* **6**, 540.

Katznelson, S., Wilkinson, A. H., Kobashigawa, J. A., *et al.* (1996). The effect of pravastatin on acute rejection after kidney transplantation—a pilot study. *Transplantation* **61**, 1469.

Kaul, T. K., Fields, B. L., Reddy, M. A. and Kahn, D. R. (1994). Cardiac operations in patients with end-stage renal disease. *Ann. Thorac. Surg.* **57**, 691.

Khauli, R. B., Steinmuller, D. R., Novick, A. C., *et al.* (1986). A critical look at survival of diabetics with end-stage renal disease. *Transplantation* **41**, 598.

Kielstein, J. T., Boger, R. H., Bode-Boger, S. M., *et al.* (1999). Asymmetric dimethylarginine plasma concentrations differ in patients with end-stage renal disease: relationship to treatment method and atherosclerotic disease. *J. Am. Soc. Nephrol.* **10**, 594.

Kim, S. B., Yang, W. S., Lee, S. K., Chi, H. S. and Park, J. S. (1998). Effect of increasing serum albumin on haemostatic factors synthesized in the liver in CAPD patients. *Nephrol. Dial. Transplant.* **13**, 2053.

Kirkman, R. L., Strom, T. B., Weir, M. R. and Tilney, N. L. (1982). Late mortality and morbidity in recipients of long-term renal allografts. *Transplantation* **34**, 347.

Klahr, S., Levey, A. S., Beck, G. J., *et al.* (1994). The effects of dietary protein restriction and blood-pressure control on the progression of chronic renal disease. Modification of Diet in Renal Disease Study Group. *N. Engl. J. Med.* **330**, 877.

Knoll, G. A. and Bell, R. C. (1999). Tacrolimus versus cyclosporin for immunosuppression in renal transplantation: meta-analysis of randomised trials. *Lancet* **318**, 1104.

Kobashigawa, J. A., Katznelson, S., Laks, H., *et al.* (1995). Effect of pravastatin on outcomes after cardiac transplantation. *N. Engl. J. Med.* **333**, 621.

Koch, M., Gradaus, F., Schoebel, F. C., Leschke, M. and Grabensee, B. (1997a). Relevance of conventional cardiovascular risk factors for the prediction of coronary artery disease in diabetic patients on renal replacement therapy. *Nephrol. Dial. Transplant.* **12**, 1187.

Koch, M., Kutkuhn, B., Grabensee, B. and Ritz, E. (1997b). Apolipoprotein A, fibrinogen, age, and history of stroke are predictors of death in dialysed diabetic patients: a prospective study in 412 subjects. *Nephrol. Dial. Transplant.* **12**, 2603.

Koch, M., Kutkuhn, B., Trenkwalder, E., *et al.* (1997c). Apolipoprotein B, fibrinogen, HDL cholesterol, and apolipoprotein(a) phenotypes predict coronary artery disease in hemodialysis patients. *J. Am. Soc. Nephrol.* **8**, 1889.

Kokado, Y., Takahara, S., Kameoka, H. and Okuyama, A. (1996). Hypertension in renal transplant recipients and its effect on long-term renal allograft survival. *Transplant. Proc.* **28**, 1600.

Koomans, H. A., Joles, J. A. and Rabelink, T. J. (1996). Tony Raine Memorial Lecture. Hypertension and the kidney: culprit and victim. *Nephrol. Dial. Transplant.* **11**, 1961.

Koyanagi, T., Nishida, H., Kitamura, M., *et al.* (1996). Comparison of clinical outcomes of coronary artery bypass grafting and percutaneous transluminal coronary angioplasty in renal dialysis patients. *Ann. Thorac. Surg.* **61**, 1793.

Kremastinos, D., Paraskevaidis, I., Voudiklari, S., *et al.* (1992). Painless myocardial ischemic in chronic hemodialysed patients: a real event? *Nephron* **60**, 164.

Krentz, A. J. and Evans, A. J. (1998). Selective imidazoline receptor antagonists for metabolic syndrome. *Lancet* **351**, 152.

Kronenberg, F., Kathrein, H., Konig, P., *et al.* (1994). Apolipoprotein (a) phenotypes predict the risk for carotid atherosclerosis in patients with end-stage renal disease. *Arterioscler. Thromb.* **14**, 1405.

Kronenberg, F., Neyer, U., Lhotta, K., *et al.* (1999). The low molecular weight apo(a) phenotype is an independent predictor for coronary artery disease in hemodialysis patients: a prospective follow-up. *J. Am. Soc. Nephrol.* **10**, 1027.

Lemmers, M. J. and Barry, J. M. (1991). Major role for arterial disease in morbidity and mortality after kidney transplantation in diabetic recipients. *Diabetes Care* **14**, 295.

Levey, A. S., Beto, J. A., Coronado, B. E., et al. (1998). Controlling the epidemic of cardiovascular disease in chronic renal disease: what do we know? What do we need to learn? Where do we go from here? National Kidney Foundation Task Force on Cardiovascular Disease. Am. J. Kidney Dis. 32, 853.

Levin, A., Singer, J., Thompson, C. R., Ross, H. and Lewis, M. (1996). Prevalent left ventricular hypertrophy in the predialysis population: identifying opportunities for intervention. Am. J. Kidney Dis. 27, 347.

Ligtenberg, G., Blankestijn, P. J., Oey, P. L., et al. (1999). Reduction of sympathetic hyperactivity by enalapril in patients with chronic renal failure. N. Engl. J. Med. 340, 1321.

Lim, P.-S., Liu, C.-S., Hong, C. J. and Wei, Y.-H. (1997). Prevalence of apolipoprotein E genotypes in ischaemic cerebrovascular disease in end-stage renal disease patients. Nephrol. Dial. Transplant. 12, 1916.

Lindholm, A., Albrechtsen, D., Frodin, L., Tufveson, G., Persson, N. H. and Lundgren, G. (1995). Ischemic heart disease—major cause of death and graft loss after renal transplantation in Scandinavia. Transplantation 60, 451.

Lindner, A., Charra, B., Sherrard, D. J. and Scribner, B. H. (1974). Accelerated atherosclerosis in prolonged maintenance hemodialysis. N. Engl. J. Med. 290, 697.

Lipkin, G. W., Tucker, B., Giles, M. and Raine, A. E. (1993). Ambulatory blood pressure and left ventricular mass in cyclosporin- and non-cyclosporin-treated renal transplant recipients. J. Hypertens. 11, 439.

Little, J., Phillips, L., Russell, L., Griffiths, A. A., Russell, G., and Davies, S. J. (1998). Longitudinal lipid profiles on CAPD: their relationship to weight gain, comorbidity, and dialysis factors. J. Am. Soc. Nephrol. 9, 1931.

London, G. M. and Druecke, T. (1997). Atherosclerosis and arteriosclerosis in chronic renal failure. Kidney Int. 51, 1678.

London, G. M., Fabiani, F., Marchais, S. J., et al. (1987). Uremic cardiomyopathy: an inadequate left ventricular hypertrophy. Kidney Int. 31, 973.

London, G. M., Guerin, A. P., Marchais, S. J., et al. (1996). Cardiac and arterial interactions in end-stage renal disease. Kidney Int. 50, 600.

Lorber, M. I., Van Buren, C. T., Flechner, S. M., et al. (1987). Pre-transplant coronary arteriography for diabetic renal transplant recipients. Transplant. Proc. 19, 1539.

Loubeyre, P., Cahen, R., Grozel, F., et al. (1996). Transplant renal artery stenosis: evaluation of diagnosis with magnetic resonance angiography compared with color duplex sonography and arteriography. Transplantation 62, 446.

Lowrie, E. G. and Lew, N. L. (1990). Death risk in hemodialysis patients: the predictive value of commonly measured variables and an evaluation of death rate differences between facilities. Am. J. Kidney Dis. 15, 458.

Lowrie, E. G. and Lew, N. L. (1992). Commonly measured laboratory variables in hemodialysis patients: relationships among them and to death risk. Semin. Nephrol. 12, 276.

Luke, R. G. (1998). Chronic renal failure: a vasculopathic state. N. Engl. J. Med. 339, 841.

Lye, W.-C., Leong, S.-O. and Lee, E. J. C. (1996). Transplant renal artery stenosis presenting with recurrent acute pulmonary oedema. Nephron 72, 302.

Macdougall, I. C., Lewis, N. P., Saunders, M. J., et al. (1990). Long-term cardiorespiratory effects of amelioration of renal anaemia by erythropoietin [published erratum appears in Lancet 1990 Mar 10;335(8689),614]. Lancet 335, 489.

Mailloux, L. U., Bellucci, A. G., Napolitano, B., Mossey, T., Wilkes, B. M. and Bluestone, P. A. (1994a). Survival estimates for 683 patients starting dialysis from 1970 through 1989: identification of risk factors for survival. Clin. Nephrol. 42, 127.

Mailloux, L. U., Bellucci, A. G., Wilkes, B. M., et al. (1991). Mortality in dialysis patients: analysis of the causes of death. Am. J. Kidney Dis. 18, 326.

Mailloux, L. U., Napolitano, B., Bellucci, A. G., Vernace, M., Wilkes, B. M. and Mossey, R. T. (1994b). Renal vascular disease causing end-stage renal disease, incidence, clinical correlates, and outcomes: a 20-year clinical experience. Am. J. Kidney Dis. 24, 622.

Mak, R. H. K. (1998). Effect of metabolic acidosis on insulin action and secretion in uremia. Kidney Int. 54, 603.

Manske, C. L., Thomas, W., Wang, Y. and Wilson, R. F. (1993). Screening diabetic transplant candidates for coronary artery disease: identification of a low risk subgroup. Kidney Int. 44, 617.

Manske, C. L., Wang, Y., Rector, T., Wilson, R. F. and White, C. W. (1992a). Coronary revascularisation in insulin-dependent diabetic patients with chronic renal failure. Lancet 340, 998.

Manske, C. L., Wilson, R. F., Wang, Y. and Thomas, W. (1992b). Prevalence of, and risk factors for, angiographically determined coronary artery disease in type 1-diabetic patients with nephropathy. Arch. Intern. Med. 152, 2450.

Manske, C. L., Wilson, R. F., Wang, Y. and Thomas, W. (1997). Atherosclerotic vascular complications in diabetic transplant candidates. Am. J. Kidney Dis. 29, 601.

Mark, A. L. (1990). Cyclosporine, sympathetic activity, and hypertension. N. Engl. J. Med. 323, 748.

Marwick, T., Hobbs, R., Vanderlaan, R. L., Steinmuller, D. and Braun, W. (1989). Use of digital subtraction fluorography in screening for coronary artery disease in patients with chronic renal failure. Am. J. Kidney Dis. 14, 105.

Maschio, G., Alberti, D., Janin, G., et al. (1996). Effect of the angiotensin-converting-enzyme inhibitor benazepril on the progression of chronic renal insufficiency. The Angiotensin-Converting-Enzyme Inhibition in Progressive Renal Insufficiency Study Group. N. Engl. J. Med. 334, 939.

Massy, Z. A., Chadefaux-Vekemans, B., Chevalier, A., et al. (1994). Hyperhomocysteinaemia: a significant risk factor for cardiovascular disease in renal transplant recipients. Nephrol. Dial. Transplant. 9, 1103.

Massy, Z. A., Guijarro, C., Wiederkehr, M. R., Ma, J. Z. and Kasiske, B. L. (1996a). Chronic renal allograft rejection: immunologic and nonimmunologic risk factors. Kidney Int. 49, 518.

Massy, Z. A. and Kasiske, B. L. (1996). Post-transplant hyperlipidemia: mechanisms and management. J. Am. Soc. Nephrol. 7, 971.

Massy, Z. A., Keane, W. F. and Kasiske, B. L. (1996b). Inhibition of the mevalonate pathway: benefits beyond cholesterol reduction? Lancet 347, 102.

Massy, Z. A., Ma, J. Z., Louis, T. A. and Kasiske, B. L. (1995). Lipid-lowering therapy in patients with renal disease. Kidney Int. 48, 188.

Massy, Z. A., Mamzer-Bruneel, M. F., Chevalier, A., et al. (1998). Carotid atherosclerosis in renal transplant recipients. Nephrol. Dial. Transplant. 13, 1792.

Mayer, A. D., Dmitrewski, J., Squifflet, J. P., et al. (1997). Multicenter randomized trial comparing tacrolimus (FK506) and cyclosporine in the prevention of renal allograft rejection: a report of the European Tacrolimus Multicenter Renal Study Group. Transplantation 64, 436.

McCune, T. R., Thacker, L. R., II, Peters, T. G., et al. (1998). Effects of tacrolimus on hyperlipidemia after successful renal transplantation: a Southeastern Organ Procurement Foundation multicenter clinical study. Transplantation 65, 87.

McLaren, A. J., Fuggle, S. V., Welsh, K. I., Gray, D. W. and Morris, P. J. (2000). Chronic allograft failure in human renal transplantation: a multivariate risk factor analysis. Ann. Surg. 232, 98.

Meyer-Lehnert, H., Bokemeyer, D., Friedrichs, U., Backer, A. and Kramer, H. J. (1997). Cellular mechanisms of cyclosporine A-associated side-effects: role of endothelin. Kidney Int. 52(Suppl. 61), S27.

Miles, A. M. V., Sumrani, N., Horowitz, R., et al. (1998). Diabetes mellitus after renal transplantation—as deleterious as non-transplant-associated diabetes? Transplantation 65, 380.

Miyata, T., van Ypersele de Strihou, C., Kurokawa, K. and Baynes, J. W. (1999). Alterations in nonenzymatic biochemistry in uremia: origin and significance of "carbonyl stress" in long-term uremic complications. Kidney Int. 55, 389.

Modena, F. M., Hostetter, T. H., Salahudeen, A. K., Najarian, J. S., Matas, A. J. and Rosenberg, M. E. (1991). Progression of kidney disease in chronic renal transplant rejection. Transplantation 52, 239.

Morris, P. J., Chan, L., French, M. E. and Ting, A. (1982). Low dose oral prednisolone in renal transplantation. Lancet 1, 525.

Mourad, G., Ribstein, J., Argiles, A., Mimran, A. and Mion, C. (1989). Contrasting effects of acute angiotensin converting enzyme inhibitors and calcium antagonists in transplant renal artery stenosis. Nephrol. Dial. Transplant. 4, 66.

Moustapha, A., Naso, A., Nahlawi, M., *et al.* (1998). Prospective study of hyperhomocysteinemia as an adverse cardiovascular risk factor in end-stage renal disease. *Circulation* **97**, 138.

Muiesan, M. L., Salvetti, M., Rizzoni, D., Castellano, M., Donato, F. and Agabiti-Rosei, E. (1995). Association of change in left ventricular mass with prognosis during long-term antihypertensive treatment. *J. Hypertens.* **13**, 1091.

Najarian, J. S., Kjellstrand, C. M. and Simmons, R. L. (1977). High-risk patients in renal transplantation. *Transplant. Proc.* **9**, 107.

Nappi, S. E., Saha, H. H. T., Virtanen, V. K., Mustonen, J. T. and Pasternack, A. I. (1999). Hemodialysis with high-calcium dialysate impairs cardiac relaxation. *Kidney Int.* **55**, 1091.

Nicholls, A. J., Catto, G. R. D., Edward, N., Engeset, J. and MacLeod, M. (1980). Accelerated atherosclerosis in long-term dialysis and transplant patients: fact or fiction? *Lancet* **1**, 276.

Nishizawa, Y., Shoji, T., Kawagishi, T. and Morii, H. (1997). Atherosclerosis in uremia: possible roles of hyperparathyroidism and intermediate density lipoprotein accumulation. *Kidney Int.* **52(Suppl. 62)**, S90.

Nygard, O., Nordrehaug, J. E., Refsum, H., Ueland, P. M., Farsatad, M. and Vollset, S. E. (1997). Plasma homocysteine levels and mortality in patients with coronary artery disease. *N. Engl. J. Med.* **337**, 230.

Odorico, J. S., Knechtle, S. J., Rayhill, S. C., *et al.* (1996). The influence of native nephrectomy on the incidence of recurrent disease following renal transplantation for primary glomerulonephritis. *Transplantation* **61**, 228.

Olbricht, C., Wanner, C., Eisenhauer, T., *et al.* (1997). Accumulation of lovastatin, but not pravastatin, in the blood of cyclosporine-treated kidney graft patients after multiple doses. *Clin. Pharmacol. Ther.* **62**, 311.

Olmer, M., Noordally, R., Berland, Y., Casanova, P., Coulange, C. and Rampal, M. (1988). Hypertension in renal transplantation. *Kidney Int.* **25(Suppl.)**, S129.

Opsahl, J. A., Husebye, D. G., Helseth, H. K. and Collins, A. J. (1988). Coronary artery bypass surgery in patients on maintenance dialysis: long-term survival. *Am. J. Kidney Dis.* **12**, 271.

Ordonez, J. D., Hiatt, R. A., Killebrew, E. J. and Fireman, B. H. (1993). The increased risk of coronary heart disease associated with nephrotic syndrome. *Kidney Int.* **44**, 638.

Owen, W. F., Lew, N. L., Liu, Y., Lowrie, E. G. and Lazarus, J. M. (1993). The urea reduction ratio and serum albumin concentration as predictors of mortality in patients undergoing hemodialysis. *N. Engl. J. Med.* **329**, 1001.

Owen, W. F. and Lowrie, E. G. (1998). C-reactive protein as an outcome predictor for maintenance hemodialysis patients. *Kidney Int.* **54**, 627.

Parfrey, P. S. and Foley, R. N. (1999). The clinical epidemiology of cardiac disease in chronic renal failure. *J. Am. Soc. Nephrol.* **10**, 1606.

Parfrey, P. S., Foley, R. N., Harnett, J. D., Kent, G. M., Murray, D. and Barre, P. E. (1996). Outcome and risk factors of ischemic heart disease in chronic uremia. *Kidney Int.* **49**, 1428.

Parfrey, P. S., Griffiths, S. M., Harnett, J. D., *et al.* (1990). Outcome of congestive heart failure, dilated cardiomyopathy, hypertrophic hyperkinetic disease, and ischemic heart disease in dialysis patients. *Am. J. Nephrol.* **10**, 213.

Parfrey, P. S., Harnett, J. D., Foley, R. N., *et al.* (1995). Impact of renal transplantation on uremic cardiomyopathy. *Transplantation* **60**, 908.

Parker, T. F., 3rd, Wingard, R. L., Husni, L., Ikizler, T. A., Parker, R. A. and Hakim, R. M. (1996). Effect of the membrane biocompatibility on nutritional parameters in chronic hemodialysis patients. *Kidney Int.* **49**, 551.

Patton, P. R., Brunson, M. E., Pfaff, W. W., *et al.* (1994). A preliminary report of diltiazem and ketoconazole: their cyclosporine-sparing effect and impact on transplant outcome. *Transplantation* **57**, 889.

Perna, A. F., Ingrosso, D., de Santo, N. G., Galletti, P., Brunone, M. and Zappia, V. (1997). Metabolic consequences of folate-induced reduction of hyperhomocysteinemia in uremia. *J. Am. Soc. Nephrol.* **8**, 1899.

Perry, I. J., Refsum, H., Morris, R. W., Ebrahim, S. B., Ueland, P. M. and Shaper, A. G. (1995). Prospective study of serum total homocysteine concentration and risk of stroke in middle-aged British men. *Lancet* **346**, 1395.

Peteiro, J., Alvarez, N., Calvino, R., Penas, M., Ribera, F. and Castro Beiras, A. (1994). Changes in left ventricular mass and filling after renal transplantation are related to changes in blood pressure: an echocardiographic and pulsed Doppler study. *Cardiology* **85**, 273.

Philipson, J. D., Carpenter, B. J., Itzkoff, J., *et al.* (1986). Evaluation of cardiovascular risk for renal transplantation in diabetic patients. *Am. J. Med.* **81**, 630.

Pirsch, J. D., Miller, J., Deierhoi, M. H., Vincenti, F. and Filo, R. S. (1997). A comparison of tacrolimus (FK506) and cyclosporine for immunosuppression after cadaveric renal transplantation. FK506 Kidney Transplant Study Group. *Transplantation* **63**, 977.

Pitt, B., Waters, D., Brown, W. V., *et al.* (1999). Aggressive lipid-lowering therapy compared with angioplasty in stable coronary artery disease. Atorvastatin versus Revascularization Treatment Investigators. *N. Engl. J. Med.* **341**, 70.

Pollini, J., Guttmann, R. D., Beaudoin, J. G., Morehouse, D. D., Klassen, J. and Knaack, J. (1979). Late hypertension following renal allotransplantation. *Clin. Nephrol.* **11**, 202.

Port, F. K. (1994). Morbidity and mortality in dialysis patients. *Kidney Int.* **46**, 1728.

Port, F. K., Wolfe, R. A., Mauger, E. A., Berling, D. P. and Jiang, K. (1993). Comparison of survival probabilities for dialysis patients vs cadaveric renal transplant recipients. *J. A. M. A.* **270**, 1339.

Pouria, S., State, O. I., Wong, W. and Hendry, B. M. (1998). CMV infection is associated with transplant renal artery stenosis. *Q. J. M.* **91**, 185.

Preston, R. A., Singer, I. and Epstein, M. (1996). Renal parenchymal hypertension: current concepts of pathogenesis and management. *Arch. Intern. Med.* **156**, 602.

Rader, D. J. and Brewer, H. B. (1992). Lipoprotein (a): clinical approach to a unique atherogenic lipoprotein. *J. A. M. A.* **267**, 1109.

Radermacher, J., Meiners, M., Bramlage, C., *et al.* (1998). Pronounced renal vasoconstriction and systemic hypertension in renal transplant patients treated with cyclosporin A versus FK506. *Transpl. Int.* **11**, 3.

Raine, A. E. (1994a). Hypertension and the kidney. *Br. Med. Bull.* **50**, 322.

Raine, A. E. (1995). Hypertension and ischaemic heart disease in renal transplant recipients. *Nephrol. Dial. Transplant.* **10(Suppl. 1)**, 95.

Raine, A. E., Bedford, L., Simpson, A. W., *et al.* (1993a). Hyperparathyroidism, platelet intracellular free calcium and hypertension in chronic renal failure. *Kidney Int.* **43**, 700.

Raine, A. E., Carter, R., Mann, J. I. and Morris, P. J. (1988). Adverse effect of cyclosporin on plasma cholesterol in renal transplant recipients. *Nephrol. Dial. Transplant.* **3**, 458.

Raine, A. E., Margreiter, R., Brunner, F. P., *et al.* (1992). Report on management of renal failure in Europe, XXII, 1991. *Nephrol. Dial. Transplant.* **7(Suppl. 2)**, 7.

Raine, A. E. and Roger, S. D. (1991). Effects of erythropoietin on blood pressure. *Am. J. Kidney Dis.* **18**, 76.

Raine, A. E. G. (1994b). Cardiovascular complications after renal transplantation. *In Kidney Transplantation*, 4th ed., (P. J. Morris, ed.), p. 339, W.B. Saunders, Philadelphia.

Raine, A. E. G., Seymour, A.-M. L., Roberts, A. F. C., Radda, G. K. and Ledingham, J. G. G. (1993b). Impairment of cardiac function and energetics in experimental renal failure. *J. Clin. Invest.* **92**, 2934.

Rajagopalan P. R., and Rapamune Global Study Group (1999). A randomized placebo-controlled trial of rapamune in primary renal allograft recipients (abstract). *J. Am. Soc. Nephrol.* **10**, 743A.

Ratcliffe, P. J., Dudley, C. R. K., Higgins, R. M., Firth, J. D., Smith, B. and Morris, P. J. (1996). Randomised controlled trial of steroid withdrawal in renal transplant recipients receiving triple immunosuppression. *Lancet* **348**, 643.

Rettig, R. (1993). Does the kidney play a role in the aetiology of primary hypertension? Evidence from renal transplantation studies in rats and humans. *J. Hum. Hypertens.* **7**, 177.

Rettig, R., Bandelow, N., Patschan, O., Kuttler, B., Frey, B. and Uber, A. (1996). The importance of the kidney in primary hypertension: insights from cross-transplantation. *J. Hum. Hypertens.* **10**, 641.

Rinehart, A. L., Herzog, C. A., Collins, A. J., Flack, J. M., Ma, J. Z. and Opsahl, J. A. (1995). A comparison of coronary angioplasty and coronary artery bypass grafting outctomes in chronic dialysis patients. *Am. J. Kidney Dis.* **25**, 281.

Rockstroh, J. K., Schobel, H. P., Vogt-Ladner, G., Hauser, I., Neumayer, H. H. and Schmieder, R. E. (1997). Blood pressure independent effects of nitrendipine on cardiac structure in patients after renal transplantation. *Nephrol. Dial. Transplant.* **12**, 1441.

Roig, E., Betriu, A. A., Castaner, A., Magrina, J., Sanz, G. and Navarro-Lopez, F. (1981). Disabling angina pectoris with normal coronary arteries in patients undergoing long-term hemodialysis. *Am. J. Med.* **71**, 431.

Ross, R. (1999). Atherosclerosis—an inflammatory disease. *N. Engl. J. Med.* **340**, 115.

Rostand, S. G. and Druecke, T. B. (1999). Parathyroid hormone, vitamin D, and cardiovascular disease in chronic renal failure. *Kidney Int.* **56**, 383.

Rostand, S. G., Gretes, J. C., Kirk, K. A., Rutsky, E. A. and Andreoli, T. E. (1979). Ischemic heart disease in patients with uremia underoing maintenance hemodialysis. *Kidney Int.* **16**, 600.

Rostand, S. G., Kirk, K. A. and Rutsky, E. A. (1984). Dialysis-associated ischemic heart disease: insights from coronary angiography. *Kidney Int.* **25**, 653.

Rostand, S. G., Kirk, K. A. and Rutsky, E. A. (1986). The epidemiology of coronary artery disease in patients on maintenance hemodialysis: implications for management. *Contrib. Nephrol.* **52**, 34.

Roxborough, H. E. and Young, I. S. (1995). Carbamylation of proteins and atherogenesis in renal failure. *Med. Hypotheses* **45**, 125.

Rozich, J. D., Smith, B., Thomas, J. D., Zile, M. R., Kaiser, J. and Mann, D. L. (1991). Dialysis-induced alterations in left ventricular filling: mechanisms and clinical significance. *Am. J. Kidney Dis.* **17**, 277.

Ruffmann, K., Mandelbaum, A., Bommer, J., Schmidli, M. and Ritz, E. (1990). Doppler echocardiographic findings in dialysis patients. *Nephrol. Dial. Transplant.* **5**, 426.

Sacks, F. M., Pfeffer, M. A., Moye, L. A., *et al.* (1996). The effect of pravastatin on coronary events after myocardial infarction in patients with average cholesterol levels. Cholesterol and Recurrent Events Trial investigators. *N. Engl. J. Med.* **335**, 1001.

Saggar-Malik, A. K., Missouris, C. G., Gill, J. S., Singer, D. R. J., Markandu, N. D. and MacGregor, G. A. (1994). Left ventricular mass in normotensive subjects with autosomal dominant polycystic kidney disease. *B. M. J.* **309**, 1617.

Sander, M., Lyson, T., Thomas, G. D. and Victor, R. G. (1996). Sympathetic neural mechanisms of cyclosporine-induced hypertension. *Am. J. Hypertens.* **9**, 121S.

Sattar, N., Packard, C. J. and Petrie, J. R. (1998). The end of triglycerides in cardiovascular risk assessment? *B. M. J.* **317**, 553.

Savage, T., Giles, M., Tomson, C. R. V. and Raine, A. E. G. (1998). Gender differences in mediators of left ventricular hypertrophy in dialysis patients. *Clin. Nephrol.* **49**, 107.

Scandinavian Simvastatin Survival Study (4S) Study Group. (1994). Randomised trial of cholesterol lowering in 4444 patients with coronary heart disease. The Scandinavian Simvastatin Survival Study (4S). *Lancet* **344**, 1383.

Schaubel, D., Desmeules, M., Mao, Y., Jeffery, J. and Fenton, S. (1995). Survival experience among elderly end-stage renal disease patients: a controlled comparison of transplantation and dialysis. *Transplantation* **60**, 1389.

Scherrer, U., Vissing, S. F., Morgan, B. J., *et al.* (1990). Cyclosporine-induced sympathetic activation and hypertension after heart transplantation. *N. Engl. J. Med.* **323**, 693.

Schleiber, S., Krauss, M., Wagner, K., *et al.* (1995). FK506 versus cyclosporin in the prevention of renal allograft rejection—Euopean pilot study: six-week results. *Transpl. Int.* **8**, 86.

Schmeider, R. E., Schlaich, M. P., Klingbeil, A. U. and Martus, P. (1998). Update on reversal of left ventricular hypertrophy in essential hypertension (a meta-analysis of all randomized double-blind studies until December 1996). *Nephrol. Dial. Transplant.* **13**, 564.

Shamlou, K. K., Drane, W. E., Hawkins, I. F. and Fennell, R. S., 3rd (1994). Captopril renography and the hypertensive renal transplantation patient: a predictive test of therapeutic outcome. *Radiology* **190**, 153.

Shapiro, R., Jordan, M., Scantlebury, V., *et al.* (1991). FK506 in clinical kidney transplantation. *Transplant. Proc.* **23**, 3065.

Shemin, D., Lapane, K. L., Bausserman, L., *et al.* (1999). Plasma total homocysteine and hemodialysis access thrombosis: a prospective study. *J. Am. Soc. Nephrol.* **10**, 1095.

Shepherd, J., Cobbe, S. M., Ford, I., *et al.* (1995). Prevention of coronary heart disease with pravastatin in men with hypercholesterolemia. West of Scotland Coronary Prevention Study Group. *N. Engl. J. Med.* **333**, 1301.

Shulman, N. B., Ford, C. E., Hall, W. D., *et al.* (1989). Prognostic value of serum creatinine and effect of treatment of hypertension on renal function: results from the Hypertension Detection and Follow-up Trial. *Hypertension* **13(Suppl. I)**, 80.

Silberberg, J., Racine, N., Barre, P. and Sniderman, A. D. (1990). Regression of left ventricular hypertrophy in dialysis patients following correction of anemia with recombinant human erythropoietin. *Can. J. Cardiol.* **6**, 1.

Silberberg, J. S., Barre, P. E., Prichard, S. S. and Sniderman, A. D. (1989a). Impact of left ventricular hypertrophy on survival in end-stage renal disease. *Kidney Int.* **36**, 286.

Silberberg, J. S., Rahal, D. P., Patton, D. R. and Sniderman, A. D. (1989b). Role of anemia in the pathogenesis of left ventricular hypertrophy in end-stage renal disease. *Am. J. Cardiol.* **64**, 222.

Sinclair, N. R. S. (1992). Low-dose steroid therapy in cyclosporine-treated renal transplant recipients with well-functioning grafts. *Can. Med. Assoc. J.* **147**, 645.

Sonksen, J., Gray, R., and Hickman, P. H. (1998). Safer non-cardiac surgery for patients with coronary artery disease. *B. M. J.* **317**, 1400.

Steinvinkel, P., Berglucn, L., Heimburger, O., Pettersson, E. and Alvestrand, A. (1993). Lipoprotein (a) in nephrotic syndrome. *Kidney Int.* **44**, 1116.

Steinvinkel, P., Heimburger, O., Jogestrand, T., Karnell, A. and Samuelsson, A. (1999a). Does persistent infection with *Chlamydia pneumoniae* increase the risk of atherosclerosis in chronic renal failure? *Kidney Int.* **55**, 2531.

Steinvinkel, P., Heimburger, O., Paultre, F., *et al.* (1999b). Strong association between malnutrition, inflammation, and atherosclerosis in chronic renal failure. *Kidney Int.* **55**, 1899.

Strandgaard, S. and Hansen, U. (1986). Hypertension in renal allograft recipients may be conveyed by cadaveric kidneys from donors with subarachnoid haemorrhage. *B. M. J.* **292**, 1041.

Sumrani, N. B., Delaney, V., Ding, Z., *et al.* (1991). Diabetes mellitus after renal transplantation in the cyclosporine era—an analysis of risk factors. *Transplantation* **51**, 343.

Surdacki, A., Wieczorek Surdacka, E., Sulowicz, W. and Dubiel, J. S. (1995). Effect of having a functioning cadaveric renal transplant on cardiovascular mortality risk in patients on renal replacement therapy. *Nephrol. Dial. Transplant.* **10**, 1218.

Sutherland, F., Burgess, E., Klassen, J., Buckle, S. and Paul, L. C. (1993a). Post-transplant conversion from cyclosporin to azathioprine: effect on cardiovascular risk profile. *Transpl. Int.* **6**, 129.

Sutherland, R. S., Spees, E. K., Jones, J. W. and Fink, D. W. (1993b). Renal artery stenosis after renal transplantation: the impact of the hypogastric artery anastomosis. *J. Urol.* **149**, 980.

Takahashi, K., Totsune, K. and Mouri, T. (1994). Endothelin in chronic renal failure. *Nephron* **66**, 373.

Tatti, P., Pahor, M., Byington, R. P., *et al.* (1998). Outcome results of the Fosinopril versus Amlodipine cardiovascular events randomized trial (FACET) in patients with hypertension and NIDDM. *Diabetes Care* **21**, 597.

Teruel, J. L., Padial, L. R., Quereda, C., Yeste, P., Marcen, R. and Ortuno, J. (1987). Regression of left ventricular hypertrophy afte renal transplantation: a prospective study. *Transplantation* **43**, 307.

Thompson, J. F., Fletcher, E. W. L., Wood, R. F. M., *et al.* (1984). Control of hypertension after renal transplantation by embolisation of host kidneys. *Lancet* **2**, 424.

Tomson, C. R. V., Channon, S. M., Parkinson, I. S., *et al.* (1988). Plasma oxalate concentration and secondary oxalosis in patients with chronic renal failure. *J. Clin. Pathol.* **41**, 1107.

Toz, H., Ozerkan, F., Unsal, A., Soydas, C. and Dorhout Mees, E. J. (1998). Dilated uremic cardiomyopathy in a dialysis patient cured by persistent ultrafiltration. *Am. J. Kidney Dis.* **32**, 664.

Tschope, W., Koch, M., Thomas, B. and Ritz, E. (1993). Serum lipids predict cardiac death in diabetic patients on maintenance hemodialysis. *Nephron* **64**, 354.

Tucker, B., Fabbian, F., Giles, M., Thuraisingham, R. C., Raine, A. E. and Baker, L. R. (1997). Left ventricular hypertrophy and ambulatory blood pressure monitoring in chronic renal failure. *Nephrol. Dial. Transplant.* **12**, 724.

Tunstall-Pedoe, H., Woodward, M., Tavendale, R., A'Brook, R. and Mluskey, M. K. (1997). Comparison of the prediction by 27 different factors of coronary heart disease and death in men and women of the Scottish heart health study: cohort study. *B. M. J.* **315**, 722.

Vallance, P., Leone, A., Calver, A., Collier, J. and Moncada, S. (1992). Accumulation of an endogenous inhibitor of nitric oxide synthesis in chronic renal failure. *Lancet* **339**, 572.

van den Dorpel, M. A., Ghanem, H., Rischen-Vos, J., Man In't Veld, A. J., Jansen, H. and Weimar, W. (1997). Conversion from cyclosporine A to azathioprine treatment improves LDL oxidation in kidney transplant recipients. *Kidney Int.* **51**, 1608.

van der Woude, F. J., van Son, W. J., Tegzess, A. M., *et al.* (1985). Effect of captopril on blood pressure and renal function in patients with transplant renal artery stenosis. *Nephron* **39**, 184.

van Guldener, C., Donker, A. J. M., Jakobs, C., Teerlink, T., de Meer, K. and Stehouwer, C. D. A. (1998a). No net renal extraction of homocysteine in fasting humans. *Kidney Int.* **54**, 166.

van Guldener, C., Janssen, M. J. F. M., Lambert, J., ter Wee, P. M., Donker, A. J. M. and Stehouwer, C. D. A. (1998b). Folic acid treatment of hyperhomocysteinemia in peritoneal dialysis patients: no change in endothelial function after long-term therapy. *Perit. Dial. Int.* **18**, 282.

van Guldener, C., Janssen, M. J. F. M., Lambert, J., *et al.* (1998c). No change in endothelial function after long-term folic acid therapy of hyperhomocysteinaemia in haemodialysis patients. *Nephrol. Dial. Transplant.* **13**, 106.

van Ypersele de Strihow, C., Vereerstraten, P., Wautheir, M., *et. al.* (1983). Prevalence, etiology and treatment of late post-transplant hypertension. *Adv. Nephrol. Necker Hosp.* **12**, 41.

Vanwalleghem, J., Coosemans, W., Raat, H., Waer, M. and Vanrenterghem, Y. (1997). Peritransplant lymphocele causing arterial hypertension by a Page kidney phenomenon. Leuven Collaborative Group for Transplantation. *Nephrol. Dial. Transplant.* **12**, 823.

Varghese, Z., Fernando, R. L., Turakjia, G., *et al.* (1999). Calcineurin inhibitors enhance low-density lipoprotein oxidation in transplant patients. *Kidney Int.* **56(Suppl.)**, 71.

Vathsala, A., Weinberg, R. B., Schoenberg, L., *et al.* (1989). Lipid abnormalities in cyclosporine-prednisone-treated renal transplant recipients. *Transplantation* **48**, 37.

Vincenti, F., Amend, W. J., Abele, J., Feduska, N. J. and Salvatierra, O. (1980). The role of hypertension in hemodialysis-associated atherosclerosis. *Am. J. Med.* **68**, 363.

Wang, C. and Salahudeen, A. K. (1995). Lipid peroxidation accompanies cyclosporine nephrotoxicity: effects of vitamin E. *Kidney Int.* **47**, 927.

Wannamethee, S. G., Shaper, A. G. and Perry, I. J. (1997). Serum creatinine concentration and risk of cardiovascular disease: a possible marker for increased risk of stroke. *Stroke* **28**, 557.

Wanner, C. and Bartens, W. (1994). Lipoprotein (a) in renal patients: is it a key factor in the high cardiovascular mortality? *Nephrol. Dial. Transplant.* **9**, 1066.

Wanner, C., Zimmermann, J., Quaschning, T. and Galle, J. (1997). Inflamation, dyslipidemia and vascular risk factors in hemodialysis patients. *Kidney Int.* **52(Suppl. 62)**, S53.

Warholm, C., Wilczek, H. and Pettersson, E. (1995). Hypertension two years after renal transplantation: causes and consequences. *Transpl. Int.* **8**, 286.

Webb, A. T., Reaveley, D. A., O'Donnell, M., O'Connor, B., Seed, M. and Brown, E. A. (1994). Lipids and lipoprotein (a) as risk factors for vascular disease in patients on renal replacement therapy. *Nephrol. Dial. Transplant.* **5**, 354.

Webb, A. T. A., Fransk, P. J., Reaveley, D. A., Greenhalgh, R. M. and Brown, E. A. (1993). Prevalence of intermittent claudication and risk factors for its development in patients on renal replacement therapy. *Eur. J. Vasc. Surg.* **7**, 523.

Weinrauch, L. A., D'Elia, J. A., Healy, R. W., *et al.* (1978). Asymptomatic coronary artery disease: angiography in diabetic patients before renal transplantation. *Ann. Intern. Med.* **88**, 346.

Welch, G. N. and Loscalzo, J. (1988). Homocysteine and atherothrombosis. *N. Engl. J. Med.* **338**, 1042.

Wheeler, D. C., Morgan, R., Thomas, D. M., Seed, M., Rees, A. and Moore, R. H. (1996). Factors influencing plasma lipid profiles including lipoprotein (a) concentrations in renal transplant recipients. *Transpl. Int.* **9**, 221.

Wickre, C. G., Norman, D. J., Bennison, A., Barry, J. M. and Bennett, W. M. (1983). Postrenal transplant erythrocytosis: a review of 53 patients. *Kidney Int.* **23**, 731.

Wilcken, D. E. L., Dudman, N. P. B., Tyrrell, P. A. and Robertson, M. R. (1988). Folic acid lowers elevated plasma homocysteine in chronic renal insufficiency: possible implications for prevention of vascular disease. *Metabolism* **37**, 697.

Wilcken, D. E. L., Gupta, V. J. and Betts, A. K. (1981). Homocysteine in the plasma of renal transplant recipients: effects of cofactors for methionine metabolism. *Clin. Sci.* **61**, 743.

Wilkinson, S. P., Stewart, W. K., Parham, D. M. and Guthrie, W. (1988). Symmetric gangrene of the extremities in late renal failure: a case report and review of the literature. *Q. J. M.* **67**, 319.

Wizemann, V., Kaufmann, J. and Kramer, W. (1992). Effect of erythropoietin on ischemia tolerance in anemic hemodialysis patients with confirmed coronary artery disease. *Nephron* **62**, 161.

Wong, W., Fynn, S. P., Higgins, R. M., *et al.* (1996). Transplant renal artery stenosis in 77 patients—does it have an immunological cause? *Transplantation* **61**, 215.

World Health Organization. (1999). 1999 World Health Organization–International Society of Hypertension Guidelines for the Management of Hypertension. Guidelines Subcommittee. *J. Hypertens.* **17**, 151.

Yang, W. S., Min, W. K., Park, J. S. and Kim, S. B. (1997). Effect of increasing serum albumin on serum lipoprotein(a) concentration in patients receiving CAPD. *Am. J. Kidney Dis.* **30**, 507.

Yasamura, T., Oka, T., Aikawa, I., Arakawa, K., Ohmori, Y. and Nakane, Y. (1981). Beneficial effect of bilateral nephrectomy on long-term survival of living related kidney allografts. *Transplant. Proc.* **21**, 1967.

Yudkin, J. S., Forrest, R. D. and Jackson, C. A. (1988). Microalbuminuria as predictor of vascular disease in non-diabetic subjects. *Lancet* **2**, 530.

Yukawa, S., Mune, M., Yamada, Y., Otani, H., Kishino, M. and Tone, Y. (1999). Ongoing trials of lipid reduction therapy in patients with renal disease. *Kidney Int.* **56(Suppl. 71)**, S141.

Zeier, M., Mandelbaum, A. and Ritz, E. (1998). Hypertension in the transplanted patient. *Nephron* **80**, 257.

Zimmermann, J., Herrlinger, S., Pruy, A., Metzger, T. and Wanner, C. (1999). Inflammation enhances cardiovascular risk and mortality in hemodialysis patients. *Kidney Int.* **55**, 648.

Infectious Complications After Renal Transplantation

J. Cohen • J. Hopkin • J. Kurtz

Introduction

The success of renal transplantation depends on a compromise between achieving sufficient immunosuppression to avoid rejection of the graft and maintaining a sufficient level of immune competence to protect the recipient from infection. In the early years of transplantation, the incidence of severe and lethal infections was high and discouraging, but with increasing experience, a compromise gradually has been reached so that renal transplantation now offers equivalent or better patient survival to hemodialysis. The problem of infection remains of considerable concern, however, and contributes substantially to the morbidity and mortality of renal transplantation. Although most infections in renal transplant recipients are caused by common pathogens, devastating opportunistic infections occur frequently enough to require a multidisciplinary approach involving infectious disease physicians and microbiologists.

Incidence

The precise incidence of posttransplant infection is unknown because the definition may vary from the clinically significant and microbiologically, serologically or histologically proven episode to a positive culture report without clinical manifestations. Death from infection is an unreliable indicator of the size of the problem not only because infection can be a terminal event in a patient dying of another cause, but also because most infections are treated successfully. Comparisons between units are hard to interpret without knowing the availability of maintenance hemodialysis facilities, which allow the irreversibly rejecting kidney to be abandoned early, or the selection criteria for transplantation of higher risk patients.

These caveats apart, the incidence of serious and lethal infection has fallen dramatically. In a study carried out in the early 1980s, Peterson and colleagues found that 32% of patients suffered a clinically significant infection; 7% of patients died, and in 87% of these deaths, infection was an important contributing factor (Peterson et al., 1982). By contrast, current studies report graft and patient survival of 85% and 95% at 1 year and 80% and 90% at 5 years, and cardiovascular events have overtaken infection as the leading cause of death (Faull et al., 1999; Hiesse et al., 1999; Shapiro et al., 1999). Nevertheless, infection remains an important cause of mortality and allograft loss, particularly in patients who have suffered primary graft failure and undergo repeat transplantation (Ojo et al., 1998). The reasons for the fall in the incidence of lethal and nonlethal infections include improvements in general clinical care arising from greater experience; improvements in methods of organ procurement, surgical technique and recipient selection and a greater awareness of the type and timing of infections. Improved tissue matching (see Chapter 10) and pregraft recipient blood transfusion may have contributed to lower rejection rates and to less intensive immunosuppression. A more conservative approach to immunosuppressive therapy is probably the most striking change in practice. Abandoning the effort to salvage the inexorably failing graft and in particular lower dose steroid therapy (Morris et al., 1982) have been shown to reduce the incidence of infection without causing poorer graft survival rates (see Chapter 15). Changing the immunosuppressive regimen needs to be monitored carefully to ensure that it does not increase unduly the risk of infection, but there is no evidence that any of the newer regimens has caused an increased incidence of infection.

Posttransplant infections can be classified by the organism, the system involved or the time of appearance in relation to surgery (Rubin et al., 1981); these are described in detail later, but a concise overview is appropriate here. Bacterial infections that occur early (<1 month) affect the urinary tract, respiratory system, wound and vascular access sites. They are common, and all may lead to septicemia. More unusual bacterial infections tend to occur later. Of the viral infections, herpes simplex virus (HSV) infections occur early, but cytomegalovirus (CMV) infection usually is not seen in the first month after transplantation. Herpes zoster may occur at any time. Nocardial, fungal, protozoal and helminthic infections all are relatively rare and present only after the early postoperative period. Overall, about 50% of infections are caused by viruses, 30% are caused by bacteria and 5% are caused by fungi. In 15% of cases, infection is polymicrobial.

Causative Factors

Renal transplant patients are susceptible to infection for three main reasons:

1. Patients have undergone a major surgical operation involving vascular and urological procedures. The transplanted organ may be contaminated during retrieval. Patients' surface defenses are breached by urinary catheters, intravenous cannulae and peritoneal dialysis catheters.

2. Patients are uremic and already immunosuppressed, are usually anemic and may suffer from coagulation defects and protein restriction effects.

3. Patients receive immunosuppressive drugs, which have broad effects on immune competence. The immunosuppressive treatment affects specific and nonspecific defense mechanisms, and prednisolone has antiinflammatory effects and delays wound healing.

Other risk factors include age (e.g., children may have particular problems) (Harmon, 1991), diabetes, hyperglycemia, poor graft function, neutropenia, hepatitis (La Quaglia et al., 1981) and splenectomy (Peters et al., 1983).

Prevention of Infection

BEFORE TRANSPLANTATION

Patients accepted into a transplant program should be screened for the presence of active infection and for evidence of exposure to several organisms that subsequently may cause problems. The two commonest sites of preexisting infection are the chest and the urinary tract. Bronchiectasis can be a considerable problem, particularly in the early posttransplant period. There is no advantage in attempting to sterilize the sputum while the patient is awaiting a graft. Sterilization is virtually impossible to maintain, and resistant organisms emerge quickly. Acute exacerbations should be treated with antibiotics and physiotherapy in the standard manner. Pneumococcal vaccination is available and safe (Immunization Practices Advisory Committee, 1982) and is indicated particularly in patients who have had a splenectomy; however, it is generally of limited value in immunosuppressed or uremic patients (Shapiro and Clemens, 1984). Patients with a history of tuberculosis should receive prophylaxis (discussed later). Chronic or repeated infection of the urinary tract should be treated actively and eradicated if possible. If eradication is not possible, bilateral nephrectomy merits careful consideration, although the procedure is hazardous in dialysis patients (Bishop *et al.*, 1977; see Chapter 4). Chronic dental or sinus infection can be an occult source of sepsis and should be corrected in all potential allograft recipients. Serological tests for evidence of past exposure to hepatitis B and C, HSV, Epstein-Barr virus (EBV), CMV, varicella-zoster virus (VZV) and human immunodeficiency virus (HIV) should be carried out and repeated at 6-month intervals. Patients who have a history of residence in or prolonged visits to areas endemic for histoplasmosis or coccidioidomycosis should have appropriate serological screening tests.

Strongyloides stercoralis is a nematode worm that may cause a fatal hyperinfection syndrome in immunosuppressed patients. Patients who are or have been residents in endemic areas of the West Indies or Far East should be screened and, if necessary, treated before the transplant (DeVault *et al.*, 1990).

Patients admitted for a transplant should be screened for nasal carriage of *Staphylococcus aureus*. Some centers treat all patients routinely with topical mupirocin while awaiting the results of the screening swabs. During the hours immediately before a transplant, every effort should be made to obtain specimens from potentially infected sites, notably the urine and dialysate fluid in patients on peritoneal dialysis.

All living related and cadaver donors should be assessed carefully for infection and screened for hepatitis B and C, CMV, EBV and HIV before transplantation. Many other infections have been reported occasionally as being transmitted from the donor to the recipient, including common aerobic bacteria, fungi, toxoplasmosis, malaria and trypanosomiasis (Gottesdiener, 1989). Although systemic infection in the donor has been regarded as an absolute contraindication to cadaveric organ transplantation, some experience suggests that this is not always the case (Little *et al.*, 1997). Considerable caution must be exercised and expert advice sought on the use of additional prophylactic antibiotic therapy that may be needed.

AT OPERATION

Most infections in the early posttransplant period are complications of the procedure itself; surgical technique is paramount in reducing the incidence of hematomas, urine leaks and lymphoceles (see Chapters 11, 28 and 29). There is general agreement that perioperative prophylactic antibiotic drugs are beneficial in reducing the incidence of wound infections (Goodman and Hargreave, 1990), although there is considerable variation in practice. The regimen depends on local bacterial epidemiology but should attempt to cover *S. aureus* and common enteric coliform bacteria. One suggestion is the combination of cefuroxime, 750 mg, and piperacillin, 4 g, for three doses with the first dose being given with the premedication. Patients allergic to penicillins can be given a single dose of vancomycin and gentamicin. Instilling antibiotics into the bladder was of no additional benefit (Salmela *et al.*, 1990).

AFTER TRANSPLANTATION

Strict *reverse-barrier* nursing of transplant recipients never has been evaluated formally, but it is unlikely to confer significant benefit. With few exceptions, infection in renal transplant recipients is due to reactivation of endogenous organisms (e.g., *Escherichia coli* septicemia, *Pneumocystis* pneumonia) or to lack of conventional preventive infection-control techniques and adequate hand washing. Barrier nursing is required, however, if the granulocyte count falls to less than 0.5×10^9 L^{-1}. Oral gastrointestinal decontamination with co-trimoxazole (trimethoprim-sulfamethoxazole) or a fluorinated quinolone (e.g., ciprofloxacin) should be used and antifungal prophylaxis (fluconazole, 200 mg daily) given.

The incidence of tuberculosis after renal transplantation varies enormously but may rise to 5% or more among individuals in a high-risk population (Garcia-Leoni *et al.*, 1990; Higgins *et al.*, 1991; Yildiz *et al.*, 1998; see Chapter 38). Tuberculosis in this setting may manifest late, even many years after the transplant; it often occurs atypically and has an appreciable mortality rate. For these reasons, we recommend chemoprophylaxis in any patient suspected to have been exposed to tuberculosis in the past. We use isoniazid alone or isoniazid and rifampicin if there is a strong history of exposure. If rifampicin is to be used, cyclosporine may be precluded (see Chapter 16). How long to continue with prophylaxis is unresolved; we normally continue it for 12 to 18 months. Atypical mycobacteria, which account for about 10% of this type of infection, may not be susceptible to isoniazid, and so the index of suspicion always should remain high.

The urinary tract is the commonest site of early infection in renal allograft recipients, and, more importantly, it is the commonest source of bacteremia (Bennett *et al.*, 1970; Peterson *et al.*, 1982). It has been suggested that urinary infection may precipitate graft rejection (Byrd *et al.*, 1978). Co-trimoxazole (Fox *et al.*, 1990; Tolkoff-Rubin *et al.*, 1982) or ciprofloxacin (Moyses-Neto *et al.*, 1997) given after removal of the urinary catheter have been shown to reduce significantly the incidence of serious urinary infection and septicemia. Co-trimoxazole also diminishes the risk of infection with *Pneumocystis carinii*, an important consideration in centers with a high incidence of this complication. There has been some concern that co-trimoxazole might cause leukopenia in transplant patients and that it might be associated with an increased risk of fungal superinfection, but a large study found no evidence of this (Maki *et al.*, 1992). We believe that co-trimoxazole, given for 1 year after transplantation (or longer in high-risk groups), is a worthwhile strategy.

Frequent follow-up is an essential part of management, especially during the first 6 months after transplantation. Patients should be told that the onset of fever should be reported without delay; fever is never insignificant in a transplant recipient.

TABLE 31–1

CAUSES OF FEVER* IN 175 RENAL ALLOGRAFT RECIPIENTS DURING A 3-YEAR PERIOD OF OBSERVATION

Cause of Fever	No. (%) of Episodes
Infection	144 (74)
Viral	107
Bacterial	27
Fungal	10
Allograft rejection	25 (13)
Malignancy	7 (4)
Drug fever	3 (2)
Others, unknown	15 (7)
Total	194 (100)

*≥38°C on 2 consecutive days. Some patients had multiple febrile episodes.
Reproduced with permission from Peterson *et al.* (1981).

Clinical Problems

FEVER AND SEPTICEMIA

Infection is the commonest cause of fever in renal transplant recipients. In an analysis of 194 episodes of fever in 174 transplant patients, infection accounted for 74% of the episodes, with allograft rejection contributing a further 13% (Peterson *et al.*, 1981; Table 31–1). The timetable of infective complications developed by Rubin *et al.* (1981; Fig. 31–1) is helpful in evaluating a patient with fever. The posttransplant course in terms of infection may be divided into three periods: (1) 0 to 6 weeks, (2) 6 weeks to approximately 6 months after the operation and (3) 6 to 12 months onward. During the first period, most infections are complications of the surgical procedure: The wound and the urinary tract are the commonest sites, and *S. aureus* and *E. coli* (and other common coliforms) are the most frequent isolates. During the second period, classic opportunist pathogens predominate: During this stage, the risk of tuberculosis, listeriosis, nontyphoid *Salmonella* (Dhar *et al.*, 1991), cryptococcal and other fungal infections and *Pneumocystis* pneumonia is highest. Primary or reactivated CMV infection also can occur. Finally, as the

intensity of immunosuppression is reduced at 6 months or more after transplant, common community-acquired infections occur (e.g., pneumococcal pneumonia or influenza).

Evaluation of the febrile patient includes a careful clinical examination and an assessment of the likelihood of noninfective causes (e.g., graft rejection, hematomas and pulmonary or peripheral venous thromboses). Appropriate investigations may be needed to confirm or refute these possibilities (see Chapters 14 and 28). Measurement of serum levels of procalcitonin has shown some promise in distinguishing between infective and noninfective conditions in the early posttransplant period (Eberhard *et al.*, 1998). If infection seems likely, the clinical and epidemiological features just noted usually help in narrowing the differential diagnosis and directing further investigation. It is helpful at this stage to form a judgment about the speed of progression of the illness; this can be useful in diagnosis and treatment. For instance, a patient 6 months posttransplant who has a 3- to 4-week history of mild fever and focal, perhaps cavitating, abnormalities on a chest radiograph is most likely to have tuberculosis or nocardiosis. There is no immediate need to begin therapy; a diagnostic bronchoscopy can be arranged and the laboratory told to look for unusual pathogens. In contrast, a patient known to have azathioprine-induced leukopenia who has an abrupt onset of high fever and diffuse patchy infiltrates 3 weeks after a transplant requires urgent treatment. In this setting, untreated gram-negative pneumonia can lead to overwhelming sepsis in a matter of hours, and empirical antibiotic therapy must begin at once.

In the febrile renal transplant patient, clinical examination and one or two simple investigations generally point to the likely site of infection, if not its cause. Management of infections at various sites is discussed in the next section. The clinical features of a patient in septic shock are not helpful in predicting the likely cause; for example, septicemia resulting from *S. aureus* or *Candida* can be indistinguishable from the classic septic shock caused by gram-negative bacteria. More helpful in deciding on an empirical regimen is a knowledge of the commonest blood culture isolates and their sensitivity patterns in a given unit. The organisms isolated most frequently are *S. aureus* and coliforms such as *E. coli*, *Klebsiella* and *Pseudomonas aeruginosa*. In neutropenic patients

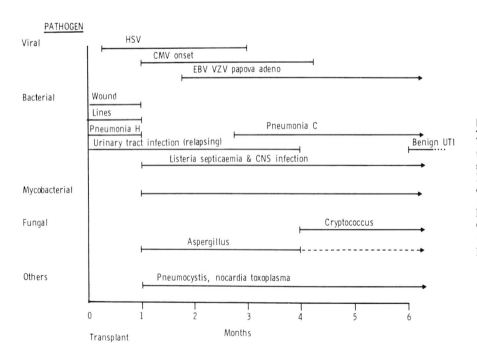

FIGURE 31–1

Timetable for the occurrence of infection in the renal transplant patient. HSV = herpes simplex virus; CMV = cytomegalovirus; EBV = Epstein-Barr virus; VZV = varicella-zoster virus; adeno = adenovirus; UTI = urinary tract infection; Pneumonia H = hospital-acquired pneumonia; Pneumonia C = community-acquired pneumonia; CNS = central nervous system. (Modified with permission from Rubin *et al.*, 1981.)

in particular, these gram-negative organisms are the most immediate threat to life, and a conventional empirical regimen is a combination of an acylureidopenicillin (such as piperacillin) and an aminoglycoside. Because of the importance of *S. aureus*, flucloxacillin should be added to this regimen. In nonneutropenic patients, flucloxacillin plus an aminoglycoside suffice. Cephalosporins are attractive because they avoid the potential nephrotoxicity of aminoglycosides and provide excellent cover against coliform infection, but some lack activity against *S. aureus*. Alternative regimens include the combination of ceftazidime and vancomycin in neutropenic patients or imipenem for nonneutropenic patients.

INTRAVASCULAR AND INTRAVENOUS LINE–ASSOCIATED INFECTIONS

Infection secondary to indwelling intravenous catheters is a common cause of fever in the early posttransplant period. The causative organisms usually are staphylococci (coagulase-negative staphylococcus and *S. aureus*), but enteric gram-negative rods and *Candida* sometimes are obtained and should never be ignored, even if the patient seems clinically well. In most hospitals, most coagulase-negative staphylococci are methicillin resistant, leaving little alternative to the use of vancomycin. *S. aureus* infections should be treated with flucloxacillin (nafcillin), unless they are shown to be methicillin resistant. The intravenous line should be removed unless there is a strong contraindication; it always should be removed in the case of *Candida* infections. Endocarditis is not a particularly common complication of renal transplantation, but when it does occur the organisms are more likely to be *S. aureus* or fungi, especially *Aspergillus* (Paterson *et al.*, 1998).

PULMONARY INFECTION

Renal transplant patients suffer not only from respiratory infections that are common to normal persons and general hospital patients but also from opportunistic infections because of their defective cellular immunity. Pneumonia is a particularly important cause of illness and death in the renal transplant group. Because of the excellent outlook for transplantation itself, considerable effort at expert diagnosis and management of complicating respiratory infections is mandatory (Fishman and Rubin, 1998).

The known opportunistic organisms include fungi (such as *P. carinii*, *Aspergillus fumigatus* and locally endemic types such as coccidioidomycosis and histoplasmosis), bacteria (*Mycobacterium*, *Nocardia*, *Legionella* and *Pseudomonas*), herpesviruses (especially CMV), protozoans (such as toxoplasmosis) and helminths (particularly *Strongyloides*). Table 31–2 is a practical rather than an exhaustive list of diagnostic possibilities.

P. carinii has been a leading cause of potentially fatal pneumonia in many immunocompromised groups. Before chemoprophylaxis programs, the annual attack rate of *Pneumocystis* in renal transplant recipients approached 20%. Opportunistic *Pneumocystis* pneumonia is probably acquired as a fresh infection from an unidentified environmental source (Hopkin, 1991). *Pneumocystis* produces a characteristically diffuse pneumonia with breathlessness, hypoxia, fever and diffuse radiographic changes. Rapid diagnosis is essential because untreated it is uniformly fatal but shows an 80% response rate to prompt treatment. Because of its high attack rate in the renal transplant group, chemoprophylaxis against this infection has become an integral part of management schedules.

TABLE 31–2
PULMONARY INFILTRATES IN THE RENAL TRANSPLANT PATIENT

Infection	Others
Bacteria	Pulmonary embolism
Pneumococcus	Cardiovascular
Staphylococcus	pulmonary edema
Gram-negative bacteria	Pulmonary vasculitis
Legionella	Drug pneumonitis
Nocardia	Tumor
Mycobacteria	
Fungi	
Pneumocystis	
Aspergillus	
Candida	
Mucor	
Cryptococcus	
Viruses	
Herpesviruses (especially cytomegalovirus)	
Parasitic	
Strongyloides	
Toxoplasma	

A. fumigatus is a hyphal saprophytic fungus in which infection is by inhalation of spores, and the lungs are the site of primary infection, although important complications such as hematogenous spread to the brain can ensue. *Aspergillus* can behave as a saprophyte in previously damaged lungs in persons with normal systemic immunity—as in allergic bronchopulmonary aspergillosis in asthmatics and mycetoma in old tuberculous cavities. In the immunocompromised, *Aspergillus* manifests as invasive aspergillosis producing pneumonia with the risk of hematogenous spread.

Nocardia asteroides is a gram-positive filamentous branching bacterium that normally is a soil saprophyte and is acquired by inhalation. Resulting disease is commoner in the immunosuppressed, including renal transplant recipients (Arduino *et al.*, 1993). The lung is the site of primary infection, where cavitating nodular shadows are most typical, but dissemination can occur to the brain and often is fatal.

Mycobacterium tuberculosis is not properly an opportunist, but its control depends heavily on effective T-cell immunity. Renal transplant patients with no clinical or radiological suggestion of tuberculous disease at the time of transplantation, but in whom previous infection is likely because of the high endemicity of tuberculosis in their country of origin (e.g., the Indian subcontinent) suffer remarkably high rates of reactivation of tuberculosis during posttransplantation immunosuppression. Of this group, 25% can develop overt tuberculosis in the first 6 months after transplantation. Pulmonary disease is commonest. Nodal, soft tissue and hectic or subacute miliary illness may occur (Higgins *et al.*, 1991), and diagnosis requires expert histology or microbiology on direct tissue samples (Yu *et al.*, 1986).

Herpes and CMV infections are discussed in detail elsewhere. Influenza and respiratory syncytial virus infections cause even more disease than is usual in the renal transplant group—with resultant pneumonias with or without secondary infection by *Pneumococcus* or *Staphylococcus*.

S. stercoralis is a helminth with a unique autoinfection life cycle. Dormant infection, often acquired many years previously, can progress dramatically during immunosuppression to produce a bronchus-obstructing and cavitating, hemorrhagic pneumonia, which can be accompanied by an enterocolitis (Morgan *et al.*, 1986).

Clinical Picture

Transplant recipients suffer simple episodes of acute bronchitis, common to everyone. The symptom of cough usually with purulent sputum may follow a simple viral rhinitis. There usually is little constitutional disturbance and few clinical and no radiographic signs in the chest; recovery may be spontaneous or follow a course of simple oral antibiotic.

More problematic is the patient with fever and radiographic pulmonary shadowing—in whom there is threat to life and the differential diagnosis is broad and includes noninfectious disease (see Table 31–2). Some general points may help in suggesting a specific diagnosis. A timetable for different infections can be constructed based on the timing of the infection after transplantation (see Fig. 31–1). Opportunistic infection is commonest during the nadir of immunosuppression between 1 and 6 months posttransplantation. Before and after this time, especially when there is good renal function accompanied by low-dose immunosuppression, infections typical of the general population, such as bacterial pneumonias, are commoner. Lymphoma, presenting in the lung, can be a rare late complication. Geographical factors may be relevant. Infection with or reactivation of endemic fungal disease, such as coccidioidomycosis or histoplasmosis, occurs in the Americas. Disseminated strongyloidiasis is seen in patients from many tropical areas but especially the West Indies and Far East (Morgan et al., 1986). Neutropenia means that infection with bacterial and fungal organisms is a special risk.

Careful clinical review is of diagnostic value. High fever suggests infection, and clinical features of chills and shivers weigh against noninfectious diagnoses, such as cardiovascular pulmonary edema, pulmonary embolism and alveolar hemorrhage. Pleurisy with pleural pain and pleural rub is not a feature of Pneumocystis pneumonia; cardiovascular pulmonary edema and alveolar hemorrhage are not features of this pneumonia. Pulmonary edema of cardiovascular origin may be suggested by marked orthopnea, the presence of gallop rhythm, elevated jugular venous pulse, peripheral edema, evidence of fluid retention from daily weighing and chart records and a chest radiograph showing a large heart and dilated pulmonary veins or septa. Such features usually establish a diagnosis of pulmonary edema, but difficulties often can be resolved by computed tomography (CT) scan or wedge pressure measurements. Hemoptysis not only may be part of an infective syndrome but also must raise the possibility of pulmonary embolism and pulmonary hemorrhage, the latter particularly on a background of glomerulonephritis or

of a falling hemoglobin level. In Pneumocystis pneumonia, fever and breathlessness often precede decisive radiographic change, which eventually is typically diffuse and bilateral; absence of physical signs in the chest is usual. Cytomegalovirus also causes a diffuse pneumonitis, which is a source of diagnostic confusion with Pneumocystis. Ill patients, with impaired consciousness, may suffer aspirational pulmonary syndromes—an acid pneumonitis or anaerobic infection. In general, the pace of the illness and character of the radiological change may provide important clues (Table 31–3).

Approach to Investigation and Management

Thorough clinical assessment, including a chest radiograph, is needed for all episodes of apparent respiratory infection in the renal transplant group. The scale of further investigation and management depends on the findings from this initial review.

A. Episodes of bronchitis with purulent sputum but no clinical and radiographic evidence of consolidation, after sputum has been obtained for microscopy and culture, should be treated with a simple oral antibiotic against Streptococcus pneumoniae and Haemophilus influenzae, such as amoxicillin and clavulanic acid, a second-generation cephalosporin or macrolide (the interaction of macrolide with cyclosporine should be remembered; see Chapter 16).

B. The patient with fever and radiographic changes requires more searching review and careful management. Computed tomography scan of the lung often refines the morphology of the pulmonary lesion; it provides (a) useful diagnostic clues and (b) a valuable guide to the best technique for invasive pulmomary samplings if needed.
  1. A febrile illness of abrupt onset (course <48 hours) with dominantly local or lobar shadowing on chest radiograph and CT scan strongly suggests bacterial pneumonia. With the likelihood of such aggressive and rapidly multiplying organisms, it is appropriate to start intravenous antibiotic treatment promptly after taking simple samples (blood, natural or hypertonic saline aerosol–induced sputum) for expert microbiology. The initial antibiotic regimen should be broad spectrum and cover Pneumococcus, Staphylococcus, Legionella and Pseudomonas. One possible regimen is a combination of cefuroxime, erythromycin and high-dose daily gentamicin.
  2. For other patients in whom the pace of the disease is less acute or the chest radiograph shows more diffuse or scattered change, the differential diagnosis enlarges. A determined investigation to produce a precise microbiological diagnosis produces the best outcome, and CT scan is valuable in planning this.
    (a) Sputum, either natural or induced by aerosolized hypertonic saline (Bigby et al., 1986), should be obtained if possible. Expert assessment of the sputum sample by fluorescent stains for mycobacteria, or DNA amplification (polymerase chain reaction) for Pneumocystis (Wakefield et al., 1991) may obviate the need for invasive samplings.
    (b) If sputum is unavailable or nondiagnostic, invasive sampling is appropriate. Invasive sampling improves diagnostic yield and clinical outcome, through application of precise effective medication.

Alveolar lavage taken by fiberoptic bronchoscopy is appropiate when the CT scan or radiograph shows diffuse or alveolar pattern changes. Some authors favor concurrent trans-

TABLE 31–3

CLINICAL AND RADIOLOGICAL FEATURES OF DIFFERENT INFECTIONS

Pace of the Illness		
Abrupt	⟶	*Insidious*
Bacterial	Pneumocystis carinii	Tuberculosis
	CMV	Nocardia
	Aspergillus	

Pattern of x-ray		
Lobar	*Scattered Nodular/ Segmental*	*Diffuse*
Bacterial	Tuberculosis	CMV
Aspergillus	Nocardia	Pneumocystis

bronchial biopsies per bronchoscope, but this poses increased risk of pneumothorax and hemorrhage, and in our experience lavage alone provides diagnostic yields greater than 75% (Hopkin *et al.*, 1983; Young *et al.*, 1984). A whole array of diagnostic techniques can be applied readily to the liquid sample, including microscopy after histochemical and immunofluorescent stains, solid-phase immunoassays (enzyme-linked immunosorbent assays) for microbial antigens and microbe-specific DNA amplifications (Kalin *et al.*, 1998). (Fig. 31–2 illustrates some typical findings in *Pneumocystis* and *Aspergillus*.)

Transthoracic or percutaneous fine-needle aspiration of pulmonary material is more appropriate when CT scan shows localized, nodular lesions (with or without cavitation, although diagnostic yields appear higher when cavitation is present) (Fishman and Rubin, 1998). Guidance of the needle by CT scan is optimal, and the same microbiological procedures can be applied to the sample as to the alveolar lavage, although less material is available. The use of modern 22- or 23-gauge needles minimizes risk of pneumothorax or bleeding; pneumothorax problems may be minimized by placing the patient with the sampled lung dependent for 1 hour postprocedure (Moore *et al.*, 1990).

Formal lung biopsy is appropriate when a patient with pneumonitis is declining, and there is still not a secure diagno-

sis. Open-lung biopsy is diagnostically effective but traumatic and usually demands postprocedure automatic ventilation. Thoracoscopic lung biopsy, if available, offers a less invasive procedure that is appropriate for diffuse or peripheral lung lesions (Ferguson and Landreneau, 1988).

Treatment in this group of patients should be dictated by the diagnostic findings. *P. carinii* is treated with co-trimoxazole intravenously or orally in a dosage of 15 or 20 mg/kg/d of trimethoprim and 75 or 100 mg/kg/d of sulfamethoxazole divided into two to four doses. If severe renal failure is present, the dosages are dictated by measuring free sulfa levels, aiming for values between 100 and 150 μg/ml, or trimethoprim levels, aiming for values between 3 and 5 μg/ml. In moderate renal impairment (creatinine clearance 15–30 ml/min), a standard dosage generally can be used for 3 days followed by a 50% dosage, but plasma levels should be tested. In all cases, treatment should continue for 2 weeks, and it seems rational to maintain the patient on chemoprophylaxis with co-trimoxazole, 480 mg twice daily by mouth (Higgins *et al.*, 1988), until the dosages of immunosuppressives have been reduced in the longer term. Response to treatment is good (>80%) when the diagnosis is made early, but some patients need temporary cessation or reduction of immunosuppressives to allow recovery from *Pneumocystis* pneumonia. Hypersensitivity to co-trimoxazole with rash or

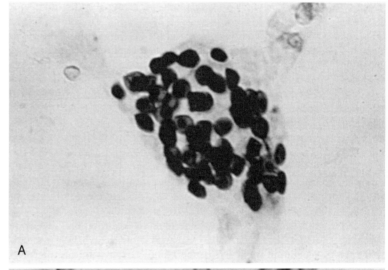

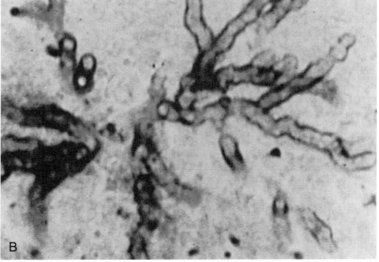

FIGURE 31–2

Typical alveolar lavage findings in pneumonias caused by *Pneumocystis carinii* (A) and *Aspergillus fumigatus* (B). (Grocott's stain; × 1,500.)

fever is the clearest indication for a change of treatment (e.g., pentamidine, 4 mg/kg/d by intravenous infusion over 1 hour) (Haverkos, 1984). Chemoprophylaxis with pentamidine can be administered effectively as an inhaled preparation, 300 mg monthly (Armstrong and Bernard, 1991), from a suitable nebulizer device (Respigard II, Mark West, Englewood, Colorado).

Aspergillus pneumonia demands prompt and vigorous treatment with amphotericin (Denning and Stevens, 1990). Liposomal formulations of amphotericin are considerably less nephrotoxic and probably of comparable efficacy, although they have not been formally evaluated in this setting. *Nocardia* is treated best with a sulfonamide such as sulfadiazine. Four to six divided doses of sulfadiazine daily may be needed as well as monitoring of serum levels (target, 100–150 µg/ml); treatment may need to be prolonged for many weeks after clinical resolution to prevent relapse.

The treatment of tuberculosis can be complicated by the influence of renal function on antituberculous drug excretion (e.g., ethambutol) and by the influence of rifampicin on the metabolism of other drugs (e.g., cyclosporine; see Chapter 16). In the treatment of established disease, the use of rifampicin, isoniazid and pyrazinamide in combination (none of whose levels are influenced seriously by impaired renal function) offers an appropriate regimen. After 2 months of triple chemotherapy, rifampicin and isoniazid can be continued for 4 more months. Easing of immunosuppressive regimens may be needed to ensure recovery.

Respiratory failure (arterial oxygen tension <8 kPa or 60 mmHg) is treated with simple oxygen supplementation (30–40%). Exhaustion or worsening blood gases frequently leads to the need for ventilation. Some patients with acute syndromes may be intubated and ventilated before diagnostic bronchoscopy is undertaken. Many patients recover despite the need for temporary ventilation.

URINARY TRACT INFECTIONS

Urinary tract infections are extremely common during the first 3 months after transplantation, occurring in 50% or more of patients (Prat *et al.*, 1985). Urinary tract infections are important because they are the most frequent source of bacteremia during this period (Peterson *et al.*, 1982). Studies on the pathogenesis and management of urinary tract infections have produced conflicting results: What seems clear is that asymptomatic bacteriuria is commoner than is clinical evidence of infection and that late infections (beyond 3–4 months) are almost invariably benign (Cuvelier *et al.*, 1985). Although urinary tract infections do not usually cause deterioration in renal function, it has been suggested that *Streptococcus faecalis* infection may act as a trigger for rejection (Byrd *et al.*, 1978).

Weeden and colleagues reported six cases of schistosomiasis in renal transplant recipients, three of whom developed urological problems caused by the infection (Weeden *et al.*, 1982). In two cases, the infection was in the transplanted ureter. These investigators recommended screening of recipients and donors from endemic areas for schistosomiasis (by cystoscopy and urine examination). Histological examination of donor ureter and recipient bladder taken at the time of surgery was the most helpful investigation in establishing the diagnosis (see Chapter 38).

WOUND INFECTION

Wound infections occur with a frequency of 1 to 10% and are almost entirely a reflection of the technical skill of the surgeon (Stephan *et al.*, 1997). The three most important sources of infection are wound hematomas secondary to inadequate hemostasis, urinary leaks and development of lymphoceles; detailed surgical aspects of this subject are discussed in Chapters 28 and 29.

Suspected wound infection should be sought actively; we have found ultrasonography and CT scanning helpful but scans using labeled white blood cells less so. Sometimes the diagnosis can be confirmed by fine-needle aspiration under radiological control, but more often formal surgical exploration is required. The usual infecting organisms are coliform bacteria (possibly carried over with the donor organ) and *S. aureus*; anaerobes are less common. Sensitivity testing dictates the correct choice of antibiotic, but as is usual in such situations, adequate drainage is more important.

CENTRAL NERVOUS SYSTEM INFECTIONS

Central nervous system infections (see Chapter 33) in renal transplant recipients occur predictably between 1 and 12 months posttransplant and are characterized by a subacute onset and the frequent lack of systemic signs. The development of fever and mild headache should be sufficient to alert the clinician to the possibility of central nervous system infection; frank meningism or focal neurological abnormalities generally are absent or develop only as a late sign. Whenever possible, a CT scan should be done as a matter of urgency and, provided that there is no contraindication, followed by a lumbar puncture. It is essential to inform the laboratory that the specimen comes from an immunosuppressed patient so that the appropriate tests can be carried out. Blood cultures should be taken in all cases of suspected central nervous system infection. In a study of 300 renal transplant recipients covering a 10-year period, 20 patients (7%) developed central nervous system infection, and of these, 9 died as a direct result (Hooper *et al.*, 1982). The list of causative organisms is short (Table 31–4).

Listeria monocytogenes

Listeria monocytogenes (Mylonakis *et al.*, 1998) may present as meningitis, brain abscess or meningoencephalitis. The cerebrospinal fluid findings may not be striking, reflecting the poor inflammatory response. In particular, the cell count may be raised only modestly, and neutrophils may predominate (despite the organism's name). Bacteria may be sparse, and the Gram-stained film must be examined carefully and specifically. Full identification of the cultures may take 48 to 72 hours. Serology is unhelpful.

The treatment for listeriosis is ampicillin, 200 mg kg^{-1} d^{-1} for 14 days; gentamicin usually is added because the drugs are synergistic *in vitro* against this organism. Clinical response to therapy can be expected in about 72 hours. Defervescence follows some days later, but the cerebrospinal fluid may remain abnormal for 1 month. In a renal transplant patient with clinical and cerebrospinal fluid findings of me-

TABLE 31–4

ORGANISMS ASSOCIATED WITH CENTRAL NERVOUS SYSTEM INFECTION IN RENAL TRANSPLANT RECIPIENTS*

Listeria	Aspergillus
Cryptococcus	Mucor
Mycobacterium	Toxoplasma
Nocardia	Strongyloides

*Placed approximately in descending order of frequency. The first three listed are the most important.

ningoencephalitis in whom cryptococcosis has been excluded (see next section) and in whom tuberculosis seems unlikely, it is reasonable to make a presumptive diagnosis of *Listeria* infection and begin empirical treatment.

Nocardiosis and Tuberculosis

Nocardiosis and tuberculosis occur most commonly as a pneumonia (see earlier) but on occasion cause isolated infections of the central nervous system. Nocardiosis (Lerner, 1996) generally presents as a cerebral abscess that is unifocal but often multilocular. There are no other distinguishing features, and the diagnosis must be confirmed by aspiration, microscopy and culture. Initial treatment is identical to that for pulmonary nocardiosis with sulfisoxazole (a loading dose of 4 g followed by 6–12 g/d in four divided doses) or co-trimoxazole (2 double-strength tablets every 8 hours or the equivalent dose intravenously). These doses need to be modified in patients with impaired renal function; drug levels of the sulfonamide should not exceed 150 μg/ml 2 hours after the dose. Although no firm data support the use of combination therapy with other antimicrobials, sensitivity testing of the isolate should be done because not all strains are reliably susceptible to all antibiotics, and problems with hypersensitivity or intolerance to first-line agents can necessitate changing the therapy. Some clinicians believe that craniotomy and drainage of the cerebral abscess is mandatory, but in our experience and that of others (Sabeel *et al.*, 1998), medical treatment alone may be effective.

The presentation of tuberculous meningitis in renal transplant patients is not different from that in the noncompromised host. Although the cerebrospinal fluid is abnormal, acid-fast bacilli are seen only in about 10 to 15% of cases subsequently proved by culture. A polymerase chain reaction assay for *M. tuberculosis* now is available fairly widely and gives a rapid answer in smear-negative cases. If the polymerase chain reaction is not available or is ambiguous, it is better to err on the side of caution and begin empirical therapy. It is usual to give adjunctive corticosteroids to patients with tuberculous meningitis (Dooley *et al.*, 1997); there are no data to suggest that renal transplant recipients already receiving corticosteroids would benefit from increasing the dose.

Cryptococcus neoformans

Cryptococcus neoformans is an encapsulated yeast that has a particular predisposition for patients with impaired cellular immunity. Although the primary route of infection is probably through the respiratory tract, the commonest clinical presentation is meningitis, with or without fungemia. Other sites that may be involved include the skin, lungs and joints or bones.

The meningitis is typically subacute in onset, heralded only by mild headache or photophobia. The cerebrospinal fluid examination reveals a modest elevation in total protein and hypoglycorrhachia; the more pronounced drop in cerebrospinal fluid glucose seen in tuberculous meningitis can be a helpful pointer. Cryptococcosis is accompanied by a cerebrospinal fluid lymphocytosis of about 0.5×10^9 L^{-1}. Cryptococci can be cultured without difficulty from cerebrospinal fluid or blood and generally are recognizable after 48 hours. Cryptococcal meningitis can be diagnosed much more rapidly by direct examination of the cerebrospinal fluid. Microscopy of fluid mixed with a drop of India ink (to act as a negative stain) reveals typical budding encapsulated yeasts in about 60% of cases. However, the diagnostic procedure of choice is the latex agglutination test for cryptococcal polysac-

charide antigen, which has a sensitivity and specificity exceeding 90%.

Treatment of cryptococcal meningitis is with intravenous amphotericin B and flucytosine, initially for 6 weeks (Bennett *et al.*, 1979). Fluconazole at a dose of 400 mg/d is likely to be equally effective but has not been tested formally in this setting. Lumbar puncture should be repeated at least once during treatment, at the end of treatment and again at 4-monthly intervals for 1 year even if the patient is asymptomatic because the relapse rate is high.

Aspergillosis, Mucormycosis and Other Mold Infections

Aspergillosis of the central nervous system generally occurs as part of a widely disseminated infection originating in the lungs. It may present as a rhinosinusitis, cerebritis or abscess, which can be single or multiple. The prognosis is poor: The mortality is greater than 75% even in patients who receive at least 14 days of amphotericin B (Denning, 1996). There are occasional reports of benefit when isolated abscesses are removed surgically.

Rhinocerebral mucormycosis (Morduchowicz *et al.*, 1986) is an uncommon mold infection that presents as fever, facial swelling, proptosis and cranial nerve lesions; it may be complicated by cerebral abscess. It is particularly common in patients with diabetic ketoacidosis and has been recognized in hemodialysis patients receiving desferrioxamine (Windus *et al.*, 1987). The treatment is amphotericin B, often with surgical débridement. There is a high mortality rate.

Dematiaceous (pigmented) molds are being recognized increasingly as causes of skin and soft tissue infections and intracranial infections in immunocompromised patients (Singh *et al.*, 1997). They seem to be more indolent than other mold infections, and medical therapy alone may be curative (Salama *et al.*, 1997).

Toxoplasmosis

Toxoplasma gondii (McCabe and Remington, 1983) is an obligate intracellular protozoal parasite that is ubiquitous in nature and causes infection in a large proportion of the world's population. The clinical picture differs according to the host range: In immunosuppressed patients, disseminated toxoplasmosis causes a syndrome similar to that due to CMV. Fever begins generally 1 to 12 months posttransplant and is associated with progressive malaise and evidence of organ involvement, in particular the lungs (Renoult *et al.*, 1997). The central nervous system involvement is well described in patients with acquired immunodeficiency syndrome (AIDS) but is uncommon in renal transplant recipients; the picture may be one of meningoencephalitis or a space-occupying lesion.

Microbiological confirmation of the diagnosis can be difficult in immunocompromised patients. The *Toxoplasma* dye test is a sensitive and specific test for acute infection but is not widely available. The presence of IgG antibodies indicates past exposure but not acute infection; immunocompromised patients may not have an IgM response. Isolation of the organisms from blood or body fluids is feasible but seldom is done in routine laboratories. The diagnosis also can be established by demonstration of tachyzoites in histological specimens and by polymerase chain reaction from biopsy samples; the presence of cysts alone is not evidence of active infection. Renal transplant recipients who have serological evidence of exposure to *Toxoplasma* and a clinical picture consistent with acute toxoplasmosis should be treated empirically. Toxoplasmosis responds well to treatment with pyrimethamine (100 mg loading dose followed by 50 mg daily plus folinic acid to protect the bone marrow) and sulfadiazine, 120 mg kg^{-1} d^{-1} in four divided doses. This regimen is continued for at least 4 weeks.

INFECTION OF THE GASTROINTESTINAL TRACT

Bacterial Infection

Classic enteric pathogens are uncommon in renal transplant recipients, although nontyphoid *Salmonella* infection can be unusually severe. Bacteremia is common, and relapses can occur many years after the transplant (Dhar *et al.*, 1991; Ejlersten and Aunsholt, 1989). Treatment must be guided by antibiotic susceptibility tests, but ciprofloxacin frequently is suitable and effective.

C. difficile is the cause of pseudomembranous colitis and antibiotic associated diarrhea. The fecal carriage rate of the organism is 2 to 5% in the general adult population, but it probably should not be considered part of the normal adult gastrointestinal flora. In long-term hospitalized patients, a colonization rate of 21% has been reported (Johnson *et al.*, 1990), but of those, only 15% developed diarrhea. Sporadic cases and outbreaks have affected renal transplant and dialysis units (Ritchie *et al.*, 1982). The severity of infection varies from asymptomatic carriage to a fatal colitis. In a 3-month prevalence study, *C. difficile* was isolated or its toxin detected in 26 of 72 patients in the Oxford Dialysis Unit and Transplant Unit (which are adjacent), and the carriage could be correlated with the length of the patient's stay. During this time, 10 patients had *C. difficile*–associated diarrhea, and 3 patients who had pseudomembranous colitis died, although this may not have been the primary cause of death. Cross-infection and antibiotic therapy appeared to be the most important factors in the spread of this organism. *C. difficile* is a particular problem in a dialysis unit that has a large continuous ambulatory peritoneal dialysis practice in which broad-spectrum antibiotic drugs are used frequently in patients admitted with peritonitis.

Treatment is with a 5-day course of metronidazole, 400 mg every 8 hours, or oral vancomycin, 125 mg every 6 hours. Relapse rates after either therapy have been reported as 15 to 50%. By typing strains employing restriction enzyme analysis of chromosomal DNA, these relapses are shown generally to be reinfections from the environment. Prevention of infection requires the following measures:

1. Use of broad-spectrum antibiotic therapy (especially second-generation and third-generation cephalosporins) should be limited.
2. Patients with diarrhea cause the greatest environmental contamination and must be isolated.
3. Sigmoidoscopes, bedpans, bedding, toilets and similarly contaminated objects should be disinfected adequately, and efficient hand-washing procedures for staff and patients should be followed.

In this context, it is important to remember that clostridia form spores that can survive 5 months in the hospital environment. It is inappropriate for immunosuppressed patients to share facilities with dialysis patients, especially those on continuous ambulatory peritoneal dialysis.

Dyspeptic symptoms are common in dialysis and transplant patients, prompting several investigators to consider the possible role of infection by *Helicobacter pylori*. No evidence has been found to suggest that this infection is commoner or more severe in these patients (Hruby *et al.*, 1997; Yildiz *et al.*, 1999).

Fungi and Parasites

Fungal infection of the upper gastrointestinal tract presents as stomatitis or esophagitis. *Candida albicans* is the commonest cause. *Candida* stomatitis should be treated with fluconazole, 100 to 200 mg daily. A patient with persistent dysphagia or retrosternal pain in association with obvious oral candidiasis can be treated empirically for *Candida* esophagitis, but if this fails or if no oral *Candida* is seen, esophagoscopy should be carried out to exclude herpetic esophagitis because the two may coexist.

Patients who harbor *S. stercoralis* may develop overwhelming hyperinfection after transplantation (Scowden *et al.*, 1978). The usual presentation is with gastrointestinal symptoms that may amount to a clinical picture of subacute obstruction. In some cases, an acute respiratory illness is caused by the migration of the worm through the lungs, although the chest film appearances can be mistaken for pulmonary edema (Weller *et al.*, 1981). Features include fever, polymicrobial gram-negative bacteremia, abdominal pain, vomiting, bloody diarrhea, jaundice and gram-negative meningitis. The diagnosis should be considered in patients coming from endemic areas, such as the West Indies or the Far East, even if residence has not been recent because the host can harbor the nematode for prolonged periods. Larvae sometimes are found in the stool or sputum, and an eosinophilia may be present. Duodenal aspiration is the best way of detecting infestation. Treatment is with ivermectin, 200 μg/kg/d for 2 days, or albendazole, 400 mg twice daily for 3 days. These courses may need to be repeated if the patient has a severe infection.

Cysts of *Cryptosporidium* can be found in the stool of renal transplant recipients (Chieffi *et al.*, 1998), but they probably are incidental and should not be attributed as the cause of diarrhea unless the patient has received unusually long or severe immunosuppression. Visceral leishmaniasis has been described in transplant recipients (Berenguer *et al.*, 1998) and should be considered in patients with the appropriate travel history.

VIRAL INFECTIONS

Viral infections in renal transplant patients may be considered in two groups. The first group are serious infections caused mainly by viruses that are latent or persistent in healthy people but reactivate after transplantation (e.g., herpes group viruses; hepatitis B, C and D and retroviruses). Some of these viruses can be transmitted to the recipient by the donated organ or transfusion of blood products. The second group are infections that are self-limiting, occur sporadically in the community and affect transplant patients in the same way as the general public (e.g., myxoviruses, paramyxoviruses and picornaviruses). In general, the most important factor contributing to posttransplant infection is the degree of immunosuppression. The greater the immunosuppression, the greater the number of infections and their severity.

Knowledge of viral infections that commonly affect transplant recipients and methods of diagnosing them is important for several reasons. A preexisting viral infection (e.g., HIV and hepatitis B carriage) may influence the decision of whether or not a patient should receive an allograft. Tests to assess susceptibility to viral infections and measures to prevent them by prior active immunization or to protect the patient from exposure to those pathogens should be part of the pretransplant workup. These tests on donor and recipient also determine the prophylactic use of antivirals or immunoglobulins in the posttransplant period. Identification of a viral pathogen may modify an aggressive search for the cause of a fever. Antiviral chemotherapy is available for some viral infections; rapid diagnosis permits early treatment.

PERSISTENT VIRAL INFECTIONS

Cytomegalovirus

Cytomegalovirus is the most important viral infection affecting transplant recipients. In Western countries, approximately 50% of patients awaiting transplantation have been infected in the past and have antibodies to CMV. In normal people, CMV infection uncommonly produces symptoms, but the virus subsequently becomes latent in monocytes, macrophages and polymorphonuclear leukocytes and tissues such as renal tubules. Cytomegalovirus infection in renal allograft recipients is more often symptomatic and can be severe or fatal. The infection is primary in a previously seronegative recipient. Secondary infection occurs in previously seropositive patients because of reactivation of the patient's own latent virus or reinfection, but it is not possible to distinguish clinically between these two possibilities.

Primary infections are associated with approximately 60% morbidity. Although secondary infections usually are asymptomatic, if illness occurs, it is more severe in recipients of seropositive kidneys, which suggests that reinfection is more likely to cause disease than is reactivation. The severity of all infections is related directly to the degree of the patient's immunosuppression, and the addition of antilymphocyte serum or OKT3 to these regimens has increased the problem.

Clinical Features

A typical symptomatic CMV infection begins as a spiking or constant fever 4 to 10 weeks after transplantation. Leukopenia, thrombocytopenia and atypical lymphocytes often are present at this time. A rise in serum aspartate aminotransferase levels and development of respiratory symptoms (dyspnea with abnormal blood gases) begin several days after the fever. Less common features are arthralgia, overt hepatitis, splenomegaly, myalgia, abdominal pain with gastrointestinal ulceration and bleeding and encephalitis. Skin vesicles are not a feature of CMV infection. A deterioration in renal function may be observed during this illness. The fever may persist for a month or more. Most patients recover. About 2% progress to develop disseminated fatal disease (Simmons *et al.*, 1977). These fatal cases failed to produce an antibody response to the virus, and at autopsy there were no signs of rejection in the transplanted kidney. The usual cause of death in CMV infection is severe pneumonitis (Fig. 31–3), which sometimes is accompanied by gastrointestinal ulceration and hemorrhage. Frequently, other opportunistic infections supervene.

Retinitis with a permanent reduction in visual acuity in at least half of patients affected is a rare manifestation in transplant recipients (Egbert *et al.*, 1980). It is recognized clinically as a perivascular infiltrate of well-demarcated granular appearance with varying amounts of exudate and hemorrhage. The lesions, caused by vasculitis, spread in a *bush fire* manner—an active advancing edge with a residual area of necrotic retina—and progress from the periphery to involve the macula.

Diagnosis

In the diagnosis of CMV, it is important to distinguish between latency, active infection (as indicated by viremia, a serological response and/or excretion of the virus) and dis-

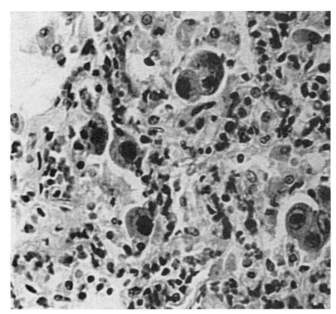

FIGURE 31–3

Histological appearance in a case of cytomegalovirus pneumonitis. Several enlarged cells with intranuclear inclusions are seen.

ease. Clinically significant disease should be confirmed by histological evidence of CMV. Culture of organs involved is important because other viruses (e.g., HSV and adenovirus) also may be isolated.

Early diagnosis of CMV disease is essential because early treatment is crucial. Survival from CMV pneumonitis, once ventilation is necessary, is rare. Cytomegalovirus can be isolated in human fibroblast cell cultures, but because it takes 5 to 28 days to produce a cytopathic effect, delay is inevitable. More rapid methods of detecting CMV are by polymerase chain reaction (Einsele *et al.*, 1991) or direct CMV-antigen detection in peripheral blood leukocytes or fine-needle aspiration biopsy specimens (van der Bij *et al.*, 1988a, 1988b). Both tests detect CMV infection about 1 week before the onset of disease and enable preemptive antiviral therapy (The *et al.*, 1992). Surveillance cultures for CMV in blood or buffy coat have a useful overall predictive value (60%) of disease (Meyers *et al.*, 1990), but the presence of CMV in urine or throat washings is less helpful.

Preemptive antiviral treatment (The *et al.*, 1992) has to be based on laboratory tests that indicate CMV activity. In CMV-seronegative recipients of a seropositive organ, a program of weekly testing for the first 2 to 3 months after transplantation, using the antigenemia assay or a qualitative polymerase chain reaction, has a positive predictive value of about 80% of detecting disease. From patient to patient with CMV disease, the level of CMV viremia varies greatly so that viral load cannot be used as a guide to disease in this group. In CMV-seropositive recipients, there is a much lower prevalence of disease, and qualitative polymerase chain reaction is not useful in predicting it. Higher levels of CMV viremia are associated with disease (Roberts *et al.*, 1998) and peak during it; also, recipients who develop disease have a rapid rise in CMV viral load when compared with recipients without disease. A quantitative CMV viremia measurement, although not useful in predicting disease, may be useful in differential diagnosis. In fatal infections, CMV has been cultured from many sites, including bone marrow, kidney, liver, lung, pancreas, large bowel and brain.

In primary and often in secondary infection, the appearance of CMV-specific IgM detected by IgM enzyme-linked immunoabsorbent antibody capture assay usually occurs within 1 to 6 days of the onset of symptoms. When detected, this is diagnostic. In the absence of CMV-specific IgM, the appearance of CMV-specific IgG in a primary infection or a greater than fourfold rise in titer is sought but may delay diagnosis for 1 to 2 weeks. The persistence of CMV-specific IgM varies from 2 weeks to many months, and its brief appearance may be the only serological marker of a secondary infection because the IgG levels may show no change.

Origin of Infection

Infection by transmission from staff or patients is unlikely. Whole-blood or leukocyte transfusions from CMV-seropositive donors can transmit the virus (Tolkoff-Rubin et al., 1978). The risk is greatest with fresh blood, and stored blood is potentially hazardous, but leukocyte-free blood appears to be safe (Brady et al., 1984). The main source of primary CMV infection is the transplanted kidney (Betts et al., 1975). This source was associated with a 63% incidence of CMV infection in previously uninfected patients at Oxford (Table 31–5). In secondary infection, the source may be the transplanted kidney or reactivation of the recipient's own virus. Restriction endonuclease analysis has been used to determine which source was responsible for infection in renal allograft recipients (Chou, 1986).

Relationship Between Cytomegalovirus, Immunosuppression and Rejection

The immunological interaction of the recipient with the transplanted kidney and the immunosuppressive therapy necessary to permit survival of the graft can activate latent CMV. With a potent regimen of high-dose steroids, azathioprine and antilymphocyte globulin, Fryd and coworkers reported a 29% incidence of overt CMV infection with a significant reduction in 1-year graft survival compared with patients who did not have clinically apparent CMV (53% vs. 79%) (Fryd et al., 1980). In contrast, the incidence of overt CMV was only 14% when low-dose steroid and azathioprine immunosuppression was given (Morris et al., 1982). Therapy for rejection episodes increases the risk of serious CMV disease. Because CMV has an immunosuppressive and an immunostimulatory effect, its precise effect on the allograft is difficult to determine. Cytomegalovirus infection may influence the graft in many ways:

1. Fatal disseminated CMV infection occurs in approximately 1 to 2% of renal transplant patients; these patients have severe depression of humoral-mediated and cell-mediated immunity, and at postmortem there are no signs of rejection in the graft.

2. In milder infections, humoral responses are normal. Similar to other febrile illnesses, the fever accompanying overt CMV may impair renal function temporarily. The role of CMV, independent of other factors, in the cause and evolution of acute and chronic renal rejection is not settled (Grattan et al., 1989; Pouteil-Noble et al., 1991a; Waltzer et al., 1987). Patients with primary CMV have significantly more rejection episodes (Ackermann et al., 1988), but in some cases this could be explained partially by the need to reduce immunosuppression to overcome the CMV infection.

3. An association between CMV viremia and glomerulopathy causing a transient rise in serum creatinine level has been reported (Richardson et al., 1981). The deterioration in renal function occurred just before detectable antibody appeared in the circulation and suggested immune complex–mediated damage to the glomerular capillaries. No tubular, vascular or interstitial signs of rejection were seen in biopsy samples of such kidneys. Herrera and colleagues subsequently cast doubt on the entity of CMV glomerulopathy and suggested that such histology represented a form of acute vascular rejection (Herrera et al., 1986).

4. Cytomegalovirus infection leads to increased expression of cell surface antigens, major histocompatibility complex (MHC) class II antigens on CD8 cells (van Es et al., 1984) and MHC class I and class II antigens on kidney cells (von Willebrand et al., 1986). The last-mentioned study suggests that the increase of MHC antigens on kidney cells could lead to rejection. In renal allograft rejection, plasma tumor necrosis factor and intercellular adhesion molecule-1 levels are elevated significantly 2 to 3 days before a clinical rejection episode (Kutukculer et al., 1995). Intercellular adhesion molecule-1 expression on vascular endothelium and tubular epithelial cells also is increased by rat CMV in a rat kidney allograft model (Yilmaz et al., 1996). These studies suggest a relationship between CMV infection, increased cytokine production, and rejection episodes. With preemptive treatment of CMV infections using a 14-day course of ganciclovir, Akposso et al. (1997) found 5-year graft and patient survival to be the same as that in uninfected transplant recipients. Limiting CMV infection might be beneficial (Akposso et al., 1997).

5. Cytomegalovirus affects immune reactions. An immunosuppressive effect, part of which is caused by reduced production of interleukin-1 (Kapasi and Rice, 1988), has been observed, and there is an inversion of the helper/suppressor (CD4/CD8) T-lymphocyte ratio. This situation increases the risk of other opportunistic infections, especially fungal (Grattan et al., 1989), supervening to the detriment of the patient.

Management

Because secondary CMV infections usually are mild and self-limiting, most do not require specific treatment, whereas primary infection does. If severe leukopenia or thrombocyto-

TABLE 31–5

EFFECT OF DONOR CYTOMEGALOVIRUS STATUS ON CYTOMEGALOVIRUS INFECTION IN 306 RENAL ALLOGRAFT RECIPIENTS AT OXFORD

| | Recipient CMV Seropositive | | Recipient CMV Seronegative | |
	Donor CMV+	Donor CMV−	Donor CMV+	Donor CMV−
Group total	84	98	60	64
No. infected	52 (62%)	52 (53%)	38 (63%)	0
	Reactivation or reinfection		Primary infection	

CMV = cytomegalovirus.

penia develops, immunosuppressive therapy may have to be reduced temporarily, despite possible hazards to the transplanted kidney. Bacterial, fungal and protozoal infections may develop, and careful clinical and laboratory monitoring of patients with overt CMV must be continued. Rejection episodes during CMV infection should not be treated with antilymphocyte globulin.

Ganciclovir, a guanine analogue that is phosphorylated by cellular enzymes to the active triphosphate form, inhibits replication of all human herpesvirus, including CMV, *in vitro* (Matthews and Boehme, 1988). Ganciclovir is phosphorylated about 10-fold more in virus-infected cells than in noninfected cells, but notwithstanding this degree of selectivity, dose-related toxicity affects the bone marrow causing neutropenia, thrombocytopenia and less often anemia. These effects are reversible on stopping the drug. In experimental animals, irreversible sterility has followed administration of the drug. Ganciclovir is excreted by the kidney, and ganciclovir-induced psychosis, especially in patients with renal insufficiency, has been reported (Combarnous *et al.*, 1994). The standard dose must be modified in patients with significant renal impairment.

Ganciclovir has been used with some success in life-threatening CMV infections (Collaborative DHPG Treatment Study Group, 1986; Snydman, 1988). There is a marked reduction of virus excretion during treatment. Clinical improvement, especially of extrapulmonary CMV disease, usually is noted (Jacobson and Mills, 1988). Response in CMV pneumonia is poorer, but survival rates of 60% have been reported in patients whose treatment started before mechanical ventilation was necessary (Reed, 1991), which is clear evidence that early antiviral treatment is essential if it is to succeed. Goodrich and associates found that early preemptive treatment with ganciclovir, started if CMV was detected, reduced dramatically the development of CMV disease in bone marrow allograft recipients (Goodrich *et al.*, 1991). These investigators advocated long-term treatment—100 days after transplantation—of patients if and when a positive surveillance culture was found. Early relapses occur in 20 to 30% of patients after treatment is stopped. Intravenous ganciclovir should be used in treating serious CMV disease, in addition to reducing immunosuppressive therapy. Although CMV resistance to ganciclovir has been reported (Erice *et al.*, 1989), it is unlikely to arise in the context of renal transplantation.

An alternative drug, foscarnet, which is active against all the herpes group viruses including CMV, may be used in these infections. This antiviral drug is a noncompetitive inhibitor of herpesvirus DNA polymerase. It is nephrotoxic, causing a reversible nephropathy manifested by a rise in serum creatinine level and renal wasting of calcium and magnesium (Deray *et al.*, 1989), and should be used with extreme caution if renal failure is present. Penile ulceration is another complication (van der Pijl *et al.*, 1990).

Prevention of Infection and Disease

Primary CMV infection in seronegative recipients can be avoided if the transfused blood and especially the transplanted kidney come from seronegative donors. Live attenuated CMV vaccine has been administered to immunize seronegative recipients in the pretransplant period. In one series (Marker *et al.*, 1981), 83% of subjects vaccinated underwent seroconversion, after which no reactivation of the vaccine virus strain has been recorded. Vaccination failed to prevent infection resulting from the CMV strain introduced with the transplanted kidney. The rationale for vaccination rests on the lower incidence of severe CMV disease in secondary, compared with primary, infection (Smiley *et al.*, 1985). In a

controlled trial (Plotkin *et al.*, 1991), this finding has been confirmed. The protection given by the vaccine against disease of at least moderate severity is 85%. Despite these early encouraging findings, currently there is no licensed CMV vaccine and there is no immediate prospect that a vaccine will become available.

Reports from many centers agree that symptomatic infection is considerably less common in secondary CMV than after primary exposure. Nevertheless, the morbidity associated with reinfection or reactivation in the severely immunosuppressed patient is considerable, especially when antilymphocyte globulin has been given. Because morbidity is reduced greatly with more moderate immunosuppression, it is important to choose the least aggressive immunosuppression regimen that does not compromise graft function and survival.

Passive immunization with high-titered CMV plasma or immune globulin or normal intravenous immune globulin has led to a significant reduction in symptomatic disease and interstitial pneumonitis in bone marrow transplant recipients, although the incidence of infection was not altered (Winston *et al.*, 1987). Similarly, high-titered CMV immune globulin given over the first 4 months after transplantation reduced CMV-related illness in CMV-seronegative recipients of organs from CMV-seropositive donors to 21% compared with 60% in the control group (Snydman *et al.*, 1987, 1991).

Antiviral drugs have been recommended for prophylaxis. Although acyclovir is ineffective in treating CMV disease, Balfour and coworkers found that high-dose acyclovir given daily (800–3,200 mg depending on renal function) for the first 12 weeks after renal transplantation significantly decreased CMV infection (especially primary) and disease (Balfour *et al.*, 1989). The efficacy of acyclovir prophylaxis has not been clearly established, however (Patel *et al.*, 1996). Valacyclovir, the acyclovir prodrug that has a higher bioavailability, has been shown to be safe and effective at reducing CMV disease after renal transplantation using a dose of 2 g given orally four times daily (with dose adjustment for reduced renal function) (Lowance *et al.*, 1999). In this study, it was noted that biopsy-proven acute graft rejection in the first 6 months was halved to 26% in those given prophylactic valacyclovir. Prophylactic regimens of ganciclovir have proved safe and effective using the oral drug (Gane *et al.*, 1997) in liver transplant recipients.

When expensive and potentially toxic drugs are to be given prophylactically, it is important to target the patients who would benefit most. These are patients at risk of primary infections and CMV-seropositive recipients being given additional immunosuppression with antilymphocytic globulin to prevent rejection. An alternative approach is the use of preemptive therapy when treatment is started after the detection of CMV viremia by weekly surveillance testing (see under diagnosis).

Herpes Simplex Virus

Primary infection with HSV is rare in transplant patients. Reactivations, about 40% of which are asymptomatic (the virus being present in throat washings or less commonly in the urine), are frequent. Warrell and colleagues found that 47% of renal transplant recipients excreted HSV (Warrell *et al.*, 1980). Reactivation is associated with a rise in antibody titer in one third of these patients. There are rare reports of transmission of virus in the grafted kidney (Dummer *et al.*, 1987; Koneru *et al.*, 1988). Infection with HSV, unless generalized, does not affect adversely allograft function.

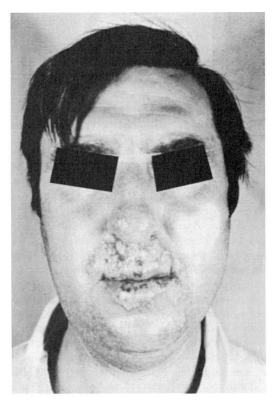

FIGURE 31–4

A case of severe mucocutaneous herpes simplex.

Clinical Features

Symptomatic HSV infection usually presents with labial and oral lesions in the first month after transplantation (Fig. 31–4). The lesions may persist longer than 1 to 2 weeks, which is the norm in a nonimmunosuppressed person. Multiple lesions are seen, as are anogenital lesions, and, occasionally, whitlows, conjunctivitis, corneal ulceration or keratitis develops. Dissemination of the infection to involve internal organs occurs rarely. Fulminant hepatitis leading to disseminated intravascular coagulation and liver failure is difficult to diagnose and usually is fatal (Kusne et al., 1991). Ulceration of the esophagus may occur, and the rectum and the ileum may be involved, causing diarrhea or hemorrhage. Fatal pneumonitis or meningoencephalitis are rare.

Diagnosis

Virus isolation from a lesion confirms HSV infection. More rapid diagnosis is possible by polymerase chain reaction for HSV DNA or specific immunofluorescence on fresh tissue scraped from a lesion or biopsy sample. Electron microscopy of vesicle fluid shows herpesvirus particles, but this method does not distinguish HSV from VZV. Throat washings and less often urine and cervical cultures may contain HSV in asymptomatic immunosuppressed patients. The antibody titer should be measured in any renal transplant patient with clinical HSV infection. Those without detectable levels at the outset, especially if there is no response within 2 weeks, are at risk of developing generalized disease. If antibody is present, most mucocutaneous lesions are likely to heal spontaneously.

Management

Asymptomatic virus excretion requires no treatment, and typical labial ulcerations (cold sores) heal spontaneously. If mucocutaneous lesions become extensive, antiviral therapy should be given as soon as lesions appear. Oral acyclovir or the better adsorbed famciclovir or valacyclovir is effective for treatment (Reichman et al., 1984) and prophylaxis (Pettersson et al., 1985). If lesions affect the eye, an ophthalmologist should be consulted.

To treat disseminated disease, systemic chemotherapy is indicated. A 5- to 7-day course of intravenous acyclovir, which may be prolonged in the case of severe generalized infection, should be given (see Appendix 1 for doses that have to be modified according to renal function). The drug is converted to the active triphosphate, and the first step of phosphorylation is carried out by virus-specific thymidine kinase, an enzyme produced by HSV-infected cells and VZV-infected cells but not by CMV-infected cells (Elion, 1982). The triphosphate derivative inhibits viral synthesis by inhibiting virus DNA polymerase and causes chain termination of viral DNA.

The blood levels achieved are 10 to 100 times that of the inhibitory dose (ID_{50}) against HSV. The half-life of acyclovir is 2 to 3 hours in the normal adult, but because approximately 70% of the drug is excreted unchanged in the urine, it is about 10 times longer in the anuric patient. Hemodialysis removes about 60% of the acyclovir present in the body (Laskin, 1984). Slow intravenous infusion of the drug is necessary because bolus administration may cause crystallization of acyclovir in the renal tubules with impairment of function. Nausea and vomiting have been noted as a side effect of acyclovir in patients with renal failure. The emergence of resistant (thymidine kinase–deficient) strains of HSV has followed one or more courses of acyclovir in immunosuppressed patients. Persistent ulceration and prolonged virus excretion may result but have not been followed by severe local or disseminated infection. These resistant strains may be treated with foscarnet or cidofovir, although both drugs are contraindicated in patients with severe renal impairment. The ultimate clinical significance of this resistance is not yet clear. Similar to all antiviral chemotherapy, early treatment is essential.

Varicella-Zoster Virus

Chickenpox is rare in graft recipients, but zoster occurs annually in approximately 3% of renal transplant patients, 10 times the rate in nonimmunocompromised people (Warrell et al., 1980). Subclinical VZV viremia can occur. Wilson and associates, using the polymerase chain reaction, found VZV in peripheral blood mononuclear cells in 7 of 37 bone marrow transplant recipients who had no manifestations of disease (Wilson et al., 1992). In two of the seven recipients, shingles appeared 60 and 130 days after the virus was detected, but the other five never developed clinical signs or symptoms.

Clinical Features

Chickenpox in the transplant recipient, as in any immunocompromised patient, is likely to be severe. The rash may become confluent, bullous, hemorrhagic or gangrenous. Pneumonitis, encephalitis or meningitis may ensue and be fatal. Zoster eruptions may be more severe and last longer in transplant recipients. Dissemination of the virus may result in satellite lesions or a generalized chickenpoxlike eruption. Meningoencephalitis is a rare complication, as is motor zoster, when that division of the affected nerve root is involved, causing weakness or paralysis. A rise in antibody to VZV without signs of disease is about twice as common as overt lesions in transplant patients. Occasionally, pain in a dermatome with no rash but accompanied by an increase in antibody is seen, *zoster sine herpete*. There is no evidence relating zoster with graft rejection.

Diagnosis

The methods of identifying VZV in a vesicle are identical to those of HSV. Because the virus is quite labile, however, isolation in cell culture frequently fails; the polymerase chain reaction on vesicle fluid or scrapings is more useful. A rise in antibody appears in response to most but not all episodes of zoster in renal transplant patients. Patients who show no serological response are likely to have recurrent or persistent eruptions or generalized infection.

Management

Chickenpox and zoster, which have an increased tendency to become generalized in immunosuppressed patients, require systemic chemotherapy with acyclovir. This treatment is effective in preventing progression of the infection (Balfour *et al.*, 1983). Treatment should be started as early as possible and may need to be continued beyond the normal 5-day course for 14 days in the absence of a serological response to the virus. When zoster affects the ophthalmic branch of the trigeminal nerve, topical antiviral eyedrops should be given in addition to systemic therapy. Adequate analgesia, expert care of eye lesions and good nursing procedures to prevent secondary bacterial infection are all important factors influencing the outcome of VZV infections in renal transplant patients.

Prevention

The immune status to VZV of allograft recipients should be determined as part of the pretransplant workup. The presence of VZV antibody by a sensitive test, such as enzyme-linked immunosorbent assay or indirect fluorescent antibody test, indicates immunity. Susceptible patients should be considered for immunization in the pretransplantation period using the live attenuated vaccine developed by Takahashi *et al.* in 1974. An 87% seroconversion rate after vaccination was found in a group of children on dialysis for chronic renal insufficiency (Broyer and Bondailliez, 1985). In children in remission from leukemia, the seroconversion rate was 88% after one dose and 98% after two doses of vaccine, and the immunity persisted for more than 10 years (Sparks and Russell, 1998). The vaccine appears to prevent clinical varicella after subsequent exposure.

If an immunocompromised patient with no history of chickenpox or vaccination and with no detectable VZV antibody has been in contact with chickenpox or zoster, zoster immune globulin should be given as soon as possible. This immune globulin attenuates but does not prevent chickenpox developing.

Epstein-Barr Virus

Epstein-Barr virus is a γ-herpes virus that has the property to cause malignant change in specific cell types and in specific circumstances. The virus is endemic in all human populations and after infection is carried lifelong as a latent infection of lymphoid cells with only occasional viral replication. The virus's oncogenic potential is associated with the latent, not reactive, infection because it is the latent genes that are able to deregulate cell growth. Epstein-Barr virus infects cells that express the CD21 receptor. This receptor, a 145-kd molecule, which also is the receptor site for the complement fragment C3d, is present on B lymphocytes and on ectocervical and pharyngeal epithelial cells (Young *et al.*, 1986).

Primary infections are uncommon after transplantation because most patients have been infected previously, but 60 to 80% of susceptible recipients undergo seroconversion. The source of the virus can be the allograft (Cen *et al.*, 1991) or, less commonly, can be unrelated to the transplant. Primary infection with EBV in a seronegative renal transplant recipient may be asymptomatic, run a typical glandular fever-type course or, rarely, be fulminant with widespread organ involvement and death (Hanto *et al.*, 1983). Early infection arising in the first 3 to 4 months after transplantation carries the greatest risk.

Reactivation of latent EBV in seropositive patients occurs commonly in the months after transplantation and is manifest by secretion of the virus into the throat from the oropharyngeal epithelia where it replicates (Sixbey *et al.*, 1984). The virus can be isolated in throat washings from 50 to 60% of immunosuppressed patients compared with 10 to 20% of normal EBV-seropositive individuals. Less often, there is a rise in antibody to EBV capsid antigen; heterophil antibody is not stimulated by EBV reactivation. Reactivations are not associated with disturbance in graft function.

The effect of immunosuppression on the cytotoxic T-cell population results in its failure to check the proliferation of EBV-infected B lymphocytes. This failure depends on the degree of immunosuppression and was found to be virtually complete in patients receiving 17.5 mg kg^{-1} d^{-1} of cyclosporine (Crawford *et al.*, 1981). The EBV-associated posttransplantation lymphoproliferative disease comprises a heterogeneous group of lymphoproliferative disorders that occur in immunocompromised individuals. Histologically the tumors range from a polymorphic proliferation of B cells to a monoclonal high-grade malignant lymphoma. Posttransplantation lymphoproliferative disease occurs in 0.5 to 1.5% of the recipients of solid organs (see Chapter 35). Primary EBV infection is an important risk factor for posttransplantation lymphoproliferative disease. The risk is three to four times higher after primary than after secondary infection, which explains its higher frequency in children. Unchecked B-lymphocyte proliferation may give rise to a glandular fever-like illness with fever and lymphadenopathy within the first year after transplantation. The histology of the lymph nodes shows benign hyperplasia, and the B cells have a normal karyotype. Untreated, the clinical course is reported to be short, fulminant and associated with a 75% mortality rate, but acyclovir therapy may be effective (Hanto *et al.*, 1983).

Polyclonal and monoclonal malignant lymphomas, which may appear at multiple sites including the central nervous system and the gut, account for 20% of cancers in renal allograft recipients (outside of Australasia; see Chapter 35) and are a later consequence of B-cell transformation. The malignant cells carry the EBV genome and express the same full range of viral latent genes *in vivo*—six viral nuclear antigens, I, 2, 3A, 3B, 3C, and LP, and two latent membrane proteins, LMP 1 and LMP 2—that are expressed *in vitro* by EBV immortalized B lymphocytes (Gratama *et al.*, 1991; Thomas *et al.*, 1990). There is good evidence for the primary role of EBV in the development of these lymphomas; LMP-1 has potent transforming effects in cell culture and is essential for EBV transformation of cells, it is abundantly expressed on the cell membranes of posttransplantation lymphoproliferative disease B cells, where it mimics activated tumor necrosis factor receptor. It binds intracellular tumor necrosis factor receptor–associated factor, and this, through a series of steps, stimulates cell growth (Liebowitz, 1998).

These tumors arise through a failure of the host's immunosurveillance rather than evasion by tumor cells not expressing immunogenic EBV-encoded antigens. The measurement, by quantitative polymerase chain reaction, of the EBV load in peripheral blood has shown that high levels are found in posttransplantation lymphoproliferative disease (Rowe et al., 1997) and that these fall in response to therapy (Green et al., 1998). Because so many latent proteins are expressed, these tumor cells might remain susceptible to virus-specific T-cell control (Rickinson, 1991; Young et al., 1989). A favorable response to reduction in immunosuppression, which is not necessarily accompanied by rejection of the allograft, and intravenous acyclovir has been reported in some patients (Starzl et al., 1984). Conventional lymphoma treatment should be combined with a discontinuation of immunosuppressive drugs (see Chapter 35). Immunotherapy using EBV-specific cytotoxic T lymphocytes, which has been successful in bone marrow transplant recipients (Heslop and Rooney, 1997), also may be considered.

Human Herpesvirus-6 and Human Herpesvirus-7

Human herpesvirus (HHV)-6 was first isolated in 1986 from peripheral blood mononuclear cells taken from six patients with lymphoproliferative diseases (Salahuddin et al., 1986). It has been shown subsequently that the primary target cells are CD4$^+$ T lymphocytes. Serologically and genomically distinct from other human herpesviruses, HHV-6 is closest to CMV, and its genome has some regions that cross-hybridize with CMV under stringent conditions (Lawrence et al., 1990). Two strains have been identified—HHV-6A and HHV-6B. The latter causes exanthem subitum (roseola infantum, sixth disease) (Yamanishi et al., 1988), but HHV-6A has not yet been associated firmly with clinical illness.

Serological surveys have shown that infection usually is acquired in the first year of life; 75% of infants have antibodies to HHV-6 by the age of 1 year (Okuno et al., 1989). Most infections are asymptomatic, but HHV-6 causes exanthem subitum as noted earlier. After infection, the virus persists in the body and frequently is shed in the saliva (Levy et al., 1990). Primary infection in older children or adults has been associated with infectious mononucleosis–like and hepatic illness (Irving and Cunningham, 1990).

In the immunosuppressed patient, HHV-6 occasionally causes life-threatening opportunistic infections. Transmitted with the donor organ, infection occurs 2 to 3 weeks after transplantation in seronegative recipients. Human herpesvirus-6 has been isolated from the blood of a liver transplant recipient who had fever and hepatitis (Ward et al., 1989). The virus also was found by immunological staining in the lungs of two bone marrow transplant recipients with interstitial pneumonia (Carrigan et al., 1991). The virus has been cultured from the blood of renal transplant recipients (Okuno et al., 1990), and it caused fatal encephalitis in a bone marrow transplant recipient (Drobyski et al., 1994). One of the problems in interpreting the relevance of HHV-6 in the posttransplant situation is that antibody titers to HHV-6, already latent in the patient, rise substantially and coincidentally with primary CMV infection (Ward et al., 1991) or immunization using live CMV vaccine. This rise is not due to cross-reacting CMV antibodies but is due to HHV-6 reactivation or reinfection. A rise in HHV-6 antibody also was seen 3 to 6 weeks after transplantation in the complete absence of CMV infection and in the presence of unchanging EBV antibody titers in five of eight patients (Ward et al., 1991).

Human herpesvirus-6 infection, primary or reactivation, occurs in about one third of solid organ donor transplants (Herbein et al., 1996). Infection usually is asymptomatic or associated with a fever and rash; as noted earlier, severe complications of HHV-6 infection are rare. Active HHV-6

increases the risk of CMV disease in CMV-seropositive transplant recipients (Dockrell et al., 1997) but does not alter the likelihood of primary CMV disease in seronegative recipients of a CMV-positive graft. Severe clinical manifestations usually are a consequence of a dual CMV/HHV-6 infection. Antiviral treatment should be targeted toward CMV; treatment also is effective against HHV-6 because its drug susceptibility resembles that of CMV. At present, there is no clear evidence that HHV-6 causes graft rejection, and in general it is not a major cause of morbidity after renal transplantation.

Human herpesvirus-7, similar to HHV-6, is a β-herpesvirus. It infects T lymphocytes, CD4 being a major component of its binding receptor, and epithelial cells of the salivary glands. Worldwide seroprevalence studies show that 75 to 98% of the population have been infected. Infection tends to occur in the second to third year of life, later than HHV-6, but has a similar spectrum of fever, rashes and seizures. Human herpesvirus-7 also has been linked rarely to an infectious mononucleosis–like illness. At present, there are only a few reports of HHV-7 in transplant recipients, and there is even less clear evidence than there is for HHV-6 of any effects of HHV-7 on the graft or the patient. As a concurrent infection with CMV, however, HHV-7 may increase the risk of CMV disease.

Human Herpesvirus 8 (Kaposi's Sarcoma–Associated Herpesvirus)

Epidemiological evidence suggests that Kaposi's sarcoma (KS) is caused by an infectious agent. Human herpesvirus-8 was identified by Chang et al. in 1994, using molecular techniques, in KS tissue from patients with AIDS. Subsequently, HHV-8 DNA has been detected in 95% of KS lesions in immunocompetent and immunocompromised individuals. In the general population HHV-8 infection is uncommon, with seroprevalence rates of 2 to 14% in different blood donor populations. The exact role of HHV-8 in the causation of KS is not yet resolved fully, and other cofactors may be required.

Transplant-associated KS occurs in 0.2 to 5% of renal transplants, a prevalence 400-fold to 500-fold higher than in a normal population of the same ethnic group. The disease is more common in Arabic, black, Greek, Jewish and Italian peoples; among Italians, 14% of blood donors are seropositive (Whitby et al., 1998). The male/female ratio of KS is 3/1.

Kaposi's sarcoma arises as a result of reactivation of persistent HHV-8 infection in a seropositive recipient (Frances et al., 1999) or after primary infection when the virus is transmitted with the donor kidney (Regamey et al., 1998). The sarcoma arises in endothelial cells and causes reddish blue macules or plaques in the skin and oropharyngeal mucosa. This nonvisceral form accounts for about 60% of cases. In the other 40%, visceral lesions are present in the gastrointestinal tract, lungs and lymph nodes. About a quarter of the visceral cases have no skin lesions, which makes their diagnosis more difficult. The mortality associated with the visceral form of KS is about 50% in the absence of, or with late, treatment.

Patients with KS should be managed by a cancer therapy unit. Local lesions may be excised, treated by radiation or treated by intralesional chemotherapy. For widespread lesions and visceral involvement, systemic chemotherapy may be used and immunosuppression should be reduced, although here is a risk that the donated organ may be lost. The role of antiviral drugs is not yet clear.

Hepatitis B Virus

Hepatitis B virus (HBV) infections usually are asymptomatic or mild in hemodialysis and renal transplant patients because of their immunocompromised state (see Chapter 32). In about 70 to 80% of hemodialysis patients, infection is followed by long-term carriage of the virus. A pool of infectious patients may arise in a unit, putting at risk uninfected patients and nonimmune staff.

Renal transplant patients with chronic HBV infection (hepatitis B surface antigen [HBsAg] positive at the time of transplantation) usually have HBV DNA present in the sera in the months after transplantation, which indicates active viral replication. They frequently have chronic hepatitis indicated by histology and/or raised serum aspartate aminotransferase and alanine aminotransferase levels. Little clinical effect is noted in the early posttransplant period, but after 2 years, there is an increase in mortality rate in HBsAg-positive patients caused by hepatic failure (Pirson et al., 1977) and intercurrent infections to which they are especially predisposed by the combination of hepatitis and immunosuppressive drugs. Fairley and coworkers assessed the risk of fatal liver disease in HBsAg-positive renal allograft recipients (Fairley et al., 1991). They found that 5 of 10 whose blood tests were positive for hepatitis B e antigen (HbeAg)/HBV DNA (indicating active viral replication and the presence of infectious virus) at the time of transplantation died of liver-related disease, compared with only 1 of 15 who were negative for these markers. This tendency for progression of liver disease to chronic active hepatitis and cirrhosis (Parfrey et al., 1985), which is unusual in patients on long-term dialysis, suggests that HBeAg/HBV DNA–positive patients would be managed better by maintenance dialysis and not transplantation. Liver biopsy before transplantation is advocated in these HbsAg-positive patients (Degos et al., 1987; Kasiske et al., 1995), with kidney transplantation only if the liver histology is normal. Hepatocellular carcinoma, which is associated with chronic HBV infection, also occurs in HBsAg carriers after renal transplantation (Schroter et al., 1982). The HBV infection is not associated with impaired graft function.

Renal transplant patients who at the time of transplantation have evidence of past HBV infection (HBsAg negative, anti–hepatitis B core antigen positive, with or without anti-HBs antibody) may undergo reverse seroconversion after immunosuppression. This reverse seroconversion results in the reemergence of HbsAg, HbeAg and HBV DNA in the blood (Dhedin et al., 1998). Although treatment of chronic hepatitis B may not have any long-term benefits in this patient group, in the short-term, lamivudine has been shown to be safe and to improve liver function and remove HBV DNA from the blood (Jung et al., 1998).

Prevention

Hepatitis B virus is spread by blood and blood products in dialysis units and has been transmitted with kidney allografts. In the absence of a policy of screening and exclusion of HBsAg-positive individuals and materials from units, HBV infections were common. The general adoption of such a policy successfully eliminated endemic HBV infections from British units (Polakoff, 1981). The HBsAg-positive patient should not be admitted to units that are HBV-free. In units that treat HBV carriers, careful attention should be paid to basic hygiene to prevent spread to uninfected patients and staff to whom hepatitis B vaccine should be given. The vaccine is effective in preventing HBV infection in vaccinees who have responded by producing anti-HBs antibody. There is a 96% seroconversion rate in normal adults (Szmuness et al., 1981), but the rate was much lower (65%) in hemodialysis patients given 3 × 40 μg doses of the vaccine, and the same dose produced seroconversion in only 32% of renal transplant patients (Grob, 1983). When necessary, patients must be immunized before transplantation and checked for responses. Vaccine boosters should be given to all responders at 5-year intervals.

Hepatitis C Virus (Non-A, Non-B Hepatitis)

The most important chronic liver disease after renal transplantation is hepatitis C (see Chapter 32). At least six genotypes of hepatitis C virus (HCV) have been described. Parenteral transmission is important in the hospital setting and in intravenous drug abusers. In half of patients infected with HCV, however, risk factors have yet to be identified. The acute infection is usually asymptomatic or mild, but the viral genome persists in the blood in about 80% of patients. Long-term sequelae of persistent infection include chronic active hepatitis, cirrhosis, which develops in about 20% and hepatoma. Carriers of the virus remain infectious.

Although HCV has not been cultured, recombinant viral antigens have been made and are used in the laboratory to detect anti-HCV antibodies (Choo et al., 1989). Screening of blood products and organ donors for antibodies to HCV is carried out to reduce the risk of posttransfusion transplantation hepatitis. Because there is a period of 3 months between exposure to the virus and seroconversion, screening tests do not completely prevent transmission of HCV by this route. The prevalence of HCV antibodies in Britain in blood donors is approximately 0.1%. This prevalence is lower than in the general population because these donors are a self-selecting low-risk group.

In renal units, before the introduction of screening HCV infection was associated with duration of dialysis and the number of transfusions received (Pouteil-Noble et al., 1991b). Prevalence rates for dialysis patients vary considerably in different parts of the world and have been quoted as between 2% and 30%. Whatever the exact figure, clusters of patients with raised serum alanine aminotransferase levels indicate that HCV hepatitis is endemic in some units (Polakoff, 1981). Studies indicate that although recipient hepatitis C status does not influence the short-term outcome after renal transplantation, long-term effects are detectable (Ali et al., 1998; Hanafusa et al., 1998; Mathurin et al., 1999).

Hepatitis C virus occasionally may be associated with type 1 membranoproliferative glomerulonephritis in the transplant recipient (Hestin et al., 1998). Hepatitis C virus should be considered in the differential diagnosis of glomerulopathy if an HCV-positive patient develops proteinuria.

Patients with chronic HCV hepatitis have been treated with interferon-α (Davis et al., 1989; Hoofnagle et al., 1986). Long-term treatment (6–12 months) leads to a rapid disappearance of HCV RNA from the blood, normalization in aspartate aminotransferase and alanine aminotransferase levels and improvement in hepatic histology in about half of those treated. After cessation of therapy, a sustained response is seen in fewer patients, especially those with a genotype I infection. Combined therapy using interferon-α and ribavirin has resulted in a higher response rate than interferon-α alone (McHutchinson et al., 1998). These therapies are not recommended in renal transplant recipients on immunosuppression, however, so that the best management strategy is to keep immunosuppression to the minimum possible and to monitor the liver histology every 3 years.

Hepatitis C virus has been transmitted by organ transplantation. Fourteen of 29 recipients of organs from HCV antibody–positive donors developed hepatitis a mean of 3.8 months after transplantation, and the infection became chronic in 12 recipients (Pereira et al., 1991). Whether HCV is acquired at the time of transplantation or previously by some other route, the outcome to the recipient is the same; 5-year patient and graft survival are similar to that in uninfected recipients. Renal transplantation is contraindicated in the presence of preexisting liver cirrhosis, however. Although it has been suggested that because of a shortage of organs those from donors who have HCV antibody could be used for HCV-positive recipients, in countries where the prevalence of HCV is low a general policy of exclusion still should be followed.

Human Immunodeficiency Virus-1

Progressive immune dysfunction is the hallmark of HIV infection. The virus infects cells that express the CD4 antigen, including T lymphocytes, macrophages and microglial cells in the central nervous system. The presence of the CD4 receptor and a coreceptor ($\alpha\beta$-chemokine receptor) (Deng et al., 1996) renders a cell susceptible to HIV infection. After infection, the virus persists in the body for life. Throughout this time, viral replication continues and, in the absence of antiviral treatment, gives rise to a constant viremia in any one person of 10^2 to 10^7 virions/ml plasma. The half-life of HIV in the blood is approximately 2 days, and a typical infected person produces about 10^8 virions/d. Human immunodeficiency virus replication is cytotoxic to the CD4$^+$ T lymphocytes in which most virus is produced. The continuous production of large quantities of virus enables frequent mutations to arise, a diversity that permits escape from immune surveillance and the development of drug resistance.

Progressive viral activity disrupts the patient's immune system, leading to secondary opportunistic infections (e.g., Pneumocystis, toxoplasmosis, candidiasis, mycobacteria, HSV and CMV) and neoplasms (e.g., KS and lymphoma). This progress is monitored best by measuring the HIV load in the plasma and by the fall in peripheral blood CD4 lymphocyte count. Infection of the microglial cells may cause a variety of neurological disorders. A wide spectrum of illness ranging from asymptomatic infection to AIDS may result. The spectrum of HIV infection has been classified by the Centers for Disease Control (1986) as follows:

Group I: Acute infection
Group II: Asymptomatic infection
Group III: Persistent generalized lymphadenopathy
Group IV:
  A. Constitutional disease (AIDS-related complex)
  B. Neurological disease (HIV encephalopathy is an AIDS-indicative disease)
  C. Secondary infectious disease:
    1. Those defining AIDS
    2. Others
  D. Malignancy secondary to HIV (defining AIDS)
  E. Other conditions

In the context of transplantation, the virus has been transmitted by blood or blood products and organs. Four recipients of kidneys from intravenous drug abusers had recurrent or continuous fevers and leukopenia and lymphopenia continuing 2 to 7 weeks after transplantation. HIV-1 antibodies appeared about 2 months after transplantation in two of the patients from whom serum was available at that time and was present in the 8-month sera of all four patients (L'Age-Stehr et al., 1985).

In the pre HIV therapy era Lang and colleagues followed 22 HIV-infected renal transplant recipients and found that 63% of those who did not return to dialysis were dead within 5 years (Lang et al., 1991). These transplant recipients had a shortening of the interval between HIV infection and the diagnosis of AIDS and an accelerated course of AIDS. Patients receiving cyclosporine fared worst. The HIV infection did not induce allogeneic unresponsiveness, and acute rejec-

tion episodes occurred. The study group concluded that dialysis was better than transplantation for HIV-infected patients with chronic renal failure.

Management

Specific treatment with a combination of antiviral drugs, selected from an ever-growing variety (nucleoside reverse transcriptase inhibitors, nonnucleoside reverse transcriptase inhibitors and protease inhibitors)—so-called highly active antiretroviral therapy—has resulted in a dramatic reduction in plasma viral load, improved CD4$^+$ T-lymphocyte count, improved quality of life and prolonged survival. A variety of drugs also are used for prophylaxis against P. carinii pneumonia and mucosal candidiasis. The management of HIV-infected persons is a highly specialized field, and expert guidance should be sought.

Diagnosis

Seroconversion usually has occurred by week 12 after infection when HIV antibodies can be detected by a variety of reliable tests. Earlier in the course of infection, a diagnosis is made by detecting HIV RNA by polymerase chain reaction or less commonly by culturing HIV or detecting viral antigen in blood from about 2 to 8 weeks after infection. These diagnoses must be confirmed by the subsequent appearance of HIV antibodies.

Prevention

Measures to prevent the spread of infection must be those of exclusion. Donors must be tested for antibodies to HIV. These antibodies serve as a marker of infectivity, but early in the course of HIV infection, there is a period of infectivity of about 1 to 2 months before antibodies develop; in the future, blood product and donor screening by polymerase chain reaction will reduce this seronegative window of infectivity. Blood and organs from high-risk donors must not be used.

Papovavirus: Human Polyomaviruses

Two polyomaviruses commonly infect humans—BK and JC (Gardner, 1977). The prevalence of antibody to these viruses in adults is 70% and 65% and is reached by the mid-teens. After inapparent infection, the virus becomes latent. Overall, about 60% of renal transplant recipients show evidence of infection or reactivation at some time after transplantation. Virus shedding in the urine occurs and may persist for many months. The presence of virus is shown in four ways: (1) Urothelial cells with basophilic intranuclear inclusions may be seen in Papanicolaou-stained urinary sediment (decoy cells), (2) the virus may be seen by electron microscopy, (3) the virus may be cultured in primary human fetal brain cells and (4) viral DNA may be detected by polymerase chain reaction.

A study of the BK-antibody status of renal donors and recipients suggests that the allograft is the usual exogenous source of the virus. At Oxford, 17 of 20 BK antibody–negative recipients of kidneys from BK antibody–positive donors underwent seroconversion after transplantation. Gardner and colleagues reported that 45% of a group of BK-seropositive recipients had a significant rise in antibody titer, indicating reactivation or reinfection (Gardner et al., 1984). Half occurred 4 to 8 weeks after transplantation, and the remainder during the following 2 years. Most polyomavirus infections are asymptomatic, but they may cause the following complications:

1. Multiplication of the virus in ureteral epithelial cells causes them to enlarge and, often in conjunction with segmental narrowing owing to ischemia and inflammation, may result in partial or complete ureteral obstruction. A temporary fall in urine output and creatinine clearance follows. Hemorrhagic cystitis can occur.

2. The JC virus is associated with progressive multifocal leukoencephalopathy (Houff et al., 1988), and this has been reported in 13 renal transplant recipients with an onset 1.0 to 2.5 years after transplantation (Walker and Padgett, 1983). JC virus causes lytic infection of myelin-producing oligodendrocytes. The scattered pin points of demyelination in the subcortical white matter enlarge and coalesce and contain enlarged abnormal astrocytes and oligodendrocytes with eosinophilic virus-packed inclusions in their nuclei. The disease begins insidiously with symptoms and signs suggesting multifocal pathology and usually progresses to death in 3 to 6 months. A definitive diagnosis can be made only histologically, but a magnetic resonance imaging study of the brain and a polymerase chain reaction test on the cerebrospinal fluid for JC DNA, which has an 88% sensitivity, usually permit a noninvasive diagnosis to be made.

3. Viral nephropathy (predominantly BK) usually mimics acute rejection clinically and is associated with a rising serum creatinine. It occurs 2 to 60 months (median, 9 months) after transplantation and leads to progressive graft dysfunction and possible loss of the graft. A feature of this condition is its association with newer immunosuppressive agents (e.g., tacrolimus and mycophenolate mofetil). Diagnosis is made by the presence of decoy cells in the urine and seeing on renal biopsy intranuclear polyomavirus inclusions, predominantly in distal tubular and collecting duct epithelial cells, surrounded by inflammation (Nickeleit et al., 2000). In the absence of an effective antiviral agent, current management relies on cautious reduction of immunosuppressive therapy. Plasma viral DNA titers decrease, but virus is not eliminated from the renal tract.

Papillomaviruses

Human papillomaviruses (HPVs) cause squamous cell proliferation and can affect a wide variety of sites in the body. These viruses replicate only in fully differentiated keratinocytes, although the viral genome is present in epithelial cells of the basal layer. The keratinocytes in which HPV replicates develop perinuclear cytoplasmic clearing and crenation of the nuclear membrane. These cells are called *koilocytes*. More than 80 HPV types have been identified by DNA hybridization; HPVs that vary by more than 10% homology are recognized as different types.

Skin Lesions

The frequency of warts, keratoses and skin cancers increases with time after renal transplantation (see Chapters 34 and 35). Barr and coworkers reported prevalences of 77%, 38% and 12% in a group of Scottish patients with functioning grafts for 5 or more years (Barr et al., 1989). Warts occur especially on sun-exposed skin resulting from ultraviolet light radiation (Boyle et al., 1984). Warts also are more resistant to treatment than those in immunocompetent people. All patients affected have a history of warts in childhood, and once warts occur in patients, they are never free of them. Flat warts, unusual warts and epidermodysplasia verruciformis, all of which are associated with specific types of HPV, have been seen in renal allograft recipients. Malignant transformation may occur in warts, more frequently in those exposed to strong sunshine (King et al., 1995). The long-term frequency of cutaneous carcinomas reaches greater than 40%.

Lesions are often multiple, and the ratio of squamous cell carcinomas to basal cell carcinomas is 15/1 (Barr et al., 1989). Using the polymerase chain reaction, DNA from epidermodysplasia verruciformis–associated HPVs has been detected in a high proportion of skin biopsy specimens from malignant and premalignant lesions—solar keratoses and Bowen's disease (de Jong-Tieben et al., 1995). Clinically, squamous cell carcinomas are difficult to distinguish from keratoacanthomas so that surveillance of all warty lesions is important. Local recurrences after removal of the squamous cell type are frequent, but metastatic spread occurred in 8% (Sheil et al., 1987).

Protection against sun exposure is important; patients should wear suitable clothing and headwear and use sun-blocking creams and lipstick. Retinoids, which should be administered under the supervision of a dermatologist (see Chapter 34), reduce the number of keratotic lesions in renal allograft recipients. The lesions tend to recur when the drug is stopped. This type of treatment may control the proliferation of premalignant and malignant lesions.

Anogenital Lesions

The high-risk HPVs, mainly types 16 and 18, are associated with anogenital and cervical neoplasia (Galloway and McDougal, 1990). Anogenital carcinomas, which are rare in the normal population, are 100-fold commoner in renal graft recipients with an incidence of 2.8% (Penn, 1986). They occur on average 7 to 8 years after transplantation. Often, there is a history of condylomata. Women, in whom lesions frequently are multiple, also have a higher incidence of these cancers than men.

A cytological survey of female graft recipients (Halpert et al., 1986) showed that the frequency of HPV infections was nine times greater and intraepithelial neoplasia of the cervix, often involving the vagina or vulva, was 16 times greater than in the general population. Infection and neoplasia were first diagnosed an average of 3.5 years and 4 years after transplantation. Alloub and colleagues in a controlled study found a fourfold increase in cervical intraepithelial neoplasia (42% vs. 10%) and a similar increase in HPV types 16 and 18 detected in a group of Scottish renal allograft recipients (Alloub et al., 1989). These investigators also noted that cervical smear tests proved an unreliable way of diagnosing intraepithelial neoplasia of the cervix. Colposcopic surveillance is preferable in patients receiving long-term immunosuppression.

Adenoviruses

Although invasive life-threatening adenovirus infections are well recognized after pediatric liver transplantation (Michaels et al., 1992), there is little evidence that infections resulting from adenoviruses are more severe in renal allograft recipients than in the normal population. Occasionally, adenoviruses, including previously unrecognized types (e.g., 34 and 35), have caused interstitial pneumonia or have been isolated from the urine, rarely in association with hemorrhagic cystitis.

SELF-LIMITING INFECTIONS
Human Parvovirus

Parvovirus B 19 causes two diseases in humans: aplastic crises in those with a shortened red blood cell survival and erythema infectiosum (fifth disease). Infections typically occur in the spring, with epidemics, which last for 2 years, developing at 4-year intervals. One infection gives life-long immunity, and about 60% of British adults have serological evidence of past infection. The incubation period is 6 days from exposure to viremia, and by day 10 there is an almost complete loss of erythroid precursors. The rash appears about day 15, by which time the patient is no longer infectious. In immunocompromised patients, including renal transplant recipients, chronic red cell aplasia that results in anemia may occur. Then the viral DNA can be detected in the blood by polymerase chain reaction. A therapeutic response is usual after a course of intravenous normal human immunoglobulin. Parvovirus B 19 infection should be considered in patients with persistent anemia.

Community Respiratory Infections

Viral respiratory infections are as common in renal transplant recipients as in the general population. The viruses responsible include influenza A and B, parainfluenza, respiratory syncytial virus, rhinoviruses and adenoviruses. When these infections are limited to the upper respiratory tract, as in the normal host, they are trivial. Lower respiratory tract involvement is commoner and more serious in immunocompromised patients, however. This is particularly the case in acute adult leukemia and after bone marrow transplantation, when mortality rises to about 50% (Couch et al., 1997). Renal transplant recipients usually are less seriously affected. There is no evidence that these infections precipitate renal rejection episodes. A feature of respiratory infections in immunocompromised individuals is their persistence as well as prolonged shedding of the virus. A consequence is the increased risk of infecting others; nosocomial acquisition has been recorded in two thirds of patients infected.

Diagnosis of respiratory viral infections is important for epidemiological study and because specific antiviral treatment is becoming available. Rapid diagnosis by detection of viral antigens in nasopharyngeal washings with a panel of fluorescence-labeled monoclonal antibodies is recommended as well as routine virus isolation in cell cultures.

Annual influenza immunization is recommended for renal transplant recipients. Serological response to the killed influenza vaccine is as good in patients receiving azathioprine as in nonimmunosuppressed people, but antibody titers were significantly lower in patients on cyclosporine (Versluis et al., 1986). Vaccination is not associated with rejection episodes (Carroll et al., 1974). In the presence of an epidemic owing to new strains of influenza A not represented in the vaccine, patients may be protected by amantadine prophylaxis. This drug also has a therapeutic effect, although resistance of the virus develops within a short time. Because amantidine is excreted in the urine, the dose needs to be adjusted for patients with poor renal function. Neuraminidase inhibitors such as zanamivir have greater efficacy for prophylaxis and for treatment and are active against influenza A and influenza B.

The antiviral ribavirin, which is approved as an aerosol treatment of severe respiratory syncytial virus infection in infants, is useful for respiratory syncytial virus and parainfluenza pneumonias in immunosuppressed patients. Aerosolized ribavirin together with intravenous immunoglobulin was effective if started early in bone marrow transplant recipients with respiratory syncytial virus disease (Whimbey et al., 1995), and the use of intravenous ribavirin looks promising (Hayden et al., 1996).

Other RNA Viruses

In immunosuppressed patients, measles can cause an unusual and fatal form of inclusion body encephalitis with an onset 2 to 5 months after the acute infection. There is a progressive deterioration in cerebral function over a period of a few weeks to 10 months (Aicardi et al., 1977; Drysdale et al., 1976).

Endogenous Retroviruses

Apart from the immunological problems occuring with cross-species transplants, for which various strategies are being developed (Lambrigts et al., 1998), there is a potential infectious disease risk associated with the use of organs from nonhuman animals (e.g., pigs) (see Chapter 42). All animals have a group of viruses that are transmitted in the germline from mother to child, as passengers in their genomes. These viruses are called endogenous retroviruses (Boeke and Stoye, 1997). Often defective, most replicate poorly if at all, do not have any biological activity and do not cause disease in their natural animal host.

With xenotransplantation, cross-species transmission occurs, and it is possible that some of these viruses may become pathogenic and cause disease in the new unnatural immunosuppressed host. Porcine endogenous retroviruses are present in many different organs, including kidney and heart, and in many breeds; they also are capable of infecting and replicating in human cells in vitro (Martin et al., 1998). It will be important, during the early xenotransplantation trials, to monitor recipients for endogenous retrovirus activity and possible disease association.

REFERENCES

Ackermann, J. R., Le For, W. M. Weinstein, S., et al. (1988). Four-year experience with exclusive use of cytomegalovirus antibody (CMV-Ab)-negative donors for CMV-Ab-negative kidney recipients. Transplant. Proc. 20(Suppl. 1), 469.

Aicardi, J., Goutieres, F., Arsenio-Nunes, M. L. and Lebon, P. (1977). Acute measles encephalitis in children with immunosuppression. Pediatrics 59, 232.

Akposso, K., Rondeau, E., Hayman, J.-P., et al. (1997). Long term prognosis of renal transplantation after pre-emptive treatment of cytomegalovirus infection. Transplantation 63, 974.

Ali, M. K., Light, J. A., Barhyte, D. Y., et al. (1998). Donor hepatitis C virus status does not adversely affect short-term outcomes in HCV+ recipients in renal transplantation. Transplantation 66, 1694.

Alloub, M. I., Barr, B. B. B., McLaren, K. M., et al. (1989). Human papillomavirus infection and cervical intraepithelial neoplasia in women with renal allografts. B. M. J. 298, 153.

Arduino, R. C., Johnson, P. C. and Miranda, A. G. (1993). Nocardiosis in renal transplant recipients. Clin. Infect. Dis. 16, 505.

Armstrong, D. and Bernard, E. (1991). Aerosol pentamidine. Ann. Intern. Med. 109, 852.

Balfour, H. H., Bean, B., Laskin, O. L., et al. (1983). Aciclovir halts progression of herpes zoster in immunocompromised patients. N. Engl. J. Med. 308, 1448.

Balfour, H. H., Chace, B. A., Stapleton, M. D., et al. (1989). A randomized placebo-controlled trial of oral aciclovir for the prevention of cytomegalovirus disease in recipients of renal allografts. N. Engl. J. Med. 320, 1381.

Barr, B. B. B., Benton, E. C., McLaren, K., et al. (1989). Human papillomavirus infection and skin cancer in renal allograft recipients. Lancet 1, 124.

Bennett, J. E., Dismukes, W. E., Duma, R. J., et al. (1979). A comparison of amphotericin B alone and combined with flucytosine in the treatment of cryptococcal meningitis. N. Engl. J. Med. 301, 126.

Bennett, W. M., Beck, C. H., Jr., Young, H. H. and Russell, P. S. (1970). Bacteriuria in the first month following renal transplantation. Arch. Surg. 101, 453.

Berenguer, J., Gomez-Campdera F., Padilla, B., et al. (1998). Visceral leishmaniasis (Kala-Azar) in transplant recipients: case report and review. Transplantation 65, 1401.

Betts, R. F., Freeman, R. B., Douglas, R. G., Jr., et al. (1975). Transmission of cytomegalovirus infection with renal allograft. Kidney Int. 8, 385.

Bigby, P. D., Margolskee, D. and Curtis, J. L. (1986). Usefulness of induced sputum in diagnosis of pneumonia in patients with AIDS. *Am. Rev. Respir. Dis.* **133**, 515.

Bishop, M. C., Moss, S. W., Oliver, D. O., *et al.* (1977). The significance of vesicoureteric reflux in nonpyelonephritic patients supported by long term hemodialysis. *Clin. Nephrol.* **8**, 354.

Boeke, J. D. and Stoye, J. P. (1997). Endogenous retrovirus. *In Retroviruses*, (J. M. Coffin, S. H. Hughes and H. E. Varmus, eds.), p. 343, Cold Spring Harbour, New York.

Boyle, J., Mackie, R. M., Briggs, J. D., *et al.* (1984). Cancer, warts and sunshine in renal transplant patients. A case control study. *Lancet* **1**, 702.

Brady, M. T., Milam, J. D., Anderson, D. C., *et al.* (1984). Use of deglycerolized red blood cells to prevent posttransfusion infection with cytomegalovirus in neonates. *J. Infect. Dis.* **150**, 334.

Broyer, M. and Bondailliez, B. (1985). Varicella vaccine in children with chronic renal insufficiency. *Postgrad. Med. J.* **61(Suppl. 4)**, 103.

Byrd, L. H., Tapia, L., Cheigh, J. S., *et al.* (1978). Association between *Streptococcus faecalis* urinary infections and graft rejection in kidney transplantation. *Lancet* **2**, 167.

Carrigan, D. R., Drobyski, W. R., Russler, S. K., *et al.* (1991). Interstitial pneumonitis associated with human herpesvirus 6 infection after marrow transplantation. *Lancet* **338**, 147.

Carroll, R. N. P., Marsh, S. D., O'Donoghue, E. P. N., *et al.* (1974). Response to influenza vaccine by renal transplant patients. *B. M. J.* **2**, 701.

Cen, H., Breinig, M. C. and Atchison, R. W. (1991). Epstein-Barr virus transmission via the donor organs in solid organ transplantation: polymerase chain reaction and restriction fragment length polymorphism analysis of IR2, IR3 and IR4. *J. Virol.* **65**, 976.

Centers for Disease Control. (1986). Classification system for human T-lymphocytic virus type III/lymphadenopathy associated virus infections. *M. M. W. R. Morb. Mortal. Wkly. Rep.* **35**, 334.

Centers for Disease Control. (1987). Revision of the CDC surveillance case definition for acquired immunodeficiency syndrome. *M. M. W. R. Morb. Mortal. Wkly. Rep.* **36(Suppl. 1S)**, 1.

Chang, Y., Cesarman, E., Pessin, M. S., *et al.* (1994). Identification of herpes-like DNA sequences in AIDS-associated Kaposi's sarcoma in transplant recipients. *Science* **266**, 1865.

Chieffi, P. P., Sens, Y. A., Paschoalotti, M. A., *et al.* (1998). Infection by *Cryptosporidium parvum* in renal patients submitted to renal transplant or hemodialysis. *Rev. Soc. Bras. Med. Trop.* **31**, 333.

Choo, Q. L., Kuo, G., Weiner, A. J., *et al.* (1989). Isolation of a cDNA clone derived from a blood-borne non-A, non-B viral hepatitis genome. *Science* **244**, 359.

Chou, S. W. (1986). Acquisition of donor strains of cytomegalovirus by renal transplant recipients. *N. Engl. J. Med.* **314**, 1418.

Collaborative DHPG Treatment Study Group. (1986). Treatment of serious cytomegalovirus infections with 9-(1,3-dihydroxy-2-propoxymethyl) guanine in patients with AIDS and other immunodeficiencies. *N. Engl. J. Med.* **314**, 801.

Combarnous, F., Fouque, D., Chossegros, P., *et al.* (1994). Neurologic side-effects of gamciclovir. *Clin. Nephrol.* **42**, 279.

Couch, R. B., Englund, J. A. and Whimby, E. (1997). Respiratory viral infections in immunocompetent and immuncompromised persons. *Am J. Med.* **102**, 2.

Crawford, D. H., Edwards, J. M. B., Sweny, P., *et al.* (1981). Studies on long-term T-cell-mediated immunity to Epstein-Barr virus in immunosuppressed renal allograft recipients. *Int. J. Cancer* **28**, 705.

Cuvelier, R., Pirson, Y., Alexandre, G. P. and van Ypersele de Stribou, C. (1985). Late urinary tract infection after transplantation: prevalence, predisposition and morbidity. *Nephron* **40**, 76.

Davis, G. L., Balart, L. A., Schiff, E. R., *et al.* (1989). Treatment of chronic hepatitis C with recombinant interferon alpha: a multi center randomized controlled trial. *N. Engl. J. Med.* **321**, 1501.

Degos, F., Debure, A. and Kries, H. (1987). Hepatitis in renal transplant recipients. *In Transplantation Reviews*, Vol. 1, (P. Morris and N. Tilney, eds.), p. 159, Grune & Stratton, London.

de Jong-Tieben, L. M., Berkhout, R. J., Smits, H. L., *et al.* (1995). High frequency of detection of epidermodysplasia verruciformis-associated human papillomavirus DNA in biopsies from malignant and premalignant skin lesions from renal transplant recipients. *J. Invest. Dermatol.* **105**, 367.

Deng, H., Liu, R., Ellmeier, W., *et al.* (1996). Identification of a major C-receptor for primary isolates of HIV-1. *Nature* **381**, 661.

Denning, D. W. and Stevens, D. A. (1990). Antifungal and surgical treatment of invasive aspergillosis: a review of 2121 published cases. *Rev. Infect. Dis.* **12**, 1147.

Denning, D. W. (1996). Therapeutic outcome in invasive aspergillosis. *Clin Infect Dis* **23**, 608.

Deray, G., Martinez, F., Katlama, C., *et al.* (1989). Foscarnet nephrotoxicity: mechanism, incidence and prevention. *Am. J. Nephrol.* **9**, 316.

DeVault, G. A., Jr., King, J. W., Rohr, M. S., *et al.* (1990). Opportunistic infections with *Strongyloides stercoralis* in renal transplantation. *Rev. Infect. Dis.* **12**, 653.

Dhar, J. M., Al-Khader, A. A., Al-Sulaiman, M., *et al.* (1991). Nontyphoid *Salmonella* in renal transplant recipients: a report of twenty cases and review of the literature. *Q. J. M.* **287**, 235.

Dhedin, N., Douvin, C., Kuentz, M., *et al.* (1998). Reverse seroconversion of hepatitis B after allogenic bone marrow transplantation. *Transplantation* **66**, 616.

Dockrell, D. H., Parada, J., Jones, M. F., *et al.* (1997). Seroconversion to human herpesvirus 6 following liver transplantation is a marker for cytomegalovirus disease. *J. Infect. Dis.* **176**, 1135.

Dooley, D. P., Carpenter, J. L. and Rademacher, S. (1997). Adjunctive corticosteroid therapy for tuberculosis: a critical reappraisal of the literature. *Clin. Infect. Dis.* **25**, 872.

Drobyski, W. R., Knox, K. K., Majewski, D., *et al.* (1994). Fatal encephalitis due to varient B human herpesvirus-6 infection in a bone-marrow transplant recipient. *N. Engl. J. Med.* **330**, 1356.

Drysdale, H. C., Jones, L. F., Oppenheimer, D. R. and Tomlinson, A. H. (1976). Measles inclusion body encephalitis in a child with treated acute lymphoblastic leukaemia. *J. Clin. Pathol.* **29**, 865.

Dummer, J. S., Armstrong, J. and Somers, J. (1987). Transmission of infection with herpes simplex virus by renal transplantation. *J. Infect. Dis.* **155**, 202.

Eberhard, O. K., Langefeld, I., Kuse, E. R., *et al.* (1998). Procalcitonin in the early phase after renal transplantation—will it add to diagnostic accuracy? *Clin. Transplant.* **12**, 206.

Editorial (1981). Pulmonary problems of the immunocompromised patient. *B. M. J.* **282**, 2077.

Egbert, P. R., Pollard, R. B., Gallagher, J. G., *et al.* (1980). Cytomegalovirus retinitis in immunosuppressed hosts: II. ocular manifestations. *Ann. Intern. Med.* **93**, 664.

Einsele, H., Steidle, M., Vallbracht, A., *et al.* (1991). Early occurrence of HCMV infection after BMT as demonstrated by PCR technique. *Blood* **77**, 1104.

Ejlertsen, T. and Aunsholt, N. A. (1989). *Salmonella* bacteremia in renal transplant recipients. *Scand. J. Infect. Dis.* **21**, 241.

Elion, G. B. (1982). Mechanism of action and selectivity of acyclovir. *Am. J. Med.* **73**, 7.

Erice, A., Chou, S., Biron, K. K., *et al.* (1989). Progressive disease due to ganciclovir-resistant cytomegalovirus in immunocompromised patients. *N. Engl. J. Med.* **320**, 289.

Fairley, C. K., Mijch, A., Gust, I. D., *et al.* (1991). The increased risk of fatal liver disease in renal transplant patients who are hepatitis Be antigen and/or HBV DNA positive. *Transplantation* **52**, 497.

Faull, R. J., Bannister, K. M., Russ, G. R., *et al.* (1999). Excellent long-term survival of low-risk, first renal allografts using cyclosporine/azathioprine double therapy. *Transplant. Proc.* **31**, 1155.

Ferguson, P. E. and Landreneau, R. J. (1988). Thoracoscopic or open lung biopsy in the diagnosis of interstitial lung disease. *Chest Surg. Clin. N. Am.* **4**, 749.

Fishman, J. A. and Rubin, R. H. (1998). Pneumonia in the organ transplant recipient. *In Pulmonary Diseases and Disorders*, 3rd Ed., (J. A. Fishman, *et al.*, eds.), p. 2153, McGraw-Hill, New York.

Fox, B. C., Sollinger, H. W., Belzer, F. O. and Maki, D. G. (1990). A prospective, randomized, double-blind study of trimethoprim-sulfamethoxazole for prophylaxis of infection in renal transplantation: clinical efficacy, absorption of trimethoprim-sulfamethoxazole, effects on the microflora, and the cost-benefit of prophylaxis. *Am. J. Med.* **89**, 255.

Frances, C., Mouquet, C. and Calvez, V. (1999). Human herpesvirus 8 and renal transplantation. *N. Engl J. Med.* **340**, 1045.

Fryd, D. S., Peterson, P. K., Ferguson, R. M., *et al.* (1980). Cytomegalovirus as a risk factor in renal transplantation. *Transplantation* **30**, 436.

Galloway, D. A. and McDougal, J. K. (1990). Human papillomaviruses and carcinomas. *Adv. Virus. Res.* **37**, 125.

Gane, E., Saliba, F., Garcia-Valdecasas, J. C., *et al.* (1997). Randomized trial of efficacy and safety of oral ganciclovir in the prevention of cytomegalovirus disease in liver transplant recipients. *Lancet* **350**, 1729.

Garcia-Leoni, M. E., Martin-Scapa, C., Rodeno, P., *et al.* (1990). High incidence of tuberculosis in renal patients. *Eur. J. Clin. Microbiol. Infect. Dis.* **9**, 283.

Gardner, S. D. (1977). The new human papovaviruses: their nature and significance. In *Recent Advances in Clinical Virology*, (A. P. Waterson, ed.), p. 93, Churchill Livingstone, Edinburgh.

Gardner, S. D., MacKenzie, E. F., Smith, C. and Porter, A. A. (1984). Prospective study of human polyomavirus BK and JC and cytomegalovirus in renal transplant recipients. *J. Clin. Pathol.* **37**, 578.

Goodman, C. M. and Hargreave, T. B. (1990). Survey of antibiotic prophylaxis in European renal transplantation practice. *Int. Urol. Nephrol.* **22**, 173.

Goodrich, J. M., Mori, M., Gleaves, C. A., *et al.* (1991). Early treatment with ganciclovir to prevent cytomegalovirus disease after allogeneic bone marrow transplantation. *N. Engl. J. Med.* **325**, 1601.

Gottesdiener, K. M. (1989). Transplanted infections: donor to host transmission with the allograft. *Ann. Intern. Med.* **110**, 1001.

Gratama, J. W., Zutter, M. M., Minarovits, J., *et al.* (1991). Expression of Epstein-Barr virus-encoded growth-transfusion-associated proteins in lymphoproliferations of bone-marrow transplant recipients. *Int. J. Cancer* **47**, 188.

Grattan, M. T., Moreno-Cabral, C. E., Starnes, V. A., *et al.* (1989). Cytomegalovirus infection is associated with cardiac allograft rejection and atherosclerosis. *J. A. M. A.* **261**, 3561.

Green, M., Cacciarelli, T. V., Mazariegos, G. V., *et al.* (1998). Serial measurements of EB viral load in peripheral blood in pediatric liver transplant recipients during treatment for PTLD. *Transplantation* **66**, 1641.

Grob, P. (1983). Hepatitis B vaccination of renal transplant and haemodialysis patients. *Scand. J. Infect. Dis.* **38(Suppl.)**, 28.

Halpert, R., Fruchter, R. G., Sedlis, A., *et al.* (1986). Human papillomavirus and lower genital neoplasia in renal transplant patients. *Obstet. Gynecol.* **68**, 251.

Hanafusa, T., Ichikawa, Y., Kishikawa, H., *et al.* (1998). Retrospective study on the impact of hepatitis C virus infection on kidney transplant patients over 20 years. *Transplantation* **66**, 471.

Hanto, D. W., Gajl-Peczalka, K. J., Frizzera, G., *et al.* (1983). Epstein-Barr virus (EBV) induced polyclonal and monoclonal B-cell lymphoproliferative diseases occurring after renal transplantation: clinical, pathologic and virologic findings and implications for therapy. *Ann. Surg.* **198**, 356.

Harmon, W. E. (1991). Opportunistic infections in children following renal transplantation. *Pediatr. Nephrol.* **5**, 118.

Haverkos, H. W. (1984). Assessment of therapy for *Pneumocystis carinii* pneumonia. *Am. J. Med.* **76**, 501.

Hayden, F. G., Sable, C. A., Connor, J. D., *et al.* (1996). Intravenous ribavirin by constant infusion for serious influenza and parainfluenza virus infection. *Antiviral Ther.* **1**, 51.

Herbein, G., Strasswimmer, J., Altieri, M., *et al.* (1996). Longitudinal study of human herpesvirus 6 infection in organ transplant recipients. *Clin. Infect. Dis.* **22**, 171.

Herrera, G. A., Alexander, R. W., Cooley, C. F., *et al.* (1986). Cytomegalovirus glomerulopathy: a controversial lesion. *Kidney Int.* **29**, 725.

Heslop, H. E. and Rooney, C. M. (1997). Adoptive cellular immunotherapy for EBV lymphoproliferative disease. *Immunol. Rev.* **157**, 217.

Hestin, D., Guillemin, F., Castin, N., *et al.* (1998). Pretransplant hepatitis C virus infection: a predictor of proteinuria after renal transplantation. *Transplantation* **65**, 741.

Hiesse, C., Kriaa, F., Eschwege, P., *et al.* (1999). Long-term results and risk factors of quadruple immunosuppression in renal transplantation. *Transplant. Proc.* **31**, 1111.

Higgins, R. M., Bloom, S. L., Hopkin, J. M. and Morris, P. J. (1988). Risks and benefits of cotrimoxazole prophylaxis for *Pneumocystis* pneumonia in renal transplantation. *Transplantation* **47**, 558.

Higgins, R. M., Cahn, A. P., Porter, D., *et al.* (1991). Mycobacterial infections after renal transplantation. *Q. J. M.* **78**, 145.

Hilts, A. E. and Fish, D. N. (1998). Dosage adjustment of antiretroviral agents in patients with organ dysfunction. *Am. J. Health Syst. Pharm.* **55**, 2528.

Hoofnagle, J. H., Mullen, K. D., Jones, D. B., *et al.* (1986). Treatment of chronic non-A, non-B hepatitis with recombinant human alpha interferon: a preliminary report. *N. Engl. J. Med.* **315**, 1575.

Hooper, D. C., Pruitt, A. A. and Rubin, R. H. (1982). Central nervous system infection in the chronically immunosuppressed. *Medicine (Baltimore)* **61**, 166.

Hopkin, J. M. (1991). *Pneumocystis carinii*, p. 1, Oxford University Press, Oxford.

Hopkin, J. M., Turney, J. H., Young, J. A., *et al.* (1983). Rapid diagnosis of obscure pneumonia in immunosuppressed renal patients by cytology of alveolar lavage fluid. *Lancet* **2**, 299.

Houff, S. A., Major, E. O., Katz, D. A., *et al.* (1988). Involvement of JC-virus in infected mononuclear cells from the bone marrow and spleen in the pathogenesis of progressive multifocal leukoencephalopathy. *N. Engl. J. Med.* **318**, 301.

Hruby, Z., Myszka-Bijak K., Gosciniak, G., *et al.* (1997). *Helicobacter pylori* infection in haemodialysis patients and renal transplant recipients. *Nephron* **75**, 25.

Immunization Practices Advisory Committee. (1982). Pneumococcal polysaccharide vaccine: recommendations of the Immunization Practices Advisory Committee. *Ann. Intern. Med.* **96**, 203.

Irving, W. L. and Cunningham, A. L. (1990). Serological diagnosis of infection with human herpesvirus type 6. *B. M. J.* **300**, 156.

Jacobson, M. A. and Mills, J. (1988). Serious cytomegalovirus disease in the acquired immune deficiency syndrome (AIDS): clinical findings, diagnosis, and treatment. *Ann. Intern. Med.* **108**, 585.

Johnson, S., Clabots, C. R., Linn, F. V., *et al.* (1990). Nosocomial *Clostridium difficile* colonization and disease. *Lancet* **336**, 97.

Jung, Y. O., Less, Y. S., Yang, W. S., *et al.* (1998). Treatment of chronic hepatitis B with Lamivadine in renal transplant recipients. *Transplantation* **66**, 733.

Kalin, M., Grandien, M. and Petrini, B. (1998). Laboratory diagnosis of respiratory infections. In *Infectious Diseases of the Respiratory Tract*, (M. Ellis, ed.), p. 3, Cambridge University Press, Cambridge.

Kapasi, K. and Rice, G. P. A. (1988). Cytomegalovirus infection of peripheral blood mononuclear cells: effects on interleukin-1 and -2 production and responsiveness. *J. Virol.* **62**, 3603.

Kasiske, B. L., Ramos, E. L., Gaston, R. S., *et al.* (1995). Evaluation of renal transplant candidates: clinical practical guidelines. *J. Am. Soc. Nephrol.* **6**, 1.

King, G. N., Healey, C. M., Glover, M. T., *et al.* (1995). Increased prevalence of dysplastic and malignant lip lesions in renal transplant recipients. *N. Engl. J. Med.* **332**, 1052.

Kondo, K., Kondo, T., Okuno, T., *et al.* (1991). Latent human herpesvirus 6 infection of human monocytes/macrophages. *J. Gen. Virol.* **72**, 1401.

Koneru, B., Tzakis, A. G., De Puydt, L. E., *et al.* (1988). Transmission of fatal herpes simplex infection through renal transplantation. *Transplantation* **45**, 653.

Kusne, S., Schwartz, M., Breinig, M. K., *et al.* (1991). Herpes simplex virus hepatitis after solid organ transplantation in adults. *J. Infect. Dis.* **163**, 1001.

Kutukculer, N., Shenton, B. K., Clark, K., *et al.* (1995). Renal allograft rejection: the temporal relationship and prediction value of plasma TNF (alpha and beta), IFN-gamma and soluble I CAM-1. *Transpl. Int.* **8**, 45.

L'Age-Stehr, J., Schwartz, A., Offerman, G., *et al.* (1985). HTLV-III infection in renal transplant recipients. *Lancet* **2**, 1361.

La Quaglia, M. P., Tolkoff-Rubin, N. E., Dienstag, J. L., *et al.* (1981). Impact of hepatitis on renal transplantation. *Transplantation* **32**, 504.

Lambrigts, D., Sachs, D. H. and Cooper, D. K. C. (1998). Discordant organ xenotransplantation in primates. *Transplantation* **66**, 547.

Lang, P., Niaudet, P. and the Groupe Cooperatif de Transplantation d'Ile de France. (1991). HIV infection in renal transplant patients. In *Transplantation and Clinical Immunology*, Vol. 23, (J. L. Jouraine, *et al.*, eds.), p. 221, Excerpta Medica, Amsterdam.

Laskin, O. L. (1984). Aciclovir: pharmacology and clinical experience. *Arch. Intern. Med.* **144**, 1241.

Lawrence, G. L., Chee, M., Craxton, M. A., *et al.* (1990). Human herpesvirus 6 is closely related to human cytomegalovirus. *J. Virol.* **64**, 287.

Lerner, P. I. (1996). Nocardiosis. *Clin. Infect. Dis.* **22**, 891.

Levy, J. A., Ferro, F., Greenspan, D. and Lennett, E. T. (1990). Frequent isolation of HHV-6 from saliva and high seroprevalence of the virus in the population. *Lancet* **335**, 1047.

Liebowitz, D. (1998). EBV and cellular signaling pathway in lymphomas from immunosuppressed patients. *N. Engl. J. Med.* **338**, 1413.

Little, D. M., Farrell, J. G., Cunningham, P. M., *et al.* (1997). Donor sepsis is not a contraindication to cadaveric organ donation. *Q. J. M.* **90**, 641.

Lowance, D., Neumayer, H.-H., Legendre, C. C., *et al.* (1999). Valaciclovir for the prevention of cytomegalovirus disease after renal transplantation. *N. Engl. J. Med.* **340**, 1462.

Maki, D. G., Fox, B. C., Kuntz, J., *et al.* (1992). A prospective, randomized, double-blind study of trimethoprim-sulfamethoxazole for prophylaxis of infection in renal transplantation: side effects of trimethoprim-sulfamethoxazole, interaction with cyclosporin. *J. Lab. Clin. Med.* **119**, 11.

Marker, S. C., Simmons, R. L. and Balfour, H. H. (1981). Cytomegalovirus vaccine in renal allograft recipients. *Transplant. Proc.* **13**, 117.

Martin, U., Kiessig, V., Blusch, J. H., *et al.* (1998). Expression of pig endogenous retrovirus by primary porcine endothelial cells and infection of human cells. *Lancet*, **352**, 692.

Matthews, T. and Boehme, R. (1988). Antiviral activity and mechanism of action of ganciclovir. *Rev. Infect. Dis.* **10(Suppl. 3)**, S490.

Mathurin, P., Mouquet, C., Poynard, T., *et al.* (1999). Impact of hepatitis B and C virus on kidney transplantation outcome. *Hepatology* **29**, 257.

McCabe, R. E. and Remington, J. S. (1983). The diagnosis and treatment of toxoplasmosis. *Eur. J. Clin. Microbiol.* **2**, 95.

McHutchinson, J. G., Gordon, S. C., Schiff, E. R., *et al.* (1998). Interferon alpha-2b alone or in combination with ribavirin as initial treatment for chronic hepatitis C. *N. Engl. J. Med.* **339**, 1485.

Meyers, J. D., Ljungman, P. and Fisher, L. D. (1990). Cytomegalovirus excretion has a predictor of cytomegalovirus disease after marrow transplantation: importance CMV viraemia. *J. Infect. Dis.* **162**, 373.

Michaels, M. G., Green, M., Wald, E. R. and Starzl, T. E. (1992). Adenovirus infections in pediatric liver transplant recipients. *J. Infect. Dis.* **165**, 170.

Moore, E. H., Shepard, J. O. McLoud, T. C., *et al.* (1990). Positional precautions in needle aspiration lung biopsy. *Radiology* **175**, 733.

Morduchowicz, G., Shmueli, D., Shapira, Z., *et al.* (1986). Rhinocerebral mucormycosis in renal transplant recipients: report of three cases, and review of the literature. *Rev. Infect. Dis.* **8**, 441.

Morgan, J. S., Schaffner, W. and Stone, W. J. (1986). Opportunistic strongyloidiasis in renal transplant recipients. *Transplantation* **42**, 518.

Morris, P. J., Chan, L., French, M. E., *et al.* (1982). Low dose oral prednisolone in renal transplantation. *Lancet* **1**, 525.

Moyses-Neto, M., Costa, R. S., Reis, M. A., *et al.* (1997). Use of ciprofloxacin as a prophylactic agent in urinary tract infections in renal transplant recipients. *Clin. Transplant.* **11**, 446.

Mylonakis, E., Hohmann, E. L. and Calderwood, S. B. (1998). Central nervous system infection with *Listeria monocytogenes*: 33 years' experience at a general hospital and review of 776 episodes from the literature. *Medicine (Baltimore)* **77**, 313.

Nickeleit, V., Klimkait, T., Binet I. F., *et al.* (2000). Testing for polyomavirus type BK DNA in plasma to identify renal allograft recipients with viral nephropathy. *N. Engl. J. Med.* **342**, 1309.

Ojo, A., Wolfe, R. A., Agodoa, L. Y., *et al.* (1998). Prognosis after primary renal transplant failure and the beneficial effects of repeat transplantation: multivariate analyses from the United States Renal Data System. *Transplantation* **66**, 1651.

Okuno, T., Higashi, K., Shiraki, K., *et al.* (1990). Human herpesvirus 6 infection in renal transplantation. *Transplantation* **49**, 519.

Okuno, T., Takahashi, K., Balachandra, K., *et al.* (1989). Seroepidemiology of human herpesvirus-6 in normal children and adults. *J. Clin. Microbiol.* **27**, 651.

Osman, H. K., Peiris, J. S., Taylor, C. E. Warwicker, P., Jarrett, R. F. and Madeley, C. R. (1996). Cytomegalovirus disease in renal allograft recipients: is human herpes virus 7 a co-factor for disease progression? *J. Med. Virol.* **48**, 295.

Parfrey, S., Farge, D., Clarke-Forbes, R. D., *et al.* (1985). Chronic hepatitis in end-stage renal disease: comparison of HBsAg-negative and HBsAg-positive patients. *Kidney Int.* **28**, 959.

Patel, R., Snydman, D. R., Rubin, R. H., *et al.* (1996). CMV prophylaxis in solid organ transplant recipients. *Transplantation* **61**, 1279.

Paterson, D. L., Dominguez, E. A., Chang, F. Y., *et al.* (1998). Infective endocarditis in solid organ transplant recipients. *Clin. Infect. Dis.* **26**, 689.

Penn, I. (1986). Cancers of the anogenital region in renal transplant recipients. *Cancer* **58**, 611.

Pereira, B. J. G., Milford, E. L., Kirkman, R. L. and Levey, A. S. (1991). Transmission of hepatitis C by organ transplantation. *N. Engl. J. Med.* **325**, 454.

Peters, T. G., Williams, J. W., Harmon, H. C., *et al.* (1983). Splenectomy and death in renal transplant patients. *Arch. Surg.* **118**, 795.

Peterson, P. K., Balfour, H. H., Jr., Fryd, D. S., *et al.* (1981). Fever in renal transplant recipients: causes, prognostic significance and changing patterns at the University of Minnesota Hospital. *Am. J. Med.* **71**, 345.

Peterson, P. K., Ferguson, R., Fryd, D. S., *et al.* (1982). Infectious diseases in hospitalized renal transplant recipients: a prospective study of a complex and evolving problem. *Medicine (Baltimore)* **61**, 360.

Pettersson, E., Eklund, B., Hockerstedt, K., *et al.* (1985). Aciclovir and renal transplantation. *Scand. J. Infect. Dis.* **47(Suppl.)**, 145.

Pirson, Y., Alexandre, G. P. J. and van Ypersele de Strihou, C. (1977). Long-term effect of HBs antigenemia on patient survival after renal transplantation. *N. Engl. J. Med.* **296**, 194.

Plotkin, S. A., Starr, S. E., Friedman, H. M., *et al.* (1991). Effect of Town live virus vaccine on cytomegalovirus disease after renal transplantation: a controlled trial. *Ann. Intern. Med.* **114**, 525.

Polakoff, S. (1981). Hepatitis in dialysis units in the United Kingdom: a Public Health Laboratory Service survey. *J. Hygiene (Camb.).* **87**, 443.

Pouteil-Noble, C., Echochard, R., Donia-Maged, A., *et al.* (1991a). Cytomegalovirus infection and rejection in renal transplantation. *In Transplantation and Clinical Immunology*, Vol. 23, (J. L. Touraine, *et al.*, eds.), p. 107, Excerpta Medica, Amsterdam.

Pouteil-Noble, C., Tardy, J. C., Chossegros, P., *et al.* (1991b). Antihepatitis C virus antibodies: prevalence and morbidity in renal transplantation. *In Transplantation and Clinical Immunology*, Vol. 23, (J. L. Touraine, *et al.*, eds.), p. 81, Excerpta Medica, Amsterdam.

Prat, V., Horcickova, M., Matousovic, K., *et al.* (1985). Urinary tract infection in renal transplant patients. *Infection* **13**, 207.

Reed, E. C. (1991). Treatment of cytomegalovirus pneumonia in transplant patients. *Transplant. Proc.* **23(Suppl. 1)**, 8.

Regamey, N., Tamm, M., Wernli, M., *et al.* (1998). Transmission of human herpesvirus 8 infection from renal transplant donors to recipients. *N. Engl. J. Med.* **339**, 1358.

Reichman, R. C., Badger, G. J., Mertz, G. J., *et al.* (1984). Treatment of recurrent genital herpes simplex infections with oral aciclovir: a controlled trial. *J. A. M. A.* **251**, 2103.

Renoult, E., Georges, E., Biava, M. F., *et al.* (1997). Toxoplasmosis in kidney transplant recipients: report of six cases and review. *Clin. Infect. Dis.* **24**, 625.

Richardson, W. P., Colvin, R. B., Cheeseman, S. H., *et al.* (1981). Glomerulopathy associated with cytomegalovirus viraemia in renal allografts. *N. Engl. J. Med.* **305**, 57.

Rickinson, A. B. (1991). Background to EBV-related lymphoproliferative diseases in transplant patients. *In Transplantation and Clinical Immunology*, Vol. 23, (J. L. Touraine, *et al.*, eds.), p. 247, Excerpta Medica, Amsterdam.

Ritchie, D. B. C., Jennings, L. C., Lynn, K. L., *et al.* (1982). *Clostridium difficile*-associated colitis: cross-infection in predisposed patients with renal failure. *N. Z. Med. J.* **95**, 265.

Roberts, T. C., Brennan, D. C., Buller, R. S., *et al.* (1998). Quantitative PCR to predict occurrence of symptomatic cytomegalovirus infection and assess response to ganciclovir therapy in renal transplant recipients. *J. Infect. Dis* **178**, 626.

Rowe, D. T., Qu, L., Reyes, J., *et al.* (1997). Use of competitive PCR to measure EBV genome load in peripheral blood in pediatric transplant patients with lymphoproliferative disorders. *J. Clin. Microbiol.* **35**, 1612.

Rubin, R. H., Wolfson, J. S., Cosimi, A. B., *et al.* (1981). Infection in the renal transplant recipient. *Am. J. Med.* **70**, 405.

Sabeel, A., Alrabiah, F., Alfurayh, O., *et al.* (1998). Nocardial brain abscess in a renal transplant recipient successfully treated with triple antimicrobials. *Clin. Nephrol.* **50**, 128.

Salahuddin, S. Z., Ablashi, D. V., Markham, P. D., *et al.* (1986). Isolation of a new virus, HBLV, in patients with lymphoproliferative disorders. *Science* **234**, 596.

Salama, A. D., Rogers, T., Lord, G. M., *et al.* (1997). Multiple *Cladosporium* brain abscesses in a renal transplant patient: aggressive management improves outcome. *Transplantation* **63**, 160.

Salmela, K., Ekland, B., Kyllonen, L., *et al.* (1990). The effects of intravesically applied antibiotic solution in the prophylaxis of infectious complication of renal transplantation. *Transpl. Int.* **3**, 12.

Schroter, G. P. J., Weil, R., Penn, I., *et al.* (1982). Hepatocellular carcinoma associated with chronic hepatitis B virus infection after kidney transplantation. *Lancet* **2**, 381.

Scowden, E. B., Shaffner, W. and Stone, W. J. (1978). Overwhelming strongyloidiasis: an unappreciated opportunistic infection. *Medicine (Baltimore)* **57**, 527.

Shapiro, E. D. and Clemens, J. D. (1984). A controlled evaluation of the protective efficacy of pneumococcal vaccine for patients at high risk of serious pneumococcal infections. *Ann. Intern. Med.* **101**, 325.

Shapiro, R., Jordan, M. L., Scantlebury, V. P., *et al.* (1999). A prospective randomized trial of tacrolimus/prednisone versus pacrolimus/prednisone/mycophenolate mofetil in renal transplant recipients. *Transplantation* **67**, 411.

Sheil, A. G. R., Flavel, S., Disney, A. P. S., *et al.* (1987). Cancer incidence in renal transplant patients treated with azathioprine or cyclosporine. *Transplant. Proc.* **19**, 2214.

Simmons, R. L., Matas, A. J., Rattazzi, L. C., *et al.* (1977). Clinical characteristics of the lethel cytomegalovirus infection following renal transplantation. *Surgery* **82**, 537.

Singh, N., Chang, F. Y., Gayowski, T., *et al.* (1997). Infections due to dematiaceous fungi in organ transplant recipients: case report and review. *Clin. Infect. Dis.* **24**, 369.

Sixbey, J. W., Nedrud, J. G., Raab-Traub, N., *et al.* (1984). Epstein-Barr virus replication in oropharyngeal epithelial cells. *N. Engl. J. Med.* **310**, 1225.

Smiley, M. C., Wlodaver, C. G., Grossman, R. A., *et al.* (1985). The role of pre-transplant immunity in protection from cytomegalovirus disease following renal transplantation. *Transplantation* **40**, 157.

Snydman, D. R. (1988). Ganciclovir therapy for cytomegalovirus disease associated with renal transplants. *Rev. Infect. Dis.* **10(Suppl. 3)**, S554.

Snydman, D. R., Werner, B. G., Heinze-Lacey, R. N., *et al.* (1987). Use of cytomegalovirus immune globulin to prevent cytomegalovirus disease in renal transplant recipients. *N. Engl. J. Med.* **317**, 1049.

Snydman, D. R., Werner, B. G., Tilney, N. C., *et al.* (1991). Final analysis of primary cytomegalovirus disease prevention in renal transplant recipients with a cytomegalovirus-immune globulin: comparison of the randomized and open-label trials. *Transplant. Proc.* **23**, 1357.

Sparks, L. and Russell, C. (1998). The new varicella vaccine: efficacy, safety and administration. *J. Pediatr. Nurs.* **13**, 85.

Starzl, T. E., Nalesnik, M. A., Porter, K. A., *et al.* (1984). Reversibility of lymphomas and lymphoproliferative lesions developing under cyclosporin-steroid therapy. *Lancet* **1**, 583.

Stephan, R. N., Munschauer, C. E. and Kumar, M. S. (1997). Surgical wound infection in renal transplantation: outcome data in 102 consecutive patients without perioperative systemic antibiotic coverage. *Arch. Surg.* **132**, 1315.

Szmuness, W., Stevens, C. E., Harley, E. J., *et al.* (1981). The immune response of healthy adults to a reduced dose of hepatitis B vaccine. *J. Med. Virol.* **8**, 123.

Takahashi, M., Otsuka, T., Okuno, Y., *et al.* (1974). Live vaccine used to prevent the spread of varicella in children in hospital. *Lancet* **2**, 1288.

The, T. H., Van der Ploeg, M., Van den Berg, A. P., *et al.* (1992). Direct detection of cytomegalovirus in peripheral blood leukocytes: a review of the antigenemia assay and polymerase chain reaction. *Transplantation* **54**, 193.

Thomas, J. A., Hotchin, N. A., Allday, M. J., *et al.* (1990). Immunohistology of Epstein-Barr virus-associated antigens in B cell disorders from immunocompromised individuals. *Transplantation* **49**, 944.

Tolkoff-Rubin, N. E., Cosimi, A. B., Russell, P. S., *et al.* (1982). A controlled study of trimethoprim-sulfamethoxazole prophylaxis of urinary tract infection in renal transplant recipients. *Rev. Infect. Dis.* **4**, 614.

Tolkoff-Rubin, N. E., Rubin, R. H., Keller, E. E., *et al.* (1978). Cytomegalovirus infection in dialysis patients and personnel. *Ann. Intern. Med.* **89**, 625.

van der Bij, W., Schirm, J., Torensma, R., *et al.* (1988a). Comparison of viremia and antigenemia for detection of cytomegalovirus in blood. *J. Clin. Microbiol.* **26**, 2531.

van der Bij, W., Torensma, R., Vanson, W. J., *et al.* (1988b). Rapid immunodiagnosis of active cytomegalovirus infection by monoclonal antibody staining of blood leukocytes. *J. Med. Virol.* **25,** 179.

van der Pijl, J. W., Frissen, P. H. J., Reiss, P., *et al.* (1990). Foscarnet and penile ulceration. *Lancet* **335**, 286.

van Es, A., Baldwin, W. M., Oljans, P. J., *et al.* (1984). Expression of HLA-DR on T-lymphocytes following renal transplantation, and association with graft rejection episodes and cytomegalovirus infection. *Transplantation* **37**, 65.

Versluis, D. J., Beyer, W. E. P., Masurel, N., *et al.* (1986). Impairment of the immune response to influenza vaccination in renal transplant recipients by cyclosporine but not azathioprine. *Transplantation* **42**, 376.

von Willebrand, E., Petterson, E., Ahonen, J., *et al.* (1986). Cytomegalovirus infection, class II antigen expression and human kidney allograft rejection. *Transplantation* **42**, 364.

Wakefield, A. E., Miller, R. M., Guiver, L. and Hopkin, J. M. (1991). DNA amplification for the diagnosis of *Pneumocystis* pneumonia from induced sputum. *Lancet* **337**, 1378.

Walker, D. L. and Padgett, B. L. (1983). Progressive multifocal leukoencephalopathy. *In Comprehensive Virology*, Vol. 18, (H. Frankel-Conrat and R. R. Wagner, eds.), p. 161, Plenum Press, New York.

Waltzer, W. C., Arnold, A. N., Anaise, D., *et al.* (1987). Impact of cytomegalovirus infection and HLA-matching on outcome of renal transplantation. *Transplant. Proc.* **19**, 4077.

Ward, K. N., Gray, J. J. and Efstathiou, S. (1989). Brief report: primary human herpesvirus 6 infection in a patient following liver transplantation from a seropositive donor. *J. Med. Virol.* **28**, 69.

Ward, K. N., Sheldon, M. J. and Gray, J. J. (1991). Primary and recurrent cytomegalovirus infections have different effects on human herpesvirus-6 antibodies in immunosuppressed organ graft recipients. *J. Med. Virol.* **34**, 258.

Warrell, M. J., Chinn, I., Morris, P. J., *et al.* (1980). The effects of viral infections on renal transplants and their recipients. *Q. J. Med.* **49**, 219.

Weeden, D., Hopewell, J. P., Moorhead, J. F., *et al.* (1982). Schistosomiasis in renal transplantation. *Br. J. Urol.* **54**, 478.

Weller, I. V., Copland, P. and Gabriel, R. (1981). *Strongyloides stercoralis* infection in renal transplant recipients. *B. M. J.* **282**, 524.

Wendt, C. H., Weisdorf, D. J., Jordan, M. C., *et al.* (1992). Parainfluenza virus respiratory infection after bone marrow transplantation. *N. Engl. J. Med.* **326**, 921.

Whimbey, E., Champlin, R. E., Englund, J. A., *et al.* (1995). Combination therapy with aerosolized ribavirin and intravenous immunoglobulin for respiratory syncytial virus disease in adult bone marrow transplant recipients. *Bone Marrow Transplant.* **16**, 393.

Whitby, D., Luppi, M., Barozzi, P., *et al.* (1998). Human herpesvirus 8 seroprevalence in blood donors and lymphoma patients from different regions of Italy. *J. Natl. Cancer Inst.* **90**, 395.

Wilson, A., Sharp, M., Koropchak, C. M., *et al.* (1992). Subclinical varicella-zoster virus viremia, herpes zoster and T-lymphocyte immunity to varicella-zoster viral antigens after bone marrow transplantation. *J. Infect. Dis.* **165**, 119.

Windus, D. W., Stokes, T. J., Julian, B. A. and Fenves, A. Z. (1987). Fatal *Rhizopus* infections in hemodialysis patients receiving deferoxamine. *Ann. Intern. Med.* **107**, 678.

Winston, D. J., Ho, W. G., Lin, C. H., *et al.* (1987). Intravenous immunoglobulin for prevention of cytomegalovirus infection and interstitial pneumonia after bone marrow transplantation. *Ann. Intern. Med.* **106**, 12.

Yamanishi, K., Shiraki, K., Kondo, T., *et al.* (1988). Identification of human herpesvirus-6 as a causal agent for exanthem subitum. *Lancet* **1**, 1065.

Yildiz, A., Besisik, F., Akkaya, V., *et al.* (1999). *Helicobacter pylori* antibodies in hemodialysis patients and renal transplant recipients. *Clin. Transplant.* **13**, 13.

Yildiz, A., Sever, M. S., Turkmen, A., *et al.* (1998). Tuberculosis after renal transplantation: experience of one Turkish centre. *Nephrol. Dial. Transplant.* **13**, 1872.

Yilmaz, S., Koshinen, P. K., Kallio, E., *et al.* (1996). Cytomegalovirus infection-enhanced chronic kidney allograft rejection is linked with intercellular adhesion molecule-1 expression. *Kidney Int.* **50**, 526.

Young, J. A., Hopkin, J. M. and Cutherbertson, W. P. (1984). Pulmonary infiltrates in immunocompromised patients: diagnosis by cytological examination of bronchoalveolar lavage fluid. *J. Clin. Pathol.* **37**, 390.

Young, L., Alfieri, C., Hennessy, K., *et al.* (1989). Expression of Epstein-Barr virus transformation-associated genes in tissues of patients with EBV lymphoproliferative disease. *N. Engl. J. Med.* **321**, 1080.

Young, L. S., Clark, D., Sixbey, J. W. and Rickinson, A. B. (1986). Epstein-Barr virus receptors on human pharyngeal epithelia. *Lancet* **1**, 240.

Yu, Y. L., Chow, W., Humphries, M. J., *et al.* (1986). Cryptic miliary tuberculosis. *Q. J. M.* **59**, 421.

Appendix 1
Principles of Antimicrobial Therapy

Antibiotic	Recommended Dose	Dialysis	Comment
Penicillins	Dose reduction for high-dose therapy (e.g., endocarditis, meningitis) in severe renal impairment For flucloxacillin, no dosage reduction unless CC <10	Penicillin G removed by HD, poorly by PD; flucloxacillin not significantly removed by HD or PD. Others variable	Penicillins can cause nephritis, seizures and coagulopathy at high drug levels. Ideal peak serum level 15–20 mg L^{-1}
Antipseudomonal penicillins			
Piperacillin	Normally 4 g q 6 h CC 20–40: 4 g q 8 h CC <20: 4 g q 12 h	2 g q 12 h in PD; 2 g q 8 h plus 1 g post-HD 100 mg L^{-1} in CAPD	
Piperacillin/ tazobactam	Normally 2.25–4.5 g q 6–8 h CC 20–80: 4.5 g q 8 h CC <20: 4.5 g q 12 h	HD 4.5 g q 12 h plus 2.25 g post-HD	Doses are expressed as total content of piperacillin and tazobactam
Ticarcillin/ clavulanic acid	Normally 3.2 g q 6–8 h CC 10–30: 1.6 g q 8 h CC <10: 1.6 g q 12 h	Dialyzed. Manufacturers not established dosage guidelines	
Cephalosporins			
Cefotaxime	Normally 1–2 g q 8 h CC <5: 1 g loading dose, then half-dose, same interval	Supplement 1 g post-HD CAPD: 1 g d^{-1}	
Ceftazidime	Normally 1–2 g q 8 h CC 30–50: 1 g q 12 h CC 15–30: 1 g q 24 h CC 5–15: 0.5 g q 24 h CC <5: 0.5 g q 48 h	Give 1 g post-HD CAPD: 0.5 g q 24 h	In severe infection doses for RF can be increased by 50%. Trough levels must be <40 mg L^{-1}
Ceftriaxone	Normally 1–4 g q 24 h CC <10: max 2 g q 24 h	HD standard dose after dialysis PD 750 mg q 12 h	Monitor levels in dialysis patients and if LF with RF
Cefuroxime	Normally 0.75–1.5 g q 8 h CC 10–20: 750 mg q 12 h CC <10: 750 mg q 24 h	Give 750 mg post-HD CAPD: 750 mg q 12 h	
Penems			
Imipenem/ cilastatin	Normally 0.5–1 g q 6–8 h CC 31–70: 500 mg q 6–8 h CC 21–30: 500 mg q 8–12 h CC 0–20: 250 mg (or 3.5 mg kg^{-1}, whichever is lower) q 12 h CC = or <5: do not use unless HD can be started within 48 h	For HD dose after dialysis and q 12 h thereafter	Doses in RF based on body weight of 70 kg. Allow proportionate reduction in doses for patients with lower weight. Increase in seizure potential if dosage too high
Meropenem	Normally unit dose, i.e., 0.5–1 g q 8 h CC 26–50: unit dose q 12 h CC 10–25: half-unit dose q 12 h CC <10: half-unit dose q 24 h	Give unit dose post-HD	Unit dose 500 mg, 1 g or 2 g depending on type and severity of infection
Monobactams			
Aztreonam	Normally 1–2 g q 8 h In RF use normal first dose, then if CC 10–30: half initial dose q 8 h CC <10: quarter initial dose q 8 h	HD supplement ⅛ initial dose post-HD	
Aminoglycosides	Use standard nomograms for loading/maintenance dosing		Check serum levels frequently. Toxicity increases with cyclosporine
Tetracyclines			
Doxycycline	Normally 200 mg on day 1, then 100 mg q 24 h	Not affected by dialysis	
Oxytetracycline	Avoid; catabolic		
Quinolones			
Ciprofloxacin	Normally 200–400 mg q 12 h IV For po, 250–750 mg q 12 h For CC <20: reduce dose by half	HD 200 mg IV or 250–500 mg po q 12 h CAPD: 200 mg IV or 250 mg po q 8–12 h	Monitor drug levels if on dialysis. Crystalluria may occur; ensure good hydration

Antibiotic	Recommended Dose	Dialysis	Comment
Levofloxacin	250–500 mg q 12–24 h IV For po 200–400 mg q 12–24 h In RF use normal first dose, then CC 20–50: half dose CC 10–19: if initial dose 250 mg give 125 mg q 48 h or if initial dose 500 mg, then quarter dose but normal interval CC <10: if initial dose 250 mg, then 125 mg q 48 h, or if initial dose 500 mg, then give 125 mg q 24 h	HD and CAPD dose for CC <10 no supplement required	See manufacturer's data for initial dosages
Norfloxacin	Normally 400 mg q 12 h po CC <30: 400 mg q 24 h	HD dose for CC <30	
Sparfloxacin	Normally 400 mg, then 200 mg q 24 h po CC <30: day 1 400 mg, day 2 give 200 mg, then 200 mg q 48 h	No data	
Macrolides			
Azithromycin	Normally 500 mg daily. No adjustment with CC >40. No data for severe RF	No data	Excreted hepatically. ESRF dosing base on extrapolation
Clarithromycin	Normally 500 mg q 12 h IV For po 250–500 mg q 12 h CC <30: reduce dose by half	No data: dose after HD	Excreted by liver and kidney. Interaction causes increased cyclosporine levels
Erythromycin	0.5–1 g q 6 h for severe infections CC <10: reduce dose by 50–75% maximum 1.5 g daily	Unaffected by HD or PD	Interaction causes increased cyclosporine levels. Ototoxicity with high doses in ESRF
Miscellaneous			
Chloramphenicol	1 g q 6–8 h	Not removed by PD or significantly by HD	Avoid in severe RF—toxic metabolites may accumulate
Clindamycin	0.6–1.2 g q 6 h	Unaffected by dialysis	Reduce dose in severe RF owing to prolonged half-life
Amoxycillin/ clavulanic acid	Normally 1.2 g q 8 h IV CC 10–30: 1.2 g IV stat, then 600 mg IV q 12 h CC <10: 1.2 g IV stat, then 600 IV q 24 h	HD decreases serum concentrations. May need additional 600 mg IV dose during and at end of dialysis	
Co-trimoxazole	Normally 960 mg q 12 h IV or PO CC 15–25: normal dose for maximum 3 d, then half dose For CC <15: do not give unless HD available, then give half standard dose	Removed by HD; dose as for CC <15	Doses are expressed as total combination of sulfamethoxazole and trimethoprim
	For PCP treatment, 120 mg kg^{-1} d^{-1} divided q 6–8 h CC 15–30: 120 mg kg^{-1} d^{-1} divided q 6–8 h for 48 h, then 60 mg kg^{-1} d^{-1} divided q 12 h CC <15: 120 mg kg^{-1} d^{-1} q 48 h	Removed by HD	High-dose therapy in RF must be monitored; ideal peak levels: trimethoprim, $\geq$ 5 mg L^{-1}; sulfamethoxazole, 100–150 mg L^{-1}. Toxicity increases with cyclosporine
Fusidic acid	500 mg q 8 h No reduction required in RF	Not significantly removed by dialysis	Do not use alone for serious *Staphylococcus* infections
Metronidazole	Usually 500 mg q 8 h No reduction required in RF	HD normal dose ensuring one dose is immediately after dialysis CAPD, PD normal dosage	
Quinupristin/ dalfopristin	Normally 7.5 mg kg^{-1} q 8–12 h	No data	Use with caution in renal impairment—insufficient data
Teicoplanin	3–6 mg kg^{-1} q 24 h. In RF do not reduce dose until day 4, then if CC 40–60: normal dose q 48 h or half dose q 24 h; CC <40: normal dose q 72 h or one third dose q 24 h	HD and CAPD dose CC <40	Serum monitoring optimizes therapy
Trimethoprim	200 mg q 12 h CC 15–25: half dose after 3 days CC <15: half dose	Dose after HD; not removed by PD	Only use in HD if plasma concentration can be estimated regularly
Vancomycin	Normally 1 g q 12 h. With RF load with 15 mg kg^{-1} then follow serum levels	Give 0.75–1 g after HD. Repeat 1 wk^{-1} or based on serum levels. Poorly removed by HD/CAPD	Nephrotoxic. Ideal peak: 30–40 mg L^{-1}; trough: 5–10 mg L^{-1}

Antibiotic	Recommended Dose	Dialysis	Comment
Antituberculous agents	Unless otherwise indicated use standard chemotherapy; ethambutol is best avoided		
Ethambutol	CC >50: normal dose CC 10–50: increase dose interval to 36 h; CC <10: increase dose interval to 48 h	For HD give 9 mg kg^{-1} d^{-1} after dialysis	Regular eye tests required
Isoniazid	CC >10: no change; CC <10: if slow acetylator, reduce dose by 100 mg	Removed by HD, PD—dose after dialysis	Ideal trough level: <1 mg L^{-1}
Pyrazinamide	Usually 25 mg kg^{-1} d^{-1} in divided doses; do not exceed 3 g d^{-1}. CC <10: 50–100% standard dose	For HD, give 40 mg kg^{-1} 24 h before thrice-weekly dialysis. CAPD, standard dose	Risk of hyperuricemia
Rifabutin	CC <30: reduce dosage by 50%	No data	
Rifampicin	No modification required in RF	Unaffected by dialysis	Interaction causes major reduction in cyclosporine levels
Streptomycin	Normally for TB treatment 1 g q 24 h IM. CC 10–50: standard dose q 24–72 h; CC <10 standard dose q 72–96 h	Removed by HD. Supplement 50% standard dose post HD. CAPD 20–40 mg L^{-1} d^{-1}	Excreted unchanged by kidneys. Avoid if possible. Important to do serum drug levels (peak >40 mcg/ml, trough <3mcg/ml)
Antiviral agents			
Aciclovir	Oral: HSV 200 mg 5 × day or CC <10: q 12 h. VZV 800 mg 5 × day or CC 10–25: 800 mg q 8 h; CC <10: 800 mg q 12 h HSV, IV 5 mg kg^{-1} q 8 h; CC 25–50: 5 mg kg^{-1} q 12 h; CC 10–25: 5 mg kg^{-1} q 24 h; CC <10: 2.5 mg kg^{-1} q 24 h	For HD and CAPD, give 2.5 mg kg^{-1} q 24 h IV for HSV or 5 mg kg^{-1} q 24 h IV for VZV; dose after dialysis	In severe infection oral HSV doses can be doubled; IV doses are for HSV; double doses for VZV
Cidofovir	Induction normally 5 mg/kg once weekly for 2 weeks, then maintenance 5 mg/kg once every 2 weeks CC < or = 55 or if proteinuria > or = 2+: contraindicated as doses unknown	To minimize potential for nephrotoxicity, administer probenicid 2 g 3 h prior to and 1 g 2 h and 8 h after administration of cidofovir. Discontinue if serum creatinine increases by >44 µmol/L or if proteinuria >2 develops. Recommended to discontinue any potential nephrotoxic agents at 7 days before starting cidofovir.	
Famciclovir	VZV treatment if immunocompromised 500 mg q 8 h CC 30–39: 250 mg q 8 h CC 10–29: 125 mg q 8 h HSV treatment if immunocompromised 500 mg q 12 h CC 30–90: 250 mg q 12 h CC 10–29: 125 mg q 12 h	For VZV, give 250 mg post-HD For HSV, give 125 mg post-HD	
Foscarnet	Induction CMV 60 mg kg^{-1} q 8 h; induction mucocutaneous HSV 40 mg kg^{-1} q 8 h. Reduce dose, same interval if: CC (ml min^{-1} kg^{-1}) 1.6–1.4: 55 or 37 mg kg^{-1}, for CMV and HSV respectively. For: CC 1.4–1.2: 49 or 33 mg kg^{-1} respectively CC 1.2–1.0: 42 or 28 mg kg^{-1} CC 1.0–0.8: 35 or 24 mg kg^{-1} CC 0.8–0.6: 28 or 19 mg kg^{-1} CC 0.6–0.4: 21 or 14 mg kg^{-1} CC <0.4: not recommended	Dialyzed. Manufacturers not established dosage guidelines	Maintain adequate hydration to prevent renal toxicity CC stated in ml min^{-1} kg^{-1}
Ganciclovir	Induction 5 mg kg^{-1} q 12 h IV for 7–14 d If CC 50–69: reduce dose 2.5 mg kg^{-1} q 24 h CC 25–49: use 2.5 mg kg^{-1} q 24 h CC 10–24: use 1.25 mg kg^{-1} q 24 h	Removed by dialysis. For HD give 1.25 mg kg^{-1} 3 times a week post-HD	Monitor white blood cells and platelets twice weekly. It has a long intracellular half-life

Antibiotic	Recommended Dose	Dialysis	Comment
Valaciclovir	HSV treatment 500 mg q 12 h CC <15: 500 mg q 24 h VZV treatment 1 g q 8 h CC 15–30: 1 g q 12 h CC <15: 1 g q 24 h	For HD dose as for CC <15 after dialysis	Doses are for treatment not prophylaxis
Oseltamivir	Treatment: 75 mg q 12 h for 5 days Prophylaxis: 75 mg q 24 h for 6 weeks CC <30: 75 mg q 24 h for 5 days CC <10: no data		
Antifungal agents			
Amphotericin B	Dosage reduction not required initially but if C >260 μmol L^{-1} discontinue or reduce dose until renal function improved	Not removed by HD	All amphotericin products, monitor serum K$^+$ and Mg^{++} regularly
Amphotericin B lipid complex	5 mg kg^{-1} q 24 h No dose alterations in RF	Can be given during HD	
Liposomal amphotericin B	Initially 1 mg kg^{-1} q 24 h and increased stepwise to 3 mg kg^{-1} q 24 h if needed. No dose alterations in RF	Start after HD complete—company recommendation	
Fluconazole	CC 11–50: day 1 normal dose IV or po, then CC 11–50: 50% dose	One dose after every dialysis	Excreted in urine as unchanged drug
Flucytosine	CC 20–40: 50 mg kg^{-1} q 12 h; CC 10–20: 50 mg kg^{-1} q 24 h; CC <10: single dose, then monitor levels	For PD: give 37.5 mg kg^{-1} d^{-1} For HD: give 25 mg kg^{-1} post-HD	Ideal peak: 25–50 mg L^{-1}; >80 is toxic. Do not use alone for serious infection
Itraconazole	IV day 1 and 2 give 200 mg q 12 h, then q 24 h CC <30: do not use IV For po 100–200 mg q 12–24 h. No dose adjustments in renal failure	Poorly dialyzed CAPD monitor levels	Interaction with rifampicin means reduced blood levels of itraconazole IV contains α-cyclodextrin
Pentamidine	For PCP treatment 4 mg kg^{-1} IV q 24 h for 14 d. CC <10: if life-threatening, 4 mg kg^{-1} q 24 h for 7–10 d, then alternate days to complete at least 14 doses	Not removed by dialysis or PD	Dosages expressed as pentamidine isethionate
Antiprotozoal agents			
Chloroquine	CC <10: Reduce dose by 50%	Not removed by HD	
Mefloquine	No dosage adjustment in RF	No data	
Proguanil	Normally 200 mg q 24 h CC 20–59: 100 mg q 24 h CC 10–19: 50 mg every second day CC <10: 50 mg once weekly	No data	In severe RF increased risk of hematological toxicity
Pyrimethamine	Treatment of toxoplasmosis 50–75 mg q 24 h for 1–3 weeks then reduce dosage by 50% weeks 4 to 5	Not removed by HD, CAPD	Reduces renal secretion of creatinine. Used in combination with second agent. In addition administer with folinic acid to prevent hematologic toxicity.
Quinine	CC 10–50: give normal dose q 12 h CC <10: give normal dose q 24 h	Removed by HD, not by PD	
Antiretroviral agents	For dosing in RF and HD, see Hilts and Fish (1998)		

CC = creatinine clearance (ml min^{-1}); HD = hemodialysis; PD = peritoneal dialysis; ESRF = end-stage renal failure; q 6 h = every 6 hours; CAPD = chronic ambulatory peritoneal dialysis; LF = liver failure; RF = renal failure; PCP = *Pneumocystis carinii* pneumonitis; HSV = herpes simplex virus; VZV = varicella-zoster virus; CMV = cytomegalovirus.

Acknowledgment: The authors thank Wendy Lawson, Senior Pharmacist, Infectious Diseases, Hammersmith Hospitals NHS Trust, for preparing the Appendix.

Liver Disease Among Renal Transplant Recipients

Svetlozar N. Natov • Brian J. G. Pereira

Clinical, Biochemical and Pathological Characteristics

INCIDENCE

Liver disease is a well-recognized complication among renal transplant recipients with a reported incidence in different studies of 1 to 67% (Allison *et al.*, 1992; Anuras *et al.*, 1977; Berne *et al.*, 1979; LaQuaglia *et al.*, 1981; Mozes *et al.*, 1978; Rao and Andersen, 1988, 1992; Sharma *et al.*, 1992; Ware *et al.*, 1975, 1979; Weir *et al.*, 1985). This wide variation mainly is due to (1) the diagnostic criteria, (2) the rigorousness with which the diagnosis has been pursued and (3) the differences in the duration of follow-up because liver disease is more likely to manifest with increasing number of years posttransplantation (Debure *et al.*, 1988). A large survey of 2,041 renal transplant recipients revealed a 16% mean incidence of posttransplant liver disease (Rao and Anderson, 1992). In different series, acute liver disease and chronic liver disease have represented varying proportions of all cases of liver dysfunction. In one study with a 37% overall incidence of liver dysfunction, 60% of the episodes of liver impairment were classified as acute, and the remaining 40% were classified as chronic (Rao and Anderson, 1992). In contrast, in another study with a similar incidence of liver disease (38%), this ratio was reversed, with acute episodes accounting for 40% of the events and chronic episodes accounting for 60% (Ware *et al.*, 1979). It is plausible that many episodes of acute liver disease that are relatively mild and resolve with no sequelae remain clinically unrecognized, and only patients with more severe acute liver injury that progresses to chronic liver disease are recognized. Likewise, some forms of chronic liver disease with a silent clinical course and no tendency to progression might be missed easily. Consequently the true incidence of posttransplant liver disease remains unknown.

CLINICAL PRESENTATION AND BIOCHEMICAL SPECTRUM

The clinical course of posttransplant liver disease among renal transplant recipients generally is indolent. The disease typically begins early in the posttransplant period (Penn *et al.*, 1969; Ware *et al.*, 1975). About 80% of patients with liver dysfunction present with clinical symptoms and/or laboratory abnormalities within 6 months (peak presentation, 8–12 weeks) from the date of transplantation (Ware *et al.*, 1975). Usually, complaints are constitutional, vague or mild and frequently absent. Symptoms and physical findings attributable to liver disease, such as jaundice, hepatosplenomegaly, vascular spiders and any other symptoms of portal hypertension, are unusual (Allison *et al.*, 1992; Anuras *et al.*, 1977; Rao *et al.*, 1993; Ware *et al.*, 1975). Jaundice is unusual among renal transplant recipients (incidence, <1–11%) (Allison *et al.*,

1992; Hamburger *et al.*, 1965; Mozes *et al.*, 1978; Ware *et al.*, 1975; Weir *et al.*, 1985) and usually is related to drug use (azathioprine being the most important), viral hepatitis or systemic infections with sepsis (Allison *et al.*, 1992; Hamburger *et al.*, 1965; Mozes *et al.*, 1978; Ware *et al.*, 1975, 1979; Weir *et al.*, 1985). In about one third of cases, no definitive cause can be implicated (Mozes *et al.*, 1978).

The presence of jaundice in renal transplant recipients with acute liver disease usually is associated with more severe liver involvement. Jaundice is commoner in patients with chronic liver disease and has been observed in about 25% of these cases, each time as a manifestation of more advanced disease (Ware *et al.*, 1975). Hepatosplenomegaly and other signs of portal hypertension usually are absent until end-stage liver disease is established (Allison *et al.*, 1992; Ware *et al.*, 1975). Although extremely rare, fulminant hepatitis presenting with rapid deterioration, jaundice, encephalopathy and fatal outcome owing to severe hepatocellular failure has been observed in renal transplant recipients (Anuras *et al.*, 1977; Dusheiko *et al.*, 1983; Ware *et al.*, 1975, 1979). Fulminant hepatitis has been encountered more commonly in recipients with hepatitis B antigenemia coinfected with delta agent or in association with hepatotoxic drugs, other forms of viral hepatitis or multiorgan failure (Kharsa *et al.*, 1987).

The reported incidence of liver function test (LFT) abnormalities among renal transplant recipients varies from 3 to 60% (Kirkman *et al.*, 1982; Mahony, 1989; Penn *et al.*, 1969; Rao and Andersen, 1988; Sharma *et al.*, 1992; Weir *et al.*, 1985), mainly in relation to the frequency and timing of testing, reporting of episodes of acute liver dysfunction, definition of chronic liver dysfunction, duration of follow-up and patient compliance with testing schedules. The time of the typical presentation of liver dysfunction is a matter of controversy. In one study, mild and transient LFT abnormalities were observed in about 75% of the cases and were commonest in the first 6 months posttransplantation (Penn *et al.*, 1969). These findings were probably not only a consequence of the high incidence of acute liver dysfunction in the early posttransplant period but also a reflection of the more comprehensive evaluation in that period. Others have noted, however, that the prevalence of LFT abnormalities increases with the time after transplantation presumably as a result of the progression of some forms of chronic liver disease to more advanced stages. In a series of 184 renal transplant recipients with grafts functioning for more than 5 years, chronically elevated aminotransferase levels were observed in only 3% of the patients in the first 4 years posttransplantation but in 14% at 7 years' follow-up. Among these patients, the elevation of the liver enzyme levels persisted in 73% of the cases (Weir *et al.*, 1985).

Liver function test abnormalities generally are not associated with clinical symptoms except in the case of advanced liver disease and liver failure (Rao and Andersen, 1988). Histological evidence of advanced liver disease can be present in the absence of abnormal LFTs. Liver function tests are an imperfect tool for the diagnosis of posttransplant liver disease.

LIVER HISTOLOGY

The clinical presentation and laboratory data do not reflect the cause and severity of posttransplantation liver disease. Liver histology is the only tool for the precise diagnosis of the wide spectrum of pathology seen among patients with posttransplant liver disease (Allison et al., 1992; Debure et al., 1988; Degos et al., 1980; Parfrey et al., 1985b; Rao et al., 1991; Ware et al., 1975). Among renal transplant recipients with evidence of chronic liver disease, liver histology provides more useful prognostic information than any biochemical test (Parfrey et al., 1985b; Rao et al., 1991; Takahara et al., 1987). A liver biopsy is recommended in all renal transplant recipients with documented abnormal LFTs with duration of 6 or more months, regardless of possible cause, unless factors that could increase the risk from the procedure (i.e., prothrombin time >15 seconds, bilirubin >10 mg/dl, clinically unstable condition or a systemic infection) are present. The commonest histological patterns of liver disease in renal transplant recipients are listed in Table 32–1.

Fat Metamorphosis

Fat metamorphosis is characterized by the presence of lipid droplets within the hepatocytes and involving a significant portion (≥30%) of the liver parenchyma.

Hepatitis

Hepatitis of varying degrees and severity is the commonest histological finding on liver biopsy. The types of hepatitis are as follows:

1. *Chronic persistent hepatitis* presents with inflammatory cell infiltration limited to the portal triad with no disruption of the limiting plate.
2. *Early chronic active hepatitis* (CAH) is notable for the extension of the inflammatory cell infiltration beyond the portal triad into the hepatic lobule and the absence of piecemeal necrosis, bridging hepatic necrosis or fibrosis. In some series, CAH has been reported as the commonest form of posttransplant liver disease (64%) (Anuras et al., 1977).
3. *Advanced chronic active hepatitis* presents with extensive cellular infiltration (lymphocytes, plasma cells and neutrophils) with disruption of the limiting plate and bridging hepatic necrosis involving multiple lobules.

Micronodular Cirrhosis

The liver parenchyma is distorted by abundant scar tissue and formation of pseudonodules.

Intrahepatic Cholestasis

Severe pericentral cholestasis without parenchymal necrosis or involvement of the portal triad dominates the histological picture. In renal transplant recipients, intrahepatic cholestasis has been observed in association with nonspecific reactive hepatitis attributable to sepsis, azathioprine therapy and viral hepatitis (Hamburger et al., 1965; Sopko and Anuras, 1978; Sparberg et al., 1969). This condition is completely reversible, although it may continue for a prolonged period (Anuras et al., 1977).

TABLE 32–1
SPECTRUM OF HISTOLOGICAL LESIONS IN LIVER BIOPSY SPECIMENS OF RENAL TRANSPLANT RECIPIENTS WITH POSTTRANSPLANT LIVER DISEASE

Fat metamorphosis
Hepatitis
  Chronic persistent hepatitis
  Early chronic active hepatitis
  Advanced chronic active hepatitis
Micronodular cirrhosis
Intrahepatic cholestasis
Hemosiderosis
Peliosis hepatitis
Nodular regenerative hyperplasia
Silicone particles
Venoocclusive disease

Hemosiderosis

Hemosiderosis presents with accumulation of excessive iron within the hepatocytes. This condition has been reported in 50% of liver biopsy specimens and is common in patients undergoing polytransfusion. Phlebotomies have resulted in diminishing the iron deposition and the degree of fibrosis but have had only a small effect on the coexisting hepatitis (Allison et al., 1992).

Peliosis Hepatis

Peliosis hepatis is characterized by irregularly dilated sinusoids, which contain erythrocytes and form cavities with irregular size, shape and distribution in the liver parenchyma. These cavities are filled with blood and often surrounded by atrophic liver cell cords that lack an endothelial lining. Bile stasis and inflammatory changes are absent. Among renal transplant recipients, peliosis hepatis has a prevalence of 3 to 12% (Degos et al., 1980; Degott et al., 1978; Ihara et al., 1982; Takahara et al., 1987). Although the cause and pathogenesis are unknown, some authors have strongly suspected the role of azathioprine therapy (Hankey and Saker, 1987; Takahara et al., 1987). All cases of peliosis hepatis in renal transplant recipients have occurred among patients treated with azathioprine (Benjamin and Shunk, 1978; Degos et al., 1980; Degott et al., 1978; Hankey and Saker, 1987; Ihara et al., 1982).

Other authors believe that peliosis hepatis may be a sequela of infections with hepatitis A virus (HAV), hepatitis B virus (HBV), hepatitis C virus (HCV), cytomegalovirus (CMV) or herpes simplex virus (HSV); malignancy; tuberculosis; diabetes; use of anabolic, androgenic and estrogenic corticosteroid agents and therapy with methyldopa or tamoxifen (Hankey and Saker, 1987). There is evidence to suggest that peliosis hepatis might not be related specifically to renal transplantation because this lesion has been observed in a patient with uremia (Trites, 1957) as well as in hemodialysis patients (Hankey and Saker, 1987), in association with exposure to vinyl chloride used in the manufacturing of dialysis circuit tubing (Hillion et al., 1983), and silicone particles, which might have fragmented from silicone-containing segments contained in older dialysis pumps (Leong et al., 1981).

Peliosis hepatis generally is considered an incidental finding with poorly defined manifestation and a benign clinical course. Peliosis hepatis might be a more serious condition than currently appreciated, however, because many reports have associated peliosis hepatis with hepatomegaly, splenomegaly, portal hypertension, liver dysfunction (particularly elevated serum alkaline phosphatase levels), liver failure and

TABLE 32–2

RELATIONSHIP BETWEEN MORPHOLOGICAL DIAGNOSIS AND SUBSEQUENT PROGRESSION TO MICRONODULAR CIRRHOSIS*

Morphological Diagnosis	Sample Size	Initial Histology: Cirrhosis Present	Follow-up Histology	
			Cirrhosis Developed	*No Cirrhosis Observed*
Fat metamorphosis	1	0	0	1
Chronic persistent hepatitis	5	0	0	5
Early CAH	15	1	9	5
Advanced CAH	8	4	4	0
Hemosiderosis	5	2	2	1
Total	34	7	15	12

*Mean interval between the initial and follow-up specimens, 4.5 ± 4.3 years.
CAH = chronic active hepatitis.
Reproduced with permission from Rao *et al.*, 1993.

intraperitoneal hemorrhage from a ruptured peliotic lesion (Degott *et al.*, 1978; Hankey and Saker, 1987).

Nodular Regenerative Hyperplasia

Nodular regenerative hyperplasia is characterized by diffuse micronodular transformation of the hepatic parenchyma without fibrous septa between the nodules (Allison *et al.*, 1992). The exact pathogenesis of this disorder has not been established. The nodular transformation is suspected to originate from obliteration of the portal veins (Wanless, 1990). Different causes have been suggested, and among these, azathioprine therapy has been cited most frequently. Nodular regenerative hyperplasia may present with clinical features of portal hypertension and mild cholestasis (Wanless, 1990).

Silicone Particles

Granular refractile silicone particles arising from peristaltic blood pump inserts, used in hemodialysis equipment before the early 1980s and deposited in the liver parenchyma, have been implicated in the occurrence of delayed hepatic dysfunction in renal transplant recipients (Hunt *et al.*, 1989). These observations were not supported by others, however (Allison *et al.*, 1992).

Venoocclusive Disease

The hallmark of venoocclusive disease is nonthrombotic obliterative occlusion of the terminal hepatic venules and sublobular veins by loose connective tissue, with adjacent sinusoidal congestion and dilatation and hepatocellular de-

generation or necrosis (Katzka *et al.*, 1986). An association with azathioprine therapy has been noted. Infection with CMV also has been implicated (Read *et al.*, 1986). Venoocclusive disease is discussed at length in the section on azathioprine hepatotoxicity.

HISTOLOGICAL PROGRESSION OF POSTTRANSPLANT LIVER DISEASE

The histological lesions on liver biopsy have great predictive value for the prognosis of posttransplant liver disease. Only certain histological forms of liver disease have been shown to be prone to morphological progression to more advanced lesions (Rao *et al.*, 1993). Rao and colleagues observed that over a mean follow-up period of 4.5 ± 4.3 years, progression to cirrhosis in the posttransplant period was commoner among patients who had pretransplant liver histology findings consistent with advanced liver disease, compared with patients who showed only mild lesions (Rao *et al.*, 1993; Table 32–2). With early institution of phlebotomy therapy, hemosiderosis was shown to be potentially curative with complete reversal of the histological lesions in 20% of the cases (Rao and Anderson, 1982). Once hepatic fibrosis develops, however, hemosiderosis progresses to cirrhosis despite the depletion of parenchymal iron (Bomford and Williams, 1976; Rao and Anderson, 1985).

Mortality in renal transplant recipients with chronic liver disease has been correlated strongly with pretransplant liver histology. Only patients with hemosiderosis, early CAH and advanced CAH progressed to liver failure and death (Table 32–3). None of the patients with histological evidence of fat metamorphosis or chronic persistent hepatitis showed

TABLE 32–3

RELATIONSHIP BETWEEN MORPHOLOGICAL DIAGNOSIS AND CLINICAL PROGRESSION TO HEPATIC FAILURE AND DEATH*

Morphological Diagnosis	Sample Size	Death from Hepatic Failure *N* (%)	Death from Other Causes *N* (%)
Fat metamorphosis	8	0	3 (37%)
Chronic persistent hepatitis	20	0	9 (45%)
Early CAH	20	7 (35%)	4 (20%)
Advanced CAH	15	9 (60%)	2 (13%)
Hemosiderosis	9	5 (55%)	2 (22%)
Total	72	21 (29%)	20 (28%)

*Mean observation, 5.7 ± 3.9 years after the biopsy.
CAH = chronic active hepatitis.
Reproduced with permission from Rao *et al.*, 1993.

evidence of clinical progression or died from liver failure during the posttransplant period (Rao *et al.*, 1993).

Drug-Induced Hepatotoxicity

AZATHIOPRINE

Azathioprine is a purine antimetabolite. It is an imidazole derivative of 6-mercaptopurine, a drug known to cause hepatic dysfunction in leukemic patients, which generally resolves with discontinuation. Azathioprine was introduced as an immunosuppressive agent in solid-organ transplantation in 1961 (Murray *et al.*, 1963). Its hepatotoxic effect, in a dose-dependent manner, was described initially in dog models. Administration for a few days at a dose 2 to 4 mg/kg was shown to cause cholestasis and hepatocellular liver injury in dogs, along with a sharp rise in the serum transaminases and alkaline phosphatase levels, which in most animals had a tendency to regress within several days. In a third of the cases, the liver injury resulted in the development of centrilobular lesions or necrosis, with a mortality rate of 33% (Starzl *et al.*, 1965).

Azathioprine-related, dose-dependent liver dysfunction has been reported in renal transplant recipients (Malekzadeh *et al.*, 1972; Sharma *et al.*, 1992; Ware *et al.*, 1979; Zarday *et al.*, 1972). Liver function test abnormalities commonly improve or resolve with a decrease in the dose of azathioprine or with its discontinuation (Malekzadeh *et al.*, 1972), and LFT abnormalities may be exacerbated with its reinstitution in about 50% of patients (Briggs *et al.*, 1973). The spectrum of azathioprine-related histological lesions in liver biopsy specimens is broad and includes peliosis hepatis (Degott *et al.*, 1978), perisinusoidal (Disse space) fibrosis (Nataf *et al.*, 1979), venoocclusive disease (Liano *et al.*, 1989), nodular regenerative hyperplasia, hepatic sinusoidal dilatation (Gerlag and van Hooff, 1987) and intrahepatic cholestasis (Haboubi *et al.*, 1988; Sparberg *et al.*, 1969; Zarday *et al.*, 1972). The pathogenesis of azathioprine hepatotoxicity is not understood completely. Azathioprine-induced direct injury of hepatic endothelial cells, hepatocytes and intralobular ducts has been implicated, however (Haboubi *et al.*, 1988; Pol *et al.*, 1996; Sparberg *et al.*, 1969; Ware *et al.*, 1979; Zarday *et al.*, 1972). The combination of azathioprine and corticosteroid therapy may favor HBV replication, whenever HBV infection is present (Farge *et al.*, 1986; Loertscher *et al.*, 1983; Strom, 1982).

The clinical presentation of azathioprine hepatotoxicity is diverse. Many reported cases are characterized by the development of moderate to severe jaundice, sometimes with marked pruritus (Hamburger *et al.*, 1965; Ware *et al.*, 1979). Clinical evidence of portal hypertension (ascites, variceal hemorrhage and severe edema) may develop in some patients. Biochemical abnormalities include hyperbilirubinemia and a cholestatic pattern of liver enzyme abnormalities (i.e., increased serum levels of alkaline phosphatase and γ-glutamyl transpeptidase).

Although some investigators have questioned the role of azathioprine hepatotoxicity in the cause of posttransplant liver disease, a study by Pol *et al.* (1996) reported that 21 (2%) of 1,035 patients who received a renal transplant at Necker Hospital in Paris between 1969 and 1992 were diagnosed with azathioprine hepatitis. The diagnosis of azathioprine-induced liver disease was based on the presence of jaundice, which disappeared after azathioprine withdrawal or dose reduction; the absence of any other overt explanation (mainly severe cirrhosis, chronic alcoholism, other hepatotoxic drug or biliovesicular disease) and the demonstration of histopathological findings consistent with intrahepatic

cholestasis, sometimes associated with centrilobular hepatocellular necrosis and vascular lesions. All of these patients were positive for viral markers of hepatotropic infection (hepatitis B surface antigen [HBsAg], HBV RNA or anti-HCV antibodies), and 18 (85%) had liver biopsy lesions consistent with chronic liver disease. In all patients, the jaundice resolved and bilirubin levels normalized within 4 to 12 weeks after dose reduction or discontinuation of azathioprine.

In two patients who underwent repeat liver biopsy 2 and 4 months after withdrawal of azathioprine, histology revealed disappearance of intrahepatic cholestasis and centrilobular hepatocellular necrosis. Rechallenge with azathioprine led to relapse of jaundice and recurrence of azathioprine-associated lesions on liver biopsy specimens. Jaundice disappeared after azathioprine discontinuation. Although this study did not address the mechanisms of azathioprine-induced hepatotoxicity, the authors speculated that active hepatotropic viral infection (HBV and/or HCV) causes liver disease and decreased catabolism of azathioprine toxic metabolites, which could predispose to azathioprine toxicity or induce it. It was concluded that azathioprine hepatitis in renal transplant recipients probably is facilitated or induced by HBV-associated or HCV-associated chronic hepatitis. Pol and colleagues recommended considering azathioprine dose reduction or withdrawal during diagnostic evaluation and treatment of viral liver disease in patients whose immunosuppressive regimens included azathioprine (Pol *et al.*, 1996).

Azathioprine-induced hepatic endothelial cell injury has been implicated in the characteristic vascular lesions observed in the liver in close relation to azathioprine therapy (i.e., peliosis hepatis, nodular regenerative hyperplasia and venoocclusive disease) (Haboubi *et al.*, 1988). The histological lesions and the clinical presentation of peliosis hepatis and nodular regenerative hyperplasia were discussed in the previous section.

Venoocclusive Disease

Venoocclusive disease is a liver complication that has been well characterized among bone marrow transplant recipients but can develop occasionally among renal transplant recipients. Liver biopsy is the only means of diagnosing venoocclusive disease. Because of the histological characteristics of this disease and the irregular distribution of the liver lesions, however, the diagnosis may be problematic. The reported incidence of 2.5% in some studies may be an overestimate and may reflect referral bias to particular centers (Liano *et al.*, 1989).

The pathogenesis of venoocclusive disease is unclear. Endothelial cell damage caused by azathioprine therapy or previous hepatotropic viral infection has been incriminated in the development of venoocclusive disease in renal transplant recipients (Haboubi *et al.*, 1988; Liano *et al.*, 1989). The role of azathioprine in the pathogenesis of venoocclusive disease seems possible but is unproven. Immunosuppression induced by azathioprine together with hepatic viral insult could be responsible for the development of venoocclusive disease (Liano *et al.*, 1989; Read *et al.*, 1986). This possibility is supported by the observation that azathioprine has been a part of the immunosuppressive regimen of all renal transplant recipients who have developed the disease.

A report of a patient with venoocclusive disease who showed improvement after azathioprine was discontinued and deterioration after it was reinstituted suggests its direct toxic effect (Katzka *et al.*, 1986). Despite the fact that most renal transplant recipients over the years have been treated with azathioprine, venoocclusive disease has been observed only rarely (Liano *et al.*, 1989). With the one exception just cited, no patient with venoocclusive disease has improved after discontinuation of azathioprine.

Venoocclusive disease has a later onset among renal transplant recipients (mean, 15 months posttransplantation; range, 8–32 months posttransplantation) as compared with bone marrow transplant recipients, in whom this disease usually develops during the first posttransplant month (Katzka et al., 1986). Venoocclusive disease is commoner in males and presents clinically with jaundice and symptoms of portal hypertension—ascites, hepatomegaly and splenomegaly (Liano et al., 1989). In some cases, mild laboratory abnormalities preceded clinical manifestations (Liano et al., 1989; Marubbio and Danielson, 1975) and were detected as early as 2 to 6 months after transplantation (Liano et al., 1989). In most cases, the initial presentation was jaundice, which occurred 6 to 108 months posttransplantation and generally was accompanied by abdominal pain and ascites and less frequently by hepatomegaly (Liano et al., 1989; Marubbio and Danielson, 1975). The prognosis is grim. Of these patients, 86% have been found to develop evidence of portal hypertension at some point during the clinical course (Katzka et al., 1986) and may progress subsequently to hepatic encephalopathy and death owing to liver failure. The mortality rate is high—55 to 70% of the reported patients died 12 to 79 months after transplantation (Liano et al., 1989).

Venoocclusive disease could be reversible or slowly progressive, with reported evolution of 138 months (Liano et al., 1989; Read et al., 1986). Although uncommon, the diagnosis of venoocclusive disease always should be considered, after excluding all other causes of liver disease, in all patients with posttransplant liver disease, particularly men, who present with mildly to moderately elevated serum levels of transaminases and alkaline phosphatase and clinical evidence of hepatomegaly and jaundice and who have been in contact with hepatotropic viruses (HBV, HCV or CMV) (Liano et al., 1989; Read et al., 1986).

There is no specific treatment for venoocclusive disease. Azathioprine should be discontinued. The use of anticoagulants has been disappointing. Portacaval shunt and liver transplantation are therapeutic options in advanced stages of venoocclusive disease. Conservative management may be compatible with long-term survival, however (Liano et al., 1989).

The hepatotoxicity of azathioprine is debatable. Although azathioprine probably can cause significant and life-threatening hepatotoxicity, it is likely that the magnitude of this problem will decrease in the future because of the rarity of this condition, the decrease in the prevalence of HBV and HCV infection among patients receiving renal replacement therapy and the replacement of azathioprine by the newer immunosuppressive agent mycophenolate mofetil.

CYCLOSPORINE-INDUCED HEPATOTOXICITY

Cyclosporine has been in use in clinical transplantation since 1978. Numerous trials have evaluated the impact of cyclosporine on graft and patient survival in renal transplantation and have reported on its adverse effects. Nephrotoxicity has been the major concern. Cyclosporine hepatotoxicity is less important (Canadian Multicentre Transplant Study Group, 1983, 1986; European Multicentre Trial Group, 1983).

The pathogenesis of cyclosporine hepatotoxicity has not been elucidated completely. Animal studies have provided some insight into the mechanisms of the hepatotoxic effects of cyclosporine. Evidence exists to suggest that the increase in total intracellular calcium concentration after hepatocyte exposure to cyclosporine is highly toxic to the hepatocyte

function and could account for cyclosporine-related hepatotoxicity (Nicchitta et al., 1985). In cyclosporine-treated rats (25 mg/kg), hypoalbuminemia, hyperbilirubinemia and hypertransaminasemia developed together with histopathological findings of centrilobular fatty changes, dilatation of endoplasmic reticulum, loss of ribosomes and occasional hepatocyte necrosis (Ryffel et al., 1983). In the isolated perfused rat liver model, cyclosporine administration was associated with a dose-dependent decrease of the bile flow, more precisely of the bile acid–dependent fraction, as a result of inhibition of bile acid secretion. Cyclosporine had no effect on alkaline phosphatase concentrations, and there were no significant differences in the transaminase levels between the cyclosporine and the control groups. Light microscopy did not reveal any histological evidence of cholestasis or hepatocellular damage (Rotolo et al., 1985).

Among renal transplant recipients, cyclosporine hepatotoxicity of different degrees of severity has been reported in 4 to 63% of the patients (Canadian Multicentre Transplant Study Group, 1983; European Multicentre Trial Group, 1983; Kahan et al., 1985; Klintmalm et al., 1981; Rotolo et al., 1985). The wide variation in the reported incidence is related largely to the definition of liver dysfunction, cyclosporine dosage, follow-up period and study population selection (Calne et al., 1978). In more recent studies, a decrease in the frequency of cyclosporine-related hepatotoxic events has been noted, presumably as a result of the lower cyclosporine dosages used in the newer immunosuppressive regimens (Canadian Multicentre Transplant Study Group, 1986; European Multicentre Trial Group, 1983). In most cases of implicated cyclosporine hepatotoxicity, the coexistence of confounding factors that could impair liver function, such as infection, hemolysis, graft-versus-host disease, congestive heart failure and drug interactions, makes it difficult to appreciate the true contribution of cyclosporine in liver injury.

Clinical cyclosporine hepatotoxicity commonly occurs early in the posttransplant period, usually within the first 3 months (Lorber et al., 1987), and presents as acute hepatic injury, mainly of cholestatic type. A possible association of cyclosporine with biliary tract disease (i.e., formation of gallstones and biliary sludge) has been reported (Lorber et al., 1987). The commonest biochemical abnormality is conjugated hyperbilirubinemia alone or in association with minimal elevation in liver enzymes. The increase in serum bilirubin appears to be dose dependent and reversible after dose adjustment or discontinuation of the drug (Canadian Multicentre Transplant Study Group, 1983).

In a large study with a 49% incidence of cyclosporine-induced hepatotoxicity, most of the patients (61%) showed elevated serum bilirubin or transaminase levels along with elevation of alkaline phosphatase and lactate dehydrogenase. Liver function test abnormalities developed during the initial 90 days posttransplantation in 94% of the cases, compared with after 90 days in only 6%. Reduction in cyclosporine dose alone resulted in resolution of LFT abnormalities in 81% of the patients, whereas another 14% experienced recurrent episodes or persistently abnormal liver biochemistry, and 5% developed biliary calculous disease (Lorber et al., 1987).

Other authors have observed that transient elevations of serum bilirubin concentrations occurred with the same frequency among cyclosporine-treated patients compared to patients whose immunosuppressive regimen did not include cyclosporine. Serum bilirubin levels were similar in these two groups, but serum aspartate transaminase (AST) levels tended to be higher among the azathioprine-treated patients when compared with patients in the cyclosporine-treated group (Najarian et al., 1985). Similarly, Moreno and colleagues reported that among renal transplant recipients without preexisting liver disease, azathioprine-treated patients had a higher incidence of posttransplant chronic liver disease compared with cyclosporine-treated patients (Moreno *et al.*, 1990).

In some studies, cyclosporine therapy in renal transplant recipients with preexisting chronic liver disease was associated with a lack of clinical evidence of progression to severe chronic liver disease and with complete normalization of the biochemical abnormalities with persistent clinical remission (Moreno *et al.*, 1990) and liver morphology, which remained unchanged over a follow-up period of 1 year (Morales *et al.*, 1989). Compared with azathioprine-treated patients, patients who received cyclosporine had slightly higher probability of remaining stable, showing no signs of progression to severe liver disease in the posttransplant period (Moreno *et al.*, 1990). Cyclosporine could modify the course of chronic liver disease after renal transplantation. Cyclosporine therapy was shown to result in clinical and histological improvement in non–renal disease patients with CAH, refractory to treatment with steroid and/or azathioprine (Hyams *et al.*, 1987). These data provide evidence against true hepatotoxic properties of cyclosporine and add strength to the contention that the drug can be used safely in patients with chronic liver disease. Whether cyclosporine therapy could be beneficial in patients with CAH is unclear.

Current data suggest that cyclosporine hepatotoxicity is a rare phenomenon, presents in the early posttransplantation period, appears to be dose dependent, typically is reversible with dose adjustment and has minor or no clinical relevance. No specific liver lesion has been linked to long-term cyclosporine therapy, and long-term cyclosporine therapy seems unlikely to produce chronic hepatotoxicity. Cyclosporine might be the drug of choice in patients with chronic liver disease undergoing renal transplantation (Moreno *et al.*, 1990).

Systemic Viral Infections Producing Hepatitis—Herpesviruses

The herpesviruses are a family of large enveloped DNA viruses that have been implicated as a primary cause of morbidity and mortality in transplant recipients. Although the herpesviruses are not primarily hepatotropic, liver involvement frequently is a part of the clinical presentation of herpesvirus-related diseases.

CYTOMEGALOVIRUS

Human CMV is a β-herpesvirus with a linear double-stranded DNA genome of 230 kb pairs. Once acquired, the virus establishes latency and may remain silent indefinitely while being excreted in saliva, urine, tears, breast milk, sperm and vaginal secretions. Apparently, any cell can be infected latently with CMV.

Host factors seem to determine the susceptibility to CMV infection and the related morbidity. The virus is transmitted with solid-organ transplantation. Preexisting immunity to CMV seems to be particularly important in the control of virus replication and spread. In renal transplant recipients, seroconversion has occurred in 36 to 95% of seronegative patients who received kidneys from seropositive donors compared with only 0 to 30% of seronegative recipients of kidneys from seronegative cadaver donors. Only seronegative recipients of organs from seropositive donors (but not seronegative recipients from seronegative donors) were found to shed CMV as a result of acquired infection and active viral replication. Seropositive renal transplant recipients can expe-

rience reactivation of endogenous latent CMV in the posttransplantation period and show evidence of CMV infection in 90 to 100%, regardless of the donor CMV status. This finding essentially implies that almost all seropositive patients experience reactivation of their own latent virus after transplantation because of pharmacological immunosuppression. Overall, CMV infections have developed in 70 to 90% of renal transplant recipients, with onset during the first 6 months posttransplantation (Natov and Pereira, 1997).

Three clearly distinguishable epidemiological patterns of CMV infection have been observed in transplant recipients:

1. *Primary infection*: Occurs in transplant recipients with no previous exposure to CMV (e.g., seronegative at the time of transplantation, who receive an organ from a seropositive donor). These patients are identified by the appearance of antibody to CMV and/or by positive cultures.

2. *Reinfection*: Occurs when seropositive transplant recipients receive an allograft from a seropositive donor and shed the virus of donor origin.

3. *Reactivation infection*: Occurs in seropositive individuals who experience reactivation of endogenous latent virus after transplantation regardless of the serological status of the donor.

Reinfection and reactivation are commonly referred to as *secondary infection* and are identified by a fourfold or higher increase in the titer of antibody to CMV.

Cytomegalovirus disease is defined as a symptomatic CMV infection characterized by fever, leukopenia and often organ-specific symptoms. The incidence of CMV disease in renal allograft recipients is 22 to 28%. A disease rate of 57% has been reported among patients who excrete the virus posttransplantation. Pretransplant immunity seems to offer some protection against the donor virus and to a certain degree may prevent its dissemination. Cytomegalovirus disease is significantly commoner among recipients with primary CMV infection (61–91%) than among recipients with secondary infection (23–42%), and CMV disease is more severe and has a significantly longer duration of fever and leukopenia in patients with primary infection than in patients with reinfection. Some investigators have observed that the incidence of CMV disease in seropositive recipients of kidneys from seropositive donors was similar to that in seropositive kidney recipients of seronegative donors (24% *vs.* 20%). Although reactivation was a mild disease with no major complications, reinfection was associated with clinically more severe disease. In contrast, others have observed that in recipients with pretransplant CMV infection, posttransplantation CMV disease occurred only among patients who received organs from seropositive donors (39%) but not among those who were transplanted with organs from seronegative donors, implying that the preexisting infection did not protect from reinfection (Natov and Pereira, 1997).

The immunosuppressed state can modulate the effects of the virus and affect the course of CMV infection. It has been shown that antilymphocyte antibody, owing to its ability to reactivate latent virus, can increase the incidence of CMV disease. In turn, the subsequent use of cyclosporine in the presence of replicating virus can play the role of a potent promoter of CMV replication and dissemination and thus can further aggravate the course of CMV disease.

Cytomegalovirus can cause acute hepatitis as the main clinical presentation of CMV disease. In the immunocompetent patient, hepatitis usually is mild and self-limiting with only mildly to moderately elevated serum levels of transaminases and alkaline phosphatase. Rarely the hepatitis can become so prominent that other causes are considered. In the immunocompromised renal transplant recipient, the diagnosis of CMV hepatitis is based on the clinical findings characteristic for a typical symptomatic CMV infection—spiking or constant fever that begins 4 to 10 weeks posttransplantation and general malaise or tiredness, often in the presence of hematological tests revealing leukopenia, thrombocytopenia and atypical lymphocytes. A few days later, these signs may be followed by the development of respiratory symptoms and less commonly by arthralgia, splenomegaly, myalgia, gastrointestinal ulcerations with bleeding and encephalitis. Cytomegalovirus retinitis is a severe late manifestation.

Acute hepatitis is common in the course of CMV infection. In one study, CMV was believed to be responsible for 47% of all episodes of acute liver disease in the posttransplant period (Ware et al., 1979). Cytomegalovirus hepatitis commonly develops 2 to 3 months after renal transplantation (Luby et al., 1974; Ware et al., 1975), which corresponds to the typical onset of CMV infection (1–4 months posttransplantation) (Rubin, 1993). In cases of overt hepatitis, jaundice and hepatomegaly are present. Laboratory tests reveal only transiently and mildly elevated alanine aminotransferase (ALT) values and rarely hyperbilirubinemia (Naraqi et al., 1978). Usually the duration of LFT abnormalities is 1 to 20 weeks, after which the liver disease resolves, consistent with the excellent prognosis of CMV-induced hepatitis. Liver histology usually shows inclusion bodies, frequently in the hepatocytes but also in the vascular endothelium and bile epithelium (Napel et al., 1984). The presence of intranuclear inclusions has been correlated with a poor inflammatory infiltration and with increased liver damage, suggesting that in the absence of a normal immune response the virus has a direct cytolytic effect on the liver. Occasionally, more commonly among liver transplant recipients than in other solid-organ transplant recipients, CMV hepatitis can develop into a more serious disease.

Most patients recover from CMV infection after a febrile period of about 1 month or more. About 2% of patients fail to respond to the virus with antibody production and progress to develop disseminated fatal disease (Simmons et al., 1977). In the rare event of lethal CMV disease, the usual cause of death is severe pneumonitis. Liver failure develops as a part of multiorgan involvement. At autopsy, the pathological findings in the liver include bile stasis, congestion, plasma infiltration, fatty metamorphosis and CMV inclusion bodies (Simmons et al., 1974).

Serological diagnosis conventionally is based on the seroconversion of a previously seronegative patient (primary infection) or on a fourfold (or higher) increase of antibody titer in the serum of a previously seropositive patient. Antibodies of IgM and IgG class can be measured by a variety of methods. Enzyme-linked immunosorbent assay (ELISA) has been found to be the most sensitive test. As a result of ineffective antiviral immune responses during immunosuppressive therapy, serological responses in transplant recipients frequently are delayed and unreliable. IgG titers do not rise for approximately 6 weeks, and transplant recipients often fail to produce IgM antibodies during the first 2 months after transplantation (Muller et al., 1993). The diagnosis of CMV infection frequently requires detection of the virus itself.

Viral cultures detect the virus and are based on the development of CMV-induced cytopathic effect in human fibroblast cell cultures. This development takes 5 to 28 days, and diagnosis inevitably is delayed. Other more rapid diagnostic methods usually are applied for diagnosis, including detection of CMV DNA by in situ hybridization or by polymerase chain reaction (PCR) and detection of early CMV antigens in infected cell cultures within 24 to 48 hours.

Treatment and prevention of CMV-induced hepatitis consists of the general principles of treatment and prevention of CMV infection with gancyclovir and intravenous administration of immune globulin, conventional management of hepatitis and aggressive supportive care in case of liver failure.

EPSTEIN-BARR VIRUS

Epstein-Barr virus (EBV) is another ubiquitous member of the herpesvirus family. It contains a double-stranded molecule of DNA, approximately 172 kb in length. Greater than 80% of all individuals have been exposed to the virus by the time they reach adulthood. Epstein-Barr virus most likely is transmitted by aerosolized particles or through mouth-to-mouth contact. Epstein-Barr virus infection may present as primary or secondary infection (reactivation). Primary infection occurs in individuals with no previous exposure to EBV and usually is defined by the appearance of antibodies to Epstein-Barr viral-capsid antigen (Schooley et al., 1983). Primary infection may develop at any age. In children, infection is most often asymptomatic. In adolescents and young adults, it usually results in infectious mononucleosis clinically presenting with sore throat, fever and cervical lymphadenopathy. Typically, EBV establishes latency but may reactivate later at any time. Reactivation refers to replication of the endogenous latent virus and manifests with EBV shedding in the saliva or cervical secretions. It is defined by a fourfold or greater rise in the titer of antibody to Epstein-Barr viral-capsid antigen or the diffuse or restricted early antigen (Schooley et al., 1983). Reactivation is much more frequent in immunosuppressed individuals. One half to two thirds of renal transplant patients excrete EBV in pharyngeal secretions, which is significantly higher than the 16 to 18% EBV excretion rate among seropositive healthy individuals (Chang et al., 1973, 1978; Cheeseman et al., 1980; Strauch et al., 1974).

During the first 2 months posttransplantation, renal transplant recipients have the same EBV excretion rate (15%) as healthy individuals (16%). Subsequently the excretion rate increases to reach its peak (87%) between the 3rd and 12th month, after which it decreases to 58% 1 to 2 years, then to 50% 2 to 10 years posttransplantation (Chang et al., 1978). Commonly the presence of EBV in these patients is not associated with clinical illness. In renal transplant recipients, the incidence of clinically manifested EBV infection (EBV disease) ranges from 0 to 30% (Marker et al., 1979; Naraqi et al., 1977; Schooley et al., 1983). Because most individuals acquire EBV early in life, in most renal transplant recipients, EBV-associated clinical illness results from reactivation of latent virus.

Epstein-Barr virus disease occurs relatively early in the posttransplant period. In one series, about two thirds of the cases of EBV-associated illness developed in the initial 6 months posttransplantation (Naraqi et al., 1977), whereas in another, all cases occurred in the first 3 months posttransplantation (Schooley et al., 1983). In a retrospective study, renal transplant recipients with an eightfold or greater rise in EBV antibody had a complicated clinical course with frequent occurrences of prolonged periods of posttransplant fever, simultaneous rise in CMV antibody levels, development of lymphoproliferative disorder and death owing to Pseudomonas sepsis (Marker et al., 1979).

Immunosuppression can modulate the course of EBV infection. Immunosuppressive regimens including, in particular, polyclonal antilymphocyte globulin, monoclonal antibody, OKT3 and cyclosporine are risk factors for the development of EBV-related lymphoproliferative disorders posttransplantation (Langnas et al., 1994; Preiksaitis et al., 1992; Rubin, 1993). Antilymphocyte antibody has the property to enhance EBV replication and consequently increases the potential for secondary infection of B cells. In turn, the subsequent use of cyclosporine blocks in a dose-dependent manner the surveillance mechanism responsible for the elimination of these transformed B cells. As a result, the immunosuppressed transplant recipient is susceptible to the development of prominent EBV-associated posttransplant lymphoproliferative disorders.

The classic presentation of EBV-induced mononucleosis is usually not seen among transplant recipients. Instead, many infectious mononucleosis–like symptoms and a variety of clinical presentations of EBV lymphoproliferative disease including tonsillitis; fever; hepatocellular dysfunction; focal involvement of the brain, lungs and gastrointestinal tract and focal disease invading the allograft have been reported (Rubin, 1993). Hepatitis commonly develops as a part of EBV disease and has a mild to moderate clinical presentation (Fuhrman et al., 1987; Markin, 1994). Jaundice can be detected in 10% of cases. Laboratory tests reveal occasional minor elevations in serum bilirubin levels, commonly ascribed to a combination of viral-induced intrahepatic cholestasis and/or ongoing hemolysis (Markin, 1994), and only mildly elevated ALT (Naraqi et al., 1978), in contrast to the marked increase seen in HBsAg-positive patients with hepatitis (Naraqi et al., 1978).

In a large series of 1,593 renal transplant recipients, lymphoproliferative disease developed in 19 patients (1.2% incidence) with a mean interval of 3.2 years after renal transplantation, and EBV was implicated as a causative agent (Hanto et al., 1983). Immunosuppressive therapies included azathioprine, prednisone, local graft irradiation and antilymphocyte globulin; only one patient received a cyclosporine-prednisone regimen. The clinical course of these patients could be classified into two different clinical syndromes. The first clinical syndrome developed soon after transplantation or antirejection therapy (mean, 9 months); was present in 8 (48%) of these patients, who were usually young (mean age, 23 years) and was characterized by a lymphoproliferative disease resembling an infectious mononucleosis–like illness with fever, sore throat and lymphadenopathy. Untreated, these patients eventually developed rapidly progressive and widely disseminated lymphoproliferative disease involving the liver, spleen and other visceral organs and resembling fatal infectious mononucleosis with a mortality rate of 75% (Hanto et al., 1983). Liver failure together with bacterial sepsis complicated the rapid and fatal course of one patient who died 10 days after presentation. Liver function tests were abnormal in another patient who had biopsy-proven lesions of polymorphic B-cell lymphoma. After transplant nephrectomy and discontinuation of immunosuppressive therapy, lesions regressed over the next 2 months. Six years later, while on hemodialysis, this patient had no evidence of disease. The second clinical syndrome occurred much later in the posttransplant period (mean, 6 years); involved the other 11 (52%) of the renal transplant recipients with lymphoproliferative disease, who were older (mean age, 48 years; range 22–68 years) and was characterized by prominent extranodal lymphoproliferation including masses developing in the central nervous system, gastrointestinal tract and liver. The clinical course was that of an aggressive, and in 91% of the cases lethal, lymphoproliferative disease. Progressive liver destruction commonly was the result of massive tumor spread to the liver and occurred in the setting of multiorgan failure (Hanto et al., 1983).

Epstein-Barr virus–associated liver disease includes a broad spectrum of histological changes. Some of the lesions, in particular after liver transplantation, may resemble the histological findings associated with infectious mononucleosis—portal inflammation consisting primarily of lymphocytes, unaffected bile ducts, hepatic arterioles and portal venules, hepatocellular ballooning and mitoses and mild canalicular cholestasis (Markin, 1994). Posttransplant lymphoproliferative disorders also may present as a prominent portal infiltrate composed of a mixture of cells ranging from small round lymphocytes to plasmatic lymphocytes and immunoblastic forms. This presentation is associated with prominent bile duct damage, infiltrates into the surrounding parenchyma across the limiting plate, focal parenchymal or prominent pericentral necrosis and steatosis. Immunoperoxidase staining reveals primarily B cells and some admixed T cells. The immune globulin–staining pattern may show a polyclonal or a monoclonal distribution of immune globulins. Although not always predictable, a positive response to decreasing immunosuppression is more likely to occur in patients who show a polyclonal distribution of immune globulin staining than among those who show a monoclonal distribution and who also are more likely to develop a systemic lymphoma.

Antiviral therapy with acyclovir or gancyclovir can halt the replication of EBV (Rubin, 1993). Preventive antiviral strategies, including antiviral therapy during periods of increased immunosuppression (especially when antilymphocyte antibody preparations are being used), seem to be justified because EBV-associated lymphoproliferative disease has been shown to develop in the subgroup of individuals with the highest degree of viral replication, which by itself is related to immunosuppressive therapy. Although of uncertain benefit, in all serious cases of EBV hepatitis, a trial of high-dose intravenous acyclovir is imperative. This trial should be done in conjunction with minimizing or discontinuing the immunosuppressive medications, particularly cyclosporine. Conventional lymphoma treatment (surgical excision, chemotherapy and radiation therapy) should be used when appropriate.

HERPES SIMPLEX VIRUS

Herpes simplex virus is another herpesvirus with a linear, double-stranded DNA molecule. Two types of HSV have been identified—HSV-1 and HSV-2, both sharing genomic sequences and antigenic properties. Herpes simplex virus can infect nearly all visceral and mucocutaneous sites. The clinical course of HSV infection depends on the age and immune status of the host, the anatomical site of infection and the antigenic type of the virus. Herpes simplex virus infection may present as primary or secondary infection. Primary infection occurs in individuals with no previous exposure to HSV, usually early in life, and in most cases has a subclinical presentation. Once acquired, HSV tends to establish latency. Subsequently, secondary infection may occur as a result of reactivation of the endogenous latent virus.

Herpes simplex virus infection is common among renal transplant recipients and has an incidence of 50 to 60% (Naraqi et al., 1977; Pass et al., 1978, 1979). Most cases occur during the first 2 months, when the degree of immunosuppression is the highest (Naraqi et al., 1977; Pass et al., 1978, 1979). Herpes simplex virus rarely causes liver disease in solid-organ transplant recipients, however. Among 3,536 liver, kidney and heart transplant recipients, the overall frequency of HSV hepatitis was found to be 0.3% with a male/female ratio of 5/7 (Kusne et al., 1991).

Herpes simplex virus hepatitis typically occurs as part of disseminated HSV infection early in the posttransplant period (median, 18 days posttransplantation; range, 5–46 days posttransplantation) (Kusne et al., 1991). Its timing precedes that of CMV hepatitis, which peaks 30 to 40 days posttransplantation. After that time, HSV infection continues to occur, although at a reduced rate (Naraqi et al., 1977). Late onset of HSV hepatitis (>2 years posttransplantation) has been documented, which indicates that a small risk of HSV hepatitis persists long after transplantation (Kusne et al., 1991).

Herpes simplex virus hepatitis commonly presents as a severe disease, with rapid, sometimes fulminant course, often with fatal outcome (Anuras and Summers, 1976; Elliot et al., 1980; Kusne et al., 1991; Naraqi et al., 1977; Taylor et al., 1981). The diagnosis is difficult and frequently delayed. Early awareness of the disease is crucial, however, because timely treatment may improve prognosis. The clinical presentation of HSV hepatitis typically includes fever (>38.5°C), stomatitis, mucocutaneous (herpetic) lesions, right upper quadrant tenderness, hepatomegaly and abdominal pain (Elliot et al., 1980; Kusne et al., 1991; Taylor et al., 1981). Pleural effusion, atelectasis and consolidation, not necessarily related to HSV pneumonia, may be present on chest radiograph. Laboratory findings include left shift with numerous band forms on the peripheral blood smear, thrombocytopenia, elevated serum transaminases and hyperbilirubinemia (Elliot et al., 1980; Kusne et al., 1991).

Herpes simplex virus hepatitis has a high mortality rate. Lethal outcome has occurred in 70% of patients (Kusne et al., 1991). The laboratory abnormalities that have been associated with fatal outcome are low platelet count, high percentage of bands on the peripheral blood smear, prolonged partial thromboplastin time (but normal prothrombin time) and a high serum creatinine at the time of diagnosis. All patients who developed hypotension, metabolic acidosis, gastrointestinal bleeding, disseminated intravascular coagulation and bacteremia and almost 90% of those with renal failure (serum creatinine >1.5 mg/dl) died.

Histologically, two distinct types of liver involvement—diffuse and focal HSV hepatitis—have been described. In the series reported by Kusne et al. (1991), 30% of patients with histologically proven hepatitis presented with diffuse HSV hepatitis; the rest had only focal involvement of the liver. All patients with diffuse hepatitis and more than half of patients with focal hepatitis died. At necropsy, 70% of patients with fatal HSV hepatitis had disseminated HSV disease involving two or more visceral organs, including lungs, trachea, larynx, esophagus, stomach, pancreas, adrenals, spleen and bladder. Evidence of disseminated intravascular coagulation was found in all patients that died. The difference in the pathogenesis between the two forms of hepatitis is poorly understood. At least in the group with diffuse hepatitis, however, the massive involvement of the liver leading to severe coagulopathy and liver failure was apparently the cause of death. Transplant recipients who present with fever, progressive transaminase elevation, abdominal symptoms and coagulopathy in the first month after transplantation always should raise the suspicion of HSV hepatitis and prompt immediate institution of intravenous acyclovir therapy at a dose of 5 mg/kg three times daily.

Prophylactic oral acyclovir administered in renal transplant recipients in the early posttransplant period has been found to be effective against HSV infection (Pettersson et al., 1985; Seale et al., 1985) and has prevented the development of HSV hepatitis (Kusne et al., 1991). Prophylaxis with oral acyclovir (200 mg three to four times daily) is recommended during the first posttransplant month (Kusne et al., 1991; Pettersson et al., 1985; Seale et al., 1985).

VARICELLA-ZOSTER VIRUS

Varicella-zoster virus (VZV) is a double-stranded DNA virus, which causes two distinct diseases—varicella (chickenpox) and herpes zoster (shingles). Varicella is the clinical presentation of a primary infection with the virus, and it is usually a benign self-limiting illness in immunocompetent patients. It is mild and common in children and more severe and rare in adults. Herpes zoster is the consequence of a recurrent (secondary) infection, which typically occurs in adults and may be quite debilitating, but in the normal host it usually is a self-limiting and relatively benign disease with good prognosis.

Among renal transplant recipients, VZV infection has an annual incidence of 0.8 to 10%, which is more than 10 times the rate among healthy individuals (Bradley et al., 1987; Lynfield et al., 1992; Naraqi et al., 1977; Parnham et al., 1995; Warrell et al., 1980; Zayas et al., 1996). Most of the cases occur in patients with negative varicella serology and represent primary infection. Some of these patients may present with reactivation of latent virus rather than with new infection because it has been shown that immunosuppression may interfere with antibody production and lead to loss of antibody among seropositive patients. It has been reported that some renal transplant recipients with previous history of chickenpox may test seronegative for VZV (Feldhoff et al., 1981; Parnham et al., 1995).

Severe pain that precedes the onset of rash by 1 to 4 days is a common presenting symptom (Parnham et al., 1995) and is believed to be a predictor of high mortality (Feldhoff et al., 1981). In the renal transplant patient, as in any immunocompromised host, disseminated VZV can lead to severe disease with visceral organ involvement, disseminated intravascular coagulation and a fatal outcome. Severe disease usually is associated with primary infection. Secondary infections are believed to have a better prognosis (Parnham et al., 1995). Clinical hepatitis usually occurs as part of multiorgan involvement in almost all patients with disseminated varicella and zoster and presents with jaundice and hepatomegaly (Lynfield et al., 1992; Parnham et al., 1995). Laboratory tests usually reveal moderate to severe elevations in serum transaminases and bilirubin (Lynfield et al., 1992; Parnham et al., 1995). Hepatic failure and/or disseminated intravascular coagulation is commonly the cause of death in fatal disseminated disease. Cases of fulminant hepatitis have been reported in bone marrow and solid-organ transplant recipients (Bensousan et al., 1995; Lynfield et al., 1992; Morishita et al., 1985). Postmortem examination has revealed multiple hemorrhages and necrosis in the liver, sometimes in the presence of disseminated intravascular coagulation with pulmonary and gastrointestinal hemorrhages (Lynfield et al., 1992).

Mortality rates among renal transplant recipients with primary VZV infection range from 0 to 80% (Bradley et al., 1987; Feldhoff et al., 1981; Lynfield et al., 1992; Parnham et al., 1995; Zayas et al., 1996). All deaths have occurred in patients with disseminated disease and visceral involvement. This wide range in mortality rates most likely is related to differences in the management of renal transplant recipients with known exposure to VZV or clinically demonstrated disease. Using higher doses of cyclosporine and having the patient remain on azathioprine therapy for 3 or more days after the onset of the viral illness have been associated with increased incidence of severe disease and greater morbidity and mortality among pediatric solid-organ transplant recipients (Feldhoff et al., 1981; McGregor et al., 1989).

Prophylaxis, early diagnosis, timely institution of treatment, discontinuation of azathioprine and modification in the immunosuppressive regimen in association with aggressive supportive care may improve prognosis and decrease mortality to 0 (Parnham et al., 1995). Prophylaxis with varicella zoster immune globulin was found to be effective in preventing VZV primary infection in 100% of the cases when administered within 72 hours of contact with varicella (Zayas et al., 1996) or was suspected to moderate the severity of the disease in cases in which primary prevention had failed (Parnham *et al.*, 1995). Once varicella is established, no proven benefit of varicella zoster immune globulin has been reported (Parnham *et al.*, 1995). Decrease in the dosage or discontinuation of azathioprine, adjustment in cyclosporine dose to keep blood levels strictly within therapeutic range and maintenance or increase of steroid dose are believed to ameliorate the clinical course of the disease and have not resulted in transplant rejection (Lynfield *et al.*, 1992; Parnham *et al.*, 1995; Zayas *et al.*, 1996). Timely institution of high-dose intravenous acyclovir therapy (10 mg/kg every 8 hours) has been associated with improved prognosis (Lynfield *et al.*, 1992; Parnham *et al.*, 1995; Zayas *et al.*, 1996). General principles applied in the treatment of hepatitis and aggressive supportive care are crucial in the management of these patients.

Not all cases of severe or fatal disease could be prevented, leading to the need for a new strategy—active immunization (Lynfield *et al.*, 1992; Zayas *et al.*, 1996). In one study from France, after administering varicella vaccine to seronegative uremic children and seropositive children with low antibody titers at least 2 months before transplantation, only a few cases of exclusively mild varicella occurred. This observation suggests that the vaccine might have played a protective role in preventing or moderating the severity of primary VZV infection (Broyer and Boudailliez, 1985).

HUMAN HERPESVIRUS 6

Human herpesvirus 6 (HHV-6) is a cytopathic lymphotropic human herpesvirus. The virus is highly prevalent in young children, with rates higher than 90% by the age of 3 (Yanagi *et al.*, 1990). More than 80% of the adult population worldwide have been infected or are currently infected with HHV-6 (Herbein *et al.*, 1996). In some series, antibody directed against HHV-6 can be detected in 85 to 100% of adults (Yanagi *et al.*, 1990). Primary infection causes exanthema subitum (roseola infantum) in infants (Yamanishi *et al.*, 1988). In older children and adults, it may present as febrile illness with lymphadenopathy (Niederman *et al.*, 1988) or infectious mononucleosis–like syndrome (Irving and Cunningham, 1990). Secondary infections resulting from viral reactivation have been suggested by serology in cardiac transplant recipients (Robert *et al.*, 1994). Different degrees of liver impairment, usually with a benign, self-limiting course but also including anecdotal cases of fulminant hepatitis, have been associated with primary HHV-6 infection among immunocompetent patients (Asano *et al.*, 1990; Dubedat and Kappagoda, 1989; Sobue *et al.*, 1991). It is difficult to determine whether these associations were causal or coincidental.

The estimated rate of detecting HHV-6 among recipients of solid-organ transplants is 14 to 82% depending on the type of the transplant (DesJardin *et al.*, 1998; Dockrell *et al.*, 1997; Morris *et al.*, 1989). The clinical significance of HHV-6 detection after organ transplantation is unclear. In the immunocompromised transplant recipient, HHV-6 usually causes asymptomatic primary and recurrent infections in the posttransplant period. Occasionally, HHV-6 infection can present as a self-limiting febrile illness with or without cutaneous rash in the absence of leukopenia or thrombocytopenia (Morris *et al.*, 1989). Cases of fulminant hepatitis and interstitial pneumonitis also have been observed (Carrigan *et al.*, 1991; Sobue *et al.*, 1991).

Severe clinical presentation during the first 3 months after organ transplantation is unusual unless there is a concomitant CMV infection (Herbein *et al.*, 1996). Clinically significant hepatitis has been reported among these patients (Herbein *et al.*, 1996). Coinfections with HHV-6 and other viruses, especially CMV, appear to be common among bone marrow and

solid-organ transplant recipients (DesJardin *et al.*, 1998; Dockrell *et al.*, 1997; Herbein *et al.*, 1996; Morris *et al.*, 1989). In these cases, it is uncertain whether the symptoms are related to reactivation of HHV-6 (DesJardin *et al.*, 1998) or to a concurrent primary infection with CMV—a well-recognized cause of fever among renal transplant recipients (Morris *et al.*, 1989). Human herpesvirus 6 has been found to have immunomodulating properties *in vitro*. Because of these immunomodulating effects, HHV-6 is likely to create a state of immunosuppression, predisposing the transplant recipient to opportunistic infection with CMV. Data on the timing of infections with HHV-6 and CMV after transplantation suggest that HHV-6 infection occurs within 4 weeks after transplantation (Herbein *et al.*, 1996), preceding CMV infection, which usually develops 4 to 6 weeks after transplantation (Snydman *et al.*, 1987). Reactivation of HHV-6 in renal transplant recipients at risk for primary CMV infection has been associated with primary CMV infection, CMV syndrome and trends for CMV-related hepatitis, CMV-related neutropenia and serious CMV disease (DesJardin *et al.*, 1998).

Gancyclovir and foscarnet are effective against HHV-6 *in vitro* (Burns and Sandford, 1990). Although no clinical studies have been conducted, a therapeutic trial with one of these medications seems to be warranted whenever HHV-6 is suspected to be implicated in the cause of a serious disease, including hepatitis of uncertain origin, developing in the early posttransplant period in a renal transplant recipient. The rest of the treatment of HHV-6-related hepatitis includes supportive care. Recovery is common, even in cases with fulminant hepatitis (Sobue *et al.*, 1991).

Hepatitis Viruses

HEPATITIS B VIRUS

Structure of Hepatitis B Virus Genome

Hepatitis B virus is a small, enveloped DNA virus, a member of the hepadnavirus family (hepatotropic DNA viruses). The virion of hepatitis B consists of surface and core. The surface incorporates the envelope protein, referred to as *HBsAg*. The core contains a DNA polymerase, double-stranded DNA, a core antigen (HBcAg) and another antigen called *e* (HBeAg), which is a protein subunit of the core. Hepatitis B surface antigen may have one of several subtype-specific antigens. The presence of these HBsAg subtypes can be used to provide additional epidemiological markers in evaluating the transmission of HBV infection.

Epidemiology

Routes of Transmission

Hepatitis B virus has ubiquitous distribution. It mainly is transmitted parenterally or by sexual contact (Kingsley *et al.*, 1990; Rosenblum *et al.*, 1992). Horizontal transmission among household contacts of HBV carriers can occur (Botha *et al.*, 1984; Tabor *et al.*, 1985). Transmission by casual contact or food has never been documented. Hepatitis B virus can be transmitted by organ transplantation (Natov and Pereira, 1997).

Prevalence

The incidence and prevalence of HBV infection (HBs-antigenemia) among dialysis patients in the United States are currently 0.06% and 1.1% and have shown a constant decrease over the years as a result of the implementation of dialysis unit precautions and hepatitis B vaccination of susceptible dialysis patients (Tokars *et al.*, 1998). The prevalence of hepatitis B surface antigenemia among renal transplant recipients reported in different studies varies from 1.8 to 18%, most likely as a result of differences in geographical areas, study populations and transplant policies (Degos *et al.*, 1988; Durlik *et al.*, 1996b; Mathurin *et al.*, 1999; Parfrey *et al.*, 1985a; Pol *et al.*, 1990; Yagisawa *et al.*, 1997).

Tests for Detection

Three antigen-antibody systems characterize HBV infection (Locarnini and Gust, 1988). The presence of HBsAg in the serum provides evidence of HBV infection and implies potential infectivity of the blood. The presence of antibody to HBsAg (HBsAb) indicates past infection with HBV or immune response to HBV vaccine. It also may represent passive antibody from hepatitis B immune globulin (HBIG). Hepatitis B e antigen is found only in HBsAg-positive individuals. It correlates with HBV replication and indicates high infectivity. The presence of antibody to HBeAg (anti-HBe) in the serum of a HBsAg carrier suggests lower titer of HBV and lower degree of infectivity. Antibody to HBcAg (anti-HBc) of IgM class indicates recent infection with HBV, whereas anti-HBc of IgG class is a marker of past infection with HBV at some undefined time.

Natural Course of Infection

Hepatitis B virus can cause acute and chronic infections. Acute infection is associated with acute hepatitis defined as a self-limiting disease characterized by acute inflammation and hepatocellular necrosis. The diagnosis rests on detecting HBsAg and anti-HBc of IgM class in the serum of a patient with clinical and laboratory evidence of acute hepatitis. More than half (50–70%) of patients with acute HBV infection do not develop clinically apparent acute hepatitis but have a silent, self-limiting infection because they are able to produce protective antibody (HBsAb and anti-HBc) and ultimately clear the virus. In most cases, acute infection with HBV has a self-limiting course. Fewer than 5% of adults (but 80–90% of infants) fail to mount an adequate immunological response to HBV infection and consequently present with persistent or chronic infection.

Among dialysis patients, as a result of an impaired immune system and inability to produce antibodies, 80% of patients who acquire the virus subsequently remain chronically infected (Fornairon *et al.*, 1996). Chronic HBV infection is accompanied by evidence of hepatocellular injury and inflammation and is associated with chronic hepatitis. The diagnosis is made by showing persistently elevated serum transaminases and HBsAg in the serum for 6 months or more. Active viral replication usually continues for many years and is manifested by the presence of HBeAg and high levels of circulating HBV DNA. Eventually, viral replication diminishes; HBeAg is replaced by anti-HBe, whereas HBsAg and anti-HBc persist. Not all patients with chronic HBV infection develop chronic hepatitis, and some ultimately enter a phase of remission with improvement in liver enzymes despite persistence of HBsAg. These individuals usually are referred to as *healthy* chronic HBsAg carriers. This terminology is in a sense misleading because these patients are at risk of reactivation of infection, and if cirrhosis has already developed, they also are at risk of developing hepatocellular carcinoma. Although the degree and the evolution of hepatocellular injury in patients with chronic HBV infection are variable, about 15 to 20% of patients who acquire the infection in adulthood and 40% of patients who become infected in childhood ultimately progress to liver cirrhosis. In some geographical regions, HBV-infected individuals develop hepatocellular carcinoma at a rate of 5.7% per year (Dusheiko, 1999).

Clinical Course of Hepatitis B Virus Among Renal Transplant Recipients

Compared with a HBsAg-negative patient, a patient who is HBsAg positive on the day of renal transplantation has a 30-fold increased relative risk of developing posttransplant chronic hepatitis (Degos *et al.*, 1980). Because of the state of immunosuppression, the clinical presentation of hepatitis B in renal transplant recipients is commonly insidious. Recognizable acute hepatitis almost never is observed, and the disease tends to be discovered in its chronic phase (Chan *et al.*, 1992). Jaundice is rarely present. Clinical symptoms are mild and consist of vague complaints of general fatigue, malaise or anorexia. The disease commonly is asymptomatic. Liver dysfunction usually presents within the first 12 months, although frank liver disease does not manifest itself until advanced stages are established, late after transplantation (Pirson *et al.*, 1977). Laboratory tests usually show only mild elevations in serum aminotransferase activity, sometimes associated with increased serum bilirubin concentrations. Occasionally, serum aminotransferases do not return to normal values but show fluctuating levels at different times (Rao *et al.*, 1991). The presence of abnormal LFTs for more than 6 months defines the liver disease as chronic.

Among HBV-infected renal transplant recipients, hepatitis B surface antigenemia commonly persists, indicating uninterrupted viral replication, most likely secondary to iatrogenic immunosuppression (Huang *et al.*, 1990; Parfrey *et al.*, 1985b), and in some studies, this has been found to predict poor prognosis (Dusheiko *et al.*, 1983; Harnett *et al.*, 1987; Scott *et al.*, 1987). Enhanced HBV replication has been associated with increased prevalence and accelerated progression of liver disease (Degos *et al.*, 1988; Harnett *et al.*, 1987). It is possible that liver injury occurs as a result of immune-mediated destruction of the liver at a time when intrahepatic viral production is at its peak. Conversely, the enhanced viral replication may arise from the increased immunological reaction to HBV-infected hepatocytes (Harnett *et al.*, 1987). Because HBV DNA concentration directly reflects the degree of viral replication, serial determinations of HBV DNA levels might be useful as a noninvasive means of monitoring liver disease activity. Peaks in HBV DNA concentrations may identify correctly transition from a relatively quiescent liver disease to an active course and alert the clinician to the need for liver biopsy or adjustment of the immunosuppressive regimen (Harnett *et al.*, 1987). A marked decline in the serum HBV DNA concentration in patients with previously diagnosed CAH may signify progression to cirrhosis and probably reflects loss of hepatic mass harboring the virus (Harnett *et al.*, 1987).

The time of acquisition of HBV infection, as ascertained by the appearance of HBsAg, seems to be of prognostic importance. The virus-host interaction is likely to be quite different depending on whether HBV is acquired in the early posttransplant period when large doses of immunosuppressive drugs are administered or HBV infection has existed for a long time before renal transplantation (Huang *et al.*, 1990). Renal transplant recipients who became HBsAg positive in the posttransplantation period as compared with patients who acquired hepatitis B surface antigenemia before transplantation have shown a higher mortality rate (Anuras *et al.*, 1977; Scott *et al.*, 1987).

The clinical presentation and the biochemical data have shown poor correlation with liver morphology. Often the histopathological findings on liver biopsy show advanced disease unexpectedly. *Silent* (i.e., in the absence of any LFT abnormalities) morphological progression of liver disease to cirrhosis is seen frequently among HBsAg-positive renal transplant recipients (Parfrey *et al.*, 1985b; Pirson *et al.*, 1977). In a few patients with biochemical evidence of hepatic dysfunction, liver biopsy failed to document any pathological changes (Parfrey *et al.*, 1985b; Pirson *et al.*, 1977). In general, LFTs appear to be poor predictors of liver disease activity, and consequently, liver biopsy is the only means for precise diagnosis and monitoring the degree of liver injury among HBsAg-positive renal transplant recipients (Harnett *et al.*, 1987; Pirson *et al.*, 1977; Rao *et al.*, 1991).

Hepatitis B may take a fulminant course with fatal outcome (Dusheiko *et al.*, 1983; Hanson *et al.*, 1985; Hung *et al.*, 1995; Kharsa *et al.*, 1987; Ware *et al.*, 1979; Yagisawa *et al.*, 1997). In these rare cases, liver histology at postmortem examination has shown massive hepatic necrosis (Dusheiko *et al.*, 1983; Hanson *et al.*, 1985). The pathogenesis of the fulminant liver failure in HBsAg-positive renal transplant recipients is not well understood. Some cases with fulminant hepatitis have been related to coinfection or superinfection with hepatitis D virus (HDV) (Kharsa *et al.*, 1987). It also has been speculated that massive hepatic necrosis could result from rapid cessation of immunosuppressive therapy with subsequent restoration of cell-mediated immunity and massive destruction of HBV-infected hepatocytes (Hanson *et al.*, 1985).

Hepatitis B surface antigen–positive renal transplant recipients have an increased incidence of hepatocellular carcinoma. This increased incidence can be attributed to the unique combination of rapid histological deterioration to liver cirrhosis, which is the most important risk factor for hepatocellular carcinoma (Colombo, 1992), and increased hepatocarcinogenesis secondary to persistent or enhanced HBV replication (Brechot, 1987; Fornairon *et al.*, 1996). Transplantation itself carries an increased risk of malignancy (Penn, 1982). Although data are inconsistent, hepatocellular carcinoma in HBsAg-positive renal transplant recipients has been reported with variable, but mostly relatively high, frequency (1–23%) (Fornairon *et al.*, 1996; Parfrey *et al.*, 1985b; Penn, 1982; Rao *et al.*, 1991; Schroter *et al.*, 1982).

In the Denver Transplant Tumor Registry, 14 cases of hepatocellular carcinoma (1%) were observed among 1,436 malignancies, which developed in 1,348 renal transplant recipients reported to the registry. The mean time between transplantation and manifestation of the tumor was 67 months (range, 13–129.5 months). One patient was documented to be HBsAg positive, but no information was available on the HBsAg status of the other 13 patients. In the series reported by Parfrey *et al.* (1985b), 14% (3 of 22) of HBsAg-positive renal transplant recipients developed hepatoma and died. Two of the patients became HBsAg positive 6 and 18 months posttransplantation. The other patient was HBsAg positive before transplantation, but chronic persistent hepatitis was already present on the initial biopsy posttransplantation. Death occurred 32 to 109 months posttransplantation (Parfrey *et al.*, 1985b). Similarly, Fornairon and coworkers observed that during a follow-up period of 125 months (range, 1–320 months) hepatocellular carcinoma occurred in 23% (8 of 35) of HBsAg-positive renal transplant recipients who had developed cirrhosis (Fornairon *et al.*, 1996). Despite discontinuation of immunosuppressive therapy and institution of chemotherapy, hepatocellular carcinoma in this population has shown an accelerated course with fatal outcome.

Factors Affecting the Course of Liver Disease Among Hepatitis B Surface Antigen–Positive Renal Transplant Recipients
Length of Follow-up

Liver disease manifests late after transplantation. A sufficiently long follow-up period is crucial for the precise assess-

ment of the relative risk of posttransplant liver disease among HBsAg-positive renal transplant recipients. Only studies with follow-up extending beyond 3 years have shown an increased incidence of liver disease in general and of more severe forms of liver disease in particular (Pirson *et al.*, 1977).

Type of Immunosuppressive Regimen

Many studies have examined the association between the type of immunosuppressive regimen and the incidence and progression of liver disease. Early series, in which patients were receiving the combination of azathioprine and prednisone, reported a high incidence of chronic liver disease among HBsAg-positive patients, which could have been related, at least in part, to the hepatotoxic effect of azathioprine and the enhanced viral replication induced by high-dose prednisone treatment (Fairley *et al.*, 1991; Hillis *et al.*, 1979; Parfrey *et al.*, 1985b). Immunosuppressive regimens using antilymphocyte preparations in addition to azathioprine and prednisone in HBsAg-positive renal transplant recipients have been associated with a high frequency of progression to liver cirrhosis and high mortality from liver disease (Hsieh *et al.*, 1996; Rao *et al.*, 1991). The use of cyclosporine in triple-therapy regimens (i.e., cyclosporine, azathioprine and prednisone) has allowed a decrease in azathioprine and prednisone doses.

Cyclosporine-based triple therapy is believed to be less hepatotoxic and to have fewer enhancing effects on viral replication and consequently to be associated with a lower incidence of posttransplant liver disease among HBsAg-positive renal transplant recipients (Hsieh *et al.*, 1996). There has been a trend toward a lower incidence of liver disease among HBsAg-positive patients in more recent studies, in which most of the patients are on triple therapy, as compared with older studies, which traditionally have used a regimen of azathioprine and prednisone (Hsieh *et al.*, 1996). A regimen of only cyclosporine and prednisone has been associated with a low (27%) incidence of chronic liver dysfunction among HBsAg-positive renal transplant recipients (Hsieh *et al.*, 1996). The combination of cyclosporine and prednisone may be the optimal immunosuppressive regimen for HBsAg-positive patients undergoing renal transplantation. Other investigators have observed no correlation, however, between the type of immunosuppressive regimen and the occurrence of hepatitis among HBsAg-positive renal transplant recipients. These investigators have been unable to show any statistically significant difference in the risk of developing chronic hepatitis and cirrhosis among patients treated with azathioprine as compared with patients treated with cyclosporine (Chan *et al.*, 1992; Huang *et al.*, 1990).

Type of Hepatitis B Virus Infection—Reactivation and *De Novo* Infection

The peculiar course of hepatitis B among renal transplant recipients commonly is attributed to the effect of immunosuppressive therapy on viral replication. Azathioprine, cyclosporine and prednisone all have been incriminated in facilitating HBV replication (Huang *et al.*, 1990; Sagnelli *et al.*, 1980). Consequently, reactivation of HBV in the posttransplant period occurs frequently among chronic HBsAg carriers. It manifests serologically with the reappearance of HBeAg and/or HBV DNA in the serum as a result of enhanced and long-lasting viral replication (Chan *et al.*, 1992; Degos *et al.*, 1988; Durlik *et al.*, 1996b; Dusheiko *et al.*, 1983; Fornairon *et al.*, 1996; Harnett *et al.*, 1987). Persistence and reactivation of viral replication posttransplantation are implicated in most cases of chronic hepatitis B among renal transplant recipients (Chan *et al.*, 1992; Degos *et al.*, 1988; Durlik *et al.*, 1996b; Dusheiko *et al.*, 1983; Fornairon *et al.*, 1996; Hanson *et al.*, 1985; Marcellin *et al.*, 1991). It appears that despite the state of iatrogenic immunosuppression, HBsAb can confer protection against hepatitis B (Chan *et al.*, 1992; Dusheiko *et al.*, 1983), which makes *de novo* HBV infection among renal transplant recipients relatively rare. As already stated, *de novo* HBV infection in the posttransplant period seems to be associated with a more aggressive clinical course and a worse prognosis (Anuras *et al.*, 1977; Scott *et al.*, 1987).

Liver Histology

Hepatitis B surface antigenemia in renal transplant recipients has been associated with more advanced histological forms of liver disease and marked tendency to morphological progression (Fornairon *et al.*, 1996; Parfrey *et al.*, 1985b; Rao *et al.*, 1991). Among renal transplant recipients with clinical evidence of posttransplant chronic liver disease, benign histological lesions (fat metamorphosis and chronic portal triaditis) were predominant on liver biopsy specimens of HBsAg-negative patients, whereas more severe histological forms of liver disease (chronic persistent hepatitis, CAH and cirrhosis) commonly were associated with the presence of hepatitis B surface antigenemia. Hepatitis B surface antigen–positive recipients, as compared with recipients who were HBsAg negative, showed not only a higher incidence of liver cirrhosis (42% *vs.* 19%) on initial liver biopsy, but also a trend toward more frequent progression to cirrhosis during histological follow-up (Rao *et al.*, 1991). Serial liver biopsies have shown that 82% of HBsAg-positive renal transplant recipients who initially presented with only benign histological lesions (virus only, reactive hepatitis or chronic persistent hepatitis) progressed to aggressive liver disease (CAH or cirrhosis) after a mean follow-up period of 83 months (Parfrey *et al.*, 1985b). Fornairon and coworkers reported an 85% rate of histological deterioration (Fornairon *et al.*, 1996). Hepatitis B surface antigen–positive renal transplant recipients appear to be at an increased risk of developing advanced stages of liver disease, in particular, liver cirrhosis (Parfrey *et al.*, 1985b). Increased HBV replication, concomitant chronic HCV infection and chronic alcohol consumption have been recognized as precipitating factors for rapid histological deterioration in HBsAg-positive renal transplant recipients (Fornairon *et al.*, 1996).

Dhar and associates did not observe any significant tendency to histological progression on serial liver biopsies performed in a group of 16 HBsAg-positive renal transplant recipients with a mean follow-up of 2.1 years (Dhar *et al.*, 1991). In patients who were HBeAg positive, reactive changes were predominant (in 85% of cases), and in only one of seven patients (15%), histological lesions were consistent with CAH. In the few cases in which histological progression did occur, however, it generally was not silent (Dhar *et al.*, 1991). Patients with CAH had persistently abnormal LFTs, cirrhotic patients showed only marginal elevations in liver biochemistry, and patients with normal liver histology had normal liver biochemical tests. A major criticism of this study is the short follow-up period, which might have not allowed enough time for morphological progression to become apparent.

In an attempt to correlate liver histopathology in HBsAg-positive renal transplant recipients with the type of immunosuppressive regimen, Stempel and colleagues reported that in a small group of HBsAg-positive renal transplant recipients receiving cyclosporine-based immunosuppressive therapy, liver biopsy specimens showed milder histological lesions than those reported in previous studies (Stempel *et al.*, 1991). Because these earlier studies had included mostly patients treated with azathioprine (known to be hepatotoxic) and prednisone (known to increase HBV replication), the authors postulated that the decrease in the doses of both medications, allowed by the introduction of cyclosporine to the immunosuppressive regimen, might have accounted for the lesser degree of liver impairment. It appears that HBsAg-positive renal transplant recipients who are treated with cyclosporine might have a lower risk of liver damage than those whose immunosuppressive regimens included azathioprine and prednisone alone. Conclusions should be guarded, however, because of the small size and the relatively short follow-up period of this study (Stempel *et al.*, 1991).

Effect of Hepatitis B Virus Infection on Posttransplantation Clinical Outcomes

The impact of HBV infection on graft and patient survival after renal transplantation has been the subject of ongoing debate since the 1970s. Many studies have shown that up to 2 years posttransplantation, hepatitis B surface antigenemia in renal transplant recipients does not affect adversely graft and patient survival (Chatterjee *et al.*, 1974; Degos *et al.*, 1988; Pirson *et al.*, 1977). Extended follow-up periods (from 3 years onward) revealed that hepatitis B surface antigenemia was associated with decreased patient survival in the late posttransplant period (Pirson *et al.*, 1977). In other studies, the decrease in patient survival among HBsAg-positive renal transplant recipients, as compared with recipients who were HBsAg negative, could be appreciated only after the follow-up period was extended beyond 5 (Sengar *et al.*, 1989) to 15 years (Gagnadoux *et al.*, 1993). It appears that hepatitis B surface antigenemia in renal transplant recipients affects adversely mostly long-term survival (>3 years posttransplantation).

Other investigators have reported significantly higher mortality rates among HBsAg-positive renal transplant recipients, as compared with recipients who were HBsAg negative, regardless of the follow-up duration (Degos *et al.*, 1988; Harnett *et al.*, 1987; White *et al.*, 1987). Similarly, Hillis and coworkers have observed accelerated mortality among renal transplant recipients who were HBsAg positive at the time of transplantation, as compared with recipients who were HBsAg negative, which began shortly after transplantation (Hillis *et al.*, 1979). This accelerated mortality was attributed to the combination of preexisting hepatitis B surface antigenemia and onset of immunosuppression induced by the institution of immunosuppressive therapy (Hillis *et al.*, 1979). The presence of hepatitis B surface antigenemia at the time of transplantation was found to be predictive of unfavorable survival (Hillis *et al.*, 1979). Likewise, Rao and associates determined that among renal transplant recipients with clinical evidence of posttransplant chronic liver disease, HBsAg-positive patients had a higher overall mortality rate than HBsAg-negative patients (Rao *et al.*, 1991). The highest mortality rate (60%) has been observed among HBsAg-positive renal transplant recipients who acquired their disease in the early posttransplant period (Scott *et al.*, 1987).

The association of hepatitis B surface antigenemia with a higher mortality among renal transplant recipients has not been observed uniformly. Several studies failed to detect any significant difference in patient survival between HBsAg-positive and HBsAg-negative renal transplant recipients (Chan *et al.*, 1992; Flagg *et al.*, 1987; Fornairon *et al.*, 1996; Huang *et al.*, 1990; Ranjan *et al.*, 1991; Rivolta *et al.*, 1987).

In some studies (Fornairon *et al.*, 1996; Parfrey *et al.*, 1985b; Pirson *et al.*, 1977; Rao *et al.*, 1991), but not all (Rivolta *et al.*, 1987; Sengar *et al.*, 1989), mortality owing to liver failure was significantly higher among HBsAg-positive renal transplant recipients as compared with HBsAg-negative recipients, frequently with more than half of all deaths in the HBsAg-positive group attributable to liver disease. The death rates from causes other than hepatitis were found to be similar among HBsAg-positive and HBsAg-negative renal transplant recipients (Pirson *et al.*, 1977). In contrast, other studies have shown that the increased mortality in HBsAg-positive renal transplant recipients was not related to hepatic dysfunction (Friedlaender *et al.*, 1989; Sengar *et al.*, 1989; White *et al.*, 1987) but to other, nonhepatic causes, such as sepsis (Nelson *et al.*, 1994), infections and vascular pathology (Hillis *et al.*, 1979). In one report, no deaths owing to liver disease were observed in a group of renal transplant recipients who were HBsAg positive at the time of transplantation (Friedlaender *et al.*, 1989).

These controversial data can be reconciled only if the increased risk of developing fatal liver disease were present exclusively in a particular subgroup of renal transplant candidates—those with active viral replication as assessed by the presence of HBeAg and/or HBV DNA (Fairley *et al.*, 1991). Consequently the wide variation in the incidence of fatal liver disease observed across studies is likely to be related to differences uniquely in the prevalence of HBeAg and/or HBV DNA. These speculations are supported by the observations that survival in HBsAg-positive renal transplant recipients with markers of active viral replication was lower (although not significantly) than in recipients without these markers. Because an excellent correlation between HBeAg and serum HBV DNA concentrations has been documented, HBeAg testing, which is relatively easy to perform, widely available and cheaper, has been recommended as a good and reliable marker of viral replication. Among chronic HBsAg carriers who undergo renal transplantation, increased mortality from liver disease may be confined to patients who are HBeAg and/or HBV DNA positive before transplantation. A policy not to transplant these patients but to treat and follow them until they become negative for these markers seems reasonable. Once this change in HBeAg and/or HBV DNA status occurs, the relative risk of fatal posttransplantation liver disease is decreased significantly (Fairley *et al.*, 1991).

Effect of Renal Transplantation on the Course of Hepatitis B Virus Infection in Dialysis Patients

Although not unanimously supported (Friedlaender *et al.*, 1989), there is evidence to suggest that HBV infection may take an accelerated course after renal transplantation (Harnett *et al.*, 1987; Parfrey *et al.*, 1985b). Harnett and colleagues showed that mortality rate in HBsAg-positive renal transplant recipients, as compared with HBsAg-positive hemodialysis patients, was significantly higher (64% *vs.* 19%) (Harnett *et al.*, 1987). This difference was attributed to deaths from liver disease (57% *vs.* 17%), implying that HBV infection among hemodialysis patients was less aggressive than that in renal transplant recipients. These observations raised the question whether HBsAg-positive end-stage renal disease (ESRD) patients should be offered renal transplantation or maintained on long-term dialysis. To date, there is no easy answer to this dilemma. Based on currently available data, several suggestions regarding management of HBsAg-positive ESRD patients have been formulated. The prevailing feeling is that transplantation should not be denied categorically to all HBsAg-positive ESRD patients. The attention has been focused on the following categories. Patients who clinically present with cirrhosis, portal hypertension or liver failure should be advised to continue on dialysis or should be offered combined liver and kidney transplantation. Patients who are older, are women or have CAH on liver histology

appear to be at an increased risk of developing cirrhosis in the posttransplant period (Rao *et al.*, 1993). The decision whether they should undergo transplantation should be made cautiously. Patients with serological markers of viral replication should be treated first with antiviral agents or interferon alfa and offered transplantation once these markers become negative.

Patients with advanced histological forms of liver disease probably fit into one of the aforementioned categories, and although they are expected to do poorly after transplantation, this may not necessarily happen. The decision whether to perform transplantation should be individualized and made in harmony with the patient's desire. Because no general principles can apply to the selection of HBsAg-positive patients for renal transplantation, each case should be decided individually with the participation of a well-informed patient capable of understanding and weighing the risks and benefits of transplantation and comparing the expected quality of life with renal transplant with the current and projected quality of life on dialysis.

Prevention and Treatment of Hepatitis B Virus Infection in End-Stage Renal Disease Patients

Hepatitis B is a preventable disease. Large-scale vaccination of all susceptible predialysis and dialysis patients can increase the percentage of immune individuals and prevent the spread of HBV infection in the ESRD population. This practice is particularly important because, owing to the existing immunosuppression, hepatitis B vaccination of renal transplant recipients is associated with a poor antibody response (18–36%) (Jacobson *et al.*, 1985; Lefebure *et al.*, 1993). Lefebure and coworkers have shown that because secondary immune responses are relatively well maintained under immunosuppression, renal transplant recipients vaccinated successfully before transplantation who had subsequently lost their protective immunity could benefit from a booster dose (Lefebure *et al.*, 1993). In this scenario, a booster injection of 40 µg given intramuscularly resulted in a rise in the HBsAb titer above protective level in 86% of patients (Lefebure *et al.*, 1993). Strict enforcement of and adherence to dialysis unit precautions are crucial in preventing the spread of HBV infection in dialysis units and consequently among renal transplant candidates.

At present, interferon alfa is the only therapy of proven benefit in the treatment of chronic viral hepatitis. This therapy is recommended early in the course of HBV infection. Because of the risk of inducing acute transplant rejection, however, interferon alfa should be avoided in renal transplant recipients. New therapeutic approaches include lamivudine and famciclovir and have shown promising preliminary results (Hoofnagle, 1997). Lamivudine is a nucleoside analogue that inhibits viral DNA synthesis. This drug was approved by the U.S. Food and Drug Administration for the treatment of chronic hepatitis B. In a small group of six HBV–positive cadaver renal transplant recipients, lamivudine therapy led to rapid disappearance of HBV DNA from the serum in all patients and normalization of ALT in four of five patients with initial elevation of ALT levels. There were no changes in renal function and no adverse effects associated with this treatment. Discontinuation of lamivudine after a 6-month course resulted in biochemical and virological relapse within weeks, which required reinstitution of lamivudine therapy (Rostaing *et al.*, 1997). Famciclovir, another nucleoside analogue with antiviral properties, is currently in phase III clinical trials and has shown promise in the treatment of chronic HBV infection.

HEPATITIS C VIRUS

Structure of Hepatitis C Virus Genome

In 1989, the HCV was cloned and identified as the major cause of parenterally transmitted non-A, non-B hepatitis (NANBH) (Choo *et al.*, 1989; Kuo *et al.*, 1989). Hepatitis C virus is a small 40- to 60-nm virus, which belongs to the Flaviviridae family. It has a lipid envelope and a single-stranded RNA viral genome of approximately 9,400 nucleotides (Choo *et al.*, 1989; Houghton *et al.*, 1991). The N-terminus encodes the basic nucleocapsid (C) followed by two glycoprotein domains, the envelope (E1) and a second envelope/nonstructural-1 (E2/NS1) region (Houghton *et al.*, 1991). Downstream to this region are the nonstructural genes NS2, NS3, NS4 and NS5. The 5′ noncoding region (5′NCR) represents the most conserved sequence, and the regions encoding the E1 and E2/NS1 are the most variable (Pereira and Levey, 1997). Sequence analysis of the viral genome has identified many distinct HCV variants. A universal system for the nomenclature of hepatitis C viral genotypes has been proposed. This system defines six major groups, which are designated as HCV types 1 through 6 (Simmonds *et al.*, 1994). Each major type consists of one or more closely related variants designated as subtypes and named *a*, *b*, *c* and so forth in order of discovery. Each subtype may include individual isolates.

Epidemiology and Clinical Manifestation

Routes of Transmission

Hepatitis C is a blood-borne infection, which accounts for more than 90% of the cases of posttransfusion hepatitis and for most of all cases of NANBH in the United States (Alter *et al.*, 1990). Blood transfusion is the most important route of transmission of HCV. Other modes of parenteral exposure (i.e., intravenous drug abuse, needle-stick injuries, professional exposure to blood) and sexual and household contacts with a person who has hepatitis C also can be implicated.

Clinical Course

The incubation period of HCV is 15 to 150 days (mean, 50 days). Clinical symptoms in patients with acute hepatitis C tend to be mild or absent. Cases of fulminant and subacute liver failure are rare but may be fatal. In transfusion-associated hepatitis C, HCV RNA levels become detectable in the serum 1 to 3 weeks after the exposure and commonly are followed by increase in serum ALT levels (Farci *et al.*, 1991). If a chronic HCV carrier state is established, HCV RNA levels usually are sustained in serum over the time (Yoshimura *et al.*, 1997). Anti-HCV antibody production typically begins at 4 weeks but can be delayed for 1 year (Aach *et al.*, 1991; Esteban *et al.*, 1990). Anti-HCV antibodies are directed toward multiple viral proteins and usually persist indefinitely or at least over a long period. Their presence is unrelated to the course or outcome of the disease (Alter *et al.*, 1992; Carrera *et al.*, 1994; Courouce *et al.*, 1995a, 1995b; Simon *et al.*, 1994).

In about half of patients, the disease takes a self-limiting course, and ALT activity returns to normal. In half of patients, ALT levels remain persistently elevated, and a relatively slow, sequential progression from acute hepatitis C to chronic HCV infection—chronic hepatitis, cirrhosis and hepatocellular carcinoma—takes place over the years (Alter, 1989). The mean interval from the time of transfusion to the diagnosis of liver disease was 10 to 13.7 years for patients with chronic hepatitis, 18.4 years for patients with CAH, 20.6 to 21.2 years for patients with cirrhosis and 28.3 to 29 years for patients with hepatocellular carcinoma (Kiyosawa *et al.*, 1990; Tong *et al.*, 1995). Regardless of the relentless progression of HCV-induced liver disease, a long-term study with an average follow-up of 18 years failed to show any increase in all-cause mortality after transfusion-associated NANBH. The frequency of death from liver disease, although low (3.3%), was significantly higher than that in the control groups (1.1% and 2.0%). It is possible that, with time, the difference between groups in all-cause mortality could reach statistical significance because an increase in mortality among subjects with transfusion-associated NANBH can be expected with the progression of liver disease (Seeff *et al.*, 1992). Longer follow-up might be required to reveal differences in mortality between groups.

Immunity

The immune mechanisms triggered by HCV infection involve humoral and cellular responses targeted at multiple determinants of the viral genome. In most cases, these responses are insufficient to provide protective immunity and fail to control the HCV infection, allowing the development of a chronic carrier state. Many studies in humans and animals have documented the development of reinfection (new infection after the previous infection has cleared) with the same or different HCV strain as well as superinfection (infection with a new HCV strain in the presence of current infection) (Kao *et al.*, 1993; Lai *et al.*, 1994; Okamoto *et al.*, 1994).

The lack of protective immunity, although incompletely elucidated, can be attributed to the following factors. First, most anti-HCV antibodies are nonneutralizing, and they do not provide immunity despite their presence. Although neutralizing antibodies to the envelope regions of HCV have been identified, they seem to circulate at a titer too low to neutralize the infecting virus and have no role in providing protective immunity (Zibert *et al.*, 1995). Second, compelling evidence is available that the cellular responses of the host are inadequate and contribute directly to the pathogenicity associated with the viral infection. Third, the existence of extrahepatic replication sites, now generally accepted, is likely to promote the chronicity of the infection. Fourth, the emergence of mutant forms able to resist neutralization has been suggested by the existence of two groups of viral particles—low-density particles (1.08–1.11 g/ml), representing the intact virions, and high-density particles (1.22–1.25 g/ml), corresponding to virions complexed with immune globulins. The presence of low-density particles (unbound forms) has been associated with a stronger infectious potency and the highest heterogeneity of the hypervariable region of the viral genome. Although providing additional evidence to the existence of neutralizing antibodies capable of complexing with the virus, this observation suggests that mutations in the hypervariable region of the viral genome may be creating mutants capable of escaping effective neutralization.

Hepatitis C Virus Genotypes—Epidemiology and Clinical Significance

The clinical significance of the genomic diversity of HCV has not been elucidated. The existing biological differences between HCV genotypes may play an important role in the epidemiology and natural history of HCV infection because genotype-related differences in disease severity, clinical outcomes and response to interferon therapy have been observed (Feray *et al.*, 1993; Mahaney *et al.*, 1994; McOmish *et al.*, 1993; Yoshioka *et al.*, 1992).

Hepatitis C virus genotypes have a distinct geographical

distribution (Choo et al., 1989; Dusheiko et al., 1994; Enomoto et al., 1990; Li et al., 1991; Mahaney et al., 1994; McOmish et al., 1993; Pol et al., 1995b; Takada et al., 1992; Tsukiyama Kohara et al., 1991). Hepatitis C virus genotype 1a is the commonest genotype in the United States and Western Europe (Choo et al., 1989; Mahaney et al., 1994; McOmish et al., 1993; Pol et al., 1995b). For the most part, HCV genotype 1b shares the geographical distribution of 1a in the United States and Europe but also is seen frequently in Japan. HCV genotype 1b is the predominant HCV genotype in Japan and the second commonest genotype in the United States (Li et al., 1991; Mahaney et al., 1994; McOmish et al., 1993). The other HCV genotypes, less frequent in the United States, typically are found in certain parts of the world. In particular, HCV genotypes 2a and 2b are seen commonly in Western Europe, Japan, China and Taiwan; 3a, in Western Europe, Thailand, Singapore, India and Bangladesh; 4a, in Middle East, Egypt and Central Africa; 5a, in South Africa and 6a, in Hong Kong (Choo et al., 1989; Dusheiko et al., 1994; Enomoto et al., 1990; Li et al., 1991; Mahaney et al., 1994; McOmish et al., 1993; Takada et al., 1992; Tsukiyama Kohara et al., 1991).

Some investigators have hypothesized that each HCV genotype has a preferential route of transmission, and the mode of acquisition of HCV infection could predict the HCV genotype distribution in high-risk populations. Significant difference has been reported between intravenous drug abusers and patients who have acquired HCV by other means. In particular, among patients who were infected with HCV by blood transfusions, 1b is the predominant HCV genotype, in contrast to intravenous drug abusers, among whom coexistence of different HCV genotypes (1b, 2b, 3 and 4) frequently is seen (Mahaney et al., 1994; Nousbaum et al., 1995; Pawlowska et al., 1997; Sallie, 1995).

Demographic differences between HCV genotypes have been noted in some but not all studies. Hepatitis C virus genotype 1b was found to be highly predominant in patients older than 40 years (Nousbaum et al., 1995; Zein et al., 1996) and in patients with HCV infection of long duration (Nousbaum et al., 1995), whereas HCV genotype 3 usually was seen in younger patients, frequently with history of drug abuse (Pontisso et al., 1995). A progressively decreasing relative prevalence of HCV genotype 1b has been observed in large reference centers in France and Italy (Nousbaum et al., 1995). In contrast, Mahaney and colleagues failed to detect any genotype-related differences among patients with HCV infection (Mahaney et al., 1994). Dusheiko and coworkers could not find any significant differences in age, serum albumin and ALT levels among patients infected with different HCV genotypes (Dusheiko et al., 1994). No significant differences in the geographical distribution of HCV genotypes across the United States (Zein et al., 1996) and no substantial changes in the spectrum of the infecting HCV genotypes have been detected over a period of 2 to 20 years. Genotype 1 has been consistently the commonest HCV genotype among patients with chronic hepatitis C in the United States across different time periods (Mahaney et al., 1994).

Several studies have attempted to correlate the severity of HCV disease to the genotype of the virus. Hepatitis C virus genotype 1b has been associated with a higher prevalence of severe liver disease (i.e., cirrhosis and hepatocellular carcinoma), a greater cytopathic effect in liver transplant recipients and a lower rate of initial and long-term sustained response to interferon alfa treatment (Brouwer et al., 1993; Feray et al., 1993; Mahaney et al., 1994; Nousbaum et al., 1995; Yoshioka et al., 1992), whereas patients infected with HCV genotypes other than 1 have shown approximately equal distribution of severe and mild liver disease (Dusheiko et al., 1994). Other investigators have reported that genotype 2 usually causes more serious liver disease (CAH or cirrhosis), despite significantly lower levels of circulating HCV RNA, and paradoxically better long-term response to treatment with interferon alfa when compared with other genotypes (Mahaney et al., 1994). Alanine aminotransferase levels were found to be higher among asymptomatic Scottish blood donors infected with HCV genotype 3 than among donors infected with HCV genotype 1 (McOmish et al., 1993). Clinical evaluation of the virulence of HCV genotypes is difficult and complex because it is conceivable that not the HCV genotype per se, but other confounding variables, such as duration of infection; viral load; mode of acquisition; reinfections; host immunity; genetic factors; age; coexisting viral, bacterial or parasitic infections and alcohol consumption, ultimately may determine the outcomes of HCV infection.

As discussed earlier, HCV infection does not provide protective immunity, and reinfection and superinfection can occur (Farci et al., 1992; Lai et al., 1994; Okamoto et al., 1994). In thalassemic children and hemophiliacs, reinfection and superinfection have been reported after multiple blood transfusions (Lai et al., 1994). Detailed epidemiological analysis has shown that the observed prevalence of mixed infections among HCV-infected individuals is lower than the estimated one, suggesting that some particular genotypes may suppress infection with other genotypes, a clinical phenomenon with conceivably significant therapeutic implications in the future (Liaw, 1995). Some investigators have suggested that the presence of multiple genotypes, rather than of a specific genotype, determines the outcomes of treatment (Okada et al., 1992). In the absence of enough data at present, the clinical significance of mixed infections is not clarified.

The genetic variations of HCV have important implications in the development of a vaccine. Because of the lack of cross-immunity between the different HCV genotypes, it is likely that a vaccine against one HCV genotype would not protect against infection with the others. To provide effective protection against the full range of HCV genotypes, it may be necessary to develop multivalent vaccines.

Tests for Detection

Tests for Antibodies to Hepatitis C Virus

The diagnosis of HCV infection is based on tests that measure anti-HCV (Pereira and Levey, 1997). Enzyme-linked immunosorbent assays and recombinant immunoblot assays (RIBA) have been in use. Enzyme-linked immunosorbent assays detect antibody to a specific HCV antigen (first-generation tests) or a combination of antigens (second-generation and third-generation tests) in a standard ELISA plate and have been used as screening tests. In contrast, RIBAs detect antibodies to one or more HCV antigens on a strip that is read visually and by virtue of their increased specificity have been considered confirmatory tests.

The first-generation anti-HCV tests (ELISA1, RIBA1) detect nonneutralizing antibodies to the C100-3 (and 5-1-1) proteins encoded by the NS3/NS4 region of the HCV prototype isolate (i.e., HCV genotype 1a). The performance of these anti-HCV tests is compromised by their genotype dependence owing to the substantial heterogeneity in C100-3 sequences of different genotypes (Nagayama et al., 1993) and the delay in antibody production to C100-3 antigen in response to HCV infection, resulting in a longer *window* period (i.e., the early stage of the infection, when viremia is present, but antibody response is not yet manifest) (Farci et al., 1991). The first-generation anti-HCV tests are no longer in use.

The second-generation tests have overcome some of these limitations. The ELISA2 includes c22 antigen from the nucleocapsid region and c200, which is a composite of c33 and c100-3 antigens from the NS3 and NS4 region. The RIBA2 uses four recombinant HCV antigens (c22, c33, c100 and 5-1-1). These tests have improved performance as a result of the increased number of incorporated antigens with highly conserved protein sequences negating any genotype dependence of the assay and a shorter window period because the production of antibodies to c22 or c33 proteins precedes by at least 1 month the production of antibodies to c100-3 (Nasoff *et al.*, 1991). With the use of second-generation tests, seroconversion can be detected 4 weeks after exposure (Aach *et al.*, 1991), and antibodies to the c22 or c33 proteins remain detectable in the serum for a longer period (Alter *et al.*, 1992).

Third-generation anti-HCV tests have become available. They incorporate an additional recombinant antigen from the NS5 region of the HCV genome, not represented in the previous tests, and an improved c33 antigen corresponding to the NS3 region, which has resulted in further improvement in sensitivity. The window period has been reduced further and was estimated at a mean of 69.8 days (Busch *et al.*, 1995).

Tests for Hepatitis C Virus RNA

Polymerase Chain Reaction. The detection of HCV RNA by reverse transcriptase PCR has been used as the gold standard to identify current HCV infection (Pereira and Levey, 1997). *Universal* primers directed to the highly conserved 5' end, which nucleotide sequence is shared by most HCV strains, are used to detect the presence of the virus. In patients with posttransfusion NANBH, high serum or plasma HCV RNA levels can occur within 1 week after exposure to the virus and weeks before the appearance of anti-HCV or the manifestation of ALT elevations (Farci *et al.*, 1991; Weiner *et al.*, 1990). The reliability of this test is limited by false-positive and false-negative results, however. Because of the extreme sensitivity of the PCR, rigorous measures are required to prevent minor contamination, which can give false-positive results. Imperfect handling and/or storage of blood samples can lead to failure to detect HCV RNA in 40% of samples and can be the cause of false-negative results (Busch *et al.*, 1992). Performance of PCR is labor intensive, protocols vary from laboratory to laboratory and the test is available in only select laboratories (Pereira and Levey, 1997).

Quantitation of Hepatitis C Virus RNA Titers. The branched-chain DNA assay (bDNA assay) is a quantitative assay for HCV RNA in which the signal/probe rather than viral nucleic acid is amplified (Lau *et al.*, 1993a; Urdea *et al.*, 1991). The lower limit of detection of the bDNA assay is 350,000 molecules/ml (Lau *et al.*, 1993a) compared with 2,000 molecules/ml for PCR (Lau *et al.*, 1993b). Although the bDNA assay is less sensitive than PCR, it is simple, automated and reproducible. Quantitative PCR also has been used to measure the level of HCV RNA in serum (Weiner *et al.*, 1990).

Tests for Hepatitis C Virus Genotypes

Precise identification of the specific viral type, subtype or isolate requires sequence analysis of the viral genome (Simmonds *et al.*, 1994). This procedure is expensive, is time-consuming and is fraught with the problem of mutations. Consequently, PCR using subtype-specific primers (Okamoto *et al.*, 1992), restriction fragment length polymorphism analysis or line probe assay based on type-specific sequence variations in the 5' untranslated region (Kurosaki *et al.*, 1993; Nakao *et al.*, 1991) has been used to identify HCV subtypes. Others have used an ELISA that detects antibodies to serotype-specific immunodominant epitopes from the NS4 region

of the HCV genome (Nagayama *et al.*, 1993; Stuyver *et al.*, 1993).

Difficulties in Interpreting Tests for Hepatitis C Virus Infection

Anti–Hepatitis C Virus–Positive, but Hepatitis C Virus RNA–Negative Patients

The anti-HCV tests that currently are licensed for clinical use detect nonneutralizing antibodies to recombinant HCV antigens (Pereira and Levey, 1997). The presence of anti-HCV does not necessarily imply the presence of HCV RNA in the serum. Hepatitis C virus RNA has been detected in 52 to 93% of dialysis patients with anti-HCV (Dussol *et al.*, 1993; Pol *et al.*, 1993). Several possibilities could account for the presence of anti-HCV in the absence of HCV RNA. First, HCV may be sequestered at sites other than the bloodstream, such as the liver or peripheral blood mononuclear cells (Dussol *et al.*, 1993; Willems *et al.*, 1994). Second, viremia could be intermittent, and HCV RNA may not be present in the plasma at the time of testing (Farci *et al.*, 1991). Thirty-five percent of HCV-infected dialysis patients showed fluctuating patterns of viremia with virus-free intervals (Umlauft *et al.*, 1997). Third, the number of copies of HCV RNA may be below the limit of detection (DuBois *et al.*, 1994). Fourth, antibody to HCV may persist after the viral RNA has disappeared. In this situation, anti-HCV–positive, but HCV RNA–negative patients might represent a group that had been infected with the virus but no longer harbor it, and for this reason they no longer are infective. Fifth, anti-HCV may have been acquired passively from blood transfusions. In this situation, anti-HCV would disappear over the next few weeks in keeping with the half-life of IgG. Sixth, false-positive results can occur owing to nonspecific reactions, a problem that has been largely resolved in the current tests.

Anti–Hepatitis C Virus–Negative, but Hepatitis C Virus RNA–Positive Patients

More than 90% of nonimmunosuppressed individuals with HCV infection test positive for anti-HCV (Alter *et al.*, 1992). Possible explanations for the presence of HCV RNA in the absence of anti-HCV include the following (Pereira and Levey, 1997). First, the anti-HCV test may not be sensitive enough to detect existing anti-HCV antibody, either because of the low titer of antibody or because the antigen used in the assay system cannot detect the serum antibody response to the particular genotype. Second, various diseases or pharmacological immunosuppression could suppress or modify the anti-HCV response. Only 83% of HCV RNA–positive dialysis patients test positive for anti-HCV. Likewise, 2.5 to 12% of dialysis patients who were anti-HCV negative by first-generation or second-generation ELISA and 28% of hemodialysis patients from an area endemic for HCV infection (Saudi Arabia) who were anti-HCV negative by third-generation ELISA tested positive for HCV RNA (al Meshari *et al.*, 1995; Pereira and Levey, 1997). Similarly, among renal transplant recipients, serological responses to HCV have been shown to be delayed or sometimes absent (Preiksaitis *et al.*, 1997). Third, the patient may be in the window period between infection and seroconversion. Fourth, after anti-HCV antibody has persisted for a certain period, it can disappear despite the persistence of HCV RNA. In addition to the aforementioned, HCV RNA has been detected in the peripheral blood mononuclear cells from hemodialysis patients without anti-HCV or HCV RNA in the serum (Oesterreicher *et al.*, 1995). The HCV RNA in these peripheral blood mononuclear cells could serve as a viral reservoir and frustrate further efforts to identify HCV infection in hemodialysis patients.

Relationship Among Serum Alanine Aminotransferase Levels, Hepatitis C Virus Infection and Liver Disease

Numerous studies have consistently found that ALT levels, in the general population as well as in ESRD patients, have limited value for the diagnosis of HCV infection. Increased ALT activity was detected in only 20% of anti-HCV–positive blood products (van der Poel et al., 1990) and 33% of anti-HCV–positive blood donors (Alter et al., 1986). Similarly, among hemodialysis patients, serum ALT levels are elevated in 4 to 67% of anti-HCV–positive patients, 12 to 31% of HCV RNA–positive patients and 33% of patients with biopsy-proven hepatitis (Ayoola et al., 1991; Colombo et al., 1992; Jeffers et al., 1990; Muller et al., 1992; Pol et al., 1993; Roger et al., 1991; Simon et al., 1994; Vasile et al., 1992). Biochemical evidence of liver disease is present in 42 to 52% of HCV RNA–positive transplant recipients (Aeder et al., 1993; Pereira et al., 1992). No association has been found between HCV genotype and liver enzyme activity (Fabrizi et al., 1997a).

The discrepancy between serum ALT levels and the presence of anti-HCV is due to several reasons. First, chronic hepatitis C characteristically has a fluctuating course with multiple peaks and troughs in ALT levels (Farci et al., 1991), and patients with normal ALT levels may have severe histological lesions. Second, HCV infection is not always associated with chronic liver disease. Only 69% of anti-HCV–positive symptom-free blood donors who underwent liver biopsy had histological evidence of chronic hepatitis, all of whom had HCV RNA in the serum (Alberti et al., 1992). It is likely that a carrier state can exist with viral replication occurring at extrahepatic sites and no apparent liver damage that can be explained by the inability of some patients to mount strong immune response to HCV and to cause hepatic injury (DuBois et al., 1994). Third, some anti-HCV–positive patients may have cleared the infection, and anti-HCV may be the remnant of past infection. Fourth, baseline ALT levels are depressed in patients on dialysis (Wolf et al., 1972). Elevated ALT levels have been observed in 4 to 23% of anti-HCV–negative dialysis patients (Colombo et al., 1992; Gilli et al., 1990; Mondelli et al., 1991; Pol et al., 1993; Vasile et al., 1992). These patients could be carriers of HCV infection in whom anti-HCV production is absent, or the liver disease might be due to a NANBH virus other than HCV or to nonviral causes. Consequently, in patients with HCV infection, liver biopsy remains the only reliable method of confirming the presence of liver disease and assessing its severity. Liver histology at the time of initial presentation has been shown to be a good predictor of intermediate and long-term outcome in transplant recipients with liver disease (Rao et al., 1993).

Liver Histology

A wide spectrum of morphological lesions has been described in liver biopsy specimens of HCV-infected renal transplant recipients. The severity of liver lesions varies considerably among studies. This variation mainly reflects the fact that liver biopsy is not used routinely for the evaluation of HCV-infected renal transplant recipients but is reserved for patients with HCV infection who manifest significant abnormalities of liver biochemistries or clinically overt liver disease. Liver biopsy often is done during episodes of laboratory or clinical exacerbation. Because criteria for performing liver biopsy have not been uniform, there is a significant selection bias in reviewing the histopathological lesions in HCV-related liver disease. When liver biopsies are performed regardless of LFT levels, in a substantial portion of patients, findings are consistent with normal histology or minimal changes. If liver biopsies are performed only in patients with abnormal LFTs, more severe lesions usually are encountered. The lack of consensus on the timing of liver biopsy results in performing biopsies in patients with different durations of HCV infection, which has an effect on the severity of the observed histological lesions. The use of different classifications for histological staging of liver lesions complicates the interpretation of liver biopsy findings further. Consequently, it is difficult to appreciate the real distribution and evolution of HCV-related liver lesions based on the published data.

The typical histological lesions found in liver biopsy specimens of HCV-infected renal transplant recipients include minimal changes, persistent chronic hepatitis, CAH and liver cirrhosis. Rarely, hepatocellular carcinoma, nodular regenerative hyperplasia, fibrosing cholestatic hepatitis and other nonspecific lesions have been observed. We have summarized the results of 13 published studies, including a total of 386 HCV-infected renal transplant recipients who underwent liver biopsy (Aroldi et al., 1998; Boletis et al., 1995; Chan et al., 1994; Fabrizi et al., 1996; Glicklich et al., 1994; Hestin et al., 1995; Kazi et al., 1994; Morales, 1995; Pol et al., 1992; Pouteil-Noble et al., 1995; Rostaing et al., 1998b; Roth et al., 1994; Weinstein et al., 1997; Table 32–4). This group is heterogeneous because the patients had significant differences in clinical presentation and laboratory data. The criteria for performing liver biopsy were not uniform. In most instances, the liver biopsy was prompted by the presence of severe disease or abnormal biochemistry. Overall, CAH and liver cirrhosis were present in 42% of the patients; only 8% had normal histology. These findings of severe liver lesions in a significant percentage of HCV-infected renal transplant recipients should be interpreted with much caution because liver biopsy was not performed routinely in any of these studies.

Serial biopsies have been reported usually in patients with clinical and biochemical evidence of progressive liver disease or with histological findings on initial liver biopsy compatible with more advanced stages of liver impairment. In these cases, findings on repeat biopsies commonly have shown histological progression of liver disease (Chan et al., 1994; Morales et al., 1993).

Prevalence of Infection Among Cadaver Organ Donors and Performance of Anti–Hepatitis C Virus Tests

The prevalence of HCV infection among cadaver organ donors varies worldwide (Gomez et al., 1991; Huang et al., 1993; Miranda et al., 1993; Pereira et al., 1994; Prados et al., 1992; Preiksaitis et al., 1997; Roth et al., 1992; Triolo et al., 1992; Vincenti et al., 1993; Wreghitt et al., 1994; Table 32–5). In 1992, we initiated a national collaborative study by eight organ procurement organizations representing different geographical regions of the United States (Pereira et al., 1994). Among 3,078 cadaver organ donors, the prevalence of a positive ELISA1 was 5.1% (range, 1.5–16.7%). Sera from these ELISA1-positive donors and 100 randomly selected ELISA1-negative cadaver organ donors were retrieved for testing by ELISA2 and PCR. The extrapolated prevalence of ELISA2 and HCV RNA among cadaver organ donors was 4.2% and 2.4%. Based on these data, we computed the sensitivity and specificity of the ELISA2 assay in detecting HCV infection to be 100% and 98.1%. Consequently, in this population the positive and negative predictive values of the ELISA2 assay

TABLE 32–4

HISTOLOGICAL LESIONS IN LIVER BIOPSY SPECIMENS OF HEPATITIS C VIRUS–INFECTED RENAL TRANSPLANT RECIPIENTS

Authors	No. Patients	ALT Levels*	Normal Histology	Minimal Changes	CPH (Lobular Hepatitis)	CAH	Cirrhosis	Others
Pol et al., 1992	32	NA	0	6 (19%)	7 (22%)	19 (59%)	0	0
Roth et al., 1994	10	↑	0	0	4 (40%)	5 (50%)	1 (10%)	0
Chan et al., 1994	13	↑	0	7 (54%)	1 (7.5%)	4 (31%)	1 (7.5%)	0
Kazi et al., 1994	6	↑	4 (66.66%)	0	0	2 (33.33%)	0 (0%)	0
Glicklich et al., 1994	29	↑ (26%)	0	3 (10%)	17 (59%)	4 (14%)	2 (7%)	3 (10%)
Morales et al., 1995	30	↑	0	0	6 (20%)	10 (33%)	7 (23%)	5 (17%)† 2 (7%)‡
Pouteil-Noble et al., 1995	81	NA	0	13 (16%)	12 (15%)	22 (27%)	8 (10%)	26 (32%)§
Hestin et al., 1995	30	mean ↑	14 (47%)	0	0	13 (43%)	3 (10%)	0
Boletis et al., 1995	37	↑ (57%)	10 (27%)	11 (30%)	6 (17%)	0	2 (5%)	3 (8%)‖ 3 (8%)¶ 2 (5%)**
Fabrizi et al., 1996	8	↑	0	0	6 (75%)	2 (25%)	0	0
Weinstein et al., 1997	2	↑	0	0	0	2 (100%)	0	0
Aroldi et al., 1998	37	↑	0	0	10 (27%)	22 (59%)	3 (8%)	2 (6%)**
Rostaing et al., 1998b	71	↑ (39%)	2 (3%)	0	41 (57%)	26 (37%)	2 (8%)	0
Total	386		30 (8%)	40 (10%)	110 (28%)	131 (34%)	29 (8%)	46 (12%)

*The numbers in brackets represent the percent of patients with abnormal ALT levels.
†Siderosis only.
‡Nodular regenerative hyperplasia.
§Predominant fibrosis.
‖Acute hepatitis.
¶Fibrosing hepatitis.
**Fibrosing cholestatic hepatitis.
ALT = alanine aminotransferase; CPH = chronic persistent hepatitis; CAH = chronic active hepatitis; NA = not available.

TABLE 32–5

PREVALENCE OF HEPATITIS C VIRUS INFECTION AMONG CADAVER ORGAN DONORS

Organ Procurement Organization	Country	Author	Study Period	No. Donors Tested	ELISA1 (%)	ELISA2 (%)	PCR (%)
U.S. National Collaborative Study	United States	Pereira et al. (1994)	1986–92	3,078	5.10	4.2	2.4
New England Organ Bank, Massachusetts			1986–92	1,012	2.90	2.4	1.7
Regional Organ Bank of Illinois, Illinois			1987–91	596	6.00	3.2	2.7
Lifelink Inc., Florida			1985–91	521	7.70	7.3	4.0
Center for Organ Recovery and Education, Philadelphia			1986–90	516	5.80	5.4	2.1
Midwest Organ Bank, Kansas			1988–90	172	4.70	4.1	2.0
Louisiana Organ Procurement Agency, Louisiana			1990–91	129	2.30	2.3	0.8
Organ Health Sciences University, Oregon			1990–91	67	1.50	NA	NA
Washington Hospital Center, Washington, D.C.			1991	66	16.70	8.3	4.2
California Transplant Donor Network, California	United States	Vincenti et al. (1993)	1989–90	205	5.90	NA	NA
University of Miami, Florida	United States	Roth et al. (1992)	1979–91	484	18.00	6.8	3.4
National Organization of Transplantation	Spain	Miranda et al. (1993)	1992	360	NA	1.6	NA
Chang Gung Memorial Hospital, Taipei	Taiwan	Huang et al. (1993)	1985–91	110	NA	11.8	11.8
S. Giovanni-Molinette Hospital, Turin	Italy	Triolo et al. (1992)	1984–90	241	NA	4.0	NA
Addenbrooke's Hospital, Cambridge	United Kingdom	Wreghitt et al. (1994)	1984–91	554	NA	1.08	NA
Hospital Alacant, Alicante	Spain	Prados et al. (1992)	1992	77	NA	3.89	3.89
Hospital Covadonga, Oviedo	Spain	Gomez et al. (1991)	1985–90	78	3.80	NA	NA

ELISA = enzyme-linked immunosorbent assay; PCR = polymerase chain reaction; NA = not available.
Reproduced with permission from Pereira and Levey, 1997.

were 55.1% and 100%. Based on these estimates, discarding organs from ELISA2-positive donors would eliminate transmission of infection, but 4.2% of anti-HCV–positive donors would be discarded, and kidneys from 1.88% of donors (anti-HCV positive, HCV RNA negative) would be wasted. Using ELISA3, Preiksaitis and coworkers reported a 3.7% prevalence of anti-HCV among cadaver organ donors in Canada (Preiksaitis et al., 1997). Because the third-generation anti-HCV tests showed high specificity in donor screening, the authors hypothesized that their use could minimize the loss of donors owing to false-positive results for anti-HCV.

Some investigators had suggested that social, demographic and clinical data could be used to predict which anti-HCV–positive donors have HCV RNA (Mendez et al., 1993; Tesi et al., 1993). Specifically, it had been suggested that anti-HCV–positive donors with no history of drug abuse or homosexual lifestyle, absence of anti-HBs or anti-HBc antibody and normal serum ALT levels were at lower risk of transmitting disease and could be used for transplantation (Mendez et al., 1993; Tesi et al., 1993). In the national collaborative study, we found that these characteristics did not distinguish anti-HCV–positive donors with and without serum HCV RNA (Pereira et al., 1994). We concluded that there are no *low-risk* anti-HCV–positive cadaver organ donors defined by clinical criteria. Another strategy to improve the prediction would be to develop confirmatory tests for use in donors with a positive ELISA2. In our study, the RIBA2, which has been suggested as a confirmatory test in blood donors, was not specific enough to distinguish ELISA2-positive organ donors with and without serum HCV RNA. Newer confirmatory tests with a greater specificity need to be developed to improve the prediction of HCV RNA among cadaver donors.

Transmission of Hepatitis C Virus by Organ Transplantation

Shortly after the introduction of the first-generation anti-HCV tests, the New England Organ Bank initiated studies to evaluate the risk of transmission of HCV infection by anti-HCV–positive cadaver organ donors. Stored sera from 716 consecutive cadaver organ donors between 1986 and 1990 (before the availability of anti-HCV tests) were screened for anti-HCV using the ELISA1, and 13 (1.8%) anti-HCV–positive

donors were identified (Pereira et al., 1991, 1992). Of the 29 recipients of organs from these anti-HCV–positive donors, 14 (48%) developed posttransplantation NANBH within a mean follow-up interval of 20 months, a prevalence that was sevenfold to eightfold higher than that among recipients of untested donors in previous studies (LaQuaglia et al., 1981; Weir et al., 1985). Of the 14 recipients who developed NANBH, 2 (14%) died from subfulminant liver failure, and 12 (86%) developed chronic liver disease. Liver pathology was available in eight patients and revealed CAH in six patients and cirrhosis in two patients. Among the 24 recipients in whom posttransplantation sera were available, 16 (67%) tested positive for anti-HCV, and 23 (96%) tested positive for HCV RNA by PCR. All 13 HCV RNA–negative recipients of organs from HCV RNA–positive donors tested positive for HCV RNA after transplantation. These observations showed unequivocally the transmission of HCV by organ transplantation. Similar studies have been undertaken by other organ procurement organizations and transplant centers (Table 32–6). Among recipients of organs from anti-HCV–positive donors, 35% (range, 0–55%) developed posttransplant liver disease, 50% (range, 14–100%) tested positive for anti-HCV after transplantation and 74% (range, 14–96%) tested positive for HCV RNA by PCR (Aeder et al., 1993; Gomez et al., 1991; Huang et al., 1993; LeFor et al., 1991; Otero et al., 1990; Pereira et al., 1991, 1992, 1995a; Pirsch et al., 1995; Prados et al., 1992; Roth et al., 1992; Tesi et al., 1994; Triolo et al., 1992; Vincenti et al., 1993; Wreghitt et al., 1994).

The differences in the rate of transmission of HCV infection by anti-HCV–positive donors reported by different centers could be due to several factors. First, clinical or laboratory evidence of liver disease and testing for anti-HCV among organ transplant recipients significantly underestimate the prevalence and transmission of HCV infection (Pereira et al., 1992). Failure to test recipients for HCV RNA at some centers could suggest erroneously a low rate of transmission of HCV infection. Second, the risk of transmission of HCV infection by anti-HCV–positive cadaver organ donors could be related to the prevalence of HCV RNA among these donors (Pereira et al., 1994). A lower prevalence of HCV RNA among anti-HCV–positive cadaver organ donors at some centers could explain the lower rate of transmission of HCV by anti-HCV–positive donors reported by these

TABLE 32–6

TRANSMISSISON OF HEPATITIS C VIRUS INFECTION BY ANTI–HEPATITIS C VIRUS–POSITIVE CADAVER ORGAN DONORS

			Posttransplant Recipients' Characteristics					
			Liver Disease		Anti-HCV		HCV RNA	
Country	Author	Study Period	N	(%)	N	(%)	N	(%)
United States	Pereira et al. (1991, 1992)	1986–90	16/29	(55)	16/24	(67)	23/24	(96)
United States	Roth et al. (1992)	1979–91	13/46	(28)	10/31	(32)	NA	
Taiwan	Huang et al. (1993)	1985–91	7/19	(37)	14/19	(74)	18/19	(95)
United States	Vincenti et al. (1993)	1990	0/7	(0)	1/7	(14)	1/7	(14)
Spain	Gomez et al. (1991)	1990	2/4	(50)	2/4	(50)	NA	
Italy	Triolo et al. (1992)	1984–90	2/13	(15)	13/13	(100)	NA	
United States	LeFor et al. (1991)		12/30	(40)	NA		NA	
United States	Aeder et al. (1993)	1988–90	5/25	(20)	11/24	(46)	13/22	(59)
United States	Tesi et al. (1994)	1990–93	18/43	(42)	15/43	(35)	21/37	(57)
United Kingdon	Wreghitt et al. (1994)	1984–91	7/15	(47)	6/15	(40)	12/14	(86)
Spain	Prados et al. (1992)	1992	2/6	(33)	5/6	(83)	5/6	(83)
United States	Pirsch et al. (1995)	1991–94	NA	NA	NA		47/61	(77)
			84/237	(35)	93/186	(50)	140/190	(74)

HCV = hepatitis C virus; NA = not available.
Reproduced with permission from Pereira and Levey, 1997.

centers (Mendez *et al.*, 1993; Roth *et al.*, 1992; Tesi *et al.*, 1993). Some authors have suggested that reduction of the viral inoculum by pulsatile perfusion of the organs as opposed to cold storage could reduce the transmission of HCV by infected organs (Roth *et al.*, 1992). This possibility remains to be proved, however.

Clinical Impact of Transmission

Long-term studies from the New England Organ Bank have compared posttransplantation clinical outcomes in the 29 recipients of organs from the 13 anti-HCV–positive cadaver organ donors (Pereira *et al.*, 1992) with 74 recipients from 37 randomly selected anti-HCV–negative donors (Pereira *et al.*, 1995a). After a median follow-up of 42 and 49 months, the relative risk of liver disease was increased fourfold among recipients from anti-HCV–positive donors (relative risk, 4.37; 95% confidence interval [CI], 1.97–9.70), and 4 (14%) of the 29 patients died owing to or with liver failure. There was no increase in graft loss (relative risk, 0.93; 95% CI, 0.51–1.70) or death (relative risk, 0.89; 95% CI, 0.41–1.93) among recipients from anti-HCV–positive donors. After extended follow-up (median, 68 months among recipients of organs from anti-HCV–positive donors and 70 months among recipients of organs from anti-HCV–negative donors), there continued to be no significant differences between groups with respect to graft loss or death. Compared with recipients of organs from anti-HCV–negative donors, the relative risk of graft loss among recipients of organs from anti-HCV–positive donors was 0.95 (95% CI, 0.54–1.67), and the relative risk of death was 1.00 (95% CI, 0.49–2.02) (Bouthot *et al.*, 1997b). Mendez and associates prospectively studied 42 anti-HCV–negative recipients of kidneys from anti-HCV–positive donors (Mendez *et al.*, 1995). After 4 years of follow-up, the prevalence of liver disease was higher than in controls, but patient survival was not significantly different. Pirsch and coworkers prospectively transplanted 69 kidneys from anti-HCV–positive donors in anti-HCV–negative recipients who were considered to have a limited life expectancy (Pirsch *et al.*, 1995). After a short follow-up, one patient died of fulminant hepatitis, and two patients developed cirrhosis. Survival among recipients from anti-HCV–positive donors was significantly lower compared with recipients from anti-HCV–negative donors. These data indicate a higher risk of liver disease but no significant adverse effect on patient or graft survival. Subfulminant hepatitis was reported only among patients who received organs from anti-HCV–positive donors.

Impact of Policies Concerning the Use of Kidneys from Donors with Hepatitis C Virus Infection

With the current shortage of cadaver kidneys and the waiting list constantly growing, it is important to consider carefully the impact of different policies concerning the use of organs from anti-HCV–positive cadaver organ donors. We calculated the impact of these policies on organ discard, transmission of HCV and acquisition of new infection after transplantation (Pereira and Levey, 1995; Table 32–7). For this discussion, we restrict consideration to policies regarding kidney donation because more data are available regarding HCV infection in kidney donors and recipients. Estimates are based on the following assumptions (Pereira and Levey, 1995): (1) Procurement of 8,161 kidneys recovered from 4,843 cadaver organ donors (1.7 kidneys per donor) in the United States in 1993 (UNOS, 1994), (2) 31,115 patients on the waiting list for kidney transplantation during that same year, (3) a 2.4% prevalence of HCV infection among cadaver organ donors (Pereira *et al.*, 1994), (4) a 100% sensitivity and 98.1% specificity of ELISA2 in detecting donors with HCV infection (Pereira *et al.*, 1994), (5) a 100% transmission of HCV infection by HCV RNA–positive donors (Pereira *et al.*, 1992, 1994), (6) a 20% prevalence of anti-HCV in dialysis patients and an 80% prevalence of HCV RNA among anti-HCV–positive patients (indicating current infection) (Morales *et al.*, 1995) and (7) no apparent clinical consequence of superinfection or mixed infection (Morales *et al.*, 1995; Natov *et al.*, 1999). We used the following definitions: (1) *Organ discard* is the loss of organs from otherwise suitable cadaver donors because of a positive test for anti-HCV, (2) *transmission of infection* is transmission of HCV RNA from donor to recipient and (3) *new infection* is acquisition of HCV RNA from the donor by a recipient who did not have HCV RNA at the time of transplantation.

Based on the aforementioned assumptions, no restrictions on the use of organs from anti-HCV–positive donors (*no restriction*; see Table 32–7) would lead to no loss of organs but transmission of infection to 2.4% of recipients (196 recipients) and new infection in 2.0% of uninfected recipients (165 recipients). In our view, the higher prevalence of liver disease and potential long-term morbidity and mortality among these recipients makes such a policy undesirable. Nonetheless, we recognize patients' autonomy to make decisions when data on morbidity and mortality are not conclusive. A nationwide moratorium on the use of kidneys from anti-HCV–positive donors (*complete restriction*; see Table 32–7) would eliminate transmission of infection but result in the discard of kidneys from 4.2% of cadaver organ donors (346 kidneys). At a time of severe shortage of cadaver organs, the loss of 346 otherwise suitable kidneys is undesirable. If use of organs from anti-HCV–positive donors were restricted to recipients with pretransplant anti-HCV (see Table 32–7), no organs would be discarded, HCV infection would be transmitted to 2.4% of recipients (196 recipients), but new infection would occur in only 0.5% (41 recipients). If, instead, organs from anti-HCV–positive donors were restricted to recipients with pretransplant HCV RNA (see Table 32–7), transmission of HCV infection to previously uninfected recipients would be eliminated, but this strategy would require pretransplant testing of potential recipients for HCV RNA by PCR. If it

TABLE 32–7

IMPACT OF POLICIES CONCERNING THE USE OF KIDNEYS FROM DONORS WITH HEPATITIS C VIRUS INFECTION

Policy	Organ Loss (%)	Transmission (%)	New Infection (%)
No restriction	0	2.4	2.0
Complete restriction	4.2	0	0
Restricted to anti-HCV–positive recipients	0	2.4	0.5
Restricted to HCV RNA–positive recipients	0	2.4	0

Reproduced with permission from Pereira and Levey, 1995.

were possible to test anti-HCV–positive donors by PCR and genotype match PCR-positive donors and recipients, superinfection with a different strain could be eliminated. Currently, there are not sufficient data to evaluate fully these latter two strategies. In our view, short-term clinical data on outcomes among anti-HCV–positive recipients of kidneys from anti-HCV–positive donors as well as the evidence that mixed infections (HCV infections with more than one HCV genotype) do not affect adversely survival among ESRD patients justify further study of the strategy of allocating kidneys from anti-HCV–positive organ donors to anti-HCV–positive transplant candidates.

Transplantation of Kidneys from Anti–Hepatitis C Virus–Positive Donors into Recipients with Pretransplantation Hepatitis C Virus Infection

In chimpanzees, previous infection with HCV does not protect from reinfection with a different strain or the same strain of the virus (Farci et al., 1992). Likewise, dialysis and transplant patients with preexisting HCV infection are not protected from superinfection with a new HCV genotype (Oldach et al., 1995; Widell et al., 1995). Two reports have shown that among HCV RNA–positive recipients of kidneys from HCV RNA–positive donors, the viral genotype present posttransplantation was the same genotype present pretransplantation and/or the genotype from the donor (Oldach et al., 1995; Widell et al., 1995). The clinical implications of superinfection in transplant recipients are not well defined. We have shown that the type of HCV infection, single versus mixed (infection with more than one HCV genotype), did not affect adversely patient survival among renal transplant candidates (Natov et al., 1999). Because of the current shortage of cadaver kidneys and to minimize the waste of kidneys from anti-HCV–positive organ donors, some transplant centers have adopted a policy to transplant kidneys from anti-HCV–positive organ donors into anti-HCV–positive recipients. In a prospective study from Spain, there were no differences in the posttransplantation prevalence of liver disease, graft survival or patient survival among 24 anti-HCV–

positive recipients who received kidneys from anti-HCV–positive donors compared with 40 anti-HCV–positive recipients of kidneys from anti-HCV–negative donors (Morales et al., 1995). Four (80%) of five anti-HCV–positive but PCR-negative recipients from PCR-positive donors acquired HCV RNA, however (Morales et al., 1995). These data suggest that superinfections do occur, but they may not have any serious clinical consequences, at least in the short-term.

Effect of Pretransplantation Anti–Hepatitis C Virus Status on Posttransplantation Clinical Outcomes

Among renal transplant recipients, the prevalence of pretransplantation anti-HCV is 11 to 49% (Fritsche et al., 1993; Huang et al., 1992; Pereira et al., 1995b; Ponz et al., 1991; Roth, 1995; Roth et al., 1994; Stempel et al., 1993; Ynares et al., 1993). Pretransplantation anti-HCV is associated with an increased risk of posttransplant liver disease, which is reported in 19 to 64% of anti-HCV–positive recipients, compared with 1 to 30% of anti-HCV–negative recipients (Fritsche et al., 1993; Lee et al., 1996; Pereira et al., 1995b; Roth et al., 1994; Stempel et al., 1993; Ynares et al., 1993; Table 32–8). Studies from the New England Organ Bank have shown that for recipients with anti-HCV before transplantation, the relative risk of posttransplantation liver disease was 5.0 (95% CI, 2.4–10.5) (Pereira et al., 1995b). Among patients with pretransplantation HCV RNA in the serum, kidney transplantation was associated with a 1.8-fold to 30.3-fold increase in viral titer, suggesting that kidney transplantation is associated with proliferation of HCV. Among patients with HCV RNA detected in the serum, however, the titer of HCV RNA did not differ between patients with and patients without posttransplantation liver disease. Other investigators have shown that the posttransplant viral load was similar in patients with mild histological changes on liver biopsy compared with patients with chronic changes (Roth et al., 1996). The transaminase patterns were not associated with the level of viral load (Roth et al., 1996). These data suggest that factors other than the viral load determine the risk of liver disease among transplant recipients with HCV infection.

TABLE 32–8
IMPACT OF PRETRANSPLANTATION ANTI–HEPATITIS C VIRUS ON GRAFT AND PATIENT SURVIVAL

Author	Study Period	Anti-HCV Status	N	Liver Disease (%)	Actuarial Graft Survival (%)*	Actuarial Patient Survival (%)*
Ynares et al., 1993	1980–81, 1986–87	ELISA1 positive	65	29	33 (10)	53 (10)
		ELISA1 negative	195	7	25 (10)	54 (10)
Fritsche et al., 1993	1979–90	ELISA2 positive	53	19	32 (10)	58 (8)
		ELISA2 negative	256	2	53 (10)	82 (8)
Roth et al., 1994	1979–91	RIBA2 positive	109	34	81 (5)	63 (5)
		RIBA2 negative	200	19	80 (5)	63 (5)
Pereira et al., 1995b	1986–90	ELISA2 positive	23	64	50†	59†
		ELISA2 negative	80	19	59†	85†
Lee et al., 1996	1979–94	ELISA1 or 2 positive	29	21	75 (5)	83 (5)
		ELISA1 or 2 negative	1,068	1	84 (5)	91 (5)
Aroldi et al., 1998	1969–89	ELISA2 positive	130	48	55 (14)	77 (14)
		ELISA2 negative	190	NA	59 (14)	85 (14)
Legendre et al., 1998	1979–94	ELISA2 positive	112	NA	40 (6.6)	87 (6.6)
		ELISA2 negative	387	NA	65 (6.7)	95 (6.7)
Mathurin et al., 1999	1972–96	ELISA2 positive	216	NA	45 (10)	55 (10)
		ELISA2 negative	216	NA	69 (10)	80 (10)

*For actuarial graft and patient survival, the numbers in parentheses indicate duration (years).
†As of 12/93.
HCV = hepatitis C virus; ELISA = enzyme-linked immunosorbent assay.

Although pretransplantation anti-HCV is associated consistently with an increased risk of posttransplantation liver disease, posttransplantation patient survival was affected adversely in only some studies (Aroldi *et al.*, 1998; Fritsche *et al.*, 1993; Lee *et al.*, 1996; Legendre *et al.*, 1998; Mathurin *et al.*, 1999; Pereira *et al.*, 1995b; Roth *et al.*, 1994; Ynares *et al.*, 1993; see Table 32–8). Studies from Roth *et al.* (1994) at the University of Miami, Ynares *et al.* (1993) at Vanderbilt University, and Stempel *et al.* (1993) at the University of California San Francisco failed to detect significant differences in patient survival between recipients with and recipients without anti-HCV before renal transplantation. In contrast, studies from Fritsche *et al.* (1993) at the Medical College of Wisconsin reported a lower 8-year patient survival among the anti-HCV–positive recipients compared with anti-HCV–negative controls. Our results from the New England Organ Bank study revealed that recipients with pretransplantation anti-HCV had a 3.3-fold higher risk of death (95% CI, 1.4–7.9) and a 9.9-fold higher risk of death owing to sepsis (95% CI, 2.6–38.3) (Pereira *et al.*, 1995b). Infection rather than liver failure was the leading cause of death among anti-HCV–positive recipients. Other, more recent studies (see Table 32–8) have found a lower survival among patients with pretransplantation anti-HCV compared with patients without anti-HCV.

The differences among studies in patient survival could be due to several factors, including (1) differences in study design, such as selection of patients and length and completeness of follow-up; (2) virus and test factors, such as sensitivity and specificity of anti-HCV test, prevalence of serum HCV RNA, genotype of infecting virus and single or mixed infection and (3) the presence and severity of pretransplant liver disease, HLA matching and immunosuppression protocols. The severity of pretransplant liver disease has been shown to be an important predictor of adverse posttransplant outcomes (Rao *et al.*, 1993).

Effect of Renal Transplantation on the Course of Hepatitis C Virus Infection in Dialysis Patients

Port and colleagues observed that in the general ESRD population, compared with wait-listed dialysis patients, patients who underwent renal transplantation had a higher relative risk of death in the first month posttransplantation (relative risk, 2.43) but a lower relative risk thereafter (relative risk, 0.96 at 1–12 months and 0.36 after 12 months) (Port *et al.*, 1993). These results showed the long-term benefit of kidney transplantation on patient survival (Port *et al.*, 1993). Evidence exists that transplantation, by virtue of the necessity for continuous immunosuppressive therapy, can worsen the course of some viral infections, including infection with HCV. As discussed earlier, in some studies, HCV infection at the time of renal transplantation was associated with an increased risk of liver disease and death in the posttransplantation period. Many studies have found that the prevalence of liver disease among anti-HCV–positive transplant recipients (19–66%) does not exceed the prevalence among anti-HCV–positive dialysis patients (18–80%), however (Alivanis *et al.*, 1991; Cordero Sanchez *et al.*, 1991; Jeffers *et al.*, 1990; Jonas *et al.*, 1992; Lilis *et al.*, 1991; Lozano *et al.*, 1991; Medici *et al.*, 1990; Mondelli *et al.*, 1990; Ponz *et al.*, 1991; Pouteil-Noble *et al.*, 1991; Schlipkoter *et al.*, 1990; Zeldis *et al.*, 1990).

Transplant physicians are faced with the dilemma whether or not to offer renal transplantation to anti-HCV–positive ESRD patients. With 41,833 patients on the renal transplant waiting list in the United States alone (UNOS Report as of 5/12/99), it is important to clarify the merits of allocation

kidneys to anti-HCV–positive patients. To evaluate the relative effect of dialysis versus transplantation on patient survival, we studied a cohort of 496 ESRD patients referred for renal transplantation between 1986 and 1990 to the transplant centers served by the New England Organ Bank. We found that the presence of anti-HCV was associated with a 1.41-fold (1.01–1.97 fold) increased risk of death, regardless of whether the patients remained on dialysis or underwent renal transplantation (Pereira *et al.*, 1998; Fig. 32–1). The HCV genotype and the type of HCV infection (mixed *vs.* single) had no significant impact on patient survival (Natov *et al.*, 1999b; Fig. 32–2). The analysis of the effect of treatment modality (dialysis *vs.* transplantation) on patient survival revealed that among the anti-HCV–positive renal transplant candidates, those who received a transplant had an initially higher risk of death (4.75 at 0–3 months and 1.76 at 4–6 months) but a lower risk thereafter (0.31 at 7 months to 4 years and 0.84 at >4 years) (Pereira *et al.*, 1998). This pattern was not affected by the HCV genotype or type of HCV infection (Natov *et al.*, 1999b). Our results show that the association between transplantation and survival was not different between anti-HCV–positive and anti-HCV–negative patients and was not influenced by the genotype or the number of infecting HCV strains. These findings suggest that the possible detrimental effect of transplantation on the course of HCV infection does not appear to outweigh its long-term beneficial effect on survival in ESRD.

In the absence of definite studies showing worse outcomes after renal transplantation, anti-HCV–positive status alone should not be considered a contraindication for renal transplantation, and anti-HCV–positive ESRD patients should be allowed to make an informed choice between dialysis and transplantation. Because the histological severity of liver damage is a strong predictor of liver failure and death after transplantation and because dialysis patients and transplant recipients can have histological evidence of liver disease in the absence of increased ALT levels, there may be merit in a policy to perform liver biopsies on anti-HCV–positive patients awaiting renal transplantation. In patients with histological evidence of liver disease, the decision to proceed with renal transplantation should be made cautiously, after considering the influence of immunosuppression on viral replication and consequent exacerbation of liver disease.

Treatment of Chronic Hepatitis C Infection in Patients with End-Stage Renal Disease—Role of Interferon Alfa and Newer Agents

The efficacy of interferon alfa therapy in chronic hepatitis C has been shown in many randomized controlled trials, and its use currently is recommended in anti-HCV–positive patients with abnormal serum aminotransferases and well-compensated chronic hepatitis on biopsy (Anonymous, 1997; Lindsay, 1997). Four forms of interferon alfa have been evaluated for clinical use in large trials: alfa-2b (most commonly used), alfa-2a, alfa-n1 and consensus interferon (Lindsay, 1997). They appear to be similarly effective. Many other α and β interferons are under evaluation (Lindsay, 1997).

Normalization of serum ALT is defined as a *biochemical response* to treatment, and clearance of HCV RNA from the serum is defined as a *virological response*. A complete biochemical and virological response by the end of the treatment is defined as *end-of-treatment response* (ETR) and at 6 or 12 months as a *sustained response* (SR) (Anonymous, 1997). Two therapeutic regimens using identical dosing (3 million units of interferon alfa administered subcutaneously three times weekly) but different duration of treatment (either 6 or 12 months) have been studied (Anonymous, 1997; Lindsay,

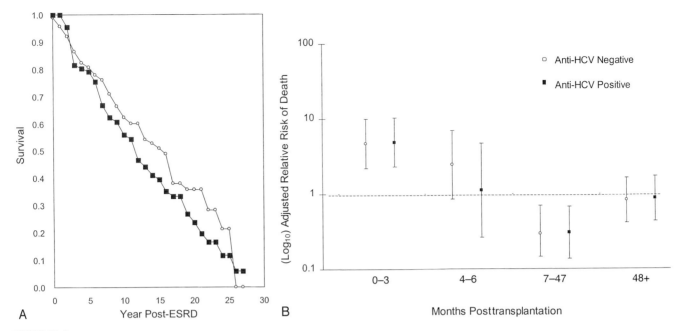

FIGURE 32–1

(A) Survival among anti-hepatitis C virus (HCV)–negative and anti-HCV–positive patients referred for renal transplantation. The unadjusted actuarial survival from the time of first initiation of renal replacement therapy (dialysis or transplantation) until death, loss to follow-up or December 31, 1995, whichever occurred first, is shown. (B) Relative risk of death for transplantation versus dialysis among anti-HCV–negative and anti-HCV–positive patients referred for renal transplantation. The relative risk of death (and the 95% confidence intervals) for different time intervals after transplantation is adjusted for age and the presence of diabetes. The relative risk of death for transplantation versus dialysis was similar for anti-HCV–positive and anti-HCV–negative patients at all intervals after transplantation. ○ = anti-HCV negative; ■ = anti-HCV positive. ESRD = end-stage renal disease. (Reproduced with permission of Pereira *et al.*, 1998.)

1997). Six-month treatment courses resulted in biochemical and virological ETR rates of 40 to 50% and 30 to 40% and biochemical and virological SR of 15 to 20% and 10 to 20% (Anonymous, 1997). The biochemical and virological responses were accompanied by histological improvement. Twelve-month treatment regimens did not produce higher biochemical or virological ETR but did increase SR rates to 20 to 30% (Anonymous, 1997). The benefits of treatment of longer duration and higher doses are being evaluated (Di Bisceglie, 1994). Although interferon alfa treatment has shown favorable biochemical and virological results, its ef-

fects on paramount clinical outcomes such as quality of life and disease progression have not been ascertained (Anonymous, 1997).

Among patients with chronic hepatitis C, the pretreatment clinical, biochemical, histological and viral characteristics that predict the success of interferon treatment have been the subject of intense investigation. Patients with lower levels of viral RNA in the serum and lower concentration of HCV antigens in the liver are more likely to respond to interferon treatment (Di Bisceglie *et al.*, 1993). Preliminary results of a large European multicenter study suggest that age less than

TABLE 32–9

INITIAL RESPONSE TO INTERFERON ALFA TREATMENT IN DIALYSIS AND TRANSPLANT PATIENTS WITH CHRONIC HEPATITIS C

Author	Study Population	N	Decrease in Serum ALT (%)*	Improvement in Liver Histology (%)*	Clearing of Serum HCV RNA (%)*
Harihara *et al.*, 1994	Tx	3	67	NA	NA
Koenig *et al.*, 1994	HD	37	71	NA	65
Rao and Anderson, 1995	HD + Tx	10	100	80	NA
Pol *et al.*, 1995a	HD	19	85	NA	53
Rostaing *et al.*, 1995	Tx	16	100	NA	0
Casanovas *et al.*, 1995	HD	10	90	NA	10
Duarte *et al.*, 1995	HD	5	100	NA	NA
Raptopoulou-Gigi *et al.*, 1995	HD	19	100	NA	77
Ozgur *et al.*, 1995	Tx	5	100	100	NA
Rodrigues *et al.*, 1997	HD	6	NA	NA	50
Yasumura *et al.*, 1997	Tx	6	100	NA	33
Umlauft *et al.*, 1997	HD	33	NA	NA	73
Rostaing *et al.*, 1998a	HD	10	NA	NA	90
Hanafusa *et al.*, 1998	Tx	10	80	NA	20

*Among patients who had an abnormal test before treatment and who completed the course of treatment.
ALT = alanine aminotransferase; HCV = hepatitis C virus; HD = hemodialysis patients; Tx = transplant recipients.

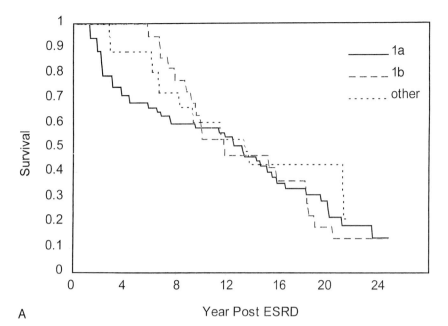

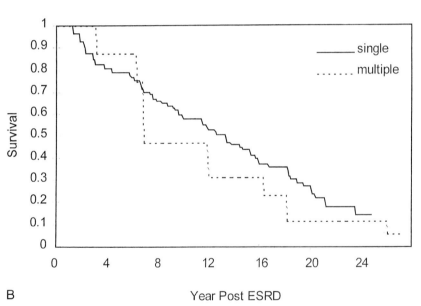

FIGURE 32–2

(A) Survival since the initiation of renal replacement therapy among renal transplant candidates infected with hepatitis C virus (HCV) genotypes 1a (heavy solid line), 1b (long dashed line), or all others (dotted line). (B) Survival since the initiation of renal replacement therapy among renal transplant candidates infected with a single (solid line) or mixed (dotted line) HCV infection. ESRD = end-stage renal disease. (Reproduced with permission of Natov et al., 1999.)

40 years, absence of cirrhosis, pretreatment ALT levels less than three times the upper limit of normal, posttransfusion rather than sporadic infection and infection with the genotypes 1, 5 and 6 are predictors of response to interferon treatment (Brouwer et al., 1993). Others have shown, however, that patients infected with genotypes 2 and 3 have a better response to interferon than those infected with genotype 1 (Chemello et al., 1994). Some of the differences in the relationship between HCV subtypes and response to interferon treatment could be related to the lack of uniformity in the viral nomenclature followed by different groups and the different types of interferon used. Nevertheless, tailoring interferon treatment based on viral type promises to be an exciting possibility.

Interferon alfa has pleiotropic effects including antiproliferative and immunomodulatory properties as well as antiviral activity (Black and Peters, 1992). Interferon alfa induces cytokine gene expression; increased cell surface expression of HLA antigens and enhanced function of natural killer cells,

cytotoxic T cells and monocytes. The use of interferon alfa as prophylaxis against CMV disease in renal transplant recipients has been associated with a high incidence of steroid-resistant allograft rejection resulting in graft loss (Kovarik et al., 1988; Kramer et al., 1985). Because interferon alfa treatment carries a risk of inducing or facilitating rejection in allograft recipients, questions have been raised regarding the efficacy, tolerance, safety and timing of interferon alfa therapy in dialysis and transplant patients.

As shown in Table 32–9, the initial response of dialysis and transplant patients to interferon alfa treatment has been encouraging with most patients showing a decrease in serum ALT levels and an improvement in liver histology (Casanovas et al., 1995; Duarte et al., 1995; Hanafusa et al., 1998; Harihara et al., 1994; Koenig et al., 1994; Ozgur et al., 1995; Pol et al., 1995a; Rao and Anderson, 1995; Raptopoulou-Gigi et al., 1995; Rodrigues et al., 1997; Rostaing et al., 1995, 1998a; Umlauft et al., 1997; Yasumura et al., 1997). As in the case with non–renal disease patients, relapses are common after stopping treatment, and long-term outcomes are not adequately defined (Pol *et al.*, 1995a; Rostaing *et al.*, 1995; Umlauft *et al.*, 1997). Although disappearance of HCV RNA from the serum is common, recurrence of viremia from extravascular sites remains a distinct possibility (Oesterreicher *et al.*, 1995; Rostaing *et al.*, 1995).

A major stumbling block to interferon alfa treatment in transplant recipients has been the occurrence of acute rejection. Most studies have observed an increased risk of acute rejection (40–100%) among transplant recipients treated with interferon alfa for chronic liver disease resulting from hepatitis C (Chan *et al.*, 1993; Harihara *et al.*, 1994; Ozgur *et al.*, 1995; Rostaing *et al.*, 1995). Rao and Anderson (1995) did not encounter allograft rejection in six renal transplant recipients treated with interferon alfa 2 to 15 years after transplantation. The absence of rejection in this study could be attributed to the fact that the patients had stable renal function for several years before the start of interferon alfa therapy and were at low risk of rejection. Others have shown irreversible rejection, however, and return to dialysis in patients treated with interferon alfa 8 years after transplantation has been documented (Harihara *et al.*, 1994; Ozgur *et al.*, 1995). Similarly, patients treated with interferon alfa to prevent posttransplantation CMV or EBV infection experienced an increased incidence of acute rejection.

Treatment with interferon alfa is associated with a flulike syndrome with asthenia, myalgia, headache, neutropenia, thrombocytopenia and depression and is related partly to the dose administered (Poynard *et al.*, 1995). Despite these side effects, the dropout rate among non–renal disease patients treated with interferon alfa has been low (Poynard *et al.*, 1995). In contrast, treatment was stopped for reasons other than transplant rejection in 0 to 54% of dialysis and transplant recipients treated with interferon alfa (Casanovas *et al.*, 1995; Koenig *et al.*, 1994; Pol *et al.*, 1995a; Rao and Anderson, 1995; Rostaing *et al.*, 1995). The reasons for this difference between non–renal disease and renal disease patients are currently unclear.

The limited efficacy of interferon alfa, its high cost, risk of acute rejection and side effects have diminished the enthusiasm for its use in transplant recipients with chronic HCV infection. The NIH Consensus Statement on management of hepatitis C currently lists renal transplant as a contraindication to treatment with interferon (Anonymous, 1997). A safer but probably less cost-effective strategy might be to treat dialysis patients with chronic hepatitis C before transplantation. Two studies in patients with chronic hepatitis C who were treated with interferon alfa while on dialysis did not observe recurrence of liver disease or an increased risk of rejection after subsequent transplantation (Casanovas *et al.*, 1995; Duarte *et al.*, 1995). In contrast, other investigators reported a high rate of relapse after transplantation (Rodrigues *et al.*, 1997) and questioned the beneficial role of this strategy. To date, data on the relapse rate in the posttransplant period are limited and controversial. Controlled studies are needed to evaluate the long-term effects of interferon alfa therapy in renal transplant candidates on the posttransplant course of liver disease, rates of transplantation, graft survival and patient survival.

Other treatment approaches to chronic hepatitis C, including steroids, ursodiol, thymosin and iron reduction therapy, have led to either disappointing or inconclusive results (Anonymous, 1997). A new oral antiviral drug, ribavirin, was introduced in clinical practice. Ribavirin is a synthetic guanosine analogue with activity against a broad spectrum of DNA and RNA viruses. It also possesses immunomodulatory properties. In several studies in non–renal disease patients, therapy with ribavirin has resulted in a decrease in serum aminotransferase concentrations in 50 to 60% of patients. If given for 12 months, this therapy has been associated with some degree of histological improvement (Di Bisceglie *et al.*, 1995). In renal transplant recipients, treatment with ribavirin failed to clear HCV RNA but was found to cause a drop in HCV RNA titers by 70 to 82% in 57% of the patients (Garnier *et al.*, 1997). Ribavirin was not associated with any detrimental side effects on graft function. The main side effect of ribavirin was dose-dependent hemolysis.

More promising results in the treatment of HCV infection have been observed with the use of ribavirin in combination with interferon alfa (Hoofnagle, 1997). Combination therapy with interferon alfa and ribavirin for 24 or 48 weeks has been shown to be superior to therapy with interferon alfa alone with respect to virological and biochemical ETR as well as SR (McHutchison *et al.*, 1998). In patients with chronic hepatitis C who relapse after treatment, this combination therapy has resulted in higher rates of sustained virological, biochemical and histological response than treatment with interferon alfa alone (Davis *et al.*, 1998). In the United States, combination therapy of oral ribavirin and subcutaneous interferon alfa-2b has been approved by the Food and Drug Administration and marketed for initial treatment and treatment of relapse of chronic hepatitis C.

GB VIRUS-C/HEPATITIS G VIRUS

Despite the development of reliable antibody assays and molecular probes for the detection of human hepatitis viruses A through E, the current serological and virological tests, in the absence of any recognizable nonviral causes for liver injury, cannot identify the cause in at least half of all cases of fulminant hepatitis (Miyakawa and Mayumi, 1997), approximately 16% of patients with posttransfusion hepatitis (Alter *et al.*, 1997a), 3% of patients with community-acquired acute hepatitis (Alter *et al.*, 1997b) and 5% of patients with chronic liver disease (Miyakawa and Mayumi, 1997). Most patients with non-A, non-B fulminant hepatic failure test negative for markers of HCV (Koretz *et al.*, 1993). The occurrence of these cases, commonly referred to as non–A through E hepatitis, has strongly suggested the existence of other, as yet unrecognized, hepatitis viruses and has encouraged the pursuit of new viral agents, which led to the discovery of the GB group of viruses (GBV)/hepatitis G.

Structure of GB Virus-C Genome

GB viruses are RNA viruses belonging to the Flavivirus family (Muerhoff *et al.*, 1995). In the late 1960s, Deinhardt and colleagues showed that an infective agent in plasma from a 34-year-old surgeon with acute hepatitis could be transmitted to marmosets and described the histology of the liver lesions caused by this agent in animals (Deinhardt *et al.*, 1967). Subsequent cross-challenge studies from this plasma suggested that the infective agent was distinct from hepatitis A, B, C, D and E. More recently, using a subtractive PCR methodology known as *representational difference analysis*, Simons and coworkers cloned two specific nucleotide sequences from the plasma of a tamarin that had been infected with pooled sera derived from serial passage in tamarins of the infective agent from the surgeon with hepatitis (Simons *et al.*, 1995b). These two agents were named *GB virus-A (GBV-A)* and *GBV-B*, after the initials of the surgeon from whom the infected serum was obtained.

Subsequent studies on serum from a West African patient with antibody to GBV-A and GBV-B revealed the presence of a nucleotide sequence with a nucleotide homology of 59% with GBV-A, 47.9% with GBV-B and 53.7% with HCV-1. The same unique sequence was identified in sera of some patients with non–A through E hepatitis (Simons *et al.*, 1995a). The nucleotide sequence of this virus, named *GBV-C*, has since been cloned and shown to contain the highly conserved RNA helicase domain characteristic of other members of the Flaviviridae family, including GBV-A, GBV-B and HCV-1 (Leary *et al.*, 1996). Linnen and associates have identified an RNA virus from the plasma of a patient with chronic hepatitis and designated it as *hepatitis G virus (HGV)* (Linnen *et al.*, 1996). Hepatitis G virus shows 95% amino acid sequence identity to GBV-C (85% at nucleotide level), suggesting that HGV and GBV-C are independent isolates of the same virus (Zuckerman, 1996); the term *GBV-C* is used hereafter.

Pathogenicity

Although GBV-C has been named a hepatitis virus and has shown a high prevalence among healthy blood donors as well as in various disease states, to date, there have been no conclusive data to show that GBV-C can cause liver disease. Earlier studies that have favored the role of GBV-C in causing hepatitis based on a higher prevalence of GBV-C RNA among volunteer blood donors with elevated ALT levels (Dawson *et al.*, 1996), patients with hepatitis of unknown cause (Fiordalisi *et al.*, 1996), chronic non–A through E hepatitis (Dawson *et al.*, 1996) and fulminant hepatitis (Heringlake *et al.*, 1996; Tameda *et al.*, 1996; Yoshiba *et al.*, 1995) have been challenged by more recent data suggesting lack of association between GBV-C and liver disease:

1. Among patients with acute hepatitis resulting from community-acquired HAV, HBV or HCV infection, biochemical markers of liver disease were similar among patients with and without GBV-C infection (Alter *et al.*, 1997b). The prevalence of chronic hepatitis among patients with HCV and GBV-C infections was similar to that among patients with HCV infection alone (Alter *et al.*, 1997b).
2. Among blood transfusion recipients, the prevalence of GBV-C RNA was not significantly different between groups with hepatitis C; non-A, non-B, non-C hepatitis or no hepatitis (Alter *et al.*, 1997a).
3. Among patients with fulminant liver failure, serum GBV-C RNA was uniformly absent in blood samples at the time of admission (i.e., before any blood transfusion) (Kanda *et al.*, 1997).
4. The prevalence of abnormal liver function tests was not significantly different between GBV-C RNA–positive and GBV-C RNA–negative cadaver organ donors (Murthy *et al.*, 1997a).
5. The prevalence of abnormal liver function tests among long-term hemodialysis patients was similar among patients with and without serum GBV-C RNA (Masuko *et al.*, 1996; Sampietro *et al.*, 1997).
6. Coinfection with GBV-C did not affect the severity of liver disease or response to interferon therapy among patients with chronic HCV–induced liver disease (Tanaka *et al.*, 1996).
7. In a study from the New England Organ Bank, the prevalence of elevated serum ALT levels among GBV-C RNA–positive patients (7%) was not different from that among GBV-C RNA–negative patients (7%) (Bouthot *et al.*, 1997a).

These studies indicate that GBV-C is unlikely to be associated with acute or chronic liver disease. Furthermore, it has been thought that GBV-C might not be a pathogen at all because except for sporadic case reports that linked the presence of serum GBV-C RNA to aplastic anemia (Byrnes *et al.*, 1996; Zaidi *et al.*, 1996), until not long ago there had been no other

data to suggest any GBV-C disease association. This lack of data might have reflected limited knowledge of GBV-C pathogenicity at that time (Mushahwar and Zuckerman, 1998). More recent studies have shown that GBV-C replicates in human liver (Mushahwar, 1998; Mushahwar *et al.*, 1998) and is involved with some cases of acute and chronic hepatitis (Fiordalisi *et al.*, 1996). There is an association between GBV-C and hepatitis C viremia and portal and periportal inflammation (Manolapoulos *et al.*, 1998). GB virus-C also replicates in the kidney, and GBV-C infection may be a risk factor for developing glomerulonephritis (Tucker *et al.*, 1998). A case of *de novo* membranoproliferative glomerulonephritis (type 1) occurring in a renal transplant recipient was associated with GBV-C infection (Berthoux *et al.*, 1999).

Epidemiology

GB virus-C has worldwide distribution. The presence of GBV-C RNA (with or without GBV-C E2 Ab) is interpreted as current infection, whereas the presence of GBV-C E2 Ab alone signifies past infection. GB virus-C exposure (a positive test for GBV-C RNA and/or GBV-C E2 Ab) refers to all patients with current or past infection.

Routes of Transmission and Prevalence

Among volunteer blood donors, the prevalence of GBV-C infection is 0.8 to 11% (Casteling *et al.*, 1998; Cheung *et al.*, 1997; Kallinowski *et al.*, 1998; Szabo *et al.*, 1997). A much higher proportion (5–16%) of them have evidence of GBV-C exposure, however (Nubling *et al.*, 1997; Pilot-Matias *et al.*, 1996; Schulte-Frohlinde *et al.*, 1998). Several lines of evidence indicate that GBV-C is a parenterally transmitted virus.

First, in animal experiments, GBV-C has been unequivocally shown to be transmitted by inoculation of infected serum (Schlauder *et al.*, 1995); an appearance of serum GBV-C RNA has been shown to coincide with transfusion-associated non–A through E hepatitis (Linnen *et al.*, 1996). Second, compared with volunteer blood donors, the prevalence of GBV-C infection is higher among populations at high risk of acquiring parentally transmitted infections such as hemophiliacs (1–24%) (Casteling *et al.*, 1998; Jarvis *et al.*, 1996; Linnen *et al.*, 1996; Tagariello *et al.*, 1996), multiply transfused individuals and commercial plasma donors (43–47%) (Neilson *et al.*, 1996; Pilot-Matias *et al.*, 1996), hemodialysis patients (3–55%) (Casteling *et al.*, 1998; Masuko *et al.*, 1996; Murthy *et al.*, 1998; Sampietro *et al.*, 1997; Sheng *et al.*, 1998; Shibuya *et al.*, 1998; Tsuda *et al.*, 1996), renal transplant recipients (14–43%) (Berthoux *et al.*, 1998; Casteling *et al.*, 1998; Fabrizi *et al.*, 1997b; Raengsakulrach *et al.*, 1997; Stark *et al.*, 1997) and intravenous drug users (16–33%) (Dawson *et al.*, 1996; Linnen *et al.*, 1996; Pilot-Matias *et al.*, 1996; Stark *et al.*, 1996). If GBV-C exposure is taken into account, the rates are even higher: 71% among commercial plasma donors and multiply transfused individuals (Pilot-Matias *et al.*, 1996), 55% among hemophiliacs (Nubling *et al.*, 1997), 21 to 44% among hemodialysis patients (Schroter *et al.*, 1999; Schulte-Frohlinde *et al.*, 1998; Seme *et al.*, 1998; Sheng *et al.*, 1998; Shibuya *et al.*, 1998; Tribl *et al.*, 1998), 28 to 53% among renal transplant recipients (Berthoux *et al.*, 1998; Dussol and Brunet, 1997; Stark *et al.*, 1997) and 74 to 100% among intravenous drug users (Nubling *et al.*, 1997; Pilot-Matias *et al.*, 1996). Third, the prevalence of GBV-C infection among cadaver organ donors is high, especially among those with serum markers of other parenterally transmitted viral infections. The prevalence of GBV-C infection among anti-HCV–positive donors (27.6%) was four times higher than that among anti-HCV–negative donors (7.3%) (Murthy *et al.*, 1997a). The prevalence of serum markers of HBV such as anti-HBs and anti-HBc antibodies was higher among donors with GBV-C infection than donors without infection. Finally, dialysis patients with GBV-C infection had received a higher number of blood transfusions and had a trend toward a longer duration of dialysis compared with patients without GBV-C infection (Murthy *et al.*, 1997b). These are both known risk factors for parenterally transmitted viral infections among dialysis patients (Pereira and Levey, 1997). These data suggest that GBV-C shares common modes of transmission with HBV and HCV and is also a parenterally transmitted virus.

Prevalence and Risk Factors Among Hemodialysis Patients

Among long-term hemodialysis patients, the prevalence of GBV-C RNA has been reported to be 3 to 55% in Asia (Masuko *et al.*, 1996; Tsuda *et al.*, 1996), 18 to 34% in the United States (Ashby *et al.*, 1996; Murthy *et al.*, 1997b) and 13 to 31% in Europe (Badalamenti *et al.*, 1996; Cabrerizo *et al.*, 1996; Charrel *et al.*, 1996; Izopet *et al.*, 1996; Sampietro *et al.*, 1997). The risk factors for GBV-C infection and the potential modes of transmission among hemodialysis patients are as yet incompletely defined. Increasing time on dialysis, higher number of blood product transfusions and glomerulonephritides as the cause of renal failure have been associated with an increased risk of GBV-C infection (Cabrerizo *et al.*, 1996; Murthy *et al.*, 1997b). In contrast to cadaver organ donors, the prevalence of GBV-C infection is not increased among anti-HCV–positive dialysis patients compared with anti-HCV negative patients. The 23% prevalence of GBV-C infection among anti-HCV–positive dialysis patients in the New England region of the United States was not significantly different from the 17% prevalence among anti-HCV–negative patients (Murthy *et al.*, 1997b). Likewise, the 45% prevalence of GBV-C infection among anti-HCV–positive dialysis patients in Miami, Florida, was not significantly different from the 32% prevalence among anti-HCV–negative patients (Ashby *et al.*, 1996). These data suggest that dialysis patients probably acquire HCV and GBV-C infection from different sources.

The reasons for the wide variation in the prevalence of GBV-C infection in different parts of the world are unclear. The highest prevalence of GBV-C infection among hemodialysis patients reported thus far (55%) was observed in Indonesia. This high prevalence is not surprising because the prevalence of anti-HCV (79%) among the same group of patients was also high—both infections are transmitted parenterally. The high prevalence of these parenterally transmitted virus infections among hemodialysis patients in this unit possibly reflects suboptimal infection control strategies in the dialysis units. Possible explanations for these differences among the different countries include variations in the prevalence of GBV-C infection among blood donors (Linnen *et al.*, 1996; Masuko *et al.*, 1996), difference in the primers used for the detection of virus and geographical differences in the prevalence of GBV-C as a result of differences in host susceptibility or virulence of different strains of GBV-C.

Prevalence Among Cadaver Organ Donors and Transmission by Organ Transplantation

A study of eight organ procurement organizations in the United States revealed that the prevalence of GBV-C RNA among cadaver organ donors between 1986 and 1992 was 8.3%, higher than the prevalence of anti-HCV by ELISA1 (5.1%), anti-HCV by ELISA2 (4.2%) or HCV RNA (2.4%) (Murthy *et al.*, 1997a). A blood alcohol level of more than 100 mg/dl and a positive anti-HCV test by ELISA2 were associ-

ated significantly with GBV-C infection among cadaver organ donors. A trend was present toward association between history of drug abuse and younger age. The odds ratio for association between GBV-C infection and HBsAb (odds ratio, 2.93) and anti-HBc (odds ratio, 3.30) was also increased. Blood product transfusions and elevated ALT levels were not associated with GBV-C infection. These data suggest that high-risk social behavior and exposure to other parenterally transmitted viral infections are associated with GBV-C infection among cadaver organ donors.

Hepatitis B virus, HCV and GBV-C probably share common routes of transmission, and as in the case of HBV and HCV, GBV-C also is likely to be transmitted by organ transplantation. Among patients who were transplanted with organs from GBV-C RNA–positive donors, there was no increase in the prevalence of posttransplantation GBV-C RNA, liver disease and NANBH. When only kidney recipients were taken into consideration, 1 of 3 (33%) recipients of kidneys from GBV-C RNA–positive donors acquired GBV-C RNA after transplantation compared with 4 of 40 (10%) recipients of kidneys from GBV-C RNA–negative donors, suggesting that GBV-C could be transmitted by organ transplantation. After a median follow-up of 6 years, there were no statistically significant differences between recipients of organs from GBV-C RNA–positive and GBV-C RNA–negative donors. Although it seems that GBV-C could be transmitted by organ transplantation, the results of this study preclude definitive conclusion. Further studies are required to determine the risk of transmission of GBV-C by organ transplantation and its role in posttransplant liver disease.

Prevalence of GB Virus-C Exposure Among Renal Transplant Candidates

We have shown that evidence of GBV-C exposure (a positive test for GBV-C RNA and/or GBV-C E2 Ab) was present in 58% of ESRD patients referred for renal transplantation to the centers served by the New England Organ Bank (Natov *et al.*, 2000). This high prevalence of GBV-C exposure is consistent with the high prevalence of GBV-C exposure among dialysis patients and renal transplant recipients reported by other investigators (17–53%) (Berthoux *et al.*, 1998; Schroter *et al.*, 1999; Schulte-Frohlinde *et al.*, 1998; Seme *et al.*, 1998; Sheng *et al.*, 1998; Shibuya *et al.*, 1998; Stark *et al.*, 1997; Tribl *et al.*, 1998). Our results confirm that testing for GBV-C RNA only grossly underestimates the true prevalence of GBV-C exposure because nearly all cases that seroconvert for GBV-C E2 Ab eventually clear the viral RNA from the blood and remain unrecognized. If only the presence of GBV-C RNA were used to appreciate the spread of GBV-C in general, all cases of past infection (GBV-C RNA–negative, but GBV-C E2 antibody–positive individuals) would have been missed. The magnitude of the spread of GBV-C can be appreciated correctly only by determining the rate of exposure to the virus (i.e., by testing for GBV-C RNA and GBV-C E2 antibody). The prevalence of GBV-C RNA in our study population was 31% compared with 58% prevalence of GBV-C exposure.

Effect of GB Virus-C Exposure and Renal Transplantation on Survival in End-Stage Renal Disease

To date, GBV-C has not been shown to affect adversely clinical outcomes among dialysis patients or renal transplant recipients. We have shown that among renal transplant candidates, GBV-C exposure was associated with a 1.28 relative risk of death, but the wide 95% CI (0.88–1.86) precluded definitive conclusions. GB virus-C exposure was not associated with a significantly increased risk of death from liver disease and/or infection (relative risk, 1.11; 95% CI, 0.58–2.11), in contrast to HCV infection, which in the same study population was associated with a 2.60-fold increase in the relative risk of death owing to liver disease or infection (Natov *et al.*, 2000).

This observation is consistent with our previous report showing lack of association of GBV-C RNA with any history or laboratory evidence of liver disease (Murthy *et al.*, 1998) and with the growing consensus that GBV-C may not be a hepatitis virus. Similar results have been reported among liver transplant recipients (Fried *et al.*, 1997; Pessoa *et al.*, 1997). Among patients who underwent liver transplantation for cryptogenic cirrhosis or for nonviral causes of end-stage liver disease, despite a high acquisition rate of GBV-C at the time of transplantation, the development of GBV-C infection did not predispose to viral hepatitis and had no adverse effect on graft or patient survival (Fried *et al.*, 1997; Pessoa *et al.*, 1997). Our results show that although the prevalence of GBV-C exposure among renal transplant recipients is high, this is not associated with increased risk of death from liver disease and/or infection. Whether GBV-C exposure increases all-cause mortality remains unresolved, however.

COINFECTIONS
Infections with Hepatitis B Virus and Hepatitis D Virus

In some studies, the aggressive nature of HBV-related liver disease and the high mortality rates among HBsAg-positive patients have been attributed to the presence of hepatitis delta virus (HDV). Hepatitis D virus, also referred to as *delta agent*, is a *defective*, single-stranded RNA virus that is highly infectious. This virus is unable to replicate on its own but can be activated by the presence of HBV and consequently can become capable of inducing hepatitis in a HBsAg-positive host. Hepatitis B virus and HDV infection may occur simultaneously, which is defined as a *coinfection*, or HDV may infect a chronic HBsAg carrier and cause *superinfection*. Coinfections usually resolve because HDV cannot outlive the transient hepatitis B surface antigenemia. In contrast, superinfections commonly lead to chronic delta hepatitis, resulting in severe disease and progression to liver cirrhosis. Hepatitis D virus superinfection always should be considered in a clinically stable HBsAg-positive patient who presents with a sudden relapse of liver disease. The serological diagnosis of HDV infection is based on measuring total antibody to HDV. A serological test is commercially available.

In the United States, the prevalence of HDV among HBsAg-positive individuals is less than 1% in the general population but greater than 10% in individuals with repeated percutaneous exposures, such as intravenous drug users and hemophiliacs. Huang and colleagues reported a 9% prevalence of HDV among HBsAg-positive renal transplant recipients (Huang *et al.*, 1990). This prevalence was higher (15%), however, if only HBsAg-positive renal transplant recipients with chronic hepatitis were taken into consideration. In Saudi Arabia, a geographical area highly endemic of HBV infection, Dhar and coworkers observed that HDV infection among HBsAg-positive renal transplant recipients was much more frequent (17%) and was associated with clinical progression of liver disease in 80% of cases (Dhar *et al.*, 1991). Histopathological findings in the patients who underwent liver biopsy were consistent with CAH (Dhar *et al.*, 1991). In contrast, many studies have failed to detect any cases of HDV infection among HBV-infected renal transplant recipients (Fornairon *et al.*, 1996; Friedlaender *et al.*, 1989; Harnett *et al.*, 1987).

Infections with Hepatitis B Virus and Hepatitis C Virus

Among renal transplant recipients, 30 to 40% of patients who are HBsAg positive are coinfected with HCV (Durlik *et al.*, 1996b; Fornairon *et al.*, 1996; Pouteil-Noble *et al.*, 1995), and 20% of patients who have HCV infection are coinfected with HBV (Pouteil-Noble *et al.*, 1995). Coinfections with HBV and HCV have been associated with an increased risk of developing posttransplant chronic liver disease and a higher incidence of severe histological lesions, particularly cirrhosis, on liver biopsy (Pouteil-Noble *et al.*, 1995; Rostaing *et al.*, 1998b; Zylberberg *et al.*, 1998) resulting from the synergistic effects of these viruses (Durlik *et al.*, 1996b; Pouteil-Noble *et al.*, 1995). Consequently, HBV/HCV coinfections are twice as common among cirrhotic patients than among noncirrhotics (Fornairon *et al.*, 1996).

Zylberberg and colleagues observed that HBV/HCV-coinfected and HBV-infected patients had similar severity of liver disease but significantly higher total Knodell, necroticoinflammatory and fibrosis scores than HCV-infected patients, suggesting that HCV had only a small additive adverse effect on liver disease among chronic HBsAg carriers (Zylberberg *et al.*, 1998). Nonetheless, cirrhosis and liver-related deaths were significantly more frequent in the HBV/HCV-coinfected group as compared with patients with HCV or HBV infection alone. There was a nonsignificant trend toward a negative impact of coinfection with HBV and HCV on patient survival after 15 years posttransplantation (Zylberberg *et al.*, 1998). These data support the notion that coinfection with HBV and HCV may be a predictor of poor clinical prognosis. Despite this association with more severe liver disease and liver-related deaths, other studies have not shown any adverse impact of HBV/HCV coinfection on graft or patient survival in the short-term (4 years after transplantation) (Durlik *et al.*, 1996a) as well as with extended follow-up to 12 years (Pouteil-Noble *et al.*, 1995). Hepatitis B virus has shown no effect on HCV replication (Pouteil-Noble *et al.*, 1995).

Infections with Hepatitis C Virus and GB Virus-C

Numerous studies have shown that 6 to 29% of patients with HCV infection are coinfected with GBV-C (Alter *et al.*, 1997a, 1997b; Berenguer *et al.*, 1996; Berthoux *et al.*, 1998; de Medina *et al.*, 1998; Fried *et al.*, 1997; Gutierrez *et al.*, 1997; Linnen *et al.*, 1996; Masuko *et al.*, 1996; Rostaing *et al.*, 1999; Schroter *et al.*, 1999; Sheng *et al.*, 1998; Tanaka *et al.*, 1996). These wide variations across studies can be explained by differences in study population and study design. We have observed that among HCV-infected renal transplant candidates, 44% were coinfected with GBV-C, and overall 70% had evidence of GBV-C exposure (Natov *et al.*, 2000). Because a significant portion of these patients had initiated dialysis treatment before the implementation of erythropoietin therapy and were likely to have been polytransfused, the higher prevalence of GBV-C coinfection among patients with HCV infection could be due to the fact that HCV and GBV-C, both blood-borne viruses, had probably shared blood transfusions as a common route of transmission. At the New England Organ Bank, coinfection with GBV-C among HCV-infected patients did not affect the severity of posttransplant liver disease, graft or patient survival (Natov *et al.*, 2000). These findings are consistent with a report from Rostaing *et al.* (1999), who observed that 28% of the HCV-infected renal transplant recipients also were positive for GBV RNA. Compared with a group of HCV-infected renal transplant recipients, who were GBV RNA negative, these patients did not present with more severe liver disease, and they had a sig-

nificantly lower degree of liver fibrosis. The authors hypothesized that possible viral interference, for which GBV-C was
thought to be responsible, could have protected the liver
from the detrimental effects of HCV. This study did not
report on patient survival. Data from patients who underwent liver transplantation for HCV-associated end-stage liver
disease have shown that coinfection with GBV-C did not
affect adversely the severity of posttransplant liver disease,
graft survival or patient survival (Berenguer et al., 1996; Fried
et al., 1997).

GB virus-C exposure among HCV-infected renal transplant recipients does not appear to be associated with increased risk of posttransplant liver disease and does not
affect adversely patient survival. Further studies are needed
before more definitive conclusions can be made, however.

REFERENCES

Aach, R. D., Stevens, C. E., Hollinger, F. B., et al. (1991). Hepatitis
C virus infection in post-transfusion hepatitis. N. Engl. J. Med.
325, 1325.

Aeder, M. I., Shield, C. F., Tegtmeier, G. E., et al. (1993). The incidence
and clinical impact of hepatitis C virus (HCV) positive donors in
cadaveric transplantation. Transplant. Proc. **25**, 1469.

Alberti, A., Morsica, G., Chemello, L., et al. (1992). Hepatitis C viraemia and liver disease in symptom-free individuals with anti-
HCV. Lancet **340**, 697.

Alivanis, P., Derveniotis, V., Dioudis, C., et al. (1991). Hepatitis C
virus in antibodies in hemodialyzed and renal transplant patients:
correlation with chronic liver disease. Transplant. Proc. **23**, 2662.

Allison, M. C., Mowat, A., McCruden, E. A. B., et al. (1992). The
spectrum of chronic liver disease in renal transplant recipients.
Q. J. M. **83**, 355.

al Meshari, K., al Ahdal, M., Alfurayh, O., Ali, A., De Vol, E. and
Kessie, G. (1995). New insights into hepatitis C virus infection of
hemodialysis patients: the implications. Am. J. Kidney Dis. **25**, 572.

Alter, H. J. (1989). Chronic consequences of non-A, non-B hepatitis.
In Current Perspectives in Hepatology (L. B. Seeff and J. H. Lewis,
eds.), p. 83, Plenum, New York.

Alter, H. J., Nakatsuji, Y., Melpolder, J., et al. (1997a). The incidence
of transfusion-associated hepatitis G virus infection and its relation to liver disease. N. Engl. J. Med. **336**, 747.

Alter, M., Hadler, S. C., Judson, F. N., et al. (1990). Risk factors for
acute non-A, non-B hepatitis in the United States and association
with hepatitis C virus infection. J. A. M. A. **264**, 2231.

Alter, M. J., Favero, M. S. and Maynard, J. E. (1986). Impact of
infection control strategies on the incidence of dialysis-associated
hepatitis in the United States. J. Infect. Dis. **153**, 1149.

Alter, M. J., Gallagher, M., Morris, T. T., et al. (1997b). Acute non-A-
E hepatitis in the United States and the role of hepatitis G virus
infection. N. Engl. J. Med. **336**, 741.

Alter, M. J., Margolis, H. S., Krawczynski, K., et al. (1992). The natural
history of community-acquired hepatitis C in the United States.
The Sentinel Countries Chronic non-A, non-B Hepatitis Study
Team. N. Engl. J. Med. **327**, 1899.

Anonymous. (1997). Management of hepatitis C. NIH Consens. Statement **15**, 1.

Anuras, S., Piros, J., Bonney, W. W., Forker, L., Colville, D. S. and
Corry, R. J. (1977). Liver disease in renal transplant recipients.
Arch. Intern. Med. **137**, 42.

Anuras, S. and Summers, R. (1976). Fulminant herpes simplex hepatitis in an adult: report of a case in renal transplant recipient.
Gastroenterology **70**, 425.

Aroldi, A., Lampertico, P., Elli, A., et al. (1998). Long-term evolution
of anti-HCV-positive renal transplant recipients. Transplant. Proc.
30, 2076.

Asano, Y., Hashikawa, T., Suga, S., Yazaki, T., Kondo, K. and Yama-
nushi, K. (1990). Fatal fulminant hepatitis in an infant with human
herpesvirus infection. Lancet **335**, 862.

Ashby, M., de Medina, M., Schluter, V., et al. (1996). Prevalence of
hepatitis G infection in chronic hemodialysis patients. J. Am. Soc.
Nephrol. **7**, 1471.

Ayoola, E. A., Huraib, S., Arif, M., et al. (1991). Prevalence and

significance of antibodies to hepatitis C virus among Saudi
haemodialysis patients. J. Med. Virol. **35**, 155.

Badalamenti, S., Sampietro, S., Corbetta, N., et al. (1996). High prevalence of HGV, a novel hepatitis virus, among hemodialysis patients. J. Am. Soc. Nephrol. **7**, 1472.

Benjamin, D. R. and Shunk, B. (1978). A fatal case of peliosis of the
liver and spleen. Am. J. Dis. Child. **132**, 207.

Bensousan, T. A., Moal, M. C., Vincent, F., Nousbaum, J. B. and
Bourbigot, B. (1995). Fulminant hepatitis revealing primary varicella in a renal graft recipient. Transplant. Proc. **27**, 2512.

Berenguer, M., Terrault, N. A., Piatak, M., et al. (1996). Hepatitis G
virus infection in patients with hepatitis C virus infection undergoing liver transplantation. Gastroenterology **111**, 1569.

Berne, T. V., Butler, J. and Silberman, H. (1979). Hepatic dysfunction
in renal transplant recipients: a serious problem. Transplant. Proc.
11, 1282.

Berthoux, P., Dejean, C., Cecillon, S., Batie, M. and Berthoux, F.
(1998). High prevalence of hepatitis G virus (HGV) infection in
renal transplantation. Nephrol. Dial. Transplant. **13**, 2909.

Berthoux, P., Laurent, B., Cecillon, S. and Berthoux, F. (1999). Membranoproliferative glomerulonephritis with subendothelial deposits (type 1) associated with hepatitis G virus infection in a renal
transplant recipient. Am. J. Nephrol. **19**, 513.

Black, M. and Peters, M. (1992). Alpha-interferon treatment of
chronic hepatitis C: need for accurate diagnosis in selecting patients. Ann. Intern. Med. **116**, 86.

Boletis, J., Delladetsima, J., Psimenou, E., et al. (1995). Liver biopsy
is essential in anti-HCV (+) renal transplant patients irrespective
of liver function tests and serology for HCV. Transplant. Proc.
27, 945.

Bomford, A. and Williams, R. (1976). Long-term results of venesection therapy in idiopathic hemosiderosis. Q. J. M. **180**, 611.

Botha, J. F., Ritchie, M. J. J., Dusheiko, G. M., Mouton, H. W. K. and
Kew, M. C. (1984). Hepatitis B virus carrier state in black children
in Ovamboland: role of perinatal and horizontal infection. Lancet
1, 1210.

Bouthot, B. A., Murthy, B. V. R., Muerhoff, A. S., et al. (1997a).
Predictors of GB Virus-C (GBV-C) Infection in Patients Referred for
Renal Transplantation, American Society of Transplant Physicians,
Chicago.

Bouthot, B. A., Murthy, B. V. R., Schmid, C. H., Levey, A. S. and
Pereira, B. J. G. (1997b). Long-term follow-up of hepatitis C virus
infection among organ transplant recipients: implications for policies on organ procurement. Transplantation **63**, 849.

Bradley, J. R., Wreghitt, T. G. and Evans, D. B. (1987). Chicken
pox in adult renal transplant recipients. Nephrol. Dial. Transplant.
1, 242.

Brechot, C. (1987). Hepatitis B virus (HBV) and hepatocellular carcinoma: HBV DNA status and its implications. J. Hepatol. **4**, 269.

Briggs, W. A., Lazarus, J. M., Birtch, A. G., Hampers, C. L., Hager,
E. B. and Merill, J. P. (1973). Hepatitis affecting hemodialysis and
transplant patients: its considerations and consequences. Arch.
Intern. Med. **132**, 21.

Brouwer, J. T., Nevens, F., Kleter, G. E. M., Elewaut, A., Adler, M.
and Brenard, R. (1993). Treatment of chronic hepatitis C: efficacy
of interferon dose and analysis of factors predictive of response:
interim report of 350 patients treated in a Benelux multicenter
study. 44th Annual Meeting of the American Association for the Study
of Liver Diseases, p. 110, Chicago.

Broyer, M. and Boudailliez, B. (1985). Varicella vaccine in children
with chronic renal insufficiency. Postgrad. Med. J. **61(Suppl. 4)**,
103.

Burns, W. H. and Sandford, G. R. (1990). Susceptibility of human
herpesvirus 6 to antivirals in vitro. J. Infect. Dis. **162**, 634.

Busch, M. P., Korelitz, J. J., Kleinman, S. H., Lee, S. R., AuBuchon,
J. P. and Schreiber, G. B. (1995). Declining value of alanine aminotransferase in screening of blood donors to prevent posttransfusion hepatitis B and C virus infection. Transfusion **35**, 903.

Busch, M. P., Wilber, J. C., Johnson, P. J., Tobler, L. and Evans, C. S.
(1992). Impact of specimen handling and storage on detection of
hepatitis C virus RNA. Transfusion **32**, 420.

Byrnes, J. J., Banks, A. T., Piatack, M., Jr. and Kim, J. P. (1996).
Hepatitis G-associated aplastic anaemia. Lancet **348**, 472.

Cabrerizo, M., Bartolome, J., Bello, E., et al. (1996). Hepatitis G virus
(HGV) infection in hemodialysis patients. J. Am. Soc. Nephrol.
7, 1478.

Calne, R. Y., White, D. J. G., Thuru, S., *et al.* (1978). Cyclosporin in patients receiving renal allografts from cadaver donors. *Lancet* **2**, 1323.

Canadian Multicentre Transplant Study Group. (1983). A randomized clinical trial of cyclosporine in cadaveric renal transplantation. *N. Engl. J. Med.* **309**, 809.

Canadian Multicentre Transplant Study Group. (1986). A randomized clinical trial of cyclosporine in cadaveric renal transplantation: analysis at three years. *N. Engl. J. Med.* **314**, 1219.

Carrera, F., Silva, J. G., Oliveira, C., Frazao, J. M. and Pires, C. (1994). Persistence of antibodies to hepatitis C virus in a chronic hemodialysis population. *Nephron* **68**, 38.

Carrigan, D. R., Drobyski, W. R., Russel, S. K., Tapper, M. A., Knox, K. K. and Ash, R. C. (1991). Interstitial pneumonitis associated with human herpes 6 infection after bone marrow transplantation. *Lancet* **338**, 147.

Casanovas, T. T., Baliellas, C., Sese, E., *et al.* (1995). Interferon may be useful in hemodialysis patients with hepatitis C virus chronic infection who are candidates for kidney transplant. *Transplant. Proc.* **27**, 2229.

Casteling, A., Song, E., Sim, J., *et al.* (1998). GB virus C prevalence in blood donors and high risk groups for parenterally transmitted agents from Gauteng, South Africa. *J. Med. Virol.* **55**, 103.

Chan, P. C., Lok, A. S., Cheng, I. K. and Chan, M. K. (1992). The impact of donor and recipient hepatitis B surface antigen status on liver disease and survival in renal transplant recipients. *Transplantation* **53**, 128.

Chan, T. M., Lok, A. S. F., Cheng, I. K. P. and Ng, I. O. L. (1993). Chronic hepatitis C after renal transplantation: treatment with alpha-interferon. *Transplantation* **56**, 1095.

Chan, T. M., Wu, P. C., Lau, J. Y., Lai, C. L., Lok, A. S. and Cheng, I. K. (1994). Clinicopathologic features of hepatitis C virus infection in renal allograft recipients. *Transplantation* **58**, 996.

Chang, R. S., Lewis, J. P. and Abildgard, C. F. (1973). Prevalence of oropharyngeal excretors of leukocyte-transforming agents among a human population. *N. Engl. J. Med.* **289**, 1325.

Chang, R. S., Lewis, J. P., Reynolds, R. D., Sullivan, M. J. and Neuman, J. (1978). Oropharyngeal excretion of Epstein-Barr virus by patients with lymphoproliferative disorders and by recipients of renal homografts. *Ann. Intern. Med.* **88**, 34.

Charrel, R., de Lamballerie, X., Dussol, B., *et al.* (1996). Prevalence of hepatitis G virus (HGV) infection among 32 transplant recipients. *J. Am. Soc. Nephrol.* **7**, 1904.

Chatterjee, S. N., Payne, J. E., Bischel, M. D., *et al.* (1974). Successful renal transplantation in patients positive for hepatitis B antigen. *N. Engl. J. Med.* **291**, 62.

Cheeseman, S. H., Henle, W., Rubin, R. H., *et al.* (1980). Epstein-Barr virus infection in renal transplant recipients. *Ann. Intern. Med.* **93**, 39.

Chemello, L., Alberti, A., Rose, K. and Simmonds, P. (1994). Hepatitis C serotype and response to interferon therapy. *N. Engl. J. Med.* **330**, 143.

Cheung, R. C., Keeffe, E. B. and Greenberg, H. B. (1997). Hepatitis G: is it a hepatitis virus? *West. J. Med.* **167**, 23.

Choo, Q., Kuo, G., Weiner, A. J., Overby, L. R., Bradley, D. W. and Houghton, M. (1989). Isolation of a cDNA clone derived from a blood-borne non-A, non-B viral hepatitis genome. *Science* **244**, 358.

Colombo, M. (1992). Hepatocellular carcinoma. *J. Hepatol.* **15**, 225.

Colombo, P., Filiberti, O., Porcu, M., *et al.* (1992). Prevalence of hepatitis C infection in a hemodialysis unit. *Nephron* **61**, 326.

Cordero Sanchez, M., Bondia Roman, A., Lopez Ochoa, J., Martin Sanchez, A. M. and Nunez Garcia, J. (1991). Anti-hepatitis C antibodies in hemodialysis. *Kidney Int.* **40**, 361.

Courouce, A. M., Barin, F., Botte, C., *et al.* (1995a). A comparative evaluation of the sensitivity of seven anti-hepatitis C virus screening tests. *Vox Sang.* **69**, 213.

Courouce, A.-M., Bouchardeau, F., Chauveau, P., *et al.* (1995b). Hepatitis C (HCV) infection in haemodialysed patients: HCV-RNA and anti-HCV antibodies (third-generation assays). *Nephrol. Dial. Transplant.* **10**, 234.

Davis, G. L., Esteban-Mur, R., Rustgi, V., *et al.* (1998). Interferon alfa-2b alone or in combination with ribavirin for the treatment of relapse of chronic hepatitis C. *N. Engl. J. Med.* **339**, 1493.

Dawson, G. J., Schlauder, G. G., Pilot-Matias, T. J., *et al.* (1996).

Prevalence studies of GB virus-C infection using reverse transcriptase-polymerase chain reaction. *J. Med. Virol.* **50**, 97.

Debure, A., Degos, F., Pol, S., *et al.* (1988). Liver disease and hepatic complications in renal transplant recipients. *Adv. Nephrol.* **17**, 375.

Degos, F., Degott, C., Bedrossian, J., *et al.* (1980). Is renal transplantation involved in post-transplantation liver disease? A prospective study. *Transplantation* **29**, 100.

Degos, F., Lugassy, C., Degott, C., *et al.* (1988). Hepatitis B virus and hepatitis B-related viral infection in renal transplant recipients. *Gastroenterology* **94**, 151.

Degott, C., Rueff, B., Kreis, H., *et al.* (1978). Peliosis hepatis in recipients of renal transplants. *Gut* **19**, 748.

Deinhardt, F., Holmes, A. W., Capps, R. B. and Popper, H. (1967). Studies on the transmission of disease of human viral hepatitis to marmoset monkeys: I. transmission of disease, serial passage and description of liver lesions. *J. Exp. Med.* **125**, 673.

de Medina, M., Ashby, M., Schluter, V., *et al.* (1998). Prevalence of hepatitis C and G virus infection in chronic hemodialysis patients. *Am. J. Kidney Dis.* **31**, 224.

DesJardin, J. A., Gibbons, L., Cho, E., *et al.* (1998). Human herpesvirus 6 reactivation is associated with cytomegalovirus infection and syndromes in kidney transplant recipients at risk for primary cytomegalovirus infection. *J. Infect. Dis.* **178**, 1783.

Dhar, J. M., Al-Khader, A. A., Al-Sulaiman, M. H. and Al-Hasani, M. K. (1991). The significance and implications of hepatitis B infection in renal transplant recipients. *Transplant. Proc.* **23**, 1785.

Di Bisceglie, A. M. (1994). Interferon therapy for chronic viral hepatitis. *N. Engl. J. Med.* **330**, 137.

Di Bisceglie, A. M., Conjeevaram, H. S., Fried, M. W., *et al.* (1995). Ribavirin as therapy for chronic hepatitis C: a randomized, double-blind, placebo-controlled trial. *Ann. Intern. Med.* **123**, 897.

Di Bisceglie, A. M., Hoofnagle, J. H. and Krawczynski, K. (1993). Changes in hepatitis C virus antigen in liver with antiviral therapy. *Gastroenterology* **105**, 858.

Dockrell, D. H., Prada, J., Jones, M. F., *et al.* (1997). Seroconversion to human herpesvirus 6 following liver transplantation is a marker of cytomegalovirus disease. *J. Infect. Dis.* **176**, 1135.

Duarte, R., Huraib, S., Said, R., *et al.* (1995). Interferon-alpha facilitates renal transplantation in hemodialysis patients with chronic viral hepatitis. *Am. J. Kidney Dis.* **25**, 40.

Dubedat, S. and Kappagoda, N. (1989). Hepatitis due to human herpesvirus-6. *Lancet* **2**, 1463.

DuBois, D. B., Gretch, D., de la Rosa, C., *et al.* (1994). Quantitation of hepatitis C viral RNA in sera of hemodialysis patients: gender-related differences in viral load. *Am. J. Kidney Dis.* **24**, 795.

Durlik, M., Gaciong, Z., Soluch, L., *et al.* (1996a). Results of kidney transplantation in HBsAg and anti-HCV seropositive renal allograft recipients. *Transplant. Proc.* **28**, 3459.

Durlik, M., Gaciong, Z., Soluch, L., *et al.* (1996b). Risk of chronic liver disease in HBsAg and/or anti-HCV-positive renal allograft recipients. *Transplant. Proc.* **28**, 50.

Dusheiko, G. (1999). Hepatitis B. In *Oxford Textbook of Clinical Hepatology*, Vol. 1, 2nd ed., (J. Bircher, J.-P. Benhamou, N. McIntyre, M. Rizzetto and J. Rodes, eds.), p. 876, Oxford University Press, Oxford.

Dusheiko, G., Schmilovitz-Weiss, H., Brown, D., *et al.* (1994). Hepatitis C virus genotypes: an investigation of type-specific differences in geographic origin and disease. *Hepatology* **19**, 13.

Dusheiko, G., Song, E., Bowiers, S., *et al.* (1983). Natural history of hepatitis B virus infection in renal transplant recipients—a fifteen-year follow-up. *Hepatology* **3**, 330.

Dussol, B. and Brunet, P. (1997). Prevalence of hepatitis G virus infection in kidney transplant recipients. *Transplantation* **64**, 537.

Dussol, B., Chicheportiche, C., Cantaloube, J. F., *et al.* (1993). Detection of hepatitis C infection by polymerase chain reaction among hemodialysis patients. *Am. J. Kidney Dis.* **22**, 574.

Elliot, W. C., Houghton, D. C., Bryant, R. E., Wicklund, R., Barry, J. M. and Bennett, W. M. (1980). Herpes simplex type 1 hepatitis in renal transplantation. *Arch. Intern. Med.* **140**, 1656.

Enomoto, N., Takada, A. and Nakao, T. (1990). There are two major types of hepatitis C virus in Japan. *Biochem. Biophys. Res. Commun.* **170**, 1021.

Esteban, J. I., Gonzales, A., Hernandez, J. M., *et al.* (1990). Evaluation of antibodies to hepatitis C virus in a study of transfusion-associated hepatitis. *N. Engl. J. Med.* **323**, 1107.

European Multicentre Trial Group. (1983). Cyclosporine in cadaveric renal transplantation: one-year follow-up of a multicenter trial. *Lancet* **2**, 986.

Fabrizi, F., Lunghi, G., Andrulli, S., *et al.* (1997a). Influence of hepatitis C virus (HCV) viraemia upon serum aminotransferase activity in chronic dialysis patients. *Nephrol. Dial. Transplant.* **12**, 1394.

Fabrizi, F., Lunghi, G., Bacchini, G., *et al.* (1997b). Hepatitis G virus infection in chronic dialysis patients and kidney transplant recipients. *Nephrol. Dial. Transplant.* **12**, 1645.

Fabrizi, F., Lunghi, G., Marai P, *et al.* (1996): Virological and histological features of hepatitis C virus (HCV) infection in kidney transplant recipients. *Nephrol. Dial. Transplant.* **11**, 159.

Fairley, C., Mijch, A., Gust, I. D., Nichilson, S., Dimitrakakis, M. and Lucas, C. R. (1991). The increased risk of fatal liver disease in renal transplant patients who are hepatitis Be antigen and/or HBV DNA positive. *Transplantation* **52**, 497.

Farci, P., Alter, H. J., Govindarajan, S., *et al.* (1992). Lack of protective immunity against reinfection with hepatitis C virus. *Science* **258**, 135.

Farci, P., Alter, H. J., Wong, D., *et al.* (1991). A long-term study of hepatitis C virus replication in non-A, non-B hepatitis. *N. Engl. J. Med.* **325**, 98.

Farge, D., Parfrey, P. S., Forbes, R. D. C., Dandavino, R. and Guttmann, R. D. (1986). Reduction of azathioprine in renal transplant patients with chronic hepatitis. *Transplantation* **41**, 55.

Feldhoff, C. M., Balfour, H. H., Simmons, R. L., Najarian, J. S. and Mauer, S. M. (1981). Varicella in children with renal transplants. *J. Pediatr.* **98**, 25.

Feray, C., Grigou, M., Samuel, D., *et al.* (1993). HCV type II has a more pathogenic course after liver transplantation. *Hepatology* **18**, 59.

Fiordalisi, G., Zanella, I., Mantero, G., *et al.* (1996). High prevalence of GB virus C infection in a group of Italian patients with hepatitis of unknown etiology. *J. Infect. Dis.* **174**, 181.

Flagg, G. L., Silberman, H., Takamoto, S. K. and Berne, T. V. (1987). The influence of hepatitis B infection on the outcome of renal allotransplantation. *Transplant. Proc.* **19**, 2155.

Fornairon, S., Pol, C., Legendre, C., *et al.* (1996). The long-term virologic and pathologic impact of renal transplantation on chronic hepatitis B virus infection. *Transplantation* **62**, 297.

Fried, M. W., Khudyakov, Y. E., Smallwood, G. A., *et al.* (1997). Hepatitis G virus co-infection in liver transplantation recipients with chronic hepatitis C and nonviral chronic liver disease. *Hepatology* **25**, 1271.

Friedlaender, M. M., Kaspa, R. T., Rubinger, D., Silver, J. and Popovtzer, M. M. (1989). Renal transplantation is not contraindicated in asymptomatic carriers of hepatitis B surface antigen. *Am. J. Kidney Dis.* **14**, 204.

Fritsche, C., Brandes, J. C., Delaney, S. R., *et al.* (1993). Hepatitis C is a poor prognostic indicator in black kidney transplant recipients. *Transplantation* **55**, 1283.

Fuhrman, S. A., Gill, R., Horwitz, C. A., *et al.* (1987). Marked hyperbilirubinemia in infectious mononucleosis. *Arch. Intern. Med.* **147**, 850.

Gagnadoux, M. F., Guest, G., Ronsse-Nussenzveig, P., Mitsioni, A. and Broyer, M. (1993). Long-term outcome of hepatitis B after renal transplantation during childhood. *Transplant. Proc.* **25**, 1454.

Garnier, J.-L., Chevallier, P., Dubernard, J.-M., Trepo, C., Touraine, J.-L. and Chossegross, P. (1997). Treatment of hepatitis C virus infection with ribavirin in kidney transplant patients. *Transplant. Proc.* **29**, 783.

Gerlag, P. G. G. and van Hooff, J. P. (1987). Hepatic sinusoidal dilatation with portal hypertension during azathioprine treatment: a cause of chronic liver disease after kidney transplantation. *Transplant. Proc.* **19**, 3699.

Gilli, P., Moretti, M., Soffritti, S., *et al.* (1990). Non-A, non-B hepatitis and anti-HCV antibodies in dialysis patients. *Int. J. Artif. Organs* **13**, 737.

Glicklich, D., Reinus, J., Greenstein, S., *et al.* (1994). Hepatitis C infection in renal transplant recipients: histology and clinical features. *J. Am. Soc. Nephrol.* **5**, 1007.

Gomez, E., Aguado, S., Gago, E., *et al.* (1991). A study of renal transplants obtained from anti-HCV positive donors. *Transplant. Proc.* **23**, 2654.

Gutierrez, R., Dawson, G. J., Knigge, M. F., *et al.* (1997). Seroprevalence of GB virus C and persistence of RNA and antibody. *J. Med. Virol.* **53**, 167.

Haboubi, N. Y., Ali, H. H., Whitwell, H. L. and Ackrill, P. (1988). Role of endothelial cell injury in the spectrum of azathioprine-induced liver disease after renal transplant: light microscopy and ultrastructural observations. *Am. J. Gastroenterol.* **83**, 256.

Hamburger, J., Crosnier, J. and Dormont, J. (1965). Experience with 45 renal homotransplantations in man. *Lancet* **1**, 985.

Hanafusa, T., Ichikawa, Y., Kishikawa, H., *et al.* (1998). Retrospective study on the impact of hepatitis C virus infection on kidney transplant patients over 20 years. *Transplantation* **66**, 471.

Hankey, G. J. and Saker, B. M. (1987). Peliosis hepatis in a renal transplant recipient and in a hemodialysis patient. *Med. J. Aust.* **146**, 102.

Hanson, C. A., Sutherland, D. E. and Snover, D. C. (1985). Fulminant hepatic failure in an HBsAg carrier renal transplant patient following cessation of immunosuppressive therapy. *Transplantation* **39**, 311.

Hanto, D. W., Gajl-Peczalska, K. J., Frizzera, G., *et al.* (1983). Epstein-Barr virus (EBV) induced polyclonal and monoclonal B-cell lymphoproliferative diseases occurring after renal transplantation. *Ann. Surg.* **198**, 356.

Harihara, Y., Kurooka, Y., Yanagisawa, T., Kuzuhara, K., Otsubo, O. and Kumada, H. (1994). Interferon therapy in renal allograft recipients with chronic hepatitis C. *Transplant. Proc.* **26**, 2075.

Harnett, J. D., Zeldis, J. B., Parfrey, P. S., *et al.* (1987). Hepatitis B in dialysis and transplant patients. *Transplantation* **44**, 369.

Herbein, G., Strasswimmer, J., Altieri, M., Woehl-Jaegle, M. L., Wolf, P. and Obert, G. (1996). Longitudinal study of human herpesvirus 6 infection in organ transplant recipients. *Clin. Infect. Dis.* **22**, 171.

Heringlake, S., Osterkamp, S., Trautwein, C., *et al.* (1996). Association between fulminant hepatic failure and a strain of GBV virus C. *Lancet* **348**, 1626.

Hestin, D., Hussenet, F., Hubert, J., *et al.* (1995). Hepatitis C following renal transplantation: histopathological correlations. *Transplant. Proc.* **27**, 2468.

Hillion, D., De Viel, E., Brgue, A., *et al.* (1983). Peliosis hepatis in a chronic hemodialysis patient. *Nephron* **35**, 205.

Hillis, W., Hillis, A. and Walker, G. (1979). Hepatitis B surface antigenemia in renal transplant recipients: increased mortality risk. *J. A. M. A.* **242**, 329.

Hoofnagle, J. H. (1997). The treatment of chronic viral hepatitis. *N. Engl. J. Med.* **336**, 347.

Houghton, M., Weiner, A., Han, J., Kuo, G. and Choo, Q. L. (1991). Molecular biology of the hepatitis C viruses: implications for diagnosis, development and control of viral disease. *Hepatology* **14**, 381.

Hsieh, H., Chen, C. H., Huang, H. F. and Tseng, Y. J. (1996). Optimal immunosuppression regimen for hepatitis B-positive kidney transplant recipients. *Transplant. Proc.* **28**, 1495.

Huang, C., Lai, M. and Fong, M. (1990). Hepatitis-B liver disease in cyclosporine-treated renal allograft recipients. *Transplantation* **49**, 540.

Huang, C. C., Lai, M. K., Lin, M. W., Pao, C. C., Fang, J. T. and Yao, D. S. (1993). Transmission of hepatitis C virus by renal transplantation. *Transplant. Proc.* **25**, 1474.

Huang, C.-C., Liaw, Y.-F., Lai, M.-K., Chu, S.-H., Chuang, C.-K. and Huang, J.-Y. (1992). The clinical outcome of hepatitis C virus antibody-positive renal allograft recipients. *Transplantation* **53**, 763.

Hung, Y. B., Liang, J. T., Chu, J. S., Chen, K. M. and Lee, C. S. (1995). Fulminant hepatic failure in a renal transplant recipient with positive hepatitis B surface antigens: a case report of fibrosing cholestatic hepatitis. *Hepatogastroenterology* **42**, 913.

Hunt, J., Farthing, M. J. G., Baker, L. R. I., Crocker, P. R. and Levison, D. A. (1989). Silicone in the liver: possible late effects. *Gut* **30**, 239.

Hyams, J. S., Ballow, M. and Leichtner, A. M. (1987). Cyclosporine treatment of autoimmune chronic active hepatitis. *Gastroenterology* **93**, 890.

Ihara, H., Ichikawa, Y., Nagano, S., Fukunishi, T. and Shinji, Y. (1982). Peliosis hepatis and nodular regenerative hyperplasia of the liver in renal transplant recipients. *Med. J. Osaka Univ.* **33**, 13.

Irving, W. L. and Cunningham, A. L. (1990). Serological diagnosis of infection with human herpesvirus type 6. *B. M. J.* **300**, 156.

Izopet, J., Rostaing, L., Sandres, K., *et al.* (1996). Impact of HGV infection in hemodialysis patients. *J. Am. Soc. Nephrol.* **7**, 1483.

Jacobson, I. M., Jaffers, G., Dienstag, J. L., et al. (1985). Immunogenicity of hepatitis B vaccine in renal transplant recipients. *Transplantation* **39**, 393.

Jarvis, L. M., Davidson, F., Hanley, J. P., Yap, P. L., Ludlam, C. A. and Simmonds, P. (1996). Infection with hepatitis G virus among recipients of plasma products. *Lancet* **348**, 1352.

Jeffers, L. J., Perez, G. O., de Medina, M. D., et al. (1990). Hepatitis C infection in two urban hemodialysis units. *Kidney Int.* **38**, 320.

Jonas, M. M., Zilleruelo, G. E., LaRue, S. I., Abitbol, C., Strauss, J. and Lu, Y. (1992). Hepatitis C infection in pediatric dialysis population. *Pediatrics* **89**, 707.

Kahan, B. D., Van Buren, C. T., Flechner, S. M., et al. (1985). Clinical and experimental studies with cyclosporine in renal transplantation. *Surgery* **97**, 125.

Kallinowski, B., Ahmadi, R., Seipp, S., Bommer, J. and Stremmel, W. (1998). Clinical impact of GB-C virus in haemodialysis patients. *Nephrol. Dial. Transplant.* **13**, 93.

Kanda, T., Yokosuka, O., Ehata, T., et al. (1997). Detection of GBV-C RNA in patients with non-A-E fulminant hepatitis by reverse-transcription polymerase chain reaction. *Hepatology* **25**, 1261.

Kao, J. H., Chen, P. J., Lai, M. Y. and Chen, D. S. (1993). Superinfection of heterologous hepatitis C virus in a patient with chronic type C hepatitis. *Gastroenterology* **105**, 583.

Katzka, D. A., Saul, S. H., Jorkasky, D., Sigal, H., Reynolds, J. C. and Soloway, R. D. (1986). Azathioprine and hepatic veno-occlusive disease in renal transplant patients. *Gastroenterology* **90**, 446.

Kazi, S., Prasad, S., Pollak, R., et al. (1994). Hepatitis C infection in potential recipients with normal liver biochemistry does not preclude renal transplantation. *Dig. Dis. Sci.* **39**, 961.

Kharsa, G., Degott, C., Degos, F., Carnot, F., Potent, F. and Kreis, H. (1987). Fulminant hepatitis in renal transplant recipients: the role of the Delta agent. *Transplantation* **44**, 221.

Kingsley, L. A., Rinaldo, C. R., Lyter, D. W., Valdiserri, R. O., Belle, S. H. and Ho, M. (1990). Sexual transmission efficiency of hepatitis B virus and HIV among homosexual men. *J. A. M. A.* **264**, 230.

Kirkman, R. L., Strom, T. B., Weir, M. R. and Tilney, N. L. (1982). Late mortality and morbidity in recipients of long-term renal allografts. *Transplantation* **34**, 347.

Kiyosawa, K., Sodeyama, T., Tanaka, E., et al. (1990). Interrelationship of blood transfusion, non-A, non-B hepatitis and hepatocellular carcinoma: analysis by detection of antibody to hepatitis C virus. *Hepatology* **12**, 671.

Klintmalm, G. B., Iwatsuki, S. and Starzl, T. E. (1981). Cyclosporin A hepatotoxicity in 66 renal allograft recipients. *Transplantation* **32**, 488.

Koenig, P., Vogel, W., Umlauft, F., Weyrer, K., Prommegger, R. and Lhotta, K. (1994). Interferon treatment for chronic hepatitis C virus infection in uremic patients. *Kidney Int.* **45**, 1507.

Koretz, R. L., Brezina, M., Polito, A. J., et al. (1993). Non-A, non-B posttransfusion hepatitis: comparing C and non-C hepatitis. *Hepatology* **17**, 361.

Kovarik, J., Mayer, G., Pohanka, E., et al. (1988). Adverse effect of low-dose prophylactic human recombinant leukocyte interferon-alpha treatment in renal transplant recipients: cytomegalovirus infection prophylaxis leading to an increased incidence of irreversible rejections. *Transplantation* **45**, 402.

Kramer, P., ten Kate, F. J. W., Bijnen, A. B., Jeekel, J. and Weimar, W. (1985). The pathology of interferon-induced renal allograft lesions. *Transplant. Proc.* **17**, 58.

Kuo, G., Choo, Q. L., Alter, H. J., et al. (1989). An assay for circulating antibodies to a major etiologic virus of human non-A, non-B hepatitis. *Science* **244**, 362.

Kurosaki, M., Enomoto, N., Marumo, F. and Sato, C. (1993). Rapid sequence variation of the hypervariable region of hepatitis C virus during the course of chronic infection. *Hepatology* **18**, 1293.

Kusne, S., Schwartz, M., Breinig, M. K., et al. (1991). Herpes simplex virus hepatitis after solid organ transplantation in adults. *J. Infect. Dis.* **163**, 1001.

Lai, M. E., Mazzoleni, A. P., Argiolu, F., et al. (1994). Hepatitis C virus in multiple episodes of acute hepatitis in polytransfused thalassaemic children. *Lancet* **343**, 388.

Langnas, A. N., Markin, R. S., Inagaki, M., et al. (1994). Epstein-Barr virus hepatitis after liver transplantation. *Am. J. Gastroenterol.* **89**, 1066.

LaQuaglia, M. P., Tolkoff-Rubin, N. E., Dienstag, J. L., et al. (1981). Impact of hepatitis on renal transplantation. *Transplantation* **32**, 504.

Lau, J. Y. N., Davis, G. L., Kniffen, J., et al. (1993a). Significance of serum hepatitis C virus RNA levels in chronic hepatitis C. *Lancet* **341**, 1501.

Lau, J. Y. N., Davis, G. L., Orito, E., Qian, K. P. and Mizokami, M. (1993b). Significance of antibody to the host cellular gene derived epitope GOR in chronic hepatitis C virus infection. *J. Hepatol.* **17**, 253.

Leary, T. P., Muerhoff, A. S., Simons, J. N., et al. (1996). Sequence and genomic organization of GBV-C: a novel member of the flaviviridae associated with human non-A-E hepatitis. *J. Med. Virol.* **48**, 60.

Lee, S. W., Kang, S. W., Choi, K. H., et al. (1996). Clinical outcomes of anti-HCV(+) renal transplant allograft recipients. *Transplant. Proc.* **28**, 1501.

Lefebure, A. F., Verpooten, G. A., Couttenye, M. M. and De Broe, M. E. (1993). Immunogenicity of a recombinant DNA hepatitis B vaccine in renal transplant recipients. *Vaccine* **11**, 397.

LeFor, W., Wright, C., Shires, D., Kahana, L., Spoto, E. and Ackermann, J. (1991). A preliminary outcome evaluation of the impact of HCV-AB studied in 521 cadaver vascular organ donors over a 6 year period. *American Society of Transplant Physicians, 10th Annual Meeting*, p. 2, Chicago.

Legendre, C., Garrigue, V., Le Bihan, C., et al. (1998). Harmful long-term impact of hepatitis C virus infection in kidney transplant recipients. *Transplantation* **65**, 667.

Leong, A. S. Y., Disney, A. P. S. and Grove, D. W. (1981). Refractile particles in liver of hemodialysis patients. *Lancet* **1**, 889.

Li, J., Tong, S., Vitvitski, L., et al. (1991). Two French genotypes of hepatitis C virus: homology of the predominant genotype with the prototype American strain. *Gene* **105**, 167.

Liano, F., Moreno, A., Matesanz, R., et al. (1989). Veno-occlusive hepatic disease of the liver in renal transplantation: is azathioprine the cause? *Nephron* **51**, 509.

Liaw, Y. F. (1995). Role of hepatitis C virus in dual and triple virus infection. [Review]. *Hepatology* 22, 1101–1108.

Lilis, D., Hadjiconstantinou, V., Kravaritis, A., et al. (1991). Prevalence of anti-HCV antibodies in four hemodialysis units in Athens. *Kidney Int.* **39**, 192.

Lindsay, K. L. (1997). Therapy of hepatitis C: overview. *Hepatology* **26(Suppl. 1)**, 71S.

Linnen, J., Wages, J., Jr., Zhang-Keck, Z. Y., et al. (1996). Molecular cloning and disease association of hepatitis G virus: a transfusion-transmissible agent. *Science* **271**, 505.

Locarnini, S. A. and Gust, I. D. (1988). Hepadnaviridae: hepatitis B virus and delta virus. In *Laboratory Diagnosis of Infectious Diseases: Principles and Practice*, Vol. 2, (A. Balow, W. J. J. Hausler and E. H. Lennette, eds.), p. 750, Springer-Verlag, New York.

Loertscher, R., Brunner, F. P., Harder, F. and Thiel, G. (1983). Withdrawal of azathioprine in renal transplant recipients with chronic active hepatitis: is it wise or not? *Nephron* **33**, 150.

Lorber, M. I., Van Buren, C. T., Flechner, S. M., Williams, C. and Kahan, B. D. (1987). Hepatobiliary and pancreatic complications of cyclosporine therapy in 466 renal transplant recipients. *Transplantation* **43**, 35.

Lozano, L., Nieto, J., Sanchez, M., Martin, J. E., Granizo, V. and Jarillo, M. D. (1991). Evaluation of incidence of hepatitis C in dialysis. *Kidney Int.* **40**, 379.

Luby, J. P., Burnett, W., Hull, A. R., Ware, A. J., Shorey, J. W. and Peters, P. C. (1974). Relationship between cytomegalovirus and hepatic function abnormalities in the period after transplantation. *J. Infect. Dis.* **129**, 511.

Lynfield, R., Herrin, J. T. and Rubin, R. (1992). Varicella in pediatric transplant recipients. *Pediatrics* **90**, 216.

Mahaney, K., Tedeschi, V., Maertens, G., et al. (1994). Genotypic analysis of hepatitis C virus in American patients. *Hepatology* **20**, 1405.

Mahony, J. F. (1989). Long-term results and complications of renal transplantation: the kidney. *Transplant. Proc.* **21**, 1433.

Malekzadeh, M. H., Grushkin, C. M., Wright, H. T. J., et al. (1972). Hepatic dysfunction after renal transplantation in childeren. *J. Pediatr.* **81**, 279.

Manolapoulos, S., Morris, A., Davis, S., Brown, D., Hajat, S. and Dusheiko, G. (1998). Influence of GB virus C viraemia on the clinical, virological and histological features of early hepatitis C-related hepatic disease. *J. Hepatol.* 28, 173.

Marcellin, P., Giostra, E., Martinot-Peignoux, M., *et al.* (1991). Redevelopment of hepatitis B surface antigen after renal transplantation. *Gastroenterology* 100, 1332.

Marker, S. C., Ascher, N. L., Kalis, J. M., Simmons, R. L., Najarian, J. S. and Balfour, H. H. (1979). Epstein-Barr virus antibody responses and clinical illness in renal transplant recipients. *Surgery* 85, 433.

Markin, R. S. (1994). Manifestations of Epstein-Barr virus-associated disorders in liver. *Liver* 14, 1.

Marubbio, A. T. and Danielson, B. (1975). Hepatic veno-occlusive disease in a renal transplant patient receiving azathioprine. *Gastroenterology* 69, 739.

Masuko, K., Mitsui, T., Iwano, K., *et al.* (1996). Infection with hepatitis GB virus C in patients on maintenance hemodialysis. *N. Engl. J. Med.* 334, 1485.

Mathurin, P., Mouquet, C., Poynard, T., *et al.* (1999). Impact of hepatitis B and C virus on kidney transplantation outcome. *Hepatology* 29, 257.

McGregor, R. S., Zitelli, B. J., Urbach, A. H., Malatack, J. J. and Gartner, J. C. J. (1989). Varicella in pediatric orthotopic liver transplant recipients. *Pediatrics* 83, 256.

McHutchison, J. G., Gordon, S. C., Schiff, E. R., *et al.* (1998). Interferon alfa-2b alone or in combination with ribavirin as initial treatment for chronic hepatitis C. *N. Engl. J. Med.* 339, 1485.

McOmish, F., Chan, S. W., Dow, B. C., *et al.* (1993). Detection of three types of hepatitis C virus in blood donors: investigation of type-specific differences in serologic reactivity and rate of alanine aminotransferase abnormalities. *Transfusion* 33, 7.

Medici, G., Vandelli, L., Savazzi, A. M. and Lusvarghi, E. (1990). Hepatitis C virus (HCV) infection on maintenance hemodialysis: biological results and clinical remarks. *J. Am. Soc. Nephrol.* 1, 368.

Mendez, R., Aswad, S., Bogaard, T., *et al.* (1993). Donor hepatitis C antibody virus testing in renal transplantation. *Transplant. Proc.* 25, 1487.

Mendez, R., El-Shahawy, M., Obispo, E., Aswad, S. and Mendex, R. G. (1995). Four years follow up of hepatitis C positive kidneys into hepatitis C negative recipients—prospective study. *J. Am. Soc. Nephrol.* 6, 1105.

Miranda, B., Sanchez, M., Sergovia, C., Felipe, C. and Matesanz, R. (1993). Characteristics of the donors in Spain 1992. *8th Congress of European Transplant Coordinators Organization,* Rodos, Greece.

Miyakawa, Y. and Mayumi, M. (1997). Hepatitis G virus—a true hepatitis virus or an accidental tourist? *N. Engl. J. Med.* 336, 795.

Mondelli, M. U., Cristana, G., Filice, G., Rondanelli, E. G., Piazza, V. and Barbieri, C. (1990). Anti-HCV positive patients in dialysis units? *Lancet* 336, 244.

Mondelli, M. U., Smedile, V., Piazza, V., *et al.* (1991). Abnormal alanine aminotransferase activity reflects exposure to hepatitis C virus in haemodialysis patients. *Nephrol. Dial. Transplant.* 6, 480.

Morales, J. M. (1995). Hepatitis C and renal transplantation: outcome of patients. *Nephrol. Dial. Transplant.* 10, 125.

Morales, J. M., Campistol, J. M., Castellano, G., *et al.* (1995). Transplantation of kidneys from donors with hepatitis C antibody into recipients with pre-transplantation anti-HCV. *Kidney Int.* 47, 236.

Morales, J. M., Munoz, M. A., Castellano, G., *et al.* (1993). Impact of hepatitis C in long-functioning renal transplants: a clinicopathological follow-up. *Transplant. Proc.* 25, 1450.

Morales, J. M., Prieto, C., Colina, F., Andres, A., Moreno, F. and Rodicio, J. L. (1989). Does ciclosporin induce clinical remission of dialysis-acquired active chronic hepatitis? *Nephron* 51, 146.

Moreno, F., Morales, J. M., Colina, F., *et al.* (1990). Influence of long-term cyclosporine therapy on chronic liver disease after renal transplantation. *Transplant. Proc.* 22, 2314.

Morishita, K., Kodo, H., Asano, S., Fijii, H., Miwa, S. and The Tokyo University Bone Marrow Transplantation Team. (1985). Fulminant varicella hepatitis following bone marrow transplantation. *J. A. M. A.* 253, 511.

Morris, D. J., Littler, E., Arrand, J. R. and Jordan, D. (1989). Human herpesvirus 6 infection in renal-transplant recipients. *N. Engl. J. Med.* 320, 1560.

Mozes, M. F., Ascher, N. L., Balfour, H. H., Simmons, R. L. and Najarian, J. S. (1978). Jaundice after renal allotransplantation. *Ann. Surg.* 188, 783.

Muerhoff, A. S., Leary, T. P., Simons, J. N., *et al.* (1995). Genomic organization of GB viruses A and B: two new members of the Flaviviridae associated with GB agent hepatitis. *J. Virol.* 69, 5621.

Muller, G. A., Braun, N., Eisele, H. and Muller, C. A. (1993). Human cytomegalovirus infection in transplantation. *Nephron* 64, 343.

Muller, G. Y., Zabaleta, M. E., Arminio, A., *et al.* (1992). Risk factors for dialysis-associated hepatitis C in Venezuela. *Kidney Int.* 41, 1055.

Murray, J. E., Merrill, J. P., Harrison, J. H., Wilson, R. E. and Dammin, G. J. (1963). Prolonged survival of human-kidney homograft by immunosuppressive drug therapy. *N. Engl. J. Med.* 268, 1315.

Murthy, B. V. R., Muerhoff, A. S., Desai, S. M., *et al.* (1997a). GB hepatitis agent among cadaver organ donors and their recipients. *Transplantation* 63, 346.

Murthy, B. V. R., Muerhoff, A. S., Desai, S. M., *et al.* (1997b). Impact of pre-transplantation GB virus-C (GBV-C) infection on the outcome of renal transplantation. *J. Am. Soc. Nephrol.* 8, 1164.

Murthy, B. V. R., Muerhoff, A. S., Desai, S. M., *et al.* (1998). Predictors of GBV-C infection among patients referred for renal transplantation. *Kidney Int.* 53, 1769.

Mushahwar, I. K. (1998). Tissue tropism of GBV-C and protective immunity of anti-GBV-C E2. *VIII International Symposium on Viral Hepatitis,* Madrid.

Mushahwar, I. K., Erker, J. C., Patterson, B. K. and Desai, S. M. (1998). Tissue tropism of GBV-C and HCV. *XIX U.S.-Japan Hepatitis Joint Panel Meeting, U.S.-Japan Cooperative Medical Science Program,* Pacific Grove, Calif.

Mushahwar, I. K. and Zuckerman, J. N. (1998). Clinical implications of GB virus C. *J. Med. Virol.* 56, 1.

Nagayama, R., Tsuda, F., Okamoto, H., *et al.* (1993). Genotype dependence of hepatitis C virus antibodies detectable by the first generation enzyme-linked immunosorbent assay with C100-3 protein. *J. Clin. Invest.* 92, 1529.

Najarian, J. S., Fryd, D. S., Strand, M., *et al.* (1985). A single institution, randomized prospective trial of cyclosporine versus azathioprine-anti-lymphocyte globulin for immunosuppression in renal allograft recipients. *Ann. Surg.* 201, 42.

Nakao, T., Enomoto, N., Takada, N., *et al.* (1991). Typing of hepatitis C virus genomes by restriction fragment length polymorphism. *J. Gen. Virol.* 72, 2105.

Napel, C. H. H., ten Houthoff, H. J. and The, T. H. (1984). Cytomegalovirus hepatitis in normal and immune-compromised hosts. *Liver* 4, 184.

Naraqi, S., Jackson, G. G., Jonasson, O. and Yamashiroya, H. M. (1977). Prospective study of prevalence, incidence, and source of herpesvirus infections in patients with renal allografts. *J. Infect. Dis.* 136, 531.

Naraqi, S., Jonasson, O., Jackson, G. G. and Yamashiroya, H. M. (1978). Clinical manifestation of infections with herpesviruses after kidney tarnsplantation: a prospective study of various syndromes. *Ann. Surg.* 188, 234.

Nasoff, M. S., Zebedee, S. L., Inchauspe, G., *et al.* (1991). Identification of an immunodominant epitope within the capsid protein of hepatitis C virus. *Proc. Natl. Acad. Sci. U. S. A.* 88, 5462.

Nataf, C., Feldmann, G., Lebrec, D., *et al.* (1979). Idiopathic portal hypertension (perisinusoidal fibrosis) after renal transplantation. *Gut* 20, 531.

Natov, S., Murthy, B. V. R., Mushahwar, I. K., *et al.* (2000). GBV-C infection and survival among renal transplant candidates (submitted for publication).

Natov, S. N., Lau, J. Y. N., Ruthazer, R., *et al.* (1999b). HCV genotype does not affect patient survival among renal transplant candidates. *Kidney Int.* 54, 700.

Natov, S. N. and Pereira, B. J. G. (1997). Transmission of disease by organ transplantation. In *Organ and Tissue Donation for Transplantation,* (J. R. Chapman, M. Deierhoi and C. Wight, eds.), p. 120, Edward Arnold, London.

Neilson, J., Harrison, P., Milligan, D. W., Skidmore, S. J. and Collingham, K. E. (1996). Hepatitis G virus in long-term survivors of haematological malignancy. *Lancet* 347, 1632.

Nelson, S. R., Snowden, S. A., Sutherland, S., Smith, H. M., Parsons, V. and Bewick, M. (1994). Outcome of renal transplantation in hepatitis BsAg-positive patients. *Nephrol. Dial. Transplant.* 9, 1320.

Nicchitta, C. V., Kanom, M. and Williamson, J. R. (1985). Cyclosporine augments receptor mediated-cellular calcium fluxes in isolated hepatocytes. *J. Biol. Chem.* **260**, 1361.

Niederman, J. C., Liu, C. R., Kaplan, M. H. and Brown, N. A. (1988). Clinical and serological features of human herpesvirus-6 infection in three adults. *Lancet* **2**, 817.

Nousbaum, J., Pol, S., Nalpas, B., *et al.* (1995). Hepatitis C virus type 1b (II) infection in France and Italy. Collaborative Study Group. *Ann. Intern. Med.* **122**, 161.

Nubling, C. M., Bialleck, H., Fursch, A. J., *et al.* (1997). Frequencies of GB virus C/hepatitis G virus genomes and of specific antibodies in German risk and non-risk populations. *J. Med. Virol.* **53**, 218.

Oesterreicher, C., Hammer, J., Koch, U., *et al.* (1995). HBV and HCV genome in peripheral blood mononuclear cells in patients undergoing hemodialysis. *Kidney Int.* **48**, 1967.

Okada, S., Akahane, Y., Suzuki, H., Okamoto, H. and Mishiro, S. (1992). The degree of variability in the amino terminal region of the E2/NS1 protein of hepatitis C virus correlates with responsiveness to interferon therapy in viremic patients. *Hepatology* **16**, 619.

Okamoto, H., Mishiro, S., Tokita, H., *et al.* (1994). Superinfection of chimpanzees carrying hepatitis C virus of genotype II/1b with that of genotype III/2a or I/1a. *Hepatology* **20**, 1131.

Okamoto, H., Sugiyama, Y., Okada, S., *et al.* (1992). Typing hepatitis C virus by polymerase chain reaction with type-specific primers: application to clinical surveys and tracing infectious sources. *J. Gen. Virol.* **73**, 673.

Oldach, D., Constantine, N., Schweitzer, E., *et al.* (1995). Clinical and virological outcomes in hepatitis C virus (HCV)-infected renal transplant recipients. *14th Annual Meeting of the American Society of Transplant Physicians*, p. 98, Chicago.

Otero, J., Roderiguez, M., Escudero, D., Gomez, E., Aguado, S. and de Ona, M. (1990). Kidney transplants with positive anti-hepatitis C virus donors. *Transplantation* **50**, 1086.

Ozgur, O., Boyacioglu, S., Telatar, H. and Haberal, M. (1995). Recombinant alpha-interferon in renal allograft recipients with chronic hepatitis C. *Nephrol. Dial. Transplant.* **10**, 2104.

Parfrey, P. S., Farge, D., Forbes, C., Dandavino, R., Kenick, S. and Guttman, R. D. (1985a). Chronic hepatitis in end-stage renal disease: comparison of HBsAg-negative and HBsAg-positive patients. *Kidney Int.* **28**, 959.

Parfrey, P. S., Forbes, R. D. C., Hutchinson, T. A., *et al.* (1985b). The impact of renal transplantation on the course of hepatitis B liver disease. *Transplantation* **39**, 610.

Parnham, A. P., Flexman, J. P., Saker, B. M. and Thatcher, G. N. (1995). Primary varicella in adult renal transplant recipients: a report of three cases plus a review of the literature. *Clin. Transplant.* **9**, 115.

Pass, R. F., Long, W. K., Whitley, R. J., *et al.* (1978). Productive infection with cytomegalovirus and herpes simplex virus in renal transplant recipients: role of source of kidney. *J. Infect. Dis.* **137**, 556.

Pass, R. F., Whitley, R. J., Whelchel, J. D., Diethelm, A. G., Reynolds, D. W. and Alford, C. A. (1979). Identification of patients with increased risk of infection with herpes simplex virus after renal transplantation. *J. Infect. Dis.* **140**, 487.

Pawlowska, M., Halota, W., Bulik, F. and Topczewska-Staubach, E. (1997). Hepatitis C virus (HCV) serotype in the asymptomatic HCV-infected patients from selected groups. *Arch. Immunol. Ther. Exp.* **45**, 455.

Penn, I. (1982). The occurrence of cancer in immune deficiencies. *Curr. Probl. Cancer* **6**, 1.

Penn, I., Hammond, W., Bell, P., *et al.* (1969). Hepatic disorders in renal homograft recipients. *Curr. Top. Surg. Res.* **1**, 67.

Pereira, B. and Levey, A. (1995). Hepatitis C infection in cadaver organ donors: strategies to reduce transmission of infection and prevent organ waste. *Pediatr. Nephrol.* **9**, S23.

Pereira, B. J. G. and Levey, A. S. (1997). Hepatitis C virus infection in dialysis and renal transplantation. *Kidney Int.* **51**, 981.

Pereira, B. J. G., Milford, E. L., Kirkman, R. L. and Levey, A. S. (1991). Transmission of hepatitis C virus by organ transplantation. *N. Engl. J. Med.* **325**, 454.

Pereira, B. J. G., Milford, E. L., Kirkman, R. L., *et al.* (1992). Prevalence of HCV RNA in hepatitis C antibody positive cadaver organ donors and their recipients. *N. Engl. J. Med.* **327**, 910.

Pereira, B. J. G., Natov, S. N., Bouthot, B. A., *et al.* (1998). Effect of

hepatitis C infection and renal transplantation on survival in end-stage renal disease. *Kidney Int.* **53**, 1374.

Pereira, B. J. G., Wright, T. L., Schmid, C. H. and Levey, A. S., for The New England Organ Bank Hepatitis C Study Group (1995a). A controlled study of hepatitis C transmission by organ transplantation. *Lancet* **345**, 484.

Pereira, B. J. G., Wright, T. L., Schmid, C. H. and Levey, A. S., for The New England Organ Bank Hepatitis C Study Group (1995b). The impact of pretransplantation hepatitis C infection on the outcome of renal transplantation. *Transplantation* **60**, 799.

Pereira, B. J. G., Wright, T. L., Schmid, C. H., *et al.* (1994). Screening and confirmatory testing of cadaver organ donors for hepatitis C virus infection: a U.S. National Collaborative Study. *Kidney Int.* **46**, 886.

Pessoa, M. G., Terrault, N. A., Ferrell, L. D., *et al.* (1997). Hepatitis G virus in patients with cryptogenic liver disease undergoing liver transplantation. *Hepatology* **25**, 1266.

Pettersson, E., Hovi, T., Ahonen, J., *et al.* (1985). Prophylactic oral acyclovir after renal transplantation. *Transplantation* **39**, 279.

Pilot-Matias, T. J., Carrick, R. J., Coleman, P. F., *et al.* (1996). Expression of the GB virus C E2 glycoprotein using the Semliki Forest virus vector system and its utility as a serologic marker. *Virology* **225**, 282.

Pirsch, J. D., Heisey, D., D'Allesandro, A. M., Knechtle, S. J., Sollinger, H. W. and Belzer, F. O. (1995). Transplantation of hepatitis C (HCV) kidneys: defining the risks. *14th Annual Meeting of the American Society of Transplant Physicians*, p. 98, Chicago.

Pirson, Y., Alexandre, G. P. and van Ypersele de Striou, C. (1977). Long-term effect of HBs antigenemia on patient survival after renal transplantation. *N. Engl. J. Med.* **296**, 194.

Pol, S., Cavalcanti, R., Carnot, F., *et al.* (1996). Azathioprine hepatitis in kidney transplant recipients: a predisposing role of chronic viral hepatitis. *Transplantation* **61**, 1774.

Pol, S., Debure, A., Degott, C., *et al.* (1990). Chronic hepatitis in kidney allograft recipients. *Lancet* **335**, 878.

Pol, S., Legendre, C., Saltiel, C., *et al.* (1992). Hepatitis C virus in kidney recipients: epidemiology and impact on renal transplantation. *J. Hepatol.* **15**, 202.

Pol, S., Romeo, R., Zins, B., *et al.* (1993). Hepatitis C virus RNA in anti-HCV positive hemodialyzed patients: significance and therapeutic implications. *Kidney Int.* **44**, 1097.

Pol, S., Thiers, V., Carnot, F., *et al.* (1995a). Efficacy and tolerance of alpha-2b interferon therapy on HCV infection of hemodialyzed patients. *Kidney Int.* **47**, 1412.

Pol, S., Thiers, V., Nousbaum, J. B., *et al.* (1995b). The changing relative prevalence of hepatitis C virus genotypes: evidence in hemodialyzed patients and kidney recipients. *Gastroenterology* **108**, 581.

Pontisso, P., Ruvoletto, M. G., Nicoletti, M., *et al.* (1995). Distribution of three major hepatitis C virus genotypes in Italy: a multicentre study of 495 patients with chronic hepatitis. *J. Viral Hepat.* **2**, 33.

Ponz, E., Campistol, J. M., Barrera, J. M., *et al.* (1991). Hepatitis C virus antibodies in patients on hemodialysis and after transplantation. *Transplant. Proc.* **23**, 1371.

Port, F., Wolfe, R., Mauger, E., Berling, D. and Jiang, K. (1993). Comparison of survival probabilities for dialysis patients vs cadaveric renal transplant recipients. *J. A. M. A.* **270**, 1339.

Pouteil-Noble, C., Tardy, J. C., Chossegros, P., Trepo, C., Aymard, M. and Touraine, J. L. (1991). Hepatitis C virus infection in renal transplantation. *Kidney Int.* **39**, 1318.

Pouteil-Noble, C., Tardy, J. C., Chossegros, P., *et al.* (1995). Co-infection by hepatitis B virus and hepatitis C virus in renal trasnplantation: morbidity and mortality in 1098 patients. *Nephrol. Dial. Transplant.* **10(Suppl. 6)**, 122.

Poynard, T., Bedrossa, P., Chevallier, M., *et al.* (1995). A comparison of three interferon alpha-2b regimens for the long-term treatment of chronic non-A, non-B hepatitis. *N. Engl. J. Med.* **332**, 1457.

Prados, M. C., Franco, A., Perdiguero, M., Munoz, C., De la Sen, M. L. and Olivares, J. (1992). Transmission of hepatitis C virus by kidney transplantation. *Transplant. Proc.* **24**, 2650.

Preiksaitis, J. K., Cockfield, S. M., Fenton, J. M., Burton, N. I. and Chui, L. W.-L. (1997). Serologic responses to hepatitis C virus in solid organ transplant recipients. *Transplantation* **64**, 1775.

Preiksaitis, J. K., Diaz-Mitoma, F., Mirzayans, F., Roberts, S. and Tyrrell, D. L. (1992). Quantitative oropharyngeal Epstein-Barr virus shedding in renal and cardiac transplant recipients: relationship to immunosuppressive therapy, serologic responses, and the risk of posttransplant lymphoproliferative disorder. *J. Infect. Dis.* **166**, 986.

Raengsakulrach, B., Ong-aj-yooth, L., Thaiprasert, T., *et al.* (1997). High prevalence of hepatitis G viremia among kidney transplant patients in Thailand. *J. Med. Virol.* **53**, 162.

Ranjan, D., Burke, G., Esquenazi, V., *et al.* (1991). Factors affecting the ten-year outcome of human renal allografts: the effect of viral infections. *Transplantation* **51**, 113.

Rao, K. V. and Anderson, W. R. (1982). Hemosiderosis: an unrecognized complication in renal allograft recipients. *Transplantation* **33**, 115.

Rao, K. V. and Anderson, W. R. (1985). Hemosiderosis and hemochromatosis in renal transplant recipients. *Am. J. Nephrol.* **5**, 419.

Rao, K. V. and Andersen, R. C. (1988). Long-term results and complications in renal transplant recipients. *Transplantation* **45**, 45.

Rao, K. V. and Anderson, W. R. (1992). Liver disease after renal transplantation. *Am. J. Kidney Dis.* **19**, 496.

Rao, K. V. and Anderson, W. R. (1995). Clinical and histological outcome following interferon treatment of chronic viral hepatitis, in uremic patients, before and after renal transplantation. *14th Annual Meeting of the American Society of Transplant Physicians*, p. 99, Chicago.

Rao, K. V., Anderson, R. W., Kasiske, B. L. and Dahl, D. C. (1993). Value of liver biopsy in the evaluation and management of chronic liver disease in renal transplant recipients. *Am. J. Med.* **94**, 241.

Rao, K. V., Kasiske, B. L. and Anderson, W. R. (1991). Variability in the morphological spectrum and clinical outcome of chronic liver disease in hepatitis B-positive and B-negative renal transplant recipients. *Transplantation* **51**, 391.

Raptopoulou-Gigi, M., Spaia, S., Garifallos, A., *et al.* (1995). Interferon-alpha2b treatment of chronic hepatitis C in haemodialysis patients. *Nephrol. Dial. Transplant.* **10**, 1834.

Read, A. E., Weisner, R. H., La Brecque, D. R., *et al.* (1986). Hepatic veno-occlusive disease associated with renal transplantation and azathioprine therapy. *Ann. Intern. Med.* **104**, 651.

Rivolta, E., De Vecchi, A., Tarantino, A., Castelnovo, C., Berardinelli, L. and Ponticelli, C. (1987). Prognostic significance of hepatitis B surface antigenemia in cadaveric renal transplant patients. *Transplant. Proc.* **19**, 2153.

Robert, C., Agut, H., Lunel-Fabiani, F. and Leger, P. (1994). Human herpesvirus-6 infection and hepatitis following heart transplantation. *Presse Med.* **23**, 1209.

Rodrigues, A., Morgado, T., Areias, J., *et al.* (1997). Limited benefit of INF-alpha therapy in renal graft candidates with chronic viral hepatitis B or C. *Transplant. Proc.* **29**, 777.

Roger, S. D., Cunningham, A., Crewe, E. and Harris, D. C. (1991). Hepatitis C virus infection in heamodialysis patients. *Aust. N. Z. J. Med.* **21**, 22.

Rosenblum, L., Darrow, W., Witte, J., *et al.* (1992). Sexual practices in the transmission of hepatitis B virus and prevalence of hepatitis Delta virus infection in female prostitutes in the United States. *J. A. M. A.* **267**, 2477.

Rostaing, L., Chatelut, E., Payen, J., *et al.* (1998a). Pharmacokinetics of alfa-interferon-2b in chronic hepatitis C virus patients undergoing chronic hemodialysis or with normal renal function: clinical implications. *J. Am. Soc. Nephrol.* **9**, 2344.

Rostaing, L., Henry, S., Cisterne, J. M., Duffaut, M., Icart, J. and Durand, D. (1997). Efficacy and safety of lamivudine on replication of recurrent hepatitis B after cadaveric renal transplantation. *Transplantation* **64**, 1624.

Rostaing, L., Izopet, J., Arnaud, C., *et al.* (1999). Long-term impact of superinfection by hepatitis G virus in hepatitis C virus-positive renal transplant patients. *Transplantation* **67**, 556.

Rostaing, L., Izopet, J., Baron, E., *et al.* (1995). Preliminary results of treatment of chronic hepatitis C with recombinant interferon alpha in renal transplant patients. *Nephrol. Dial. Transplant.* **10**, 93.

Rostaing, L., Izopet, J., Cisterne, J.-M., *et al.* (1998b). Impact of hepatitis C virus duration and hepatitis C virus genotypes on renal transplant patients: correlation with clinicopathological features. *Transplantation* **65**, 930.

Roth, D. (1995). Hepatitis C virus: the nephrologist's view. *Am. J. Kidney Dis.* **25**, 3.

Roth, D., Fernandez, J. A., Babischkin, S., *et al.* (1992). Detection of hepatitis C infection among cadaver organ donors: evidence for low transmission of disease. *Ann. Intern. Med.* **117**, 470.

Roth, D., Zucker, K., Cirocco, R., *et al.* (1994). The impact of hepatitis C virus infection on renal allograft recipients. *Kidney Int.* **45**, 238.

Roth, D., Zucker, K., Cirocco, R., *et al.* (1996). A prospective study of hepatitis C virus infection in renal allograft recipients. *Transplantation* **61**, 886.

Rotolo, F. S., Branum, G. D., Bowers, B. A. and Meyers, W. C. (1985). Effect of cyclosporine on bile secretion in rats. *Am. J. Surg.* **151**, 35.

Rubin, R. (1993). Infectious disease complications of renal transplantation. *Kidney Int.* **44**, 221.

Ryffel, B., Donatsch, P., Madorin, M., *et al.* (1983). Toxicological evaluation of cyclosporin A. *Arch. Toxicol.* **53**, 107.

Sagnelli, E., Mauzillo, G., Maio, G., *et al.* (1980). Serum levels of hepatitis B surface and core antigens during immunosuppressive treatment of HBsAg positive chronic active hepatitis. *Lancet* **2**, 395.

Sallie, R. (1995). Hepatitis C: IIb (IV) or not IIb (IV) that is the question. *Hepatology* **22**, 671.

Sampietro, M., Badalamenti, S., Graziani, G., *et al.* (1997). Hepatitis G virus in hemodialysis patients. *Kidney Int.* **51**, 348.

Schlauder, G. G., Dawson, G. J., Simons, J. N., *et al.* (1995). Molecular and serological analysis in the transmission of the GB hepatitis agents. *J. Med. Virol.* **46**, 81.

Schlipkoter, U., Roggendorf, M., Ernst, G., *et al.* (1990). Hepatitis C virus antibodies in haemodialysis patients. *Lancet* **335**, 1409.

Schooley, R. T., Hirsh, M. S., Colvin, R. B., *et al.* (1983). Association of herpesvirus infections with T-lymphocyte-subset alterations, glomerulopathy, and opportunistic infections after renal transplantation. *N. Engl. J. Med.* **308**, 307.

Schroter, G. P. J., Weil, R. I., Penn, I., Speers, W. C. and Waddell, W. R. (1982). Hepatocellular carcinoma associated with chronic hepatitis B virus infection after kidney transplantation. *Lancet* **2**, 381.

Schroter, M., Feucht, H. H., Schafer, P., Zollner, B. and Laufs, R. (1999). GB virus C/hepatitis G virus infection in hemodialysis patients: determination of seroprevalence by a four-antigen recombinant immunoblot assay. *J. Med. Virol.* **57**, 230.

Schulte-Frohlinde, E., Schmolke, S., Reindl, W., *et al.* (1998). Significance of antibodies to recombinant E2 protein of hepatitis G virus in hemodialysis patients. *J. Viral Hepat.* **5**, 341.

Scott, D., Mijch, A., Lucas, C. R., Marshall, V., Thomson, N. and Atkins, R. (1987). Hepatitis B and renal transplantation. *Transplant. Proc.* **19**, 2159.

Seale, L., Jones, C. J., Kathpalia, S., *et al.* (1985). Prevention of herpesvirus infections in renal allograft recipients by low-dose oral acyclovir. *J. A. M. A.* **254**, 3435.

Seeff, L. B., Buskell-Bales, Z., Wright, E. C., *et al.* (1992). Long-term mortality after transfusion-associated non-A, non-B hepatitis. *N. Engl. J. Med.* **327**, 1906.

Seme, K., Pollak, M., Jeverica, S., Koren, A. and Sasa Zuzek-Resek, S. (1998). Prevalence of hepatitis G virus infection in Slovenian hemodialysis patients as determined by the detection of viral genome and E2 antibodies. *Nephron* **79**, 426.

Sengar, D. P. S., Couture, R. A., Lazarovitz, A. I. and Jindal, S. L. (1989). Long-term patient and renal allograft survival in HBsAg infection: a recent update. *Transplant. Proc.* **21**, 3358.

Sharma, R. K., Elhence, R., Kher, V., Naik, S. R. and Bhandari, M. (1992). Liver disease in renal transplant recipients. *Transplant. Proc.* **24**, 1915.

Sheng, L., Widyastuti, A., Kosala, H., *et al.* (1998). High prevalence of hepatitis G virus infection compared with hepatitis C virus infection in patients undergoing chronic hemodialysis. *Am. J. Kidney Dis.* **31**, 218.

Shibuya, A., Takeuchi, A., Kamata, K., Saigenji, K., Kobayashi, N. and Yoshida, A. (1998). Prevalence of hepatitis G virus RNA and anti-E2 in Japanese haemodialysis population. *Nephrol. Dial. Transplant.* **13**, 2033.

Simmonds, P., Alberti, A., Alter, H. J., *et al.* (1994). A proposed system for the nomenclature of hepatitis C virus genotypes. *Hepatology* **19**, 1321.

Simmons, R. L., Lopez, C. L., Balfour, H., Kalis, J., Rattazzi, L. C. and Najarian, J. S. (1974). Cytomegalovirus: clinical virological correlations in renal transplant. *Ann. Surg.* **180**, 623.

Simmons, R. L., Matas, A. J., Ratazzi, L. C., Balfour, H. H. J., Howard, R. J. and Najarian, J. S. (1977). Clinical characteristics of the lethal cytomegalovirus infection following renal transplantation. *Surgery* **82**, 537.

Simon, N., Courouce, A. M., Lemarrec, N., *et al.* (1994). A twelve year natural history of hepatitis C virus infection in hemodialyzed patients. *Kidney Int.* **46**, 504.

Simons, J. N., Leary, T. P., Dawson, G. J., *et al.* (1995a). Isolation of novel virus-like sequences associated with human hepatitis. *Nat. Med.* **1**, 564.

Simons, J. N., Pilot-Matias, T. J., Leary, T. P., *et al.* (1995b). Identification of two flavivirus-like genomes in the GB hepatitis agent. *Proc. Natl. Acad. Sci. U. S. A.* **92**, 3401.

Snydman, D. R., Werner, B. G., Heinze-Lacey, B., *et al.* (1987). Use of cytomegalovirus immune globulin to prevent cytomegalovirus disease in renal-transplant recipients. *N. Engl. J. Med.* **317**, 1049.

Sobue, R., Miyazaki, H., Okamoto, M., *et al.* (1991). Fulminant hepatitis in primary human herpesvirus-6 infection. *N. Engl. J. Med.* **324**, 1290.

Sopko, J. and Anuras, S. (1978). Liver disease in renal transplant recipients. *Am. J. Med.* **64**, 139.

Sparberg, M., Simon, N. and Del Greco, F. (1969). Intrahepatic cholestasis due to azathioprine. *Gastroenterology* **57**, 439.

Stark, K., Bienzle, U., Hess, G., Engel, A. M., Hegenscheid, B. and Schluter, V. (1996). Detection of the hepatitis G virus genome among injecting drug users, homosexual and bisexual men, and blood donors. *J. Infect. Dis.* **174**, 1320.

Stark, K., Meyer, C. G., Tacke, M., *et al.* (1997). Hepatitis G virus RNA and hepatitis G virus antibodies in renal transplant recipients: prevalence and risk factors. *Transplantation* **64**, 608.

Starzl, T. E., Faris, T. D., Hennan, T. J., *et al.* (1965). Factors determining short and long survival after orthotopic liver homotransplantation in the dog. *Surgery* **58**, 131.

Stempel, C., Lake, J., Ferrell, L., *et al.* (1991). Effect of cyclosporine on the clinical course of HBsAg-positive renal transplant patients. *Transplant. Proc.* **23**, 1251.

Stempel, C. A., Lake, J., Kuo, G. and Vincenti, F. (1993). Hepatitis C—its prevalence in end-stage renal failure patients and clinical course after kidney transplantation. *Transplantation* **55**, 273.

Strauch, B., Andrews, L., Siegel, N. and Miller, G. (1974). Oropharyngeal excretion of Epstein-Barr virus by renal transplant recipients and other patients treated with immunosuppressive drugs. *Lancet* **1**, 234.

Strom, T. (1982). Hepatitis B, transfusions and renal transplantation five years later. *N. Engl. J. Med.* **307**, 1141.

Stuyver, L., Rossau, R., Wyseur, A., *et al.* (1993). Typing of hepatitis C virus isolates and characterization of new subtypes using a line probe assay. *J. Gen. Virol.* **74**, 1093.

Szabo, A., Viazov, S., Heemann, U., Kribben, A., Philipp, T. and Roggendorf, M. (1997). GBV-C/HGB infection in renal dialysis and transplant patients. *Nephrol. Dial. Transplant.* **12**, 2380.

Tabor, E., Bayley, A. C., Cairns, L. and Gerety, R. J. (1985). Horizontal transmission of hepatitis B virus among childern and adults in five villages in Zambia. *J. Med. Virol.* **15**, 113.

Tagariello, G., Infantolino, D., Biasin, M. R., Davoli, P. G. and Traldi, A. (1996). Hepatitis G viral RNA in Italian haemophiliacs with and without hepatitis C infection. *Lancet* **348**, 760.

Takada, N., Takase, S., Enomoto, N., *et al.* (1992). Clinical backgrounds of the patients having different types of hepatitis C virus genomes. *J. Hepatol.* **14**, 35.

Takahara, S., Ihara, H., Ichikawa, Y., *et al.* (1987). Prospective study and long-term follow-up of liver damage in renal transplant recipients. *Transplant. Proc.* **19**, 2221.

Tameda, Y., Kosaka, Y., Tagawa, S., *et al.* (1996). Infection with GB virus C (GBV-C) in patients with fulminant hepatitis. *J. Hepatol.* **25**, 842.

Tanaka, E., Alter, H. J., Nakatsuji, Y., *et al.* (1996). Effect of hepatitis G virus infection on chronic hepatitis C. *Ann. Intern. Med.* **125**, 740.

Taylor, R. J., Saul, S. H., Dowling, J. N., Hakala, T. R., Peel, R. L. and Ho, M. (1981). Primary disseminated herpes simplex infection with fulminant hepatitis following renal transplantation. *Arch. Intern. Med.* **141**, 1519.

Tesi, R., Waller, K., Morgan, C., *et al.* (1994). Transmission of hepatitis C by kidney transplantation—the risks. *Transplantation* **57**, 826.

Tesi, R. J., Waller, M. K., Morgan, C. J., *et al.* (1993). Use of low-risk HCV-positive donors for kidney transplantation. *Transplant. Proc.* **25**, 1472.

Tokars, J. I., Miller, E. R., Alter, M. J. and Arduino, M. J. (1998). National surveillance of dialysis associated diseases in the United States, 1995. *ASAIO J.* **44**, 98.

Tong, M. J., el-Farra, N. S., Reikes, A. R. and Co, R. L. (1995). Clinical outcomes after transfusion-associated hepatitis C. *N. Engl. J. Med.* **332**, 1463.

Tribl, B., Oesterreicher, C., Pohanka, E., Sunder-Plassmann, G., Petermann, D. and Muller, C. (1998). GBV-C/HGV in haemodialysis patients: anti-E2 antibodies and GBV-C/HGV-RNA in serum and peripheral blood mononuclear cells. *Kidney Int.* **53**, 212.

Triolo, G., Squiccimarro, G., Baldi, M., *et al.* (1992). Antibodies to hepatitis C virus in kidney transplantation. *Nephron* **61**, 276.

Trites, A. E. W. (1957). Peliosis hepatis. *Arch. Pathol.* **63**, 183.

Tsuda, F., Hadiwandowo, S., Sawada, N., *et al.* (1996). Infection with GB virus C (GBV-C) in patients with chronic liver disease or on maintenance hemodialysis in Indonesia. *J. Med. Virol.* **49**, 248.

Tsukiyama Kohara, K., Kohara, M., Yamaguchi, K., *et al.* (1991). A second group of hepatitis C viruses. *Virus Genes* **5**, 243.

Tucker, T. J., Smuts, H. E. M., Kirsch, P. E., Eickhaus, P., Robson, S. C. and Swanepoel, C. (1998). The hepatitis G virus? GBV-C is associated with glomerulonephritis. *S. Afr. Med. J.* **88**, 286.

Umlauft, F., Gruenewald, K., Weiss, G., *et al.* (1997). Patterns of hepatitis C viremia in patients receiving hemodialysis. *Am. J. Gastroenterol.* **92**, 73.

UNOS. (1994). UNOS update. Annual Report. **10**, 27.

Urdea, M. S., Horn, T., Fultz, T. J., *et al.* (1991). Branched DNA amplication multimers for the sensitive, direct detection of human hepatitis viruses. *Nucl. Acids Symp. Ser.* **24**, 197.

van der Poel, C. L., Reesink, H. W., Schaasberg, W., *et al.* (1990). Infectivity of blood seropositive for hepatitis C virus antibodies. *Lancet* **335**, 558.

Vasile, A., Allegra, V., Canciani, D., Forchi, G. and Mengozzi, G. (1992). Prospective and retrospective assessment of clinical and laboratory parameters in maintenance hemodialysis patients with and without HCV antibodies. *Nephron* **61**, 318.

Vincenti, F., Lake, J., Wright, T., Kuo, G., Weber, P. and Stempel, C. (1993). Nontransmission of hepatitis C from cadaver kidney donors to transplant recipients. *Transplantation* **55**, 674.

Wanless, I. R. (1990). Micronodular transformation (nodular regenerative hyperplasia) of the liver: a report of 64 cases among 2,500 autopsies and a new classification of benign hepatocellular nodules. *Hepatology* **11**, 787.

Ware, A. J., Luby, J. P., Eigenbrodt, E. H., Long, D. L. and Hull, A. R. (1975). Spectrum of liver disease in renal transplant recipients. *Gastroenterology* **68**, 755.

Ware, A. J., Luby, J. P., Hollinger, B., *et al.* (1979). Etiology of liver disease in renal transplant patients. *Ann. Intern. Med.* **91**, 364.

Warrell, M. J., Chinn, I., Morris, P. J. and Tobin, J. O. (1980). The effects of viral infection on renal transplants and their recipients. *Q. J. M.* **49**, 219.

Weiner, A. J., Kuo, G., Bradley, D. W., *et al.* (1990). Detection of hepatitis C viral sequences in non-A, non-B hepatitis. *Lancet* **335**, 1.

Weinstein, T., Zevin, D., Ori, Y., *et al.* (1997). Hepatitis C infection in renal transplant recipients in Israel. *Transplant. Proc.* **29**, 2696.

Weir, M. R., Kirkman, R. L., Strom, T. B. and Tilney, N. L. (1985). Liver disease in recipients of long-surviving renal allografts. *Kidney Int.* **28**, 839.

White, A. G., Kumar, M. S. A., Stranneegard, O. and Abouna, G. M. (1987). Renal transplantation in hepatitis B surface antigen-positive patients. *Transplant. Proc.* **19**, 2150.

Widell, A., Mansson, S., Persson, N. H., Thysell, H., Hermodsson, S. and Blohme, I. (1995). Hepatitis C superinfection in hepatitis C virus (HCV)-infected patients transplanted with an HCV-infected kidney. *Transplantation* **60**, 642.

Willems, M., Peerlinck, K., Moshage, H., *et al.* (1994). Hepatitis C virus-RNAs in plasma and in peripheral blood mononuclear cells of hemphiliacs with chronic hepatitis C: evidence for viral replication in peripheral blood mononuclear cells. *J. Med. Virol.* **42**, 272.

Wolf, P. L., Williams, D., Coplon, N. and Coulson, A. S. (1972). Low aspartate transaminase activity in serum of patients undergoing chronic hemodialysis. *Clin. Chem.* **18**, 567.

Wreghitt, T. G., Gray, J. J., Allain, J.-P., *et al.* (1994). Transmission of hepatitis C virus by organ transplantation in the United Kingdom. *J. Hepatol.* **20**, 768.

Yagisawa, T., Toma, H., Tanabe, K., *et al.* (1997). Long-term outcome of renal transplantation in hepatitis B surface antigen-positive patients in cyclosporin era. *Am. J. Nephrol.* **17**, 440.

Yamanishi, K., Okuno, T., Shiraki, K., *et al.* (1988). Identification of human herpesvirus-6 as a causal agent for exanthem subitum. *Lancet* **1**, 1065.

Yanagi, K., Harada, S., Ban, F., Oya, A., Okabe, N. and Tobinai, K. (1990). High prevalence of antibody to human herpesvirus-6 and decrease in titer with increase in age in Japan. *J. Infect. Dis.* **161**, 153.

Yasumura, T., Nakajiama, H., Hamashima, T., *et al.* (1997). Long-term outcome of recombinant INF-α treatment of chronic hepatitis C in kidney transplant recipients. *Transplant. Proc.* **29**, 784.

Ynares, C., Johnson, H. K., Kerlin, T., Crowe, D., MacDonell, R. and Richie, R. (1993). Impact of pretransplant hepatitis C antibody status upon long-term patient and renal allograft survival—a 5- and 10-year follow-up. *Transplant. Proc.* **25**, 1466.

Yoshiba, M., Okamoto, H. and Mishiro, S. (1995). Detection of GBV-C hepatitis virus genome in serum from patients with fulminant hepatitis of unknown aetiology. *Lancet* **346**, 1131.

Yoshimura, E., Hayashi, J., Ueno, K., *et al.* (1997). No significant changes in levels of hepatitis C virus (HCV) RNA by competitive polymerase chain reaction in blood samples from patients with chronic HCV infection. *Dig. Dis. Sci.* **42**, 772.

Yoshioka, K., Kakumu, S., Wakita, T., *et al.* (1992). Detection of hepatitis C virus by polymerase chain reaction and response to interferon-alpha therapy: relationship to genotypes of hepatitis C virus. *Hepatology* **16**, 293.

Zaidi, Y., Chapman, C. S. and Myint, S. (1996). Aplastic anaemia after HGV infection. *Lancet* **348**, 471.

Zarday, Z., Veith, F. J., Gliedman, M. L. and Soberman, R. (1972). Irreversible liver damage after azathioprine. *J. A. M. A.* **222**, 690.

Zayas, E., Gonzalez Caraballo, Z., Morales Otero, L. and Santiago Delpin, E. A. (1996). Varicella zoster in a transplant program: experience with 15 cases and 70 contacts. *Transplant. Proc.* **28**, 3296.

Zein, N. N., Rakela, J., Krawitt, E. L., *et al.* (1996). Hepatitis C virus genotypes in the United States: epidemiology, pathogenicity, and response to interferon therapy. *Ann. Intern. Med.* **125**, 634.

Zeldis, J. B., Depner, T. A., Kuramoto, I. K., Gish, R. G. and Holland, P. V. (1990). The prevalence of hepatitis C virus antibodies among hemodialysis patients. *Ann. Intern. Med.* **112**, 958.

Zibert, A., Schreier, E. and Roggendorf, M. (1995). Antibodies in human sera to hypervariable region 1 of hepatitis C virus can block viral attachment. *Virology* **208**, 653.

Zuckerman, A. J. (1996). Alphabet of hepatitis viruses. *Lancet* **347**, 558.

Zylberberg, H., Landau, A., Carnot, F., *et al.* (1998). Impact of co-infection by hepatitis B virus and hepatitis C virus in renal transplantation. *Transplant. Proc.* **30**, 2820.

Neurological Complications

Michael Donaghy

Clinical Approach to Neurological Problems in Transplant Recipients

Neurological problems are major contributors to morbidity and mortality in transplant recipients. Most problems occur months or years after engraftment and may never come to the attention of the transplant surgeon. A range of neurological disease is possible in transplant recipients with a noteworthy incidence of a few particular conditions: cerebral lymphoma, stroke, infections and drug complications. Diagnosis and treatment are undertaken best in conjunction with a neurologist acquainted with transplantation. Often, additional advice must be sought from neuroradiology, infectious disease, neurosurgical, neuropathological and oncological consultants. An accurate yet prompt diagnosis may prove elusive, but this quest is crucial for initiating prompt and suitable therapy—particularly for infections. Diagnostic confusion can be caused by the residue of prior neurological disease, from the coexistence of multiple diagnoses and from suppression of normal inflammatory responses by immunosuppression. Neurological disease can result from the disease process initially causing renal failure, such as systemic lupus erythematosus, systemic vasculitis or diabetes mellitus.

The first diagnostic step requires the patient's problem to be assigned to one of these broad syndromes: diffuse encephalopathy, focal cerebral abnormality, seizure disorder or peripheral nerve damage. Then one should seek the disease entities encountered most commonly in transplant recipients within that particular syndrome (Table 33–1). Certain disorders are particularly common perioperatively, including damage to peripheral nerves and electrolyte disturbances.

DIFFUSE ENCEPHALOPATHY

Diffuse encephalopathy varies in its severity and manifestations, ranging from slight confusion or somnolence to complete coma. It may be accompanied by headache, personality change, meningismus or seizures depending on the cause of encephalopathy. Cyclosporine toxicity most commonly becomes symptomatic within the first 3 months after transplantation and causes various patterns of encephalopathy, including tremor, seizures and visual disturbances (Kahan *et al.*, 1987). Tacrolimus (FK506) can produce a similar encephalopathy. OKT3 monoclonal antibody treatment of acute rejection can produce temporary aseptic meningitis occasionally accompanied by mild encephalopathy. Infective meningoencephalitis is an important cause of diffuse encephalopathy, but signs of meningeal irritation often are absent in the immunosuppressed transplant recipient (Hooper *et al.*, 1982). *Listeria monocytogenes* infection produces a meningoencephalitis that may develop over a few days and often includes signs of brain stem dysfunction, such as eye movement disorders or dysarthria. *Cryptococcus neoformans* meningitis usually develops more than 6 months after engraftment with an insidious clinical progression. Patients may develop an en-

cephalopathy resulting from the remote effects of systemic sepsis, and this may be accompanied by seizures or focal signs (Jackson *et al.*, 1986). So-called rejection encephalopathy has occurred during episodes of acute graft rejection particularly in young patients and usually involves convulsions, headache and confusion (Gross *et al.*, 1982). It is unclear whether rejection encephalopathy is a discrete entity or merely reflects cumulative physiological, pharmacological and metabolic insults, including hypertension, at the time of acute graft rejection. Hypertensive encephalopathy usually is associated with retinopathy and papilledema. Postoperative hyponatremia can induce seizures, but this is more frequent after liver rather than renal transplantation.

Treatable causes frequently underlie encephalopathy in transplant recipients; prompt and thorough investigation is mandatory. Computed tomography (CT) or magnetic resonance imaging (MRI) studies of the brain ensure that multiple mass lesions are not masquerading as a diffuse encephalopathy, a particular problem with multifocal cerebral lymphoma. If the brain scan is normal, the cerebrospinal fluid should be examined for tuberculosis, fungi and conventional bacteria. Simultaneous cerebrospinal fluid and blood glucose

TABLE 33–1

NEUROLOGICAL SYNDROMES IN TRANSPLANT RECIPIENTS

Diffuse Encephalopathy
Cyclosporine toxicity
Tacrolimus toxicity
OKT3 antibody meningoencephalopathy
Meningitis/encephalitis (e.g., *Listeria, Cryptococcus*)
Electrolyte disturbances
Rejection encephalopathy
Hypertensive encephalopathy
Remote effect of systemic sepsis
Multifocal cerebral lymphoma

Focal Central Nervous System Abnormalities
Cerebral lymphoma
Cerebral infarction/hemorrhage
Focal cerebral infection (e.g., aspergillosis, nocardiosis)
Central pontine myelinolysis

Seizures
Cyclosporine toxicity
Hypomagnesemia
Hyponatremia
Rejection encephalopathy
Cerebral lymphoma
Focal cerebral infection
Meningitis/encephalitis

Peripheral Nerve Syndromes
Perioperative femoral nerve damage
Perioperative lumbosacral plexopathy in diabetics
Guillain-Barré syndrome
Tacrolimus neuropathy
Critical illness polyneuropathy

estimations should be performed on fluoride-preserved specimens; a blood/cerebrospinal fluid ratio greater than 2/1 strongly points to meningeal infection or malignant meningitis and is a valuable clue if microscopy is inconclusive. Only rarely do the clinical and laboratory parameters point so convincingly to cyclosporine toxicity, hypertension or hyponatremia that other diagnostic tests can be foregone. Cyclosporine blood levels may not be available sufficiently promptly to avoid initiating trials of therapy for potential alternative diagnoses. Hyponatremia can itself be a nonspecific feature of chronic meningitis or other intracranial disease and should not be accepted as the definitive and only explanation for an encephalopathy.

FOCAL CEREBRAL NEUROLOGICAL ABNORMALITIES

Focal cerebral neurological abnormalities may be encountered in transplant recipients and include hemiparesis, dysphasia and homonymous visual field loss. Focal disorders causing disturbances of memory, speech or spatial orientation may be misinterpreted as diffuse encephalopathies. Ischemic stroke is encountered commonly during the long-term follow-up of transplant recipients and usually occurs with an abrupt neurological deficit; usually headache is absent or relatively mild (Adams *et al.*, 1986). The risk of primary cerebral lymphoma is increased greatly in transplant recipients. Cerebral dysfunction generally has been progressively worsening for weeks or months by the time of diagnosis; headache seems to be a relatively late feature (Hochberg and Miller, 1988). Cerebral lymphoma may be multifocal, masquerading as a diffuse encephalopathy.

Focal cerebral infections in transplant recipients are usually due to aspergillosis or, less often, toxoplasmosis or nocardiosis. Aspergillosis usually occurs within 6 months immediately after transplantation (Hooper *et al.*, 1982). Headache and fever are not reliable indicators of these cerebral infections. Central pontine myelinolysis usually presents with tetraparesis that progresses over hours to days. If the cranial musculature also is affected, causing loss of speech, it may simulate coma by causing a *locked-in state*. Central pontine myelinolysis is less common in recipients of renal transplants than recipients of liver transplants. It usually occurs in the postoperative period a few days after too rapid correction of chronic hyponatremia (Wszolek *et al.*, 1989). Benign intracranial hypertension, also known as *pseudotumor cerebri*, causing headache and papilledema, has been reported in children after renal transplantation and may be related to cyclosporine administration (Sheth *et al.*, 1994).

Transplant recipients with focal neurological disturbances should be investigated initially by CT or MRI. The CT scan may show no abnormalities during the first 48 hours after an ischemic stroke. Focal mass lesions usually require neurosurgical biopsy with histological and microbiological examination of the specimen.

SEIZURES

Seizures occur regularly in transplant recipients. Cyclosporine reduces seizure thresholds (Kahan *et al.*, 1987). Seizures are particularly frequent in hypomagnesemic patients also receiving cyclosporine (Thompson *et al.*, 1984). Multiple interacting factors often combine to cause epileptic seizures in transplant recipients (Gilmore, 1988). Patients should be investigated with CT or MRI studies of the brain to detect focal lesions, such as cerebral lymphoma, infection or infarction. Blood levels of cyclosporine, sodium and magnesium should be estimated, and the possibilities of meningeal

infection, systemic sepsis, graft rejection and hypoglycemia in transplanted diabetics should be considered.

PERIPHERAL NERVE DISEASE

Peripheral nerve disease is relatively uncommon in renal transplant recipients. It usually results from perioperative trauma to the lumbosacral plexus. Femoral nerve lesions usually occur postoperatively with unilateral weakness of knee extension, loss of the patellar reflex and sensory disturbance on the anterior thigh or medial calf. These abnormalities may not be apparent until the patient attempts to walk postoperatively. Usually the intrapelvic femoral nerve has been compressed by self-retaining retractor blades. To avoid this compression, the surgeon should check that the femoral artery remains pulsatile after positioning these retractor blades during engraftment (Meech, 1990; Pontin *et al.*, 1978; Vasiri *et al.*, 1981). These femoral nerve lesions usually resolve, but this takes some months and can be incomplete.

Diabetics undergoing renal transplantation appear to be vulnerable to a presumed ischemic lesion of the lumbosacral plexus when the internal iliac artery is used for revascularization of the graft (Hefty *et al.*, 1990). This lesion presents postoperatively with buttock pain and weakness of the leg below the knee; recovery may occur but may be incomplete. Limb paresthesias are common in patients taking cyclosporine. A true polyneuropathy is rarely, if ever, attributable to this drug, however; neurotoxic effects of other drugs or metabolic conditions are difficult to exclude in the few postulated cases (Blin *et al.*, 1989; Walker and Brochstein, 1988). Subacute tetraparesis caused by Guillain-Barré syndrome has followed renal transplantation and is thought to result from transmitted cytomegalovirus infection or reactivation of latent cytomegalovirus infection (Bale *et al.*, 1980; Donaghy *et al.*, 1989). Chronic polyneuropathy has been recorded in liver transplant recipients receiving tacrolimus (Bronster *et al.*, 1995), and it remains to be seen whether this also occurs in renal transplant recipients receiving tacrolimus.

Cerebral Lymphoma

A markedly increased incidence of lymphoproliferative disorders has been noted since the early days of transplantation (Hoover and Fraumeni, 1973; Penn, 1984). It was recognized immediately that primary lymphomas of the central nervous system account for much of this increase (Schneck and Penn, 1971), an impression repeatedly confirmed by more contemporary studies (Hochberg and Miller, 1988; see Chapter 35). The background incidence of primary cerebral lymphoma also is increasing rapidly in the immunocompetent normal population (Eby *et al.*, 1988; Jellinger and Paulus, 1992). This situation may predispose immunosuppressed transplant recipients to further increases in incidence in the future. At present, the risk of cerebral lymphoma in transplant recipients is estimated at 2%—30 to 350 times higher than in the immunocompetent population.

Cerebral lymphoma generally arises as a primary tumor in transplant recipients; cerebral or meningeal spread from systemic lymphoma is encountered much less commonly. Histologically, non-Hodgkin's monoclonal B-lymphocyte proliferations account for most primary central nervous system lymphomas. Epstein-Barr virus is suspected strongly to play an important role in the production of cerebral lymphoma, based on serum antibody responses and immunostaining and DNA hybridization studies of biopsy specimens (Bashir *et al.*, 1989; Hanto *et al.*, 1983; Ho *et al.*, 1985; Hochberg *et al.*, 1983). Analysis of data pooled from earlier reports shows a median interval of 9 months between transplantation and development of primary cerebral lymphoma in transplant recipients (range, 5.5–46 months) (Hochberg and Miller, 1988). It is not known whether the widespread introduction of cyclosporine since the mid-1980s has influenced the incidence or timing of cerebral lymphoma in renal transplant recipients.

Primary cerebral lymphoma is unifocal in two thirds of patients and affects the cerebral hemispheres approximately 3.5 times as frequently as it affects the brain stem or cerebellum (Hochberg and Miller, 1988; Murray et al., 1986). Cerebral lymphoma is multifocal in one third of the patients. Cerebral lymphoma can invade the meninges, but malignant meningitis more often reflects spread from a systemic primary. Patients usually present with neurological deficits that worsen over a few weeks or months. Focal symptoms and signs may include hemiparesis, aphasia, hemianopia and cerebellar ataxia. Other patients, particularly those with multifocal cerebral lymphoma, may present with features more suggestive of a diffuse encephalopathy, such as personality or intellectual change or seizures. Headache usually is a late symptom, often reflecting raised intracranial pressure or meningeal involvement (Hochberg and Miller, 1988). Less frequent neurological presentations of lymphomas include malignant meningitis, spinal cord lesions resulting from localized intradural masses and visual disturbance resulting from ocular deposits (Hochberg and Miller, 1988).

Primary intracerebral lymphoma usually is visualized by CT or MRI brain scans. Contrast enhancement improves the sensitivity of CT scans in detecting lymphoma and particularly reveals the smaller lesions in multifocal disease. Intracerebral lymphoma usually is located periventricularly and appears as a homogeneously contrast-enhancing mass with relatively little surrounding edema. This appearance is in contrast to the ring-enhancing lesions with marked edema typically seen with malignant glioma or in secondary carcinomatous deposits. Gadolinium-enhanced MRI is the most sensitive way to detect intracerebral lymphoma and offers a satisfactory alternative to myelography in detecting spinal meningeal deposits. Diffuse lymphomatous involvement of the meninges may be detected by cytological examination of the cerebrospinal fluid; multiple specimens may be required before histological confirmation is forthcoming. The cerebrospinal fluid glucose level usually is reduced in lymphomatous meningitis.

A suspected diagnosis of primary intracerebral lymphoma should be confirmed by prompt neurosurgical biopsy and neuropathological examination. It is important to avoid high-dose steroid therapy before obtaining the biopsy specimen; dexamethasone often shrinks cerebral lymphomas within a few days and can interfere with the reliability of histological diagnosis (DeAngelis et al., 1990; Singh et al., 1982). Neurosurgeons should not aim to resect primary intracerebral lymphoma because this does not enhance long-term survival, and there is substantial immediate morbidity after attempts to resect deep-seated tumor masses (DeAngelis et al., 1990).

The author's views on the treatment and prognosis of primary intracerebral lymphoma are based largely on studies in patients who have not been immunosuppressed for the purposes of transplantation. The effects of continued immunosuppressant drug therapy on the efficacy of treatment or on survival when cerebral lymphoma occurs in transplant recipients are unknown. Steroids combined with cranial radiotherapy may give dramatic initial responses, with regression of tumor on brain scans and substantial clinical improvement, but the median survival is 10 to 18 months. Improved median survival of 42 months has been reported when high-dose cytosine arabinoside and intrathecal methotrexate are combined with radiotherapy (DeAngelis et al., 1990). Intraarterial methotrexate before radiotherapy produces tumor response in 85% of patients, but this combined therapy carries a high risk years later of severe leukoencephalopathy, with dementia, ataxia and incontinence, especially in older patients (DeAngelis, 1999). DeAngelis (1991) considered that chemotherapy should be started before radiotherapy for the best results. Optimal treatment regimens for intracerebral lymphoma currently are being sought, and patients with cerebral lymphoma should be managed by an oncologist experienced in this area.

Cerebrovascular Disease

Stroke is a major cause of morbidity and mortality after transplantation in the early months and in the later years of otherwise successful transplants. In the early days of transplantation, a 6-year follow-up study found that ischemic stroke accounted for 3% of deaths, a risk estimated to be more than 100 times higher than for the normal population (Ibels et al., 1974). A later series found that stroke accounted for 12% of deaths during 10 years of follow-up, and stroke or transient cerebral ischemic attacks occurred in 8.5% of the 10-year survivors (Mahoney et al., 1982). In comparison with ischemic stroke, subarachnoid hemorrhage occurs infrequently in transplant recipients, even in recipients with underlying polycystic renal disease who are at risk of cerebral aneurysm (Adams et al., 1986). Overall, thromboembolic disease was second only to sepsis as a cause of death in the early years after transplantation (Blohme and Ahlmen, 1977; Rao et al., 1976), but it is now the major cause of death and continues to be a prominent cause of illness in patients who survive with a functioning graft more than 10 years (Rao, 1987; see Chapter 30).

Various risk factors contribute to the huge increase in stroke after transplantation (Adams et al., 1986; see Chapter 30). Transplant recipients older than age 40 years are at particular risk (Adams et al., 1986; Ibels et al., 1974). One study noted an increased stroke risk in patients whose renal failure originally was due to hypertension (Ibels et al., 1974). This association was not found in another survey, however, that noted a clear association of ischemic stroke with underlying polycystic renal disease, a condition in which hypertension is common (Adams et al., 1986). Diabetes mellitus and systemic lupus erythematosus also predispose a patient to stroke after transplantation (Adams et al., 1986).

Hyperlipidemia occurs in renal failure and after transplantation and could cause accelerated atherosclerosis (Ibels et al., 1975; see Chapter 30). Atherosclerosis may be accelerated by long-term prednisolone therapy. This effect might prove to be less in the modern era of cyclosporine and tacrolimus immunosuppression, which allows a lower long-term dosage of prednisolone. As yet, no epidemiological studies have assessed possible changes in the incidence of thromboembolic disease as a result of the introduction of cyclosporine.

Ischemic stroke usually presents with the relatively abrupt onset of a focal neurological deficit, such as hemiparesis, speech disturbance, clumsiness and hemianopia. Headache may be present but usually is not severe. Computed tomography scan of the brain often shows no abnormalities in the first 24 to 48 hours after stroke. If the neurological deficit recovers within 24 hours, it is termed a *transient cerebral ischemic attack* rather than a completed stroke. It is particularly important to recognize transient ischemic attacks, to investigate for potentially treatable risk factors and to initiate low-dose aspirin therapy (75–300 mg daily) as prophylaxis against future stroke.

Potentially treatable or reversible risk factors include hypertension, smoking, diabetes mellitus, syphilis, polycythemia and thrombocythemia. Anticardiolipin antibodies should be sought particularly if there is a history of systemic lupus erythematosus. If multiple strokes occur, if there is fever, if there has been prominent headache preceding the stroke or if a markedly lymphocytic cerebrospinal fluid is associated with a stroke, infection or cerebral vasculitis should be considered. The fungal infections aspergillosis and mucormycosis can present as stroke after hyphal invasion of cerebral arteries with distal embolization. Cerebral vasculitis has occurred in an immunosuppressed transplant recipient (Rothenberg, 1985).

Atheromatous internal carotid artery stenosis should be excluded in transplant recipients affected by stroke. Duplex scanning of the carotids can be done in most patients; whether one should proceed to angiography in the presence of a doubtful duplex scan is questionable, bearing in mind the attendant stroke rate of angiography. In the general population with stroke associated with internal carotid artery stenosis exceeding 75%, carotid endarterectomy is known to produce a small but significant improvement in long-term, stroke-free survival (European Carotid Surgery Triallists' Collaborative Group, 1991; North American Symptomatic Carotid Endarterectomy Trial Collaborators, 1991). It is uncertain whether the recommendations from these trials can be translated automatically to the population of renal transplant recipients who have been affected by stroke. Transplant recipients would be expected to have high risks of stroke in other cerebral arterial territories, of ischemic coronary artery disease and of other serious medical and perioperative disorders. All of these factors that affect long-term prognosis could offset the small long-term benefits otherwise expected from carotid endarterectomy. In the absence of definitive information regarding the transplant population, the decision regarding carotid endarterectomy should be made on the usual grounds.

Rejection Encephalopathy

An entity of rejection encephalopathy has been proposed on the basis of observations in 13 patients who exhibited a reversible acute neurological syndrome that coincided with severe acute rejection of the transplanted kidney (Gross et al., 1982). The young transplant patient may be particularly susceptible; 11 of these patients were less than 20 years of age. The patients developed varying combinations of convulsions, headache, confusion, disorientation and irritability, and one had papilledema. Simultaneous acute rejection was defined by presence of graft swelling and tenderness, fever, weight gain and hypertension. The encephalopathic patients did not exhibit a different degree of hypertension than nonencephalopathic patients with acute graft rejection. Only one patient was receiving cyclosporine, a recognized precipitant of seizures in transplant recipients.

No differences in blood biochemical parameters or medication schedule were identified between encephalopathic and nonencephalopathic patients except that the rise in serum creatinine level was higher in those with encephalopathy. Computed tomography scans of the brain sometimes showed edema of the cerebral white matter. The cerebrospinal fluid pressure was invariably raised, although the constituents usually were normal. Electroencephalography showed nonspecific slow wave activity.

Gross and colleagues emphasized that resolution of this encephalopathy is commensurate with vigorous immunosuppressive treatment of graft rejection (Gross et al., 1982). It is unclear whether so-called rejection encephalopathy should be regarded as a direct consequence of severe graft rejection or merely a reflection of the accumulation of metabolic, pharmacological and physiological insults occurring during severe graft rejection. Patients who develop encephalopathy in the context of acute graft rejection should be evaluated for possible cyclosporine toxicity, electrolyte disorders, fluid overload, severe uremia, systemic sepsis and malignant hypertension. If more than a few weeks have elapsed after transplantation, neurological infections and cerebral lymphoma should be considered.

Neurological Infection

A wide range of neurological infection occurs in transplant recipients (Gallis et al., 1975; Hooper et al., 1982; Peterson and Anderson, 1986; see Chapter 31). Diagnosis can be difficult and requires close cooperation between the transplant clinician, neurologist, microbiologist and neuropathologist. In an early study covering the 1970s, 7% of renal transplant recipients developed central nervous system infection over a 10-year period, with nearly half dying as a result (Hooper et al., 1982). Cryptococcus, Aspergillus and Listeria infections accounted for 90% in this series. Since then, cyclosporine immunosuppression has been widely introduced, with the impression that the range of central nervous system infection has widened. In particular, infections with Nocardia and Toxoplasma seem to be diagnosed more commonly. Intracranial infection should be suspected in transplant recipients with combinations of headache, fever, confusion, impaired consciousness, focal deficits or seizures. Investigation depends first on CT or MRI brain studies to detect focal lesions amenable to biopsy and second on cerebrospinal fluid examination if there is no cerebral mass lesion providing a contraindication to lumbar puncture.

Three main syndromes of central nervous system infection are encountered. First, meningitis may be due to Listeria, Cryptococcus or conventional bacterial infection. Less frequently, meningitis is due to tuberculosis or coccidioidomycosis in endemic areas, such as Arizona (Cohen et al., 1982). Aseptic meningitis may follow a few days after OKT3 monoclonal antibody therapy for acute graft rejection or after administration of high-dose intravenous immunoglobulin and usually resolves after headache for a few more days; occasionally a mild encephalopathy with confusion may occur (Coleman and Norman, 1990; Martin et al., 1988). Second, focal brain abscesses can be due to Aspergillus or Nocardia and less frequently to mucormycosis or Candida. Mucormycosis is particularly common in transplanted diabetics. It starts in the paranasal sinuses producing periorbital edema and proptosis and subsequently may invade the intracavernous carotid artery, leading to cerebral artery emboli and strokes (Carbone et al., 1985). Third, diffuse encephalitis may be due to Aspergillus or Toxoplasma and less frequently progressive multifocal leukoencephalopathy or cytomegalovirus; herpes encephalitis is uncommon in the immunosuppressed.

Repeated cerebrospinal fluid examinations or brain biopsy of focal lesions usually is required to establish the microbiological diagnosis. Most of the infections described produce a predominantly lymphocytic cerebrospinal fluid pleocytosis, often with a low glucose level. Serological tests for a range of fungal infections should be performed on serum and cerebrospinal fluid. Cryptococcal antigen may be detected immunologically in the cerebrospinal fluid. The cerebrospinal fluid should be examined microscopically by Gram stain, Ziehl-Nielsen staining and ink stain. Cultures should be set up for conventional bacteria, tuberculosis and fungi. Specific antimicrobial therapy is undertaken with the guidance of an infectious disease consultant (see Chapter 31). In patients acutely ill with meningitis, *blind* ampicillin treatment for *Listeria* should be started immediately after lumbar puncture, pending accurate diagnosis. Occasionally, blind therapy has to be initiated for a probable diagnosis of fungal infection, *Nocardia* or tuberculosis.

Listeria monocytogenes

L. monocytogenes causes meningitis and, less frequently, meningoencephalitis or focal cerebral infection (Stamm *et al.*, 1982). Fever and headache develop subacutely; focal neurological deficits, impaired consciousness and signs of meningism are encountered in less than half (Pollock *et al.*, 1984). *Listeria* infection may present at any time after transplantation but rarely within the first month (Hooper *et al.*, 1982). The cerebrospinal fluid white blood cell count usually is raised to a few hundred per cubic millimeter, but this can vary from less than 10/mm³ to many thousands per cubic millimeter and be predominantly polymorphonuclear or lymphocytic.

The cerebrospinal fluid glucose level is reduced in approximately half of patients (Stamm *et al.*, 1982). Diagnosis is easiest in patients with purely meningitic syndromes in whom there is a high chance of positive cultures from blood and/or cerebrospinal fluid. Confirmation of the diagnosis may prove difficult in patients with focal neurologic signs, but particular suspicion of listeriosis should be raised by a combination of brain stem dysfunction and cellular cerebrospinal fluid. Combined ampicillin and gentamicin therapy is recommended. The combination of trimethoprim and sulfamethoxazole is an alternative option (Peterson and Anderson, 1986). A quarter of renal transplant recipients with listeriosis may die as a result (Stamm *et al.*, 1982).

Cryptococcus neoformans

C. neoformans usually produces an indolent chronic lymphocytic meningitis and rarely presents earlier than 6 months after transplantation (Hooper *et al.*, 1982). Headache and fever, often mild, are the usual symptoms. Focal signs or significantly altered consciousness is rare. The cerebrospinal fluid pressure often is increased, and it may contain 500 lymphocytes/mm³ with a low glucose level. It may take some time to culture the organism from cerebrospinal fluid, and immunological detection of cerebrospinal fluid cryptococcal antigen is recommended as a quick, reliable diagnostic method. Antifungal treatment with intravenous amphotericin B and/or fluconazole eradicates the infection in most patients without necessitating a reduction in immunosuppression that might jeopardize graft survival (Hooper *et al.*, 1982; Watson *et al.*, 1985).

Cytomegalovirus

Proven cytomegalovirus encephalitis is rare in transplant recipients, although it often is suspected (Bamborschke *et al.*, 1992). Clinical experience of this condition has been derived mainly from acquired immunodeficiency syndrome (AIDS) patients (Holland *et al.*, 1994). Patients usually present with a meningoencephalitis in which confusion and memory loss are prominent. Other features, such as headache or retinitis, are only variably present. Magnetic resonance imaging brain scan can be normal or show atrophy, white matter abnormalities or meningeal enhancement. Cerebrospinal fluid can be normal or lymphocytic, and a positive polymerase chain

reaction seems to be a reliable indicator of central nervous system infection (Cohen, 1996). This diagnosis is important because of the prospect for treatment with ganciclovir or foscarnet and the need to reduce the immunosuppressant drug regimen (Holland *et al.*, 1994; Watson *et al.*, 1985). The prognosis of cytomegalovirus encephalitis is poor in AIDS patients.

Aspergillus fumigatus

A. fumigatus of the brain usually develops within the first few months after renal transplantation (Hooper *et al.*, 1982). Most patients develop sudden focal neurological deficits or seizures, are febrile and have evidence of lung involvement (Beal *et al.*, 1982). Computed tomography brain scans may show focal lesions with relatively little mass effect or contrast enhancement. The cerebrospinal fluid sometimes contains an excess of lymphocytes with a normal glucose concentration. The strokelike onset of symptoms reflects invasion of cerebral blood vessels by fungus with distal embolization. The cerebral lesions may be multiple. Purely meningitic syndromes may occur, but meningitis usually results from rupture of cerebral abscesses into the subarachnoid space. Lung or cerebral biopsy is required for diagnosis. Downward deterioration is rapid, and most patients with cerebral involvement die despite antifungal therapy with amphotericin B (Beal *et al.*, 1982; Hooper *et al.*, 1982; Weiland *et al.*, 1983).

Nocardia asteroides

Brain abscess from *N. asteroides* can occur in transplant recipients, frequently disseminated from a pulmonary focus of infection. Clusters of patients with nocardial infection may occur in transplant units (Baddour *et al.*, 1986). The cerebral hemispheres are involved most frequently, causing aphasia, hemiparesis, visual field loss or confusion in the context of headache and fever. Brain stem or spinal cord lesions can occur. Associated subcutaneous lesions may be palpable, and biopsies can be performed easily. Aspiration of cerebral abscesses generally is recommended as treatment and may be necessary to establish the diagnosis. Aspiration should be combined with high-dose sulfonamide therapy.

Progressive Multifocal Leukoencephalopathy

Progressive multifocal leukoencephalopathy is a rare and fatal condition producing widespread demyelination within the central nervous system, particularly in the immunosuppressed. The clinical presentation varies. Usually the onset is insidious. Diffuse cerebral hemisphere involvement may present with dementia, blindness or bilateral weakness. More focal presentations cause hemiparesis, hemianopia and sometimes epilepsy. Patients with progressive multifocal leukoencephalopathy usually die within months to a year after a relentlessly progressive decline. Occasionally the decline may be more abrupt after an explosive onset, and there have been rare survivors for some years or remissions. Diagnosis is suggested by MRI, which shows diffuse demyelination, particularly in the subcortical white matter. Any mass effect, if present, usually is minor, and gadolinium contrast enhancement is unusual. The cerebrospinal fluid, cell and protein content usually is normal. Progressive multifocal leukoencephalopathy is caused by papovavirus infection, usually with JC virus but sometimes SV40 virus. Polymerase chain reaction detects JC virus DNA in most cerebrospinal fluid samples from patients with this condition (Perrons *et al.*, 1996). There has been no convincing evidence that antiviral treatments alter the relentless downhill course of the condition.

Side Effects of Immunosuppressant Drugs

Cyclosporine and tacrolimus most commonly cause neurological side effects, particularly markedly in liver transplant recipients. These side effects range from tremors, fits or paresthesia to a serious leukoencephalopathy. High-dose steroid therapy may cause mood alteration and occasionally psychosis requiring major tranquilizers if the steroid dosage cannot be reduced safely. Steroid-induced myopathy has become rarer because cyclosporine has allowed long-term dosages to be lower. Steroid-induced myopathy occurs much less commonly with prednisolone compared with fluorinated steroids, such as dexamethasone.

CYCLOSPORINE

Neurological complications have been attributed to cyclosporine in approximately 20% of renal transplant recipients (Kahan et al., 1987; O'Sullivan, 1985). Cyclosporine-related neurological side effects are commoner in liver transplant recipients, possibly as a result of associated hypocholesterolemia and hyponatremia (Adams et al., 1987; De Groen et al., 1987). Limb tremor is the commonest side effect, occurring in 20%. It usually is most marked within the first 3 months and rarely is noteworthy a few years after transplantation (Kahan et al., 1987). Many patients report burning paresthesia of the limbs while taking cyclosporine, but clinical and electrophysiological evaluation usually does not reveal evidence of peripheral neuropathy. If neuropathy is present in such patients, it is usually attributable to prolonged uremia before transplantation or other predisposing conditions; it is debatable whether neuropathy is caused directly by cyclosporine (Blin et al., 1989; Walker and Brochstein, 1988). Visual hallucinations or cortical blindness may be associated with high blood cyclosporine levels (Katirji, 1987; Stein et al., 1992). Depression, somnolence and other psychological disorders occasionally develop in cyclosporine recipients (Kahan et al., 1987). Tremors, paresthesia and visual hallucinations usually are dose-related side effects of cyclosporine and improve or resolve on lowering the dosage. Many instances of tremor and paresthesia are not sufficiently disabling or troublesome to warrant stopping or reducing effective immunosuppressive therapy.

Leukoencephalopathy is a rare but potentially serious side effect of cyclosporine therapy. It seems to be commonest in bone marrow and liver transplant recipients (Atkinson et al., 1984; De Groen et al., 1987; Stein et al., 1992). The relatively higher cholesterol level in the blood of renal transplant recipients may protect against encephalopathy; in contrast, hypocholesterolemia appears to predispose to encephalopathy in transplant recipients (De Groen et al., 1987). Confusion, coma, cortical blindness, cerebellar syndromes, hemiplegias and flaccid quadriparesis have all been described in cyclosporine recipients. The multifocal disorder including varying combinations of these features has been termed *cerebrocerebellar syndrome* (Stein et al., 1992). These features usually develop within the first 3 months of cyclosporine therapy. Mutism and migraine headaches have been attributed to cyclosporine in liver transplant recipients, but as yet such complications have not been reported in renal transplantation (Steiger et al., 1994; Valldeoriola et al., 1996). Blood cyclosporine levels usually are elevated but can be normal. Computed tomography or MRI brain studies show diffuse white matter abnormalities. The cerebrospinal fluid protein sometimes is ele-

vated. The neurological syndrome and brain imaging abnormalities usually resolve after stopping cyclosporine or after dosage reduction if blood levels were particularly high.

Cyclosporine is responsible for precipitating seizures in some patients, particularly those who also are hypomagnesemic (Adams et al., 1987; Thompson et al., 1984). The overall incidence of seizures is unknown and is influenced by coincidental factors, such as hyponatremia, graft rejection, hypertension and high-dose steroid therapy. Other coincidental factors need to be considered when seizures occur, including hyponatremia, graft rejection, hypotension, high-dose steroid therapy, cerebral infections and lymphomas. Pharmacological data suggest that seizures occur in 1.5% of cyclosporine-treated renal transplant recipients (O'Sullivan, 1985). Chronic aluminum overload after prolonged renal dialysis before transplantation may predispose to seizures (Nordal et al., 1985). Seizures in patients taking cyclosporine should be prevented initially by correcting associated precipitating factors and reducing the dosage if blood cyclosporine levels are high. If seizures persist despite these measures, the choice of an appropriate anticonvulsant drug becomes difficult. The enzyme-inducing effects of phenytoin, carbamazepine and phenobarbitone pose problems in achieving adequately immunosuppressive blood levels of cyclosporine (Gilmore, 1988; Walker and Brochstein, 1988). Valproate sodium is the recommended anticonvulsant in patients receiving cyclosporine (Hillebrand et al., 1987).

TACROLIMUS

Tacrolimus is used as an alternative immunosuppressant to cyclosporine (both are calcineurin inhibitors) and usually is a satisfactory replacement in cases of severe cyclosporine-associated neurological side effects. Tacrolimus has neurotoxic side effects in 20 to 30% of patients, however, and most experience regarding side effects comes from liver transplantation (Mueller et al., 1994; Wijdicks et al., 1994). Side effects usually occur within the first months of therapy and are commoner at higher doses. Speech disturbances, generalized seizures, tremor and ataxia, encephalopathy, nightmares and agitation have occurred. Most complications resolve with dosage reduction, but mild tremor or speech disturbance may persist.

A leukoencephalopathy can occur with white matter abnormalities on MRI affecting the parietooccipital regions and centrum semiovale. It closely resembles cyclosporine-associated leukoencephalopathy and occurs in adults and children (Small et al., 1996; Torocsik et al., 1999). This syndrome usually presents with occipital headache, nausea and vomiting, followed by a seizure, and visual disturbances may occur. Tacrolimus blood levels may be high, although not invariably, and the disorder resolves with dosage reduction. A severe demyelinating sensorimotor peripheral neuropathy resembling chronic inflammatory demyelinating polyneuropathy has been associated with tacrolimus (Bronster et al., 1995).

OKT3 ANTIBODIES

OKT3 monoclonal antibody therapy for acute rejection has been followed by aseptic meningitis 2 to 7 days later. Such patients develop varying degrees of fever, photophobia and headache associated with an aseptic cerebrospinal fluid pleocytosis. These features may occur in 14% of patients treated with OKT3. The syndrome resolves spontaneously even if OKT3 therapy is continued (Martin et al., 1988). A single instance of reversible encephalopathy with prominent myoclonic jerking has been recorded after OKT3 administration (Coleman and Norman, 1990).

Central Pontine Myelinolysis

Central pontine myelinolysis involves acute or subacute demyelination of the mid–brain stem, principally affecting the corticospinal tracts as they traverse the pons (Wright *et al.*, 1979). Over a matter of hours or a few days, patients develop symmetrical limb weakness with extensor plantar responses. The bulbar and facial musculature also may be paralyzed. In severe cases, a locked-in state develops in which the patient remains fully conscious, but no voluntary movements are possible apart from vertical eye movements. This state can be misinterpreted as coma. Death commonly ensues, and the remainder of patients are chronically disabled. Full recovery is rare. This demyelination of the brain stem is rarely shown by CT scanning, but MRI shows the lesion (Miller *et al.*, 1988).

An association of central pontine myelinolysis with hyponatremia has long been noted, particularly in the context of thiazide diuretic therapy, liver disease in alcoholics and inappropriate antidiuretic hormone secretion. The condition has occurred in renal transplant recipients (Norenberg *et al.*, 1982; Schneck, 1966) but appears to be commoner after liver transplantation (Wszolek *et al.*, 1989). Central pontine myelinolysis often has been noted a few days after correction of chronic hyponatremia with intravenous fluids at daily rates exceeding 12 mmol sodium/L. Because many cases of this disastrous neurological disorder appear to be iatrogenic, it is recommended that the serum sodium concentration be increased by less than 8 mmol/L/d (Norenberg *et al.*, 1982; Sterns *et al.*, 1986; Wszolek *et al.*, 1989). Renal transplant recipients potentially are vulnerable to central pontine myelinolysis, particularly postoperatively, and care should be taken in regard to the rate of correction of electrolyte disturbances in patients with chronic hyponatremia.

REFERENCES

Adams, D. H., Ponsford, S., Gunson, B., *et al.* (1987). Neurological complications following liver transplantation. *Lancet* **1**, 949.

Adams, H. P., Dawson, G., Coffman, T. J. and Corry, R. J. (1986). Stroke in renal transplant recipients. *Arch. Neurol.* **43**, 113.

Atkinson, K., Biggs, J., Darveniza, P., Boland, P., Concannon, A. and Dodds, A. (1984). Cyclosporine-associated central nervous system toxicity after allogeneic bone marrow transplantation. *Transplantation* **38**, 34.

Baddour, L. M., Baselski, V. S., Herr, M. J., Christensen, G. D. and Bisno, A. L. (1986). Nocardiosis in recipients of renal transplants: evidence for nosocomial transmission. *Am. J. Infect. Control* **14**, 214.

Bale, J. F., Rote, N. S., Bloomer, L. C. and Bray, P. F. (1980). Guillain-Barré-like polyneuropathy after renal transplant: possible association with cytomegalovirus infection. *Arch. Neurol.* **37**, 784.

Bamborschke, S., Wullen, T., Huber, M., *et al.* (1992). Early diagnosis and successful treatment of acute cytomegalovirus encephalitis in a renal transplant recipient. *J. Neurol.* **239**, 205.

Bashir, R. M., Harris, N. L., Hochberg, F. H. and Singer, R. M. (1989). Detection of Epstein-Barr virus in CNS lymphomas by in-situ hybridization. *Neurology* **39**, 813.

Beal, M. F., O'Carroll, C. P., Kleinman, G. M. and Grossman, R. I. (1982). Aspergillosis of the nervous system. *Neurology* **32**, 473.

Blin, O., Desnuelle, C., Pellissier, J. F., *et al.* (1989). Neuropathie péripherique et ciclosporine. *Therapie* **44**, 55.

Blohme, I. and Ahlmen, J. (1977). Late complications after successful renal transplantation. *Scand. J. Urol. Nephrol.* **42(Suppl.)**, 173.

Bronster, D. J., Yonover, P., Stein, J., Scelsa, S. N., Miller, C. M. and Sheiner, P. A. (1995). Demyelinating sensorimotor polyneuropathy after administration of FK506. *Transplantation* **59**, 1066.

Carbone, K. M., Pennington, L. R., Giminez, L. F., Burrow, C. R. and Watson, A. J. (1985). Mucormycosis in renal transplant patients—a report of two cases and review of the literature. *Q. J. M.* **224**, 825.

Cohen, B. A. (1996). Prognosis and response to therapy of cytomega-

lovirus encephalitis and meningomyelitis in AIDS. *Neurology* **46**, 444.

Cohen, I. M., Galgiani, J. N., Potter, D. and Ogden, D. A. (1982). Coccidioidomycosis in renal replacement therapy. *Arch. Intern. Med.* **142**, 489.

Coleman, A. E. and Norman, D. J. (1990). OKT3 encephalopathy. *Ann. Neurol.* **28**, 837.

DeAngelis, L. (1991). Primary central nervous system lymphoma: a new clinical challenge. *Neurology* **41**, 619.

DeAngelis, L. M., Yahalom, J., Heinemann, M.-H., Cirrincione, M. S., Thaler, H. T. and Krol, G. (1990). Primary CNS lymphoma: combined treatment with chemotherapy and radiotherapy. *Neurology* **40**, 80.

DeAngelis, L. (1999). Primary central nervous system lymphoma. *J. Neurol. Neurosurg. Psychiatry* **66**, 699.

De Groen, P. C., Aksamit, A. J., Rakela, J., Forbes, G. S. and Krom, R. A. F. (1987). Central nervous system toxicity after liver transplantation: the role of cyclosporine and cholesterol. *N. Engl. J. Med.* **317**, 861.

Donaghy, M., Gray, J. A., Squier, W., *et al.* (1989). Recurrent Guillain-Barré syndrome after multiple exposures to cytomegalovirus. *Am. J. Med.* **87**, 339.

Eby, N. L., Grufferman, S., Flannelly, C. M., Schold, S. C., Vogel, F. S. and Burger, P. C. (1988). Increasing incidence of primary brain lymphoma in the US. *Cancer* **62**, 2461.

European Carotid Surgery Triallists' Collaborative Group. (1991). MRC European carotid surgery trial: interim results for symptomatic patients with severe (70–99%) or with mild (0–29%) carotid stenosis. *Lancet* **337**, 1235.

Gallis, H. A., Berman, R. A., Cate, T. R., Hamilton, J. D., Gunnells, J. C. and Stickel, D. L. (1975). Fungal infection following renal transplantation. *Arch. Intern. Med.* **135**, 1163.

Gilmore, R. L. (1988). Seizures and antiepileptic drug use in transplant patients. *Neurol. Clin.* **6**, 279.

Gross, M. L. P., Sweny, P., Pearson, R. M., Kennedy, J., Fernando, O. N. and Moorhead, J. F. (1982). Rejection encephalopathy. *J. Neurol. Sci.* **56**, 23.

Hanto, D. W., Gajl-Peczalska, J. G., Frizzera, G., *et al.* (1983). Epstein-Barr virus (EBV) induced polyclonal and monoclonal B-cell lymphoproliferative diseases occurring after renal transplantation. *Ann. Surg.* **198**, 356.

Hefty, T. R., Nelson, K. A., Hatch, T. R. and Barry, J. M. (1990). Acute lumbosacral plexopathy in diabetic women after renal transplantation. *J. Urol.* **1043**, 107.

Hillebrand, G., Castro, L. A., Van Scheidt, W., Beukelmann, D., Land, W. and Schmidt, D. (1987). Valproate for epilepsy in renal transplant recipients receiving cyclosporine. *Transplantation* **43**, 915.

Ho, M., Miller, G., Atchison, R. W., *et al.* (1985). Epstein-Barr virus infections and DNA hybridization studies in protransplantation lymphoma and lymphoproliferative lesions: the role of primary infection. *J. Infect. Dis.* **152**, 876.

Hochberg, F. H. and Miller, D. C. (1988). Primary central nervous system lymphoma. *J. Neurosurg.* **68**, 835.

Hochberg, F. H., Miller, G., Schooley, R. T., Hirsch, M. S., Feorino, P. and Henle, W. (1983). Central nervous system lymphoma related to Epstein-Barr virus. *N. Engl. J. Med.* **309**, 745.

Holland, N. R., Power, C., Mathews, V. P., Glass, J. D., Forman, M. and McArthur, J. C. (1994). Cytomegalovirus encephalitis in acquired immunodeficiency syndrome (AIDS). *Neurology* **44**, 507.

Hooper, D. C., Pruitt, A. A. and Rubin, R. H. (1982). Central nervous system infections in the chronically immunosuppressed. *Medicine* **61**, 166.

Hoover, R. and Fraumeni, J. F. (1973). Risk of cancer in renal transplant recipients. *Lancet* **2**, 55.

Ibels, L. S., Simons, L. A., King, J. O., Williams, P. F., Neale, F. C. and Stewart, J. H. (1975). Studies on the nature and causes of hyperlipidemia in uremia, maintenance hemodialysis and renal transplantation. *Q. J. M.* **176**, 601.

Ibels, L. S., Stewart, J. H., Mahoney, J. F. and Sheil, A. G. R. (1974). Deaths from occlusive arterial disease in renal allograft recipients. *B. M. J.* **3**, 552.

Jackson, A. C., Gilbert, J. J., Young, G. B. and Bolton, C. F. (1986). The encephalopathy of sepsis. *Can. J. Neurol. Sci.* **12**, 303.

Jellinger, K. A. and Paulus, W. (1992). Primary central nervous system lymphomas—an update. *J. Cancer Res. Clin. Oncol.* **119**, 7.

Kahan, B. D. (1989). Cyclosporine. *N. Engl. J. Med.* **321**, 1725.

Kahan, B. D., Flechner, S. M., Lorber, M. I., Golden, D., Conley, S. and Van Buren, C. T. (1987). Complications of cyclosporine-prednisone immunosuppression in 402 renal allograft recipients exclusively followed at a single center for from one to five years. *Transplantation* **43**, 197.

Katirji, M. B. (1987). Visual hallucinations and cyclosporine. *Transplantation* **43**, 768.

Mahoney, J. F., Sheil, A. G. R., Etheridge, S. B., Storey, B. G. and Stewart, J. H. (1982). Delayed complications of renal transplantation and their prevention. *Med. J. Aust.* **2**, 426.

Martin, M. A., Massanari, R. M., Nghiem, D. D., Smith, J. L. and Corry, R. J. (1988). Nosocomial aseptic meningitis associated with administration of OKT3. *J. A. M. A.* **259**, 2002.

Meech, P. R. (1990). Femoral neuropathy following renal transplantation. *Aust. N. Z. J. Surg.* **60**, 117.

Miller, G. M., Baker, H. L., Okazaki, H. and Whisnant, J. P. (1988). Central pontine myelinolysis and its imitators. *Radiology* **168**, 795.

Mueller, A. R., Platz, K. P., Bechstein, W., *et al.* (1994). Neurotoxicity after orthotopic liver transplantation. *Transplantation* **58**, 155.

Murray, K., Kun, L. and Cox, J. (1986). Primary malignant lymphoma of the central nervous system: results of treatment of 11 cases and review of the literature. *J. Neurosurg.* **65**, 600.

Nordal, K. P., Talseth, T., Dahl, F., *et al.* (1985). Aluminium overload, a predisposing condition for epileptic seizures in renal transplant patients treated with cyclosporine? *Lancet* **2**, 153.

Norenberg, M. D., Leslie, K. O. and Robertson, A. S. (1982). Association between rise in serum sodium and central pontine myelinolysis. *Ann. Neurol.* **11**, 128.

North American Symptomatic Carotid Endarterectomy Trial Collaborators. (1991). Beneficial effect of carotid endarterectomy in symptomatic patients with high-grade carotid stenosis. *N. Engl. J. Med.* **325**, 445.

O'Sullivan, D. P. (1985). Convulsions associated with cyclosporin A. *B. M. J.* **290**, 858.

Palmer, B. F. and Toto, R. D. (1991). Severe neurologic toxicity induced by cyclosporine A in three renal transplant patients. *Am. J. Kidney Dis.* **18**, 116.

Penn, J. (1984). Cancer in immunosuppressed patients. *Transplant. Proc.* **2**, 492.

Perrons, C. J., Fox, J. D., Lucas, S. B., *et al.* (1996). Detection of polyomaviral DNA in clinical samples from immunocompromised patients: correlation with clinical disease. *J. Infect.* **32**, 205.

Peterson, P. K. and Anderson, R. C. (1986). Infection in renal transplant recipients: current approaches to diagnosis, therapy and prevention. *Am. J. Med.* **81(Suppl. 1A)**, 2.

Pollock, S. S., Pollock, T. M. and Harrison, M. J. G. (1984). Infection of the central nervous system by *Listeria monocytogenes*: a review of 54 adult and juvenile cases. *Q. J. M.* **211**, 331.

Pontin, A. R., Donaldson, R. A. and Jacobson, J. E. (1978). Femoral neuropathy after renal transplantation. *S. Afr. Med. J.* **53**, 376.

Rao, K. V. (1987). Renal transplantation: complications and results in the second decade. *Transplant. Proc.* **19**, 3758.

Rao, K. V., Smith, E. J., Alexander, J. W., Fidler, J. P., Pemmaraju, S. R. and Pollack, V. E. (1976). Thromboembolic disease in renal allograft recipients. *Arch. Surg.* **111**, 1086.

Rifkind, D., Marchioro, T. L., Schneck, S. A. and Hill, R. B. (1967). Systemic fungal infections complicating renal transplantation and immunosuppressive therapy. *Am. J. Med.* **43**, 28.

Rothenberg, R. J. (1985). Isolated angiitis of the brain. *Am. J. Med.* **79**, 629.

Rubin, A. M. and Kang, H. (1987). Cerebral blindness and encephalopathy with cyclosporin-A toxicity. *Neurology* **37**, 1072.

Schneck, S. A. (1966). Neuropathological features of human organ transplantation: II. Central pontine myelinolysis and neuroaxonal dystrophy. *J. Neuropathol. Exp. Neurol.* **25**, 18.

Schneck, S. A. and Penn, I. (1971). De-novo brain tumors in renal transplant recipients. *Lancet* **1**, 983.

Sheth, K. J., Kivlin, J. D., Leichter, H. E., Pan, C. G. and Multauf, C. (1994). Pseudotumour cerebri with vision impairment in two children with renal transplantation. *Paediatr. Nephrol.* **8**, 91.

Singh, A., Strobos, R. J., Singh, B. M., *et al.* (1982). Steroid-induced remissions in CNS lymphoma. *Neurology* **32**, 1267.

Small, S. L., Fukui, M. B., Bramblett, G. T., and Eidelman, B. H. (1996). Immunosuppression-induced leukoencephalopathy from tacrolimus (FK506). *Am. Neurol.* **40**, 575.

Stamm, A. M., Dismukes, W. E., Simmons, B. P., *et al.* (1982). Listeriosis in renal transplant recipients: report of an outbreak and review of 102 cases. *Rev. Infect. Dis.* **4**, 665.

Steiger, M. J., Farrah, T., Rolles, K., Harvey, P., and Burroughs, A. K. (1994). Cyclosporin-associated headache. *J. Neurol. Neurosurg. Psychiatry* **57**, 1258.

Stein, D. P., Lederman, R. J., Vogt, D. P., Carey, W. D. and Brougham, T. A. (1992). Neurological complications following liver transplantation. *Ann. Neurol.* **31**, 644.

Sterns, R. H., Riggs, J. E. and Schochet, S. S. (1986). Osmotic demyelination syndrome following correction of hyponatremia. *N. Engl. J. Med.* **314**, 1535.

Thompson, C. B., June, C. H., Sullivan, K. M. and Thomas, E. D. (1984). Association between cyclosporine neurotoxicity and hypomagnesaemia. *Lancet* **2**, 1116.

Torocsik, H. V., Curless, R. G., Post, J., Tzakis, A. G. and Pearse, L. (1999). FK506-induced leukoencephalopathy in children with organ transplants. *Neurology* **52**, 1497.

Valldeoriola, F., Graue, F., Rimola, A., *et al.* (1995). Cyclosporine-associated mutism in liver transplant patients. *Neurology* **46**, 252.

Vasiri, N. D., Barton, C. H., Ravikumar, G. R., Martin, D. G., Ness, R. and Staiki, J. (1981). Femoral neuropathy: a complication of renal transplantation. *Nephron* **28**, 30.

Walker, R. W. and Brochstein, J. A. (1988). Neurologic complications of immunosuppressive agents. *Neurol. Clin.* **6**, 261.

Watson, A. J., Russell, R. P., Cabreja, R. F., Braverman, R. and Whelton, A. (1985). Cure of cryptococcal infection during continued immunosuppressive therapy. *Q. J. M.* **217**, 169.

Weiland, D., Ferguson, R. M., Peterson, P. K., Snover, D. C., Simmons, R. L. and Najarian, J. S. (1983). Aspergillosis in 25 renal transplant patients. *Ann. Surg.* **198**, 622.

Wijdicks, E. F., Weisner, R. H., Dahlke, L. J., and Krom, R. A. (1994). FK506-induced neurotoxicity in liver transplantation. *Ann. Neurol.* **35**, 498.

Wright, D. G., Laureno, R. and Victor, M. (1979). Pontine and extrapontine myelinolysis. *Brain* **102**, 361.

Wszolek, Z. K., McComb, R. D., Pfeiffer, R. F., *et al.* (1989). Pontine and extrapontine myelinolysis following liver transplantation: relationship to serum sodium. *Transplantation* **48**, 1006.

Nonmalignant and Malignant Skin Lesions in Renal Transplant Patients

Cristina Bordea • Vanessa A. Venning • Fenella Wojnarowska

Introduction

Skin problems are a common and important consequence of renal transplantation and a cause of concern to patients and physicians. Patients present with skin manifestations of their drug regimens and problems arising as a consequence of immunosuppression. The use of steroids and cyclosporine is associated with important dermatological side effects, but there is insufficient experience with newer immunosuppressives (mycophenolate mofetil, tacrolimus) to identify major new cutaneous side effects. The state of nonspecific immunosuppression renders the transplant recipient susceptible to many bacterial, viral and fungal infections and predisposes the patient to the development of premalignant and malignant skin lesions. There is a similar profile of drug cutaneous side effects in renal transplant recipients of all racial groups, but the consequences of immunosuppression differ markedly with racial group, skin type and geographical location (Table 34–1). In patients of Northern European ancestry, the dominant long-term problem is nonmelanoma skin cancer, which is commonest in such patients living near the equator. The problem of skin cancers in renal transplant recipients is of growing importance, and skin cancers are a significant cause of morbidity and, more rarely, mortality. In tropical and subtropical areas, infections predominate, and Kaposi's sarcoma

is seen. In practice in the Oxford Renal Transplant Centre Dermatology Clinic, the commonest skin problems are malignant and premalignant lesions, warts, fungal infections, acne and folliculitis.

Drug Side Effects
CORTICOSTEROIDS

The commonest cutaneous changes after renal transplantation are due to the cushingoid side effects of corticosteroids. The frequency of these side effects has been recorded in a study of the skin findings in 200 renal transplant recipients (Koranda et al., 1974), and their occurrence has been confirmed by many subsequent studies worldwide (Barba et al., 1996; Chugh et al., 1994; Seckin et al., 1998). Purpura and some redistribution of body fat occurred in greater than 90% of patients, and more than half developed atrophic friable skin with poor wound healing. Striae frequently were extensive over the abdomen, buttocks and thighs and capable of producing slowly healing ulcers. Other frequent findings were facial erythema, telangiectasia, generalized skin dryness, and rough skin over the upper arms and thighs (keratosis pilaris) caused by blockage of the hair follicle orifices by keratin plugs. The last-mentioned finding is common in

TABLE 34–1

FREQUENCY OF SKIN LESIONS IN DIFFERENT POPULATIONS AND DIFFERENT GEOGRAPHICAL LOCATIONS

Country	Latitude (°)	Authors	No. Patients	Percent of Patients with Skin Manifestations (Absolute Numbers)							
				Herpesvirus (Herpes Simplex and Zoster)	Human Papillomavirus	Fungal and Yeast Infections	Bacterial Infections	Solar Keratoses	Nonmelanoma Skin Cancer (SCC/BCC)	Melanoma	Kaposi's Sarcoma
Sweden	60	Blohme and Larko, 1990	98		55	7		29	24 (7/16)		
Scotland	55	Bunney et al., 1990	162	1	33	10		7	1 (1/1)		
Italy Adults	45	Barba et al., 1996	285		31	23	5	6	4 (5/8)		<1
Children	45	Menni et al., 1991	32	6	12	6	6				
New Zealand	40	Hepburn et al., 1994	52		75	10		40	17 (17/14)*	2	
Turkey	40	Seckin et al., 1998	80	8	48	59	18	5	3 (2/1)		3
Iran	35	Amiransari et al., 1995	107	15	28	39		8	0 (0/1)*		5 patients*
India	30	Chugh et al., 1994	157	14	8	74	9		<1 (1/10)		
Puerto Rico (Hispanic)	20	Lugo-Janer et al., 1991b	82	4	28	>48	17	10	9 (8/0)	1	0
India	15	Vijaykumar et al., 1998	340		31	62	16		0	0	0

Italics indicate manifestation in local transplant population but not in this series.
SCC = squamous cell carcinoma; BCC = basal cell carcinoma.

healthy persons, but showers of new lesions may appear during steroid therapy. The development of these familiar cushingoid changes in part depends on the duration and dosage of steroid therapy, but there also is marked variation in individual susceptibility.

Corticosteroids stimulate the pilosebaceous unit, possibly through an androgen-mediated mechanism, and this is responsible for the appearance of hirsutism and steroid acne (Fig. 34–1). Visible fine hairs over the arms, back and cheeks were reported in 49% of Koranda's series. In some patients, this hair growth is reversible as the prednisolone dosage is lowered, but in doses around 20 mg/d, localized hirsutism frequently is persistent. Steroid acne may develop within 2 to 3 weeks of the start of treatment, and although it generally remits as the prednisolone dosage is lowered, it can be persistent on maintenance doses. The condition resembles acne vulgaris, affecting only androgen-dependent areas of skin bearing sebaceous glands (i.e., face, chest, back and upper arms). A point of distinction from acne vulgaris is the scarcity of open comedones (blackheads), the predominant lesions being discrete superficial monomorphic papulopustules, chiefly distributed over the facial convexities (Ebling and Cunliffe, 1992). Severe forms of acne also may occur, with deep-seated inflammatory nodulocystic lesions capable of scarring. Perioral dermatitis, which is characterized by redness and papulopustules around the mouth and nose, occurs in transplant recipients receiving systemic steroids (Adams et al., 1982).

Management

Most steroid side effects require no specific treatment and tend to improve as steroid doses are lowered to maintenance levels. There is some evidence that topical tretinoin (0.05%) is capable of reversing aspects of corticosteroid-induced skin atrophy (de Lacharriere et al., 1990), but this agent often is tolerated poorly because of its irritant effect. General dryness of the skin can be counteracted by the use of emollients, such as aqueous cream or emulsifying ointment. First-line treatment for steroid acne is the use of topical agents, such as 5% benzoyl peroxide or topical retinoids (tretinoin, isotretinoin or adapalene). Topical antibiotics, such as tetracycline, erythromycin and clindamycin, also may be tried. More severe cases require oral antibiotics. Normally, minocycline, 100 mg once daily, is the drug of choice because of increased patient compliance, although doxycycline and oxytetracycline are alternatives, given as a 3- to a 12-month course. In severe cases, isotretinoin is given at a dose of 0.5 or 1 mg/kg for a minimum of 4 months, although cheilitis, paronychia and effects on lipids are sometimes troublesome.

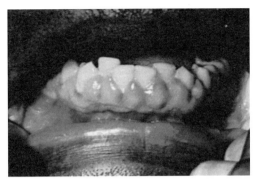

FIGURE 34–2

Gingival hypertrophy in a patient on cyclosporine alone.

CYCLOSPORINE

The skin is one of the principal sites of accumulation of cyclosporine (Neiderberger et al., 1984), and mucocutaneous side effects of cyclosporine have been recognized since the introduction of this drug, the commonest being gum hypertrophy (Tyldesley and Rotter, 1984; Fig. 34–2) and hypertrichosis (Canafax and Ascher, 1983; Fig. 34–3). Gum hyperplasia has a reported frequency of 8 to 70% (Daley et al., 1986; Tyldesley and Rotter, 1984). Nifedipine produces similar gum hyperplasia and is synergistic (Slavin and Taylor, 1987). The onset may be within the first month of cyclosporine treatment, but there is a sharp increase in incidence around 3 to 6 months (Bencini et al., 1986a). Clinically, soreness of the gums may precede hyperplasia, and although initially confined to the anterior interdental papillae, the whole gum subsequently may become hyperplastic. The changes may be more severe in patients with poor oral hygiene (Tyldesley and Rotter, 1984), although they also occur in otherwise

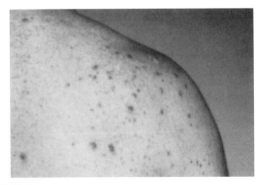

FIGURE 34–1

Steroid acne with monomorphic inflamed lesions with few comedones (see color plate).

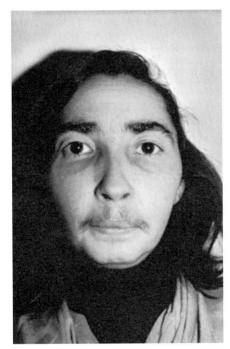

FIGURE 34–3

Hypertrichosis in a 35-year-old woman on cyclosporine alone 3 months after transplantation (see color plate).

healthy mouths (Bencini *et al.*, 1986a). It has been suggested that children are more susceptible (Menni *et al.*, 1991).

Hypertrichosis of some degree probably develops in 100% of cyclosporine-treated patients (Lindholm *et al.*, 1988); cosmetically significant hypertrichosis has been reported in 60% during the first 6 months of treatment (Bencini *et al.*, 1986a). In some women, this hypertrichosis results in a severe cosmetic problem. Keratosis pilaris may precede the appearance of thick pigmented hair over the trunk, back, shoulders, arms, neck, forehead and cheeks. Severe hypertrichosis appears to be commoner in dark-skinned subjects, a finding that suggests that some people may be genetically predisposed to the development of side effects (Bencini *et al.*, 1986a). It does not appear to be an androgen-mediated side effect because cyclosporine-induced hypertrichosis is not confined to androgen-dependent areas of skin (Mortimer *et al.*, 1983) and is independent of sex hormone levels (Lindholm *et al.*, 1988).

Bencini and colleagues described many other skin lesions, all of pilosebaceous origin, occurring in cyclosporine-treated renal transplant recipients: epidermal (pilar) cysts in 28% of patients, keratosis pilaris in 21%, sebaceous hyperplasia in 10% and acne in 15% (Bencini *et al.*, 1986a). Multiple epidermal cysts, 3 to 5 mm in diameter, occur on the cheeks and forehead, often in association with hypertrichosis, and appear to be due to obstruction of the infundibular portion of the follicle duct by hyperkeratosis. The tendency is for a reduction in number and size of cysts over time, in contrast to the hypertrichosis that shows no tendency to remit. Sebaceous hyperplasia presents as yellowish papules over the face and forehead in male patients. Acne, well recognized in patients treated with corticosteroids alone or in combination with cyclosporine, has been described in a patient receiving cyclosporine as the sole immunosuppressive agent (Bencini *et al.*, 1986b).

The principal target organ for cyclosporine in the skin appears to be the pilosebaceous unit, a structure also modified by corticosteroids, making differentiation between the effects of the two drugs difficult; in many cases, they appear to be acting synergistically. Reduced clearance of prednisolone during cyclosporine treatment may account for some of this synergy (Ost, 1984).

Management

There is no specific treatment for gum hyperplasia, although some investigators stress the importance of good oral hygiene and antiseptic mouthwashes in primary prevention. In severe cases, gingivectomy may be indicated (Tyldesley and Rotter, 1984).

A few patients develop hypertrichosis of such severity as to be a major cosmetic problem. When treatment is required, the hair may be removed by any method acceptable to the patient. Only electrolysis is permanent, although it is slow and time-consuming; some units offer electrolysis for this problem (see Chapter 40). There is currently much interest in laser hair removal, but although laser removal often is rapid, there is little evidence on long-term efficacy. Temporary measures include depilatory creams, shaving, plucking and waxing (mass plucking). Repeated plucking and waxing have the disadvantage of making successful electrolysis slightly more difficult later. An alternative in fair-skinned women is to bleach the hairs. Hypertrichosis is dose dependent and is reversible with reduction of the dosage or cessation of treatment.

TACROLIMUS

Tacrolimus (FK506) is used in renal transplantation, and data from hepatic and renal transplantation suggest that skin problems are slightly commoner than with cyclosporine, although hirsutism and gingival hypertrophy are less than with cyclosporine (Spencer *et al.*, 1997). Pruritus is the commonest adverse reaction, and alopecia, sweating and many diverse skin eruptions have been reported (Fujisawa, unpublished data).

MYCOPHENOLATE MOFETIL

Mycophenolate mofetil is used in renal transplantation and seems to have a low incidence of skin side effects because fewer side effects were documented compared with azathioprine (Simmons *et al.*, 1997). There is increased susceptibility to herpes simplex and zoster compared with placebo and an association with nonmelanoma skin cancers (European Mycophenolate Mofetil Cooperative Study Group, 1995; Mathew, 1998; Simmons *et al.*, 1997; Sollinger *et al.*, 1995; The Tricontinental Mycophenolate Mofetil Renal Transplantation Study Group, 1996).

Infections

Skin infections are a common sequela to renal transplantation and may be caused by bacteria, fungi, viruses or parasites. They appear to be common in patients treated with combined prednisolone and cyclosporine (Bencini *et al.*, 1986a) as well as in patients managed with conventional prednisolone and azathioprine immunosuppression. Their incidence depends on geographical location (see Table 34–1).

BACTERIAL INFECTIONS
Pyogenic Bacteria

Bacterial infections of the skin are common in renal transplant recipients, and patients are at continuing risk of these infections. Bencini and coworkers found 16 bacterial lesions among 105 transplant recipients, although the prevalence seems to depend greatly on geographical location (commonest in tropical and subtropical areas) (Bencini *et al.*, 1983; see Table 34–1). Apart from wound infections, the range of clinical lesions encountered in transplant patients includes impetigo, folliculitis, furuncles, abscesses, cellulitis and erysipelas, and the lesions tend to run a more severe and protracted course than usual (Haim *et al.*, 1973). Similar to in normal subjects, group A streptococci and *Staphylococcus aureus* are the commonest causative organisms, although the possibility of unusual pathogens should be borne in mind, particularly in cases of cellulitis. The resident skin flora of transplant recipients is similar to that of normal persons with no increased carriage of potential pathogens (Noble *et al.*, 1974).

Management

In view of the risk of serious infections, antibiotic treatment should be started promptly on clinical grounds but only after obtaining appropriate specimens for bacteriological confirmation. Topical fusidate (Fucidin) or mupirocin is rapidly curative in minor impetigo, although in most cases systemic flucloxacillin is indicated. Lesions containing pus (e.g., furuncles and abscesses) require drainage (unless discharge occurs spontaneously) combined with appropriate antibiotics. Antiseptic baths help prevent recurrent furunculosis, and nasal carriage of staphylococci can be eradicated temporarily by topical, but not systemic, antibiotic agents in patients in whom this is a predisposing factor.

Deeper seated infections, such as cellulitis and erysipelas, require prompt parenteral benzyl penicillin. Bacterial confirmation may be difficult but should be attempted because gram-negative organisms and fungi rarely can produce a cellulitis indistinguishable from streptococcal disease. Investigation should include skin swabs, aspiration of any blister fluid and needle aspiration of injected saline for culture. Serial serological testing for antibodies specific for *Streptococcus pyogenes* may be indicated. Any potential portal of entry (e.g., interdigital cracks owing to fungal infection) should be treated.

Mycobacteria

Atypical mycobacterial infections occasionally occur in renal transplant patients and produce exceptionally disseminated nodular skin lesions. *Mycobacterium marinum* (Gombert *et al.*, 1981) and *Mycobacterium chelonei* (Proby *et al.*, 1991) have been reported. Culture and isolation from biopsy or aspirated material is essential for precise diagnosis, and because prolonged culture with fastidious temperature requirement is needed, the clinical suspicion should be made clear to the pathologist. These organisms vary in their resistance to standard antituberculous drugs and may prove extremely persistent.

FUNGAL INFECTIONS

Fungal and yeast infections are common and affect most renal transplant recipients in tropical and subtropical countries (see Table 34–1). Although many are minor, some are severe and life-threatening (Lugo-Janer *et al.*, 1991a). Superficial infections by fungi and yeasts are extremely common in the immunocompromised host. Although none are serious, such infections may be a considerable nuisance to some patients, and physicians caring for renal transplant patients should be able to recognize and treat them. Treatment is more difficult than in immunocompetent patients.

Candida

Infections by *Candida albicans* usually are superficial and localized, although skin lesions also may accompany systemic candidiasis. The yeast thrives in moist intertriginous sites, such as the inframammary folds, groin, vulva and digital web spaces, producing the familiar well-demarcated glazed erythema, satellite lesions and curdy plaques. Vesicles and superficial pustules occasionally may be present. Obesity, diabetes and occlusion (e.g., under rings) are additional predisposing factors. Angular cheilitis and stomatitis are other common presentations (Haim *et al.*, 1973). Chronic paronychia, with a tender heaped up nail fold, usually is associated with *C. albicans* infection, although other *Candida* species (e.g., *Candida parapsilosis*) may be found. Frequent hand wetting and loss of the protective cuticle are important predisposing factors. Acute purulent exacerbations of chronic paronychia, with extreme tenderness of the nail fold, usually are due to *S. aureus*. *Candida* invasion of the nail may occur in immunocompromised patients producing whitish discoloration in a friable dystrophic nail. This condition often is indistinguishable clinically from dermatophyte nail infection (Lugo-Janer *et al.*, 1991a).

Management

Culture of *Candida* from skin swabs helps confirm the clinical diagnosis. *Candida* intertrigo responds to any of the topical imidazole preparations (e.g., miconazole nitrate cream) or nystatin. Careful drying of the skin folds and

weight reduction, when appropriate, help prevent recurrence. Oral candidiasis may be treated with local nystatin or an oral gel preparation of an imidazole. There is sufficient absorption from such imidazole preparations to cause serious drug interactions; particularly dangerous is interaction with warfarin. Treatment with systemic fluconazole may require double the usual dose, and there are interactions with cyclosporine (see Chapter 16).

Chronic paronychia frequently is a stubborn problem in immunocompetent patients. Hand wetting and damage to the cuticle should be avoided, and frequent liberal application of an imidazole cream around the nail fold serves a barrier function as well as therapy for *Candida*. Acute purulent exacerbations require treatment with oral flucloxacillin or erythromycin; however, erythromycin has an interaction with cyclosporine (Chapter 16). The management of nail infections is considered later.

Pityriasis Versicolor

The yeastlike fungus *Pityrosporum orbiculare* produces a distinctive eruption with multiple minimally scaly macular lesions widely scattered over the trunk and upper arms known as *pityriasis versicolor* (Fig. 34–4). The macules may be hyperpigmented or hypopigmented and usually are asymptomatic apart from their appearance. The prevalence of pityriasis versicolor in renal transplant patients is reported to be 18 to 25% in different regions compared with 0.5% in healthy subjects in a temperate zone (Amiransari *et al.*, 1995; Chugh *et al.*, 1994; Koranda *et al.*, 1974; Lugo-Janer *et al.*, 1991a). The diagnosis usually is clinically obvious but may be confirmed by microscopy of potassium hydroxide–treated skin scrapings to show the hyphae and spores. This organism is sensitive to many antifungal agents, including Whitfield's ointment, topical terbinafine and the imidazoles. The frequently widespread distribution means that treatment is simpler and cheaper using a lotion, such as selenium sulfide shampoo, rubbed onto wet skin and left for 5 minutes or overnight before washing off. This procedure must be repeated daily for 7 days, then weekly for a few weeks and thereafter at less frequent intervals. Ketoconazole shampoo or cream also can be used. Systemic itraconazole interacts with cyclosporine and is best avoided. Relapses are common. Persistence of hypopigmentation for many months is common and does not imply failure of treatment, although lesions with scaling usually harbor fungus.

Dermatophyte Infections

The skin of patients who are chronically immunosuppressed more frequently is colonized with potentially patho-

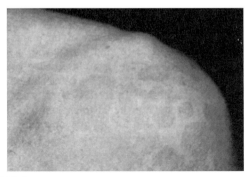

FIGURE 34–4

Pityriasis versicolor: pigmented macular lesions with superficial scaling over the shoulder region (see color plate).

genic fungi than that of healthy control subjects (Koranda *et al.*, 1974; Shuttleworth *et al.*, 1987b). The rate of dermatophyte carriage on clinically normal skin was estimated as 12% in renal transplant patients, compared with 6.8% in a control population (Koranda *et al.*, 1974). There are more fungal infections in males and in warm climates (Lugo-Janer *et al.*, 1991a; see Table 34–1). Problems resulting from dermatophytes reported in renal transplant patients include tinea corporis, tinea pedis and scalp infections and infection of the nails, although presumably infection at any site is possible. Skin infections may be clinically typical (i.e., annular lesions with scaling at the margins), although extensive skin involvement, Majocchi's granuloma or atypical nodular lesions have been reported (Bergfield and Roenigk, 1978; Dymock, 1979; Sequeira *et al.*, 1998; Fig. 34–5). Nails infected with dermatophyte fungi typically are yellowish, crumbly and distorted, with heaped up debris under the free edge. The appearance may be indistinguishable clinically from other causes of nail dystrophy. The presence of dermatophytes elsewhere (e.g., groin and toe webs) may aid diagnosis. Fingernail infections and involvement of multiple nails are seen more commonly in immunocompromised patients than in other patients.

Management

Whenever fungal infection is a possibility, appropriate specimens (scales, nail clippings or scrapings taken with a scalpel blade) should be treated with potassium hydroxide and subjected to microscopy to look for fungal hyphae. Fresh clippings or scrapings should be sent for fungal culture. Mycological confirmation of the diagnosis before treatment is essential to rule out noninfective causes of nail dystrophy and to differentiate dermatophyte from *Candida* infection.

Topical imidazoles and terbinafine are used in the treatment of dermatophyte infection of skin because they bring about quick clearance and have high cure rates. Treatment two to three times daily should be continued until 2 weeks after clinical cure is apparent. Topical nail preparations may contain rather than eliminate nail infections.

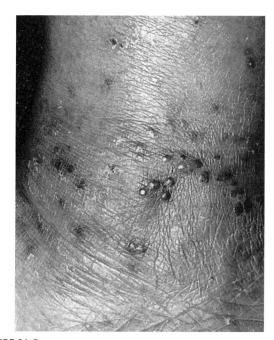

FIGURE 34–5

Dermatophyte infection shows grouped papules on the lower leg; biopsy and culture were needed to confirm the diagnosis.

Extensive, nodular and granulomatous infections all require systemic treatment. Nail infections respond only to systemic treatment. Immunosuppressed patients usually require double the conventional doses of systemic antifungal drugs, there are potential drug interactions and the long-term cure rates are unknown. Systemic treatment is offered for nail infections only when there are symptoms such as pain resulting from pressure of footwear on a grossly thickened toenail or fingernail infections causing pain through lifting of the nail or producing severe cosmetic handicap. Griseofulvin, 1 g daily, was the conventional treatment for dermatophyte infections but is ineffective for *Candida* infections. Prolonged courses are required—1 to 2 months for the skin, a minimum of 6 months for fingernail infections and 12 months or longer for toenails—and in the immunocompetent patient griseofulvin has been replaced by newer antifungal drugs. Terbinafine, 250–500 mg daily, is used, until clinical cure in skin infections and for a minimum of 3 months in nail infections. In contrast to the azole antifungals, terbinafine should not affect blood levels of cyclosporine. Itraconazole interacts with cyclosporine and is best avoided.

Cryptococcal Infections

Impaired cellular immunity predisposes to infection by *Cryptococcus neoformans*. Cutaneous involvement by *Cryptococcus* usually accompanies disseminated systemic infection, although in a series from India in which 2% of patients had the disease, only half had skin nodules (Chugh *et al.*, 1994). Primary cutaneous cryptococcosis occurs rarely and usually is the result of inoculation of the pathogen because of injury (Shuttleworth *et al.*, 1989). The skin lesions accompanying systemic cryptococcosis are described variously as papulonodular, acneiform and ulcerative and more rarely as an acute cellulitis resembling bacterial infection (Jennings *et al.*, 1981). Biopsy and aspiration of subcutaneously injected sterile saline provides material for histological examination and culture. The management of cryptococcosis is discussed in Chapter 31. In areas of the world where such organisms are endemic, *Histoplasma capsulatum* and other species also must be included in the differential diagnosis of acute cellulitis (Farr *et al.*, 1981). Other rare deep cutaneous mycoses encountered in renal transplant recipients include mycetomas (Kish *et al.*, 1983), chromoblastomycosis (Wackym *et al.*, 1985) and *Cladophialophora bantiana* (Jacyk *et al.*, 1997).

VIRAL INFECTIONS

Two groups of viruses affecting skin are important in renal transplant patients: the herpesviruses and the human papillomaviruses (HPV).

Herpesviruses

Immunosuppression can lead to reactivation of latent infection by various members of the herpesvirus group. Herpes simplex and varicella-zoster viruses produce severe infections in the immunocompromised host (see Chapter 31). Human herpesvirus type 8 is believed to be associated with Kaposi's sarcoma (see Chapter 35).

Herpes simplex may present with persistent small single or grouped erosions in renal transplant recipients and require systemic treatment with aciclovir or valaciclovir (dose adjusted for renal function). If minor topical acyclovir may suffice. Herpes zoster presents with blisters, which may be purpuric in a localized dermatomal distribution. The blisters usually but not invariably are preceded and accompanied by pain and itch. Treatment requires prompt systemic antiviral therapy, intravenous acyclovir, followed by oral valaciclovir for 2 weeks (dose adjusted for renal function).

Human herpesvirus type 8 is believed to be associated with Kaposi's sarcoma. Kaposi's sarcoma presents in the skin with purple plaques, which sometimes may resemble bruises, and nodules. This infection is commonest in the Mediterranean and Middle East (see Table 34–1). Kaposi's sarcoma is discussed in detail in Chapter 35.

Cytomegalovirus

Cytomegalovirus infection involving the skin is unusual, and no specific lesion exists. Plaques, nodules, vesicobullous lesions, cutaneous vasculitis, oral lesions and perineal ulceration have been described (Horn and Hood, 1990; Lescher, 1988; Minars et al., 1977).

Epstein-Barr Virus

Oral hairy leukoplakia, a persistent hypertrophic white plaque on the border of the tongue, is associated with opportunistic Epstein-Barr virus infection. Originally described in patients infected with human immunodeficiency virus (HIV), this lesion is no longer regarded as specific for HIV and appears to be associated with immunosuppression in general, including transplant recipients (Greenspan et al., 1989; Itin et al., 1988, 1991; Kanitakis et al., 1991).

Human Papillomaviruses

The heterogeneous group of HPV includes the causative organisms for common warts, plantar warts, flat warts and genital warts. Interest has been focused on HPV because of evidence pointing to the possible oncogenicity of certain types (discussed subsequently).

Epidemiology and Clinical Features

The prevalence of warts in renal transplant recipients varies in different series (see Table 34–1). In the early studies, 31 to 87% of renal transplant recipients were affected (Boyle et al., 1984; Gassenmaier et al., 1986; Rudlinger et al., 1986; Spencer and Anderson, 1970). In more recent studies, there is geographical variation, with the highest prevalence recorded in New Zealand (Hepburn et al., 1994). Warts were less common in children than adults (Barba et al., 1996; Menni et al., 1991).

The number of patients with warts and the number of warts per patient correlate with the duration of immunosuppression (Barba et al., 1996; Blohme and Larko, 1990; Chugh et al., 1994; Hepburn et al., 1994; Lugo-Janer et al., 1991b; Seckin et al., 1998). They also occur more commonly in transplant patients with a history of high sun exposure (Boyle et al., 1984; McLelland et al., 1988; Shuttleworth et al., 1987a), which accords with the high rates in New Zealand (Hepburn et al., 1994). In one series, warts were commoner in persons with a history of burning and failure to tan on sun exposure (McLelland et al., 1988). Sun exposure also plays a role in determining the distribution of warts, with sun-exposed areas having the highest numbers of warts (Barba et al., 1996; Chugh et al., 1994; Hepburn et al., 1994; Lugo-Janer et al., 1991b) and sun protection reducing the numbers (Barba et al., 1996). Although warts predominate on sun-exposed skin, they are not confined to these sites.

Warts are almost always multiple and sometimes very numerous (Barba et al., 1996; Blohme and Larko, 1990; Chugh et al., 1994; Hepburn et al., 1994; Lugo-Janer et al., 1991b; Menni et al., 1991; Seckin et al., 1998). Common warts are the most frequent clinical type and usually are multiple and may number many dozens of lesions (Fig. 34–6). Other clinical types observed in transplant recipients include flat warts, unusual wart lesions with a pityriasis versicolor–like appearance, plantar warts (Lutzner et al., 1981) and genital warts (Barba et al., 1996; Bunney et al., 1990; Rudlinger et al., 1986). In our experience, warts presenting on severely sun-damaged skin may be difficult to distinguish clinically from other keratotic lesions, including solar keratoses, keratoacanthomas and squamous cell carcinomas. All these lesions may coexist. Warts in transplant recipients show little tendency to remit and appear more resistant to treatment than usual.

Virology

There are more than 70 HPV types, some of which have been recognized only in immunosuppressed patients. In broad terms, HPV types 2 and 4 are found in common warts; types 1, 2 and 4 in plantar warts; types 3 and 10 in flat (plane) warts; types 5, 8 and others in epidermodysplasia verruciformis and types 6, 11, 16, 18 and others in genital warts. Human papillomavirus types 5, 8, 16, 18 and others are associated with squamous cell carcinomas. The number of HPV types identified is increasing rapidly, but the significance of many types is unclear.

Many HPV types have been identified within warts from renal transplant recipients. The commonest types are HPV 2, 3 and 4, with HPV types 1, 5, 6, 8, 10, 11, 16 and 18 occurring less frequently (Bunney et al., 1990; Euvrard et al., 1989; Gassenmaier et al., 1986; Hepburn et al., 1994; Lutzner et al., 1980; Pfister et al., 1979; Rudlinger et al., 1986, 1988; Van der Leest et al., 1987; Wilson et al., 1989). Unusual types, such as HPV type 49 (Favre et al., 1989) and a novel variant of HPV type 1 (Wilson et al., 1989), are reported. More than one HPV type can occur in a single patient (Hepburn et al., 1994; Van der Leest et al., 1987), and infections can occur at sites not normally associated with certain HPV types. For example, HPV types 1 and 4, usually associated with plantar warts, and HPV types 6, 11, 16 and 18, usually confined to mucosal lesions, all have been identified in skin warts from transplant recipients. The rare type, HPV 5, has been associated in transplant recipients with warts and with plaques of warts resembling those seen in patients with epidermodysplasia verruciformis (discussed later) (Hepburn et al., 1994; Lutzner et al., 1980). It appears that transplant recipients are susceptible to infections with diverse HPV types including rare types, that multiple infections are possible and that the site specificity of certain HPV types differs from the normal population.

There is good reason to consider certain types of HPV infection potentially oncogenic (discussed subsequently), but

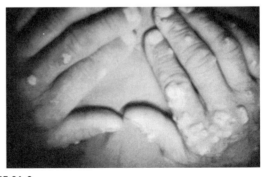

FIGURE 34–6

Extensive common warts on the hands of a renal transplant recipient (see color plate).

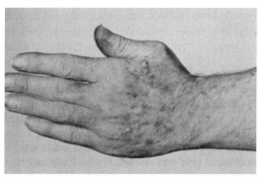

FIGURE 34–7

"Transplant hand": Sun-damaged skin on the hand of a renal transplant recipient shows solar keratosis (see color plate).

the presence of viral warts does not correlate directly with the presence of skin cancers (Barba *et al.*, 1996; Hepburn *et al.*, 1994), and warts are common in renal transplant recipient populations in which skin cancers are rare (Barba *et al.*, 1996; Chugh *et al.*, 1994; Lugo-Janer *et al.*, 1991b; Seckin *et al.*, 1998).

Management

In many transplant patients, the lesions are typical clinically and present no problem with diagnosis. On severely sun-damaged skin, however, multiple keratotic lesions including warts, solar keratoses, keratoacanthomas and squamous cell carcinomas (Fig. 34–7) may coexist and be difficult to distinguish clinically from one another. In such doubtful cases, biopsy may be helpful, although some lesions appear to be mixed histologically, with dysplasia coexisting with viral changes in a single lesion (Blessing *et al.*, 1989). In view of the suggestion that warts may be a risk factor for the development of squamous cell carcinoma, Boyle and coworkers argued that efforts should be made to eradicate the lesions, particularly those on sun-exposed skin (Boyle *et al.*, 1984). There is little evidence so far that treating the lesions eradicates virus from the skin, and treatment should be directed primarily at dealing with symptomatic lesions.

Treating the warts rarely results in cure. Painting the warts with keratolytic paints or gels (e.g., 16% salicylic acid) daily and paring with a blade may provide cosmetic improvement because they are flatter and less noticeable. Cryosurgery using liquid nitrogen occasionally is effective, but recurrence is common; repeated treatments usually are required. Although surgical intervention for warts normally is limited to curettage, in renal transplant patients there is a case for formal excision for any diagnostically doubtful lesions to ensure an adequate specimen for histological evaluation.

PARASITIC INFESTATIONS

Scabies is the commonest infestation affecting 3% of Turkish and 12% of Indian patients (Seckin *et al.*, 1998; Vijaykumar *et al.*, 1998), although it is reported rarely. Scabies may present the typical clinical picture of intense generalized pruritus with burrows and other lesions that characteristically favor the hands, feet and genitals but spare the head and neck. There may be papular lesions. The intense itching sometimes can be masked in patients taking prednisolone, however, and the clinical picture may be atypical in other respects. The distribution of lesions can be unusual, with face and scalp involvement (Venning and Millard, 1992) or a flexural predilection (Anolik and Rudolph, 1976), and exceptionally heavy

mite infections are possible, producing widespread scaling mimicking chronic eczema (Norwegian or crusted scabies) (Dymock, 1979; Wolf *et al.*, 1985). The epidermal scales harbor numerous mites, seen readily on light microscopy; such patients are highly infectious and in a hospital setting they may become the focus of a local epidemic. More than one application of a scabicide (e.g., permethrin 5%) to the whole body including the head is likely to be required to achieve cure. All contacts must be treated simultaneously to prevent reinfection.

Inflammatory Diseases

The expression of preexisting or new inflammatory diseases may be influenced by immunosuppression in renal transplant recipients.

SEBORRHEIC DERMATITIS

Seborrheic dermatitis (seborrheic eczema) is a well-recognized manifestation of immunosuppression in HIV infection and is associated with *pityrosporum ovale* infection and occurs in renal transplant recipients, with a reported incidence of 4 to 14% (Barba *et al.*, 1996; Lugo-Janer *et al.*, 1991b). Seborrheic dermatitis presents with pruritus and scaling. It may affect the face, particularly the eyebrows and nasolabial folds, the ears and scalp. Involvement of the groin, other body folds and genitals can be troublesome and complicated by secondary infection with *S. aureus*. Treatment is with topical steroids in combination with antiyeast preparations, for example, hydrocortisone and clotrimazole or miconazole for the face and these or more potent steroids for other regions (e.g., clobetasone and tetracycline and nystatin, betamethasone and clotrimazole or fucidin if there is bacterial infection).

PSORIASIS

Preexisting psoriasis often ceases to be a problem after transplantation because of the initial major immunosuppression and later presumably because of the use of cyclosporine, a recognized (second line) treatment for psoriasis. If psoriasis is persistent and does not respond to simple topical measures, increasing the dose of cyclosporine should be considered. Phototherapy must be used with great caution because of the photocarcinogenesis, which is particularly marked if psoralens and ultraviolet A (PUVA) therapy is used.

ECZEMAS

Endogenous eczemas, such as atopic eczema, lichen simplex, pompholyx eczema and discoid eczema, seem to be rare in renal transplant recipients, presumably because of immunosuppression, but some cases are reported (Lugo-Janer *et al.*, 1991b). Similarly the exogenous eczema, contact dermatitis, is rare.

URTICARIA AND TYPE I ALLERGY

Preexisting idiopathic urticaria and angioedema often are less troublesome during periods of high immunosuppression, but as the doses are lowered, these conditions may require treatment. Cetirizine is the antihistamine of choice in renal transplant recipients because this has the least potential for interaction with cyclosporine. Type I allergy to foods (e.g., nuts, fruits, shellfish) persists, and the need for availability of emergency adrenaline is not abolished by immunosuppression.

PYODERMA GANGRENOSUM

Haim and colleagues reported a case of protracted penile ulceration compatible with pyoderma gangrenosum (Haim *et al.*, 1973). The ulcers remitted after rejection of the renal transplant and withdrawal of immunosuppressive drugs.

Noninflammatory Changes

TELANGIECTASIA AND POIKILODERMA OF CIVATTE

Marked telangiectasias are seen in some renal transplant recipients and are partially due to systemic steroids (see earlier) and in some cases to nifedipine (Tsele and Chu, 1992; Fig. 34–8). It may be that the two drugs are synergistic. Some women have marked photo-induced changes with telangiectasia on the side of the neck with sparing of the V under the chin; this change is known as *poikiloderma of Civatte* and has been reported from New Zealand in almost 10% of patients (Hepburn *et al.*, 1994). Treatment is difficult, but laser therapy may be helpful.

SEBORRHEIC WARTS

Seborrheic warts (seborrheic keratoses) are seen commonly in the normal population, have been reported in renal transplant recipients and are observed commonly in our clinic (Hepburn *et al.*, 1994; Seckin *et al.*, 1998). It is unclear whether these are commoner in renal transplant recipients. Their importance lies in their frequent confusion with dysplastic lesions. They vary in color from skin colored to deep brown or black. They are raised plaques with an irregular warty surface and may have a greasy appearance. These warts are always multiple and vary in size from a few millimeters to a few centimeters. They are removed easily by curettage, which also allows histological confirmation of the diagnosis, or they may be treated with cryosurgery.

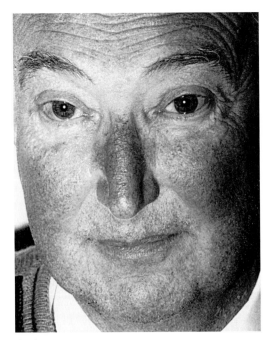

FIGURE 34–8

Extensive telangiectasia in a transplant recipient who had taken nifedipine for many years.

ACANTHOSIS NIGRICANS

Koranda and coworkers reported that 20 of 200 renal transplant recipients had acanthosis nigricans (Koranda *et al.*, 1974). Only two patients were obese, and none had concurrent evidence of internal malignancy. There has been a subsequent report from Puerto Rico of a single patient with acanthosis nigricans (Lugo-Janer *et al.*, 1991b).

NAIL CHANGES

Nail disorders of many kinds are common (Barba *et al.*, 1996; Seckin *et al.*, 1998). Transverse white banding of the fingernails has been described in two renal transplant recipients (Held *et al.*, 1989; Linder, 1978), in both cases in association with acute rejection. This description differs from the pallor of the nails in uremia or hypoalbuminemia, which is due to alteration of nail-bed collar (pseudoleukonychia) rather than the nail plate itself (true leukonychia) (Held *et al.*, 1989). Nail brittleness and splitting (onychoschizia) has been described in childhood renal transplant recipients (Menni *et al.*, 1991).

Premalignant and Malignant Skin Conditions

In the long-term after kidney transplantation, skin cancers represent the commonest malignancy in patients of European descent (Bouwes Bavinck *et al.*, 1996; Disney *et al.*, 1997; Gaya *et al.*, 1995; London *et al.*, 1995; Penn, 1994a; see Table 34–1 and Chapter 35). The first report of an increased risk of skin cancer in transplant patients was published by Walder *et al.* in 1971. These authors described the occurrence of multiple skin cancers in 14% of a group of Australian patients who received a kidney transplant 4 to 45 months previously and who were treated with azathioprine and prednisolone, none of whom had had skin cancer before transplantation. The clinical features described in the article summarize well the main characteristics of skin cancers developing in this group of patients: reversal of the squamous cell carcinoma/basal cell carcinoma ratio reported in the general population, tendency for the lesions to be multiple, increased age at transplantation of the patients who subsequently developed skin cancer, presence of atypical *recurrent keratoacanthomas* and increased prevalence of keratoses on sun-exposed sites with rapid evolution of some of them into squamous cell carcinomas (Walder *et al.*, 1971).

Multiple reports have been published from transplant centers across the world that investigated the incidence and/or prevalence and clinical features of skin cancers in renal transplant recipients. Comparisons between results published from different centers have to take into account differences in the study design. A summary of published data is presented in Table 34–2. The cumulative incidence rises with the time after transplantation yet varies with the level of sun exposure. In the area of Queensland in Australia, a country situated at approximately 20° latitude in the Southern Hemisphere, the cumulative incidence of basal cell carcinoma and/or squamous cell carcinoma rose from 7% at 1 year to 45% at 11 years and 70% at 20 years after transplantation (Bouwes Bavinck *et al.*, 1996). Comparatively the cumulative incidence for basal cell carcinoma and/or squamous cell carcinoma in the Netherlands, a country situated at approximately 50° latitude North, was 0.2%, 16% and 41% at the same time points (Hartevelt *et al.*, 1990).

The premalignant and malignant skin conditions that have been reported to occur most frequently in transplant recipients include solar keratosis, keratoacanthoma, Bowen's disease, basal cell carcinoma, squamous cell carcinoma, malig-

TABLE 34–2

STUDIES ON THE INCIDENCE AND PREVALENCE OF SKIN CANCER IN RENAL TRANSPLANT RECIPIENTS

Authors	Center	No. Patients	Length of Immuno-suppression*	Prevalence/Incidence	Relative Risk†	Mean (SD) Time to Presentation	Tumors Recorded; Comments
Europe							
Shuttleworth et al., 1987a	Cardiff, UK	85	2–20 y	25%	NA	12.5 y (5.25 y)	SK, Bowen's, SCC, BCC
McLelland et al., 1988	London, UK	121	5.9 y (5.2 y)	9.9%	NA	5.9 y (5.2 y)	SK, Bowen's, SCC, BCC, MM
Brown et al., 1988	Belfast, N. Ireland	223	6.6 y [2–21 y]	5.8% / 0.45%/y	NA	NA	SCC, BCC, KA; SCC/BCC = 3.5/1
Liddington et al., 1989	Oxford, UK	598	0–13 y	5%	NA	7.05 y [3.6–11 y]	Bowen's, SCC, BCC, KA, MM
Hartevelt et al., 1990	Leiden, Netherlands	764	8.7 y [1–21 y]	3,500/100,000† / 6.15% / 3.3 BCC/1,000 patient-years / 7.6 SCC/1,000 patient-years	253 (SCC) / 10 (BCC)	9.1 y	SCC, BCC
Blohme and Larko, 1990	Göteborg, Sweden	98	10–23 y	37%	3.5	NA	SK, Bowen's, SCC, BCC, sweat gland carcinoma, malignant histiocytoma
Vogt et al., 1990	Hanover, Germany	598	3.48 y [1 mo–5.6 y]	1 case of SCC lip	NA	NA	SCC
Glover et al., 1994	London, UK	219	4.78 y [3 mo–21.6 y]	21.9%	NA	4.78 y [3 mo–21.6 y]	Bowen's, SCC, BCC
Thiel et al., 1994	Basel, Switzerland	350	10 y	17% (cyclosporine group) / 15% (azathioprine group)	NA	NA	SCC, BCC, MM, sarcoma
London et al., 1995	Leeds, UK	918	NA	6% at 10 y / 30% at 20 y	162 (SCC)	7.75 y [2 mo–19.75 y]	SCC, BCC
Gaya et al., 1995	London, UK	274	2,622 patient-years	6.9%	19.4	9.5 y	SCC, BCC, MM
Alamartine and Bertoux, 1995	St. Etienne, France	560	NA	3.3%	NA	4.3 y (2.9 y)	SCC, BCC
Benalia et al., 1995	Paris, France	915	NA	3.5%	NA	NA	NA
Ferrandiz et al., 1995	Barcelona, Spain	81	1–4 y	14.8%	NA	1.4 y [6 mo–3 y]	SK, SCC, BCC
America							
Cohen et al., 1987	Wisconsin, US	580	12.5 y	4.5%	NA	6.5 y [9 mo–15.8 y]	Bowen's, SCC, BCC, MM, Kaposi's sarcoma
Gupta et al., 1986	Ontario, Canada	523	NA	7.5%	3.2	7.2 y [2–15.1 y]	SCC, BCC, MM, Kaposi's sarcoma. SCC/BCC = 2.3/1
Venkateswara and Andersen, 1988	Minnesota, US	57	1.06 y (0.18)	10.5%	NA	NA	SCC, BCC
Lugo-Janer et al., 1991	Puerto Rico	82	2.9 y [0.08–13.8]	12%	NA	6.1 y	SK, SCC, MM (no cases of BCC observed)
Barrett et al., 1993	Ohio, US	876	3.5 y	5.36%	NA	7 y	SCC, BCC, MM, Kaposi's sarcoma, Merkel's cell tumor
Australia							
Sheil et al., 1993	ANZDATA	6,596	NA	20%	NA	NA	SCC, BCC, MM
Hepburn et al., 1994	Christchurch, New Zealand	52	9.6 y (5.9)	19.2%	NA	9.6 y (5.9 y)	SCC, BCC, MM
Bouwes Bavinck et al., 1996	Queensland, Australia	1,098	8.8 y (5.2)	7% at 1 y / 45% at 11 y / 70% at 20 y	NA	4.6 y (4.3 y)	SCC, BCC, MM; SCC/BCC = 1.5/1
Others							
Suzuki et al., 1994	Japan	374	3,391 patient-years	1.06%	NA	NA	NA

*Mean (standard deviation) or interval (in brackets) of exposure to immunosuppression.
†Overall relative risk for the skin cancers analyzed, unless particular type specified.
SK = solar keratosis; SCC = squamous cell carcinoma; BCC = basal cell carcinoma; MM = malignant melanoma; KA = keratoacanthoma; NA = data not available.

nant melanoma and Kaposi's sarcoma. Cases of angiosarcoma, Merkel's cell carcinoma (Gooptu et al., 1997; Penn, 1994a), sebaceous carcinoma (Blohme and Larko, 1990; Penn, 1994a) and a pure cutaneous plasma cell tumor also have been reported (Whittam et al., 1996). Of these, squamous cell carcinoma was the commonest in long-term retrospective studies (Liddington et al., 1989; London et al., 1995; Sheil et al., 1992) and was the most frequently presenting tumor (Bordea et al., 1998). In a prospective study of a Hispanic transplant population, basal cell carcinoma occurred more often than squamous cell carcinoma for the first 3 years after transplantation (Ferrandiz et al., 1995).

The squamous cell carcinoma/basal cell carcinoma ratio reverses compared with the general population, from 1/4 to 1.5/1 in Australia (Bouwes Bavinck et al., 1996) and from 1/8 to 3.6/1 in the Netherlands (Hartevelt et al., 1990). The reversal is less pronounced in Australia and New Zealand than in Europe (see Table 34–2). The latent period between transplantation and presentation with skin cancer varies from a few months to more than 20 years (see Table 34–2). With a few exceptions, it appears that the mean latent period is shorter in areas with high levels of sun exposure.

Renal transplant patients present with skin cancers approximately 20 to 30 years earlier than their nonimmunosuppressed counterparts. In the nonimmunosuppressed population in the United Kingdom, the mean age at presentation is 70 years for basal cell carcinoma and 73 years for squamous cell carcinoma (Ko et al., 1994). In our transplant population, the mean age at presentation with skin cancer was 56 years (Bordea et al., 1998). Similar results have been reported from the United States (Cohen et al., 1987). Calculating the relative risk (i.e., how many times the incidence of skin cancer is increased in the study population in comparison to the general population) was possible only in a few centers that provided control population data. The relative risk of developing skin cancer after transplantation ranged from 3.5 in Sweden (Blohme and Larko, 1990) to 20 in Australia (Hardie et al., 1980). The increased risk of skin cancer in transplant recipients is due almost entirely to the increased occurrence of squamous cell carcinoma. The risk of squamous cell carcinoma after transplantation ranged from 18.4-fold in Canada (Gupta et al., 1986) to 253-fold in the Netherlands (Hartevelt et al., 1990). The risk of skin cancer is higher in men than in women (Bouwes Bavinck et al., 1996; Gaya et al., 1995). It is not clear whether the increased risk in men is due to differences in the levels of sun exposure or whether other factors might be involved; one study that specifically investigated the history of sun exposure in male and female transplant patients found similar levels of exposure in the two groups. The relative risk of basal cell carcinoma was not increased in transplant patients (Gupta et al., 1986; Hardie, 1995; Kinlen et al., 1979) except for a Dutch study that found a relative risk of 10 (Hartevelt et al., 1990). The incidence of malignant melanoma also is increased in transplant patients, although at lower levels than squamous cell carcinoma (4.4-fold in Australia [Sheil and Disney, 1991] and 8.3-fold in the United Kingdom [Kinlen et al., 1979]).

Most skin cancers occur on sun-exposed areas, pointing to the effect of ultraviolet (UV) exposure in the pathogenesis (Hartevelt et al., 1990; Liddington et al., 1989). An increased frequency of squamous cell carcinoma was noticed in low-risk areas in renal transplant patients, however (Liddington et al., 1989). Squamous cell carcinomas are located preferentially on the face and dorsum of hands, whereas basal cell carcinomas develop frequently on the face and trunk but never are diagnosed on the back of hands (Hartevelt et al., 1990). A rare site for squamous cell carcinoma development is the eye (Gaya et al., 1995; Touzeau et al., 1999).

Many patients have multiple tumors at the time of diagnosis. Over time, in our experience, almost two thirds of the patients developed more than one skin cancer, and in this group one patient had 50 skin tumors removed with lesions occurring as frequently as once a month. Cases have been reported of patients with more than 100 cancers each (Penn, 1994a). Hyperkeratoses develop frequently on sun-exposed sites, some of which undergo malignant change, and in some patients multiple squamous cell carcinomas develop in the hyperkeratotic areas (Marshall, 1974; Walder et al., 1971). The dorsum of the hands and forearms sometimes take on a characteristic appearance described as *transplant hand*; this presents as a "dry and somewhat scaly skin with increasing numbers of either verrucae planae or actinic keratoses, or both" (Blohme and Larko, 1990; see Fig. 34–7). The changes on the dorsum of the hands can be so severe as to require complete resurfacing with skin graft harvested from a non–sun-exposed site.

The clinical course of squamous cell carcinoma is more aggressive in transplant patients, multiple lesions developing in the same patient and having an increased tendency to recur and metastasize (Sheil et al., 1993). Of the 3,087 transplant patients with cancer reported from around the world to the Cincinnati Tumor Transplant Registry (CTTR), 179 (5.8%) developed lymph node metastases (Penn, 1994a). Of these, 75% were from squamous cell carcinomas; 17%, from melanomas; 7%, from Merkel's cell tumors and 1%, from basal cell carcinomas. Of the patients, 5% died of their skin cancers, with 61% of deaths caused by squamous cell carcinomas; 34%, melanomas; 4%, Merkel's cell tumors and 1% (one patient), basal cell carcinoma (Penn, 1994a). Most cases of aggressive squamous cell carcinoma occurred in Australia (Sheil et al., 1993).

In pediatric (<18 years old) renal transplant recipients, skin and lip skin cancers represented only 19% of the posttransplant malignancies. Almost 20% of these presented in childhood, and of these, half were malignant melanomas (Penn, 1994b).

Premalignant Skin Tumors

SOLAR KERATOSIS

Solar keratoses present as localized areas of adherent hyperkeratosis on sun-exposed skin and are associated histologically with dysplastic changes in the basal epidermis, together with evidence of solar damage. The reported incidence of solar keratosis after transplantation in the United Kingdom varied from 7.4% (Boyle et al., 1984) to 22.3% (Shuttleworth et al., 1987a). In a New Zealand renal transplant population, with an average 9.5 years of continuous immunosuppression, the prevalence of solar keratoses was 42.3% (Hepburn et al., 1994).

The lesions may appear 2 to 6 months after transplantation. In nonimmunosuppressed patients, the malignant potential of solar keratoses is regarded as low, although a slow-growing squamous cell carcinoma may develop after a prolonged latency. In transplant recipients, keratoses tend to be multiple, tend to recur after conservative treatment and may evolve rapidly into squamous cell carcinoma (Walder et al., 1971). Efforts should be made to treat as many solar keratoses as possible by cryosurgery, topical 5% 5-fluorouracil cream (see under Management), curettage or cautery. Topical and systemic retinoids are discussed subsequently. Patients should be advised about sun protection and should be examined regularly for recurrences and/or malignant change.

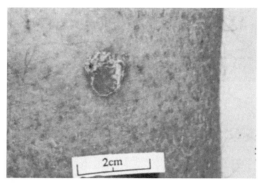

FIGURE 34–9

Typical annular lesion of porokeratosis showing the distinctive keratotic edge and slightly atrophic center (see color plate).

BOWEN'S DISEASE

Typically presenting as a persistent scaly erythematous plaque on exposed or covered skin, Bowen's disease represents true carcinoma *in situ* and has malignant potential. Bowen's disease occurs in transplant recipients, although the frequency is not well documented. McLelland *et al.* (1988) reported a prevalence of 5.8%. In our series, the prevalence reached 9% (Bordea *et al.*, 1998). In our experience, the lesions may be atypical clinically and present as banal keratotic lesions for which the differential diagnosis must include solar keratosis, keratoacanthoma, warts and squamous cell carcinoma. Bowen's disease can be treated by twice-weekly or three-times-weekly applications of topical 5% 5-fluorouracil cream, excision, cryosurgery or curettage. The choice of the method of treatment depends on the size and number of lesions, anatomical site and patient's health status.

POROKERATOSIS

Porokeratosis is an unusual condition that is characterized by annular lesions with a distinctive raised keratotic edge (Fig. 34–9). The variant repeatedly described in transplant patients (Bencini *et al.*, 1986a) and in other immunosuppressed patients (Lederman *et al.*, 1986) consists of multiple small (1–2 cm) lesions distributed widely on the limbs (disseminated superficial actinic porokeratosis). Reactivation of previously quiescent porokeratosis of Mibelli (another variant of the condition) also has been described in a transplant recipient (MacMillan and Roberts, 1975). The cause of porokeratosis is unknown, but it has been proposed that the keratotic edge arises from proliferation of an abnormal clone of epidermal cells; UV exposure and acquired immunosuppression may be important factors in permitting such clonal proliferation. Rarely, porokeratosis of Mibelli has transformed into a squamous cell carcinoma, although this complication never has been described in a renal transplant recipient. Treatment is unsatisfactory; emollients, mild keratolytics and cryosurgery all have been tried.

Malignant Skin Tumors
KERATOACANTHOMA

Common in the nonimmunosuppressed population, keratoacanthoma presents as a firm, rapidly growing, dome-shaped tumor of 1 to 2.5 cm in diameter with a central keratin-filled crater (Fig. 34–10). They occur mainly on sun-exposed areas but can develop on any hairy cutaneous site.

Although keratoacanthomas are normally self-limiting and regress spontaneously, any rapidly growing skin lesion occurring in a transplant patient is an indication for surgical excision. It is difficult to know what is the prevalence of true keratoacanthomas in renal transplant recipients because some squamous cell carcinomas may have been misdiagnosed as keratoacanthoma. The recommended treatment is excision with histological examination.

SQUAMOUS CELL CARCINOMA

In renal transplant recipients, squamous cell carcinoma usually presents as a rapidly growing, raised, keratotic lesion with or without central ulceration, often sore and with an indurated base (Fig. 34–11; see also Fig. 35–3). If a central ulcer is present, the border does not always resemble the classic description. Some patients may present with multiple lesions within the same area (Fig. 34–12). Squamous cell carcinoma is a true, invasive carcinoma of the surface epidermis, which can spread to the lymph nodes and in some cases cause death. The recommended treatment is surgical excision to ensure histological clearance of the tumor. After surgery, patients need to be followed up for local recurrence and lymph node metastases.

BASAL CELL CARCINOMA

Basal cell carcinoma is a relatively slowly developing tumor with a tendency toward local invasion and tissue destruction, although the metastatic potential is extremely low. Five types of basal cell carcinoma can occur: noduloulcerative (Fig. 34–13), pigmented, morphealike or fibrosing, superficial and fibroepithelioma. In contrast to squamous cell carcinoma, the clinical appearance of basal cell carcinoma in transplant patients is similar to that in nonimmunosuppressed patients. The treatment of choice is surgery. Curettage and cryotherapy are alternative options.

MALIGNANT MELANOMA

Four clinicopathological variants of malignant melanoma are described: superficial spreading melanoma, nodular mel-

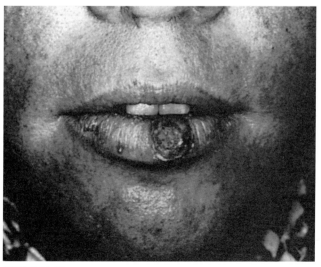

FIGURE 34–10

A keratoacanthoma on the lip of a young man 5 years after renal transplantation. The lesion had first appeared 6 weeks previously, rapidly reaching the appearance shown.

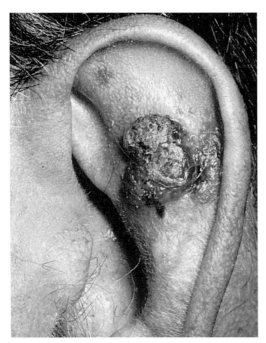

FIGURE 34–11

Squamous cell carcinoma on the ear.

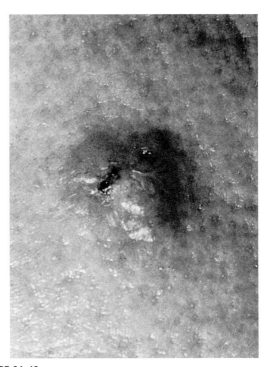

FIGURE 34–13

Nodular basal cell carcinoma with some early ulceration on the face.

anoma, lentigo maligna melanoma and acral lentiginous or palmoplantar melanoma. With the exception of amelanotic melanoma lesions, all variants present as a changing pigmented lesion, which is not typical of other benign nevi found on the patient's skin. Changes can affect size, shape and color. There can be signs of inflammation, oozing or

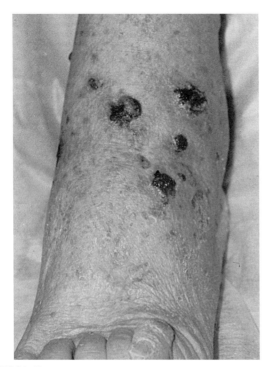

FIGURE 34–12

Multiple squamous cell carcinomas on the leg of a woman with signs of lymphedema.

bleeding, itch or altered sensation. Particular attention must be paid to examining pigmented lesions in transplant patients to detect any early changes. Any suspicious lesion must be excised and examined histologically.

Risk Factors and Pathogenesis

Ultraviolet exposure, immunosuppressive drug treatment, genetic factors and possibly virus infection with HPV are thought to contribute to the pathogenesis of skin cancers in renal transplant recipients.

Ultraviolet Exposure

In immunocompetent and immunosuppressed patients, most skin cancers develop on sun-exposed areas. The incidence of skin cancer is highest in white patients living in tropical and subtropical climates. Epidemiological studies show a relationship between skin cancer and sun exposure. Nonmelanoma skin cancers are related to cumulative exposure, whereas melanomas (with the exception of lentigo malignant melanoma) appear to be related to exposure in childhood or intermittent high-dose exposure (Young and Walker, 1995).

It is believed that UV acts by initiating a cascade of events in the skin, starting with absorption by a chromophore or chromophores locally and ending in immunomodulation. Among the first changes, membrane damage, induction of cytoplasmic transcription factors, DNA damage and isomerization of urocanic acid (Fabo and Noonan, 1983; Fabo et al., 1983) appear to play an important part. Ultraviolet radiation can reduce the number of Langerhans' cells and impair their ability to stimulate proliferative T-cell responses in vitro (Baadsgaard et al., 1989). It is possible that antigens encountered through UV-exposed skin are presented differently, or not at all, from those encountered through normal skin. It is reasonable to speculate that these defects might contribute further to the breakdown of immunosurveillance already impaired by immunosuppressive drugs and enhance the development of premalignant and malignant lesions.

Immunosuppressive Drugs

Azathioprine increases the speed of UV-induced skin cancer development in animal models (Kelly *et al.*, 1987). Other effects of azathioprine include chromosome breaks (Jensen, 1967) and inhibition of repair of UV-induced damage (Kelly *et al.*, 1986). The development of tumors in immunosuppressed patients who have not been treated with azathioprine suggests that chemical carcinogenesis is not the only factor involved, however.

Systemic administration of cyclosporine in immunosuppressive doses in animal models of chemically induced carcinogenesis had no effect on tumor incidence and latency but caused more malignant squamous cell carcinomas than in animals subjected to carcinogen treatment only (Berger, 1991). In models of UV-induced carcinogenesis, however, systemic administration of cyclosporine or azathioprine increased the incidence and reduced the mean tumor latency period (Berger, 1991). *In vitro* studies have shown that cyclosporine has the ability to inhibit antigen-processing and accessory functions of epidermal Langerhans' cells (Dupuy *et al.*, 1991; Furue and Katz, 1988). Some investigators have found a decrease in the number of Langerhans' cells in the skin of transplant recipients (Bergfelt, 1993; Petzelbauer and Wolff, 1992; Servitje *et al.*, 1991; Sontheimer *et al.*, 1984), detectable 3 days after starting the treatment (Gabel *et al.*, 1987). Topical as well as systemic corticosteroids are known to deplete epidermal Langerhans' cells (Ashworth *et al.*, 1988; Belsito *et al.*, 1982; Berman *et al.*, 1983) and impair their antigen-presenting capacity (Aberer *et al.*, 1984; Ashworth *et al.*, 1988; Belsito *et al.*, 1982).

There has been much discussion about the risk associated with different immunosuppressive regimens. Disney and co-workers found that skin cancer occurred significantly more frequently in patients treated with both cyclosporine and azathioprine than with either of this drugs alone (Disney *et al.*, 1997). In the group of patients treated with cyclosporine only, the incidence was slightly higher for the first 6 years after transplantation, after which it reached levels similar to the group treated with azathioprine alone. In a randomized comparison of two cyclosporine regimens, patients who received the low-dose cyclosporine had significantly fewer warts and premalignant and malignant skin lesions but had more rejection episodes (Dantal *et al.*, 1998).

Human Papillomavirus

Human papillomavirus long has been recognized as the causative agent of common warts and condyloma acuminatum. Human papillomavirus is a small, nonenveloped DNA virus of the Papovaviridae family (Shah and Howley, 1996). The first evidence that HPV infection is associated with squamous cell carcinoma of the skin was found in patients with the rare, genetically determined condition epidermodysplasia verruciformis. Epidermodysplasia verruciformis is characterized by the development of numerous flat wartlike lesions, which in 30 to 50% of patients progress to squamous cell carcinomas 20 to 30 years later. A specific group of closely related HPV types, the epidermodysplasia verruciformis group, especially HPV 5 and HPV 8, have been isolated from greater than 90% of squamous cell carcinomas from these patients (Orth, 1987). A role for HPV analogous to that of epidermodysplasia verruciformis–related skin cancer seems plausible. After transplantation, there is an increase in viral

skin infections (see Table 34–1), and the tumors with the highest incidence are those thought to arise from oncogenic viruses. Clinically, squamous dysplasia and squamous cell carcinoma develop in close proximity and are usually preceded by viral wart lesions (Hartevelt *et al.*, 1990). In some patients, the skin changes resemble those of patients with epidermodysplasia verruciformis. Histologically, viral warts and keratotic skin lesions often display varying degrees of epidermal dysplasia, and some squamous cell carcinomas retain HPV-associated features on microscopic examination (Benton *et al.*, 1992). Lutzner *et al.* (1983) identified HPV 5 from *in situ* and invasive squamous cell carcinomas and viral warts on sun-exposed skin of a renal transplant recipient. Other groups have later confirmed the finding and reported the presence of other HPV types. With the use of polymerase chain reaction techniques and combinations of primers, it is possible to detect HPV DNA in 91% of squamous cell carcinomas (de Villiers *et al.*, 1997). Five viral types (HPV 20, HPV 23, HPV 38, DL40 and DL267) were detected in 73% of the nonmelanoma skin cancers tested and often were found in combination with other HPV types within the same lesion (de Villiers *et al.*, 1997). A high prevalence of HPV DNA in renal transplant–associated basal cell carcinoma (65%) and squamous cell carcinoma (83%) has been reported by other investigators (Surentheran *et al.*, 1998). In addition to epidermodysplasia verruciformis HPV types, which were predominant, mucosal types have been detected (Surentheran *et al.*, 1998). With regard to mechanisms of viral-induced oncogenesis, the cutaneous types of HPV appear to have different transformation strategies when compared with the mucosal (genital) types of HPV. In particular, HPV 8 E6 gene appears not to form complexes with p53, and HPV 8 E7 does not bind to the cellular retinoblastoma protein (Pfister, 1992). At this stage, the molecular mechanisms of HPV-induced carcinogenesis are not established.

Management

Potential renal transplant recipients in populations *at risk* must be informed about the risk of skin problems and in particular skin cancers before they decide to undergo organ transplantation. Efforts must be made to reduce sun exposure, and patients need to be educated about the dangers of UV exposure so that they understand the rationale and avoid further damage. To be of maximum benefit, sun protection measures should start as early as possible (as soon as the patients are accepted for transplantation). Advice should be centered on sun avoidance: appropriate clothing (wide-brimmed hats, long-sleeved shirts, long trousers), avoidance of sunbathing and when feasible a change of outdoor activities so that midday sun is avoided. Sun-barrier creams providing broad-spectrum protection against UVA and UVB are appropriate, but they should not be regarded as a substitute for sun avoidance (Venning, 1988). The principal effect of sun-barrier creams is to diminish the inflammatory response, and there is a risk that patients may feel encouraged to spend longer periods than otherwise exposed to the sun. Additional preventive measures include reduction of immunosuppression to a minimum compatible with good graft function and regular review of the skin during the lifetime of their transplant by an experienced clinician.

Reference has been made to the treatment of individual premalignant or malignant skin lesions. The clinical appearance of skin cancers in renal transplant patients does not always resemble that in immunocompetent patients. Nonsurgical methods can be considered for premalignant lesions and nonspecific keratoses if a clinical diagnosis can be made confidently. If in doubt, biopsy or surgical excision with histological examination is preferred. This approach provides histological diagnosis, assessment of aggressiveness and confirmation of the adequacy of excision. Some patients with multiple lesions, especially on the dorsum of hands, may require excision of a larger area and reconstruction of the defect with a skin graft harvested from a non–sun-exposed site. Patients who have had squamous cell carcinomas removed need to be checked for lymph node metastases. In our experience, metastatic spread is uncommon and has occurred only with skin cancers that are known to have a high risk of metastatic spread in immunocompetent patients (e.g., sebaceous carcinoma, Merkel's cell tumor, malignant melanoma and squamous cell carcinoma of the lip and ear).

A proportion of renal transplant patients progressively develop widespread and numerous warty skin lesions that include viral warts, solar keratoses, keratoacanthoma, Bowen's disease and frankly malignant lesions. Such patients present a difficult management problem and may benefit from medical treatment-prophylaxis.

Retinoids

Topical Retinoic Acid

Several studies have shown the efficacy of all *trans*-retinoic acid (tretinoin [Retin-A] cream) in the treatment of solar keratoses (Barranco *et al.*, 1970; Robinson and Kligman, 1975). Topical tretinoin with low-dose etretinate (10 mg/d), administered to renal transplant patients with frequently occurring dysplastic skin lesions halved the rate of development of new squamous cell carcinomas. The clinical effect was associated with an increase in the number of Langerhans' cells (Rook *et al.*, 1995). In contrast, there is no evidence that topical retinoic acid has any benefit in prevention of occurrence or recurrence of solar keratoses (Purcell *et al.*, 1986). Topical 0.025% tretinoin gel in combination with topical interferon-β produced complete regression of flat warts in 62% of patients (Schreiner *et al.*, 1995).

Systemic Retinoids

Medical prophylaxis together with treatment of established skin lesions is a useful alternative to surgery in some patients, although this approach still is being evaluated. Synthetic analogues of vitamin A, the retinoids isotretinoin (13-*cis*-retinoic acid) and etretinate, are known to suppress epithelial dysplasia and neoplasms in nontransplant patients (Kraemer *et al.*, 1988; Moriarty *et al.*, 1982). Oral etretinate, 1 mg/kg/d, cleared established warty and dysplastic lesions and partially suppressed the development of new lesions when used over a 6-month period (Shuttleworth *et al.*, 1988). Kelly and associates reported similar results using etretinate, 50 mg/d, in four transplant recipients over a 12-month period (Kelly *et al.*, 1991). Low-dose etretinate (0.3 mg/kg/d) over 3 to 26 months produced a significant reduction in the number of skin cancers during the first 6 months of treatment and a trend toward a longer term reduction at 18 months of treatment (Gibson *et al.*, 1998). Mucocutaneous side effects were well tolerated, and no abnormalities of renal function, liver function, hematological parameters or significant changes in cyclosporine were observed. Etretinate has now been replaced by its metabolite acitretin.

Acitretin (Neotigason) is a second-generation monoaromatic retinoid and is the main acid derivative and active metabolite of etretinate. Short-term treatment with acitretin, 0.5 mg/kg/d, reduced temporarily the development of new squamous cell carcinomas (Vandeghinste *et al.*, 1992) and the number of keratotic skin lesions (Bouwes Bavinck *et al.*, 1995),

but these recurred after discontinuation of treatment. Long-term prophylactic treatment with acitretin, 0.3 mg/kg/d, reduced significantly the development of new nonmelanoma skin cancers in renal transplant patients during the period of treatment, with well-tolerated side effects (McKenna and Murphy, 1999).

Low-dose isotretinoin (0.2–0.4 mg/kg) in combination with calcitriol (0.5–1 μg/d) produced at least a 60% decrease in the number of lesions in 8 of 11 patients with multiple actinic keratoses transforming into early malignancies, with mild side effects (Skopinska *et al.*, 1997). There are no published reports of the use of isotretinoin in transplant recipients. In contrast to etretinate, isotretinoin does not increase natural killer cell numbers (Anolik *et al.*, 1998; McKerrow *et al.*, 1988), and this has been proposed as a theoretical advantage in terms of safety to the graft. In our experience in Oxford, both drugs suppressed neoplasms in small numbers of patients. Possible mechanisms by which retinoids may reduce the development of skin cancer include inhibition of tumor initiation and promotion, induction of normal cell differentiation and immunomodulation (Holliday *et al.*, 1992). Neither etretinate (Shuttleworth *et al.*, 1988) nor isotretinoin (Marcussen and Tyden, 1988; Tam and Cooper, 1987) appears to affect kidney graft function or survival.

Side effects are usual and sometimes troublesome. Drying of the mucous membranes leading to desquamation causes sore, cracked lips in most patients. Skin dryness, pruritus and hair changes are observed less frequently. Reversible biochemical changes including hyperlipidemia, chiefly affecting triglyceride levels, and disturbances of liver enzymes are relatively common and require monitoring. Bones and joints are affected in a few patients, causing myalgia, arthralgia and reduced exercise tolerance. More serious is the risk of skeletal hyperostosis, and radiographs of any symptomatic sites are indicated. All retinoids are highly teratogenic, and in view of the long half-life, acitretin is contraindicated in female patients who may wish to conceive in the next few years. Active contraception is mandatory (for duration, see manufacturers' recommendations), and pregnancy should be excluded before starting treatment.

The antineoplastic effects of retinoids are reversible, and on cessation of treatment new lesions develop. One possible concern has been that the rate of tumor development may be accelerated in the immediate posttreatment period (Kelly *et al.*, 1991; Kraemer *et al.*, 1988), although experience at the Oxford Transplant Centre has not provided convincing evidence of a rebound phenomenon when retinoids are withdrawn. Because of their side effects, retinoids are best reserved for patients with multiple warty dysplastic lesions and malignancies requiring repeated surgical treatment.

REFERENCES

Aberer, W., Stingl, L., Pogantsch, S., *et al.* (1984). Effect of glucocorticosteroids on epidermal cell-induced immune responses. *J. Immunol.* **133**, 792.

Adams, S. J., Davison, A. M., Cunliffe, W. J. and Giles, G. R. (1982). Perioral dermatitis in renal transplant recipients maintained on corticosteroids and immunosuppressive therapy. *Br. J. Dermatol.* **106**, 589.

Alamartine, E. and Bertoux, F. (1995). Tumours in kidney-transplanted patients: a comprehensive one-centre study. *Transplant. Proc.* **27**(2), 1761.

Amiransari, B., Khallili, M., Anssarin, H., Bassiri, A. and Simforoosh, N. (1995). Cutaneous manifestations in renal transplant patients. *Transplant. Proc.* **27**, 2743.

Anolik, J. H., DiGiovanna, J. J. and Gaspari, A. A. (1998). Effect of isotretinoin on natural killer cell activity in patients with xeroderma pigmentosum. *Br. J. Dermatol.* **138**, 236.

Anolik, M. A. and Rudolph, R. I. (1976). Scabies simulating Darier's disease in an immunosuppressed host. *Arch. Dermatol.* **112**, 73.

Ashworth, J., Booker, J. and Breathnach, S. M. (1988). Effects of topical corticosteroid therapy on Langerhans cell antigen presenting function in human skin. *Br. J. Dermatol.* **118**, 457.

Baadsgaard, O., Lisby, S., Wantzin, S., et al. (1989). Rapid recovery of Langerhans cells alloreactivity, without induction of autoreactivity, after in vivo ultraviolet A, but not ultraviolet B exposure of human skin. *J. Immunol.* **142**, 4213.

Barba, A., Tessari, G., Boschiero, L. and Chieregato, G. C. (1996). Renal transplantation and skin diseases: review of the literature and results of a 5-year follow-up of 285 patients. *Nephron* **73**, 131.

Barker, J. N. and MacDonald, J. P. (1988). Eruptive dysplastic naevi following renal transplantation. *Clin. Exp. Dermatol.* **13**, 123.

Barranco, V. P., Olson, R. I. and Everett, M. A. (1970). Response of actinic keratoses to topical vitamin A acid. *Cutis* **6**, 681.

Barrett, W. L., First, M. R., Aron, B. S., et al. (1993). Clinical course of malignancies in renal transplant recipients. *Cancer* **72**, 2186.

Belsito, D. V., Flotte, T. J., Lim, H. W., et al. (1982). Effect of glucocorticoids on epidermal Langerhans cells. *J. Exp. Med.* **155**, 291.

Benalia, H., Mouguet, C., Luciani, J., et al. (1995). Incidence of cutaneous tumours in kidney transplant patients: a 20 year follow up. *Transplant. Proc.* **27**(2), 1769.

Bencini, P. L., Crosti, C., Montagnino, G. and Sala, F. (1986a). Porokeratosis and immunosuppression. *J. Am. Acad. Dermatol.* **14**, 682.

Bencini, P. L., Montagnino, G., Crosti, C., Sala, F. and De Vecchi, A. (1986b). Acne in a renal transplant patient treated with cyclosporin A. *Br. J. Dermatol.* **114**, 396.

Bencini, P. L., Montagnino, G., De Vecchio, A., et al. (1983). Cutaneous lesions in renal transplant recipients. *Nephron* **34**, 79.

Bencini, P. L., Montagnino, G., Sala, F., De Vecchi, A., Crosti, C. and Tarantino, A. (1986c). Cutaneous lesions in 67 cyclosporin-treated renal transplant recipients. *Dermatologica* **172**, 24.

Benton, E. C., Shahidullah, H. and Hunter, J. A. (1992). Human papillomavirus in the immunosuppressed. *Papillomavirus Rep.* **3**, 23.

Berger, M. R. (1991). Animal models of cancer caused by immunosuppression. *In Cancer in Organ Transplant Recipients*, (D. Schmahl and I. Penn, eds.), p. 3, Springer-Verlag, Berlin.

Bergfelt, L. (1993). Langerhans cells, immunomodulation and skin lesions: a quantitative, morphological and clinical study. *Acta Derm. Venereol. Suppl. (Stockh.)* **180(Suppl.)**, 1.

Bergfield, W. F. and Roenigk, H. H. (1978). Cutaneous complications of immunosuppressive therapy: review of 215 renal transplant patients. *Cutis* **22**, 169.

Berman, B., France, D. S., Martinelli, G. P., et al. (1983). Modulation of expression of epidermal Langerhans cell properties following in situ exposure to glucocorticosteroids. *J. Invest. Dermatol.* **80**, 168.

Blessing, K., McLaren, K. M., Benton, E. C., et al. (1989). Histopathology of skin lesions in renal allograft recipients—an assessment of viral features and dysplasia. *Histopathology* **14**, 129.

Blohme, I. and Larko, O. (1984). Premalignant and malignant skin lesions in renal transplant patients. *Transplantation* **37**, 165.

Blohme, I. and Larko, O. (1990). Skin lesions in renal transplant patients after 10–23 years of Immunosuppressive therapy. *Acta Derm. Venereol. (Stockh.)* **70**, 491.

Bordea, C., Wojnarowska, F. T., Redburn, J. and Morris, P. J. (2000). Skin cancer in renal transplant patients: a 21-year retrospective analysis (D. Phil. thesis, Oxford University, submitted).

Bouwes Bavinck, J. N., Hardie, D. R., Green, A., et al. (1996). The risk of skin cancer in transplant patients in Queensland, Australia. *Transplantation* **61**, 715.

Bouwes Bavinck, J. N., Tieben, L. M., Woude, F. K. V. D., et al. (1995). Prevention of skin cancer and reduction of keratotic skin lesions during acitretin therapy in renal transplant recipients: a double-blind, placebo-controlled study. *J. Clin. Oncol.* **18**, 1933.

Boyle, J., Mackie, R. M., Briggs, J. D. and Junor, B. J. R. (1984). Cancer, warts and sunshine in renal transplant patients. *Lancet* **70**, 702.

Brown, J. H., Hutchinson, T., Kelly, A. M. T., et al. (1988). Dermatologic lesions in a transplant population. *Transplantation* **46**, 530.

Bunney, M. H., Benton, E. H., Barr, B. B., Smith, I. W., Anderton, J. L. and Hunter, J. A. (1990). The prevalence of skin disorders in renal allograft recipients receiving cyclosporin A compared with those receiving azathioprine. *Nephrol. Dial. Transplant.* **5**, 379.

Canafax, D. M. and Ascher, N. L. (1983). Cyclosporin immunosuppression. *Clin. Pharmacol.* **2**, 515.

Chugh, K. S., Sharma, S. C., Singh, V., Sahuja, V. and Gupta, K. L. (1994). Spectrum of dermatological lesions renal allograft recipients in a tropical environment. *Dermatology* **188**, 108.

Cohen, E. B., Komorowski, R. A. and Clowry, L. C. (1987). Cutaneous complications in renal transplant recipients. *Am. J. Clin. Pathol.* **88**, 32.

Daley, T. D., Wysocki, G. P. and Day, C. (1986). Clinical and pharmacological correlation in cyclosporin induced gingival hyperplasia. *Oral Surg. Oral Med. Oral Pathol.* **62**, 417.

Dantal, J., Hourmant, M., Cantarovich, D., et al. (1998). Effects of long-term immunosuppression in kidney-graft recipients on cancer incidence: randomised comparison of two cyclosporine regimens. *Lancet* **351**, 623.

de Lacharriere, O., Escoffier, C., Gracia, A.-M., et al. (1990). Reversal effects of topical retinoic acid on the skin of kidney transplant recipients under systemic corticotherapy. *J. Invest. Dermatol.* **95**, 516.

de Villiers, E.-M., Lavergne, D., McLaren, K. and Benton, E. C. (1997). Prevailing papillomavirus types in non-melanoma carcinomas of the skin in renal allograft recipients. *Int. J. Cancer* **73**, 356.

Disney, A. P. S., Russ, G. R., Walker, R. and Sheil, A. G. R. (1997). *ANZDATA Registry Report 1997*, Australia and New Zealand Transplant Registry, Adelaide, South Australia.

Dupuy, P., Bagot, M., Michel, L., et al. (1991). Cyclosporine A inhibits the antigen-presenting functions of freshly isolated human Langerhans cells in vitro. *J. Invest. Dermatol.* **96**, 408.

Dymock, R. B. (1979). Skin diseases associated with renal transplantation. *Aust. J. Dermatol.* **20**, 61.

Ebling, F. J. G. and Cunliffe, W. J. (1992). *In Textbook of Dermatology*, 5th ed., (R. H. Champion, J. L. Burton and F. J. G. Ebling, eds.), p. 1736, Blackwell Scientific Publications, Oxford.

European Mycophenolate Mofetil Cooperative Study Group. (1995). Placebo controlled study of mycophenolate mofetil combined with cyclosporin and corticosteroids for prevention of acute rejection. *Lancet* **345**, 1321.

Euvrard, S., Chardonnet, Y., Hermier, C., Viac, J. and Thivolet, J. (1989). Verrues et carcinomes épidermoides après transplantation rénale. *Ann. Dermatol. Venereol.* **116**, 201.

Fabo, E. C. D. and Noonan, F. P. (1983). Mechanism of immune suppression by ultraviolet radiation in vivo: I. evidence for the existence of a unique photoreceptor in skin and its role in photoimmunology. *J. Exp. Med.* **157**, 84.

Fabo, E. C. D., Noonan, F. P., Fisher, M., et al. (1983). Further evidence that the photoreceptor mediating UV-induced systemic immune suppression is urocanic acid. *J. Invest. Dermatol.* **80**, 319.

Farr, B., Beacham, B. E. and Atuk, N. O. (1981). Cutaneous histoplasmosis after renal transplantation. *South. Med. J.* **74**, 635.

Favre, M., Obalek, S., Jablonska, S. and Orth, G. (1989). Human papillomavirus Type 49, a type isolated from flat warts of renal transplant patients. *J. Virol.* **63**, 4909.

Ferrandiz, C., Fuente, M. J., Ribera, M., et al. (1995). Epidermal dysplasia and neoplasia in kidney transplant recipients. *J. Am. Acad. Dermatol.* **33**, 590.

Floersheim, G. L. and Bollag, W. (1972). Accelerated rejection of skin allografts by vitamin A acid. *Transplantation* **15**, 564.

Furue, M. and Katz, S. (1988). The effect of cyclosporine on epidermal cells: I. cyclosporine inhibits accessory cell functions of epidermal Langerhans cells in vitro. *J. Immunol.* **140**, 4139.

Gabel, H., Jontell, M., Ohman, C. and Brynger, H. (1987). Epidermal Langerhans cells in the early phase of immunosuppression. *Transplant. Proc.* **19(1 Pt. 2)**, 1205.

Gassenmaier, A., Fuchs, P., Schell, H. and Pfister, H. (1986). Papillomavirus DNA in warts of immunosuppressed renal allograft recipients. *Arch. Dermatol. Res.* **278**, 219.

Gaya, S. B. M., Rees, A.J., Lechler, R. I., et al. (1995). Malignant disease in patients with long-term renal transplants. *Transplantation* **59**, 1705.

Gibson, G. E., O'Grady, A., Kay, E. W. and Murphy, G. M. (1998). Low-dose retinoid therapy for chemoprophylaxis of skin cancer in renal transplant recipient. *J. Eur. Acad. Dermatol. Venereol.* **10**, 42.

Gissmann, L. and Schwarz, E. (1985). *In Papilloma Viruses, Ciba Foundation Symposium No. 120*, (D. Evered and S. Clarke, eds.), p. 191, Pitman, London.

Glover, M. T., Niranjan, N., Kwan, J. T. C., et al. (1994). Non-melanoma skin cancer in renal transplant recipients: the extent of the problem and a strategy for management. *Br. J. Plast. Surg.* **47**, 86.

Gombert, M. E., Goldstein, E. J. C., Corrado, M. L., Stein, A. J. and Butt, K. M. H. (1981). Disseminated *Mycobacterium marinum* infection after renal transplantation. *Ann. Intern. Med.* **94**, 486.

Gooptu, C., Woollons, A., Ross, J., et al. (1997). Merkel cell carcinoma arising after therapeutic immunouppression. *Br. J. Dermatol.* **137**, 637.

Greenspan, D., Greenspan, J. S., de Souza, Y. G., Levy, J. A. and Ungar, A. M. (1989). Oral hairy leukoplakia in an HIV-negative renal transplant recipient. *J. Oral Pathol. Med.* **18**, 32.

Gupta, A. K., Cardella, C. J. and Haberman, H. F. (1986). Cutaneous malignant neoplasms in patients with renal transplants. *Arch. Dermatol.* **122**, 1288.

Haim, S., Friedman-Birnbaum, R., Better, O. S. and Tuma, S. (1973). Skin complications in immunosuppressed patients: follow up of kidney recipients. *Br. J. Dermatol.* **89**, 169.

Hardie, I. R. (1995). Skin cancer in transplant recipients. *Transplant. Rev.* **9**, 1.

Hardie, I. R., Strong, R. W., Hartley, L. C. J., et al. (1980). Skin cancer in caucasian renal allograft recipients living in a subtropical climate. *Surgery* **87**, 177.

Hartevelt, M. M., Bouwes Bavinck, J. N., Kootte, A. M. M., et al. (1990). Incidence of skin cancer after transplantation in The Netherlands. *Transplantation* **49**, 506.

Held, J. L., Chew, S., Grossman, M. E. and Kohn, S. R. (1989). Transverse striate leukonychia associated with acute rejection of renal allograft. *J. Am. Acad. Dermatol.* **20**, 513.

Hepburn, D. J., Dakshinamurthy, D., Bailey, R. R. and Macdonald, K. J. S. (1994). Cutaneous manifestations of renal transplantation in a New Zealand poulation. *N. Z. Med. J.* **107**, 497.

Holliday, M., Ho, K. K. and Barnetson, R. S. C. (1992). Regulation of the skin immune system by retinoids during carcinogenesis. *J. Invest. Dermatol.* **99(Suppl.)**, 83S.

Horn, T. D. and Hood, A. F. (1990). Cytomegalovirus is predictably present in perineal ulcers from immunosuppressed patients. *Arch. Dermatol.* **126**, 642.

Itin, P., Rufli, T., Huser, B. and Rudlinger, R. (1991). Oral hairy leukoplakia in renal transplant recipients. *Hautarzt* **42**, 487.

Itin, P., Rufli, T., Rudlinger, R., et al. (1988). Oral hairy leukoplakia in an HIV-negative renal transplant recipient: a marker for immunosuppression. *Dermatologica* **177**, 126.

Jacyk, W. R., Du Bruyn, J. H., Holm, N., Gryffenberg, H. and Karusseit, V. O. (1997). Cutaneous infection due to *Cladophialophora bantiana* in a patient receiving immunosuppressive therapy. *Br. J. Dermatol.* **136**, 428.

Jennings, H. S., Bradsher, R. W., McGee, Z. A., Johnson, H. K. and Alford, R. H. (1981). Acute cryptococcal cellulitis in renal transplant recipients. *South. Med. J.* **74**, 1150.

Jensen, M. K. (1967). Chromosome studies in patients treated with azathioprine and amethopterin. *Acta Med. Scand.* **182**, 445.

Kanitakis, J., Euvrard, S., Lefrancois, N., et al. (1991). Oral hairy leukoplakia in an HIV-negative renal transplant recipient. *Br. J. Dermatol.* **124**, 483.

Kelly, G. E., Meikle, W. and Sheil, A. G. R. (1987). Effects of immunosuppressive therapy on the induction of skin tumours by ultraviolet irradiation in hairless mice. *Transplantation* **44**, 429.

Kelly, G. E., Sheil, A. G. R., Wass, J., et al. (1986). Effects of ultraviolet irradiation and immunosuppressive therapy on mouse epidermal cell kinetics. *Br. J. Dermatol.* **114**, 196.

Kelly, J. W., Sabto, J., Gurr, F. W. and Bruce, F. (1991). Retinoids to prevent skin cancer in renal transplant recipients. *Lancet* **338**, 1407.

Kinlen, L. J., Sheil, A. G. R., Peto, J. and Doll, R. (1979). Collaborative United Kingdom–Australasian study of cancer in patients treated with immunosuppressive drugs. *B. M. J.* **2**, 1461.

Kish, L. S., Taylor, J. S., Bergfield, W. F. and Hall, G. S. (1983). *Petriellidium (Allescheria) boydii* mycetoma in an immunosuppressed host. *Cleve. Clin. Q.* **50**, 209.

Ko, C. B., Walton, S., Keczkes, K., et al. (1994). The emerging epidemic of skin cancer. *Br. J. Dermatol.* **130**, 269.

Koranda, F. C., Dehmel, E. M., Kahn, G. and Penn, I. (1974). Cutaneous complications in immunosuppressed renal homograft recipients. *J. A. M. A.* **229**, 419.

Kraemer, K. H., Di Giovanna, J. J., Maoshell, A. N., Tarone, R. E. and Peck, G. L. (1988). Prevention of skin cancer in xeroderma pigmentosum with isotretinoin. *N. Engl. J. Med.* **318**, 1633.

Kripke, M. L. and Morison, W. L. (1985). Modulation of immune function by UV radiation. *J. Invest. Dermatol.* **85**, 62s.

Lederman, J. S., Sober, A. J. and Lederman, G. S. (1986). Porokeratosis and immunosuppression *J. Am. Acad. Dermatol.* **14**, 683.

Lescher, J. L. (1988). Cytomegalovirus infections and the skin. *J. Am. Acad. Dermatol.* **18**, 1333.

Liddington, M., Richardson, A. J., Higgins, R. M., et al. (1989). Skin cancer in renal transplant recipients. *Br. J. Surg.* **76**, 1002.

Linder, M. (1978). Striped nails after kidney transplant. *Ann. Intern. Med.* **88**, 809.

Lindholm, A., Pousette, A., Carlstrom, K. and Klintmalm, G. (1988). Cyclosporin-associated hypertrichosis is not related to sex hormone levels following renal transplantation. *Nephron* **50**, 199.

London, N. J., Farmery, S. M., Will, E. J., et al. (1995). Risk of neoplasia in renal transplant patients. *Lancet* **346**, 403.

Lugo-Janer, G., Pedraza, R., Morales Otero, L. A., et al. (1991a). Superficial mycoses in renal transplant recipients *Transplant. Proc.* **23**, 1787.

Lugo-Janer, G., Sanchez, J. L. and Santiago-Delpin, E. (1991b). Prevalence and clinical spectrum of skin diseases in kidney transplant recipients. *J. Am. Acad. Dermatol.* **24**, 410.

Lutzner, M., Croissant, O., Ducasse, M.-F., Kreis, H., Crosnier, J. and Orth, G. (1980). A potentially oncogenic human papillomavirus (HPV 5) found in two renal allograft recipients. *J. Invest. Dermatol.* **75**, 353.

Lutzner, M. A. (1983). The human papillomaviruses. *Arch. Dermatol.* **119**, 631.

Lutzner, M. A., Croissant, O., Ducasse, M. F., Kreis, H., Crosnier, J. and Orth, G. (1981). An unusual wart-like skin lesion found in a renal allograft recipient. *Arch. Dermatol.* **117**, 43.

Lutzner, M. A., Orth, G., Dutronquay, V., Ducasse, M.-F., Kreis, H. and Crosnier, J. (1983). Detection of human papillomavirus type-5 DNA in skin cancers of an immunosuppressed renal allograft recipient. *Lancet* **2**, 422.

MacMillan, A. L. and Roberts, S. O. B. (1975). Porokeratosis of Mibelli after renal transplantation. *Br. J. Dermatol.* **90**, 45.

Marcussen, J. A. and Tyden, G. (1988). Acne conglobata in transplant patients treated with isotretinoin. *Br. J. Dermatol.* **118**, 310.

Marshall, V. (1974). Premalignant and malignant skin tumors in immunosuppressed patients. *Transplantation* **17**, 272.

Mathew, T. H., for the Tricontinental Mycophenolate Mofetil Renal Transplantation Study Group. (1998). A blinded long-term randomized multicentre study of mycophenolate mofetil in cadaveric renal transplantation. *Transplantation* **65**, 1450.

McKenna, D. B. and Murphy, G. M. (1999). Skin cancer chemoprophylaxis in renal transplant recipients: 5 years of experience using low-dose acitretin. *Br. J. Dermatol.* **140**, 656.

McKerrow, K. J., Mackie, R. M., Lesko, M. J. and Pearson, C. (1988). The effect of oral retinoid on the normal immune system. *Br. J. Dermatol.* **119**, 313.

McLelland, J., Rees, A., Williamsom, G. and Chu, T. (1988). The incidence of immunosuppression related skin disease in long term transplant patients. *Transplantation* **46**, 871.

Menni, D., Beretta, D., Piccinno, R. and Ghio, L. (1991). Cutaneous and oral lesions in 32 children after renal transplantation. *Pediatr. Dermatol.* **8**, 194.

Minars, N., Silverman, J. F., Escobar, M. and Martinez, J. (1977). Fatal cytomegalic inclusion disease: associated skin manifestations in a renal transplant recipient. *Arch. Dermatol.* **113**, 1569.

Moriarty, M., Dunn, J., Darragh, A., Lambe, R. and Brick, I. (1982). Etretinate in the treatment of actinic keratosis. *Lancet* **1**, 364.

Mortimer, P. S., Thompson, J. F., Dawber, R. P. R., Ryan, T. J. and Morris, P. J. (1983). Hypertrichosis and multiple cutaneous squamous cell carcinomas in association with cyclosporin A therapy. *J. Roy. Soc. Med.* **76**, 786.

Neiderberger, W., Lemaire, M., Maurer, G., Nussbaumer, K. and Wagner, O. (1984). Distribution and binding of cyclosporin in blood and tissues. *In Cyclosporin*, (B. D. Kanan, ed.), p. 203, Grune & Stratton, Orlando.

Noble, W. C., Rebel, M. H. and Smith, I. (1974). An investigation of the skin flora of dialysis and transplant patients. *Br. J. Dermatol.* **91**, 201.

Orth, G. (1987). The papillomaviruses. *In The Papovaviridae*, Vol. 2, (N. P. Salzman and P. M. Howley, eds.), p. 199, Plenum Press, New York.

Ost, L. (1984). Effects of cyclosporin on prednisolone metabolism. *Lancet* **1**, 451.

Penn, I. (1994a). Occurrence of cancers in immunosuppressed organ transplant recipients. *In Clinical Transplants*, (T. A. Cecka, ed.), p. 99, UCLA Tissue Typing Laboratory, Los Angeles.

Penn, I. (1994b). Posttransplant malignancies in pediatric organ transplant recipients. *Transplant. Proc.* **26**, 2763.

Petzelbauer, P. and Wolff, K. (1992). Effects of cyclosporine A on resident and passenger immune cells of normal human skin and UV-induced erythema reactions. *Br. J. Dermatol.* **127**, 560.

Pfister, H. (1992). Human papillomaviruses and skin cancer. *Semin. Cancer Biol.* **3**, 263.

Pfister, H., Gross, G. and Hagedorn, M. (1979). Characterization of human papilloma virus 3 in warts of a renal allograft patient. *J. Invest. Dermatol.* **73**, 349.

Phillips, M. E. and Ackerman, A. B. (1982). "Benign" and "malignant" neoplasms associated with verrucae vulgares. *Am. J. Dermatopathol.* **4**, 61.

Proby, C. M., Murdoch, M. E. and Leigh, I. M. (1991). Persistent cutaneous *Mycobacterium chelonei* infection. *Br. J. Dermatol.* **125**, 52.

Purcell, S. M., Pierce, D. K., Dixon, S. L., et al. (1986). Chemoprevention of actinic keratoses with topical all trans retinoic acid. *J. Invest. Dermatol.* **86**, 501.

Robinson, T. A. and Kligman, A. M. (1975). Treatment of solar keratoses of the extremities with retinoic acid and 5-fluorouracil. *Br. J. Dermatol.* **92**, 703.

Rook, A. H., Jaworsky, C., Nguyen, Y., et al. (1995). Beneficial effect of low-dose systemic retinoid in combination with topical tretinoin for the treatment and prophylaxis of premalignant and malignant skin lesions in renal transplant recipients. *Transplantation* **59**, 714.

Rudlinger, R., Bunney, M. H., Smith, I. W. and Hunter, J. A. A. (1988). Detection of human papilloma virus type 5 DNA in a renal allograft patient in Scotland. *Dermatologica* **177**, 280.

Rudlinger, R., Smith, I. W., Bunney, M. H. and Hunter, J. A. A. (1986). Human papillomavirus infections in a group of renal transplant recipients. *Br. J. Dermatol.* **115**, 681.

Schreiner, T., Broska, J. and Fierlbeck, G. (1995). Topical application of tretinoin, interferon beta and their combination in the treatment of warts. *J. Dermatol. Treat.* **6**, 17.

Seckin, D., Oguz Gulec, T., Demirag, A. and Bilgin, N. (1998). Renal transplantation and skin disease. *Transplant. Proc.* **30**, 802.

Sequeira, M., Burdick, A. E., Elgart, G. W. and Berman, B. (1998). New-onset Majocchi's granuloma in two kidney transplant recipients under tacrolimus treatment. *J. Am. Acad. Dermatol.* **38**, 486.

Servitje, O., Seron, D., Ferrer, I., et al. (1991). Quantitative and morphometric analysis of Langerhans cells in non-exposed skin in renal transplant patients. *J. Cutan. Pathol.* **18**, 106.

Shah, K. V. and Howley, P. M. (1996). Papillomaviruses. *In Fields' Virology*, (B. N. Fields, D. M. Knipe, P. M. Howley, et al., eds.), p. 2077, Lippincott-Raven, Philadelphia.

Sheil, A. G. R., Disney, A. P., Mathew, T. H., et al. (1993). De novo malignancy emerges as a major cause of morbidity and late failure in renal transplantation. *Transplant. Proc.* **25**(1 Pt. 2), 1383.

Sheil, A. G. R., Disney, A. P. S., Mathew, T. H., et al. (1992). Malignancy following renal transplantation. *Transplant. Proc.* **24**, 1946.

Sheil, A. G. R. and Disney, A. P. S. D. (1991). *ANZDATA 14th Report*, Australia and New Zealand Transplant Registry, Adelaide, South Australia.

Shuttleworth, D., Marks, R., Griffin, P. J. A. and Salaman, J. R. (1987a). Dysplastic epidermal change in immunosuppressed patients with renal transplants. *Q. J. M.* **64**, 609.

Shuttleworth, D., Marks, R., Griffin, P. J. A. and Salaman, J. R. (1988). Treatment of cutaneous neoplasia with etretinate in renal transplant recipients. *Q. J. M.* **68**, 717.

Shuttleworth, D., Philpot, C. M. and Knight, A. G. (1989). Cutaneous cryptococcosis: treatment with oral fluconazole. *Br. J. Dermatol.* **120**, 683.

Shuttleworth, D., Philpot, C. M. and Salaman, J. R. (1987b). Cutaneous fungal infection following renal transplantation: a case control study. *Br. J. Dermatol.* **117**, 585.

Simmons, W. D., Rayhill, S. C. and Sollinger, H. W. (1997). Preliminary risk-benefit assessment of mycophenolate mofetil in transplant rejection. *Drug Saf.* **17**, 75.

Singer, A. and Campion, M. J. (1985). Human papillomavirus. *Br. J. Hosp. Med.* **32**, 104.

Skopinska, M., Majewski, S., Bollag, W. and Jablonska, S. (1997). Calcitriol and isotretinoin combined therapy for precancerous and cancerous skin lesions. *J. Dermatol. Treat.* **8**, 5.

Slavin, J. and Taylor, J. (1987). Cyclosporin, nifedipine and gingival hyperplasia. *Lancet* **2**, 739.

Sollinger, H. W., for the U.S. Renal Transplant Mycophenolate Mofetil Study Group. (1995). Mycophenolate mofetil for the prevention of acute rejection in primary cadaveric renal allograft recipients. *Transplantation* **60**, 225

Sontheimer, R. D., Bergstresser, P. R., Gailiunas, P., et al. (1984). Perturbation of Langerhans cells in immunosuppressed human renal allograft recipients. *Transplantation* **37**, 168.

Spencer, C. M., Goa, K. L. and Gillis, J. C. (1997). Tacrolimus: an update of its pharmacology and clinical efficacy in the management of organ transplantation. *Drugs* **54**, 925.

Spencer, E. S. and Anderson, H. K. (1970). Clinically evident, nonterminal infection with herpes viruses and the wart virus in immunosuppressed renal allograft recipients. *B. M. J.* **3**, 251.

Surentheran, T., Harwood, C. A., Spink, P. J., et al. (1998). Detection of HPV DNA in non-melanoma skin cancer from immunocompetent and immunosuppressed individuals. *In Human Papillomaviruses in Dermatology: Satellite Symposium of the International Investigative Dermatology Meeting*, p. 7, Vaals, Netherlands.

Suzuki, S., Tanaka, K., Ohsaka, Y., et al. (1994). Development of de novo malignancies following renal transplantation: a single centre study. *Transplant. Proc.* **26**(2), 938.

Tam, M. and Cooper, A. (1987). The use of isotretinoin in a renal transplant with acne. *Br. J. Dermatol.* **116**, 463.

The Tricontinental Mycophenolate Mofetil Renal Transplantation Study Group. (1996). A blinded randomized clinical trial of mycophenolate mofetil for the prevention of acute rejection in cadaveric renal transplantation. *Transplantation* **61**, 1029.

Thiel, G., Bock, A., Spondlin, M., et al. (1994). Long-term benefits and risks of cyclosporine A (Sandimmune—an analysis at 10 years). *Transplant. Proc.* **26**(5), 2493.

Touzeau, O., Borderie, V. M. and Lacroche, L. (1999). Carcinoma of the corneoscleral limbus in a patient treated with cyclosporine after heart transplantation. *N. Engl. J. Med.* **341**, 374.

Tsele, E. and Chu, A. C. (1992). Nifedipine and telangiectasias. *Lancet* **339**, 365.

Tyldesley, W. R. and Rotter, E. (1984). Gingival hyperplasia induced by cyclosporin A. *Br. Dent. J.* **157**, 305.

Vandeghinste, N., Bersaque, J. D., Geerts, M. L. and Kint, A. (1992). Acitretin as cancer chemoprophylaxis in a renal transplant recipient. *Dermatology* **185**, 307.

Van der Leest, R. J., Zachiw, K. R., Ostraw, R. S., Bender, M., Pass, F. and Faras, A. J. (1987). Human papillomavirus heterogeneity in 36 renal transplant recipients. *Arch. Dermatol.* **123**, 354.

Venkateswara, R. K. and Andersen, R. C. (1988). Long-term results and complications in renal transplant recipients. *Transplantation* **45**, 45.

Venning, V. (1988). Renal transplantation and the skin. *Lancet* **1**, 294.

Venning, V. A. and Millard, P. M. (1992). Recurrent scabies with unusual clinical features in a renal transplant recipient. *Br. J. Dermatol.* **126**, 204.

Vijaykumar, R., Fernando, E., Rajendran, S., Jayakumar, M. and Muthusethupathi, M. A. (1998). Dermatological manifestations in renal transplant recipients. *Transplant. Proc.* **30**, 3136.

Vogt, P., Frei, U., Repp H., et al. (1990). Malignant tumours in renal transplant recipients receiving cyclosporine: survey of 598 first-kidney transplantations. *Nephrol. Dial. Transplant.* **5**, 282.

Wackym, P. A., Gray, G. F., Richie, R. E. and Gregg, C. R. (1985). Cutaneous chromomycosis in renal transplant recipients. *Arch. Intern. Med.* **145**, 1036.

Walder, B. K., Robertson, M. R. and Jeremy, D. (1971). Skin cancer and immunosuppression. *Lancet* **2**, 1282.

Whittam, L. R., Coleman, R. and MacDonald, D. M. (1996). Plasma cell tumour in a renal transplant recipient. *Clin. Exp. Dermatol.* **21**, 367.

Wilson, C. A. B., Holmes, S. C., Campo, M. S., et al. (1989). Novel variants of human papillomavirus type 2 in warts from immunocompromised individuals. *Br. J. Dermatol.* **121**, 571.

Wolf, R., Wolf, D., Viskoper, R. J. and Sandbank, M. (1985). Norwegian type scabies mimicking contact dermatitis. *Postgrad. Med.* **78**, 228.

Young, A. R. and Walker, S. L. (1995). Photoprotection from UVR-induced immunosuppression. *In Photoimmunology*, (J. Krutmann and C. A. Elmets, eds.), p. 285, Blackwell Scientific Publications, Oxford.

Cancer in Dialysis and Transplant Patients

A. G. R. Sheil

Introduction

The concept that cancer arises in aberrant cells that normally are eliminated by the immune system was proposed by Thomas (1959) and elaborated by Burnet (1967). A good deal of laboratory evidence in animals supported this concept, but information in humans was scanty until the widespread use of immunosuppressive drugs for transplantation and other purposes. The first indication that immunosuppressed transplant recipients were susceptible to cancer came with the transplantation of apparently normal kidneys removed from donors dying with cancer. It was soon recognized that such organs could harbor malignant cells that could proliferate in the recipient, causing death (Martin *et al.*, 1965; McPhaul *et al.*, 1965). A few years later, the first reports of cancer arising *de novo* in transplant recipients appeared (Doak *et al.*, 1968; Penn *et al.*, 1969). Later the suggestion came that patients on dialysis programs, many awaiting transplantation, are at heightened risk of cancer development (Matas *et al.*, 1975). This chapter discusses cancer in dialysis patients and organ transplant recipients as well as the management of patients with past or present cancer who may need transplantation.

Cancer in Dialysis Patients

Cancers affecting renal function are commoner in patients on dialysis than in the general population. In some patients, cancers such as multiple myeloma are the direct cause of renal failure. In others, renal failure results when attempted cure of renal or ureteric malignancies involves removal of all functioning renal tissue. In other cases, patients have conditions that cause renal failure that also are associated with a high incidence of malignancy, such as analgesic nephropathy. Patients on long-term dialysis may acquire a form of cystic disease of the kidneys associated with a high incidence of malignancy (Dunnill *et al.*, 1977).

There has been controversy over whether dialysis patients are more susceptible to malignancy other than that affecting the renal tract. Several authors (Herr *et al.*, 1979; Lidner *et al.*, 1981; Matas *et al.*, 1975; Miach *et al.*, 1976; Sutherland *et al.*, 1977) concluded that there is an increased incidence of malignancy in chronic renal failure. Others found no increase (Slifkin *et al.*, 1977) or increase in a specific class of cancer only (Kinlen *et al.*, 1980). Kinlen and colleagues found an increased incidence of non-Hodgkin's lymphoma but not of other types of cancer (Kinlen *et al.*, 1980). These authors concluded that the unusual opportunity for detecting cancer in hemodialysis patients may account for some of the reported excesses.

Details of cancers that occur in dialysis patients are monitored by the Australia and New Zealand Combined Dialysis and Transplant Registry. The 1997 Registry report (Sheil, 1997) comprises 21,093 patients on dialysis for a mean of 2.2 years. Of these patients, 595 (3%) developed malignancies involving the skin, and a further 533 (2.5%) patients developed malignancies of other organs. All malignancies were diagnosed for the first time while patients were on dialysis and excluded cancers that were the reason for patients needing dialysis. Although 26% of malignancies other than skin involved the kidney, bladder and ureter (a total of 149 cancers), most did not. The rate of cancer development (excluding renal tract) is approximately 1.5 times that expected in the age-matched general population. Although this increase is significant ($P<0.001$), it is modest. The duration of dialysis is an important consideration, however, particularly because of the propensity for long-term dialysis patients to develop the cystic disease of the kidney that is associated with malignancy, mentioned previously. In Japan, a country with a large prolonged-dialysis population, 2% of patients develop renal cell cancer (Ishikawa, 1991). An analysis of deaths caused by cancer in Japan revealed that dialysis patients were at increased risk of cancer mortality compared with the general population (males relative risk [RR], 2.48, $P<0.05$; females RR, 3.99, $P<0.05$) (Iseki *et al.*, 1993).

Cancer in Renal Transplant Recipients
TRANSFERRED CANCER

A large proportion of patients who receive organ grafts from cancer-affected donors develop cancer in the organ graft and systemically (Penn, 1977a). In rare cases when this happens, cessation of immunosuppressive therapy and removal of the allograft results in rejection of the cancer with apparent cure (Wilson *et al.*, 1968; Zukoski *et al.*, 1970). Most patients with transferred cancer go on to die of malignancy, however (Penn, 1980).

Potential organ donors found to have cancer should be excluded. Because of the severe shortage of donor organs, however, exceptions are made for donors with low-grade cancers of the skin or carcinoma *in situ* of the uterine cervix because such tumors rarely metastasize. The organs of donors with primary intracerebral malignancy (except for cancers with a high histological grade of malignancy or that have been operated on previously) also are used for transplant because of the rarity of metastasis (Chui *et al.*, 1999), but transfer of cancer from such donors is documented, and extreme caution is urged (International Consensus Document, 1997). In every instance, clinicians must make every effort to exclude the presence of cancer in an organ donor; these efforts should include early postmortem search for tumor in cadaveric donors. Despite careful efforts, some grafts are implanted from donors subsequently discovered to have metastatic malignancy (Healey and Davis, 1998). Such grafts should be removed as soon as is practical. The possibility of tumor (and infectious agent) transfer with organ grafts must be explained to potential recipients and included in informed consent documents to be signed by them. Even with these precautions, litigation by cancer-affected recipients has occurred, and the legal position of those deciding to use the organs of donors with cancer or those implanting them remains to be determined in all countries.

DE NOVO CANCER

That *de novo* cancer is a complication in immunosuppressed transplant recipients is widely recognized. Single-center or registry reports record nonskin cancer incidences of 2 to 8% of transplant populations, and this has led some authors to believe that the risk is small (Macleod and Catto, 1988). The method of calculating risk as a percentage of a transplant population greatly underestimates the long-term threat to immunosuppressed transplant recipients, however, because transplant populations are biased toward the larger numbers of recently transplanted patients and against the fewer long-surviving patients. There are increasing numbers of reports of significant incidences (34–50%) of cancer in immunosuppressed transplant recipients followed for 20 years or more posttransplant (Gaya et al., 1995; Montagnino et al., 1996; Slavis et al., 1990), with reports from Australia and New Zealand of incidences 30 years after cadaveric donor renal transplant of skin cancer in 75% of patients, nonskin cancer in 33% of patients, and some form of cancer (skin or nonskin) in 80% of patients (Sheil, 1997; Fig. 35–1).

Etiology

Several different mechanisms may contribute to the increased risk of cancer in immunosuppressed allograft recipients. The relative importance of these mechanisms vary with the type of cancer.

Impaired Immune Surveillance

It is widely held that abnormal cells arise frequently in normal individuals, as originally proposed by Ehrlich (1909), and that some such cells, arising by somatic mutation or viral infection, may become autonomous, thus establishing neoplasia. It has been suggested that the immune system is important in eliminating such spontaneous potential neoplasms (Thomas, 1959). Loss or impairment of a surveillance mechanism for neoplastic mutant cells has been postulated as a cause of cancer (Burnet, 1967; Keast, 1970). There is considerable controversy concerning the importance of immune surveillance in cancer etiology in laboratory and clinical work. Support for the importance of immune surveillance in protection against cancer in humans comes from the increased tumor development that occurs with some congenital or acquired immunodeficiency diseases (Kersey et al., 1973) including acquired immunodeficiency syndrome (AIDS) (Waterson, 1983), the experience with transplanted malignancy referred to previously, the increasing incidence of cancer in immunosuppressed transplant recipients and experimental work confirming a positive effect of immune suppression on tumor recurrence (Freise et al., 1999).

It is likely that immunosuppressive agents act as potentiating agents for other oncogenic stimuli, such as oncogenic viruses, chemical carcinogens and ultraviolet (UV) light. It has been suggested that immunosuppressive agents with powerful antilymphocyte activity, such as cyclosporine, antilymphocyte globulin (ALG), antithymocyte globulin and OKT3, may enhance viral oncogenesis because of the alteration of function or elimination of T lymphocytes, as discussed subsequently under oncogenic viruses. A clear potentiating effect of ALG on cancer development was shown when ALG was used in conjunction with oncogenic viruses (Allison et al., 1967; Law et al., 1968) or chemical carcinogens (Balner and Dersjant, 1969; Cerilli and Treat, 1969; Rabbat and Jeejeebhoy, 1970).

The immunosuppressive agent cyclosporine, introduced into clinical practice in 1978 (Calne et al., 1978), is in widespread use. Considerable interest exists as to whether there may be an altered pattern or incidence of malignancy resulting from immunosuppression with cyclosporine. Early reports (Penn, 1987; Vogt et al., 1990) confirmed that malignant complications occur in patients taking cyclosporine for immunosuppression. Although Penn (1987) recorded high incidences of Kaposi's sarcoma and non-Hodgkin's lymphoma, Vogt et al. (1990) recorded heterogeneous malignancies occurring in 18 (3%) of 598 renal transplant recipients. In Australia, the rate of development and types of nonskin cancer occurring in cyclosporine-treated patients were no different from those in azathioprine-treated patients or in patients treated with combinations of these agents. Skin cancers in patients treated with a combination of cyclosporine and azathioprine were more frequent, however (Sheil, 1997).

Direct Neoplastic Action of Immunosuppressive Drugs

As well as contributing to oncogenesis through immune inhibition, immunosuppressive agents may be directly oncogenic. The commonly used immunosuppressants for renal transplantation are cyclosporine, azathioprine and corticoste-

FIGURE 35–1

Risk of cancer posttransplant (1965 to March 31, 1997) in recipients of primary cadaveric and living unrelated renal grafts where patients and grafts survived at least 90 days after transplant. The percentage probability that patients will develop cancer each year after cadaveric donor renal transplantation. The graphs are for nonskin cancer, skin cancer, and any cancer. The number of patients surviving beyond 10 years is 1,611 and beyond 20 years is 188. (Reproduced with permission from Sheil, 1997.)

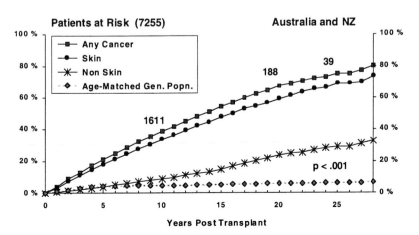

roids. Other agents used less frequently include antilympho-cyte agents, chlorambucil, cyclophosphamide, actinomycins and radiotherapy. A variety of newer agents, such as tacrolimus, sirolimus and the antimetabolite mycophenolate mofetil, as well as a range of immunosuppressive antibodies, have been introduced. Allograft recipients often are treated with a wide variety of antibiotic, antihypertensive, antidiabetic, antiepileptic, sedative and other agents, some of which are known to have carcinogenic effects.

Of the most commonly used immunosuppressives, prednisone has been shown to have no effect on chromosome numbers or morphology. Azathioprine has been shown to cause chromosome breaks and nuclear abnormalities in humans and animals (Jensen, 1967). No direct oncogenic effect has been shown, however. Cyclosporine did not show malignant potential in extended toxicology experiments in animals (Beveridge, 1983). Cyclosporine has enhanced the growth of malignant cells *in vitro* (Hojo *et al.*, 1999), however, possibly by evoking increased production of transforming growth factor-β (Nabel, 1999), a property shared with tacrolimus (Han *et al.*, 1995).

The advent of each new, powerful immunosuppressive agent carries the threat of enhanced risk of malignant complications in transplant recipients. Reports of increased cancer risk have been frequent, appearing soon after the introduction of each agent, including OKT3 (Canfield *et al.*, 1992), cyclosporine (Calne *et al.*, 1979) and tacrolimus (Newell *et al.*, 1996), almost always with reference to posttransplant lymphoproliferative disease (PTLD). With rare exceptions, each new agent has been used in conjunction with other immunosuppressive agents, however, and matched, concurrent, control patients are difficult to obtain. There is now a widespread belief that the intensity of immunosuppression in a general sense is the determining factor rather than specific agents. In concert with this conclusion, the greatest incidence of PTLD is in the early months after transplant, when immunosuppression is most severe, with reduced incidence thereafter (Opelz and Henderson, 1993). Regarding maintenance immunosuppression in the long term, the intuitive practice of clinicians to maintain the lowest doses compatible with a rejection-free course to diminish immunosuppression complications, including cancer, is supported by a randomized comparison of a standard-dose cyclosporine–treated renal transplant group and a low-dose group, with significantly fewer cancers developing in the low-dose group (Dantal *et al.*, 1998).

Oncogenic Viruses

Oncogenic viruses are well recognized in experimental work (Allison *et al.*, 1967; Schwartz and Beldotti, 1965). A combination of some viruses and bacterial endotoxin in animals increases the incidence of lymphomas and sarcomas (Keast, 1970), and the synergism between a plasmodium and a virus has been shown to increase the incidence of malignant lymphomas in mice (Wedderburn, 1970).

Transplant recipients are susceptible to viral infections, some of which are potentially oncogenic in humans, including Epstein-Barr virus (EBV), cytomegalovirus, herpes simplex, herpes zoster, hepatitis C and human papillomaviruses (HPVs). The common types of malignancy encountered in transplant recipients (lymphomas and cancers of the skin, lip and uterine cervix) are those in which oncogenic viruses are thought likely to have a causative role (Penn, 1977a). The short induction period between transplantation and appearance of some malignancies is in favor of viral oncogenesis because viral transformation could take place from the time of starting immunosuppression.

Kinlen and colleagues concluded that virus infection is almost certainly involved in the development of non-Hodgkin's lymphoma, Kaposi's sarcoma and hepatoma (Kinlen *et al.*, 1983). Epstein-Barr virus has a recognized association with PTLD, as reviewed later. Other cancers in transplant recipients that have been associated with viral infections include cancers of the vulva, vagina and uterine cervix with HPV and herpes simplex virus (Alloub *et al.*, 1989; Gissmann *et al.*, 1983; Sillman *et al.*, 1984), hepatoma with hepatitis B virus (Beasley, 1982) and hepatitis C virus (DiBisceglie, 1997) and Kaposi's sarcoma with human herpesvirus 8 (Kedda *et al.*, 1996). The likelihood of a viral cause in some skin cancers (HPV, EBV or herpesviruses) is discussed later in the section on those malignancies.

Chronic Antigenic Stimulation and Immune Regulation

The continuing presence of foreign allograft antigens in the recipient may be important in cancer causation. Many authors have shown that chronic lymphoid stimulation results in a high incidence of malignant lymphomas (Armstrong *et al.*, 1962; Schwartz and Beldotti, 1965; Smithers and Field, 1969; Walford, 1966). The mechanism may be a direct consequence of protracted antigenic stimulation of the lymphoreticular system. Schwartz (1972) presents persuasive arguments for a mechanism that normally controls the extent of immune reactions in a feedback relationship. In situations of partial immunosuppression, which exist in most human allograft recipients, incomplete development of an immune response fails to stimulate full feedback inhibition of lymphoreticular activity. Continued stimulation of lymphoid tissue may lead to hyperplasia and ultimately neoplasia. Alternatively, hyperplasia may lead to derepression of a latent virogene, allowing viral proliferation and resulting in malignant transformation. The importance of the presence of viable antigen in the development of neoplasia in human allograft recipients is suggested by McEwan and Petty (1972) and Kinlen *et al.* (1979), who found a much lower incidence of cancer in patients treated with immunosuppressive agents but without transplants than in transplant recipients.

Uremia

Uremic individuals and dialysis patients have defective humoral and cell-mediated immunity (Merrill, 1968; Wilson *et al.*, 1965). These defects have been implicated in the increased cancer risk of patients on dialysis described previously and may contribute to the continuing cancer risk after transplantation.

Genetic Predisposition

Genetic differences are important in determining susceptibility or resistance to a variety of naturally occurring or virus-induced leukemias and tumors in mice (Kersey *et al.*, 1973). That many transplant recipients do not develop cancer also implies that genetic influences determine individual susceptibility. With skin cancer, genetic influences similar to those that pertain in the general population are demonstrable, as discussed later.

Donor-Recipient Interactions

Complex donor-recipient interactions are involved in cancer development in transplant recipients, best recognized with non-Hodgkin's lymphoma but also apparent in cancer affecting bone marrow recipients (Witherspoon *et al.*, 1994) and perhaps of importance with many cancers. Although the increased incidence of non-Hodgkin's lymphoma after heart transplantation compared with renal (Opelz and Henderson, 1993) or liver transplantation (Sheil et al., 1997) as well as a greater incidence after heart-lung or lung transplantation is thought to be due to the more aggressive immunosuppressive therapy used for recipients of thoracic organ transplants, there is a strong preferential location of lymphomas in the heart or lung after heart, heart-lung or lung transplants and in the kidney after renal transplant (Opelz and Henderson, 1993). Local lymphoid tissue in or near the transplanted organs may be at increased risk of malignant transformation because of its first-line-of-defense situation. Also to be considered, however, is whether the lymphoid tissues that transform to neoplasia are donor or recipient derived. Theoretically, it could be either because donor-derived cells survive long-term in immunosuppressed transplant recipients (Starzl et al., 1992) and are subjected to the same risk factors (immunological reactions, immunosuppression, other pharmacological agents and environment). Donor-derived lymphomas have been reported (Armes et al., 1994; Hjelle et al., 1989; Meduri et al., 1991; Spiro et al., 1993), and it has been shown that lymphoid cells of an EBV-positive donor can persist in the graft transplanted to an EBV-negative recipient and lead to an EBV-associated posttransplant lymphoma (Mentzer et al., 1996).

Environment and Other Local and General Influences Determining the Patterns of Cancers for Transplant Units and Countries

A range of factors related to the location where recipients receive their transplant could be involved in cancer development and influence the pattern of cancers that occur. A striking illustration of environmental effect is the association of skin cancers in white recipients with sun exposure. Also, UV light has immunosuppressive properties that may influence the development of other cancers. Non-Hodgkin's lymphoma has been shown to be related to UV light exposure in the general population in England and Wales (Bentham, 1996). Other local influences include viral infections encountered by patients before or after transplant; local practice in viral infection prevention, detection and therapy; the organ transplanted and the immunosuppressive therapy used and its dosage. The local factors operate against a background of general influences, such as age, sex and genetic diversity as well as the duration of time after transplantation. Of all these influences, none acts in isolation; there is a complex interaction of them all, which determines for each individual center the final incidence and pattern of posttransplant cancer for that center.

Types of Cancer

The distribution of malignancies recorded in transplant recipients differs from that of the age-matched general population. The nonskin cancers that have occurred in Australia and New Zealand are shown in Table 35–1. Here, a RR of 1.0 reflects the expected incidence of cancer; numbers greater than and less than 1.0 reflect the degree of increased or decreased risk for that cancer.

Table 35-1 shows that most cancers that occur in the general population have been recorded in cadaveric donor renal graft recipients. Ten percent of the transplant population is affected, representing a continuous increase (Sheil et al., 1997). Because most transplant recipients are relatively young, the occurrence of any cancer should be rare. For most malignancies, the frequency of occurrence is increased

compared with that in the age-matched general population. Overall the increased RR for nonskin malignancies is 3.2 (females RR, 3.9; males, RR 2.7).

The cancers with the greatest increased risk have in common an established or suspected viral component to the cause. For cadaveric donor graft recipients, they include lymphomas (RR, 8.4), Kaposi's sarcoma (RR, 82.6), leukemia (RR, 3.3), hepatoma (RR, 7.3), cancer of the esophagus (RR, 5.8), cervical cancer (in situ RR, 7.6; invasive RR, 3.1), cancer of the vulva and vagina (RR, 41.0) and cancer of the penis (RR 24.2). There are increased risks in the native renal tracts of renal transplant recipients, as discussed subsequently, and an increase in malignancies affecting the endocrine glands (RR, 5.3). After excluding all of the above-mentioned lymphoid and renal tract cancers, however, the frequency of other nonskin cancer is still twice that of the age-matched population in Australia and New Zealand (Sheil, 1999), inferring either more widespread viral involvement in cancer development than currently is recognized or that the originally postulated immunosuppressive inhibition of immune elimination of naturally occurring malignant mutations is operative. Among the relatively few cancers so far without significantly increased incidence is that of the female breast (RR, 1.0), as originally pointed out by Penn (1977a). The only two cancers with significantly reduced incidence in renal transplant recipients are those of the prostate (RR, 0.6) and ovary (RR, 0.4), perhaps reflecting a decreased hormonal drive in these patients.

Analysis of the cancers occurring in recipients of living related donor renal grafts shows a reduced proportion of patients affected (6.7% vs. 10%). These patients are younger with somewhat shorter follow-up, however. When compared with the age-matched general population, the RR is increased compared with cadaver donor graft recipients (5.4 vs. 3.2), a difference that is statistically significant ($P<0.02$). There are no striking differences in the distribution of malignancies recorded in living related donor graft recipients except that alimentary tract cancers constitute a much smaller proportion of cancers recorded (8% vs. 18%). The increased risk of cancer in living related donor graft recipients may reflect greater susceptibility of younger patients to viral infections or to the effects of immunosuppressive agents or that greater proportions of these recipients survive with functioning grafts, exposing them to the effects of continued immunosuppression, antigenic stimulation and viral exposure.

Genitourinary Malignancies

The most frequent malignancies are those of the genitourinary system. These malignancies constitute one third of the total. The female genital tract is particularly at risk, contributing approximately one half of the genitourinary malignancies. Squamous cell carcinomas of the vulva and vagina and in situ and invasive carcinomas of the uterine cervix have greatly increased RRs. These cancers have an association with HPV infections. The considerably increased RRs for bladder (RR, 7.19), kidney (RR, 6.9) and ureter (RR, 300.0) malignancies no doubt reflect, in part, the serious urinary tract abnormalities common in these patients. Retained native kidneys represent a definitive threat because the cause of renal failure may have been a condition known to predispose to malignancy, such as analgesic nephropathy (Kleim et al., 1996), and because the retained kidneys may have developed the condition of acquired cystic disease with its malignant potential. For the latter reason, renal cell cancer is the commonest malignancy after renal transplantation in Japan (Hoshida et al., 1997). Penn and Brunson (1988) recorded a further increase in incidence of renal malignancies in patients treated

TABLE 35–1

AUSTRALIA AND NEW ZEALAND RISK OF CANCER* AFTER CADAVERIC DONOR RENAL TRANSPLANTATION†

Site of Cancer	Cancer Observed	Cancer Expected	Risk Ratio	95% Confidence Interval
Alimentary tract	184	80.53	2.30	1.97–2.31
Buccal cavity	34	13.61	2.5	1.73–3.49
Pharynx	5	2.40	2.1	0.68–4.86
Esophagus	19	3.25	5.8	3.52–9.13
Stomach	10	7.56	1.3	0.63–2.43
Small intestine	3	0.73	4.1	0.85–12.01
Colon	58	25.73	2.3	1.71–2.91
Rectum and anus	25	17.87	1.4	0.91–2.07
Liver	12	1.65	7.3	3.76–12.70
Gallbladder and extrahepatic bile ducts	5	2.21	2.3	0.73–5.28
Pancreas	13	5.51	2.4	1.26–4.03
Respiratory	88	37.76	2.30	1.87–2.87
Larynx	7	2.93	2.4	0.96–4.92
Trachea, bronchus and lung	76	33.35	2.3	1.80–2.85
Pleura	5	1.48	3.4	1.10–7.88
Bone	3	0.69	4.3	0.90–12.71
Connective Tissue	1	3.03	0.3	0.01–1.84
Breast	52	49.63	1.00	0.78–1.37
Female	50	49.27	1.0	0.75–1.34
Male	2	0.36	5.6	0.67–20.07
Genitourinary	313	81.78	3.8	3.42–4.28
Cervix–in situ	66	4.06	7.6	2.57–20.68
Cervix–invasive	14	4.45	3.1	1.72–5.28
Uterus	11	7.66	1.4	0.72–2.57
Ovary	2	5.26	0.4	0.05–1.37
Vulva and vagina	43	1.05	41.0	29.64–55.16
Prostate	23	37.95	0.6	0.38–0.91
Testis	5	3.11	1.6	0.52–3.75
Penis	8	0.33	24.2	10.47–47.77
Bladder	66	8.80	7.5	5.80–9.54
Kidney	63	9.06	7.0	5.34–8.90
Ureter	12	0.04	300.0	155.03–524.05
Central nervous system	7	7.51	0.9	0.37–1.92
Other than lymphoma	7	7.51	0.9	0.37–1.92
Endocrine glands	19	3.60	5.3	3.18–8.24
Thyroid	16	3.58	4.5	2.55–7.26
Parathyroid	2	0.01	200.0	24.20–722.50
Other endocrine	1	0.02	50.0	1.25–278.60
Lymphoma	123	14.63	8.4	6.99–10.03
Central nervous system	17	0.01	>1000	939.00–>10,000
Non-Hodgkin's	103	12.82	8.03	6.56–9.75
Hodgkin's	3	1.81	1.7	0.34–4.84
Multiple myeloma	9	3.63	2.5	1.13–4.71
Leukemia	29	8.68	3.3	2.24–4.80
Kaposi's sarcoma	19	0.23	82.6	49.73–129.00
Malignant melanoma	104	32.50	3.2	3.17–3.88
Miscellaneous	78	12.03	6.5	5.13–8.09
Total	1,029‡	318.51	3.2	3.04–3.43

*Nonmelanotic skin cancers are not included.
†Data for the period 1965 through September 1998 (n = 9,200).
‡The 1,029 cancers occurred in 925 (10%) patients.
The data reported here have been supplied by ANZDATA Registry (The Queen Elizabeth Hospital, 28 Woodville Road, Woodville South, Adelaide, South Australia, 5011). The interpretation and reporting of these data are the responsibility of the editor and in no way should be seen as an official policy or interpretation of the ANZDATA Registry.

with cyclosporine. Penn and Brunson (1988) indicated that the possibility that renal adenocarcinoma may be a complication of the nephrotoxicity of cyclosporine must be considered.

Alimentary Tract Malignancies

Malignancies involving the digestive organs are a second major group and constitute 20% of the total. One half involve the large bowel. The entire gastrointestinal tract and its accessory organs are at increased risk, however, particularly the

esophagus (RR, 5.04) and liver (RR, 5.67). Malignancies in which the increased risk has not yet reached statistical significance are the pharynx, small intestine, rectum and anus and gallbladder and bile ducts.

Posttransplant Lymphoproliferative Disease and Malignant Lymphoma

Posttransplant lymphoproliferative disease is the commonest neoplasia occurring in the early posttransplant course of graft recipients. Posttransplant lymphoproliferative disease affects approximately 1% of renal transplant recipients (Sheil *et al.*, 1997), the greatest incidence being in the first posttransplant year (0.2%) with reduced incidence thereafter (0.04%/y) (Opelz and Henderson, 1993). Posttransplant lymphoproliferative disease occurs especially in situations of intense immunosuppression with powerful agents such as cyclosporine, tacrolimus or OKT3, particularly when used for the treatment of resistant rejection episodes. Cyclosporine has been shown to enhance EBV infection of lymphocyte cultures *in vitro* (Bird *et al.*, 1981). Recipients of cardiac allografts are at heightened risk, possibly because of the aggressive immunosuppression used. Child graft recipients also are at risk, as discussed subsequently. Posttransplant lymphoproliferative disease may regress completely in some patients with reduction of immunosuppressive therapy (Starzl *et al.*, 1984) with or without added antiviral therapy (Hanto *et al.*, 1981), or it may progress inexorably on to a fatal outcome with or without evolution to non-Hodgkin's lymphoma.

In the early reports of malignancies after renal transplantation, when immunosuppression was largely azathioprine/prednisone based, non-Hodgkin's lymphoma contributed approximately 40% of all nonskin cancers (Penn, 1975; Schneck and Penn, 1971). With the passage of time and concomitant diagnosis of other forms of malignancy, the proportion constituted by lymphomas fell. By 1981 (Penn, 1981), it was 29%, and in 1988 (Penn and Brunson, 1988), it was 12%. Similarly, in Australia and New Zealand, non-Hodgkin's lymphoma now constitutes only 12% of all nonskin malignancies (Sheil *et al.*, 1997). Since the introduction of cyclosporine and tacrolimus, it appears that a similar pattern of incidence may occur. In patients treated with cyclosporine, non-Hodgkin's lymphoma accounts for almost 40% of nonskin malignancies (Penn and Brunson, 1988), and high incidences have been reported in tacrolimus-treated recipients (Newell *et al.*, 1996). Just as in the precyclosporine era the proportion of lymphomas fell progressively, it is likely that a similar reduction will occur with the passage of time in the present era.

Registry reports from different countries have concluded that cyclosporine has no specific role in lymphoma causation (Opelz and Henderson, 1993; Sheil *et al.*, 1997), and workers now believe that posttransplant lymphoproliferative disease and the malignant lymphomas are an inevitable consequence of effective immunosuppressive therapy regardless of the particular immunosuppressive agents used. Similar to other posttransplant malignancies, a range of environmental, genetic and other factors probably is involved in the cause of posttransplant lymphoproliferative disease. For example, North American transplant recipients are at increased risk compared with European transplant recipients (Opelz and Henderson, 1993). Non-Hodgkin's lymphoma in the general population has been linked to UV light exposure (Bentham, 1996) and to the occurrence of skin cancer (Adami *et al.*, 1995).

Powerful immunosuppression is thought to inhibit T cell–dominated immune responses and to set the scene for unbridled B-lymphocyte cell proliferation now thought to be in response to latent or primary EBV infection (Bird and McLachlan, 1980; Crawford *et al.*, 1980; Hanto *et al.*, 1983; Nagington and Gray, 1980; Nalesnik *et al.*, 1988; Thiru *et al.*, 1981). A human and viral T cell–suppressive, B cell–stimulatory cytokine (interleukin-10) has been implicated (Birkeland *et al.*, 1999; Moore *et al.*, 1991). Epstein-Barr virus is ubiquitous, with 95% of the adult population having serological evidence of prior exposure with resulting latent infection and the possibility of reactivation. It is estimated that approximately 50% of children are EBV negative at the time of transplantation, with susceptibility to primary infection

from environmental exposure or directly from a virus-positive graft or blood transfusion (Dunn and Kreuger, 1998). Epstein-Barr virus has been linked to Burkitt's lymphoma (Henle *et al.*, 1968) and nasopharyngeal carcinoma as well as immunoblastic lymphomas in persons affected with human immunodeficiency virus (HIV) (List *et al.*, 1987). The implication of EBV with lymphoproliferative disorders in transplant recipients has led to a successful search for similar involvement in patients with primary lymphoma of the central nervous system in the absence of immunosuppression (Hochberg *et al.*, 1983).

It has been surmised that the polyclonal proliferative B-cell response to EBV ultimately could allow development of a monoclonal lymphoma (Klein and Purtilo, 1981) after perhaps passing through stages of multiclonality and oligoclonality (Cleary and Sklar, 1984). Although this sequence of events is the likely explanation for some of the malignant lymphomas that occur in the early posttransplant months, it is unlikely that it accounts for all malignant lymphomas, particularly those occurring remote from the transplant time.

The widespread lymphoproliferative response to EBV infection has histological features (in removed lymphatic tissue) ranging from polymorphic B-cell hyperplasia to monomorphic lymphoma. In some of these patients, lymphoproliferation results in tumor masses, in which the lymphoid cells usually are of a polyclonal type. In about one third of patients (Hanto *et al.*, 1983; Starzl *et al.*, 1984), however, the lesions are monoclonal, the hallmark of malignant lymphomas. The commonest of the malignant lymphomas are large cell lymphomas described as immunoblastic and including plasmacytoid, clear cell, polymorphous and epithelioid cell varieties. The whole range of malignant lymphomas has been recorded, however, including lymphoblastic lymphomas, Hodgkin's disease and a variety of poorly defined malignancies. Hodgkin's disease accounts for only 2% of lymphomas in organ transplant recipients compared with 34% in the general population (Penn, 1981). Approximately half of patients with lymphoma have localized disease, and half have disseminated disease (Penn, 1981). In patients with localized disease, the area most commonly affected is the central nervous system. When there is disseminated disease, the liver, spleen, lymph nodes and bone marrow usually are involved as well as the central nervous system. One third of recipients with disseminated disease have involvement of the renal allograft.

The frequency with which the lymphomas that occur in transplant recipients involve the central nervous system is unusual, in that approximately 40% of lymphomas in transplant recipients involve the brain or spinal cord, compared with only 2% of such malignancies in the general population. Lymphomas involving the central nervous system frequently are multicentric. It has been suggested that the known weak immunological reactions of the normal brain may allow neoplastic cells to flourish here in the immunosuppressed individual (Schneck and Penn, 1971).

Carcinoma of the Lung and Leukemia

Two other malignancies occurring with steadily increasing frequency are carcinoma of the lung and leukemia. These cancers constitute 8% (carcinoma of the lung) and 3% (leukemia) of malignancies.

Kaposi's Sarcoma

Kaposi's sarcoma is an unusual malignancy that contributes a variable proportion to *de novo* cancer in organ transplant recipients. Genetic predisposition is a dominant factor with this malignancy. Kaposi's sarcoma affects immunosuppressed transplant recipients of African, Arabic, Italian, Jewish or Greek ancestry (Penn, 1995a), no matter where these patients receive transplants, the incidence in any transplant population depending largely on the proportion of patients with Mediterranean heritage in that population. In Western countries, Kaposi's sarcoma affects approximately 0.25% of renal allograft recipients, contributing 2 to 3% of all cancers, whereas in Saudi Arabia, the condition affects approximately 5% of recipients, contributing 40 to 70% of all cancers (Al-Sulaiman and Al-Khader, 1994; Qunibi et al., 1988). Kaposi's sarcoma is exceedingly rare in Japan (Hoshida et al., 1997). Men are affected three times as frequently as women (Penn, 1995a). Almost one half of cases occur within the first year after transplantation (Penn, 1995a). With Kaposi's sarcoma, the complex interplay of risk factors is apparent because herpesviruses are implicated with some certainty (Chang et al., 1994) as well as immunosuppression, as immunosuppression withdrawal sometimes results in complete regression (Penn, 1995a). The specific herpesvirus involved, human herpesvirus type 8, can be transmitted by renal allografts (Regamey et al., 1998).

Kaposi's sarcoma has a multicentric origin and is characterized by tumors with endothelium-lined vascular spaces, spindle-shaped cells, extravasated red cells and clusters of inflammatory cells. Of transplant patients with this cancer, 60% have involvement of the skin and/or the oropharyngolaryngeal mucosa (Penn, 1980). In these sites, the lesions appear as circumscribed purplish macules or as granulomas that fail to heal. The remaining patients have visceral involvement, particularly of the gastrointestinal tract or respiratory system. Although patients with visceral involvement often fail to respond to therapy, approximately 40% of patients with nonvisceral lesions have complete or partial remission of cancer after cessation or reduction of immunosuppressive therapy (Penn, 1995a). Reduced immunosuppression results in most patients (around 60%) (Penn, 1995a) losing their grafts to rejection, however.

Skin Cancer

The commonest malignancies encountered in allograft recipients are skin cancers (Penn et al., 1971; Walder et al., 1971; see Chapter 34). Transplant recipients living in geographical areas established as *high risk* for skin cancer in the general population suffer considerable morbidity and some mortality as a result of skin lesions.

Walder and associates described in Australian recipients the rapid evolution of cutaneous hyperkeratoses into squamous cell carcinomas, the tendency for skin cancers to be multiple and the more frequent occurrence as well as tendency of recurrence of keratoacanthomas (Walder et al., 1971). Walder and associates pointed out that squamous cell carcinomas occurred with a greater incidence than basal cell carcinoma, which is the reverse of what occurs in the general population (Walder et al., 1971).

The premalignant and malignant skin conditions that occur in transplant recipients include keratoacanthomas, Bowen's disease, basal cell carcinoma, squamous cell carcinoma and malignant melanoma. Conditions that have occurred in patients in Australia and New Zealand are listed in Table 35–2. The apparent decreased incidence in recipients of living donor grafts is accounted for by the younger age and shorter follow-up of these patients compared with recipients of cadaveric donor grafts. When these factors are taken into account, there is no significant difference in skin cancer incidences between living donor and cadaveric donor recipients.

The commonest skin malignancy is squamous cell carci-

TABLE 35–2

AUSTRALIA AND NEW ZEALAND SKIN PRECANCER AND CANCER IN PATIENTS AFTER RENAL TRANSPLANTATION

	Beyond 3 Months' Posttransplant	
	Living Related Donor	*Cadaveric Donor*
Precancer		
Keratoacanthoma	18	489
Bowen's disease	26	583
Cancer		
SCC	79 (58%)	1,644 (55%)
BCC	47 (34%)	1,137 (38%)
Melanoma	8 (6%)	87 (3%)
Other	3 (2%)	106 (4%)
Total cancers	137	2,974
Total patients with cancer	105 (9%)	2,031 (24%)
Patients at risk	1,178	8,618
Patient-years of risk	8,005	68,580

SCC = squamous cell carcinoma; BCC = basal cell carcinoma.

The data reported here have been supplied by ANZDATA Registry (The Queen Elizabeth Hospital, 28 Woodville Road, Woodville South, Adelaide, South Australia, 5011). The interpretation and reporting of these data are the responsibility of the editor and in no way should be seen as an official policy or interpretation of the ANZDATA Registry.

noma. Squamous cell carcinoma occurs with some increased frequency in low-risk areas, but in high-risk areas its frequency is calculated to be at least 20 times that expected in a comparable population (Hardie et al., 1980). Although squamous cell carcinoma occurs mostly on parts of the body exposed to the sun, this is not always the case. Some patients develop almost generalized squamous cell carcinomas of the skin and require repeated operations for removal of lesions (Fig. 35–2). In some transplant patients, squamous cell carcinomas involving the vulva or vagina occur. Although some of the vulval and vaginal lesions have an origin in viral warts (Caterson et al., 1984), most do not. With squamous cell carcinoma, there is a tendency for lesions to be multiple, aggressive and prone to recurrence and metastasis (Sheil, 1977; Fig. 35–3). In a 1991 report (Sheil, 1991), the rates of metastases and deaths of patients with squamous cell cancers were 8% and 4%, compared with metastatic rates of 0.6% in a series in the general population in Australia (Nixon et al., 1986). Patients with skin cancer also are more likely to develop other more fulminant types of cancer than are allograft recipients without skin cancer (Sheil, 1977).

Although it is not clear whether the risk of basal cell carcinoma is increased in transplant recipients compared with the general population, it seems likely that malignant melanoma is occurring with increased frequency (Greene et al., 1981; Kinlen et al., 1983; Sheil, 1991). In the report by Sheil (1991), 10 (0.4%) of 4,594 transplant recipients developed melanoma, an incidence four times that expected in the age-matched general Australian population, which is already at high risk for malignant melanoma. These lesions were aggressive with metastatic and death rates at that time of 29% and 20%.

With skin cancer, the disproportionate increase in squamous cell carcinoma suggests that, similar to lymphoreticular malignancies, factors other than decreased immunosurveillance are operative in the cause. Closely linked environmental and genetic influences are at play. In countries with extended sunlight hours, the incidence of skin cancer can reach 75% of all white patients who survive with functioning grafts for 20 years or more posttransplant (Bouwes-Bavinck et al., 1996). In patients with similar European heritage but with

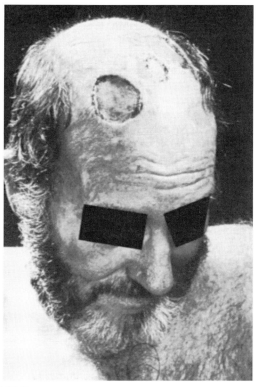

FIGURE 35-2

This patient began to develop squamous cell carcinomas of the scalp 4 years after cadaveric donor transplantation. The lesions became multiple and recurrent, requiring repeated operations. Ultimately the whole scalp required formal removal.

less UV light exposure, such as in Denmark (Hartevelt *et al.*, 1990) or Northern England (London *et al.*, 1995), the incidence is approximately half of this figure. The entwining of genetic and environmental factors is well illustrated because nonwhite recipients in countries with extended sunlight hours are at greatly reduced risk (Lugo-Janer *et al.*, 1991; Roeger *et al.*, 1992), and skin cancer is exceedingly rare in countries such as Saudi Arabia (Al-Sulaiman and Al-Khader, 1994), Japan (Hoshida *et al.*, 1997) and Pakistan (Lal *et al.*, 1998).

In whites, the UV component of sunlight causing damage to DNA is the prime risk factor. Pretransplant sun exposure is important (Kelly *et al.*, 1987). Ultraviolet light effects may be enhanced in immunosuppressed transplant recipients because antimetabolite immunosuppressive agents such as azathioprine and mycophenolate mofetil inhibit DNA synthesis (Wheeler *et al.*, 1972), and it seems likely that this would impair DNA repair synthetic mechanisms. The two major metabolites of azathioprine, 6-mercaptopurine and methyl-nitro-thio-imidazole, have strong photooxidative activities in the presence of UV light that may cause photosensitization and photoallergy (Trush *et al.*, 1982).

Viral involvement in cancer development seems likely. Human papillomavirus has been implicated in the cause of skin cancers in immunosuppressed renal allograft recipients (Bouwes-Bavinck *et al.*, 1993; Lutzner *et al.*, 1983). Epstein-Barr virus has been implicated in skin cancers developing in renal (Thomas *et al.*, 1995) and cardiac graft recipients (Ternesten-Bratel *et al.*, 1998). There is a definite viral association when squamous cell carcinoma develops from warts. Approximately 40% of transplant recipients develop these lesions (Koranda *et al.*, 1974; Spencer and Anderson, 1970).

In nearly every affected patient, there is a history of warts as a child, suggesting that development after transplantation is the result of reactivation of latent viruses rather than from a primary infection. Koranda *et al.* (1974) and Mullen *et al.* (1976) described patients with widespread warts suggestive of epidermodysplasia verruciformis who developed multiple squamous cell carcinomas and proposed that these cancers might be virally induced, activated by immunosuppression. Koranda's patients showed malignant transformation only in sites exposed to the sun, suggesting interaction between various carcinogenic stimuli (Koranda *et al.*, 1974). In these cases and in cancers complicating vulval warts, HPV and herpesviruses are involved. There have been isolated reports of HPV association with basal cell carcinoma in immunosuppressed transplant recipients (Obasek *et al.*, 1988).

Other factors may be involved in the cause of skin malignancies in transplant recipients. There are reduced numbers of Langerhans' cells in the skin (Sontheimer *et al.*, 1984), these cells having a known immunological function. Advancing age and skin cancers before transplant are recognized risk factors (Roeger *et al.*, 1992). The combination of cyclosporine with azathioprine for immunosuppression is emerging as a risk factor (Glover *et al.*, 1997; Sheil, 1997). Defense against skin cancer has been linked to HLA antigens and the degree of HLA matching of the recipient with the donor (Bouwes-Bavinck *et al.*, 1991).

Time of Cancer Presentation

Transplant recipients constitute a group of humans subjected by need to the most rapidly effective oncogenic influences recognized. Other known carcinogens, such as tobacco,

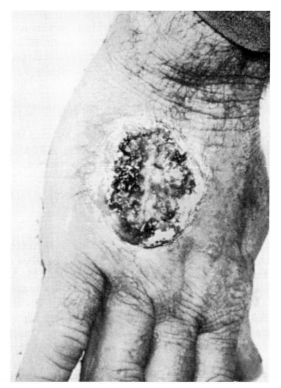

FIGURE 35-3

This patient scratched his hand on a piece of wire. Within 6 weeks, this aggressive squamous cell carcinoma developed. Although there were no involved lymph glands at the time of presentation, lymph glands became involved 6 months later. Despite block dissection, metastases became systemic, causing death 1 year later.

UV light, ionizing radiation and aniline dyes, have long latent periods between exposure and development of malignancy.

The pattern of posttransplant cancer evolves with the time interval posttransplant. Although all varieties of cancer can occur within the early months posttransplant, non-Hodgkin's lymphoma has its peak incidence within 1 year of transplant with decreased frequency thereafter. Because the heightened risks of lymphomas (Hoover and Fraumeni, 1983), skin cancers (Sheil, 1991) and other malignancies (Sheil, 1991) persist indefinitely, however, the average times of appearance of these cancers lengthen gradually in concert with the progressively lengthening mean follow-up period for transplant recipients. In Australia with patient follow-up of 0 to 31 years (mean, 7.9 years), the current mean time of appearance for lymphomas, Kaposi's sarcoma and cancers of the endocrine glands is approximately 6 years after transplant; for cancers affecting the respiratory tract, 8 years; for breast cancer, genitourinary system cancers and leukemia, 8.8 years and for cancers of the alimentary tract, 10.4 years. For skin malignancy, average time of diagnosis is 7.6 years posttransplant (Sheil, 1997).

CANCER DEVELOPMENT AND SURVIVAL AFTER TRANSPLANTATION

It might be expected that renal transplant recipients who develop cancer would survive less well than other recipients who do not. The relationship between cancer development and survival after renal transplantation is complex, however. The incidence of cancer increases with time after transplantation (Hoover and Fraumeni, 1983; Sheil, 1977, 1991; Sloan et al., 1977), affecting recipients who are otherwise doing well. Also, some of the cancers that occur posttransplant, such as skin cancers and cancers of the uterine cervix, are controlled by therapy. Others, including some lymphomas, appear amenable to treatment if diagnosis and therapy are early. In contrast, visceral cancers and cancers affecting the blood are highly malignant. The result of these disparate influences is that in the early posttransplant years, patient survival and continued graft function for patients with cancer are better than for patients without cancer (Sheil, 1977; Sheil et al., 1979; Sloan et al., 1977). Later, beyond 7 or 8 years after transplantation, graft and patient survivals worsen rapidly in patients with cancer because of death owing to cancer and because of withdrawal of immunosuppressive therapy in an attempt to control cancer (Sheil et al., 1979).

Factors that could explain the paradox in the early posttransplant years of improved survival and better graft function of patients who develop cancer compared with those who do not include the possibilities that routine immunosuppressive therapy may result in more profound inhibition of the immune response in some patients or that such patients may have reduced innate ability to mount immune responses. In either case, although tolerance of the renal allograft is improved, there could be decreased ability to withstand viral oncogenesis or to eliminate malignant clones. Recipients surviving with good graft function are those most likely to be exposed for long periods to immunosuppressive therapy, chronic antigenic stimulation from the graft and viral and environmental influences.

Prevention

Clinicians caring for potential transplant recipients must appreciate the threat of cancer development after transplantation and do whatever is possible regarding prevention. Be-

fore transplantation, all steps should be taken to exclude malignancy in each patient. Tobacco smoking should be prohibited. All patients, especially in high-risk areas for skin malignancy, must be forewarned of the potential dangers of skin cancers and advised on preventive measures, including the protection of exposed skin areas with appropriate clothing and barrier creams. Patients should see dermatologists experienced with the care of transplant recipients. Existing skin lesions should be treated.

In female patients, pelvic examinations and uterine cervical smears must be performed before transplantation and regularly thereafter. Patients with persistent cellular dysplasia or in situ cancer of the cervix uteri should be treated by cervical cone biopsy, and patients with invasive cancer should be treated by hysterectomy.

The immune status of patients regarding a wide range of viruses, including hepatitis B and C, cytomegalovirus, HIV, EBV, herpes simplex and herpes zoster, should be established. Donor viral studies should be routine to avoid viral transmission. After transplantation, it is common to employ prophylactic antiviral agents to treat patients at high risk of viral infection (McDiarmid et al., 1998), such as cytomegalovirus-negative or EBV-negative recipients who receive organs from donors positive for these agents or recipients receiving powerful immunosuppression to treat rejection (Hibberd, 1992). The monitoring of patients at high risk by quantitative viral polymerase chain reaction tests, to allow preemptive therapy, is being pursued (Green et al., 1996).

Management

After transplantation, clinicians constantly must be alert that patients may have symptomatic or nonsymptomatic cancer because early diagnosis and effective treatment are important. Comprehensive and regular clinical reviews by transplantation clinicians, dermatologists and, for female recipients, gynecologists, together with appropriate investigations, should be pursued.

Benign and premalignant skin lesions are treated by cautery, freezing or excision. All persisting skin, lip, vulval or anal lesions should undergo biopsy or excision. All malignant lesions must be excised widely, with reparative skin grafts if necessary. With squamous cell carcinoma or malignant melanoma of the skin, draining lymph nodes may require block dissection should metastatic involvement be present at the time of initial presentation.

In patients with rapid, recurrent development of squamous cell carcinoma or patients with generalized carcinomatous changes in the skin, change or withdrawal of immunosuppressive therapy must be considered. To date, no satisfactory solution for these patients has been found. When cyclosporine has been substituted for azathioprine as the primary immunosuppressant, the results have been disappointing, usually with continued squamous cell carcinoma development. Squamous cell carcinomas have been reported to develop in patients for the first time after conversion from azathioprine to cyclosporine when conversion was for reasons other than skin cancer (Thompson et al., 1985). Substitution of agents such as chlorambucil or cyclophosphamide for azathioprine and/or cyclosporine has sometimes been followed by regression of skin changes but usually has resulted sooner or later in rejection of the allograft. Patients who elect cessation of immunosuppressive therapy—especially when removal of the allograft after rejection is required—have a dramatic reduction or cessation of development of skin lesions. It is unusual for patients to accept this option, however, with its attendant need for return to dialysis.

Attention has focused on the use of retinoids for prevention and control of squamous cell cancers in transplant recipients (Kelly *et al.*, 1991; Shuttleworth *et al.*, 1988) as well as the general population (Hong *et al.*, 1990; Lippman and Meyskens, 1987). A trial of systemic and topical administration of retinoids in renal transplant recipients resulted in remarkable amelioration of existing skin lesions with a reduction in the rate of appearance of new lesions (Rook *et al.*, 1995). Although continued systemic therapy has proved difficult because of side effects such as headache, dry skin and mucous membranes and elevated levels of serum triglycerides, prolonged topical applications may prove useful (Rook *et al.*, 1995).

Should metastases to lymph nodes develop from squamous cell carcinoma or malignant melanoma, block dissection of the draining lymph nodes may result in cure. Most clinicians also reduce, change or stop immunosuppression. When metastases become systemic, prognosis is grave because the likelihood of successful treatment with antineoplastic agents is remote after allograft removal.

For malignancies involving the viscera, it is usual to treat localized lesions by standard excision or radiotherapy appropriate for young patients in the general population, while immunosuppressive therapy is maintained. If metastases occur, most clinicians withdraw immunosuppressive drugs, excise metastases if these appear single or localized, institute therapy with antineoplastic drugs and remove the allograft if and when rejection occurs.

With lymphomas, particularly in the early posttransplant course, appropriate therapy is the cessation or severe reduction of immunosuppression (Starzl *et al.*, 1984) because B-cell proliferation may not have progressed to the stage of monoclonal malignancy. Most authors recommend additional treatment with antiviral agents such as acyclovir (Hanto *et al.*, 1981) or ganciclover (Cacciarelli *et al.*, 1998). These methods also may be successful with localized Kaposi's sarcoma. Treatment with interferon alfa and intravenous immune globulin has been successful (Cantarovich *et al.*, 1998; Shapiro *et al.*, 1988), as has the administration of EBV-specific donor T cells in bone marrow graft recipients (Papadopoulos *et al.*, 1994). Protocols involving monoclonal antibodies directed against the CD20 B lymphocyte–associated surface membrane antigen, which is expressed widely in normal and malignant B cells, are being explored (Kaminski *et al.*, 1993).

In general, localized lymphoma is treated when possible by excision or, when this is not possible, by radiotherapy. When lymphoma occurs late after transplantation and is multicentric, it is usual to withdraw immunosuppression, treat with antineoplastic agents or radiotherapy as appropriate for the histological type of malignancy and deal with rejection in the organ graft if it occurs. Other cancers of the immune system and blood (multiple myeloma and varieties of leukemia) are treated with appropriate antineoplastic agents, but in Australia (Sheil, 1991), most patients have succumbed to cancer.

Transplantation in Patients with Previous Cancer

With the known predisposition of immunosuppressed transplant recipients to malignant disease, the question arises whether it is safe for patients who have had prior malignancy to undergo transplantation. Penn (1995b) reviewed 350 patients with preexisting renal cancers who went on to renal transplantation: 279 (80%) had symptomatic neoplasms involving one or both kidneys; of these, 76 had Wilms' tumors (54% bilateral) treated by nephrectomy before transplanta-

tion, of whom 11 (14%) developed recurrence after transplantation. Ten (91%) patients with recurrence had had pretransplant nephrectomy performed less than 2 years earlier. Follow-up averaged 59 months posttransplantation. Of the 203 other patients treated before transplantation (i.e., with symptomatic, non-Wilms' cancers), 129 had unilateral cancers, of which 28 (22%) recurred. Seventy-four had bilateral cancers, and 31 (42%) recurred. Follow-up for this group of patients averaged 46 months posttransplantation. Although 34 (58%) patients with recurrences had been treated by nephrectomy 2 years or less before transplantation, some recurrences occurred in patients treated more than 5 years before transplantation. The remaining 71 patients (with nonsymptomatic cancers) had incidental renal tumors discovered at the time of bilateral nephrectomy, most at intervals 2 years before transplantation to the time of transplantation (average 6 months), and 8 had tumors discovered posttransplantation (average 3 months). None developed recurrences with an average follow-up of 3 years.

In an earlier review, Penn (1983) discussed patients with malignancies other than renal treated before transplantation. Of 119 patients with epithelial tumors involving the breast or a wide variety of internal organs, 18 (14%) developed recurrence or metastases, mostly from tumors of the breast, bladder or colorectum. Although the same general rule of fewer recurrences with greater time from treatment of the cancer applied, 5 (28%) of the 17 recurrences occurred in patients who had been treated an average of 7 years before transplantation. Duration of follow-up of these patients averaged almost 4 years. There were 22 patients with prior lymphopoietic malignancies. The disease persisted or recurred in 11 (50%) recipients. Most of the recurrences were in patients who had multiple myeloma. Nine of the 11 patients were not treated or were not in remission at the time of transplantation or the existing malignancies had not been recognized at the time of transplantation. Generally, recurrences did not occur in patients treated 2 years before transplantation or who were in remission at the time of transplantation. Four patients had Hodgkin's disease treated an average of 5 years before transplantation, and none had recurrences; average follow-up was 3 years.

Of patients with skin cancer in Penn's (1983) review, the incidence of recurrence after transplantation was high (58%), and there was no correlation between the time of treatment before transplantation and the likelihood of recurrence. Of the six patients who had melanoma, three had recurrences. The three recurrences were in patients treated 21, 48 and 120 months before transplantation.

Currently, most clinicians offer transplantation to patients in renal failure after treatment of low-grade cancers, such as skin cancers or *in situ* cancers of the uterine cervix, and maintain on dialysis, for at least 2 years, patients who have had other cancers treated successfully. Patients with a cancer that has a poor prognosis in the general population probably should not be referred for transplantation at least until several years have passed from the time of successful treatment of malignancy.

REFERENCES

Adami, J., Frisch, M., Yuen, J., *et al.* (1995). Evidence of an association between non-Hodgkin's lymphoma and skin cancer. *B. M. J.* **310**, 1491.

Allison, A. S., Berman, L. D. and Levey, R. H. (1967). Increased tumour induction by adenovirus type 12 in thymectomized mice and mice treated with anti-lymphocyte serum. *Nature* **215**, 185.

Alloub, M. I., Barr, B. B. B., McLaren, K. M., *et al.* (1989). Human papillomavirus infection and cervical intraepithelial neoplasia in women with renal allografts. *B. M. J.* **298**, 153.

Al-Sulaiman, M. H. and Al-Khader, A. A. (1994). Kaposi's sarcoma in renal transplant recipients. *Transplant. Sci.* **4**, 46.

Armes, J. E., Angus, P., Southey, M. C., *et al.* (1994). Lymphoproliferative disease of donor origin arising in patients after orthotopic liver transplantation. *Cancer* **74**, 2436.

Armstrong, M. Y. K., Schwartz, R. S. and Beldotti, L. (1962). Neoplastic sequelae of allogenic disease: 111 histological events following transplantation of allogenic spleen cells. *Transplantation* **5**, 1380.

Balner, H. and Dersjant, H. (1969). Increased oncogenic effect of methylcholanthrene after treatment with anti-lymphocyte serum. *Nature* **224**, 376.

Beasley, R. P. (1982). Hepatitis B virus as the etiological agent in hepatocellular carcinoma: epidemiologic considerations. *Hepatology* **2**, 553.

Bentham, G. (1996). Association between incidence of non-Hodgkin's lymphoma and solar ultraviolet radiation in England and Wales. *B. M. J.* **312**, 1128.

Beveridge, T. (1983). Cyclosporin-A: an evaluation of clinical results. *Transplant. Proc.* **15**, 433.

Bird, A. G. and McLachlan, S. M. (1980). Cyclosporin A and Epstein-Barr virus. *Lancet* **2**, 418.

Bird, A. G., McLachlan, S. M. and Britton, S. (1981). Cyclosporine A promotes spontaneous outgrowth in vitro of Epstein-Barr virus induced-cell lines. *Nature* **289**, 300.

Birkeland, S. A., Bendtzen, K., Moller, B., *et al.* (1999). Interleukin-10 and posttransplant lymphoproliferative disorder after kidney transplantation. *Transplantation* **67**, 876.

Bouwes-Bavinck, J. N., Gissmann, L., Claas, F. H. J., *et al.* (1993). Relation between skin cancer, humoral responses to human papillomaviruses, and HLA class II molecules in renal transplant recipients. *J. Immunol.* **151**, 1579.

Bouwes-Bavinck, J. N., Hardie, D. R., Green, A., *et al.* (1996). The risk of skin cancer in renal transplant recipients in Queensland, Australia. *Transplantation* **61**, 715.

Bouwes-Bavinck, J. N., Vermeer, B. J., van der Woude, F. J., *et al.* (1991). Relation between skin cancer and HLA antigens in renal-transplant recipients. *N. Engl. J. Med.* **325**, 843.

Burnet, F. M. (1967). Immunological aspects of malignant disease. *Lancet* **1**, 1171.

Cacciarelli, T. V., Green, M., Jaffe, R., *et al.* (1998). Management of posttransplant lymphoproliferative disease in pediatric liver transplant recipients receiving primary tacrolimus (FK506) therapy. *Transplantation* **66**, 1047.

Calne, R. Y., Rollis, K., Thiru, S., *et al.* (1979). Cyclosporin A initially as the only immunosuppressant in 34 recipients of cadaveric organs: 32 kidneys, 2 pancreases and 2 livers. *Lancet* **2**, 1033.

Calne, R. Y., Thiru, S., McMaster, P., *et al.* (1978). Cyclosporin A in patients receiving renal allografts from cadaver donors. *Lancet* **2**, 1323.

Canfield, C. W., Hudnall, S. D., Colonna, J. O., *et al.* (1992). Fulminant Epstein-Barr virus-associated post-transplant lymphoproliferative disorders following OKT3 therapy. *Clin. Transplant.* **6**, 1.

Cantarovich, M., Barkun, J. S., Clark Forbes, R. D., *et al.* (1998). Successful treatment of post-transplant lymphoproliferative disorder with interferon-alpha and intravenous immunoglobulin. *Clin. Transplant.* **12**, 109.

Caterson, R. J., Furber, J., Murray, J., *et al.* (1984). Carcinoma of the vulva in two young renal allograft recipients. *Transplant. Proc.* **16**, 559.

Cerilli, G. J. and Treat, R. C. (1969). The effect of antilymphocyte serum on the induction and growth of tumour in the adult mouse. *Transplantation* **8**, 774.

Chang, Y., Cesarman, E., Pessin, M. S., *et al.* (1994). Identification of herpesvirus-like DNA sequences in AIDS-associated Kaposi's sarcoma. *Science* **266**, 1865.

Chui, A. K. K., Herbertt, K., Wang, L. S., *et al.* (1999). Risk of tumour transmission in transplantation from donors with primary brain tumours—an Australian and New Zealand Registry Report. *Transplant. Proc.* **31**, 1266.

Cleary, M. L. and Sklar, J. (1984). Lymphoproliferative disorders in cardiac transplant recipients are multiclonal lymphomas. *Lancet* **2**, 489.

Crawford, D. H., Thomas, J. A., Janossy, G., *et al.* (1980). Epstein-Barr virus nuclear antigen positive lymphoma after Cyclosporin A treatment in patient with renal allograft. *Lancet* **1**, 1355.

Dantal, J., Hourmant, M., Cantarovich, D., *et al.* (1998). Effect of long term immunosuppression in kidney-graft recipients on cancer incidence: randomised comparison of two cyclosporin regimens. *Lancet* **531**, 623.

DiBisceglie, A. M. (1997). Hepatitis C and hepatocellular carcinoma. *Hepatology* **26**, 34S.

Doak, P. B., Montgomerie, J. L., North, J. D. K., *et al.* (1968). Reticulum cell sarcoma after renal homotransplantation and azathioprine and prednisone therapy. *B. M. J.* **4**, 746.

Dunn, S. P. and Krueger, L. J. (1998). Immunosuppression of paediatric liver transplant recipients: minimising the risk of posttransplant lymphoproliferative disorders. *Transplant. Immunol. Lett.* **14**, 5.

Dunnill, M. S., Millard, P. R. and Oliver, D. (1977). Acquired cystic disease of the kidneys: a hazard of long-term intermittent maintenance haemodialysis. *J. Clin. Pathol.* **30**, 868.

Ehrlich, P. (1909). Ueber den jetzigen stand der karzinomforchung. *Ned. Tijdschr. Geneeskd.* **1**, 273.

Freise, C. E., Ferrell, L., Liu, T., *et al.* (1999). Effect of systemic cyclosporine on tumour recurrence after liver transplantation in a model of hepatocellular carcinoma. *Transplantation* **67**, 510.

Gaya, S. B. M., Rees, A. J., Lechler, G., *et al.* (1995). Malignant disease in patients with long-term renal transplants. *Transplantation* **59**, 1705.

Gissman, L., Wolnik, H., Ikenberg, H., *et al.* (1983). Human papillomavirus types 6 and 11 DNA sequence in genital and laryngeal papillomas and in some cervical cancers. *Proc. Natl. Acad. Sci. U. S. A.* **80**, 560.

Glover, M. T., Deeks, J. T., Raftery, M. J., *et al.* (1997). Immunosuppression and risk of non-melanoma skin cancer in renal transplant recipients. *Lancet* **349**, 398.

Green, M., Reyes, J., Todo, R., *et al.* (1996). Use of quantitative competitive PCR (QC-PCR) to guide preemptive therapy (PT) against EBV associated post-transplant lymphoproliferative disorders (PTLD) after intestinal transplantation (ITx) in children. *Transplant. Proc.* **28**, 2759.

Greene, M. H., Young, T. I. and Clark, W. H., Jr. (1981). Malignant melanoma in renal transplant recipients. *Lancet* **1**, 1196.

Han, C. W., Imamura, M., Hashino, S., *et al.* (1995). Differential effects of the immunosuppressants cyclosporin A, FK 506 and KM 2210 on cytokine gene expression. *Bone Marrow Transplant.* **15**, 733.

Hanto, D., Frizzera, G., Gajl-Peczalska, K., *et al.* (1981). EBV in the pathogenesis of polyclonal "post-transplant lymphoma." *Transplant. Proc.* **13**, 764.

Hanto, D. W., Gajl-Peczalska, K. J., Frizzera, G., *et al.* (1983). Epstein-Barr virus induced polyclonal and monoclonal B-cell lymphoproliferative diseases occurring after renal transplantation: clinical, pathologic and virologic findings and implications for therapy. *Ann. Surg.* **198**, 356.

Hardie, I. R., Strong, R. W., Hartley, L. C. J., *et al.* (1980). Skin cancer in caucasian renal allograft recipients living in a subtropical climate. *Surgery* **87**, 177.

Hartevelt, M. M., Bavinck-Bouwes, J. N., Kootte, A. M. M., *et al.* (1990). Incidence of skin cancer after renal transplantation in The Netherlands. *Transplantation* **49**, 506.

Healey, P. J. and Davis, C. L. (1998). Transmission of tumours by transplantation. *Lancet* **352**, 2.

Henle, G., Henle, W. and Diehl, V. (1968). Relation of Burkitt's tumor-associated herpes-type virus to infectious mononucleosis. *Proc. Natl. Acad. Sci. U. S. A.* **59**, 94.

Herr, H. W., Engen, D. E. and Hostetler, J. (1979). Malignancy in uremia: dialysis versus transplantation. *J. Urol.* **121**, 584.

Hibberd, P. L. (1992). Symptomatic cytomegalovirus disease in the cytomegalovirus antibody sero-positive renal transplant recipient treated with OKT3. *Transplantation* **53**, 68.

Hjelle, B., Evans-Holm, M., Yen, T. S., *et al.* (1989). A poorly differentiated lymphoma of donor origin in a renal allograft recipient. *Transplantation* **47**, 945.

Hochberg, F. H., Miller, G., Schooley, R. I., *et al.* (1983). Central-nervous-system lymphoma related to Epstein-Barr virus. *N. Engl. J. Med.* **309**, 745.

Hojo, M., Morimoto, T., Maluccio, M., *et al.* (1999). Cyclosporine induces cancer progression by a cell-autonomous mechanism. *Nature* **397**, 530.

Hong, W. K., Lippman, S. M., Itri, L. M., *et al.* (1990). Prevention of second primary tumors with isotretinoin in squamous-cell carcinoma of the head and neck. *N. Engl. J. Med.* **323**, 795.

Hoover, R. and Fraumeni, J. F. (1983). Risk of cancer in renal-transplant recipients. *Lancet* **2**, 69.

Hoshida, Y., Tsukuma, H., Yasunaga, Y., *et al.* (1997). Cancer risk after renal transplant in Japan. *Int. J. Cancer* **71**, 517.

International Consensus Document. (1997). Standardization of organ donor screening to prevent transmission of neoplastic diseases. Select Committee of Experts in the organisational aspects of cooperation in Organ Transplantation, Council of Europe. *Transplant. Newsletter* **2**, 4.

Iseki, K., Osawa, A. and Fukiyama, K. (1993). Evidence for increased cancer deaths in chronic dialysis patients. *Am. J. Kidney Dis.* **22**, 308.

Ishikawa, I. (1991). Uremic acquired renal cystic disease. *Nephron* **58**, 257.

Jensen, M. K. (1967). Chromosome studies in patients treated with azathioprine and amethopterin. *Acta Med. Scand.* **182**, 445.

Kaminski, M. S., Zasadny, K. R., Francis, I. R., *et al.* (1993). Radioimmunotherapy of B-cell lymphoma with [131I] anti-B1 (anti-CD20) antibody. *N. Engl. J. Med.* **329**, 459.

Keast, D. (1970). Immunosurveillance and cancer. *Lancet* **2**, 710.

Kedda, M. A., Margolius, L., Kew, M. C., *et al.* (1996). Kaposi's sarcoma-associated herpesvirus in Kaposi's sarcoma occurring in immunosuppressed renal transplant recipients. *Clin. Transplant.* **10**, 429.

Kelly, G. E., Mahony, J. F., Sheil, A. G. R., *et al.* (1987). Risk factors for skin carcinogenesis in immunosuppressed kidney transplant recipients. *Clin. Transpl.* **1**, 271.

Kelly, J. W., Sabto, J., Gurr, F. W., *et al.* (1991). Retinoids to prevent skin cancer in organ transplant recipients. *Lancet* **338**, 1407.

Kersey, J. H., Spector, B. D. and Good, R. A. (1973). Immunodeficiency and cancer. *Adv. Cancer Res.* **18**, 211.

Kinlen, L., Doll, R. and Peto, J. (1983). The incidence of tumours in human transplant recipients. *Lancet* **1**, 1196.

Kinlen, L. J., Eastwood, J. B., Kerr, D. N. S., *et al.* (1980). Cancer in patients receiving dialysis. *B. M. J.* **2**, 1401.

Kinlen, L. J., Sheil, A. G. R., Peto, J., *et al.* (1979). Collaborative United Kingdom-Australasian study of cancer in patients treated with immunosuppressive drugs. *B. M. J.* **2**, 1461.

Kleim, V. , Thon, W., Krautzig, S., *et al.* (1996). High mortality from urothelial carcinoma despite regular tumor screening in patients with analgesic nephropathy after renal transplantation. *Transpl. Int.* **9**, 231.

Klein, G. and Purtilo, D. (1981). Summary: symposium on Epstein-Barr virus induced lymphoproliferative diseases in immuno deficient patients. *Cancer Res.* **41**, 4302.

Koranda, F. C., Dehmel, E. M., Kahn, G., *et al.* (1974). Cutaneous complications in immunosuppressed renal homograft recipients. *J. A. M. A.* **229**, 419.

Lal, M., Alamdar, S., Ali, B., *et al.* (1998). Postrenal transplant malignancies in a living-related donor program. *Transplant. Proc.* **30**, 822.

Law, L. W., Ting, R. C. and Allison, A. C. (1968). Effects of antilymphocyte serum on induction of tumours and leukaemia by murine sarcoma virus. *Nature* **220**, 611.

Lidner, A., Farewell, V. T. and Sherrard, D. J. (1981). High incidence of neoplasia in uremic patients receiving long-term dialysis. *Nephron* **27**, 292.

Lippman, S. M. and Meyskens, F. L., Jr. (1987). Treatment of advanced squamous cell carcinoma of the skin with isotretinoin. *Ann. Intern. Med.* **107**, 499.

List, A. F., Greco, F. A. and Vogler, L. B. (1987). Lymphoproliferative diseases in immuno-compromised hosts: the role of Epstein-Barr virus. *J. Clin. Oncol.* **5**, 1673.

London, N. J., Farmery, S. M., Well, E. J., *et al.* (1995). Risk of neoplasia in transplant patients. *Lancet* **346**, 403.

Lugo-Janer, G., Sanchez, J. L. and Santiago-Delpin, E. (1991). Prevalence and clinical spectrum of skin diseases in kidney transplant recipients. *J. Am. Acad. Dermatol.* **24**, 410.

Lutzner, M. A., Orth, G. and Dutronquay, V. (1983). Detection of human papillomavirus type 5 DNA in skin cancers of an immunosuppressed renal allograft recipient. *Lancet* **2**, 422.

Macleod, A. M. and Catto, G. R. (1988). Cancer after transplantation: the risks are small. *B. M. J.* **297**, 4.

Martin, D. C., Rubini, M. and Rosen, V. J. (1965). Cadaveric renal homotransplantation with inadvertent transplantation of carcinoma. *J. A. M. A.* **192**, 752.4

Matas, A. J., Simmons, R. L., Kjellstrand, C. M., *et al.* (1975). Increased incidence of malignancy during chronic renal failure. *Lancet* **1**, 883.

McDiarmid, S. V., Jordan, S., Lee, G. S., *et al.* (1998). Prevention and pre-emptive therapy of posttransplant lymphoproliferative disease in paediatric liver recipients. *Transplantation* **66**, 1604.

McEwan, A. and Petty, L. G. (1972). Oncogenicity of immunosuppressive drugs. *Lancet* **1**, 326.

McPhaul, J. J., McIntosh, D. A. and Hall, W. (1965). Tissue transplantation still vexes. *N. Engl. J. Med.* **272**, 105.

Meduri, G., Fromentin, L., Vieillefond, A., *et al.* (1991). Donor-related non-Hodgkin's lymphoma in a renal allograft recipient. *Transplant. Proc.* **23**, 2649.

Mentzer, S. J., Longtine, J., Fingeroth, J., *et al.* (1996). Immunoblastic lymphoma of donor origin in the allograft after lung transplantation. *Transplantation* **61**, 1720.

Merrill, J. P. (1968). The immunologic capability of uremic patients. *Cancer Res.* **28**, 1449.

Miach, P. J., Dawborn, J. K. and Xipell, J. (1976). Neoplasia in patients with chronic renal failure on long-term dialysis. *Clin. Nephrol.* **5**, 101.

Montagnino, G., Lorca, E., Tarantino, A., *et al.* (1996). Cancer incidence in 854 kidney transplant recipients from a single institution: comparison with normal population and with patients under dialytic treatment. *Clin. Transpl.* **10**, 461.

Moore, K. W., Russet, F. and Banchereau, J. (1991). Evolving principles in immunopathology: interleukin 10 and its relationship to Epstein-Barr virus protein BCFR1. *Semin. Immunopathol.* **13**, 157.

Mullen, D. L., Silverberg, S. G., Penn, I., *et al.* (1976). Squamous cell carcinoma of the skin and lip in renal homograft recipients. *Cancer* **37**, 729.

Nabel, G. J. (1999). A transformed view of cyclosporine. *Nature* **397**, 471.

Nagington, J. and Gray, J. (1980). Cyclosporin A, immunosuppression, Epstein-Barr antibody and lymphoma. *Lancet* **1**, 536.

Nalesnik, M. A., Jaffe, R., Starzl, T. E., *et al.* (1988). The pathology of post transplant lymphoproliferative disorders occurring in the setting of cyclosporine A prednisone immunosuppression. *Am. J. Pathol.* **133**, 173.

Newell, K. A., Alonso, E. M., Whittington, P. F., *et al.* (1996). Post-transplant lymphoproliferative disease in pediatric liver transplantation. *Transplantation* **62**, 370.

Nixon, R. L., Dorevitch, A. P. and Marks, R. (1986). Squamous cell carcinoma of the skin: accuracy of clinical diagnosis and outcome of follow-up in Australia. *Med. J. Aust.* **144**, 235.

Obasek, S., Favre, M., Jabsosnska, S., *et al.* (1988). Human papillomavirus type 2-associated basal cell carcinoma in two immunosuppressed patients. *Arch. Dermatol.* **124**, 930.

Opelz, G. and Henderson, R. (1993). Incidence of non-Hodgkin's lymphoma in kidney and heart transplant recipients. *Lancet* **342**, 1514.

Papadopoulos, E. B., Ladanyi, M., Emanuel, D., *et al.* (1994). Infusions of donor leukocytes to treat Epstein-Barr virus-associated lymphoproliferative disorders after allogenic bone marrow transplantation. *N. Engl. J. Med.* **330**, 1185.

Penn, I. (1975). Incidence of malignancies in transplant recipients. *Transplant. Proc.* **7**, 323.

Penn, I. (1977a). Development of cancer as a complication of clinical transplantation. *Transplant. Proc.* **9**, 1121.

Penn, I. (1977b). Transplantation in patients with primary renal malignancies. *Transplantation* **24**, 424.

Penn, I. (1980). Some contributions of transplantation to our knowledge of cancer. *Transplant. Proc.* **12**, 676.

Penn, I. (1981). Malignant lymphomas in organ transplant recipients. *Transplant. Proc.* **13**, 736.

Penn, I. (1983). Kaposi's sarcoma in immunosuppressed patients. *J. Clin. Lab. Immunol.* **12**, 1.

Penn, I. (1987). Cancers following cyclosporine therapy. *Transplantation* **43**, 32.

Penn, I. (1995a). Sarcomas in organ allograft recipients. *Transplantation* **60**, 1485.

Penn, I. (1995b). Primary kidney tumors before and after renal transplantation. *Transplantation* **59**, 480.

Penn, I. and Brunson, M. E. (1988). Cancers after cyclosporine therapy. *Transplant. Proc.* **3**, 885.

Penn, I., Halgrimson, C. G. and Starzl, T. E. (1971). De novo malignant tumors in organ transplant recipients. *Transplant. Proc.* **3**, 773.

Penn, I., Hammond, W., Brettschneider, L., *et al.* (1969). Malignant lymphomas in transplantation patients. *Transplant. Proc.* **1**, 106.

Qunibi, W., Akhtar, M., Sheth, K., *et al.* (1988). Kaposi's sarcoma: the most common tumor after renal transplantation in Saudi Arabia. *Am. J. Med.* **84**, 225.

Rabbat, A. G. and Jeejeebhoy, H. F. (1970). Heterologous antilymphocyte serum (ALS) hastens the appearance of methylcholanthrene-induced tumours in mice. *Transplantation* **9**, 164.

Regamey, N., Tamm, M., Wernli, M., *et al.* (1998). Transmission of human herpesvirus 8 infection from renal-transplant donors to recipients. *N. Engl. J. Med.* **339**, 1358.

Roeger, L. S., Sheil, A. G. R., Disney, A. P. S., *et al.* (1992). Risk factors associated with the development of squamous cell carcinomas in immunosuppressed renal transplant recipients. *Clin. Transpl.* **6**, 202.

Rook, A. H., Jaworsky, C., Nguyen, T., *et al.* (1995). Beneficial effect of low-dose systemic retinoid in combination with topical tretinoin for the treatment and prophylaxis of premalignant and malignant skin lesions in renal transplant recipients. *Transplantation* **59**, 714.

Schneck, S. A. and Penn, I. (1971). De novo brain tumours in renal transplant recipients. *Lancet* **1**, 983.

Schwartz, R. S. (1972). Immunoregulation, oncogenic viruses and malignant lymphomas. *Lancet* **1**, 1266.

Schwartz, R. S. and Beldotti, L. (1965). Malignant lymphomas following allogenic disease: transition from an immunological to a neoplastic disorder. *Science* **149**, 1511.

Shapiro, R. S., Chauvenet, A., McGuire, W., *et al.* (1988). Treatment of B-cell lymphoproliferative disorders with interferon alfa and intravenous gamma globulin. *N. Engl. J. Med.* **318**, 1334.

Sheil, A. G. R. (1977). Cancer in renal allograft recipients in Australia and New Zealand. *Transplant. Proc.* **9**, 1133.

Sheil, A. G. R. (1991). *In The XIV Report of the Australia and New Zealand Combined Dialysis and Transplant Registry*, (A. P. S. Disney, ed.), p. 100, Queen Elizabeth Hospital, Woodville, South Australia.

Sheil, A. G. R. (1997). Cancer report 1997. *In The Twentieth Annual Report: Australia and New Zealand Dialysis and Transplant Registry*, (A. P. S. Disney, ed.), p. 138, Queen Elizabeth Hospital, Adelaide, South Australia.

Sheil, A. G. R. (1999). Patterns of malignancies following renal transplantation. *Transplant. Proc.* **31**, 1263.

Sheil, A. G. R., Disney, A. P. S., Mathew, T. H., *et al.* (1997). Lymphoma incidence, cyclosporine and the evolution and major impact of malignancy following organ transplantation. *Transplant. Proc.* **29**, 825.

Sheil, A. G. R., Mahony, J. F., Horvath, J. S., *et al.* (1979). Cancer and survival after cadaveric donor renal transplantation. *Transplant. Proc.* **11**, 1052.

Shuttleworth, D., Marks, R., Griffin, P. J. A., *et al.* (1988). Treatment of cutaneous neoplasia with etretinate in renal transplant recipients. *Q. J. M.* **257**, 717.

Sillman, F., Stanck, A., Sedlis, A., *et al.* (1984). The relationship between human papillomavirus and lower genital intraepithelial neoplasia in immunosuppressed women. *Am. J. Obstet. Gynaecol.* **150**, 300.

Slavis, S. A., Novick, A. C., Steinmuller, D. R., *et al.* (1990). Outcome of renal transplantation in patients with a functioning graft for 20 years or more. *J. Urol.* **144**, 20.

Slifkin, R. F., Goldberg, J., Neff, M. S., *et al.* (1977). Malignancy in end-stage renal disease. *Trans. Am. Soc. Artif. Intern. Organs* **23**, 34.

Sloan, G. M., Cole, P. and Wilson, R. E. (1977). Risk indicators of de novo malignancy in renal transplant recipients. *Transplant. Proc.* **9**, 1129.

Smithers, D. W. and Field, E. O. (1969). Immunosuppression and cancer. *Lancet* **1**, 672.

Sontheimer, R. D., Bergstresser, P. R., Gailiunas, P., *et al.* (1984). Perturbation of epidermal Langerhans cells in immunosuppressed human renal allograft recipients. *Transplantation* **37**, 168.

Spencer, E. S. and Anderson, H. K. (1970). Clinically evident, nonterminal infections with herpes viruses and the wart virus in immunosuppressed renal allograft recipients. *B. M. J.* **3**, 251.

Spiro, I. J., Yandell, D. W., Li, C., *et al.* (1993). Brief report: lymphoma of donor origin occurring in the porta hepatis of a transplanted liver. *N. Engl. J. Med.* **329**, 27.

Starzl, T. E., Demetris, A. J., Murase, N., *et al.* (1992). Cell migration, chimerism, and graft acceptance. *Lancet* **339**, 1579.

Starzl, T. E., Porter, K. A., Iwatsuki, S., *et al.* (1984). Reversibility of lymphomas and lymphoproliferative lesions developing under cyclosporin-steroid therapy. *Lancet* **1**, 583.

Sutherland, G. A., Glass, J. and Gabriel, R. (1977). Increased incidence of malignancy in chronic renal failure. *Nephron* **18**, 182.

Ternesten-Bratel, A., Kjellstrom, C. and Ricksten, A. (1998). Specific expression of Epstein-Barr virus in cutaneous squamous cell carcinomas from heart transplant recipients. *Transplantation* **66**, 1524.

Thiru, S., Calne, R. Y. and Nagington, J. (1981). Lymphoma in renal allograft patients treated with cyclosporin A as one of the immunosuppressive agents. *Transplant. Proc.* **13**, 359.

Thomas, D. W., Ramsahoye, B., Jasani, B. and Lim, S. (1995). Epstein-Barr virus in squamous cell carcinoma after renal transplantation. *Transplantation* **60**, 390.

Thomas, L. (1959). *In Cellular and Humoral Aspects of the Hypertensive States*, (H. S. Lawrence, ed.), p. 529, Cassell, London.

Thompson, J. F., Allen, R., Morris, P. J., *et al.* (1985). Skin cancer in renal transplant patients treated with cyclosporin. *Lancet* **1**, 158.

Trush, M. A., Mimnaugh, E. G. and Gram, T. E. (1982). Activation of pharmacologic agents to radical intermediates. *Biochem. Pharmacol.* **31**, 3335.

Vogt, P., Frei, U., Repp, H., *et al.* (1990). Malignant tumours in renal transplant recipients receiving cyclosporin: survey of 598 first-kidney transplantations. *Nephrol. Dial. Transplant.* **5**, 282.

Walder, B. K., Robertson, M. R. and Jeremy, D. (1971). Skin cancer and immunosuppression. *Lancet* **2**, 1282.

Walford, R. L. (1966). Increased incidence of lymphoma after injections of mice with cells differing at weak histocompatibility loci. *Science* **152**, 78.

Waterson, A. P. (1983). Acquired immune deficiency syndrome. *B. M. J.* **286**, 743.

Wedderburn, N. (1970). Effect of concurrent malarial infection on development of virus-induced lymphoma in Balb-C mice. *Lancet* **2**, 1114.

Wheeler, G. P., Bowdon, B. J. and Adamson, D. J. (1972). Comparison of the effects of several inhibitors of the synthesis of nucleic acids upon the viability and progression through the cell cycle of cultures H. Ep. No. 2 cells. *Cancer Res.* **32**, 2661.

Wilson, R. E., Hager, E. B., Hampers, C. L., *et al.* (1968). Immunologic rejection of human cancer transplanted with a renal allograft. *N. Engl. J. Med.* **278**, 479.

Wilson, W. E. C., Kirkpatrick, C. H. and Talmage, D. W. (1965). Suppression of immunologic responsiveness in uraemia. *Ann. Intern. Med.* **62**, 1.

Witherspoon, R. P., Deeg, H. J. and Store, R. (1994). Secondary malignancies after marrow transplantation for leukemia or aplastic anemia. *Transplantation* **57**, 1413.

Zukoski, C. F., Killen, D. A., Ginn, E., *et al.* (1970). Transplanted carcinoma in an immunosuppressed patient. *Transplantation* **9**, 71.

Renal and Pancreas Transplantation for Diabetic Nephropathy

Eli A. Friedman • Amy L. Friedman • Bruce G. Sommer

Diabetes Prevalence and Type

Diabetes mellitus leads the causes of end-stage renal disease (ESRD) in the United States, Japan and most nations in industrialized Europe. As tabulated in the United States Renal Data System (USRDS) 1999 Report, of 79,102 patients begun on therapy for ESRD during 1997, 33,096 (41.8%) had diabetes, an *incidence* rate of 120 per 1 million population (USRDS, 1999; Fig. 36–1). Reflecting their relatively higher death rate compared with patients with other causes of ESRD, the *prevalence* of diabetic ESRD patients in the United States on December 31, 1997, was 33.2% (100,892 of 304,083 patients) (USRDS, 1999). Glomerulonephritis and hypertensive renal disease rank below diabetes in frequency of diagnosis among new ESRD patients, substantiating the following statement by Mauer and Chavers (1985): "Diabetes is the most important cause of ESRD in the Western world."

According to the *National Diabetes Fact Sheet* (Centers for Disease Control, 1998), more than 16 million people in the United States have diabetes, of whom one third are unaware of their disorder. During 1999, in the United States, it was estimated that 798,000 people would have newly diagnosed diabetes, and 187,000 people would die from diabetes. Depending on age, race and gender, diabetes in 1996 ranked from eighth (white men 45–65 years old) to fourth (black

women ≥45 years old) leading cause of death (National Center for Health Statistics, 1999). Health care expenditures for diabetes in the United States range from $98 billion to $150 billion annually. The full impact of diabetic complications is unassessed but includes in addition to 33,096 new cases of ESRD, 56,000 lower limb amputations and 24,000 cases of blindness (American Diabetes Association, 1999).

Excessive morbidity and mortality encountered in the treatment of patients with diabetes and failed kidneys previously discouraged and presently retards their acceptance for renal transplantation because of the consensus belief that rehabilitation in these patients is poor. Current understanding of the importance of careful medical regulation of hypertension and hyperglycemia has improved the peritransplant and posttransplant outcome in diabetic recipients to the extent that renal transplantation is viewed as the preferred therapy for ESRD in diabetes.

Medicare statistics counted diabetic nephropathy as the diagnosis listed for 1,607 of 8,058 (20.7%) kidney transplants performed in 1989 in the United States; the proportion of kidney recipients with diabetes rose to 24.1% (2,896 of 11,996) in 1996. In Europe, the proportion of kidney transplants performed in diabetic recipients is smaller (about 18%). Accompanying the growing acceptance of kidney transplantation in diabetics was a mounting success rate in the 1990s of pancreatic transplants in type 1 diabetes, converting what previously was considered experimental surgery into established therapy (see later).

The American Diabetes Association (1999) reclassified diabetes; the intent of the new diagnostic criteria is to help remedy the problem of undiagnosed diabetes as well as to transform a system of diagnosis based on treatment to one based on disease cause. As outlined by the American Diabetes Association, there are four major categories of diabetes: (1) type 1 (absolute insulin deficiency), (2) type 2 (insulin resistance with an insulin secretory defect), (3) other specific types and (4) gestational diabetes mellitus. Key changes from former diagnostic criteria are the fasting glucose level (≥126 mg/dl) for diagnosis of diabetes plus the suggestion that oral glucose tolerance tests are not essential for routine practice to make the diagnosis of diabetes.

Because the severity and type of diabetes can change over time, it is important to ensure the early recognition and management of glycemic disorders. Screening programs that employ fasting plasma glucose concentrations of greater than or equal to 110 mg/dl as a marker of insulin resistance should help identify not only patients with hyperglycemia, but also patients with insulin resistance without significant hyperglycemia. If hemoglobin A_{1c} levels are normal, patients in this category are at increased risk for developing diabetes-induced macrovascular complications and may benefit from active intervention to reduce cardiac risk factors (Peters and Schriger, 1998).

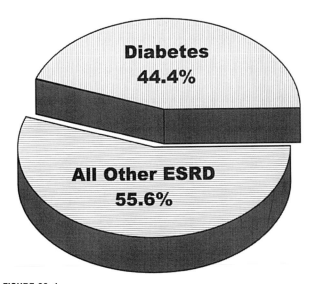

FIGURE 36–1

End-stage renal disease (ESRD) is the termination of progressive diabetic nephropathy. Diabetes heads the list of incident ESRD cases reported to the United States Renal Data System (USRDS), accounting for 44.4% of newly treated patients in 1997. (Data from USRDS by authors.)

Type 1 diabetes is a synonym for insulin-dependent diabetes mellitus (IDDM, juvenile diabetes), and *type 2 diabetes* is a synonym for non–insulin-dependent diabetes mellitus (NIDDM, maturity-onset diabetes); there are multiple difficulties with efforts to segregate diabetes in clinical practice into these two main types. It is not unusual to follow the course of patients who evolve over several years from purportedly type 2 to type 1 diabetes. The confounding term *type 1½ diabetes* has been proposed to cover the blurry interface between type 1 and type 2 diabetes (Juneja and Palmer, 1999). Careful studies of nonobese adults with onset of diabetes before age 40 permit confident classification in only 25% of subjects (Dussoix *et al.*, 1997).

Fewer than 10% of diabetics in the United States are thought to have type 1 diabetes. Laboratory confirmation of type 1 diabetes according to the National Diabetes Data Group is provided by low plasma insulin levels, circulating islet cell antibody (ICA) titers and characteristic HLA DR types (DR3, DR4, DQβ). Using these criteria in 100 consecutive patients aged 13 to 70 years at the time of starting insulin therapy, Wilson and colleagues found that 70 patients in their series who were diagnosed before the age of 40 fit the National Diabetes Data Group stereotype for type 1 diabetes relatively well; 88% of those who were younger than age 20 at diagnosis were ICA positive, one third were DR3/DR4 heterozygotes and only 6% had neither high-risk antigen (Wilson *et al.*, 1985). There was difficulty, however, in adopting National Diabetes Data Group guidelines to patients older than age 40 at diagnosis; only one fifth were ICA positive, and less than one third were DR3/DR4 heterozygotes.

More than 90% of diabetic Americans have type 2 diabetes (NIDDM) (American Diabetes Association, 1988), defined by the American Diabetes Association as afflicting people who are "usually older than 30 years at diagnosis, obese, and have relatively few classic symptoms. They are not prone to ketoacidosis except during periods of stress. Although not dependent on exogenous insulin for survival, they may require it for adequate control of hyperglycemia." Longitudinal studies of patients with type 2 diabetes reveal that insulin resistance is a necessary prelude, but hyperglycemia does not develop unless there is a defect (inherited or acquired) in insulin resistance (Anonymous, 1989). Pointing out the interrelationship between glucose intolerance with hyperinsulinemia, hyperlipidemia and hypertension, Reaven (1988) proposed the term *syndrome X* to tie together the metabolic perturbations that result in coronary artery disease and other vascular disorders in diabetes. Throughout the world, a pandemic of type 2 diabetes is emerging as a major health care crisis (Berger *et al.*, 1999; Rosenbloom *et al.*, 1999). The direct and indirect costs attributed to diabetes in 1997 totaled $44.1 billion and comprised $7.7 billion for diabetes and acute glycemic care, $11.8 billion because of the excess prevalence of related chronic complications, and $24.6 billion because of the excess prevalence of general medical conditions (American Diabetes Association, 1998; Scheen, 1999).

Complicating the care of diabetic patients is the extensive overlap in presenting signs and symptoms, which often blurs the distinction between diabetes types. At one extreme of the diagnostic spectrum, maturity-onset diabetes of the young (MODY) is an entity simulating type 1 diabetes that occurs as an autosomal dominant abnormality in whites, leading to macrovascular and microvascular disorders (Tattersall and Mansell, 1991). Patients with MODY are insulinopenic and hypersensitive to sulfonylureas. In Japan, type 2 diabetes occurs frequently in patients younger than age 30 who are nonobese (Takahashi *et al.*, 1990); Nagai (1982) reported that of 551 patients diagnosed as diabetic before the age of 30,

337 (61.2%) had type 2 diabetes. Diabetic retinopathy and nephropathy are as frequent in Japanese patients with young-onset type 2 diabetes as in patients with type 1 diabetes. According to Abourizk and Dunn (1990), "Clinicians treating diabetic patients encounter numerous insulin-taking diabetic subjects who clinically are neither IDDM nor NIDDM." Based on a review of 348 consecutive diabetic patients of mean age 53 years, evaluated in Hartford, Connecticut, diabetes type could not be established in 35% of whites, 57% of blacks, and 59% of Hispanics (Abourizk and Dunn, 1990). Calling for a new classification of diabetes, Abourizk and Dunn (1990) remarked that current criteria for assigning diabetes types "have been neither useful for clinicians nor illuminating for researchers." Throughout the world, most (80–100% depending on race [all full-blooded Native Americans with diabetes have type 2]) patients with diabetes have type 2 diabetes. In type 1 diabetes and type 2 diabetes, renal failure secondary to nodular and diffuse intercapillary glomerular sclerosis may develop, and in each diabetes type, a sequence of microalbuminuria, followed by fixed proteinuria, then azotemia, has been described (Christensen *et al.*, 1987; Mogensen, 1992; Mogensen *et al.*, 1983).

Natural History of Diabetic Nephropathy

Building on studies in the Pima Indian tribe (Bennett, 1999) and black Americans living in Brooklyn, New York (Palmisano and Lebovitz, 1990), knowledge of the time course of renal disease in type 2 diabetes has expanded to permit a longitudinal picture equivalent to the careful observational reports of type 1 diabetic children and young adults. Previous extrapolations drawn from animal models, mainly streptozotocin-induced diabetic rats and alloxan-induced diabetic dogs, are flawed by differences between species—nodular intercapillary glomerulosclerosis is not a component of induced diabetes in rats, the animal model employed most frequently (van Zwieten, 1999). Five progressive stages of renal involvement in type 1 diabetes are proposed by Mogensen (1999).

STAGE 1: ACUTE RENAL HYPERTROPHY AND HYPERFUNCTION

At initial diagnosis of type 1 diabetes, although blood pressure is normal, increased kidney and glomerular size and elevated glomerular filtration rate (GFR) by 20 to 50% are noted universally (Mogensen and Christensen, 1984). Increased inulin clearances first were recognized in the 1930s and 1940s (Cambier, 1934; Spuhler, 1946) and subsequently confirmed as glomerular hyperfiltration using radionuclide techniques (Ditzel and Schwartz, 1967; Fiaschi *et al.*, 1952; Mogensen, 1971). Nephromegaly is the hallmark of developing glomerulopathy (Baumgartl *et al.*, 1998). No single mechanism explains both the increase in renal size and the glomerular hyperfiltration, although a correlation with hyperglycemia has been noted (Wiseman *et al.*, 1984; Fig. 36–2). That hyperglycemia and hyperfiltration may be linked is suggested by the observation that GFR starts to decline within 8 days of initiation of insulin therapy (Christiansen *et al.*, 1981, 1982; Mogensen and Anderson, 1975; Wiseman *et al.*, 1985) and falls further during 3 months of therapy (Mogensen and Anderson, 1975). Typical insulin therapy yielding good-to-fair glucose control is associated with a persistently elevated GFR in 25 to 40% of patients, however (Mogensen and Christensen, 1984; Mogensen *et al.*, 1981, 1983; Wiseman *et al.*, 1984), and it is this subgroup of patients with hyperfil-

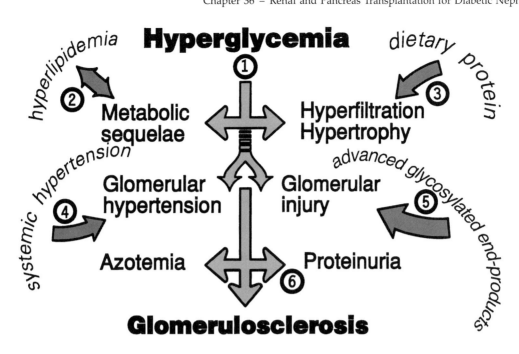

FIGURE 36–2

Postulated pathogenesis of diabetic glomerulopathy includes hemodynamic and metabolic perturbations. Potential intervention points in the sequence are numbered: (1) Establishment of euglycemia prevents all microvascular and macrovascular complications in animal models of diabetes. Whether in human diabetes some organ damage is predetermined genetically, even in the absence of hyperglycemia, is unknown. (2) Control of hyperlipidemia in nephrosis and post–kidney transplant patients retards macrovascular complications. That plasma lipid reduction is beneficial in type 1 diabetes and/or type 2 diabetes is inferred from evidence-based trials in other disorders. (3) Reduction in dietary protein retards progression of nephropathy in animal models of diabetes and has been shown to slow the rate of glomerular filtration rate loss in type 1 diabetes. (4) Reduction in blood pressure is a mainstay of the clinical regimen for all stages of diabetic nephropathy. Advocacy of angiotensin-converting enzyme inhibitors as first-line therapy in hypertensive diabetics with or without clinical nephropathy is the stated policy of the American Diabetes Association. (5) Clinical trials of drugs (aminoguanidine) to block formation of advanced glycosylated end products have been inconclusive in terms of retarding progression of nephropathy in type 1 diabetes and type 2 diabetes or in reducing mortality in diabetic ESRD patients on hemodialysis. (6) Erythropoietin effectively raises red cell mass, improving well-being and work effort in the anemia of renal insufficiency.

tration who go on to manifest reductions in GFR (Azevedo and Gross, 1991; Jones et al., 1991; Mogensen and Christensen, 1984), culminating in clinical nephropathy (proteinuria and azotemia) (Mogensen, 1986; Mogensen and Christensen, 1984; Mogensen et al., 1988). Most (60–70%) patients with type 1 diabetes do not progress to clinical nephropathy (Mogensen and Christensen, 1984), supporting the inference that glomerular hyperfiltration probably is not an independent risk factor for development of progressive nephropathy (Lafferty and Brenner, 1990; Messent et al., 1991).

Healthy adults excrete less than 25 mg of albumin daily. Microalbuminuria—urinary protein losses ranging from 30 to 200 mg/d—is a sign of renal damage in diabetes of both types, hypertension and other renal disorders that predicts renal insufficiency and ultimately ESRD. The Albustix test—commonly employed for screening for proteinuria—detects protein excretion greater than 250 mg/24 h, about 50% of which is albumin, defining the lower limit of macroalbuminuria. Otherwise, asymptomatic diabetic patients may excrete more than 30 mg of albumin daily, a previously undetected preclinical component of diabetic nephropathy. Microalbuminuria not only predicts subsequent nephropathy but also is a harbinger of death from cardiovascular disease (Dinneen and Gerstein, 1997). Evidence indicates the benefit of initiation of treatment with an angiotensin-converting enzyme (ACE) inhibitor in a *renoprotective regimen* in normotensive microalbuminuric patients with type 1 or type 2 diabetes (Ravid et al., 1998).

STAGE 2: NORMOALBUMINURIA

Almost all patients are normoalbuminuric (albumin excretion rate <20 µg/min [29 mg/d]) for the first 5 years of type 1 diabetes. Glomerular filtration rate is 20 to 50% greater than normal for age in this stage. Because the exact onset of type 2 diabetes is difficult to document, urinary protein studies are lacking in this stage. On renal biopsy specimens, mild thickening of the glomerular basement membrane first is noted 18 to 24 months after onset of type 1 diabetes and may be pronounced after 3.5 to 5 years (Osterby, 1974; Osterby and Gundersen, 1975). Glomerular basement membrane thickening is present in diabetics who do not go on to develop nephropathy (Osterby, 1983). The glomerular mesangial matrix expands after 2 to 3 years (Osterby, 1973) and increases out of proportion to the increase in glomerular volume. Exercise-induced microalbuminuria may be the only clinical evidence of renal involvement during this stage (Vittinghus and Mogensen, 1981), which extends 4 to 15 years after diagnosis. Biopsy specimens of kidneys from nondiabetic donors transplanted into diabetic recipients show the same changes of mesangial matrix expansion and glomerular basement membrane thickening within 3 to 5 years posttransplant (Mauer et al., 1989).

STAGE 3: INCIPIENT DIABETIC NEPHROPATHY: THE MICROALBUMINURIC STAGE

Microalbuminuria (albumin excretion rate 20–200 µg/min [30–300 mg/d]) is typical after 6 to 15 years in about 35% of type 1 diabetic patients and an unknown interval in type 2 patients (Parving et al., 1988; Viberti and Keen, 1984). Initially, microalbuminuria may be present intermittently with wide variation in daily total protein excretion. The amount of microalbuminuria is exacerbated by hypertension, uncontrolled hyperglycemia, strenuous exercise, urinary tract infections, hypervolemia and dietary protein loads. Daily fluctuations in albuminuria yield a coefficient of variation greater than 45% (Chachati et al., 1987; Cohen et al., 1987b; Gatling et al., 1988; Rowe et al., 1985).

After microalbuminuria becomes constant, most patients follow a progressive downhill course, unless intervention takes place (Mathiesen et al., 1984; Mogensen, 1987; Mogensen and Christensen, 1984; Parving et al., 1982; Viberti et al., 1982). Typically, albumin excretion increases by about 25 μg/min per year, whereas GFR remains normal or elevated (Mogensen, 1971). Once the microalbuminuria exceeds 70 μg/min, however, GFR declines at a widely variable rate. About 40% of patients with type 1 diabetes have persistent hypertension (>140–160/90 mm Hg) plus microalbuminuria (Borch-Johnsen, 1988); both signs herald the near-term development of clinical nephropathy (Norgaard et al., 1990). Glomerular morphology may be normal or abnormal in this stage, which is termed *incipient nephropathy* (Chavers et al., 1989). By the time the GFR has fallen to subnormal levels, morphological changes in glomeruli are a constant finding.

STAGE 4: PROTEINURIA, OVER NEPHROPATHY: CLINICAL PROTEINURIA, FALLING GLOMERULAR FILTRATION RATE

During the fourth stage, the impact of progressive renal destruction becomes clinically evident. For about 30 to 40% of patients with either type 1 or type 2 diabetes, signs attributable to proteinuria (300–25,000 mg/d), including a nephrotic syndrome (proteinuria ≥3.5 g/d, hypoalbuminemia and hyperlipidemia) and/or hypertension, are detected because of patient complaint or at a routine physical examination. Serum albumin levels in the diabetic nephrotic syndrome usually are higher than in other nephrosis, perhaps because glycated albumin is more likely than normal albumin to permeate capillary membranes.

Glomeruli in proteinuric diabetes of both types show diffuse intercapillary glomerulosclerosis accompanied by mesangial expansion and a thickened glomerular basement membrane (Mauer et al., 1984; Steffes et al., 1989); typical Kimmelstiel-Wilson lesions of nodular glomerulosclerosis are seen in only about 50% of cases (Gellman et al., 1959). Because of the salutary effect sustaining normotension and improving metabolic control, this stage, which previously lasted no longer than 1 or 2 years, may be protracted to 10 years or longer. The natural history of nephropathy in both major types of diabetes is being rewritten continuously because of application of effective renoprotective measures (Christensen et al., 1999; Frankel, 1998; Gaede et al., 1999; Gerstein, 1999).

STAGE 5: END-STAGE RENAL DISEASE

Although the subset of ESRD patients with diabetes has progressively increased absolutely since the mid-20th century (type 2 diabetes is now pandemic) (Ritz, 1999; Rosenbloom et al., 1999), the relative proportion (attack rate) of all diabetic patients who ultimately become uremic is declining. Medical texts of the 1960s and 1970s described the rapid and inexorable deterioration of diabetic individuals once proteinuria was discovered. These earlier observations state that after 20 to 30 years of type 1 diabetes, about 30 to 40% of patients manifest irreversibly failed kidneys (Balodimus, 1971). By the

1990s, however, proteinuric type 1 and type 2 diabetic patients commonly experience pre-ESRD intervals of a decade or longer. Uremic symptoms and signs in diabetic patients are manifested at higher creatinine clearances than in nondiabetic subjects; renal replacement therapy usually is needed within 3 to 5 years after onset of the nephrotic syndrome. Uremia therapy often is postponed for years with correction of anemia (erythropoietin) and dietary and fluid restrictions.

Renal Involvement in Type 2 Diabetes

Any effort to construct a time scale for stages of type 2 diabetes is made imprecise by the inability to specify a starting date for the disease in most patients (Ritz et al., 1999). Although type 2 diabetes may present in hyperosmolar coma or as a cause of gradual weight loss, it is more characteristic to discover type 2 diabetes in an unsuspecting individual with other complaints. Harris and colleagues in a study of cohorts of type 2 diabetes patients in Wisconsin and Western Australia, concluded that the onset of type 2 diabetes may occur 9 to 12 years before a clinical diagnosis is established (Harris et al., 1992). At a minimum, 50% of patients with type 2 diabetes are unaware that they have diabetes (Harris et al., 1987). It follows that the prevalence of clinical nephropathy in type 2 diabetes—which also is not defined clearly—is underreported at 2.5 to 10% (Damsgaard and Mogensen, 1986; Fabre et al., 1982; Herman and Teutsch, 1985; Marks, 1965). Prospective studies of populations at high risk for type 2 diabetes, such as black Americans (Cowie et al., 1989; Herman and Teutsch, 1985), Hispanics (Cowie et al., 1989; Herman and Teutsch, 1985; Pugh et al., 1988) and some Native American tribes (e.g., Pima) (Hasslacher et al., 1989; Knowles et al., 1978; Kunzelman et al., 1989; Nelson et al., 1988, 1989; Ritz et al., 1991), indicate that the interval between clinical recognition of type 2 diabetes and onset of ESRD ranges from 5 to 15 years; the older the patient at diagnosis of diabetes, the more rapid the progression to ESRD (Nolph et al., 1988). Elderly people who develop type 2 diabetes also risk GFR reduction as a result of advancing age (Davies and Shock, 1950; Lindeman et al., 1985; Rowe et al., 1976) and atherosclerosis (Takazakura et al., 1972).

Glomerular hyperfiltration and microalbuminuria, previously thought absent in type 2 diabetes, have been detected in a small proportion of Pima Indians (Myers et al., 1991), black Americans (Lebovitz and Palmisano, 1990; Palmisano and Lebovitz, 1989; Palmisano and Sachmechi, 1987), and white Americans (Berionade, 1986; Bruton et al., 1990; Nowack et al., 1992). Discrepancies between these and previous reports may relate to differences in ethnic groups, variation in technique for determining GFR or evaluation at different stages of type 2 diabetes. Microalbuminuria is present in 20 to 37% of patients with newly diagnosed type 2 diabetes (Damsgaard and Mogensen, 1986; Fabre et al., 1982; Gall et al., 1991; Uusitupa et al., 1987). Elderly people with diabetes may have other causes for microalbuminuria, including hypertension, urinary tract infection and nondiabetic glomerulopathy (Parving et al., 1990). The predictive value of microalbuminuria in type 1 diabetes may be true for type 2 diabetes, as evidenced by a four times increased risk of progression to macroalbuminuria discerned in a prospective study of 76 Danish subjects with NIDDM followed for 9 years (Mogensen, 1984). Urinary albumin concentration may remain normal after many years of having type 2 diabetes (Mogensen, 1983).

Microalbuminuria is a marker for increased risk of death from cardiovascular disease in type 2 diabetes (Jarrett et al., 1984; Mogensen, 1984; Schmitz and Vaeth, 1988; Yudkin et

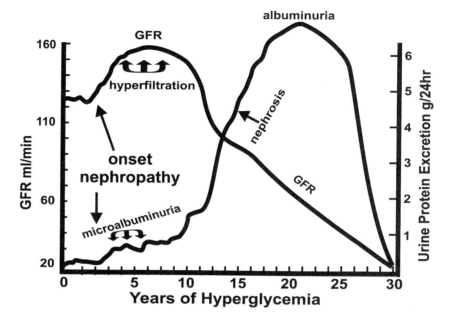

FIGURE 36–3

Early nephropathy in type 1 diabetes and type 2 diabetes is delineated by glomerular hyper-filtration and microalbuminuria. Thereafter, in-exorable decline in glomerular filtration rate (GFR) is associated with increasing amounts of albuminuria, typically reaching nephrotic range losses (>3.5 g/d). The natural history of diabetic nephropathy is changing as effective antihypertensive drugs are employed and hy-perglycemia is lessened to the extent that the relationship between duration of diabetes and decline in residual GFR is changing for the bet-ter.

al., 1988), similar to findings in the nondiabetic population (Yudkin et al., 1988). Diabetic glomerulosclerosis can be in-ferred from a typical clinical course expressing transition from microalbuminuria, through fixed proteinuria, to a ne-phrotic syndrome (proteinuria >3.5 g/d). Additional support for the diagnosis of diabetic nephropathy rather than some other cause of renal disease is the presence of coincident retinopathy, a universal finding in a nephrotic diabetic pa-tient. Conversely, failure to detect retinopathy is reason to suspect that the observed renal syndrome is not due to diabe-tes. A kidney biopsy, although unnecessary for most typical nephrotic diabetics, may unmask, in unusual presentations, nephropathy unrelated to diabetes (absence of retinopathy, small kidneys, red cell casts). Before the importance of blood pressure normalization to survival in diabetic nephropathy was appreciated, uremia usually followed nephrosis within 1 to 3 years. Only 28% of patients with type 1 diabetes survived for 10 years after the onset of *clinical* proteinuria in a 1961 study, an era when neither dialysis nor kidney transplantation was available (Caird, 1961; Fig. 36–3).

Histopathology of Diabetic Glomerulopathy

During the course of diabetic nephropathy, glomerular hypertrophy, especially in the glomeruli least affected by glomerulopathy, is prominent. Fluorescence microscopy of glomeruli from long-term diabetics shows deposition of albu-min and immunoglobulins in a ribbonlike pattern along tu-bular basement membranes and Bowman's capsule, probably reflecting passive entrapment of plasma proteins rather than an active immune process. Similar findings have been re-ported in skin and muscle, in which its significance is equally obscure (Miller and Michael, 1976).

As shown in Figures 36–4 and 36–5, kidney biopsy speci-mens in azotemic type 1 diabetes and type 2 diabetes consis-tently show mesangial expansion, glomerular basement membrane thickening, and afferent and efferent arteriolo-sclerosis. Diabetes of long duration results in glomerular obliteration by combined diffuse and nodular intercapillary glomerulosclerosis. It has not proved possible to correlate glomerular basement membrane thickening and decreased GFR, amount of albuminuria or level of hypertension (Mauer et al., 1985). Mauer and colleagues were able to identify a

relationship between mesangial expansion and the severity of clinical diabetic nephropathy, however, leading to the spec-ulation that mesangial expansion induces glomerular func-tional deterioration by restricting glomerular capillary vascu-lature and its filtering surface (Mauer et al., 1985). In most studies, the longer the duration of diabetes, the greater the risk of contracting nephropathy.

Once proteinuria develops in diabetes, renal function (GFR) may be lost at varying rates. To anticipate when ESRD will occur, deteriorating GFR in a patient can be charted accurately by plotting the inverse (reciprocal) of serum creati-nine against time. As GFR falls below 20 ml/min, the patient (both type 2 diabetes and type 1 diabetes) becomes catabolic and prone to multiple intercurrent disorders. A minor head cold, for example, easily tolerated by a diabetic with normal renal function, may confine an azotemic diabetic to bed for a week. Orthostatic hypotension, bowel malfunction (obstipa-tion alternating with explosive nocturnal diarrhea) and rap-idly progressing vision loss amplify the morbidity of renal insufficiency.

Because of contemporaneous multisystem failure, it usu-ally is necessary to institute dialysis therapy at a higher creatinine clearance in a diabetic than in a nondiabetic pa-tient. Maintenance hemodialysis, although rarely required in nondiabetic patients whose creatinine clearance is greater than about 5 ml/min (approximately equivalent to a serum creatinine of 8–12 mg/dl), often is necessary in diabetic ne-phropathy when creatinine clearance falls to about 10 ml/min (serum creatinine concentration of approximately 4–8 mg/dl). Maintenance of euglycemia becomes difficult as re-nal function deteriorates in type 1 diabetes and type 2 diabe-tes. Diminished renal catabolism of administered insulin in type 1 diabetes and endogenous insulin (and other small peptide hormones) in type 2 diabetes may cause episodic profound hypoglycemia after the injection of formerly safely tolerated doses of insulin or oral hypoglycemic agents.

Renal disorders other than diabetic nephropathy occur in type 1 diabetes and type 2 diabetes with the same frequency as in nondiabetic individuals. A presumption of diabetic nephropathy may be misleading to the extent that coincident disorders remain undiagnosed. For example, type 2 diabetes and polycystic kidney disease may lead to ESRD in midlife. Failure to discover the polycystic disease confounds subse-

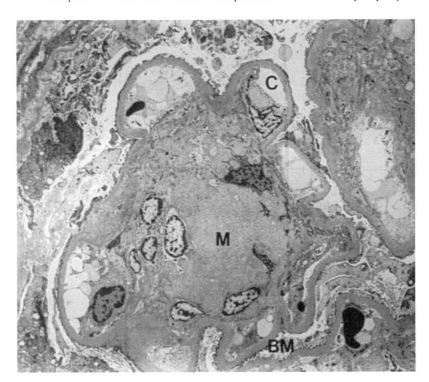

FIGURE 36–4

Electron photomicrograph of glomerulus in type 1 diabetes shows a thick glomerular basement membrane (BM) and expanded mesangium (M) encroaching on capillaries (C). These findings are characteristic of nephropathy in type 1 diabetes and type 2 diabetes.

quent management of hematuria (ruptured renal cyst), hepatomegaly (cystic) and other organ derangement not induced by diabetes. Distinguishing renal damage caused by hypertension from that caused by diabetes may be difficult, even with a renal biopsy. Hypertension is noted in 50 to 70% of patients with type 2 diabetes at the time of diagnosis. It has proved complicated to segregate the effect of protracted blood pressure elevation on worsening proteinuria or deteriorating GFR (Panzram, 1987; Ritz et al., 1991a; Standl et al., 1989). Confounding the problem is the fact that hypertension, itself a cause of ESRD, often is noted in the absence of renal disease and has been related to obesity, advancing age and hyperinsulinism (DeFronzo and Ferranini, 1991).

Genetic Predisposition to Diabetic Nephropathy

Epidemiological studies suggest that not only is diabetes an inherited disorder, at least in predisposition, but also hypertension and nephropathy are inherited. For example, diabetic subjects with a family history of essential hypertension have a higher incidence of nephropathy (Krolewski et al., 1988; Mangili et al., 1988; Viberti et al., 1987). The diabetic sibling of a patient with type 1 diabetes and nephropathy has a 72% cumulative risk of developing diabetic nephropathy, as contrasted with the diabetic sibling of a patient with type 1

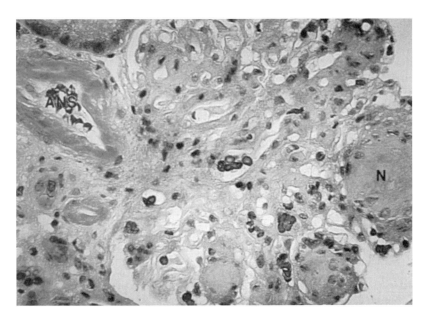

FIGURE 36–5

Light photomicrograph of glomerulus from an azotemic patient with type 2 diabetes shows diffuse and nodular glomerulosclerosis. Arteriolonephrosclerosis (ANS) and multiple nodules (N) are evident. Nodular (Kimmelstiel-Wilson lesion) and diffuse glomerulosclerosis are characteristic findings in the nephropathy of type 1 diabetes and type 2 diabetes.

diabetes who does not have nephropathy (Quinn *et al.*, 1996). Essential hypertension is associated with increased activity of the erythrocyte sodium-lithium countertransport system (Ibsen *et al.*, 1982), and patients who manifest glomerular hyperfiltration also have increased activity of this membrane transport system (Carr *et al.*, 1990). It follows that in diabetes, a genetic or familial tendency to hypertension may increase the risk of phenotypic expression of hypertension and/or nephropathy. Challenges to this thesis center on the fact that the mechanisms for increased sodium-lithium countertransport activity in hypertension and in diabetes are dissimilar (Jensen *et al.*, 1990; Rutherford *et al.*, 1990).

More recent inquiries infer that although there is good correlation between sodium-lithium countertransport activity and hypertension, the relationship in diabetes is weak and probably not significant (Van Norren *et al.*, 1998). As observed by Viberti (1999), a genetic dissection of a complex trait such as diabetic nephropathy, which is likely to involve an interaction between more than one gene, environmental factors and compensatory factors, may prove difficult.

Pathogenesis of Diabetic Nephropathy

Hyperglycemic rats (see later) and diabetic patients manifest metabolic and hemodynamic abnormalities that cause vasculopathy and renal injury. No consistently reliable signs or tests signal the time, however, when functional perturbations begin to induce macrovasculopathy and/or microvasculopathy. Partisans expound the relative importance of capillary hypertension and hyperglycemia in the pathogenesis of microvasculopathy.

Clinical trials of enhanced metabolic regulation of hyperglycemia in type 1 and type 2 diabetes dismissed all doubt from the indictment of hyperglycemia as a major cause of human diabetic nephropathy. Although earlier studies in humans linked the prevalence of microalbuminuria and late diabetic complications to inferior glycemic control, broadly based prospective trials—especially the Diabetes Control and Complications Trial (DCCT)—won the argument (DCCT Research Group, 1986). Striving for normoglycemia employing intensive diabetes therapy in the DCCT produced a 39% reduction in the occurrence of microalbuminuria and a 54% reduction in the occurrence of albuminuria (DCCT Research Group, 1995; Delahanty, 1998; Di Landro *et al.*, 1998). By one projection, comprehensive treatment of type 2 diabetes, maintaining a hemoglobin A_{1c} value of 7.2%, would reduce the cumulative incidence of blindness, ESRD and lower-extremity amputation by 72%, 87% and 67% (Eastman *et al.*, 1997).

Kidney and pancreas transplantation offers evidence that hyperglycemia is a major, if not sole, determinant of diabetic glomerulopathy. First, at the onset of diabetic nephropathy, sustained euglycemia reduces the enlarged kidney size typical of early hyperfiltration (Tuttle *et al.*, 1991). Second, early glomerulopathy is reversible in a euglycemic environment, as shown by the disappearance of glomerulosclerosis in two cadaveric donor kidneys obtained from a diabetic after transplantation into nondiabetic recipients (Abouna *et al.*, 1986). Third, recurrent intercapillary glomerulosclerosis and renal failure can destroy kidneys obtained from nondiabetics when transplanted into diabetics (Maryniak *et al.*, 1985). Fourth, kidneys transplanted into recipients who have become diabetic only after transplantation (steroid diabetics) may show characteristic nodular intercapillary glomerulosclerosis subsequently. Finally, a decade of euglycemia afforded by a pancreas transplant reverses renal biopsy–proven nodular intercapillary glomerulosclerosis in type 1 diabetics (Fioretto *et al.*, 1999).

Proposed explanations for how hyperglycemia causes tissue injury include the accumulation of sorbitol and advanced glycosylation end products. Hyperlipidemia, a confounding variable present in most adult diabetics, is a risk for accelerated atherosclerosis resulting in injury to small and large blood vessels. No single mechanism accounts for seemingly disparate reports linking solely hemodynamic or metabolic perturbations to the kidney in diabetes. As shown in Figure 36–6, many suspected mechanisms might lead to kidney and other microvascular damage.

The possible role of the sorbitol pathway in this process is controversial (Frank, 1994; Hotta, 1997). Intracellular glucose is metabolized, in part, to sorbitol through the enzyme aldose reductase. Accumulation of sorbitol within the cells results in a rise in cell osmolality and a decrease in intracellular *myo*-inositol; these changes, in turn, lead to a decrease in sodium–potassium–adenosine triphosphatase activity and a possible shift in the redox potential within cells. In type 2 diabetes, a high serum level of aldose reductase correlated with development of active proliferative diabetic retinopathy in a 10-year prospective observational study comprising 97 subjects (Nishimura *et al.*, 1997).

Sorbitol production in experimental diabetes is enhanced markedly by hyperglycemia. An intriguing hint of the potential value of blocking aldose reductase is afforded by extraction from a Brazilian natural medicine for diabetes (made from the leaves of *Myricia multiflora* DC) of new glucosides, myrciaitrin 1 and myrciaphenone, which are potent inhibitors of aldose reductase and α-glucosidase (Yoshikawa, 1998). Sorbinil, an aldose reductase inhibitor, minimizes albuminuria and glomerular basement membrane thickening in streptozotocin-induced diabetic rats treated for 5 months; it also reduces renal cortical activity of glucosyl-galactosyl-hydroxylysyl-glucohydrolase, an enzyme involved in the catabolism of collagen disaccharide units (Kassab *et al.*, 1994).

Other drugs that block aldose reductase activity include carboxylic acid derivatives (tolrestat and ponalrestat) and flavonoids. Clinical trials in the 1990s assessed the efficacy of sorbinil, tolrestat and ponalrestat in the treatment of diabetic retinopathy, neuropathy and nephropathy. In one study, tolrestat (200 mg/d) given to 20 patients with type 1 diabetes after 6 months of placebo (Pedersen *et al.*, 1991) reversed glomerular hyperfiltration, reduced the GFR from 156 to 124 mL/min ($P<0.001$) and decreased urinary albumin excretion from 197 to 158 mg/d ($P<0.001$). Urinary albumin excretion was measured in 16 diabetic subjects treated for 12 months with tolrestat, 200 mg daily, or ascorbic acid, 500 mg twice daily. Although ascorbic acid decreased urinary albumin excretion rate after 9 months, tolrestat had no effect on proteinuria or other measured variables (McAuliffe *et al.*, 1998). Aldose reductase inhibitors have not been shown convincingly to be beneficial except perhaps in some patients with diabetic neuropathy.

Inferences from experiments in induced-diabetic rats suggest that plasma hyperviscosity and/or elevated circulating thromboxane and platelet-derived growth factors may be responsible for small vessel injury under defined circumstances. An unsubstantiated, although intriguing, approach to retarding diabetic microvasculopathy is to reduce erythrocyte stiffness, a hemorrheologic alteration universally noted in diabetes, by administration of pentoxifylline (Solerte and Ferrari, 1985; Solerte *et al.*, 1987).

Advanced Glycosylated End Products

In the healthy state, reducing sugars such as glucose react nonenzymatically and reversibly with free amino groups in

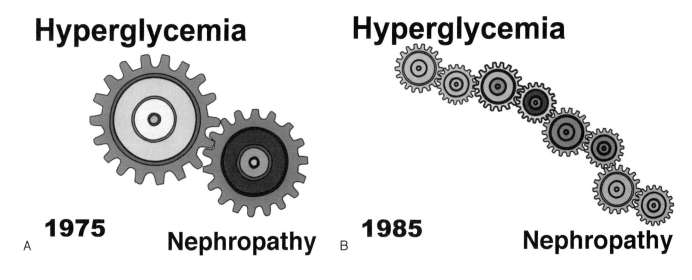

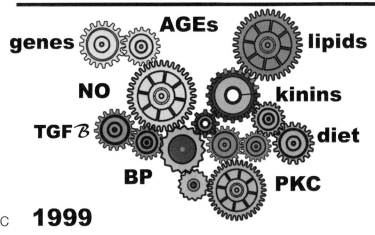

FIGURE 36–6

(A) A long-contested relationship between hyperglycemia and renal disease in diabetes was proposed in the 1970s. (B) By the mid-1980s, it was evident that numerous intermediate steps were involved in linking ambient glucose levels to tissue injury. (C) Presently, several candidate mechanisms have been proposed to explain the microvasculopathy and macrovasculopathy of diabetes. (AGEs = advanced glycosylated end products; NO = nitric oxide; TGF-β = transforming growth factor-β; BP = blood pressure, PKC = protein kinase C.)

proteins to form small amounts of stable Amadori products through Schiff base adducts. With aging, spontaneous further irreversible modification of proteins by glucose results in the formation of advanced glycosylated end products (AGEs), a heterogeneous family of biologically and chemically reactive compounds with cross-linking properties (Porte and Schwartz, 1996). High ambient glucose concentrations present in diabetes (Brownlee, 1994; Vlassara, 1996) amplify this process of protein modification. Circulating AGE peptides (molecular weight 2,000–6,000) cross-link with collagen, promoting diabetic microvascular complications, increasing vascular permeability, procoagulant activity, adhesion molecule expression and monocyte influx, contributing to vascular injury. Specific receptors binding AGEs are located on endothelial cells (Schmidt et al., 1995). Plasma and tissue levels of AGEs increase progressively as diabetic patients develop renal failure (Makita et al., 1994). Although neither hemodialysis nor peritoneal dialysis decreases these *toxic* levels to normal, after restoration of half-normal glomerular filtration by renal transplantation, AGE levels fall sharply to within the normal range within 8 hours.

Advanced glycosylated end product formation promotes diabetic complications by changing the structure and function of extracellular matrix in the glomerular mesangium and elsewhere. In type IV collagen from basement membrane, for example, AGE formation decreases binding of the noncollagenous NC1 domain to the helix-rich domain, interfering with lateral association of these molecules into a normal lattice structure (Tsilbary et al., 1988; Charonis and Tsilbary, 1992). Advanced glycosylated end products are toxic as a result of their interference with vital nitric oxide–mediated processes, including neurotransmission, wound healing, blood flow in small vessels and decreased cell proliferation (Ono et al., 1998).

Aminoguanidine, a compound similar to α-hydrazinohistidine, known to reduce diabetes-induced vascular leakage, is being evaluated as an AGE blocker potentially bypassing the necessity to attain euglycemia (Brownlee, 1989). Aminoguanidine diminishes proteinuria, mesangial matrix expansion, matrix gene expression and basement membrane thickness in diabetic rats (Brownlee, 1994). Glomeruli and tubules in aminoguanidine-treated rats show reduced deposition of AGEs, a benefit related directly to the duration of therapy;

experimental diabetic neuropathy and heart disease are prevented by aminoguanidine.

Aminoguanidine acts by preventing formation of reactive AGEs and their subsequent cross-linking with albumin, leading to a reduction in AGE levels, while blocking synthesis of nitric oxide (Yang *et al.*, 1998). Initial clinical trials of aminoguanidine in type 1 diabetes and type 2 diabetes as well as in diabetic hemodialysis patients have been inconclusive because of hepatotoxicity (type 1 diabetes) and problems with experimental design. Derivative trials are in the planning stage.

Clinical Management

Extrarenal comorbidity consumes most of the time devoted to management of a diabetic patient experiencing progressive nephropathy. Coordinating management of diabetic retinopathy, cardiovascular disease and peripheral vascular disease as well as the myriad manifestations of diabetic sensory and motor neuropathy forces the responsible internist or nephrologist into the role of medical team manager. Whenever multiple disciplines converge in the care of a single patient, there is risk of placing the patient in a tug of war between conflicting, although not necessarily different, plans of therapy. Whether one or another antihypertensive or hypolipidemic drug is prescribed is less important than whether the patient's blood pressure and plasma lipids are normalized. Lacking a team leader, patient care can drift, leading to missed or duplicate tests and procedures performed in the midst of confusion and rising anxiety. A schema for comprehensive diabetic management is provided in Figure 36–7, and the professional collaborators required for idealized care are shown in Figure 36–8.

Diabetes and hypertension are common conditions. Hypertension and diabetes mellitus—both associated with high morbidity and mortality—occur together in 50% of diabetics, resulting in a 7.2-fold increase in crude mortality. Whether

associated with nephropathy in type 1 diabetes or type 2 diabetes, hypertension escalates mortality to 37 times greater than that of a healthy population (MacLeod and McLay, 1998). The life-preserving benefits of blood pressure reduction in overt diabetic nephropathy, established by Parving (1998a), with ACE inhibitors and/or non–ACE inhibitors (frequently in combination with diuretics), include (1) reduced albuminuria, (2) delayed progression of nephropathy, (3) postponed renal insufficiency and (4) improved survival in type 1 and type 2 diabetics. Additionally, treatment of diabetics with isolated systolic hypertension induces a sharp reduction in fatal and nonfatal cardiovascular events (Parving, 1998b).

After onset of ESRD, uncontrolled hypertension adds a significant risk to patient and kidney graft survival in diabetic kidney transplant recipients (Friedman *et al.*, 1985). Mainly as a result of regulation of hypertension, mortality in advanced diabetic nephropathy improved from 50 to 70% in the decade when antihypertensive therapy was not routine (Krolewski *et al.*, 1985) to 18% when effective treatment of hypertension became routine. Effective reduction in blood pressure can be achieved by combinations of diuretics, vasodilators, β-blockers, calcium channel blockers and renin antagonists. Systemic hypertension is injurious to the kidney because dilated afferent glomerular arterioles transmit systemic blood pressure to glomeruli, increasing further the glomerular capillary hypertension already present secondary to hyperfiltration and/or glomerular hypertrophy (Hostetter, 1990). Care of the diabetic patient mandates blood pressure control to slow progression of diabetic renal disease (Mogensen, 1990).

In type 1 diabetes, treatment of hypertension in the microalbuminuric stage significantly slows or arrests progression (Christensen and Mogensen, 1986); once proteinuria becomes constant, the rate of further decline of GFR can be reduced (Parving *et al.*, 1989). Parving and coworkers, in a landmark study of six hypertensive adults with nephrotic-

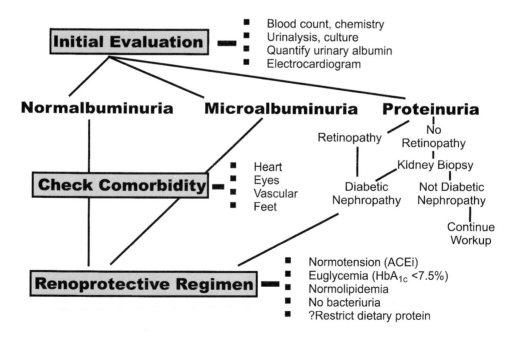

FIGURE 36–7

Assessing renal integrity in diabetes. Outlined steps in management of newly evaluated diabetic patients focus on proteinuria as a key variable determining testing and referral. The concept of a renoprotective regimen involves minimizing injury by treating urinary infection and reducing risks attributable to hypertension, hyperglycemia and hyperlipidemia. (ACEi = angiotensin-converting enzyme inhibitors; HbA_{1c} = glycosylated hemoglobin A.)

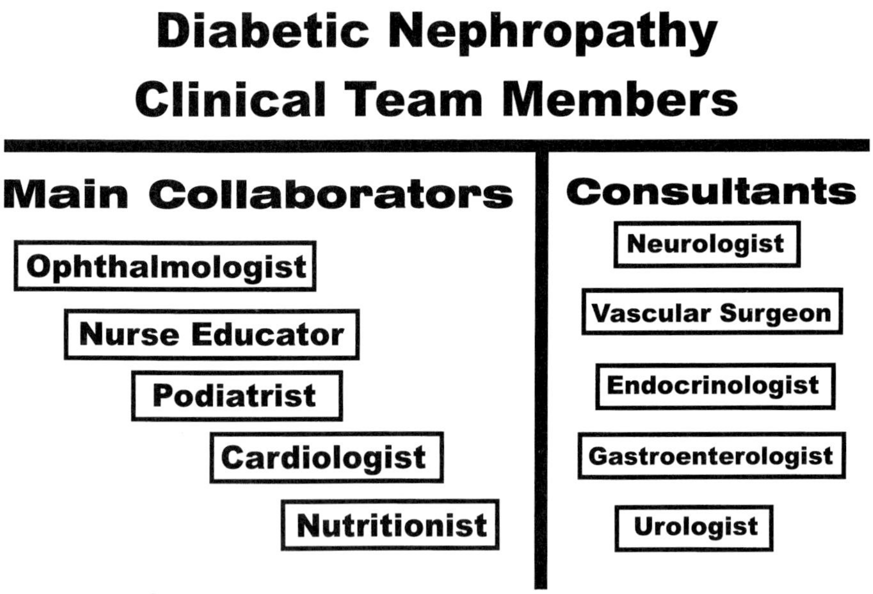

Diabetic Nephropathy
Clinical Team Members

Main Collaborators

Ophthalmologist

Nurse Educator

Podiatrist

Cardiologist

Nutritionist

Consultants

Neurologist

Vascular Surgeon

Endocrinologist

Gastroenterologist

Urologist

FIGURE 36–8

Successful management of diabetic patients with advancing nephropathy and/or end-stage renal disease requires the skills of multiple specialists. A team captain, or a *clinical care coordinator,* is essential to assist in scheduling what can seem to be an un-ending sequence of tests, clinic visits and procedures. By default, the nephrologist usually is designated as the main physician once renal insufficiency clearly indicates the necessity for uremia therapy.

range proteinuria resulting from type 1 diabetes, observed that treatment with metoprolol, hydralazine and furosemide for 28 to 86 months reduced mean blood pressure from 162/103 to 144/95 mm Hg, resulting in a 60% reduction in the rate of fall of GFR from 1.23 to 0.49 ml/min per month and a reduction in albumin excretion by 5 to 10% per year (Parving *et al.*, 1983). Using a similar antihypertensive regimen, Mathiesen and associates reduced hypertensive blood pressures from 143/96 to 129/84 mm Hg in 10 patients with type 1 diabetes who were followed for 32 to 91 months with a 75% decrease in the rate of decline of GFR from 0.89 to 0.22 ml/min per month (Mathiesen *et al.*, 1989b). Antihypertensive therapy in patients with type 1 diabetes and clinical or advanced nephropathy for longer than 8 years improved survival greatly from 48 to 87% (Working Group on Hypertension in Diabetes, 1987). In this collaborative trial, target blood pressure reduction was to at least 140/90 mm Hg; current thinking argues, however, for sustaining antihypertensive therapy "... at a blood pressure level less than that conventionally considered hypertensive" (Plouin *et al.*, 1992). Reduction of arterial pressure to 140/90 mm Hg slows decline in renal function in diabetic nephropathy, with the inference that decreasing arterial pressure to less than 130/85 mm Hg affords greater protection against the progression of diabetic nephropathy. Gaining this degree of blood pressure reduction almost always necessitates more than one antihypertensive drug as well as a cooperative patient.

ANGIOTENSIN-CONVERTING ENZYME INHIBITORS

Angiotensin-converting enzyme inhibitors are highly effective in retarding progression of kidney damage in rats (Anderson *et al.*, 1989). Not all antihypertensive drugs reduce proteinuria and retard glomerular injury in rats, a particular benefit of treatment with ACE inhibitors (Zatz *et al.*, 1985). A special advantage for ACE inhibitors has been linked to their purported reduction of intraglomerular pressure. Enalapril improved renal function and retarded histological damage in five of six nephrectomized rats, however, despite continued elevation of glomerular capillary pressure (Fogo *et al.*, 1986).

Multiple studies document the value of ACE inhibitors in hypertensive diabetic patients with incipient nephropathy. Angiotensin-converting enzyme inhibitors slow the fall of GFR by about 50% during the first 2 years of follow-up

(Marre *et al.*, 1987). Combining an ACE inhibitor with a calcium antagonist permits equivalent blood pressure reduction by lower doses of both drugs, attenuating albuminuria and the rate of decline of GFR with a lower side-effect profile than that of either agent alone (Bakris *et al.*, 1992). To date, however, no evidence indicates that treatment with an ACE inhibitor decreases the risk of or the time to development of ESRD above other antihypertensive drug combinations. Whether treatment with an ACE inhibitor holds special advantage over other classes of antihypertensive drugs in terms of renoprotective effect in diabetic nephropathy is judged a *major controversy* by the International Society of Hypertension (Johnston *et al.*, 1992). In advanced diabetic nephropathy, reductions in proteinuria and reduction in the rate of GFR loss followed treatment with an ACE inhibitor (Taguma *et al.*, 1985). In prospective studies, because of their efficacy, relative lack of side effects and good metabolic profile during treatment, ACE inhibitors ranked as first-line treatment in type 1 diabetes (Mogensen, 1992) and type 2 diabetes (Savage and Schrier, 1992).

SELECTION OF ANTIHYPERTENSIVE DRUGS

Selection of specific drugs for treatment of hypertensive diabetic patients can be confusing. Markets for ACE inhibitors and calcium channel blockers exceed $2 billion each fostering extensive advertising campaigns targeting physicians. The stressful decision process involves choosing among drug classes, then picking a unique molecular configuration within a class. Head-to-head prospective trials of ACE inhibitors versus calcium channel blockers have been completed. In the Appropriate Blood Pressure Control in Diabetes (ABCD) trial in hypertensive patients with type 2 diabetes, the incidence of cardiovascular events over a 5-year follow-up was compared for enalapril versus nisoldipine, a long-acting calcium antagonist (Estacio and Schrier, 1998). The study randomized diabetic patients for moderate blood pressure control (target diastolic pressure 80–89 mm Hg) or intensive control (target diastolic pressure 75 mm Hg). In 470 hypertensive patients, the incidence of fatal and nonfatal myocardial infarctions was significantly ($P = 0.001$) higher among patients receiving nisoldipine (n = 25) compared with patients receiving enalapril (n = 5). A similar outcome was reported in the Fosinopril versus Amlodipine Cardiovascular Events Randomized Trial (FACET), sustaining the impression that ACE inhibitors may be preferable to calcium antagonists for managing hypertension in diabetic patients (Poulter, 1998).

Parving (1998a), who initially showed the salutary renoprotective effect of reducing hypertensive blood pressure in diabetic patients (before introduction of ACE inhibitors or calcium channel blockers), interpreted the ABCD and FACET results as follows: "[T]he combination of a calcium antagonist with an ACE inhibitor is a rational therapeutic choice in patients with coexisting hypertension and diabetes." Other investigators, reflecting majority thinking, reached a differing conclusion: "Angiotensin-converting enzyme inhibitors and low-dose diuretics may be more effective than calcium antagonists for prevention of cardiovascular events in hypertensive patients with diabetes or impaired glucose control" (Pahor et al., 1998).

Approximately 15% of diabetic patients in our clinic discontinue enalapril, captopril or other ACE inhibitors because of troublesome side effects, particularly hyperkalemia and a dry, nonproductive cough. Of these patients, perhaps half tolerate blood pressure reduction with an angiotensin II receptor antagonist, such as lovasartin, candisartan or irbesartan (Paster et al., 1998). Whether angiotensin II receptor antagonists retard progression of diabetic nephropathy is undetermined, although they are well tolerated and safe in hemodialysis patients (Saracho et al., 1998).

Based on interpretation of available evidence, after prescribing an ACE inhibitor (switching to an angiotensin II receptor antagonist for patients intolerant to an ACE inhibitor), our second-choice drug for diabetic nephropathy is a calcium antagonist, alone or in combination with or without diuretics. For resistant hypertension, we next add β-blockers, central α$_2$-adrenergic agonists (e.g., clonidine including transdermal patch preparations) and peripheral vasodilators (prazosin, hydralazine or minoxidil) in a trial-and-error approach. For most patients with type 2 diabetes, obesity is a coincident disorder for which a weight reduction program and physical training are established to enhance insulin sensitivity and improve hyperlipidemia (Henry et al., 1986).

Hyperlipidemia is recognized as a risk factor for progression of nephropathy in diabetes that is independent of hyperglycemia and hypertension. In type 2 diabetes, the combination of high normal–range blood pressure with moderately elevated levels of total cholesterol and hemoglobin A$_{1c}$ defines a group at high risk for progression to diabetic nephropathy as well as symptomatic arteriosclerotic cardiovascular disease (Ravid et al., 1998). Hypertensive blood pressures should be corrected in type 1 diabetes and type 2 diabetes at all levels of renal function. Vision loss progresses more rapidly in hypertensive than in normotensive diabetics. Uncontrolled hypertension adds a significant risk to patient and kidney graft survival in diabetic kidney transplant recipients (Friedman et al., 1985).

Systemic hypertension is thought to be injurious because dilated afferent glomerular arterioles of the diabetic kidney (related to hyperglycemia and other metabolic and hormonal factors) permit transmission of systemic blood pressure to the glomeruli, increasing further glomerular capillary hypertension already present secondary to hyperfiltration and/or glomerular hypertrophy (Hostetter, 1990; Hostetter et al., 1981; Zatz et al, 1985). Kidneys with unilateral renal artery stenosis are protected from the effect of systemic blood pressure and exhibit minimal if any morphological changes of diabetes, whereas the contralateral kidney with a patent artery shows typical diabetic nephropathy (Berionade et al., 1987).

DIETARY PROTEIN RESTRICTION

In the healthy state (Bosch et al., 1983; Maschio et al., 1986) and in diabetes, the amount of dietary protein intake modulates renal hemodynamics (Kupin et al., 1987). Ingestion of a high-protein diet increases the risk of nephropathy in type 1 diabetes (Krolewski et al., 1985). Moderate and severe protein restriction early in the course of diabetes normalizes glomerular hypertension (Rennke et al., 1986; Wen et al., 1985; Zatz et al., 1985) because of decreased fractional clearance of albumin (Bending et al., 1988; Cohen et al., 1987a) and IgG (Bending et al., 1988). In a prospective, randomized, controlled study (Zeller et al., 1991), 20 subjects with type 1 diabetes and clinical proteinuria (mean 3144 ± 417 mg/d) or renal impairment (iothalamate clearance 46 ± 4.8 ml/min/1.73 m^2) were given a 0.6 g/kg/d protein diet for a mean of 34.7 months. There was a fourfold decrease in the rate of fall of GFR compared with that in 15 controls. After 3 months, mean protein excretion fell by 24% (760 mg) in the study group and rose by 22% (928 mg) in controls. At the conclusion of the trial, reduction in proteinuria in the study population was only 6% (196 mg), whereas controls had a 24% (1,024 mg) increase. Other studies in type 1 diabetes patients with advanced nephropathy reported twofold to fourfold reductions in the rate of fall of GFR (Barsotti et al., 1988; Evanoff et al., 1987, 1989; Pedersen et al., 1989; Viberti et al., 1988; Wiseman et al., 1987) and significant decrease in proteinuria. The amount of urinary proteinuria in the nephrotic syndrome of type 1 diabetes is reduced by dietary protein restriction (El Nahas et al., 1984; Kaysen et al., 1986), but similar positive results have not been obtained in type 2 diabetes. In one study of 13 patients with type 2 diabetes and renal insufficiency after a mean of 12.2 ± 12.9 months on a 30 g protein, 350 mg phosphorus diet, only 2 patients showed improvement in GFR (Kaysen et al., 1986).

As a generalization, neither optimal timing nor the extent of dietary protein restriction has been determined for type 1 diabetes or type 2 diabetes. Based on the fragmentary evidence cited previously, we recommend a 0.6 to 0.8 g/kg/d protein diet in type 1 diabetes and type 2 diabetes once proteinuria is greater than or equal to 1 g/d and/or a falling GFR is noted, provided that overall nutritional status is satisfactory. The American Diabetes Association advises an 0.8 g/kg/d protein diet in "diabetics who have or are at risk for nephropathy" (Wylie-Rosett, 1988). Protein restriction is not advocated in type 1 diabetes or type 2 diabetes when microalbuminuria is the only perturbation attributed to diabetes.

Although conclusions of four prospective, randomized and controlled trials are inconsistent when analyzed individually, a meta-analysis indicated that a low-protein diet reduced the risk of renal failure or death in nondiabetic patients by 33% (Pedrini et al., 1996). The same meta-analysis of five studies in type 1 diabetes found that dietary protein restriction significantly slowed decline in renal function by 44%, while reducing urinary protein excretion. Similarly, substantial protein restriction in a primary care practice for type 2 diabetic patients reduced proteinuria (Pijls et al., 1999).

Gaining compliance with a prescribed dietary protein intake of 0.8 g/kg/d in which protein is replaced isocalorically by unsaturated fat and carbohydrate is the key difficulty in application of a low-protein diet. Few, even highly motivated, patients remain on the diet after 6 months. Similar to smoking cessation and weight reduction, the good effect of a protein-restricted diet remains an illusory goal in practice.

GLYCEMIC CONTROL

Studies in streptozotocin-induced diabetic rats indicate that (1) glomerular basement membrane thickening increases

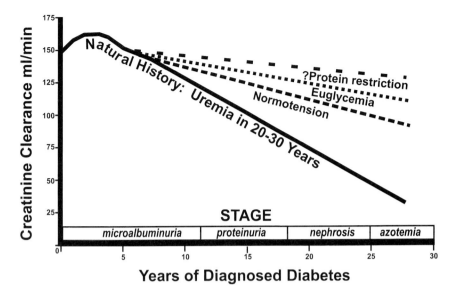

FIGURE 36–9

Retarding diabetic nephropathy. Favorable change in the slope of declining kidney function in diabetic nephropathy (type 1 and type 2 diabetes) resulting from normalizing blood pressure and blood glucose is depicted. The extent of delay of end-stage renal disease is unknown, although a decade or longer of stable azotemia is not unusual.

proportional to the severity of hyperglycemia (Fox *et al.*, 1977); (2) histopathological changes of nephropathy reverse with either insulin therapy or transplantation of islets of Langerhans and (3) regression of mesangial expansion and glomerular basement membrane thickening follows transplantation of affected kidneys into nondiabetic, isogeneic recipients (Mauer *et al.*, 1975a, 1975b; Weil *et al.*, 1975). Several studies in humans correlate the prevalence of microalbuminuria (Gatling *et al.*, 1988; Mogensen, 1976; Nelson *et al.*, 1989; Wiseman *et al.*, 1984) and late diabetic complications with poor glycemic control (Hasslacher and Ritz, 1987; Mathiesen *et al.*, 1989b; Rosenstock *et al.*, 1986; Skyler, 1979). The interval between onset of diabetes and the start of clinical proteinuria is shortened by poor glycemic control (Hasslacher and Ritz, 1987), and the risk of developing macroalbuminuria is four to five times greater in patients with poor control (Mauer *et al.*, 1981; Nyberg *et al.*, 1987). Figure 36–9 depicts key components of treatment strategies to slow the course of progressive kidney disease in diabetes.

Demographics of Diabetic Nephropathy

Previously, it was thought that renal failure is common (30–40%) in type 1 diabetes and relatively rare in type 2 diabetes (Grenfell and Watkins, 1986). More recent reports of a single population followed longitudinally indicate an approximately equal risk of nephropathy in both major diabetes types. Humphrey and coworkers observed an equivalent rate of renal failure over 30 years in cohorts of 1,832 type 2 diabetes and 136 type 1 diabetes patients in Rochester, Minnesota (Humphrey *et al.*, 1989). A long-term European study in Heidelberg reached the same conclusion, noting that a serum creatinine level greater than 1.4 mg/dl was present in 59% of type 1 diabetes and 63% of type 2 diabetes subjects (Hasslacher *et al.*, 1989).

Racial variables are evident in high-risk groups, including blacks, Hispanics and some Native Americans, all of whom have higher attack rates for diabetes and diabetic nephropathy; in all instances, the excess is in type 2 diabetes. Reported analyses of ESRD therapy that segregate patients by race and diabetes type are flawed largely by counting all insulin-treated subjects as having type 1 diabetes. We surveyed the race and gender of 232 of 1,450 (16%) diabetic patients undergoing maintenance hemodialysis at 14 centers in Brooklyn in 1986 and found the largest patient subset consisted of 87

black women, who comprised 37.5% of the total study population (Lowder *et al.*, 1988). Most surveyed diabetic patients on hemodialysis (139 or 59.9%) had type 2 diabetes; diabetes type could not be judged in 24 (10.3%) patients. Renal failure takes about 20 years to develop in type 1 diabetes. The mean interval between diagnosis of diabetes and performance of the patient's first hemodialysis in our Brooklyn series was 14.9 ± 9.3 years. Patients with type 1 diabetes whose onset was before age 20 had the longest interval (20.5 ± 5.9 years) to onset of hemodialysis ($P<0.01$), whereas patients with type 1 diabetes with onset after age 20 began hemodialysis after a mean of 15.3 ± 8.6 years, which was not significantly different from the overall mean.

Uremia Therapy

Nearly half of all diabetic uremic patients in the United States require treatment for ESRD without adequate preparation (i.e., established vascular or peritoneal access, tissue typing for kidney transplantation and education regarding options in therapy) (Ifudu *et al.*, 1999). Similar failed planning has been reported in France (Chantrel *et al.*, 1999) and Germany (Ritz *et al.*, 1999). As an expedient solution to the urgent need for treatment, about 75% of diabetic patients who develop ESRD are treated first with maintenance hemodialysis, approximately 15 to 20% of patients are treated with peritoneal dialysis and only 8 to 15% of patients receive a kidney transplant (Table 36–1). Before the necessity for blood pressure control was appreciated, hemodialysis was a disastrous therapy in diabetic ESRD patients that neither prolonged useful life nor attained rehabilitation (Ghavamian *et al.*, 1972), leading to the consensus that diabetic nephropathy should be excluded from ESRD therapy. Sutherland and colleagues at the University of Minnesota showed the value of combining initial hemodialysis with subsequent kidney transplantation, leading to their policy that "virtually every diabetic patient with renal failure referred to the University of Minnesota was accepted for transplantation, regardless of age, associated complications, or availability of a related donor" (Sutherland *et al.*, 1982). Once apprehension over treating diabetic ESRD patients dissipated, step-by-step continuing improvement in survival and life quality has been attained by hemodialysis, peritoneal dialysis and kidney transplantation, affording a choice among satisfactory treatments to the diabetic patient (Fig. 36–10).

TABLE 36–1

OPTIONS IN THERAPY FOR THE DIABETIC PATIENT WITH UREMIA

Hemodialysis
  Home hemodialysis
  Facility hemodialysis
Peritoneal dialysis
  Intermittent
  Continuous ambulatory
  Continuous cyclic (machine)
Kidney transplantation
  Living donor kidney
  Cadaver donor kidney
Kidney and pancreas transplantation
Kidney and pancreatic islet transplantation*

*Investigational.

HEMODIALYSIS

Because a diabetic patient is burdened by extensive systemic vascular disease and other comorbid disorders, establishment of a hemodialysis regimen is more difficult than in an age-matched and gender-matched nondiabetic individual (Table 36–2). Starting with surgical construction of a vascular access to the circulation, which may require preparatory endarterectomy of atherosclerotic plaques, almost every aspect of the hemodialysis regimen is a greater stress to a diabetic patient. Discovery of calcification of hand arteries is a warning sign that diversion of arterial blood flow may jeopardize the integrity of one or more fingers. Access complications, including gangrene of the hand (Tzamaloukas et al., 1991), ischemic monomelic neuropathy and repetitive thrombosis, cause various steal syndromes, limiting effective blood flow. Older diabetic patients usually require a synthetic (Dacron) prosthetic vascular graft placed in the mid or upper arm, an access choice more likely to fail than in nondiabetic patients (Mayers et al., 1992).

Timed observation of diabetic patients undergoing hemodialysis at a planned extracorporeal blood flow of 300 to 500

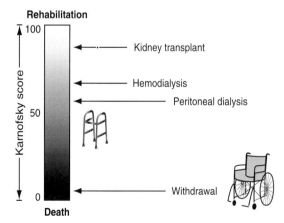

FIGURE 36–10

End-stage renal disease (ESRD) in diabetic nephropathy. Although no prospective randomized trials of uremia therapy in ESRD resulting from diabetes have been conducted, consensus thinking is that a kidney transplant permits the most complete return to former life functions. Whether hemodialysis is truly superior to peritoneal dialysis as depicted is debated. The Karnofsky score is a means of quantifying activity, with 100 being perfect health and 0 being death. Scores below 70 indicate the need for assistance in the normal chores of daily life.

TABLE 36–2

CONCERNS WHEN STARTING HEMODIALYSIS IN DIABETIC NEPHROPATHY

General
Periodic measurement of efficacy of dialysis nitrogenous solute extraction according to the National Kidney Foundation–Dialysis Outcomes Quality Initiative (urea reduction ratio >70%, or KT/V >1.3, where K = surface area of dialyzer, T = duration of dialysis treatment and V = volume of body water content) (Callahan et al., 1999). Monitor serum albumin concentration and hematocrit

Establishment of Vascular Access
Internal arteriovenous fistula
Bovine carotid arteriovenous heterograft
Teflon arteriovenous graft
Jugular percutaneous double–lumen catheter

Metabolic Regulation
Frequent finger-stick glucose measurements (type 1)
Fractional insulin doses or insulin pump (type 1 and type 2)
Educate regarding diet and exercise (type 1 and type 2)
Normalize weight (type 1 and type 2)
Frequent hemoglobin A_{1c} measurements
Hypolipidemic regimen if indicated

Propensity to Hypotension
Approximate (dry) weight
Minimize intradialytic weight gain
Target hematocrit at 34–38%
Bicarbonate-based, *normal*-sodium dialysate
Gradual ultrafiltration

Preservation of Vision
Strive for normotention and normoglycemia
Continuing surveillance by ophthalmologist
Low heparin dosage
Two or more pillows for head elevation during active retinopathy

Preservation of Lower Extremities
Wearing heel *booties*
Doppler flow evaluation of leg vessels
Collaboration with podiatrist (shoes, nails)

Obstipation Complicating Use of Phosphate Binders
High fiber diet
Prescribe detergent with antacid gel for phosphate sorption
Metoclopramide, cisapride
Cascara

Depression
Membership in American Association of Kidney Patients
Membership in American Diabetes Association
Full explanation of therapeutic options and plans
Periodic meetings with family and/or significant other

ml/min for 4 to 6 hours, three times each week, disclosed that the scheduled duration of dialysis often is not attained because of episodic hypotension and inferior access blood flow (Riggs et al., 1989). One consequence of reducing dialysis time is an increase in mortality (Berger and Lowrie, 1991; Held et al., 1991); survival of diabetic patients on maintenance hemodialysis is inferior to that of nondiabetic patients of both sexes and in all age groups. The striking toll of diabetic vasculopathy is illustrated by the half-time survival of diabetics on hemodialysis in one large series of 3 years versus 7.5 years for nondiabetic patients (Kjellstrand et al., 1980). This disparity in survival continues, according to the USRDS, which reported that fewer than 60% of diabetic patients live more than 2 years after starting maintenance hemodialysis, whereas fewer than 5% survive after 10 years of hemodialysis or peritoneal dialysis (USRDS, 1999). Limiting the utility of maintenance hemodialysis is the reality that only a few of those who survive attain satisfactory rehabilitation. In Brooklyn, for example, in a survey of 232 diabetic patients undergoing hemodialysis at 13 facilities, only 7 patients returned to full-time employment, whereas 64.9% were so disabled that they required assistance to accomplish routine activities (Lowder et al., 1988).

A prescient marker of poor survival in diabetic hemodialysis patients is a low serum albumin concentration (Lowrie and New, 1990). After correction of the low serum albumin of diabetic patients using proportional hazards analysis, much, but not all, of their increased mortality disappears. Throughout the 1990s, there has been encouraging continuous improvement in survival of diabetic ESRD patients treated by dialysis, but according to the 1999 USRDS report, diabetic dialysis patients die at a sharply higher rate compared with all dialysis patients.

PERITONEAL DIALYSIS

Continuous ambulatory peritoneal dialysis (CAPD) is the technique employed most frequently for peritoneal dialysis in the diabetic uremic patient, accounting for about 15% of all newly treated diabetic ESRD patients (Table 36–3). At slightly lower cost than hemodialysis, CAPD offers advantages of freedom from a machine, performance at home, rapid training, reduced cardiovascular stress and avoidance of heparin, when compared with hemodialysis. Continuous ambulatory peritoneal dialysis can be learned as a home regimen by motivated diabetic patients, even those who are blind, in 10 to 15 days, although the typical patient requires about 4 weeks. Patients learn to exchange 2 to 3 L of commercially prepared sterile dialysate solution three to five times daily. Fingerstick blood glucose measurements are required several times each day as a guide to the quantity of insulin administered. Insulin, antibiotics and other drugs are added by the patient to each dialysate exchange as needed. Fluid overload in intravascular and extracellular compartments is removed by switching to dialysate with a higher glucose concentration (4.5%) than the routinely used 1.5%.

Wide variation in the prescription (frequency and volume of exchanges) for peritoneal dialysis exchanged is practiced, including performing most exchanges during nighttime sleep, by addition of a mechanical cycler, in a variation termed *continuous cyclic peritoneal dialysis*. Continuous ambulatory peritoneal dialysis and continuous cyclic peritoneal dialysis place the diabetic patient at risk for peritonitis as well as a gradual decrease in peritoneal surface area, which may prove to be insufficient for adequate dialysis. Not all nephrologists regard CAPD as a suitable therapy; it is applied to a greater or lesser proportion of diabetic ESRD patients according to the bias of the individual nephrologist. Legrain et al. (1984) at one extreme endorse CAPD as a *first-choice treatment*, but less enthusiastic reports, such as that from Rubin and Hsu (1991), recount poor technique and poor patient survival in diabetic patients treated with CAPD in Mississippi. Only 34% of diabetic patients continued CAPD after 2 years in the series by Rubin and Hsu (1991), with about 18% remaining on peritoneal dialysis at 3 years.

Superior survival in diabetic ESRD patients treated by hemodialysis compared with peritoneal dialysis is reported consistently by the USRDS as classified by gender, race or age. In the United States, peritoneal dialysis patients experience a higher death rate than hemodialysis patients secondary to cardiovascular disease and cerebrovascular disease. By contrast, employing the Cox proportional hazards statistical method for unequal group analysis in 389 patients accepted

TABLE 36–3

CONCERNS ABOUT CONTINUOUS AMBULATORY PERITONEAL DIALYSIS IN DIABETIC NEPHROPATHY

General
Periodic measurement of efficacy of dialysis nitrogenous solute extraction according to the National Kidney Foundation–Dialysis Outcomes Quality Initiative (weekly KT/V >2.0, where K = surface area of dialyzer, T = duration of dialysis treatment and V = volume of body water content). For patients without residual urine volume excretion, more frequent exchanges at higher volume may be necessary to provide sufficient dialysis (Tzamaloukas et al., 1998). Monitor serum albumin concentration and hematocrit

Establishment of Peritoneal Access
Bathe with antimicrobial (hexachlorophene) soap
Direction
Tunnel
Type of catheter
Instruction regarding dialysate-drainage connection

Metabolic Regulation
Frequent finger-stick glucose measurements (type 1)
Fractional insulin doses or insulin pump (type 1 and type 2)
Educate regarding diet and exercise (type 1 and type 2)
Normalize weight (type 1 and type 2)
Frequent hemoglobin A_{1c} measurements
Hypolipidemic regimen if indicated

Propensity to Hyperlipidemia
Minimize excess calories
Minimize insulin
Hypolipidemic drugs

Preservation of Vision
Strive for normotension and normoglycemia
Continuing surveillance by ophthalmologist
Low heparin dosage
Two or more pillows for head elevation during active retinopathy

Preservation of Lower Extremities
Wearing heel *booties*
Doppler flow evaluation of leg vessels
Collaboration with podiatrist

Obstipation Complicating Use of Phosphate Binders
Prescribe detergent with antacid gel for phosphate sorption
Metoclopramide, cisapride
Cascara

Depression
Membership in American Association of Kidney Patients
Membership in American Diabetes Association
Full explanation of therapeutic options and plans
Periodic meetings with family and/or significant other

for renal replacement therapy in Leicester between 1974 and 1985 (Burton and Walls, 1987), no statistically significant differences between the relative risk of death for patients on CAPD (1.0), patients on hemodialysis (1.30) and patients who received a kidney transplant (1.09) were detected. Continuous ambulatory peritoneal dialysis, the authors concluded, "is at least as effective as haemodialysis or kidney transplantation in preserving life" (Burton and Walls, 1987). The Canada–United States (CANUSA) comparison of peritoneal dialysis and hemodialysis found superior survival of diabetic ESRD patients treated by peritoneal dialysis (Churchill, 1998; Churchill et al., 1997, 1998).

KIDNEY TRANSPLANTATION

End-stage renal disease in diabetes presents a major challenge in surgical management. The transplant team at the

University of Minnesota recognized early the therapeutic potential of renal transplantation in uremic patients with type 1 diabetes (Kelly *et al.*, 1967; Najarian *et al.*, 1979). Currently, renal transplantation is established as the treatment of choice for the uremic diabetic patient (Sutherland *et al.*, 1982). Long-term survival of the uremic diabetic patient with a well-functioning renal transplant is much better than that achieved in diabetic patients using other forms of renal replacement therapy (Khauli *et al.*, 1986; Reltig and Levinsky, 1991). Since 1980, the results of renal transplantation in diabetic patients have been about equal to those achieved in nondiabetic patients (Sutherland *et al.*, 1982). Diabetic patients should not be excluded categorically from transplantation because of anticipated problems with infection and wound healing. Diabetic patients are not significantly more prone, as previously thought, than nondiabetic patients to major complications after transplant surgery, provided that modifications are made before, during and after the transplantation procedure to adjust to their unique problems (Paterson *et al.*, 1987; Table 36–4).

Renal transplantation has the potential to place stress on the cardiovascular system as a result of the intentional volume expansion that takes place during the surgical procedure. Careful attention must be devoted to presurgical evaluation of the cardiovascular system in the diabetic patient before kidney and/or pancreas whole-organ transplantation. For some uremic diabetic patients, the discovery of severe coronary artery disease prompts revascularization of the myocardium by coronary artery bypass graft surgery or angioplasty as a condition to reconsideration of kidney transplantation (Braun *et al.*, 1983).

Coronary angiography was employed by Khauli and associates for preliminary screening for the presence and severity of coronary artery disease and left ventricular dysfunction in 48 diabetic patients scheduled for a kidney transplantation (Khauli *et al.*, 1983). In 23 patients, kidney transplantation was preceded by a myocardial revascularization procedure without a death. Two-year patient and graft survival for living donor and cadaver donor recipients given standard immunosuppression with azathioprine and prednisone was 81% and 68% for living donor recipients and 61% and 32% for cadaver donor recipients. Khauli and associates believe it wise to "discourage transplantation" in patients who have "the simultaneous presence of >70 per cent arterial stenosis and left ventricular dysfunction" (Khauli *et al.*, 1983). Philipson and colleagues studied 60 diabetic patients being considered for a kidney transplant and concluded that "patients with diabetes and end-stage renal disease who are at highest risk for cardiovascular events can be identified, and these patients probably should not undergo renal transplantation" (Philipson *et al.*, 1986). Only 7 of the 60 patients had a negative thallium stress test, 4 of whom received a kidney transplant, without subsequent cardiovascular events. Of the 53 diabetic patients with positive or nondiagnostic stress thallium tests, cardiac catheterization was used to identify 26 patients with mild or no coronary disease or left ventricular dysfunction; 16 patients in this group received transplants with no cardiovascular events. Moderate heart disease was noted in 10 patients, of whom 8 received transplants and 2 died of heart disease; of 13 patients with severe coronary artery disease or left ventricular malfunction, 8 died before receiving a transplant, 3 from cardiovascular disease. Perhaps the most important aspect of this series was the finding that 38% of diabetic ESRD patients had coronary artery disease.

Contemporary cardiac evaluation, including a thorough history and physical examination, should include an electrocardiogram, echocardiogram, thallium stress test, and, if needed, coronary artery catheterization and Holter monitoring (Corry *et al.*, 1987; Gill *et al.*, 1987). Arrhythmias on minimal exercise, electrocardiogram changes on stress and an ischemic myocardium with occluded coronary vessels are reasons to decline the transplant option in ESRD management. Data generated from these tests aid the transplant team in adjusting the degree of volume expansion during the operation.

Symptomatic peripheral vascular disease should be evaluated preoperatively with noninvasive Doppler flow studies and, in some instances, angiography to help determine where the renal allograft should be placed. Arteries found to be supplying a lower extremity with marginal peripheral flow must not be used to revascularize an organ allograft because the extremity may be placed in jeopardy (Fanning *et al.*, 1986). We have found that diabetic transplant recipients frequently have atherosclerotic narrowing of the internal iliac artery, forcing use of the external iliac artery for the arterial anastomosis. At the time of transplant surgery, a local proximal endarterectomy of the external iliac artery is required in instances of severe atherosclerotic narrowing.

With careful evaluation of the coronary and peripheral vascular systems before renal transplantation, there is a high incidence of extremity amputation and cardiovascular death in diabetic renal allograft recipients followed for 3 or more years, owing to progression of diabetic macrovasculopathy and microvasculopathy (Abendroth *et al.*, 1990; Gonzalez-Carrillo *et al.*, 1982). Patient survival in diabetic recipients older than age 40 is lower, generally less than that of younger diabetic renal transplant recipients, owing to cardiovascular death (Yuge and Cecka, 1992). The increased risk of cardiovascular death posttransplant in older diabetic patients also is present in the same patient managed by dialytic therapy. Overall, as depicted in Figures 36–11 and 36–12, survival in ESRD in diabetes is better with a kidney transplant than with dialysis. Reflecting multiple incremental improvements in overall care, the 2-year survival during maintenance hemodialysis or after a cadaveric kidney transplant is increasing continuously (Fig. 36–13).

TABLE 36–4

ASSESSMENT OF COMORBID RISKS IN DIABETIC PATIENTS WITH UREMIA

Cystopathy: cystometrogram, urine culture, residual volume
Heart disease: electrocardiogram, exercise stress test, coronary angiography
Gastrointestinal disease (gastroparesis, obstipation, diarrhea): abdominal radiography
Respiratory disease: vital capacity
Preservation of vision: visual acuity, fluorescein angiography
Bone consequences of uremia: metabolic radiographic bone survey, plasma aluminum level, bone scan
Limb preservation: podiatric assessment, Doppler flow studies of limb perfusion
Dental assessment
Social worker and nurse educator's assessment of potential for self-care

Posttransplant Management

Posttransplant management of the diabetic renal transplant recipient often is complex, as in the case of distinguishing between acute allograft rejection, acute tubular necrosis and cyclosporine drug nephrotoxicity in an oliguric newly transplanted patient. Interpretation of renal scans, sonograms, biopsy specimens and tests of glomerular and tubular function still is largely an art based on experience.

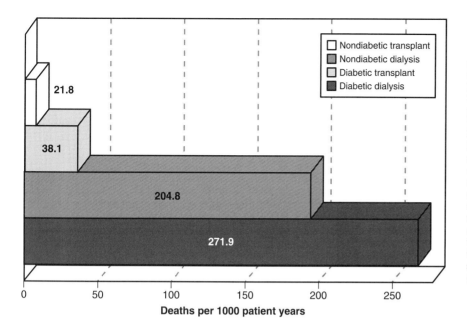

Deaths per 1000 patient years

FIGURE 36–11

End-stage renal disease (ESRD) death rates: 1995–1997. From composite death rates reported by the United States Renal Data System (USRDS) in 1999, several inferences can be drawn: (1) Mortality of ESRD patients during dialysis (combined peritoneal dialysis and hemodialysis) treatment is greater than after a kidney transplant. Whether treated by dialysis or a kidney transplant, the death rate of diabetic ESRD patients is higher than for nondiabetic ESRD patients. Because assignment to therapy was not randomized, and appreciating that patients chosen for a kidney transplant were younger and healthier than the residual pool of dialysis patients, caution should be applied in interpreting these data. (Data from USRDS.)

Metabolic control of plasma glucose concentration is best effected by frequent—hourly when needed—measurements of glucose and an intravenous infusion of insulin. Postoperative protracted gastric atony from gastroparesis may delay resumption of oral feeding. Administration of a liquid suspension of metoclopramide before meals usually enhances gastric motility, improving gastric emptying. Bethanechol, which may be given in combination with metoclopramide, also improves gastric motility. Constipation, sometimes evolving into obstipation, is a frequent problem after transplantation; to resume spontaneous defecation, early ambulation, stool softening agents and suspension of cascara are effective. At the other extreme, explosive and continuous

liquid diarrhea, a manifestation of autonomic neuropathy, may enervate and dehydrate the postoperative diabetic patient. Loperamide, given hourly in doses of 4 mg/h, almost always halts the diarrhea. Urinary retention, a functional outflow obstruction, also is a manifestation of autonomic neuropathy expressed as diabetic cystopathy. Insistence on frequent voiding, self-application of manual external pressure above the pubic symphysis (Credé's maneuver) and administration of oral bethanechol usually permit resumption of spontaneous voiding. Rarely, repeated self-catheterization is required for an unresponsive atonic bladder.

Diabetic recipients of renal transplants generally require longer hospitalizations than do nondiabetic patients (Naj-

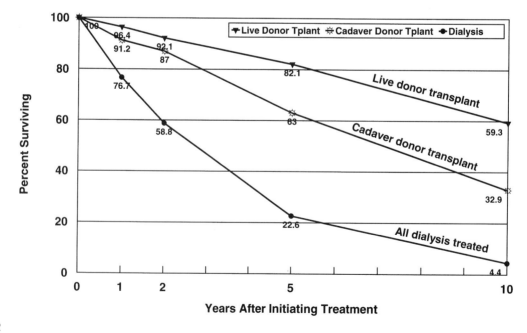

FIGURE 36–12

Survival for 10 years for diabetic and nondiabetic renal transplant recipients of living related and cadaver donor kidneys is compared with survival on dialytic therapy as reported by the United States Renal Data System (USRDS). Results for continuous ambulatory peritoneal dialysis and maintenance hemodialysis are pooled because outcome is not statistically different between these two modalities. Fewer than 5% of diabetic end-stage renal disease patients treated by either form of dialysis survive a decade. (Reproduced with permission of USRDS, 1999.)

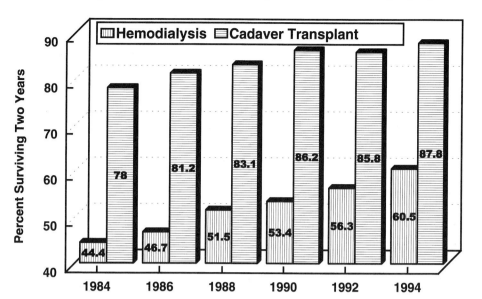

FIGURE 36–13

After 2 years of end-stage renal disease therapy, survival of diabetic patients treated by hemodialysis and kidney transplantation is improving continuously as reported by the United States Renal Data System (USRDS). (Data from USRDS.)

arian *et al.*, 1979). Wide swings in glucose concentration, including alternating hypoglycemia and hyperglycemia up to hyperosmolar nonketonic coma, are life-threatening to the diabetic recipient, particularly immediately postoperatively and during times of high-dose steroid administration for rejection treatment. Insulin requirements may increase sharply in type 1 diabetes and type 2 diabetes during the postoperative course, then fall as corticosteroid doses are reduced and glucose-containing parenteral fluids are withdrawn.

Impotence—of neuropathic, vasculopathic or psychogenic origin—is common in diabetic dialysis patients and, in a few patients, may improve after a successful kidney transplant. Use of a penile prosthesis or precoital intrapenile injections of prostaglandins may be appropriate for rehabilitation when impotence persists. In the absence of overt cardiac disease, sildenafil (Viagra) has a role.

Subjective assessment of their own quality of life by diabetic renal transplant recipients compares favorably with that of the general population in the United States. Nevertheless, rehabilitation of the diabetic patient with ESRD can be blocked by vision loss and debilitating, painful motor and autonomic neuropathy. The renal transplant team depends on collaboration with an ophthalmologist skilled in laser surgery and a podiatrist experienced in preventive management of diabetic feet. With early renal transplantation before initiation of a dialysis regimen, many diabetic patients become increasingly disabled because of progressive extrarenal disease processes (Sutherland, 1988).

An additional threat to renal allograft integrity is imposed by recurrent diabetic glomerulopathy first detectable as glomerular basement membrane thickening with mesangial expansion after 2 years (Osterby *et al.*, 1991) and later as characteristic glomerulosclerosis in long-term type 1 diabetes transplant recipients (Bohman *et al.*, 1984; Mauer *et al.*, 1989). After as short an interval as 5 years, diabetic renal transplant recipients, especially those who have not attained relatively tight glucose control, may manifest a nephrotic syndrome again followed by progressive azotemia and ESRD. Najarian and coworkers provided encouraging evidence that survival of diabetic kidney transplant recipients may exceed 10 years (Najarian *et al.*, 1989). Of 265 ESRD patients with type 1 diabetes who were given a renal transplant between December 1966 and April 1978, 100 were alive with a functioning graft 10 years later (actual patient and primary graft survivals

of 40% and 32%). For HLA-identical recipients of living related donor kidneys, the actual 10-year functional graft survival was 62%. Cardiovascular disease, which caused 10 of 23 deaths in the second decade after kidney transplantation, continued as the most frequent cause of death in diabetic renal graft recipients.

PANCREAS TRANSPLANTATION

A logical extension of renal transplantation in uremic patients with type 1 diabetes is a curative (for type 1 diabetes) concurrent pancreatic allograft. Combining pancreas and kidney transplants does not raise immediate perioperative mortality; however, perioperative morbidity is increased (USRDS, 1992). Pancreas transplantation is a *life-enriching* procedure because patients with type 1 diabetes discontinue self-administered insulin injections and experience an improved sense of well-being. The primary objective of pancreatic transplantation is to halt, or at least retard, progression of diabetic microvascular and macrovascular extrarenal complications.

Surgical Considerations

In contrast to renal transplantation, the surgical approach to whole-organ pancreatic transplantation has not evolved into a single ideal technique (Figs. 36–14 and 36–15). The pancreas is a fragile, finicky gland with substantial intolerance to trauma, hypoperfusion or duct obstruction. Such insult may cause acute pancreatitis, pseudocyst formation or leakage of digestive pancreatic enzymes intraabdominally or cutaneously (pancreatic fistula), all feared complications associated with excessive morbidity and mortality. Justification of the anticipated benefits must suffice to persuade the surgeon to initiate deliberate manipulation and dissection of the gland in association with planned ischemia because both accompany pancreatic transplantation. Surgical concerns focus on minimizing technical deleterious consequences of transplantation, obviating rejection and expediting diagnosis of adverse episodes that do occur.

As for a kidney transplant (discussed earlier), detection and management of vascular disease of the coronary, cerebrovascular or peripheral beds is a major determinant of longevity in the recipient. Although criteria vary widely among transplant programs, it is crucial that the intended pancreas recipient not have such advanced disease that perioperative

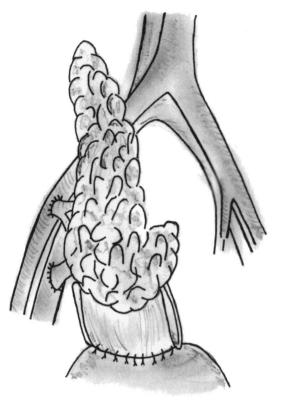

FIGURE 36–14

Pancreas transplant. Drainage of proteolytic enzymes from the exocrine pancreas is a major concern in choosing the site for allograft placement. In the United States, direct attachment to the urinary bladder is popular. Pancreaticoduodenal transplantation with urinary bladder exocrine drainage in right iliac fossa. End-to-side anastomosis of portal vein to external iliac vein for venous drainage and end-to-side anastomosis of iliac artery extension graft from splenic artery and superior mesenteric artery to external iliac artery for arterial inflow.

survival is unlikely. We consider objective cardiac assessment of left ventricular function and coronary arterial flow within 6 to 12 months of transplantation mandatory. It is rare that a diabetic potential pancreas recipient is able to perform sufficient physical activity to achieve a diagnostic stress level. Significant heart disease often remains unnoticed as a consequence of autonomic neuropathy.

Although algorithms designed to evaluate cardiac integrity have been proposed, in the current managed care era we do not dictate the evaluation process to the patient's primary care physician or cardiologist. Each of the commonly employed techniques has limitations. Coronary angiography is overly sensitive and may show anatomical lesions that do not have clinical significance, whereas noninvasive nuclear isotope or ultrasound examinations may miss subtle myocardial disease. At a minimum, we request assessment of the left ventricular ejection fraction and coronary vascular supply. When abnormalities are identified, coronary angiography is performed.

The first reported transplant of pancreatic tissue was by Hedon (1893), who claimed to prevent the development of diabetes in a dog by grafting of a portion of native pancreas before total resection of the organ. In 1922 with the discovery of insulin by Banting and Best, the acute mortality of diabetics from the metabolic derangements caused by diabetes pushed pancreatic transplantation far away from the fore-

front of diabetes care (Gayet and Guillaumie, 1927). The use of insulin extended the life of individuals with diabetes dramatically; however, the secondary ravages of the disease became evident during the next 10 years and became the major cause of subsequent mortality and morbidity. The inability to maintain normal glycemic conditions with the intermittent exogenous delivery of insulin and the development of secondary complications, especially ESRD owing to diabetes, led to the application of kidney transplantation for treatment of diabetic nephropathy (Najarian et al., 1979). This treatment did not restore normal metabolism for the diabetic, however, and metabolic control often was made more difficult with the restored normal renal breakdown of insulin and the necessity of steroids as immunosuppressive agents.

Forty years after Gayet and Guillaumie (1927) performed the first successful transplantation of an immediately vascularized pancreatic allograft in a dog model, Largiarder et al. (1967) and Lillehei et al. (1970) worked out the surgical techniques of pancreas transplantation in large animal models. These studies led to the first clinical attempts at pancreatic transplantation. On December 17, 1966, at the University of Minnesota, a team led by Kelly and Lillehei performed the first reported vascularized pancreas transplant in a human (Kelly et al., 1967). The body and tail of a cadaveric pancreas was used, and the pancreatic duct was ligated. This allograft was placed in the left iliac fossa, and a simultaneously transplanted kidney was placed in the opposite side. The patient became normoglycemic and insulin independent immediately. This team subsequently went on to perform a series of 13 more pancreatic transplants between 1966 and 1973. Twelve of these transplants were pancreatic duodenal

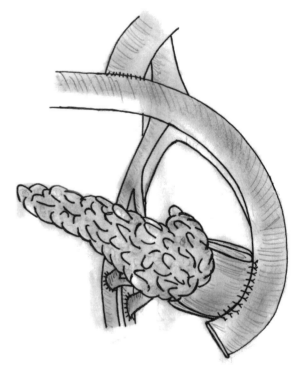

FIGURE 36–15

Pancreas transplant. Techniques using a direct pancreas-to-bowel connection are widely employed. Pancreaticoduodenal transplantation with enteric exocrine drainage to Roux-en-Y jejunal limb. End-to-side anastomosis of portal vein to external iliac vein for venous drainage and end-to-side anastomosis of iliac artery extension graft from splenic artery and superior mesenteric artery to external iliac artery for arterial inflow.

grafts, which were anastomosed through a duodenal Roux-en-Y. Only one of these pancreatic allografts functioned for more than 1 year (Lillehei et al., 1976).

Gliedman and associates recognized the septic complications associated with a bowel anastomosis in the immunosuppressed recipient and joined the severed duct of the segmental pancreatic allografts to the recipient's ureter (Gliedman et al., 1973). Long-term pancreatic graft function was achieved in two of the six patients in the series for 2 and 4 years after transplantation. Gliedman and associates also were among the first to report on the use of urinary amylase as a potential marker for pancreatic graft rejection (Gliedman et al., 1973). Groth and coworkers in the 1970s introduced clinical pancreatic transplantation using segmental grafts with enteric exocrine drainage (Groth et al., 1982). At the same time, Dubernard and colleagues in Lyon, France, used a novel technique of occluding the pancreatic duct by injecting it with the polymer neoprene in vascularized segmental grafts (Dubernard et al., 1978).

In the 1970s, after the report by Ballinger and Lacy (1972) that islet transplantation as free individual grafts could be used to achieve normoglycemia in rats with streptozotocin-induced diabetes, the incentive to perform whole clinical pancreas transplantation declined. The technical and immunological failures associated with the procedure led to a mortality and morbidity rate that surpassed most other organ transplants during that time (Collin, 1978). For most transplant centers, the poor results could not be justified for a procedure that was not regarded as life saving. Trials of islet transplantation in humans met with varying and transient success, however (Pipeleers and Pipeleers-Marichal, 1977). The long-term goal to achieve a euglycemic state in the diabetic was a long way from being achieved.

Dubernard's simple application of ductal obstruction to the technique of pancreas transplantation renewed interest in segmental and whole-organ clinical pancreas transplantation. This technique proved to be relatively safe, had less infectious complications associated with it and was adopted by several institutions as the technique of choice. It was found later in long-term clinical trials of this technique that ductal injection eventually induced global pancreatic fibrosis, which involved the insulin-producing islet cells, leading to the return of diabetes (Feitosa Tajra et al., 1998).

The management of the pancreatic allograft duct has proved to be the Achilles' heel of pancreas transplantation, as was the biliary duct in liver transplantation (Starzl et al., 1977). Currently the most popular techniques for management of the pancreatic duct are enteric drainage, bladder drainage and, to a lesser extent, polymer injection (DiCarlo et al., 1998). Bladder drainage was popularized by Corry et al. (1986) and Cook et al. (1983) in the mid-1980s using a cuff of duodenal tissue surrounding the ampulla of Vater or a composite graft of the donor's duodenum attached to the pancreas and joining it directly to the recipient's bladder. A byproduct of this technique has been the ability to measure urinary amylase easily, as suggested by Gliedman et al. (1973), as a possible signal for graft rejection. Although the initial experience in pancreatic transplantation used the physiological drainage of exocrine secretions into the bowel, the technique was fraught with septic complications, including intraabdominal and wound infections.

Urinary drainage, ultimately leading to the duodenovesical anastomosis, helped pancreas transplantation to become more successful and was adopted by most clinical pancreatic transplantation centers worldwide. The advent of bladder drainage complications related to activated pancreatic enzymes in the urinary tract and chronic loss of bicarbonate necessitated the conversion of some recipients to enteric drainage. The ease of the conversion process and the relative lack of complications renewed interest in primary enteric anastomosis for the pancreatic allograft (Burke et al., 1990). Although bladder drainage continues to be the most used technique, enteric drainage quickly is becoming the procedure of choice (Douzdjian et al., 1993; Gruessner et al., 1997). Evaluations of large groups of pancreas transplant recipients have suggested that enteric drainage provides a trend toward increased long-term survival without the bladder-specific complications, including dysuria, hematuria and metabolic acidosis, associated with the bladder drainage techniques (Sugitani et al., 1998). Whole-organ pancreatic transplantation, over use of the segmental pancreas, is currently the procedure of choice for pancreas transplantation because of the technical ease of the donor and recipient operation and the larger islet dose for the recipient (DiCarlo et al., 1998).

In all of these described surgical techniques, pancreatic venous drainage by the donor portal vein is systemic by the recipient's iliac vein. Experimental work in dogs shows that systemic vascular drainage is associated with hyperinsulinemia and increased lipogenesis in arterial walls and in striated muscles (Konigsrainer et al., 1998). Calne (1984) reported first on a technique of portal venous drainage for segmental pancreas grafts. Pancreas transplantation with portal venous drainage and enteric exocrine drainage has been championed by Graber et al. (1993). In this technique, the portal vein draining the pancreas is anastomosed to a tributary of the recipient's superior mesenteric vein, and the arterial inflow to the pancreas is gained by way of a graft to the common iliac artery of the recipient (Graber et al., 1993). Exocrine drainage from the pancreas is completed through a Roux-en-Y anastomosis from the duodenum of the donor to the jejunum of the recipient. Vascular complications after pancreas transplantation have been common in the past and include thrombosis, hemorrhage, stenosis, aneurysm formation and arterial-venous fistula formation. Refinements in vascular techniques and newer immunosuppressive agents have led to a dramatic decline in vascular-related complications, however. Routine use of an arterial graft for inflow, anastomosis of the portal vein after complete mobilization of the recipient's iliac vein and limited use of vein extension grafts have decreased the incidence of most vascular complications (Bynon et al., 1993; Gruessner et al., 1997). Whether pancreatic venous drainage into the portal system proves to be the procedure of choice remains to be evaluated.

In another pioneering study, Sutherland and colleagues at the University of Minnesota in 1979 began a series of living related donor pancreatic transplants (Sutherland et al., 1980). The surgical technique included enteric drainage of a distal segment of pancreatic allograft removed from the living related donor. Donor mortality in the series has been 0 and the incidence of surgical complications approximately 10 to 15%. Living related donor pancreas transplantation provides an attractive option for a limited group of diabetic patients (i.e., diabetic patients who should avoid high immunosuppression, patients who are highly sensitized and have a low probability of receiving a cadaver graft, recipients with a donor who is a nondiabetic nonidentical twin and uremic patients who want one operation with no waiting time to remain or to become dialysis-free as well as insulin independent) (Humar et al., 1997). The group in Minnesota has found that living related pancreas transplants can be performed safely in all recipient categories—pancreas transplant alone, pancreas transplantation after a kidney transplant or simultaneous pancreas-kidney transplantation. All living related pancreas donors must meet strict criteria, including being at least 10 years older in age than the age of onset of diabetes in the sibling recipient, no immediate family member is diabetic

TABLE 36–5

VARIABLES IN MORBIDITY IN DIABETIC KIDNEY TRANSPLANT RECIPIENTS: COMORBIDITY INDEX*

Persistant angina or evolving myocardial infraction
Other cardiovascular problems (severe hypertension, symptomatic congestive heart failure, cardiomyopathy)
Active respiratory disease
Symptomatic autonomic neuropathy (gastroparesis, obstipation, diarrhea, cystopathy, orthostatic hypotension)
Neurological problems, cerebrovascular accident or stroke residual
Musculoskeletal disorders, including all varieties of renal bone disease
Infections including AIDS but excluding vascular access site or peritonitis
Hepatitis, hepatic insufficiency, enzymatic pancreatic insufficiency
Hematological problems other than anemia
Spinal abnormalities, lower back problems or arthritis
Vision impairment (minor to severe—decreased acuity to blindness)
Limb amputation (minor to severe—finger to lower extremity)
Mental or emotional illness (neurosis, depression, psychosis)

*To obtain a numerical comorbidity index for an individual patient, rate each variable from 0 to 3 (0 = absent, 1 = mild [of minor import to patient's life], 2 = moderate and 3 = severe). By proportional hazard analysis, the relative significance of each variable can be isolated from the other 12.
AIDS = acquired immunodeficiency syndrome.

other than the recipient and all donors must have a post intravenous glucose first-phase insulin level above the 30th percentile for the normal range. No donor meeting these strict criteria has become hyperglycemic after hemipancreatectomy, and long-term follow-up shows them to be metabolically stable (Kendall *et al.*, 1989; Seaquist and Robertson, 1992).

The Minnesota group has reported on development of a technique for simultaneous kidney and segmental pancreas transplantation from living related donors (Gruessner and Sutherland, 1996). The experience with living related pancreas transplant shows higher long-term function for technically successful pancreatic grafts compared with those from cadaver donors. The living related donor pancreas recipient requires less immunosuppression and was found to have

fewer rejection episodes (Sutherland *et al.*, 1994). Since the 1980s, the technical aspects of using segmental allografts from living donors have improved and provide the potential recipient with the multiple previously stated benefits, while preserving a limited cadaver pancreas pool for other recipients.

Although pancreas transplantation is not a benign procedure and remains a difficult *cure* for the ravages of diabetes, the surgical procedure remains the only treatment that promises hope for exogenous insulin independence and freedom from the debilitating secondary complications of diabetes mellitus. Central to life prolongation after onset of uremia in diabetes is recognition and management of comorbid extrarenal disease (see Table 36–4). Relative severity of diabetic ESRD patients can be compared using a simple rating system termed the *comorbidity index* (Table 36–5).

Outcome of Pancreas Transplantation

Whole-pancreas transplantation is an uncommon approach to management of type 1 diabetes. The world's largest cumulative experience is available from the International Pancreas Transplant Registry (IPTR) and includes a total of 11,442 transplants (8,839 from the United States) (Gruessner and Sutherland, 1999). Whether limited by the shortage of cadaver organs, availability of suitable preuremic candidates, lack of enthusiasm by transplant teams or all of the above, solitary pancreas transplantation (pancreas transplant alone [PTA]) is performed rarely, representing only 4% of reported cases. One-year allograft survival (64%) is lowest in PTA (Fig. 36–16). Cadaveric pancreas transplantation performed in a recipient with a functioning renal allograft (pancreas after kidney [PAK]) is considered by many to represent the most reasonable strategy for candidates with access to a living kidney donor, although two separate operations are required. In our experience, the waiting time preceding transplantation of both organs is minimized under allocation schemes requiring diabetics to wait for cadaveric kidneys as long as other renal recipients. Although higher pancreatic graft survival is reported for simultaneous cadaveric pancreas and kidney (SPK) recipients than PAK recipients (83% *vs.* 71%), intergroup differences such as (1) duration of pretransplant maintenance dialysis, (2) duration of state of immunosuppression before pancreas transplantation and (3) HLA iden-

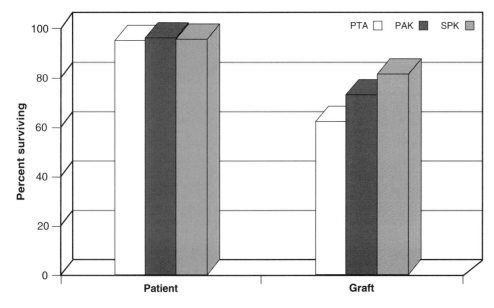

FIGURE 36–16

Patient and allograft survival at 1 year for pancreas and kidney transplantation in diabetic recipients. Although there is no difference in patient survival according to the sequence of grafting, pancreas graft survival is distinctly superior after a simultaneous pancreas and kidney transplant (SPK) than after a pancreas after a kidney transplant (PAK) or a pancreas transplant alone (PTA). Data are from the International Pancreas Transplant Registry (Gruessner and Sutherland, 1998).

TABLE 36–6

SURGICAL COMPLICATIONS OF PANCREAS TRANSPLANTATION

	Enteric Drainage	Bladder Drainage	Duct Injection
Fibrosis	+	+	+ + +
Septic complications: peritonitis, abscess, mycotic aneurysm	+ +	+ +	+
Bladder related: dysuria, hematuria, metabolic acidosis, recurrent urinary tract infections	0	+ +	0
Thrombosis	+	+	+
Exocrine anastomotic leak	+ +	+	0
Pseudocysts (Candinas et al., 1994; Patel *et al.*, 1991)	+	+	+
Bleeding	+	+	+

tity or difference of renal and pancreatic donors likely contribute to the discrepancy.

International Pancreas Transplant Registry data show that primary pancreatic duct management in the United States is limited almost exclusively to bladder or enteric drainage, with the latter increasingly popular. New confidence in the enteric drainage approach is reflected in a conversion rate from bladder to enteric drainage of 8% in technically successful SPK within 1 year and 11% at 2 years. Results from the most recent era (1994–1998) show virtually identical graft survival at 1 year (83% *vs.* 82%) for SPK transplants. Thrombosis (6.3% in SPK) is the commonest technical cause of graft failure for all three grafting sequences followed by infections and pancreatitis, leak and bleeding (Table 36–6). Immunological pancreatic allograft loss from rejection and autoimmunity is declining in frequency as the impact of enhanced immunosuppressive strategies is felt (Fig. 36–17). Nevertheless the advantage of the SPK approach versus PAK, presumably owing to the legitimacy of interpreting a kidney biopsy as an indicator of pancreatic rejection, remains evident from the lower rate of immunological organ loss in this category.

Pancreas transplantation performed in patients with extensive extrarenal disease has neither arrested nor reversed diabetic retinopathy, diabetic cardiomyopathy or extensive peripheral vascular disease (Ramsay *et al.*, 1988). Nevertheless, most importantly, a functioning pancreas transplant frees patients with type 1 diabetes from the daily burden of balancing diet, exercise and insulin dosage (Katz *et al.*, 1991; Piehlmeier *et al.*, 1992). From December 1966 through December 1990, the IPTR lists a total of 3,082 pancreas transplants, of which a detailed analysis was possible in 2,087 (Sutherland, 1991). Overall, 1-year recipient and graft functional survival rates were 89% and 62%. Individual programs attained better results as exemplified by the Goteborg team, who reported 67 transplants, of which 50 were combined with kidney transplants and 17 were pancreas after kidney transplants, with 1-year patient and graft survival rates of 95% and 83% (Olausson *et al.*, 1991).

Pancreas Transplantation for Type 2 Diabetes

Virtually every component of the American Diabetes Association's definition of type 2 diabetes represents at least a relative practical contraindication to pancreas transplantation. Most patients with type 2 diabetes are older than age 40 at the time end-organ damage and/or ESRD develops. In view of current limited expectations for full rehabilitation, most experts would consider earlier pancreas transplantation generally inappropriate. Advanced (relatively) age in type 2 diabetes usually is associated with substantive extrarenal diabetic vasculopathy, which is a reason for exclusion by many pancreas transplant programs. Obesity, the other key

FIGURE 36–17

Immunological pancreas allograft loss by era in diabetic recipients. Steady improvements in immunosuppressive strategies have resulted in decreasing graft loss in simultaneous pancreas and kidney transplant (SPK), pancreas after kidney transplant (PAK) and pancreas transplant alone (PTA). Data are from the International Pancreas Transplant Registry (Gruessner and Sutherland, 1998).

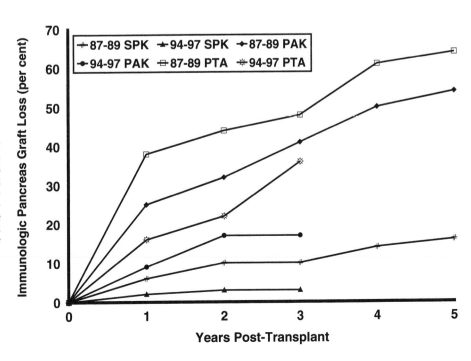

defining property of type 2 diabetes, is strongly associated with increased morbidity and mortality from all surgical procedures and specifically after pancreas transplantation (Odorico *et al.*, 1998). Obesity raises the rate of technical complications because of increased difficulty in obtaining adequate anatomical visualization, poor healing and associated perioperative complications such as deep venous thrombosis. Diabetic patients with exogenous obesity greater than 20% of normal weight, including most type 2 patients, are not offered a pancreas transplant. Insulin resistance represents the key theoretical contraindication to pancreas transplantation in type 2 diabetes patients. It is argued that exposure of donor β cells to the type 2 diabetes environment leads to their overstimulation and ultimate exhaustion, meaning functional graft loss (Sasaki *et al.*, 1998). In view of the limited supply of high-quality cadaver pancreas glands, the prevailing practice of limiting their use to type 1 diabetics is understandable and consistent with the goal of maximizing duration of graft function.

Despite the rhetoric, clinical results of inadvertent pancreas transplantation for type 2 diabetes have surpassed expectations. Sasaki and colleagues reported their experience with 13 simultaneous pancreas-kidney transplant recipients (Sasaki *et al.*, 1998). Elevated C-peptide levels in recipients—establishing their diabetes as type 2—were identified only retrospectively; transplant candidacy had been assessed purely on clinical criteria. Graft survival in these type 2 diabetic recipients was 100% with a mean follow-up of 45.5 months. Our experience with a single patient also identified as having type 2 diabetes after inadvertent pancreas transplantation has been similarly encouraging; the recipient lost a primary pancreas graft to venous thrombosis but is insulin independent 6 months after transplantation of a second pancreas.

The current critical organ shortage precludes routine pancreas transplantation in type 2 diabetes patients because most have become poor candidates for extensive surgery by the time any permutation of the procedure would be appropriate. Nevertheless, encouraging results of the initial experience justify further exploration of pancreas transplantation in type 2 diabetes patients.

Transplantation of Pancreatic Islets

In contrast to most clinical disease states managed with organ replacement therapy, the therapeutic goal of pancreatic transplantation (i.e., restoration of euglycemia) might be attained by transplantation of a portion of the whole pancreas, the islets of Langerhans. Obviating the risks of a major surgical procedure by simple injection of a small-volume suspension of islets is appealing. Clinical success, indicated not only by some signs of persistent islet function, but also by true insulin independence, has been achieved in only a small fraction of diabetic islet recipients. Despite this reality, enthusiasm for this conceptual approach to amelioration of diabetes drives researchers to pursue what many consider the *Holy Grail* of endocrinology.

Although the intact pancreas is fragile, the islets it harbors are more durable. Viable, insulin-producing islets can be isolated with a relatively simple and reproducible technique using enzymatic digestion of the whole-organ stroma in rats, dogs and primates. With some technical modifications, human islets also are culled from normal pancreas glands procured from cadaver donors (Marshak *et al.*, 1999) or resected for disease (Rabkin *et al.*, 1997). As long as the whole gland is resected and handled according to general principles of organ procurement (i.e., minimal warm ischemia, prompt cooling and perfusion with University of Wisconsin solution),

its endocrine component is tolerant of cold ischemia. Once isolated, fresh islets can be transported safely across great distances (Rabkin *et al.*, 1997). The key implication of this flexibility is that the isolation laboratory need not be located at or even in proximity to the transplant center.

Regardless of the original source, selection of the heterotopic site to host the islets remains problematic. Access to oxygen, nutrients and hormonal stimuli and a means of egress for hormonal products are conditions of islet viability. The recipient organ must tolerate the presence of the islets without developing an inflammatory or obliterative response. A wide range of sites including the peritoneum (Sutherland, 1994), thymus (Posselt *et al.*, 1992; Tuch *et al.*, 1999), testicle (Ar'Rajab *et al.*, 1994), spleen (Gray, 1990), kidney capsule (Leow *et al.*, 1994) and liver (Stevens *et al.*, 1994) have supported long-term survival of engrafted islets in rats, dogs and primates. Of these sites, only the last two have practical potential for human application; the liver has been preferred for clinical trial.

In the most straightforward scenario, islets isolated from pancreas glands removed to treat the symptoms of chronic pancreatitis are autotransplanted during a second procedure in the same patient. This elegant approach to prevention of the endocrine insufficiency that results from 40 to 100% of pancreatectomies (Fournier *et al.*, 1998) is reported in more than 150 patients (Robertson *et al.*, 1998), all with intrahepatic implantation of the islets. Access to the portal venous system is achieved through the inferior mesenteric vein, through small mesenteric tributaries or through a transsplenic approach and has been sporadically associated with significant technical complications including splenic infarction (White *et al.*, 1999). From this finite experience, it is clear that technically successful primary instillation of suspended islets into the portal venous system can be limited by long-term progressive graft loss. With no immunological basis for gradual islet destruction, exposure to factors associated with the ectopic location such as nutritional toxins, intestinal bacteria and endotoxins must be implicated in the failure to achieve prolonged graft survival.

After initial engraftment, islet longevity also depends on successful evasion of two unique types of immunological attack. Most potential recipients must depend on a genetically dissimilar islet donor. In other allogeneic solid-organ transplants, immunosuppressive medications to prevent rejection are tolerated with manageable side effects. Although limited, the reported experience with islet allotransplantation into nondiabetic recipients confirms the suitability of similar immunosuppressive strategies. Insulin independence was achieved in 60% of 15 patients who underwent hepatectomy and pancreatectomy with combined liver and islet allotransplantation (Carroll *et al.*, 1995; Tzakis *et al.*, 1990). Despite these encouraging results, widespread application remains unlikely under the best of circumstances. Human pancreas donors are scarce; only 5,791 were available in the United States in 1998 (USRDS, 1998). Even if all 4,573 donors from whom whole-organ pancreas grafts were not procured became islet donors, the availability of allogeneic islets would fall far short of the huge pool of uremic diabetic recipients who might benefit.

Newly transplanted islets are subject to recurrence of the same T cell–mediated autoimmune β cell destruction that originally caused the host's type 1 diabetes. Recipients of pancreatic segments from identical twins can experience rapidly recurrent diabetes without any evidence of rejection, implicating strongly such an autoimmune mechanism in the graft failure (Sibley *et al.*, 1985). More recently, the use of *gentle* immunosuppression may have protected one identical twin recipient of a simultaneous pancreas-kidney graft from autoimmune-mediated insulitis (Benedetti *et al.*, 1999). Immunosuppression also protects islets embedded within pancreatic allografts to some extent, although Esmatjes and colleagues have identified the diabetic immunomarker antibodies to islet cells and to glutamic acid decarboxylase in 22% and 14% of patients with functioning grafts (Esmatjes *et al.*, 1998). For unclear reasons, however, isolated islet allografts are more susceptible to injury. Antiislet antibodies have been associated with a significantly increased risk of islet graft loss (Jaeger *et al.*, 1997, 1998; Roep *et al.*, 1999). There is little doubt that autoimmunity currently plays a limiting role in the progressive loss of insulin production after clinical islet allotransplantation.

No other area seems quite as appropriate for exploratory attempts to use living tissue from another species (*xenotransplantation*) as islet transplantation. With a noninvasive transplant procedure and graft loss marked by minimal clinical consequences other than the onset of hyperglycemia, the risk/benefit ratio seems entirely favorable. The achievement of Thomas and colleagues of stable, long-term acceptance of xenogeneic islets in diabetic monkeys without chronic immunosuppression is exciting (Thomas *et al.*, 1999). The demonstration that a porcine retrovirus was capable of infecting human cells (Patience *et al.*, 1997) raised worldwide alarm, however, and precipitated virtual arrest of all clinical xenotransplant trials (Bach and Fineberg, 1998; Bach *et al.*, 1998; Butler, 1999). Analysis of the infectious risks to individual patients and humans as a whole is under way. General agreement that such research should be conducted with stringent controls and closed, carefully surveyed animal herds has tempered enthusiasm for this approach, generating a warning from the U.S. Food and Drug Administration (Paradis *et al.*, 1999). Nevertheless, the impact of a successful immunosuppressive strategy for xenotransplantation would be so broad that animal research continues.

Diabetics and physicians should remain undaunted by the clinical failure to date to achieve long-term survival of any xenograft. The paucity of human tissue serves as powerful motivation to investigators trying to overcome the obstacle of rejection. Within a strictly controlled environment, xenotransplantation is likely to become a component of cost-effective therapy for diabetes (Fig. 36–18).

A different strategy to maintain long-term function uses techniques to isolate islets from immune attack, rather than preventing it. Immunoisolation barriers usually have been synthesized from alginate/poly-l-lysine encapsulation of the islets, permitting entry of nutrients, exit of hormonal products and defense against recognition and attack by components of the immune system. Intriguing demonstration of prolonged glucose regulation in small animals (O'Shea *et al.*, 1984) has been extended to cynomolgus monkeys (Sun *et al.*, 1996). A report of the *in vitro* use of capsules made of confluent chondrocytes shows that this approach has significant potential (Pollok *et al.*, 1999). Other imaginative approaches,

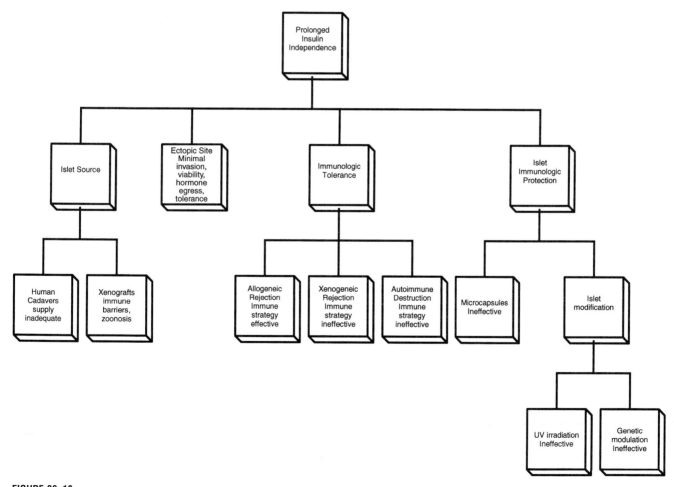

FIGURE 36–18

Achieving successful islet transplantation: status in 2000. Significant obstacles to achieving clinically prolonged insulin independence after islet transplantation remain.

TABLE 36–7

EVALUATING END-STAGE RENAL DISEASE OPTIONS FOR DIABETIC PATIENTS

	Peritonal Dialysis	Hemodialysis	Kidney Transplant	Pancreas and Kidney Transplant
Extensive extrarenal disease	No limitation	Severe orthostatic hypotension may curtail blood flow rate during hemodialysis. Peripheral vascular disease may prevent establishment of suitable vascular access.	Excluded in severe cardiovascular disease. Correction of coronary artery disease is an enabling step	Strong reluctance to subject patients with severe systematic vasculopathy to the stress of long major surgery
Geriatric patients	No limitation	No limitation	Arbitary exclusion as determined by program. Age 70 is approximate upper limit for transplant surgery. Exceptions made	Generally restricted to recipients <50 years old
Complete rehabilitation	Few individuals return to gainful employment	Few individuals return to gainful employment	Best with living related donor transplants. Return to home, school and work obligations common. Common so long as graft functions	Without question, a functioning pancreas plus a functioning kidney facilitates near-complete return to preuremia activity. Does not restore lost vision or reverse peripheral vascular disease
Death rate	Much higher than for nondiabetic individuals and greater than for hemodialysis treatment in U.S. Improved substantially since the 1980s	Much higher than for nondiabetic individuals, 2–5 times greater than for demographic and risk matched kidney transplant recipients. Improving	Higher than for nondiabetic kidney graft recipients. Lower with related than with unrelated donors. Improving	Debatable but probably higher than for kidney transplant alone. Approximately 90% of recipients are alive at 1 year with about 80% having a functioning pancreas
First year survival	About 75%	About 78%	>92%	>90%
Survival to second decade	Almost never, few transfer to hemodialysis	<5%	About 1 in 5 cadaver kidney recipients and 1 in 3 live donor kidney recipients	Insufficient experience. Currently a rare event
Progression of complications	Death due to cardiovascular disease commonest. Usual and unremitting. Hyperglycemia and hyperlipidemia accentuated	Death due to cardiovascular disease commonest. Usual and unremitting. May benefit from metabolic control	Partially ameliorated by correction of azotemia. No evidence that retinopathy, heart disease or peripheral vascular disease is retarded	Neuropathy and retinopathy slowed by functioning pancreas and kidney in type 1 diabetic subjects. Too few data to permit conclusion in type 2 recipients
Special advantage	Can be self-performed. Avoids swings in solute and intravascular volume level. Freedom to travel	Can be self-performed. Efficient extraction of solute and water in hours. Widely available throughout U.S. and Canada	Cures uremia. Freedom to travel. Permits return to former lifestyle so long as allograft functions well	Startling improvement possible with restoration of robust health if extrarenal complications have not progressed pretransplant
Disadvantage	Peritonitis. Hyperinsulinemia, hyperglycemia, hyperlipidemia. Long hours of treatment. More days hospitalized than either hemodialysis or transplant	Blood access a hazard for clotting, hemorrhage and infection. Cyclical hypotension, weakness. Aluminum toxicity from phosphate binders, amyloidosis	Cosmetic disfigurement, hypertension, personal expense for cytotoxic drugs. Induced malignancy. HIV and other viral (cytomegalovirus) transmission	Difficult surgery with frequent rehospitalizations during first year. Bladder exocrine drainage may be complicated by dysuria, hematuria and nocturnal pain
Patient acceptance	Variable, usual compliance with passive tolerance for regimen	Variable, often noncompliant with dietary, metabolic or antihypertensive component of regimen	Enthusiastic during periods of good renal allograft function	Exalted when pancreas proffers euglycemia. Reversal of lifestyle, particularly removal of dietary restriction, can be startling
Bias in comparison	Delivered as first choice by enthusiasts, although emerging evidence indicates substantially higher mortality than for hemodialysis	Treatment by default. Often complicated by inattention to progressive cardiac and peripheral vascular disease. Depersonalized in large corporate dialysis centers	All kidney transplant programs preselect patients with fewest complications	Exclusion of potential recipients >50 years old favorably prejudices outcome
Relative cost	About equivalent to hemodialysis and more expensive than a transplant over 5-year cost basis	Less expensive than kidney transplant in first year, subsequent years more expensive	After first year, kidney transplant lowest cost option when compared with peritoneal dialysis or hemodialysis	Pancreas and kidney engraftment most expensive uremia therapy for diabetic patient

HIV = human immunodeficiency virus.

such as islet immunomodulation before transplantation through tissue culture, antibody application and ultraviolet irradiation (Lau *et al.*, 1984), have failed to progress to clinical applicability.

Future Management of Diabetes

A fresh approach to attaining euglycemia is being pursued. After elucidation of the function of the insulin receptor, a search was initiated through 50,000 compounds to unearth any that might stimulate the receptor's phosphorylating action, activating its intrinsic tyrosine kinase. A nonpeptidyl five-ringed quinone (L-783,281) extracted from the Kenyan fungus *Pseudomassaria* was discovered to have the capacity to mimic insulin action in biochemical and cellular assays, acting as an *insulin pill* (Zhang *et al.*, 1999). In two mutant mouse models of diabetes, L-783,281 administered orally lowered blood glucose levels by 50%—equivalent to the reduction attained with current oral antidiabetic therapies. The novel concept of cell receptor modification to alter downstream signaling molecules is being extended to bone marrow (Guinan *et al.*, 1999) and solid-organ transplant recipients in what has been termed the *new immunology* (Schwartz, 1999). For patients with diabetes, there is reasonable promise of long-term successful *tolerance* of kidney and pancreas allografts in patients whose vasculopathy is best managed by organ substitution.

In 2000, the ESRD patient with type 1 diabetes is well advised to consider a simultaneous kidney-pancreas transplant as preferred therapy, offering an opportunity to cure an inexorable disease. Either insulin receptor stimulation or restoration of islet function by injecting allogeneic or xenogeneic polymer-coated islet β cells, discontinuing the major surgery required for segmental pancreas or whole-pancreas grafting, would simplify or eliminate the stress of surgery, while attaining the same objective.

Conclusions

A functioning kidney transplant provides the uremic diabetic patient a greater probability for survival with good rehabilitation than does CAPD or maintenance hemodialysis (Table 36–7). There are no reports, however, of prospective controlled studies of dialysis versus kidney transplantation in diabetic patients whose therapy was assigned randomly. For the few (<10%) diabetic ESRD patients who have type 1 diabetes, a combined simultaneous pancreas-kidney transplantation should be considered to effect a cure of the diabetes so long as the pancreas functions. No matter which ESRD therapy has been elected, optimal rehabilitation in diabetic ESRD patients requires that ongoing effort, throughout the course of uremia therapy, be devoted to recognition and management of comorbid conditions. End-stage renal disease therapy, whether CAPD, hemodialysis or a kidney (and pancreas) transplant, must be individualized to the patient's specific medical and family circumstances. Rehabilitation is greater in diabetic kidney transplant recipients than during CAPD or maintenance hemodialysis. Subjective appraisal—mainly by nondiabetic patients—ranks life quality equivalent in all three modalities.

Reassessment is required for all conclusions pertaining to survival, morbidity and rehabilitation in ESRD derived before introduction of erythropoietin, which is now given to more than 88% of U.S. dialysis patients. The impact of erythropoietin is so great that new baselines for *usual outcome* must be drawn for CAPD and hemodialysis in diabetic and nondiabetic patients. Some well-dialyzed diabetic hemodialy-

sis patients with normal hematocrit values might opt rationally not to have a cadaveric transplant until drugs less toxic than those currently used for immunosuppression are introduced.

Attention to control of hypertension and hyperlipidemia slows the course of macrovascular disease, particularly of the coronary arteries, which threatens long-term survival of diabetic kidney recipients. Pretransplant and repetitive posttransplant cardiac evaluation is mandatory to identify and correct silent coronary artery disease that may be severe and life-threatening. Outcome (survival) is improving continuously in ESRD treatment in diabetes, by dialytic therapy, by renal transplantation and, in type 1 diabetes, by combined pancreas-kidney transplantation. This inexorable progress in therapy reflects multiple small advances in understanding of the pathogenesis of extrarenal microvasculopathy and macrovasculopathy of an inexorable disease, coupled with safer immunosuppression. It is not irrational to predict that before 2010, protocols now under investigation for normalizing hyperglycemia in diabetes will preempt completely the microvasculopathy and macrovasculopathy known as diabetic nephropathy.

REFERENCES

Abendroth, D., Landgraf, R., Illner, W. D. and Land, W. (1990). Beneficial effects of pancreatic transplantation in insulin-dependent diabetes mellitus patients. *Transplant. Proc.* **22**, 696.

Abouna, G., Adnani, M. S., Kumar, M. S. and Samhan, S. A. (1986). Fate of transplanted kidneys with diabetic nephropathy. *Lancet* **1**, 622.

Abourizk, N. N. and Dunn, J. C. (1990). Types of diabetes according to National Diabetes Data Group classification. *Diabetes Care* **13**, 1120.

Amair, P., Khanna, R., Leibel, B., *et al.* (1982). Continuous ambulatory peritoneal dialysis in diabetic end-stage renal disease. *N. Engl. J. Med.* **306**, 625.

American Diabetes Association. (1988). *Physician's Guide to Insulin-Dependent (Type I) Diabetes: Diagnosis and Treatment*, 2nd ed., American Diabetes Association, Alexandria, Virginia.

American Diabetes Association. (1998). Economic consequences of diabetes mellitus in the U.S. in 1997. *Diabetes Care* **21**, 296.

American Diabetes Association. (1999). Clinical practice recommendations. *Diabetes Care* **22(Suppl. 1)**, S1.

Andersen, S., Rennke, H. G., Garcia, D. L. and Brenner, B. M. (1989). Short- and long-term effects of antihypertensive therapy in the diabetic rat. *Kidney Int.* **36**, 526.

Anonymous. (1989). Type 2 diabetes or NIDDM: looking for a better name. *Lancet* **1**, 589.

Ar'Rajab, A., Dawidson, I. J., Harris, R. B. and Sentementes, J. T. (1994). Immune privilege of the testis for islet xenotransplantation (rat to mouse). *Transplant. Proc.* **26**, 3446.

Azevedo, M. J. and Gross, J. L. (1991). Follow up of glomerular hyperfiltration in normoalbuminuric type 1 (insulin-dependent) diabetic patients. *Diabetologia* **34**, 611.

Bach, F. H. and Fineberg, H. V. (1998). Call for moratorium on xenotransplants. *Nature* **391**, 326.

Bach, F. H., Fishman, J. A., Daniels, N., *et al.* (1998). Uncertainty in xenotransplantation: individual benefit versus collective risk. *Nat. Med.* **4**, 141.

Bakris, G. L., Barnhill, B. W. and Sadler, R. (1992). Treatment of arterial hypertension in diabetic humans: importance of therapeutic selection. *Kidney Int.* **41**, 912.

Ballard, D. J., Humphrey, L. L., Melton, L. J., 3d, *et al.* (1988). Epidemiology of persistent proteinuria in type II diabetes mellitus. *Diabetes* **37**, 4052.

Ballinger, W. F. and Lacy, P. E. (1972). Transplantation of intact pancreatic islets in rats. *Surgery* **72**, 175.

Balodimus, M. C. (1971). Diabetic nephropathy. In *Joslin's Diabetes*, (A. Marble, P. White, R. F. Bradley and L. P. Krall, eds.), p. 526, Lea & Febiger, Philadelphia.

Bank, N., Klose, R., Aynedjian, H. S., Nguyen, D. and Sablay, L. B.

(1987). Evidence against increased glomerular pressure initiating diabetic nephropathy. *Kidney Int.* **31**, 898.

Barsotti, G., Ciardella, F., Morelli, E., Cupisti, A., Mantovanelli, A. and Giovanetti, S. (1988). Nutritional treatment of renal failure in type 1 diabetes. *Clin. Nephrol.* **29**, 280.

Baumgartl, H. J., Banholzer, P. , Sigl, G., Haslbeck, M. and Stadl, E. (1998). On the prognosis of IDDM patients with large kidneys: the role of large kidneys for the development of diabetic nephropathy. *Nephrol. Dial. Transplant.* **13**, 630.

Bending, J. J., Dodds, R. A., Keen, H. and Viberti, G. C. (1988). Renal response to restricted protein intake in diabetic nephropathy. *Diabetes* **37**, 1641.

Bending, J. J., Viberti, G. C., Watkins, P. J. and Keen, H. (1986). Intermittent clinical proteinuria and renal function in diabetes: evolution and the effect of glycemic control. *B. M. J.* **292**, 83.

Benedetti, E., Dunn, T., Massad, M. G., et al. (1999). Successful living related simultaneous pancreas-kidney transplant between identical twins. *Transplantation* **67**, 915.

Bennett, P. H. (1999). Type 2 diabetes among the Pima Indians of Arizona: an epidemic attributable to environmental change? *Nutr. Rev.* **57(5 Pt. 2)**, S51.

Berger, B., Stenstrom, G. and Sundkvist, G. (1999). Incidence, prevalence, and mortality of diabetes in a large population: a report from the Skaraborg Diabetes Registry. *Diabetes Care* **22**, 773.

Berger, E. E. and Lowrie, E. G. (1991). Mortality and the length of dialysis. *J. A. M. A.* **265**, 909.

Berionade, V. (1986). Creatinine clearance in non-insulin dependent diabetes mellitus. *Kidney Int.* **31**, 179.

Berionade, V. C., Lefebvre, R. and Falardeau, P. (1987). Unilateral nodular diabetic glomerulosclerosis: recurrence of an experiment of nature. *Am. J. Nephrol.* **7**, 55.

Bohman, S. O., Wilczek, H., Tyden, G., Jaremko, G., Lundgren, G. and Groth, C. G. (1984). Recurrence of diabetic nephropathy in human renal allografts: preliminary report of a biopsy study. *Transplant. Proc.* **16**, 649.

Borch-Johnsen, K. (1988). Incidence of nephropathy in insulin-dependent diabetes as related to mortality. *In The Kidney and Hypertension in Diabetes Mellitus*, (C. E. Mogensen, ed.), p. 33, Martinus Nijhoff, Boston.

Bosch, J. P., Sacaggi, A., Lauer, A., Ronco, C., Belledonne, M. and Glabman, S. (1983). Renal functional reserve in humans. *Am. J. Med.* **75**, 943.

Braun, W. E., Phillips, D. and Vidt, D. G. (1983). The course of coronary artery disease in diabetics with and without renal allografts. *Transplant. Proc.* **15**, 1114.

Brownlee, M. (1989). Pharmacological modulation of the advanced glycosylation reaction. *Prog. Clin. Biol. Res.* **304**, 235.

Brownlee, M. (1994). Glycation and diabetic complications. *Diabetes* **43**, 836.

Bruton, B. L., Perusek, M. C., Lancaster, J. L., Kopp, D. T. and Tuttle, K. R. (1990). Effects of glycemia on basal and amino-acid stimulated (AA-S) renal hemodynamics and kidney size in non-insulin dependent diabetes (NIDD). *J. Am. Soc. Nephrol.* **1**, 623.

Burke, G. W., Gruessner, R., Dunn, D. L. and Sutherland, D. E. (1990). Conversion of whole pancreaticoduodenal transplants from bladder to enteric drainage for metabolic acidosis or dysuria. *Transplant. Proc.* **22**, 651.

Burton, P. R. and Walls, J. (1987). Selection-adjusted comparison of life-expectancy of patients on continuous ambulatory peritoneal dialysis, haemodialysis, and renal transplantation. *Lancet* **1**, 1115.

Butler, D. (1999). FDA warns on primate xenotransplants. *Nature* **398**, 549.

Bynon, J. S., Stratta, R. J., Taylor, R. J., Lowell, J. A. and Cattral, M. (1993). Vascular reconstruction in 105 consecutive pancreas transplants. *Transplant. Proc.* **25**, 3288.

Caird, R. I. (1961). Survival of diabetics with proteinuria. *Diabetes* **10**, 178.

Callahan, M. B., Bender, K. and McNeely, M. (1999). The role of the health care team in the implementation of the National Kidney Foundation-Dialysis Outcomes Quality Initiative: a case study. *Adv. Ren. Replace. Ther.* **6**, 42.

Calne, R. Y. (1984). Paratopic segmental pancreas grafting a technique with portal venous drainage. *Lancet* **1**, 595.

Cambier, P. (1934). Application de la theorié de Rehberg a l'etude clinique des affections rénales et du diabetes. *Ann. Med.* **35**, 273.

Candinas, D., Schlumpf, R., Roethlin, M., Weder, W. and Largiader, F. (1994). Impact of pancreatic pseudocysts in segmental duct-occluded pancreas transplants on graft function. *Transplant. Proc.* **26**, 456.

Carr, S., Mbanya, J. C., Thomas, T., et al. (1990). Increase in glomerular filtration rate in patients with insulin-dependent diabetes and elevated erythrocyte Na-Li countertransport. *N. Engl. J. Med.* **322**, 500.

Carroll, P. B., Rilo, H. L. and Alejandro, R. (1995). Long-term (>3-year) insulin independence in a patient with pancreatic islet cell transplantation following upper abdominal exenteration and liver replacement for fibrolamellar hepatocellular carcinoma. *Transplantation* **59**, 875.

Cecka, J. M. and Terasaki, P. I. (1992). The UNOS Scientific Renal Transplant Registry—1991. *In Clinical Transplants 1991*, (P. I. Terasaki, ed.), p. 1, UCLA Tissue Typing Lab, Los Angeles.

Centers for Disease Control and Prevention. (1998). *National Diabetes Fact Sheet: National Estimates and General Information on Diabetes in the United States*, revised edition, U.S. Department of Health and Human Services, Centers for Disease Control and Prevention, Atlanta, Ga.

Chachati, A., von Frenckell, R., Foidart-Willems, J., Godon, J. P. and Lefebvre, P. J. (1987). Variability of albumin excretion in insulin-dependent diabetics. *Diabet. Med.* **4**, 437.

Chantrel, F., Enache, I., Bouiller, M., et al. (1999). Abysmal prognosis of patients with type 2 diabetes entering dialysis. *Nephrol. Dial. Transplant.* **14**, 129.

Charonis, A. S. and Tsilbary, E. C. (1992). Structural and functional changes of laminin and type IV collagen after nonenzymatic glycation. *Diabetes* **41**, 52, 49.

Chavers, B. M., Bilous, R. W., Ellis, E. N., Steffes, M. W. and Mauer, S. M. (1989). Glomerular lesions and urinary albumin excretion in type 1 diabetes without overt proteinuria. *N. Engl. J. Med.* **320**, 966.

Cheigh, J., Raghavan, J., Sullivan, J., Tapia, L., Rubin, A. and Stenzel, K. H. (1991). Is insufficient dialysis a cause for high morbidity in diabetic patients? *J. Am. Soc. Nephrol.* Abstract 2, **317**.

Christensen, C. K., Christiansen, J. S., Schmitz, A., Christensen, T., Hermansen, K. and Mogensen, C. E. (1987). Effect of continuous subcutaneous insulin infusion on kidney function and size in IDDM patients: a 2 year controlled study. *J. Diabetes Complications* **1**, 91.

Christensen, C. K. and Mogensen, C. E. (1986). Acute and long term effect of antihypertensive treatment on exercise-induced albuminuria in incipient diabetic nephropathy. *Scand. J. Clin. Lab. Invest.* **46**, 553.

Christensen, P. K., Rossing, P., Nielsen, F. S. and Parving, H. H. (1999). Natural course of kidney function in Type 2 diabetic patients with diabetic nephropathy. *Diabet. Med.* **16**, 388.

Christiansen, J. S., Frandsen, M. and Parving, H.-H. (1981). The effect of intravenous insulin infusion on kidney function in insulin-dependent diabetes mellitus. *Diabetologia* **20**, 199.

Christiansen, J. S., Gammelgaard, J., Tronier, B., Svendsen, P. A. and Parving, H.-H. (1982). Kidney function and size in diabetics before and during insulin treatment. *Kidney Int.* **21**, 683.

Churchill, D. N. (1998). Implications of the Canada-USA (CANUSA) study of the adequacy of dialysis on peritoneal dialysis schedule. *Nephrol. Dial. Transplant.* **13(Suppl. 6)**, 158.

Churchill, D. N., Thorpe, K. E., Nolph, K. D., Keshaviah, P. R., Oreopoulos, D. G. and Page, D. (1998). Increased peritoneal membrane transport is associated with decreased patient and technique survival for continuous peritoneal dialysis patients. The Canada-USA (CANUSA) Peritoneal Dialysis Study Group. *J. Am. Soc. Nephrol.* **9**, 1285.

Churchill, D. N., Thorpe, K. E., Vonesh, E. F. and Keshaviah, P. R. (1997). Lower probability of patient survival with continuous peritoneal dialysis in the United States compared with Canada. Canada-USA (CANUSA) Peritoneal Dialysis Study Group. *J. Am. Soc. Nephrol.* **8**, 965.

Cohen, D., Dodds, R. and Viberti, G. C. (1987a). Effect of protein restriction in insulin-dependent diabetics at risk of nephropathy. *B. M. J.* **294**, 795.

Cohen, D. L., Close, C. F. and Viberti, G. C. (1987b). The variability of overnight urinary albumin excretion in insulin-dependent diabetic and normal subjects. *Diabet. Med.* **4**, 437.

Collin, J. (1978). Current state of transplantation of the pancreas. *Ann. R. Coll. Surg. Engl.* **60**, 21.

Cook, K., Sollinger, H. W., Warner, T., Kamps, D., and Belzer, F. O. (1983). Pancreaticocystostomy: an alternative method for exocrine drainage of segmental pancreatic allografts. *Transplantation* **35**, 634.

Corry, R. J., Nghiem, D. D., Schanbacher, B., *et al.* (1987). Critical analysis of mortality and graft loss following simultaneous renal-pancreatic duodenal transplantation. *Transplant. Proc.* **19**, 2305.

Corry, R. J., Nghiem, D. D., Schulak, J. A., Beutel, W. D. and Gonwa, T. A. (1986). Surgical treatment of diabetic nephropathy with simultaneous pancreatic duodenal and renal transplantation. *Surg. Gynecol. Obstet.* **162**, 547.

Cowie, C. C., Port, F. K., Wolfe, R. A., Savage, P. J., Moll, P. P. and Hawthorne, V. M. (1989). Disparities in incidence of diabetic end stage renal disease according to race and type of diabetes. *N. Engl. J. Med.* **321**, 1074.

Damsgaard, E. M. and Mogensen, C. E. (1986). Microalbuminuria in elderly hyperglycemic patients and controls. *Diabet. Med.* **3**, 430.

Davies, D. F. and Shock, N. W. (1950). Age changes in glomerular filtration rate, effective renal plasma flow, and tubular excretory capacity in adult males. *J. Clin. Invest.* **29**, 496.

DCCT Research Group. (1986). The Diabetes Control and Complications Trial (DCCT): design and methodologic considerations for the feasibility phase. *Diabetes* **35**, 530.

DCCT Research Group. (1988). Weight gain associated with intensive therapy in the Diabetes Control and Complications Trial. *Diabetes Care* **11**, 567.

DCCT Research Group (1995). Effect of intensive therapy on the development and progression of diabetic nephropathy in the Diabetes Control and Complications Trial. The Diabetes Control and Complications (DCCT) Research Group. *Kidney Int.* **47**, 1703.

DeFronzo, R. J. and Ferranini, E. (1991). Insulin resistance: a multifaceted syndrome responsible for NIDDM, obesity, hypertension, dyslipidemia and atherosclerotic cardiovascular disease. *Diabetes Care* **14**, 173.

Delahanty, L. M. (1998). Implications of the diabetes control and complications trial for renal outcomes and medical nutrition therapy. *J. Ren. Nutr.* **8**, 59.

DiCarlo, V., Castoldi, R., Cristallo, M., *et al.* (1998). Techniques of pancreas transplantation through the world: an IPITA Center study. *Transplant. Proc.* **30**, 231.

Di Landro, D., Catalano, C., Lambertini, D., *et al.* (1998). The effect of metabolic control on development and progression of diabetic nephropathy. *Nephrol. Dial. Transplant.* **13(Suppl. 8)**, 35.

Dinneen, S. and Gerstein, H. C. (1997). The association of microalbuminuria and mortality in non-insulin-dependent diabetes mellitus: a systematic overview of the literature. *Arch. Intern. Med.* **157**, 1413.

Ditzel, J. and Schwartz, M. (1967). Abnormally increased glomerular filtration rate in short-term insulin-treated diabetic subjects. *Diabetes* **16**, 2647.

Douzdjian, V., Abecassis, M. M., Cooper, J. L., Smith, J. L. and Corry, R. J. (1993). Incidence, management and significance of surgical complications after pancreatic transplantation. *Surg. Gynecol. Obstet.* **177**, 451.

Drury, P. L., Watkins, P. J., Viberti, G. C., Walker, J. D. (1989). Diabetic nephropathy. *Br. Med. Bull.* **45**, 127.

Dubernard, J. M., Traeqer, J., Neyra, P., Touraine, J. L., Tranchant, D. and Blanc-Brunat, N. (1978). A new preparation of segmental pancreatic grafts for transplantation: trials in dogs and in man. *Surgery* **84**, 633.

Dussoix, P., Vaxillaire, M., Iynedjian, P. B., *et al.* (1997). Diagnostic heterogeneity of diabetes in lean young adults: classification based on immunoligical and genetic parameters. *Diabetes* **46**, 622.

Eastman, R. C., Javitt, J. C., Herman, W. H., *et al.* (1997). Model of complications of NIDDM: II. analysis of the health benefits and cost-effectiveness of treating type 2 diabetes with the goal of normoglycemia. *Diabetes Care* **20**, 735.

Edelstein, D. and Brownlee, M. (1992). Mechanistic studies of advanced glycosylation end product inhibition by aminoguanidine. *Diabetes* **41**, 26.

El Nahas, A. M., Masters-Thomas, A., Brady, S. A., *et al.* (1984). Selective effects of low protein diets in renal diseases. *B. M. J.* **289**, 1337.

Esmatjes, E., Rodriguez-Villar, C., Ricart, M. J., *et al.* (1998). Recurrence of immunological markers for type 1 (insulin-dependent) diabetes mellitus in immunosuppressed patients after pancreas transplantation. *Transplantation* **66**, 128.

Estacio, R. O. and Schrier, R. W. (1998). Antihypertensive therapy in type 2 diabetes: implications of the appropriate blood pressure control in diabetes (ABCD) trial. *Am. J. Cardiol.* **82**, 9R.

Evanoff, G., Thompson, C., Brown, J. and Weinman, E. (1989). Prolonged dietary protein restriction in diabetic nephropathy. *Arch. Intern. Med.* **149**, 1129.

Evanoff, G. V., Thompson, C. S., Brown, J. and Weinman, E. J. (1987). The effect of dietary protein restriction on the progression of diabetic nephropathy: a 12 month follow-up. *Arch. Intern. Med.* **147**, 492.

Fabre, J., Balant, L. P., Dayer, P. G., Fox, H. M. and Vernet, A. T. (1982). The kidney in maturity onset diabetes: a clinical study of 510 patients. *Kidney Int.* **21**, 730.

Fanning, W. J., Henry, M. L., Sommer, B. G., *et al.* (1986). Lower extremity and renal ischemia following renal transplantation. *Vasc. Surg.* **23**, 231.

Feitosa Tajra, L. C., Dawhara, M., Benchaib, M., LeFrancois, N., Martin, X. and Dubernard, J. M. (1998). Effect of surgical technique on long-term outcome of pancreatic transplantation. *Transpl. Int.* **11**, 295.

Fiaschi, E., Grassi, B. and Andres, G. (1952). La Funzione Renale Nel Diabete Mellito. *Ressegna Di Fisiopatologia clinica E Terapeutica* **24**, 372.

Fioretto, P., Steffes, M. W., Sutherland, D. E., Goetz, F. C. and Mauer, M. (1999). Reversal of lesions of diabetic nephropathy after pancreas transplantation. *N. Engl. J. Med.* **339**, 69.

Fogo, A., Yoshida, Y. and Ichikawa, I. (1986). Angiotensin converting enzyme inhibition (CEI) suppresses accelerated growth of glomerular cells in vivo and vitro. *Kidney Int.* **33**, 296.

Fournier, B., Andereggen, E., Buhler, L., *et al.* (1998). Evaluation à long-terme de 9 autotransplantations d'ilots de Langerhans après resection du pancreas. *Schweiz. Med. Wochenschr.* **128**, 856.

Fox, C. J., Darby, S. C., Ireland, J. T. and Sonksen, P. H. (1977). Blood glucose control and glomerular capillary basement membrane thickening in experimental diabetes. *B. M. J.* **2**, 605.

Frank, R. N. (1994). The aldose reductase controversy. *Diabetes* **43**, 169.

Frankel, D. H. (1998). Blood-pressure control preserves renal function. *Lancet* **351**, 1562.

Friedman, E. A., Chou, L. M., Beyer, M. M., Butt, K. M. H. and Manis, T. (1985). Adverse impact of hypertension on diabetic recipients of transplanted kidneys. *Hypertension* **7(6 Pt. 2)**, 1131.

Gaede, P., Vedel, P., Parving, H.-H. and Pedersen, O. (1999). Intensified multifactorial intervention in patients with type 2 diabetes mellitus and microalbuminuria: the Steno type 2 randomised study. *Lancet* **353**, 617.

Gall, M. A., Rossing, P., Skott, P., *et al.* (1991). Prevalence of micro- and macroalbuminuria, arterial hypertension, retinopathy and large vessel disease in European type 2 (non-insulin dependent) diabetic patients. *Diabetologia* **34**, 655.

Galler, M., Backenroth, R., Folkert, V. W. and Schlondorff, D. (1982). Effect of converting enzyme inhibitors on prostaglandin synthesis by isolated glomerular and aortic strips from rats. *J. Pharmacol. Exp. Ther.* **220**, 23.

Gatling, W., Knight, C., Mullee, M. A. and Hill, R. D. (1988). Microalbuminuria in diabetes: a population study of the prevalence and assessment of three screening tests. *Diabet. Med.* **5**, 343.

Gayet, R. and Guillaumie, M. (1927). La regulation de la secretion interne pancreatique par un processus humoral, demontrée par des transplantations de pancreas. *Compt. Ren. Soc. Biol.* **97**, 1613.

Gellman, D. D., Pirani, C. L., Soothill, J. F., Muehrcke, R. C., Maduros, W. and Kark, R. M. (1959). Structure and function in diabetic nephropathy: the importance of diffuse glomerulosclerosis. *Diabetes* **8**, 251.

Gerstein, H. C. (1999). Preventive medicine in a diabetes clinic: an opportunity to make a difference. *Lancet* **353**, 606.

Ghavamian, M., Gutch, C. F., Kopp, K. F. and Kolff, W. J. (1972). The sad truth about hemodialysis in diabetic nephropathy. *J. A. M. A.* **222**, 1386.

Gill, J. B., Ruddy, T. D., Newell, J. B., *et al.* (1987). Prognostic importance of thallium uptake by the lungs during exercise in coronary artery disease. *N. Engl. J. Med.* **317**, 1485.

Gliedman, M. L., Gold, M., Whittaker, J., *et al.* (1973). Clinical segmental pancreatic transplantation with ureter-pancreatic duct anastomosis for exocrine drainage. *Surgery* **74**, 171.

Gonzalez-Carrillo, M., Moloney, A., Bewick, M., *et al.* (1982). Renal transplantation in diabetic nephropathy. *B. M. J.* **285**, 1713.

Graber, A. O., Shokouh-Amiri, H., Grewal, H. P. and Britt, L. G. (1993). A technique for portal pancreatic transplantation with enteric drainage. *Surg. Gynecol. Obstet.* **177**, 417.

Gray, D. W. (1990). Islet isolation and transplantation techniques in the primate. *Surg. Gynecol. Obstet.* **170**, 225.

Grenfell, A. and Watkins, P. J. (1986). Clinical diabetic nephropathy: natural history and complications. *Clin. Endocrinol. Metab.* **15**, 783.

Groth, C. G., Collste, H., Lundgren, G., *et al.* (1982). Successful outcome of segmental human pancreatic transplantation with enteric exocrine diversion after modifications in technique. *Lancet* **2**, 522.

Gruessner, A. C. and Sutherland, D. E. R. (1998). Pancreas transplants for United States (US) and non-US cases as reported to the International Pancreas Transplant Registry (IPTR) and to the United Network for Organ Sharing (UNOS). *In Clinical Transplants 1997*, (J. M. Cecka and P. I. Terasaki, eds.), p. 45, UCLA Tissue Typing Laboratory, Los Angeles.

Gruessner, A. C. and Sutherland, D. E. R. (1999). Analysis of United States (US) and non-US pancreas transplants as reported to the International Pancreas Transplant Registry (IPTR) and to the United Network for Organ Sharing (UNOS). *In Clinical Transplants 1998*, (J. M. Cecka and P. I. Terasaki, eds.), p. 53, UCLA Tissue Typing Laboratory, Los Angeles.

Gruessner, R. W. G. and Sutherland, D. E. R. (1996). Simultaneous kidney and segmental pancreas transplants from living related donors—the first two successful cases. *Transplantation* **61**, 1265.

Gruessner, R. W. G., Sutherland, D. E. R., Troppmann, C., *et al.* (1997). The surgical risk of pancreas transplantation in the cyclosporine era: an overview. *J. Am. Coll. Surg.* **185**, 128.

Guinan, E. C., Boussiotis, V. A., Neuberg, D., *et al.* (1999). Transplantation of anergic histoincompatible bone marrow allografts. *N. Engl. J. Med.* **340**, 1704.

Harris, M. I., Hadden, W. C., Knowles, W. C. and Bennett, P. H. (1987). Prevalence of diabetes and impaired glucose tolerance and plasma glucose levels in the United States population aged 20–74 years. *Diabetes* **36**, 523.

Harris, M. I., Klein, R., Welborn, T. A. and Knuiman, M. W. (1992). Onset of NIDDM occurs at least 4–7 yr before clinical diagnosis. *Diabetes Care* **15**, 815.

Hasslacher, C. and Ritz, E. (1987). Effect of control of diabetes mellitus on progression of renal failure. *Kidney Int.* **32(Suppl. 22)**, 53.

Hasslacher, C. H., Ritz, E., Wahl, P. and Michael, C. (1989). Similar risks of nephropathy in patients with type I or type II diabetes mellitus. *Nephrol. Dial. Transplant.* **4**, 859.

Hebert, L. A., Falkenhain, M. E., Nahman, N. S., Jr., Cosio, F. G. and O'Dorisio, T. M. (1999). Combination ACE inhibitor and angiotensin II receptor antagonist therapy in diabetic nephropathy. *Am. J. Nephrol.* **19**, 1.

Hedon, E. (1893). Sur la consommation du sucre chez le chien après l'extirpation du pancréas. *Arch. Physiol. Norm. Pathol.* **5**, 154.

Held, P. J., Levin, N. W., Bovbjerg, R. R., Pauly, M. V. and Diamond, L. H. (1991). Mortality and duration of hemodialysis treatment. *J. A. M. A.* **265**, 871.

Henry, R. R., Wallace, P. and Olefsky, J. M. (1986). Effects of weight loss on mechanisms of hyperglycemia in obese non-insulin dependent diabetes mellitus. *Diabetes* **35**, 990.

Herman, W. H. and Teutsch, S. M. (1985). Kidney disease associated with diabetes. *In Diabetes in America*, NIH publication no. 85-1468, p. 1, U.S. Government Printing Office, Washington, D.C.

Hostetter, T. H. (1990). Pathogenesis of diabetic glomerulopathy: hemodynamic considerations. *Semin. Nephrol.* **10**, 219.

Hostetter, T. H., Troy, J. L. and Brenner, B. M. (1981). Glomerular hemodynamics in experimental diabetes. *Kidney Int.* **19**, 410.

Hotta, N. (1997). New concepts and insights on pathogenesis and treatment of diabetic complications: polyol pathway and its inhibition. *Nagoya J. Med. Sci.* **60**, 89.

Humar, A., Gruessner, R. W. and Sutherland, D. E. (1997). Living related donor pancreas and pancreas-kidney transplantation. *Br. Med. Bull.* **53**, 879.

Humphrey, L. L., Ballard, D. J., Frohnert, P. P., Chu, C. P., O'Fallon, W. M. and Palumbo, P. J. (1989). Chronic renal failure in non-insulin-dependent diabetes mellitus. *Ann. Intern. Med.* **10**, 788.

Ibsen, K. K., Jensen, H. A., Wieth, J. C. and Funder, J. (1982). Essential hypertension: sodium-lithium countertransport in erythrocytes from patients and from children having one hypertensive parent. *Hypertension* **4**, 703.

Ifudu, O., Dawood, M., Iofel, Y., Valcourt, J. S. and Friedman, E. A. (1999). Delayed referral of black, hispanic, and older patients with chronic renal failure. *Am. J. Kidney Dis.* **33**, 728.

Jaeger, C., Brendel, M. D., Hering, B. J., *et al.* (1997). Progressive islet graft failure occurs significantly earlier in autoantibody-positive than in autoantibody-negative IDDM recipients of intrahepatic islet allografts. *Diabetes* **46**, 1907.

Jaeger, C., Brendel, M. D., Hering, B. J., *et al.* (1998). IA-2 antibodies are only positive in association with GAD 65 and islet cell antibodies in islet transplanted insulin-dependent diabetes mellitus patients. *Transplant. Proc.* **30**, 659.

Jarrett, R. J., Viberti, G. C., Argyropoulos, A., Hill, R. D., Mahmud, U. and Murrells, T. J. (1984). Microalbuminuria predicts mortality in non-insulin dependent diabetes. *Diabet. Med.* **1**, 17.

Jensen, J. J., Mathiesen, E. R., Norgaard, K., *et al.* (1990). Increased blood pressure and sodium-lithium countertransport activity are not inherited in diabetic nephropathy. *Diabetologia* **33**, 619.

Johnston, C. I., Cooper, M. E. and Nicholis, G. M. (1992). Meeting report of the International Society of Hypertension Conference on Hypertension and Diabetes. *J. Hypertens.* **10**, 393.

Jones, S. L., Wiseman, M. J. and Viberti, G. C. (1991). Glomerular hyperfiltration as a risk factor for diabetic nephropathy: five year report of a prospective study. *Diabetologia* **34**, 59.

Juneja, R., Palmer, J. P. (1999). Type 1½ diabetes: myth or reality? *Autoimmunity* **29**, 65.

Kassab, J. P., Guillot, R., Andre, J., *et al.* (1994). Renal and microvascular effects of an aldose reductase inhibitor in experimental diabetes: biochemical, functional, and ultrastructural studies. *Biochem. Pharmacol.* **48**, 1003.

Katz, H., Homan, M., Velosa, J., *et al.* (1991). Effects of pancreas transplantation on postprandial glucose metabolism. *N. Engl. J. Med.* **325**, 1278.

Kaysen, G., Gambertoglio, J., Jiminez, I., Jones, H. and Huthchinson, F. N. (1986). Effects of dietary protein intake on albumin homeostasis in nephrotic patients. *Kidney Int.* **29**, 572.

Kelly, W. D., Lillehei, R. C., Merkel, F. K., *et al.* (1967). Allotransplantation of the pancreas and duodenum along with the kidney in diabetic nephropathy. *Surgery* **61**, 827.

Kendall, D. M., Sutherland, D. E. R., Goetz, F. C. and Najarian, J. S. (1989). Metabolic effect of hemipancreatectomy in living related pancreas transplant donors: preoperative prediction of postoperative oral glucose tolerance. *Diabetes* **38**, 101.

Khauli, R. B., Novick, A. C., Braun, W. E., Steinmuller, D., Buszta, C. and Goormastic, M. (1983). Improved results of 54 renal transplantation in the diabetic patient. *J. Urol.* **130**, 867.

Khauli, R. B., Steinmuller, D. R., Novick, A. C., *et al.* (1986). A critical look at survival of diabetics with end-stage renal disease: transplantation versus dialysis therapy. *Transplantation* **41**, 598.

Kjellstrand, C. M., Goetz, F. C. and Najarian, J. S. (1980). Transplantation and dialysis in diabetic patients: an update. *In Diabetic Renal Retinal Syndrome*, (E. A. Friedman and F. A. L'Esperance, Jr., eds.), p. 345, Grune & Stratton, New York.

Knowles, W. C., Bennett, P. H., Hamman, R. F. and Miller, M. (1978). Diabetes incidence and prevalence in Pima Indians: a 19-fold greater incidence than in Rochester, Minnesota. *Am. J. Epidemiol.* **108**, 497.

Konigsrainer, A., Foger, B., Steurer, W., *et al.* (1998). Influence of hyperinsulinemia of lipoproteins after pancreas transplantation with systemic insulin drainage. *Transplant. Proc.* **30**, 637.

Krolewski, A. S., Canessa, M., Warren, J. H., *et al.* (1988). Predisposition to hypertension and susceptibility to renal disease in insulin-dependent diabetes mellitus. *N. Engl. J. Med.* **318**, 140.

Krolewski, A. S., Warram, J. H., Christlieb, A. R., Busick, E. J. and Kahn, C. R. (1985). The changing natural history of nephropathy in type 1 diabetes. *Am. J. Med.* **78**, 785.

Kunzelman, C. L., Knowles, W. C., Pettit, D. J. and Bennett, P. H. (1989). Incidence of proteinuria in type 2 diabetes in the Pima Indians. *Kidney Int.* **35**, 681.

Kupin, W. L., Cortes, P., Dumler, S., Feldcamp, C. S., Kilates, M. C.

and Levin, N. W. (1987). Effect on renal function on change from high to moderate protein intake in type 1 diabetic patients. *Diabetes* **36**, 73.

Laffel, L. M., McGill, J. B. and Gans, D. J. (1995). The beneficial effect of angiotensin-converting enzyme inhibition with captopril on diabetic nephropathy in normotensive IDDM patients with microalbuminuria. North American Microalbuminuria Study Group. *Am. J. Med.* **99**, 497.

Lafferty, H. M. and Brenner, B. M. (1990). Are glomerular hypertension and "hypertrophy" independent risk factors for progression of renal disease? *Semin. Nephrol.* **3**, 294.

Largiader, F., Lyons, G. W., Hidalgo, F., *et al.* (1967). Orthotopic allotransplantation of the pancreas. *Am. J. Surg.* **113**, 70.

Lau, H., Reemtsma, K. and Hardy, M. A. (1984). Prolongation of rat islet allograft survival by direct ultraviolet irradiation of the graft. *Science* **223**, 607.

Lebovitz, H. E. and Palmisano, J. (1990). Cross-sectional analysis of renal function in black Americans with non-insulin dependent diabetes mellitus. *Diabetes Care* **13(Suppl. 4)**, 1186.

Legrain, M., Rottembourg, J., Bentchikou, A., *et al.* (1984). Dialysis treatment of insulin dependent diabetic patients: ten years experience. *Clin. Nephrol.* **21**, 72.

Leow, C. K., Shimizu, S., Gray, D. W. and Morris, P. J. (1994). Successful pancreatic islet autotransplantation to the renal subcapsule in the cynomolgus monkey. *Transplantation* **57**, 161.

Lillehei, R. C., Ruiz, J. O., Acquino, C. and Goetz, F. C. (1976). Transplantation of the pancreas. *Acta Endocrinol.* **83(Suppl. 205)**, 303.

Lillehei, R. C., Simmons, R. L., Najarian, J. S., *et al.* (1970). Pancreaticoduodenal allotransplantation: experimental and clinical experience. *Ann. Surg.* **172**, 405.

Lindblad, A. S., Nolph, K. D., Novak, J. W. and Friedman, E. A. (1988). A survey of the NIH CAPD registry population with end-stage renal disease attributed to diabetic nephropathy. *J. Diabetic Complications* **2**, 227.

Lindeman, R. D., Tobin, J. D. and Shock, N. W. (1985). Longitudinal studies on the rate of decline in renal function with age. *J. Am. Geriatr. Soc.* **33**, 278.

Lowder, G. M., Perri, N. A. and Friedman, E. A. (1988). Demographics, diabetes type, and degree of rehabilitation in diabetic patients on maintnance hemodialysis in Brooklyn. *J. Diabetic Complications* **2**, 218.

Lowrie, E. G. and New, N. L. (1990). Death risk in hemodialysis patients: the predictive value of commonly measured variables and an evaluation of death rate differences between facilities. *Am. J. Kidney Dis.* **15**, 458.

Lyons, T. J., Dailie, K. E., Dyer, D. G., Dunn, J. A. and Baynes, J. W. (1991). Decrease in skin collagen glycation with improved glycemic control in patients with insulin-dependent diabetes mellitus. *J. Clin. Invest.* **87**, 1910.

MacLeod, M. J. and McLay, J. (1998). Drug treatment of hypertension complicating diabetes mellitus. *Drugs* **56**, 189.

Makita, Z., Bucala, R., Rayfield, E. J., *et al.* (1994). Reactive glycosylation end products in diabetic uraemia and treatment of renal failure. *Lancet* **343**, 1519.

Makita, Z., Radoff, S., Rayfield, E. J., *et al.* (1991). Advanced glycosylation end products in patients with diabetic nephropathy. *N. Engl. J. Med.* **325**, 836.

Mangili, R., Bending, J. J., Scott, G., Li, L. K., Gupta, A. and Viberti, G. (1988). Increased sodium-lithium countertransport activity on red cells of patients with insulin-dependent diabetes and nephropathy. *N. Engl. J. Med.* **318**, 146.

Marks, H. H. (1965). Longevity and mortality of diabetics. *Am. J. Public Health* **55**, 416.

Marre, M., Leblanc, H., Suarez, L., Thanh-Tam, G., Menard, J. and Possa, P. (1987). Converting enzyme inhibition and kidney function in normotensive diabetic patients with persistent microalbuminuria. *B. M. J.* **294**, 1448.

Marshak, S., Leibowitz, G., Bertuzzi, F., *et al.* (1999). Impaired beta-cell functions induced by chronic exposure of cultured human pancreatic islets to high glucose. *Diabetes* **48**, 1230.

Maryniak, R. K., Mendoza, N., Clyne, D., Balakrishnan, K., Weiss, M. A. (1985). Recurrence of diabetic nodular glomerulosclerosis in a renal transplant. *Transplantation* **39**, 35.

Maschio, G., Oldrizi, L. and Rugiu, C. (1986). The effects of dietary protein restriction on the course of early chronic failure. *Contemp. Issues Nephrol.* **14**, 203.

Mathiesen, E. R., Borch-Johnsen, K., Jensen, D. V. and Deckert, T. (1989a). Improved survival in patients with diabetic nephropathy. *Diabetologia* **32**, 884.

Mathiesen, E. R., Oxenboll, B., Johansen, K., Svendsen, P. A. and Deckert, T. (1984). Incipient nephropathy in type 1 (insulin-dependent) diabetes. *Diabetologia* **26**, 406.

Mathiesen, E. R., Ronn, B., Jensen, T., Storm, B. and Deckert, T. (1989b). Microalbuminaria is prior to elevation of blood pressure in diabetic nephropathy. *In First Workshop on Blood Pressure and Diabetic Nephropathy: Pathogenesis and Treatment*, EDNSG, Pisa, Italy.

Mauer, S. M. and Chavers, B. M. (1985). A comparison of kidney disease in type I and type II diabetes. *Adv. Exp. Med. Biol.* **189**, 299.

Mauer, S. M., Goetz, F. C., McHugh, L. E., *et al.* (1989). Long-term study of normal kidneys transplanted into patients with type i diabetes. *Diabetes* **38**, 516.

Mauer, S. M., Steffes, M. W. and Brown, D. M. (1975a). Animal models of diabetic nephropathy. *Adv. Nephrol.* **8**, 280.

Mauer, S. M., Steffes, M. W. and Brown, D. M. (1981). The kidney in diabetes. *Am. J. Med.* **70**, 603.

Mauer, S. M., Steffes, M. W. and Brown, D. M. (1985). Effects of mesangial localization of polyvinyl alcohols on glomerular basement membrane thickness. *Kidney Int.* **5**, 751.

Mauer, S. M., Steffes, M. W., Ellis, E. N., Sutherland, D. E., Brown, D. M. and Goetz, F. C. (1984). Structural-functional relationships in diabetic nephropathy. *J. Clin. Invest.* **74**, 1143.

Mauer, S. M., Steffes, M. W., Sutherland, D., Najarian, J., Michael, A. F. and Brown, D. M. (1975b). Studies of the rate of regression of the glomerular lesions in diabetic rats treated with pancreatic islet transplantation. *Diabetes* **24**, 280.

Mayers, J. D., Markell, M. S., Cohen, L., *et al.* (1992). Hospital admission for hemodialysis vascular access (HVA) related complications in diabetic patients. Presented at annual meeting of the *American Society for Artificial Internal Organs*, Nashville, Tennessee.

Mazze, R. S., Sinnock, P., Deeb, L. and Brimberry, J. L. (1985). An epidemiological model for diabetes mellitus in the United States: five major complications. *Diabetes Res. Clin. Pract.* **1**, 185.

McAuliffe, A. V., Brooks, B. A., Fisher, E. J., Molyneaux, L. M. and Yue, D. K. (1998). Administration of ascorbic acid and an aldose reductase inhibitor (Tolrestat) in diabetes: effect on urinary albumin excretion. *Nephron* **80**, 277.

Messent, J., Jones, S., Wiseman, M. and Viberti, G. C. (1991). Glomerular hyperfiltration and albuminuria—an 8 year prospective study. *Diabetologia* **34(Suppl. 2)**, AI.

Miller, K. and Michael, A. F. (1976). Immunopathology of renal extracellular membranes in diabetes mellitus: specificity of tubular basement-membrane immunofluorescence. *Diabetes* **25**, 701.

Mogensen, C. E. (1971). Glomerular filtration rate and renal plasma flow in normal and diabetic man during elevation of blood sugar levels. *Scand. J. Clin. Lab. Invest.* **28**, 177.

Mogensen, C. E. (1976). Renal function changes in diabetes. *Diabetes* **25**, 872.

Mogensen, C. E. (1982). Long term anti-hypertensive treatment inhibiting progression of diabetic nephropathy. *B. M. J.* **285**, 685.

Mogensen, C. E. (1983). A complete screening of urinary albumin concentration in an unselected diabetic outpatient clinic population (1082 patients). *Diabetic Nephropathy* **2**, 11.

Mogensen, C. E. (1984). Microalbuminuria predicts clinical proteinuria and early mortality in maturity-onset diabetes. *N. Engl. J. Med.* **310**, 356.

Mogensen, C. E. (1986). Early glomerular hyperfiltration in insulin-dependent diabetics and late nephropathy. *Scand. J. Clin. Lab. Invest.* **46**, 201.

Mogensen, C. E. (1987). Microalbuminuria as a predictor of clinical diabetic nephropathy. *Kidney Int.* **31**, 673.

Mogensen, C. E. (1990). Prevention and treatment of renal disease in insulin-dependent diabetes mellitus. *Semin. Nephrol.* **10**, 260.

Mogensen, C. E. (1992). Angiotensin converting enzyme inhibitors and diabetic nephropathy. *B. M. J.* **304**, 327.

Mogensen, C. E. (1999). Microalbuminuria, blood pressure and diabetic renal disease: origin and development of ideas. *Diabetologia* **42**, 263.

Mogensen, C. E. and Andersen, M. J. F. (1975). Increased kidney size and glomerular filtration rate in untreated juvenile diabetes: normalization by insulin treatment. *Diabetologia* **11**, 221.

Mogensen, C. E. and Christensen, C. K. (1984). Predicting diabetic nephropathy in insulin-dependent patients. *N. Engl. J. Med.* **311**, 89.

Mogensen, C. E., Christensen, C. K., Christiansen, J. S., Boye, N., Pedersen, M. M. and Schmitz, A. (1988). Early hyperfiltration and late, renal damage in insulin-dependent diabetes. *Pediatr. Adolesc. Endocrinol.* **17**, 197.

Mogensen, C. E., Christensen, C. K. and Vittinghus, E. (1983). The stages in diabetic renal disease with emphasis on the stage of incipient diabetic nephropathy. *Diabetes* **32(Suppl. 2)**, 64.

Mogensen, C. E., Steffes, M. W., Deckert, T. and Christiansen, J. S. (1981). Functional and morphological renal manifestations in diabetes mellitus. *Diabetologia* **21**, 89.

Myers, B. D., Nelson, R. G., Williams, G. W., *et al.* (1991). Glomerular function in Pima Indians with non-insulin dependent diabetes mellitus of recent onset. *J. Clin. Invest.* **88**, 524.

Nagai, N. (1982). Clinical statistics of 551 patients with diabetes mellitus found before 30 years of age. *J. Tokyo Wom. Med. Coll.* **52**, 904.

Najarian, J. S., Kaufman, D. B., Fryd, D. S., *et al.* (1989). Long-term survival following kidney transplantation in 100 type 1 diabetic patients. *Transplantation* **1**, 106.

Najarian, J. S., Sutherland, D. E. R., Simmons, R. L., *et al.* (1979). Ten year experience with renal transplantation in juvenile onset diabetes. *Ann. Surg.* **190**, 487.

National Center for Health Statistics. (1999). *Health, United States, 1998*, Public Health Service, Hyattsville, Md.

National Diabetes Data Group. (1979). Classification and diagnosis of diabetes mellitus and other categories of glucose intolerance. *Diabetes* **16**, 283.

Nelson, R. G., Kunzelman, C. L., Pettit, D. J., Saad, M. F., Bennett, P. H. and Knowles, W. C. (1989). Albuminuria in type 2 (non-insulin dependent) diabetes mellitus and impaired glucose tolerance in Pima Indians. *Diabetologia* **32**, 870.

Nelson, R. G., Newman, J. M., Knowles, W. C., *et al.* (1988). Incidence of end-stage renal disease in type 2 (non-insulin dependent) diabetes mellitus in Pima Indians. *Diabetologia* **31**, 730.

Nicholls, K. and Mandel, T. E. (1989). Advanced glycosylation end-products in experimental murine diabetic nephropathy: effect of islet isografting and of aminoguanidine. *Lab. Invest.* **60**, 486.

Nishimura, C., Hotta, Y., Gui, T., *et al.* (1997). The level of erythrocyte aldose reductase is associated with the severity of diabetic retinopathy. *Diabetes Res. Clin. Pract.* **37**, 173.

Nolph, K. D., Lundblad, A. S. and Novak, J. W. (1988). Current concepts: continuous ambulatory peritoneal dialysis. *N. Engl. J. Med.* **318**, 1595.

Norgaard, K., Feldt-Rasmussen, B., Borch-Johnsen, K., Saelan, H. and Deckert, T. (1990). Prevalence of hypertension in type 1 (insulin-dependent) diabetes mellitus. *Diabetologia* **33**, 407.

Nowack, R., Raum, E., Blum, W. and Ritz, E. (1992). Renal hemodynamics in recent onset type II diabetes. *Am. J. Kidney Dis.* **20**, 342.

Nyberg, G., Bhlome, G. and Norden, G. (1987). Input of metabolic control on progression of clinical diabetic nephropathy. *Diabetologia* **30**, 82.

Odorico, J. S., Becker, Y. T., Van der Werf, W., *et al.* (1998). Advances in pancreas transplantation: the University of Wisconsin experience. *In Clinical Transplants 1997*, (Cecka, J. M. and Terasaki, P. I. eds.), UCLA Tissue Typing Laboratory, Los Angeles.

Olausson, M., Nyberg, G., Norden, G., Frisk, B. and Hedman, L. (1991). Outcome of pancreas transplantations in Goteberg, Sweden 1985–1990. *Diabetologia* **34(Suppl. 1)**, S1.

Ono, Y., Aoki, S., Ohnishi, K., *et al.* (1998). Increased serum levels of advanced glycation end-products and diabetic complications. *Diabetes Res. Clin. Pract.* **41**, 131.

O'Shea, G. M., Goosen, M. F. and Sun, A. M. (1984). Prolonged survival of transplanted islets of Langerhans encapsulated in a biocompatible membrane. *Biochim. Biophys. Acta* **804**, 133.

Osterby, R. (1973). A quantitative electron microscopic study of mesangial regions in glomeruli from patients with short term juvenile diabetes mellitus. *Lab. Invest.* **29**, 99.

Osterby, R. (1974). Early phases in the development of diabetic glomerulopathy: quantitative electron microscopic study. *Acta Med. Scand.* **574(Suppl.)**, 3.

Osterby, R. (1983). Basement membrane morphology in diabetes mellitus. *In Diabetes Mellitus: Theory and Practice*, (M. Ellenberg and H. Rigkin, eds.), p. 323, Medical Examination Publishing, New York.

Osterby, R. and Gundersen, H. J. G. (1975). Glomerular size and structure in diabetes mellitus: 1. early abnormalities. *Diabetologia* **11**, 225.

Osterby, R., Nyberg, G., Hedman, L., Karlberg, I., Persson, H. and Svalander, C. (1991). Kidney transplantation in type 1 (insulin-dependent) diabetic patients. *Diabetologia* **9**, 668.

Pahor, M., Psaty, B. M. and Furberg, C. D. (1998). New evidence on the prevention of cardiovascular events in hypertensive patients with type 2 diabetes. *J. Cardiovasc. Pharmacol.* **32(Suppl. 2)**, S18.

Palmisano, J. J. and Lebovitz, H. E. (1989). Renal function in black Americans with type II diabetes. *J. Diabetic Complications* **3**, 40.

Palmisano, J. J. and Lebovitz, H. E. (1990). Cross-sectional analysis of renal function in black Americans with NIDDM. *Diabetes Care* **13(Suppl. 4)**, 1186.

Palmisano, J. and Sachmechi, I. (1987). Renal function in type 2 diabetes. *Diabetes* **36(Suppl. 2)**, 206A.

Panzram, G. (1987). Mortality and survival in type 2 (non-insulin dependent) diabetes mellitus. *Diabetologia* **30**, 123.

Paradis, K., Langford, G., Long, Z., *et al.*, the XEN 111 Study Group, and Otto, E. (1999). Search for cross-species transmission of porcine endogenous retrovirus in patients treated with living pig tissue. *Science* **285**, 1236.

Parving, H., Oxenboll, B., Svendsen, P. A., Christiansen, J. S. and Andersen, A. R. (1982). Early detection of patients at risk of developing diabetic nephropathy: a longitudinal study of urinary albumin excretion. *Acta Endocrinol. (Copenh.)* **100**, 550.

Parving, H.-H. (1998a). Calcium antagonists and cardiovascular risk in diabetes. *Am. J. Cardiol.* **82**, 42R.

Parving, H.-H. (1998b). Is antihypertensive treatment the same for type 2 diabetes and type 1 diabetes patients? *Diabetes Res. Clin. Pract.* **39(Suppl.)**, S43.

Parving, H.-H. (1999). Diabetic hypertensive patients: is this a group in need of particular care and attention? *Diabetes Care* **22(Suppl. 2)**, B76.

Parving, H.-H., Andersen, A. R., Hommel, E. and Smidt, U. (1985). Effects of long term antihypertensive treatment on kidney function in diabetic nephropathy. *Hypertension* **7(Suppl. II)**, 114.

Parving, H.-H., Andersen, A. R., Smidt, U. M., Hommel, E., Mathiesen, E. R. and Svendsen, P. A. (1987). Effect of antihypertensive treatment on kidney function in diabetic nephropathy. *B. M. J.* **294**, 1443.

Parving, H.-H., Andersen, A. R., Smidt, U. M. and Svendsen, P. A. A. (1983). Early aggressive anti-hypertensive therapy reduces rate of decline in kidney function in diabetic nephropathy. *Lancet* **2**, 1175.

Parving, H.-H., Gall, M.-A., Skott, P., Jorgensen, H. E., Jorgensen, F. and Larsen, S. (1990). Prevalence and causes of albuminuria in non-insulin dependent diabetic (NIDDM) patients. *Kidney Int.* **37**, 243.

Parving, H.-H., Hommel, E., Mathiesen, E., *et al.* (1988). Prevalence of microalbuminuria, arterial hypertension, retinopathy and neuropathy in patients with insulin-dependent diabetes. *B. M. J.* **296**, 156.

Parving, H.-H., Hommel, E., Nielsen, M. D. and Giese, J. (1989). Effect of captopril on blood pressure and kidney function in normotensive insulin-dependent diabetics with nephropathy. *B. M. J.* **299**, 533.

Paster, R. Z., Snavely, D. B., Sweet, A. R., *et al.* (1998). Use of losartan in the treatment of hypertensive patients with a history of cough induced by angiotensin-converting enzyme inhibitors. *Clin. Ther.* **20**, 978.

Patel, B. K., Garvin, P. J., Aridge, D. L., Chenoweth, J. L. and Markivee, C. R. (1991). Fluid collections developing after pancreatic transplantation: radiologic evaluation and intervention. *Radiology* **181**, 215.

Paterson, A. D., Dornan, T. L., Peacock, I., Burden, R. P., Morgan, A. G. and Tattersall, R. B. (1987). Cause of death in diabetic patients with impaired renal function: an audit of a hospital diabetic clinic population. *Lancet* **1**, 313.

Patience, C., Takeuchi, Y. and Weiss, R. A. (1997). Infection of human cells by an endogenous retrovirus of pigs. *Nat. Med.* **3**, 282.

Pedersen, M. M., Christiansen, J. S. and Mogensen, C. E. (1991).

Reduction of glomerular hyperfiltration in normoalbuminuric IDDM patients by 6 months of aldose reductase inhibition. *Diabetes* **40**, 527.

Pedersen, M. M., Mogensen, C. E., Jorgensen, S. F., Moller, B., Lykhe, G. and Pederson, O. (1989). Renal effects from limitation of high dietary protein in normoalbuminuric diabetic patients. *Kidney Int.* **27**, S115.

Peters, A. L. and Schriger, D. C. (1998). The new diagnostic criteria for diabetes: the impact on management of diabetes and macrovascular risk factors. *Am. J. Med.* **1051**(1A), 155.

Pedrini, M. T., Levey, A. S., Lau, J., Chalmers, T. C. and Wang, P. H. (1996). The effect of dietary protein restriction on the progression of diabetic and nondiabetic renal disease: a meta-analysis. *Ann. Intern. Med.* **124**, 627.

Philipson, J. D., Carpenter, B. J., Itzkoff, J., *et al.* (1986). Evaluation of cardiovascular risk for renal transplantation in diabetic patients. *Am. J. Med.* **81**, 630.

Piehlmeier, W., Bullinger, M., Nusser, J., *et al.* (1992). Quality of life in diabetic patients prior to or after pancreas transplantation in relation to organ function. *Transplant. Proc.* **24**, 871.

Pijls, L. T. J., de Vried, H., Donker, A. J. M. and van Eijk, J. T. M. (1999). The effect of protein restrictioin on albuminuria in patients with type 2 diabetes mellitus: a randomized trial. *Nephrol. Dial. Transplant.* **14**, 1445.

Pipeleers, D. G. and Pipeleers-Marichal, M. (1977). Transplantation of pancreatic islets. *Diabetes Metab.* **3**, 273.

Plouin, P.-F., Azizi, M. and Day, M. (1992). Treatment of hypertension in diabetes: threshold of intervention and therapeutic options. *Diabetes Metab.* **18**, 182.

Pollok, J. M., Begemann, J. F., Kaufmann, P. M., *et al.* (1999). Long-term insulin-secretory function of islets of Langerhans encapsulated with a layer of confluent chondrocytes for immunoisolation. *Pediatr. Surg. Int.* **15**, 164.

Porte, D., Jr. and Schwartz, M. W. (1996). Diabetes complications: why is glucose potentially toxic? *Science* **272**, 699.

Posselt, A. M., Barker, C. F., Friedman, A. L. and Naji, A. (1992). Prevention of autoimmune diabetes in the BB rat by intrathymic islet transplantation at birth. *Science* **256**, 1321.

Poulter, N. R. (1998). Calcium antagonists and the diabetic patient: a response to recent controversies. *Am. J. Cardiol.* **12**, 82.

Pugh, J. A., Stern, M. P., Haffner, S. M., Eifler, C. W. and Zapata, M. (1988). Excess incidence of end stage renal disease in Mexican Americans. *Am. J. Epidemiol.* **127**, 135.

Quinn, M., Angelico, M. C., Warram, J. H. and Krolewski, A. S. (1996). Familial factors determine the development of diabetic nephropathy in patients with IDDM. *Diabetologia* **39**, 940.

Rabkin, J. M., Leone, J. P., Sutherland, D. E., et al. (1997). Transcontinental shipping of pancreatic islets for autotransplantation after total pancreatectomy. *Pancreas* **15**, 415.

Rabkin, R., Petersen, J., Kitaji, J., Marck, B., Murphy, W. and Muirhead, E. E. (1984). Effect of antihypertensive therapy on the kidney in spontaneously hypertensive rats with diabetes. *Kidney Int.* **25**, 205.

Ramsay, R. C., Goetz, F. C., Sutherland, D. E., *et al.* (1988). Progression of diabetic retinopathy after pancreas transplantation for insulin-dependent diabetes mellitus. *N. Engl. J. Med.* **318**, 208.

Ravid, M., Brosh, D., Levi, Z., Bar-Dayan, Y., Ravid, D. and Rachmani, R. (1998). Use of enalapril to attenuate decline in renal function in normotensive, normoalbuminuric patients with type 2 diabetes mellitus: a randomized, controlled trial. *Ann. Intern. Med.* **128**(12 Pt. 1), 982.

Reaven, G. M. (1988). Banting Lecture 1988: role of insulin resistance in human disease. *Diabetes* **37**, 1595.

Reltig, R. A. and Levinsky, N. G. (eds.). (1991). *Institute for Medicine (U.S.): Kidney Failure and the Federal Government Access to Kidney Transplantation*, p. 167, National Academy of Sciences, Washington, D.C.

Rennke, H. G., Sandstrom, D., Zatz, R., Meyer, T. W., Cowan, R. S. and Brenner, B. M. (1986). The role of dietary protein in the development of glomerular structural abnormalities in long term experimental diabetes mellitus. *Kidney Int.* **29**, 289.

Riggs, J. E., Moss, A. H., Labosky, D. A., Liput, J. H., Morgan, J. J. and Gutmann, L. (1989). Upper extremity ischemic monomelic neuropathy: a complication of vascular access procedures in uremic diabetic patients. *Neurology* **39**, 997.

Ritz, E. (1999). Nephropathy in type 2 diabetes. *J. Intern. Med.* **245**, 111.

Ritz, E., Hasslacher, C. and Beutel, G. (1991a). Hypertension and diabetic nephropathy. *J. Nephrol.* **1**, 11.

Ritz, E., Koch, M., Fliser, D. and Schwenger, V. (1999). How can we improve prognosis in diabetic patients with end-stage renal disease? *Diabetes Care* **22(Suppl. 2)**, B80.

Ritz, E., Nowack, D., Fliser, D., Koch, M. and Tschope, W. (1991b). Type II diabetes mellitus: is the renal risk adequately appreciated? *Nephrol. Dial. Transplant.* **6**, 679.

Robertson, G. S., Dennison, A. R., Johnson, P. R., *et al.* (1998). A review of pancreatic islet autotransplantation. *Hepatogastroenterology* **45**, 226.

Robison, W. G., Jr., Tillis, T. N., Laver, N. and Kinoshita, J. H. (1990). Diabetes-related histopathologies of the rat retina prevented with an aldose reductase inhibitor. *Exp. Eye Res.* **50**, 355.

Roep, B. O., Stobbe, I., Duinkerken, G., *et al.* (1999). Auto- and alloimmune reactivity to human islet allografts transplanted into type 1 diabetic patients. *Diabetes* **48**, 484.

Rosenbloom, A. L., Joe, J. R., Young, R. S. and Winter, W. E. (1999). Emerging epidemic of type 2 diabetes in youth. *Diabetes Care* **22**, 345.

Rosenstock, J., Friberg, T. and Raskin, P. (1986). Effect of glycemic control on microvascular complications in patients with type I diabetes mellitus. *Am. J. Med.* **81**, 1012.

Rowe, D. J. F., Bagga, H. and Betts, P. B. (1985). Normal variations in rate of albumin excretion and albumin to creatinine ratios in overnight and daytime urine collections in non-diabetic children. *B. M. J.* **291**, 693.

Rowe, J. W., Andres, R., Tobin, J. D., Norris, A. H. and Shock, N. W. (1976). The effect of age on creatinine clearance in men: a cross-sectional and longitudinal study. *J. Gerontol.* **31**, 155.

Rubin, J. and Hsu, H. (1991). Continuous ambulatory peritoneal dialysis: ten years at one facility. *Am. J. Kidney Dis.* **17**, 165.

Rutherford, P. A., Thomas, T. H. and Wilkinson, R. (1990). The mechanism of raised sodium-lithium countertransport in type I diabetes mellitus is different from that in essential hypertension. *Diabet. Med.* **7(Suppl. 2)**, 1A.

Saracho, R., Martin-Malo, A., Martinez, I., Aljama, P. and Montenegro, J. (1998). Evaluation of the Losartan in Hemodialysis (ELHE) Study. *Kidney Int.* **68(Suppl.)**, S125.

Sasaki, T. M., Gray, R. S., Ratner, R. E., *et al.* (1998). Successful long-term kidney-pancreas transplants in diabetic patients with high C-peptide levels. *Transplantation* **65**, 1510.

Savage, S. and Schrier, R. W. (1992). Progressive renal insufficiency: the role of angiotensin converting enzyme inhibitors. *Adv. Intern. Med.* **37**, 85.

Scheen, A. J. (1999). The epidemic of metabolic diseases, a major problem of public health. *Rev. Med. Liege* **54**, 87.

Schmidt, A. M., Hori, O., Chen, J. X., *et al.* (1995). Advanced glycation end products interacting with their endothelial receptor induce expression of vascular cell adhesion molecule-1 (VCAM-1) in cultured human endothelial cells and in mice. *J. Clin. Invest.* **96**, 1395.

Schmitz, A. and Vaeth, M. (1988). Microalbuminuria—a major risk factor in non-insulin dependent diabetes: a 10 year followup study of 503 patients. *Diabet. Med.* **5**, 126.

Schwartz, R. S. (1999). The new immunology—the end of immunosuppressive drug therapy? *N. Engl. J. Med.* **340**, 754.

Seaquist, E. R. and Robertson, R. P. (1992). Effects of hemipancreatectomy on pancreatic alpha and beta cell function in healthy human donors. *J. Clin. Invest.* **89**, 1761.

Sibley, R., Sutherland, D. E. R., Goetz, F. and Michael, A. F. (1985). Recurrent diabetes mellitus in the pancreas iso- and allograft: a light and electron microscopic and immunohistochemical analysis of four cases. *Lab. Invest.* **53**, 132.

Skyler, J. S. (1979). Complications of diabetes mellitus: relationship to metabolic dysfunction. *Diabetes Care* **2**, 499.

Solerte, S. B. and Ferrari, E. (1985). Diabetic retinal vascular complications, erythrocyte filtrability and pentoxifylline: results of a 2 year follow-up study. *Pharmatherapeutica* **4**, 341.

Solerte, S. B., Fioravanti, M., Patti, A. L., *et al.* (1987). Pentoxifylline, total urinary protein excretion rate and arterial blood pressure in long-term insulin-dependent diabetic patients with overt nephropathy. *Acta Diabetol.* **24**, 229.

Spuhler, O. (1946). *Zur Physio-Pathologie der Niere*, p. 45, Hans Huber, Bern.

Standl, E., Steigler, H., Roth, R., Shultz, K. and Lemacher, K. (1989). On the impact of hypertension on the prognosis of NIDDM: results of the Schwabing-GP program. *Diabetes Metab.* **15**, 352.

Starzl, T. E., Putnam, C. W., Hansbrough, J. F., Porter, K. A. and Reid, H. A. (1977). Biliary complications after liver transplantation: with special reference to the biliary cast syndrome and techniques of secondary duct repair. *Surgery* **81**, 212.

Steffes, M. W., Osterby, R., Chavers, B. and Mauer, S. M. (1989). Mesangial expansion as a central mechanism for loss of kidney function in diabetic patients. *Diabetes* **38**, 1077.

Stevens, R. B., Lokeh, A., Ansite, J. D., Field, M. J., Gores, P. F. and Sutherland, D. E. (1994). Role of nitric oxide in the pathogenesis of early pancreatic islet dysfunction during rat and human intraportal islet transplantation. *Transplant. Proc.* **26**, 692.

Sugitani, A., Gritsch, H. A., Shapiro, R., Bonham, C. A., Egidi, C. A. and Corry, R. J. (1998). Surgical complications in 123 consecutive pancreas transplant recipients: comparison of bladder and enteric drainage. *Transplant. Proc.* **30**, 293.

Sun, Y., Ma, X., Zhou, D., *et al.* (1996). Normalization of diabetes in spontaneously diabetic cynomologus monkeys by xenografts of microencapsulated porcine islets without immunosuppression. *J. Clin. Invest.* **98**, 1417.

Sutherland, D. E. (1991). Report from the International Pancreas Transplant Registry. *Diabetologia* **34(Suppl. 1)**, S28.

Sutherland, D. E. (1994). Intraperitoneal transplantation of microencapsulated canine islet allografts with short-term, low-dose cyclosporine for treatment of pancreatectomy-induced diabetes in dogs. *Transplant. Proc.* **26**, 804.

Sutherland, D. E. R. (1988). Who should get a pancreas transplant? *Diabetes Care* **11**, 681.

Sutherland, D. E. R., Goetz, F. C. and Najarian, J. S. (1980). Living related donor segmental pancreatectomy for transplantation. *Transplant. Proc.* **12(Suppl. 2)**, 19.

Sutherland, D. E. R., Gruessner, R., Dunn, D., Moudry-Munns, K., Gruessner, A. and Najarian, J. S. (1994). Pancreas transplantation from living-related donors. *Transplant. Proc.* **26**, 443.

Sutherland, D. E. R., Morrow, C. E., Fryd, D. S., Ferguson, R., Simmons, R. L. and Najarian, J. S. (1982). Improved patient and primary renal allograft survival in uremic diabetic recipients. *Transplantation* **34**, 319.

Taguma, Y., Kitamoto, Y., Futaki, G., *et al.* (1985). Effect of captopril on heavy proteinuria in azotemic diabetics. *N. Engl. J. Med.* **313**, 1617.

Takahashi, C., Nagai, N., Ujihara, N., *et al.* (1990). Clinical profile of Japanese dialysis patients with diabetic nephropathy, diagnosed as having diabetes before the age of thirty. *Diabetes Res. Clin. Pract.* **10**, 127.

Takazakura, E., Wasabu, N., Handa, A., Takada, A., Shinoda, A. and Takeuchi, J. (1972). Intrarenal vascular changes with age and disease. *Kidney Int.* **2**, 224.

Tamborlane, W. V., Puklin, J. E., Bergman, M., *et al.* (1982). Long term improvement of metabolic control with the insulin pump does not reverse diabetic microangiopathy. *Diabetes Care* **5**, 58.

Tattersall, R. B. and Mansell, P. I. (1991). Maturity onset-type diabetes of the young (MODY): one condition or many? *Diabet. Med.* **8**, 402.

Thomas, F. T., Ricordi, C., Contreras, J. L., *et al.* (1999). Reversal of naturally occurring diabetes in primates by unmodified islet xenografts without chronic immunosuppression. *Transplantation* **67**, 846.

Tsilbary, E. C., Charonis, A. S., Reger, L. A., *et al.* (1988). The effect of nonenzymatic glycosylation on the binding of the main noncollagenous NC1 domain to type IV collagen. *J. Biol. Chem.* **263**, 4302.

Tuch, B. E., Wright, D. C., Martin, T. E., *et al.* (1999). Fetal pig endocrine cells develop when allografted into the thymus gland. *Transplant. Proc.* **31**, 670.

Tuttle, K. R., Bruton, L., Perusek, M. C., Lancaster, J. L., Kopp, D. T. and DeFronzo, R. (1991). Effect of strict glycemic control on renal hemodynamic response to amino acids and renal enlargement in insulin-dependent in insulin-dependent diabetes mellitus. *N. Engl. J. Med.* **324**, 1626.

Tzakis, A. G., Ricordi, C. and Alejandro, R. (1990). Pancreatic islet transplantation after upper abdominal exenteration and liver replacement. *Lancet* **336**, 402.

Tzamaloukas, A. H., Murata, G. H., Harford, A. M., et al. (1991). Hand gangrene in diabetic patients on chronic dialysis. *Trans. Am. Soc. Artif. Intern. Organs* **37**, 638.

Tzamaloukas, A. H., Murata, G. H., Piraino, B., *et al.* (1998). Peritoneal urea and creatinine clearances in continuous peritoneal dialysis patients with different types of peritoneal solute transport. *Kidney Int.* **53**, 1405.

USRDS. (1991). *Annual Data Report*, The National Institutes of Health, National Institute of Diabetes and Digestive and Kidney Diseases, Bethesda, Md.

USRDS. (1992). *Annual Data Report*, The National Institutes of Health, National Institute of Diabetes and Digestive and Kidney Diseases, Bethesda, Md.

USRDS. (1998). *Annual Data Report*, The National Institutes of Health, National Institute of Diabetes and Digestive and Kidney Diseases, Bethesda, Md.

USRDS. (1999). *Annual Data Report*, The National Institutes of Health, National Institute of Diabetes and Digestive and Kidney Diseases, Bethesda, Md.

Uusitupa, M., Siitonen, O., Penttila, I., Aro, A. and Pyorala, K. (1987). Proteinuria in newly diagnosed type II diabetic patients. *Diabetes Care* **10**, 191.

Van Norren, K., Thien, T., Berden, J. H., Elving, L. D. and De Pont, J. J. (1998). Relevance of erythrocyte Na + / Li + countertransport measurement in essential hypertension, hyperlipidaemia and diabetic nephropathy: a critical review. *Eur. J. Clin. Invest.* **28**, 339.

van Zwieten, P. A. (1999). Diabetes and hypertension: experimental models for pharmacological studies. *Clin. Exp. Hypertens.* **21**, 1.

Vasquez, B., Flock, E. V., Savage, P. J., *et al.* (1984). Sustained reduction of proteinuria in type 2 (non-insulin dependent) diabetes following diet-induced reduction of hyperglycemia. *Diabetologia* **26**, 127.

Viberti, G. (1999). Why do we have to invoke genetic susceptibility for diabetic nephropathy? *Kidney Int.* **55**, 2526.

Viberti, G. and Keen, H. (1984). The patterns of proteinuria in diabetes mellitus: relevance to pathogenesis and prevention of diabetic nephropathy. *Diabetes* **33**, 686.

Viberti, G., Keen, H. and Wiseman, M. J. (1987). Raised arterial pressure in parents of proteinuric insulin-dependent diabetics. *B. M. J.* **295**, 515.

Viberti, G. C, Bilous, R. W., Mackintosh, B., Bending, J. J. and Keen, H. (1983). Long term correction of hyperglycemia and progression of renal failure in insulin dependent diabetes. *B. M. J.* **286**, 598.

Viberti, G. C., Dodds, R. A. and Bending, J. J. (1988). Non-glycemic intervention in diabetic nephropathy: the role of dietary protein intake. *In The Kidney and Hypertension in Diabetes*, (C. E. Mogensen, ed.), p. 205, Martinus Nijhoff, Boston.

Viberti, G. C., Hill, R. D., Jarrett, R. J., Argyropoulous, A., Mahmud, U. and Keen, H. (1982). Microalbuminuria as a predictor of clinical nephropathy in insulin-dependent diabetes mellitus. *Lancet* **1**, 1430.

Viberti, G. C. and Walker, J. D. (1988). Diabetic nephropathy: etiology and prevention. *Diabetes Metab. Rev.* **4**, 147.

Vittinghus, E. and Mogensen, C. E. (1981). Albumin excretion and renal haemodynamic response to physical exercise in normal and diabetic man. *Scand. J. Clin. Lab. Invest.* **4**, 627.

Vlassara, H. (1996). Protein glycation in the kidney: role in diabetes and aging. *Kidney Int.* **49**, 1795.

Weil, R., Nozawara, M., Koss, M., *et al.* (1975). Pancreatic transplantation in diabetic rats: renal function, morphology, ultrastructure and immunohistology. *Surgery* **78**, 142.

Wen, S-F., Huang, T-P. and Moorthy, A. V. (1985). Effects of low-protein diet on experimental diabetic nephropathy in the rat. *J. Lab. Clin. Med.* **106**, 589.

White, S. A., Robertson, G. S., Davies, J. E., Rees, Y., London, N. J. and Dennison, A. R. (1999). Splenic infarction after total pancreatectomy and autologous islet transplantation into the spleen. *Pancreas* **18**, 419.

Wiseman, M., Viberti, G., Mackintosh, D., *et al.* (1984). Glycemia, arterial pressure and microalbuminuria in type 1 (insulin-dependent) diabetes mellitus. *Diabetologia* **26**, 401.

Wiseman, M. J., Redmond, S., House, F. *et al.* (1985). The glomerular hyperfiltration of diabetes is not associated with elevated plasma levels of glucagon and growth hormone. *Diabetologia* **28**, 718.

Wiseman, M. J., Bognetti, E., Dodds, R., *et al.* (1987). Changes in renal function in response to protein restricted diet in type 1 (insulin-dependent) diabetic subjects. *Diabetologia* **30**, 154.

Wilson, R. M., Van der Minne, P., Deverill, I., *et al.* (1985). Insulin dependence: problems with the classification of 100 consecutive patients. *Diabet. Med.* **2**, 167.

Working Group on Hypertension in Diabetes. (1987). Statement on hypertension in diabetes mellitus: Final report. *Arch. Intern. Med.* **147**, 830.

Wylie-Rosett, J. (1988). Evaluation of protein in dietary management of diabetes mellitus. *Diabetes Care* **11**, 143.

Yang, C. W., Yu, C. C., Ko, Y. C. and Huang, C. C. (1998). Aminoguanidine reduces glomerular inducible nitric oxide synthase (iNOS) and transforming growth factor-beta 1 (TGF-beta 1) mRNA expression and diminishes glomerulosclerosis in NZB/W F1 mice. *Clin. Exp. Immunol.* **113**, 258.

Yudkin, J. S., Forrest, R. D., Jackson, C. A. (1988). Microalbuminuria as predictor of vascular disease in non-diabetic subjects. Islington Diabetes Survey. *Lancet* **2**, 530.

Yoshikawa, M., Shimada, H., Nishida, N., *et al.* (1998). Antidiabetic principles of natural medicines. II. Aldose reductase and alpha-glucosidase inhibitors from Brazilian natural medicine, the leaves of Myrcia multiflora DC. (Myrtaceae): structures of myrciacitrins I and II and myrciaphenones A and B. *Chem. Pharm. Bull.* (Tokyo) **46**, 113.

Yuge, J. and Cecka, J. M. (1992). Sex and age effects in renal transplantation. *In: Clinical Transplants 1991* (P. I. Terasaki, ed.), UCLA Tissue Typing Lab, Los Angeles, CA, p. 261.

Zatz, R., Meyer, T. W., Rennke, H. G. and Brenner, B. M. (1985). Predominance of hemodynamic rather than metabolic factors in the pathogenesis of diabetic nephropathy. *Proc. Natl. Acad. Sci. U. S. A.* **82**, 5963.

Zeller, K., Whittaker, E., Sullivan, L., *et al.* (1991). Effect of restricting dietary protein on the progression of renal failure in patients with insulin-dependent diabetes mellitus. *N. Engl. J. Med.* **324**, 78.

Zhang, B., Salituro, G., Szalkowski, D., *et al.* (1999). Discovery of a small molecule insulin mimetic with antidiabetic activity in mice. *Science* **284**, 974.

Renal Transplantation in Children

Richard N. Fine • Geeta Bajaj

Incidence of End-Stage Renal Disease

The incidence of treated end-stage renal disease (ESRD) (counts of new patients per 1 million population) continues to increase worldwide. Interest in the incidence of chronic renal failure in children was stimulated in the last quarter of the 20th century by the need to determine the facilities required to care for children with ESRD. The first reports in the early 1970s from North America and Europe suggested an incidence of 1 to 5 children/1 million total population. The differences depended to some extent on whether children presenting at less than age 1 year were included in the analyses and at which chronological or developmental age a child with ESRD was deemed to be an adult (Holliday and Potter, 1970; Meadow *et al.*, 1970; Scharer, 1971). The reported upper age cutoff for pediatric patients among the ESRD registries worldwide ranges from 15 to 19 years. The United States Renal Data System (USRDS) defines pediatrics as all patients less than age 20 years old.

There have been many prospective and retrospective analyses of the incidence of chronic renal failure in many centers serving as the only referral for a defined area. In these studies, the incidence ranged from 1 to 5 children/1 million total population to 4 to 5 children/1 million total population (Alexander, 1984; Arbus *et al.*, 1986; Helin and Winberg, 1980; Leumann, 1976; Mongeau *et al.*, 1978; Potter *et al.*, 1980). More than half the children with ESRD were between the ages of 11 and 16 years, whereas the incidence of ESRD in infants less than 1 year old is possibly of the order of 0 to 2/1 million total population (Alexander, 1984; Potter *et al.*, 1980). Many pediatric facilities care for older adolescents based on developmental age at presentation rather than chronological age (Fine, 1979).

A retrospective survey of 26 university hospitals, 40 children's hospitals and 245 general hospitals with pediatric units in the former Federal Republic of Germany for the years 1972–1977 was undertaken by a group of pediatric nephrologists under the auspices of the *Arbeitsgemeinschaft fur Padiatrische Nephrologie* to define the incidence and prevalence of chronic renal failure, preterminal renal failure and terminal renal failure. During the 6-year period, the incidence of terminal renal failure in children 0 to 16 years old was 5.05 children/1 million population of the same age. The incidence varied according to the age groups 0 to 5 years, 5 to 10 years and 10 to 16 years and was 1.61, 4.03 and 8.15 children/1 million population of the same age. The proportion of children with terminal renal failure who received ESRD care (dialysis and/or transplantation) increased with age from 32% in the 0- to 5-year-old category, to 72% in the 5- to 10-year-old category to 87% in the 10- to 16-year-old category (Pistor *et al.*, 1985a, 1985b). These data indicate that the incidence of ESRD in children is underestimated when children receiving ESRD care are the only ones included in the computation.

The incidence of ESRD in a specific locale may be influenced by the prevalence of specific disease entities or the availability of sophisticated equipment and expertise to care for the critically ill neonate with neonatal asphyxia. For example, in Finland, the congenital nephrotic syndrome accounts for a significant number of children with ESRD, whereas in Sweden, 21% of children with chronic renal failure had nephronophthisis (Helin and Winberg, 1980). In Argentina, an endemic hemolytic-uremic syndrome (HUS) is common (Gianantonio *et al.*, 1968). In Denmark, Belgium and the Netherlands, 7%, 9% and 12% of the children starting renal replacement therapy in the years 1977–1983 had HUS, whereas only 2% and 3% of the children from Spain and the United Kingdom starting treatment during the same period had this syndrome (Broyer *et al.*, 1985). Although renal failure is common in patients admitted to a neonatal intensive care unit, the infants either die or recover; it does not seem that a significant number develop ESRD and influence the incidence figures (Alexander, 1984; Anand *et al.*, 1978; Norman and Asadi, 1979).

Synthesis of the information available indicates that the annual incidence of ESRD in children is 1 to 5/1 million total population. If all infants less than 1 year old as well as adolescents 16 to 21 years old are included, the incidence is at least 5/1 million total population.

A report of the European Dialysis Transplant Association (EDTA), detailing demography of dialysis and transplantation in children in Europe in 1984, showed that the access of children to care varied (Broyer *et al.*, 1986). Of the 33 countries providing data on renal replacement therapy to the EDTA, 18 did not report acceptance of any child in the 0- to 4-year-old age group during the year ending December 31, 1984. Five countries did not report accepting any child less than 15 years old for renal replacement therapy during the same period. The overall acceptance rate for children less than 15 years old beginning renal replacement therapy during the year varied from 0.5 children/1 million child population in Greece to 11.6/1 million child population in Israel (Broyer *et al.*, 1985). With the emergence of the USRDS, meaningful data on the incidence of ESRD in patients 0 to 19 years old have become available in the United States. In the 1998 Annual Report (USRDS, 1998), the mean incidence for the years 1994–1996 for pediatric patients less than 19 years old was 13/1 million children/year. According to the 1998 USRDS report, the pediatric annual incidence for the 1995–1996 period increased compared with the 1993–1994 period. The increase was thought to be due to the inclusion of non-Medicare patients in 1994–1995 reported by the U.S. Health Care Financing Administration rather than an increase in the diagnosis and treatment for younger patients.

Within the pediatric ESRD population, there are large variations in the incidence rates of ESRD by age and race of the patients included in the pediatric population. The incidence in the United States ranged from 9/1 million population in the 0 to 4 years old age group to 30/1 million in the 15- to 19-years-old age group. The pediatric treated patient ESRD incidence rates per 1 million U.S. population per year for the 1994–1996 period were 11 for white Americans, 26 for black Americans, 14 for Asian/Pacific Islanders and 21 for Native Americans. Similar to the variation in European countries, there is a variation in incidence in different states: Florida had an incidence of 9.3 and Northern California had an incidence of 4.9 new patients/1 million children per year. The incidence of ESRD in a pediatric population depends on the age of the patients to be included in the pediatric population as well as the locale investigated.

Etiology

The unique characteristics of children and adolescents necessitate the determination of the precise cause of the pathological process producing irreversible renal function impairment in a child. Many diseases that lead to chronic renal failure in children are hereditary. Identifying the specific cause in the proband may facilitate identification of occult disease in relatives. The presence of a hereditary disease should be considered when evaluating potential living related donors. Certain disease entities have the propensity to recur in the allograft. Delineation of the specific primary renal disease permits appropriate counseling regarding the risk of recurrence. Prospective and retrospective epidemiological studies detailing the cause of chronic renal failure in various catchment areas are valid only if accurate data are available.

Habib and colleagues reviewed the cause of chronic renal failure in 270 children who were seen during a 10-year period at the Hôpital des Enfants Malades in Paris (Habib et al., 1973). The authors defined five main categories of renal disease that accounted for 259 cases: glomerular nephropathies (26%), hereditary nephropathies (23%), renal hypoplasia (22%), urinary tract malformations (21%) and vascular nephropathies (4%). A congenital nephropathy accounted for 66% of the 270 cases of chronic renal failure.

Mongeau and associates were able to delineate the cause of chronic renal failure in 71 of 77 children who presented to the Hôpital Sainte-Justive in Montreal during a 6-year period and defined four main disease categories: urinary tract malformations (39%), chronic glomerulonephritis (24%), renal dysplasia-hypoplasia (23%) and hereditary nephropathies (14%) (Mongeau et al., 1978). Of the remaining six patients not included in the four categories, three had HUS, one had bilateral Wilms' tumor, one had systemic lupus erythematosus and one had idiopathic Fanconi's syndrome.

Helin and Winberg (1980), in a retrospective study of chronic renal failure in 77 children in the period 1974–1977 in Sweden, detailed four main disease categories: obstructive anomalies (30%), glomerulonephritides (27%), nephronophthisis (21%) and focal or asymmetrical parenchymal defects (hypoplasia, dysplasia, aplasia, cystic disease) (12%). Of the remaining eight patients (10%), placed in a miscellaneous category, two had cystinosis, two had HUS, two had undefined hereditary nephropathy, one had bilateral Wilms' tumor and one had Laurence-Moon-Biedl syndrome.

The report of the EDTA Pediatric Registry (Broyer et al., 1985) categorized the primary renal disease of 1,946 children starting therapy in the period 1980–1983 as follows: glomerulonephritis (24.3%), pyelonephritis and intestinal nephritis (24.0%), hereditary nephritis and familial diseases (15.1%), multisystem diseases (10.5%), hypoplasia (7.5%), vascular diseases (2.8%), other diseases (9.0%) and cause unknown (6.8%). The 1998 report of the USRDS described the causes of renal failure in pediatric patients (0–19 years old) from 1992–1996 as follows: glomerulonephritis (31.7%); cystic, congenital or hereditary diseases (24.4%); collagen vascular dis-

eases (24.4%); hypertension (5%) and cause unknown (8.1%) (USRDS, 1998).

The North American Pediatric Renal Transplant Cooperative Study (NAPRTCS) was initiated in 1987 with the goal of registering 80% of the renal transplants performed in the United States and Canada in pediatric patients less than 18 years old. During an 11-year period (January 1987–January 1998), 6,038 renal transplants were reported for 5,516 pediatric patients from 75 participating centers in the United States and Canada. Table 37–1 shows the diagnosis of the primary renal disease in these recipients. Four specific entities (aplastic, hypoplastic or dysplastic kidneys; obstructive uropathy; focal segmental glomerulosclerosis (FGS) and reflux nephropathy) account for half the recipients. The commonest glomerular disease was FGS. Approximately 50% of the diagnoses were confirmed by biopsy or nephrectomy tissue specimens (North American Pediatric Renal Transplant Cooperative Study, 1998).

The cause of the primary renal disease varies with the age of the child. This variation was indicated by the data of Potter et al. (1980), which delineated the cause of chronic renal failure in 154 children according to three different age groups. Most of the children with obstructive uropathy were in the adolescent age group at the time dialysis was required, whereas Wilms' tumor occurred exclusively in children less than 5 years old. Similarly, a comparison of the distribution of primary renal diseases in children less than 5 years old with the total data of the EDTA Pediatric Registry (Doncker-

TABLE 37–1

PRIMARY RENAL DISEASE IN 5,516 PEDIATRIC PATIENTS RECEIVING A RENAL TRANSPLANT IN NORTH AMERICA

Diagnosis	No. Patients	%
Aplastic, hypoplastic or dysplastic kidneys	571	15.2
Obstructive uropathy	476	12.7
Focal segmental glomerulosclerosis	526	14.0
Reflux nephropathy	129	3.4
Systemic immunological disease	282	7.5
Chronic glomerulonephritis	143	3.8
Congenital nephrotic syndrome	88	2.3
Syndrome of agenesis of abdominal musculature	82	2.2
Medullary, cystic disease or juvenile nephronophthisis	79	2.1
Hemolytic-uremic syndrome	122	3.3
Polycystic kidney disease	114	3.0
Cystinosis	60	1.6
Membranoproliferative glomerulonephritis type I	38	1.0
Pyelonephritis or interstitial nephritis	70	1.9
Renal infarct	68	1.8
Familial nephritis	71	1.9
Idiopathic crescentic glomerulonephritis	79	2.1
Membranoproliferative glomerulonephritis type II	75	2.0
Oxalosis	22	0.6
Wilms' tumor	26	0.7
Drash syndrome	22	.6
Membrane nephropathy	17	.5
Sickle cell nephropathy	14	.4
Diabetic glomerulonephritis	5	.1
Other	314	8.4
Unknown	255	6.8

Reproduced with permission from the North American Pediatric Renal Transplant Cooperative Study (1999).

wolcke *et al.*, 1982) indicated a lower incidence in the glomer-ulonephritis and urinary tract malformation categories and higher incidence in the systemic and vascular disease catego-ries in the younger age group of patients.

In contrast, the data from NAPRTCS (1998) note that urinary tract malformations (aplastic, hypoplastic or dysplas-tic kidneys and obstructive uropathy) have a higher inci-dence in recipients in the 0- to 1-year-old and 2- to 5-year-old age categories than older recipient groups (Table 37–2). Specific median age data for all ESRD pediatric patients (n = 5,155) reported to the USRDS from 1992–1996 verify that patients with congenital diseases have a lower median age at ESRD than patients with glomerular diseases (Table 37–3).

These studies indicate that the cause of the primary renal disease producing chronic renal failure in children differs from that reported in adult patients (see Chapter 4). Primar-ily, there is an increased incidence of congenital and heredi-tary disease causing chronic renal failure in the pediatric age group and virtually no diabetic nephropathy.

Factors Influencing Acceptability for Transplantation

RECIPIENT AGE

The outcome of renal transplantation in children less than 1 year old had been dismal before the report by So *et al.* in 1987 (Table 37–4). Cerilli and coworkers reported the success-ful transplantation with a cadaver donor graft of a 9-month-old girl who developed ESRD as a result of HUS (Cerilli *et al.*, 1972). At the time of the report, the patient was 13 months posttransplant and said to be progressing normally except for a slightly decreased growth rate. DeShazo and colleagues reported their experience from Minnesota of cadaver donor transplantations in four infants, 6 weeks to 12 months old (DeShazo *et al.*, 1974). The death of all four infants after transplantation led these investigators to conclude that the virtue of attempting transplantation in infants less than 1 year old required reevaluation.

Kwun and associates transplanted successfully a 3-month-old infant (who developed ESRD secondary to cortical necro-sis resulting from shock consequent to a large subcapsular hematoma of the liver) with both kidneys from an anenceph-alic newborn (Kwun *et al.*, 1978). At 22 months of age, the child was developmentally retarded, and although growth

TABLE 37–2

AGE DISTRIBUTION OF PRIMARY RENAL DISEASE IN PEDIATRIC TRANSPLANT RECIPIENTS IN NORTH AMERICA

Diagnosis	0–1 (n=127) (%)	2–5 (n=344) (%)	6–12 (n=763) (%)	13–17 (n=795) (%)
Aplastic, hypoplastic or dysplastic kidneys	28	24	17	11
Obstructive uropathy	19	23	17	14
Focal segmental glomerulosclerosis	1	8	13	12
Other	52	45	53	63

Reproduced with permission from the North American Pediatric Renal Transplant Cooperative Study (1999).

TABLE 37–3

INCIDENCE OF REPORTED END-STAGE RENAL DISEASE THERAPY IN THE UNITED STATES

Primary Disease Groups	Total (1993–1997)	Incidence (%)	Age Median (y)
Total no. patients with end-stage renal disease	5,431	100	14
Diabetes	89	1.6	16
Hypertension	244	4.5	18
Glomerulonephritis	1,620	30.1	16
Goodpasture's syndrome	37	0.7	16
Focal glomerulosclerosis or focal glomerular nephritis	555	10.3	15
Membranous nephropathy	29	0.5	16
Membranoproliferative glomerulonephritis	138	2.5	16
All other glomerulonephritis	81	10.4	16
Cystic kidney diseases	1,410	26.2	10
Interstitial nephritis	494	9.2	14
Analgesic nephropathy	48	0.0	15
All other interstitial nephritis	106	3.9	15
Obstructive nephropathy	176	3.3	12
Collagen vascular diseases	283	9.8	16
Lupus erythematosus	252	6.5	17
Scleroderma	5	0.0	18
Wegener's granulomatosis	40	0.7	16
Hemolytic-uremic syndrome or thrombotic thrombocytopenic purpura	106	2.0	8
Polyarteritis	4	0.2	11
Henoch-Schönlein purpura	45	0.8	14
Malignancies	11	0.3	3
Renal and urinary tract neoplasms	37	0.7	6
Lymphomas	1	<0.1	5
Metabolic diseases	32	1.1	10
Amyloidosis	4	0.1	19
Gouty or uric acid nephropathy	176	3.3	12
Oxalate nephropathy	8	0.2	10
Cystinosis	38	0.6	12
Congenital or other hereditary	64	19.3	2
Congenital obstructive uropathy	362	5.0	11
Renal dysgenesis, agenesis or dysplasia	481	2.7	8
Alport's syndrome	148	2.7	16
Sickle-cell disease	17	0.3	19
AIDS-related	23	0.4	16
Other end-stage renal disease	16	0.5	7
Cause unknown	387	7.2	15
Missing information	442	7.4	13

AIDS = acquired immunodeficiency syndrome.
Reprinted with permission from U.S. Renal Data Systems (1999).

velocity after transplantation was normal, no catch-up growth had occurred. These workers related their experience with cadaver donor transplantation in two additional infants 4 weeks old and 8 months old. The 4-week-old infant died of sepsis in the postoperative period after thrombosis of an anencephalic graft, and the 8-month-old infant had a normal functioning graft 4 weeks posttransplant. The success experi-enced by Kwun *et al.* (1978) prompted them to advocate transplantation in infants with ESRD because they believed

TABLE 37-4

TRANSPLANTATION IN INFANTS LESS THAN 1 YEAR OLD

Author	Age (mo)	Primary Renal Disease	Donor	Function (mo)	Outcome
Goodwin *et al.* (1963)	6 d	Prune-belly syndrome	C, An	NF	Died
Cerilli *et al.* (1972)	5	HUS	C	13	Alive
DeShazo *et al.* (1974)	12	—	C	—	Alive
	5	—	C	—	Died
	4	—	C	—	Died
	1.5	—	C	—	Died
Lawson *et al.* (1975)	8 d	—	C	NF	Died
	9	—	LD	—	Died
	12	—	C	—	Died
Kwun *et al.* (1978)	1	PKD	C, An	NF	Died
Moel and Butt (1981)	3	CN	C, An	6 R	Died
	8	OU	C	42 R	Died
Campbell *et al.* (1984)	17 d	CN	C	3 R	Alive
So *et al.* (1987)	11.5	Hypoplasia	C	89 R	Alive
	11.5	Hypoplasia	LD	52	Alive
	6	Hypoplasia	LD	44	Alive
	6.5	Oxalosis	LD	23 RO	Alive
	6	CN	LD	39	Alive
	10	OU	LD	36	Alive
	11	Oxalosis	LD	14 RO	Died
	7	Oxalosis	LD	32	Alive
	8	Hypoplasia	LD	24	Alive

An = anencephalic; C = cadaver; CN = cortical necrosis; HUS = hemolytic-uremic syndrome; NF = nonfunction; PKD = polycystic-kidney disease; OU = obstructive uropathy; R = rejection; RO = recurrent oxalosis; and LD = living donor.

that long-term dialysis "rarely results in adequate growth and development." A follow-up report by Moel and Butt (1981) from the Downstate Medical Center, Brooklyn, New York, indicated that the 3-month-old infant at transplantation had died later at 3.5 years of age with hypertensive encephalopathy and that the 8-month-old infant's graft was lost through rejection 6 months posttransplant.

Before the report of So *et al.* (1987), of 13 infants who received 12 cadaver donor and 1 living related donor grafts, only 1 was alive with a functioning graft at the time of the report (see Table 37-4). The report of So *et al.* (1987) was more encouraging. Of the nine infants who received eight living related donor and one cadaver donor graft, only one infant died, and six of the primary grafts were functioning 24 to 52 months posttransplant. At the time of the report, the two patients who lost the primary grafts at 23 and 89 months posttransplant were retransplanted successfully (see Table 37-4). The series from Minnesota was updated by a report by Najarian *et al.* (1992). In the period 1970–1991, 28 kidney transplants (27 primary transplants and 1 retransplant) were performed from 23 living related donors and 5 cadaver donors in infants less than 1 year old (mean age, 7 ± 2 months; range, 6 weeks–12 months). The 1-year and 5-year graft survival rates for the living related donor grafts were 96% and 63%, whereas the 1-year and 5-year graft survival rates for the cadaver donor grafts were both 20%. These data indicate that living related donor transplantation in infants less than 1 year old can have a successful outcome.

Rizzoni and colleagues reported their experience with 31 transplants in 19 children less than 5 years old (Rizzoni *et al.*, 1980). Combining their data with data from the literature, a total of 72 children (<5 years old) received 92 grafts from 32 living related donors and 60 cadaver donors. At the time of the reports, 19 (26%) children had died, and 43 (60%) children had functioning grafts. There was a striking difference in outcome depending on donor source. Of 32 living related donor grafts, 24 (75%) were functioning, whereas only 19 (32%) of 60 cadaver donor grafts were functioning. The ad-

vantage of living related donor transplantation and the poor outcome with cadaver donor transplantation in children less than 5 years old was substantiated further by reports of Hodson *et al.* (1978) and Moel and Butt (1981) (see Table 37-4).

Subsequent reports detailing the results of transplantation in young children were more encouraging. Trompeter and coworkers described the results from Guy's Hospital of 16 grafts (13 cadaver donors and 3 living related donors) in 15 children less than 5 years old at transplantation (Trompeter *et al.*, 1983). Although the mean follow-up interval was only 1 to 2 years, 11 (75%) patients were surviving with functioning grafts, and 4 (25%) patients had died. Postoperative growth was said to be encouraging, especially after initiation of alternate-day steroid therapy. Perusal of the growth data indicates, however, that only 4 of 10 children with a graft functioning for longer than 3 months were growing above the 3rd percentile growth curve, and only 4 of the 10 children appeared to be exhibiting catch-up growth.

Arbus and colleagues reported their experience with 39 cadaver donor grafts in 28 children less than 6 years old (Arbus *et al.*, 1983). After a mean follow-up period of 40 months, 19 (68%) patients had functioning grafts, and 6 (21%) had died. The causes of graft failure were primary nonfunction (25%), vascular thrombosis (25%), recurrent HUS (20%), rejection (15%) and death (15%). Posttransplant growth appeared to parallel the pretransplant growth curve in most children (±80%). Only four (22%) of the children were growing above the 10th percentile growth curve.

Kalia and associates described the results of 14 renal transplants in 13 children less than 5 years old (Kalia *et al.*, 1988). Of recipients, 11 were alive at the time of the report, and 9 had a functioning graft. A cadaver donor was used in six cases and living related donor in eight. Graft survival at 1 year was 92%, and at 2 to 5 years it was 73%. Sustained catch-up growth was reported in all recipients with successful grafts, and with one exception all school-aged children were functioning at an age-appropriate grade level.

Koffman and coworkers updated the data from Guy's Hospital in children less than 5 years old (Koffman et al., 1989). Thirty-six children (mean age, 3 years, 11 months) received 44 renal allografts from 40 cadaver donors and 4 living related donors. The 5-year patient survival rate was 78%, and graft survival rate was 64% for first grafts. Seven first grafts were lost from rejection and three from vascular problems. Retransplantation results were disappointing, with only three of eight being successful.

From the analysis of the preceding data, it was difficult to advocate renal transplantation in young children with ESRD as the preferred treatment. The short-term outcome of cadaver donor transplantation in infants less than 1 year old was dismal. Similarly, except for the reports of Trompeter et al. (1983), Arbus et al. (1983), Brodehl et al. (1986), Kalia et al. (1988) and Koffman et al. (1989), the results of cadaver donor transplantation in children 1 to 6 years old have been disappointing. The long-term results of the reports of Trompeter et al. (1983) and Arbus et al. (1983) were difficult to assess because the mean follow-up period was only 14 and 40 months. The report of Koffman et al. (1989) is relatively optimistic, however.

The outcome of living related (parental) donor transplantation in children 1 to 5 years old was more encouraging. Combining the reports of Hodson et al. (1978) and Miller et al. (1982) from Minnesota indicated that 18 of 28 (64%) initial living related donor grafts were functioning at the time of the reports and that only 5 (18%) of the children had died. The follow-up periods were 13 to 75 months and 20 to 112 months in the two reports.

The reports of Trompeter et al. (1983), Arbus et al. (1983), Hodson et al. (1978) and Miller et al. (1982) stressed the degree of linear growth achieved after successful transplantation as an advantage of this treatment. Perusal of the growth curves of the recipients included in these reports as well as the data of Rizzoni et al. (1980) and Brodehl et al. (1986) indicates that few children had sustained catch-up growth after transplantation. In most recipients, posttransplant growth paralleled the growth curve at the time of transplantation or showed evidence of further reduction in growth velocity.

So and colleagues noted accelerated growth in five of nine infants with good primary graft function who were transplanted at less than 1 year old (So et al., 1987). Four of the five recipients had normal stature 2 to 4 years after transplantation.

The impact of renal transplantation on psychomotor development is difficult to assess. Serial measurements were included in the report of So et al. (1987). Of the 10 children with functioning grafts reported by Rizzoni and associates, 7 were attending regular school, 2 were attending a school for handicapped children and 1 was in nursery school (Rizzoni et al., 1980). Intellectual assessment of 15 children with functioning grafts by Arbus and coworkers revealed that 6 were high average, 5 were average, 3 were low average and 1 was mildly retarded (Arbus et al., 1983). Miller and colleagues indicated that all recipients had delayed psychomotor development at the time of transplantation (Miller et al., 1982). After transplantation, 8 of 10 recipients with a functioning graft were said to be functioning "at close or at normal levels." Specific developmental test results were available in four recipients: Two recipients were functioning at a normal level for chronological age, and two were retarded.

Of the nine infants transplanted by So and colleagues, four showed clear developmental delay before transplantation (So et al., 1987). Seven recipients were reassessed 3 to 22 months posttransplantation, and five had normal motor and cognitive development.

Further data have been more encouraging. Briscoe and coworkers reported the outcome of renal transplantation in 21 children less than 2 years old and compared the results with the outcome of children 2 to 18 years old who received transplants between January 1980 and January 1990 (Briscoe et al., 1992). The 5-year actuarial patient survival rates for living related donor and cadaver donor recipients were 85% and 70%, and the 5-year graft survival rates were 86% and 38%. Patient survival was statistically superior in the older recipients of living related donor and cadaver donor grafts. There was no statistically significant difference in graft survival rates when comparing recipients less than 2 years old with recipients greater than 2 years old.

Salvatierra and associates reported successful transplantation of nine hemodynamically stable infants with adult-size kidneys (Salvatierra et al., 1998). The mean serum creatinine level 12 months posttransplant was $0.49 + 0.16$ mg/dl.

The 1998 NAPRTCS report indicates that the 4-year graft survival rates for living related donor grafts in the 0- to 1-year-old, 2- to 5-year-old, 6- to 12-year-old and 13- to 20-year-old old age groups were similar; however, there was a significant decrease in the 0- to 1-year-old age group (45%) compared with the other three age groups (61–68%) with a cadaver donor graft. Despite newer immunosuppression strategies, graft survival rates in recipients less than 2 years old are suboptimal if the graft is from a cadaver donor. Such data have led to a recommendation accepted by many that transplantation be deferred until the recipient is at least 2 years old with a weight of 10 kg unless a living related donor is available.

The EDTA Registry reported data on 296 children less than 2 years old from 24 countries who began renal replacement therapy in the period 1969–1988. During the periods 1978–1982, 1983–1985 and 1986–1988, the incidence of children less than 2 years old starting renal replacement therapy increased from 3.6 to 4.4 to 8.9%. The 3-year patient survival for children less than 2 years old starting renal replacement therapy improved from 65% in 1978 to 1982 to 78% in 1986 to 1988.

One-year graft survival rates were 54% for recipients transplanted at less than 2 years old compared with 65% for recipients transplanted at greater than 2 years old. Graft failure was caused by thrombosis in 23% of recipients who were less than 5 years old at transplantation compared with 11% in pediatric recipients greater than 10 years old. The combined data from Europe are similar to data from North America regarding treatment of children with ESRD who are less than 2 years old.

The optimal management for the young child with ESRD is difficult to determine. If a living related donor is available, transplantation is an acceptable option. From the current available information, it is not possible to predict the long-term outcome of such an undertaking. Cadaver donor transplantation for children less than 1 year old is controversial. With the availability of some form of continuous peritoneal dialysis, such children can be managed until an adequate assessment of psychomotor development can be made. If the infant is thriving with continuous peritoneal dialysis, it seems reasonable to defer transplantation until a later date. Cadaver donor transplantation is a reasonable alternative to dialysis in children 2 to 5 years old. With the availability of continuous peritoneal dialysis as an alternative to long-term hemodialysis, the urgency to transplant young children because of the difficulties with dialysis is obviated.

Kohaut and associates reported the course of three infants in whom continuous ambulatory peritoneal dialysis (CAPD) was begun during the first 3 months of life (Kohaut et al., 1985). Living related donor transplantation was undertaken at 13 to 15 months of age. At the time of the report, all three grafts were functioning 15 to 19 months posttransplant with a serum creatinine level of 0.6 mg/dl. The height of the three recipients was within the normal range, and developmental examination revealed no abnormalities.

DONOR AGE

Anencephalic Donors

Goodwin and coworkers reported the use of anencephalic kidneys for transplantation into a 6-day-old infant with prune-belly syndrome (Goodwin et al., 1963). Specific data are available regarding transplantation of one or both kidneys from anencephalic donors to 29 recipients aged 6 days to 50 years (Table 37–5). An additional 18 transplants using anencephalic donors have been identified by the Eurotransplant Registry (Kinnaert et al., 1984) that probably included the cases reported by Dreikorn et al. (1977), Brodehl et al. (1986) and possibly two of the five cases reported by Gomez-Campdera et al. (1990). A total of 43 recipients have received one or both kidneys from an anencephalic donor; however, sufficient data are available to analyze outcome only in 37 recipients (Kinnaert et al., 1984; see Table 37–5).

Of the 37 grafts, 16 (43%) never functioned, primarily because of poor perfusion secondary to vascular thrombosis.

An additional eight (22%) grafts functioned for 5 months or less, all of which were lost as a result of rejection. Only one third of the anencephalic grafts sustained long-term (>1 year) function.

The longest survivor is a 4-year-old boy with prune-belly syndrome who was transplanted with both kidneys from an anencephalic donor by Martin et al. (1969). In a follow-up report by Iitaka et al. (1978), the recipient was 9.5 years posttransplant with a serum creatinine level of 0.5 mg/dl, and his height was between the 10th and 25th percentile for chronological age. The other 12 long-term functioning anencephalic grafts were as follows: in a 3-month-old infant reported originally by Kwun et al. (1978) and subsequently by Moel and Butt (1981), who survived 3.5 years with both kidneys from an anencephalic donor before dying secondary to hypertensive encephalopathy despite adequate graft function; in two pediatric recipients who were surviving 1.5 and 3 years at the time of the report by Iitaka et al. (1978) and in nine other recipients (Gomez-Campdera et al., 1990; Kinnaert et al., 1984), eight of whom were surviving 1.5 to 7 years with a functioning graft.

In addition to the significant incidence of primary nonfunction, the problems surrounding anencephalic donors are emphasized in the report of Iitaka et al. (1978). Of 14 potential anencephalic donors, 8 could not be used. Four anencephalic newborns deteriorated rapidly, and the kidneys were consid-

TABLE 37–5
TRANSPLANTATION OF KIDNEYS FROM ANENCEPHALIC DONORS

Author	Recipient Age	Primary Renal Disease	Outcome Allograft	Recipient
Goodwin et al. (1963)	6 d	Prune-belly syndrome	NF	Died
Fine et al. (1970)	2 y	CN	NF	Alive
LaPlante et al. (1970)	2 y	PKD	NF	Alive
King et al. (1971)	6 y	OU	2 m	Died
	15 y	CGN	NF	Alive
Lawson et al. (1973)	8 d	PKD	NF	Died
Salvatierra and Belzer (1975)	1.5 y	—	3 m	Died
Dreikorn (1977)	44 y	CGN	2 d R	Alive
Iitaka et al. (1978)	4 y	Prune-belly syndrome	9.5 y	Alive
	18 y			
	11 y	MPGN	3 y	Alive
	5 y	MCD	1.5 y	Alive
	19 y	OU	1 m R	Alive
	14 y	RPGN	NF	Alive
		OU	NF	Alive
Moel and Butt (1981)	3 m	CN	3.5 y R NF	Died
			NF	
	1 m	PKD	NF	Died
	17 m	HUS		Alive
	21 m	Dysplasia		Alive
Arbut et al. (1983)	—	—	NF	—
Shapira et al. (1985)	4.5 y	Wilms' tumor	1 y	Alive
Brodehl et al. (1986)	2.5 y	Dysplasia	F	Alive
Holzgreve et al. (1987)	4 y	—	1 10/12 y	Alive
		—	1 10/12 y	
	9 y			Alive
	25 y*			
Leunissen et al. (1989)	27 y*	CGN	5 m R	Alive
Gomez-Campdera et al. (1990)	13 y	Oxalosis	R	Died
	16 y	OU	5 y	Alive
	23 y	CGN	NF	Alive
	50 y	NS	2 y	Alive
	8 y	MCD	2 y	Alive

*2 kidneys en bloc.
CGN = chronic glomerulonephritis; CN = cortical necrosis; HUS = hemolytic-uremic syndrome; MCD = medullary cyst disease; MPGN = membranoproliferative glomerulonephritis; NS = nephrosclerosis; OU = obstructive uropathy; PKD = polycystic kidney disease; R = rejected; RPGN = rapidly progressive glomerulonephritis.

ered unsuitable for transplantation. In three instances, a suitable histocompatible recipient could not be found, and in one donor a solitary kidney could not be perfused at the time of harvesting. The latter situation emphasized the potential for urinary tract malformations in anencephalics, in whom the incidence of such malformations has been reported to be 26.8% (Naeye et al., 1971).

Spees and colleagues detailed the potential suitability of anencephalic donors by reviewing autopsy material on 174 anencephalics (Spees et al., 1984). The overall incidence of renal and urogenital abnormalities was 11.5%, which is only slightly higher than the 8.4% incidence in 2,153 consecutive autopsies of infants and children reported by Rubenstein et al. (1961). A review of the case histories revealed that only 34.5% of the 174 anencephalic cases would have qualified as heart-beating donors, of which 93% could have donated at least one kidney. An additional potential complication of anencephalic donors was the development of proteinuria and focal glomerulosclerosis in one recipient reported by Leunissen et al. (1989) that was attributable to hyperfiltration.

Although a few long-term successes have occurred using grafts from anencephalic donors, the high rate of primary nonfunction should discourage the use of such donors. The difficulties encountered in attempting to harvest such kidneys, from ethical and technical viewpoints, as well as the potential for urinary tract malformations are additional problems that complicate the use of anencephalic donors.

The difficulties in harvesting organs from anencephalic donors if one waits for brain stem activity to cease before declaring brain death was emphasized by Peabody et al. (1989). Six potential anencephalic donors were given intensive care from birth, and six others received care only when signs of imminent death were apparent to determine if the former would yield acceptable organs for transplantation within the first week of life. Only two infants met the criteria for brain death, and no solid organs were procured. Delay in initiating intensive care resulted in organs not suitable for transplantation.

An alternative method reported by Holzgreve et al. (1987) yielded viable kidneys that were transplanted successfully into three recipients. The anencephalic infants were intubated immediately after birth and given ventilatory support until the kidneys were removed 45 to 60 minutes after delivery. If this method were to be used in the United States, the current definition of brain death for anencephalics would have to be modified (Botkin, 1988; Landwirth, 1988; Sounding Board, 1989).

Pediatric Donors

A brief analysis in the 11th report of the Human Renal Transplant Registry (Barnes et al., 1973) indicated that the survival rate of first cadaver grafts from donors 6 to 50 years old was superior to that of donors in the 0- to 5-years-old or greater than 50-years-old groups. These data call into question the use of kidneys from donors in the last two age groups.

Darmady (1974) analyzed the results of 6,883 kidney transplants from the Human Renal Transplant Registry according to donor age. There was a significant improvement in graft survival in the 11- to 20-year-old and 21- to 30-year-old donor age groups when compared with older donors. A stepwise decline in graft survival rates was shown when the data were analyzed according to donor age by Morling and colleagues, who analyzed the outcome of 355 first and second cadaver donor transplants performed in Copenhagen according to donor age (Morling et al., 1975). In both of these studies, pediatric donors less than 10 years old were not included. In contrast, Solheim and coworkers failed to show

any difference in graft survival rates with increasing donor age when evaluating 219 cadaver donor transplants performed in Oslo that were divided into three donor groups: less than 20 years old, 20 to 49 years old and less than 50 years old (Solheim et al., 1976).

The use of pediatric donors less than 10 years old is still controversial. Kelly and associates transplanted five pediatric cadaver kidneys from donors 5 months old to 7 years old into recipients 1.5 to 29 years old, and only one of the five kidneys provided adequate function (Kelly et al., 1967). Fine and colleagues transplanted four kidneys from donors 2 to 5 years old into adolescent recipients 12 to 17 years old and obtained adequate function in three grafts (creatinine clearance 100 ml/min/1.73 m²) (Fine et al., 1969b). Anatomical hypertrophy of the three functioning grafts was shown radiographically. A comparison of the outcome of pediatric cadaver kidneys from donors 0 to 5 years old with donors 6 to 10 years old and 11 to 20 years old was undertaken by the Human Renal Transplant Registry (Merkel et al., 1974). The survival rate for the 0- to 5-year-old donor graft was less than that for the other two age groups, which had comparable survival rates. The pediatric recipient who received a graft from a pediatric donor 0 to 5 years old had a poorer outcome than pediatric recipients receiving grafts from pediatric donors 6 to 10 years old.

van Speybroeck and coworkers noted no deleterious effect on 1-year and 2-year graft survival rates from using kidneys from cadaver donors 1 to 15 years old (van Speybroeck et al., 1979). The data of these investigators indicated improved graft survival rates when pediatric cadaver kidneys were transplanted into younger recipients. Similarly, Boczko and associates noted improved graft survival rates when transplanting 31 pediatric cadaver kidneys from donors 1.5 to 9 years old into adult recipients in comparison with 141 adult cadaver donor kidneys into adult recipients (Boczko et al., 1978).

Additional data failed to clarify definitively the suitability of pediatric kidneys. Glass and colleagues analyzed the results of 502 renal transplants performed at the Downstate Medical Center in New York (Glass et al., 1979). Sixty-five grafts from pediatric donors were divided into three age groups—0 to 5, 6 to 10 and 11 to 15 years old—and their outcomes were compared with those obtained in recipients of adult (>16 years old) donor grafts. There was no statistically significant difference in the results between the three pediatric donor groups and adult donor group, prompting these investigators to urge that "brain-dead pediatric patients of any age should be considered to be potential cadaveric kidney donors."

In 1981, a report from the same institution detailed the results of 440 consecutive cadaver-donor grafts according to the decade of donor age (Hong et al., 1981). At 24 months posttransplant, the 0- to 10-year-old and greater than 51-year-old donor groups had a 30% graft survival rate, whereas the other age groups had a 50 to 60% graft survival rate. Primary nonfunction contributed to the poor graft survival rate in the 0- to 10-years-old age group, which was particularly apparent with infant kidneys.

The report by van der Vliet et al. (1982) analyzed the results from the Eurotransplant Registry of cadaver donor transplants in the years 1967–1981. The 5-year graft survival rate of 5,993 grafts from donors 11 to 50 years old was almost identical (43.3%) to that of 626 grafts from donors less than 11 years old (43.6%). These workers concluded that pediatric donors can be a valuable source of cadaver kidneys for transplantation.

An additional report on the influence of cadaver donor age on renal graft survival (Wetzels et al., 1986) analyzed 36 recipients who received cadaver kidneys from donors less than 11 years old and compared the results with 374 recipients who received cadaver kidneys from donors 11 to 51 years old and 21 recipients who received cadaver kidneys from donors greater than 51 years old. All recipients were greater than 16 years old. Graft survival at 1 year posttransplant was significantly worse in the younger age group (45.6%) than in the older age groups (75.5% and 75.9%). Renal artery stenosis and kidney loss resulting from technical failures were more frequent in the grafts from the younger donors. The reasons for these discrepant data regarding pediatric cadaver donors are not apparent; however, the proportion of donors less than 5 years old, especially if a significant number of donors were less than 1 year old, could account for the varying results.

Although Murray et al. (1967) reported that a single free kidney from infants undergoing ureterosubarachnoid shunting for hydrocephalus provided adequate function in adult recipients, Meakins et al. (1972), Kinne et al. (1974) and Anderson et al. (1974) in the early 1970s suggested that en-bloc transplantation of both pediatric cadaver kidneys into adult recipients was advantageous. Schneider and coworkers detailed the long-term success with 21 double pediatric cadaver kidneys from donors 6 months old to 10 years old that were transplanted into recipients 5 to 51 years old (Schneider et al., 1983). There was no difference in outcome when compared with age-matched control recipients of adult donor cadaver kidneys. No increased incidence of vascular or technical problems was noted. Eight of the 11 functioning double pediatric grafts were surviving at 7 to 11 years.

Kootstra et al. (1978) transplanted 24 single kidneys from donors 1.5 to 10 years old and Boczko et al. (1978) transplanted 31 single kidneys from donors 1.5 to 9 years old into adult recipients (Boczko et al., 1978). The single pediatric kidneys provided adequate function in the adult recipients. Silber (1974) reported serial measurements of four kidneys from pediatric donors 4 to 5 years old that were transplanted into adult recipients. At the time of transplantation, the longitudinal axis of the kidneys measured from 10.1 to 10.8 cm; 5 to 9 months posttransplant, the grafts increased in size to 13.2 to 13.6 cm. One can conclude that a single kidney from a pediatric donor greater than 1.5 years old can provide adequate function for an adult recipient, although Salvatierra and Belzer (1975) considered the minimum donor age to be 10 months. Pediatric donors less than 1 year old would increase the number of kidneys available for transplantation (Bart et al., 1981). The incidence of complications, especially primary nonfunction and vascular thrombosis, that occur with the use of such kidneys dictates that kidneys from infants less than 1 year old should be avoided, however, except under the special circumstances of an infant recipient. Because of the increased incidence of vascular thrombosis with cyclosporine (Ettenger and Fine, 1986), we were reluctant to use pediatric cadaver donors less than 5 years old when cyclosporine was an initial immunosuppressive agent because of the potential additive risk of vascular thrombosis.

Multiple reports address the following issues: Does the outcome of transplantation of pediatric cadaver donors in adult recipients justify the use of such donors? Is there a lower pediatric cadaver donor age limit that is acceptable? Should pediatric cadaver donors be used preferentially for pediatric recipients? Are there specific complications associated with the use of pediatric cadaver kidneys?

Smith and colleagues assessed the outcome of 67 pediatric grafts from donors less than 16 years old that were transplanted into adult recipients using cyclosporine-prednisone immunosuppression (Smith et al., 1988). The 1-year graft survival rate of 54% for donors less than 10 years old indi-

cated inferior results. Trevino and coworkers transplanted 100 patients with kidneys from donors 5 months to 16 years old (kidneys from donors <2 years old were transplanted en bloc) with a 4-year graft survival rate of 64%, indicating pediatric cadaver donors were an excellent donor kidney source (Trevino et al., 1988). These workers indicated that a higher incidence of acute tubular necrosis occurred with the pediatric donor kidneys. Similarly, Hayes and associates noted comparable results with adult donors with 126 single kidneys from donors 9 months old to 16 years old transplanted into adult recipients, although the incidence of urological complications was 23.5% in the recipients of grafts from donors 0 to 2 years old, in contrast to an overall 5% urological complication rate (Hayes et al., 1988).

Because of the increasing need for cadaver donor kidneys, there have been continued efforts to make maximal use of kidneys from young pediatric cadaver donors. Bretan and colleagues described their experience with en-bloc pediatric kidneys from donors younger than 60 months old with non-sensitized primary adult recipients using quadruple immunosuppression with OKT3 (Bretan et al., 1997). The graft survival rates at 12 months and 24 months were 100% and 85%. All grafts were said to function immediately, and there were no technical losses.

Gruessner and colleagues noted a 5-year graft survival rate of 52% for 131 grafts from recipients less than 10 years old compared with 55% for adult donors (Gruessner et al., 1990). Rao and associates noted no difference in graft survival rates of 17 recipients who received grafts from cadaver donors less than 10 years old compared with older pediatric and adult donors (Rao et al., 1990). Tellis and coworkers noted no difference in graft survival rate when kidneys from donors 2 to 7 years old were transplanted into adult recipients compared with donors greater than 7 years old using azathioprine-prednisone or azathioprine-cyclosporine-prednisone immunosuppression (Tellis et al., 1990). Abouna and coworkers noted a 60% 1-year graft survival rate for 20 grafts from pediatric donors less than 5 years old transplanted into adult recipients with a mean cold ischemia time of 48 ± 13 hours (Abouna et al., 1991).

In contrast, Opelz (1988b) analyzed 4,230 transplants from pediatric donors and noted significant improvement with increasing donor age. Kidneys from donors less than 3 years old yielded the poorest results regardless of recipient age. Data from Eurotransplant (Groenwood et al., 1989) indicated that graft survival rates were especially poor (50% at 1 year) when kidneys from donors less than 5 years old were transplanted into recipients less than 5 years old. The 5-year graft survival rates of 53 pediatric recipients who received grafts from donors greater than 10 years old, 5 to 10 years old and less than 5 years old were 87%, 55% and 44% in the report of Hoyer et al. (1990), which was statistically poorer for the younger donors (P<0.001). Ruder and colleagues noted poorer 1-year graft survival rates in pediatric recipients of 18 donors less than 6 years old (39%) compared with 42 donors greater than 6 years old (90%), concluding that pediatric donors less than 6 years old carry an increased risk for graft failure (Ruder et al., 1989). Focusing on 44 recipients less than 6 years old, So and associates reported a 40% 1-year graft survival rate for 10 grafts from recipients less than 4 years old compared with 59% for 34 grafts from recipients greater than 4 years old, using quadruple immunosuppression (So et al., 1990).

In an attempt to analyze the effect of donor age on graft survival in pediatric cadaver renal transplant recipients, Harmon and colleagues evaluated the outcome of 787 cadaver donor transplants in children less than 18 years old reported to NAPRTCS in the years 1987–1990 (Harmon et al., 1992).

Graft survival was poorest from donors less than 5 years old with the increase in graft failure attributed to vascular thrombosis and primary nonfunction. A later report of the NAPRTCS (1998) shows the continued adverse impact of young (<5 years old) age on graft survival rates at 5 years. This effect is independent of recipient age.

Although current practice is to limit use of pediatric donors less than 3 years old and to be less than enthusiastic about use of pediatric donors 3 to 6 years old, in pediatric recipients it is important to recognize that a substantial number of kidneys (±50%) from such young donors provide adequate (albeit less than that achieved from older donors) function in pediatric recipients. One additional note of caution with pediatric cadaver kidneys is the potential for the development of proteinuria and FGS as a result of hyperfiltration. Hayes and coworkers reported the finding of FGS on graft biopsy specimens at 13 ± 6 months posttransplant from 7 of 10 adult recipients of a graft from a pediatric cadaver donor less than 6 years old (Hayes *et al.*, 1991). Protein excretion and serum creatinine levels were significantly higher in these recipients than in a control population. These workers concluded that adult recipients of pediatric cadaver donor grafts may be at greater risk for development of FGS than recipients of adult donor kidneys.

Adult Donors

The report by Miller *et al.* (1982), of transplanting 12 children weighing 5,400 to 8,800 g, and the report of So *et al.* (1987), of transplanting an additional 8 children less than 1 year old and weighing 5,000 to 7,700 g with grafts from adult donors, indicate the technical feasibility of using adult kidneys for transplantation into small recipients. The series from Minnesota has increased to 23 living related or living unrelated adult donor kidneys transplanted into infants less than 1 year old. McMahon and colleagues reported parental donors for seven recipients weighing less than 10 kg; six of seven survivors had excellent graft function 7 to 62 months posttransplant without any technical complications (McMahon *et al.*, 1989). Despite the technical feasibility of using an adult kidney in a small child, we occasionally have used pediatric cadaver kidneys for a child weighing less than 10 kg.

If immunological considerations dictate the use of adult kidneys in small children, this can be accomplished. The 1998 NAPRTCS annual report stated a 78% 5-year graft survival rate for living related donor grafts in infants less than 2 years old and a 51% 5-year graft survival rate for cadaver-donor grafts. Salvatierra and colleagues studied hemodynamic changes induced by adult-sized kidney transplantation in nine hemodynamically stable and optimally hydrated infants (Salvatierra *et al.*, 1998; Salvatierra and Sarwal, 2000). One-year graft survival and patient survival in the nine infants were 100% with a mean serum creatinine level at 12 months of age of 0.49 ± 0.16 mg/dl. The authors recommend aggressive intravolume maintenance to avoid low flow to the kidney that may induce acute tubular necrosis, vascular thrombosis or primary nonfunction.

Nghiem and colleagues evaluated the growth and function of 21 pairs or *en-bloc* kidneys transplanted into adult recipients (Nghiem *et al.*, 1995). The investigators reported that *en-bloc* kidneys grew at a statistically significant rate ($P<0.001$) as determined by diethylenetriaminepentaacetic acid, glomerular filtration rate (GFR) and kidney volumes. The resistive indices remained at normal range (0.60–0.63), and recipients' blood pressure was normal at greater than 6 months' follow-up.

Gourlay and associates reported their experience of transplanting 83 adults with pediatric cadaver donors aged 5 months to 10 years; 100 adults who received adult cadaver kidneys acted as controls (Gourlay *et al.*, 1995). Actual patient and graft survival rates at 1 and 3 years were 91% and 77% (1 year) and 86% and 68% (3 years) for recipients of pediatric kidneys compared with 97% and 92% (1 year) and 90% and 80% (3 years) for recipients of adult kidneys. Serum creatinine level was equal in the two groups at 1-year follow-up ($P=0.63$). As noted previously, living related donor grafts from adult donors have an excellent survival rate when transplanted into recipients less than 2 years old.

MENTAL AND NEUROLOGICAL STATUS

The infant with significant developmental delay and the child with severe mental retardation who present with progressive renal insufficiency or ESRD pose difficult problems for the health care team. The major issues raised include the following: Would preemptive introduction of ESRD care prevent or reverse the degree of intellectual impairment associated with uremia? Should the life of a child with severe mental retardation be prolonged by the extraordinary therapeutic modalities involved in ESRD care? To what extent would the rigors of the treatment regimen adversely influence the consciousness of the retarded child?

Although the adverse impact of uremia on the functioning of the nervous system has been appreciated in the past, it is only more recently that the magnitude of the problem has been noted in children. Baluarte and coworkers described a distinct syndrome in six children, aged 26 months old to 10 years old, with congenital renal disorders that was characterized by myoclonus, dysarthria, seizures, dementia and coma (Baluarte *et al.*, 1977). The syndrome was evident when there was significant renal functional impairment (5–10 ml/min/ 1.73 m²) and was unremitting, despite dialysis and successful transplantation. Bale and colleagues noted similar neurological abnormalities of seizures and intellectual impairment in three children with congenital renal abnormalities (Bale *et al.*, 1980). The findings were observed initially when the GFR was 15 to 25 ml/min/1.73 m². Aluminum intoxication was implicated by Baluarte *et al.* (1977); however, the cerebrospinal fluid aluminum concentration was measured in one child by Bale *et al.* (1980) and found to be normal.

The magnitude of the problem was emphasized by the report of Rotundo *et al.* (1982), who undertook a retrospective analysis of 23 children with chronic renal failure diagnosed before 1 year of age. Of the 23 children, 20 had progressive encephalopathy characterized by developmental delay (19), microcephaly (15), hypotonia (13), seizures (13) and dyskinesia (11). A specific cause was not identified; however, four patients developed central nervous system symptoms before receiving any oral aluminum therapy, and all patients had symptoms before initiation of dialysis. All of the patients reported by Rotundo *et al.* (1982) had associated significant growth impairment, and 15 of the 20 patients with progressive encephalopathy had progressive reduction in head size.

The relationship between the onset of chronic renal failure during the first year of life and subsequent developmental delay was emphasized by the report of McGraw and Haka-Ikse (1985), who studied 12 boys with onset of chronic renal failure at less than 1 month old. Developmental testing at 13 to 54 months old in 10 of the 12 patients revealed the following: normal in 2 of 10 (20%), developmental quotient (DQ) 60 to 80 in 3 of 10 (30%), DQ 40 to 60 in 4 of 10 (40%) and DQ less than 40 in 1 of 10 (10%). Serial head circumference measurements were less than 2 standard deviations (SD) below the mean in 9 of 12 patients, and 9 of 12 patients had a history of seizures. Linear growth retardation was present in eight (67%) patients. A progressive neurological disorder occurred in one patient that did not remit after successful transplantation.

These reports implicate the adverse impact of uremia on the developing brain because all patients had evidence of renal functional impairment during the first year of life. An additional etiological possibility is the toxic effect of aluminum on the developing brain. All of the patients described in the report of McGraw and Haka-Ikse (1985) had received aluminum-containing phosphate binders; 4 of the 20 patients reported by Rotundo et al. (1982) had not received aluminum-containing compounds.

The report by Freundlich et al. (1985) described elevated aluminum levels in the brain of two infants with chronic renal failure who died in the first year of life without receiving aluminum-containing phosphate binders and implicated the infants' formula as the source of the high aluminum levels in the brain. The latter could implicate aluminum toxicity in the cause of the neurological manifestations in infants with chronic renal failure who did not receive aluminum-containing phosphate binders. Although an unequivocal relationship between neurological impairment and aluminum toxicity does not exist, it would be prudent to avoid aluminum-containing compounds in infants with chronic renal failure and use calcium carbonate as the primary phosphate-binding agent (Salusky et al., 1986). Bale et al. (1980) and Rotundo et al. (1982) suggested that earlier initiation of dialysis and/or transplantation should be considered in infants with congenital renal abnormalities to avoid these neurological sequelae.

A follow-up report to that of McGraw and Haka-Ikse (1985) from the same institution (Geary and Haka-Ikse, 1989) was considerably less pessimistic regarding neurological development of infants with chronic renal failure. Thirty-three children with chronic renal failure detected in the first year of life were tested for neurological function on two occasions approximately 2 years apart. Aluminum usage was exceptional, and assiduous attempts were made to optimize caloric intake. Initially, 11 of 33 children had a DQ less than 80; 10 of 11 children were mildly delayed, and 1 child was moderately delayed in development. When last evaluated, 10 of 33 children had a DQ less than 80; 8 of 10 children were mildly delayed, and 2 of 10 children were moderately delayed. The latter two patients had cerebrovascular accidents. This incidence ($\pm 30\%$) was much lower than that previously reported of 60 to 85% (Polinsky et al., 1987).

These workers ascribed the lower incidence of neurological developmental delay in infants with chronic renal failure to (1) a virtual elimination of the use of aluminum-containing phosphate binders; (2) an aggressive approach to optimize nutrition and (3) a postponement of transplantation, provided that growth and development were satisfactory. Neurological development in infants transplanted during the first year of life has been favorable. So and coworkers indicated that seven of nine infants who were transplanted during the first year of life and followed for 4 months to 7.5 years had normal mental development, and five of nine had normal motor development (So et al., 1987). Because decreased head circumference in infants with chronic renal failure was associated with neurodevelopmental delay (Rotundo et al., 1982), Najarian and colleagues evaluated head circumference in eight infant recipients who were transplanted during the first year of life before and after transplantation (Najarian et al., 1992). The SD score (SDS) for head circumference improved from -2.0 ± 0.52 to -0.7 ± 1.5 posttransplant. The SDS was unchanged in one, decreased in one and improved in six of the eight infants after transplantation. Although neurodevelopmental delay is a potential complication of chronic renal failure in infants, the incidence is substantially less than that reported initially, and most importantly improvement is likely to continue after successful renal transplantation.

Polinsky and associates suggested that the effects of severe chronic renal failure, when present from infancy, on neurological development would be answered better by adopting a more uniform approach to the evaluation and reporting of data such as (1) timing of neuological and developmental assessments with regard to the stage of management of renal disease; (2) types of testing performed and (3) rates of head growth, levels of renal function, nutritional status and psychosocial status of the patients before and at the time of testing (Polinsky et al., 1987).

The current approach to the infant with chronic renal failure is careful surveillance of growth and head circumference with the intent to initiate dialysis once growth deviates from the normal curve. Developmental testing in infants is not sufficiently precise to warrant therapeutic intervention on the basis of only deviant test results. It is thought that abnormalities of growth and head circumference are more precise indicators of the adverse effects of uremia. Whether or not the earlier initiation of ESRD care in these infants would prevent the development of the neurological sequelae of uremia remains to be delineated.

There are no definitive answers to the other two philosophical questions. Observation of children with mild-to-moderate degrees of mental retardation has indicated that they do not respond as well to the imposed constraints of ESRD care as children with normal intellectual capacity (Francis et al., 1970). The family of a mentally retarded child should be given a dispassionate assessment of the various therapeutic options. If the family decides against ESRD care, it is imperative that the health care team provide continued psychoemotional and medical support. Abandonment of the child and family after the decision not to embark on ESRD care would lead the family to question the wisdom of their decision.

If the child presents with a history of long-standing chronic renal failure that had its onset in infancy and the child is mentally retarded, it is appropriate to assume that the child's intellectual impairment is not related to a sudden decline in renal function. It is important, however, to detail the premorbid mental capacity of the child with the sudden onset of ESRD who appears to be functioning at a subnormal level. The uremic milieu depresses cognitive function, and the reality of ESRD produces psychological depression. A detailed analysis of the child's intellectual functioning in the premorbid state is vital before counseling the family regarding the potential therapeutic options.

PSYCHOEMOTIONAL STATUS

The major difficulty in caring for a child with ESRD and psychoemotional problems is the inability to ensure compliance with the therapeutic regimen. Korsch et al. (1978) reported a 19% noncompliance rate and Beck et al. (1980) a 43% noncompliance rate with medications after renal transplantation in pediatric recipients. In more than two thirds of the recipients, the graft was lost or permanently damaged. The difficulty in dealing with the psychoemotionally disturbed recipient is emphasized by the detection of repeated noncompliance in 50% of the recipients who were retransplanted after initial graft loss from noncompliance (Negrete et al., 1980) as well as the fact that extensive counseling reduced noncompliance from a 43% to a 19% incidence rate only (Beck et al., 1980). Detailed analysis of the noncompliant patient indicated that adolescence, female sex, family instability (Beck et al., 1980) and low self-esteem on personality testing (Korsch *et al.*, 1978) were predisposing factors. The lack of uniform success after psychotherapeutic intervention in the noncompliant patient (Beck *et al.*, 1980) and the devastating effect on graft function emphasize the impact of this problem.

Identification of the potential noncompliant patient is mandatory for development of innovative approaches to this problem. Surveillance for noncompliant behavior must continue throughout the posttransplant period. Potter and coworkers reported graft loss as a result of noncompliance in recipients with a functioning graft for greater than 10 years (Potter *et al.*, 1986).

During the 9-year period from September 1980 to September 1989, 209 renal transplants were performed in 177 pediatric recipients at the University of California Los Angeles (UCLA) Center for Health Sciences. Of the 177 recipients, 159 had a functioning graft for greater than 1 month and were considered to be at risk for noncompliance. Using the criteria of unexplained graft dysfunction, weight loss, decreased cushingoid appearance and low cyclosporine levels, noncompliance was noted in 52 (33%) recipients. In 33 of 52 recipients, noncompliance was documented by the patient admitting such behavior, and in 16 recipients it was suspected but not confirmed (Korsch *et al.*, 1993).

Meyers and coworkers reported noncompliance in 12 of 56 children and adolescents after renal transplantation (Meyers *et al.*, 1996). They identified the following risk factors: adolescent age group, female sex, difficulty in reaching the center, lower socioeconomic status, lack of social support, family instability, inappropriate health beliefs, past noncompliance, complexity of prescribed medication and time after initial graft survival. The authors suggested that compliance may be improved by providing information on an ongoing basis to comply with medication, by paying attention to medication and by increasing the frequency of clinic visits.

The 1998 NAPRTCS data attribute less than 2% of graft failures to noncompliance. Intermittent and permanent discontinuation of immunosuppressive medications may contribute to the incidence of chronic rejection as the primary cause of graft failure.

PREEXISTING MALIGNANCY

Wilms' tumor is the principal malignancy requiring ESRD care in pediatric patients (see also Chapter 35). Penn (1979) reviewed the course of renal transplantation in 20 patients—80% of whom had bilateral involvement. Recurrences of the tumors or metastases occurred in 47% of children who received a graft within 1 year after primary treatment of the tumor. No recurrence or metastasis was evident if transplantation was delayed for greater than 1 year after initial treatment. Patient survival at 2 years posttransplantation was 75% with unilateral involvement and 38% with bilateral involvement. Death was attributable primarily to overwhelming sepsis. Previous chemotherapy and irradiation have been causally related to the incidence of sepsis (DeMaria *et al.*, 1979). Transplantation in children with Wilms' tumor should be deferred for at least 1 year after primary treatment of the tumor to detect persistence of the malignancy and to avoid the risk of overwhelming sepsis after transplantation that may be related to the tumoricidal immunosuppression.

Pais and coworkers reviewed 26 previously reported cases of ESRD secondary to Wilms' tumor who were transplanted and added three additional cases from their experience (Pais *et al.*, 1992). Of the 29 cases, only 4 were transplanted since 1980. The actuarial patient survival for the 29 cases at 2 years was 45%. These workers reemphasized the virtue of waiting

at least 1 year for completion of treatment for the tumor before proceeding with transplantation. For 14 patients in whom the delay was less than 1 year, the recurrence rate and mortality rate were 62% and 79% compared with 13% and 27% in the 15 patients in whom the delay exceeded 1 year.

The incidence of Wilms' tumor as the primary renal disease in children undergoing transplantation undoubtedly is understated from the 29 cases reported in the literature. The 1998 report of the NAPRTCS indicated that in 5,516 recipients transplanted in North America during a 10-year period the primary renal disease was Wilms' tumor in 32 cases (NAPRTCS, 1998).

Because two of the three patients reported by Pais and coworkers had lung metastasis before transplantation, these investigators were interested in the impact of pretransplant metastasis on the posttransplant course (Pais *et al.*, 1992). All four patients who had pretransplant abdominal metastasis died of active metastatic disease, whereas two of three patients with lung metastasis were alive and well. Lung metastasis probably should not be a contraindication to proceeding with renal transplantation, provided that the metastatic disease has been treated and the patient is free of identifiable metastatic disease for at least 1 year after treatment.

Few children with primary nonrenal malignancies have undergone renal transplantation. Fine *et al.* (1977a) transplanted two children (with rhabdomyosarcoma and neuroblastoma), Makker and Kirson (1980) transplanted one child (Burkitt's lymphoma), Brouhard *et al.* (1988) transplanted one child (hepatoblastoma) and Gruber *et al.* (1991) transplanted one child (unidentified cancer) with primary nonrenal pretransplant malignancies. At the time of the reports, the primary malignancy had not recurred. The outcome of the patient reported by Gruber *et al.* (1991) was not provided. The presence of a primary nonrenal malignancy is not a contraindication to renal transplantation in children.

BLADDER ADEQUACY

The presence of an abnormal lower urinary tract is not a contraindication to transplantation (see also Chapter 12). Warshaw and colleagues described the results of transplantation in 52 children whose primary disease was obstructive uropathy (Warshaw *et al.*, 1980). Corrective procedures alone were performed in 16, urinary diversion alone was performed in 10 and a combination of corrective and diversionary procedures was performed in 26 patients before the development of ESRD. Of the 52 patients with abnormal lower urinary tracts, Warshaw and colleagues used the bladder without significant complications in 45 recipients, 39 of whom had prior corrective lower urinary tract surgery or bladder defunctionalization (Warshaw *et al.*, 1980). Firlet (1976) described a previously defunctionalized bladder in five children with excellent results, and Butt *et al.* (1976) noted satisfactory bladder function after transplantation in two children with posterior urethral valves and previously defunctionalized bladder.

Children with chronic renal failure who have had previous diversionary procedures can benefit from undiversion once it is established that no further salutary effect on renal function can be gained by the urinary diversion. Gonzalez and associates described the outcome of undiversion in 13 children aged 5 months old to 16 years old (Gonzalez *et al.*, 1984). No accelerated deterioration of renal function was noted over a mean follow-up period of 25 months. Nine of the 13 children subsequently underwent transplantation. Ten children had positive urine cultures before undiversion. All nine children who required transplantation maintained sterile urine from the time of undiversion until transplantation, and three of the four who did not require transplantation maintained sterile urine. Minor complications requiring reoperation occurred in three patients. These workers advocate undiversion before transplantation as a method to increase the bladder capacity of a previously defunctionalized bladder and to eradicate infection before transplantation. Assiduous attempts should be made to use a previously defunctionalized bladder at the time of transplantation.

If the bladder is not usable, an ileal conduit or nonrefluxing colon can be used. An ileal loop was employed in seven recipients by Warshaw et al. (1980). Firlet and Merkel (1977) described an ileal conduit in five pediatric recipients. All conduits functioned without evidence of ureteroileal obstruction, significant infection or stomal stenosis. An alternative to an ileal conduit in recipients with unusable bladders was described by Levitt et al. (1979). The graft ureter was anastomosed to an existing cutaneous ureterostomy in two recipients with good results. If the recipient has a neurogenic bladder, posttransplant clean intermittent catheterization can be offered in lieu of a diversionary procedure. Despite an initial hesitancy to employ this approach because of the fear of infection, it may prove to be eminently satisfactory.

An increased incidence of posttransplant urological complications and urinary tract infections was noted by Warshaw et al. (1980) in recipients with abnormal bladders. Graft function was not adversely affected, however. Similarly, Kreiger et al. (1980) reported an identical success rate in pediatric patients with normal lower urinary tracts. No increased incidence of urinary tract infections after transplantation in the patients with abnormal bladders was observed by Kreiger et al. (1980). Analyses by Hatch (1994), Fontaine et al. (1998) and Koo et al. (1999) have noted long-term (5–10 years) graft survival rates of 73 to 81% in pediatric recipients with dysfunctional bladders.

Currently the options identified in the aforementioned reports for patients with ESRD and a dysfunctional bladder are as follows: (1) use of the native bladder with frequent emptying; (2) intermittent catheterization of the native bladder; (3) augmented cystoplasty with ileum, colon or stomach and subsequent intermittent catheterization or spontaneous voiding; (4) incontinent conduit with ileum or sigmoid colon and (5) continent diversion with a Mitrofanoff stoma via the ureter or appendix. Complications of these procedures include frequent urinary tract infections (>80%); hyperchloremic acidosis and hematuria-dysuria syndrome, especially if the stomach is used.

POTENTIAL FOR RECURRENCE OF PRIMARY RENAL DISEASE

Potential involvement of the graft with a similar pathological process that affected the recipient's native kidneys is an important consideration when evaluating a child for renal transplantation—perhaps of greater importance than in the adult. In adults, recurrent disease accounts for less than 2% of all graft failure (Mathew, 1988), whereas in children it may account for 5 to 15% of graft loss (Broyer et al., 1992b; McEnery et al., 1992). Three main categories of disease affecting the native kidneys can involve the graft: primary glomerulonephritis, generalized systemic diseases that secondarily involve the kidney and inherited metabolic disease with deposition of abnormal metabolites in the kidney.

Specific confirmation of recurrent glomerulonephritis often is difficult. First, a specific histological diagnosis of the recipient's primary renal disease frequently is not available. If a renal biopsy specimen was not obtained early in the course of the recipient's evolving renal disease, it may be impossible subsequently to delineate a specific pathological

entity. At the time ESRD develops, there is frequently significant distortion of the glomerular architecture to obviate the possibility of discerning specific histological characteristics.

Second, immunological damage of the graft glomeruli can mimic various primary glomerular diseases (Porter et al., 1967). Transplant glomerular disease (Hsui et al., 1980) or graft glomerulonephropathy (Olsen et al., 1974) is associated with glomerular lesions that are similar to lesions seen in patients with FGS and/or mesangiocapillary glomerulonephritis (Cameron, 1982). Such transplant glomerulopathy, also called *rejection glomerulopathy*, is believed to be the consequence of chronic vascular rejection (Ramos, 1991).

Finally, de novo glomerulonephritis can develop in the graft. Membranous glomerulonephritis is the primary *de novo* disease that has been reported to occur in grafts. There are at least 95 documented cases of *de novo* membranous glomerulonephritis (Truong et al., 1989). Its incidence has been reported to range from approximately 2 to 10% (Couchoud et al., 1995; Montagnino et al., 1989; Nast and Cohen, 1992; Truong et al., 1989). A cooperative study in France reported 19 cases of *de novo* membranous glomerulonephritis in 1,000 graft biopsies (Charpentier et al., 1982). There may be a higher incidence in children. Antignac and colleagues found that 9% of routine transplant biopsies in children showed features of membranous glomerulonephritis (Antignac et al., 1988).

Many investigators have presented comprehensive reviews of the literature regarding recurrent glomerulonephritis in renal transplant recipients (Cameron, 1982, 1991; Cameron and Turner, 1977; Charpentier et al., 1999; Mathew, 1988, 1991; Ramos, 1991). Despite a relatively high incidence of histological recurrence of the glomerular lesion, the frequency of graft loss attributable to recurrence is low (10%).

Focal glomerulosclerosis is the commonest specific primary glomerular disease resulting in ESRD in children. It accounts for 12% of ESRD in North American children undergoing renal transplantation (NAPRTCS, 1998) and remains the recurrent disease of greatest concern in pediatric renal transplantation. Focal glomerulosclerosis recurs in approximately 30% of cases and leads to graft loss in one half to two thirds of those afflicted (Table 37–6). There are moderate differences from study to study, however. Leumann and colleagues surveyed 17 European centers and accumulated data on 27 children with FGS who received renal grafts (Leumann et al., 1980). Recurrence was documented in 10 (37%) with resultant graft loss in 5 (18.5%). Many single-center reports from pediatric facilities detail the course of patients whose

TABLE 37–6

RECURRENCE RATES AND GRAFT LOSS FROM RECURRENT DISEASE IN CHILDREN

Disease	Recurrence Rate (%)	Clinical Severity	Recipients with Recurrence Whose Graft Failed (%)
FGS	25–30	High	40–50
MPGN type I	70	Mild	12–30
MPGN type II	100	Low	10–20
SLE	5–40	Low	5
HSP	55–85	Low–mild	5–20
HUS			
Classical	12–20	Moderate	0–10
Atypical	±25	High	40–50

FGS = focal glomerulosclerosis; HSP = Henoch-Schönlein purpura; HUS = hemolytic-uremic syndrome; MPGN = membranoproliferative glomerulonephritis; SLE = systemic lupus erythematosus.

primary disease was FGS after renal transplantation. Malek-zadeh *et al.* (1979) noted a recurrence rate of 5.6% (1 of 18); Currier *et al.* (1979), a recurrence rate of 17% (2 of 12) and Striegel *et al.* (1986), a recurrence rate of 50% (12 of 24).

In a series of reports from the Hôpital des Enfants Ma-lades, the recurrence rate remained consistent over time. Habib *et al.* (1982) observed a recurrence rate of 33% (8 of 24); Broyer *et al.* (1987a), a rate of 33% (14 of 43) and Gagna-doux *et al.* (1999), a rate of 34% of all grafts (106 grafts in 101 patients with FGS). Other studies show the same general recurrence rate with moderate variation. Ingulli and Tejani (1991) observed a recurrence rate of 14% in 42 pediatric transplants, whereas Senggutuvan *et al.* (1990) noted a rate of 22% in 13 of 59 allografts. A large multicenter study conducted under the auspices of the NAPRTCS showed biopsy-proven recurrence of 20.5% in 27 of 132 North Ameri-can children whose original disease was FGS (Tejani and Stablein, 1992). In this study, the 95% confidence interval was 14 to 27%.

The reasons for the variations in the incidence of recur-rence are still unknown, but it is likely that the differences in patient demographics and the criteria used to document recurrence can account for some of the variation. Three fac-tors have been implicated as being highly predictive of recur-rence: (1) duration of original disease, (2) presence of mesan-gial proliferation in the native kidney and (3) age of the patient at the onset of the original disease.

Leumann *et al.* (1980) noted that the duration of the origi-nal disease was less than 3 years in 9 of 10 patients with recurrence, and Striegel *et al.* (1986) reported that the dura-tion of the original disease was less than 36 months in 9 of 11 patients with recurrence, whereas only 3 of 13 patients whose original disease had a duration of greater than 36 months had recurrence. Broyer and colleagues noted that the mean duration of the original disease was much shorter in the 14 recipients who developed recurrence (2.1 *vs.* 5.5 years) (Broyer *et al.*, 1987a). In their updated report, this group found that 53% of patients developed recurrence when the time to ESRD was less than 4 years, but only 25% developed recurrence when there was a longer course (Gagnadoux *et al.*, 1993). The NAPRTCS multicenter study found that the only significant risk factor was the time from the diagnosis of FGS to ESRD. The mean (52 months) and median (38 months) for patients without recurrence were significantly longer than the mean (38 months) and median (28 months) for patients with recurrence ($P<0.05$) (Tejani and Stablein, 1992). These data tend to confirm the impression that chil-dren with a more *explosive* form of FGS have an increased risk of recurrence (Tejani and Stablein, 1992). A review by Charpentier *et al.* (1999) emphasizes further the risk factors for recurrence of FGS for patients less than 15 years old, initial malignant course and presence of mesangial prolifera-tion (Charpentier *et al.*, 1999).

Maizel and coworkers related recurrence to the presence of mesangial proliferation in addition to FGS (Maizel *et al.*, 1981). A 50% incidence of recurrence was noted with the presence of mesangial proliferation in the native kidney. Sim-ilarly, Habib and associates reported that 5 of 8 recipients with recurrence had mesangial proliferation, whereas only 3 of 15 recipients without recurrence showed this lesion in the native kidneys (Habib *et al.*, 1982). The report of Striegel *et al.* (1986), which included some of the patients reported by Maizel *et al.* (1981), confirmed the importance of mesangial proliferation as a predictive factor. Only 2 of 10 (20%) patients with pure FGS had recurrence, whereas 5 of 8 (63%) patients with FGS and focal mesangial proliferation and 5 of 6 (83%) with FGS and diffuse mesangial proliferation developed re-currence.

In their updated series, Gagnadoux and colleagues from the Hôpital des Enfants Malades found a 70% recurrence rate when the biopsy specimen showed diffuse mesangial proliferation versus 41% when this was absent (Gagnadoux *et al.*, 1993). Other studies have attached less significance to this finding. In their large multicenter study, for example, Tejani and Stablein (1992) found that among patients with no mesangial proliferation, 20% developed recurrence, whereas only 25% with mesangial proliferation developed recurrence. Senggutuvan and coworkers found that mesangial prolifera-tion and the rapidity of disease progression to ESRD were only moderately predictive of recurrence and relatively un-helpful in specific instances (Senggutuvan *et al.*, 1990).

The age at onset of the original disease appears to be an important consideration in many studies. Recurrence of FGS is primarily, but not solely, a pediatric problem. In the study of Senggutuvan *et al.* (1990), 50% of children experienced recurrence, but only 11% of adolescents and adults experi-enced recurrence. Children less than 6 years old appeared to be at increased risk. Similarly, studies from New York (Ingulli and Tejani, 1991) and Milan (Banfi *et al.*, 1990) suggest that young children are at greatest risk for recurrence. Paradoxi-cally, young age at onset was not of predictive value in the French study (Gagnadoux *et al.*, 1993) or the multicenter NAPRTCS study (Tejani and Stablein, 1992). In the French experience, the highest rate of recurrence (52%) was observed in children greater than 6 years old. A consideration of all these data would suggest that only when two or more of the predictive factors (mesangial proliferation, rapidity of progression to ESRD and young age at onset) are present can recurrence be predicted with any confidence.

Another factor that has been suggested to influence recur-rence of FGS is the degree of histocompatibility between donor and recipient. Zimmerman (1980) noted a higher recur-rence rate in recipients of a living related donor compared with cadaver donor grafts (65% *vs.* 35%) and a recurrence rate in 11 HLA-identical sibling grafts of 82%. In the report of Malekzadeh *et al.* (1979), the one instance of recurrence was in a parental graft, and in the report of Striegel *et al.* (1986), 7 of 12 initial grafts affected by recurrence were from a living related donor. All four retransplant recipients in the latter report who developed recurrences had cadaver donors.

Later studies suggest that concordance of histocompatibil-ity matching may not be as important as previously thought. The NAPRTCS multicenter study (Tejani and Stablein, 1992) found no significant increase in recurrence in recipients of living related donor transplants when compared with recipi-ents of cadaver donor grafts. Similarly, this study and the study of Senggutuvan *et al.* (1990) found no association be-tween HLA matching and recurrence. From these data, it would appear appropriate not to decree the use of living related donor kidneys in children with ESRD resulting from FGS. Kidneys from living related donors represent an ever-increasing percentage of organs for children (McEnery *et al.*, 1992). In children with ESRD resulting from FGS, the 2-year graft survival of living related donor transplants is 10% better than that of cadaver donor transplants (Tejani and Stablein, 1992). Living related donor transplantation appears to be an appropriate consideration, particularly if there is an inordi-nate wait for a cadaver donor organ.

Another consideration in recurrence is the race of the recipient. The NAPRTCS multicenter study (Tejani and Sta-blein, 1992) found that black American children had only a 9% recurrence rate, whereas white children had a 23% recur-rence rate, and Latinos had a 26% recurrence rate. These findings could help explain the low incidence of recurrence in the study of Ingulli and Tejani (1991) because their patient population had a high proportion of black American children.

After one graft loss from recurrence, the risk of recurrence in a subsequent graft is approximately 85% (Cameron, 1991); however, recurrence is not inevitable. Stephanian and associates found that the best predictor of recurrent FGS in subsequent transplants was the fate of the primary allograft (Stephanian *et al.*, 1992). Patients with rapid recurrence and progression of the primary allograft had a high likelihood of recurrence and graft loss in subsequent transplants. Patients who had FGS recurrence but long-term function with a first transplant tended to be free of recurrence or to have prolonged function with recurrence in subsequent transplants.

Recurrence of FGS in subsequent grafts (Malekzadeh *et al.*, 1979; Pinto *et al.*, 1981; Streigel *et al.*, 1986) has implicated the presence of a circulating factor or factors as being responsible for the primary disease in patients who manifest recurrence. Numerous circulating factors have been identified as being important in the pathogenesis of minimal change nephrotic syndrome or FGS (Savin *et al.*, 1996). Some are thought to be elaborated by or in some other manner related to aberrant cellular immunological activity. Of particular interest is the finding of Savin *et al.* (1996) that *in vitro* incubation of isolated glomeruli with the sera of some patients with FGS results in a marked increase in protein permeability. The sera of patients with recurrent FGS frequently show this activity. It appears possible that patients can be identified who are likely to exhibit recurrence. Rational intervention strategies then can be defined.

Graft loss associated with recurrence occurred in five of eight children in the series reported by Habib *et al.* (1982), in the one child reported by Malekzadeh *et al.* (1979) and in 14 of 16 grafts (four retransplants) in the series reported by Striegel *et al.* (1986). The NAPRTCS multicenter study found that 10 (37%) of 27 children with recurrence experience graft failure directly attributable to recurrent FGS (Tejani and Stablein, 1992). Despite the morbidity attendant to recurrence and the potential for graft loss, the varying incidence of recurrence and the inability to predict unequivocally and prospectively which patients will manifest recurrence dictate that children with FGS should not be excluded as transplant candidates. If recurrence develops in an initial graft, however, caution is advised when considering retransplantation. Two of the 12 patients with recurrence reported by Streigel *et al.* (1986) and 2 of the 14 patients reported by Broyer *et al.* (1987b) had clinical remission spontaneously or with immunosuppressive treatment and long-term graft function.

Other series have described some cases of spontaneous remission, although these appear to be the exception rather than the rule (Franco *et al.*, 1987; Stephanian *et al.*, 1992). One should be cautious in predicting the outcome of recurrence of the nephrotic syndrome after transplantation. Recurrence of the nephrotic syndrome has not yet been reported in the familial steroid-resistant nephrotic syndrome or in the Drash syndrome (diffuse mesangial sclerosis) (Gagnadoux *et al.*, 1993). Children with congenital nephrotic syndrome generally do not develop posttransplant recurrence (Hoyer *et al.*, 1973); some reports suggest recurrence may occur, albeit infrequently (Flynn *et al.*, 1992; Lane *et al.*, 1991).

Currently, there is no definitive method to treat and reverse recurrent FGS. There had been initial hope that cyclosporine treatment for immunosuppression would help ameliorate the recurrence. As a general rule, however, cyclosporine in the usual doses has not substantially prevented recurrent disease in pediatric renal transplantation (Banfi *et al.*, 1990; Cameron, 1991; Vincenti *et al.*, 1989). Similarly, there had been hope that plasma exchange could remove the putative circulating substance causing FGS recurrence, reversing the proteinuria. Our group obtained complete and lasting remission of the nephrotic syndrome with plasmapheresis in two recipients who had FGS in their native kidneys and immediate recurrence of the nephrotic syndrome (Laufer *et al.*, 1988).

Other studies have reported limited numbers of cases wherein transient or complete remission has occurred after plasma exchange (Dantal *et al.*, 1991; Franco *et al.*, 1987; Munoz *et al.*, 1985). Many studies have not found plasmapheresis, by itself, to be of significant long-term value (Cameron, 1990; Dantal *et al.*, 1991; Pinto *et al.*, 1981). Many different approaches and combinations have been studied, with varying degrees of success. Dantal and coworkers have used immunoabsorption of a patient's plasma with a protein A column successfully to control proteinuria in recurrent FGS (Dantal *et al.*, 1990). We have used plasmapheresis in conjunction with high-dose cyclosporine in 11 pediatric recipients with 12 allografts and severe recurrence of the nephrotic syndrome. This treatment combination was successful in achieving long-term complete or partial remission in 10 of the 12 transplants with minimal or no impairment in renal function (Mowry *et al.*, 1993).

In some cases, it may be possible to omit the plasma exchange and use only high-dose cyclosporine to achieve remission of posttransplant FGS recurrence (Ingulli *et al.*, 1990). Cochat and associates employed early plasma exchange and 8 weeks of cyclophosphamide, in addition to the usual posttransplant regimen of cyclosporine and prednisone, in three patients with severe recurrence (Cochat *et al.*, 1993). Two of the three patients achieved a complete remission, whereas the third experienced a late relapse after complete remission. The late relapse was controlled by another course of plasma exchange and cyclophosphamide. One of these patients experienced a significant bacterial infection after the first course of combined treatment.

Other approaches that have been taken, with some degree of success, include plasmapheresis in combination with angiotensin-converting enzyme inhibitors (Artero *et al.*, 1992) and oral meclofenamate, a nonsteroidal antiinflammatory drug that may work by altering glomerular hemodynamics (Torres *et al.*, 1984). Each of these approaches has some limitations in efficacy or in undesired side effects. Controlled trials are necessary to delineate the optimal approach.

Histological evidence of recurrence regularly occurs in patients with membranoproliferative glomerulonephritis (MPGN) type II and, to a lesser extent, in patients with MPGN type I. Pennisi and colleagues reported that two children with MPGN type II had histological recurrence of intramembranous deposits, whereas the grafts of only one of nine recipients with MPGN type I showed subendothelial deposits (Pennisi *et al.*, 1978a). No relationship between histological recurrence and decreased graft function was noted.

Reports from the Hôpital des Enfants Malades (Broyer *et al.*, 1987b; Gagnadoux *et al.*, 1993) noted recurrence of MPGN type I in 10 of 13 (77%) patients who underwent graft biopsy. Three of these patients lost grafts as a result of recurrence. Approximately 30% of patients with recurrence of type I MPGN lose the allografts as a result of the recurrence (Ramos, 1991). One estimate of loss from recurrence in pediatric patients was 12% (Cameron, 1991). Some of the discrepancies in the literature about recurrence rates and graft loss owing to recurrence may be caused by an overestimation of the recurrence of MPGN type I. The histological appearance resembles closely that of transplant glomerulopathy (described earlier).

All nine patients with MPGN type II (dense-deposit disease) as the original disease reported by Gagnadoux *et al.* (1993) manifested histological recurrence of the disease in the graft. Graft loss was attributable to recurrence in two patients. Similarly, all three patients with MPGN type II reported by Najarian et al. (1986) developed recurrence that resulted in graft loss in two patients. The recurrence rate appears to be virtually 100% in children. The incidence of graft loss appears to vary from 10 to 20% of those with recurrence (Gagnadoux et al., 1993; Mathew, 1991). The severity of recurrence and the ultimate failure rate are significantly higher when the original disease is rapidly progressive and the biopsy specimens of the native kidney and the transplant feature epithelial crescents (Cameron, 1991; Eddy et al., 1984). Treatment of allograft failure from recurrent MPGN type II (with crescents) has been generally disappointing (Mathew, 1991); however, Oberkircher and coworkers treated one 5-year-old child successfully with plasmapheresis and high-dose corticosteroids with a successful outcome (Oberkircher et al., 1988).

Of the systemic glomerular diseases, systemic lupus erythematosus and Henoch-Schönlein purpura are the two entities that require consideration in pediatric patients. There have been no reports of recurrence of systemic lupus erythematosus in pediatric recipients, and in our experience with more than 20 patients we have not observed any instance of recurrence. The report of Amend et al. (1981) of recurrence of systemic lupus erythematosus in 2 of 21 adult recipients and that of Moorthy et al. (1986) of recurrence of systemic lupus erythematosus in 1 of 18 adult recipients indicate the potential for such a phenomenon. Nyberg and colleagues performed biopsies in 16 patients with systemic lupus erythematosus 6 months to 11 years after transplant and found that 7 showed histological changes of recurrent systemic lupus erythematosus (Nyberg et al., 1992). Six of these patients showed clinical signs of renal involvement. Renal manifestations improved with increased immunosuppressive therapy, and only one graft was lost to recurrent systemic lupus erythematosus. Most instances of such recurrence are clinically mild, but significant proteinuria and deterioration of graft function occasionally can occur (Ramos, 1991). Augmented immunosuppression therapy may be helpful when clinically significant recurrence supervenes (Fernandez et al., 1990).

An extensive experience with renal transplantation in children with IgA nephropathy and Henoch-Schönlein purpura has been reported by Gagnadoux et al. (1993) and Levy et al. (1982). Deposition of IgA in the mesangium was noted in 5 of 8 patients with IgA nephropathy and 11 of 13 children with Henoch-Schönlein purpura in whom biopsies were performed 1 to 3 years posttransplant. Only one patient in each group had graft loss in these conditions. We have seen no graft loss or clinically significant disease in children with either of these conditions. Similarly, Bunchman and colleagues failed to observe any evidence of recurrence in 14 patients with Henoch-Schönlein purpura who received 20 grafts (6 of the grafts were lost owing to rejection) (Bunchman et al., 1987).

Graft loss secondary to recurrent Henoch-Schönlein purpura has been reported in children (Baliah et al., 1974). At least seven pediatric renal transplant recipients whose original disease was Henoch-Schönlein purpura have had recurrence and subsequent allograft failure (Cameron, 1991). In one series of 17 children whose original disease was Henoch-Schönlein purpura, 5 developed clinical and histological recurrences in their transplants, and 2 of these lost their graft as a result of recurrent disease. An additional four patients had histological recurrences without evidence of clinical involvement. The overall recurrence rate was 75% in recipients of living related donor transplants but 0% in cadaver donor transplant recipients (Hasegawa et al., 1989). The association between recurrent purpura and recurrent graft involvement has led to the recommendation that transplantation should be deferred until active clinical purpura has abated for 6 to 12 months (Cameron, 1982).

Hemolytic-uremic syndrome is the commonest cause of primary acute renal failure in children. In 90% of the cases, the children are less than 5 years old (Herdman and Uriza, 1975). With intensive supportive care, especially the early initiation of dialysis, the mortality rate has decreased considerably. Some children fail to recover adequate renal function after the initial clinical manifestations with resultant ESRD. Some children are left with significant residual renal functional impairment that culminates in ESRD at a later date. End-stage renal disease more commonly follows atypical HUS. This condition is characterized by the lack of a diarrheal prodrome, a relatively frequent but not invariable incidence of hypocomplementemia and often a familial pattern of involvement (Kaplan et al., 1992).

The NAPRTCS registry indicated that 145 children with HUS received kidney transplants in the years 1987–1992, or 3% of the total number of children receiving transplants in North America (see Table 37–1). Assessing the true significance of recurrent HUS is difficult because the histological and the hematological features can appear in severe vascular rejection and because cyclosporine and perhaps antilymphocyte globulin (ALG) occasionally can produce a similar picture.

Hebert and coworkers, employing rigid criteria, observed recurrent HUS in 50% of patients (Hebert et al., 1986). Because of the potential for recurrence, these workers suggested that ALG and cyclosporine be avoided. Cyclosporine may be especially problematic because of its effect on vascular prostacyclin and thromboxane balance, predisposing the patient to graft thrombosis. This effect had led some groups to avoid cyclosporine and others to use it only in low doses. At UCLA, we have deferred transplantation until all clinical manifestations have abated completely and have used cyclosporine in doses somewhat reduced from those of our usual protocols. The patients treated in this way have well-functioning grafts, although there is some biopsy evidence of mild cyclosporine-associated glomerulopathy in the form of thrombosis.

Bassani and associates, in a study of 18 children with classic endemic HUS who received kidney transplants, found that none fulfilled the criteria required for the diagnosis of recurrence in the allograft and that only 3 had a suggestion of recurrence with less rigorous criteria (Bassani et al., 1991). Cyclosporine therapy proved to be the pivotal factor in optimizing graft outcome. These investigators concluded that the results of renal transplantation in patients with classic diarrhea-associated HUS were as good as in patients with other types of renal disease and that there was no contraindication to cyclosporine or living donor transplantation.

Eijgenraam and associates found recurrence of HUS in only 2 of 24 allografts (Eijgenraam et al., 1990). The overall graft outcome of children whose original disease was HUS did not differ from that of children whose ESRD was caused by other conditions. The only factor that appeared to affect graft outcome adversely was a short interval between the onset of the syndrome and the subsequent first renal transplantation. In analyzing these studies, it is important to distinguish between children who had classic HUS (i.e., with a diarrheal prodrome) and children who had an atypical form. Recurrences are seen predominantly in children with atypical HUS; patients with autosomal recessive or dominant inherited HUS are at particularly great risk for posttransplant recurrence (Kaplan, 1992). It is important to characterize the original episode of the syndrome before deciding on the appropriateness of a living related donor (Kaplan, 1992).

The two metabolic diseases resulting in ESRD in children that require consideration are cystinosis and oxalosis. Mahoney and colleagues described the results of renal transplantation in four cystinotic children with grafts from parental donors (Mahoney et al., 1970). No recurrence of Fanconi's syndrome was noted 32 months posttransplant. Serial graft biopsy findings revealed cystine accumulation in the interstitium and occasionally in the mesangium but not in the tubular or glomerular epithelial cells as occurs in the native cystinotic kidney. Similar findings were noted by Malekzadeh and coworkers in six children with cystinosis who received cadaver donor grafts (Malekzadeh et al., 1977). The cystine content of white blood cells and cultured skin fibroblasts remained elevated after transplantation, despite adequate graft function.

Data accumulated by the EDTA Pediatric Registry (Broyer et al., 1981a) on 47 children with cystinosis who were transplanted revealed improved 1-year patient and graft survival rates (89% and 82% vs. 81% and 67%) when compared with rates of children with other primary renal diseases. Similar improvement in graft survival rates was noted at a single pediatric center by Broyer and colleagues, who related the phenomenon to reduced activity of cystinotic immunocompetent cells (Broyer et al., 1981b).

In general, the extrarenal manifestations of cystinosis persist after transplantation. The ocular involvement varies with occasional improvement in visual acuity. Persistent impairment or further deterioration resulting in blindness (Broyer et al., 1981a, 1981b) occurred in 3 of 17 cystinotic patients who had a functioning graft for 11 years (Broyer et al., 1987b).

Corneal transplantation is sometimes necessary (Almond et al., 1993). Photophobia was noted to resolve almost completely in three patients by Langlois et al. (1981) and one patient by Mahoney et al. (1970) after transplantation. In our experience, the degree of photophobia has remained unchanged or worsened. Although hypothyroidism did not develop in any of nine children after transplantation reported by Langlois et al. (1981), we noted it in one child 6 years posttransplant. Broyer and colleagues indicated that half of their cystinotic patients with functioning grafts required supplemental thyroid treatment (Broyer et al., 1987b).

Almond and coworkers noted that four of seven children developed posttransplant hypothyroidism requiring replacement (Almond et al., 1993). Children who are hypothyroid before transplantation require continued thyroid supplementation posttransplant. A particularly ominous complication is neurological impairment. Almond and coworkers described one patient who developed polyneuropathy (Almond et al., 1993). We observed two patients with neurological involvement. One had symptoms of progressive multifocal leukoencephalopathy and died as a result of this condition. Most patients with cystinosis appear to have some neurological deficits, primarily motor incoordination and hypotonia. Progressive neurological involvement may occur in young adults (Trauner et al., 1988).

Most cystinotic children are severely growth retarded before transplantation, and although growth occurs after transplantation, their ultimate adult height is stunted severely (Malekzadeh et al., 1977). Broyer and coworkers indicated that the final adult height of their cystinotic patients with a functioning graft was 130 to 135 cm for girls and 140 to 145 cm for boys (Broyer et al., 1987b). Pubertal development has occurred in cystinotic children after transplantation (Broyer et al., 1981a, 1981b; Malekzadeh et al., 1977).

Trials are ongoing to attempt to deplete the intracellular cystine concentration and deter the progression to ESRD

(Gahl et al., 1986a). Markello and associates found that with early (<2 years) and adequate cysteamine treatment, renal failure may be deferred until late adulthood (Markello et al., 1993). Untreated children or children in whom therapy was begun late were likely to require ESRD therapy by the end of the first decade of life. Despite the inability of successful transplantation to correct the primary metabolic defect, transplantation appears to be the preferred management once ESRD has occurred.

A survey (Gahl et al., 1986b) of 43 medical centers in the United States detailed the clinical findings of 80 cystinotic patients greater than 10 years old to identify the long-term extrarenal consequences of cystinosis. Of these 80 patients, 72 had received a renal graft, and the oldest graft recipient was 26 years old. A high percentage of patients had persistent extrarenal manifestations: requirement of thyroid replacement therapy (75%), splenomegaly (27%), hepatomegaly (42%), photophobia (86%), decreased visual acuity (32%) and corneal ulcerations (15%). In addition, 5 patients developed insulin-dependent diabetes mellitus posttransplant, and 13 patients had various neurological abnormalities, ranging from mild weakness to substantial impairment of speech, swallowing and walking. Based on the results of the survey, these investigators suggested that consideration be given to cystine-depleting agents after kidney transplantation in an attempt to prevent progression of the nonrenal complications of cystinosis.

According to an analysis of the EDTA Pediatric Registry (Broyer et al., 1992b), there were 36 first renal allografts in pediatric patients with primary hyperoxaluria or oxalosis since 1971. In the NAPRTCS database (see Table 37–1), 16 patients (1%) with oxalosis received kidneys in the period 1987–1992. Results from the EDTA Pediatric Registry cited a 3-year graft survival of 23% for patients receiving a living donor transplant and 18% for patients receiving a cadaver donor graft; 40% of the recipients had died (Broyer et al., 1990).

Patients with oxalosis have been regarded as *untransplantable* because of recurrence with oxalate deposition in the graft. In 1984, Scheinman et al. reported improved results in six children with oxalosis. They minimized oxalate deposition in the graft using peritransplant dialysis to lower oxalate levels aggressively. Living related donor grafts were preferred to ensure immediate graft function with a brisk diuresis. These and other anecdotal reports (Leumann et al., 1978; Whelchel et al., 1983) stressed the posttransplant use of pyridoxine, magnesium, orthophosphate supplementation and noncalciuric thiazide diuretics. A study from the University of Minnesota reported nine grafts (seven living related donors) in seven children, with three deaths and only four grafts surviving for more than 2.5 years (Katz et al., 1989). Despite the potential for some long-term graft success in children with oxalosis, the chances of recurrence are significant.

Combined (Watts et al., 1985) or staged (McDonald et al., 1989) liver and kidney transplantation offers new potential for improved outcome. The allografted liver can provide the deficient enzyme alanine–glyoxylate aminotransferase to metabolize glyoxalate and to help mobilize tissue oxalate, whereas the well-functioning renal transplant can excrete the mobilized plasma oxalate without resultant nephrocalcinosis (Watts et al., 1991). Perioperative hemodialysis appears necessary to help remove the body burden of oxalate. Although morbidity and mortality from infection, biliary leakage and other causes are still significant, success and full rehabilitation are possible (Watts et al., 1991). To be maximally successful, combined transplantation needs to be pursued early in the evolution of chronic renal failure, with plasma oxalate concentration serving as a valuable guide in assessing the imminence of the oxalotic phase of the illness (Watts *et al.*, 1991).

The optimal management of these children still is not clear. Treatment with renal transplantation alone can be successful even if hepatic alanine–glyoxylate aminotransferase levels remain abnormally low or are located in inappropriate subcellular locations (Katz *et al.*, 1992). Short-term results with combined liver and kidney transplantation (Watts *et al.*, 1991) are roughly comparable to those of kidney transplant alone performed at the University of Minnesota (Katz *et al.*, 1989). One set of recommendations suggests that kidney transplantation should be performed early, before the onset of renal failure, when the body's oxalate burden is relatively low (Watts *et al.*, 1988). Liver transplantation should be reserved for patients with evidence of markedly increased tissue oxalate stores and for patients on dialysis for more than 1 year (Katz *et al.*, 1992). The optimal approach awaits long-term follow-up.

PRIOR METHODS OF DIALYSIS

The renaissance of peritoneal dialysis as a primary method of dialysis for children with ESRD has occurred with the development of the home-based modalities of CAPD and continuous cycling peritoneal dialysis (CCPD). In our experience, more than 90% of all pediatric patients beginning dialysis since 1981 at our institution have been trained for CAPD and/or CCPD. According to the NAPRTCS database, 42% of children received peritoneal dialysis before being transplanted in the period 1987–1992. Another 28% received hemodialysis, and 5% received both methods.

The emergence of CAPD and CCPD raised the following questions regarding transplantation in children using these modalities: (1) Is graft survival affected by the prior dialytic modality? (2) Are there specific posttransplant complications related to the use of CAPD and/or CCPD? (3) Does a prior episode of peritonitis preclude proceeding with transplantation, and if not, what time interval is required after treatment of an episode of peritonitis before proceeding with transplantation? (4) If posttransplant dialysis is required, can peritoneal dialysis be resumed, or is initiation of hemodialysis mandatory? (5) What is the optimal management of the peritoneal catheter after transplantation?

Stefanidis and coworkers showed comparable actuarial graft survival rates in children undergoing CAPD compared with a concurrent group of pediatric graft recipients who had received prior hemodialysis (Stefanidis *et al.*, 1983). No other comparative data are available for pediatric patients. Guillou and associates noted a markedly decreased 1-year cadaver donor graft survival rate (33.5%) in 37 adult CAPD patients compared with a 63.5% survival rate in 79 adult hemodialysis patients (Guillou *et al.*, 1984). These workers related the low graft survival rate in the CAPD patients to improved immunological status as indicated by a higher OKT4/OKT8 ratio in the CAPD patients. Conversely, Evangelista and colleagues noted a 72% 2-year graft survival rate for adult recipients undergoing CAPD compared with a 2-year survival rate of 58% in patients maintained on hemodialysis (Evangelista *et al.*, 1985). In our experience (Leichter *et al.*, 1986b), no adverse effect on graft survival was apparent, although comparative data with other dialytic modalities were not available. Gagnadoux and coworkers noted that the modalities of treatment before transplantation had no influence on graft survival (Gagnadoux *et al.*, 1993).

Posttransplant ascites in pediatric CAPD recipients was noted initially by Watson *et al.* (1984). The incidence apparently varies in different centers. It occurred in only 1 of 44 children in 14 European pediatric centers, whereas 20 of 42 recipients in three North American pediatric centers developed ascites (Scharer and Fine, 1985). In our experience, the incidence of posttransplant ascites was 27% (Leichter *et al.*, 1986b). Malagon and Hogg (1987) described an incidence of 13% (3 of 23 patients). The pathogenesis of posttransplant ascites in CAPD patients is unclear; however, drainage through the *in-situ* peritoneal catheter on one or more occasions usually is curative.

The potential for infectious complications related to using the peritoneum for dialysis or as a result of leaving the peritoneal catheter *in situ* after transplantation has been a major area of concern. In our experience, only 5 patients developed peritonitis after 48 renal transplants (Leichter *et al.*, 1986b). If only the time interval that the catheters were in place after transplantation is used, the incidence was one episode every 37.8 patient months. Similarly the international survey (Scharer and Fine, 1985) noted nine episodes of peritonitis in 6 of 96 patients. No patient death was attributable to peritonitis in either report; however, four of six patients ultimately lost their grafts according to the international survey. Leichter and coworkers indicated that in their series no graft was lost as a result of an infectious complication (Leichter *et al.*, 1986b). In the series of Malagon and Hogg (1987), 3 of 23 patients (13%) developed infections that potentially were related to peritoneal dialysis. None had symptoms of peritonitis, although two had *Staphylococcus epidermidis* septicemia.

The incidence of exit-site (11%) and tunnel (9%) infections after transplantation is low (Leichter *et al.*, 1986b). After antibiotic treatment, the catheters were removed unless further dialysis was required.

No data indicate that prior episodes of peritonitis in pediatric patients adversely affect transplant outcome (Leichter *et al.*, 1986b; Scharer and Fine, 1985). In our experience, a recent episode of peritonitis in a child awaiting a transplant does not preclude the transplant. Potential recipients should be treated appropriately for 10 to 14 days, with negative peritoneal fluid culture findings without antibiotic treatment before transplantation. The perioperative peritoneal cell count should not suggest peritonitis. We have performed transplantation while patients were still receiving antibiotic treatment for peritonitis without adverse consequences. The peritoneal fluid cultures were sterile, and cell counts were in the normal range. The patients had been receiving antibiotics for at least 5 days. This is a significant issue because the incidence of CAPD and/or CCPD is increasing in the pediatric population with ESRD, and the potential to limit access to available cadaver kidneys exists if rigid criteria requiring prolonged infection-free intervals after an episode of peritonitis are used. If there is a chronic exit-site infection present at the time of surgery, the catheter should be removed and appropriate parenteral antibiotic drugs administered. An overt tunnel infection should be treated before transplantation.

Peritoneal dialysis after transplantation, if required, is not associated with any increased complications (Scharer and Fine, 1985; Leichter *et al.*, 1986b; Malagon and Hogg, 1987). Initiation of hemodialysis is not required after transplantation except if the graft is placed intraperitoneally.

HUMAN IMMUNODEFICIENCY VIRUS STATUS

Four reports (Connor *et al.*, 1988; Ingulli *et al.*, 1991; Rousseau *et al.*, 1988; Strauss *et al.*, 1989) have documented the increasing incidence (2.8–9.1%) of renal disease in patients with human immunodeficiency virus (HIV) infection. Of the 33 HIV-positive patients with documented renal disease in the four reports, 14 (42%) developed ESRD. At least three patients (Ingulli *et al.*, 1991) underwent dialysis, and no patient was reported to have undergone transplantation.

The initial report of HIV infection in a pediatric posttransplant patient was by Malekzadeh *et al.* (1987a). An 11-year-old boy developed Kaposi's sarcoma 5 years posttransplantation with a cadaver donor kidney. Subsequently, Tzakis and associates reported the occurrence of HIV infection in 25 recipients of whole-organ grafts, of which 10 were children (Tzakis *et al.*, 1990). Two of the pediatric HIV-positive patients were kidney recipients. Both were alive at the time of the report, although one lost a kidney at 8 months posttransplant and was currently on dialysis. Human immunodeficiency virus infection was present before transplantation in one patient and was acquired perioperatively in the other patient.

In general, the outlook for the pediatric allograft recipient who is HIV positive is better than that of the adult recipient. Of the 15 adult whole-organ recipients, 5 died, whereas only 1 of 10 pediatric recipients died. Additional data are required before a definitive recommendation can be made regarding the advisability of transplanting a pediatric patient who is HIV positive.

Factors Affecting Allograft Survival in Children

HLA MATCHING

During the precyclosporine era, it generally was accepted that optimal matching of HLA antigens improved living related donor and cadaver donor transplant outcome (see also Chapter 10). Although some have questioned the value of HLA matching in the cyclosporine era, multicenter reports, such as those from the Collaborative Transplant Study with 10,000 first cadaver grafts, show statistically and clinically significant matching effects. The Collaborative Transplant Study reported a 17% 1-year graft survival advantage when grafts were matched fully at the HLA-B and HLA-DR loci compared with totally mismatched grafts (88% *vs.* 71%) (Opelz, 1987). To assess long-term graft outcome, HLA matching also has been examined using graft half-life, that is, the period of time it takes for half the allografts in a given group to fail. Numerous studies show that the half-life of well-matched grafts is significantly greater than that of more poorly matched ones (i.e., optimal matching extends long-term graft survival) (Gjerston *et al.*, 1991). Most studies show little difference in half-lives between the match grades intermediate between the best and worst matching.

A strong matching influence is present in retransplantation. The Collaborative Transplant Study showed a 23% 1-year survival advantage for grafts completely matched at the HLA-B and HLA-DR loci compared with those completely mismatched. The Collaborative Transplant Study also showed that matching for HLA-A as well as for HLA-B and HLA-DR was important. Fully matched grafts had a 2-year cumulative survival of 82%, whereas totally mismatched transplants had a 2-year cumulative survival of only 49% (Opelz, 1989).

Further studies extend and modify these conclusions. Analysis of data from the United Network for Organ Sharing (UNOS) suggests that black American transplant recipients derive little or no benefit when HLA-B and HLA-DR antigens are matched, possibly caused, in part, by the difficulty in defining precisely many of the histocompatability antigens in the black American population at that time (Cicciarelli and Cho, 1992). In white recipients, by comparison, there was a highly significant matching effect between best-matched and worst-matched grades. This effect was observed first 3 months after transplant and persisted through 3 years of follow-up. At 3 years, there was a 20% difference in graft survival from best-matched to worst-matched transplants (Cicciarelli and Cho, 1992). When class I or class II HLA antigens are defined more precisely, the correlation between graft outcome and histocompatability matching improves dramatically (Opelz *et al.*, 1991). There may be a stronger effect of matching for class II antigens early in the posttransplant course (Cicciarelli and Cho, 1992). Some suggestion exists of a *threshold matching effect*, whereby the best results are in patients with four or more HLA-A, HLA-B and HLA-DR matches; the poorest results are in the zero, one or two antigen-matched transplants (Cicciarelli and Cho, 1992). Multivariate analysis of UNOS data suggests that, with the exception of donor race, HLA matching has the strongest influence on graft outcome (Cicciarelli and Cho, 1992).

In pediatric cadaver transplantation, the NAPRTCS database suggests that HLA-B and HLA-DR matching confer a small degree of improvement to graft outcome at 3 years (67% *vs.* 62% for HLA-B and HLA-DR matching) (McEnery *et al.*, 1992). Optimal matching appears to be most important for the young recipient. The 1998 NAPRTCS report concluded that no differences were seen in the 1- and 2-year graft survival rates of poorly HLA matched, anti–T cell–induced recipients, whereas HLA matching has been important in the outcome in the non–anti–T cell–induced recipient group ($P<0.04$). The UCLA Transplant Registry reports that for 1- to 5-year-old and 6- to 10-year-old recipients, first cadaver graft survival is 9% higher at 6 months with 0 to 1 HLA-B and HLA-DR mismatched grafts (75% *vs.* 66% in the 1- to 5-year-old recipients; 87% *vs.* 78% in the 6- to 10-year-old recipients) (Yuge and Cecka, 1991). With regard to donor age, HLA-B and HLA-DR matching has a beneficial effect in all donor age groups, but the effect appears to be largest in kidneys from donors 1 to 5 years old (Yuge and Cecka, 1991). When better matched, the youngest donor age category still yields a relatively low 1-year graft survival rate (65%) (Yuge and Cecka, 1991). Prolonged cold ischemia time (i.e., >30 hours) produces an 18% decrease in 1-year graft survival in donors 1 to 5 years old compared with adult donors. It may be counterproductive to share such small kidneys over long distances for the sake of good HLA matching.

The value of HLA matching continues to be debated because of the concern that the advantages of better matching may be outweighed by the disadvantages associated with extra storage time required to transplant organs that are shared over long distances. A report on more than 500 six–HLA antigen-matched cadaveric kidneys shared between distant centers showed that the 2-year survival rate of these organs was 87%. This result was superior to the 76% 2-year graft survival rate observed in a control group that was not well matched but was not transported over long distances. In this report, optimal matching seemed to neutralize the deleterious effect of high levels of anti-HLA antibodies, with a 2-year graft survival rate of 83% in highly presensitized patients. An insufficient number of six-antigen matches were available for analysis in pediatric recipients to corroborate the beneficial effect noted in adult recipients (Takemoto *et al.*, 1991).

The quality of the HLA match has implications for the transplant recipient if the graft subsequently is rejected. Patients rejecting a first renal transplant are more likely to develop high levels of antibodies to HLA antigens subsequently if the kidney had been poorly matched (Sanfilippo *et al.*, 1987). For this reason, patients who received first allografts with better histocompatibility matching spend significantly shorter times on the list awaiting retransplantation.

Most children with ESRD require multiple transplants over their lifetime. It is prudent to optimize HLA matching whenever possible to prolong graft function as well as to maintain the best prospect for future retransplantation. This point is emphasized in Chapter 10.

BLOOD TRANSFUSION

The availability of recombinant human erythropoietin (rHuEpo) and the improved graft survival rates with introduction of newer immunosuppressive agents such as cyclosporine in pediatric recipients have led to a substantial reduction in the therapeutic need for blood transfusion and the elective use of blood transfusion to improve graft survival. The 1998 report of the NAPRTCS indicated that 41% of living related donor and 25% of cadaver donor recipients have had no transfusions before transplantation (NAPRTCS, 1998).

In the precyclosporine era, large studies established that blood transfusions powerfully enhanced renal allograft outcome (Opelz et al., 1973). The mechanism of the transfusion effect is elusive, although many lines of evidence point to an active immunological process down-regulating the response to the allograft. As renal transplant management improved in the 1980s, the transfusion effect became less prominent (Tiwari, 1985), and reports emerged stressing that cyclosporine diminished further the relative contribution of blood transfusion to improvements in graft survival (Kahan et al., 1983). Currently the transfusion effect appears to be absent in all recipients except children less than 15 years old, in whom a small effect is noted (Ahmed and Terasaki, 1992).

The controversy regarding blood transfusion has been complicated by the development and proven efficacy of rHuEPO to minimize or eliminate transfusion requirements (Eschbach et al., 1987). The virtual elimination of transfusion should help eliminate significant anti-HLA sensitization. Early studies suggest that rHuEPO during dialysis does not compromise early graft function (Ettenger et al., 1991a). In the dialysis patient with a high percentage of panel reactive antibody, the elimination of blood transfusion decreases the titer of anti-HLA antibodies and may decrease some aspects of nonspecific cell-mediated immunity (Grimm et al., 1990).

In the precyclosporine era, transfusions from a potential living donor, so-called donor-specific transfusions led to superior results. The disadvantage of donor-specific transfusions is the potential generation of anti-HLA antibodies. Such sensitization occurs in 10 to 30% of patients receiving donor-specific transfusions but can be reduced to less than 10% with concomitant azathioprine administration (Anderson et al., 1984). In haploidentical living related transplantation, there appears to be no significant graft survival differences between donor-specific transfusions with noncyclosporine immunosuppression and no donor-specific transfusions and cyclosporine immunosuppression (Potter et al., 1991).

Donor-specific transfusion in pediatric recipients was described by Potter et al. (1985). These workers report a 93% 5-year actuarial graft survival rate in 37 recipients of a living related donor graft after donor-specific transfusion. Both graft failures were the result of recurrence of FGS in the graft. Sensitization after donor-specific transfusion, resulting in a positive crossmatch and obviating the use of the specific donor-specific transfusion donor, was shown to occur with an incidence of 26%. This incidence subsequently was reduced to 11%, with the concurrent administration of azathioprine at the time of donor-specific transfusion. Ettenger and coworkers (1983) initially noted a high sensitization rate with donor-specific transfusions in children. Later, we found a reduction in the incidence of sensitization to 5% with low-dose stored whole blood or concurrent azathioprine adminis-

tration. Only 1 of 13 recipients subjected to either of the protocols lost a graft as a result of rejection. This finding seems to indicate that these methods do not modify the salutary effects of donor-specific transfusions.

The long-term efficacy of donor-specific transfusions in pediatric recipients was not established by the report of Potter et al. (1985) because 17 of the 35 recipients with a functioning graft were less than 2 years posttransplant, and 8 of the 35 had a serum creatinine level greater than 2.0 mg/dl. Broyer and associates have reported excellent short-term results using donor-specific transfusions in 20 pediatric recipients (Broyer et al., 1987b). The 3-year graft survival rate was 90%.

A less optimistic effect of donor-specific transfusions in pediatric recipients was reported by Chavers et al. (1987). The 24-month graft survival rate in 16 recipients who received donor-specific transfusions with concomitant azathioprine therapy was only 75%, and 2 of the 12 functioning grafts manifested chronic rejection 1 to 1.5 years posttransplant. These investigators noted biopsy-proven acute tubular necrosis in three recipients that occurred in the immediate posttransplant period. Chavers and colleagues urge early biopsy to distinguish acute tubular necrosis from accelerated rejection in pediatric recipients subjected to donor-specific transfusion protocols (Chavers et al., 1987).

Data from the NAPRTCS (1998) indicate that the 4-year graft function rate is superior in recipients of living related donor or cadaver donor grafts who received no or one to five prior pretransplant lifetime transfusions compared with recipients receiving more than five blood transfusions. There is no consensus for abandoning blood transfusions in nontransfused pediatric recipients, however, owing to lack of sufficient data, arising from different observations made in different studies. Purposeful blood transfusion as a prerequisite for transplantation has a limited number of advocates with current immunosuppression.

BILATERAL NEPHRECTOMY AND SPLENECTOMY

Bilateral nephrectomy is not a prerequisite before renal transplantation and should be reserved for specific indications. The adverse effects of the renoprival state on erythropoietin production (Van Ypersele de Strihou and Stragier, 1969) and vitamin D metabolism (Oettinger et al., 1974) as well as the salutary effects of minimal urinary output on the management of the child undergoing dialysis dictate a conservative approach to the performance of a bilateral nephrectomy in ESRD. Renin-dependent hypertension unresponsive to newer antihypertensive medication (e.g., angiotensin II receptor blockers, angiotensin-converting enzyme inhibitors, minoxidil, nifedipine and α-blockers), persistent massive proteinuria in children with the nephrotic syndrome and persistent clinical pyelonephritis are the primary indications for this procedure. Persistent vesicoureteral reflux or hydronephrosis secondary to previous ureterovesical or ureteropelvic junction obstruction are not necessarily indications for kidney removal. Attempts to salvage a minimally functioning kidney should be made in each instance.

Bennett (1976) reported a decreased graft survival rate in nephrectomized patients. The reason for this adverse effect on survival was not apparent. Our experience with pediatric recipients has not shown that bilateral nephrectomy influences graft survival adversely. According to the NAPRTCS database, prior nephrectomy did not affect 3-year graft outcome significantly, but it was associated with higher rates of acute tubular necrosis. This association was true for recipients of living donor (8.4%) and cadaver donor (27%) transplants. If the indications for bilateral nephrectomy are present, especially uncontrollable hypertension and persistent massive proteinuria, an alternative to surgical removal is percutaneous transluminal embolization (Thompson *et al.*, 1983).

In the past, splenectomy was advocated as a procedure before transplantation for adjunctive immunosuppression. The reports of overwhelming sepsis in splenectomized pediatric recipients (Cerilli and Jones, 1977; McEnery and Flanagan, 1977) indicated that the procedure should be undertaken with caution in children. The long-term potential adverse consequences of splenectomy in pediatric recipients has been emphasized by Potter and colleagues, who reported death from sudden overwhelming infection in three splenectomized children at 4, 8 and 13 years after transplantation (Potter *et al.*, 1986).

A renaissance in adjunctive splenectomy was stimulated by the controlled study indicating improved graft survival in splenectomized recipients receiving antilymphocyte globulin (ALG) (Fryd *et al.*, 1981). The data were reanalyzed in 1984, and the differences in survival rates between splenectomized and nonsplenectomized patients was no longer significant (Sutherland *et al.*, 1985). Neither the aforementioned study nor any other controlled study of splenectomy and renal transplantation involved pediatric patients. Because the improvement in graft survival was not present and the risk to the splenectomized recipient was considerable, this procedure generally has been avoided in pediatric recipients. Postsplenectomy prophylactic antibiotic therapy can minimize the potential for overwhelming sepsis; however, such a therapeutic approach assumes patient compliance.

RETRANSPLANTATION

Fine and coworkers evaluated the factors affecting the outcome in pediatric recipients of 75 retransplants from cadaver donors in the precyclosporine era (Fine *et al.*, 1979). The survival rate at 5 years posttransplant for second and third grafts was similar to that obtained for first grafts ($\pm 45\%$). All three fourth grafts failed within the first transplant month.

The primary factor influencing graft survival was recipient sensitization. The survival rate for nonpresensitized (<5%) and moderately presensitized (5–50%) recipients was significantly better than that of highly presensitized recipients (>50%) recipients. The HLA-A and HLA-B antigen compatibility led to improved survival rates in the highly presensitized recipient. This group recommended that only three or four HLA-A and HLA-B antigen matched grafts be used for retransplantation in the highly presensitized recipient (Fine *et al.*, 1979).

So and colleagues described their experience with 66 retransplants (32 cadaver donor, 27 living related HLA-nonidentical donor, 6 living related HLA-identical donor and 1 living unrelated donor) in children (So *et al.*, 1985). They found that overall graft and patient survival rates after retransplantation did not differ from their experience with primary grafts. Graft survival rates after retransplantation were improved, however, if the primary graft functioned for greater than 1 year and if the failed graft did not require transplant nephrectomy before retransplantation. No data were provided to account for the mechanism by which the *in situ* failed graft had a salutary effect on retransplantation. When both factors were present, graft outcome for second grafts was excellent. The report by So *et al.* (1985) was the first to describe extensive experience with retransplantation in children using living related donors.

Similar to with adults, results with retransplantation have changed in the cyclosporine era. Proportional hazards analy-

sis identified previous transplantation as a factor that increased the risk of subsequent graft failure in pediatric cadaver renal transplantation (McEnery *et al.*, 1992). The NAPRTCS database found that the graft survival at 3 years was 65% for first transplants but only 56% for retransplants. Similarly, at UCLA, cadaver graft survival for first transplants using sequential immunosuppression (discussed later) was 94% at 1 year and 91% at 2 years. Retransplant survival rates employing the same immunosuppressive regimen were 82% at 1 year and 70% at 2 years (Ettenger *et al.*, 1991b). Although these results represented a significant improvement over results with other immunosuppressive protocols, primary transplant outcome was still dramatically better than the outcome in retransplant recipients.

Results with living related donor retransplantation in children do not show this same effect. Three-year graft survival rates were identical (81%) in primary transplant and retransplant recipients in the NAPRTCS database.

Laufer and associates described five patients with living related donor grafts from HLA-identical siblings after rejection of one to five prior cadaver donor grafts (Laufer *et al.*, 1987). Four of the recipients had greater than 50% panel reactive antibodies immediately before transplantation, and two had greater than 90% at sometime during their course of ESRD. Four of the five recipients had functioning grafts at 1.5 to 8.5 years after transplant, whereas one lost a graft 2.5 years after transplant in conjunction with systemic cytomegalovirus (CMV) infection. Human leukocyte antigen–identical sibling grafts may provide prolonged function in high-risk recipients who have rejected one or more previous cadaver donor grafts.

Tejani and Sullivan (1996) reported their experience with repeat transplants over a 10-year period. Their analysis concluded that graft survival of a living related donor repeat transplant was similar to that of primary transplant, and young donor age was a significant deterrent to long-term (5 years) graft survival.

RECIPIENT AGE

As discussed in some detail earlier, the outcome of renal transplantation in children less than 6 years old was suboptimal and in children less than 1 year old dismal. New developments have improved the clinical picture to some degree. Nevertheless, young recipient age and particularly a recipient age of 2 years or younger is associated with a significant decrease in cadaver allograft survival (McEnery *et al.*, 1992).

Transplantation in infants less than 1 year old previously was associated with an 85% mortality rate (discussed earlier). Reports from the University of Minnesota have documented excellent short-term results in infants less than 1 year old, however, primarily with kidneys from living related donors (Najarian *et al.*, 1992). In North America, results do not reach this benchmark, although they are improving. The NAPRTCS reported that in children less than 2 years old, the 2-year graft survival rate for living related donor kidneys was 71%, whereas for cadaver donor kidneys it was only 46% at 1 year (McEnery *et al.*, 1992). Reasons cited for differences between the University of Minnesota reports and the multicenter NAPRTCS data include differences in surgical and pediatric nephrology experience, use of very young donor kidneys (discussed later), differences in immunosuppressive regimens and differences in experience of transplant centers in the treatment of very young transplant recipients (Warady, 1992). Schurman and coworkers studied the effect of center volume on pediatric renal transplantation (Schurman *et al.*, 1999). Their analysis of the NAPRTCS data showed superior graft survival in the high-volume centers at 3 months posttransplant, which appeared predominantly to be the result of lower rates of cadaver donor graft thrombosis and acute tubular necrosis. These investigations found, however, that the effect of center volume on graft survival was significant only with the exclusion of T-cell induction from the proportional hazards model ($r = 0.81$ and $RR = 0.70$ for the moderate and high volume groups, $P < 0.02$).

Results for graft survival in children 6 years old and younger have improved significantly. At UCLA, the 1-year cadaver graft survival rate in this age group increased from 33% in the years 1980–1985 to 90% in the years 1985–1988 (Ettenger et al., 1989). So and associates reported a 1-year graft survival rate of 82% in children less than 3 years old using a newer immunosuppressive protocol (So et al., 1990). Key factors for success appear to be (1) a multidisciplinary team approach, (2) careful intraoperative fluid management, (3) kidneys that are relatively large (discussed subsequently), (4) intraperitoneal placement of the graft when necessary with vascular anastomosis to the common iliac artery or aorta, (5) measures to avoid delayed graft function and (6) cyclosporine therapy in a sequential regimen (i.e., using an anti–T cell preparation and avoiding cyclosporine until graft dysfunction abates, as discussed later) (Ettenger et al., 1991b; Rosenthal et al., 1990; So et al., 1990).

Achieving successful transplant outcome in young children is complicated by many unique metabolic, technical and immunological considerations. Children appear to metabolize cyclosporine more rapidly than do adults, making target cyclosporine blood levels more difficult to achieve. This rapid metabolism is age related, with the youngest children metabolizing cyclosporine most rapidly (Neiberger et al., 1987). Smaller children and infants may require particularly large oral doses of cyclosporine when calculated per kilogram body weight because of impaired absorption owing to the limited surface area of the small intestines (Whitington et al., 1990).

From a technical standpoint, small children present multiple challenges. Vascular thrombosis can account for 15% of graft loss in children (Harmon et al., 1991). Vascular thrombosis occurs with increased frequency in living related donor transplantation when the recipient is less than 6 years old (Harmon et al., 1991). Long anastomosis times, common in the very small recipient, and resultant prolonged early graft dysfunction can reduce allograft survival in recipients treated with cyclosporine (Canadian Multicenter Transplant Study Group, 1983).

Early acute tubular necrosis has a profound negative impact on graft outcome. In children, early acute tubular necrosis is associated with only a 53% functional graft survival rate at 2 years, whereas in the absence of acute tubular necrosis, the 2-year graft survival rate is 74% (McEnery et al., 1992). The other technical challenge is the placement of large kidneys into small children. Although this placement may result in improved graft survival and renal function (Ettenger et al., 1989), it may present some formidable demands (Rosenthal et al., 1990). Young children may be more immunologically reactive than older children or adults, as measured by nonspecific cellular immune assays (discussed subsequently). This increased reactivity suggests that younger children may have an increased propensity for rejection and require potent immunosuppressive strategies to optimize graft survival. In addition, young children may manifest only subtle clinical findings while rejecting a large kidney (Bunchman et al., 1990). Bunchman and coworkers suggested that the clinical marker of acute rejection (i.e., a rise in serum creatinine) is a poor diagnostic indicator of rejection in small children because the large transplanted kidney may undergo extensive renal damage as a result of rejection before a rise in the serum creatinine level (Bunchman et al., 1990). It is easy to understand why graft loss from rejection is quite high in young children.

DONOR AGE

In cadaver donor pediatric renal transplantation, the conventional wisdom had been to use kidneys from young donors for young recipients. This practice formed the basis for the UNOS and United Kingdom Transplant Service Support Authority (UKTSSA) organ allocation systems for pediatric recipients to give children expedited access to cadaver kidney transplants. Under this system, children 15 years old and younger received preferential access to grafts from donors less than 10 years old (Ettenger, 1992). Because of this policy, children with ESRD in the United States and the United Kingdom were heavily reliant on pediatric cadaver donors. Donors 10 years old and younger have provided almost 40% of the cadaver grafts for pediatric recipients, with donors less than 5 years old accounting for 25% of all pediatric cadaver transplants (McEnery et al., 1992). Nevertheless, a large body of accumulated evidence supports the conclusion that kidneys from cadaver donors less than the age of 6 years have graft survival rates 20 to 40% lower than those from adolescents or adults.

Results using donors 6 to 10 years old fall somewhere in between these two extremes. Data from the NAPRTCS indicate that at 1 year, graft survival rates from donors 0 to 5 years old, 6 to 10 years old, and greater than 10 years old are approximately 63%, 73% and 80%; at 3 years, the graft survival rate for the youngest donor age group is 57%, whereas it ranges from 64 to 68% in the older groups (Alexander et al., 1989; McEnery et al., 1992). Other studies have shown similar findings (discussed earlier). Results are particularly poor when cadaver donor kidneys from young donors (≤ 3 years old) are placed in young recipients (Arbus et al., 1991). In addition to differences in graft outcome, larger kidneys result in better short-term renal function than smaller kidneys from young donors (Ettenger et al., 1989).

There are multiple interrelated reasons why kidneys from very young donors result in poor graft outcome even in the cyclosporine era. Technical issues are important. The inverse linear relationship between graft thrombosis and donor age in pediatric cadaver renal transplantation (Harmon et al., 1991) suggests that vascular anastomoses with small organs are challenging. The small absolute size of the transplanted arteries and veins and a possible increased responsiveness to vasospastic stimuli may contribute to an increased risk of thrombosis (Harmon et al., 1991). As noted earlier, longer anastomosis times, which often occur when small organs are used, are associated highly with acute tubular necrosis and decreased graft outcome when cyclosporine is used from the outset after transplantation. This finding is probably due, at least in part, to the fact that one of cyclosporine's toxic effects is a dramatic increase in renal afferent arteriolar vasoconstriction and a decrease in renal blood flow (Thiel, 1986).

Technical problems are important, but they may not be the only salient considerations. Although kidneys from young donors can functionally hypertrophy over the long-term (Silber, 1974), the same small kidneys may be acutely vulnerable to permanent parenchymal damage from severe episodes of rejection by virtue of their small renal mass and vasculature (Cecka and Terasaki, 1990). This concern is particularly relevant for young recipients because, as discussed elsewhere in this chapter, they may be strongly immunologically responsive with a propensity to vigorous rejection. Kidneys from young donors may be more sensitive to the ravages of prolonged cold ischemia time.

According to the UCLA Kidney Transplant Registry, young donors (1–5 years old) had only a 4% lower survival rate than kidneys from adult donors when kidneys had less than 18 hours of cold ischemia time. This difference increased to 18% (56% *vs.* 74%) with greater than 30 hours of cold ischemia time (Yuge and Cecka, 1991). Perhaps for similar reasons, kidneys from donors less than 15 years old transported over long distances had significantly reduced graft outcome (Cecka, 1989). The reasons for this marked response are not known, but many relate to irrecoverable ischemic damage to kidneys with small renal mass (Cecka and Terasaki, 1990).

Shoskes and Halloran (1991) showed that ischemia causes an interferon-γ dependent up-regulation of major histocompatibility complex (MHC) class I and class II antigens. It is possible that this MHC antigen up-regulation makes these kidneys with long cold ischemia times more immunogenic and vulnerable to rejection. The same laboratory has shown that kidneys from young germ-free mice manifest significant up-regulation of MHC antigen expression when the young mice are transferred to a nonsterile environment and become colonized with bacteria (Cockfield *et al.*, 1990). There are no data on MHC antigen expression on kidneys from young human donors, but these animal studies suggest that many circumstances may make such small kidneys more immunogenic. That this may be the case in humans is suggested by the finding that pediatric recipients of kidneys from young donors have a significant increase in the frequency of rejection episodes (McEnery *et al.*, 1992).

Gellert and coworkers evaluated graft survival and renal function of cadaver donor grafts according to donor age in pediatric recipients (Gellert *et al.*, 1996). Their study concluded that graft survival and function in children with a pediatric or an adult graft may not differ because graft function adapts to the requirement of the recipient.

Berg and colleagues evaluated the potential for adult donor grafts to increase the absolute GFR when a child recipient grows (Berg *et al.*, 1997). They reported that absolute GFR and effective renal plasma flow (ml/min) of grafts from donors less than 20 years old (all cadaver donor grafts) increased during a 5-year follow-up period, resulting in a constant relative GFR and effective renal plasma flow. In contrast, GFR and effective renal plasma flow of grafts from donors greater than 20 years old remained constant. During follow-up, there was a significant decline in relative values. Child donor grafts seem better able to increase their function with the growth of the child recipient than adult grafts.

Hemodynamic factors may play a role in the relatively poor outcome obtained with very young donor kidneys. Studies in animals (Okuda *et al.*, 1987) and anecdotal reports in clinical situations suggest an enhanced susceptibility to the development of glomerulosclerosis in kidneys from young donors as well as in kidneys with decreased nephron mass (Hayes *et al.*, 1991; Leunissen *et al.*, 1989). It appears that after a critical reduction in renal mass, progressive destruction of remnant glomeruli occurs, possibly involving hyperfiltration of residual renal units. Although this effect may result in proteinuria and possibly decreased GFR (Hayes *et al.*, 1991), diminished graft survival does not appear in the short-term. Proteinuria and diminished graft function are probably the indications of potential problems with long-term graft outcome. By this reasoning, nephron *underdosing* with single kidneys from young donors may lead to relatively poor long-term graft outcome (Brenner *et al.*, 1992), particularly in growing children.

Because of the problems inherent in transplanting kidneys from young donors to pediatric recipients, the UNOS has changed its sharing algorithm. The new sharing protocol avoids giving children a disproportionate share of small kidneys. Preliminary UNOS data show that using this new algorithm, 1-year cadaver renal allograft outcome in children has improved from 73 to 82% (P<0.007). Although other factors in addition to larger donors may have had a role in this improvement, it seems likely that optimizing donor size had an important role in this improvement in pediatric cadaver donor renal transplant outcome. The UKTSSA have adopted a similar policy, and pediatric recipients (<18 years old) have priority for well-matched kidneys, either adult or pediatric, over adult recipients.

RECIPIENT IMMUNE RESPONSIVENESS

An individual's nonspecific immune responsiveness strongly affects the ability to reject an allograft. This nonspecific immune response differs from person to person and can be quantitated using many tests of immune function. Assays include spontaneous blastogenesis, levels of activated and total T lymphocytes, ratio between CD4 and CD8 cells and lymphocyte proliferative response to mitogen stimulation (Kerman, 1989). Patients with high indices of nonspecific immunity in these tests have an increased propensity to reject and a poor graft outcome.

Young children appear to have a heightened nonspecific immune reactivity when compared with older children or adults. The immunological defects often observed in adult dialysis patients appear to be absent in children (Drachman *et al.*, 1989). Children less than 6 years old on dialysis have higher indices of nonspecific cellular immune responsiveness than older children or young adults; these indices include spontaneous blastogenesis; number of total T lymphocytes (i.e., CD3-bearing and CD4-bearing lymphocytes), B lymphocytes and immature activated lymphocytes and increased CD4/CD8 ratio (Ettenger *et al.*, 1987).

Pediatric kidney and liver transplant recipients show similar patterns. Young transplant recipients (<2 years old) have higher numbers of CD2$^+$, CD3$^+$, CD4$^+$ and CD8$^+$ lymphocytes than older children. There is a downward trend in each of these lymphocyte subset populations until the age of 5 years, when values are similar to those reported in adults (Schroeder *et al.*, 1991). All of these tests, when increased, indicate increased propensity for rejection (Kerman *et al.*, 1983; Uittenbogaart *et al.*, 1980). It is possible that this elevation in immunological responsiveness and propensity for rejection is common to all young children because increased numbers of CD4$^+$ T lymphocytes (Denny *et al.*, 1992) and increased CD4/CD8 ratios (Denny *et al.*, 1992; Yanase *et al.*, 1986) are present in normal young children and vary inversely with age.

These aforementioned findings suggest that young children may be at a higher risk for immunological rejection than older children and may require more intensive immunosuppression (Ettenger *et al.*, 1992b). That this view may be valid is supported by information from at least two large databases: the UCLA Transplant Registry and the EDTA. These analyses have found that pediatric renal transplant recipients have higher graft losses as a result of rejection than do adults of all ages (Cho *et al.*, 1990).

Technical Considerations

Except for small children (<20 kg), the technical aspects of renal transplantation in children are similar to those in adults. In the small child, the primary technical consideration is the placement of the graft. Can the graft be placed extraperitoneally with vascular anastomosis to the iliac and/or hypogastric vessels, or is a transabdominal approach required with use of the aorta and vena cava? Although some surgeons (see Chapter 9) have advocated the transabdominal approach when placing adult kidneys into children weighing less than 20 kg, it has been our experience that this approach is not always required.

Rosenthal and coworkers examined technical factors contributing to successful transplantation in 17 children less than 6 years old in the years 1985–1989 at UCLA (Rosenthal et al., 1990). The patients weighed 10 to 19 kg (mean, 14.1 kg). Only 3 of the 17 children required intraperitoneal placement. Children weighing greater than 15 kg almost always can have the grafts placed extraperitoneally even when the kidney is anastomosed to the aorta and the vena cava. When the child weighs 10 to 15 kg, the approach depends on the size discrepancy between donor and recipient. Of the nine patients who weighed 10 to 15 kg in our series, the kidneys were placed extraperitoneally in six, even though the aorta was used in two and the vena cava in four of these six (Rosenthal et al., 1990). For children weighing 9 to 20 kg, an alternative is to use a transperitoneal approach to place the kidneys retroperitoneally in anatomical position (Frawley and Farnsworth, 1990). Recipients weighing less than 10 kg are best approached transperitoneally with the kidney placed intraperitoneally behind the right colon (Starzl et al., 1964). Ureteral reimplantation usually is accomplished by means of ureteroneocystostomy, unless the bladder is inadequate. Use of an ileal conduit is acceptable under the circumstances as discussed in Chapters 11 and 12.

Precise intraoperative fluid management and maintenance of adequate intravascular volume are essential if posttransplant acute tubular necrosis is to be avoided. This practice is particularly crucial when placing an adult kidney into a relatively small child. An adult donor kidney may sequester 150 to 250 ml of blood. To prevent hypotension, this amount should be administered as a bolus of isotonic crystalloid or colloid before unclamping of the renal vessels. Central venous pressure and arterial blood pressure should be monitored closely during surgery.

Many centers assess peripheral perfusion using core and toe temperature monitoring. The intraoperative central venous pressure should be maintained at 10 to 14 cm H_2O, and the child's mean arterial pressure should be maintained at greater than 70 mm Hg before vascular clamps are removed. Occasionally, such aggressive fluid therapy can be harmful, particularly in a child whose myocardial function is suboptimal. Appropriate inotropic support sometimes is necessary. An inotropic agent such as dopamine can facilitate renal vasodilatation, and if the mean arterial blood pressure is relatively low despite an adequate central venous pressure, the inotropic support can be raised to achieve appropriate blood pressure. For all of these reasons, we institute intravenous dopamine at 2 to 4 μg/kg/min at the start of surgery. Furosemide (2–4 mg/kg) and mannitol (0.5–1.0 g/kg) may be given during creation of the vascular anastomosis to facilitate urine output. All urine output must be replaced intravenously immediately so that the child does not become hypovolemic.

As with introperative fluid management, it is important postoperatively that small patients receiving relatively large kidneys maintain appropriate intravascular volumes and adequate blood pressures. The central venous pressure should be maintained in the range of 6 to 10 cm H_2O. Insensible fluid losses should be calculated and administered as 5% dextrose in water (use either 400 ml/m² body surface area or 40 ml/100 kcal metabolized). The urine output should be replaced with an electrolyte solution approximating the electrolyte composition of the urine; this is usually 0.33% or

0.45% saline, without 5% dextrose. Because urine volumes often can be prodigious after transplantation, it is important to omit the dextrose in the urine replacement to avoid hyperglycemia. Potassium supplementation should be administered. Patients with well-functioning transplants may become hypokalemic because of urinary losses. Occasionally, total urine replacement may not be sufficient to maintain the central venous pressure and vascular volume in the desired range because of third space losses, development of occult postdialysis ascites in patients previously maintained on peritoneal dialysis or early recurrence of the nephrotic syndrome. Supplemental fluid boluses (10 ml/kg of normal saline or 5% albumin solution in saline) may be required to support blood pressure, to reestablish acceptable central venous pressure and to restore appropriate urine output.

If the child is fluid overloaded, it may be appropriate to replace only a portion of the urine output for a few hours until the central venous pressure is reestablished at a desired level. It is then appropriate to restore isovolumetric urine replacement to maintain the euvolemic state. Early initiation of dialysis may be appropriate for the patient in marked congestive heart failure or for one with acute tubular necrosis and electrolyte abnormalities that must be corrected. Hemodialysis or peritoneal dialysis may be performed safely. It is important to avoid overly aggressive ultrafiltration fluid removal because this can exacerbate ongoing acute tubular necrosis.

As the renal function improves and the patient begins oral intake, the kidney begins to concentrate the urine. Reduced fluid administration can be maintained by mouth by the second or third postoperative day.

Immunosuppression

Similar to in adult transplantation, clinical immunosuppression evolved dramatically in the 1990s. The mainstays of immunosuppression in children today are corticosteroids, azathioprine and cyclosporine (Tejani et al., 1993).

CORTICOSTEROIDS

Glucocorticosteroids such as prednisone are given at relatively low doses in children (0.2–2 mg/kg/d) to prevent rejection episodes (Ettenger et al., 1990; see also Chapter 15). At higher doses (3–10 mg/kg/d), oral prednisone or parenteral methylprednisolone reverses acute cellular rejection episodes (Ettenger and Rosenthal, 1992). Glucocorticosteroids may inhibit gene transcription by causing corticosteroid receptors or corticosteroid-induced proteins to bind to DNA in the area of the glucocorticoid response elements (Beato, 1989). The corticosteroids decrease macrophage production of interleukin (IL)-1 and inhibit transcription of message for IL-6 by peripheral blood mononuclear cells (Zanker et al., 1990). In antirejection doses, corticosteroids cause lympholysis by direct effects on the lymphocyte membrane. Corticosteroids also cause sequestration of circulating T cells and inhibition of cytotoxic T cells. Corticosteroids antagonize neutrophil and monocyte chemotaxis and stabilize lysosomal membranes. Corticosteroids are absorbed rapidly from the gastrointestinal tract with peak plasma concentration occurring within 1 to 3 hours. Prednisone is metabolized to prenisolone in the liver. Plasma concentrations of corticosteroids are influenced by drugs that induce or inhibit hepatic enzymes that affect metabolism.

The primary mechanism of action of corticosteroids is the prevention of IL-2 and IL-6 production by macrophages (Snyder et al., 1982). Corticosteroids block the initial phase of the immune response by inhibiting the transcription of the IL-1β gene (Yamanto, 1985) and by inducing rapid degradation of IL-1 mRNA (Knudsen et al., 1987; Lee et al., 1988). This rapid degradation, in turn, inhibits the IL-1-dependent release of IL-2 from activated T cells. Corticosteroids also inhibit IL-6 transcription (Fowler et al., 1990) by antigen-presenting cells, preventing the generation of important co-stimulator signals for T-cell activation (Cupps and Fauci, 1982).

Corticosteroids bind to the intracytoplasmic and intranuclear receptor proteins (Baxter and Forsham, 1972; Fauci, 1978; O'Malley, 1971). The receptor steroid complex is activated after it dissociates from the heat-shock protein. The complex translocates across the nuclear membrane to bind specific DNA sites reversibly, the corticosteroid response elements that are similar to the activator protein 1 sequence of the cytokine gene enhancer regions (Tsai et al., 1988), inhibiting gene transcription. Corticosteroids also induce lipocortin, a potent inhibitor of phospholipase A with potent antiinflammatory effects (Flower, 1985). Peripheral lympholysis in host tissue is another immunosuppressive mechanism of action of corticosteroids (Fauci, 1985).

Corticosteroids are absorbed rapidly from the gastrointestinal tract with peak plasma concentrations occurring within 1 to 3 hours (Walker and d'Aprice, 1988). Prednisone is metabolized to prednisolone in the liver. Plasma concentrations of corticosteroids are influenced by drugs that induce or inhibit hepatic metabolism.

Toxic effects of steroids have been well documented. The most important in the pediatric age group is their effect on growth. Other side effects include hypertension, hyperglycemia, hyperlipidemia, cushingoid facies, acne, hypertrichosis, osteoporosis, aseptic necrosis, delayed wound healing, myopathy, peptic ulcer disease, personality changes and pseudotumor cerebri.

The superior immunosuppressive efficacy of cyclosporine and the well-known toxicity of long-term steroid therapy have prompted trials of corticosteroid-free immunosuppression. Reported benefits of eliminating corticosteroids from the immunosuppressive regimens have included an improvement in growth velocity hypertension (Hricik et al., 1992), hyperlipidemia (Hricik et al., 1993) and glucose intolerance (Hricik et al., 1991). Results from a metaanalysis of seven prospective, randomized controlled trials of corticosteroid-free immunosuppression after renal transplantation (Hricik et al., 1993) showed that, collectively, success was achieved in 47% of 681 patients, but the rate varied widely from 40 to 85%. These authors suggested that the elimination of corticosteroids was associated with an increased short-term risk of acute allograft rejection without adversely affecting graft and patient survival. In contrast, the Canadian Multicenter Transplant Study found no difference in the rate of acute rejection, but the actuarial 5-year graft survival was significantly lower in the corticosteroid withdrawal group (Sinclair, 1992).

The incidence and degree of steroid side effects have been shown to be decreased by the use of alternate-day steroid dosing. Jabs and colleagues reported data from the NAPRTCS about the use of alternate-day steroids (Jabs et al., 1996). At 12 months posttransplant, only 21% of children were on alternate-day steroids. Use of alternate-day steroids was not associated with any deleterious effect on graft function 12 to 48 months posttransplantation in the children registered in the NAPRTCS database.

The use of deflazacort in pediatric renal transplant patients has been shown to have a beneficial effect on growth. Deflazacort is an oxazoline analogue of prednisolone (Nathanson et al., 1967) that has lower effects on calcium, phosphorus and glucose metabolism (Canniggia et al., 1977) at equieffective antiinflammatory and immunosuppressive doses. The antiinflammatory and immunosuppressive potency of deflazacort has been established to be 20% less than that of prednisone (Hahn et al., 1981; Nathanson et al., 1967).

Ferraris and coworkers studied 14 pediatric renal transplant recipients with living related donor, haploidentical match with stable renal function (Ferraris et al., 1996). Switching from methylprednisolone to deflazacort was not associated with an increased incidence of rejection episodes. There was no significant change in serum creatinine and calculated creatinine clearance during deflazacort therapy. The growth velocity increased from 3.7 ± 0.6 to 8.4 ± 0.5 cm/g ($P<0.01$) in eight pubertal and prepubertal children and the weight/height ratio decreased from $20.0 \pm 0.7.1\%$ to $12.5 \pm 6.5\%$ ($P<0.01$). The cell-mediated lympholysis decreased from $13.9 \pm 1.3\%$ to $6.26 \pm 0.33\%$ during deflazacort therapy. Only a slight change in mixed lymphocyte culture (MLC) reactivity was seen. The same authors reported an increase in serum growth hormone, linear growth velocity, and a decrease in the weight/height ratio with the use of deflazacort in children with successful renal transplantation (Ferraris et al., 1992).

Corticosteroids are used for maintenance immunosuppression and treatment of acute cellular rejection. In the perioperative period, intravenous methylprednisolone in a dose of 2.5 mg/kg/d is used starting 1 day before transplant. The dose is reduced gradually to 1.5 mg/kg/d by postoperative day 7. The intravenous route is changed to oral as soon as the patient can take oral medications. The NAPRTCS reports that at 30 days posttransplant, the average dose of corticosteroids is 0.63 mg/kg/d (Stablein and Sullivan, 1996). Target prednisone doses are as follows: 0.33 mg/kg/d at 1 to 2 months, 0.25 mg/kg/d at 3 months, 0.18 to 0.2 mg/kg/d at 3 to 4 months and 0.13 to 0.18 mg/kg/d at 6 months posttransplant.

The most frequent treatment for acute cellular rejection is a brief course of increased corticosteroids, often called *pulse therapy.* The dose is 5 to 30 mg/kg/d intravenously with a maximum of 1 g/d for 3 to 5 days. Other regimens include 500 mg/m² of oral prednisone therapy over 1 week and 2 mg/kg/d of oral prednisone for 1 to 2 weeks followed by a slow taper. No data indicate the superiority of one particular regimen. We use intravenous methylprednisolone for 3 consecutive days followed by two additional doses on alternate days. After this, maintenance oral corticosteroid immunosuppression is restarted at slightly higher levels than existed just before the rejection episode.

The use of corticosteroid alternate-day therapy has been associated with a decrease in the incidence of hypertension, an improvement in glucose tolerance, a decrease in the serum cholesterol level, a reduction in cushingoid appearance and an improvement in growth velocity (Broyer et al., 1992a; Pennisi et al., 1978b). Others prefer to continue daily low-dose (0.10–0.12 mg/kg/d) corticosteroids indefinitely because of concerns about rejection and medication noncompliance (Ettenger et al., 1990). Some investigators have found that alternate-day steroid therapy may be associated with decreased compliance and impaired allograft function, although others have not noted this (Potter et al., 1975; Reimold, 1973).

Long-term corticosteroid therapy in pediatric patients causes numerous side effects. Of most concern is growth failure (see elsewhere in this chapter) and susceptibility to infection. Other important side effects include delayed wound healing, hypertension, obesity, hyperlipidemia, cushingoid facies, acne, hypertrichosis, cataracts, osteoporosis, aseptic necrosis, myopathy, hyperglycemia, peptic ulcer disease, pancreatitis, personality changes and pseudotumor cerebri.

An alternate approach to corticosteroid therapy that may lead to decreased side effects is with deflazacort. Ferraris and coworkers tested this agent on nine stable renal transplant recipients 9 to 15 years old (Ferraris *et al.*, 1992). Methylprednisolone (0.2 mg/kg/d) was replaced with deflazacort (0.3 mg/kg/d). Creatinine clearance values remained stable, and there were no obvious rejection episodes. The cushingoid appearance diminished significantly in all of the patients, the growth velocity SDS increased from -4.5 to -3.0, and mean growth velocity increased from 1.5 to 3 cm/y. Growth hormone secretion rates improved. If larger studies validate these findings, deflazacort or other agents with less corticosteroid toxicity may be of value in maintenance immunosuppressive therapy for the pediatric renal transplant recipient. Deflazacort is not available in Europe and North America.

AZATHIOPRINE

Azathioprine was the keystone of immunosuppression treatment for renal transplantation since its discovery in 1961 (Hitchings and Elion, 1969; see also Chapter 15). In 1977, McGeown *et al.* first introduced a combination of azathioprine and low-dose corticosteroids. Azathioprine, in conjunction with prednisone, was the standard regimen of maintenance immunosuppression in children for many years. Azathioprine's active metabolites include 6-mercaptopurine and 6-thionosinic acid. These impair synthesis of DNA and RNA by blocking synthesis of adenine and guanine nucleic acids. 6-Thionosinic acid can be incorporated into nucleic acids and leads to chromosome breaks. Azathioprine has antiproliferative effect on dividing B and T lymphocytes by interfering with their nucleotide synthesis during their proliferative cycle.

Azathioprine functions as a prodrug and requires activation by the liver. It is excreted through the biliary system. It is well absorbed from the gastrointestinal tract with a peak plasma concentration achieved within about 2 hours of oral administration. When given alone in pediatric transplantation (e.g., HLA identical sibling donor and cyclosporine intolerance), the dose of azathioprine is 2 mg/kg/d to a maximum of 150 mg with a downward dose adjustment if bone marrow suppression (neutropenia, thrombocytopenia or macrocytic anemia) or other side effects occur. When used in a triple-therapy protocol, dosages usually range from 1 to 2 mg/kg/d. The NAPRTCS registry (1996) indicates that approximately 88% of pediatric recipients receive azathioprine at an initial dose of 2.2 mg/kg/d. At 60 months, the percentage receiving azathioprine is similar, with a median dose of 1.63 mg/kg/d. There is minimal difference in the dosage of azathioprine between living related donor and cadaver donor recipients.

The most important side effects (besides dose-related bone marrow toxicity) are idiosyncratic toxicities to the bone marrow and liver (Maddocks *et al.*, 1986). Other side effects include pancreatitis, alopecia, nausea, vomiting and increased risk of infection and neoplasia. Initial stages in azathioprine metabolism are mediated by xanthine oxidase. Xanthine oxidase inhibitors (e.g., allopurinol) administered concurrently with azathioprine may be dangerous because they can lead to markedly elevated immunosuppressive effects and hematological toxicity.

Azathioprine is selected most often for children together with prednisone and cyclosporine in a triple-therapy regimen. Data on the efficacy of triple-therapy compared with a cyclosporine-prednisone regimen in children are sparse. Azathioprine in triple therapy is meant to permit lower doses of cyclosporine. In a NAPRTCS survey of maintainence immunosuppression in children, recipients of cadaver donor grafts and living related donor grafts were receiving significantly less cyclosporine at 30 days posttransplant if they were on triple therapy. Triple therapy was associated with a significantly lower mean serum creatinine level at 6 months posttransplant in cadaver donor graft recipients but not in recipients of living related donor transplants (Tejani *et al.*, 1993). The investigators concluded that triple therapy is appropriate for pediatric recipients of cadaver donor kidneys but provides no benefit over cyclosporine-prednisone in children receiving kidneys from living donors.

Azathioprine, the 5-imidazole derivative of 6-mercaptopurine, was synthesized first in the early 1950s by Hitchings and Elion (1969). Azathioprine is converted to thionosinic acid monophosphate (TIMP) intracellularly. TIMP inhibits phosphoribosyl-pyrophosphate aminotransferase, the first step in *de novo* purine synthesis (Winkelstein, 1979). *In vivo*, its metabolities are incorporated into developing strands of DNA; this inhibits the synthesis and metabolism of purine and alters the synthesis of RNA (Hitchings and Elion, 1969). Azathioprine has antiproliferative effect on dividing B and T lymphocytes by interfering with nucleotide synthesis during their proliferative cycle. Azathioprine acts distally in the lymphocyte activation cascade by reducing the availability of purines required by rapidly dividing cells to synthesize DNA and RNA. The drug inhibits the primary immune responses with little effect on secondary responses and is useful in preventing acute rejection but not in reversing the process.

Azathioprine functions as a prodrug and requires activation by the liver. It is excreted through the biliary system. Azathioprine is well absorbed from the gastrointestinal tract with a peak plasma concentration achieved within about 2 hours of oral administration (Walker and d'Aprice, 1988). Azathioprine is used as one of the triple-therapy immunosuppressives along with cyclosporine and corticosteroids. The dose is 1 to 2 mg/kg/d when used in a triple therapy protocol.

The side effects of azathioprine include an idiosyncratic and a dose-related bone marrow toxicity, which hierarchically affects the formed elements (Maddocks *et al.*, 1986). That is, neutrophils are affected more than erythrocytes, and erythrocytes are affected more than platelets. The bone marrow toxicity is particularly evident in some ethnic groups, such as Asians, because of gene polymorphisms in the azathioprine metabolic enzyme pathway that can predispose to the development of marked cytopenias (Demattos *et al.*, 1996). Other side effects include nausea, vomiting, pancreatitis, alopecia, increased risk of infection and neoplasia. Xanthine oxidase inhibitors administered concurrently with azathioprine significantly increase hematological toxicity and immunosuppressive effects of azathioprine. The dose of azathioprine should be reduced by 66 to 75% if such drugs are required concomitantly (Walker and d'Aprice, 1988).

MYCOPHENOLATE MOFETIL

Mycophenolate mofetil acts as an immunosuppressive through its active protein mycophenolic acid (see also Chapter 18). Mycophenolic acid is a potent and specific inhibitor of the *de novo* purine synthesis pathway. Intracellularly, mycophenolic acid binds to and inhibits uncompetitively and reversibly inosine monophosphate dehydrogenase. This action, in turn, blocks the generation of guanosine necleotides and subsequently T-cell and B-cell proliferation (Allison and Eugui, 1993). T and B lymphocytes preferentially use the *de novo* pathway of purine synthesis and are particularly sensitive to the inhibitory action of the drug. *In vitro* mycophenolate mofetil clocks the proliferation of T and B lymphocytes and generation of cytotoxic T cells after stimulation by mitogens (Platz *et al.*, 1991).

Three randomized, double-blind, multicenter trials in the United States, Europe, Australia and Canada, comprising 1,493 renal transplant recipients, compared mycophenolate mofetil in doses of 2 and 3 g daily with placebo or azathioprine, given in combination with cyclosporine, corticosteroids and ALG (only in the United States). The patient survival rates were similar in all the groups, and graft survival rates with mycophenolate mofetil were marginally better than with either placebo or azathioprine. The safety profile was similar to azathioprine except that the incidence of diarrhea was slightly higher (European Mycophenolate Mofetil Cooperative Study Group, 1995; Halloran, 1996; Solinger, 1995; Tricontinental Mycophenolate Mofetil Renal Transplantation Study Group, 1996).

The Mycophenolate Mofetil Acute Renal Rejection Study group (1998) compared the safety and efficacy of the addition of mycophenolate mofetil to the treatment regimen of an early first acute cellular rejection. The study concluded that mycophenolate mofetil administered in combination with pulse steroids decreased significantly the subsequent use of antilymphocyte therapy in the treatment of acute renal allograft rejection. At 6 months, 16.8% required ALG in the mycophenolate mofetil group versus 41.7% in the azathioprine group.

In a short-term study by Hueso *et al.* (1998), the use of mycophenolate mofetil in 16 patients (first cadaver donor renal transplant) with suspected cyclosporine nephrotoxicity allowed cyclosporine dose reduction, which improved renal function, reduced TGF-β production and allowed better control of hypertension without triggering acute rejection.

Ettenger and coworkers studied 37 (16 living related donor and 21 cadaver donor) pediatric renal transplant patients (Ettenger *et al.*, 1997). Sequential therapy with ALG was followed by mycophenolate mofetil, cyclosporine and corticosteroids. Mycophenolate mofetil was administered in doses ranging from 8 to 30 mg/kg/bid. They currently recommend a dose of 600 mg/M²/bid (i.e., 1200 mg/M²/day). The incidence of clinical acute rejection episodes was 13% and increased to 19% with inclusion of data from routine 1-year surveillance biopsies. The results of the Pediatric Mycophenolate Mofetil Study Group of 18% rejection episodes in the cadaver donor recipients were significantly better than 60% in the NAPRTCS data (1996). The increased infection rate, especially with CMV, indicates a need to increase CMV prophylaxis with mycophenolate mofetil. A controlled trial studying the effect on graft survival is required before mycophenolate mofetil is routinely used in pediatric recipients.

CYCLOSPORINE

Cyclosporine is recognized as a major advance in transplantation (see also Chapter 16). Although there was significant improvement in graft survival in the years before cyclosporine's introduction, the use of cyclosporine has improved graft survival more. Overall, cadaver allograft survival has improved from a 1-year rate of 55 to 60% in the precyclosporine era to 75 to 85% currently.

Cyclosporine is a cyclic decapeptide with a molecular weight of 1202 daltons extracted from the fungus perfecti *Tolypocladium inflatum gams*. Seven of the 11 amino acids are N-methylated, conferring an overall hydrophobic character with a hydrophilic site (Borel *et al.*, 1976). It has potent *in vitro* and *in vivo* immunosuppressive activity. Cyclosporine is a prodrug that binds first to a cytosolic immunophilin (cyclophilin) to create a drug/protein complex that inhibits calcineurin activity. Calcineurin is a calcium-activated and

calmodulin-activated phosphatase that has many actions in T cells. It inhibits T-cell synthesis of lymphokines and primary humoral signals for the activation and proliferation cascades that induce cell-mediated cytotoxicity and humoral immunity—IL-2, IL-3, interferon-γ, IL-6 and IL-7 (Handschumacher *et al.*, 1984).

Cyclosporine specifically inhibits the activation of the gene for the cytokine IL-2, may partially reduce the synthesis of IL-2 receptors and inhibits events in the lymphocyte activation attendant to binding IL-2 to IL-2 receptors. Cyclosporine is thought to act by blocking the activation of a DNA binding protein necessary to activate the promoter sequences for the IL-2 gene in the lymphocyte, especially the helper T cells. Cyclosporine is an effective immunosuppressant because it acts at a proximal site in the lymphocyte activation cascade (Fischer *et al.*, 1989; Schreiber *et al.*, 1991).

Cyclosporine displays distinct pharmacokinetic properties in children as compared with adult transplant recipients (Kahan *et al.*, 1986). Pharmacokinetic studies of cyclosporine in children after renal transplant indicated a higher clearance rate (11.8 ml/min/kg) compared with 5.7 ml/min/kg for adult patients, a shorter half-life 7.3 hours compared with 10.7 hours in adults and comparable bioavailability (30.8% compared with 27.5% for adult populations) (Kahan *et al.*, 1986). A kinetic analysis by Neiberger *et al.* (1987) using a two-compartment model confirmed that the equilibration and the elimination periods were much shorter in children than in adults, reflecting faster drug elimination. The volume of distribution as a steady-state also was significantly greater in children.

When cyclosporine first came into use, children did not have the same rapid gains in graft survival that were seen in adults (Fine and Ettenger, 1988). This difference appears to relate, at least in part, to an age-related decreased absorption and increased metabolism of cyclosporine. The pharmacokinetic studies described previously validate the clinical impression that children (particularly young children) require higher doses of cyclosporine at more frequent intervals to achieve trough blood levels comparable to those obtained in adult recipients (Hoyer *et al.*, 1984; Klare *et al.*, 1984). Hoppu *et al.* (1991) studied cyclosporine pharmacokinetics in children 1.1 to 2.5 years old and found that the mean calculated dose necessary to achieve desired steady-state blood levels was 5 mg/kg/d intravenously or 21 mg/kg/d orally. Cyclosporine blood levels and consequently the degree of immunosuppression often are inadequate when administering conventional adult dosing schedules.

Offner and colleagues related cyclosporine dosing to body surface area rather than weight in young children (Offner *et al.*, 1987). They specify a starting dose of 500 mg/m², tapered by 50 mg/m² weekly to a maintenance dose of 300 mg/m². This regimen has led to excellent graft survival of 84% at 2 years and 78% at 3 years. According to this formula, an infant may require initial doses of 20 to 30 mg/kg to achieve appropriate cyclosporine levels, and this is indeed the case (Ettenger *et al.*, 1990; Hoppu *et al.*, 1991). It often is necessary to administer cyclosporine to young children at a three times a day schedule to optimize the area under the curve (AUC) and to establish appropriate immunosuppression.

The clinical use of cyclosporine is hindered by its pharmacokinetic variability (Klintmalm *et al.*, 1985), which requires close monitoring of blood levels to avoid toxicity or underdosing. Trough concentrations are helpful in extreme cases of poor gastrointestinal absorption or rapid drug metabolism but are of limited value to predict adverse events or the actual exposure to the drug (Grevel *et al.*, 1989). Abbreviated AUC profiles have been proposed, but data with cyclosporine lack correlation between the predicted and measured cyclosporine AUC with this method (Gaspari *et al.*, 1993). There are insufficient data to show that monitoring cyclosporine levels with AUC measurements results in better allograft outcome (but see Chapter 16).

The absorption of cyclosporine from the gastrointestinal tract is incomplete and variable. A peak plasma concentration usually is reached 2 to 6 hours after a single oral dose, and the half-life is 10 to 27 hours (Lemaire et al., 1990). It is metabolized primarily in the liver through the cytochrome P450–111 system. The levels of cyclosporine are affected by drugs that induce or inhibit the cytochrome P450 system (see Table 37–1). The microemulsion form of cyclosporine (Neoral) is better absorbed and well tolerated, and 1/1 dose ratio conversion from cyclosporine to Neoral is not associated with increased rate of side effects.

Cyclosporine has numerous adverse effects. The most significant of these is nephrotoxicity, which occurs in three clinical settings. Nephrotoxicity occurring immediately after transplantation as an additive effect on renal ischemia may help explain the relatively poor graft survival rate that occurs when cyclosporine is used from the outset in patients whose grafts had increased reanastomosis times and initial nonfunction (Canadian Mulitcentre Transplant Study Group, 1983). The consequences of vasoconstriction for early graft function may be reduced by avoiding perioperative intravenous cyclosporine and by delaying early perioperative use until the likelihood of vasoconstrictive ischemic injury is less likely. This delayed use of cyclosporine is achieved by the use of antibody induction followed by maintenance immunosuppression in a sequential quadruple-therapy regimen.

Acute cyclosporine nephrotoxicity occurs in greater than 30% of patients within the first 6 months after renal transplantation and may be difficult to distinguish from mild acute rejection. The diagnosis is based mainly on a combination of clinical and histological features supplemented by monitoring of cyclosporine blood levels (Alexopoulos et al., 1991). Patients with cyclosporine toxicity frequently are asymptomatic and afebrile; the rise in serum creatinine usually is slow, and many episodes are accompanied by only a small change in urinary volume. The most important clue indicating cyclosporine toxicity is the slow rise in serum creatinine versus a rapid increase in serum creatinine in acute rejection. The diagnostic test is renal allograft biopsy.

Long-term administration of cyclosporine produces an insidious deterioration in renal function with more extensive histological change. Renovascular resistance is elevated twofold, largely owing to an increase in preglomerular resistance, and there is a gradual erosion of renal functional reserve (Mobb et al., 1992; Myers et al., 1991). Morphological changes include an occlusive afferent arteriolopathy with sclerosis of glomeruli, and ischemic nephrons are associated with patchy fibrosis of the surrounding interstitium. The incidence and severity of chronic cyclosporine nephrotoxicity after renal transplantation have declined markedly as the induction and maintenance doses of cyclosporine have been reduced. Chronic cyclosporine toxicity is an uncommon cause of late renal allograft loss (Hong et al., 1992; Vanrentergham et al., 1990). Progression to dialysis is reported in 4% of heart transplant recipients by 4.5 years posttransplant, and a similar decline is seen in pediatric and adult liver transplant recipients, with GFR falling to less than 18 ml/min/1.73 m² in more than half of the patients at follow-up (Greenberg et al., 1990).

Cyclosporine appears to have other effects on the kidney as well. In a few patients, it may cause a de novo thrombotic microangiopathy (Buturovic et al., 1990). In these patients, the original disease was not HUS. This thrombotic microangiopathy often may be related to a cyclosporine-mediated reduction in renal prostacycline synthesis. In pediatric renal transplantation, it is important to recognize that this entity exists and to differentiate it from HUS recurrence. In this de novo entity, some investigators have recommended the infusion of fresh frozen plasma and the discontinuation of cyclosporine, whereas others have continued cyclosporine at lower doses with eventual recovery (Buturovic et al., 1990).

Hypomagnesemia may be seen in the early posttransplant period as a result of cyclosporine-induced renal magnesium wasting (Barton et al., 1987). Hypomagnesemia may predispose the patient to seizures or aggravate a preexisting seizure diathesis. Cyclosporine also may cause a type IV renal tubular acidosis with hyperkalemia. This condition is thought to be related to impaired aldosterone synthesis and metabolism.

Cyclosporine has many other side effects. Hypertension is seen in more than 80% of cyclosporine-treated pediatric renal allograft recipients and is thought to be secondary to increased renal sodium reabsorption (Hoyer et al., 1990; Jarowenko et al., 1987). The use of calcium channel blockers is common to treat posttransplant hypertension because these agents may oppose cyclosporine-induced afferent arteriolar vasoconstriction. Because the combined use of calcium channel blockers and cyclosporine predisposes to gingival hyperplasia, an angiotensin receptor antagonist is used frequently to treat posttransplant hypertension.

Hepatotoxicity can occur with mild cholestasis and elevated transaminase levels in a dose-related fashion (Lorber et al., 1987). There may be an increased rate of cholelithiasis; this can occur in children as well as adults (Diaz-Gonzalez et al., 1991). Cyclosporine neurotoxicity may manifest infrequently as tremors, seizures, cortical blindness, cerebellar edema, structural central nervous system changes and coma. This form of neurotoxicity has been linked to the presence of low cholesterol levels and is seen more frequently in liver than in kidney transplant recipients (DeGroen et al., 1987).

Cosmetic side effects include hypertrichosis and gingival hyperplasia (Butler et al., 1987). Gingival hyperplasia is particularly common in young children and may be related to high salivary concentrations of cyclosporine (DeCamargo, 1989). Children treated with cyclosporine alone or in combination with calcium channel blockers should have close periodontal follow-up. Acne may be aggravated by cyclosporine. Some pediatric patients may develop changes in facial appearance during treatment with cyclosporine. This appearance is characterized by prominent supraorbital ridges and eyebrows, coarse skin, thick lips and maxillary and mandibular changes resulting in retrognathia (Crocker et al., 1993).

Matas and coworkers studied retrospectively 234 pediatric renal transplant patients using induction therapy with delayed introduction of cyclosporine (Matas et al., 1996). Their multivariate analysis for risk factors for biopsy-proven rejection in the first 3 months and in the first 6 months revealed that cyclosporine trough levels at 1 month was the crucial factor. Recipients with cyclosporine levels less than 100 ng/ml (high-performance liquid chromatography) had 2.24 times the risk of rejection versus recipients with blood levels greater than 100 ng/ml.

Cyclosporine may be used in quadruple sequential therapy. Sequential therapy is an induction program in which initial immunosuppression is accomplished with an anti–T cell preparation for a varied length of time. Cyclosporine is withheld until posttransplant graft dysfunction begins to resolve (e.g., the serum creatinine level falls to 2 mg/dl). In children, induction therapy has the additional advantage of providing augmented immunosuppression.

Cyclosporine is used as a maintenance immunosuppressive drug to prevent allograft rejection. It was first used in a triple-therapy regimen in pediatric transplantation in 1982. In the perioperative period, in a living related donor transplant, cyclosporine is usually started 1 day before transplantation with a loading dose of 10 mg/kg. Thereafter, in the immediate postoperative period, it is administered in an intravenous dose of 2.5 to 5 mg/kg/d. This is one third the oral dose, taking into account the limited bioavailability of oral cyclosporine. The dose is changed to an oral dose of 10 to 15 mg/kg/d as soon as the patient is ready for oral medications but, as mentioned earlier, many units prefer to use a dosage based on surface area rather than weight. Cyclosporine is administered every 12 hours for children and every 8 hours for infants. Cyclosporine blood levels must be followed daily during initiation of therapy because wide changes may occur when tissue stores are saturated. Dosage of cyclosporine depends on blood trough levels (Table 37–7).

The clinical use of cyclosporine is hindered by its pharmacokinetic variability (Klintmalm et al., 1985; see earlier), which requires close monitoring of blood levels to avoid toxicity or underdosing. Trough levels are helpful in extreme cases of poor gastrointestinal absorption or rapid drug metabolism but are of limited value to predict adverse events of the actual exposure to the drug (Grevel et al., 1989). Abbreviated AUC has been proposed, but data with cyclosporine lack correlation between the predicted and measured cyclosporine AUC with this method (Gaspari et al., 1993).

Because of the difficulties with use of cyclosporine in young children, many pediatric centers employ induction therapy with an anti–T cell preparation for a fixed time in the peritransplant period (usually 10–14 days) (Almond et al., 1992). A variant is sequential therapy. Sequential therapy is an induction program in which initial immunosuppression is accomplished with an anti–T cell preparation for a varied length of time. Cyclosporine is withheld until posttransplant graft dysfunction begins to resolve (e.g., the serum creatinine level falls to 2 mg/dl). Because the anti–T cell preparation is potent yet not nephrotoxic, this program allows the medical team to avoid cyclosporine, with its propensity to reduce renal blood flow, during the early phase of graft dysfunction, when acute tubular necrosis can be prolonged by renal blood flow reduction. An anti–T cell preparation can allow the medical team a rejection-free period during which the recipient can be stabilized hemodynamically. This rejection-free period is a valuable time for establishing and optimizing the maintainence immunosuppressive medications (Ettenger et al., 1992b).

In children, induction therapy or sequential therapy has the additional advantage of providing augmented immunosuppression; this appears to be particularly useful in light of the finding that children appear to be vigorous immune responders (discussed previously). In adult studies, monoclonal antibody therapy (i.e., OKT3) may be associated with significant reduction in acute rejection episodes and steroid-resistant rejection episodes (Goldman et al., 1991; Kreis et al., 1991).

According to a NAPRTCS report, 45% of children receiving renal transplants in the United States in the years 1987–1989 underwent some form of induction therapy (Alexander et al., 1989). Polyclonal preparations (i.e., ALG or Minnesota

TABLE 37–7
TARGET BLOOD TROUGH LEVELS FOR CYCLOSPORINE

Posttransplant	HPLC (ng/ml)	TDX (ng/ml)
Day 0–week 6	200–300	300–500
Week 7–month 3	150–250	275–450
Month 3–year 4	100–200	200–450

HPLC = high-performance liquid chromatography.

antilymphoblast globulin) were used six to seven times more frequently than was OKT3. The median time course for induction therapy with a polyclonal preparation was 9 days, whereas for OKT3 it was 10 days. The median dosage for the polyclonal preparations was approximately 15 mg/kg/d; for OKT3, the median dose was 0.1 mg/kg.

In the NAPRTCS report, induction therapy was associated with a significantly decreased rejection rate in the first 100 days after transplantation. As a general rule, induction therapy appeared to defer rather than decrease rejection episodes. By 1 year posttransplant, there were equivalent rejection rates when comparing patients who received induction therapy with those who did not (Alexander et al., 1989). The report published by the NAPRTCS (McEnery et al., 1992) shows that early use of an anti–T cell biological agent is associated with a significantly improved cadaver graft survival rate in children ($P = 0.004$).

Single-center studies suggest that some form of induction may improve graft survival in children. At the University of Minnesota, a fixed course of Minnesota antilymphoblast globulin has been shown to improve pediatric allograft outcome. Sequential therapy improved patient and allograft outcome significantly in 131 pediatric renal transplants (Almond et al., 1992). The 1- and 5-year cumulative allograft survival rates in the 49 cadaver transplants in this study were 92% and 74%. Sequential therapy was particularly beneficial for recipients less than 6 years old, boosting the cadaver graft survival at 1 year from 48 to 78% (So et al., 1990).

As noted earlier, long-term cyclosporine carries with it the potential for chronic nephrotoxicity. For this reason, it was the conventional wisdom that cyclosporine doses should be lowered to the greatest extent possible. We have observed many children with low cyclosporine blood levels, however, who have had slowly rising serum creatinine levels and evidence on renal biopsy of low-level acute rejection activity.

Basadonna and coworkers found that recipients who have experienced one or more rejection episodes are more likely to develop chronic rejection (Basadonna et al., 1993). In this series, patients experiencing more than one acute rejection episode or who experience their first rejection episode greater than 60 days after transplantation have a particularly high incidence of chronic rejection. It appears to be important to strike a long-term balance in the dose of cyclosporine between the high dose that results in severe chronic nephrotoxicity and the low dose that may predispose the patient to *smoldering* acute and/or chronic rejection. This *therapeutic window* often is difficult to discern.

The oral liquid form of cyclosporine has been nearly replaced by oral capsules in 100-mg and 25-mg dosage strengths. This much easier to use preparation is appreciated by parents and adolescents and may improve compliance. The liquid form still is used by younger patients who cannot swallow capsules and allows small dose changes so important in these recipients.

Cyclosporine is metabolized by the P450 cytochrome system in the liver. All drugs that induce or inhibit the cytochrome P450 system affect and/or alter the blood levels of cyclosporine. Many agents can affect cyclosporine's absorption, distribution and metabolism. If treatment with these drugs is required, the patient must be monitored closely, and appropriate cyclosporine dosage adjustments must be made. Families must be cautioned to consult the transplant team before starting new medications prescribed by other health care professionals. Studies are ongoing to assess the effect of growth hormone on cyclosporine levels. Drugs that can lower cyclosporine levels frequently used by pediatric patients include the anticonvulsants phenytoin, carbamazepine and phenobarbital and the antituberculous drugs isoniazid and rifampin. Cholestyramine and mineral oil may interfere with absorption of cyclosporine. Commonly used agents in children that increase gastrointestinal motility and cause diarrhea, such as the oral antibiotics dicloxacillin and ampicillin-sulbactam and supplemental oral phosphate and magnesium, can lower cyclosporine levels precipitously and cause rejection. Drugs that increase cyclosporine levels frequently given to pediatric patients include the antibiotics erythromycin and ciprofloxacin; certain calcium channel blocking agents including verapamil, diltiazem and nicardipine and antifungals such as ketoconazole and fluconazole. Steroid hormones, such as high-dose methylprednisolone, and certain oral contraceptive agents, such as levonorgestrel and ethinyl estradiol, also may increase cyclosporine levels. Metaclopramide may increase cyclosporine absorption.

TACROLIMUS

Tacrolimus is a polycyclic macrolide produced by a strain of *Streptomyces tsukubaensis* (Tanaka *et al.*, 1987; see also Chapter 17). It acts by inhibiting the production of IL-2, IL-3 and interferon-γ by T cells *in vitro* (Kay *et al.*, 1989). The drug is believed to act on T lymphocytes during the initial hours of the GO state of activation by a mechanism similar to that of cyclosporine. Tacrolimus binds to intracellular cytoplasmic receptors known as *immunophilins*, particularly the FKBP12 binding protein (Yoshimura and Oka, 1990). The tacrolimus-FKBP12 complex binds to and inhibits calcineurin. It blocks the phosphate activity of calcineurin and prevents dephosphorylation of the cytoplasmic subunit of a transcription factor, nuclear factor of activated T cells (NF-AT), which normally enters the nucleus and activates expression of T-cell activation lymphokine gene (Northrop *et al.*, 1994).

Tacrolimus has 10 to 100 times the potency of cyclosporine in *in vitro* models of immunosuppression (Yoshimura and Oka, 1990). Tacrolimus is metabolized by the cytochrome P450 3A enzyme in the liver and has drug interactions similar to cyclosporine. As primary immunosuppressive therapy, tacrolimus requires larger doses in children than in adults and is given pretransplant at an oral dose of 0.15 mg/kg. Postoperatively, tacrolimus is given as an intravenous infusion in a dose of 0.05 to 0.10 mg/kg/d. The dose is changed to 0.15 mg/kg/dose orally twice a day as soon as the patient is ready for oral medication (Shapiro, 1998). The target whole blood levels are listed in Table 37–8.

As rescue therapy, oral tacrolimus is used in a dose of 0.15 mg/kg twice a day. The goal is to achieve a level of 15 to 25 ng/ml until the rejection episode is reversed. Thereafter the dose of tacrolimus and steroids is reduced gradually. If the indication for initiation of tacrolimus is cyclosporine toxicity, the recommended dose of tacrolimus is one fourth to one half the dose used for refractory rejection to maintain target levels of 5 to 9 ng/ml.

Tacrolimus was first approved by the U.S. Food and Drug Administration in 1994 for liver transplant recipients and in 1997 for kidney transplant recipients; it has been in clinical use since February 1989 (Starzl *et al.*, 1989). In one of the first controlled trials performed in liver transplant recipients (Todo *et al.*, 1991), no significant difference was found in

TABLE 37–8
TARGET WHOLE-BLOOD LEVELS FOR TACROLIMUS

Posttransplant (wk)	IMX (ng/ml)
0–2	20–25
2–4	15–20
4–12	10–15
>12	5–9

patient survival between cyclosporine and tacrolimus arms, but 61% of patients given tacrolimus were free of rejection as compared with 18% in the cyclosporine group at 1-year follow-up. The adverse effects were the same in both groups.

Shapiro *et al.* (1999) used tacrolimus-based immunosuppression in 81 (41% living related donor and 59% cadaver donor) pediatric renal transplant recipients in the years 1989–1996. Of patients, 64% were undergoing first transplant. The 1 and 4 years actuarial patient survival rates were 99% and 94%. Graft survival rates were 98% and 84% at 1 and 4 years. The mean tacrolimus dose was 0.18 ± 0.12 mg/kg/d, and the mean level was 9.9 ± 4.6 ng/ml by whole-blood analysis.

The use of tacrolimus in pediatric recipients facilitated the withdrawal of corticosteroids in 73% of patients, although corticosteroids had to be restarted in 10% of the recipients. The incidence of posttransplant lymphoproliferative disease (PTLD) was 4%, which was much lower than observed previously by the same authors. The authors explain the reduction in the incidence of PTLD as resulting from the following reasons: (1) aggressive policy of tapering steroids and tacrolimus and maintaining low trough level of 5 to 9 ng/ml; (2) Epstein-Barr virus prophylaxis with CMV IgG and ganciclovir for high-risk patients and improved monitoring using Epstein-Barr virus serology and polymerase chain reaction to detect primary Epstein-Barr virus. Tacrolimus-induced posttransplant diabetes mellitus was seen in 10% of the recipients but was readily reversible with gradual dose reduction of tacrolimus and tapering or discontinuing corticosteroids. Posttransplant diabetes mellitus occurs secondary to a direct, reversible effect of tacrolimus in the beta cells of the islets, leading to a decrease in insulin secretion (Tamura *et al.*, 1995). Nephrotoxicity and neurotoxicity were similar to that described with cyclosporine qualitatively and quantitatively (Shapiro *et al.*, 1990).

Tacrolimus has been used as salvage therapy for refractory allograft rejection. Tacrolimus was used in 24 pediatric renal transplant recipients for refractory rejection episodes. The 74% of the patients with refractory rejection were reversed successfully (Jordan *et al.*, 1997). The NAPRTCS (North American Pediatric Renal Transplant Cooperative Study) data show that 10.8% of pediatric recipients in 1997 received tacrolimus-based immunosuppression compared with 79.6% who received cyclosporine (Benfield et al; 1999).

SIROLIMUS

Sirolimus is a macrolide antibiotic isolated from *Streptomyces hygroscopicus* (see also Chapter 19). It is structurally similar to tacrolimus. Sirolimus is a potent inhibitor of T-cell activation. Sirolimus suppresses IL-2-driven or IL-4-driven T-cell proliferation (Calne *et al.*, 1989). Combined treatment with sirolimus and cyclosporine has been reported to act synergistically in prolonging allograft survival in mice (Morris *et al.*, 1990). *In vitro* synergy studies show that sirolimus potentiates the action of cyclosporine (Kahan *et al.*, 1991).

Cyclosporine and tacrolimus selectively block the transcriptional activation of several cytokine genes, inhibiting cytokine production. Sirolimus acts at a later stage in T-cell cycle progression by blocking cytokine-mediated signal transduction pathways. The immunosuppressive mechanism of sirolimus is different from that of cyclosporine and tacrolimus. It is to be expected that the side-effect profile of sirolimus is different from cyclosporine and tacrolimus (Sigal and Dumont, 1992).

In a phase I randomized, double-blind, placebo-controlled study of 16 patients with renal transplants by Brattstorm and colleagues, 12 received sirolimus, and 4 received placebo (Brattstorm *et al.*, 1997). A single dose of 3 to 15 mg/m² was administered orally. Sirolimus was absorbed rapidly with peak whole-blood concentration between 0.5 and 2 hours in all but two patients. The concentration of sirolimus in plasma was below the limit of detection at 6 to 12 hours after the administration of the dose. The whole-blood concentration and the AUC correlated reasonably with the dose. Sirolimus is metabolized extensively, primarily by cytochrome P450 3A4 in the liver and the small intestine (Sattler *et al.*, 1992). Coadministration of sirolimus with cyclosporine may require dose adjustment because they are both metabolized by the cytochrome P450 system. The study events reported were mild dizziness, mild epistaxis and mild elevation in liver enzymes and amylase level.

In another phase I trial, sirolimus facilitated rapid corticosteroid withdrawal from a cyclosporine-based immunosuppressive regimen in stable renal transplant patients (Murgia *et al.*, 1996). The combination of sirolimus with tacrolimus is antagonistic in view of its competition for the FK binding protein.

Evidence suggests that sirolimus may have a unique effect in inhibiting the vasculopathic proliferative lesions associated with immune injury in experimental models of chronic rejection (Morris *et al.*, 1995) and may down-regulate the expression of cytokines and chemokines crucial for chronic transplant injury (Wasowska *et al.*, 1996). This drug may be a prototype of a new class of drugs that inhibit growth factor–mediated events relevant to progressive deterioration of graft function.

A phase III trial of sirolimus has been initiated for pediatric renal transplant recipients by the NAPRTCS. The immunosuppression is a quadruple therapy: induction with anti–IL-2 receptor antibody (basiliximab) followed by either sirolimus, cyclosporine and corticosteroid or mycophenolate mofetil, cyclosporine and corticosteroid. The aim of the study is to ascertain that with more effective immunosuppression, there would be fewer acute rejection episodes, and steroid withdrawal might be facilitated.

ANTILYMPHOCYTE GLOBULIN

Polyclonal antilymphocyte antibody preparations were developed independently by Waksman *et al.* (1961) and Woodruff and Anderson (1963; see also Chapter 20). These preparations were used to induce inhibition in lymphocyte function. Polyclonal immunoglobulins are obtained by injecting animals (mainly horses and rabbits) with human lymphoid cells—B lymphoblasts, peripheral T lymphocytes or thymus lymphocytes—then separating the resulting immune sera to obtain purified globulin fractions.

The polyclonal antibodies achieve immunosuppression by inducing complement-mediated lympholysis, opsonization of lymphocytes and modification of T-cell surface antigens, blocking lymphocyte function (Abouna *et al.*, 1993). These polyclonal antibodies bind to lymphocytes and result in rapid, profound lymphopenia. The number of circulating T cells gradually increases after discontinuation of treatment, although the proliferative response of T cells continues to be impaired.

Antilymphocyte globulin (ALG) is infused over 4 hours through an inline filter into a central vein to minimize local and systemic reactions. Antilymphocyte globulin therapy is monitored by the biological effect on T cells to maintain circulating CD3 lymphocyte numbers at 50 to 100 cells/μl 1 hour after infusion (Kreis *et al.*, 1981). The dosage is 15 mg/kg/dose intravenously for 10 to 14 days. When ALG is used as induction therapy, cyclosporine usually is introduced when serum creatinine is less than 2 mg/dl. Because the ALG is derived from sera pooled from the multiple animals,

there is significant batch-to-batch variability. The antibodies are directed against not only the T cells involved in cellular rejection, but also a variety of T-cell and non–T cell antigens (Cosimi, 1983). Large doses of immunoglobulins are required to achieve the desired clinical effect because only a small amount of total antibody infused reacts with cells of interest. Antilymphocyte globulin also is used for corticosteroid-resistant acute cellular rejection episodes.

Polyclonal immune globulin preparations vary in their constituent antibodies, and treatment may be variable in terms of efficacy and in the incidence and nature of adverse reactions. The potential adverse effects include fever, chills, thrombocytopenia, leukopenia, hemolysis, rash, serum sickness, respiratory distress and rarely anaphylaxis. These adverse reactions may be prevented by premedication with antihistamines and acetaminophen.

MONOCLONAL ANTIBODIES (OKT3)

Muromonab-CD3 is a murine monoclonal anti–T cell antibody directed against the CD3 antigen present on the cell surface of all mature human T lymphocytes (Storm, 1987; see also Chapter 20). Orthoclonal monoclonal antibody OKT3 specifically binds to one of the 20-kd subunits of CD3. The CD3 antigen is associated closely with the T-lymphocyte antigen receptor complex that functions in the recognition of foreign antigens. Binding of OKT3 to the CD3 complex results in the blockade of the antigen receptor complex. OKT3 binding to the lymphocyte cells interferes with the activation, proliferation and differentiation of cytotoxic lymphocytes in response to class I and class II MHC antigens (Kreis *et al.*, 1991; Strom, 1987).

Monoclonal antibodies have several advantages over polyclonal ALG, including more precise specificity of antilymphocyte reactivity, much less batch-to-batch variability that is inherent with ALG preparations and the need to administer much less foreign protein through a peripheral vein. The two notable limitations of OKT3 therapy are development of antimurine antibodies, which restricts a second course of OKT3 therapy, and the adverse reaction routinely experienced with the first dose of OKT3.

OKT3 is administered as an intravenous bolus in a dosage of 5 mg for 10 to 14 days. The intravenous administration of OKT3 leads to the opsonization of T cells and the rapid removal of CD3+ cells from the circulation by reticuloendothelial cells (Cosimi *et al.*, 1981). Numerous adverse effects have been associated with the use of OKT3. A flulike syndrome is well recognized after administration of the first and, to a much lesser extent, the second dose of OKT3 therapy. The onset of symptoms is rapid within a few hours of administration of OKT3; the symptom complex includes fever, chills, headache, dyspnea, chest pain, bronchospasm, nausea, vomiting and diarrhea. Hypotension and hypertension may be seen. The severity of symptoms can be reduced by premedication with steroids and antihistamines, close attention to meticulous fluid balance and surveillance for infectious complications. Life-threatening edema first reported with the use of OKT3 is now prevented by ensuring that the patient has no evidence of volume overload and that the weight of the patient is within 3% of the lowest weight.

OKT3 was introduced as an induction therapy in the attempt to block the initial insult to the target organ by T lymphocytes as well as to attenuate the frequency and severity of rejection episodes that threaten allograft survival. OKT3 was used first in 1980 in a cadaver donor renal allograft recipient at the Massachusetts General Hospital for the treatment of acute rejection.

Similar to the induction therapy based on ALG, most

immunosuppressive regimens combine azathioprine and corticosteroid with the delayed addition of cyclosporine to avoid overimmunosuppression and possible cyclosporine-related nephrotoxicity (Hanto et al., 1994). OKT3 has been used as sequential therapy with cyclosporine, corticosteroid and azathioprine in adult and pediatric renal transplant recipients. The positive impact of OKT3 on the reduction of acute rejection in adult patients (Norman et al., 1988) was not observed in some of the pediatric studies, however (Bartosh et al., 1993). These studies are in contrast to the NAPRTCS data, in which the incidence of acute rejection episodes was significantly reduced with the use of induction therapy (Stablein and Sullivan, 1996).

OKT3 has been used for treatment of allograft rejection unresponsive to pulse methylprednisolone or polyclonal ALG. Goldstein and coworkers reported reversal rates of 65% for OKT3 primary and rescue therapy (Goldstein et al., 1991). In pediatric recipients, OKT3 has been used mainly as rescue therapy for steroid-resistant and/or ALG-resistant rejection.

Different studies and authors report a wide range (27–100%) of development of anti-OKT3 antibodies in the use of OKT3. The use of OKT3 leads to anti-OKT3 antibody formation in 100% of patients. Coadministration of other immunosuppressive agents reduces the formation of antibodies significantly, however (Norman et al., 1991). The presence of low titer of anti-OKT3 does not preclude treatment with OKT3, although higher doses may be necessary to achieve clinical effect. The presence of high titer of anti-OKT3 antibodies (>1/1000) is a contraindication for reuse of OKT3 (Morris et al., 1995). Based on the current literature, the use of monoclonal antibody therapy with OKT3 is recommended for steroid-resistant rejection.

Appropriate immunological monitoring is crucial to the success of OKT3 in children. Regular measurement of the number of $CD3^+$ T cells gives an indication of the effectiveness of OKT3. Most centers aim to achieve a target of less than $20/mm^3$ CD3-bearing T cells as an absolute number or less than 10% of the total number of peripheral lymphocytes (Ettenger et al., 1992c). If the $CD3^+$ T-cell numbers fail to drop or if they show a secondary rise after transiently reaching this goal, the administered dose is ineffective or inadequate, and increased doses may be required. A subgroup of children has been identified who repopulate $CD3^+$ cells so quickly that they require twice-daily dosing with OKT3 (Ettenger et al., 1992c). Other centers monitor OKT3 serum levels, which should remain greater than 800 to 1,000 ng/ml (Ettenger et al., 1992c; Goldstein et al., 1986).

A suboptimal response to OKT3 usually is caused by the presence of anti-OKT3 antibodies. These antibodies may be directed against the combining site of the OKT3 molecule (so-called antiidiotype antibodies), or they may be directed against species-specific determinants on the OKT3 molecule (antimurine antibody). Using an enzyme-linked immunoabsorbent assay technique, antiidiotypic antibodies generally are present in a low titer (<1/100), whereas antimouse antibodies often are present at high-titer levels (1/1000). Leone et al. (1987) found anti-OKT3 antibody in 90% of tested children after OKT3 administered for rejection, whereas our group (Ettenger et al., 1988) found their presence in only 27% of the children treated. When we administered OKT3 in sequential therapy, we found that 43% of the children developed anti-OKT3 antibody; 25% had low-titer antibody, whereas 18% developed high-titer antibody (Ettenger et al., 1992c).

The degree of anti-OKT3 sensitization varies widely in other reported pediatric series. Although Schroeder and associates found only a 27% incidence after rejection treatment (Schroeder et al., 1991), a follow-up study by Leone et al.

(1990) found a rate of 85%. With induction therapy, Niaudet et al. (1990) found a 94% incidence of anti-OKT3 antibodies by the enzyme-linked immunoabsorbent assay technique (Niaudet et al., 1990). Bartosh and coworkers found an incidence of 58%, which is more similar to ours (Bartosh et al., 1992).

ANTI–INTERLEUKIN-2 RECEPTOR ANTIBODY

Significant side effects are seen with mouse CD3 monoclonal antibody because it interacts with all T lymphocytes (Soulillou, 1994). Research has been focused on the development of increasingly selective monoclonal antibodies with the potential to regulate specific immunological responses through functional receptors, reducing side effects (see also Chapter 20).

During transplant rejection, cytokine IL-2 induces the rapid proliferation of T lymphocytes by binding to its high-affinity receptor on the surface of antigen-activated T lymphocytes. The predominant role of the IL-2/IL-2 (CD25) receptor pathway in T-lymphocyte proliferation and the selective expression of CD25 on activated T lymphocytes led to the identification of CD25 as a potential target for monoclonal antibody therapy (Kirkman et al., 1985).

Basiliximab is a chimeric (human and mouse) CD25 monoclonal antibody. Preclinical studies have shown that the high affinity of the murine variable region is maintained after chimerization and that basiliximab competes effectively with IL-2 and inhibits IL-2-driven proliferative responses (Amlot et al., 1995). Phase I and II trials have shown that basiliximab has a long mean terminal half-life of 1 to 2 weeks, and minimal immunogenicity is well tolerated in human allograft recipients and provides CD25 suppression, the duration of which is dose dependent (Kovarik et al., 1996).

In a phase III study using chimeric (human and mouse) CD25 antibody (basiliximab), a 32% reduction in the proportion of patients with biopsy-proven acute rejection episodes with basiliximab compared with placebo (24%) was reported (Nashan et al., 1997). Graft survival rates 12 months after transplantation were similar in the two groups, however. In a phase III trial with a humanized monoclonal antibody (daclizumab), only 28% of patients given daclizumab had one or more episodes of biopsy-proven acute rejection compared with 47% in the placebo group (P<0.001). The number of rejections per patient was also significantly lower, and the time to biopsy-proven acute rejection was significantly longer in the patients in the daclizumab group as compared with placebo. There was no significant difference in graft survival at 12 months between the treatment groups (Nashan et al., 1999). A phase III trial in pediatric recipients is ongoing.

The beneficial effect of these anti–IL-2 receptor antibodies on acute rejection may reflect the complementary modes of action of basiliximab and daclizumab and cyclosporine. Cyclosporine prevents IL-2 gene activation, whereas anti–IL-2 receptor monoclonal antibodies block the stimulation of T lymphocytes by IL-2 (Kupiec-Weglinski et al., 1988).

The most frequently reported adverse effect with the use of anti–IL-2 receptor antibody is infection (Nashan et al., 1997, 1999). The incidence of infection is comparable to that observed with conventional triple-therapy immunosuppression regimens, however. The cytokine release syndrome observed with OKT3 is not seen with the use of anti–IL-2 receptor antibody. There is no reported increased incidence of PTLD with the use of anti–IL-2 receptor antibodies.

Basiliximab is used in a dose of 12 mg/m². The maximum dose is 20 mg. The first dose is administered 2 hours preoperatively intravenously over 30 minutes, and the second dose is administered on postoperative day 4. Daclizumab is administered in a dose of 1 mg/kg intravenously over 15 minutes. Five doses are given at 2-weekly intervals. The first dose is administered immediately before transplantation.

SIDE EFFECTS OF ANTIBODIES

Agents such as OKT3 and ALG that result in nonspecific and profound immunosuppression have many important implications in pediatric renal transplantation. The side effects of the polyclonal preparations are well known in children because these agents have been in wide use for a long time. Because the various available polyclonal preparations are so heterogeneous and difficult to standardize, side effects are varied. Side effects include neutropenia, thrombocytopenia, serum sickness, allergic reactions and increased susceptibility to infections including CMV and Epstein-Barr virus infections and lymphoproliferative disorders (discussed later).

OKT3 has several significant adverse side effects that occur primarily with the first few doses. These side effects appear to be due to transient activation of T lymphocytes on their initial encounter with OKT3. This T-cell activation leads to release of cytokines such as tumor necrosis factor (Gaston et al., 1991). These cytokine-related effects subside once circulating $CD3^+$ cells are depleted. Noncardiogenic pulmonary edema is a serious first-dose effect and may be exacerbated by fluid overload (Ettenger et al., 1992c; Ortho Multicenter Transplant Study Group, 1985). Other first-dose effects include fever, chills, bronchospasm, diarrhea, headache, vomiting, polyserositis and aseptic meningitis. Cytokine release may be implicated in the transient worsening of graft function commonly seen during OKT3 treatment.

The severe early complications included cerebral edema, pulmonary edema, seizure and arrhythmias. An episode of fatal cerebral edema unaccompanied by any central nervous system structural abnormality prompted us to reduce the first two doses of OKT3 in the induction period. With this measure, pulmonary edema was observed in one patient when the standard dose of 5 mg of OKT3 was given on the third day. The administration of high-dose corticosteroids 1 to 3 hours before OKT3 administration is of some help in ameliorating some of the early adverse side effects (Chatenoud et al., 1991). Other measures such as indomethacin (First et al., 1992) or agents that block OKT3-mediated tumor necrosis factor-α release (Gaston et al., 1991) may be helpful in ending these side effects.

Of the pediatric transplant recipients at UCLA who received sequential therapy with OKT3, 15% developed an infectious complication. Although many agents can be responsible for such infections after sequential therapy, CMV infection has emerged at UCLA as a particularly vexing problem. This situation is not surprising given the dependence on cadaver donor transplantation at our center and the preference for the cadaver donors greater than 6 years old because of the associated improved graft survival (discussed earlier). Cytomegalovirus-seronegative patients receiving kidneys from CMV-seropositive donors are at a significantly higher risk of serious disease compared with seropositive recipients. The acquisition of anti-CMV antibody increases with age. Broyer and colleagues found that only 28% of children less than 10 years old were seropositive, whereas almost 60% of those 16 to 20 years old had acquired antibody (Broyer et al., 1987b).

Certain agents have been shown to be effective in preventing primary symptomatic CMV infections. Snydman and associates showed that CMV hyperimmune globulin given prophylactically decreased the severity of CMV disease in seronegative patients receiving lymphoblasts or OKT3 for rejection (Snydman et al., 1991). This study included many pediatric patients. Prophylactic oral acyclovir has been given

successfully in adult renal transplant recipients on sequential therapy (Fletcher et al., 1991).

Another strategy is to use high doses of standard intravenous immune globulin. Certain lots of standard intravenous immune globulin have anti-CMV titers that are half those of the hyperimmune preparations. These lots may be effective in reducing the severity of CMV disease in children at high risk for primary infection. We have employed a protocol under which seven high doses of standard intravenous immune globulin have been administered over 16 weeks to seronegative children receiving sequential therapy and a seropositive cadaver renal transplant. A total of 23 children at risk for primary CMV infection have been treated—87% have had no clinical infection, whereas 9% have had mild symptoms, and only 1 (4%) has had severe CMV disease (Firzli and Ettenger, 1990, unpublished observations). Whatever the strategy chosen, it seems appropriate to initiate some form of anti-CMV prophylaxis as well as other more commonly used antiinfective prophylactic strategies (Mauer et al., 1992) if one is to minimize the increased infection risk that is inherent when using monoclonal or polyclonal agents in children.

Postoperative Medical Complications

INFECTION

The risk of infection, including opportunistic infection, in the renal transplant patient is determined primarily by the interaction of two factors: the epidemiological exposures the patient encounters and the patient's net state of immunosuppression (see also Chapter 31). The immunosuppressive regimens currently employed are accompanied by a well-defined temporal sequence of infections (Rubin, 1993). In the renal transplant patient, three time periods may be specified. In the first month posttransplant, more than 95% of infectious disease syndromes are bacterial in nature. The fact that opportunistic infections are not present in the first month posttransplant, when the dose of immunosuppression is highest, suggests that the duration of immunosuppression rather than the daily dose administered is the major determinant. In the period 1 to 6 months posttransplant, viral infections, most commonly CMV and opportunistic infections with *Pneumocystis carinii*, *Listeria monocytogenes* and *Aspergillus fumigatus*, are common. More than 6 months posttransplant, 75% of recipients have infections similar to the general population; 25% have chronic viral infection or opportunistic infection.

Infections occur with increased frequency and severity in the immunocompromised host, as described in detail in Chapter 31. Bacterial infections account for significant mortality after renal transplantation in children (Avner et al., 1981; Broyer et al., 1987b; Najarian et al., 1986; Potter et al., 1986).

The herpesviruses—CMV, herpesvirus hominids and varicella zoster—are the most frequent viral agent group affecting the graft recipient. Human CMV generally is considered to be the most frequently occurring opportunistic pathogen and the most important infectious agent in renal transplantation. Fine and associates initially reported the occurrence of the CMV syndrome in pediatric recipients (Fine et al., 1972).

The CMV syndrome was manifested by prolonged fever, leukopenia, thrombocytopenia, pulmonary symptoms and hepatic dysfunction. Decreased graft function has been associated with CMV infection (Lopez et al., 1974). Because it takes 2 to 3 weeks to culture the virus from the throat, urine, blood and bone marrow aspirate or to show a rise in the CMV antibody titer, it frequently is difficult to differentiate involvement of this virus from other infections or rejection during the early posttransplant clinical course. Differentiation of CMV infection from rejection is imperative. Reduction in the dosage of corticosteroids and possibly other immunosuppressive agents hastens resolution of the CMV symptoms, whereas increased dosage of corticosteroids or providing other antirejection treatment results in further viral dissemination and prolongs or increases the severity of the clinical abnormalities.

The incidence of individual immune reactivity in pediatric graft recipients increases with age (Broyer *et al.*, 1987a); a higher percentage of young pediatric recipients are CMV negative (no antibody to CMV) at the time of transplantation. Broyer *et al.* (1987a) noted that the incidence of CMV positivity in recipients less than 5 years old was 29.4%, whereas it was 59.3% in those 16 to 20 years old (Broyer *et al.*, 1987a). This finding is important because of the demonstration that transplantation of a kidney from a CMV-positive donor into a CMV-negative recipient is associated with a significant incidence of posttransplant primary CMV infection (Weir *et al.*, 1987). Serial determinations of CMV reactivity of potential recipients before transplantation and assessment of the CMV reactivity of all potential donors are mandatory. Avoidance of transplanting a CMV-positive kidney into a CMV-negative recipient might reduce the incidence of primary CMV infection after transplantation. The CMV status of the donor also appears to be important. Iragorri and colleagues found that the factor that correlated most highly with the development of CMV infection in pediatric renal transplant recipients was seropositivity in the donor (Iragorri *et al.*, 1993). A retrospective analysis of 142 pediatric renal transplant recipients showed that a CMV-seropositive donor represents a risk factor for CMV disease regardless of the recipient's CMV serological status (Bock *et al.*, 1997).

New sensitive techniques permit the recognition of CMV infection at a relatively early stage in children. Direct detection of CMV antigens in peripheral blood leukocytes has proved to be an important step forward in the rapid and early diagnosis of CMV infection. This antigenemia assay is based on the monoclonal antibody–aided demonstration of CMV antigen using immunoperoxide or immunofluorescent staining for the lower matrix phosphoprotein pp65. The antigenemia assay is a quantitiative test and has several advantages for monitoring of active CMV disease: It is rapid (4-5 hours), it has high sensitivity (80–90% for infection, 99–100% for disease) and it has high specificity (93–95%). These techniques include the development of anti-CMV IgM antibody in previously seronegative children and the recognition of CMV antigen or DNA in the blood (Ho, 1991). Reliable quantification of the polymerase chain reaction signal is not routinely available, however, and the antigenemia assay may be superior for monitoring purposes.

Ganciclovir has become the mainstay of treatment for CMV. Experience with children is limited. The recommended dosage in children is 5 mg/kg every 12 hours, with strict dosage adjustments for diminution of renal function (Nevins and Dunn, 1992). Neutropenia and thrombocytopenia are the most frequent adverse effects, but liver enzyme and serum creatinine elevations may occur. In preliminary data, there have been no fatalities when ganciclovir has been administered in transplanted children, and in children who relapsed, recovery occurred with retreatment (Nevins and Dunn, 1992).

Cytomegalovirus prophylaxis in children has been discussed earlier. Hyperimmune CMV globulin was beneficial in children who participated in the randomized trial of Snydman *et al.* (1991). In eight children in the placebo control group, seven developed CMV syndrome, and three died. In the group treated with hyperimmune CMV globulin, only 5 of 13 developed CMV syndrome, and no patients died (Har-

mon, 1991). Based on these and other studies, appropriate prophylaxis, by immune globulin or antiviral chemotherapy, is warranted in the child at risk for primary infection (Gagnadoux *et al.*, 1993; Hibberd and Rubin, 1991).

The NAPRTCS (Bock *et al.*, 1997) retrospective analysis data show that 12 months posttransplant incidence of patients hospitalized with CMV was 56%. Prophylaxis with anti-CMV IgG reduced the risk of CMV hospitalization significantly (*P*<0.03). The prophylatic use of antiviral agents was associated with a decreased risk of major organ involvement during the CMV infection (*P*<0.005). Graft survival was significantly better for patients who received any form of prophylaxis compared with patients without any prophylaxis (88% *vs.* 52%, *P*<0.001).

Lowance *et al.* (1999) reported the results of the International Valacyclovir CMV Prophylaxis Transplant Study group. Treatment with valacyclovir orally for 90 days posttransplant reduced the incidence or delayed the onset of CMV disease in seronegative patients (*P*<0.001) and seropositive patients (*P* = 0.03). Despite these data with valacyclovir, ganciclovir still remains the standard of treatment for CMV disease.

Fine and colleagues reported the benign course of varicella in an 8-year-old graft recipient who was receiving 5 mg of prednisone and 50 mg of azathioprine daily (Fine *et al.*, 1969a). Hurley and associates reported two cases of varicella in 76 pediatric recipients over a 5-year period (Hurley *et al.*, 1980). One recipient died with massive upper gastrointestinal bleeding. Feldhoff and coworkers described 19 episodes of varicella in 160 pediatric recipients during an 11-year period (Feldhoff *et al.*, 1981). Eight of the recipients had severe infection, and one died. These investigators correlated the continuation of azathioprine with severity of infection. It was recommended that azathioprine be discontinued with the onset of symptoms and that it not be reinstituted until 24 to 48 hours after new crops of vesicles cease.

If a child without humoral immunity to varicella zoster is exposed to chickenpox, he or she should receive varicella-zoster immune globulin (Mauer *et al.*, 1992) preferably within 72 hours of the exposure. If chickenpox develops, intravenous acyclovir needs to be instituted without delay. Lynfield and coworkers reported their experience with eight children with renal transplants who required hospitalization for primary varicella (Lynfield *et al.*, 1992). Despite treatment with high-dose intravenous acyclovir, two died. Harmon *et al.* (1991) reported good results with intravenous acyclovir. similar experience. Despite varicella-zoster immune globulin prophylaxis and early aggressive acyclovir treatment, chickenpox can have serious and even fatal consequences.

Kashtan and coworkers reported the outcome of varicella in 66 pediatric renal transplant recipients in the years 1984–1996 (Kashtan *et al.*, 1996). They treated these patients with discontinuation of azathioprine and hospitalization with administration of intravenous acyclovir (500 mg/m² every 8 hours with dose adjustment for renal function), and azathioprine was resumed at 50% of the original dose when all lesions were crusted and increased to full dose in 3 to 5 days. Varicella-zoster immune globulin was administered in 27 of 69 cases. No deaths occurred in patients treated with this regimen. Acute rejection followed chickenpox in 3 of 68 cases in the study, and no grafts were lost as a result of these rejection episodes.

Varicella can be fatal and can have serious implications in children who have no history of the disease or who have no humoral immmunity to varicella despite treatment with varicella-zoster immune globulin and acyclovir. Based on the aforementioned studies, Broyer and associates suggested that pretransplant assessment of immunity to varicella should be undertaken, and children without humoral antibodies for varicella should be vaccinated before transplantation (Broyer et al., 1987b). This group started routine active immunization against varicella to seronegative children before renal transplant as soon as the vaccine was available in 1980. Such a procedure led to a dramatic decline in the incidence of posttransplant varicella infection. The varicella vaccine (Gershon et al., 1986) is not approved for use in all areas of the world.

Broyer et al. in 1997 reported the long-term results of varicella vaccination in 704 pediatric renal transplant recipients in the period 1973–1992. Patients were divided into three groups: group A, 49 naive patients; group B, 415 patients with a history of varicella and positive serology and group C, 212 patients who received varicella immunization. A total of 22 naive patients developed varicella at a mean time interval of 4.5 ± 3.8 years posttransplant. Four of 415 patients in group B developed varicella. In the vaccinated group C, the prevalence of varicella was 12%, which was significantly lower than in the group of naive patients ($P<0.001$).

Furth and colleagues reported 44 of 2,320 pediatric renal transplant recipients requiring hospitalization for varicella in the prevaccine era (Furth et al., 2000). Three of 44 patients developed varicella in the first posttransplant year; 3 had graft failure, and 1 died within the follow-up period. The cause of death was sleep apnea 4 years after varicella infection. There was no evidence of increased risk of acute rejection episodes or long-term allograft dysfunction as sequelae of varicella in the first posttransplant year. No mortality related to varicella was reported in the first year posttransplant.

The effect of varicella zoster immunity in recipients treated with cyclosporine was detailed in a longitudinal study of pediatric recipients by Trachtman et al. (1986). Humoral and cell-mediated immunity to varicella zoster was assessed serially in 25 renal graft recipients 4 to 21 years old who received cyclosporine and prednisone. Humoral immunity to varicella zoster remained intact posttransplant, whereas cell-mediated immunity declined in the immediate posttransplant period and returned gradually to pretreatment values by 9 to 12 months. The clinical significance of these data could not be assessed because only one recipient was exposed to varicella, received varicella-zoster immune globulin prophylaxis and subsequently developed mild varicella. These workers concluded that their data would not preclude live-attenuated varicella vaccine pretransplant in susceptible recipients who are going to receive cyclosporine immunosuppression. The 33% prevalence rate of susceptibility indicates the urgent need to make the vaccine universally available. A study is under way by the NAPRTCS to assess the safety and efficacy of varicella vaccine posttransplant in patients without adequate protection against varicella.

Influenza, a common respiratory virus, has been shown to cause substantial morbidity and mortality in immunosuppressed transplant recipients (Mauch et al., 1999). Edvardson and coworkers prospectively studied the efficacy of influenza vaccine in 47 ± 18 pediatric renal transplant recipients in two phases: 1990–1991 and 1991–1992 (Edvardson et al., 1996). Influenza vaccination produced equivalent humoral immunity in transplant recipients and normal subjects, indicating that vaccination was as effective in this population as in normal subjects. Vaccination did not increase the frequency of acute allograft rejection. These authors recommend that routine vaccination against influenza is safe, may protect against infection and should be performed annually in this high-risk population. Furth and coworkers reported that pediatric renal transplant recipients develop an adequate antibody response to pneumococcal vaccine and retain adequate

serum antibody levels 1 year after vaccination (Furth et al., 1996). For some serotypes, however, 40% of patients may not retain protective levels of antibody.

Pulmonary involvement after transplantation is a potentially devastating infectious complication. The infectious agent can be bacterial (Legionella), viral (CMV), fungal (Nocardia, Candida, Aspergillus) or parasitic (Pneumocystis). Because it is difficult to differentiate the causative organism on the basis of radiological appearance, it is frequently necessary to perform a transtracheal aspiration or open-lung biopsy. At times, more than one agent (CMV and Pneumocystis) is involved. The prophylactic administration of trimethoprim-sulfamethoxazole preparations has reduced the occurrence of Pneumocystis significantly in the immunocompromised host (Hughes, 1977; N Engl J Med, 1993).

Hepatic dysfunction (see also Chapter 32) after transplantation may be related to azathioprine toxicity (Malekzadeh et al., 1972), viral hepatitis, CMV, herpesvirus hominus or hepatitis A, B or C (Aronoff et al., 1973; Ware et al., 1975). Children who develop persistent hepatitis B antigenemia during dialysis are acceptable candidates for transplantation (Fine et al., 1977b), although the potential for transmission of the virus should be considered and appropriate precautions taken because more than 90% are hepatitis E antigen positive (Ettenger et al., 1980). No evidence of progressive liver disease has occurred in pediatric recipients with persistent antigenemia (Fennell et al., 1981; Fine et al., 1977b) as has been reported in adult patients. We are aware, however, of two patients who died of hepatic failure after having hepatitis B infection as pediatric renal transplant recipients more than 15 years previously. It is possible that a long period is necessary for progressive liver disease to evolve into hepatitis B. This appears to be the experience at other large pediatric centers as well (Mauer et al., 1992). It is important to immunize children with ESRD with hepatitis vaccine.

Until the development in 1989 of an assay to detect antibody against the recombinant viral antigen of hepatitis C (c100–3) (Choo et al., 1989), the cause of liver disease in most ESRD patients was not clear. Since then, the role of hepatitis C virus (HCV) in acute and chronic liver disease and hepatocellular carcinoma has become better understood (Bruix et al., 1989; Columbo et al., 1989). The transmission of HCV by the transfusion of blood products has been shown unequivocally, and preliminary data suggest that sexual, vertical and intrafamilial spread also occur (Giovannini et al., 1990; Hess et al., 1989; Perez-Romero et al., 1990).

Organ transplantation can transmit HCV. Hepatitis C developed in 14 of 29 (48%) recipients of organs from donors positive for anti-HCV antibodies, a prevalence 7.4 times the 6.5% prevalence after transplantation from untested donors that was reported previously (Pereira et al., 1991). The liver disease began in these recipients a mean of 3.8 months posttransplantation and became chronic in 12 patients. The other two patients had subfulminant hepatic failure. Liver disease was more frequent in the patients who had received antilymphocyte preparations. The more severe course and more rapid progression of posttransplantation liver disease may be due to the impairment of host defenses by immunosuppression. As in the case of CMV and HIV, donors can be pretested for HCV, and if positive, their kidneys are not used for transplantation.

Studies using polymerase chain reaction showed the presence of HCV RNA in serum specimens and have reemphasized the risk of HCV transmission by an affected allograft. When an organ from an HCV RNA–positive donor was transplanted into an HCV RNA–negative recipient, the incidence of posttransplant HCV infection was 100% (Pereira et al., 1991). The U.S. Public Health Service (1991) recommends limiting the use of organs from anti-HCV positive donors for only life-saving procedures (liver, heart or lung transplants) and not for renal transplantation.

A more subtle finding is the effect that HCV infection may have on immunosuppression in cyclosporine-treated patients. We have observed that children with evidence of mild HCV infection may have an unexpectedly high level of cyclosporine metabolites in relation to the parent compound when cyclosporine blood levels are monitored (Sanchez and Ettenger, unpublished observations). When cyclosporine levels are measured, it is important not to rely solely on polyclonal antibody–based testing because of the potential overestimation of immunosuppression. We noted an increased incidence of rejection when we relied on polyclonal-based testing and found that it was important to use tests of cyclosporine blood levels that measured only parent compound (e.g., high-pressure liquid chromatography).

The HIV epidemic has involved the renal graft recipient. At least one pediatric graft recipient has developed acquired immunodeficiency syndrome (AIDS) and Kaposi's sarcoma (Malekzadeh et al., 1987b). Transmission of HIV after transplantation of kidneys from infected donors has been reported (L'Age-Stehr et al., 1985; Neumayer et al., 1986; Prompt et al., 1985). At present, we are testing all pediatric recipients awaiting transplantation. If a potential recipient is HIV positive, we believe that with our current state of knowledge and the lack of a definitive anti-HIV agent that transplantation in such HIV-positive potential recipients is contraindicated.

HYPERTENSION

The prevalence of posttransplant hypertension in pediatric recipients was found to be 86% in 86 and 75 recipients reported by Ingelfinger (1984) and Tejani (1983) and 85% in 334 pediatric cadaver donor recipients reported by Broyer et al. (1987a; see also Chapter 30). Stablein and Sullivan (1996) for the NAPRTCS report that 70% of cadaver donor pediatric transplant recipients and about 55% of living related donor recipients were on antihypertensive therapy 7 years post-transplant. An elevated blood pressure occurs under varying circumstances in pediatric graft recipients (Malekzadeh et al., 1975). In the immediate posttransplant period, hypertension usually is related to hypervolemia, especially in the patient with acute tubular necrosis and minimal urinary output. Hypertension is a frequent concomitant occurrence with acute rejection and usually resolves with reversal of the rejection episode. Similarly, varying degrees of hypertension accompany chronic rejection. Control of hypertension is required with antihypertensive medication, and lack of control may be related to the rapidity of deterioration of graft function. Opelz and colleagues showed a striking association between systolic and diastolic blood pressure levels and graft survival and found that posttransplant blood pressure was a highly significant predictor of long-term graft survival (Opelz et al., 1998).

The causes of persistent posttransplant hypertension in the 109 affected pediatric recipients reported by Broyer et al. (1987a) were as follows: chronic rejection (59%); renal artery stenosis (20.5%); native kidney (4.5%); recurrence of primary renal disease (4.5%), which included MPGN (4 cases), FGS (4 cases) and periarteritis nodosa (1 case); nonviable kidney (1.5%) and no obvious cause (10%). There was no evidence that a large kidney transplanted into a small child who was then potentially exposed to hypoperfusion accounted for any increased frequency of hypertension. The onset of hypertension in association with declining renal function during the initial 3 to 12 months posttransplant, or any time thereafter, may indicate the development of renal artery stenosis (Ma-

lekzadeh et al., 1975). The clinical findings frequently mimic those of acute rejection.

The incidence of renal artery stenosis was 12% in the report of Broyer et al. (1987a) and 6.9% in the report of Malekzadeh et al. (1987b); however, renal artery stenosis was not noted in any recipient of a living related donor graft in the report of Broyer et al. (1987a), and if only the 400 cadaver donor grafts were included, the incidence was 8%. In both reports (Broyer et al., 1987a; Malekzadeh et al., 1987b), grafts from pediatric cadaver donors less than 2 years old were identified as a significant risk factor for the development of renal artery stenosis. Eleven of 31 grafts with renal artery stenosis were from donors in this age group in the report of Malekzadeh et al. (1987b). An additional risk factor identified by Broyer et al. (1987a) was a urinary leak.

Diagnosis of renal artery stenosis is by angiography, and the therapeutic options include surgical repair, transluminal angioplasty (Barth et al., 1981) and antihypertensive drug therapy. Surgical repair was successful in 14 of 21 (66%) attempts in the report of Malekzadeh et al. (1987b) and in 5 of 10 (50%) cases in the report of Broyer et al. (1987a). The incidence of graft loss associated with surgical intervention was 25% and 50% in the latter two reports. Transluminal angioplasty was attempted in eight recipients in the report of Broyer et al. (1987a) and in four recipients in the report of Malekzadeh et al. (1987b), with a success rate of 37.5% and 25% and a graft loss in 12.5% and 25%. Antihypertensive therapy was the sole treatment in 25 recipients reported by Broyer et al. (1987a).

Complete healing with the disappearance of the stenosis on repeat angiography occurred in nine (36%) recipients; improvement in the degree of hypertension was noted in an additional five (20%) recipients, loss of grafts in two (8%) recipients and persistence of hypertension in eight recipients. Because the conservative approach appears to yield results equal to or better than those obtained with the two invasive procedures, the conservative approach should be the treatment of choice for renal artery stenosis, resorting to either invasive procedure only if significant evidence of end-organ disease is present in association with an inability to control the level of hypertension adequately. Diagnostic angiography is probably indicated only if it is necessary to distinguish between renal artery stenosis and rejection or if a therapeutic invasive procedure is contemplated.

The development of hypertension in the recipient with intact native kidneys presents a difficult diagnostic dilemma. Differential plasma renin determinations generally are not helpful in delineating the cause of the hypertension (Curtis et al., 1981). Broyer and associates indicated that in 10 pediatric recipients hypertension was believed to be related to the native kidney when the ratio of vena cava and renal veins to kidney transplant renin was greater than 2 (Broyer et al., 1987a). Native kidney removal should be considered only if the hypertension fails to respond to antihypertensive agents such as nifedipine, captopril and minoxidil (Curtis et al., 1981); the embolization of native kidneys (discussed in Chapter 28) may be an approach particularly appropriate for the hypertensive child.

Although angiotensin-converting enzyme inhibitors are effective in lowering blood pressure in graft recipients, it is important to be aware of their potential deleterious effect on graft function. Reduction in renal function has been described in recipients with renal artery stenosis, which is attributable to the intrarenal hemodynamic effects of captopril (Curtis et al., 1983). We observed similar findings in recipients who were hypertensive without demonstrable renal artery stenosis. If the serum creatinine level increases concomitant with captopril therapy, it is important to discontinue the captopril and to obtain serial determinations of graft function before initiating additional diagnostic or therapeutic strategies.

Gagnadoux and colleagues treated 27 pediatric recipients with renal artery stenosis with captopril (Gagnadoux et al., 1985). In 12 (44%) patients, treatment was effective without concomitant change in renal function. In the remaining cases, 50% had a moderate and 50% had a severe reduction in graft function associated with blood pressure control. Captopril dosage did not appear to be a risk factor for precipitating a decline in graft function; however, preexisting renal function impairment and greater than 75% narrowing of the renal artery stenosis were identified as risk factors. One risk factor was sodium depletion primarily related to diuretic administration. Of 14 recipients who manifested a decline in graft function after captopril treatment in a setting of sodium depletion, 11 received captopril after salt repletion and/or discontinuation of diuretics without manifesting any subsequent decline in graft function.

Surveillance for the development of hypertension in the pediatric recipient with prompt therapeutic intervention is imperative because of the potential for catastrophic complications. Of the 299 (12%) recipients with posttransplant hypertension, 39 had significant complications, including hypertensive encephalopathy (25) resulting in prolonged coma (10), cerebral hemorrhage (7) resulting in death (3) or severe neurological impairment (3) and death from congestive heart failure and pulmonary edema (3) (Broyer et al., 1987a). Sixteen (46%) of the 35 hypertensive complications occurred in close juxtaposition to increased corticosteroid therapy for rejection.

Previous investigations of ambulatory blood pressure monitoring have indicated that casual blood pressure measurements taken at home or in the office are not representative of average blood pressure in children with chronic renal failure or posttransplantation (Lingens et al., 1997). Krull and coworkers performed ambulatory blood pressure monitoring in 84 children at median intervals of 9.4 years posttransplant (Krull et al., 1993). Of 84 patients, 71 were on antihypertensive treatment. Of patients, 20% were still found to have blood pressure greater than 2 SD above normal blood pressure levels on antihypertensive therapy.

Lingens and colleagues studied 27 children with ambulatory blood pressure monitoring and found a reduced nocturnal dip in blood pressure associated with an underlying renovascular or renoparenchymal pathology (Lingens et al., 1997). Ambulatory blood pressure monitoring detected attenuated or inverse nocturnal dipping of mean arterial blood pressure in 30% of patients with renal transplant. Calzolan and associates studied 30 patients, 20 on antihypertensive therapy and 10 not on antihypertensive therapy, with ambulatory blood pressure monitoring (Calzolan et al., 1998). Using casual blood pressure data, 10 of 20 (50%) were high normal or hypertensive compared with 15 of 20 (75%) who were high normal or hypertensive using ambulatory blood pressure monitoring. Similarly, of the 10 patients not on any antihypertensive therapy, 3 of 10 (33%) were high normal or hypertensive with casual blood pressure monitoring and 4 of 10 (40%) were high normal or hypertensive with ambulatory blood pressure monitoring. Close monitoring with ambulatory blood pressure monitoring is desirable in children who are at greater risk of developing hypertension posttransplant. Hypertension is common in children receiving cyclosporine immunosuppression, occurring in 80% of patients (Hoyer et al., 1990). Its pathogenesis and management were discussed earlier.

CORTICOSTEROID TOXICITY

The development of posterior subcapsular lenticular opacities is related to the dosage of corticosteroids in pediatric

recipients (Fine et al., 1975). An incidence of 55% has been reported in pediatric recipients with a functioning graft for more than 1 year (Wilson and Fine, 1979). Visual impairment is rare; however, once it occurs, cataract removal is necessary.

Excessive weight gain after transplantation is partially attributable to the appetite-stimulating effects of corticosteroids. In the adolescent recipient, obesity has adverse psychoemotional effects. It is understandable that the child who had a severely restricted dietary intake during the course of chronic renal failure as well as during the period of dialysis would have the tendency to eat excessively once the restraints were removed.

Hyperlipidemia was present in two thirds of the pediatric graft recipients studied by Pennisi et al. (1976). About 50% of the patients studied by Saldanha et al. (1976) had abnormal lipoprotein electrophoretic patterns evenly divided between types II and IV. A direct correlation between the degree of hypercholesterolemia and corticosteroid dosage was reported by Pennisi et al. (1976). This relationship was not substantiated by the data of Broyer et al. (1987b). Because there is a potential relationship between hyperlipidemia and premature cardiovascular disease, it seems prudent to attempt to maintain the serum lipid levels within normal limits posttransplantation. The risk factors for accelerated atherosclerosis were assessed by Goldstein et al. (1984). Assay of apolipoproteins AI, AII and B revealed a uniform increase in AI and AII as well as an increase in the AII/B ratio, with only an increase in apolipoprotein B in patients manifesting hypercholesterolemia. The AI/B ratio was normal or decreased in the latter recipients and increased in others. These apolipoprotein data indicated that two thirds of the recipients had negative risk factors for development of accelerated atherosclerosis. Exercise may be effective adjunctive therapy (Goldberg et al., 1979) in recipients with increased factors.

Little is known about the long-term cardiovascular status of pediatric renal transplant recipients in whom newer modes of immunosuppression were employed. It is worrisome to observe that in all time periods after successful transplantation, the mean serum cholesterol levels in pediatric renal transplant recipients at UCLA exceeded the 185 mg/dl at-risk level for children (Ettenger et al., 1990). Because cardiovascular disease is one of the greatest causes of posttransplant morbidity, it may be important to address this in the pediatric transplant recipient as well.

We examined lipid profiles in children on cyclosporine-based immunosuppression and found that greater than 60% had significant elevation in total cholesterol, low-density lipoprotein cholesterol or triglyceride levels. These elevations did not correlate with corticosteroid dosage, cyclosporine dosage or body mass index (Sager and Ettenger, unpublished observations). Given these findings and the risk of cardiovascular disease, it seems appropriate to consider trials in children of lipid-lowering agents.

New immunosuppressive agents have been added to the therapeutic arsenal. These agents are in different phases of trials and probably will result in major changes in immunosuppressive protocols in the future. There is no evidence that tacrolimus (Shapiro et al., 1991) or mycophenolate mofetil (Hoffmann-La Roche, unpublished data) affects lipoprotein metabolism. Results suggest an asssociation between sirolimus treatment and increases in cholesterol concentrations (Murgia et al., 1996).

ASEPTIC NECROSIS

Aseptic necrosis of bone has been reported to develop in 11 of 171 (6%) pediatric recipients by Uittenbogaart et al. (1978), in 11 of 100 (11%) pediatric recipients by Potter et al.

(1978) and in 6 of 29 (21%) pediatric recipients by Hely *et al.* (1982). However, the prevalence is currently lower with the increased use of steroid-sparing regimens. Any bone may be affected; however, the femoral heads (hips) or femoral condyles (knees) are involved most commonly, with multiple bone involvement a common occurrence. Of the 28 recipients affected in the three reports detailing aseptic necrosis in pediatric recipients, one femoral head was involved in 6 patients, both femoral heads in 3, both femoral condyles in 7 and both femoral heads and femoral condyles in 6; multiple bone involvement occurred in 6, including the femoral heads in 3. Of the 28 recipients, 18 had at least involvement of the femoral head.

Pain was usually the initial clinical manifestation, and symptoms antedated radiological confirmation by 9 months. Occasionally, asymptomatic evidence of aseptic necrosis was detected by routine radiological examination.

The cause of aseptic necrosis is unknown; however, a relationship to corticosteroid therapy has been postulated. In the three reports detailing aseptic necrosis in pediatric graft recipients, no correlation between corticosteroid dosage and development of aseptic necrosis was found. Preexistent or persistent secondary hyperparathyroidism also has been implicated in the development of aseptic necrosis. Although all patients had evidence of preexisting renal osteodystrophy in the report of Uittenbogaart *et al.* (1978), the posttransplant serum calcium and phosphorus levels were not significantly different from levels of recipients without aseptic necrosis. Potter and coworkers noted lower serum phosphorus levels in their recipients who developed aseptic necrosis, however (Potter *et al.*, 1978). It has been our impression that the incidence of aseptic necrosis has decreased concomitant with a reduction in the dosage of corticosteroids given to patients as well as an improvement in management of pretransplant osteodystrophy. Prevention of aseptic necrosis by minimizing the dosage of corticosteroids prescribed and effecting a resolution of osseous disease before transplantation is advisable.

Once aseptic necrosis occurs, treatment is directed toward alleviation of symptoms. Adjustment of the corticosteroid dosage once aseptic necrosis has evolved is of little therapeutic benefit. No specific therapy is usually necessary, unless the femoral head is involved. In our experience, total hip replacement is the treatment of choice for aseptic necrosis of the femoral head that is associated with continued symptoms. It is advantageous to proceed with surgery before the patient develops psychological morbidity from persistent symptoms.

DE NOVO MALIGNANCY

The incidence of malignancy after transplantation in pediatric recipients has not been described in detail. Data on the incidence of malignancies in long-term survivors are lacking (Donckerwolcke and Kinderziekenhuis, 1991). Specific reports from pediatric centers in the United States, Canada, Europe and Australia detailing the incidence and type of malignancy are listed in Table 37–9. The three cases with lymphoma reported by Najarian *et al.* (1986) were related to Epstein-Barr virus infection. Two of the three patients in these cases had received total lymphoid radiation.

The 1998 report of the NAPRTCS identified 92 malignancies in 5,173 children receiving renal transplants during the 10-year period 1987-1997 (NAPRTCS, 1998). Of the 92 malignancies, 71 were confirmed. Of the 71 confirmed cases, 15 were nonlymphoproliferative, and 56 were proliferative. Of the lymphoproliferative cases, 36 were PTLD, 14 were lymphoma, 5 were immunoblastic sarcoma and 1 was leukemia. The nonlymphoproliferative diagnoses included carcinoma

TABLE 37–9

MALIGNANCY IN PEDIATRIC ALLOGRAFT RECIPIENTS

Author	No. Patients	Follow-up (y)	Malignancy (No. Cases)
Weil *et al.* (1976)	57	13	Reticulum cell sarcoma of brain
Martin *et al.* (1979)	77	12.5	None
Arbus *et al.* (1980) Chantler *et al.* (1980)	78	10	Hepatocarcinoma
Novello and Fine (1982)	75	10	Rhabdomyosarcoma
	257	14.5	Lymphoangiomatosis Rhabdomyosarcoma of prostate Adenocarcinoma of thyroid Carcinoma *in situ* of cervix (2) Basal cell carcinoma of skin (2)
Potter *et al.* (1986)	203	20	Skin cancer
Najarian *et al.* (1986)	304	18	Lymphoma (3)
Broyer *et al.* (1987b)	358	11	None

(10), sarcoma (3), melanoma (1) and neuroblastoma (1). The diagnosis was made less than 1 to 18 months posttransplant, and 8 of the 16 recipients were surviving 6 to 54 months posttransplant.

Posttransplant lymphoproliferative disease has generated great concern in the transplant community and particularly in pediatrics. At one large center, the frequency of PTLD was 4% in children and 0.8% in adults (Ho *et al.*, 1988). Much evidence links Epstein-Barr virus infection with its development. Patients with primary Epstein-Barr virus infections seem to be at greatest risk (Melosky *et al.*, 1992). In one study, 43% of patients who developed tumors had primary Epstein-Barr virus infections compared with only 8% in a population of patients without tumors ($P > 0.01$) (Ho *et al.*, 1985).

Fewer than 10% of adult transplant candidates are seronegative for Epstein-Barr virus and at risk for primary infection after transplantation (Ho, 1987). Young children are more likely to be seronegative (>80%) for Epstein-Barr virus and are at a greater risk for developing PTLD because pretransplant seronegative status for EBV is identified as one of the risk factors (Nalensik *et al.*, 1988).

Posttransplant lymphoproliferative disease appears to be a condition involving several sequential stages: (1) moderate proliferation of many B-cell clones; (2) oligoclonal proliferation of B cells and plasma cells and organ infiltration and (3) oligoclonal or monoclonal proliferation of B cells and plasma cells, in enormous amount, with escape from all regulatory influences. The two initial stages appear to be reversible, provided that immunosuppression is reduced. The last stage seems to be irreversible, even with the more aggressive therapies given in lymphomas (Touraine *et al.*, 1985). Early diagnosis of this condition is crucial for a complete recovery. The average time of occurrence of PTLD has decreased from 42 months to 11 months as a result of more potent immunosuppressive drugs used today. Posttransplant lymphoproliferative disease in children commonly presents in the head and neck region (Hammer *et al.*, 1998; Lattyak *et al.*, 1998). It may also present as a benign infectious mononucleosis–like syndrome, as an extranodal tumor mass in the gastrointestinal or central nervous system or as diffuse disease involving multiple systems.

Patients at risk for primary infection are identified by measuring pretransplant sera for antibodies to Epstein-Barr virus. Should a vaccine against the virus be developed, seronegative transplant recipients would be candidates for immunization. Posttransplant close monitoring by polymerase chain reaction helps in early diagnosis and early intervention. The other risk factor identified is the mismatch between donor and recipient (i.e., CMV-seropositive donor and CMV-seronegative recipient) (Walker, 1995). The other preventive strategy may be to select an appropriate donor and recipient match. This strategy may not be feasible, however, with an acute shortage of organs for transplantation. Morbidity resulting from EBV may be reduced by administration of immunoglobulins or specific antivirals, or both, in the immediate posttransplant period (Ho, 1995).

Sequential therapy in children has raised concern about the development of PTLD because there appears to be a relationship to intensive immunosuppression (Melosky et al., 1992), especially in heart transplant recipients (Swinnen et al., 1990). In an analysis of our experience with sequential therapy, we found that the cumulative doses of OKT3 were far below those reported by Swinnen et al. (1990), even when normalized by weight (Ettenger et al., 1992b). Nevertheless, others have reported the occurrence of PTLD in children (Ettenger et al., 1992a). It is likely that the posttransplant malignancies in general and lymphoproliferative syndrome specifically are related most closely to the intensity of the immunosuppression (Penn, 1990). Although one of the principles of sequential therapy is augmented immunosuppression, prudence and restraint are indicated when treating recalcitrant rejection episodes.

Growth and Pubertal Development

The anticipation that a successful renal transplant would be accompanied by significant improvement in growth velocity has not uniformly come to fruition. Pennisi and coworkers assessed growth in 41 long-term (3–8 years posttransplant) graft recipients receiving daily corticosteroids (Pennisi et al., 1978c). Normal growth was noted in only 12.5% of the recipients. The factors implicated in the lack of uniform increase in linear height posttransplantation have been growth potential at the time of transplantation, chronological age at the time of transplantation, graft function and corticosteroid dosage.

Bosque and associates evaluated growth of 46 children with a bone age of less than 15 years who received an initial renal transplant between 1975 and 1980 (Bosque et al., 1983). All recipients were maintained on alternate-day therapy after 6 months posttransplant. The average growth for the 46 children was normal after transplantation with a mean SDS of $+0.7 \pm 0.3$ (standard error of the mean) for boys and -0.3 ± 0.3 (standard error of the mean) for girls, and 25 of the children exhibited accelerated growth. At the time of the report, most of the children were growth retarded with a mean SDS between -2.0 and -3.0. In 11 prepubertal children, these workers found no relationship among GFR, alternate-day therapy dose or plasma phosphate level and posttransplant growth.

The lack of correlation among corticosteroid dosage, graft function and growth in prepubertal recipients was confirmed by van Diemen-Steenvoorde and coworkers in an analysis of long-term growth from three centers in the Netherlands (van Diemen-Steenvoorde et al., 1987). Despite normal growth after transplantation in 60% of the prepubertal recipients, 55% were growth retarded at the initiation of puberty. The reports of Bosque et al. (1983) and van Diemen-Steenvoorde et al. (1987) challenged the concept that corticosteroid dosage and level of graft function are important factors influencing posttransplant growth.

Grushkin and Fine (1973) initially documented that chil-

dren with a bone age of less than 12 years at transplantation grew minimally, if at all, after transplantation. This finding subsequently was confirmed by Pennisi et al. (1978c) in recipients receiving daily corticosteroids and by Hoda et al. (1975) in recipients receiving alternate-day therapy. Data from the EDTA Pediatric Registry (Donckerwolcke et al., 1978) and the report of Bosque et al. (1983) have been contradictory. The report of van Diemen-Steenvoorde et al. (1987) noted that recipients who had entered puberty before transplantation and had a bone age of 13.8 ± 1.4 years at the time of transplantation had a significant height increment after transplantation. Substantial growth was noted after transplantation, despite a bone age greater than 12 years. Aschendorff et al. (1990) evaluated the final adult height in 20 adolescents with a chronological age of 10.5 to 17 years and a bone age of greater than 12 years at transplantation who were treated with cyclosporine-prednisone or azathioprine-prednisone. The annual growth rate in the cyclosporine group (3.0 cm/y) was double that of the azathioprine group (1.4 cm/y), and the predicted adult height was exceeded by 1.3 cm in the cyclosporine group but was missed by 3.9 cm in the azathioprine group. Target heights were not achieved in either group. The reasons for these discrepant data are not apparent; however, it appears that the bone age at transplantation may be less crucial for posttransplant growth in the cyclosporine era than previously indicated.

Ingelfinger and coworkers noted improved growth after transplantation in children who received a graft before age 7 years (Ingelfinger et al., 1981). The importance of chronological age was verified by Miller et al. (1982). Six of 10 children transplanted between 11 and 45 months old had either normal or catch-up growth after transplantation. These investigators advocated early transplantation in young children with chronic renal failure to maximize posttransplant growth potential.

The adverse effect of impaired graft function on growth after transplantation was initially emphasized by Pennisi et al. (1979). Recipients with a GFR less than 60 ml/min/1.73 m^2 grew poorly after transplantation. Measurement of somatomedin activity in graft recipients has shown a good correlation with GFR. Relatively minimal reduction in graft function may mediate growth impairment by decreased somatomedin activity.

The precise mechanism by which corticosteroids suppress growth is unknown. Corticosteroids suppress pituitary growth hormone (GH) release, down-regulate hepatic GH receptors, inhibit insulin–like growth factor (IGF) bioactivity and alter levels of insulin–like growth factor (Tonshoff and Mehls, 1996). An additional mechanism postulated for steroid-induced growth inhibition is a direct inhibitory effect on cartilage in reducing collagen synthesis and bone formation (Allen and Goldberg, 1992). In an animal model, administration of dexamethasone led to 40 to 60% reduction in the insulin–like growth factor-I mRNA levels, suggesting that corticosteroid-induced reduction of local insulin–like growth factor-I production is at the transcriptional level, resulting in growth retardation (Adams et al., 1988).

The introduction of alternate-day therapy has been associated with improvement in growth velocity (McEnery et al., 1973; Potter et al., 1975; Reimold, 1973). Broyer and coworkers undertook a controlled study to ascertain the impact of alternate-day therapy versus daily corticosteroid therapy in pediatric recipients (Broyer et al., 1992a). Recipients were randomly assigned to daily or alternate-day corticosteroid therapy at 14 to 27 months posttransplant. The daily dose of 0.25 mg/kg was abruptly switched to 0.625 mg/kg on alternate days for 3 to 6 months, then tapered to 0.5 mg/kg on alternate days. At 1 year, the SDS was $+0.41 \pm 0.42$ SD/year in the alternate-day therapy group compared with -0.12 ± 0.53 SD/year in those receiving daily corticosteroids. Graft function was not altered by the introduction of alternate-day therapy; consequently, it appears to be effective in reducing the inhibitory effects of corticosteroids on growth velocity.

Jabs and colleagues analyzed the effects of alternate-day steroid dosing on growth in 337 children with functioning grafts 12 months posttransplantation (Jabs et al., 1996). The mean change in the SDS from 1 to 24 months posttransplant was significantly greater in children on alternate-day dosing (0.5 ± 0.06) than in those on daily dosing (0.1 ± 0.03). Other factors in this study associated with better growth were recipient age less than 13 years, lower total steroid dose over 48 hours and lower serum creatinine (all $P<0.001$). Also the decline in graft function did not differ between those on alternate-day steroid therapy and those on daily steroid therapy.

Maxwell and associates studied growth after renal transplantation in children of pubertal age (59 grafts in 54 recipients) (Maxwell et al., 1998). Immunosuppression consisted of azathioprine, cyclosporine and alternate-day steroid by 10 to 12 weeks posttransplant. The mean height SDS at transplant was -1.8 ± 0.2 and increased significantly thereafter to -0.6 ± 0.3 at 5 years posttransplant ($P<0.001$). The greatest improvement in height SDS in the first year was seen in children with the highest GFR ($r=0.429$, $P=0.002$) and in those who were shortest at the time of transplant ($r=0.356$, $P=0.009$).

Because most children are growth retarded at the time of transplantation, it is imperative that successful renal transplantation promotes accelerated or catch-up growth if ultimate adult height is to be within the normal range (Fig. 37–1). The most important factors determining the potential for achieving accelerated growth posttransplant are age at the time of transplantation, graft function, corticosteroid dosage (Fennell et al., 1986; Harmon and Jabs, 1992) and perturbations of growth factors.

The potential salutary effect of cyclosporine on posttransplant growth is difficult to assess because of the relatively short follow-up period of the data reported. Preliminary information has been encouraging. A synopsis of the data reported in the literature regarding growth in pediatric recipients receiving cyclosporine indicates that all authors are enthusiastic (Brodehl et al., 1987; Ellis et al., 1985; Klare et al., 1984; Knight et al., 1985; MacDonald et al., 1986; Offner et al., 1991; Tejani et al., 1986). A final assessment awaits further information.

The data from NAPRTCS (1998) show that at transplantation, the mean height deficit (SDS score) for all patients was -2.00 SD below the appropriate age-adjusted and sex-adjusted levels. The mean height deficit was more marked in males (-2.07) than in females (-1.89). Recipients less than 2 years old at the time of transplantation had an increase in height compared with other children the same age of about 0.25 SD in the first 6 months posttransplant, and greater than 0.75 SD by 12 months. Recipients between 2 and 5 years at the time of transplantation achieved acceleration on linear growth more slowly with a mean increase in height of 0.66 SD at 2 years posttransplantation. Children greater than 6 years old showed no improvement in height deficit at 4 years of follow-up posttransplant growth. These data substantiate the importance of age at the time of transplantation as a significant factor for posttransplant growth.

The availability of cyclosporine has facilitated the potential to eliminate corticosteroids posttransplant and assess the impact on growth. Klare et al. (1984), Knight et al. (1985) and Tejani et al. (1986) noted short-term accelerated growth using cyclosporine as the initial sole immunosuppressive agent or

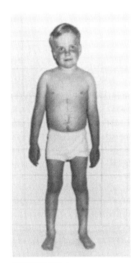
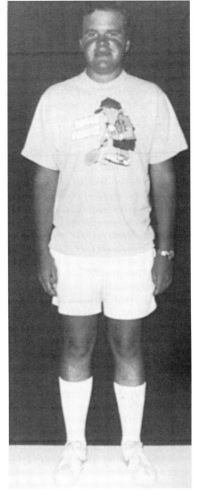

FIGURE 37–1

The picture on the left shows a 6-year-old boy shortly after a successful kidney transplant from his father. The picture on the right shows the same boy 11 years later, demonstrating the potential for growth in pediatric recipients.

discontinuing prednisone at some time interval after transplantation.

A follow-up report by Klare et al. (1991) on 33 pediatric recipients indicated that 70% of the patients were treated successfully without corticosteroids during a 9-year period with an 85% primary graft survival rate. These workers concluded that all prepubertal children with good renal function could achieve catch-up rates when treated without corticosteroids.

In a follow-up report to that of Knight et al. (1985), Hodson et al. (1989) indicated that of 20 transplants in which cyclosporine was the initial sole immunosuppressant, 13 recipients were maintained on monotherapy for greater than 1 year. Ten of the 13 (77%) showed catch-up growth (change in SDS of $>+0.5$), in contrast to only 3 of 26 (12%) requiring prednisone. At the time of the report, 6 of the 20 grafts were lost (70% survival rate), and 9 of the 20 (45%) were maintained on cyclosporine alone.

Reisman and associates noted improved growth after discontinuing prednisone in 7 of 16 recipients who were followed for a mean duration of 2 years after discontinuation (Reisman et al., 1990). Nine of 16 (56%) patients had an acute rejection episode, 6 of whom had a permanent decrease in graft function. This report emphasized the potential adverse impact on graft function of discontinuing prednisone.

Ghio and coworkers discontinued prednisone at 6 months posttransplant in 29 pediatric recipients (Ghio et al., 1992). Despite a rejection rate of 29% after cessation of prednisone, 20 of 24 patients (83%) in whom prednisone was discontinued remained off prednisone for a mean follow-up period of 30 ± 17 months. Linear growth significantly improved after stopping prednisone with a mean improvement of height SDS of +1.38 in the prepubertal and +1.60 in the pubertal recipients. Three recipients who manifested a rejection episode after initial cessation of corticosteroids and had corticosteroids reintroduced subsequently were able to discontinue corticosteroid therapy without any adverse consequences.

Either cyclosporine monotherapy or discontinuation of corticosteroids definitely is associated with a significant improvement in growth velocity and a positive change in the height SDS in renal allograft recipients. The potential for graft dysfunction is not inconsequential, and to date, no method has been delineated to detect a priori recipients who will manifest graft dysfunction in the absence of concomitant corticosteroid therapy.

The importance of growth factors in posttransplant growth was noted initially by Pennisi et al. (1979), who observed subnormal somatomedin activity in 7 of 10 recipients and an inadequate GH response to hypoglycemia in 4 of 8 recipients. Rees and colleagues described decreased GH secretion in 8 of 17 recipients with normal insulinlike growth factor-I levels (Rees et al., 1988). Tejani and coworkers reported that 4 of 21 recipients receiving greater than 5 mg of daily prednisone failed to show a normal GH response to levodopa (Tejani et al., 1989). Jabs and associates described abnormal GH secretion in six of eight poorly growing renal allograft recipients (Jabs et al., 1990). In 40 pubertal renal allograft recipients, Schaefer and coworkers correlated the peak GH amplitude during spontaneous GH secretion with height velocity (Schaefer et al., 1991). There was an inverse correlation with peak amplitude and corticosteroid dosage, leading these investigators to conclude that pubertal growth failure was related to corticosteroid-induced GH hyposecretion.

Fine and colleagues studied the effect of recombinant human growth hormone (rhGH) in 13 children with renal transplantation (Fine et al., 1992). They observed that levodopa and propranolol–induced GH secretion test was consistent with GH deficiency in 6 of 13 recipients. The mean serum insulinlike growth factor levels increased significantly from 1.14 + 0.47 at baseline to 2.38 + 1.14 (P = 0.001) after 6 months. Hokken-Koelega and colleagues in their study of GH treatment in 11 prepubertal children posttransplant reported pretreatment levels of insulinlike growth factor-II to be normal and levels of insulinlike growth factor-I at the upper limit of the normal range or above normal (Hokken-Koelega et al., 1996).

Guest and associates observed no difference in GH peak in response to the glucagon-propranolol test in 74 children posttransplant (Guest et al., 1998). Only four children had a peak response below 10 mg/ml. Growth hormone peak was not significantly different between prepubertal and early prepubertal children.

In an animal model, Kovacs and associates showed that the growth-depressing and catabolic effects of corticosteroids could be overcome with concomitant rhGH (Kovacs et al., 1991a). Before the more extensive report of Kovacs et al. (1991b), clinical studies were initiated to determine the efficacy of rhGH on improving the growth velocity of pediatric renal allograft recipients. The initial five reports (Bartosh et al., 1992; Fine et al., 1991; Johansson et al., 1990; Rees et al., 1990; Van Dop et al., 1992) verified the salutary effects of rhGH on improving growth velocity in pediatric allograft recipients. The data from three controlled studies are shown in Table 37–10. A major concern has been the precipitation of graft dysfunction by rhGH. The data indicate that 27% of the recipients experience graft dysfunction after rhGH treatment; however, the mean GFR has not changed after treatment (Table 37–11). Guest and coworkers showed that the risk of acute rejection was not increased in children who had no or only one episode before starting GH treatment, whereas the patients with more than one episode of rejection had a significant risk of developing another episode (Guest et al., 1998). Growth hormone increases muscle mass. Estimation of GFR by methods other than inulin clearance may be affected by the use of GH in these patients. Different studies have used different methods to estimate and determine GFR, and that data may not be comparable. In addition, owing to the natural history of chronic rejection, it may be difficult to prove the role of GH in causing graft dysfunction posttransplant. Resolution of this issue awaits the performance of a controlled study using more sophisticated methodology for assessing graft function before and serially after rhGH treatment under the auspices of the NAPRTCS.

After successful transplantation, puberty proceeds. Pennisi and associates evaluated pubertal development in 24 children who had a bone age of less than 12 years at the time of transplantation (Pennisi et al., 1977c). During the 3.5- to 8-year follow-up period, 10 recipients remained prepubertal, 9 initiated and were progressing through puberty and 5 had progressed to normal pubertal development.

Subsequently, van Diemen-Steenvoorde and coworkers assessed sexual maturation in 68 long-term pediatric graft recipients (van Diemen-Steenvoorde et al., 1987). The onset of puberty was at a chronological age of 14.6 ± 1.9 years in boys and 13.3 ± 1.9 years in girls. Height velocity during puberty was normal in 62.5% of the recipients, and no difference in pubertal growth was noted in recipients transplanted before or after the onset of puberty. The duration of pubertal development after transplantation was noted to be normal. Despite these excellent pubertal growth data, one third of the recipients attained an adult height greater than 2 SD below

TABLE 37–10

RECOMBINANT HUMAN GROWTH HORMONE TREATMENT POSTTRANSPLANT

Author	No. Patients	Prior 12 Months (cm/y [range])	rhGH 12 Months (cm/y [range])	P value
Maxwell et al. (1996)	16	4.0 (0.8–8.1)	8.3 (3–12.5)	<0.001
Hokken-Koelega (1996)	11	1.5 (0.7)	5.3 ± 1.0/6 m	<0.001
Guest et al. (1998)	41	4.1 ± 2.0	7.7 ± 2.5	<0.0001

NOTE. Data are from three controlled studies.
rhGH = recombinant human growth hormone.

TABLE 37–11

RECOMBINANT HUMAN GROWTH HORMONE POSTTRANSPLANT IMPACT ON ALLOGRAFT FUNCTION

| Author | No. Patients | Mean Calculated Creatinine Clearance (ml/min/1.73 m² [range]) | |
		Pre-rhGH	*12 mo. rhGH*
Rees *et al.* (1990)	6 Prepubertal	66 (27–108)	64 (11–110)
	6 Pubertal		
Johnsson *et al.* (1990)	15 Prepubertal	70 (35–90)	65 (0–94)
	13 Pubertal	62 (23–108)	72 (11–110)
Fine *et al.* (1991)	9	58 (35–111)	57 (5–94)
		57 ± 22	56 ± 26
Van S (1991)	17 Prepubertal	71	64
	19 Pubertal	67	68
Van Dop *et al.* (1992)	9	0.79	0.53
Bartosh *et al.* (1992)	5	47 ± 22	35 ± 18
		51 ± 22	58 ± 29
Benfield *et al.* (1993)	10	77	59
Jabs *et al.* (1993)	8		
Tonshoff *et al.* (1993)	17	59	49
Janssen *et al.* (1993)	19	64	58
		85	78
Hokken-Koelega (1994)	16		
Chavers *et al.* (1995)	8	56 ± 27	58 ± 20
Maxwell (1995)	16	52 (18–117)	59 (15–113)
Hokken-Koelega (1996)	11	66 (13)	80 (30)
Guest *et al.* (1998)	41	67 ± 26	64 ± 26

rhGH = recombinant human growth hormone.

the mean. The investigators emphasized that the loss of growth potential during pubertal development after transplantation has a significant influence on ultimate adult height.

In female recipients who are pubertal before transplantation and become amenorrheic during the course of chronic renal failure, menses usually returns within 6 to 12 months after successful transplantation. Pubertal female recipients should be given appropriate contraceptive information in the early posttransplant period because of the potential for pregnancy (Fine, 1982; Korsch et al., 1980).

Ferraris and associates examined pubertal development in 12 male patients after transplantation (Ferraris et al., 1980). Genital maturation was delayed significantly in comparison to chronological age and bone age. The Tanner stage of puberty correlated best with bone age. Serum testosterone and luteinizing hormone concentrations were normal; serum follicle-stimulating hormone concentration was normal in recipients with a serum creatinine level less than 2.0 mg/dl and elevated in recipients with a greater reduction in graft function. The pituitary-testicular axis was normal in recipients with good renal function. All androgens produced by the adrenal gland were decreased, presumably because of concomitant corticosteroid therapy. The efficacy of using exogenous androgen therapy could be considered in recipients with significantly delayed pubertal development after successful transplantation.

Fine and associates observed that 5 of 13 pediatric recipients studied manifested progression of pubertal development after the initiation of rhGH (Fine et al., 1992). They observed that many patients had an advancement in Tanner stage with rhGH and faster development of pubic hair, but these were not conclusive for testicular volume and breast development. Guest and coworkers in their study found no conclusive evidence of the effect of GH on pubertal development posttransplant (Guest et al., 1998).

Long-Term Outcome

It is difficult to predict the long-term outcome for graft survival in pediatric recipients of current renal allografts from previous data because recipient management and immunosuppressive regimens have fluctuated dramatically. Data from the precyclosporine era reported by Najarian et al. (1986) of 210 living related donor recipients and 78 cadaver donor recipients indicated 10-year actuarial survival rates of 52% and 47%. Sixteen HLA-identical sibling grafts had a 90% 10-year actuarial survival rate. Similarly, Broyer and coworkers noted a 10-year actuarial survival rate for 335 cadaver donor grafts of 40% (Broyer et al., 1987b).

Potter et al. (1991) updated their data (Potter et al., 1986) on the long-term outcome of 37 children 3 to 16 years old who received 23 living related and 14 cadaver donor grafts before 1970. Patient survival was 78% at 10 years and 68% at 22 to 26 years after initial transplantation. Graft survival rates were 56% at 10 years, 31% at 20 years and 23% at 22 to 26 years. At 20 years, 35% of the living related and 21% of the cadaver donor grafts were functioning. Actuarial graft survival rates for 23 retransplants was 49% at 10 years and 37% at 15 years.

Brodehl and associates compared the long-term outcome of 112 recipients treated with cyclosporine with 77 recipients treated with azathioprine who were transplanted in the period 1973–1990 (Brodehl et al., 1992). The actuarial survival rate at 8 years was 60% for the cyclosporine group and 40% for the azathioprine group. Analysis of 32 recipients who received cyclosporine and 34 recipients who received azathioprine and survived greater than 5 years indicated improved subsequent survival rates and graft function rates (GFR) in the azathioprine group. The net effect is overall long-term improvement in the graft survival rates after the introduction of cyclosporine; however, long-term survivors treated with azathioprine may have more stable graft function.

Graft loss from chronic rejection and/or patient death

results in subsequent attrition despite long-term adequate function. Indolent immunological attack of the graft probably occurs in every recipient, and the pediatric recipient can anticipate the need for multiple grafts to achieve longevity. The contribution of glomerular hyperperfusion to the decline in graft function remains to be delineated (Feehally et al., 1986). If currently ongoing controlled trials substantiate the contention that limitation of protein intake reduces the adverse effects of glomerular hyperperfusion, consideration should be given to limiting protein intake in pediatric graft recipients in an attempt to achieve sustained long-term function. Such limitation of protein intake should not affect adversely the growth of the recipient.

The long-term quality of life in pediatric recipients with a functioning graft for greater than 10 years was assessed by questionnaire in the report of Morel et al. (1991). There was a 100% response to the 57 questionnaires. In general, 89% were satisfied with life, and only 4% indicated that health problems often interfere with social life. There was dissatisfaction with body appearance in 32% with the major concern being short stature and the effects of brittle bones. Nevertheless, the long-term quality of life appears excellent in pediatric allograft recipients.

Most recent data from the NAPRTCS (1998) show the estimated graft survival probabilities and standard error as 0.911 ± 0.006, 0.84 ± 0.008 and 0.785 ± 0.01 at years 1, 3 and 5 for recipients of living donor organs. Comparable estimates for recipients of cadaver donor organs are 0.818 ± 0.008, 0.72 ± 0.01 and 0.64 ± 0.11.

REFERENCES

Abouna, G. M., Al-Abdullah, I. H., Kelly, S. D., et al. (1993). Randomized clinical trial of antithymocyte globulin induction in renal transplantation comparing a fixed daily dose with adjustment according to T cell monitoring. *Transplantation* **56**, 827.

Abouna, G. M., Kumar, M. S., Samhan, M., et al. (1991). Transplantation of small pediatric cadaver kidneys into adult recipients. *Transplant. Proc.* **23**, 2604.

Adams, M., Wesner, H. and Farnsworth, W. (1988). Dexamethasone reduces steady state insulin like growth factor I MRNA levels in rat neuronal and glial cells in primary culture. *Endocrinology* **123**, 2565.

Ahmed, Z. and Terasaki, P. I. (1992). Effect of transfusions. *In Clinical Transplants 1991*, (P. I. Terasaki and J. M. Cecka, eds.), p. 305, UCLA Tissue Typing Laboratory, Los Angeles.

Alexander, S. R. (1984). Treatment of infants with ESRD. *In End Stage Renal Disease in Children*, (R. N. Fine and A. B. Gruskin, eds.), p. 17, W.B. Saunders, Philadelphia.

Alexander, S. R., Arbus, G. S., Butt, K. M. H., et al. (1989). The 1989 Report of the North American Pediatric Renal Transplant Cooperative Study. *Pediatr. Nephrol.* **4**, 542.

Alexopoulos, E., Leontsini, M., Daniilidis, M., et al. (1991). Differentiation between renal allograft rejection and cyclosporin toxicity: a clinicopathological study. *Am. J. Kidney Dis.* **18**, 108.

Allen, D. B. and Goldberg, B. D. (1992). Stimulation of collagen synthesis and linear growth by growth hormone glucocorticoid treated children. *Pediatrics* **89**, 416.

Allison, A. C. and Eugui, E. M. (1993). Immunosuppressive and other effects of mycophenolic acid and an ester prodrug, mycophenolate mofetil. *Immunol. Rev.* **136**, 5.

Almond, P. S., Matas, A. J., Gillingham, K., et al. (1992). Pediatric renal transplants—results with sequential immunosuppression. *Transplantation* **53**, 46.

Almond, P. S., Matas, A. J., Nakhleh, R. E., et al. (1993) Renal transplantation for infantile cystinosis: long-term follow-up. *J. Pediatr. Surg.* **28**, 232.

Amend, W. J. C., Jr., Vincenti, F., Feduska, N. J., et al. (1981). Recurrent systemic lupus erythematosus involving renal allografts. *Ann. Intern. Med.* **94**, 444.

Amlot, P. L., Rawlings, E., Fernando, O. et al. (1995). Prolonged action of a chimeric interleukin 2 receptor(CD 25) monoclonal antibody in use in cadaveric renal transplantation. *Transplantation* **60**, 748.

Anand, S. K., Northway, J. D. and Crussi, F. G. (1978). Acute renal failure in newborn infants. *J. Pediatr.* **92**, 985.

Andersen, O. S., Jonasson, O. and Merkel, F. K. (1974). En bloc transplantation of pediatric kidneys into adult patients. *Arch. Surg.* **108**, 35.

Anderson, C. B., Tyler, J. D., Sicard, G. A., et al. (1984). Pretreatment of renal allograft recipients with immunosuppression and donor-specific blood. *Transplantation* **38**, 664.

Antignac, C., Hinglais, N., Gubler, M. C., et al. (1988). De-novo membranous glomerulonephritis in renal allografts in children. *Clin. Nephrol.* **30**, 1.

Arbus, G. S., Galiwango, J., DeMaria, J. E., et al. (1980). The first 10 years of the dialysis-transplantation programme at The Hospital for Sick Children. *Can. Med. Assoc. J.* **120**, 659.

Arbus, G. S., Geary, D. F., McLorie, G. A., et al. (1986). Pediatric renal transplants: a Canadian perspective. *Kidney Int.* **30**, S31.

Arbus, G. S., Hardy, B. E., Balfe, J. W., et al. (1983). Cadaveric renal transplants in children under 6 years of age. *Kidney Int.* **24**, S111.

Arbus, G. S., Rochon, J. and Thompson, D. (1991). Survival of cadaveric renal transplant grafts from young donors and in young recipients. *Pediatr. Nephrol.* **5**, 152.

Aronoff, A., Gault, M. H., Huang, S. N., et al. (1973). Hepatitis with Australia antigenemia following renal transplantation. *Can. Med. Assoc. J.* **103**, 43.

Artero, M., Biava, C., Amend, W., et al. (1992). Recurrent focal glomerulosclerosis: natural history and response to therapy. *Am. J. Med.* **92**, 375.

Aschendorff, C., Offner, G., Winkler, L., et al. (1990). Adult height achieved in children after kidney transplantation. *Am. J. Dis. Child.* **144**, 1138.

Avner, E. D., Harmon, W. E., Grupe, W. E., et al. (1981). Mortality of chronic hemodialysis and renal transplantation in pediatric end-stage renal disease. *Pediatrics* **67**, 412.

Bale, J. F., Jr., Siegler, R. L. and Bray, P. (1980). Encephalopathy in young children with moderate chronic renal failure. *Am. J. Dis. Child.* **134**, 581.

Baliah, T., Kim, K. H., Anthone, S., et al. (1974). Recurrence of Henoch-Schönlein purpura glomerulonephritis in transplanted kidneys. *Transplantation* **18**, 343.

Baluarte, H. J., Gruskin, A. B., Hiner, L. B., et al. (1977). Encephalopathy in children with chronic renal failure. *Proc. Clin. Dial. Transplant. Forum* **7**, 95.

Banfi, G., Colturi, C., Montagnino, G., et al. (1990). The recurrence of focal segmental glomerulosclerosis in kidney transplant patients treated with cyclosporine. *Transplantation* **50**, 594.

Barnes, B. A., Bergan, J. J., Braun, W. E., et al. (1973). The 11th Report of the Human Renal Transplant Registry. *J. A. M. A.* **226**, 1197.

Bart, K. J., Macon, E. J., Whittier, F. C., et al. (1981). Cadaveric kidneys for transplantation: a paradox of shortage in the face of plenty. *Transplantation* **31**, 379.

Barth, K. H., Brusilow, S. W., Kaufman, S. L., et al. (1981). Percutaneous transluminal angioplasty of homograft renal artery stenosis in a 10 year old girl. *Pediatrics* **67**, 675.

Barton, C. H., Vaziri, N. D., Martin, D. C., et al. (1987). Hypomagnesemia and renal magnesium wasting in renal transplant recipients receiving cyclosporine. *Am. J. Med.* **83**, 693.

Bartosh, S., et al. (1992). Effects of growth hormone administration in pediatric renal allograft recipients. *Pediatr. Nephrol.* **6**, 68.

Bartosh, S. M., Aronson, A. J., Swanson-Pervitt, E. E., Jr., et al. (1993). OKT3 induction in pediatric transplantation. *Pediatr. Nephrol.* **7**, 45.

Basadonna, G. P., Matas, A. J., Gillingham, K. J., et al. (1993). Early versus late acute renal allograft rejection: impact on chronic rejection. *Transplantation* **55**, 993.

Bassani, C. E., Ferraris, J., Gianantonio, C. A., et al. (1991). Renal transplantation in patients with classical hemolytic-uremic syndrome. *Pediatr. Nephrol.* **5**, 607.

Baxter, J. D. and Forsham, P. H. (1972). Tissue effects of glucocorticoids. *Am. J. Med.* **53**, 573.

Beato, M. (1989). Gene regulation by steroid hormones. *Cell* **56**, 335.

Beck, D. E., Fennell, R. S., Yost, R. L., et al. (1980). Evaluation of an educational programme on compliance with medication regimens in paediatric patients with renal transplants. *J. Pediatr.* **96**, 1094.

Benfield, M. R., Stablein, D. and Tejani, A. (1999). Trends in immuno-suppressive therapy: a report of the North American Pediatric Renal Transplant Cooperative Study (NAPRTCS). *Pediatr. Transplant.* **3**, 27. PMID: 10359028; UI: 99285523.

Ben-Maimon, C. S., Burke, J. F., Besarab, A., *et al.* (1991). Evidence against chronic progressive cyclosporine nephrotoxicity. *Transplant. Proc.* **23**, 1260.

Bennett, W. M. (1976). Cost-benefit ratio of pretransplant bilateral nephrectomy. *J. A. M. A.* **235**, 1703.

Berg, U. B. and Bohlin, A.-B. (1992). Renal function following kidney transplantation in children treated with cyclosporine. *Pediatr. Nephrol.* **6**, 339.

Berg, U. B., Bohlin, A. and Tyden, G. (1997). Influence of donor and recipient ages and sex on graft function after pediatric renal transplantation. *Transplantation* **64**, 1424.

Bock, G. H., Sullivan, E. K., Miller, D., *et al.* (1997). Cytomegalovirus infections following renal transplantation—effects of antiviral prophylaxis: a report of the North American Pediatric Renal Transplant Cooperative Study (NAPRTCS). *Pediatr. Nephrol.* **11**, 665.

Boczko, S., Tellis, V. and Veith, F. J. (1978). Transplantation of children's kidneys into adult recipients. *Surg. Gynecol. Obstet.* **146**, 387.

Borel, J. F., Feurer, C., Gubler, H. U., *et al.* (1976). Biological effects of cyclosporin A: a new antilymphocytic agent. *Agents Actions* **6**, 468.

Bosque, M., Munian, A., Bewick, M., *et al.* (1983). Growth after renal transplants. *Arch. Dis. Child.* **58**, 110.

Botkin, J. R. (1988). Anencephalic infants as organ donors. *Pediatrics* **82**, 250.

Brattstrom, C., Sawe, J., Tyden, G., *et al.* (1997). Kinetics and dynamics of single oral doses of sirolimus in sixteen renal transplant recipients. *Ther. Drug Monit.* **19**, 397.

Brenner, B. M., Cohen, R. A. and Milford, E. L. (1992). In renal transplantation, one size may not fit all. *J. A. M. A.* **3**, 162.

Bretan, P. N., Jr., Friese, C., Goldstein, R. B., *et al.* (1997). Immunologic and patient selection strategies for successful utilization of less than 15 kg pediatric donor kidneys—long term experience with 40 transplantss. *Transplantation* **62**, 233.

Briscoe, D. M., Kim, M. S., Lillehei, C., *et al.* (1992). Outcome of renal transplantation in children less than two years of age. *Kidney Int.* **42**, 657.

Brodehl, J., Bokenkamp, A., Hoyer, P. F., *et al.* (1992). Long-term results of cyclosporin A therapy in children. *J. Am. Soc. Nephrol.* **2**, S246.

Brodehl, J., Offner, G. and Hoyer, P. F. (1987). Cyclosporine in pediatric kidney transplantation. *In Advances in Nephrology,* (J. Hamburger, J. Crosnier, J. P. Grunfeld and M. D. Maxwell, eds.), p. 335, Year Book Medical Publishers, Chicago.

Brodehl, J., Offner, G., Pichlmayr, R., *et al.* (1986). Long-term results of cyclosporin A therapy in children. *Transplant. Proc.* **4**, 8.

Brouhard, B. H., Winsett, O. E., Kalia, A., *et al.* (1988). Treatment of hepatoblastoma in an infant before successful renal transplantation. *Transplantation* **46**, 316.

Broyer, M., Brunner, F. P., Brynger, H., *et al.* (1986). Demography of dialysis and transplantation in children under 6 years of age. *Nephrol. Dial. Transplant.* **1**, 9.

Broyer, M., Brunner, F. P., Brynger, H., *et al.* (1990). Kidney transplantation in primary oxalosis: data from the EDTA registry. *Nephrol. Dial. Transplant.* **5**, 332.

Broyer, M., Donckerwolcke, R. A., Brunner, F. P., *et al.* (1981a). Combined report on regular dialysis and transplantation of children in Europe 1980. *Proc. Eur. Dial. Transplant. Assoc.* **18**, 60.

Broyer, M., Gagnadoux, M. F., Beurton, D. M., *et al.* (1980). Importance of HLA-A, B matching in kidney transplantation in children. *Transplantation* **30**, 310.

Broyer, M., Gagnadoux, M. F., Guest, G., *et al.* (1987b). Kidney transplantation in children: results of 383 grafts performed at Enfants Malades Hospital from 1973–1984. *In Advances in Nephrology,* (J. Hamburger, J. Crosnier, J. P. Grunfeld and M. D. Maxwell, eds.), p. 307, Year Book Medical Publishers, Chicago.

Broyer, M., Guest, G. and Gagnadoux, M. F. (1992a). Growth rate in children receiving alternate-day corticosteroid treatment after kidney transplantation. *J. Pediatr.* **120**, 721.

Broyer, M., Guest, G., Gagnadoux, M. F., *et al.* (1987a). Hypertension following renal transplantation in children. *Pediatr. Nephrol.* **1**, 16.

Broyer, M., Guillot, M., Gubler, M. C., *et al.* (1981b). Infantile cystinosis: a reappraisal of early and late symptoms. *In Advances in Nephrology,* (J. Hamburger, J. Crosnier, J. P. Grunfeld and M. D. Maxwell, eds.), p. 137, Year Book Medical Publishers, Chicago.

Broyer, M., Rizzoni, G., Brunner, H., *et al.* (1985). Combined report on regular dialysis and transplantation of children in Europe, XIV, 1984. *Proc. Eur. Dial. Transplant. Assoc.* **22**, 55.

Broyer, M., Selwood, N. and Brunner, F. (1992b). Recurrence of primary renal disease on kidney graft: a European pediatric experience. *J. Am. Soc. Nephrol.* **2**, S55.

Broyer, M., Tete, M. J., Guest, G., *et al.* (1997). Varicella and zoster in children after kidney transplantation: long term results of vaccination. *Pediatrics* **99**, 35.

Bruix, J., Barrera, J. M., Calvert, X., *et al.* (1989). Prevalence of antibodies to hepatitis C virus in Spanish patients with hepatocellular carcinoma and hepatic cirrhosis. *Lancet* **2**, 1004.

Buckels, J. A. C., MacKintoch, P. and Barnes, A. D. (1981). Controlled trial of low- versus high-dose oral steroid therapy in 100 cadaveric renal transplants. *Proc. Eur. Dial. Transplant. Assoc.* **18**, 394.

Bunchman, T., Sibley, R., Mauer, S. M., *et al.* (1987). Anaphylactoid purpura (AP) with nephritis: can patients at risk for renal failure be identified? *Kidney Int.* **31**, 192.

Bunchman, T. E., Fryd, D. S., Sibley, R. K., *et al.* (1990). Manifestations of renal allograft rejection in small children receiving adult kidneys. *Pediatr. Nephrol.* **4**, 255.

Butler, R. T., Kalkwarf, K. L. and Kaldahl, W. B. (1987). Drug-induced gingival hyperplasia: phenytoin, cyclosporine, and nifedipine. *J. Am. Dent. Assoc.* **114**, 56.

Butt, K. M., Myer, A., Kountz, S. L., *et al.* (1976). Renal transplantation in patients with posterior urethral valves. *J. Urol.* **116**, 708.

Buturovic, J., Kandus, A., Malovrh, M., *et al.* (1990). Cyclosporine-associated hemolytic uremic syndrome in four renal allograft recipients: resolution without specific therapy. *Transplant. Proc.* **22**, 1726.

Calne, R., Lim, S., Samaan, A., *et al.* (1989). Rapamycin for immunosuppression of organ allografting. *Lancet* **2**, 227.

Calne, R. Y., Rolles, K., Dunn, D. C., *et al.* (1979). Cyclosporin A initially as the only immunosuppressant in 34 recipients of cadaveric organs: 32 kidneys, 2 pancreases, and 2 livers. *Lancet* **2**, 1033.

Calzolari, A., Giordano, U., Matteuci, M. C., *et al.* (1998). Hypertension in young patients after renal transplantation. *Am. J. Hypertens.* **11**, 497.

Cameron, J. S. (1982). Glomerulonephritis in renal transplants. *Transplantation* **34**, 237.

Cameron, J. S. (1990). Ask the expert. *Pediatr. Nephrol.* **3**, 300.

Cameron, J. S. (1991). Recurrent primary disease and de novo nephritis following renal transplantation. *Pediatr. Nephrol.* **5**, 412.

Cameron, J. S. and Turner, D. R. (1977). Recurrent glomerulonephritis in allografted kidneys. *Clin. Nephrol.* **7**, 47.

Campbell, D. A., Dafoe, D. C., Roloff, D. W., *et al.* (1984). Cadaveric renal transplantation in a 2.2-kilogram neonate. *Transplantation* **38**, 197.

Canadian Multicentre Transplant Study Group. (1983). A randomized clinical trial of cyclosporine in cadaveric renal transplantation. *N. Engl. J. Med.* **309**, 809.

Canniggia, A., Marchetti, M., Gennari, C., *et al.* (1977). Effects of a new glucocorticoid, oxazacort, on some variables connected with bone metabolism in man: a comparison with prednisone. *Int. J. Pharmacol.* **15**, 126.

Cecka, J. M. (1989). Donor and preservation factors. *In Clinical Transplants 1988,* (P. Terasaki, ed.), p. 399, UCLA Tissue Typing Laboratory, Los Angeles.

Cecka, J. M. and Terasaki, P. I. (1990). Matching kidneys by size in renal transplantation. *Clin. Transplant.* **4**, 82.

Cerilli, G. J., Nelsen, C. and Dorfmann, L. (1972). Renal homotransplantation in infants and children with the hemolytic-uremic syndrome. *Surgery* **71**, 66.

Cerilli, J. and Jones, L. (1977). A reappraisal of the role of splenectomy in children receiving renal allografts. *Surgery* **82**, 510.

Chan, L., French, M. E., Oliver, O. O., *et al.* (1981). High- and low-dose prednisolone. *Transplant. Proc.* **13**, 336.

Chantler, C., Carter, J. E., Bewick, M., *et al.* (1980). 10 years' experience with regular hemodialysis and renal transplantation. *Arch. Dis. Child.* **55**, 435.

Charpentier, B., Hiesse, L., Marchand, S., *et al.* (1999). De novo and recurrent disease: recurrent glomerulopathies. *Transplant. Proc.* **31**, 264.

Charpentier, B., Levy, M. and the CSIF. (1982). Cooperative study of de novo extramembranous glomerulonephritis in renal allografts in humans: a report of 19 new cases in 1550 renal transplant patients of the transplantation group of the Ile de France. *Nephrologie* 3, 158.

Chatenoud, L., Legendre, C., Ferran, C., *et al.* (1991). Corticosteroid inhibition of the OKT3-induced cytokine-related syndrome-dosage and kinetics pre-requisites. *Transplantation* 51, 334.

Chavers, B. M., Doherty, L., Nevins, T. E., *et al.* (1995). Effects of growth hormone on kidney function in pediatric transplant recipients. *Pediatr. Nephrol.* 9, 176.

Chavers, B. M., Nevins, T. E., Knaack, M. *et al.* (1987). Early acute tubular necrosis, late rejection in pediatric renal transplantation with donor-specific transfusion. *Transplant. Proc.* 19, 1526.

Cho, Y. W., Terasaki, P. I. and Graver, B. (1990). Fifteen year kidney graft survival. *In Clinical Transplants 1989*, (P. I. Terasaki, ed.), p. 325, UCLA Tissue Typing Laboratory, Los Angeles.

Choo, Q. L., Kuo, G., Weiner, A. J., *et al.* (1989). Isolation of a cDNA clone derived from a blood-borne non-A, non-B viral hepatitis genome. *Science* 244, 359.

Cicciarelli, J. and Cho, Y. (1992). HLA matching: univariate and multivariate analyses of UNOS registry data. *In Clinical Transplants 1991*, (P. I. Terasaki and J. M. Cecka, eds.), p. 325, UCLA Tissue Typing Laboratory, Los Angeles.

Cochat, P., Kassir, A., Colon, S., *et al.* (1993). Recurrent nephrotic syndrome after transplantation: early treatment with plasmapheresis and cyclophosphamide. *Pediatr. Nephrol.* 7, 50.

Cockfield, S. M., Urmson, J., Pleasants, J. R., *et al.* (1990). The regulation of expression of MHC products in mice: factors determining the level of expression in kidneys of normal mice. *J. Immunol.* 144, 2967.

Columbo, M., Kuo, G., Choo, Q. L., *et al.* (1989). Prevalence of antibodies to hepatitis C virus in Italian patients with hepatocellular carcinoma. *Lancet* 2, 1006.

Conley, S. B., Flechner, S. M., Rose, G., *et al.* (1985). Use of cyclosporine in pediatric renal transplant recipients. *J. Pediatr.* 106, 45.

Connor, E., Gupta, S., Joshi, V., *et al.* (1988). Acquired immunodeficiency syndrome associated renal disease in children. *J. Pediatr.* 113, 39.

Cosimi, A. B. (1983). The clinical usefulness of antilymphocyte antibodies. *Transplant. Proc.* 15, 583.

Cosimi, A. B., Colvin, R. B., Burton, R. H., *et al.* (1981). Use of monoclonal antibodies to T cell subsets for immunological monitoring and treatment in recipients of renal allografts. *N. Engl. J. Med.* 305, 308.

Couchoud, C., Pouteil-Noble, C., Colon, S., *et al.* (1995). Recurrence of membranous nephropathy after renal transplantation: incidence and risk factor in 1614 patients. *Transplantation* 59, 1275.

Crocker, J. F. S., Dempsey, T., Schenk, M. E., *et al.* (1993). Cyclosporin A toxicity in children. *Transplant. Rev.* 7, 72.

Cupps, T. R. and Fauci, A. S. (1982). Corticosteroids mediate immune regulation in man. *Immunol. Rev.* 65, 133.

Currier, C. B., Jr., Papadopoulou, Z., Helfrich, G. B., *et al.* (1979). Successful renal transplantation in focal segmental glomerulosclerosis. *Transplant. Proc.* 11, 49.

Curtis, J. J., Lucas, B. A., Kotchen, T. A., *et al.* (1981). Surgical therapy for persistent hypertension after renal transplantation. *Transplantation* 31, 125.

Curtis, J. J., Luke, R. G., Whelchel, J. D., *et al.* (1983). Inhibition of angiotensin-converting enzyme in renal transplant recipients with hypertension. *N. Engl. J. Med.* 308, 377.

Dantal, J., Baatard, R., Hourmant, M., *et al.* (1991). Recurrent nephrotoxic syndrome following renal transplantation in patients with focal glomerulosclerosis. *Transplantation* 52, 827.

Dantal, J., Testa, A., Bigot, E., *et al.* (1990). Disappearance of proteinuria after adsorption in a patient with focal glomerulosclerosis. *Lancet* 2, 190.

Darmady, E. M. (1974). Transplantation and the ageing kidney. *Lancet* 2, 1046.

Dawidson, I., Rooth, P., Fry, W. R., *et al.* (1989). Prevention of acute cyclosporine-induced renal blood flow inhibition and improved immunosuppression with verapamil. *Transplantation* 48, 575.

DeCamargo, P. M. (1989). Cyclosporin- and nifedipine-induced gingival enlargement: an overview. *J. West. Soc. Periodont.* 37, 57.

DeGroen, P. C. (1988). Cyclosporine, low-density lipoprotein, and cholesterol. *Mayo Clin. Proc.* 63, 1012.

DeGroen, P. C., Aksamit, A. J., Rakela, J., *et al.* (1987). Central nervous system toxicity after liver transplantation: the role of cyclosporine and cholesterol. *N. Engl. J. Med.* 317, 861.

DeMaria, J. E., Hardy, B. E., Brezinski, A., *et al.* (1979). Renal transplantation in patients with bilateral Wilms' tumor. *J. Pediatr. Surg.* 14, 577.

Demattos, A. M., Olyaei, A. J. and Bennett, W. M. (1996). Pharmacology of immunosuppressive medications used in renal diseases and transplantation. *Am. J. Kidney Dis.* 28, 631.

Denny, T., Yogev, R., Gelman, R., *et al.* (1992). Lymphocyte subsets in healthy children during the first 5 years of life. *J. A. M. A.* 267, 1484.

DeShazo, C. V., Simmons, R. L., Bernstein, D. M., *et al.* (1974). Results of renal transplantation in 100 children. *Surgery* 76, 461.

Diaz-Gonzalez, M. E., Mendoza, S. A., Griswald, W. R., *et al.* (1991). Symptomatic cholelithiasis in pediatric renal transplant recipients. *Pediatr. Nephrol.* 5, 15.

Donckerwolcke, R. A., Broyer, M., Brunner, F., *et al.* (1982). Combined report on regular dialysis and transplantation of children in Europe XI. *Proc. Eur. Dial. Transplant. Assoc.* 19, 61.

Donckerwolcke, R. A., Chantler, C., Broyer, M., *et al.* (1980). Combined report on regular dialysis and transplantation of children in Europe, 1979. *Proc. Eur. Dial. Transplant. Assoc.* 17, 87.

Donckerwolcke, R. A., Chantler, C., Brunner, F. P., *et al.* (1978). Combined report on regular dialysis and transplantation of children in Europe, 1977. *Proc. Eur. Dial. Transplant. Assoc.* 15, 77.

Donckerwolcke, R. A. and Kinderziekenhuis, W. (1991). Long-term complications of renal transplantation. *Child. Nephrol. Urol.* 11, 179.

Drachman, R. B., Schlesinger, M., Shapira, H., *et al.* (1989). The immune status of uraemic children/adolescents with chronic renal failure and renal replacement therapy. *Pediatr. Nephrol.* 3, 305.

Dreikorn, K., Rohl, L. and Horsch, R. (1977). The use of double renal transplants from paediatric cadaver donors. *Br. J. Urol.* 49, 361.

Eddy, A., Sibley, R., Mauer, S. M., *et al.* (1984). Renal allograft failure due to recurrent dense intramembranous deposit disease. *Clin. Nephrol.* 21, 305.

Edvardson, V. O., Flynn, J. T., Deforest, A., *et al.* (1996). Effective immunization against influenza in pediatric renal transplant recipients. *Clin. Transplant.* 10, 556.

Ehrich, J. H. H., *et al.* (1992). Renal replacement therapy for end-stage renal failure before 2 years of age. *Nephrol. Dial. Transplant.* 7, 1171.

Eijgenraam, F. J., Donckerwolcke, R. A., Monnens, L. A. H., *et al.* (1990). Renal transplantation in 20 children with hemolytic-uremic syndrome. *Clin. Nephrol.* 33, 87.

Ellis, D., Avner, E. D., Rosenthal, J. T., *et al.* (1985). Renal function and somatic growth in pediatric cadaver renal transplantation with cyclosporine-prednisone immunosuppression. *Am. J. Dis. Child.* 139, 1161.

Emmel, E. A., Verweij, C. L., Durand, D. B., *et al.* (1989). Cyclosporin A specifically inhibits function of nuclear proteins involved in T cell activation. *Science* 246, 1617.

Eschbach, J. W., Egrie, J. C., Downing, M. R., *et al.* (1987). Correction of the anemia of end-stage renal disease with recombinant human erythropoietin: results of a combined phase I and II clinical trial. *N. Engl. J. Med.* 316, 73.

Ettenger, R., Cohen, A., Nast, C., *et al.* (1997). Mycophenolate mofetil as a maintenance immunosuppression in pediatric renal transplantation. *Transplant. Proc.* 29, 340.

Ettenger, R., Marik, J. and Rosenthal, J. T. (1992b). Sequential therapy in pediatric cadaveric renal transplantation: a critical analysis. *J. Am. Soc. Nephrol.* 2, S304.

Ettenger, R. B. (1992). Children are different: the challenges of pediatric renal transplantation. *Am. J. Kidney Dis.* 20, 668.

Ettenger, R. B., Blifeld, C., Prince, H., *et al.* (1987). The pediatric nephrologist's dilemma: growth after renal transplantation and its interaction with age as a possible immunologic variable. *J. Pediatr.* 111, 1022.

Ettenger, R. B. and Fine, R. N. (1986). Pediatric renal transplantation. *In Renal Transplantation*, (M. R. Garavoy and R. D. Guttman, eds.), p. 399, Churchill Livingstone, New York.

Ettenger, R. B., Grimm, P. and Firzli, E. S. (1992a). Kidney transplantation in children. *In Handbook of Kidney Transplantation*, (G. M. Danovitch, ed.), p. 305, Little, Brown, Boston.

Ettenger, R. B., Jordan, S. C., Malekzadeh, M. M., *et al.* (1981). *In Developments in Nephrology: Pediatric Nephrology, Proc. Vth Int. Pediatr. Nephrol. Symp.*, Vol. 3, (A. B. Gruskin and M. E. Norman, eds.), p. 364, Martinus Nijhoff, Boston.

Ettenger, R. B., Kerman, R., Arnett, J., *et al.* (1983). Sensitization following donor-specific transfusions for living-related renal transplantation. *Transplant. Proc.* **15**, 943.

Ettenger, R. B., Marik, J. and Grimm, P. C. (1991a). The impact of recombinant human erythropoietin therapy on renal transplantation. *Am. J. Kidney Dis.* **18(Suppl. 1)**, 57.

Ettenger, R. B., Marik, J., Rosenthal, J. T., *et al.* (1988). OKT 3 for rejection, reversal in pediatric renal transplantation. *Clin. Transplant.* **2**, 180.

Ettenger, R. B. and Rosenthal, J. T. (1992). Renal transplant rejection. *In Current Therapy in Allergy, Immunology and Rheumatology*, 4th ed., (L. M. Lichtenstein and A. S. Fauci, eds.), p. 88, Mosby-Year Book, St. Louis.

Ettenger, R. B., Rosenthal, J. T., Marik, J. L., *et al.* (1989). Successful cadaveric renal transplantation in infants and young children. *Transplant. Proc.* **21**, 1707.

Ettenger, R. B., Rosenthal, J. T., Marik, J. L., *et al.* (1990). Cadaver renal transplantation in children: results with long-term cyclosporine immunosuppression. *Clin. Transplant.* **4**, 329.

Ettenger, R. B., Rosenthal, J. T., Marik, J. L., *et al.* (1991b). Improved cadaveric renal transplant outcome in children. *Pediatr. Nephrol.* **5**, 137.

Ettenger, R. B., Schroeder, T. and Superina, R. (1992c). Monoclonal antibody therapy in pediatric transplantation. *Transplant. Proc.* **24(Suppl. 1)**, 1.

Ettenger, R. B., Tong, M. J., Landing, B. H., *et al.* (1980). Hepatitis B infection in pediatric dialysis and transplant patients: significance of e antigen. *J. Pediatr.* **97**, 550.

European Multicentre Trial. (1982). Cyclosporin A as sole immunosuppressive agent in recipients and kidney allografts from cadaver donors: preliminary results of a European Multicentre Trial. *Lancet* **2**, 57.

European Mycophenolate Mofetil Cooperative Study Group. (1995). Placebo controlled study of mycophenolate mofetil combined with cyclosporine and corticosteroids for prevention of acute rejection. *Lancet* **345**, 1321.

Evangelista, J. B., Jr., Bennett-Jones, D., Cameron, J. S., *et al.* (1985). Renal transplantation in patients treated with haemodialysis and short term and long term continuous ambulatory peritoneal dialysis. *Br. M. J.* **291**, 1004.

Fauci, A. S. (1978). Mechanisms of the immunosuppressive and anti-inflammatory effects of glucocorticoids. *J. Immunopharmacol.* **1**, 1.

Fauci, A. S. (1985). The effect of hydrocortisone on the kinetics of normal lymphocytes. *Blood* **46**, 235.

Feehally, J., Bennett, S. E., Harris, K. P. G., *et al.* (1986). Is chronic renal transplant rejection a nonimmunological phenomenon? *Lancet* **2**, 486.

Feldhoff, C. M., Balfour, H. H., Simmons, R. L., *et al.* (1981). Varicella in children with renal transplants. *J. Pediatr.* **98**, 25.

Fennell, R. S., III, Andres, J. M., Pfaff, W. W., *et al.* (1981). Liver dysfunction in children and adolescents during hemodialysis and after renal transplantation. *Pediatrics* **67**, 855.

Fennell, R. S., III, Love, J. T., Carter, R. L., *et al.* (1986). Statistical analysis of statural growth following kidney transplantation. *Eur. J. Pediatr.* **145**, 86.

Fernandez, J. A., Milgrom, M., Burke, G. W., *et al.* (1990). Recurrence of lupus nephritis in a renal allograft with histologic transformation of the lesion. *Transplantation* **50**, 1056.

Ferraris, J., Saenger, P., Levine, L., *et al.* (1980). Delayed puberty in males with chronic renal failure. *Kidney Int.* **18**, 344.

Ferraris, J. R., Day, P., F., Gutman, R., *et al.* (1992). Effect of therapy with a new glucocorticoid deflazacort, on linear growth and growth hormone secretion after renal transplantation. *J. Pediatr.* **121**, 809.

Ferraris, J. R., Day, P., Gutman, R., *et al.* (1992). Effect of therapy with a new glucocorticoid, deflazacort, on linear growth and growth hormone secretion after renal transplantation. *J. Pediatr.* **121**, 809.

Ferraris, J. R., *et al.* (1996). Immunosuppressive activity of deflazacort in pediatric renal transplantation. *Transplantation* **62**, 417.

Filo, R. S., Smith, E. J. and Leapman, S. B. (1980). Therapy of acute cadaveric renal allograft rejection with adjunctive antithymocyte globulin. *Transplantation* **30**, 455.

Fine, R. N. (1979). Transplantation in children. *In Kidney Transplantation: Principles and Practice*, 1st ed., (P. J. Morris, ed.), p. 353, Academic Press, London.

Fine, R. N. (1982). Pregnancy in renal allograft recipients. *Am. J. Nephrol.* **2**, 117.

Fine, R. N., Brennan, L. P., Edelbrock, H. H., *et al.* (1969b). Use of pediatric cadaver kidneys for homotransplantation in children. *J. A. M. A.* **210**, 477.

Fine, R. N., Edelbrock, H. H., Riddell, H., *et al.* (1977a). Renal transplantation in children. *Urology* **9**, 61.

Fine, R. N. and Ettenger, R. B. (1988). Renal transplantation in children. *In Kidney Transplantation: Principles and Practice*, 3rd ed., (P. J. Morris, ed.), p. 635, W.B. Saunders, Philadelphia.

Fine, R. N., Grushkin, C. M., Malekzadeh, M., *et al.* (1972). Cytomegalovirus syndrome following renal transplantation. *Arch. Surg.* **105**, 564.

Fine, R. N., Korsch, B. M., Stiles, Q., *et al.* (1970). Renal homotransplantation in children. *J. Pediatr.* **76**, 347.

Fine, R. N., Malekzadeh, M. H., Pennisi, A. H., *et al.* (1977b). HBs antigenemia in renal allograft recipients. *Ann. Surg.* **185**, 411.

Fine, R. N., Malekzadeh, M. H., Pennisi, A. J., *et al.* (1979). Renal retransplantation in children. *J. Pediatr.* **95**, 244.

Fine, R. N., Offner, G., Wilson, W. A., *et al.* (1975). Posterior subcapsular cataracts: post-transplantation in children. *Ann. Surg.* **182**, 585.

Fine, R. N., Wright, J. R., Jr., Lieberman, E., *et al.* (1969a). Azathioprine and varicella. *J. A. M. A.* **207**, 147.

Fine, R. N., Yadin, O., Moulten, L., *et al.* (1992). Extended recombinant human growth hormone treatment after renal transplantation in children. *J. Am. Soc. Nephrol.* **2**, S274.

Fine, R. N., *et al.* (1991). Recombinant human growth hormone treatment of children following renal transplantation. *Pediatr. Nephrol.* **5**, 147.

Firlit, C. F. (1976). Use of defunctionalized bladders in pediatric renal transplantation. *J. Urol.* **116**, 634.

Firlit, C. F. and Merkel, F. K. (1977). The application of ileal conduits in pediatric renal transplantation. *J. Urol.* **118**, 647.

First, M. R., Schroeder, T. J., Hariharan, S., *et al.* (1992). The effect of indomethacin on the febrile response following OKT3 therapy. *Transplantation* **53**, 91.

First, M. R., Schroeder, T. J., Hurtubise, P. E., *et al.* (1989). Successful retreatment of allograft rejection with OKT3. *Transplantation* **47**, 88.

Fischer, G., Whitman, L. E., Lang, K., *et al.* (1989). Cyclophilin and peptidyl proyl cis-trans isomerases are probably identical proteins. *Nature* **337**, 476.

Fletcher, C. V., Englund, J. A., Edleman, C. K., *et al.* (1991). Pharmacologic basis for high-dose oral acyclovir prophylaxis of cytomegalovirus disease in renal allograft recipients. *Antimicrob. Agents Chemother.* **35**, 938.

Flower, R. J. (1985). Background and discovery of lipocortins. *Agents Actions* **17**, 255.

Flynn, J. T., Schulman, S. L., *et al.* (1992). Treatment of steroid-resistant post-transplant nephrotic syndrome with cyclophosphamide in a child with congenital nephrotic syndrome. *Pediatr. Nephrol.* **6**, 553.

Folman, R., Arbus, G. S., Churchill, B., *et al.* (1978). Recurrence of the hemolytic uremic syndrome in a 3 1/2 year old child, 4 months after second transplantation. *Clin. Nephrol.* **10**, 121.

Fontaine, E., Gagnadoux, M. F., Niaudet, P., *et al.* (1998). Renal transplantation in children with augmentation cystoplasty: long-term results. *J. Urol.* **159**, 2110.

Fowler, B., Weltz, G., Nieder, R. J., *et al.* (1990). Evidence that glucocorticoids block expression of the human interleukin-6 gene by accessory cells. *Transplantation* **49**, 183.

Francis, V. R., Fine, R. N. and Korsch, B. M. (1970). Physiologic and social adjustment to external hemodialysis and renal homotransplantation in 42 children. *Proc. Eur. Dial. Transplant. Assoc.* **7**, 366.

Franco, A., Peres, R., Anaya, F., *et al.* (1987). Spontaneous remission of proteinuria in recurrent focal glomerulosclerosis: reappraisal of plasma exchange treatment. *Clin. Nephrol.* **28**, 118.

Frawley, J. E. and Farnsworth, R. H. (1990). Adult donor kidney transplantation in small children: a surgical technique. *Aust. N. Z. J. Surg.* **60**, 911.

Freundlich, M., Zilleruelo, G., Arbitol, C., *et al.* (1985). Infant formula as a cause of aluminum toxicity in neonatal uraemia. *Lancet* **2**, 527.

Fryd, D. S., Sutherland, D. E. R., Simmons, R. L., *et al.* (1981). Results of a prospective randomized study on the effect of splenectomy versus no splenectomy in renal transplant patients. *Transplant. Proc.* **13**, 48.

Furth, S. L., Neu, A. M., Case, B., *et al.* (1996). Pneumococcal polysaccharide vaccine in children with chronic renal disease: a prospective study of antibody response and duration. *J. Pediatr.* **128**, 99.

Furth, S. L., Sullivan, E. K., Neu, A. M., *et al.* (1997). Varicella in the first year after transplantation: a report of the North American Pediatric Renal Transplant Cooperative Study. *Pediatr. Transplant.* **1**, 37.

Gagnadoux, M. F., Niaudet, P., Bacri, J. L., *et al.* (1985). Nonimmunological risk factors in pediatric renal transplantation. *Transplant. Proc.* **17**, 187.

Gagnadoux, M. F., Niaudet, P. and Broyer, M. (1993). Nonimmunological risk factors in paediatric renal transplantation. *Pediatr. Nephrol.* **7**, 89.

Gagnadoux, M. F., Niaudet, P., Droz, D., *et al.* (1999). Risk of primary disease recurrence in pediatric renal transplantation. *Transplant. Proc.* **31**, 235.

Gahl, W., Reed, G., Thoene, J., *et al.* (1986a). *Am. Pediatr. Soc.* **20**, 264A.

Gahl, W. A., Schneider, J. A., Thoene, J. G. and Chesney, R. (1986b). Course of nephropathic cystinosis after age 10 years. *J. Pediatr.* **109**, 605.

Gaspari, F., Ruggeneati, P., Torre, L., *et al.* (1993). Failure to predict cyclosporine area under the curve using a limited sampling strategy. *Kidney Int.* **44**, 436.

Gaston, R. S., Dejerhoi, M. H., Patterson, T., *et al.* (1991). OKT3 first dose reaction: association with T cell subsets and cytokine release. *Kidney Int.* **39**, 141.

Geary, D. F. and Haka-Ikse, K. (1989). Neurodevelopment progress of young children with chronic renal disease. *Pediatrics* **84**, 68.

Gellert, S., Devaux, S., Schonberger, B., *et al.* (1996). Donor age and graft function. *Pediatr. Nephrol.* **10**, 716.

Gershon, A. A., Steinberg, S. P. and Gelb, L. (1986). Live attenuated varicella vaccine use in immunocompromised children and adults. *Pediatrics* **78**, 757.

Ghio, L., Tarantino, A., Edefonti, A., *et al.* (1992). Advantages of cyclosporine as sole immunosuppressive agent in children with transplanted kidneys. *Transplantation* **54**, 834.

Gianantonio, C. A., Vitacco, M., Mendilaharzu, F., *et al.* (1968). The hemolytic-uremic syndrome: renal status of 76 patients at long-term follow-up. *J. Pediatr.* **72**, 757.

Giovannini, M., Tagger, A., Ribero, M. L., *et al.* (1990). Maternal-infant transmission of hepatitis C virus and HIV infections: a possible interaction. *Lancet* **335**, 1166.

Gjertson, D. W., Terasaki, P. I., Takemoto, S., *et al.* (1991). National allocation of cadaveric kidneys by HLA matching: projected effect on outcome and costs. *N. Engl. J. Med.* **324**, 1032.

Glass, N. R., Stillman, R. M., Butt, J. M. H., *et al.* (1979). Results of renal transplantation using pediatric cadaver donors. *Surgery* **85**, 504.

Goldberg, A. P., Haigers, J. M., Delmez, J. A., Heath, G. W. and Harter, H. R. (1979). Exercise training improves abnormal lipid and carbohydrate metabolism in hemodialysis patients. *ASAIO Trans.* **25**, 431.

Goldman, M., Abramowicz, D., DePauw, L., *et al.* (1991). Beneficial effects of prophylactic OKT3 in cadaver kidney transplantation: comparison with cyclosporin A in a single center prospective randomized study. *Transplant. Proc.* **23**, 1046.

Goldstein, G., Fuccello, A. J., Norman, D. J., *et al.* (1986). OKT3 monoclonal antibody plasma levels during therapy and the subsequent development of host antibodies to OKT3. *Transplantation* **42**, 507.

Goldstein, G., Norman, D. J., Shield, C. F., *et al.* (1991). OKT 3 monoclonal antibody reversal of acute renal allograft rejection unresponsive to conventional immunosuppressive treatments. *In Transplantation: Approaches to Graft Rejection*, (H. T. Meryman, ed.), p. 239, Alan R. Liss, New York.

Goldstein, S., Duhamel, G., Laudat, M. H., *et al.* (1984). Plasma lipids, lipoproteins and apolipoproteins AI, AII and B in renal transplanted children: what risk for accelerated atherosclerosis? *Nephron* **38**, 87.

Gomez-Campdera, F. J., Robles, N. R., Anaya, F., *et al.* (1990). Kidney transplantation from anencephalic donors: report of 5 cases and a review of the literature. *Child Nephrol. Urol.* **10**, 143.

Gonzalez, R., LaPointe, S., Sheldon, C. A., *et al.* (1984). Undiversion in children with renal failure. *J. Pediatr. Surg.* **19**, 632.

Goodwin, W. E., Kaufman, J. J., Mims, M. M., *et al.* (1963). Human renal transplantation: I. clinical experiences with six cases of renal homotransplantation. *J. Urol.* **89**, 13.

Gourlay, W., Stothers, L., McLoughin, M. G., *et al.* (1995). Transplantation of pediatric cadaver kidneys into adult recipients. *J. Urol.* **153**, 322.

Gradus (Ben-Ezer), D. and Ettenger, R. (1982). Renal transplantation in children. *Pediatr. Clin. North Am.* **29**, 1013.

Greenberg, A., Thompson, M. E., Griffith, B. J., *et al.* (1990). Cyclosporin toxicity in cardiac allograft patients—a seven year follow up. *Transplantation* **50**, 589.

Grevel, J., Welsh, M. S. and Kahan, B. D. (1989). Cyclosporin monitoring in renal transplantation: area under the curve monitoring is superior to trough level monitoring. *Ther. Drug Monit.* **11**, 246.

Grimm, P. C., Sinai-Trieman, L., Sekiya, N. M., *et al.* (1990). Effects of recombinant human erythropoietin on HLA sensitization and cell-mediated immunity. *Kidney Int.* **38**, 12.

Groenwoud, A. F., Persijn, G. G., Amaro, J. D., *et al.* (1989). Influence of immunosuppressive therapy: HLA matching and donor age on long-term cadaveric pediatric renal allograft survival. *Transplant. Proc.* **21**, 1683.

Gruber, S. A., Chavers, B., Skjei, K. L., *et al.* (1991). De novo cancer after pediatric kidney transplantation. *Transplant. Proc.* **23**, 1373.

Gruessner, R. W., Matas, A. J., Dunn, D. L., *et al.* (1990). A comparison of pediatric versus adult cadaver donor kidneys for transplantation. *Transplant. Proc.* **22**, 361.

Grushkin, C. M. and Fine, R. N. (1973). Growth in children following renal transplantation. *Am. J. Dis. Child.* **125**, 514.

Guest, G., Berard, E., Crosnier, H., *et al.* (1998). Effects of growth hormone in short children after renal transplantation. *Pediatr. Nephrol.* **12**, 437.

Guillou, P. J., Will, E. J., Davidson, A. M., *et al.* (1984). CAPD—a risk factor in renal transplantation? *Br. J. Surg.* **71**, 878.

Habib, R., Broyer, M. and Benmaiz, H. (1973). Chronic renal failure in children. *Nephron* **11**, 209.

Habib, R., Hebert, D., Gagnadoux, M. F., *et al.* (1982). Transplantation in idiopathic nephrosis. *Transplant. Proc.* **14**, 489.

Hahn, B., Pletscher, S. and Munian, M. (1981). Immunosuppressive effects of deflazacort: a new glucocorticoid with bone sparing and carbohydrate sparing properties, comparison with prednisone. *J. Rheumatol.* **8**, 783.

Halloran, P. (1996). A pooled analysis of three randomized double blind clinical studies in prevention of rejection with mycophenolate mofetil in renal allograft recipients (the one year analysis). *American Society of Transplant Physicians 15th Annual Meeting*, p. 166, Dallas.

Halpert, E., Tunnessen, W. W., Fivush, B., *et al.* (1991). Cutaneous lesions associated with cyclosporine therapy in pediatric renal transplant recipients. *J. Pediatr.* **119**, 489.

Hammer, G. B., Cao, S., Boltz, M. G., *et al.* (1998). Post transplant lymphoproliferative disease may present with severe airway obstruction. *Anaesthesiology* **89**, 263.

Handschumacher, R. E., Harding, M. W., Rice, J., *et al.* (1984). Cyclophilin—a specific cytosolic binding protein for cyclosporin A. *Science* **226**, 544.

Hanto, D. W., Jendrisak, M. D., So, S. K. S., *et al.* (1994). Induction immunosuppression with antilymphocyte globulin or OKT 3 in cadaver kidney transplantation. *Transplantation* **57**, 377.

Hardy, M. A., Nowygrod, R., Elberg, A. and Appel, G. (1980). Use of ATG in treatment of steroid-resistant rejection. *Transplantation* **29**, 162.

Harmon, W. E. (1991). Opportunistic infections in children following renal transplantation. *Pediatr. Nephrol.* **5**, 118.

Harmon, W. E., Alexander, S. R., Tejani, A., *et al.* (1992). The effect of donor age on graft survival in pediatric cadaver renal transplant recipients—a report of the North American Pediatric Renal Transplant Cooperative Study. *Transplantation* **54**, 232.

Harmon, W. E. and Jabs, K. (1992). Factors affecting growth after renal transplantation. *J. Am. Soc. Nephrol.* **12**, S295.

Harmon, W. E., Stablein, D., Alexander, S. R., *et al.* (1991). Graft thrombosis in pediatric renal transplant recipients. *Transplantation* **51**, 406.

Hasegawa, A., Kawamura, T., Ito, H., *et al.* (1989). Fate of renal grafts with recurrent Henoch-Schönlein purpura nephritis in children. *Transplant. Proc.* **21**, 2130.

Hatch, D. A. (1994). Kidney transplantation in patients with an abnormal lower urinary tract. *Urol. Clin. North Am.* **21**, 311.

Hayes, J. M., Novick, A. C., Streem, S. B., *et al.* (1988). The use of single pediatric cadaver kidneys for transplantation. *Transplantation* **45**, 106.

Hayes, J. M., Steinmuller, D. R., Streem, S. B., *et al.* (1991). The development of proteinuria and focal-segmental glomerulosclerosis in recipients of pediatric donor kidneys. *Transplantation* **52**, 813.

Hebert, D., Sibley, R. K. and Mauer, S. M. (1986). Recurrence of hemolytic uremic syndrome in renal transplant recipients. *Kidney Int.* **30**, S51.

Helin, I. and Winberg, J. (1980). Chronic renal failure in Swedish children. *Acta Paediatr. Scand.* **69**, 607.

Hely, D., Fennell, R. S., III, Petty, W., *et al.* (1982). Osteonecrosis of the femoral head and condyle in the post transplantation courses of children and adolescents. *Int. J. Pediatr.* **3**, 297.

Herdman, R. C. and Uriza, R. E. (1975). Coagulopathy in renal disease—including uremic syndrome. *In Pediatric Nephrology,* (M. I. Rubin and T. M. Barrat, eds.), p. 189, Williams & Wilkins, Baltimore.

Hess, G., Massing, A., Rossol, S., *et al.* (1989). Hepatitis C virus and sexual transmission. *Lancet* **2**, 987.

Hibberd, P. L. and Rubin, R. H. (1991). Prevention of cytomegalovirus infection in the pediatric renal transplant patient. *Pediatr. Nephrol.* **5**, 112.

Higgins, R. M., Bloom, S. L., Hopkin, J. M., and Morris P. J. (1989). The risks and benefits of low-dose cotrimoxazole prophylaxis for Pneumocystis pneumonia in renal transplantation. *Transplantation* **47**, 558.

Hitchings, G. H. and Elion, G. B. (1969). Chemical immunosuppression and transplantation. *Acc. Chem. Res.* **2**, 202.

Ho, M. (1987). Infection and organ transplantation. *In Anesthesia and Organ Transplantation,* (S. Gelman, ed.), W.B. Saunders, p. 49, Philadelphia.

Ho, M. (1991). Human cytomegalovirus infections in immunosuppressed patients. *In Cytomegalovirus—Biology and Infection,* 2nd ed., (M. Ho, ed.), p. 249, Plenum, New York.

Ho, M. (1995). Risk factors and pathogenesis of post transplant lymphproliferative disorders. *Transplant. Proc.* **27(Suppl. 1)**, 38.

Ho, M., Jaffe, R., Miller, G., *et al.* (1988). The frequency of Epstein-Barr virus infection and associated lymphoproliferative syndrome after transplantation and its manifestations in children. *Transplantation* **45**, 719.

Ho, M., Miller, G., Atchison, R., *et al.* (1985). Epstein-Barr virus infections and DNA hybridization studies in post-transplantation lymphoma and lymphoproliferative lesions: the role of primary infection. *J. Infect. Dis.* **152**, 876.

Hoda, Q., Hasinoff, D. J. and Arbus, G. S. (1975). Growth following renal transplantation in children and adolescents. *Clin. Nephrol.* **3**, 6.

Hodson, E. M., Knight, J. F., Sheil, A. G. R., *et al.* (1989). Cyclosporin A as sole immunosuppressive agent for renal transplantation in children: effect on catch-up growth. *Transplant. Proc.* **21**, 1687.

Hodson, E. M., Knight, J. F., Sheil, A. G. R., *et al.* (1990). End-stage renal failure in children: 16 years' experience at one Australian centre. *Med. J. Aust.* **152**, 245.

Hodson, E. M., Najarian, J. S., Kjellstrand, C. M., *et al.* (1978). Renal transplantation in children ages 1 to 5 years. *Pediatrics* **61**, 458.

Hokken-Koelega, A. C. S., Stignen, T., DeJong, R. C., *et al.* (1996). A placebo controlled, double blind trial of growth hormone treatment in prepubertal children after renal transplant. *Kidney Int.* **49**, S53.

Holzgreve, W., Beller, F. K., Buchholz, B., *et al.* (1987). Kidney transplantation from anencephalic donors. *N. Engl. J. Med.* **316**, 1069.

Holliday, M. D. and Potter, D. E. (1970). Treatment of chronic uremia in childhood. *Adv. Pediatr.* **17**, 81.

Hong, J. H., Shirani, K., Arshad, A., *et al.* (1981). Influence of cadaver donor age on the success of kidney transplantation. *Transplantation* **32**, 532.

Hong, J. H., Sumrani, N., Delaney, V., *et al.* (1992). Causes of late renal allograft failure in the cyclosporin era. *Nephron* **62**, 272.

Hoppu, K., Koskimies, O., Holmberg, C., *et al.* (1991). Pharmacokinetically determined cyclosporine dosage in young children. *Pediatr. Nephrol.* **5**, 1.

Hoyer, J. R., Kjellstrand, C. M., Simmons, R. L., *et al.* (1973). Successful renal transplantation in three children with congenital nephrotic syndrome. *Lancet* **1**, 1410.

Hoyer, P. F., Offner, G., Oemar, B. S., *et al.* (1990). Four years' experience with cyclosporin A in pediatric kidney transplantation. *Acta Pediatr. Scand.* **79**, 622.

Hoyer, P. F., Offner, G., Wonigeit, K., *et al.* (1984). Dosage of cyclosporin A in children with renal transplants. *Clin. Nephrol.* **22**, 68.

Hricik, D. E., Bartucci, M. R., Mayes, J. T., *et al.* (1993). The effects of steroid withdrawal on the lipoprotein profiles of cyclosporin treated kidney and pancreas transplant recipients. *Transplantation* **54**, 868.

Hricik, D. E., Bartucci, M. R., Moir, E. J., *et al.* (1991). Effects of steroid withdrawal on post-transplant diabetes mellitus in cyclosporin treated renal transplant recipients. *Transplantation* **51**, 374.

Hricik, D. E., Lautmas, J., Bartucci, M. R., *et al.* (1992). Variable effects of steroid withdrawal on blood pressure reduction in cyclosporine treated renal transplant recipients. *Transplantation* **53**, 1232.

Hsui, H. C., Suzuki, Y., Churg, J., *et al.* (1980). Ultrastructure of the glomerular basement membrane in long-term renal allografts with transplant glomerular disease. *Histopathology* **4**, 351.

Hueso, M., Bover, J., Seron, D., *et al.* (1998). Low dose cyclosporin and mycophenolate mofetil in renal allograft recipients with suboptimal renal function. *Transplantation* **66**, 1727.

Hughes, W. T. (1977). *Pneumocystis carinii* pneumonia. *N. Engl. J. Med.* **297**, 1381.

Hurley, J. K., Greenslade, T., Lewy, P. R., *et al.* (1980). Varicella-zoster infections in pediatric renal transplant recipients. *Arch. Surg.* **115**, 551.

Iitaka, K., Martin, L. W., Cox, J. A., *et al.* (1978). Transplantation of cadaver kidneys from anencephalic donors. *J. Pediatr.* **93**, 216.

Ingelfinger, J. R. (1984). Hypertension in children with ESRD. *In End-Stage Renal Disease in Children,* (R. N. Fine and A. B. Gruskin, eds.), p. 340, W.B. Saunders, Philadelphia.

Ingelfinger, J. R., Grupe, W. E., Harmon, W. E., *et al.* (1981). Growth acceleration following renal transplantation in children less than 7 years of age. *Pediatrics* **68**, 255.

Ingulli, E. and Tejani, A. (1991). Incidence, treatment, and outcome of recurrent focal segmental glomerulosclerosis post-transplant in 42 allografts in children—a single-center experience. *Transplantation* **51**, 401.

Ingulli, E., Tejani, A., Butt, K. M. H., *et al.* (1990). High-dose cyclosporine therapy in recurrent nephrotic syndrome following renal transplantation. *Transplantation* **49**, 219.

Ingulli, E., Tejani, A., Fikrig, S., *et al.* (1991). Nephrotic syndrome associated with acquired immunodeficiency syndrome in children. *J. Pediatr.* **119**, 710.

Iragorri, S., Pillay, D., Scrine, M., *et al.* (1993). Prospective cytomegalovirus surveillance in pediatric renal transplantation patients. *Pediatr. Nephrol.* **7**, 55.

Jabs, K. L., Sullivan E. R., Avner E. D., *et al.* (1996). Alternate dosing improves growth without adversely affecting graft survival or long term graft function. *Transplantation* **61**, 31.

Jabs, K. L., Van Dop, C. and Harmon, W. E. (1990). Endocrinologic evaluation of children who grow poorly following renal transplantation. *Transplantation* **49**, 71.

Jarowenko, M. K., Flechner, S. M., Van Buren, C. T., *et al.* (1987). Influence of cyclosporin on post transplant blood pressure response. *Am. J. Kidney Dis.* **10**, 98.

Johansson, G., *et al.* (1990). Recombinant human growth hormone treatment in short children with chronic renal disease, before transplantation or with functioning renal transplants: an interim report on five European studies. *Acta Pediatr. Scand.* **370(Suppl.)**, 36.

Jordan, M. L., Naraghi, R., Shapiro, R., *et al.* (1997). Tacrolimus rescue therapy for renal allograft rejection—five years experience. *Transplantation* **63**, 223.

Kahan, B. D., Gibbons, S., Tejpal, N., *et al.* (1991). Synergistic interaction of cyclosporine and rapamycin to inhibit immune performances of normal human peripheral blood lymphocytes in vitro. *Transplantation* **51**, 232.

Kahan, B. D., Kramer, W. G., Wideman, C., *et al.* (1986). Demographic factors affecting the pharmacokinetics of cyclosporin estimated by radio-immunoassay. *Transplantation* **41**, 455.

Kahan, B. D., Van Buren, C. T., Flechner, S. M., *et al.* (1983). Cyclosporine immunosuppression mitigates immunologic risk factors in renal allotransplantation. *Transplant. Proc.* **15**, 2469.

Kahan, B. D., *et al.* (1986). Analysis of pharmacokinetic profiles in 232 renal and 87 cardiac allograft recipients treated with cyclosporin. *Transplant. Proc.* **18**, 115.

Kalia, A., Brouhard, B. H., Travis, L. B., *et al.* (1988). Renal transplantation in the infant and young child. *Am. J. Dis. Child.* **142**, 47.

Kaplan, B. S. (1992). Hemolytic-uremic syndrome in children. *Curr. Opin. Pediatr.* **4**, 254.

Kaplan, B. S., Levin, M. and de Chadarevian, J. P. (1992). The hemolytic-uremic syndrome. *In Pediatric Kidney Disease*, (C. M. Edelman, J. Bunstein, S. R. Meadow, A. Spitzer and L. B. Travis, eds.), p. 1383, Little, Brown, Boston.

Kashtan, C. E., Cook, M., Chavers, B. M., *et al.* (1996). Outcome of chicken pox in 66 pediatric renal transplant recipients. *J. Pediatr.* **131**, 874.

Katz, A., Freese, D. and Danpure, C. J. (1992). Success of kidney transplantation in oxalosis is unrelated to residual hepatic enzyme activity. *Kidney Int.* **42**, 1408.

Katz, A., Kim, Y., Scheinman, J. I., *et al.* (1989). Long-term outcome of kidney transplantation in children with oxalosis. *Transplant. Proc.* **21**, 2033.

Kay, J. E., Benzie, C. R., Goodier, M. R., *et al.* (1989). Inhibition of T lymphocyte activation by the immunosuppressive drug FK506. *Immunology* **67**, 473.

Kelly, W. D., Lillehei, R. C., Aust, J. B., *et al.* (1967). Allotransplantation of the pancreas and duodenum along with the kidney in diabetic nephropathy. *Surgery* **62**, 704.

Kerman, R. H. (1989). Immune monitoring considerations in transplantation. *In Principles of Organ Transplantation*, (M. W. Flye, ed.), p. 135, W.B. Saunders, Philadelphia.

Kerman, R. H., Van Buren, C. T., Payne, W., *et al.* (1983). Monitoring of T-cell subsets and immune events in renal allograft recipients. *Transplant. Proc.* **15**, 1170.

Kiberd, B. A. (1989). Cyclosporine-induced renal dysfunction in human renal allograft recipients. *Transplantation* **48**, 965.

King, L. R., Gerbie, A. G., Idriss, F. S., *et al.* (1971). Human renal transplantation with kidney grafts from the newborn. *Invest. Urol.* **8**, 622.

Kinnaert, P., Persijn, G., Cohen, B., *et al.* (1984). Transplantation of kidneys from anencephalic donors. *Transplant. Proc.* **16**, 71.

Kinne, D. W., Spanos, P. K., DeShazo, M. M., *et al.* (1974). Double renal transplants from pediatric donors to adult recipients. *Am. J. Surg.* **127**, 292.

Kinukawa, T., Iwaki, Y. and Teraskai, P. (1983). *9th Ann. Sci. Meet. Am. Soc. Transplant. Surg.* Chicago.

Kirk, A. J. B., Omar, I., Bateman, D. N., *et al.* (1989). Cyclosporine-associated hypertension in cardiopulmonary transplantation. *Transplantation* **48**, 428.

Kirkman, R. L., Barret, L. V., Gaulton, G. N., *et al.* (1985). Administration of an anti-interleukin-2 receptor monoclonal antibody prolongs cardiac allograft survival in mice. *J. Exp. Med.* **162**, 358.

Klare, B., Strom, T. M., Hahn, H., *et al.* (1991). Remarkable long-term prognosis and excellent growth in kidney-transplant children under cyclosporine monotherapy. *Transplant. Proc.* **23**, 1013.

Klare, B., Walter, J. V., Hahn, H., *et al.* (1984). Cyclosporin in renal transplantation in children. *Lancet* **2**, 692.

Klintmalm, G. B. G., Sawe, J., Ringden, O., *et al.* (1985). Cyclosporine plasma levels in renal transplant patients. Association with renal toxicity and allograft rejection. *Transplantation* **39**, 132.

Knight, J. F., Roy, L. P. and Sheil, A. G. (1985). Catch-up growth in children with successful renal transplants immunosuppressed with cyclosporin alone. *Lancet* **1**, 159.

Knudsen, P. J., Dianarello, C. H. and Storm, T. B. (1987). Glucocorticoids inhibit transcriptional and post-transcriptional expression of interleukin-1 in U937 cells. *J. Immunol.* **139**, 4129.

Koffman, C. G., Rigden, S. P. A., Bewick, M., *et al.* (1989). Renal transplantation in children less than 5 years of age. *Transplant. Proc.* **21**, 2001.

Kohaut, E. C., Whelchel, J. R., Waldo, F. B., *et al.* (1985). Living-related donor renal transplantation in children presenting with end-stage renal disease in the first months of life. *Transplantation* **40**, 725.

Koo, H. P., Bunchman, T. E., Flynn, J. T., *et al.* (1999). Renal transplantation in children with severe lower urinary tract dysfunction. *J. Urol.* **161**, 240.

Kootstra, G., West, J. C., Dryburgh, P., *et al.* (1978). Pediatric cadaver kidneys for transplantation. *Surgery* **83**, 333.

Kopp, J. B. and Klotman, P. E. (1990). Cellular and molecular mechanisms of cyclosporine nephrotoxicity. *J. Am. Soc. Nephrol.* **1**, 162.

Korsch, B. M., Fine, R. N. and Negrete, V. F. (1978). Noncompliance in children with renal transplants. *Pediatrics* **61**, 872.

Korsch, B. M., Klein, J. D. and Negrete, V. F. (1980). Physical and psychological follow-up on offspring of renal allograft recipients. *Pediatrics* **65**, 275.

Korsch, B. M., Negrete, V. F. and Fine, R. (1993). Clinical implications of non-compliance in children and adolescents with end-stage renal disease in pediatric nephrology. *In Renal Disease Dynamics*, (J. Strauss, ed.), p. 159, University of Miami Press, Coral Gables, Fla.

Kovacs, G., Fine, R. N., Worgall, S., *et al.* (1991a). Recombinant human growth hormone overcomes the growth-suppressive effect of methylprednisolone in uremic rats. *Pediatr. Nephrol.* **5**, 552.

Kovacs, G., Fine, R. N., Worgall, S., *et al.* (1991b). Growth hormone prevents steroid-induced growth depression in health and in uremia. *Kidney Int.* **40**, 1032.

Kovarik, J. M., Rawlings, E., Sweny, P., *et al.* (1996). Prolonged immunosuppressive effect and minimal immunogenicity from chimeric (CD25) monoclonal antibody SDZCH1621 in renal transplantation. *Transplant. Proc.* **28**, 913.

Kreiger, J. N., Brem, A. S. and Kaplan, M. R. (1980). Urinary tract infection in pediatric renal transplantation. *Urology* **15**, 362.

Kreis, H., Legendre, C. and Chatenoud, L. (1991). OKT3 in organ transplantation. *Transplant. Rev.* **5**, 181.

Kreis, H., Mansouri, R., DeCamps, J. *et al.* (1981). Antilymphocyte globulin in cadaver kidney transplantation: a randomized trial based on T cell monitoring. *Kidney Int.* **19**, 438.

Krull, F., Hegerhorst, A., Offner, G., *et al.* (1993). 24 hour blood pressure monitoring for control of antihypertensive therapy in pediatric kidney transplant recipients. *Transplant. Proc.* **25**, 2575.

Kupiec-Weglinski, J. W., Hahn, H., Kirkman, R., et al. (1988). Cyclosporine potentiates the immunosuppressive effects of anti-interleukin 2 receptor monoclonal antibody therapy. *Transplant. Proc.* **20**, 207.

Kwun, Y. A., Butt, K. M. H., Kim, K. H., *et al.* (1978). Successful renal transplantation in a 3-month-old infant. *J. Pediatr.* **92**, 426.

L'Age-Stehr, J., Schwarz, A., Offermann, G., *et al.* (1985). HTLV-III infection in kidney transplant recipients. *Lancet* **2**, 1361.

Landwirth, J. (1988). Should anencephalic infants be used as organ donors? *Pediatrics* **82**, 257.

Lane, P. H., Schnaper, H. W., Vernier, R. L., *et al.* (1991). Steroid-dependent nephrotic syndrome following renal transplantation for congenital nephrotic syndrome. *Pediatr. Nephrol.* **5**, 300.

Langlois, R. P., O'Regan, S., Pelletier, M., *et al.* (1981). Kidney transplantation in uremic children with cystinosis. *Nephron* **28**, 273.

LaPlante, M. P., Kaufman, J. J., Goldman, R., *et al.* (1970). Kidney transplantation in children. *Pediatrics* **46**, 665.

Lattyak, B. V., Rosenthal, P., Mudge, C., *et al.* (1998). Post transplant lymphoproliferative disorder presenting in the Head and Neck. *Laryngoscope* **108**, 1195.

Laufer, J., Ettenger, R. B., Ho, W. G., *et al.* (1988). Plasma exchange for recurrent nephrotic syndrome following renal transplantation. *Transplantation* **46**, 540.

Laufer, J., Ettenger, R. B., Marik, J., *et al.* (1987). Retransplantation with HLA-identical living-related allografts in children. *Transplantation* **44**, 322.

Lawson, R. K., Bennett, W. M., Campbell, R. A., *et al.* (1973). Hyperacute renal allograft rejection in the human neonate. *Invest. Urol.* **10**, 444.

Lawson, R. K., Talwalkar, Y. B., Musgrave, J. E., *et al.* (1975). Renal transplantation in pediatric patients. *J. Urol.* **113**, 225.

Lee, S. W., Tson, A. P. and Chou, H. (1988). Glucocorticoids selectively inhibit the transcription of the interleukin 1 beta gene and decrease the stability of interleukin 1 beta mRNA. *Proc. Natl. Acad. Sci. U. S. A.* **8**, 1204.

Leithner, C., Sinzinger, H., Pohanka, E., *et al.* (1982). Recurrence of haemolytic uraemic syndrome triggered by cyclosporin A after renal transplantation. *Lancet* **7**, 1470.

Leichter, H. E., Ettenger, R. B., Jordan, S. C., *et al.* (1986a). Short-course antithymocyte globulin for treatment of renal transplant rejection in children. *Transplantation* **41**, 133.

Leichter, H. E., Salusky, I. B., Ettenger, R. B., *et al.* (1986b). Experience with renal transplantation in children undergoing peritoneal dialysis (CAPD/CCPD). *Am. J. Kidney Dis.* **3**, 181.

Lemaire, M., Fahr, A. and Maurer, G. (1990). Pharmacokinetics of cyclosporin: inter- and intra-individual variation and metabolic pathways. *Transplant. Proc.* **22**, 1110.

Leone, M., Alexander, S., Barry, J., *et al.* (1987). OKT3 monoclonal antibody in pediatric kidney transplant recipients with recurrent and resistant allograft rejection. *J. Pediatr.* **111**, 45.

Leone, M., Barry, J., Alexander, S., *et al.* (1990). Monoclonal antibody OKT3 therapy in pediatric kidney transplant recipients. *J. Pediatr.* **116**, S86.

Leumann, E. P. (1976). Die chronische Niereninsuffizienz in Kindesalter. Ergebnisse einer Schweizerischen rundfrage. *Schweiz Med. Wochenschr.* **106**, 244.

Leumann, E. P., Briner, J., Donckerwolcke, R. A. M., *et al.* (1980). Recurrence of focal segmental glomerulosclerosis in the transplanted kidney. *Nephron* **25**, 65.

Leumann, E. P., Wegmann, W. and Largiader, F. (1978). Prolonged survival after renal transplantation in primary hyperoxaluria of childhood. *Clin. Nephrol.* **9**, 29.

Leunissen, K. M. L., Bosman, F. T., Kootstra, G., *et al.* (1989). Focal glomerulosclerosis in neonatal kidney grafts. *Nephron* **51**, 29.

Levitt, S. B., Coberwal, D., Kogan, S. J., *et al.* (1979). Use of preexisting ureterocutaneous anastomosis as conduit in renal allotransplantation. *Urology* **13**, 377.

Levy, M., Ami Moussa, R., Habib, R., *et al.* (1982). Anaphylactoid purpura nephritis and transplantation. *Kidney Int.* **22**, 326.

Lewis, R., Potbielski, J., Sprayberry, S., *et al.* (1993). Stability of renal allograft glomerular filtration rate associated with long-term use of cyclosporine A. *Transplantation* **55**, 1014.

Lingens, N., Dobos, E., Witte, K., *et al.* (1997). Twenty four-hour ambulatory blood pressure profiles in pediatric patients after renal transplantation. *Pediatr. Nephrol.* **11**, 23.

Lingens, N., Soergel, M., Loirat, C., *et al.* (1995). Ambulatory blood pressure monitoring in pediatric patients treated by regular hemodialysis and peritoneal dialysis. *Pediatr. Nephrol.* **9**, 167.

Lopez, C., Simmons, R. L., Mauer, S. M., *et al.* (1974). Association of renal allograft rejection with virus infections. *Am. J. Med.* **56**, 280.

Lorber, M. J., van Buren, C. T., Fleckner, S. M., *et al.* (1987). Hepatobiliary and pancreatic complications of cyclosporine therapy in 466 renal transplant recipients. *Transplantation* **43**, 35.

Lowance, D., Neumayer, M. M., Legendre, C. M., *et al.* (1999). Valacyclovir for the prevention of CMV disease after renal transplantation. *N. Engl. J. Med.* **340**, 1462.

Luke, R. (1987). Hypertension in renal transplant recipients. *Kidney Int.* **31**, 1024.

Lynfield, R., Herrin, J. T. and Rubin, R. H. (1992). Varicella in pediatric renal transplant recipients. *Pediatrics* **90**, 216.

MacDonald, A. S., Crocker, J. F. S., Belitsky, P., *et al.* (1986). Cyclosporine therapy in pediatric renal transplantation. *Transplant. Proc.* **18**, 153.

Maddocks, J. L., Lennard, L., Amess, J., *et al.* (1986). Azathioprine and severe bone marrow depression. *Lancet* **1**, 156.

Mahoney, C. P., Striker, G. E., Hickman, R. O., *et al.* (1970). Renal transplantation for childhood cystinosis. *N. Engl. J. Med.* **283**, 397.

Maizel, S. E., Sibley, R. K., Horstoman, J. P., *et al.* (1981). Incidence and significance of recurrent focal segmental glomerulosclerosis in renal allograft recipients. *Transplantation* **32**, 512.

Makker, S. P. and Kirson, I. J. (1980). Renal transplantation in a child with Burkitt's lymphoma. *Arch. Intern. Med.* **140**, 278.

Malagon, M. and Hogg, R. J. (1987). Renal transplantation after prolonged dwell peritoneal dialysis in children. *Kidney Int.* **31**, 981.

Malekzadeh, M., Grushkin, C. M., Stanley, P., *et al.* (1987b). Renal artery stenosis in pediatric transplant recipients. *Pediatr. Nephrol.* **1**, 22.

Malekzadeh, M. H., Brennan, L. P., Payne, V. C., Jr., *et al.* (1975). Hypertension after renal transplantation in children. *J. Pediatr.* **86**, 370.

Malekzadeh, M. H., Church, J. A., Siegel, S. E., *et al.* (1987a). Human immunodeficiency virus-associated Kaposi's sarcoma in a pediatric renal transplant recipient. *Nephron* **42**, 62.

Malekzadeh, M. H., Grushkin, C. M., Wright, H. T., Jr., *et al.* (1972). Hepatic dysfunction after renal transplantation in children. *J. Pediatr.* **81**, 279.

Malekzadeh, M. H., Heuser, E. P., Ettenger, R. B., *et al.* (1979). Focal glomerulosclerosis and renal transplantation. *J. Pediatr.* **95**, 249.

Malekzadeh, M. H., Neustien, H. B., Schneider, J. A., *et al.* (1977). Cadaver renal transplantation in children with cystinosis. *Am. J. Med.* **63**, 525.

Malekzadeh, M. H., Pennisi, A. J., Phillips, L., *et al.* (1978). Growth and endocrine function in children with cystinosis following renal transplantation. *ASAIO Trans.* **24**, 278.

Markello, T. C., Bernardini, I. M. and Gahl, W. A. (1993). Improved renal function in children with cystinosis treated with cysteamine. *N. Engl. J. Med.* **328**, 1157.

Martin, L. W., Gonzalez, L. L., West, C. D., *et al.* (1969). Homotransplantation of both kidneys from an anencephalic monster to a 17 pound boy with Eagle-Barret syndrome. *Surgery* **66**, 603.

Martin, L. W., McEnery, P. T., Rosenkrantz, J. G., *et al.* (1979). Renal homotransplantation in children. *J. Pediatr. Surg.* **14**, 571.

Matas, A. J., Gillingham, K. J., Chavers, B. M., *et al.* (1996). The importance of cyclosporine levels in pediatric kidney transplantation. *Clin. Transplant.* **10**, 482.

Matas, A. J., Tellis, V. A., Quinn, T., *et al.* (1985). Treatment of renal transplant rejection episodes in patients receiving prednisone and azathioprine. *Transplantation* **40**, 35.

Mathew, T. H. (1988). Recurrence of disease following renal transplantation. *Am. J. Kidney Dis.* **12**, 85.

Mathew, T. H. (1991). Recurrent disease after renal transplantation. *Transplant. Rev.* **5**, 31.

Mauch, T. J., Bralton, S., Myers, T., *et al.* (1999). Influenza B virus infection in pediatric solid organ transplant recipients. *Pediatrics* **94**, 225.

Mauer, S. M., Nevins, T. E. and Ascher, N. (1992). In *Pediatric Kidney Disease* (C. M. Edelman, ed.), p. 941, Little, Brown, Boston.

Maxwell, H., Dalton, R. N., Nair, D. R. *et al.* (1996). Effect of recombinant human growth hormone on renal function in children with renal transplants. *J. Pediatr.* **128**, 177.

Maxwell, H., Haffner, D. and Rees, L. (1998). Catch up growth occurs after renal transplantation in children of pubertal age. *J. Pediatr.* **133**, 435.

McDonald, J. C., Landerame, M. D., Rohr, M. S., *et al.* (1989). Reversal by liver transplantation of the complications of primary hyperoxaluria as well as the metabolic defect. *N. Engl. J. Med.* **321**, 1100.

McEnery, P. T. and Flanagan, J. (1977). Fulminant sepsis in splenectomized children with renal allografts. *Transplantation* **24**, 154.

McEnery, P. T., Gonzales, I. F., Martin, L. W., *et al.* (1973). Growth and development of children with renal transplants: use of alternate-day steroid therapy. *J. Pediatr.* **83**, 806.

McEnery, P. T., Stablein, D. M., Arbus, G., *et al.* (1992). Renal transplantation in children: a report of the North American Pediatric Renal Transplant Cooperative Study. *N. Engl. J. Med.* **326**, 1727.

McGeown, M. G., Kennedy, J. A., Loughridge, W. G., *et al.* (1977). One hundred kidney transplants in the Belfast city hospital. *Lancet* **11**, 648.

McGraw, M. E. and Haka-Ikse, K. (1985). Neurologic-developmental sequelae of chronic renal failure in infancy. *J. Pediatr.* **106**, 579.

McMahon, Y., MacDonell, R.C., Jr. and Richie, R. E. (1989). Is kidney transplantation in the very small child (less than 10 kg) worth it? *Transplant. Proc.* **21**, 2003.

McNally, P. G. and Feehally, J. (1992). Pathophysiology of cyclosporine A nephrotoxicity: experimental and clinical observation. *Nephrol. Dial. Transplant.* **7**, 791.

Meadow, R., Cameron, J. S. and Ogg, C. (1970). Regional service for acute and chronic dialysis of children. *Lancet* **2**, 707.

Meakins, J. L., Smith, E. J. and Alexander, J. W. (1972). En bloc transplantation of both kidneys from pediatric donors into adult patients. *Surgery* **71**, 72.

Melosky, B., Karim, M., Chris, A., *et al.* (1992). Lymphoproliferative disorders after renal transplantation in patients receiving triple or quadruple immunosuppression. *J. Am. Soc. Nephrol.* **2**, S290.

Merkel, F. K., Ing, T. S., Ahmadian, Y., *et al.* (1974). Transplantation in and of the young. *J. Urol.* **111**, 679.

Meyers, K. E., Thomson, P. D., and Weiland, H. (1996). Noncompliance in children and adolescents after renal transplantation. *Transplantation* **62**, 186.

Miller, L. C., Bock, G. H., Lum, C. T., *et al.* (1982). Transplantation of adult kidney into the very small child: long-term outcome. *J. Pediatr.* **100**, 675.

Mobb, G. E., Veitch, P. S. and Bell, P. R. (1992). Cyclosporin A abolishes renal reserve capacity. *Renal Fail.* **14**, 175.

Moel, D. T. and Butt, K. M. H. (1981). Renal transplantation in children less than 2 years of age. *J. Pediatr.* **99**, 535.

Moen, T., Albrechtsen, D., Flatmark, A., *et al.* (1980). Importance of HLA-DR matching in cadaveric renal transplantation. *N. Engl. J. Med.* **303**, 850.

Mongeau, J. G., Robitaille, P. and Grall, M. M. (1978). Chronic renal failure in children. *Can. Med. Assoc. J.* **118**, 907.

Montagnino, G., Colturi, C., Banfi, G., *et al.* (1989). Membranous nephropathy in cyclosporine-treated renal transplant recipients. *Transplantation* **47**, 725.

Moorthy, A. V., Zimmerman, S. W., Mejia, G., *et al.* (1986). Recurrence of lupus nephritis (LN) after renal transplantation (RTX). *J. Am. Soc. Nephrol.* 307A.

Morel, P., Almond, P. S., Matas, A. J., *et al.* (1991). Long-term quality of life after kidney transplantation in childhood. *Transplantation* **52**, 47.

Morling, N., Ladegoged, J., Lange, P., *et al.* (1975). Kidney transplantation and donor age. *Tissue Antigens* **6**, 163.

Morris, M. C., Chanbers, T. L., Evans, P. W. G., *et al.* (1982). Oxalosis in infancy. *Arch. Dis. Child.* **57**, 224.

Morris, P. J. (1981). Cyclosporin A. *Transplantation* **32**, 349.

Morris, R., Gregory, C. R., Huang, X., *et al.* (1995). Studies in experimental models of chronic rejection: use of rapamycin (sirolimus) and isoxazole derivatives (leflunomide and its analogues) for the suppression of graft vascular disease and obliterative bronchiolitis. *Transplant. Proc.* **27**, 2068.

Morris, R. E., Wu, J. and Shorthouse, R. (1990). A study of the contrasting effects of cyclosporin, FK506, and rapamycin on the suppression of allograft rejection. *Transplant. Proc.* **22**, 1638.

Mowry, J., Marik, J., Cohen, A., *et al.* (1993). Treatment of recurrent focal segmental glomerulosclerosis with high-dose cyclosporine-A and plasmapheresis. *Transplant. Proc.* **25**, 1345.

Munoz, J., Sanchez, M., Perez-Garcia, R., *et al.* (1985). Recurrent focal glomerulosclerosis in renal transplants proteinuria relapsing following plasma exchange. *Clin. Nephrol.* **24**, 213.

Murgia, M. G., Jordan, S. and Kahan, B. D. (1996). The side effect profile of sirolimus: a phase I study in quiescent cyclosporin prednisone treated renal transplant patients. *Kidney Int.* **49**, 209.

Murray, J. E., Wilson, R. E. and O'Connor, N. E. (1967). Evaluation of long-functioning human kidney transplants. *Surgery* **124**, 509.

Mycophenolate Mofetil Acute Rejection Study Group. (1998). Mycophenolate mofetil for the treatment of a first acute renal allograft rejection. *Transplantation* **65**, 235.

Myers, B. D. and Newton, L. (1991). Cyclosporin induced chronic nephropathy: An obliterative microvascular renal injury. *J. Am. Soc. Nephrol.* **2(Suppl.)**, 545.

Myers, B. D., Newton, L. and Oyer, P. (1991). The case against the indefinite use of cyclosporine. *Transplant. Proc.* **23**, 41.

Myers, K. E. C., Thomson, P. D. and Weiland, H. (1991). Noncompliance in children and adolescents after renal transplantation. *Transplantation* **62**, 186.

Naeye, R. L., Pa, H. and Blanc, W. A. (1971). Organ and body growth in anencephaly: a quantitative, morphological study. *Arch. Pathol.* **91**, 140.

Najarian, J. S., Almond, P. S., Mauer, M., *et al.* (1992). Renal transplantation in the first year of life: the treatment of choice for infants with end-stage renal disease. *J. Am. Soc. Nephrol.* **2**, S228.

Najarian, J. S., So, S. K., Simmons, R. L., *et al.* (1986). The outcome of 304 primary renal transplants in children. *Ann. Surg.* **3**, 246.

Nalensik, M. A., Makowka, L. and Starzl, T. E. (1988). The diagnosis and treatment of post transplant lymphoproliferative disorders. *Curr. Surg.* **25**, 365.

Nashan, B., Light, S., Hardie, I. R., *et al.*, for the Daclizumab Double Therapy Group. (1999). Reduction of acute renal allograft rejection by daclizumab. *Transplantation* **67**, 110.

Nashan, B., Moore, R., Amlot, P., *et al.*, for the CHIB 201 International Study Group. (1997). Randomized trial of basiliximab versus placebo for control of acute cellular rejection in renal allograft recipients. *Lancet* **350**, 1193.

Nast, C. C. and Cohen, A. H. (1992). Pathology of kidney transplantation. In *Handbook of Kidney Transplantation*, (G. M. Danovitch, ed.), p. 263, Little, Brown, Boston.

Nathanson, G., Winters, G. and Testa, E. (1967). Steroids possessing nitrogen atoms: synthesis of new highly active corticoids (17a, 16a-d) oxazoline steroids. *J. Med. Chem.* **10**, 799.

Neiberger, R., Weiss, R., Gomez, M., *et al.* (1987). Elimination kinetics of cyclosporin following oral administration to children with renal transplant. *Transplant. Proc.* **19**, 1525.

Neumayer, H. H., Wagner, K. and Kresse, S. (1986). HTLV-III antibodies in patients with kidney transplants or on haemodialysis. *Lancet* **1**, 497.

Nevins, T. E. and Dunn, D. L. (1992). Use of ganciclovir for cytomegalovirus infection. *J. Am. Soc. Nephrol.* **2**, S270.

Nghiem, D. D., Hsia S., and Schlosser, JD. (1995). Growth and function of en bloc infant kidney transplants: preliminary study. *J. Urol.* **153**, 326.

Niaudet, P., Jean, G., Broyer, M., *et al.* (1990). Prophylactic use of OKT3 in pediatric kidney transplant recipients. *J. Am. Soc. Nephrol.* **1**, 766.

Norman, D. J. and Leone, M. R. (1991). The role of OKT3 in clinical transplantation. *Pediatr. Nephrol.* **5**, 130.

Norman, D. J., Shield, C. F., Barry, J., *et al.* (1988). Early use of OKT 3 monoclonal antibody in renal transplantation to prevent rejection. *Am. J. Kidney Dis.* **11**, 107.

Norman, M. E. and Asadi, F. K. (1979). A prospective study of acute renal failure in the newborn infant. *Pediatrics* **63**, 475.

North American Pediatric Renal Transplant Cooperative Study Annual Report. (1992). *J. Am. Soc. Nephrol.* 12 suppl, S213–311.

North American Pediatric Renal Transplant Cooperative Study Annual Report. (1997). *Pediatr. Transplant* **1**, 146–162.

Northrop, J. P., Ho, S. N., Chen, L., *et al.* (1994). NF-AT components define a family of transcription factors targeted in T cell activation. *Nature* **369**, 497.

Novello, A. C. and Fine, R. N. (1982). Renal transplantation in children—a review. *Int. J. Pediatr. Nephrol.* **3**, 87.

Nyberg, G., Blohme, I., Persson, H., *et al.* (1992). Recurrence of systemic lupus erythematosus in transplanted kidneys: a follow-up transplant biopsy study. *Nephrol. Dial. Transplant.* **7**, 1116.

Oberkircher, O. R., Enama, M., West, J. C., *et al.* (1988). Regression of recurrent membranoproliferative glomerulonephritis type II in a transplanted kidney after plasmapheresis therapy. *Transplant. Proc.* **20(Suppl.)**, 418.

Oettinger, C. W., Merrill, R., Blanton, T., and Briggs, W. (1974). Reduced calcium absorption after nephrectomy in uremic patients. *N. Engl. J. Med.* **291**, 458.

Offner, G., Aschendorff, C. and Brodehl, J. (1991). Growth after renal transplantation: an update. *Pediatr. Nephrol.* **5**, 472.

Offner, G., Hoyer, P. F., Brodehl, J., *et al.* (1987). Cyclosporin A in pediatric kidney transplantation. *Pediatr. Nephrol.* **1**, 125.

Okuda, S., Motomura, K., Sanai, T., *et al.* (1987). Influence of age on deterioration of the remnant kidney in uninephrectomized rats. *Clin. Sci.* **72**, 571.

Olsen, S., Bohman, S. O. and Posborg-Petersen, V. (1974). Ultrastructure of the glomerular basement membrane in long-term renal allografts with transplant glomerular disease. *Lab. Invest.* **30**, 176.

O'Mallery, B. N. (1987). Mechanism of action of steroid hormones. *N. Engl. J. Med.* **284**, 370.

O'Malley, B. W. (1971). Unified hypothesis for early biochemical sequence of events in steroid hormone action. *Metabolism* **20**, 981.

Opelz, G., Sengar, D. P., Mickey, M. R. Terasaki, P. I. (1973). Effect of blood transfusions on subsequent kidney transplants. *Transplant. Procs.* **5**, 253.

Opelz, G. (1987). Effect of HLA matching in 10,000 cyclosporine-treated cadaver kidney transplants. Collaborative Transplant Study. *Transplant. Proc.* **19**, 641.

Opelz, G. (1988a). Importance of HLA antigens splits for kidney transplant matching. *Lancet* **2**, 61.

Opelz, G. (1988b). Influence of recipient and donor age in pediatric renal transplantation. Collaborative Transplant Study. *Transpl. Int.* **1**, 95.

Opelz, G. (1989). Influence of HLA matching on survival of second kidney transplants in cyclosporine-treated recipients. *Transplantation* **47**, 823.

Opelz, G., Mytilineos, J., Scherer, S., *et al.* (1991). Survival of DNA HLA-DR typed and matched cadaver kidney transplants. Collaborative Transplant Study. *Lancet* **2**, 461.

Opelz, G., Wujciak T. and Ritz, E. (1998) Association of chronic kidney graft failure with recipient blood pressure. *Kidney Int.* **53**, 217.

Ortho Multicenter Transplant Study Group. (1985). A randomized clinical trial of OKT3 monoclonal antibody for acute rejection of cadaveric renal transplants. *N. Engl. J. Med.* **313**, 337.

Pais, E., Pirson, Y., Squifflet, J. P., *et al.* (1992). Kidney transplantation in patients with Wilms' tumor. *Transplantation* **53**, 782.

Paller, M. S. and Murray, B. M. (1985). Renal dysfunction in animal models of cyclosporine toxicity. *Transplant. Proc.* **17(Suppl. 1)**, 155.

Peabody, J. L., Emery, J. R. and Ashwal, S. (1989). Experience with anencephalic infants as prospective organ donors. *N. Engl. J. Med.* **321**, 344.

Penn, I. (1979). Renal transplantation for Wilm's tumor: report of 20 cases. *J. Urol.* **122**, 793.

Penn, I. (1990). Cancers complicating organ transplantation. *N. Engl. J. Med.* **323**, 1767.

Pennisi, A. J., Costin, G., Phillips, L. S., *et al.* (1979). Somatomedin and growth hormone studies in pediatric renal allograft recipients who receive daily prednisolone. *Am. J. Dis. Child.* **133**, 950.

Pennisi, A. J., Fiedler, J., Mickcy, R., *et al.* (1975). Hyperlipidemia in pediatric renal allograft recipients. *J. Pediatr.* **87**, 249.

Pennisi, A. J., Heuser, E. T., Malekzadeh, M. N., *et al.* (1978a). Renal transplantation in children with membranoproliferative glomerulonephritis. *VIIth Int. Cong. Nephrol.*, Montreal.

Pennisi, A. J., Heuser, E. T., Mickey, M. R., *et al.* (1976). Hyperlipidema in pediatric hemodialysis and renal transplant patients associated with coronary artery disease. *Am. J. Dis. Child.* **130**, 957.

Pennisi, A. J., Malekzadeh, M. H., Uittenbogaart, C. H., *et al.* (1978b). Alternate day corticosteroid therapy in pediatric serial transplant recipients. *VIIth Int. Cong. Nephrol.*, Montreal.

Pennisi, A. J., Phillips, L. S., Costin, G., *et al.* (1978c). Linear growth in long-term renal allograft recipients. *Clin. Nephrol.* **8**, 415.

Pereira, B. J. G., Milford, E. L., Kirkman, R. L., *et al.* (1991). Transmission of hepatitis C virus by organ transplantation. *N. Engl. J. Med.* **325**, 454.

Perez-Romero, M., Sanchez-Quijano, A. and Lissen, E. (1990). Transmission of hepatitis C virus. *Ann. Intern. Med.* **113**, 411.

Pinto, J., Laurda, G., Cameron, J. S., *et al.* (1981). Recurrence of focal segmental glomerulosclerosis in renal allografts. *Transplantation* **32**, 83.

Pistor, K., Obling, H. and Scharer, K. (1985a). Children with chronic renal failure in the Federal Republic of Germany: I. epidemiology, modes of treatment, survival. *Clin. Nephrol.* **23**, 272.

Pistor, K., Scharer, K., Obling, H., *et al.* (1985b). Children with chronic renal failure in the Federal Republic of Germany: II. primary renal diseases, age and intervals from early renal failure to renal death. *Clin. Nephrol.* **23**, 278.

Platz, K. P., Sollinger, H. W., Hullert, D. A., *et al.* (1991). RS-61443: a new, potent immunosuppressive agent. *Transplantation* **51**, 27.

Polinsky, M. S., Kaiser, B. A., Stover, J. B., *et al.* (1987). Neurologic development of children with severe chronic renal failure from infancy. *Pediatr. Nephrol.* **1**, 157.

Porter, K. A., Dossetor, J. E., Marchioro, T. L., *et al.* (1967). Human renal transplants: I. glomerular changes. *Lab. Invest.* **16**, 153.

Potter, D., Feduska, N., Melzer, J., *et al.* (1986). Twenty years of renal transplantation in children. *Pediatrics* **77**, 465.

Potter, D., Garovoy, M., Hopper, S., *et al.* (1985). Effect of donor-specific transfusions on renal transplantation in children. *Pediatrics* **76**, 402.

Potter, D. E., Genant, H. K. and Salvatierra, O., Jr. (1978). Avascular necrosis of bone after renal transplantation. *Am. J. Dis. Child.* **132**, 1125.

Potter, D. E., Holliday, M. A., Piel, C. F., *et al.* (1980). Treatment of end-stage renal disease in children: a 15-year experience. *Kidney Int.* **18**, 103.

Potter, D. E., Holliday, M. A., Wilson, C. J., *et al.* (1975). Alternate day steroids for children after renal transplantation. *Transplant. Proc.* **7**, 79.

Potter, D. E., Najarian, J., Belzer, F., *et al.* (1991). Long-term results of renal transplantation in children. *Kidney Int.* **40**, 752.

Prompt, C. A., Reis, M. M., Grillo, F. M., *et al.* (1985). Transmission of AIDS virus at renal transplantation. *Lancet* **2**, 672.

Ptachcinski, R. J., Bur, G. J., Rosenthal, J. T., *et al.* (1986). Cyclosporine pharmacokinetics in children following cadaveric renal transplantation. *Transplant. Proc.* **4**, 766.

Ramos, E. L. (1991). Recurrent diseases in the renal allograft. *J Am. Soc. Nephrol.* **2**, 109.

Rao, K. V., Kasiske, B. L., Odlund, M. D., *et al.* (1990). Influence of cadaver donor age on post-transplant renal function and graft outcome. *Transplantation* **49**, 91.

Rees, L., Greene, S. A., Adlard, P., *et al.* (1988). Growth and endocrine function after renal transplantation. *Arch. Dis. Child.* **63**, 1326.

Rees, L., *et al.* (1990). Treatment of short stature in renal disease with recombinant human growth hormone. *Arch. Dis. Child.* **65**, 856.

Reimold, E. W. (1973). Intermittent prednisolone therapy in children and adolescents after renal transplantation. *Pediatrics* **52**, 235.

Reisman, L., Lieberman, K. V., Burrows, L., *et al.* (1990). Follow-up cyclosporine-treated pediatric renal allograft recipients after cessation of prednisone. *Transplantation* **49**, 76.

Reznik, V. M., Berger, J. S., Lyoni Jones, K., *et al.* (1989). Cyclosporine induces abnormal facial bone growth in children: a preliminary study. *Pediatr. Nephrol.* **3**, 296.

Reznik, V. M., Griswold, W. R., Halasz, N. A., *et al.* (1987a). Cyclosporine (C.S.A.)-induced changes in the facial appearance of pediatric renal transplant recipients. *Kidney Int.* **31**, 467.

Reznik, V. M., Lyoni Jones, K., Durham, B. L., *et al.* (1987b). Changes in facial appearance during cyclosporin treatment. *Lancet* **2**, 1405.

Rizzoni, G., Malekzadeh, M. H., Pennisi, A. J., *et al.* (1980). Renal transplantation in children less than 5 years of age. *Arch. Dis. Child.* **55**, 532.

Rooth, P., Dawidson, I., Diller, K., *et al.* (1988). Protection against cyclosporine-induced impairment of renal microcirculation by verapamil in mice. *Transplantation* **45**, 433.

Rosenthal, J. T., Ettenger, R. B., Ehrlich, R., *et al.* (1990). Technical factors contributing to successful kidney transplantation in small children. *J. Urol.* **144**, 116.

Ross, W. B., Roberts, D., Griffin, P. J. A., *et al.* (1986). Cyclosporin interaction with danazol and norethisterone. *Lancet* **1**, 330.

Rotundo, A., Nevins, T. E., Lipton, M., *et al.* (1982). Progressive encephalopathy in children with chronic renal insufficiency in infancy. *Kidney Int.* **21**, 486.

Rousseau, E., Russo, P., Lapointe, N., *et al.* (1988). Renal complications of acquired immunodeficiency syndrome in children. *Am. J. Kidney Dis.* **11**, 48.

Rubenstein, M., Meyer, R. and Bernstein, J. (1961). Congenital abnormalities of the urinary system: I. a postmortem survey of developmental anomalies and acquired congenital lesions in a children's hospital. *J. Pediatr.* **58**, 356.

Rubin, R. (1993). Infectious diseases complication of renal transplantation. *Kidney Int.* **44**, 221.

Ruder, H., Schaefer, F., Gretz, N., *et al.* (1989). Donor kidneys of infants or very young children are unacceptable for transplantation. *Lancet* **2**, 168.

Saldanha, L. F., Hurst, K. S., Amend, J. C., Jr., *et al.* (1976). Hyperlipidemia after renal transplantation in children. *Am. J. Dis. Child.* **130**, 951.

Salusky, I. B., Coburn, J. W., Foley, J., *et al.* (1986). Effects of oral calcium carbonate on control of serum phosphorus and changes in plasma aluminum levels after discontinuation of aluminum-containing gels in children receiving dialysis. *J. Pediatr.* **108**, 767.

Salvatierra, O., Jr. and Belzer, R. O. (1975). Pediatric cadaver kidneys: their use in renal transplantation. *Arch. Surg.* **110**, 181.

Salvatierra, O., Iwaki, Y., Vincenti, F., *et al.* (1982). Update of the University of California at San Francisco experience with donor-specific blood transfusions. *Transplant. Proc.* **14**, 363.

Salvatierra, O., Singh, T., Shifrin, R., *et al.* (1998). Successful transplantation of adult sized kidneys into infants requires maintenance of high aortic blood flow. *Transplantation* **66**, 819.

Salvatierra, O., Vicenti, F., Amend, W., *et al.* (1980). Deliberate donor-specific blood transfusions prior to living-related renal transplantation. *Ann. Surg.* **192**, 543.

Salvatierra, O., Jr. and Sarwal, M. (2000). Renal perfusion in infant recipients of adult-sized kidneys is a critical risk factor. *Transplantation* **70**, 412.

Sanfilippo, F., Goeken, N., Niblack, G., *et al.* (1987). The effect of first cadaver renal transplant HLA-A,B match on sensitization levels and retransplant rates following graft failure. *Transplantation* **43**, 240.

Sattler, M., Guengerich, F. P., Yun, C. H., *et al.* (1992). Cytochrome P-450 3A enzymes are responsible for biotransformation of FK506 and rapamycin in man and rat. *Drug Metab. Dispos.* **20**, 753.

Savin, V. J., Sharma, R., Sharma, R., *et al.* (1996). Circulating factor associated with increased glomerular permeability to albumin in recurrent focal segmental glomerulosclerosis. *N. Engl. J. Med.* **334**, 878.

Schaefer, F., Stanhoper, R., Preece, M. A., *et al.* (1991). Pulsatile growth hormone secretion in peripubertal patients with chronic renal failure. *J. Pediatr.* **119**, 568.

Scharer, K. (1971). Incidence and causes of chronic renal failure in children. *Proc. Eur. Dial. Transplant. Assn.* **8**, 211.

Scharer, K. and Fine, R. N. (1985). Renal transplantation in children treated by CAPD: a report on a cooperative study. *In CAPD in Children*, (R. N. Fine, K. Scharer and O. Mehls, eds.), p. 212, Springer-Verlag, Heidelberg.

Scheinman, J. I., Najarian, J. S. and Mauer, S. M. (1984). Successful strategies for renal transplantation in primary oxalosis. *Kidney Int.* **25**, 804.

Schneider, J. R., Sutherland, D. E., Simmons, R. L., *et al.* (1983). Long-term success with double pediatric cadaver donor renal transplants. *Ann. Surg.* **4**, 439.

Schreiber, S. L., Lin, J., Albers, M. W., *et al.* (1991). The immunophilin ligand complexes as probes of intracellular signaling pathways. *Transplant. Proc.* **23**, 2839.

Schroeder, T. J., First, M. R., Mansour, M. E., *et al.* (1990). Anti-murine antibody formation following OKT3 therapy. *Transplantation* **49**, 48.

Schroeder, T. J., Ryckman, F. C., Hurtubise, P. E., *et al.* (1991). Immunologic monitoring during and following OKT3 therapy in children. *Clin. Transplant.* **5**, 191.

Schurman, S. J., Stablein, D. M., Perlman, S. A., *et al.* (1999). Center volume effects in pediatric renal transplantation: a report of the North American Pediatric Renal Transplant Cooperative Study (NAPRTCS).

Senggutuvan, P., Cameron, J. S., Hartley, R. B., *et al.* (1990). Recurrence of focal segmental glomerulosclerosis in transplanted kidneys: analysis of incidence and risk factors in 59 allografts. *Pediatr. Nephrol.* **4**, 21.

Shapira, Z., Yussim, A., Savir, A., *et al.* (1985). The use of the portal system for the transplantation of a neonate kidney graft in a child with Wilms' tumor. *J. Pediatr. Surg.* **20**, 549.

Shapiro, R. (1998). Tacrolimus in pediatric renal transplantation: a review. *Pediatr. Transplant.* **2**, 270.

Shapiro, R., Fung, J. J., Jain, A. B., *et al.* (1990). The side effects of FK506 in humans. *Transplant. Proc.* **22**, 35.

Shapiro, R., Scantlebury, V. P., Jordan, M. L., *et al.* (1999). Pediatric renal transplantation under tacrolimus based immunosuppression. *Transplantation* **67**, 299.

Shoskes, D. A. and Halloran, P. F. (1991). Ischemic injury induces altered MHC gene expression in kidney by an interferon-gamma-dependent pathway. *Transplant. Proc.* **23**, 599.

Sigal, N. H. and Dumont, F. J. (1992). Cyclosporin A, FK506, and rapamycin pharmacologic probes of lymphocyte signal transduction. *Ann. Rev. Immunol.* **10**, 519.

Silber, S. J. (1974). Renal transplantation between adults and children: differences in renal growth. *J. A. M. A.* **228**, 1143.

Sinclair, N. R. (1992). Low-dose steroid therapy in cyclosporine-treated renal transplant recipients with well-functioning grafts. The Canadian Multicentre Transplant Study Group. *J. Med. Assoc. J.* **147**, 645.

Slomowitz, L. A., Wilkinson, A., Hawkins, R., *et al.* (1990). Evaluation of kidney function in renal transplant patients receiving long-term cyclosporine. *Am. J. Kidney Dis.* **15**, 530.

Smith, A. Y., Kerman, R. H., Van Buren, C. T., *et al.* (1988). Pediatric cadaveric kidneys in recipients treated with cyclosporine. *Transplant. Proc.* **20**, 215.

Snyder, D. S. and Unanue, E. R. (1982). Corticosteroids inhibit immune macrophages immunoglobulin expression and interleukin-1 production. *Immunology* **129**, 1803.

Snydman, D. R., Verner, B. G., Tilney, N. L., *et al.* (1991). Final analysis of primary cytomegalovirus disease prevention in renal transplant recipients with a cytomegalovirus-immune globulin: comparison of the randomised and open-label trials. *Transplant. Proc.* **23**, 1357.

Snydman, D. R., Werner, B. G. and Heinze-Lacey, B. (1987). Prevention of kidney transplant associated primary cytomegalovirus disease with an intravenous cytomegalovirus immune globulin (CMVIa-IV): an interim analysis. *Am. Soc. Transpl. Phys. 5th Ann. Meeting*, Chicago.

So, S., Chang, P. N., Najarian, J. S., *et al.* (1987). Growth and development in infants after renal transplantation. *J. Pediatr.* **110**, 343.

So, S. K., Gillingham, K., Cook, M., *et al.* (1990). The use of cadaver kidneys for transplantation in young children. *Transplantation* **50**, 979.

So, S. K., Simmons, R. L., Fryd, D. S., *et al.* (1985). Improved results of multiple renal transplantation in children. *Surgery* **98**, 729.

Solheim, B. G., Thorsby, E., Osbakk, T. A., *et al.* (1976). Donor age and cumulative kidney graft survival. *Tissue Antigens* **7**, 251.

Solinger, H. (1995). Mycophenolate mofetil for the prevention of acute rejection in primary cadaveric renal allograft recipients. *Transplantation* **60**, 225.

Sommer, B. G., Henry, M. L. and Ferguson, R. M. (1986). Sequential conventional immunotherapy with maintenance cyclosporine following renal transplantation. *Transplant. Proc.* **18**, 569.

Soulillou, J. P. (1994). Relevant targets for therapy with monoclonal antibodies in allograft transplantation. *Kidney Int.* **46**, 540.

Sounding Board. (1989). Anencephalic newborns: can organs be transplanted before brain death? *N. Engl. J. Med.* **321**, 388.

Spees, E. K., Clark, G. B. and Smith, M. T. (1984). Are anencephalic neonates suitable as kidney and pancreas donors? *Transplant. Proc.* **1**, 57.

Stablein, D. M. and Sullivan, E. K. (1996). Renal transplantation, dialysis, chronic renal insufficiency. The 1996 Annual Report of the North American Renal Transplant Cooperative Study.

Stablein, D. M., Sullivan, E. K. and Donaldson, L. (1998). Renal transplantation, dialysis, chronic renal insufficiency. The 1998 Annual Report of the North American Renal Transplant Cooperative Study.

Starzl, T. E., Marchioro, T. L., Morgan, M. W., *et al.* (1964). A technique for use of adult renal homografts in children. *Surg. Gynecol. Obstet.* **119**, 106.

Starzl, T. E., Marchioro, T. L. and Porter, K. A. (1967). The use of heterologous antilymphoid agents in canine renal and liver homotransplantation and in human renal homotransplantation. *Surg. Gynecol. Obstet.* **124**, 301.

Starzl, T. E., Todo, S., Fung, J., *et al.* (1989). FK506 for liver, kidney, and pancreas transplantation. *Lancet* **28**, 1000.

Stefanidis, C. J., Balfe, J. W., Arbus, G. S., *et al.* (1983). Renal transplantation in children treated with continuous ambulatory peritoneal dialysis. *Perit. Dial. Bull.* **3**, 5.

Stephanian, E., Matas, A. J., Mauer, S. M., *et al.* (1992). Recurrence of disease in patients retransplanted for focal segmental glomerulosclerosis. *Transplantation* **53**, 755.

Stiller, C. and Opelz, G. (1991). Should cyclosporine be continued indefinitely? *Transplant. Proc.* **23**, 36.

Strauss, J., Abitbol, C., Zilleruelo, G., *et al.* (1989). Renal disease in children with the acquired immunodeficiency syndrome. *N. Engl. J Med.* **321**, 625.

Striegel, J. E., Sibley, R. K., Fryd, D. S., *et al.* (1986). Recurrence of focal segmental sclerosis in children following renal transplantation. *Kidney Int.* **30**, S44.

Strom, T. B. (1987). Towards more selective therapies to block graft rejection. *AKF Nephrol. Lett.* **4**, 13.

Strom, T. B. and Kelley, V. E. (1989). Toward more selective therapies to block undesired immune responses. *Kidney Int.* **35**, 1026.

Sutherland, D. E. R., Fryd, D. S., So, S. R. S., *et al.* (1985). The long-term effect of splenectomy versus no splenectomy on renal allograft survival: reanalysis of a randomized prospective study. *Transplant. Proc.* **17**, 136.

Swinnen, L. J., Costanzo-Nordiu, M. R., Fisher, M. S., *et al.* (1990). Increased incidence of lymphoproliferative disorder after immunosuppression with the monoclonal antibody OKT3 in cardiac-transplant recipients. *N. Engl. J. Med.* **323**, 1723.

Takemoto, S., Carnahan, E. and Terasaki, P. I. (1991). A report of 504 six antigen-matched transplants. *Transplant. Proc.* **23**, 1318.

Tamura, K., Fujimura, T., Tsutsumi, T., *et al.* (1995). Inhibition of insulin production by FK506 is caused at the transcriptional level in pancreatic beta cells when FKBPI2 content is relatively high. *Transplant. Proc.* **27**, 357.

Tanaka, H., Kuroda, A., Marsawa, *et al.* (1987). Structure of FK506: a novel immunosuppressant isolated from streptomyces. *J. Am. Soc. Nephrol.* **109**, 5031.

Tejani, A. (1983). Post-transplant hypertension and hypertensive encephalopathy in renal allograft recipients. *Nephron* **34**, 73.

Tejani, A., Butt, K. M., Khawar, M. R., *et al.* (1986). Cyclosporine experience in renal transplantation in children. *Kidney Int.* **30**, S35.

Tejani, A., Butt, K. M. H., Rajpot, D., *et al.* (1989). Strategies for optimizing growth in children with kidney transplants. *Transplantation* **47**, 229.

Tejani, A. and Stablein, D. H. (1992). Recurrence of focal segmental glomerulosclerosis post-transplantation: a special report of the North American Pediatric Renal Transplant Cooperative Study. *J. Am. Soc. Nephrol.* **2**, S258.

Tejani, A., Stablein, D., Fine, R. N., *et al.* (1993). Maintenance immunosuppression therapy and outcome of renal transplantation in North American children: a report of the North American Pediatric Renal Transplantation Cooperative Study. *Pediatr. Nephrol.* 7, 132.

Tejani, A. and Sullivan, E. K. (1996). Factors that impact on the outcome of second renal transplants in children. *Transplantation* **62**, 606.

Tellis, V. A., Greenstein, S. M., Schechner, R. S., *et al.* (1990). Pediatric donors: still successful in adults. *Transplant. Proc.* **22**, 363.

Thiel, G. (1986). Experimental cyclosporine A nephrotoxicity: a summary of the International Workshop (Basel, April 24–26, 1985). *Clin. Nephrol.* **25(Suppl. 1)**, 205.

Thompson, J. F., Fletcher, E. W. L., Chalmers, D. H. K., *et al.* (1983). Bilateral renal embolization for the control of hypertension in transplant patients. *Br. J. Surg.* **70**, 681.

Ting, A. and Morris, P. J. (1978). Matching for B-cell antigens of the HLA-DR series in cadaver renal transplantation. *Lancet* **1**, 575.

Tiwari, J. L. (1985). Review: kidney transplantation and transfusion. *In Clinical Transplants 1985*, (P. I. Terasaki, ed.), p. 257, UCLA Tissue Typing Laboratory, Los Angeles.

Todo, S., Fung, J. J., Tzakis, A. J., *et al.* (1991). One hundred ten consecutive primary orthotopic liver transplants under FK506 in adults. *Transplant. Proc.* **23**, 1397.

Tonshoff, B. and Mehls, O. (1996). Interaction between glucocosteroids and the somatotrophic axis. *Acta Pediatr.* **417**, 72.

Torres, V. E., Velosa, J. A., Holley, K. E., *et al.* (1984). Meclofenamate treatment of recurrent idiopathic nephrotic syndrome with focal segmental glomerulosclerosis after renal transplantation. *Mayo Clin. Proc.* **59**, 146.

Touraine, J. L., Bosi, E., El Yafi, M. S., *et al.* (1985). The infectious lymphoproliferative syndrome in transplant patients under immunosuppressive treatment. *Transplant. Proc.* **17**, 96.

Toussaint, C., Goffin, Y., Potvliege, P., *et al.* (1976). Kidney transplantation in primary oxalosis. *Clin. Nephrol.* **5**, 239.

Trachtman, H., Hammerschlag, M. R., Tejani, A., *et al.* (1986). A longitudinal study of varicella immunity in pediatric renal transplant recipients. *J. Infect. Dis.* **154**, 335.

Trauner, D. A., Chase, C., Scheller, J., *et al.* (1988). Neurologic and cognitive deficits in children with cystinosis. *J. Pediatr.* **112**, 912.

Trevino, G., Dickerman, J. T., Coggins, W., *et al.* (1988). The optimal use of pediatric donors for renal transplantation. *Transplant. Proc.* **20**, 359.

Tricontinental Mycophenolate Mofetil Renal Transplantation Study Group. (1996). A blinded, randomized clinical trial of mycophenolate mofetil for the prevention of acute rejection in cadaveric renal transplantation. *Transplantation* **61**, 1029.

Trompeter, R. S., Haycock, G. B., Bewick, M., *et al.* (1983). Renal transplantation in very young children. *Lancet* **1**, 373.

Truong, L., Gelfand, J., D'Agati, V., *et al.* (1989). De novo membranous glomerulonephropathy in renal allografts: a report of ten cases and review of the literature. *Am. J. Kidney Dis.* **14**, 131.

Tsai, N. Y., Carlstedt-Duke, J. and Weigal, N. L. (1988). Molecular interactions of steroid hormone receptor with its enhancer element: evidence for receptor dimer function. *Cell* **55**, 361.

Tzakis, A. G., Cooper, M. H., Dummer, J. S., *et al.* (1990). Transplantation in HIV + patients. *Transplantation* **49**, 354.

Uittenbogaart, C. H., Isaacson, A. S., Stanley, P., *et al.* (1978). Aseptic necrosis after renal transplantation in children. *Am. J. Dis. Child.* **132**, 765.

Uittenbogaart, C. H., Robinson, B. J., Malekzadeh, M. H., *et al.* (1979). Use of antithymocyte globulin (dose by rosette protocol) in pediatric renal allograft recipients. *Transplantation* **28**, 291.

Uittenbogaart, C. H., Robinson, B. J., Malekzadeh, M. H., *et al.* (1980). Pretransplant T cell levels and renal allograft survival. *Surgery* **87**, 432.

United States Public Health Service. (1991). Agency guidelines for screening donors of blood, plasma, organs, tissues and semen for evidence of hepatitis B and hepatitis C. *Morb. Mortal. Wkly. Rep. M. M. W. R.* **40(Suppl. RR4)**.

United States Renal Data Systems. (1990). *USRDS 1990 Annual Data Report*, p. 1, The National Institutes of Health, National Institute of Diabetes and Digestive and Kidney Diseases, Bethesda, Md.

United States Renal Data Systems. (1991). *USRDS 1991 Annual Data Report*, p. 1, The National Institute of Diabetes and Digestive and Kidney Diseases, Bethesda, Md.

United States Renal Data Systems (1998). Part II. Living unrelated donor rate grew 46% annually from 1993–1996; hospitalizations higher for pediatric HD vs. PD patients. *Nephrol. News Issues* **12**, 62.

van der Vliet, J. A., Cohen, B. and Koostra, G. (1982). Transplantation of pediatric cadaver kidneys. *Transplant. Proc.* **14**, 74.

van Diemen-Steenvoorde, R. and Donckerwolcke, R. A., (1988). Growth and sexual maturation in children after kidney transplantation. *Acta Paediatr. Scand.* **343 (Suppl.)**, 109.

Van Dop, C., Jabs, K. L., Donoroje, P. A., *et al.* (1992). Accelerated growth rates in children treated with growth hormone after renal transplantation. *J. Pediatr.* **120**, 244.

Vanrenterghem, Y., Waer, M., Roels, L., *et al.* (1990). Long term prognosis of cadaveric renal allograft transplanted with cyclosporine as basic immunosuppression. *Transplant. Proc.* **22**, 1691.

van Speybroeck, J. V., Feduska, N., Amend, W., *et al.* (1979). The influence of donor age on graft survival. *Am. J. Surg.* **137**, 374.

Van Ypersele de Strihou, C. and Stragier, A. (1969). Effect of bilateral nephrectomy on transfusion requirements of patients undergoing chronic dialysis. *Lancet* **2**, 705.

Vincenti, F., Biava, C., Tomlanovitch, S., *et al.* (1989). Inability of cyclosporine to completely prevent the recurrence of focal glomerulosclerosis after kidney transplantation. *Transplantation* **47**, 595.

Waksman, B. H., Arbouys, S. and Aranson, B. G. (1961). The use of specific "lymphocyte" antisera to inhibit hypersensitive reactions of the delayed type. *J. Exp. Med.* **114**, 997.

Walker, R. (1995). Pretransplant assessment of the risk for post transplant lymphoproliferative disorder. *Transplant. Proc.* **27(Suppl. 1)**, 41.

Walker, R. G. and d'Aprice, A. J. F. (1988). Azathioprine and steroids. *In Kidney Transplantation: Principles and Practice*, (P. J. Morris, ed.), p. 319, W.B. Saunders, Philadelphia.

Warady, B. (1992). Treatment of infants with end-stage renal disease. *Curr. Opin. Pediatr.* **4**, 264.

Ware, A. J., Luby, J. P. and Eigenbrodt, E. H. (1975). Spectrum of liver disease in renal transplant recipients. *Gastroenterology* **68**, 755.

Warshaw, B. L., Edelbrock, H. H., Ettenger, R. B., *et al.* (1980). Renal transplantation in children with obstructive uropathy. *J. Urol.* **123**, 737.

Wasowska, B., Hancock, W., Onodera, K., *et al.* (1996). Rapamycin plus cyclosporin A—a novel regimen to prevent chronic allograft rejection in sensitized hosts. *American Society of Transplant Physicians Annual Meeting*, p. 120, Dallas.

Watson, A. R., Vigneux, A., Bannatyne, R. M. and Balfe, J. W. (1986). Peritonitis during continuous ambulatory peritoneal dialysis in children. *Can. Med. Assoc. J.* **134**, 1019.

Watts, R. W. E., Calne, R. Y., William, R., *et al.* (1985). Primary hyperoxaluria (type I): attempted treatment by combined hepatic and renal transplantation. *Q. J. M.* **57**, 697.

Watts, R. W. E., Morgan, S. H., Danpure, C. J., *et al.* (1991). Combined hepatic and renal transplantation in primary hyperoxaluria type I: clinical report of nine cases. *Am. J. Med.* **90**, 179.

Watts, R. W. E., Morgan, S. H., Purkiss, P., *et al.* (1988). Timing of renal transplantation in the management of pyridoxine-resistant type I primary hyperoxaluria. *Transplantation* **45**, 1143.

Weil, R., III, Putman, C. W., Porter, K. A., *et al.* (1976). Transplantation in children. *Surg. Clin. North Am.* **56**, 467.

Weir, M. R., Irwin, B. C., Maters, A. W., *et al.* (1987). Incidence of cytomegalovirus disease in cyclosporine-treated renal transplant recipients based on donor/recipient pretransplant immunity. *Transplantation* **43**, 187.

Wetzels, J. F. M., Hoitsman, A. J. and Koene, R. A. P. (1986). Influence of cadaver donor age on renal graft survival. *Clin. Nephrol.* **25**, 256.

Whelchel, J. D., Alison, D. V., Luke, R. G., *et al.* (1983). Successful renal transplantation in hyperoxaluria. *Transplantation* **35**, 161.

Whitington, P. F., Emond J. C., Whitington, S. H., *et al.* (1990). Small-bowel length and the dose of cyclosporine in children after liver transplantation. *N. Engl. J. Med.* **332**, 733.

Wilson, W. A. and Fine, R. N. (1979). Long-term follow-up of cataracts in children after renal transplantation. *Am. Ophthalmol Soc.* **1**, 8.

Winkelstein, A. (1979). The effect of azathioprine and 6 mercaptopurine on immunity. *J. Immunopharmacol.* **1**, 429.

Woodruff, M. F. A. and Anderson, N. A. (1963). Effect of lymphocyte depletion by thoracic duct fistula and administration of acute antilymphocyte serum on the survival of skin homograft in rats. *Nature* **200**, 702.

Yamanto, R. R. (1985) Steroid receptor regulated transcription of specific genes and gene networks. *Ann. Rev. Genet.* **19**, 209.

Yanase, Y., Tango, T., Okumura, K., *et al.* (1986). Lymphocyte subsets identified by monoclonal antibodies in healthy children. *Pediatr. Res.* **20**, 1147.

Yoshimura, N. and Oka, T. (1990). FK506, a new immunosuppressive agent: a review. *J. Immunopharmacol.* **10**, 32.

Yuge, J. and Cecka, J. M. (1991). Pediatric recipients and donors. *In Clinical Transplants 1990*, (P. Terasaki, ed.), p. 425, UCLA Tissue Typing Laboratory, Los Angeles.

Zankar, B., Walz, G., Wieder, K. J., *et al.* (1990). Evidence that glucocorticosteroids block expression of the human interleukin-6 gene by accessory cells. *Transplantation* **49**, 183.

Zimmerman, C. E. (1980). Renal transplantation for focal segmental glomerulosclerosis. *Transplantation* **29**, 172.

38

Renal Transplantation in Developing Countries

M. Rafique Moosa • Abdul Aziz Walele • Abdallah S. Daar

Introduction

Renal transplantation is the only viable therapeutic option for most patients with irreversible renal failure in developing countries. The high cost of dialysis limits this form of treatment to a privileged few, making a successful renal transplant a greater necessity than elsewhere. The struggling economies of most developing countries have many other priorities, and the question of whether dialysis and transplantation are justified at all has been raised but remains largely rhetorical. If transplants are to be done, the timing of transplantation must be optimized, graft function must be maximized and costs and complications must be minimized. Many developing countries are beset by problems, including political and military violence, economic upheavals, corruption and unstable governments. There are major demands on available resources, and generally less than 5% of gross national product (GNP) is spent on health. In the United States, 14.3% of GNP is spent on health care, whereas Pakistan spends 1.1% (Rizvi *et al.*, 1990), and India spends 1.5% (Chugh and Jha, 1995; Weening *et al.*, 1998). Many health problems in developing countries are related to poverty, malnutrition, lack of potable water and infections.

Malaria and human immunodeficiency virus (HIV) infection, especially in sub-Saharan Africa, put enormous strains on limited health care budgets. Within these limitations, nephrologists have to manage patients with irreversible renal failure. Proponents of renal transplantation argue that transplantation should be encouraged because it is the most cost-effective form of renal replacement therapy, with the best promise of improved quality of life and an excellent chance of rehabilitation. Rizvi and Naqvi (1995) argued that curbing transplantation until other health issues are addressed should be avoided because the delivery of health services is notoriously poor. It has been estimated that 80% of the world's population live in developing countries and consume 15% of world resources (Fig. 38–1). The World Bank classification of countries by economic groupings, based on GNP per capita (World Bank, 1997), is (1) *low income*, less than $785 (U.S. dollars); (2) *lower middle income*, $786 to $3,125; (3) *upper middle income*, $3,126 to $9,655 and (4) *high income*, greater than $9,656. The countries with low-income and middle-income economies are referred to as *developing countries*. The disparity between *emerging* market economies of developing countries and established market economies of developed countries continues to widen (Grunberg, 1996). Nowhere is this disparity more striking than in the differential resources spent on health.

The availability and rate of transplant activity vary considerably; however, demand exists even in the poorest nations. Kidney transplants were performed in 95% of 44 countries surveyed by Kazim *et al.* (1992)—most were performed in the more developed countries.

Most uremic patients are unlikely to receive treatment because with poverty there is a struggle to provide the most basic medical care. With many developing countries having virtually no dialysis activity or cadaver donor programs, the only hope for patients with irreversible renal failure is a living related donor transplant. On a worldwide basis, the number of patients with end-stage renal disease (ESRD) starting dialysis increased by more than 33-fold in the years 1975–1989, but the number of transplants increased only 5-fold in the same period. Of all the transplants worldwide, less than 10% are performed in developing countries, which rely heavily, and in some cases exclusively, on living related donors. The marked discrepancy between the number of patients with ESRD and the number of patients who receive transplants continues to grow at an alarming rate. In developing countries, the discrepancy between what is technically possible and what is economically viable is striking with regard to renal replacement treatment; in Pakistan, 400 kid-

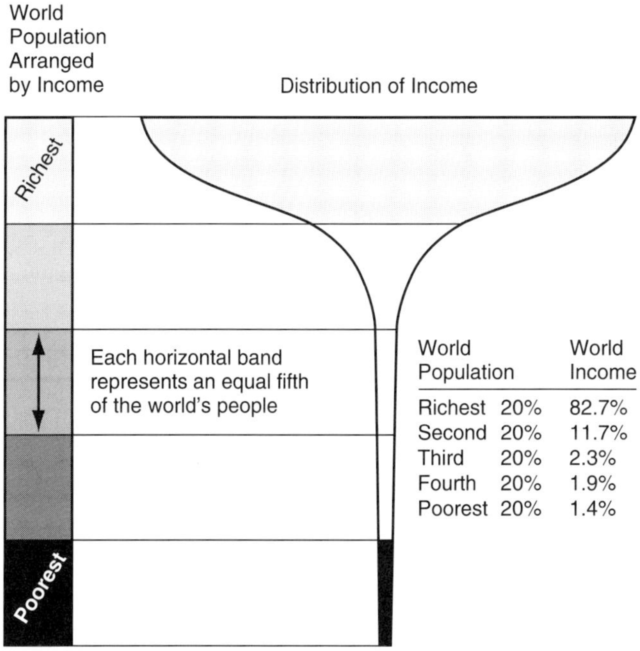

FIGURE 38–1

The champagne glass of world poverty. The discrepancy in the wealth of the rich and poor countries of the world is extremely large and continues to grow, largely as a result of the indebtedness of the poorest countries, resulting in the stem of the glass becoming thinner. The poorest 60% of the world's population are almost equally poor. (Anonymous, 1999b; reproduced with permission from the *British Medical Journal*.)

TABLE 38–1

INCIDENCE OF END-STAGE RENAL FAILURE IN SELECTED DEVELOPING COUNTRIES COMPARED WITH UNITED STATES

Country/Region	pmp*	Year Reported	Reference
Algeria	34	1996	Abomelha, 1996
Bahrain	100	1998	Al Arrayed, 1998
Egypt	200	1992	Barsoum, 1992b
India	100	1990	Yadav, 1990
Jordan	120	1999	Said, 1999
Kenya	90	1988/95	McLigeyo et al., 1988; Were and McLigeyo, 1995
Libya	200	1996	Abomelha, 1996
Morocco	120	1999	Bourquia, 1999
Oman	90–100	1993	Aghanashinikar et al., 1993
Pakistan	100	1992	Naqvi et al., 1992
Reunion	188	1998	Albitar et al., 1998
Saudi Arabia	80	1996	Abomelha, 1996
South Africa	240	1995	Meyers, 1995
South America	60–100	1992	Martinez and Donkervoort, 1992
Sudan	100	1996	Abomelha, 1996
Syria	75	1997	Ayash, 1997
Tunisia	48	1996	Abomelha, 1996
Uruguay	90	1994	Fernandez et al., 1995
Yemen	385	1996	Sheiban and Al-Garba, 1999
United States	*276*	*1996*	Anonymous, 1999a

*pmp = per 1 million population.

ney transplants are done annually, representing less than 10% of the number of patients who require treatment (Rizvi et al., 1998b).

End-Stage Renal Disease in Developing Countries—Comparison with Developed Countries

INCIDENCE

The incidence of ESRD is 48 to 240 per 1 million population, compared with 76 to 268 per 1 million population in the developed regions of North America (USRDS, 1998), Europe (Mallick et al., 1995) and the Asia-Pacific region (Ota, 1998;

Table 38–1). End-stage renal disease in developing countries seems to be at least as common, if not commoner, than in developed countries (McLigeyo et al., 1988). In the absence of formal registry data, the extent of the problem and the causes are difficult to establish with certainty (Chugh and Jha, 1995; Kang et al., 1992). If the incidence is higher, this may be due to the higher incidence of glomerulonephritis in tropical countries and the predisposition of some populations to hypertension (Basinda et al., 1988). The figures given probably underestimate the true incidence because most of the people live in rural areas, where there is limited access to health care and patients do not reach urban dialysis facilities (Chugh and Jha, 1995).

The incidence of ESRD is steadily increasing in the United States; since 1987, it has increased at a rate of 6% per year.

TABLE 38–2

DEMOGRAPHY OF PATIENTS RECEIVING RENAL REPLACEMENT THERAPY

Country	No. Patients	Mean Age (y)	Males (%)	Reference
Brazil	1,563	38 (CAD)* 33 (LRD)	63	Sasso et al., 1990
India (1)	265	36	80	Kathuria et al., 1995
India (2)	310	—	93	Chugh et al., 1993
Kenya	77	30	64	McLigeyo et al., 1988
Malaysia	37	37	64	Lei et al., 1992
Morocco	2,000	51	59	Bourquia, 1999
Nigeria	368	<40	73	Mabayoje et al., 1992
Oman/UAE	130	38	62	Salahudeen et al., 1990
Pakistan (1)	500	32	78	Rizvi et al., 1998
Pakistan (2)	79	43	61	Kumar et al., 1992
Qatar	187	41	55	Rashid et al., 1998
Reunion	767	52	41	Albitar et al., 1998
South Africa	7,331	40–59*	59	du Toit et al., 1994
Slovenia	151	35	70	Kandus et al., 1992
Turkey (1)	520	35	77	Yildiz et al., 1998
Turkey (2)	562	32	80	Kekec et al., 1992
United States	*79,102*	*61*	*53*	USRDS, 1999

*Peak ages.
CAD = cadaveric donor; LRD = living related donor.

TABLE 38–3

CAUSES OF CHRONIC RENAL FAILURE IN SELECTED DEVELOPING COUNTRIES*

Country	CGN	HTN	ADPKD	IPN	Other	Diabetes	SLE
Kenya[1] (n = 77)	44	22	—	—	35	—	—
Brazil[2] (n = 1,563)	43	13	—	—	32	4	—
India† (n = 405)	49	—	4.3	43	—	12	—
Pakistan[3] (n = 79)	44	8.8	—	10	14	14	—
Philippines† (n = 872)	52	—	4.3	24	—	11	1
South East Asia† (n = 248)	55	—	3	1	—	14	1
Kuwait† (n = 501)	50	2.8	3	23	17	2.6	—
Republic of South Africa[4] (n = 5,560)	32	28	7	11	15	0.01	0.23
Nigeria[5] (n = 368)	5.9	61	4.4	—	14	11	3.7
Reunion[6] (n = 657)	13	28	9.6	8.7	7.5	33.6	—

*Incidence in percentages.
[1]McLigeyo et al., 1988.
[2]Kathuria et al., 1995.
[3]Kumar et al., 1992.
[4]du Toit et al., 1994.
[5]Mabayoje et al., 1992.
[6]Albitar et al., 1998.
†Remaining data from Daar, 1994.
CGN = chronic glomerulonephritis; HTN = hypertension; ADPKD = autosomal dominant kidney disease; IPN = interstitial nephritis/chronic pyelonephritis; SLE = systemic lupus erythematosus.

There is no clear explanation for this growth, although the increase in the incidence of diabetes mellitus may be a major contributing factor (USRDS, 1999). Whether developing countries are experiencing a similar trend is uncertain. More recent estimates of ESRD incidence in developing countries are somewhat higher than the 1987 estimate of 80 per 1 million population, suggesting perhaps a modest increase. In the United States, compared with whites, the point prevalence rate for ESRD was 4.5-fold higher for black Americans and 3.7-fold higher for Native Americans. Minority groups in developed countries appear to have been affected disproportionately by this increase (USRDS, 1999). Although differences between black Americans and blacks in the developing world are vast, it is possible that a similar undocumented process is occurring in developing countries.

DEMOGRAPHICS
Age

A marked difference exists in the mean age of patients initiated on renal replacement therapy in developing countries compared with Europe and the United States (Table 38–2). In 1997, the mean age of a patient starting renal replacement therapy in the United States was 61 years, whereas in some developing countries, the mean age is 30 years. In the United States, the incidence of ESRD is rising most rapidly in the greater than 75 years old age group, suggesting that the mean age is set to increase in other industrialized countries (USRDS, 1999). A possible explanation for the younger presentation in developing countries is that inadequate preventive and curative medical care allow more rapid development of ESRD (Chugh and Jha, 1995).

Gender

Another important difference that has emerged is the marked male predominance in the incidence of renal replacement therapy compared with industrialized countries. In the United States, men account for 53% of patients started on treatment. In developing countries, men account for 93% of patients receiving treatment. The incidence of chronic renal failure is unlikely to be considerably higher in men, and

the marked discrepancies probably reflect social and cultural factors that favor men.

CAUSES OF CHRONIC RENAL FAILURE

There are clear-cut regional and racial differences in the causes of ESRD (Tables 38–3 and 38–4).

Hypertension

The prevalence of hypertension in developing countries varies from 1% in certain African countries to 30% in Brazil. In sub-Saharan Africa, hypertension is the commonest cause of ESRD in blacks (Seedat et al., 1984); in South Africa, hypertension accounts for 37% of black compared with 8% of white ESRD patients (Seedat, 1999). As in the United States, where hypertension is commoner in black Americans, it occurs at an earlier age in blacks than in whites and is more commonly associated with end-organ damage (Milne et al., 1989; USRDS, 1999). Renal failure is most commonly associated with malignant hypertension but may occur with less severe hypertension (Milne, 1997). Malignant hypertension occurs relatively more commonly in black than white patients and often is the initial presentation in African patients (Milne et al., 1989), in whom its hallmark of fibrinoid necrosis was detected on histology in 92% of cases reported by Isaacson

TABLE 38–4

GEOGRAPHICAL VARIATIONS IN COMMON CAUSES OF END-STAGE RENAL FAILURE

Region	Disease
Sub-Saharan Africa	Hypertension
Pacific Rim countries	IgA nephropathy
Middle East	Urinary stones
South Africa (whites)	Analgesic nephropathy
China	Systemic lupus erythematosus
Balkan States	Balkan endemic nephropathy
Mediterranean basin	Familial Mediterranean fever
Egypt	Schistosomiasis

Reproduced with permission of Daar, 1994.

et al. (1991). These histological findings contrast with those of Pitcock *et al.* (1976), who could not show fibrinoid necrosis in black Americans and believed that the diagnostic lesion was subintimal musculomucoid hyperplasia.

An important consideration in the treatment of patients with renal failure resulting from malignant hypertension is the potential for recovery. In a study reported by James *et al.* (1995), 12 of 54 (22%) patients with malignant hypertension presenting with uremia recovered sufficient renal function to allow the discontinuation of intermittent peritoneal dialysis treatment after 2.7 months. The longest delay of recovery in that series was 12 months, although other reports exist of delays of 25 months. Recovery of renal function was associated with acute oligoanuria and higher initial blood pressure. It would be advisable to delay transplantation for 3 to 6 months (where possible), to exclude potential return of kidney function.

The use of antihypertensive medication in South Africa has led to a decrease of 25% in the incidence of stroke and myocardial infarction, but over the same period there was a 45% increase in the incidence of ESRD, mainly resulting from hypertension and diabetes (Seedat, 1998). This suggestion that blood pressure control does not result in improved renal outcome, especially in black patients, implies that other factors may play a role, including the erroneous diagnosis of primary renal disease. Nephrologists were twice as likely to label a black person as having hypertensive renal disease than a white person who presented with the same clinical picture (Pernerger *et al.*, 1995). Studies suggest that black patients are more susceptible to renal injury from hypertension than white patients (McClellan *et al.*, 1998; Tierney *et al.*, 1989). The Multiple Risk Factor Intervention Trial (MRFIT) suggested that good blood pressure control resulted in stabilization or improvement in renal function in nonblack, but not in black, patients (Walker *et al.*, 1992). Many other explanations based on genetic and physiological differences have been forwarded. (For a detailed discussion, see Seedat, 1998.)

Glomerulonephritis

The incidence and pattern of glomerulonephritis varies in different regions (Date *et al.*, 1987; Seggie *et al.*, 1984). Chronic glomerulonephritis accounts for most causes of ESRD, but because biopsies seldom are performed on end-stage kidneys, the underlying cause is not often established. In a large clinicopathological study of 2,827 patients with renal disease reported by Date *et al.* (1987) from India, nephrotic syndrome was found to be the commonest clinical presentation of renal disease. Minimal change disease, focal segmental glomerulosclerosis, mesangiocapillary glomerulonephritis, membranous glomerulonephritis, lupus glomerulonephritis and diabetic glomerulosclerosis accounted for 83% of all cases presenting with nephrotic syndrome. Membranous glomerulonephritis was the commonest cause of nephrotic syndrome in adults greater than 40 years old. Amyloidosis was rare. In certain tropical areas where quartan malaria is endemic, the incidence of nephrotic syndrome is 20 to 60 times that in the United States (Kibukamusoke *et al.*, 1999). The other frequent clinical presentation of renal disease was acute nephritis resulting from diffuse proliferative glomerulonephritis, crescentic glomerulonephritis or mesangial proliferative glomerulonephritis, which together account for 88% of all cases. Patients with small kidneys and patients with classic diabetic nephropathy did not undergo renal biopsy. Patients with chronic renal failure with normal-sized kidneys were more likely to have focal segmental glomerulosclerosis than any other histology. The elevated antistreptococcal antibodies in almost 50% of patients with nephritis seem to confirm the

predisposition of individuals in the tropics to infections. This predisposition is borne out in the experience of Seggie *et al.* (1984), who reported on the pattern of glomerulonephritis presenting as nephrotic syndrome in Zimbabwe and reviewed the African experience.

In the Zimbabwean experience, β-hemolytic streptococcal, hepatitis B virus (HBV) and syphilitic infections accounted for 45 of 98 (46%) patients who underwent renal biopsies. Despite being an endemic area, malaria was the cause of nephrotic syndrome in only one patient (Seggie *et al.*, 1984). In Nigeria (Hendrickse *et al.*, 1972) and Uganda (Kibukamusoke *et al.*, 1999), however, *Plasmodium malariae* plays a more important role in nephrotic syndrome. The features of glomerulonephritis in other parts of Africa were (1) its higher incidence compared with temperate climates; (2) the observation that minimal change was a rare cause of nephrotic syndrome in children, which usually was associated with HBV infection (Coovadia *et al.*, 1979; van Buuren *et al.*, 1999) and (3) the high prevalence in older adults of idiopathic and postinfectious proliferative glomerulonephritis (Brown *et al.*, 1977; Kung'u and Sitati, 1980; Seedat, 1979).

In Seggie's series of 27 patients diagnosed with poststreptococcal infection, 11 (41%) were complications of scabies infection (Seggie *et al.*, 1984). The four patients with syphilitic nephrotic syndrome responded rapidly to penicillin therapy. Noninfectious causes of nephrotic syndrome were rare and included diabetic nephropathy, amyloid and polyarteritis nodosa. Of 68 patients within this cohort, who were followed for 6 to 30 months, 22 (32%) died as a result of end-stage kidney failure because of the lack of renal replacement therapy facilities in Zimbabwe.

Although most patients in Zimbabwe had evidence of schistosomiasis, this was not significantly different in patients with glomerulonephritis compared with normal controls (Seggie *et al.*, 1984). There was no characteristic histological pattern identified with schistosomiasis, although diffuse or mesangial proliferative glomerulonephritis was shown in most of the patients. Immunological staining of the glomeruli for specific schistosomal antigens was consistently negative. Glomerular disease associated with schistosomiasis has been well documented in Egypt and India (Barsoum, 1993; Chugh and Sakhuja, 1990; see later).

IgA Nephropathy

IgA nephropathy is characterized by the mesangial deposition of IgA, usually with C3. Prevalence varies in different geographical regions (Berger, 1969; Glassock *et al.*, 1991). It is a common cause of primary glomerular disease in South East Asia (45% of patients), relatively uncommon in North America (5%) and Europe (11%) and rare in black Africans (D'Amico, 1987; Swanepoel *et al.*, 1989). The disease often goes unrecognized in many patients (D'Amico, 1987). It has been estimated that IgA nephropathy is the commonest primary glomerulonephritis in the world (D'Amico, 1987). Although it has a benign course in most patients, it has been estimated that it accounts for about 10% of patients on maintenance hemodialysis in many countries (Julian, 1998). Renal function deteriorates progressively, leading to ESRD in approximately 20% of patients after 20 years of overt disease (Julian, 1998; Lai and Wang, 1994). IgA nephropathy presents in most patients with either asymptomatic microscopic hematuria and proteinuria or macroscopic hematuria (Julian, 1998; Swanepoel *et al.*, 1989) and has a tendency to recur in a transplanted kidney (Berger, 1988; see also Chapter 4), although this occurs over 1 to 4 years and seldom results in the loss of the graft (Cameron and Turner, 1977). Limited evidence suggests that it may be safe to transplant kidneys with mesangial IgA deposits into patients who do not have IgA-related disease; the mesangial deposits disappear (Silva et al., 1982). There is currently no specific therapy for IgA nephropathy, but when it is associated with crescentic nephritis, pulse steroid therapy, cytoreductive therapy and plasma exchange may be considered. These therapies may be used for clinical exacerbation of the disease in the absence of crescentic changes.

Diabetic Nephropathy

Diabetic nephropathy is the commonest cause of ESRD in the United States, Japan and industrialized Europe (Ismail et al., 1999). In the United States, diabetic nephropathy accounts for 40% of patients in the Medicare ESRD program (USRDS, 1999). In contrast, it accounts for less than 3 to 14% of patients receiving treatment for ESRD in developing countries, with occasional exceptions (see Table 38–3). This sharp contrast may be due to bias against selection of these patients for renal replacement therapy rather than rarity of diabetic nephropathy among patients from developing countries (Albitar et al., 1998; Alzaid et al., 1994).

A report from India discusses the experience of diabetic nephropathy in a Third World setting. Chugh and coworkers profiled 250 adults with type 2 diabetic nephropathy and found that glycemic control was poor in most (54%) (Chugh et al., 1989). Patients developed proteinuria 9.5 years after the diagnosis of diabetes. Renal failure occurred in 82% of cases and at a mean of 10.5 years after the diagnosis of diabetes. Comparing their experience with that of Fabre et al. (1982), who studied 510 patients in a First World setting, Chugh et al. (1989) found that the Indian patients had more severe proteinuria: the number with nephrotic-range proteinuria was 18% compared with 4% in Fabre's series. A similar observation was made by Samanta et al. (1986), who established that Asians with type 2 diabetes developed proteinuria more frequently than whites. Genetic factors seem to play an important role in the predisposition to diabetic nephropathy, as evidenced by the racial differences in the development of diabetic nephropathy (Friedman, 1989) and the high concordance rate in families (Borch-Johnsen et al., 1992). Hypertension was present in 61% of Chugh's cohort of type 2 diabetics, similar to the incidence reported by Parving et al. (1993) from Scandinavia but less than the 84% incidence reported from Switzerland by Fabre et al. (1982). The hypertensive patients had higher creatinine values compared with normotensive patients, attesting to the important role of hypertension in the progression of renal failure. End-stage renal disease occurred 12 years after the onset of diabetes in the Indian experience. This time is considerably sooner than the 22 years reported by Kussman et al. (1976). The more rapid progression to ESRD compared with their counterparts in Western countries likely is due to the poorer glycemic and blood pressure control (Chugh et al., 1989; Parving et al., 1993).

The reason for the underrepresentation of diabetics in renal replacement therapy programs in developing countries is either that they are not started on dialysis or that they have a poorer outcome on dialysis and after renal transplantation (Friedlander and Hricik, 1997). In industrialized countries, dialysis patients with diabetes have higher first-year mortality than nondiabetics, although the figures show an overall improvement in the 1990s. Diabetics who undergo transplantation also have a higher morbidity and mortality when compared with nondiabetic controls (Breyer, 1998). The best treatment for diabetic ESRD is a kidney transplant. For living related donor transplants, 2-year graft survival and patient survival are comparable to that of nondiabetic transplant patients. The increased morbidity and mortality rate in diabetics is related to the complications of atherosclerosis, which exceed those of patients who do not have nephropathy. Malnutrition and infections (serious problems in developing countries) compromise the survival of patients with diabetic ESRD (Breyer, 1998).

Irreversible Acute Renal Failure as a Cause of End-Stage Renal Failure

It is not always the case that patients with acute renal failure recover renal function albeit with subtle permanent changes (Bhandari and Turner, 1996). Some acutely uremic patients fail to recover completely, however, and may remain dialysis dependent. The frequency of ESRD varies, depending on the cause and the course of the acute renal failure. Acute tubular necrosis is the commonest cause of acute renal failure and fails to resolve in 1 to 6% of cases (Bonomini et al., 1984; Kjellstrand et al., 1984). Of patients with acute renal failure resulting from parenchymal disease, 41% develop irreversible disease. Inhabitants of developing countries are especially prone to acute renal failure, with medical causes being the dominant subgroup. Within this subgroup, infections and toxins present in herbal remedies were the leading causative factors (Gold, 1980; Seedat and Nathoo, 1993). Infections spread by the fecal-oral route, such as typhoid fever, gastroenteritis and Escherichia coli septicemia, appear to be on the increase (Chugh et al., 1989; Seedat and Nathoo, 1993).

Nephrotoxins are an important cause of acute and chronic renal failure in developing countries, where physicians need to be aware of the nephrotoxic potential of drugs, plants and snake venom. This knowledge may allow the judicious application of countermeasures as well as supportive measures. Nephrotoxic plants and agents include (1) impila (Callilepsis laureola), found in Africa and associated with liver damage; (2) marking-nut tree, which can cause acute renal failure in lumberjacks accidentally exposed to the sap, which can be absorbed through the skin (Abuelo, 1990) and (3) snakebite, which is an important cause of acute renal failure in tropical countries, especially in India and Brazil (Abuelo, 1990; Nelson, 1989; Warrell, 1993). The mechanism of acute renal failure after snakebite varies. Snake venom may cause hemolysis and rhabdomyolysis, activate complement and the coagulation cascade, lower the blood pressure, disturb neuromuscular function and cause renal tubular damage directly (Abuelo, 1990). The spectrum of renal manifestations includes glomerulonephritis (puff adder and saw-scaled vipers), hemolytic-uremic syndrome (gwardar and other species), acute cortical necrosis (several species) and acute tubular necrosis (rattlesnake, Russell's viper, among others) (Abuelo, 1990).

Cortical necrosis is an important cause of irreversible renal failure in developing countries (Chugh et al., 1994). Women are particularly prone to the development of acute renal cortical necrosis, although self-induced abortion as a cause is now less frequent, largely as a result of the liberalization of abortion laws in some developing countries (Seedat and Nathoo, 1993). Obstetrical causes were responsible for almost 60% of acute cortical necrosis in a report of 113 cases from India (Chugh et al., 1994). Anuria, present in 80% of the patients, was an important clue to the diagnosis. Histological examination of the kidney confirmed diffuse cortical necrosis in two thirds of cases and patchy changes in the rest. Dialysis support could be withdrawn in only 19 of 113 (17%) patients (all of whom had evidence of patchy cortical necrosis). Of the 19 patients in whom dialysis was discontinued, 7 progressed to ESRD over the subsequent 3 to 12 months.

Diarrheal disease, which is a particular problem in tropical countries (Rashid *et al.*, 1993), is responsible for most prerenal failure, which accounts for 60% of acute renal failure (Chugh *et al.*, 1989). In this stage, aggressive rehydration may prevent progression to acute renal failure, which has a considerably less favorable prognosis. Prevention of acute renal failure should be given higher priority. Reducing the incidence of acute renal failure requires increasing education levels, improving nutritional status, improving hygiene and sanitation and ensuring a reliable supply of potable water, achievable only if socioeconomic conditions improve (Seedat and Nathoo, 1993). After renal transplantation, patients should be warned to avoid traditional medicines, which may contain toxic substances.

Human Immunodeficiency Virus–Associated Nephropathy

The HIV/acquired immunodeficiency syndrome (AIDS) pandemic is sweeping across developing countries, especially sub-Saharan Africa, at an alarming rate. The World Health Organization estimated that by the year 2000, of the 30 to 40 million people infected with HIV, 90% would be in the developing world. For nephrologists and transplant physicians, the HIV/AIDS pandemic has several implications. Human immunodeficiency virus and AIDS are associated with several forms of renal disease, of which the most serious is HIV-associated nephropathy (Ray, 1999). Human immunodeficiency virus–associated nephropathy is characterized by a combination of several pathological entities that include collapsing focal segmental sclerosis, glomerular visceral epithelial cell hypertrophy, tubulointerstitial infiltration with edema and fibrosis, and microcystic tubular dilatation (Cohen and Nast, 1988; D'Agati and Appel, 1997). These morphological changes are accompanied by enlargement of the kidneys and rapid progression to ESRD. In the United States, HIV-associated nephropathy is now the third leading cause of renal failure in young black Americans (Winston *et al.*, 1999). Human immunodeficiency virus–associated nephropathy has a poor prognosis, suggesting that it is a late rather than an early manifestation of HIV-1 infection (Winston *et al.*, 1999). In contrast to idiopathic focal segmental glomerulosclerosis, HIV-associated nephropathy behaves aggressively and causes ESRD within 1 year (Langs *et al.*, 1990). Although these patients receive dialysis treatment in Western countries, few of them would be offered treatment in developing countries. In developed countries, there has been controversy as to whether these patients should be offered renal transplantation.

The high prevalence of HIV infection within a community implies that a significant number of potential organ donors will have to be rejected if they test positive. There are several reports of patients seroconverting after the purchase of kidneys for unconventional living unrelated donor kidney transplants (Chevalier *et al.*, 1991; Salahudeen *et al.*, 1990). Perhaps the most important implication of the HIV/AIDS epidemic is that valuable financial and human resources are diverted to caring for HIV/AIDS patients (Stoneburner *et al.*, 1994). This diversion of resources precludes the institution or expansion of potentially life-saving renal replacement therapy programs (Plot and Tezzo, 1990).

Hepatitis B Virus Infection

The highest prevalence of chronic HBV infection occurs in developing countries. In Hong Kong, the HBV seropositivity is 9.5% in the general population and 13.5% in the dialysis population (Cheng, 1992), whereas in Saudi Arabia it is 8.3% and 87.9%, respectively (Dhar *et al.*, 1991). Hepatitis B virus infection is an important cause of nephrotic syndrome, especially in children. In South Africa, it accounts for 40% of nephrotic syndrome in black children and usually is steroid resistant (Bhimma *et al.*, 1997; Gilbert and Wiggelinkhuizen, 1994). Most patients have a benign course, but HBV-associated nephropathy is an important cause of ESRD (Bhimma *et al.*, 1997; Lai *et al.*, 1991) in adults and to a lesser extent in children (Bhimma *et al.*, 1997; Gilbert and Wiggelinkhuizen, 1994; Lai *et al.*, 1991). Although interferon has been shown to be effective in treating nephrotic syndrome, it requires prolonged treatment, which is expensive and has a high relapse rate (Lai *et al.*, 1991). Interferon is not affordable to most people who might benefit.

Many potential organ donors would be positive for HBV and be excluded from donation (Cheng, 1992). One group from Hong Kong reported transplanting hepatitis B surface antigen (HBsAg)–positive kidneys into five patients who had been exposed to the antigen previously, either naturally or through immunization. They passively immunized four patients. None of the recipients became chronic carriers or developed chronic hepatitis over a mean follow-up of 50 months (Cheng, 1992). Dhar and colleagues reported similar experience from Saudi Arabia (Dhar *et al.*, 1991). If organs from donors who are positive for HBsAg and negative for HBeAg and delta particle are to be used in patients who are immune or have HBsAg, it seems prudent to cover the recipient with hyperimmunoglobulin and booster vaccination before transplantation (Daar, 1994). Other important considerations of HBV-seropositive patients are the infective threat that they pose to staff and other patients and the additional costs and care required by these patients, who need to be isolated.

Recurrence

An important reason for establishing the underlying cause of chronic renal failure is that certain diseases are more likely to recur in a transplanted kidney. Focal segmental glomerulosclerosis, membranous glomerulonephritis, mesangiocapillary glomerulonephritis, IgA nephropathy and diabetic nephropathy may recur. Some diseases take several years to develop, whereas others, such as mesangiocapillary glomerulonephritis type II, recur rapidly, although it results in graft loss in only 10 to 20% of cases. Focal segmental glomerulosclerosis also predictably recurs in young individuals in whom the native kidneys were lost after an aggressive clinical course. Graft loss occurs in 50% of cases, and in this situation a living related donor transplant possibly should be avoided (Cameron, 1994; Ramos and Tisher, 1994; see also Chapter 4).

Replacement Therapy Options in Developing Countries

The management of ESRD poses complex medical, social, moral and economic challenges for patients and communities in developing nations. Life-saving therapy entails the institution of dialysis and/or transplantation. In developing countries, most patients with ESRD are offered only conservative treatment because of the lack of access to dialysis and transplantation. In Latin America, a report from São Paulo, Brazil (Sesso *et al.*, 1996), showed that 26% of patients did not receive any form of renal replacement therapy. Reports indicate that most of sub-Saharan Africa (Assounga, 1999; Swanepoel, 1999; Were, 1999) has no effective renal replacement therapy program. In Egypt, 60% (Barsoum, 1992b); Southern India, 66% (Rao *et al.*, 1998); Pakistan, 75% (Naqvi *et al.*,

1998); Romania, 73% (Ursea *et al.*, 1997) and Albania, 89% (Khan *et al.*, 1996) of the incident ESRD population do not receive any form of renal replacement therapy. Acceptance rates for renal replacement therapy in the developed world are 61 to 99% (Schena, 1997).

HEMODIALYSIS

In developed countries, 56 to 60% of ESRD patients receive dialysis (Geerling *et al.*, 1994; USRDS, 1994). In some countries the figure is higher. The situation in developing countries is different (Fig. 38–2). The problems facing the initiation of such programs include the following:

Prohibitive capital expenses of setting up dialysis units (Arije *et al.*, 1995b; Chugh and Jha, 1995)

Lack of trained staff to care for patients (McLigeyo *et al.*, 1988)

Technical problems, including erratic power supply, unreliable water supply and mechanical breakdowns (Arije *et al.*, 1995b)

Shortage of reagents and spares (Arije *et al.*, 1995b; McLigeyo *et al.*, 1988)

Access of patients to long-term dialysis. With almost two thirds of the population in developing countries situated in rural areas and treatment centers almost exclusively in urban areas, patients have to travel great distances, which essentially precludes their inclusion in long-term dialysis programs (Chugh and Jha, 1995; McLigeyo *et al.*, 1988).

The reported mortality of patients receiving hemodialysis is high in some developing countries. Of 77 patients undergoing dialysis in Kenya in the period 1984–1986, 65% died while on dialysis over a mean period of 3 months (McLigeyo *et al.*, 1988). Other centers have reported much better results, however, with patient survival in Egypt being 85% (Barsoum, 1992b) and in Uruguay 91% (Fernandez *et al.*, 1995) at 1 year. The long-term outcome of maintenance dialysis as the treatment modality of choice shows patient survival to range from 10 to 15% at 3 years in India (Divakar *et al.*, 1998) and 25 to 52% at 5 years in Egypt (Barsoum, 1992b), South Africa (du Toit *et al.*, 1994) and Taiwan (Lai *et al.*, 1992). In the

absence of an established renal transplant program, it is not viable economically to maintain large numbers of patients on a maintenance hemodialysis program in a developing country (McLigeyo *et al.*, 1988). In South Africa, national guidelines set by the Department of Health preclude patients from the renal replacement therapy program if they are not suitable transplant candidates for any reason.

PERITONEAL DIALYSIS

Peritoneal dialysis is an efficient form of renal replacement therapy (Oeopoulos, 1999) that does not require the capital expenses of hemodialysis. In most instances, it is less expensive than hemodialysis (Barsoum, 1992b; Were and McLigeyo, 1995). Other advantages of peritoneal dialysis are that it is more physiological than intermittent hemodialysis and requires less stringent dietary and fluid restrictions. It is more appropriate for certain classes of patients, such as diabetics and children. Some developing countries have made peritoneal dialysis the leading form of dialysis; 93% of dialysis patients in Mexico receive peritoneal dialysis, and many South American countries are expanding their peritoneal dialysis programs (Chugh and Jha, 1995). In South Africa, the number of patients on hemodialysis has been increasing at a faster rate than patients on peritoneal dialysis, yet in 1994, 32% of patients were on peritoneal dialysis (du Toit *et al.*, 1994). In other developing countries, peritoneal dialysis is grossly underused: In India, less than 1% of ESRD patients receive peritoneal dialysis. This underuse in developing countries is partly due to physician bias (Abu-Aisha and Paul, 1994; Chugh and Jha, 1995). Other reasons are as follows:

Patients are less educated and less compliant.

The risk of peritoneal infection is high in the hot, humid climate and poor sanitary conditions that prevail.

Economic necessity forces all family members to work, leaving the patient with no assistance if required (Abu-Aisha and Paul, 1994; Chugh and Jha, 1995).

The lack of skilled personnel results in high rates of infection (Arije *et al.*, 1995a).

Cost of antibiotics is high (Arije *et al.*, 1995a).

FIGURE 38–2

The dialysis activity of several developing countries (approximately 1994) is compared with that of the United States. (Data from various registry and published data as well as estimates.)

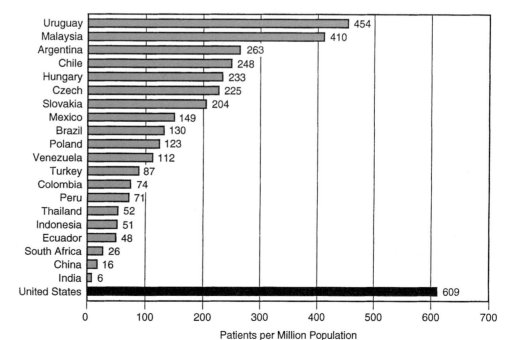

Recurrent peritonitis and other technical problems were major limitations to the use of peritoneal dialysis in the management of uremic patients in Nigeria (Arije *et al.*, 1995a), where there has been no improvement in peritonitis rates since the report by Ojogwu in 1983. South Africa reported a substantial reduction in the incidence of acute peritonitis from 2.2 episodes per patient per year in 1984 to 0.7 episodes in 1994 (du Toit *et al.*, 1994). Despite its lower cost, financial constraints were one of the main reasons for discontinuing treatment in 35% of the African patients.

RENAL TRANSPLANTATION

There is a worldwide shortage of organs, and the gap between supply and demand (especially after the introduction of cyclosporine in the 1980s) grows inexorably. The most striking feature of renal replacement therapy programs in developing countries is the emphasis, and in some cases exclusive reliance, on living related donor transplantation. Transplantation often occurs without the benefit of backup dialysis facilities and largely in the absence of a cadaver donor program (Daar, 1991a; Naqvi and Rizvi, 1995). Lack of resources, cultural factors and ignorance all contribute to the ongoing shortage of organs (Naqvi and Rizvi, 1995). Patients who previously would not have been considered for transplantation (e.g., diabetics, elderly and children) are now on waiting lists.

The number of transplants performed per 1 million population correlates with the socioeconomic status of a country (Chugh and Jha, 1996). Of all renal transplants that have been performed around the world, most (>90%) have been in developed countries (Chevalier *et al.*, 1991), which perform on average 20 to 40 transplants per 1 million population per year. This figure compares with 1 to 5 per 1 million population in most developing countries, where only 2% of the estimated need for organ transplantation is met. Under these circumstances, the purchase of kidneys from living nonrelated donors has flourished. (For a detailed discussion of this subject, see Chapter 41.)

Donors

The incidence of ESRD is estimated at anywhere from 100 to 200 per 1 million population per year. The maximum yield of cadaver donors (in Spain) is about 30 per 1 million population, and is considerably less in most countries. It appears that all countries need to use living donors. The use of living nonrelated donors has been suggested as one possible solution to ameliorate the situation (Daar, 1991b), and although this source had fallen into disrepute because of exploitation by a few, it remains an important potential source of organs. Daar and colleagues, for the purpose of simplifying the discussion of the ethical issues involved, have classified living donation into six categories: (1) genetically related, (2) emotionally related, (3) altruistic strangers, (4) gray basket, (5) rampant commercialism and (6) criminally coerced (Daar *et al.*, 1997; Daar, 1998).

Living Related Donors

In the absence of long-term dialysis and cadaver donor programs, living related donor transplantation is the only option available to patients in most developing countries (Chugh and Jha, 1996; De Villa *et al.*, 1997; Martinez and Donkervoort, 1992; Naqvi *et al.*, 1992; Sesso *et al.*, 1990). The patient's situation usually is handled sympathetically in the extended family systems that characterize many of these countries, making available to the patients many potential genetically related donors.

The workup of potential donors requires careful attention. In a report from Pakistan (Naqvi *et al.*, 1998), some of the problems of living related donors experienced in a developing country were highlighted. Although the average number of potential donors per recipient was six, this advantage was dissipated quickly. The structure of most Pakistani society is feudal and tribal in rural areas. Communities live in extended family setups under the patronage of a single elder, making the number of potential family donors quite large. Medical problems excluded 40% of potential donors, however. Hypertension was the commonest, usually undetected, problem. Other problems included urological ones, renal calculi, diabetes mellitus, ischemic heart disease and hepatitis. This array of problems reflects the limited access to health information and care common in developing countries. Approximately 25% of potential donors refused to donate for social reasons as a result of ignorance and misconceptions. Families refused to allow a breadwinner from donating for fear of incapacity and loss of family income. There was the perception that the donation would leave the male breadwinner permanently disabled. In the case of women, the perception was that the operation reduced her fertility and compromised her capacity to run a household. In a society where arranged marriages are the norm, organ donation by a woman reduced greatly the chances of finding a suitable partner (Naqvi *et al.*, 1998). The fact that more women were prepared to donate was considered to be more a reflection of their lack of empowerment in a male-dominated society than perhaps true altruism. With an adult literacy rate of only 25%, increasing awareness of health issues in a predominantly rural society is fraught with difficulty (Naqvi *et al.*, 1992).

Spousal Donors

Spousal organ donation can be an extremely rewarding form of treatment, with most donors expressing satisfaction with their decision and improvement in family relationships (Terasaki *et al.*, 1997). Evidence from several sources has established the success of spousal transplants. The 3-year survival rates for spousal transplants were 85% compared with 81% for living unrelated donors and 82% for parental donors (Terasaki *et al.*, 1995, 1997). Results of spousal transplants could be improved by a further 10% if the recipient had received donor-specific blood transfusions previously (Barry *et al.*, 1985; Haberal *et al.*, 1995b; Terasaki *et al.*, 1995). Spousal donations are an important source of kidneys in developing countries as well (Haberal *et al.*, 1995b). About two thirds of donations are from wives to husbands, which is approximately the same ratio as in Western countries (Daar, 1991b; Kathuria *et al.*, 1995; Naqvi and Rizvi, 1995). Throughout the world, an attempt should be made, preferably by a trained psychologist, to establish truly informed and uncoerced consent whenever a wife is to donate to a husband.

The benefits of spousal renal donor transplants extend beyond the restoration of renal function in the recipient. Terasaki and coworkers surveyed 176 spousal renal donors and obtained an overwhelmingly positive response (Terasaki *et al.*, 1997). There were improvements in marital, sexual and filial relationships, and all respondents, with a single exception, would recommend donation to a spouse. The countries with the highest spousal renal donor transplants in Asia are India (5.2% of transplants), Korea (3.6%) and Hong Kong (3.2%) (Chugh and Jha, 1996).

Emotionally Related Donors

In the absence of a suitable relative, an altruistic living donation by a close friend generally would be acceptable today, provided that the donor is motivated by genuine concern for the patient's welfare (Chugh and Jha, 1996; Naqvi and Rizvi, 1995).

Donors in Unconventional Renal Transplantation and Paired Kidney Exchange Donor Transplantation

For a discussion of donors in unconventional renal transplantation and paired kidney exchange donor transplantation, see Chapter 41.

Non–Heart-Beating Donors

Non–heart-beating donors are another potential source of organs. In countries where cadaver donor programs have not been instituted or where family members are reluctant to permit the removal of organs from a brain-dead donor who is warm to the touch and has a heartbeat and respiratory movements, consideration may be given to using non–heart-beating donors. The use of kidneys from non–heart-beating donors has been achieved with some success (James *et al.*, 1995). Although the incidence of delayed graft function was high (85%), the long-term patient and graft survival were comparable to matched controls (Kootstra *et al.*, 1992). The best mean creatinine values were 10% better in the control group who received kidneys from heart-beating donors. In developing countries, where the concept of brain death is not accepted fully, the harvesting of organs from non–heart-beating donors could be the first step toward the implementation of a cadaver donor program (Kootstra *et al.*, 1992; Naqvi and Rizvi, 1995). However, to date there have been no serious attempts to adopt this form of cadaveric donation in developing countries.

Cadaver Donors

Ignorance appears to be the major limiting factor inhibiting the institution and growth of cadaver organ donation programs in many developing countries (Cheng, 1992). Most religious commentators, including Islamic, Christian, Hindu, Judaic and Buddhist, support transplantation (Daar, 1997; Habgood *et al.*, 1997). Saudi Arabia is an excellent example of a conservative Muslim country that has implemented a cadaver donor program successfully (Shaheen *et al.*, 1996). The success of such a program requires several factors to be addressed (Chugh and Jha, 1996).

Education. A concerted education campaign is required to increase public awareness of the need for organ donation so as to change negative public attitudes that hinder discussion of this subject by family members. In developing countries, low adult literacy rates hinder education drives. In many South East Asian countries, organ donation is considered a *Western concept* that has not yet gained acceptance in these communities (Cheng, 1992).

Attitude. The attitude of indifferent health care professionals has been identified as a major limiting factor, and changing such indifferent attitudes should be given priority (Cheng, 1992; Naqvi and Rizvi, 1995).

Legal aspects. Recognition of the concept of brain death and the enactment of laws that allow the use of organs from cadaveric donors are important. Many developing countries do not have such laws, including Pakistan, Bangladesh and Malaysia. In 1995, India passed the Human Organ Transplantation Act (HOTA), which banned trade

in organs, recognized brain death and simultaneously promoted cadaver organ donation (Daar, 1997a; Naqvi and Rizvi, 1995).

Resources. Adequate resources in terms of finance personnel and services are crucial. Cadaver donor programs tend to be more expensive than living donor transplants and are constrained in countries where health resources are stretched to the limit (Chugh and Jha, 1996). Access to intensive care facilities is required to allow the ventilation of donors. The severe shortage of intensive care unit beds in developing countries can be a major limitation (De Villa *et al.*, 1997; Naqvi and Rizvi, 1995b). A reliable tissue-typing laboratory is essential.

TRANSPLANT ACTIVITY

No country in the world can claim to have enough donors for its transplantation needs. At best, 45 to 50% of the prevalent ESRD population have functioning grafts in developed countries. In developing countries, the situation is much worse, with renal replacement therapy and transplant activity being well below the need (Chugh and Jha, 1995). The number of transplant centers throughout the developing world has continued to increase, however, since the 1980s.

Latin America

Latin America has experienced a phenomenal increase in transplant activity. In the period 1980–1990, the number of kidneys transplanted increased by 242%. This region is the fastest growing in terms of number of transplants, new units established and progress with cadaver organ donation. What makes the achievement more remarkable is that it occurred during a decade of economic recession in the region. The Latin American Registry includes 21 countries, a regional population of 470 million, representing approximately 10% of the world transplant activity (Santiago-Delphin, 1997). The registry was created in 1991 and had recorded 46,697 renal transplants by 1997 (Santiago-Delphin and Garcia, 1999). Brazil, with the region's largest population, performed the greatest number of transplants; Chile had the highest renal transplant rate of 16 per 1 million inhabitants in 1997 (Santiago-Delphin and Garcia, 1999). Another important development has been an increase in the number of cadaver donors, which by 1990 accounted for 42% of all transplants (Martinez and Donkervoort, 1992). Currently, cadaver and living donor transplants are approaching parity in Latin America. Argentina, Brazil, Chile and Colombia have continued to increase cadaver donor transplant activity. Argentina pioneered organ transplantation in the region and leads with successful legislative changes. This change is evident by the significant increase in cadaver organ procurement rate of 3.9 to 13 per 1 million population in the period 1991–1995 (Neustadt *et al.*, 1996)—a major improvement. In the Latin American region, Cuba is one country that stands out impressively for its organized cadaver transplant program (Magrans *et al.*, 1996; Marmol *et al.*, 1996; Santiago-Delphin and Garcia, 1999) with a health care system that generally is acknowledged as one of the greatest achievements of its political revolution. Of Cuban transplant activity, 80% is from cadaver organ donation (Santiago-Delphin and Garcia, 1999). During the years 1990–1994, the donor rate increased from 9.5 to 13.8 per 1 million population, whereas its cadaver transplantation rate increased from 14 to 18 per 1 million population (Magrans *et al.*, 1996).

Many of the problems encountered in Latin America are not unique and are shared by countries elsewhere (Martinez and Donkervoort, 1992). These problems include the *lack* of:

Organized regional or national coordinating centers. The supply of organs could be increased by the introduction of transplant coordinators to organize and facilitate the logistics of organ procurement. Currently the programs rely on the enthusiasm of the transplant team, who receive no additional remuneration for the extra work performed.

Education of key personnel in the intensive care units who fail to identify potential donors. The general public appears to have a sympathetic attitude, but the donation rate remains low.

Financial resources to provide appropriate immunosuppression. Improvements in the socioeconomic situation should lead to the creation of a network of organ procurement and transplantation ideally supported financially by national health care administration and health insurers.

Adequate legislation in some of the countries, making it difficult to promote cadaver donation.

Asia Pacific Region

Combining the registry report of 12 Asian developing countries (Ota, 1999) with individual country reports (Naqvi et al., 1998; Tagaki, 1997) shows that a total of 29,027 kidney transplants were performed in the period 1993–1997. The Peoples' Republic of China is exceptional in undertaking the greatest number of cadaver donor transplants in the region (Ota, 1999)—its main source of organs is reported to be from judicially executed prisoners (Cheng et al., 1991). Excluding China's controversial contribution, living related donor transplantation accounts for 90% of transplants in the region. India undertakes the greatest number of living donor transplants. Of the 7,742 living donor transplants undertaken in Asia in the 2-year period 1996–1997, 83% were living related donor transplants and 17% were living unrelated donor transplants (Ota, 1999). Cadaver donation is underdeveloped in most of Asia, where brain death has not yet been generally accepted. Efforts are being made to increase this source, however, despite social and cultural inhibitions (Chugh and Jha, 1995; Ota, 1998, 1999; Park, 1998). Many of these countries do not have organ procurement organizations that are supported by the necessary legislation.

Singapore was one of the earliest Asian countries to introduce legislation on organ transplantation (Kaur, 1998), starting with the Medical Therapy, Education and Research Act, an *opting-in* law, in 1972. This act facilitated the procurement of only 97 cadaver kidney transplants over a 15-year period. As a result the HOTA (Human Organ Transplant Act), a presumed consent *opting-out* law, was introduced in 1987. This act made provision for the procurement of organs from cadavers, defined death to include brain death criteria and banned commercialism. The HOTA seemed to have increased the number of cadaver organs in its early years, but this number has since plateaued. Hong Kong has had a cadaver organ procurement program using brain-death criteria since 1980 (Cheng, 1992). Despite this program, a donor shortage persists, owing to a lack of awareness by the public and particularly by health professionals as well as (probably) cultural and religious factors. Since 1981, Taiwan has had a significant cadaver donor program resulting from active organ procurement using brain-death criteria, although the laws were enacted only in 1987 (Tagaki, 1997). In Korea, 29% of the prevalent renal replacement therapy population have functioning renal allografts from predominantly living donors, and Korea plans to introduce a national organ sharing system (Kim, 1996).

Commercialism had earned India a poor reputation (Chugh and Jha, 1996), but in 1995, it passed the HOTA, which banned trade in organs and simultaneously legalized brain-death criteria and cadaver organ donation (Daar, 1997a). Since then, there has been a slow but steady increase in cadaver donation, including the occasional donation of hearts and livers.

The annual number of renal transplants has increased over the years in Asia, but great potential remains for further growth. This growth can be achieved through legal and social acceptance of the brain-death concept, the establishment of organ procurement organizations and, most important, education of the public and health care providers through systematic support from the authorities.

Middle East and Afro-Arab Region

Progress continues to be made in the Middle East and Afro-Arab region, where most countries now have kidney transplant programs (Fig. 38–3). Similar to most developing countries, living related donors account for most transplants. The data from 16 countries (Abomelha, 1996) showed that 6,408 renal transplants were performed by 1997; some of these took place in neighboring countries. The number of patients receiving renal replacement therapy appears small, considering that the regional ESRD incidence ranges from 34 to 200 per 1 million population. The renal transplant rate ranges from 1 to 15 per 1 million population, with a regional average of 2 per 1 million population. The history of renal transplantation in the region has followed fairly distinct patterns (Daar, 1991a). Initially, transplantation of cadaver donors was undertaken in Europe and America. Local living related transplant programs then were established, followed by local experience with imported cadaver kidneys. During this period, commercialized living unrelated donor transplantation undertaken in neighboring countries thrived. More recently, the region has seen progress because almost all Middle Eastern countries now have successful transplant programs. Countries with cadaver programs include Saudi Arabia (Al-Khader, 1999; Loges de Cordier et al., 1997; Shaheen et al., 1996), Oman (Abomelha, 1996; Aghanashinikar et al., 1993; Kehinde, 1998), Jordan (Abomelha, 1996), Kuwait (Abomelha, 1996), Turkey (Erek, 1999; Haberal et al., 1995a, 1998), Lebanon (Abomelha, 1996; Kamel et al., 1993, 1998) and Tunisia (Abomelha, 1996; El Matri et al., 1993). An exemplary experience is that of Cyprus (Kyriakides et al., 1993), with an ESRD incidence of 80 per 1 million population and a transplantation rate of 60 per 1 million population, of which cadaver donors make up one third. This active cadaver program was achieved through intensive public education. Saudi Arabia also has made major strides in developing a cadaver donor program through public education and excellent coordinators. This program has been achieved through the efforts of its procurement agency, the Saudi Centre for Organ Transplantation.

The lack of cadaver donor programs has persisted despite support from religious authorities (Daar, 1997b; Salahi et al., 1998). As a result, many patients, against the wishes of their local transplant teams, have gone abroad to obtain living nonrelated donor kidneys through commerce in India, Egypt, Iraq and possibly Iran (Akpolat and Ozturk, 1998; Chugh and Jha, 1996; Daar, 1997b; Salahi et al., 1998; Salahudeen et al., 1990). On the whole, donors have come from the following sources: 56% living related donors, 34% living nonrelated donors and 10% cadaver donors. The practice of commercial living nonrelated donor transplantation has been reported to have a negative impact on the development of local transplant programs in the region (Abouna, 1993). Since the early discussions of this issue (Daar, 1989), the flow of patients resorting to commercial living nonrelated donor transplants in the region has persisted. Iran reports the largest experience

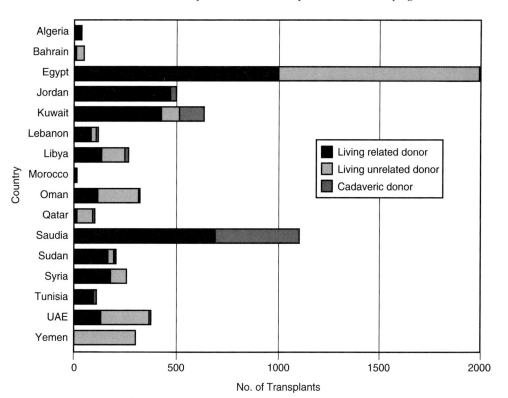

FIGURE 38–3

Total transplant activity in the Afro-Arab region as of December 31, 1992. The most striking feature of this region is that cadaveric donor transplantations formed only 10% of all transplants, with only Saudi Arabia performing any significant number of these transplants. The large number of living unrelated transplants in Egypt was due to commercial activity that has been curtailed to some extent now (Abomelha, 1996).

of living nonrelated donor transplants (Ahmad *et al.,* 1995a; Reissi *et al.,* 1995; Simforoosh *et al.,* 1992), but local transplant teams are said to be uninvolved in commercial arrangements.

Africa and Indian Ocean Islands

Africa has a population of nearly 700 million. There is little available information because there are no reliable registries (Youmbissi, 1999). Except for North Africa (Barsoum, 1992b; El Matri *et al.,* 1993; Zaid *et al.,* 1993), the Indian Ocean Islands (Albitar *et al.,* 1998) and South Africa (du Toit et al., 1994; Naicker, 1996), there is no significant renal replacement therapy in Africa (Assounga, 1999; Swanepoel, 1999; Were, 1999). Some countries provide renal support and follow-up to a small number of patients who have undergone transplantation abroad. In 1984, Kenya initiated small-scale dialysis with a view toward transplantation abroad (McLigeyo *et al.,* 1988; see later), and Tanzania adopted a similar strategy (Basinda *et al.,* 1988), but both programs have remained rudimentary. In Nigeria, of an estimated 2,600 patients with ESRD seen at a single institution in Lagos over a 5-year period, only 14% were able to undergo dialysis because they had to cover their own costs, of about $100 (U.S. dollars) per session, in a country where the annual per capita income was $300. In this series, only 7 of 368 patients could afford living related donor transplantation abroad (Mabayoje *et al.,* 1992). As in many other developing countries, most of these patients presented in the terminal stages of disease.

The incidence of ESRD in Reunion Island (Indian Ocean), with a population of 650,000, was 188 per 1 million population in 1996 (Albitar *et al.,*1998). During that year, 125 patients started dialysis, and 767 patients were on renal replacement therapy, of whom 110 had received renal allografts, predominantly living related. Although only 14% of ESRD patients had a functioning renal transplant, the provision of renal replacement therapy to so many with ESRD is impressive by African standards. In sub-Saharan Africa, South Africa is the

only country that has an effective transplant program, with 85% of transplants being cadaveric in origin (du Toit *et al.,* 1994; Naicker, 1996; Odell *et al.,* 1992). Spanning three decades, more than 4,000 kidney transplants were undertaken in 13 centers throughout South Africa. The ESRD incidence ranges from 80 per 1 million population in white South Africans to 240 per 1 million population in black South Africans (Naicker, 1996). The overall renal replacement therapy rate is 17 per 1 million population, ranging from 8 per 1 million population in the black population to 41 per 1 million population in the white population. During the 10-year period 1984-1994, the acceptance rate for black patients on renal replacement therapy increased by 175%, whereas the rate increased by 30% for white patients (du Toit *et al.,* 1994). South Africa presently provides transplant expertise to patients from Namibia, Botswana, Zimbabwe, Lesotho, Swaziland and Mauritius.

Central and Eastern Europe

After the collapse of communism, many countries suffered adverse socioeconomic conditions, and this was reflected in the effective renal replacement therapy rates (Rutkowski *et al.,* 1998). The former Soviet Union (Rutkowski *et al.,* 1998), Poland (Rutkowski *et al.,* 1997), Romania (Ursea *et al.,* 1997) and Albania (Khan *et al.,* 1996) had renal replacement therapy rates comparable to developing countries, whereas Czechoslovakia and Hungary fared better. The region has made rapid progress since 1993, however, not only in renal services, but also in improvements in the quality of life of patients. Central and Eastern Europe provides renal replacement therapy, predominantly dialysis, at an annual rate of 220 per 1 million population (Rutkowski *et al.,* 1997, 1998; Ursea *et al.,* 1997). In Poland, reflecting the regional experience, transplantation accounted for 8% of the renal replacement therapy population (Rutkowski *et al.,* 1997). Since 1990, the number of transplant units in the region has increased by 148%, but the number of transplants has increased only by 44%.

TRANSPLANT OUTCOME
Patient Survival

Egypt (Barsoum, 1992b), India (Divakar et al., 1998), United Arab Emirates (Masri et al., 1993), Turkey (Akpolat and Ozturk, 1998), Iran (Reissi et al., 1995), Saudi Arabia (Alshaibani et al., 1998), Tunisia (Ben Abdallah et al., 1997), Pakistan (Naqvi and Rizvi, 1995b; Rizvi et al., 1998b), Taiwan (Lai et al., 1992) and Korea (Park et al., 1992b, 1992c, 1998) reported living donor transplantation patient survival ranging from 72 to 100% at 5 years (Table 38–5). The survival decreased to 67 to 86% at 10 years in reports from Saudi Arabia (Alshaibani et al., 1998) and Korea (Park et al., 1992b, 1992c, 1998). There are fewer reports of long-term outcome in living nonrelated donor transplantation, but poorer results have been reported for commercial transplants in the past. Patient survival of 86% at 2 years was reported from Saudi Arabia in patients transplanted abroad; this rate compared with 100% and 95% 2-year patient survival for living related donor and cadaver donor transplants in patients transplanted locally (Chaballout et al., 1995). Rahbar et al. (1993) reported 91% 5-year patient survival in Iranian living nonrelated donor transplants. Patient survival with cadaver donor transplants was 71 to 94% at 5 years in reports from South Africa (du Toit et al., 1994), Cyprus (Kyriakides et al., 1993), Saudi Arabia (Alshaibani et al., 1998), Taiwan (Lai et al., 1992) and Korea (Park et al., 1998). This rate decreased to 29 to 90% at 10 years in reports from South Africa (Margolius and Botha, 1999) and Saudi Arabia (Alshaibani et al., 1998).

Graft Survival

Comparing graft outcome from different regions is difficult because of the many variables.

Living Donors

The graft survival of living donor transplants was 47 to 95% at 5 years in reports from South Africa (du Toit et al., 1994), Cyprus (Kyriakides et al., 1993), Lebanon (Kamel et al., 1998), United Arab Emirates (Masri et al., 1993), Saudi Arabia (Alshaibani et al., 1998), Tunisia (Ben Abdallah et al., 1997), Pakistan (Naqvi and Rizvi, 1995b; Rizvi et al., 1998b), Taiwan (Lai et al., 1992) and Korea (Park et al., 1998). The graft survival in HLA-identical donor transplants was 90 to 95% at 5 years in reports from Lebanon (Kamel et al., 1998) and Pakistan (Rizvi et al., 1998b). This rate decreased to 73% at 10 years in reports from Korea (Park et al., 1992b, 1992c, 1998). The graft survival in HLA-haploidentical and poorly matched donor transplants was 47 to 90% at 5 years in reports from Lebanon (Kamel et al., 1998), Pakistan (Naqvi and Rizvi, 1995b; Rizvi et al., 1998b) and Korea (Park et al., 1992b, 1992c, 1998).

Living Nonrelated Donors

In the larger series of living nonrelated donor transplants from developing countries, graft survival ranged from 81 to 88% at 5 years in reports from Lebanon (Kamel et al., 1998), Iran (Reissi et al., 1995), Korea (Park et al., 1992b, 1992c, 1998) and Brazil (Goldani et al., 1991). This rate decreased to 47% at 10 years in reports from Korea (Park et al., 1992b, 1992c).

Cadaver Donors

China has the highest cadaver transplant activity in the Asian-Pacific region, although its unconventional organ source is highly controversial. In 1992, a Chinese report revealed a poor graft survival rate of 26% at 5 years during the precyclosporine era (before 1985), but this had improved to 41% at 5 years with cyclosporine immunosuppression. In more recent series in developing countries, cadaver donor graft survival ranged from 55 to 72% at 5 years in reports from South Africa (du Toit et al., 1994), Cyprus (Kyriakides et al., 1993) and Saudi Arabia (Alshaibani et al., 1998). This rate decreased to 29 to 58% at 10 years in reports from South Africa (du Toit et al., 1994) and Saudi Arabia (Alshaibani et al., 1998).

Comparative Survival on Transplantation and Dialysis

Several reports exist from developing countries of patient survival on maintenance dialysis as the primary therapeutic modality. Survival ranged from 10 to 15% at 3 years in India (Divakar et al., 1998) to 25 to 52% at 5 years in Egypt (Barsoum, 1992b), South Africa (du Toit et al., 1994) and Taiwan (Lai et al., 1992). The poor outcomes on dialysis in India partly reflect poorer patient selection because most of the patients would have failed to qualify for transplantation (Rao et al., 1998). In the Philippines, survival is better with transplantation than with dialysis (Naidas, 1998), but in one report there was no difference (Lai et al., 1992), although the quality of life was better with transplantation.

Posttransplant Complications

Recipients of renal allografts in developing countries may be more prone to certain complications. Contributing to the risk for infections are protein-calorie malnutrition, tropical climate, poverty, lower socioeconomic status, lack of hygiene, poor sanitation, lack of potable water, presence of parasites and perhaps genetic factors (Cantarovich et al., 1992; Ianhez et al., 1992; Rizvi et al., 1990, 1998a). Other factors are listed in Table 38–6.

INFECTIONS

Infections are a major cause of morbidity and of graft and patient loss (see also Chapter 31). The incidence of infections after renal transplantation is related to the degree of immunosuppression and the duration of treatment. Incidence also is related to nosocomial hazards, including invasive procedures, catheters and environmental contamination with potentially hazardous pathogens, such as *Pseudomonas, Aspergillus* and *Pneumocystis*. In a study from Pakistan, infection was the commonest cause of patient loss—contributing 74% of deaths with functioning grafts and 23% of deaths with failed grafts. Almost half of patients with infections required hospitalization, adding further to the cost of treatment (Rizvi et al., 1998a) (Fig. 38–4). Bacterial infections were the commonest (43%), followed by viral (34%), protozoan (13%) and fungal (9%) infections (Rizvi et al., 1990, 1998a). In terms of specific infections, urinary tract infections are the commonest reported, followed by respiratory tract infections (Rizvi et al., 1991). Malaria is the commonest parasitic infection in the general population, whereas tuberculosis is still a major killer in many developing countries (Moosa and Bouwens, 1997) and not uncommonly flares up after the institution of immunosuppression (Erken et al., 1992; Rizvi et al., 1990, 1991; Sidabutar et al., 1992).

Bacterial Infections

Urinary tract infections account for 81% of bacterial infections. Rostami et al. (1992) reported from Iran that the classic

TABLE 38–5

IMMUNOSUPPRESSIVE REGIMENS USED IN SELECTED DEVELOPING COUNTRIES AND OUTCOMES

Country (Period)	No. Transplants	Donor Type	Immuno-suppression*	% Survival (at year indicated) Patient	Graft	Reference
Australian Aborigines (1971–1990)	48	CD	NS	—	79(1) + 53(3)	Kirubakaran and Pugsley, 1992
Bangladesh (1982–1992)	68 / 26	LRD / LURD	Aza / CsA†	—	96(1) + 81(3)	Rashid et al., 1992
Brazil (1970–1989)	687 / 60 / 239	LRD / LURD / CD	NS	— / — / —	70(1) + 49(5)	Goldani et al., 1991
(1987–1989)	1,051 / 467 / 45	LD / CD / ?	CsA (42%) / CsA (75%)	89(2) / 80(2)	76(2) / 61(2)	Sesso et al., 1990
Egypt (1994)	45	LRD	Aza (Good matches) CsA	92(1) + 86(5)	89(1) + 73(5)	Barsoum, 1994
(1992)	130 / 15	LURD(C) / CD	CsA			
	30 / 124	LRD / LURD(C)	CsA / CsA	88(1) + 80(4)	86(1) + 58(4)	Barsoum, 1992b
India (1985–1988)	153 / 303	LRD / LURD(C)	Aza / CsA (low dose)	— / —	83(1) / 83(1)	Thiagarajan et al., 1990
Iran (1989–1994)	16 / 180	LRD / LURD	CsA / CsA	91)5)	88(5)	Reissi et al., 1995
(1984–1992)	220 / 241	LRD / LURD(C)	CsA / CsA	— / —	83(1) + 69(3) / 76(1) + 70(3)	Simforoosh et al., 1992
Kuwait (1985–1990)	53	LURD(C)	NS	90(2)	90(2)	Johny et al., 1990
Mexico (1967–1991)	282 / 10 / 46	LRD / LURD / CD	CsA 1984† (Aza in HLA identical LRD)	86(1) + 68(5)	77(1) + 60(5)	Bordes-Aznar et al., 1992
Pakistan (1975–1996)	500	LRD	CsA 1990	93(1) + 83(5)	90(1) + 78(5)	Rizvi et al., 1998b
(1985–1994)	300	LRD	NS	90(1) + 74(5)	87(1) + 70(5)	Naqvi and Rizvi, 1995b
Philippines (1969–1992)	1,024	LRD / CAD	CsA† (1983) / CsA†	90(1) / 75(1) + 71(3)	90(1) / 62(1) + 56(3)	Liquete and Ona, 1992
Saudi Arabia (1999)	~2,500 / 910	LRD / CD	CsA / CsA	96(1) + 95(1)	90(1) + 78(1)	Al-Khader, 1999
(1995)	46 / 60 / 44	LRD / CD / LURD(C)	NS	100(1) / 95(1) / 86(1)	90(1) / 78(1) / 72(1)	Chaballout et al., 1995
Singapore (1985–1992)	47 / 157	LRD / CD	CsA / CsA	95(1) + 88(7)	86(1) + 77(7) / 98(1) + 92(6)	Vathsala et al., 1992
Slovenia (1986–1991)	83 / 65	CD / LRD	CsA / CsA	91(1) + 88(3) / 95(1) + 93(5)	73(1) + 73(3) / 90(1) + 90(3)	Kandus et al., 1992
South Africa (1993)	241	CD	CsA	75(3)	60(3)	Naicker, 1996
Sri Lanka (1985–1992)	105	LRD	CsA†	71(1) + 47(4)	71(1) + 47(4)	Sheriff et al., 1992
Taiwan (1968–1992)	~1,000	LRD / CD	NS	92(1)	82(1)	Lee, 1992
Turkey (1985–1989)	80	LURD	NS	95(1-3)	80(1-3)	Daar, 1991
(1975–1993)	766 / 230	LRD / CD	CsA (1985) / CsA	Aza: 60(10) / CsA: 87(1) + 72(5)	Aza: 42(10) / CsA: 66(1) + 37(5)	Haberal et al., 1995a
(1985–1992)	391	LRD	DST + Aza or + CsA	DST 98(1) -DST 94(1)	92(1) / 72(1)	Hamaloglu et al., 1992
UAE (1991)	89	LURD(C)	CsA	94(1) + 84(3)	92(1) + 83(3)	Weber et al., 1998
UAE/Oman (1984–1988)	130	LURD(C)	CsA	82(1) + 81(3.75)	77(1) + 75(3.75)	Salahudeen et al., 1990

*Regimen predominantly used.
†Cyclosporine discontinued at 3 to 12 months.
CD = cadaveric donor; LRD = living related donor; LURD = living unrelated donor; LURD(C) = commercial living unrelated donor; Aza = azathioprine; CsA = cyclosporine as part of triple or dual therapy; NS = not specified; DST = donor-specific blood transfusion.

TABLE 38–6

RISK FACTORS FOR POSTTRANSPLANT INFECTIVE COMPLICATIONS IN DEVELOPING COUNTRIES

High adult illiteracy
Poor health education
Influence of quack and indigenous medicine
Environmental pollution
Prevalence of communicable diseases
Lack of potable water supply and sewage disposal

Reproduced with permission of Rizvi *et al.*, 1990.

symptoms of urinary tract infection were almost consistently absent, with the diagnosis being made on the presence of bacteriuria. The commonest organisms isolated were *E. coli* and *Klebsiella* species. Although the response to antibiotic treatment is good, relapses are common. Urinary tract infection may be associated with acute rejection episodes (Walele, 1998).

Pneumonia (excluding tuberculosis) occurred in 16% of 110 South African renal allograft recipients reported by Edelstein *et al.* (1995) at a mean of 91 days posttransplantation. The patients responded to second-generation and third-generation cephalosporins, and none succumbed to their illness. No cases of *Pneumocystis carinii* or fungal pneumonia were diagnosed, although bronchoscopy was not done routinely. The reduced doses of steroids, which are part of triple therapy, did not appear to have reduced the incidence of infections compared with standard therapy with higher dose steroids and azathioprine. Acute rejection was a risk factor for the development of pneumonia.

Salmonella infection has been reported to be a problem in several developing countries, including Egypt, Pakistan and Indonesia (Barsoum, 1992b; Gueco *et al.*, 1989; Rizvi *et al.*, 1991; Rostami *et al.*, 1992). Barsoum (1992b) instituted routine Widal agglutination testing before renal transplantation. Antibodies to *Salmonella* species were detected in 42% of all cases, with *S. typhi* being the commonest. Salmonellosis caused a febrile illness 10 months after transplantation, all in patients who had been seronegative previously, indicating that the infection was acquired *de novo* (Barsoum, 1992b). Nontyphoid *Salmonella* can present as a febrile illness associated with bacteremia and as an acute gastroenteritis. The

latter has to be differentiated from disease caused by *Campylobacter jejuni* and *Listeria monocytogenes*. Patients usually responded well to antimicrobial therapy, but recurrences were frequent, and seeding to the cardiovascular system was a risk (Sia and Paya, 1998). Of greater concern was the observation that *Salmonella* infection was thought to have induced at least four acute rejection episodes in the seven Egyptian cases. There was no significant difference in patient or graft survival if patients were Widal seropositive to start with, however. In developing countries, blood cultures should be done early if salmonellosis is suspected and appropriate antibiotic therapy instituted (Barsoum, 1992b).

Tuberculosis

Tuberculosis is one of the oldest known diseases, and there has been a worldwide resurgence, largely as a result of the HIV/AIDS epidemic. *Mycobacterium tuberculosis* infects an estimated 8 to 10 million new patients and claims 2 to 3 million lives each year, a problem so serious that the World Health Organization declared tuberculosis a global public health emergency (Ludre *et al.*, 1992; World Health Organization, 1994). Developing countries, especially in sub-Saharan Africa, have been particularly devastated by the dual pestilences of AIDS and tuberculosis.

In developing countries, the incidence of tuberculosis posttransplant is considerably higher than that in industrialized countries; malnutrition, overcrowding, poverty and illiteracy contribute to this high incidence (Moosa and Bouwens, 1997; Table 38–7). Tuberculosis is commoner in patients on hemodialysis; in India and New York, there was a 10-fold and 15-fold increase, respectively, in the incidence compared with the general population (Daar, 1994). In countries of the Indian subcontinent, 12% of renal transplant patients (Naqvi *et al.*, 1997; Sakhuja *et al.*, 1996) develop tuberculosis compared with 1.7% in the United Kingdom (Higgins *et al.*, 1991). The interval between development of tuberculosis posttransplantation varies from 1 month to 10 years (Lubani *et al.*, 1989; Naqvi *et al.*, 1997). In Pakistan, 63% (Naqvi *et al.*, 1997); India, 58% (Sakhuja *et al.*, 1996) and Turkey, 82% (Yildiz *et al.*, 1998a) of patients who developed tuberculosis did so within the first year posttransplant.

Tuberculous interstitial nephritis is an unusual form of the disease that has been described after transplantation by Al-Sulaiman *et al.* (1990) of Saudi Arabia and Goncalves *et al.* (1992) of Brazil. The diagnosis was made by the histological findings of granulomas in the graft. In contrast to the Brazil group, the Saudi group did not detect acid-fast bacilli and

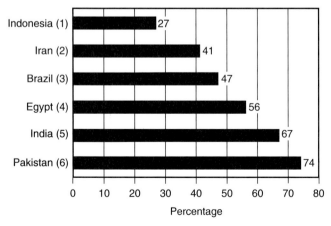

FIGURE 38–4

Infection is the leading cause of mortality in renal allograft recipients in developing countries. 1 = Sidabutar *et al.*, 1999; 2 = Rostami *et al.*, 1992; 3 = Sesso *et al.*, 1990; 4 = Barsoum, 1992b; 5 = Prakash *et al.*, 1999; 6 = Rizvi *et al.*, 1998.

TABLE 38–7

INCIDENCE AND MEAN LATENT PERIOD TO DIAGNOSIS OF TUBERCULOSIS AFTER RENAL TRANSPLANTATION IN SELECTED DEVELOPING COUNTRIES

Country/Region	Incidence %	Latent period (range) (mo.)	Reference
South America	2.3	—	Cantarovich *et al.*, 1992
South Africa	1.7, 4.5, 6.6	15.3 (2–78)	Moosa and Bouwens, 1997
India	11.8	20.7 (1–84)	Sakhuja *et al.*, 1996
Pakistan	12.4	(1–108)	Naqvi *et al.*, 1997
Saudi Arabia	3.5	16.6 (1–84)	Qunibi *et al.*, 1990
Turkey	4.2	44.4 (3–111)	Yildiz *et al.*, 1998
Mexico	5.0	45.4	Zaragoza *et al.*, 1996
Philippines	3.1	13.4 (3–38)	Gueco *et al.*, 1989

caseation in their cases. In developing countries, tuberculosis may be transmitted to the recipient from an incidentally infected donor, and measures should be taken to reduce this likelihood by donor screening (Daar, 1994).

The disease typically presents with the classic symptoms of cough, fever, anorexia and weight loss. The classic features of tuberculosis often are obscured by the immunosuppression, and a high index of suspicion should be maintained (Coutts *et al.*, 1979; Malhotra *et al.*, 1986; Moosa and Bouwens, 1997). The extrapulmonary forms of tuberculosis are particularly difficult to diagnose (Coutts *et al.*, 1979). Transplant patients are prone to developing extrapulmonary and disseminated forms of tuberculosis. In a review of the subject, Qunibi *et al.* (1990) found a 39% incidence of disseminated disease and a higher incidence in their own series from Saudi Arabia. Sakhuja *et al.* (1996) reported a similarly high incidence (28%) in India. In South Africa, however, only 12% of cases had disseminated disease (Moosa and Bouwens, 1997).

For patients with pulmonary tuberculosis, the presence of *M. tuberculosis* can be confirmed by examination of the sputum for acid-fast bacilli. Examining three sputum specimens instead of one increases the yield. The gold standard for diagnosis is culture of *M. tuberculosis* from the appropriate specimen, but this takes a long time and is relatively expensive. The polymerase chain reaction test for tuberculosis has failed to live up to expectations mainly because of a high false-positive rate (Moosa and Bouwens, 1997; Schluger *et al.*, 1999).

An important tool for the diagnosis of pulmonary tuberculosis is the chest radiograph. In postprimary tuberculosis, apical cavitation is the typical radiological finding. The predominant radiological pattern with therapeutic or HIV-induced immunosuppression was focal pulmonary opacities in 81% of cases. Apical cavitation occurred in less than 10% in the report by Moosa and Bouwens (1997). Apical cavitation occurs as a result of an interaction between large amounts of tubercle bacilli and infiltrating lymphocytes; vast amounts of cytokines are released with consequent necrosis and liquefaction (Balasubramanian *et al.*, 1994; Moosa and Bouwens, 1997). In immunosuppressed patients, this process is dampened, and this may explain the low incidence of cavitation.

The tuberculosis skin test has limited diagnostic value in developing countries, where tuberculosis is endemic and most of the population has been exposed to the tubercle bacillus (Qunibi *et al.*, 1990; Tokat *et al.*, 1996). A positive skin test implies infection and not disease, regardless of the degree of positivity. Tokat *et al.* (1996) reported that most of their Turkish renal transplant patients were anergic. In severely immunosuppressed patients, the test often is falsely negative (Cook, 1991).

The diagnosis of tuberculosis may be difficult to prove, with the result that many units resort to a therapeutic trial of antituberculosis agents. Patients with typical features who responded to treatment are considered to have tuberculosis (Higgins *et al.*, 1991; Malhotra *et al.*, 1986; Sakhuja *et al.*, 1996). In view of the potentially serious adverse effects of antituberculosis chemotherapy, every attempt should be made to confirm the diagnosis (Moosa and Bouwens, 1997). The introduction of the triple immunosuppressive regimen including cyclosporine did not lead to a significant decline in the incidence of tuberculosis, despite reduction in the amount of steroids used (John *et al.*, 1994; Moosa and Bouwens, 1997; Sakhuja *et al.*, 1996). A report suggested that, under cyclosporine, the interval between transplantation and the development of tuberculosis was reduced considerably (John *et al.*, 1994), but this is not a consistent finding (Higgins *et al.*, 1991; Moosa and Bouwens, 1997). The treatment of

acute graft rejection appears to precipitate the development of tuberculosis in some cases (Costa *et al.*, 1999; Edelstein *et al.*, 1995; Hall *et al.*, 1994).

Successful treatment requires adequate doses of drugs for an adequate period of time. Patients with renal allografts who develop tuberculosis respond well to conventional therapy but often relapse (Cook, 1991), especially with inadequate therapy. The choice of drugs determines the duration of therapy. If the combination of isoniazid and rifampicin is used with another agent, usually pyrazinamide, 6 months of therapy should be adequate. If any regimen is used that does not include isoniazid and rifampicin, treatment should be continued for a minimum of 9 to 12 months (Moosa and Bouwens, 1997). Drug interaction is a problem. Rifampicin and, to a lesser extent, isoniazid are potent inducers of the liver cytochrome P-450 enzyme system, markedly increasing the elimination of cyclosporine and steroids. The dose of the immunosuppressive drugs may need to be increased severalfold to maintain therapeutic levels. Alternatively a regimen that excludes rifampicin should be employed (Moosa and Bouwens, 1997) and maintained for a minimum of 9 to 12 months. With prolonged therapy, compliance is always a potential problem. A developing country innovation, directly observed therapy, has ensured the success of intermittent therapy where other techniques have failed (Wilkinson, 1994; Wilkinson and de Cock, 1996). The increase in multidrug resistance is another major problem facing developing countries (Moosa and Bouwens, 1997).

The use of chemoprophylaxis is unresolved in the absence of controlled studies. Many centers use isoniazid when a transplant patient has historical or radiological evidence of tuberculosis (Costa *et al.*, 1999; Higgins *et al.*, 1991; Moosa and Bouwens, 1997). Others believe that the risk of tuberculosis is small when low doses of steroids are used and that the use of prophylaxis is not justified (Qunibi *et al.*, 1990). For reasons that are unclear, bacille Calmette-Guérin vaccination has not been effective in protecting adults from developing tuberculosis, and it cannot be relied on to protect the renal transplant recipient. The development of an effective vaccine would go a long way toward addressing the plight of millions of people in developing countries who live with the threat of the disease (Malin and Young, 1996).

The mortality of disseminated tuberculosis is high in transplant recipients in developing countries. There are reports of mortality approaching 40% in the disseminated form of the disease compared with 11% in the isolated form (Qunibi *et al.*, 1990). Relapse of tuberculosis is uncommon if the disease is treated adequately (Sakhuja *et al.*, 1996).

Protozoan Infections

Malaria

Malaria, caused by the protozoan parasite *Plasmodium*, is the commonest parasitic infection in developing countries, where it continues to have a major influence on social and economic development (Cantarovich *et al.*, 1992). Four species affect humans, of which *P. falciparum* is the most lethal. The disease, especially *P. falciparum*, has resisted attempts at eradication and continues to gain new territory. It is particularly prevalent in sub-Saharan Africa, where it infects 250 million people and causes about 2 million childhood deaths annually. Global mortality is 1% (Daar, 1994).

Malaria may occur in renal transplant patients after the bite of an infected female anopheline mosquito or the transfusion of infected blood (Cantarovich *et al.*, 1992; Ona, 1992). There are isolated reports of the protozoan being transmitted by the kidney graft; this occurred despite flushing of the kidneys because the schizonts adhere to the vascular endothelium (Holzer et al., 1985). The diagnosis of malaria after a kidney transplant can be difficult because the features mimic those of acute rejection. Suspicion should be raised if the renal function normalizes after pulse methylprednisolone treatment in the presence of ongoing fever. Clinical features that should alert the clinician to the diagnosis of malaria include varying combinations of abdominal pain, vomiting, diarrhea, jaundice, cough, stupor, coma, orthostatic hypotension, hepatosplenomegaly and worsening anemia (Daar, 1994). In a developing country, the most cost-efficient diagnostic test is the examination of thick and thin blood films for the parasite. Repeated examinations of blood films are essential, preferably by a skilled technologist. An indirect fluorescent antibody test for malaria also is available.

The treatment for all forms of malaria (except chloroquine-resistant falciparum malaria) is chloroquine phosphate. Chloroquine-resistant *P. falciparum* is treated with a combination of quinine and other agents, such as pyrimethamine and doxycycline. The severely ill patient is treated with intravenous quinine. The maintenance dose should be reduced in severe renal failure (Eiam-Ong and Sitprija, 1998). For patients from endemic areas, a high index of suspicion is necessary to institute early treatment. The problem is the patient from a nonendemic region, in whom a travel history is missed. Patients who never have been exposed to malaria generally have a more serious course of disease than patients living in endemic areas. Patients not living in endemic areas who plan to travel to endemic areas should be advised to take appropriate precautions because they are more prone to developing fulminant forms of malaria. There generally are no contraindications to the use of malaria chemoprophylaxis in renal transplant patients. Recommendations on specific prophylaxis vary from region to region and from time to time (Behrnes and Curtis, 1993). Expert advice should be sought before visiting a particular region. Patients traveling to malaria endemic areas should be advised that personal protection measures, such as the covering of the arms and legs, insect nets and repellents and avoiding nocturnal excursions to avoid mosquito bites, are important to prevent malaria (Durrheim et al., 1998). Currently, no effective vaccine is available for the prevention of malaria, but there are possibilities on the horizon (Eiam-Ong and Sitprija, 1998).

Chagas' Disease

American trypanosomiasis (Chagas' disease) is endemic in South America. It is caused by the extracellular protozoan *Trypanosoma cruzi*, and it represents the commonest protozoan disease in this region. It usually is transmitted by the feces of blood-sucking insects or by blood transfusion. It also may be acquired congenitally. The disease may present with acute, subacute or chronic clinical features. The acute presentation is a febrile illness in children associated with vomiting, diarrhea and chagoma. The subacute and chronic forms present with myocarditis and heart failure, with the chronic form being complicated by megacolon and megaesophagus. The diagnosis is relatively easy to confirm using a range of available serological tests. Specific and effective treatment for acute Chagas' disease is with nifurtimox (nitrofurazone). In addition to killing the promastigotes in blood, this agent prevents seroconversion and reduces morbidity and mortality. The infection has been transmitted with a donor kidney. Cantarovich et al. (1992) reported 26 patients who received organs from Chagas-seropositive donors. Only three recipients developed parasitemia, of whom two remained asymptomatic. The third patient developed features of acute Chagas' disease 145 days after renal transplantation. All the

patients responded to specific therapy with no short-term or long-term sequelae. In view of the low transmission rate and availability of effective treatment, the use of organs from potential seropositive donors should not be excluded. In a region where 20% of the population is infected, reactivation of Chagas' disease in the recipient is a potential problem. In another report of 35 transplant patients who were seropositive preoperatively, 13 had evidence of reactivation of parasitemia, and all responded to specific therapy. Fatalities have been described, however, usually with meningoencephalitis as the major clinical manifestation. Serial monitoring for parasitemia and serology should be standard practice in endemic areas. Prophylaxis should be considered in patients who receive heavy immunosuppression (Cantarovich et al., 1992).

Toxoplasmosis

Toxoplasmosis is caused by the intracellular protozoan *Toxoplasma gondii*, and it is endemic in many countries. The cysts of *T. gondii* remain dominant in host tissue for life but cause disease when patients are immunosuppressed. The parasite can be transmitted by blood transfusion, and it has been transmitted with renal allografts (Anthony, 1972; Reynolds et al., 1966). There are reports of seronegative patients who received kidneys from *Toxoplasma*-seropositive patients; all four such patients developed disseminated disease, and two died. The clinical features are variable but include fever, lymphadenopathy and neurological syndromes. With the parasite's predilection for muscle tissue, cardiac allograft recipients are particularly at risk. Diagnosis is by appropriate immunofluorescent antibody test (Cantarovich et al., 1992). Treatment includes pyrimethamine and sulfadiazine, although spiromycin has been used. Co-trimoxazole is not an alternative to these drugs. As for reactivation, in a report of eight patients who were seropositive before transplantation and followed for 18 months, only one patient showed an increased titer on indirect hemagglutination. The patient remained asymptomatic and required no specific therapy. In endemic areas, however, the disease should be sought actively postoperatively in patients presenting with severe febrile illness, especially if major neurological manifestations are present after heavy immunosuppression. In a review of the subject, Renoult and colleagues established that 86% of patients presented within 3 months of transplantation with fever, neurological disturbances and pneumonia as the main clinical manifestations (Renoult et al., 1999). The mortality rate in this report was 86%, with the diagnosis being made postmortem in almost 50%. Of the 11 patients given specific therapy, 10 (91%) survived. Early diagnosis and prompt therapy are essential for successful management.

Helminthic Infestations

Schistosomiasis

Urinary schistosomiasis is caused by *Schistosoma haematobium*, which is endemic in Africa and southwestern Asia (Husain, 1994). The intestinal forms of schistosomiasis are prevalent in Africa, parts of the Middle East, the Caribbean and South America and are caused by *Schistosoma mansoni*, whereas *Schistosoma japonica* is confined to the Far East. Urinary schistosomiasis is prevalent in almost all children in endemic areas (Daar, 1994). The urinary abnormalities are caused by the granulomatous reaction excited by the deposition of large numbers of eggs in the bladder and ureter of the host over a period of several years. The net result of this inflammatory process is fibrosis, calcification, obstruction and functional abnormalities (Barsoum, 1993). Calculi, bacterial infections and squamous cell bladder carcinoma may complicate the disease further (Barsoum, 1993). Urinary schistosomiasis contributes to the high prevalence of chronic renal failure in certain endemic areas (Barsoum, 1992a). Schistosomiasis also may cause renal disease by immunological mechanisms. Nephrotic syndrome is prevalent in Egypt in regions with high endemicity of *S. haematobium*, although evidence has implicated *S. mansoni* as well (Daar, 1994). Mesangial proliferative glomerulonephritis is the commonest lesion and is associated with IgM and C3 deposits (Sobh *et al.*, 1990). The intestinal forms of schistosomiasis seen in Brazil and caused by *S. mansoni* are associated most commonly with mesangiocapillary glomerulonephritis and focal segmental glomerulosclerosis, although most other types of glomerulopathy have been described. Immune complex deposits with IgM, IgA, IgG and IgE have been described. A strong association has been found between the mesangiocapillary glomerulonephritis of hepatointestinal schistosomiasis and different *Salmonella* strains (Barsoum, 1993).

Patients with urinary schistosomiasis can be transplanted successfully. Graft and patient survival are no different compared with controls, but urological complications can occur in 15% of patients. The risk of reactivation is low, provided that patients receive antischistosomal chemotherapy before transplantation. These patients are at increased risk of bladder carcinoma, and cystoscopy should be part of the long-term follow-up plan (Barrou *et al.*, 1997). In endemic areas, potential donors should be screened carefully. Potential donors with only a history of infection but no cystoscopic or radiological abnormalities should be accepted; potential donors showing structural changes—even small sandy patches on cystoscopy—probably should be excluded because progression may lead to further urinary tract damage.

Strongyloidiasis

Strongyloidiasis is a nematode infestation that is a potentially devastating disease in immunosuppressed patients. It was reviewed extensively previously (Daar, 1988), but in the interim there have been few reports in transplant recipients. Nevertheless, strongyloidiasis should be kept in mind, especially in the tropics (Cantarovich *et al.*, 1992). Briefly, because of the organism's capacity to multiply repeatedly within the host without external reinfection (in contrast to *Schistosoma*), a state of hyperinfestation may occur years after exposure. In the immunosuppressed patient, this hyperinfestation may take a fulminant course (e.g., pneumonia, respiratory failure, severe diarrhea or intestinal obstruction) accompanied by polybacterial gram-negative septicemia and disseminated intravascular coagulopathy. Eosinophilia should alert the clinician to the possibility of *Strongyloides* infestation because the worm may not be found in the stool unless it is concentrated after incubation. The worm also may be found in duodenal aspirates, and in severe cases larvae may be present in sputum or bronchial aspirates. In the severely ill patient, respiratory support, therapy for disseminated intravascular coagulopathy and broad-spectrum antibiotic drugs may be needed, in addition to specific therapy with thiabendazole or mebendazole. In endemic areas, it is advisable to give prophylactic thiabendazole or mebendazole on several occasions to ensure eradication of migrating larvae and adult worm. *Strongyloides* may be transmitted with a kidney graft.

Fungal Infections

Hot climate, high humidity, low socioeconomic status, clothing habits and poor personal hygiene are said to be some of the factors contributing to the high frequency of fungal infections in patients in developing countries. In addition, immunosuppressive therapy, prolonged antibiotic therapy, leukopenia as well as the metabolic consequences of malnutrition, diabetes mellitus and uremia predispose these patients to mycotic infections (Chugh *et al.*, 1992, 1993). Chugh and coworkers categorized fungal infections into superficial and systemic infections (Chugh *et al.*, 1992).

In the Indian experience, superficial fungal infection occurred in most transplanted patients. Of the 157 patients followed for a 2-year period, 74% had fungal infections of the skin and superficial mucosa. The greatest incidence (83%) was after 12 months of maintenance immunosuppressive therapy. *Tinea versicolor* was the commonest fungal infection, accounting for three fourths of all these infections. *Candida* infection of the gastrointestinal tract occurred in 7% of patients (this is similar to the 3–5% in developed countries [Hibberd and Rubin, 1994]) and generally responded well to oral nystatin or ketoconazole. *Candida* urinary tract infection in 3.4% of patients was related almost invariably to the prolonged use of an indwelling urinary catheter. These patients responded well to removal of the catheter and amphotericin B bladder irrigation.

Chugh and coworkers identified systemic fungal infections in 19 of 310 (6.1%) Indian patients over a 15-year period (Chugh *et al.*, 1992). By comparison, the incidence of fungal infections in developed countries seems to be decreasing rapidly: the reported incidence was 45% in 1967 (Rifkind *et al.*, 1967), 12% in 1975 (Gallis *et al.*, 1975) and 1.4% in 1982 (Peterson *et al.*, 1982). The infections observed most commonly by Chugh *et al.* (1992) were *Cryptococcus neoformans* (42%), *Candida albicans* (37%), *Mucor* species (11%) and *Aspergillus flavus* (5.5%). The patients generally were well stabilized on maintenance immunosuppression, and graft function was normal in 68% of patients at the time of diagnosis. Additional risk factors were diabetes mellitus, leukopenia, recent pulse therapy for acute rejection and concomitant bacterial infections. None of the patients had concomitant cytomegalovirus (CMV) infection, which was found by Jayakumar and associates to be a risk factor in their Indian patients (Jayakumar *et al.*, 1998). Most systemic fungal infections (63%) reported by Chugh *et al.* (1992) occurred greater than 12 months posttransplantation. This timing contrasts with timing of nosocomial fungal infections reported in developed countries, where most infections occur in the first 2 months posttransplantation, when patients are maximally immunosuppressed (Hadley and Karchmer, 1995). In Chugh's patients, the commonest presenting feature was fever unresponsive to antibiotics. Of 19 patients, 16 (84.2%) presented with fever.

Patients with cryptococcal infections presented with features of meningitis, with other organ involvement in 78% of cases. The diagnosis of cryptococcal infection was confirmed on positive latex agglutination test or culture of the organism from cerebrospinal fluid, blood or urine. Systemic candidiasis presented most commonly with clinical features of pyelonephritis affecting the graft. The diagnosis can be confirmed with culture of *C. albicans* in the blood or urine. Cavernous sinus thrombosis was the typical complication with which two patients with rhinocerebral mucormycosis presented. The diagnosis was suspected clinically because patients had periorbital cellulitis and black necrotic pus discharging from the nasal mucosa and palate that characteristically showed *Mucor* when the mucosal tissue was examined. It was not stated whether these two patients were hyperglycemic. Both cases were fatal. In a review of mucormycosis in renal transplant patients by Carbone *et al.* (1985), 20 cases were reported, of whom 70% presented with rhinocerebral disease and 70% were diabetic. In Chugh's series, aspergillosis presented as a lung infiltrate in two patients who had symptoms of cough and expectoration. *A. flavus* was cultured in the blood of both patients. Diagnosis was made by examination of lung tissue.

Treatment of systemic fungal infections is based on amphotericin B with or without flucytosine in certain diseases. Newer agents have been used with some success in cryptococcal infection (Terrell and Hughes, 1992). All three patients in Chugh's series who received fluconazole recovered. Fluconazole is prohibitively expensive, and although it has proved to be effective in many infections and can be administered orally, amphotericin B remains the cornerstone of antifungal therapy for the time being (Terrell and Hughes, 1992). Drug interactions may influence cyclosporine levels profoundly, requiring drastic cyclosporine dosage reduction (Canafax *et al.*, 1991); the combination of cyclosporine with amphotericin B has a particularly detrimental effect on renal function (Hibberd and Rubin, 1994).

The prognosis of systemic fungal infections is poor. Of the 19 patients in Chugh's series, 12 (63%) died. Jayakumar *et al.* (1998) reported a similar mortality in their patients. The poor outcome may be related to the delay in diagnosis and treatment because of a low index of suspicion and the unusual manifestations of these infections. The series of patients with mucormycosis reported by Carbone *et al.* (1985) had a 50% mortality despite treatment.

Considering the poor outcome of fungal infections and the difficulties in using antifungal agents, prevention must be given particular attention. The efficacy of antifungal chemoprophylaxis has not been proved in solid-organ transplantation, however (Paya, 1993). Nevertheless, chemoprophylaxis is practiced widely and consists in the main of oral nystatin, which is employed to prevent oral and esophageal candidiasis (Hadley and Karchmer, 1995; Hibberd and Rubin, 1994; Paya, 1993).

Viral Infections

Of renal transplant patients, 60 to 90% have serological evidence of CMV infection in the first year posttransplantation. Of these, 35% develop overt disease, and 2% die as a result of CMV-related complications (Mancilla *et al.*, 1992). The frequency of CMV infection and disease varies (Table 38–8). Cuhadaroglu and colleagues reporting from Turkey found that 60 (27.5%) of 218 serially transplanted patients were CMV IgG positive (Cuhadaroglu *et al.*, 1992). Of these patients, 42 (70%) had been treated for rejection, and 14 (23%) had received OKT3 and plasmapheresis, supporting the importance of immunosuppression in the development of CMV disease (Cuhadaroglu *et al.*, 1992). Reactivation and *de novo* infection are the two epidemiological patterns of CMV infection recognized. Transmission of CMV from an infected donor to an unexposed recipient may occur. In this situation, *matching* of the donor to the recipient is important. In the event of a CMV IgG-seronegative patient receiving an organ

from an IgG-seropositive donor, immunoprophylaxis with CMV hyperimmune globulin has been recommended (Cuhadaroglu *et al.*, 1992). Acyclovir is a safe and relatively inexpensive alternative form of prophylaxis (Mancilla *et al.*, 1992), but its efficacy has been questioned. Symptomatic CMV disease occurs in the first 4 months posttransplantation when immunosuppression is most intense. It usually manifests as a febrile illness, with neutropenia, thrombocytopenia, pneumonia, hepatitis or gastrointestinal ulceration. Chorioretinitis is characteristic of CMV infection and has to be excluded (Sia and Paya, 1998). It also may predispose to other opportunistic infections, such as *P. carinii*, *Aspergillus* and *Listeria* (Peterson and Anderson, 1986; Rubin and Tolkoff-Rubin, 1988; Rubin *et al.*, 1999).

Invasive CMV disease typically is associated with the presence of CMV inclusion bodies detected by immunohistochemistry or DNA hybridization techniques in tissue specimens. Newer diagnostic techniques that are being evaluated rely on the detection of CMV antigenemia and polymerase chain reaction–based detection of CMV DNA (Sia and Paya, 1998). These tests may allow the disease to be monitored. Serology, although suggestive, is not always a reliable guide to active infection.

The modern treatment of CMV infection is with ganciclovir or foscarnet. Diagnosed and treated early, CMV infection has a good outcome. The prognosis of CMV disease in developing countries seems to be considerably worse than the 2% reported in developed countries (Davis, 1990; Snydman *et al.*, 1991; see Table 38–8). Barsoum (1992b) from Egypt reported an increase of cellular rejection episodes for patients with CMV disease.

LIVER DISEASE

Liver disease complicates 9 to 34% of renal transplants in reports from industrialized countries (see also Chapter 32). Hepatitis C virus (HCV) is a major cause of liver-related morbidity and mortality. Other causes of liver dysfunction after renal transplantation include HBV (see earlier), Epstein-Barr virus (EBV) and CMV infections as well as drugs, including alcohol, cyclosporine and azathioprine. Drugs were responsible for approximately half of all cases of liver dysfunction in some series (Morales, 1998; Pereira, 1998).

Hepatitis C Virus Infection

Hepatitis C virus is an RNA virus that first was recognized and cloned in 1989 (Pereira, 1998; Pereira and Levey, 1997). Since that time, HCV has been found to be more prevalent in dialysis and transplant patients than in the general population. The prevalence of HCV averages 30% in these patients but varies geographically and with the generation of anti–HCV antibody test employed. The highest prevalences have been reported in developing countries (Huraib *et al.*, 1995; Muller *et al.*, 1992; Sheu *et al.*, 1992). The incidence and prevalence of HCV in developed countries is diminishing at a steady rate, but little is known about the epidemiological behavior of HCV in developing countries (Pereira and Levey, 1997).

Hepatitis C virus infection usually is acquired on dialysis before the patient receives renal transplantation. The risk factors that predispose patients to HCV infection include the number of blood transfusions, the duration of dialysis therapy, retransplantation and hemodialysis (as compared with peritoneal dialysis) (Morales, 1998; Pereira and Levey, 1997). Ongoing HCV infection is present in 8 to 85% of these patients as established by HCV RNA. Liver biopsy specimens frequently show chronic hepatitis, but cirrhosis and liver

TABLE 38–8

CYTOMEGALOVIRUS IN RENAL TRANSPLANT PATIENTS

Country	No.	Infection (%)	Disease (%)	Mortality (%)	Reference
Mexico	123	—	7.3	22	Mancilla *et al.*, 1992
Turkey	218	27.5	6.4	28.5	Cuhadaroglu *et al.*, 1992
Egypt	154	87.3	44.7	18.5	Barsoum, 1992b

failure are rare in hemodialysis patients (Goffin *et al.*, 1995; Morales, 1998).

The issue of transplanting recipients with HCV-seropositive donors is controversial. Several series have shown that HCV infection in recipients is accompanied by biochemical liver abnormalities and more aggressive histopathological changes compared with HCV-seronegative controls (Pereira and Levey, 1997; Roth *et al.*, 1994; Vosnides, 1997). Morales (1998) showed progression of liver disease posttransplant on repeat liver biopsy specimens in 11 of 15 patients who were HCV positive. Vosnides (1997) showed progressive fibrosis in 13 patients who underwent repeat liver biopsies. In contrast, several groups failed to show the serious adverse events described. Fourteen HCV-infected patients were subjected to pretransplant liver biopsies as well as posttransplant virology and biochemical studies (Goral and Helderman, 1998). All patients did well despite evidence of increased viral replication and elevation of liver enzymes. Haem and coworkers followed 62 HCV-seropositive renal transplant patients for a mean of 72 months (Haem *et al.*, 1996). Despite 42% of the patients having chronic active hepatitis, the patient and graft survival were no different compared with HCV-seronegative patients (Goral and Helderman, 1998; Haem *et al.*, 1996). Despite the controversy, the survival of HCV-seropositive transplant patients was better than that of dialysis patients, and transplantation is the preferred treatment (Goral and Helderman, 1998). Rao and Ma (1996) observed an increase in the number of potentially serious infections, including those of the bloodstream, central nervous system and lungs. Morales (1998) reported an increase in the number of CMV, tuberculosis, *P. carinii* pneumonia and sepsis cases. It is postulated that these complications may be due to an immunodeficiency state induced by HCV. The New England Organ Bank reported a 10-fold increased risk of death resulting from sepsis in recipients who had anti-HCV antibodies (Pereira *et al.*, 1995).

Treatment of HCV is difficult and potentially dangerous. Interferon alfa can trigger acute rejection, and its use cannot be recommended generally in renal transplant recipients (Berthoux, 1995; Morales, 1998; Rostaing *et al.*, 1995). Interferon alfa is expensive and not readily affordable by patients in developing countries. Approximately 50% of patients respond to treatment, which is usually for 6 months, but 50% of these relapse when treatment is stopped (Berthoux, 1995; Pereira and Levey, 1997). A safer alternative to interferon alfa is ribavirin, which can be used alone or with interferon alfa (Berthoux, 1995; Morales, 1998). A significant increase in HCV RNA titers posttransplantation is strong evidence that immunosuppression promotes viral replication (Pereira *et al.*, 1995, 1999). Decreasing immunosuppression is the most important therapeutic approach in renal transplant patients and the only one available to many patients in developing countries (Morales, 1998).

The survival of renal failure patients with HCV is better with transplantation than with dialysis, provided that patients do not have advanced liver disease (Pereira *et al.*, 1999). Several recommendations have been made for the management of these patients before and after transplantation. These recommendations include the performance of liver biopsies for patients who are HCV seropositive and who are HCV RNA positive or have elevated alanine aminotransferase (ALT) levels. Patients who have evidence of cirrhosis should be offered dialysis where feasible. Patients with chronic active hepatitis may be offered interferon alfa where available. All other patients can undergo transplantation safely (Morales, 1998).

Avoiding blood transfusion at all stages minimizes the risk of HCV infection, especially in the absence of screening for HCV. After transplantation, overimmunosuppression should be avoided. Careful follow-up and the avoidance of alcohol and other hepatotoxic drugs is recommended (Morales, 1998).

Hepatitis B Virus Infection

There has been a dramatic reduction in the incidence of HBV infection in dialysis patients because of isolation and systematic vaccination policies. Hepatitis B virus continues to be a serious problem in developing countries, however (Morales, 1998). Although there is a high carrier rate of 80% after HBV infection in dialysis patients, the disease is seldom serious, although liver disease occurs frequently. The survival of HBV-infected dialysis patients is similar to that of uninfected patients (Morales, 1998). There may be progression of liver disease posttransplantation, however, in HBsAg-positive patients, particularly in older patients, female patients and patients who have chronic active hepatitis (Rao *et al.*, 1993). Patients with cirrhosis may go on to develop hepatocellular carcinoma, especially if there is coinfection with HCV (Fornainron *et al.*, 1996; Morales, 1998; Rao *et al.*, 1993). Reports on the outcome of HBsAg-positive renal allograft recipients are contradictory, with some reports of a higher mortality and others disputing this (Huang and Lai, 1992; Pol *et al.*, 1990). Barsoum (1992b) from Egypt reported that anti-HbsAg–seropositive recipients had significantly better patient and graft survival compared with seronegative recipients. The discrepancies may be related to two important considerations—the preexisting liver status as established by liver biopsy and the HBeAg status of the recipient. Dhar *et al.* (1991) reported from Saudi Arabia that all HbsAg-seropositive patients who were presented for renal transplantation underwent liver biopsies. Patients who had evidence of cirrhosis were excluded from transplantation, and of these patients, 4 of 27 (15%) died of liver failure within 2 years. All three patients who had chronic active hepatitis and were transplanted did poorly, with two patients developing chronic liver disease and one patient losing his kidney as a result of rejection. Of the 10 patients with minimal or reactive changes only on liver histology, repeat biopsies done 6 years posttransplantation showed chronic active hepatitis in 25% (Dhar *et al.*, 1991). In the rest, the histology remained unchanged. In the same report from Saudi Arabia, 80% of pretransplant patients who had HBeAg and antibodies to the delta particle progressed to chronic active hepatitis. Morales (1998) recommended that HbsAg-seropositive patients with severe liver disease should be advised against kidney transplantation as well as patients who are HBeAg or HBV DNA positive because such patients, who have active viral replication after transplantation, are at great risk of developing fulminant liver disease (Fairley *et al.*, 1991). There have been several reports of high mortality associated with hepatitis B surface antigenemia (Pirson *et al.*, 1977; Rao *et al.*, 1991). Morales (1998) reported a 64% 10-year patient survival compared with 80% among HbsAg-negative patients. The usual causes of death were liver failure and infection.

Preventive measures that should be instituted during dialysis include isolation of HBV patients and vaccination of all seronegative patients. Patients with chronic liver disease should be encouraged to remain on dialysis. The high-risk groups described above also should be considered in this category (Rao *et al.*, 1993). Other patients should be managed depending on liver histology and the evidence of viral replication. Patients who are HBV DNA or HBeAg positive and patients with severe chronic active hepatitis are at greatest risk of liver failure and should be excluded from renal transplantation (Morales, 1998). A *nonaggressive* immunosuppressive regimen should be employed in patients who undergo transplantation (Morales, 1998). When immunosuppression is withdrawn, it should be done slowly to prevent massive hepatic necrosis and concomitant liver failure, which have been reported during rapid withdrawal (Daar, 1994).

Other Viruses

Hepatitis E virus, which is spread by the fecal-oral route, is common in developing countries. Lack of hygiene and poor sanitation have made hepatitis E virus endemic in India, Bangladesh and Indonesia. Major outbreaks of the disease have been reported in Algeria, Ghana and Ethiopia (Robson et al., 1994). The disease caused by hepatitis E virus usually is benign, with fulminant hepatic failure being reported in only 0.5 to 3% of cases. Hepatitis E behaves in a similar fashion to hepatitis A in not progressing to chronic liver disease. It has not been identified as a problem in transplant or dialysis patients.

Hepatitis G virus (HGV) is the newest addition to the known members of the Flaviviridae family; it is detected in 1 to 2% of the general population. Hepatitis G virus can cause clinical hepatitis, but the extent to which it causes hepatocellular injury is uncertain. There is speculation that HGV causes little inflammation in the liver, and its association with chronic liver disease may reflect its parenteral transmissibility along with HBV and HCV (Charlton et al., 1998). A study in Hungarian children revealed a significantly higher incidence of HGV RNA positivity of those on dialysis and after transplantation. Of 27 patients on all forms of treatment for ESRD, 5 had HGV RNA, of whom 4 were from the group of 12 transplant recipients. In a control group of 40 children with urinary tract infection, only one was positive (Szabo et al., 1998). Another group reported a high prevalence of HGV RNA in pediatric transplant patients (Kudo et al., 1996). Immunosuppression may play a role in the high incidence and persistence of HGV infection (Szabo et al., 1997). Little is known currently about the epidemiology and clinical features of the disease. There is mounting evidence, however, that the virus is transmitted by blood and blood products (Kudo et al., 1996; Masuko et al., 1996). There are many unanswered questions about this virus and its pathogenicity.

GASTROINTESTINAL COMPLICATIONS

Poor socioeconomic conditions appear to contribute to the high gastrointestinal morbidity seen in posttransplant patients in developing countries. Over a period of 10 years, 166 of 265 (62.6%) renal allograft recipients in India developed gastrointestinal complications (Kathuria et al., 1995). This incidence is considerably higher than the incidence of 3 to 37% reported from developed countries (Benoit et al., 1993; Hadjivannakis et al., 1971; Kathuria et al., 1995; Moore and Hume, 1969). The main difference in the Indian series was the high incidence of acute diarrhea: 125 of 265 (47.2%) patients had 132 episodes. Of the 47 stool samples examined, bacteria were responsible for most (57.4%) of the episodes, followed by parasites (27.7%), fungi (8.5%) and viruses (2.1%). Most patients became ill in the second month after transplantation (Kathuria et al., 1995).

Esophageal candidiasis occurred in 19 of 265 (7%) patients. Predisposing factors included diabetes mellitus, triple immunosuppression and bone marrow suppression. Odynophagia was the commonest presenting symptom (74%) of esophageal candidiasis. Esophageal candidiasis was present on endoscopy in 4 of 19 patients who presented only with oral candidiasis. The patients were treated with oral nystatin with or without ketoconazole. Amphotericin B also was used in some patients. The overall mortality rate was 26%, and this increased to 100% in patients in whom esophageal candidiasis was part of disseminated disease. Besides being caused by candidiasis, esophagitis caused by reflux and CMV infection was documented.

Upper gastrointestinal bleeding is another serious complication, which occurred in 6% of the Indian cohort, with most (47%) of the bleeds occurring within 6 months. Most of the bleeds were due to gastric erosions. Patients did not receive prophylaxis unless there was preoperative evidence of disease. Patients were managed with blood transfusions, H₂-receptor blockers or omeprazole, with or without antacids. The mortality was 40% in this group of patients with upper gastrointestinal bleeding. Despite the additional costs, it appears to be advisable to maintain patients on routine prophylaxis against peptic ulcer disease in the early period posttransplantation to reduce the incidence of peptic ulcer disease and the risk of gastrointestinal bleeding (Troppman et al., 1995). H₂-receptor blockers and antacids should be used for the first 8 weeks when immunosuppression is at its most intense, although others advocate longer treatment (Reese et al., 1991).

Ischemic colitis and acute pancreatitis, although rare, had 100% and 60% mortality rates in this Indian series. Tuberculosis affecting the peritoneum and gut (3%) was not unexpected in a country where the disease is endemic. The presentation can be varied, and a high index of suspicion is required in posttransplant patients who have fevers and abdominal complaints, especially if this presentation is associated with an abnormal chest radiograph. Patients generally respond to standard antituberculous therapy, although the duration of therapy is controversial, with recommendations varying from 6 to 18 months (Higgins et al., 1991; Kathuria et al., 1995; Malhotra, 1994).

MALIGNANCIES

Kaposi's Sarcoma

Kaposi's sarcoma is the commonest malignancy in renal transplant patients in Saudi Arabia, Egypt and the nonwhite population of South Africa (Bakr et al., 1997; Margolius, 1996; Qunibi et al., 1988; see also Chapters 34 and 35). In Saudi Arabia, Kaposi's sarcoma accounts for 87% of all malignancies in transplant recipients. The incidence more than doubled after introduction of cyclosporine, and the disease occurs earlier than it did in the azathioprine era (Penn, 1999). The mean time to the development of Kaposi's sarcoma is 21 months, but it may occur 2.5 months posttransplantation. Kaposi's sarcoma is one of the earliest malignancies to develop after transplantation. The disease typically presents in the lower limbs, with painless reddish blue eruptions that may ulcerate. Histological examination shows typical spindle cells in the presence of vascular endothelial proliferation. Besides the skin, the lesions may also occur in the oropharynx and conjunctivae. Visceral involvement, especially of the lungs and gastrointestinal system, usually is a serious complication but may have a fair prognosis with appropriate treatment (Margolius, 1996). Evidence suggests that the development of Kaposi's sarcoma depends on immunosuppression and infection by human herpesvirus-8 (Alkan et al., 1997; Boshoff and Weiss, 1997). The virus has been detected in virtually all Kaposi's sarcoma tissue whether of endemic (African), epidemic (AIDS) or iatrogenic origin (Boshoff et al., 1995; Brooks et al., 1997).

The role of human herpesvirus-8 in the pathogenesis of Kaposi's sarcoma opens new possibilities for treatment in the future. Treatment presently consists of reduction of immunosuppression in patients with cutaneous involvement and complete withdrawal when visceral involvement is present (Montagnino *et al.*, 1994; Qunibi *et al.*, 1988). The reduction of immunosuppression results in clearing of human herpesvirus-8 from previously infected tissue (Moosa *et al.*, 1998). Withdrawal of immunosuppression usually results in graft loss, but reduction of immunosuppression may be achieved with successful maintenance of the graft. The success of this treatment varies, with 24 to 75% of patients undergoing partial or complete remission of Kaposi's sarcoma (Montagnino *et al.*, 1994; Qunibi *et al.*, 1988). Radiotherapy may be useful for treating localized lesions. Chemotherapy has been used for patients who have visceral disease and do not respond to withdrawal of immunosuppressive therapy. Antiviral drugs and a variety of cytotoxic agents have been used with varying success (Margolius, 1996). Patients who have been cured of Kaposi's sarcoma face an uncertain future. If grafts are rejected, they need to be maintained on dialysis; retransplantation and further immunosuppression should not be undertaken without careful consideration because the disease has recurred when immunosuppression was reintroduced (Al-Sulaiman *et al.*, 1992).

Posttransplantation Lymphoproliferative Disorder

Posttransplantation lymphoproliferative disorder is an uncommon B-cell malignancy that occurs in patients exposed to exogenous immunosuppression together with EBV infection. In one of the first communications from a developing country, Quintanilla-Martinez *et al.* (1998) reported the presence of this lesion in 8 (2%) of 390 renal allograft recipients in Mexico. Seven of the eight (88%) patients presented with gastrointestinal disease. The gut involvement is considerably higher than the 12 to 21% reported in large series from developed countries (Nalesnik, 1990; Penn, 1987). Epstein-Barr virus type A was shown in seven of eight patients. Epstein-Barr virus type A may contribute to the development of posttransplantation lymphoproliferative disorder by immortalizing and inducing autonomous B-cell proliferation (Frank *et al.*, 1995). Although 25% of cases had deletion of the *LMP-1* gene in EBV, the significance of this phenomenon in the development of posttransplantation lymphoproliferative disorder is uncertain. The prognosis in Egyptian patients who had gastrointestinal involvement was extremely poor, with five of seven succumbing to the disease (Bakr *et al.*, 1997).

Other Malignancies

In Egypt, Kaposi's sarcoma accounted for 50% of 22 malignancies developing in 950 patients (Bakr *et al.*, 1997). Bladder carcinoma comprised 14% of all malignancies and occurred only in patients with a history of urinary schistosomiasis. The patients were treated with radical surgery or intravesical bacille Calmette-Guérin. Of the three patients, two survived, although graft function was impaired. Other malignancies noted were lymphoma, nasopharyngeal carcinoma, basal cell carcinoma of the lip, hepatoma, colon carcinoma and malignant fibrous histiocytoma. Mortality of all patients with malignancies (including Kaposi's sarcoma) was 41%. They also noted a doubling of the incidence of carcinoma in patients on cyclosporine (1.4% *vs.* 2.7%) and a reduction in the interval between transplantation and the development of carcinoma (4.9 months on cyclosporine *vs.* 76 months on azathioprine). The pattern of malignancies in renal transplant populations in developing countries seems to differ from that reported in industrialized countries, with an excess of Kaposi's sarcoma and few skin and lip malignancies being reported.

Special Considerations in Transplantation
PREGNANCY AFTER RENAL TRANSPLANTATION

Correction of the uremic state by a functioning renal allograft often restores fertility in women of reproductive age, and 2 to 3% become pregnant in Western countries (Lindheimer and Katz, 1992; Sturgiss and Davison, 1992). Average fertility rates are higher in developing countries than industrialized countries (De Villa *et al.*, 1997). Saber *et al.* (1995) from Brazil reported a pregnancy rate of 14% in 136 renal allograft recipients of childbearing age, the Omani group reported a rate of 31% in 80 female patients (Al Hassani *et al.*, 1995) and Al-Khader (1999) from Saudi Arabia reported a rate of almost 50%. All reports suggest that with extra care, pregnancy can be undertaken successfully after renal transplantation (see Chapter 39).

Problems encountered by Saber *et al.* (1995) included hypertension in 67%, but this was controlled easily. Preeclampsia was rare. Infections, predominantly of the urinary tract, occurred in 86% of the pregnancies. No rejection episodes or graft loss was documented during the pregnancy or the immediate postpartum period; graft and patient survival were no different compared with controls. The incidence of obstetrical problems was high, however. Prematurity occurred in 67% of patients compared with 5% in the general population. The reason could be the high incidence of urinary tract infections and premature rupture of membranes. Obstetrical intervention for uncontrolled hypertension and fetal distress also could account for prematurity (Saber *et al.*, 1995). The incidence of cesarean sections (76%) (Saber *et al.*, 1995) and small-for-dates infants (64%) was increased (Al-Khader, 1999), but no congenital abnormalities were detected in any of the infants reported. The available information suggests that pregnancy after a successful renal transplant is safe if the patient has normal renal function and delays conception for 1 year posttransplantation. Careful management by a multidisciplinary group is essential (Saber *et al.*, 1995).

TRANSPLANTATION IN CHILDREN AND THE ELDERLY
Children

In contrast to developed countries, children form a much larger proportion of the population in developing countries (Al-Khader, 1999; see also Chapter 37). The incidence of ESRD of 7 per 1 million child population in these countries is similar to or slightly higher than that reported from developed countries (Al-Khader, 1999; Eke and Eke, 1994; Garcia *et al.*, 1992a, 1992b; Grunberg, 1996). The causes of ESRD in children are most commonly congenital abnormalities of the urinary tract (40%) and chronic glomerulonephritis (33%) (Al-Khader, 1999; Garcia *et al.*, 1992a, 1992b; Saieh, 1990). In Saudi Arabia, consanguineous marriages contribute to the high incidence of hereditary diseases in children (Al-Khader, 1999). In Nigeria, almost 50% of obstructive uropathy was due to meatal stenosis resulting from poorly performed circumcisions, representing an important preventable cause of renal failure (Eke and Eke, 1994). In societies with limited access to diagnostic facilities, renal disease in children may go undiagnosed, and the incidence may be underestimated. In developing countries, the meager resources are used generally for the care of adults (Grunberg, 1996; Saieh, 1990). Children are not only actively discriminated against, but also there are reports alleging that pediatric dialysis facilities have been taken over for adults. Poorly paid health care workers try to assist children who not only have to battle with a chronic illness, but also suffer further because they miss a great deal of schooling, lack independence and have to make frequent visits to the hospital. These problems contribute to feelings of poor self-worth, and the children and their families require psychological support (Saieh, 1990) if it is available.

Peritoneal dialysis is particularly suitable for children but is limited in developing countries because of socioeconomic and sanitary considerations (Grunberg, 1996; Grunberg and Verocay, 1987; Saieh, 1990). When intermittent peritoneal dialysis has been used in carefully selected patients, it has been successful, with high rates of rehabilitation (Saieh, 1990). Hemodialysis is used rarely in the treatment of uremic children. In good hands, however, children less than 12 years old can tolerate treatment with few complications and with a good chance of rehabilitation (Saieh, 1990).

A well-functioning renal allograft is the best treatment for a child with ESRD—perhaps even more so than in an adult. It offers the recipient the opportunity of a better quality of life, improved growth and psychomotor development as well as the reestablishment of social and psychological functioning. With the low incidence of cadaver donor transplantation in developing countries, living related donor transplantation is the main option for these children. In a study of 31 living related donor transplants in 27 children reported from Latin America, preemptive transplants were undertaken in 6. The mothers were donors in 66% and the fathers in 10% (Saieh, 1990). Data from the United Network for Organ Sharing (UNOS) show that children have a 20% greater chance of rejecting a kidney from the father than the mother (Cecka et al., 1997). The 2-year patient and graft survival were 68% (because no dialysis facilities were available to children whose grafts failed) (Saieh, 1990). One of the largest pediatric series from a developing country reported the outcome of primary living related donor transplants undertaken in 119 children in the years 1970–1990 in southern Brazil (Garcia et al., 1992a, 1992b). Graft survival was 70% at 1 year and 50% at 4 years. Ahmad et al. (1995) reported on the Iranian experience of renal transplantation in 26 pediatric patients. Four patients had not received maintenance dialysis before transplantation. Living related donors were used in 11 recipients, living unrelated donors were used in 11 recipients and cadaver donors were used in 4 recipients. Postoperative acute renal failure occurred in 12 patients, but further details are lacking. The 1-year graft survival was 86% in cases of living donor kidneys and 75% in cases of cadaver donor kidneys. The authors reported that few compliance problems were encountered because of parental devotion in donating organs and in the care of the patient.

Prevention of renal disease must be a priority in children (Saieh, 1990). The appropriate management of urinary tract infection in children can lead to the detection of vesicoureteric reflux and urological abnormalities, which are the commonest cause of chronic renal failure in children (Henning et al., 1988). Pediatric nephrologists in developing countries make a strong plea for the elimination of discriminatory practices against children (Saieh, 1990) and claim "the same rights for subjects who were living in the same country but with the unique difference of age and size" (Grunberg, 1996).

Elderly

The elderly constitute an increasingly greater proportion of the world population, a phenomenon well recognized in developed countries. It is estimated that in 2000, 229 million people aged 65 years or older are living in developing countries compared with 167 million in industrialized countries (Andrews, 1988; Mets, 1993; United Nations Organization,

1979). Experience in the United States indicates that the incidence of ESRD increases with age. Currently, ESRD is increasing most rapidly in persons greater than 65 years old at a rate of 5 to 8% per annum. Persons aged greater than 65 years constitute 48% of new patients in the USA developing ESRD (USRDS, 1999).

Industrialized countries such as the United Kingdom in the past have discriminated against persons greater than 55 years old (Berlyne, 1982; Rennie et al., 1985). In Sweden, only 4 of 10 patients greater than 70 years old received treatment (Kjellstrand, 1988). Among developing countries, a report from South Africa indicated that the number of patients greater than 60 years of age starting renal replacement therapy of any kind was 8% of all ESRD patients in 1994 (du Toit et al., 1994). In 1991, 15% of patients on renal replacement therapy in Tehran were greater than 50 years old (Rahbar et al., 1993), whereas in the same year patients greater than 65 years old comprised 26% of new patients starting hemodialysis in Uruguay, increased from 8% a decade earlier (Fernandez et al., 1995).

In a report from the Brazilian Transplant Registry, patients greater than 65 years old accounted for 0.7% of 1,563 transplants done (Sesso et al., 1990). This low figure is comparable to that reported from many industrialized countries (Marcias-Nunez and Cameron, 1992). The transplant rate varies greatly, but countries with well-developed renal replacement therapy programs, such as Germany and the Netherlands, transplant a relatively small number of patients aged greater than 55 years. The reason for the low incidence of transplantation in the elderly may be that the use of a scarce resource in someone whose life expectancy may be shorter than that of the graft may be considered to be wasteful (Marcias-Nunez and Cameron, 1992). Although controversial, available data suggest that cumulative patient and graft survival are comparable to that of younger patients (Sumrani et al., 1991), with a significantly lower incidence of acute rejection being reported in some studies (Hestin et al., 1994; Vela et al., 1994). In a report from Iran, the 1-year patient and graft survival were 88% and 76% in transplant recipients aged greater than 50 years compared with 97% and 89% patient and graft survival in transplant recipients aged less than 50 years (Rahbar et al., 1993).

In many cultures, the elderly are an integral part of an extended family, in which they are treated with respect and reverence. In this situation, the question arises whether organs procured from elderly family members may be used when no other suitable donors are available. Rizvi et al. (1998a) in Pakistan used kidneys from living donors aged up to 74 years. They found that the kidneys from the 56 donors aged greater than 50 years had a poorer survival rate compared with the 444 donors aged less than 50 years (Table 38–9). The 1-year and 5-year graft survival rates were 92% and 80% for donor age less than 50 years and 86% and 68% for donor age greater than 50 years. No comment was made

TABLE 38–9
SURVIVAL OF GRAFTS FROM ELDERLY DONORS

Country	Age Group (No. Patients)	Graft Survival % (At year indicated)		Reference
		Elderly	*Controls*	
India	>60 (27)	86 (1)	88	Kumar et al., 1994
Pakistan	>50 (56)	86 (1)	92	Rizvi et al., 1998
		68 (5)	80	
Greece	>60 (?)	84 (3)	87	Kostakis et al., 1997

on the number of rejection episodes or the reasons for the apparently poorer survival rates. A more favorable outcome was reported by Kumar *et al.* (1994) from India, who compared the results of 27 donors aged greater than 60 years with 25 donors aged less than 45 years. The 1-year graft survival rates were 86% and 88% in the elderly and younger donors, respectively. There was no difference in the incidence of acute tubular necrosis (Kumar *et al.*, 1994). These findings are consistent with those reported by Kostakis *et al.* (1997) in Greece and Sumrani *et al.* (1993) in New York. In Slovenia, living related donors were aged up to 79 years, including 50 parents and one grandparent (Kandus *et al.*, 1992). The mean age of the donors was 52 years, and the mean age of the recipients was 31 years. Parents were the largest source of living donors (77%) in Slovenia, compared, for example, with 8% in the Philippines (De Villa *et al.*, 1997). Although the outcome in recipients of older kidneys was not analyzed specifically, the overall patient and graft survival were 95% and 90% at 1 year, which is comparable to that reported from developed countries (Kandus *et al.*, 1992). In the face of a desperate shortage of organs and the fact that living donor transplantation is the only option for many patients in developing countries, there is no current evidence to suggest that the healthy elderly should be excluded from donating (Hestin *et al.*, 1994; Sumrani *et al.*, 1991; Vela *et al.*, 1994).

RACE AND ETHNICITY

Race and ethnicity have some bearing on the rates of ESRD, renal replacement therapy and outcome (see Chapter 39). In the United States, the point prevalence of ESRD was 4.5-fold higher in black Americans and 3.7-fold higher in Native Americans compared with their white counterparts (USRDS, 1999). Black patients have lower transplantation rates than their white counterparts, however (USRDS, 1998). Figures from the 1970s showed the less well educated, those with poor financial resources and racial and ethnic minorities are less likely to be listed for transplantation before starting on dialysis (Opelz *et al.*, 1977). The transplantation rate was 54% lower in black women aged 45 to 64 years and 60% lower in young black men aged 20 to 44 years compared with their white counterparts. The national average cadaver donor transplant rate in young men was 6.2 per 100 dialysis patient-years for black recipients compared with 14.4 per 100 dialysis patient-years for white recipients.

Early graft survival in black American patients has improved as a result of optimal immunosuppressive regimens, but long-term graft survival has remained significantly lower than in their white counterparts (Zeigler *et al.*, 1997). Reduction in the rate of acute rejection improved outcome in black American patients. Comparing equivalent immunosuppressive protocols for cadaver transplants, race alone was not a predictor of outcome. The poor outcome in black patients appears to be related to poor HLA matching and unfavorable socioeconomic status (Zeigler *et al.*, 1997). Poor HLA matching was an important predictor for patients of low socioeconomic standing with poor health coverage (Butkus *et al.*, 1992). Race may be a surrogate marker for low socioeconomic status, poor health coverage and perhaps other factors such as compliance.

Poor graft and patient survival have been documented in the Aboriginal populations of Australia (Disney, 1995; Morris, 1998). Treatment of ESRD in this population by dialysis and transplantation is difficult for social, cultural, geographic and economic reasons, and survival is worse than that observed in other Australian populations with ESRD.

Early experience with transplantation in South Africa revealed a significant difference in graft survival in black patients between living related donor and cadaver donor transplants at 5 years: 66% versus 28% (Modiba *et al.*, 1989). In a later report, the number of black patients transplanted increased from 12 to 32% of the total transplants in the period 1986–1994 (Kahn *et al.*, 1997). In this latter study, again, in black patients, a significant difference was observed in graft survival between living related donor and cadaver donor transplants at 3 years: 83% versus 43% (Kahn *et al.*, 1997). Overall, black patient survival was 82% and 65% at 1 year and 3 years, whereas graft survival was 67% and 47% at 1 year and 3 years. The cumulative graft survival for 761 cadaver donor renal transplants was not significantly different in black, white and mixed-race groups at 3 years. In black renal transplant recipients, the graft survival at 5 years was similar regardless of the race of the donor organ (black donors, 40%; white donors, 54% and mixed-race donors, 41%). An earlier South African study of 225 primary cadaver donor renal transplants compared 1-year graft survival in white and nonwhite patients in the precyclosporine and postcyclosporine eras (Moosa *et al.*, 1992). In the precyclosporine period, graft survival was 46% and 44% at 1 year in white and nonwhite patients. With cyclosporine use, graft survival was 68% and 71% at 1 year in white and nonwhite patients. Both studies reported no differences in graft survival because of race or socioeconomic status in South Africans; this is in contrast to observations for predictors of graft survival in black Americans.

Many transplant units in developed countries have a significant number of patients from developing countries. The impact of ethnicity and race of these immigrant communities on renal replacement therapy in their adopted countries is strikingly apparent (Ready, 1998; Ready *et al.*, 1992). Patients from South Asian immigrant communities are overrepresented on renal transplant waiting lists in the United Kingdom. They represent 25% of patients on the Birmingham Renal Failure Programme, disproportionately higher than their 14% ethnic representation in the region. The annual growth rate of the waiting list in Birmingham in the period 1990–1996 was 6.4%, but the rate was 24% for South Asian patients. An important contributing factor appears to be the lack of suitable cadaver donors as a result of ethnic distributions in ABO blood group and HLA tissue types. Blood group B occurs in 35% of South Asians but in only 8% of the United Kingdom donor pool and the general United Kingdom white population that largely makes up the donor pool. Many HLA-A, HLA-B and HLA-DR antigens occur frequently in South Asians but rarely in white donors. These ethnic differences limit the chance of good ABO and HLA matching in South Asian recipients for transplantation. A solution to these biological differences is to increase the rate of organ procurement within the South Asian community. A survey showed that culture and religion play a less prohibitive part in determining the level of cadaver organ procurement within this community than was suggested previously (Randhawa, 1998). The approach to resolving this impasse is to promote organ donation more persuasively within the Asian community.

A study from the Netherlands, which has a socialized health service providing uniform access to all, revealed no differences in overall graft survival between non-European and European recipients of primary cadaver renal transplants (Roodnat *et al.*, 1999). Analysis of the non-European recipients, predominantly first-generation immigrants from developing countries, revealed a significant racial influence on graft survival. Four categories of non-European races—Asian, Turkish, Arab and African—were analyzed. Compared with Asians (reference category), Arab recipients had the highest relative risk (RR = 4.0) followed by Africans

(RR = 2.3) for death or transplant failure. There was excellent graft survival in Asian recipients. Factors thought to explain these differences included genetic factors, practical communication difficulties and compliance issues; these were unrelated to socioeconomic circumstances because all race and ethnic groups had equal access to health care.

Asian patients in the United States have superior graft survival compared with other ethnic groups (Cecka *et al.*, 1992). Although there were no differences in patient survival, graft survival was 84% at 1 year in 1,004 Asian first cadaver transplant recipients compared with 79% at 1 year in 16,878 white transplant recipients. The graft survival differences were apparent within the first 3 months, and they did not differ significantly between Asians transplanted in Asia or the United States.

Race and ethnicity as determinants of transplant outcome probably reflect underlying genetic differences in immune response, drug metabolism or HLA matching. The differences also may reflect socioeconomic differences in populations and their compliance rates. Further studies are needed to clarify these issues.

IMPACT OF NONCOMPLIANCE

A great challenge for transplant teams is to ensure maximal survival of patients and grafts by obtaining maximal follow-up and drug compliance. Most reports on compliance issues in transplant patients are from developed countries. The adverse impact of noncompliance in renal transplant patients first was reported by Owens *et al.* in 1975. Clinical noncompliance was identified as behavior that resulted in rejection episodes (minor noncompliance) or graft loss (major noncompliance). In a prospective follow-up of 531 renal transplant patients in the United States, noncompliance was the third leading cause of graft failure after irreversible graft rejection in compliant patients and systemic infection (Didlake *et al.*, 1988). Irreversible rejection in compliant patients was the leading cause of graft failure in the first year. Rejection, both compliance and noncompliance related, occurred with equal frequency in the second posttransplant year, and in the third posttransplant year, noncompliance was responsible for 24% of graft losses. All graft losses that occurred in the fourth and subsequent years were related to noncompliance. Graft failure resulting from noncompliance was reported to occur in 24 to 78% of patients in their second or subsequent years (Didlake *et al.*, 1988; Kiley *et al.*, 1993). It is suggested that noncompliance be considered with any late acute rejection episode (De Geest *et al.*, 1995; Didlake *et al.*, 1988; Dunn *et al.*, 1990). Subclinical noncompliance with medication in the absence of graft rejection or graft loss is 22 to 65% (De Geest *et al.*, 1995; Siegal *et al.*, 1999; Sketris *et al.*, 1994).

Although no single factor appears to predominate, gender, age, race, marital status, employment, social support and duration posttransplant all seem to influence compliance (De Geest *et al.*, 1995; Didlake *et al.*, 1988; Kiley *et al.*, 1993; Siegal *et al.*, 1999; Sketris *et al.*, 1994). Male patients were frequently noncompliant with medication, whereas female patients were noncompliant with diet (Siegal *et al.*, 1999). Young (De Geest *et al.*, 1995; Didlake *et al.*, 1988), single or unmarried adults (De Geest *et al.*, 1995) tend to be more noncompliant, a profile that probably reflects poor social support. Black race by itself has not been shown to have an independent impact on the long-term graft survival (Butkus *et al.*, 1992); however, some reports indicate that black recipients tend to be relatively more noncompliant (De Geest *et al.*, 1995; Didlake *et al.*, 1988; Sketris *et al.*, 1994). Although psychiatric patients may have clear reasons for noncompliant behavior, this usually is iden-

tifiable before transplantation. Contrary to expectations, noncompliance also occurs in well-educated patients in gainful employment, with good health coverage (Siegal *et al.*, 1999). Reports have shown that compliance behavior is not modified by the source of donor kidney (Didlake *et al.*, 1988; Sketris *et al.*, 1994), but it has been speculated that one of the reasons for the excellent graft survival in spousal transplants may be better compliance.

The reasons given by patients in the developed world for their poorly compliant behavior appear to be more obvious than demographic characteristics would suggest: forgetfulness, cosmetic effects, cumbersome prescriptions, quantity of medication and inconvenient dosage schedules (Sketris *et al.*, 1994). In developing countries, a study of compliant behavior from South Africa assessed the perception, knowledge and attitude of pediatric transplant patient families (Meyers *et al.*, 1996). The noncompliant group more often missed their clinic visits despite similar distances traveled, forgot to take their medication and took more than the necessary medications. They also remembered fewer medication names and knew less about their disease, their graft and immunosuppression than the compliant patients. Despite the poor compliance behavior, ongoing education was considered to be important by 85% of the families.

A few studies from developing countries reported on the impact of noncompliance and related factors in transplant patients. A retrospective study of 77 pediatric patient families in South Africa reported that 22% were noncompliant with the prescribed medication, dosages or clinic visits (Meyers *et al.*, 1995). In pediatric patient families, social class correlated with noncompliance. Although 91% of black patient families were of the poorest social class, race corrected for social class failed to reach significance as a predictor of noncompliance. Noncompliance did not correlate with patient gender, parental marital status, family's distance from the transplant center or preemptive transplantation. Graft loss and mortality was significantly higher and the average graft survival was shorter in the noncompliant group. The 2.5-year graft survival in compliant patients was 71% compared with 42% in the noncompliant group. A study from Puerto Rico compared 12 compliant and noncompliant renal transplant patients (Rodriquez *et al.*, 1991); 8 noncompliant patients lost their grafts, and 2 died, whereas there were no events in the compliant group. Transport, financial, family and behavioral problems were significantly commoner in noncompliant patients. The risk factors for noncompliance in these patients were a lower socioeconomic status, psychosocial problems such as depression, family problems and consistent pretransplant noncompliant behavior. In a report from Taiwan, noncompliance was the third commonest cause of graft loss after graft rejection and infection; 82% of noncompliant patients lost their graft (Lee, 1992). In rural communities of developing countries, it is generally presumed that low socioeconomic status and access to health care may have a negative impact on graft survival. A South African study comparing urban and rural patients and their cadaver graft survival showed, however, that there was no significant difference in 5-year graft survival in the two groups (Pontin *et al.*, 1997). The study supported transplantation of rural patients and their referral back to peripheral centers for follow-up.

Economic and Social Considerations
COST AND ECONOMIC CONSIDERATIONS

Cost has significant implications on the future of renal transplantation in developing countries, where transplantation is constrained heavily by financial resources. There are striking differences in the provision of renal replacement therapy in different regions. The relationship between transplant activity and per capita income of countries in the developing world shows strikingly that cost and economic considerations have a major bearing on delivery (Fig. 38–5). A similar relationship was shown in Latin America (Martinez and Donkervoort, 1992).

The cost of renal replacement therapy depends on the importation of dialysis equipment, dialysate fluid, disposables and immunosuppressive therapy, specifically cyclosporine, for transplantation. Several reports confirm that transplantation is less expensive than dialysis in the developing world (Barsoum, 1992b; Chugh and Jha, 1995; Naqvi and Rizvi, 1995; Rizvi and Naqvi, 1995).

In Taiwan (Hu *et al.*, 1998), the average cost of transplantation in the first year was approximately 70% that of hemodialysis, decreasing to 38% in subsequent years. Another report (Were and McLigeyo, 1995) compared the annual maintenance cost between the different treatment modalities in Nigeria. Peritoneal dialysis was 70% the cost of hemodialysis, and a living related donor kidney transplant was 50% the cost of hemodialysis in the first year, decreasing to 10% in subsequent years. The distinct advantage of transplantation resulting from prolonged graft survival is improved quality of life (Lai *et al.*, 1992; Parfrey *et al.*, 1989; Park *et al.*, 1992a). Transplantation affords the patient more freedom with rehabilitation to gainful employment. The transplant becomes economically beneficial if the graft survives longer than the break-even cost of transplantation to maintenance dialysis. In Taiwan, a break-even cost saving was achieved after 1.5 years on cyclosporine-based regimens, whereas in the United States this was achieved after 4.6 years (Eggers, 1992). Donor selection that offers the best graft survival confers the greatest cost-effectiveness. Genetic and emotionally related living donors offer better graft survival and greater cost-effectiveness than cadaver donors do.

In the case of living donor transplantation, considerable costs can be saved if a patient receives a graft without prior dialysis. For patients with a living donor, early preemptive transplantation is an ideal choice for primary treatment of ESRD in developing countries. Avoiding hemodialysis not only saves costs, but also avoids the inconvenience and discomfort of dialysis and protects the patient from undue exposure to blood products (Evans, 1986; John *et al.*, 1998). A report from Pakistan on the impact of pretransplant hemodialysis revealed that dialysis for less than 3 months pretransplant conferred significantly better graft survival than treatment longer than 12 months (Rizvi *et al.*, 1998a). In Lucknow, India, a study of cost-containment strategies noted that decreasing the waiting period and the duration on dialysis before transplantation was a major cost-saving intervention

(Shrivastava *et al.*, 1998b). The report favored preemptive transplantation as a cost-effective approach for living related transplants. In a study from Vellore, South India, a group of 43 preemptive renal transplant recipients had significantly less morbidity than those transplanted from dialysis (John *et al.*, 1998). Before transplantation, these patients had higher hemoglobin and serum albumin levels and had considerably less HBV (5% *vs.* 16%) and tuberculosis (2% *vs.* 10%) infection. In the first year, rejection episodes were similar in the two groups. The incidence of hypertension and posttransplant diabetes was similar. As expected, there was considerable cost savings advantage, which amounted to $2,000 (U.S. dollars) per patient per year. A report from the Philippines compared the cost-effectiveness of preemptive renal transplantation with maintenance hemodialysis and peritoneal dialysis (Naidas, 1998). The probability of surviving 8 years was 78% with preemptive renal transplantation, 48% with hemodialysis and 36% with peritoneal dialysis. The reports of preemptive renal transplantation from developed countries confirm comparable (Katz *et al.*, 1991; Migliori *et al.*, 1999) or superior (Roake *et al.*, 1996) results. Because patients were highly motivated, they made considerable financial and emotional input, and noncompliance was rare (John *et al.*, 1998; Katz *et al.*, 1991).

Overall, renal transplantation is less expensive than dialysis in developing countries. The absence of government support and the high cost of imported medication make treatment affordable to only a few affluent individuals, however, including those with family support or those with assistance from employers (Chugh and Jha, 1995; Dalela *et al.*, 1992). Schemes to reduce costs include cyclosporine withdrawal at 3 to 12 months, maintaining patients on azathioprine and steroids (Morris *et al.*, 1982). Another strategy has been to combine cyclosporine with ketoconazole or diltiazem, both of which increase cyclosporine levels, allowing dose and cost reduction.

POSSIBLE NEGATIVE CONSEQUENCES OF TRANSPLANTATION

In some countries, the introduction of organ transplantation has had major negative consequences. From Egypt, Barsoum (1992b) described the situation in dire terms:

> During no other period in the history of medicine has any procedure created such social chaos as did renal transplantation in the Third World. The reason is simply the premature adoption of such a highly sophisticated therapy at an individual level rather than a national level. Health politicians are generally reluctant to face the innumerable religious, ethical, cultural, financial and technical issues entailed in a national transplant program. These issues would entail a national transplant program that must involve the use of cadaver organs.

FIGURE 38–5

Renal transplant activity and gross national product (GNP) per capita of selected countries. A clear relationship between these parameters is shown. (Transplant activity obtained from published data and GNP data from the World Bank [1997] *World Bank Atlas*).

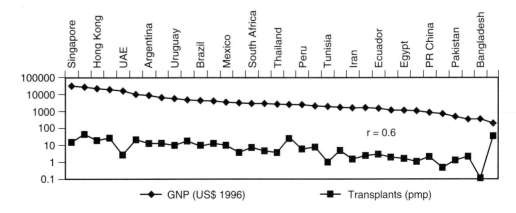

Although this is perhaps an uncommonly voiced view, transplantation can be a disruptive influence when introduced without due planning in poor countries. In many parts of the developing world, however, transplantation seems to be increasing, and regional transplant societies are growing.

INFLUENCING PUBLIC ATTITUDES

Whether in the Far East (Cheng, 1992), South America (Martinez and Donkervoort, 1992) or Africa (Brink and Pike, 1992; Pike *et al.*, 1992), the attitude of the public seems to support organ donation. Despite this supportive attitude, the number of cadaver donors has failed to increase significantly. Al-Khader (1999) reported that family consent for organ procurement was obtained in only 34% of cases in Saudi Arabia, one of the developing countries most successful in the introduction of cadaveric donation. It has been suggested that better use of the media is required to highlight the plight faced by desperate patients and the fact that considerable foreign exchange may be saved if local expertise is nurtured and local facilities are improved (Naqvi *et al.*, 1992). This suggestion was confirmed in a report from Saudi Arabia in which the National Kidney Foundation used the media to educate the public on organ donation. Using electronic and print media, the National Kidney Foundation increased public awareness of organ donation, from virtually nil to 82% of those surveyed over a 2-year period (Aswad *et al.*, 1992). The media can be a double-edged sword, however, as experienced in the United States. *Saturation campaigns* raised public awareness on the need for organ donation but also fostered a crucial misunderstanding of the complexity of the field, raising unrealistic expectations in the public mind (Rapaport *et al.*, 1990). In poorer countries, where the bulk of the population may have limited access to the media and where adult illiteracy rates are high, alternative methods of influencing public opinion on transplantation and organ donation need to be considered.

Transplant coordination is still in its infancy in developing countries. With an understanding of local sociocultural beliefs and a sensitivity to the needs and concerns of families, transplant coordinators could form a vital link between the community and the transplant team (De Villa *et al.*, 1997; Kyriakides *et al.*, 1989). With the growth of cadaver donor programs, the transplant coordinator will play a growing role in the identification and care of potential donors and their families. De Villa and coworkers, from the Philippines, stressed the importance of government support for organ procurement efforts and the enactment of national laws and policies that facilitate transplantation (De Villa *et al.*, 1997).

SOCIOCULTURAL ISSUES

As the technical problems of organ transplantation have been resolved by experience, research and serendipity, sociocultural issues are beginning to gain attention. Religion plays an important role in organ transplantation (Daar, 1994; Gabr, 1999). Daar and Marshall (1998) noted how certain social and cultural influences affect transplant-related behavior.

The uneducated patient who develops renal failure may have no equivalent terminology in his or her vernacular to describe the concept. The patient may not associate kidney function with urine formation, which may be considered a bladder function. Kidney failure may be considered the consequence of a variety of misdemeanors. Gold and colleagues found that some uremic patients with edema consider this to be due to sexual intercourse with a mourning widow or because the patients offended ancestral sensibilities in another fashion (Gold *et al.*, 1978). Black patients consult

their traditional healers first and are subjected to certain rituals and are prescribed herbs that frequently aggravate the situation (Gold *et al.*, 1978). The bewildered patient, who is often unsophisticated, poorly educated and has little understanding of biology, seeks a second opinion from a Western-trained physician when he or she feels that traditional medicine has failed. The patient is faced with the daunting task of resolving the dichotomous assessment of the traditional healer, who previously has served the patient faithfully, and that of the modern physician, whose medicine is new to the patient. The natural history of kidney disease given by the physician may not be understood, in contrast to that given by the traditional healer (Aluwihare and Daar, 2000).

REFERENCES

Abomelha, M. S. (1996). Renal failure and transplantation activity in the Arab World. Arab Society of Nephrology and Renal Transplantation. *Nephrol. Dial. Transplant.* **11**, 28.
Abouna, G. M. (1993). Negative impact of trading in human organs on the development of transplantation in the Middle East. *Transplant. Proc.* **25**, 2310.
Abu-Aisha, H. and Paul, T. T. (1994). CAPD: is it a viable mode of RRP in Saudi Arabia? *Saudi J. Kidney Dis. Transplant.* **5**, 154.
Abuelo, J. G. (1990). Renal failure caused by chemicals, foods, plants, animal venoms, and misuse of drugs: an overview. *Arch. Intern. Med.* **150**, 505.
Aghanashinikar, P. N., Daar, A. S., Marhuby, H., *et al.* (1993). Omani experience with a heterogeneous group of kidney transplant recipients over a 10-year period. *Transplant. Proc.* **25**, 2359.
Ahmad, E., Malek Hossieni, S. A., Nekatzgoo, N., *et al.* (1995b). A report of 26 cases of renal transplantation in children. *Transplant. Proc.* **27**, 2570.
Ahmad, E., Malek Hosseini, S. A., Salahi, H., Javid, R., Ghahramani, N. and Nezakatgoo, N. (1995a). Experience with 300 renal transplants in Shiraz, Iran. *Transplant. Proc.* **27**, 2767.
Akpolat, T. and Ozturk, M. (1998). Commerce in renal transplantation. *Nephrol. Dial. Transplant.* **30**, 710.
Al Arrayed, A. (1998). Renal replacement in Bahrain. *Saudi J. Kidney Dis. Transplant.* **9**, 457.
Albitar, S., Bourgeon, B., Genin, R., *et al.* (1998). Epidemiology of ESRD in Reunion Island. *Nephrol. Dial. Transplant.* **13**, 1143.
Al Hassani, M. K., Sharma, U., Mohsin, P., Al Maiman, Y., Nanda Kumar, M. and Daar, A. S. (1995). Pregnancy in renal transplantation recipients: outcome and complications in 44 pregnancies. *Transplant. Proc.* **27**, 2585.
Alkan, S., Karcher, D. S., Ortiz, A., Khalil, S., Akhtar, M. and Ali, M. A. (1997). Human herpesvirus-8/Kaposi's sarcoma–associated herpesvirus in organ transplant patients with immunosuppression. *Br. J. Haematol.* **96**, 412.
Al-Khader, A. A. (1999). Cadaveric renal transplantation in the Kingdom of Saudi Arabia. *Nephrol. Dial. Transplant.* **14**, 846.
Alshaibani, K., Raza, S., Alfurayh, O., *et al.* (1998). The kidney transplant program at King Faisal Specialist Hospital and Research Center: results of the last ten years. *Transplant. Proc.* **30**, 3103.
Al-Sulaiman, M. H., Dhar, J. M., Al-Hasani, M. K., Haleem, A. and Al-Khader, A. A. (1990). Tuberculous interstitial nephritis after kidney transplantation in Saudi Arabia. *Transplantation* **50**, 162.
Al-Sulaiman, M. H., Monsu, D. H., Dhar, J. M., *et al.* (1992). Does regressed posttransplant Kaposi's sarcoma recur following reintroduction of immunosuppression? *Am. J. Nephrol.* **12**, 384.
Aluwihare, A. P. R. and Daar, A. S. (2000). Surgery of advanced disease and late presentation. In *Oxford Texbook of Surgery*, 2nd ed., (P. J. Morris and W. C. Wood, eds.), Oxford University Press, New York and Oxford.
Alzaid, A. A., Sobkhi, S. and De Silva, V. (1994). Prevalence of microalbuminuria in Saudi Arabians with non-insulin dependent diabetes mellitus: a clinic based study. *Diabetes Res. Clin. Pract.* **26**, 115.
Andrews, G. R. (1988). Health and the ageing population. Ciba Foundation Symposium. J. Wiley, Chichester.
Anonymous. (1999a). Healthy people 2010 objectives: chronic kidney disease. Draft chapter. http://www.niddk.nih.gov/federal/kuh-dic/kidsub/2010.htm. Accessed 5 May 1999.

Anonymous. (1999b). The champagne glass of world poverty. *B. M. J.* **318**, ii.

Anthony, C. (1972). Disseminated toxoplasmosis in a liver transplant patient. *J. Am. Med. Womens Assoc.* **27**, 601.

Arije, A., Akinlade, K. S., Kadiri, S. and Akinkugbe, O. O. (1995a). The problems of peritoneal dialysis in the management of chronic uraemia in Nigeria. *Trop. Geogr. Med.* **47**, 74.

Arije, A., Kadiri, S., Akinkugbe, O. O. and Osobamiro, O. (1995b). Hemodialysis in Ibadan: a preliminary report on the first 100 dialyses. *Afr. J. Med. Sci.* **24**, 255.

Assounga, A. G. (1999). Management of renal failure in Central Africa in 1997. *Kidney Int.* **55**, 2121.

Aswad, S., Souqiyyeh, M. Z. and Huraib, S. (1992). The role of the media in cadaver transplantation in a developing country. *Transplant. Proc.* **24**, 2049.

Ayash, Z. (1997). Renal replacement therapy in Syria. *Saudi J. Kidney Dis. Transplant.* **8**, 436.

Bakr, M. A., Sobh, M., el Agroudy, A., *et al.* (1997). Study of malignancy among Egyptian kidney transplant recipients. *Transplant. Proc.* **29**, 3067.

Balasubramanian, V., Wieghaus, E. H., Taylor, B. T., *et al.* (1994). Pathogenesis of tuberculosis: pathway to apical localisation. *Tubercle Lung Dis.* **75**, 168.

Barrou, B., Bitker, M. O., Boyer, C., Sylla, C. and Chatelain, C. (1997). Results of renal transplantation in patients with *Schistosoma* infection. *J. Urol.* **157**, 1232.

Barry, J. M., Hefty, T., Fischer, S. M. and Norman, D. J. (1985). Donor specific blood transfusions and successful spousal kidney transplantation. *J. Urol.* **133**, 1024.

Barsoum, R. S. (1992a). Schistosomiasis. *In Oxford Textbook of Clinical Nephrology*, (J. S. Cameron, A. M. Davison, J. P. Grunfeld, D. Kerr and E. Ritz, eds.), p. 1729, Oxford University Press, Oxford.

Barsoum, R. S. (1992b). The Egyptian transplant experience. *Transplant. Proc.* **24**, 2417.

Barsoum, R. S. (1993). Schistosomal glomerulopathy. *Kidney Int.* **44**, 1.

Barsoum, R. S. (1994). Renal transplantation in a developing country. *Afr. J. Health Sci.* **1**, 30.

Barsoum, R. S. (1998). Haemodialysis: cost-conscious end-stage renal failure management. *Nephrology* **4**, S96.

Basinda, S. L., Maro, E. E., McLarty, D. G., Young, A. E. and Wing, A. J. (1988). Ten Tanzanian transplants: problems and perspectives. *Postgrad. Med. J.* **64**, 778.

Behrnes, R. H. and Curtis, C. F. (1993). Malaria in travellers: epidemiology and prevention. *B. M. J.* **49**, 363.

Ben Abdallah, T., El Younsi, F., Ben Hamida, F., *et al.* (1997). Results of 144 consecutive renal transplants from living related donors. *Transplant. Proc.* **29**, 3071.

Benoit, G., Moukarzel, M. and Verdelli, G. (1993). Gastrointestinal complications in renal transplantation. *Transpl. Int.* **6**, 45.

Berger, J. (1969). IgA deposits in renal disease. *Transplant. Proc.* **1**, 939.

Berger, J. (1988). Recurrence of IgA nephropathy in renal allografts. *Am. J. Kidney Dis.* **12**, 371.

Berlyne, G. M. (1982). Over 50 and uraemic = death. *Nephron* **31**, 190.

Berthoux, F. (1995). Hepatitis C virus infection and disease in renal transplantation. *Nephron* **71**, 386.

Bhandari, S. and Turney, J. H. (1996). Survivors of acute renal failure who do not recover renal function. *Q. J. M.* **89**, 415.

Bhimma, R., Coovadia, H. M. and Adhikari, M. (1997). Nephrotic syndrome in South African children: changing perspectives over 20 years. *Pediatr. Nephrol.* **11**, 429.

Bonomini, V., Stefoni, S. and Vangelista, A. (1984). Long-term patient and renal prognosis in acute renal failure. *Nephron* **36**, 172.

Borch-Johnsen, K., Nørgaard, K. and Hommel, E. (1992). Is diabetic nephropathy an inherited complication? *Kidney Int.* **41**, 719.

Bordes-Aznar, J., Pena, J. C., Herrera-Accosta, J., *et al.* (1992). Twenty-four-year experience in kidney transplantation at one single institution in Mexico City. *Transplant. Proc.* **24**, 1794.

Boshoff, C. and Weiss, R. A. (1997). Aetiology of Kaposi's sarcoma: current understanding and implications for therapy. *Mol. Med. Today* **3**, 488.

Boshoff, C., Whitby, D., Hatzioannou, T., *et al.* (1995). Kaposi's sarcoma associated herpesvirus in HIV-negative Kaposi's sarcoma. *Lancet* **345**, 1043.

Bourquia, A. (1999). Renal replacement therapy in Morocco. *Saudi J. Kidney Dis. Transplant.* **10**, 66.

Breyer, J. (1998). Diabetic nephropathy. *In Primer on Kidney Diseases*, 2nd ed., (A. Greenberg, A. K. Cheung, T. M. Coffman, R. J. Falk and J. C. Jennette, eds.), p. 215, Academic Press, San Diego.

Brink, J. and Pike, R. (1992). Transplantation in developing countries. *S. Afr. Med. J.* **82**, 149.

Brooks, L. A., Wilson, A. J. and Crook, T. (1997). Kaposi's sarcoma-associated herpesvirus (KSHV)/human herpesvirus 8 (HHV8)—a new human tumour virus. *J. Pathol.* **182**, 262.

Broumand, B. (1997). Living donors: the Iran experience. *Nephrol. Dial. Transplant.* **12**, 1830.

Brown, K. G. E., Abrahams, C. and Meyers, A. M. (1977). The nephrotic syndrome in Malawian Blacks. *S. Afr. Med. J.* **52**, 275.

Butkus, D. E., Meydrech, E. F. and Raju, S. S. (1992). Racial differences in the survival of cadaveric renal allografts: overriding effects of HLA matching and socio-economic factors. *N. Engl. J. Med.* **327**, 840.

Cameron, J. S. (1994). Recurrent renal disease after renal transplantation. *Curr. Opin. Nephrol. Hypertens.* **3**, 602.

Cameron, J. S. and Turner, D. R. (1977). Recurrent glomerulonephritis in allografted kidneys. *Clin. Nephrol.* **7**, 47.

Canafax, D. M., Graves, N. M., Hilligoss, D. M., *et al.* (1991). Increased cyclosporine levels as a result of simultaneous fluconazole and cyclosporine therapy in renal transaplant recipients: a double-blind, randomized pharmacokinetic and safety study. *Transplant. Proc.* **23**, 1041.

Cantarovich, F., Vazquez, M., Garcia, W. D., Abbud, F. M., Herrera, C. and Villegas, H. A. (1992). Special infections in organ transplantation in South America. *Transplant. Proc.* **24**, 1902.

Carbone, K. M., Pennington, L. R., Gimenez, L. I., Burrow, C. R. and Watson, A. J. (1985). Mucormycosis in renal transplant patients: a report of two cases and review of the lierature. *Q. J. M.* **224**, 825.

Cecka, J. M., Gjerston, D. and Terasaki, P. I. (1992). Superior renal allograft survival among Asian recipients. *Transplant. Proc.* **24**, 1431.

Cecka, J. M., Gjertson, D. W. and Terasaki, P. I. (1997). Pediatric renal transplantation: an overview of the UNOS data. United Network for Organ Sharing. *Pediatr. Transplant.* **1**, 55.

Chaballout, A., Said, R., Alboghdadly, S., Huraib, S. and Selim, H. (1995). Living-related, cadaveric and living unrelated donor kidney transplants: a comparison study at the King Fahad Hospital, Riyadh. *Transplant. Proc.* **27**, 2775.

Charlton, M. R., Brandwagen, D, Wiesner, R. H., *et al.* (1998). Hepatitis G virus infection in patients transplanted for cryptogenic cirrhosis. *Transplantation* **65**, 73.

Cheng, I. K. P. (1992). Special issues related to transplantation in Hong Kong. *Transplant. Proc.* **24**, 2423.

Cheng, I. K. P., Lai, K. N., Au, T. C., Chan, G. P., Poon, G. P. and Chan, Y. T. (1991). Comparisons of the mortality and morbidity rates between proper and unconventional renal transplantation using organs from executed prisoners. *Transplant. Proc.* **23**, 2533.

Chevalier, C., Busson, M., Hors, J. and Foulon, G. (1991). Medical care of end-stage renal disease in 52 countries: evolution since 1975 and potential activity for the next 5 years. *Transplant. Proc.* **23**, 2529.

Chugh, K. S. and Jha, V. (1995). Differences in the care of ESRD patients worldwide: required resources and future outlook. *Kidney Int.* **50(Suppl.)**, S7.

Chugh, K. S. and Jha, V. (1996). Commerce in transplantation in Third World countries. *Kidney Int.* **49**, 1181.

Chugh, K. S., Jha, V., Sakhuja, V. and Joshi, K. (1994). Acute renal cortical necrosis—a study of 113 patients. *Ren. Fail.* **16**, 37.

Chugh, K. S., Kumar, R., Sakhuja, V., Pereira, B. J. and Gupta, A. (1989). Nephropathy in type 2 diabetes mellitus in Third World countries—Chandigarh study. *Int. J. Artif. Organs* **12**, 299.

Chugh, K. S. and Sakhuja, V. (1990). Glomerular diseases in the tropics. *Am. J. Nephrol.* **10**, 437.

Chugh, K. S., Sakhuja, V., Jain, S., *et al.* (1992). Fungal infections in renal allograft recipients. *Transplant. Proc.* **24**, 1940.

Chugh, K. S., Sakhuja, V., Jain, S., *et al.* (1993). High mortality in systemic fungal infections following renal transplantation in third-world countries. *Nephrol. Dial. Transplant.* **8**, 168.

Chugh, K. S., Sakhuja, V., Malhotra, H. S. and Pereira, B. J. G. (1989). Changing trends in acute renal failure in third world countries. *Q. J. M.* **272**, 1117.

Cohen, A. H. and Nast, C. C. (1988). HIV-associated nephropathy: a unique glomerular, tubular and interstitial lesion. *Mod. Pathol.* **1**, 87.

Cook, C. C. (1991). Immunosuppression and *Mycobacterial* sp. infection. *Q. J. M.* **78**, 97.

Coovadia, H. M., Adhikari, M. and Morel-Maroger, L. (1979). Clinicopathological features of the nephrotic syndrome in South African children. *Q. J. M.* **49**, 77.

Costa, J. M. N., Meyers, A. M. and Botha, J. R. (1999). Mycobacterial infections in recipients of kidney allografts: a seventeen year experience. *Acta Med. Port.* **1**, 51.

Coutts, I. I., Jegarajah, S. and Stark, J. E. (1979). Tuberculosis in renal transplant patients. *Br. J. Dis. Chest* **74**, 141.

Cuhadaroglu, S., Tokyay, R., Velidedeoglu, E. and Haberal, M. (1992). The incidence of cytomegalovirus infection in kidney recipients. *Transplant. Proc.* **24**, 1924.

Daar, A. S. (1988). Renal transpantation in developing countries. *In Kidney Transplantation*, 3rd ed., (P. J. Morris, ed.), p. 709, W.B. Saunders, Philadelphia.

Daar, A. S. (1989). Ethical issues—a Middle East perspective. *Transplant. Proc.* **21**, 1402.

Daar, A. S. (1991a). Organ donation—world experience: the Middle East. *Transplant. Proc.* **23**, 2505.

Daar, A. S. (1991b). The case for using living non-related donors to alleviate the world wide shortage of cadaver kidneys for transplantation. *Ann. Acad. Med. Singapore* **20**, 443.

Daar, A. S. (1994). Transplantation in developing countries. *In Kidney Transplantation*, 4th ed., (P. J. Morris, ed.), p. 478, W.B. Saunders, Philadelphia.

Daar, A. S. (1997a). An emerging transplant force—developing countries: Middle East and the Indian subcontinent. *Transplant. Proc.* **29**, 1577.

Daar, A. S. (1997b). The response to the challenge of organ shortage in the Middle East region: a summary. *Transplant. Proc.* **29**, 3215.

Daar, A. S. (1997c). A survey of religious attitudes towards donation and transplantation. *In Procurement and Preservation and Allocation of Vascularized Organs*. (G. M. Collins, J. M. Dubernard, W. Land and G. G. Persijn, eds.), pp. 333–338, Kluwer Academic Publishers, Dordecht.

Daar, A. S. (1998a). Paid organ donation: the Grey Basket concept. *J. Medical Ethics.* 1998 Dec; 24(6):365–8.

Daar, A. S. (1998b). An overview of transplantation issues in the Middle East. *Transplant. Proc.* **30**, 3638.

Daar, A. S., Land, W., Yahya, T. M., Schneewind, K., Gutman, T. and Jakobsen, A. (1997). Living-donor renal transplantation: evidence-based justification for an ethical option. *Transpl. Rev.* **11**, 95.

Daar, A. S. and Marshall, P. (1998). Culture and psychology in organ transplantation. *World Health Forum* **19**, 124.

D'Agati, V. and Appel, G. B. (1997). HIV infection and the kidney. *J. Am. Soc. Nephrol.* **8**, 138.

Dalela, D., Bhandari, M., Kumar, A., Kher, V. and Sharma, R. K. (1992). Creation of low-cost model of renal transplantation suitable for developing countries. *Transplant. Proc.* **24**, 2129.

D'Amico, G. (1987). The commonest glomerulonephritis in the world: IgA nephropathy. *Q. J. M.* **64**, 709.

Date, A., Raghavan, R., John, T. J., Richard, J., Kirubakaran, M. G. and Shell, T. (1987). Renal disease in adult Indians: a clinicopathological study. *Q. J. M.* **64**, 729.

Davis, C. L. (1990). The prevention of cytomegalovirus disease in renal transplantation. *Am. J. Kidney Dis.* **16**, 175.

Dean, M. (1991). Is your treatment economic, effective, efficient? *Lancet* **337**, 480.

De Geest, S., Borgermans, L., Gemoets, H., *et al.* (1995). Incidence, determinants and consequence of sub-clinical non-compliance with immunosuppressive therapy in renal transplant recipients. *Transplantation* **59**, 340.

De Villa, V., Alonzo, H., Tejada, F., *et al.* (1997). Characterization of kidney allograft donation in the Philippines. *Transplant. Proc.* **29**, 1584.

Dhar, J. M., Al-Khader, A. A., Al-Sulaiman, M. H. and Al-Hasani, M. K. (1991). The significance and implications of hepatitis B infection in renal tranplant recipients. *Transplant. Proc.* **23**, 1785.

Didlake, R. H., Dreyfus, K., Kerman, R. H., Van Buren, C. T. and Kahan, B. D. (1988). Patient non-compliance: a major cause of late graft failure in cyclosporine-treated renal transplants. *Transplant. Proc.* **20**, 63.

Disney, A. (1995). Demographic and survival of patients receiving renal replacement therapy for chronic renal failure in Australia and New Zealand: report on dialysis and rernal transplantation treatment from the Australia and New Zealand dialysis and transplant registry. *Am. J. Kidney Dis.* **25**, 165.

Divakar, D., Thiagarajan, C. M. and Reddy, K. C. (1998). Ethical aspects of renal transplantation in India. *Transplant. Proc.* **30**, 3626.

Donnelly, P., Oman, P., Henderson, R. and Opelz, G. (1996). Living donor kidney transplantation in pre-dialysis patients: experience of marginal donors in Europe and the United States. *Transplant. Proc.* **28**, 3566.

Dunn, J., Golden, D., Van Buren, C. T., Lewis, R. M., Lawen, J. and Kahan, B. (1990). Causes of graft loss beyond two years in the cyclosporine era. *Transplantation* **49**, 349.

Durrheim, D. N., Braack, L. E., Waner, S. and Gammon, S. (1998). Risk of malaria in visitors to the Kruger National Park, South Africa. *J. Travel Med.* **5**, 173.

du Toit, E. D., Pascoe, M., MacGregor, K. and Thompson, P. D., SADTR. (1994). Combined report on maintenance dialysis and transplantation in the Republic of South Africa. Cape Town, South Africa.

Edelstein, C. L., Jacobs, J. C. and Moosa, M. R. (1995). Pulmonary complications in 110 consecutive renal transplant recipients. *S. Afr. Med. J.* **85**, 160.

Eggers, P. (1992). Comparison and treatment cost between dialysis and transplantation. *Semin. Nephrol.* **12**, 284.

Eiam-Ong, S. and Sitprija, V. (1998). Falciparum malaria and the kidney: a model of inflammation. *Am. J. Kidney Dis.* **32**, 375.

Eke, F. U. and Eke, N. N. (1994). Renal disorders in children. *Pediatr. Nephrol.* **8**, 383.

El Matri, A., Ben Abdallah, T., Ben Maiz, H., *et al.* (1993). Organ transplantation in Tunisia. *Transplant. Proc.* **25**, 2350.

Erek, E. (1999). Nephrology, dialysis and transplantation in Turkey. *Nephrol. Dial. Transplant.* **14**, 851.

Erken, U., Erken, E., Tansug, Z. and Turkyilmaz, R. (1992). Triple-drug regimen for first kidney transplants in developing countries. *Transplant. Proc.* **24**, 1843.

Evans, R. (1986). Cost-effectiveness analysis of transplantation. *Surg. Clin. North Am.* **66**, 603.

Fabre, J., Balant, L. P., Dayer, P. G., Fox, H. W. and Vernet, A. T. (1982). The kidney in maturity onset diabetes mellitus: a clinical study of 510 patients. *Kidney Int.* **21**, 730.

Fairley, C. K., Mijch, A., Gust, I. D., Nichilson, S., Dimitrakakis, M. and Lucas, C. R. (1991). The increased risk of fatal liver disease in renal transplant patients who are hepatitis B antigen and/or HBV DNA positive. *Transplantation* **52**, 497.

Fenton, S., Desmeules, M., Copleston, P., *et al.* (1995). Renal replacement therapy in Canada. *Am. J. Kidney Dis.* **25**, 134.

Fernandez, J. M., Schwedt, E., Ambrosoni, P., Gonzalez, F. and Mazzuchi, N. (1995). Eleven years of chronic hemodialysis in Uruguay: mortality time course. *Kidney Int.* **47**, 1721.

Fornainron, S., Pol, S., Legendre, C. H., *et al.* (1996). The long-term virologic and pathologic impact of renal transplantation on chronic hepatitis B virus infection. *Transplantation* **62**, 297.

Frank, D., Cesarman, E., Liu, Y., Michler, R. and Knowles, D. (1995). Post-transplant lymphoproliferative disorders frequently contain type A and not type B Epstein-Barr virus. *Blood* **85**, 1396.

Friedlander, M. A. and Hricik, D. E. (1997). Optimizing end-stage renal disease therapy for the patient with diabetes mellitus. *Semin. Nephrol.* **17**, 331.

Friedman, E. A. (1989). Race and diabetic nephropathy. *Transplant. Proc.* **19**, 77.

Gabr, M. (1999). Organ transplantation in developing countries. *World Health Forum* **19**, 120.

Gallis, H. A., Berman, R. A., Cate, T. R., Hamilton, J. D., Gunnells, J. C. and Stickels, D. L. (1975). Fungal infections follwing renal transplantation. *Arch. Intern. Med.* **23**, 1517.

Garcia, C. D., Goldani, J. C. and Garcia, V. D. (1992a). Twenty years of pediatric renal replacement therapy in the state of Rio Grande do Sul, Brazil. *Transplant. Proc.* **24**, 1804.

Garcia, C. D., Goldani, J. C. and Garcia, V. D. (1992b). Pediatric dialysis in the state of Rio Grande do Sul, Brazil. *Pediatr. Nephrol.* **6**, 74.

Geerling, W., Tufveson, G., Ehrich, J. H. H., *et al.* (1994). Report on the management of renal faillure in Europe, XXIII. *Nephrol. Dial. Transplant.* **9**, 6.

Gilbert, R. D. and Wiggelinkhuizen, J. (1994). The clinical course of hepatitis B virus-associated nephropathy. *Pediatr. Nephrol.* **8**, 11.

Glassock, R. J., Adler, S. G., Ward, H. J. and Cohen, A. H. (1991). Primary glomerular disease. *In The Kidney,* 4th ed. (B. M. Brenner and F. C. Rector, eds.), p. 1182, W.B. Saunders, Philadelphia.

Goffin, E., Pirson, Y. and Van Ypersele de Strihou, C. (1995). Implications of chronic hepatitis B or hepatitis C infection for renal transplant candidates. *Nephrol. Dial. Transplant.* **10**, 88.

Gold, C. H. (1980). Acute renal failure from herbal and patent remedies in blacks. *Clin. Nephrol.* **14**, 134.

Gold, C. H., Mokone, S. M. and Mongangane, H. (1978). The impact of renal failure on the South African black and his attitude towards haemodialysis. *S. Afr. Med. J.* **53**, 755.

Goldani, J. C., Bianchini, A. C., Mattos, A. and Garcia, V. D. (1991). Renal transplantation in the state of Rio Grande do Sul, Brazil. *Transplant. Proc.* **23**, 2541.

Goncalves, A. R. P., Caetano, M. A., Paula, F. J., Lanhez, L. E., Saldanha, L. B. and Sagga, E. (1992). Tuberculous interstitial granulomatous nephritis (TB-IGN) in renal transplants (Tx): report of 3 cases. *Transplant. Proc.* **24**, 1911.

Goral, S. and Helderman, J. H. (1998). Hepatitis C and renal transplantation: the controversy continues. *Kidney Int.* **53**, 1419.

Grunberg, J. (1996). The challenge of care of children with renal disease in developing countries: a Latin American outlook. *Indian Pediatr.* **33**, 91.

Grunberg, J. and Verocay, M. C. (1987). Pediatric CAPD in developing countries. *In Chronic Ambulatory Peritoneal Dialysis (CAPD) and Chronic Cyclic Peritoneal Dialysis (CCPD) in Children,* (R. N. Fine, ed.), p. 21, Martinus Nijhoff, Boston.

Gueco, I., Saniel, M., Mendoza, M., Alano, F. and Ona, E. (1989). Tropical infections after renal transplantation. *Transplant. Proc.* **21**, 2105.

Haberal, M., Bilgin, N., Arslan, G., Buyukpamukcu, N., Karamehmetoglu, M. and Telatar, H. (1998). Twenty-two years of experience in transplantation. *Transplant. Proc.* **30**, 683.

Haberal, M., Demirag, A., Cohen, B., *et al.* (1995a). Cadaver kidney transplantation in Turkey. *Transplant. Proc.* **27**, 2768.

Haberal, M., Velidedeoglu, E., Arslan, G., Bilgin, N., Buyukpamukcu, N. and Karamehmetoglu, M. (1995b). The effect of DST in kidney transplantation between spouses. *Transplant. Proc.* **27**, 2576.

Habgood, The Right Reverend Lord, Spagnola, A. G., Sgreccia, E. and Daar, A. S. (1997). Religious views on organ and tissue donation. *In Organ and Tissue Donation for Transplantation,* (J. R. Chapman, M. Deirhoi, C. Wright, eds.), pp. 23–33, Arnold, London.

Hadjivannakis, E. J., Evans, D. B., Smellie, W. A. and Calne, R. Y. (1971). Gastrointestinal complications after renal transplantation. *Lancet* **2**, 781.

Hadley, S. and Karchmer, A. W. (1995). Fungal infections in solid organ transplant recipients. *Infect. Dis. Clin. North Am.* **9**, 1045.

Haem, J., Berthoux, P., Grattard, F., *et al.* (1996). Clear evidence of the existence of healthy carriers of hepatitis C virus among renal transplant recipients. *Transplantation* **61**, 886.

Hall, C. M., Wilcox, P. A., Swanepoel, C. R., *et al.* (1994). Mycobacterial infection in renal transplant recipients. *Chest* **106**, 435.

Hamaloglu, E., Tokyay, R., Arslan, G., Bilgin, N., Buyukpamukcu, N. and Haberal, M. (1992). Living related donor transplantation at a Turkish center. *Transplant. Proc.* **24**, 1848.

Hawkins, B. R., on behalf of the Collaborative Study Transplant contributors in Hong Kong. (1998). No difference in the causes of graft failure in living related and cadaver kidney transplantation in Hong Kong Chinese. *Transplant. Proc.* **30**, 3090.

Hendrickse, R. G., White, H. G., Edington, G. M., Houba, V., Glasgow, E. G. and Adeniyi, A. (1972). Quartan malarial nephrotic syndrome. *Lancet* **1**, 1143.

Henning, P., Tomlinson, L., Ridgen, S. P. A., Haycock, G. B. and Chanther, C. (1988). Long term outcome of treatment of end-stage renal failure. *Arch. Dis. Child.* **63**, 35.

Hestin, D., Frimat, L., Hubert, J., Renoult, E., Huu, T. C. and Kessler, M. (1994). Renal transplantation in patients over 60 years old. *Clin. Nephrol.* **42**, 232.

Hibberd, P. L. and Rubin, R. H. (1994). Clinical aspects of fungal infection in organ transplant recipients. *Clin. Infect. Dis.* **19(Suppl. 1)**, S33.

Higgins, R. M., Cahn, A. P., Porter, D., *et al.* (1991). Mycobacterial infections after renal transplantation. *Q. J. M.* **78**, 145.

Holzer, B. R., Gluck, Z., Zambeli, D. and Fey, M. (1985). Transmission of malaria by renal transplantation. *Transplantation* **39**, 315.

Hu, R.-H., Lee, P.-H., Tsai, M.-K. and Lee, C.-Y. (1998). Medical cost difference between renal transplantation and haemodialysis. *Transplant. Proc.* **30**, 3617.

Huang, C. C. and Lai, M. K. (1992). The clinical outcome of hepatitis C virus antibody-positive renal allograft recipients. *Transplantation* **53**, 763.

Huraib, S., Al-Rashed, R., Aldrees, A., Aljefry, M., Arif, M. and Al-Faleh, F. A. (1995). High prevalence of and risk factors in hepatitis C in renal haemodialysis patients in Saudi Arabia: a need for new dialysis strategies. *Nephrol. Dial. Transplant.* **10**, 470.

Husain, I. (1994). Urinary schistosomiasis (bilharzia). *In Oxford Textbook of Surgery,* (P. J. Morris and R. Mall, eds.), Oxford University Press, Oxford.

Ianhez, L. E., Sampaio, M., Fonseca, J. A. and Sabbaga, E. (1992). The influence of socioeconomic conditions in renal posttransplant infection. *Transplant. Proc.* **24**, 3100.

Isaacson, C., Milne, F. J., Van Niekerk, I., Kenyon, M. R. and Mzamane, V. A. (1991). The renal histopathology of essential hypertension in black South Africans. *S. Afr. Med. J.* **80**, 173.

Ismail, N., Becker, B., Srtzelczyk, P. and Ritz, E. (1999). Renal disease and hypertension in non-insulin diabetes mellitus. *Kidney Int.* **55**, 1.

James, S. H., Meyers, A. M., Milne, F. J. and Reinach, S. G. (1995). Partial recovery of renal function in black patients with apparent end-stage renal failure due to primary malignant hypertension. *Nephron* **71**, 29.

Jayakumar, M., Gopalakrishnan, N., Vijayakumar, R., Rajendran, S. and Muthusethupathi, M. A. (1998). Systemic fungal infections in renal transplant recipients at Chennai, India. *Transplant. Proc.* **30**, 3135.

John, A. G., Rao, M. and Jacob, C. K. (1998). Preemptive live-related renal transplantation. *Transplantation* **66**, 204.

John, G. T., Vincent, L., Jayaseelan, L., *et al.* (1994). Cyclosporine immunosuppression and mycobacterial infection. *Transplantation* **58**, 247.

Johny, K. V., Nesim, J., Namboori, N. and Gupta, R. K. (1990). Values gained and lost in live unrelated renal transplantation. *Transplant. Proc.* **22**, 915.

Julian, B. A. (1998). IgA nephropathy and related disorders. *In Primer on Kidney Diseases,* 2nd ed. (A. Greenberg, A. K. Cheung, T. M. Coffman, R. J. Falk and J. C. Jennette, eds.), p. 170, Academic Press, San Diego.

Kahn, D., McCurdie, F., Pontin, A. R., Swanepoel, C. R., Rayner, B. L. and van Zyl-Smit, R. (1997). Results of renal transplantation in black patients in South Africa. *Transplant. Proc.* **29**, 3721.

Kamel, G., Stephan, A., Barbari, A., *et al.* (1998). Transplantation at Rizk Hospital: ten years' experience. *Transplant. Proc.* **30**, 3114.

Kamel, G., Stephan, A., Salme, P. and Zeineh, S. (1993). Renal transplantation: the Lebanese experience. *Transplant. Proc.* **25**, 2356.

Kandus, A., Buturovic, P. J., Malovrh, M. and Bren, A. F. (1992). Kidney transplantation in Slovenia from 1986 through 1991. *Transplant. Proc.* **24**, 2430.

Kang, Z., Fang, G. and Chen, W. (1992). A comparative study of the outcome of renal transplantation in peritoneal dialysis and hemodialysis patients. *Chin. Med. Sci. J.* **7**, 49.

Kasiske, B., London, W. and Ellison, M. D. (1998). Race and socioeconomic factors influencing early placement on the kidney transplant waiting list. *J. Am. Soc. Nephrol.* **9**, 2142.

Kathuria, P., Sakhuja, V., Gupta, K. L., *et al.* (1995). Gastrointestinal complications after renal transplantation: 10 year data from a North Indian Transplant Center. *ASAIO J.* **41**, M698.

Katz, S. M., Kerman, R. H., Golden, D., *et al.* (1991). Pre-emptive transplantation: an analysis of benefits and hazards in 85 cases. *Transplantation* **51**, 1411.

Kaur, M. (1998). Organ donation and transplantation in Singapore. *Transplant. Proc.* **30**, 3631.

Kazim, E., Rukmani, M., Fernandez, S. N., *et al.* (1992). Buying a kidney: The easy way out? *Transplant. Proc.* **24**, 2112.

Kehinde, E. O. (1998). Attitude to cadaver organ donation in Oman: preliminary report. *Transplant. Proc.* **30**, 3624.

Kekec, R., Tavli, S. and Haberal, M. (1992). Infections after kidney transplantation. *Transplant. Proc.* **24**, 1932.

Khan, I. H., Thereska, N., Barbullushi, M. and MacLeod, A. M. (1996). The epidemiology of chronic renal failure and provision of renal services in Albania. *Nephrol. Dial. Transplant.* **11**, 1751.

Kibukamusoke, J. W., Hutt, M. S. R. and Wilks, N. E. (1999). The nephrotic syndrome in Uganda and its association with quartan malaria. *Q. J. M.* **36**, 393.

Kiley, D. J., Lam, C. S. and Pollak, R. (1993). A study of treatment compliance following kidney transplantation. *Transplantation* **55**, 51.

Kim, M. J. (1996). Nephrology and renal replacement therapy in South Korea: a brief report of the Korean Society of Nephrology and Transplantation. *Nephrol. Dial. Transplant.* **11**, 979.

Kirubakaran, M. G. and Pugsley, D. J. (1992). Morbidity and mortality among Australian Aboriginal transplant recipients. *Transplant. Proc.* **24**, 1808.

Kjellstrand, C. M. (1988). Giving life-giving death: ethical problems of high technology medicine. *Acta Med. Scand.* **75**, 5.

Kjellstrand, C. M., Ebben, J. and Davin, T. (1984). Time of death, recovery of renal function, development of chronic renal failure and the need for chronic haemodialysis in patients with acute tubular necrosis. *Trans. ASAIO* **27**, 45.

Kootstra, G., Wynen, R. and van Hoof, J. P. (1992). The non-heart-beating kidney donor: of any help in developing countries? *Transplant. Proc.* **24**, 2040.

Kostakis, A., Bokos, J., Staniadiades, D., Zanos, G. and Bolestis, J. (1997). The 10 year single centre experience using elderly donors for living related kidney transplantation. *Geriatr. Nephrol. Urol.* **7**, 127.

Kudo, T., Morishma, T., Tsuzuki, K., Orito, E. and Mizokami, M. (1996). Hepatitis G virus in immunosupressed paediatric allograft recipients. *Lancet* **348**, 751.

Kumar, A., Kumar, R. V., Srinadh, E. S., *et al.* (1994). Should elderly donors be accepted in a living related renal transplant program? *Clin. Transplant.* **8**, 523.

Kumar, H., Alam, F. and Naqvi, S. A. (1992). Experience of haemodialysis at the Kidney Centre. *J. Pak. Med. Assoc.* **42**, 234.

Kung'u, A. and Sitati, S. M. (1980). Glomerulonephritis in Kenya: a histological study. *East Afr. Med. J.* **57**, 525.

Kussman, M. J., Goldstein, H. and Gleason, R. E. (1976). The clinical course of diabetic nephropathy. *J. A. M. A.* **236**, 1861.

Kyriakides, G. K., Hadjigavriel, M., Hadjicostas, P., Nicolaides, A. and Kyriakides, M. (1993). Renal transplantation in Cyprus. *Transplant. Proc.* **25**, 2361.

Kyriakides, G. K., Hadjigavriel, M., Pierides, A., Chouris, S., Kyriakides, M. and Varnavides, A. (1989). Renal transplantation in a developing country (Cyprus). *Transplant. Proc.* **21**, 2182.

Lai, K. N., Li, P. K. T., Lui, S. E., *et al.* (1991). Membranous nephropathy related to hepatitis B virus adults. *N. Engl. J. Med.* **324**, 1457.

Lai, K. N. and Wang, A. Y. M. (1994). IgA nephropathy: common nephritis leading to end-stage renal failure. *Int. J. Artif. Organs* **17**, 457.

Lai, M. K., Huang, S. H., Chu, S. H., Chuang, C. K. and Huang, J. Y. (1992). Two-hundred and thirty cases of kidney transplantation: single center experience in Taiwan. *Transplant. Proc.* **24**, 1452.

Langs, C., Gallo, G. and Schacht, R. (1990). Rapid renal failure in AIDS-associated focal glomerulosclerosis. *Arch. Intern. Med.* **150**, 287.

Layafette, R. A., Mayer, G. and Meyer, T. W. (1992). Angiotensin II blockade limits glomerular injury in rats with reduced renal mass. *J. Clin. Invest.* **90**, 766.

Lee, C. J. (1992). Organ transplantation in Taiwan. *Transplant. Proc.* **24**, 1824.

Lei, C., Abdullah, K., Morad, Z. and Suleiman, A. B. (1992). Surgical complications of living unrelated kidney transplantations in a Third-World country. *Transplant. Proc.* **24**, 1815.

Lindheimer, M. D. and Katz, A. I. (1992). Pregnancy in the renal transplant patient. *Am. J. Kidney Dis.* **19**, 173.

Liquete, R. M. O. R. and Ona, E. T. (1992). Transplant practices in the Philippines. *Transplant. Proc.* **24**, 1809.

Loges de Cordier, M. B., al-Sebayel, M., Kiziliski, T., *et al.* (1997). Donor retrieval patterns in a Saudi multi-organ transplant center. *Transplant. Proc.* **29**, 3064.

Lubani, M. M., Doudin, K. I., Sharda, D. C., *et al.* (1989). Congenital chloride diarrhoea in Kuwaiti children. *Eur. J. Pediatr.* **148**, 333.

Ludre, P., Ten Dam, G. and Kochi, A. (1992). Tuberculosis: a global review of the situation. *Bull. World Health Organ.* **70**, 149.

Mabayoje, M. O., Bamgboye, E. L., Odutola, T. A. and Mabadeje, A. F. B. (1992). Chronic renal failure at the Lagos University Teaching Hospital: a 10-year review. *Transplant. Proc.* **24**, 1851.

Magrans, C., Manalich, J., Alfonzo, J., Almaguer, M. and Herrera, R. (1996). Organ procurement for transplantation in Cuba. *Transplant. Proc.* **28**, 3353.

Malhotra, H. S., Dash, S. C., Dhawan, I. K., *et al.* (1986). Tuberculosis and renal transplantation—observations from an endemic area of tuberculosis. *Postgrad. Med. J.* **62**, 359.

Malhotra, K. K. (1994). Tuberculosis in maintenance hemodialysis and renal transplant patients. *In Asian Nephrology*, (K. S. Chugh, ed.), p. 597, Oxford University Press, Delhi.

Malhotra, K. K., Dash, S. C., Dhawan, I. K., Bhuyan, U. N. and Gupta, A. (1986). Tuberculosis and renal transplantation— observations from an endemic area of tuberculosis. *Postgrad. Med. J.* **62**, 359.

Malin, A. S. and Young, A. E. (1996). Designing a vaccine for tuberculosis. *B. M. J.* **312**, 1495.

Mallick, N. P., Jones, E. and Selwood, N. (1995). The European (European Dialysis and Transplantation Association-European Renal Association) Registry. *Am. J. Kidney Dis.* **25**, 176.

Mancilla, E., Alberu, J., Alessio-Robles, L., *et al.* (1992). Prevalence of clinically overt cytomegalovirus disease in kidney transplant patients. *Transplant. Proc.* **24**, 1919.

Marcias-Nunez, J. F. and Cameron, J. S. (1992). Treatment of end-stage renal disease: the elderly. *In Oxford Textbook of Clinical Nephrology*, (J. S. Cameron, A. M. Davison, J. P. Grunefeld and D. Kerr, eds.), p. 1621, Oxford University Press, Oxford.

Margolius, L. P. (1996). Kaposi's sarcoma and other malignancies in renal transplant recipients. *Transpl. Rev.* **10**, 129.

Margolius, L. P. and Botha, J. R. (1999). The 4th decade of renal transplantation: where have we come? *Kidney Int.* **55**, 2125.

Marmol, A., Herrera, R. and Moreno, D. (1996). Organ procurement and renal transplantation in Cuba. *Transplant. Proc.* **28**, 3356.

Martinez, L. and Donkervoort, S. C. (1992). Special issues related to transplantation in South America. *Transplant. Proc.* **24**, 2414.

Masri, M. A., Shakuntala, R. V., Dhawan, I. K., *et al.* (1993). Transplantation in the United Arab Emirates. *Transplant. Proc.* **25**, 2358.

Masuko, K., Mitsui, T., Iwano, K., *et al.* (1996). Infection with the hepatitis GB virus C in patients on maintenance haemodialysis. *N. Engl. J. Med.* **334**, 1485.

McClellan, W., Tuttle, E. and Issa, A. (1998). Racial differences in the incidence of end-stage renal disease (ESRD) are not entirely explained by differences in the prevalence of hypertension. *Am. J. Kidney Dis.* **12**, 285.

McLigeyo, S. O., Otieno, L. S., Kinuthia, D. M., Ongeri, S. K., Mwongera, F. K. and Wairagu, S. G. (1988). Problems with a renal replacement programme in a developing country. *Postgrad. Med. J.* **64**, 783.

Mets, T. F. (1993). The disease pattern of elderly medical patients in Rwanda, central Africa. *J. Trop. Med. Hyg.* **96**, 291.

Meyers, A. M. (1995). The treatment of end-stage renal failure in South Africa. *Hospital Supplies* May, 6.

Meyers, K. E. C., Thompson, P. D. and Weiland, H. (1996). Noncompliance in children and adolescents after renal transplantation. *Transplantation* **62**, 186.

Meyers, K. E. C., Weiland, H. and Thomson, P. D. (1995). Paediatric renal transplantation non-compliance. *Pediatr. Nephrol.* **9**, 189.

Migliori, R. J., Simmons, R. L., Payne, W. D., *et al.* (1999). Renal transplantation done safely without prior chronic dialysis therapy. *Transplantation* **43**, 51.

Milne, F. J. (1997). The treatment of severe hypertension. *Hypertension: South African perspective* July, 17.

Milne, F. J., James, S. H. and Veriawa, Y. (1989). Malignant hypertension and its renal complications in black South Africans. *S. Afr. Med. J.* **76**, 164.

Modiba, M. C. M., Mzamane, D. V. A., Pantanowitz, D., Botha, J. R., Meyers, A. M. and Myburgh, J. A. (1989). Renal transplantation in black South Africans: the Baragwanath experience. *Transplant. Proc.* **21**, 2010.

Montagnino, G., Bencini, P. L., Tarontino, A., *et al.* (1994). Clinical features and cause of Kaposi's sarcoma in kidney transpalnt patients: report of 13 cases. *Am. J. Nephrol.* **14**, 121.

Moore, T. C. and Hume, D. M. (1969). The period and nature of hazard in clinical renal transplantation. *Ann. Surg.* **170**, 1.

Moosa, M. R. and Bouwens, C. (1997). Tuberculosis in renal allograft recipients: the South African experience. *Transpl. Rev.* **11**, 84.

Moosa, M. R., Grobbelaar, C., Swanevelder, S. A. and Edelstein, C. L. (1992). The influence of race and the impact of socioeconomic and clinical factors on primary renal allograft survival. *Transplant. Proc.* **24**, 1754.

Moosa, M. R., Treurnicht, F. K., van Rensberg, E. J., Schneider, J. W., Jordaan, H. F. and Engelbrecht, S. (1998). Detection and subtyping of human herpesvirus-8 in renal transplant patients before and after remission of Kaposi's sarcoma. *Transplantation* **66**, 214.

Morales, J. M. (1998). Renal transplantation in patients positive for hepatitis B or C. *Transplant. Proc.* **30**, 2064.

Morris, P. J. (1998). Renal transplantation in indigenous populations. *Nephrology* **4**, S106.

Morris, P. J., Johnson, R. J., Fuggle, S. V., Belger, M. A., Briggs, J. D., on behalf of the HLA Task Force of the Kidney Advisory Group of the United Kingdom Transplant Service Authority (UKTSSA). (1982). Analysis of factors that affect outcome of primary cadaveric renal transplantation in the UK. *Lancet* **354**, 1147.

Muller, G. Y., Zabaleta, M. E., Armino, A., *et al.* (1992). Risk factors for dialysis-associated hepatitis C in Venezuela. *Kidney Int.* **41**, 1055.

Naicker, S. (1996). Nephrology in South Africa. *Nephrol. Dial. Transplant.* **11**, 30.

Naidas, O. D. (1998). Cost effective analysis of alternative treatments of end-stage renal disease: Philippine experience. *Transplant. Proc.* **30**, 3617.

Nalesnik, M. A. (1990). Involvement of the gastrointestinal tract by Epstein-Barr virus-associated post-transplant lymphoproliferative disorders. *Am. J. Surg. Pathol.* **14(Suppl. 1)**, 92.

Naqvi, A., Akhtar, F., Naqvi, R., *et al.* (1997). Problems of diagnosis and treatment of tuberculosis following renal transplantation. *Transplant. Proc.* **29**, 3051.

Naqvi, A. and Rizvi, A. (1995). Renal transplantation in Pakistan. *Transplant. Proc.* **27**, 2778.

Naqvi, A. A. (1995). Ethical issues in renal transplantation in developing countries. *J. Pak. Med. Assoc.* **45**, 233.

Naqvi, S. A., Hussain, M., Askari, H., *et al.* (1992). Economics of renal rehabilitation in Pakistan: a case for increasing transplantation activity. *Transplant. Proc.* **24**, 2125.

Naqvi, S. A. and Rizvi, S. A. (1995a). Ethical issues in renal transplantation in developing countries. *Br. J. Urol.* **76(Suppl. 2)**, 97.

Naqvi, S. A. and Rizvi, S. A. H. (1995b). Renal transplantation in Pakistan. *Transplant. Proc.* **27**, 2778.

Naqvi, S. A. A., Mazhar, F., Ahmed, R., Jamal, H. and Rizvi, A. (1998). Limitation in selection of donors in a living-related renal transplant programme. *Transplant. Proc.* **30**, 2286.

Nelson, B. K. (1989). Snake envenomation: incidence, clinical presentation and management. *Med. Toxicol. Adverse Drug Exp.* **4**, 17.

Neustadt, D., Fagalde, A., Cambariere, R. and Piulats, E. (1996). The "Republica Argentina organ procurement development organization model": collaborative study. *Transplant. Proc.* **28**, 3360.

Odell, J. A., Brink, J. G., Terblanche, J. and Kahn, D. (1992). Transplantation of solid organs in South Africa. *S. Afr. Med. J.* **82**, 427.

Oeopoulos, D. G. (1999). The optimization of continuous ambulatory peritoneal dialysis. *Kidney Int.* **55**, 1131.

Ojogwu, L. I. (1983). Peritoneal dialysis in the management of hypertensive acute oliguric renal failure. *Trop. Geogr. Med.* **35**, 385.

Ona, E. T. (1992). Early pitfalls in renal transplantation. *Transplant. Proc.* **24**, 1280.

Opelz, G., Mickey, M. R. and Terasaki, P. I. (1977). Influence of race on kidney transplant survival. *Transplant. Proc.* **9**, 137.

Ota, K. (1998). Strategies for increasing transplantation in Asia and prospects of organ sharing: the Japanese experience. *Transplant. Proc.* **30**, 3650.

Ota, K. (1999). Asian Transplant Registry. *Transplant. Proc.* **31**, 2005.

Owens, M. L., Maxwell, J. G., Goodnight, J. and Wolcott, M. W. (1975). Discontinuance of immunosuppression in renal transplant patients. *Arch. Surg.* **110**, 1450.

Parfrey, P. S., Vavasour, H., Bullock, M., Henry, S., Harnett, J. D. and Gault, M. H. (1989). Development of a health questionnaire specific for end-stage renal disease. *Nephron* **52**, 28.

Park, H., Bang, W. R., Kim, S. J., *et al.* (1992a). Quality of life of ESRD patients: development of a tool and comparison between transplant and dialysis patients. *Transplant. Proc.* **24**, 1435.

Park, K. (1998). Prospects of organ sharing and strategies for increasing transplants in Asia. *Transplant. Proc.* **30**, 3647.

Park, K., Kim, Y. S. and Kim, S. I. (1992b). Analysis of risk factors affecting the outcome of primary living donor renal transplantation in Korea. *Transplant. Proc.* **24**, 2426.

Park, K., Kim, Y. S., Kim, S. I., Kim, M. S. and Moon, J. I. (1998). Single center experience of 1500 kidney transplants. *Transplant. Proc.* **30**, 3088.

Park, K., Suh, J. S., Kim, S. I., *et al.* (1992c). Single center experience of 600 living donor transplants: univariate analysis of risk factors affecting outcome. *Transplant. Proc.* **24**, 1447.

Parving, H.-H., Smidt, U. M., Hommel, E., *et al.* (1993). Effective antihypertensive treatment postpones renal insuffiency in diabetic nephropathy. *Am. J. Kidney Dis.* **22**, 188.

Paya, C. V. (1993). Fungal infections in solid-organ transplantation. *Clin. Infect. Dis.* **16**, 677.

Penn, I. (1987). Cancers following cyclosporine therapy. *Transplantation* **43**, 32.

Penn, I. (1999). The changing pattern of posttransplant malignancies. *Transplant. Proc.* **23**, 1102.

Penn, I. and Brunson, M. E. (1988). Cancers after cyclosporine therapy. *Transplant. Proc.* **3**, 885.

Pereira, B. J. G. (1998). Renal transplantation in patients positive for hepatitis B or C. *Transplant. Proc.* **30**, 2070.

Pereira, B. J. G. and Levey, A. S. (1997). Hepatitis C virus infection in dialysis and renal transplantation. *Kidney Int.* **51**, 981.

Pereira, B. J. G., Natov, S. N., Bouthot, B. A., *et al.* (1999). Effect of hepatitis C infection and renal transplantation on survival in end-stage renal disease. *Kidney Int.* **53**, 1374.

Pereira, B. J. G., Wright, T. L. and Schmid, C. H. (1995). A controlled study of hepatitis C transmission by organ transplantation. The New England Organ Bank Hepatitis C Study Group [published errata appears in *Lancet* 1995, **345**:662]. *Transplantation* **60**, 799.

Pernerger, T. V., Whelton, P. K., Klag, M. J. and Rossiter, K. A. (1995). Diagnosis of hypertensive end-stage renal disease: effect of the patient's race. *Am. J. Epidemiol.* **141**, 10.

Peterson, P. K. and Anderson, R. C. (1986). Infection in renal transplant recipients: current approaches to diagnosis, therapy and prevention. *Am. J. Med.* **81**, 2.

Peterson, P. K., Ferguson, R., Fryd, D. S., Balfour, H. H., Rynasiewicz, J. and Simmons, R. L. (1982). Infectious diseases in hospitalised renal transplant recipients: a prospective study of a complex and evolving problem. *Medicine* **61**, 360.

Pike, R., Odell, J. A. and Kahn, D. (1992). Public attitudes to organ donation in South Africa. *Transplant. Proc.* **24**, 2102.

Pirson, Y., Alexandre, G. P. J. and Van Ypersele de Strihou, C. (1977). Long-term effect of HBs antigenemia on patient survival after renal transplantation. *N. Engl. J. Med.* **296**, 194.

Pitcock, J. A., Johnson, J. G., Hatch, F. E., Acchiardo, S., Muirhead, E. E. and Brown, N. (1976). Malignant hypertension in blacks: malignant intrarenal arterial disease observed by light and electron microscopy. *Hum. Pathol.* **7**, 333.

Plot, P. and Tezzo, R. (1990). The epidemiology of HIV and other sexually transmitted infections in the developing world. *Scand. J. Infect. Dis.* **69(Suppl.)**, 89.

Pol, S., Debure, A. and Degott, C. (1990). Chronic hepatitis in kidney allograft recipients. *Lancet* **335**, 878.

Pontin, A. R., Juszkiewics, P., Pascoe, M. and Kahn, D. (1997). Results of renal allograft survival comparing locally domiciled transplant patients and distant domiciled transplant patients. p. 44, XVIIth Congress of the Southern African Transplantation Society, Cape Town.

Prakash, S. K., Sahl, U. S., Gedela, S. R., Tripathi, K. and Agrawal, D. K. (1999). Infection in renal allograft transplantation recipients. *Transplant. Proc.* **24**, 1943.

Quintanilla-Martinez, L., Lome-Maldonaldo, C., Schwarzmann, F., *et al.* (1998). Post-transplantation lymphoproliferative disorders in Mexico: an aggressive clonal disease associated with Epstein-Barr virus type A. *Mod. Pathol.* **11**, 200.

Qunibi, W., Akhtar, M., Sheth, K., *et al.* (1988). Kaposi's sarcoma: the most common tumor after renal transplantation in Saudi Arabia. *Am. J. Med.* **84**, 225.

Qunibi, W. Y., al Sibai, M. B., Taher, S., *et al.* (1990). Mycobacterial infection after renal transplantation—report of 14 cases and review of the literature. *Q. J. M.* **77**, 1039.

Rahbar, K., Nobakht, A. and Nasrollahi, A. (1993). Renal transplantation and dialysis in a geriatric population in Tehran, Iran. *Transplant. Proc.* **25**, 2362.

Ramos, E. L. and Tisher, C. C. (1994). Recurrent diseases in the kidney transplant. *Am. J. Kidney Dis.* **24**, 142.

Randhawa, G. (1998). An exploratory study examining the influence of religion on attitudes towards organ donation among the Asian population in Luton, UK. *Nephrol. Dial. Transplant.* **13**, 1949.

Rao, K. V., Kasiske, B. L. and Anderson, W. R. (1991). Variability in the morphological spectrum and clinical outcome of chronic liver disease. *Transplantation* **51**, 391.

Rao, M., Juneja, R., Maria Shirly, R. B. and Jacob, C. K. (1998). Haemodialysis for end-stage renal disease in Southern India—a perspective from a tertiary referral care center. *Nephrol. Dial. Transplant.* **13**, 2494.

Rao, V. K., Anderson, S., Kasiske, B. L. and Dahl, D. C. (1993). Value of liver biopsy in the evaluation and management of chronic liver disease in renal transplant recipients. *Am. J. Med.* **94**, 241.

Rao, V. K. and Ma, J. (1996). Chronic viral hepatitis enhances the risk of infection but not acute rejection in renal transplant recipients. *Transplantation* **62**, 1765.

Rapaport, F. T., Waltzer, W. C. and Anaise, D. (1990). How can one balance duty to all cultures and ethnic groups with effective procurement and equitable distribution of organs for clinical transplantation? New evidence of the key importance of local primacy for a successful organ donation effort. *Transplant. Proc.* **22**, 1007.

Rashid, A., Abboud, O., Taha, M. and El-Sayed, M. (1998). Renal replacement therapy in Qatar. *Saudi J. Kidney Dis. Transplant.* **9**, 36.

Rashid, H. U., Hossain, R. M. and Khanam, A. (1993). Outcome of acute renal failure in adults in a teaching hospital in Bangladesh. *Ren. Fail.* **15**, 603.

Rashid, H. U., Rasul, G., Rahman, M., Jinnat, S. and Wahab, M. A. (1992). Experience of kidney transplantation in Bangaldesh. *Transplant. Proc.* **24**, 1831.

Ray, P. E. (1999). Looking into the past and future of human immuno-deficiency virus nephropathy. *Kidney Int.* **55**, 1123.

Ready, A. (1998). Transplanting an ethnic community: approaches to the crisis. *Nephrol. Dial. Transplant.* **13**, 2490.

Ready, A. R., Trafford, J., Hooker, A. and Briggs, D. (1992). Impact of a large non-indigenous population on the renal transplant waiting list. *Transplant. Proc.* **24**, 1435.

Reese, J., Burton, F., Lingle, D., *et al.* (1991). Peptic ulcer disease following renal transplantation in the cyclosporine era. *Am. J. Surg.* **162**, 558.

Reissi, D., Bardideh, A., Samadzadeh, B. and Razi, A. (1995). Kidney transplantation in Kermanshah, Iran: a 5-year experience. *Transplant. Proc.* **27**, 2765.

Rennie, D., Rettig, R. A. and Wing, A. J. (1985). Limited resources and the treatment of end-stage renal failure in Britain and the United States. *Q. J. M.* **56**, 321.

Renoult, E., Georges, E., Biava, M. F., *et al.* (1999). Toxoplasmosis in kidney transplant recipients: a report of six cases and review. *Clin. Infect. Dis.* **24**, 625.

Reynolds, E., Wall, K. and Pfeiffer, R. (1966). Generalised toxoplasmosis following renal transplantation. *Arch. Intern. Med.* **118**, 401.

Rifkind, D., Marchioro, T. L., Schneck, S. A. and Hill, R. B. (1967). Systemic fungal infections complicating renal transplantation and immunosuppressive therapy. *Am. J. Med.* **43**, 28.

Rizvi, A., Naqvi, A., Hussain, I., *et al.* (1990). Problems of renal transplantation in Pakistan. *Transplant. Proc.* **22**, 2269.

Rizvi, A., Naqvi, A., Hussain, I., *et al.* (1991). Problems with immuno-suppression in developing countries. *Transplant. Proc.* **23**, 2204.

Rizvi, A., Naqvi, A., Hussain, Z., *et al.* (1998a). Factors influencing graft survival in living-related donor kidney transplantation at a single center. *Transplant. Proc.* **30**, 712.

Rizvi, S. A., Naqvi, S. A., Hussain, Z., *et al.* (1998b). Factors influencing renal transplantation in a developing country. *Transplant. Proc.* **30**, 1810.

Rizvi, S. A. H. and Naqvi, A. (1995). The need to increase transplantation activity in developing countries. *Transplant. Proc.* **27**, 2739.

Roake, A. J., Cahill, A. P., Gray, C. M., Gray, D. W. R., Morris, P. J., *et al.* (1996). Pre-emptive cadaveric renal transplantation: clinical outcome. *Transplantation* **62**, 1411.

Robson, S. C., Schoub, B. and Abdool Karim, S. S. (1994). Viral hepatitis B—an overview. *S. Afr. Med. J.* **84**, 530.

Rodriquez, A., Diaz, M., Colon, A. and Santiago-Delphin, E. A. (1991). Psychosocial profile of non-compliant patients. *Transplant. Proc.* **23**, 1807.

Roodnat, J. I., Zietse, R., Rischen-Vos, J., *et al.* (1999). Effect of race on kidney transplant survival in non-European recipients. *Transplant. Proc.* **31**, 312.

Rostaing, L., Izopet, J., Baron, E., Duffart, M., Puel, J. and Durand, D. (1995). Treatment of chronic hepatitis C with recombinant interferon alpha in kidney transplant recipients. *Transplantation* **59**, 1426.

Rostami, M., Ali Askari, M. and Shojan, S. (1992). Determination of the causes of fever in allograft recipients in Western Iran (Bakhtaran). *Transplant. Proc.* **24**, 1935.

Roth, D., Zucker, K., Cirocco, R., *et al.* (1994). The impact of hepatitis C virus infection on renal allograft recipients. *Kidney Int.* **45**, 238.

Rubin, R. H., Cosimi, A. B. and Tolkoff-Rubin, N. E. (1999). Infectious disease syndromes attributable to cytomegalovirus and their significance among renal transplant patients. *Transplantation* **24**, 458.

Rubin, R. H. and Tolkoff-Rubin, N. E. (1988). Opportunistic infections in renal allograft recipients. *Transplant. Proc.* **20**, 12.

Rutkowski, B., Puka, J., Lao, M., *et al.* (1997). Renal replacement therapy in an era of socio-economic changes—report from the Polish Registry. *Nephrol. Dial. Transplant.* **12**, 1105.

Rutkowski, R., Ciocalteu, A., Djukanovic, L., *et al.* (1998). Central and Eastern Europe Advisory Board in chronic renal failure: evolution of renal replacement therapy in Central and Eastern Europe seven years after political and economic liberation. *Nephrol. Dial. Transplant.* **13**, 860.

Saber, L. T., Duarte, G., Costa, J. A., Cologna, A. J., Garcia, T. M. and Ferraz, A. S. (1995). Pregnancy and kidney transplantation: experience in a developing country. *Am. J. Kidney Dis.* **25**, 465.

Said, R. (1999). Renal replacement therapy in Jordan. *Saudi J. Kidney Dis. Transplant.* **10**, 64.

Saieh, A. C. (1990). The management of end-stage renal disease in underdeveloped countries: a moral and an economic problem. *Pediatr. Nephrol.* **4**, 199.

Sakhuja, V., Jha, V., Varma, P. P., Joshi, K. and Chugh, K. S. (1996). The high incidence of tuberculosis among renal transplant recipients in India. *Transplantation* **61**, 211.

Salahi, H., Ghahramani, N., Malek-Hosseini, S. A., *et al.* (1998). Religious sanctions regarding cadaver organ transplantation in Iran. *Transplant. Proc.* **30**, 769.

Salahudeen, A. K., Woods, H. F., Pingle, A., *et al.* (1990). High mortality among recipients of bought living-unrelated donor kidneys. *Lancet* **336**, 725.

Samanta, A., Burden, A. C., Feehally, J. and Walls, J. (1986). Diabetic renal disease: differences between Asians and white patients. *B. M. J.* **293**, 696.

Santiago-Delphin, E. A. (1997). The organ shortage: a public health crisis: what are Latin American governments doing about it? *Transplant. Proc.* **29**, 3203.

Santiago-Delphin, E. A. and Garcia, V. D. (1999). Latin American Transplant Registry VIIIth Report. *Transplant. Proc.* **31**, 214.

Schena, F. P. (1997). Report on the first meeting of the chairmen of the national and international registries. *Kidney Int.* **52**, 1422.

Schluger, M. W., Kinney, D., Naskin, T. J., *et al.* (1999). Clinical utility of the polymerase chain reaction in the diagnosis of infections due to *Mycobacterium tuberculosis*. *Chest* **105**, 1116.

Seedat, Y. K. (1979). Clinicopathological features of the nephrotic syndrome in the Africans and Indians of South Africa. *S. Afr. Hosp. Med.* **5**, 222.

Seedat, Y. K. (1998). Why has improved hypertension treatment not reduced the incidence of end-stage renal failure? *Hypertens. South Afr. Perspect.* **6**, 5.

Seedat, Y. K. (1999). Prevalence of hypertension in South Africa. *Hypertens. South Afr. Perspect.* **7**, 2.

Seedat, Y. K., Naicker, S., Rawat, R. and Parsoo, I. (1984). Racial differences in the causes of end-stage renal failure in Natal. *S. Afr. Med. J.* **65**, 956.

Seedat, Y. K. and Nathoo, B. C. (1993). Acute renal failure in blacks and Indians in South Africa—comparison after 10 years. *Nephron* **64**, 198.

Seggie, J., Davies, P. G., Ninin, D. and Henry, J. (1984). Patterns of glomerulonephritis in Zimbabwe: survey of disease characterised by nephrotic syndrome. *Q. J. M.* **209**, 109.

Sesso, R., Ancao, M. S., Draibe, S. A., Sigulem, D. and Ramos, O. L. (1990). Survival analysis of 1563 renal transplants in Brazil: report of the Brazilian Registry of Renal Transplantation. *Nephrol. Dial. Transplant.* **5**, 956.

Sesso, R., Frassinetti Fernandes, P., Ancao, M., *et al.* (1996). Acceptance for chronic dialysis treatment: insufficient and unequal. *Nephrol. Dial. Transplant.* **11**, 982.

Shaheen, F. A. M., Souqiyyeh, M. Z., Attar, M. B. and Al-Swailem, A. R. (1996). The Saudi Center for Organ Transplantation: an ideal model for Arab countries to improve treatment of end-stage organ failure. *Transplant. Proc.* **28**, 247.

Sheiban, A.-K. and Al-Garba, A. S. (1999). Yemen nephrology—revisited. *Saudi J. Kidney Dis. Transplant.* **10**, 183.

Sheriff, R., de Abrew, K., Jayasekara, G., *et al.* (1992). Living related donor kidney transplantation in Sri Lanka. *Transplant. Proc.* **24**, 1816.

Sheu, J. C., Lee, S. H., Wang, A. Y. M, Shih, L. N. and Chen, D. S. (1992). Prevalence of anti-HCV and HCV viraemia in haemodialysis patients in Taiwan. *J. Med. Virol.* **37**, 108.

Shrivastava, A., Bhandari, M., Kumar, A., Singh, P. and Sharma, R. K. (1998a). Quest for organ donors: ethical considerations in India. *Transplant. Proc.* **30**, 3629.

Shrivastava, A., Singh, M., Bhandari, M. and Kumar, A. (1998b). Economics of organ transplantation in India. *Transplant. Proc.* **30**, 3121.

Sia, I. G. and Paya, C. V. (1998). Infectious complications following renal transplantation. *Surg. Clin. North Am.* **78**, 95.

Sidabutar, R. P., Sumardjono, N. A. and Suhardono. (1992). Infection in kidney transplantation recipients in Indonesia. *Transplant. Proc.* **24**, 1934.

Siegal, B., Greenstein, S. M. and the Collaborative Study Group. (1999). Profiles of non-compliance in patients with a functioning renal transplant: a multicenter study. *Transplant. Proc.* **31**, 1326.

Silva, F. G., Chander, P., Pirani, C. L. and Hardy, M. A. (1982). Disappearance of glomerular mesangial IgA deposits after renal allograft transplantation. *Transplantation* **33**, 214.

Simforoosh, N., Bassiri, A., Amiransari, B. and Gol, S. (1992). Living-unrelated renal transplantation. *Transplant. Proc.* **24**, 2421.

Singh, P., Srivastava, A. and Kumar, A. (1998). Current status of transplant coordination and organ donation in India. *Transplant. Proc.* **30**, 3627.

Sketris, I., Waite, N., Grobler, K., West, M. and Gerus, S. (1994). Factors affecting compliance with ciclosporin in adult renal transplant patients. *Transplant. Proc.* **26**, 2538.

Snydman, D. R., Werner, B. G., Tilney, N. L., *et al.* (1991). Final analysis of primary cytomegalovirus disease prevention in renal transplant recipients wirth a cytomegalovirus-immune globulin: comparison of the randomised and open-label trials. *Transplant. Proc.* **23**, 1357.

Sobh, M., Moustafa, F., El Arbagy, A., El Din, M. S., Shamaa, S. and Amer, G. (1990). Nephropathy in asymptomatic patients with active *Schistosomiasis mansoni* infection. *Int. Urol. Nephrol.* **22**, 37.

Stoneburner, R. L., Sato, P., Burton, A. and Mertens, T. (1994). The global HIV pandemic. *Acta. Paediatr.* **400(Suppl.)**, 1.

Sturgiss, S. N. and Davison, J. M. (1992). Effect of pregnancy on long-term function of renal allografts. *Am. J. Kidney Dis.* **19**, 167.

Sumrani, N., Daskalakis, P., Miles, A. M., Hong, J. H. and Somner, B. G. (1993). The influence of donor age on function of renal allografts from living related donors. *Clin. Nephrol.* **39**, 260.

Sumrani, N., Delaney, V., Ding, Z. K., *et al.* (1991). Renal transplantation from elderly living donors. *Transplantation* **51**, 305.

Swanepoel, C. R. (1999). Renal failure in the Southern zone of Afran. *Kidney Int.* **55**, 2121.

Swanepoel, C. R., Madaus, S., Cassidy, M. J., *et al.* (1989). IgA nephropathy—Groote Schuur Hospital experience. *Nephron* **53**, 61.

Szabo, A., Sallay, P., Kribben, A., *et al.* (1998). Hepatitis G virus infection in children on dialysis and after renal transplantation. *Pediatr. Nephrol.* **12**, 93.

Szabo, A., Viavoz, S., Heemann, U., Kribben, A., Phillip, T. and Roggendorf, M. (1997). GBV-C/HGV infection in renal dialysis and transplant patients. *Nephrol. Dial. Transplant.* **12**, 2380.

Tagaki, H. (1997). Organ transplantation in Japan and Asian countries. *Transplant. Proc.* **29**, 3199.

Terasaki, P. I., Cecka, J. M., Gjertson, D. W. and Cho, Y. W. (1997). Spousal and other living renal donor transplants. *Clin. Transplant.* **269**, 84.

Terasaki, P. I., Cecka, J. M., Gjertson, D. W. and Takemoto, S. (1995). High survival rates of kidney transplants from spousal and living unrelated donors. *N. Engl. J. Med.* **333**, 333.

Terrell, C. L. and Hughes, C. E. (1992). Antifungal agents used for deep-seated mycotic infections. *Mayo Clin. Proc.* **67**, 69.

Thiagarajan, C. M., Reddy, K. C., Shunmugasundaram, D., *et al.* (1990). The practice of unconventional renal transplantation (UCRT) at a single centre in India. *Transplant. Proc.* **22**, 912.

Tierney, W. M., McDonald, C. J. and Luft, F. C. (1989). Renal disease in hypertensive adults: effect of race and type II diabetes mellitus. *Am. J. Kidney Dis.* **13**, 485.

Tokat, Y., Kilic, M., Kursat, S., *et al.* (1996). Tuberculosis after renal transplantation. *Transplant. Proc.* **28**, 2353.

Troppman, C., Papalous, B. E., Chiou, A., *et al.* (1995). Incidence, complications, treatment and outcome of ulcers of the upper gastrointestinal tract after renal transplantation. *J. Am. Coll. Surg.* **180**, 433.

United Nations Organization. (1979). Age and sex composition by population, by country, 1960–2000. UNO, New York.

Ursea, N., Mircescu, G., Constantinovici, N. and Verzan, C. (1997). Nephrology and renal replacement therapy in Romania. *Nephrol. Dial. Transplant.* **12**, 684.

U.S. Renal Data System. (1994). USRDS 1994 annual data report. National Institutes of Health, National Institutes of Diabetes and Digestive and Kidney Diseases, Bethesda, Md.

U.S. Renal Data System. (1998). USRDS 1998 annual data report. National Institutes of Health, National Institute of Diabetes and Digestive and Kidney Diseases, Bethesda, Md.

U.S. Renal Data System. (1999). USRDS 1999 annual data report. The National Institutes of Health, National Institute of Diabetes and Digestive and Kidney Diseases, Bethesda, Md.

van Buuren, A. J., Bates, W. D. and Muller, N. (1999). Nephrotic syndrome in Namibian children. *S. Afr. Med. J.* **89**, 1088.

Vathsala, A., Woo, K. T. and Lim, C. H. (1992). Renal transplantation in Singapore. *Transplant. Proc.* **24**, 1819.

Vela, C., Cristol, J. P., Hauet, T., Iborra, F., Chong, G. and Mourad, G. (1994). La transplantation rénal chez le sujet de pens de 60 ans: analyses de résultats à propos de 57 patients. *Nephrologie* **15**, 381.

Vosnides, G. G. (1997). Hepatitis C in renal transplantation (clinical conference). *Kidney Int.* **52**, 843.

Walele, A. A. (1998). Urinary tract infections in renal transplant recipients. Dissertation, University of Cape Town, Cape Town.

Walker, G., Neaton, J. D., Cutler, J. A., Neuwirth, W. M. and Cohen, J. (1992). Renal function changes in hypertensive members of the Multiple Risk Factor Intervention Trial. *J. A. M. A.* **268**, 3038.

Warrell, D. A. (1993). Venomous bites and stings in the tropical world. *Med. J. Aust.* **159**, 773.

Weber, G., Schwartz, E., Schlaeffer, F., Lang, R. and Alkan, M. (1998). Imported severe falciparum malaria in Israel. *J. Travel Med.* **5**, 97.

Weening, J. J., Brenner, B. M., Dirks, J. H. and Schrier, R. W. (1998). Toward global advancement of medicine: the International Society of Nephrology experience. *Kidney Int.* **54**, 1017.

Were, A. J. and McLigeyo, S. O. (1995). Cost consideration in renal replacement therapy in Kenya. *East Afr. Med J.* **72**, 69.

Were, A. J. O. (1999). Renal failure in Africa. *Kidney Int.* **55**, 2121.

Wilkinson, D. (1994). High compliance tuberculosis treatment programme in a rural community. *Lancet* **343**, 647.

Wilkinson, D. and de Cock, K. M. (1996). Tuberculosis control measures in South Africa: time for a new paradigm? *S. Afr. Med. J.* **86**, 33.

Winston, A., Klotman, M. E. and Klotman, P. E. (1999). HIV-associated nephropathy is a late, not early, manifestation of HIV-1 infection. *Kidney Int.* **55**, 1036.

World Bank. (1997). *World Bank Atlas,* 29th ed. The World Bank, Washington, D.C.

World Health Organization. (1994). TB: a global emergency. (WHO/TB/94.177). WHO, Geneva.

Xiao, X., Li, Y., Ao, J. and Chen, Y. (1992). Analysis of prognostic factors affecting renal allograft survival. *Transplant. Proc.* **24**, 1442.

Yadav, R. V. (1990). Transplantation as a health priority in India. *Transplant. Proc.* **22**, 908.

Yildiz, A., Sever, M. S., Turkmen, A., *et al.* (1998). Tuberculosis after renal transplantation: experience of one Turkish centre. *Nephrol. Dial. Transplant.* **13**, 1872.

Youmbissi, T. J. (1999). Renal failure in Africa. *Kidney Int.* **555**, 2119.

Zaid, D., Ramdani, B., Terrab, S., *et al.* (1993). Renal transplantation in Morocco: 101 transplants in 94 patients. *Transplant. Proc.* **25**, 2354.

Zaragoza, R. M., Hernandez, A., Trevino, M., Diliz, H. S. and Alvarez, L. (1996). Tuberculosis and renal transplantation. *Transplant. Proc.* **28**, 3309.

Zeigler, S. T., Gaston, R. S., Rhynes, V. K., *et al.* (1997). Renal transplantation in African-American recipients: three decades at a single center. *Transplant. Proc.* **29**, 3726.

39

Results of Renal Transplantation

Peter J. Morris

Introduction

Although much of this book discusses the many problems of renal transplantation and their prevention and management, it is only when the overall results of renal transplantation are reviewed, not only in terms of patient and graft survival but also patient rehabilitation, that the remarkable achievements of renal transplantation in the management of end-stage renal failure are placed in true perspective. Each edition of this book has presented a continuing improvement in cadaveric graft survival as illustrated by the United Network of Organ Sharing (UNOS) Registry in the United States (Fig. 39–1). Patient survival, which has been approximately 90% or better at 1 year for some time, has not improved much, mainly because of the higher risk patients now undergoing transplantation. Many of the results of renal transplantation in different situations are described in different chapters. In this chapter, the results of living related, living unrelated and cadaver renal transplantation are summarized, paying particular attention to the many factors that influence graft survival. I have drawn extensively on data from several registries of renal transplantation, including the UNOS, the Collaborative Transplant Study (CTS), the European Dialysis and Transplant Association (EDTA) and the United Kingdom Transplant Service Support Authority (UKTSSA). The results of transplantation in children have been described fully in Chapter 37 and are not discussed further.

Patient and Graft Survival
LIVING RELATED DONORS
Monozygotic Twins

Monozygotic twins are the ideal donor and recipient because of their genetic identity for major and minor histocompatibility antigens. Transplantation between identical twins has not been uniformly successful, however, because failures occur as a result of technical problems or recurrent glomerulonephritis. Tilney *et al.* (1975) reviewed the results of 28 identical twin transplants at the Peter Bent Brigham Hospital, where the first pioneering transplant between identical twins was performed in 1954. Two deaths occurred within 2 weeks of transplantation, one from infarction of the kidney and one from septicemia secondary to a perinephric infection. Seven other patients developed recurrent nephritis at 6 months to 10 years posttransplantation; five patients died of the recurrent disease because of lack of maintenance dialysis to which these patients could be returned. An analysis of the Brigham experience of 30 identical twin transplants (Tilney, 1986), in which follow-up extended to 27 years, showed a 25-year patient survival rate of around 65% and a graft survival rate of around 55% (Fig. 39–2). Eight of the 11 graft failures were due to recurrent nephritis, occurring 3 months to 20 years posttransplantation. In general, the recipients remained in excellent health; cardiovascular disease took its toll as time progressed, primarily in the more elderly recipients.

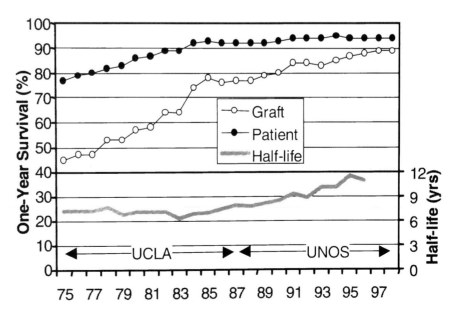

FIGURE 39–1

The changing results of kidney transplants in the United States as reported by the UCLA Registry and in more recent years by UNOS. (Reproduced with permission of Cecka, 2000.)

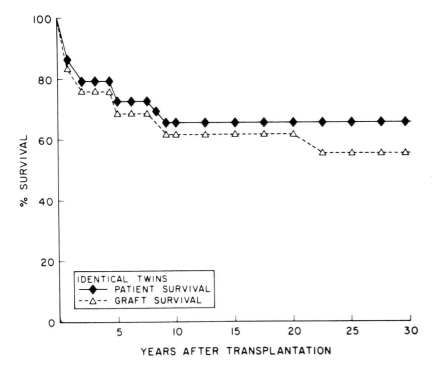

FIGURE 39–2

The survival of patients and grafts after identical twin transplants at the Brigham Hospital. (Reproduced with permission of Tilney, 1986.)

The EDTA Registry has reported 41 renal transplants between monozygotic twins. Glomerulonephritis was the original cause of renal failure in 24 of these patients. Of 41 patients, 36 were alive with functioning grafts 12 to 174 months posttransplantation. Two grafts failed from recurrent disease, two grafts failed from *de novo* glomerulonephritis and one recipient died in a traffic accident (Kramer *et al.*, 1982). One donor developed renal failure secondary to the same glomerulonephritis as in the original recipient. There seems to be a case for using some immunosuppression in identical twin recipients when the original disease is a type of glomerulonephritis with a high recurrence rate (see Chapter 4), but how much and what type of immunosuppression should be used are uncertain. There are no data concerning outcome of renal transplants in monozygotic twins in this situation in the cyclosporine era.

Family Donors

Although living related donors were a significant source of kidneys in the Western world, especially in the United States, in the early years of transplantation, the improved results of cadaver transplantation with cyclosporine had led to a decline in the proportion of living related donor transplants in the Western world. The ever-increasing shortage in cadaver donors in relation to the demand has led, however, to a reappraisal of policies that tend to preclude living related transplantation because of the inherent risk to the donor, especially in Europe. A family donor is defined as a first-degree relative—a sibling, a parent or a child—although more distant relatives (e.g., cousin or uncle) are used more frequently. There has been a dramatic increase in the use of living unrelated donors, mostly, but not always, spouse-to-spouse transplants; these donors generally are described as emotionally related donors.

Within the family, the HLA-identical sibling transplant is the ideal donor-recipient combination for transplantation (apart from the rare instance of an identical twin transplant). In the azathioprine era, the results of HLA-identical transplants were excellent (Salvatierra *et al.*, 1977; Simmons *et al.*,

1977), with a 90 to 95% 1-year graft survival rate. There has been some improvement in the cyclosporine era with the CTS Registry reporting a 1-year graft survival of around 95% and a 5-year graft survival of 85% (Fig. 39–3). In the azathioprine era, loss of kidneys secondary to rejection was reported (d'Apice *et al.*, 1976; Dick *et al.*, 1972; Salaman *et al.*, 1976), presumably caused by prior sensitization against minor histocompatibility antigens. No such cases have been reported in the cyclosporine era, although rejection still is seen. Today, recurrent glomerulonephritis is the main cause of graft failure in HLA-identical sibling transplants. In a study of 60 recipients of HLA-identical living related sibling grafts, 33 with chronic glomerulonephritis and 27 with non-glomerular disease, approximately 30% of recipients with glomerulonephritis had failed at 10 years from recurrent disease compared with none with nonglomerular disease (Andresdottir *et al.*, 1999).

Controversy exists as to whether cyclosporine should be used in HLA-identical sibling transplants, bearing in mind the possible long-term nephrotoxic effects of cyclosporine and the excellent results achieved with azathioprine and prednisolone. This concept was disputed by Flechner and colleagues, who maintained that cyclosporine led to less loss of kidneys from chronic rejection and that there was no evidence of nephrotoxicity at least 3 years posttransplantation (Flechner *et al.*, 1987). It is reasonable to conclude today that the concern about cyclosporine and long-term nephrotoxicity in this situation is not borne out by experience, and graft survival appears to be a little better in the cyclosporine era (Cecka, 2000; Opelz *et al.*, 1999; see Fig. 39–3). Current policy with HLA-identical sibling transplants in Oxford is to use the current triple-therapy protocol (see Chapter 16) but to discontinue steroids within 6 months of transplantation and to maintain whole-blood trough levels of cyclosporine at 100 to 150 ng/ml. Azathioprine is continued at 1.5 mg/kg, but if any problem occurs with leukopenia, this dosage is reduced further or discontinued.

As has been noted, the outcome of 1-haplotype-identical living related transplants between siblings, parent to child and child to parent, has improved dramatically over many

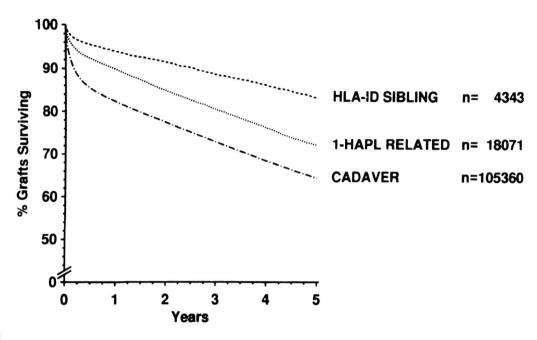

FIGURE 39–3

Survival of primary kidney grafts according to relationship in the CTS Registry (1987–1997). (Reproduced with permission of Opelz *et al.*, 1999.)

years. This improvement was due in the first instance to donor-specific transfusion, with or without azathioprine, and subsequently to the introduction of cyclosporine (Anderson *et al.*, 1987; Cheigh *et al.*, 1987; Flechner *et al.*, 1984; Groth *et al.*, 1987; Iwaki and Terasaki, 1986; Norman *et al.*, 1987; Sanfilippo and Vaughn, 1987; Terasaki *et al.*, 1985). The controversies referred to in the previous edition of this text—whether donor-specific transfusions are any more effective than random transfusions and whether transfusions are still necessary in the cyclosporine era—no longer remain so. The general consensus in the University of California Los Angeles (UCLA) and UNOS registries in North America and the CTS in Europe was that neither donor-specific nor random transfusion influences survival of 1-haplotype-disparate living related grafts (Ahmed and Terasaki, 1992; Opelz, 1993b).

Salvatierra, who introduced the donor-specific transfusion protocol into living related transplantation, still believes that donor-specific transfusion under azathioprine before transplantation and combined with a sequential cyclosporine protocol results in a better graft survival. Salvatierra and coworkers reported a 98% 4-year graft survival rate in 71 recipients of 1-haplotype-disparate and 2-haplotype-disparate living related transplants compared with a 65% 4-year graft survival in historical groups treated with cyclosporine but not given donor-specific transfusion (Salvatierra *et al.*, 1991). Groth *et al.* (1987) reported earlier that the outcome of 1-haplotype-disparate living related transplants was equal to that of HLA-identical siblings with cyclosporine, regardless of whether transfusions were given to the recipient before transplantation. At present, it does not seem that random or donor-specific transfusions are necessary in recipients of living related transplants treated with a cyclosporine-based protocol. Nevertheless, an open mind should be kept about the role of donor-specific transfusions in view of the enormous literature on antigen-induced specific unresponsiveness (see Chapter 23). This question can be resolved only by a large prospective multicenter trial of donor-specific transfusions in haplotype-disparate living related transplants.

Although there has been reluctance in the past to use 2-

haplotype-disparate sibling donors, the advent of cyclosporine has changed those policies. Good early results reported in this situation (Salvatierra, 1986; Sanfilippo and Vaughan, 1987; Sodal *et al.*, 1987) continue to be borne out (Kaufman *et al.*, 1993; Salvatierra *et al.*, 1991; Sanfilippo *et al.*, 1990), although these results were achieved with donor-specific and/or random transfusions before transplantation. There no longer seems to be a major contraindication in the cyclosporine era to transplantation between 2-haplotype-disparate siblings, although it still is unclear whether blood transfusion is beneficial before transplantation. Prior transfusion may allow selection of a donor to which the recipient will be relatively unresponsive with a subsequent transplant. In a CTS analysis, there is a hierarchy of survival: Graft survival was best in HLA-identical transplants, followed by 1-haplotype-disparate sibling transplants, with 2-haplotype-disparate sibling transplants being distinctly worse (Fig. 39–4).

LIVING UNRELATED DONORS

In the third edition of this book, the question of living unrelated donors was considered for the first time. At that time, preliminary data from several units reported excellent early results in recipients of living unrelated or distantly related kidneys from emotionally related donors (e.g., spouses) (Belzer *et al.*, 1987; Kumar *et al.*, 1987; Reding *et al.*, 1987; Sodal *et al.*, 1987). In the 1990s, there was a rapid increase in experience of living unrelated transplantation, and the graft survival rate in these recipients of living unrelated kidneys is equivalent in North America to that of the 1-haplotype-disparate living related transplant survival rate and superior to the cadaver graft survival rate (Cecka, 2000; Cecka and Terasaki, 1993; Kaufman *et al.*, 1993; Pirsch *et al.*, 1991; Fig. 39–5). Similarly, in Korea, the graft survival rate of living unrelated transplants is similar to that of 1-haplotype-disparate living related transplants (Park *et al.*, 1993). In contrast, the earlier CTS data from Europe showed no difference in graft survival rates between living unrelated transplants and cadaver transplants (Opelz, 1993b). A more recent large analysis from the CTS shows that overall living unre-

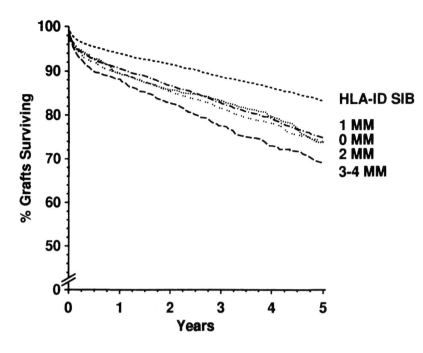

HLA-ID SIB   n=4343

1 MM   n=2749
0 MM   n= 605
2 MM   n=3859
3-4 MM   n= 910

FIGURE 39–4

Analysis of kidney transplants between siblings from the CTS Registry (1987–1997). 0 MM = transplants with no mismatch between donor and recipient (i.e., HLA compatible, but the siblings were not HLA identical). (Reproduced with permission of Opelz *et al.*, 1999.)

lated graft survival is superior to cadaver transplantation but that there is a distinct impact of fortuitous matching for HLA on graft outcome (Opelz *et al.*, 1999; Fig. 39–6).

There are major potential ethical problems with living unrelated donors (Morris, 1985, 1987), but the Transplantation Society does not prohibit such transplants, provided that the Society's guidelines are adhered to strictly (Council of the Transplantation Society, 1986). These issues were discussed in detail by Daar and Sells (1990) and are discussed further in Chapter 41.

CADAVER DONORS

Since the first edition of this book, there has been a marked increase in the number of kidney transplants performed throughout the world. Although this increase initially was due to an increase in cadaver transplantation, more recent years have seen the number of cadaver transplants remaining relatively stable or falling (with the marked excep-

tion of Spain), while the number of living donors has risen markedly, especially in European countries where previously the proportion of living donor transplants was relatively low.

Although improvements in graft survival had been noted in previous editions, predominantly resulting from the transfusion effect and possibly HLA matching (Morris, 1984), there has been a continuing increase in graft survival during the cyclosporine era (Cecka, 2000; Hariharan *et al.*, 2000; Table 39–1; see Fig. 39–1). The 1-year survival rate of first cadaver grafts approaches 90%, and the 1-year survival rate of second grafts is not much less, although that of third or more grafts is significantly less (Cecka, 1999). Patient survival after cadaver transplantation, which improved dramatically in the late 1970s in experienced units, has become generally excellent with most national or regional registries reporting 1-year patient survival rates of at least 90% with 5-year patient survival rates of around 80%.

In the second edition, it was noted that an analysis by Vollmer *et al.* (1983) of patients with end-stage renal failure

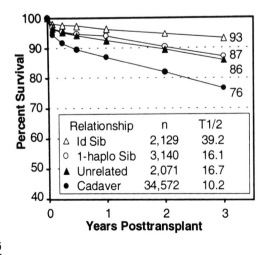

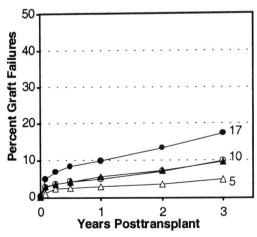

FIGURE 39–5

Graft survival and graft failure rates for living related and living unrelated grafts in the UNOS Registry between 1994 and 1998. T1/2 = half-life. (Reproduced with permission of Cecka, 2000.)

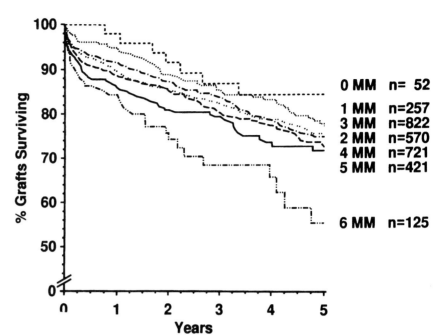

FIGURE 39-6

The influence of matching for HLA in transplants between living unrelated donors and recipients from the CTS Registry (1987–1997) (*P*<0.001). (Reproduced with permission of Opelz *et al.*, 1999.)

in the Northwest Kidney Center Program based in Seattle showed a significantly better survival rate after living related transplantation than after cadaver transplantation or with dialysis. No difference was found in patient survival rates after cadaver transplant or with dialysis after factors such as the period spent on dialysis before transplantation and the age and morbidity of the patient at the start of treatment were taken into account, however. This analysis did not address the quality of life after the respective treatments, but it did not support an argument in favor of cadaver transplantation over dialysis purely on the basis of patient survival. In the previous edition, I suggested that it would be surprising if a similar analysis today did not show that cadaver transplantation was a better approach to the treatment of end-stage renal failure than dialysis in terms only of patient survival. In terms of potential quality of life, there is little doubt that living related or cadaver transplantation is superior to dialysis (discussed later).

Now an important study from the U.S. Renal Data System Coordinating Center and the Department of Biostatistics at the University of Michigan (Wolfe *et al.*, 1999) shows that long-term survival of patients on the waiting list for cadaver transplantation was much better if the patient received a transplant. Wolfe and colleagues confirmed that overall survival of patients on dialysis was superior in patients who were placed on the waiting list for a transplant (annual death rate, 6.3 per 100 patient-years) compared with patients not placed on the list (annual death rate, 16.1 per 100 patient-years), reflecting the selection of healthier patients for possible transplantation (Wolfe *et al.*, 1999). In an intention-to-treat analysis of patients waiting on dialysis for a first cadaver transplant, Wolfe and colleagues showed that although there was a greater risk of death in the first few months posttransplantation, as time passed there was an increasingly better survival of patients who were transplanted (Wolfe *et al.*, 1999; Fig. 39–7). This improved survival was present in all age groups, although more marked in younger patients as well as in black Americans and diabetics. Overall the projected years of life of patients on the waiting list who did not receive a transplant was 10 years compared with 20 years in patients who received a first cadaver transplant. This important study should have a major impact on treatment programs for end-stage renal failure.

Factors Influencing Patient and Graft Survival

Many factors influence patient and graft survival after renal transplantation, and all of these are discussed in different chapters so that only the major factors involved are summarized here.

TABLE 39–1

PROJECTED HALF-LIVES OF RENAL TRANSPLANTS PERFORMED IN THE YEARS 1988–1995 IN THE UNITED STATES, BEFORE AND AFTER CENSORING OF DATA OF PATIENTS WHO DIED WITH FUNCTIONING GRAFTS

Donor	Projected Half-Lives							
	1988	*1989*	*1990*	*1991*	*1992*	*1993*	*1994*	*1995*
Before Censoring								
Living	12.7	15.0	14.8	14.8	16.9	16.7	21.8	21.6
Cadaver	7.9	8.7	8.8	9.7	9.6	10.3	11.0	13.8
After Censoring								
Living	16.9	20.8	19.9	21.5	21.9	22.9	35.0	35.9
Cadaver	11.0	12.0	12.5	14.5	14.2	15.1	17.4	19.5

Adapted with permission of Harihan *et al.*, 2000.

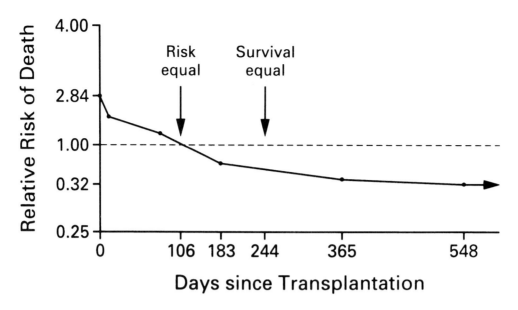

FIGURE 39–7

Adjusted relative risk of death among 23,275 recipients of a first cadaver transplant. The reference group was the 46,164 patients on dialysis who were on the waiting list (relative risk, 1.0). Patients in both groups had equal lengths of follow-up since placement on the waiting list. Values were adjusted for age, sex, race, cause of end-stage renal disease, year of placement on the waiting list, geographical region and time from first treatment for end-stage renal disease to placement on the waiting list. The points at which the risk of death and the likelihood of survival were equal in the two groups are indicated. The log scale was used. (Reproduced with permission of Wolfe et al., 1999.)

IMMUNOSUPPRESSION

Without some form of immunosuppression, there would be no transplantation except between monozygotic twins. Azathioprine and steroids were the backbone of transplantation for virtually 20 years, but the realization that low doses of steroids were as effective as high doses in the late 1970s resulted in a significant decrease in patient mortality rate and morbidity (see Chapter 15). Heterologous antilymphocyte globulin has been employed for many years either prophylactically to prevent rejection or to treat acute rejection episodes. Heterologous antilymphocyte globulin can be replaced by monoclonal antibody therapy, which is considered as the second generation of biological antilymphocyte reagents (see Chapter 20).

Cyclosporine-based protocols (see Chapter 16) are the backbone of immunosuppressive therapy today, although the advent of tacrolimus, mycophenolate and sirolimus is having an impact on the use of cyclosporine (see Chapters 17–19). Many other forms of immunosuppression have been used over the years, such as splenectomy, thymectomy, thoracic duct drainage, local graft irradiation and cyclophosphamide (see Chapter 21). All, for the most part, have become part of the rapidly evolving history of renal transplantation. Total lymphoid irradiation (see Chapter 22), although a potent immunosuppressive therapy, probably has been made redundant by the advent of cyclosporine. The three well-documented cases of donor-specific tolerance in a recipient of a renal allograft were treated with total lymphoid irradiation (Strober et al., 1989). The *holy grail* of tolerance induction in a human recipient of a renal transplant is coming closer (see Chapter 23).

MATCHING FOR HLA

Matching for HLA has been discussed in detail in Chapter 10. Donors and recipients of cadaver transplants in large bodies of data (e.g., CTS, UNOS and UKTSSA registries) show better short-term and long-term graft survival rates based on matching for HLA-A, HLA-B and HLA-DR (Cecka, 2000; Morris et al., 1999; Opelz et al., 1999; Figs. 39–8, 39–9 and 39–10). The recognition that matching for HLA-DR alone exerts an influence on the outcome of cadaver renal transplantation (Opelz et al., 1999), as first pointed out many years ago (Ting and Morris, 1978), even with cyclosporine immunosuppression, is important in that it allows the application of matching more readily to cadaver transplantation (Taylor et al., 1994).

BLOOD TRANSFUSIONS BEFORE TRANSPLANTATION

The transfusion effect probably was the most significant factor in the improved graft survival seen in living related and cadaver transplantation before the advent of cyclosporine therapy. The transfusion effect, the continuing existence of which was doubtful at the time of the last edition of this book, appeared to have disappeared as shown in the UCLA and UNOS registries and in the CTS (Ahmed and Terasaki, 1992; Gjertson, 1993; Opelz, 1993b). A prospective study of the effect of transfusions before transplantation in nontransfused recipients (Opelz et al., 1997), all of whom were receiving cyclosporine therapy, did show improved graft outcome in the patients who were deliberately transfused, however. Data from the UNOS also suggest a modest transfusion effect in the cyclosporine era in white recipients (Cicciarelli, 1990). There is a place still for careful and large randomized prospective trials of transfusions before cadaver and living donor transplantation in nontransfused recipients. One trial has been performed in the United States in non–HLA identical living donor transplants in which donor-specific transfusion was given 24 hours before transplantation, but no effect was seen (Alexander et al., 1999). It would appear that the title of one of the first articles on transfusions in renal transplantation, "The Paradox of Blood Transfusions in Renal Transplantation" (Morris et al., 1968), remains apt today.

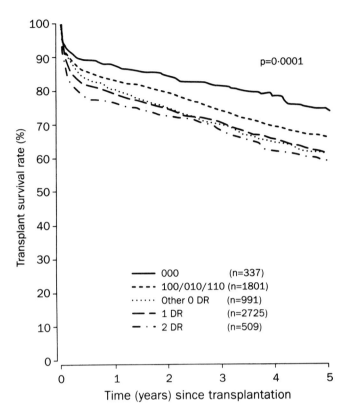

FIGURE 39-8

Survival of first cadaver renal allografts according to the number of mismatches between donor and recipient at the HLA-A, HLA-B and HLA-DR loci from UKTSSA (e.g., 010 = no mismatch at the HLA-A locus, 1 mismatch at the HLA-B locus and no mismatch at the HLA-DR locus). (Reproduced with permission of Morris *et al.*, 1999.)

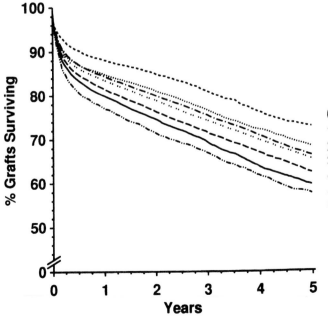

0 MM n= 4303
1 MM n= 6547
2 MM n=13765
3 MM n=19427
4 MM n=14496
5 MM n= 7125
6 MM n= 2250

FIGURE 39-9

The effect of HLA matching at the HLA-A, HLA-B and HLA-DR loci on outcome of first cadaver grafts from the CTS Registry (*P*<0.0001). (Reproduced with permission of Opelz *et al.*, 1999.)

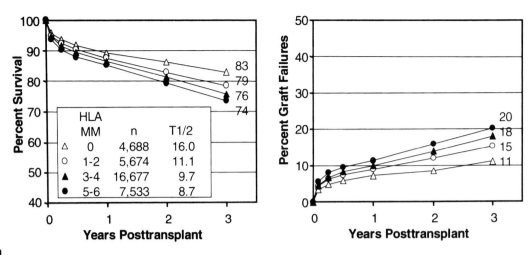

FIGURE 39–10

The effect of HLA matching at the HLA-A, HLA-B and HLA-DR loci on cadaver graft survival from the UNOS Registry (1994–1998). (Reproduced with permission of Cecka, 2000.)

SEX OF DONORS AND RECIPIENTS

The sex of the recipient first was claimed by Opelz and Terasaki (1977) to influence the effect of matching for HLA in cadaver transplantation in that graft outcome in male recipients was influenced by better compatibility between donor and recipient. These workers were unable to show any influence of mismatching for sex between donor and recipient, failing to confirm the suggestion of Oliver (1974) that there may be sex-linked histocompatibility antigens in humans. Subsequent analyses of the UCLA Registry data (Cecka, 1986; Kennealy, 1985) showed that there was no difference in graft survival between female and male recipients, despite a greater incidence of preformed lymphocytotoxic antibodies in female recipients. A further analysis of the UNOS Registry showed that the sex of the donor and recipient did not influence the short-term outcome of renal allografts, but transplants from female donors into male recipients had the worst 10-year graft survival rate (Terasaki et al., 1993). Of particular interest was the superior graft survival rate in mothers receiving a kidney from a child compared with that in fathers (the contrary of what might be expected), suggesting some form of enhanced suppression in mothers previously exposed during pregnancy to allogeneic histocompatibility antigens of the eventual kidney donor.

Another retrospective study was reported by Burlingham et al. (1998) of graft outcome in 1-haplotype-disparate sibling-to-sibling transplants in which the recipient received a kidney with a mismatch for the noninherited maternal or the paternal HLA antigen haplotype. Graft outcome at 5 years and at 10 years was significantly better in the siblings exposed to the noninherited maternal antigen than in siblings exposed to a noninherited paternal antigen, the so called *NIMA effect* (noninherited maternal antigen). This study suggested that a degree of unresponsiveness to maternal antigens not passed onto the fetus *in utero* had induced some specific unresponsiveness. A similar analysis from the CTS Registry did not confirm this finding, however (Opelz, 1999).

No evidence of a sex-linked histocompatibility antigen was found in that male-to-female transplants did no worse than female-to-male; in fact, the opposite occurred. Kidneys from male donors had significantly higher graft survival rates than kidneys from female donors, especially donors older than age 30, with cyclosporine immunosuppression (Gjertson, 1993). The deleterious influence of the female sex of the donor on graft survival appeared to be abrogated by matching for HLA-A and/or HLA-B, especially in patients receiving a second graft. The kidney from a female donor may fail earlier because of its smaller nephron mass and is therefore more likely to be exposed to nephron overload or hyperperfusion (Terasaki et al., 1994).

BLOOD GROUPS OF DONORS AND RECIPIENTS

Opelz and Terasaki (1977) first pointed out that the effect of HLA matching is influenced by the ABO blood group of the recipient because the matching influence was seen only in non-O recipients. This study tended to confirm the earlier observation of Joysey et al. (1973) that O recipients showed a better graft outcome than non-O recipients. An analysis of the UCLA Registry data shows that any advantage of the O recipient over the non-O recipient has been lost with cyclosporine (Cecka, 1986). There is a suggestion that kidneys from type O donors transplanted to non-O recipients had a better 1-year graft survival rate than O kidneys transplanted to O recipients.

These comments apply to ABO-compatible grafts, the accepted criterion for renal transplantation. Because of the concern about the larger size of waiting lists and the longer time on the waiting list of blood group O recipients, most national bodies (e.g., UKTSSA) restrict the use of O-type kidneys to O-type recipients except for highly sensitized patients or HLA-6 antigen matches. The outcome of ABO-incompatible grafts has been discussed in Chapter 10; with the exception of A_2-to-O type transplants, the usual outcome has been hyperacute rejection. An analysis of 113 ABO-incompatible grafts from the CTS group (Opelz, 1993b) showed that although greater than 50% of the grafts failed immediately or soon after transplantation, 40% survived for 3 years. Insufficient numbers were available to allow evaluation of the various incompatible subgroups (e.g., A_2 to O, B to O, AB to O). There were also 42 ABO-incompatible living related grafts in the CTS Registry, and nearly 70% were functioning at 1 year. This group presumably was made up largely of patients from Brussels who had been prepared with splenectomy, plasmapheresis and cyclophosphamide (see Chapter 10). Alkhunaizi and colleagues reported 15 A_2 kidneys transplanted in O or B recipients with only one failure in a patient with a high anti-A_1 titer who did not undergo plasma exchange in advance (Alkhunaizi et al., 1999). The data concerning cadaver ABO-incompatible grafts are of considerable interest and need more detailed evaluation.

RECIPIENT AGE

Since the first report of an acceptable outcome to renal transplantation in the elderly (Ost *et al.*, 1980) and the widespread introduction of cyclosporine-based immunosuppressive protocols, most units have adapted a much more liberal approach to the selection of elderly recipients for transplantation. The results of renal transplantation in the elderly (arbitrarily defined as >55, >60 or >65 years old in various reports) have continued to confirm the validity of such policies (Barry *et al.*, 1996; Benedetti *et al.*, 1994; Cantarovich *et al.*, 1994; Fauchald *et al.*, 1988; Fryd *et al.*, 1987b; Hirati *et al.*, 1996; Ismail *et al.*, 1994; Lauffer *et al.*, 1988; Mandelbaum *et al.*, 1987; Okiye *et al.*, 1983; Pirsch *et al.*, 1989, 1992; Roodnet *et al.*, 1999; Roza *et al.*, 1989; Tesi *et al.*, 1994). Although there is a higher mortality rate in the early years posttransplantation, which is reflected by a poorer graft survival (Fig. 39–11), rejection is less common than in younger patients and rarely a major problem (Jassal *et al.*, 1997). Cardiovascular disease, including pulmonary embolism, and infection are the two major causes of death in this age group. It is unusual for a graft to be lost from irreversible rejection. Bearing in mind the shortage of cadaver kidneys for renal transplantation, it is important to select elderly patients who are relatively low-risk recipients (Nyberg *et al.*, 1995a; Schulak *et al.*, 1990) and to use lower levels of immunosuppression. Nyberg and coworkers pointed out that some of their elderly patients lost muscular strength after transplantation, which they did not regain, emphasizing that rehabilitation after transplantation is not as good as that in the younger patient (Nyberg *et al.*, 1995b). The study by Wolfe *et al.* (1999), referred to earlier, points out that older patients have a survival advantage with a transplant compared with survival on dialysis. This study confirmed the same suggestion from an earlier Canadian study (Schaubel *et al.*, 1995).

DONOR AGE

Although it was observed in the 1970s that the older the donor, the poorer the survival of the graft (Darmady, 1974), this has become more evident since the introduction of cyclosporine. This poorer survival may be due to the higher nonfunction rate of kidneys from older donors in the presence of cyclosporine; it also reflects the use of more marginal kidneys from older donors in recent years.

The increasing age of donors is associated with reduced 1-year graft survival in many, but not all, single-center reports (Alexander and Vaughn, 1991; Langle *et al.*, 1992; Pirsch *et al.*, 1992; Rao *et al.*, 1990); in Oxford, increasing donor age has a major influence on graft outcome. The registry analyses all confirm that kidneys from elderly donors have a poorer long-term graft survival rate (Cecka, 2000; Morris *et al.*, 1999; see Fig. 39–11). An increasing body of evidence shows that renal function as judged by plasma creatinine level or creatinine clearance is poorer in recipients of kidneys from older donors (Ablaza *et al.*, 1993; Higgins *et al.*, 1995; Isoniemi *et al.*, 1992; Kasiske, 1988; Koffman *et al.*, 1993; Nghiem *et al.*, 1993; Rao *et al.*, 1990; Sumari *et al.*, 1991). This association with donor age and renal function is well illustrated in data from the Oxford Centre (Fig. 39–12).

Donor age has been shown to have a powerful association with long-term graft survival by Thorogood *et al.* (1992) using data from the Eurotransplant Registry. In a model that took into account HLA matching and other factors, such as diabetes, in the recipient, donor age was the most important vari-

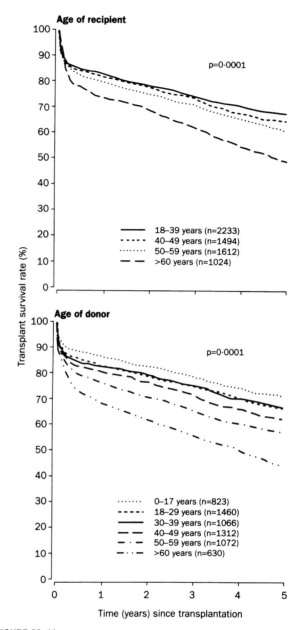

FIGURE 39–11

Survival of first cadaver transplants according to the age of the recipient and the age of the donor from UKTSSA. (Reproduced with permission of Morris *et al.*, 1999.)

able associated with the graft half-life. The influence of donor age overcame the effects of HLA-matching effect in patients. The mean graft half-life in patients with a well-matched graft from an elderly donor was 6.9 years (n = 48; 95% confidence interval, 4.8–9.9), whereas the half-life of an unmatched graft from a younger donor was 51% higher at 10.4 years (n = 588, 95% confidence interval, 8.6–12.5).

In another more recent multivariate analysis of outcome of first cadaver renal transplants in the United Kingdom, kidneys from donors greater than 50 years old fared less well at all time points after transplantation (Morris *et al.*, 1999). The deleterious impact of an elderly kidney on outcome was as great as the beneficial effect of a kidney matched at HLA-A, HLA-B and HLA-DR. Similar data have been reported

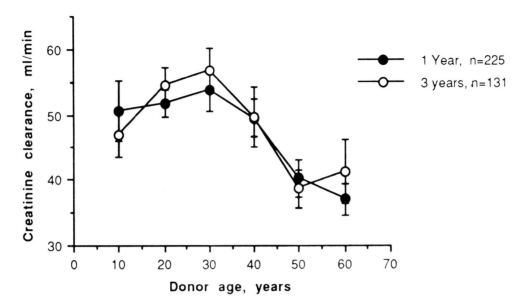

FIGURE 39–12

Creatinine clearance in recipients of cadaver renal transplants at Oxford in whom the kidney was functioning at 1 and 3 years posttransplantation, based on the age of the donor. (Reproduced with permission from Higgins *et al.*, 1995.)

from the UNOS (Chertow *et al.*, 1996; Cho and Terasaki, 1997).

Reduced graft function with increasing donor age is likely caused by reduction in renal reserve and nephron mass that occurs with normal human aging (Anderson and Brenner, 1986; Terasaki *et al.*, 1994). The extent of interstitial fibrosis, tubular atrophy and glomerulosclerosis is correlated with donor age before and after transplantation (Curschellas *et al.*, 1991; Gaber *et al.*, 1995; Isoniemi *et al.*, 1992). The average rate of loss of creatinine clearance from a normal human kidney greater than age 30 years is similar to that in a transplant population, at about 0.3 ml/min per year (Davies, 1950). Gaber and colleagues showed that when more than 20% of donor glomeruli are sclerosed, there is an increased risk of delayed graft function and poor outcome (Gaber *et al.*, 1995). Similar data have been presented in marginal donors, in which increasing degrees of glomerulosclerosis, interstitial fibrosis, tubular atrophy and arteriosclerosis in the donor kidney were associated with a poor outcome (Randhawa *et al.*, 2000). Pokorna and colleagues in a study of procurement biopsy specimens from 200 consecutive donors believe that the biopsy provides only limited information for the decision whether or not to proceed with transplantation of a kidney from a marginal donor (Pokorna *et al.*, 2000).

If normal aging of the kidney were to progress at a natural rate, there would be no major effect on survival. It may be that long-term graft survival depends on other factors, such as chronic vascular rejection or stimuli of interstitial fibrosis and glomerulosclerosis. Kidneys from older donors may be particularly vulnerable to the effects of other scarring processes because of reduced renal reserve or preexisting interstitial renal disease. For these reasons, there have been some studies of transplantation of both kidneys from an elderly donor into a single recipient, the results suggesting that this approach may be accompanied by a better outcome (Lee *et al.*, 1999; Dietl *et al.*, 2000; Lu *et al.*, 2000).

Kidneys from young donors also do poorly, especially kidneys from very young donors (Hayes *et al.*, 1988; Holzgreve *et al.*, 1987; Ildstad *et al.*, 1990; Ploeg *et al.*, 1987; Wengerter *et al.*, 1986). Ildstad *et al.* (1990) reported a 1-year graft survival rate of kidneys from donors less than 12 months

old, including anencephalic donors, of only 19%. The pediatric kidney does no better in the pediatric recipient than in the adult recipient (but perhaps for different reasons). There is an increasing tendency to try to transplant kidneys from older pediatric donors or adult donors into pediatric recipients because graft survival is better. Kidneys from the very young donor (e.g., <5 years old) may be implanted *en bloc* into adult donors with a reasonable expectation of a good result (see Chapter 11).

Donor age is an important factor in determining graft survival, and the use of kidneys from the very young and the very old should be avoided if possible. In older donors, immediate histology of the kidney may help to select kidneys that can be used with a reasonable expectation of a favorable outcome (Gaber *et al.*, 1995), although the correlation between histology and outcome is inexact (Pokorna *et al.*, 2000). There also is an increasing tendency to match older kidneys with older recipients, but such a policy makes the careful selection of low-risk older recipients more important, as discussed in the previous section. As shown in the UKTSSA analysis (Morris *et al.*, 1999), the effects of recipient age and donor age are independent of each other (Fig. 39–13).

TIME ON DIALYSIS

An early EDTA analysis showed that graft survival was better in patients who had been on dialysis for a long time (Jacobs *et al.*, 1977). This better survival rate might have been due to the death of poor-risk patients on dialysis before transplantation, to better matching of long-term well-dialyzed patients or to a greater likelihood of transfusions in patients on long-term dialysis. An increasing number of patients are now being transplanted before needing dialysis, and not only is there no evidence that graft survival in these two groups is worse than in patients on hemodialysis (Fryd *et al.*, 1987a; Tegzess *et al.*, 1987), but also a study from Oxford suggested that patients who were transplanted before requiring dialysis had a better graft outcome than a matched group of patients transplanted on dialysis, all patients being on cyclosporine (Roake *et al.*, 1996). This trend coincides with the use of cyclosporine, and it is not possible to distinguish

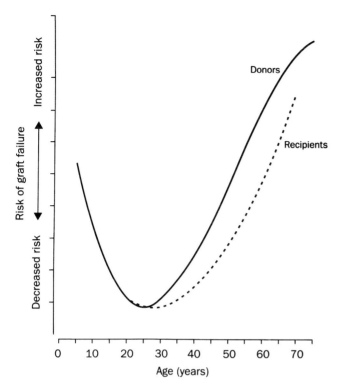

FIGURE 39–13

The pattern of risk of graft failure according to the age of the donor and recipient developed from a multifactorial Cox model with donor's age fitted as linear quadratic and cubic terms and recipient's age fitted as linear and quadratic terms based on the analysis presented in Figure 39–11. (Reproduced with permission of Morris *et al.*, 1999.)

any possible beneficial effect of long-term dialysis from that offered by cyclosporine.

BILATERAL NEPHRECTOMY

Several early analyses suggested that patients who have had a bilateral nephrectomy before transplantation have a better graft survival rate after transplantation (American College of Surgeons/NIH Organ Transplant Registry, 1975b; Sanfilippo *et al.*, 1984). This finding was attributed to the more frequent blood transfusions required by anephric patients on hemodialysis. An additional factor might be due to a reduction in the severity of hypertension after transplantation and a later reduction in cardiovascular mortality. Because bilateral nephrectomy before transplantation is an extremely uncommon practice now, this is no longer an important factor in determining graft survival.

INITIAL FUNCTION

Although there was some evidence in the precyclosporine era that delay in onset of function of the transplanted kidney was related to long-term impairment of renal function and graft survival (Davidson *et al.*, 1977), this had always been a subject of some controversy. This subject has attracted considerable interest with the use of cyclosporine, especially because there is evidence that cyclosporine nephrotoxicity may be enhanced in an ischemic kidney (see Chapter 16). In most reports, delayed graft function (usually defined as the need for dialysis in the first week posttransplantation) is associated with poorer graft survival (Belitsky *et al.*, 1987; Cecka, 2000;

Giral-Classe *et al.*, 1998; McLaren *et al.*, 1999; Moreso *et al.*, 1999; Nicholson *et al.*, 1996; Ohshima *et al.*, 1987; Ojo *et al.*, 1997; Perez-Fontan *et al.*, 1998; Pfaff *et al.*, 1998; Shoskes and Cecka, 1997, 1998; Taylor *et al.*, 1987; Tejani *et al.*, 1999). Although delayed graft function in the above-cited reports is an independent factor influencing graft outcome, there also is an increased incidence of acute rejection in many instances, and the combination of delayed graft function and acute rejection leads to the worst graft survival of all. In some reports, delayed graft function is not associated with poorer graft survival unless associated with acute rejection (Douzdjian *et al.*, 1997; Marcen *et al.*, 1998; Senel *et al.*, 1998; Troppmann *et al.*, 1995). An analysis of delayed graft function in Oxford showed that delayed graft function had a significant impact on graft survival, especially if associated with acute rejection in the first 3 months posttransplantation (McLaren *et al.*, 1999; Fig. 39–14).

Delayed graft function relates to subsequent renal function, and impairment of initial renal function, evident as early as the fifth transplant day by a serum creatinine level greater than 2.5 mg dl^{-1}, correlates with a poorer 1-year graft survival rate and poorer renal function at 1 year in surviving grafts (Belitsky *et al.*, 1987; Toyotome *et al.*, 1986), as does the level of renal function on the first day posttransplantation (Lim and Terasaki, 1992). Later analyses from the UCLA and UNOS registries confirmed that there is a striking correlation between graft survival at 3 years and 10 years posttransplantation and the serum creatinine level on discharge from the hospital as well as between the 10-year graft survival and the need for dialysis in the first week posttransplantation (Cecka and Terasaki, 1993; Terasaki *et al.*, 1993). Ten-year graft survival was 48% when no dialysis was required but 29% if dialysis was required. Other factors in this study influencing renal function in the initial period after transplantation were recipient weight, cold ischemia time and donor age (Cecka and Terasaki, 1993). Data from the UNOS confirm earlier findings (Cecka, 1999).

RACE

It was suggested in the azathioprine era that black recipients had significantly lower graft survival rates than white recipients and that kidneys from black donors seemed not to survive as well in recipients of either race (Opelz *et al.*, 1977). A later analysis by Perdue and Terasaki (1982) suggested that other factors, such as the center effect, were responsible for the apparent poorer survival of grafts in black recipients and of kidneys from black persons in recipients of either race. Similarly, at that time, no effect of race was found in the data of the SEOPF (Southeastern Organ Procurement Foundation) (McDonald *et al.*, 1981).

A thorough analysis of UCLA Registry data (Galton, 1985) confirmed that graft survival was lower in black American recipients than white or Latino recipients and that kidneys from black Americans had a worse graft survival rate regardless of whether they were in black or white recipients. Stratification of the data for a center effect confirmed that this was a significant factor in the different survival figures, but also suggested that other factors were important. These factors included the five times greater frequency of malignant hypertension in black recipients than in white recipients, better HLA-A and/or HLA-B and HLA-DR matching in white recipients and a lower transfusion rate in black recipients. Cyclosporine might alter the outcome of transplantation in blacks, as suggested by early data from Harbor-UCLA Medical Center, in which 1-year cadaver graft survival for black American recipients was around 90% (Ward *et al.*, 1987).

A considerable body of single-center and registry data is

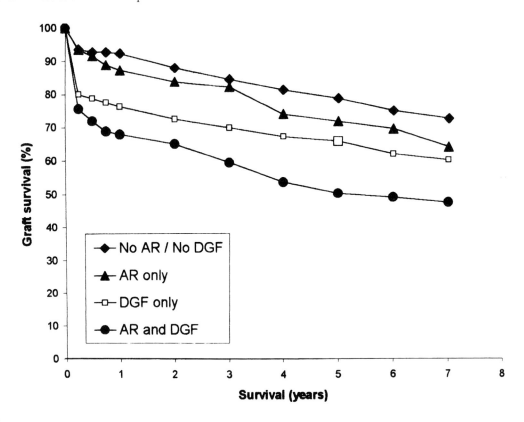

FIGURE 39–14

Kaplan-Meier actuarial survival curves for various combinations of acute rejection (AR) and delayed graft function (DGF). Acute rejection occurred in the first 3 months posttransplantation and was confirmed by biopsy. Delayed graft function was defined as the need for dialysis in the first week posttransplantation. Numbers at risk initially in individual groups: AR − DGF −, n = 235; AR − DGF +, n = 80; AR + DGF −, n = 260; AR + DGF +, n = 106. (Reproduced with permission of McLaren *et al.*, 1999.)

available, all of which confirm that the outcome of cadaver renal transplants is inferior in black recipients, even in the cyclosporine era (Butkus, 1991). Data from the UNOS, UCLA and CTS registries continue to confirm the much poorer graft survival in black recipients, regardless of whether the donor was black or white (Cecka, 2000; Cecka and Terasaki, 1993; Koyama *et al.*, 1994; Opelz, 1993b; Terasaki *et al.*, 1993; Fig. 39–15). In contrast, transplants in Asian recipients appear to

have a superior graft survival to that of white recipients (Cecka, 2000; Cho and Terasaki, 1996; Opelz, 2000; Fig. 39–15).

The survival of black HLA-identical sibling transplants is the same as that for whites, in marked contrast to 1-haplo-type-matched black sibling transplants, which is much poorer and on the same level as black cadaver graft survival (Cecka and Terasaki, 1993; Laskow *et al.*, 1992). The reasons

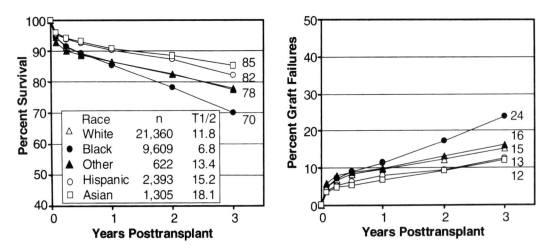

FIGURE 39–15

Survival of kidney grafts according to the race of the recipient from the UNOS Registry (1994–1998). (Reproduced with permission of Cecka, 2000.)

for the poorer graft survival in black recipients are uncertain and cannot be reconciled easily with the previous hypotheses of poor compliance, center effect and poorer matching.

ASSOCIATED DISEASE

The presence of comorbid disease, such as cardiovascular, pulmonary or diabetes-related conditions, decreases patient survival and occasionally graft survival. The original disease causing end-stage renal failure might be expected to influence graft survival. Patients with diabetic nephropathy invariably have lower graft survival rates than patients with glomerulonephritis, pyelonephritis or polycystic disease as the cause of end-stage renal failure. Similarly, patients with systemic lupus erythematosus have been said to have a lower graft survival rate than other patients with major diseases (Cats and Galton, 1985; Mitsuishi and Cecka, 1993), but this no longer seems to be evident (Cecka, 1999). Patients with Fabry's disease and oxalosis in the UNOS data have 5-year graft survival rates of approximately 60% (Cecka, 1999). Poorer graft survival rate in diabetic patients is apparent in the UNOS, EDTA and UKTSSA registries but was not seen in the enormous Minneapolis experience, in which graft survival in diabetic patients was no different at 1 and 6 years than that in nondiabetic patients (Basadonna et al., 1993).

By investigating all new patients with diabetic end-stage renal failure for coronary artery disease, including the use of angiography, Lorber and colleagues showed that 32% of patients with significant coronary artery disease were suitable for coronary artery surgery (Lorber et al., 1987). In their diabetic group as a whole, patient survival was 92% at 1 and 4 years posttransplantation, which they attributed to the prevention of deaths from myocardial infarction in the early years posttransplantation. A more aggressive approach to associated disease may be indicated in patients presenting with end-stage renal failure who are candidates for transplantation, especially with respect to the investigation and treatment of coronary artery disease.

REJECTION

Rejection episodes requiring treatment during the first hospitalization after transplantation or in the first 6 months after transplantation are associated with a poorer graft survival rate at 1 and 3 years than in patients with no rejection episodes. Rejection episodes appear to be a major determinant of graft outcome in the UNOS Registry data (Hariharan et al., 2000; Koyama and Cecka, 1993; Matas et al., 2000). The association between the graft outcome and the early rejection course of the graft was first noted in the 1960s (Williams et al., 1967); currently, with far more potent immunosuppression, it remains a major determinant of graft outcome in the long-term (Cecka, 2000; Hariharan et al., 2000; Terasaki et al., 1993; Fig. 39–16; see Fig. 39–14). As discussed in the previous section, this association is more striking in kidneys that have delayed graft function after transplantation. Nevertheless the incidence of acute rejection as a surrogate marker of long-term graft survival has proved to be disappointing in the modern multicenter trials of new immunosuppressive agents, in which a reduced incidence of acute rejection has not been reflected in general by improved graft survival. To some extent, this result is due to the histological classification of rejection used in these trials (Bates et al., 1999; see Chapter 24). The minor grades of rejection with no vascular changes and that respond to treatment satisfactorily do not appear to be associated with poorer graft survival.

Another observation is that the impact of rejection on graft survival in cadaver transplantation is greater when the kidney was from a young or old donor, suggesting that the decreased nephron mass in such kidneys might make them more susceptible to the damage produced by the rejection reaction. It was confirmed that matching for HLA-A, HLA-B and HLA-DR influenced strongly the incidence of early rejection episodes, especially matching for HLA-DR. These observations from the UNOS Registry and other centers concerning the significant impact of early rejection episodes on graft outcome (Christianns et al., 1991; Groenewoud, 1987; Hariharan et al., 2000; Lundgren et al., 1986; Taylor et al., 1994; Vanrentergehm et al., 1987; see Chapter 10) suggest that attempts to reduce the incidence of early rejection episodes by better matching, particularly for HLA-DR, or more potent immunosuppression might be rewarding in terms of better long-term graft survival, provided that the side effects of more potent immunosuppression do not outweigh any potential benefits.

PRESERVATION AND ISCHEMIC TIMES

Although there has been some renewed interest in pump preservation and its possible use in the evaluation of mar-

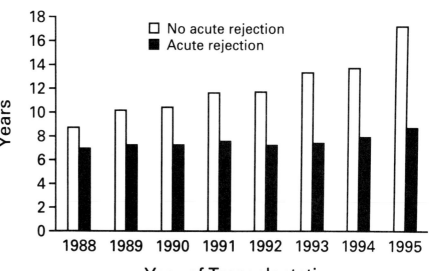

FIGURE 39–16

Projected half-lives of grafts from cadaver donors according to the presence or absence of clinical acute rejection during the first year posttransplantation in transplants performed in the period 1988–1995 from UNOS. (Reproduced with permission of Hariharan et al., 2000.)

ginal kidneys (Daemen *et al.*, 1999), cold storage of the kidney after perfusion with a variety of preservation solutions is the normal practice (see Chapter 9). Although Collins and EuroCollins solutions have been the most commonly used preservation solutions for many years, the University of Wisconsin (UW) solution has become increasingly popular and is now used by most North American units and approximately 50% of units in Europe. Although a randomized prospective multicenter trial of UW versus EuroCollins solution in Europe (Ploeg *et al.*, 1992) showed that delayed graft function was commoner in the EuroCollins group and that 1-year graft survival rate was better in the UW group (88% *vs.* 83%; *P* = 0.04), the UCLA Registry data and the CTS data failed to confirm these findings, at least with preservation up to 24 hours (Opelz, 1993a; Zhou and Cecka, 1993). After 24 hours of preservation or cold ischemia, the use of UW solution was associated with a better 1-year graft survival rate in the CTS data. The duration of cold ischemia appeared to be associated with a poorer graft outcome, particularly in the case of the younger donor, whereas the older donor kidney had a poorer outcome regardless of the duration of cold ischemia (Zhou and Cecka, 1993). More recent analyses confirm that outcome is poorer with prolonged ischemia times (>20–30 hours). In an analysis of more than 3,000 kidney pairs in which one of each pair had at least 10 hours greater cold ischemia time, the kidneys with the longer ischemia time had a greater incidence of delayed graft function, rejection and primary nonfunction (Cecka, 2000). Histological evidence of ischemia/reperfusion injury in approximately 50% of biopsy specimens of cadaver transplants obtained about 30 minutes posttransplantation, but not in biopsy specimens of living donors (Koo *et al.*, 1998; see Chapter 25), has led to renewed interest in reducing cold ischemia times to a minimum. These changes occur on top of those occurring as a result of brain death (Koo *et al.*, 1999).

COMPLIANCE WITH IMMUNOSUPPRESSIVE TREATMENT

There is a growing awareness of noncompliance with immunosuppression that may result in rejection and graft loss (Santiago-Delpin *et al.*, 1989; Schweizer *et al.*, 1990). This subject has been reviewed extensively by Colon *et al.* (1991); it is a problem that is probably much greater than most clinicians realize. Santiago-Delpin and colleagues described noncompliance as the "most important problem with which they are currently involved" in Puerto Rico (Santiago-Delpin *et al.*, 1989). Noncompliance rates in reports range from 5 to 43% (Beck *et al.*, 1980; Didlake *et al.*, 1988). As Colon and colleagues suggested in their review, prospective studies are needed that assess compliance over extended periods and compare it over various aspects of treatment (Colon *et al.*, 1991). Both types of studies need to be associated with detection techniques, such as blood levels and pill counting. Raiz and colleagues suggested that compliance with medication after transplantation is associated with subjective rather than objective variables (e.g., patients' positive feelings for their physicians and the experience of transplantation) (Raiz *et al.*, 1999). Noncompliance is a factor that cannot be evaluated accurately at present, but it is an important determinant of graft outcome and an important factor determining the outcome of clinical trials, as pointed out by Matas (1999).

CENTER EFFECT

The center effect has been one of the most significant factors influencing graft survival (Cicciarelli, 1985; Gilks *et al.*, 1984; Opelz *et al.*, 1975; Taylor *et al.*, 1985). The likelihood of survival with a functioning graft after transplantation depended more on the center in which the patient was to be treated than any of the factors already discussed. Numerous attempts have been made to explain the center effect, including different transfusion policies, different criteria for patient acceptance, different HLA-matching policies and different waiting times for transplantation as a result of race, sensitization, original disease and sex—everything that is known to influence graft survival.

The difference between the best and the worst cadaver 1-year graft survival figures was of the order of 40% in all these earlier analyses. Whether this wide range of results still exists in the cyclosporine era is not known, but almost certainly it does not. Mickey (1986) found no change, other than that the results in all centers had improved by about 10% regardless of whether they were centers with bad, average or good survival figures. The United Kingdom Transplant Service Registry showed a dramatic decrease in the range of 1-year graft survival figures in the period 1978–1984, by which time cyclosporine was being used by all units. In 1978, the range of 1-year graft survival was 60 to 78%, whereas in 1984, it was 75 to 82% (Bradley *et al.*, 1986a). An audit by the UKTSSA analyzed cadaver transplants performed in 31 centers in the years 1981–1986 and 1987–1991. In the first period, the range of graft survivals at 1 year was 57 to 85% with 27 of 33 centers having a graft survival rate of 70 to 80%. The patient survival rate at 1 year ranged from 68 to 94% with 19 centers being 90% or greater. In the second period, the 1-year graft survival rate was 75 to 95% with 24 of 31 centers having a 1-year graft survival of 80% or better. The patient survival rate was 79 to 96% with 23 centers being 90% or greater (UKTSSA Renal Transplant Audit, 1993). A more recent UKTSSA audit of renal transplantation showed that the center effect was less apparent, with the range of 1-year graft survival being around 10% (range 80–90%), which was not significant (unpublished data).

Although there are considerable differences between centers in the different factors that can influence graft survival, the center effect cannot be explained on this basis alone. In an earlier study, Taylor and colleagues spent several days in each of a selected number of centers in the United Kingdom with good, average and bad results. They evaluated prospectively 50 consecutive transplants in detail and concluded that clinical care was of considerable importance in explaining the center effect but that it was impossible to assess this in any objective way (Taylor *et al.*, 1985). Burdick and Williams (1986) showed in their own center that there was a difference in graft outcome depending on whether the patient lived in the city or in the country.

Mickey (1986) addressed the center effect in detail, considering only transplants performed in the period 1983–1984, and confirmed that a wide range of results occurs for first-cadaver transplants regardless of whether or not cyclosporine is given. Mickey believed that the center effect could not be explained on the basis of the differences in centers for factors known to influence graft survival. He also showed that the center effect is not confined to the early posttransplantation period but continues for grafts functioning at 3 months. Of considerable relevance was Mickey's examination of the results of HLA-identical sibling transplants in which no center effect was apparent, but the numbers were not adequate to exclude the existence of a center effect.

The analysis of the center effect from the UNOS Registry in the early 1990s (Cho and Cecka, 1993; Gjertson, 1993) confirmed that the center effect still existed in the United States and was a dominant influence on graft outcome. Cho and Cecka (1993) assigned 115 centers in North America to one of four groups by ordering weighted scores based on the

TABLE 39–2

GRAFT SURVIVAL AND HALF-LIVES OF CADAVER GRAFTS BASED ON THE GROUPING OF CENTERS ACCORDING TO A WEIGHTED OUTCOME

| Centers | Graft Survival (%) | | | |
	6 mo	1 y	3 y	Half-Life (y)
Group I	89	88	80	15.3
Group II	87	84	73	10.1
Group III	82	80	69	9.8
Group IV	77	75	64	8.3

Derived from data from Cho and Cecka, 1993.

estimated 6-month graft survival rates and half-lives in the period 1987–1992 (Table 39–2). Group I centers had a better 6-month graft survival rate and a longer half-life than groups II, III and IV. First, there was no difference between the centers in the outcome of living related transplants. Second, there was no correlation between graft survival at 6 months and half-lives projected for grafts surviving 6 months. Third, group IV centers (those with the poorest short-term and long-term graft survival rates) transplanted more elderly and more hospitalized patients and used more kidneys with prolonged ischemia times, kidneys from very young or old donors and kidneys from black donors. This analysis illustrated for the first time that case mix can be responsible for the center effect, at least in part. In support of this study is a more recent analysis of UNOS data, which shows that most transplant centers achieved survival rates not significantly different from their expected survival rates and that center effects were most apparent in the first year posttransplantation (Lin et al., 1998). The most recent analysis of the center effect by Terasaki and Cecka (2000) examined the difference in a graft outcome between large and small centers. Ten-year graft survival rates at larger centers were no more than 5% greater than at smaller centers. Larger centers had better results in diabetic recipients, with older donors, with living unrelated donors, in regrafts and in sensitized recipients.

Although the center effect does exist, it is a less important influence on the outcome of renal transplantation, and to a large extent it is explained by case mix of the usual factors known to influence graft outcome. Nevertheless one is left with the unavoidable conclusion that factors that are impossible to evaluate, such as preoperative selection, surgical techniques and postoperative care and follow-up, must also be important, which is not surprising.

SENSITIZATION AND REGRAFTS

The presence of sensitization as determined by lymphocytotoxic panel reactivity did not appear to influence the outcome of first-cadaver grafts but did exert a deleterious influence on second and third grafts (Iwaki et al., 1986). A more recent UNOS analysis of all cadaver grafts showed an association between the degree of sensitization and graft outcome (Cecka, 2000). Similarly, more recent CTS data showed a poorer graft outcome in recipients with greater than 50% panel reactivity, unless the recipient received a kidney with no HLA mismatches (Opelz et al., 1999). Sequential grafts in general have a poorer outcome than first grafts (Bradley et al., 1986b). The influence of peak or current preformed antibodies is complicated by the approach each unit takes to the interpretation of the crossmatch between recipient and donor (see Chapter 10). The presence of high levels of panel-reactive cytotoxic antibodies has been shown to be associated with

the occurrence of never-functioning kidneys, the incidence of which increases with sequential grafts. This difference in the incidence of never-functioning kidneys accounts entirely for the different graft survival figures for first, second and third grafts (Iwaki et al., 1986) and suggests that hyperacute rejection, albeit modified, has occurred in many of these patients with never-functioning kidneys. At Oxford, where a sophisticated level of pretransplant antibody screening of all recipients together with a similar level of sophistication in the crossmatch before transplantation exists, the outcome of patients with regrafts is identical overall to that of first-cadaver grafts (see Chapter 10 and Fig. 10–9). Nevertheless, in the CTS data, second grafts do not do as well as first grafts (Opelz, 1993b). In the UNOS data, not only do sequential grafts have a poorer outcome than first grafts, but also patients who are sensitized do less well than nonsensitized patients, with the peak antibody reactivity being most predictive of graft outcome (Cecka, 2000; Ogura, 1993; Opelz, 1999). The outcome in the sensitized patient depends on a variety of factors, such as the class and the specificity of the antibody, the crossmatch and the technique used for crossmatching and a first graft versus a regraft.

Many factors influence the fate of a second or subsequent graft (Morris et al., 1981), but in general in the azathioprine era the fate of a second graft depended on the source of the first and the second graft, the cause of graft loss and the duration of the first graft. Although there is disagreement about some of these points, a second–living related graft would do nearly as well as a first-related graft, whereas a second-cadaver graft would tend to have a higher failure rate than a first-cadaver graft. A second-cadaver graft after a first-related graft would do as well as a first-cadaver graft, whereas a second-related graft after a first-cadaver graft would do as well as a first-cadaver graft. If the first graft is lost by rejection within the first few months posttransplantation, a second graft would have a worse chance than a first graft, but if the first graft is lost some years after transplantation, a second graft has an equal chance of doing well (Ascher et al., 1979; Husberg and Starzl, 1974; Kountz et al., 1972; Opelz et al., 1976).

The influence of duration of the first graft on the outcome of a second graft was shown by the EDTA analysis in the precyclosporine era (Jacobs et al., 1977): Second-graft survival at 1 year was 57% if the first graft functioned for more than 1 year but only 37% if the first graft failed from rejection within 3 months of transplantation. Subsequent examination of the UCLA Registry data showed the same differences, but cyclosporine appeared to have improved the regraft survival figure in patients losing their kidneys within 3 months of transplantation as well as after 3 months (Cicciarelli, 1985). This analysis showed a marked effect of matching for HLA-A and/or HLA-B in so-called responder patients—those who had lost the first kidneys in the first 3 months.

Analysis of the UCLA and UNOS Registry data confirmed that loss of grafts at any time up to 6 months was associated with a significantly poorer graft survival of a retransplant than if the first graft had survived for longer than 6 months (Mitsuishi and Cecka, 1992). Similarly, recipients who had lost grafts within 6 months but were sensitized (panel-reactive antibody >10%) had a poorer regraft survival than nonsensitized recipients. In contrast, regrafts in patients whose first graft lasted more than 6 months showed a similar survival whether sensitized or not. Overall, the survival rate of regrafts has improved steadily in the UCLA and UNOS registries, more than the rate for first grafts, but there is a 10% difference in 1-year graft survival rates between first grafts and regrafts. As pointed out in Chapter 10, the survival of regrafts and grafts in sensitized patients can be similar to that of first grafts, provided that there is adequate characterization of the class and specificity of antibodies in the recipient and a sensitive crossmatch technique.

TRANSPLANTATION FOR CONGENITAL AND METABOLIC DISORDERS

Renal transplantation has been performed in a variety of congenital and metabolic diseases in sufficient numbers to assess the outcome of grafts in these situations. Diabetes mellitus is the commonest of these metabolic disorders requiring transplantation (see Chapter 36). The number of diabetic patients being accepted for treatment for end-stage renal failure is increasing steadily each year. For example, in Europe, the number of diabetic patients has increased from less than 2% of all new patients in 1973 to more than 7% in 1981, and this figure continues to increase; it is 23% in Finland (Ekstrand et al., 1987). In the UNOS Registry, diabetes is responsible for 36% of white patients receiving a renal transplant in the United States, which is the commonest cause of end-stage renal failure (Mitsuishi and Cecka, 1993). The results of renal transplantation in patients with diabetic nephropathy have been poor in the past. For example, in the precyclosporine era, the American College of Surgeons/NIH Organ Transplant Registry (1975a) reported that of patients receiving cadaver grafts, 62% were alive and 35% of the grafts were functioning at 1 year, whereas of patients receiving a living related graft, 80% were alive and 62% of the grafts were functioning at 1 year. These results were much worse than those in nondiabetic patients.

Since 1975, the results of transplantation in diabetic patients have improved considerably as units have gained more experience in the care of these patients (see Chapter 36). This improvement was stimulated by the superb results of the Minneapolis Unit that were achieved with conventional immunosuppression (Najarian et al., 1980, 1989). The UCLA Registry reported 1-year cadaver graft survival of 50% and greater than 80% for HLA-identical siblings in diabetic patients (Cats and Galton, 1985). Since cyclosporine became available, the results of transplantation in diabetic patients have improved further, perhaps because of the steroid-sparing property of cyclosporine. The Minneapolis group found no difference in a prospective trial of cyclosporine versus conventional therapy with antilymphocyte globulin or in the development of diabetes-related complications (Pescovitz et al., 1987). With current immunosuppressive protocols, the 1-year and 6-year graft survival rates are similar in diabetic and nondiabetic recipients, although living related donor transplant recipients have a better outcome than cadaver recipients (Basadonna et al., 1993; Frey et al., 1992).

The UNOS analysis of the period 1987–1992 shows that, with the exception of patients whose renal failure was due to IgA nephropathy (who did better), there was no difference in cadaver graft survival rates at 1 year; about 80% survived regardless of the cause of end-stage renal failure. By 3 years, the graft survival rate at 1 year ranged from 77% for IgA nephropathy to 62% for nephrosclerosis and around 67% for insulin-dependent diabetes (Mitsuishi and Cecka, 1993). In the diabetic group in the UNOS data, a better graft survival rate was observed in recipients who were HLA-DR3/4 (as expected, being most of the recipients) compared with those who were not HLA-DR3/4. As stressed in Chapter 36, transplantation is now the treatment of choice for diabetic patients with end-stage renal failure. There is an enhanced survival in diabetic patients who are transplanted in comparison with those on the waiting list but not transplanted, as discussed earlier (Wolfe et al., 1999).

Of the other metabolic and congenital disorders causing end-stage renal failure, information is available about many patients with end-stage renal failure resulting from Alport's syndrome, amyloidosis, cystinosis, Fabry's disease, familial nephritis, gout, medullary cystic disease, exalosis and systemic lupus erythematosus (American College of Surgeons/NIH Organ Transplant Registry, 1975a; Cecka, 1999; Groth and Ringden, 1984; Mitsuishi and Cecka, 1993). The results of renal transplantation are similar to those of the commoner causes of end-stage renal failure, with the exception of Fabry's disease and oxalosis (see Chapter 4), but UNOS data show a much improved outcome in these conditions (Cecka, 1999). Cats and Galton (1985) found a consistently lower graft survival rate in patients with systemic lupus erythematosus in an analysis of the UCLA Registry data. A previous analysis of UNOS data confirmed the poorer graft survival rates in patients with systemic lupus erythematosus (Mitsuishi and Cecka, 1993), but a more recent analysis showed similar survival at 5 years after transplantation to most other causes of end-stage renal failures (Cecka, 1999). White patients with HLA-DR2/3 had a significantly better graft survival rate than recipients without these antigens. Nephrosclerosis as a cause of renal failure in transplant recipients was associated with poorer graft survival in blacks, but not in whites.

In patients with Fabry's disease, the high failure rate was not due to recurrent renal damage so that it is not possible to exclude such patients from renal transplantation. More recent UNOS data show much improved survival. Oxalosis has been considered an unsuitable condition for transplantation because recurrence of oxalosis is common and early, and little palliation is achieved in such cases. There has been a considerable improvement in outcome in more recent years, however (Cecka, 1999; see Chapter 4).

Rehabilitation and Quality of Life

Patient and graft survival cannot be considered in isolation from the quality of life after transplantation. The potential not only to keep a patient alive but also to restore him or her to a relatively normal existence makes renal transplantation the preferable form of treatment for end-stage renal failure. Rehabilitation of patients on dialysis and after transplantation was assessed carefully by Jacobs et al. (1977) in an analysis of European centers. At that time, rehabilitation was best after a living donor transplant, with 77.9% of patients fully employed, whereas the percentage of patients fully employed after cadaver transplantation was 64.7%, almost identical to that of patients on home dialysis, 64.6%. If all patients were included except those who were medically unable to work, 91.6% of patients after cadaver transplant were in full-time or part-time work or were capable of full-time work. The rate of rehabilitation was shown to increase markedly after cadaver transplantation with the passage of time. For example, 37.6% of patients were fully employed 4 to 6 months posttransplantation, whereas 60.5% were fully employed after 1 year and 71% after 2 years.

A later analysis from the United States of the quality of life of patients with end-stage renal disease (Evans et al., 1985) found that 79% of transplant patients were able to function at near-normal levels compared with 47 to 59% of patients on dialysis, depending on the type of dialysis. Approximately 75% of the transplant recipients were able to work, compared with 25 to 59% of the dialysis patients. Subjective assessments were made of life satisfaction, well-being and psychological effect as an evaluation of quality of life. Transplant patients did not differ much from the general population in this regard but were superior to patients on dialysis. Assessment of quality of life is not straightforward, however (Evans, 1990). The general availability of erythropoietin has improved markedly the quality of life of patients on hemodialysis compared with the past.

After a successful renal transplant, a patient may be restored virtually to a normal life, with the proviso that immunosuppressive drugs are necessary, usually for the life of the graft, although there are reports of the cessation of azathioprine and steroids without rejection of the graft (Sheriff *et al.*, 1978; Uehling *et al.*, 1976). An analysis by Simmons and Abress (1987) of patients treated at Minneapolis in a controlled trial of cyclosporine and steroids versus azathioprine, steroids and antilymphocyte globulin showed that in terms of physical, emotional and some aspects of social well-being, patients treated with cyclosporine had a significantly more favorable quality of life than patients on azathioprine therapy.

An analysis of work disability, functional limitations and health status of recipients after kidney transplantation suggested that transplantation is not a panacea (Manninen *et al.*, 1993) and that many patients, regardless of graft outcome and disease diagnosis, report defects in their functional ability and overall state of health. Nevertheless, after transplantation, a patient's lifestyle can return to normal, and there often is a personality change in the patient with a successful transplant. Many patients become achievers, in that they rapidly gain promotion in positions in which they had been relatively stationary before the onset of the illness leading to transplantation. Many patients take a much greater interest in community affairs, having a definite feeling of debt to the community that has enabled the facilities to be provided that allow them to live.

PREGNANCY

One of the most impressive aspects of successful renal transplantation in the young person is the ability of the male patient to father a child and the female patient to give birth to a healthy child (Fig. 39–17). Approximately 1 in 50 women of childbearing age with a functioning transplant becomes pregnant, and several thousand successful pregnancies have occurred (Bumgardner and Matas, 1992; Hou, 1985). In the United States, a National Transplant Pregnancy Register has been established in Philadelphia and is accumulating valuable data (Armenti *et al.*, 2000). A similar register has been established in the United Kingdom by UKTSSA, and data are being accumulated rapidly. These data are particularly important in the assessment of new drugs. Although the incidence of spontaneous abortion may be higher than normal in these patients, there is no evidence of an increased incidence of congenital anomalies in pregnancies carried successfully to term (Davison, 1991). There is a definite risk of rejection associated with pregnancy (about 9%), and permanent impairment of renal function occurs in 15% of patients, but this seems to occur mostly in women with relatively poor renal function in the allograft before conception (Armenti *et al.*, 1998, 2000; Bumgardner and Matas, 1992; Davidson and Lindheimer, 1982; Fine, 1982; Penn *et al.*, 1980). There is a 40 to 50% incidence of prematurity and an incidence of growth retardation of 20% in offspring.

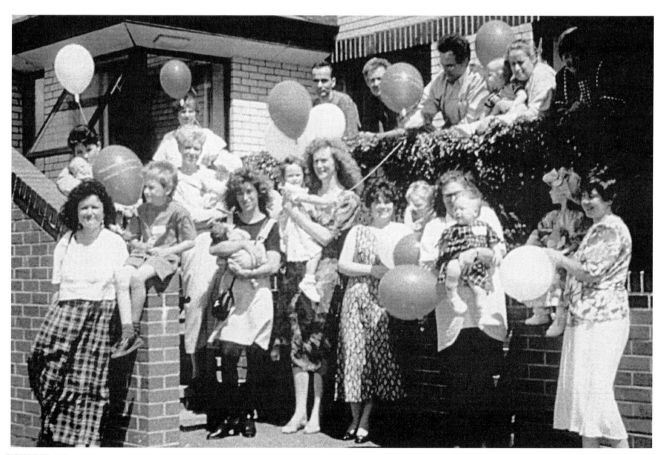

FIGURE 39–17

Some of the mothers transplanted at the Oxford Transplant Centre with their children born after their kidney transplant.

The ideal timing of pregnancy is 2 to 5 years posttransplantation, when renal function is relatively normal and stable. At a later stage, renal function is likely to be impaired, and further deterioration with pregnancy is possible. The presence of hypertension at the time of conception represents a risk to mother and fetus. A successful outcome of pregnancy in the renal transplant patient is likely if the serum creatinine level is less than 150 μmol L⁻¹ (1.5 mg dl⁻¹). A high serum creatinine at any time before or during the pregnancy is associated with a higher risk of graft loss postpartum (Armenti et al., 2000). In the presence of good renal function, repeat pregnancies are not contraindicated. Scott et al. (1986) reported a woman with a renal transplant who completed five pregnancies successfully without any deterioration of renal function.

BODY MASS INDEX

Obesity is recognized as an increasingly important independent factor influencing patient and graft survival after transplantation. A link between increased body mass index and short-term graft survival was noted by Cho and colleagues (1995), and soon after reports appeared of greater patient mortality related to obesity (body mass index >30) (Halme et al., 1997; Modlin et al., 1997). Mild obesity before transplantation (body mass index >25) was noted to be associated independently with poorer patient and graft survival after transplantation (Meier-Kriesche et al., 1999). This effect could be related to increased death resulting from cardiovascular disease, decreased kidney size compared with recipient size or influence on immunosuppressive drug concentrations. Potential overweight recipients before transplantation must be encouraged to lose weight; similarly, after transplantation, all recipients should be advised about an appropriate caloric intake.

Long-Term Outcome of Renal Transplantation

The results of renal transplantation presented throughout this book and in this chapter have tended to concentrate on 1-year graft survival figures; graft survival at 1 year reflects graft survival at 10 years (Table 39–3). Takiff et al. (1986), in an analysis of 14,000 patients who had a renal transplant before 1976 in the precyclosporine era, found 10-year graft survival rates of 67% in HLA-identical siblings, 38% in parental transplants and 20% in cadaver donors. In the long-term, histocompatibility was the most important factor influencing graft outcome. Other factors shown to influence long-term survival were transfusions, transplant number, HLA-A and/or HLA-B mismatches, cold ischemia time, original disease, recipient race and quality of graft function at 1 month.

Lee and colleagues described the outcome of 283 primary renal grafts performed at Richmond in the period 1962–1975 (Lee et al., 1987). Of these, 141 (83 from living related donors and 58 from cadaver donors) grafts survived 10 years. After 10 years, losses continued equally caused by rejection and death of the patient. Cardiovascular morbidity was significant in young patients previously transplanted as teenagers. The causes of death after 10 years were distributed evenly among cardiovascular disease, infection, neoplasm and hepatic failure. Although rehabilitation was considered good in these patients, there is no question that the long-term renal transplant patient remains at considerable risk. Similar data were reported by Mahoney et al. (1986) in an analysis of patients surviving with a cadaver graft for at least 10 years. The continuing morbidity and mortality rates were considerable.

In the cyclosporine era, results have steadily improved, as described by Hariharan et al. (2000) and depicted by the improving predicted half-lives for living and cadaver transplants in Table 39–1 from the same study. Factors that influenced outcome have been discussed, but the key factors are HLA matching, race, center, original disease, early renal function and early rejection (Terasaki et al., 1993). These factors have not changed in more recent years, although the predicted survival is now higher in all of the above-mentioned groups (Cecka, 2000).

Conclusions

Dialysis and transplantation are costly treatments, and every Western country, faced with rapidly rising medical costs, has reflected on the cost-effectiveness of expensive therapies (Levinsky, 1992). Inevitably the spotlight falls on dialysis and transplantation: Is this cost justified? Unquestionably the treatments are expensive, and costs vary from nation to nation. Assuming that one considers treatment of patients with end-stage renal failure justified, transplantation is by far the cheaper option available. In developing countries, renal transplantation is almost the only option available because often long-term dialysis is not available. Of patients with the potential for full-time work, most are restored to full-time work after living donor and cadaver transplantations. In such situations, a productive member of society is reestablished, with the consequent saving in pensions or benefits to surviving family members. The demonstration that survival is enhanced by transplantation compared with dialysis in nearly all patient groups, as discussed earlier, provides more objective evidence of the key role that transplantation should play in the management of end-stage renal failure.

The justification for the treatment of end-stage renal failure by an integrated program of dialysis and transplantation seems self-evident. The primary aim is to achieve a successful

TABLE 39–3

ACTUAL VERSUS PREDICTED GRAFT SURVIVAL*

Donor	Actual Graft Survival at 10 Years for Transplants in the Years 1975–1980		Predicted Graft Survival at 10 Years for Transplants in the Years 1987–1990	
	Survival (%)	*Half-life (y)*	*Survival (%)*	*Half-life (y)*
HLA-identical sibling	69	24 ± 1.7	79	32.9 ± 7.5
Parent	43	11.8 ± 0.7	51	11.2 ± 1.3
First cadaver	25	7.9 ± 0.2	44	10.3 ± 0.4

*Actual graft survival at 10 years of transplants performed in the years 1975–1980 in the precyclosporine era are given in the left half of the table; predicted graft survival at 10 years for transplants performed in the years 1987–1990 based on actual 1-, 2- and 3-year graft survival rates are given on the right side.
Data derived with permission from UNOS Registry data.

transplant, using dialysis to maintain patients while awaiting a transplant and for patients who are unsuitable for transplant for medical or immunological reasons. Because a large proportion of patients with end-stage renal failure who are suitable for transplantation are relatively young, achievement of a successful renal transplant in these patients is one of the more satisfying areas of medical practice today.

REFERENCES

Ablaza, V., Morris, M., Badosa, F., Anderson, L., Raja, R. and Mital, D. (1993). Kidneys from cadaveric donors over 60 years of age. *Transplant. Proc.* **25**, 1554.

Ahmed, Z. and Terasaki, P. I. (1992). Effect of transfusions. *In Clinical Transplants 1991*, (P. I. Terasaki, ed.), p. 305, UCLA Tissue Typing Laboratory, Los Angeles.

Alexander, J. W., Light, J. A., Donaldson, L. A., *et al.* (1999). Evaluation of pre- and posttransplant donor-specific transfusion/cyclosporine A in non-HLA identical living donor kidney transplant recipients. Cooperative Clinical Trials in Transplantation Research Group. *Transplantation* **68**, 1117.

Alexander, J. W. and Vaughn, W. K. (1991). The influence of donor age on outcome. *Transplantation* **51**, 135.

Alkhunaizi, A. M., de Mattos, A. M., Barry, J. M., Bennett W. M. and Norman, D. J. (1999). Renal transplantation across the ABO barrier using A2 kidneys. *Transplantation* **67**, 1319.

American College of Surgeons/NIH Organ Transplant Registry. (1975a). Renal transplantation in congenital and metabolic diseases. *J. A. M. A.* **233**, 148.

American College of Surgeons/NIH Organ Transplant Registry. (1975b). The 12th Report of the Human Renal Transplant Registry. *J. A. M. A.* **233**, 787.

Anderson, C. B., Tyler, J. D., Rodey, G. E., *et al.* (1987). Preoperative immunomodulation of renal allograft recipients by concomitant immunosuppression and donor-specific transfusions. *Transplant. Proc.* **19**, 1494.

Anderson, S. and Brenner, B. M. (1986). The effect of aging on the renal glomerulus. *Am J. Med.* **80**, 435.

Andresdottir, M. B., Hoitsma, A. J., Assmann, K. J., Koene, R. A. and Wetzels, J. F. (1999). The impact of recurrent glomerulonephritis on graft survival in recipients of human histocompatibility leucocyte antigen-identical living related donor grafts. *Transplantation* **68**, 623.

Armenti, V. T., Moritz, M. J. and Davison, J. M. (1998). Drug safety issues in pregnancy following transplantation and immunosuppression. *Drug Saf.* **19**, 219.

Armenti, V. T., Moritz, M. J., Jarrell, B. E. and Davison, J. M. (2000). Pregnancy after transplantation. *Transplant. Rev.* **14**, 1.

Ascher, N. L., Ahrenholz, D. H., Simmons, R. L. and Najarian, J. S. (1979). 100 second renal allografts from a single transplantation institution. *Transplantation* **27**, 30.

Barry, J. M., Lemmers, M. J., Meyer M. M., *et al.* (1996). Cadaver kidney transplantation in patients more than 65 years old. *World J. Urol.* **14**, 243.

Basadonna, G., Matas, A. J., Gillingham, K., *et al.* (1993). Kidney transplantation in patients with type I diabetes: 26 year experience at the University of Minnesota. *In Clinical Transplants 1992*, (P. I. Terasaki and J. M. Cecka, eds.), p. 227, UCLA Tissue Typing Laboratory, Los Angeles.

Bates, W. D., Davies, D. R., Welsh, K., *et al.* (1999). An evaluation of the Banff classification of early renal allograft biopsies and correlation with outcome. *Nephrol. Dial. Transplant.* **14**, 2364.

Beck, D., Fennell, R., Yost, R., *et al.* (1980). Evaluation of an educational programme on compliance with medication regimens in paediatric patients with renal transplants. *J. Pediatr.* **96**, 1094.

Belitsky, P., MacDonald, P., Gajewski, J., *et al.* (1987). Significance of delayed function in cyclosporine-treated cadaver kidney transplant. *Transplant. Proc.* **19**, 2096.

Belzer, F. O., Kalayoghi, M. and Sollinger, H. W. (1987). Donor-specific transfusion in living-unrelated renal donor-recipient combination. *Transplant. Proc.* **19**, 1514.

Benedetti, E., Matas, A. J., Hakim, N., *et al.* (1994). Renal transplantation for patients 60 years old: a single-institution experience. *Ann. Surg.* **220**, 445.

Bradley, B. A., Gilks, W., Gore, S. M., Klouda, P. T. and Selwood, W. H. (1986a). *In Clinical Transplants 1986*, (P. I. Terasaki, ed.), p. 93, UCLA Tissue Typing Laboratory, Los Angeles.

Bradley, B. A., Selwood, N. H., Klauda, P. T., *et al.* (1986b). Kidney transplants in the United Kingdom. *In Clinical Transplants 1986*, (P. I. Terasaki, ed.), p. 47, UCLA Tissue Typing Laboratory, Los Angeles.

Bumgardner, G. L. and Matas, A. J. (1992). Transplantation and pregnancy. *Transplant. Rev.* **6**, 139.

Burdick, J. F. and Williams, G. M. (1986). What causes center effects in kidney transplantation. *Ann. Surg.* **203**, 311.

Burlingham, W. J., Grailer, A. P., Heisey, D. M., *et al.* (1998). The effect of tolerance to noninherited maternal HLA antigens on the survival of renal transplants from sibling donors. *N. Engl. J. Med.* **339**, 1657.

Butkus, D. E. (1991). Primary renal cadaveric allograft survival in blacks—is there still a significant difference? *Transplant. Rev.* **5**, 91.

Cantarovich, D., Baatard, R., Baranger, T., *et al.* (1994). Cadaveric renal transplantation after 60 years of age: a single center experience. *Transpl. Int.* **7**, 33.

Cats, S. and Galton, J. (1985). Effects of original disease in kidney transplant outcome. *In Clinical Kidney Transplants 1985*, (P. I. Terasaki, ed.), p. 111, UCLA Tissue Typing Laboratory, Los Angeles.

Cecka, J. M. (1986). The roles of sex, race and ABO groups. *In Clinical Transplants 1986*, (P. I. Terasaki, ed.), p. 199, UCLA Tissue Typing Laboratory, Los Angeles.

Cecka, J. M. (1999). The UNOS Scientific Renal Transplant Registry. *In Clinical Transplants 1998*, (J. M. Cecka and P. I. Terasaki, eds.), p. 1, UCLA Tissue Typing Laboratory, Los Angeles.

Cecka, J. M. (2000). The UNOS Scientific Renal Transplant Registry. *In Clinical Transplants 1999*, (J. M. Cecka and P. I. Terasaki, eds.), p. 1, UCLA Immunogenetic Center, Los Angeles.

Cecka, J. M. and Terasaki, P. I. (1993). The UNOS Scientific Renal Transplant Registry. *In Clinical Transplants 1992*, (P. I. Terasaki and J. M. Cecka, eds.), p. 1, UCLA Tissue Typing Laboratory, Los Angeles.

Cheigh, J. S., Suthanthiran, M., Stubenbord, W. T., *et al.* (1987). Optimization of donor specific blood transfusion in kidney transplantation. *Transplant. Proc.* **19**, 2250.

Chertow, G. M., Milford, E. L., Meckenzie, H. S. and Brenner, B. M. (1996). Antigen-independent determinants of cadaveric kidney transplant failure. *J. A. M. A.* **276**, 1732.

Cho, Y. W. and Cecka, J. M. (1993). Center effect in the UNOS Renal Transplant Registry. *In Clinical Transplants 1992*, (P. I. Terasaki and J. M. Cecka, eds.), p. 333, UCLA Tissue Typing Laboratory, Los Angeles.

Cho, Y. W. and Terasaki, P. I. (1996). Comparison of kidney graft survival in Asian and Caucasian patients transplanted in the United States. *Transplant. Proc.* **28**, 1571.

Cho, Y. W. and Terasaki, P. I. (1997). Impact of new variables reported to the UNOS registry. *In Clinical Transplants 1997*, (J. M. Cecka and P. I. Terasaki, eds.), p. 305, UCLA Tissue Typing Laboratory, Los Angeles.

Cho, Y. W., Terasaki, P. I. and Cecka, J. M. (1995). New variables reported to the UNOS Registry and their impact on cadaveric renal transplant outcomes—a preliminary study. *In Clinical Transplants 1995*, (J. M. Cecka and P. I. Terasaki, eds.), p. 405, UCLA Tissue Typing Laboratory, Los Angeles.

Christiaans, M. H., Van den Berg Loonen, P., Pettenburg, H. G. and Leunissen, K. M. (1991). More favorable clinical course in kidney allograft recipients due to HLA-B + DR matching. *Transplant. Proc.* **23**, 2674.

Cicciarelli, J. S. (1985). Transplant center and kidney graft survival. *In Clinical Transplants 1984*, (P. I. Terasaki, ed.), p. 285, UCLA Tissue Typing Laboratory, Los Angeles.

Cicciarelli, J. S. (1990). UNOS Registry data: effect of transfusions. *In Clinical Transplants 1990*, (P. I. Terasaki, ed.), p. 407, UCLA Tissue Typing Laboratory, Los Angeles.

Colon, E. A., Popkin, M. K., Matas, A. J. and Collies, A. L. (1991). Overview of noncompliance in renal transplantation. *Transplant. Rev.* **5**, 175.

Council of the Transplantation Society. (1986). Commercialization in transplantation: the problems and some guidelines for practice. *Transplantation* **41**, 1.

Curschellas, E., Landmann, J., Durig, M., *et al.* (1991). Morphological findings in "zero-hour" biopsies of renal transplants. *Clin. Nephrol.* **36**, 215.

Daar, A. S. and Sells, R. S. (1990). Living nonrelated donor renal transplantation—a reappraisal. *Transplant. Rev.* **4**, 128.

d'Apice, A. J. F., Morris, P. J., Kincaid-Smith, P., Mathew, T. H. and Marshall, V. C. (1976). Possible rejection of an HLA-identical sibling renal allograft. *Med. J. Aust.* **1**, 195.

Daemen, J. H., de Vries, B., Oomen, A. P., DeMeester, J. and Kootstra, G. (1997). Effect of machine perfusion preservation on delayed graft function in non-heart beating donor kidneys—early results. *Transpl. Int.* **10**, 317.

Darmady, E. M. (1974). Transplantation and the aging kidney. *Lancet* **2**, 1046.

Davidson, J. M. and Lindheimer, M. D. (1982). Pregnancy in renal transplant recipients. *J. Reprod. Med.* **27**, 613.

Davidson, J. M., Uldall, P. R. and Taylor, R. M. (1977). Relation of immediate posttransplant renal function to long-term function in cadaver kidney recipients. *Transplantation* **23**, 310.

Davies, D. F. (1950). Age changes in glomerular filtration rate, effective renal plasma flow, and tubular excretory capacity in adult males. *J. Clin. Invest.* **29**, 496.

Davison, J. M. (1991). Dialysis, transplantation and pregnancy. *Am. J. Kidney Dis.* **17**, 127.

Dick, H. M., Boyd, G. A., Briggs, J. D., Wood, R. F. M. and Bell, P. R. F. (1972). Severe rejection of an HLA-identical sibling renal transplant. *Tissue Antigens* **2**, 480.

Didlake, R., Dreyfus, K., Kerman, R., *et al.* (1988). Patient noncompliance: a major cause of late graft failure in cyclosporine treated transplants. *Transplant. Proc.* **20**, 63.

Dietl, K. A., Wolters, H., Marschall, B., *et al.* (2000). Cadaveric "two-in-one" kidney transplantation from marginal donors: experience of 26 cases after 3 years. *Transplantation* **70**, 790.

Douzdjian, V., Bhaskar, S., Baliga, P. K. and Rajagopalan, P. R. (1997). Graft outcome in cadaver renal transplants treated with full-dose cyclosporine induction without antibody. *Clin. Transpl.* **11**, 294.

Ekstrand, A., Gronhagen-Riska, C., Groop, L., Salmela, K., Kuhlback, B. and Ahomen, J. (1987). Results of kidney transplantation in patients with diabetic nephropathy. *Transplant. Proc.* **19**, 1535.

Evans, R. (1990). Quality of life assessment and the treatment of end-stage renal disease. *Transplant. Rev.* **4**, 28.

Evans, R. W., Manninea, D. L., Garrison, L. P., *et al.* (1985). The quality of life of patients with end stage renal disease. *J. Med.* **312**, 553.

Fauchald, P., Albrechtsen, D., Leivestad, T., *et al.* (1988). Renal replacement therapy in elderly patients. *Transpl. Int.* **1**, 131.

Fine, R. N. (1982). Pregnancy in renal allograft recipients. *Am. J. Nephrol.* **2**, 117.

Flechner, S. M., Kerman, R. M., van Buren, C. and Kahan, B. D. (1984). Successful transplantation of cyclosporin-treated haploidentical living related recipients without transfusions. *Transplantation* **37**, 73.

Flechner, S. M., Kerman, R. M., van Buren, C. T., Lorber, M., Barker, C. J. and Kahan, B. D. (1987). Does cyclosporin improve the results of HLA-identical renal transplantation? *Transplant. Proc.* **19**, 1485.

Frey, D. J., Matas, A. J., Gillingham, K. J., *et al.* (1992). Sequential therapy—a prospective randomized trial of MALG *vs.* OKT3 for prophylactic immunosuppression in cadaveric renal allograft recipients. *Transplantation* **54**, 50.

Fryd, D., Migliori, J. S., Ascher, N. L., *et al.* (1987a). Can renal transplantation be done safely without prior dialysis therapy? *Transplant. Proc.* **19**, 1557.

Fryd, D. S., So, S. K. S., Kruse, L., *et al.* (1987b). Improving results of renal transplantation with multidrug therapy in patients over fifty years of age. *Clin. Transplant.* **1**, 75.

Gaber, L. W., Moore, L. W., Alloway, R. R., *et al.* (1995). Glomerulosclerosis as a determinant of posttransplant function of older donor renal allografts. *Transplantation* **60**, 334.

Galton, J. (1985). Racial effect on kidney transplantation. *In Clinical Kidney Transplants 1985*, (P. I. Terasaki, ed.), p., 153, UCLA Tissue Typing Laboratory, Los Angeles.

Gilks, W. R., Selwood, N. and Bradley, B. A. (1984). The variation among transplant center results in the United Kingdom and Ireland from 1977 to 1981. *Transplantation* **38**, 235.

Giral-Classe, M., Hourmant, M., Cantarovich, D., *et al.* (1998). De-

layed graft function of more than six days strongly decreases long-term survival of transplanted kidneys. *Kidney Int.* **54**, 972.

Gjertson, D. W. (1993). Multifactorial analysis of renal transplants accepted to the United Network for Organ Sharing Registry. *In Clinical Transplants 1992*, (P. I. Terasaki and J. M. Cecka, ed.), p. 299, UCLA Tissue Typing Laboratory, Los Angeles.

Groenewoud, A. F. (1987). The impact of HLA-DR incompatibilities on likely graft function and the number of rejection treatments. *Transplant. Proc.* **19**, 683.

Groth, C. and Ringden, R. (1984). Transplantation in relation to the treatment of inherited disease. *Transplantation* **38**, 319.

Groth, C. G., Fehrmman, A., Ringden, O. and Lundgren, G. (1987). Related donor kidney transplantation is the best form of treatment for uremia. *Transplant. Proc.* **19**, 2278.

Guttman, R. D. (1987). A perspective on long-term outcome in organ transplantation. *Transplant. Proc.* **19**, 67.

Halme, L., Eklund, B., Kyllonen, L. and Salmela, K. (1997). Is obesity still a risk factor in renal transplantation? *Transpl. Int.* **10**, 284.

Hariharan, S., Johnson, C. P., Bresnahan, B. A., *et al.* (2000). Improved graft survival after renal transplantation in the United States, 1988 to 1996. *N. Engl. J. Med.* **342**, 605.

Hayes, J. M., Novick, A. C., Streem, S. B., *et al.* (1988). The use of single paediatric cadaver kidneys for transplantation. *Transplantation* **45**, 106.

Hestin, D., Frimat, L., Hubert, J., *et al.* (1994). Renal transplantation in patients over sixty years of age. *Clin. Nephrol.* **42**, 232.

Higgins, R. M., Sheriff, R., Bittar, A. A., *et al.* (1995). The quality of function of renal allografts is associated with donor age. *Transpl. Int.* **8**, 221.

Hirati, M., Cho, Y. W., Cecka, J. M. and Terasaki, P. I. (1996). Patient death after renal transplantation—an analysis of its role in graft outcome. *Transplantation* **61**, 1479.

Holzgreve, W., Beller, F. K., Buchholz, B., *et al.* (1987). Kidney transplantation from anencephalic donors. *N. Engl. J. Med.* **316**, 1069.

Hou, S. (1985). Pregnancy in women with chronic renal disease. *N. Engl. J. Med.* **312**, 836.

Husberg, B. S. and Starzl, T. E. (1974). The outcome of kidney transplantation. *Arch. Surg.* **108**, 584.

Ildstad, S. T., Tollerud, D. J., Noseworthy, J., Ryckman, F., Sheldon, C. A. and Martin, L. W. (1990). The influence of donor age on graft survival in renal transplantation. *J. Pediatr. Surg.* **25**, 134.

Ismail, N., Hakim, R. M. and Helderman, J. H. (1994). Renal replacement therapies in the elderly: Part II. renal transplantation. *Am. J. Kidney Dis.* **23**, 1.

Isoniemi, H. M., Krogerus, L., von Willebrand, E., Taskinen, E., Ahonen, J. and Hayrey, P. (1992). Histopathological findings in well functioning, long term renal allograft. *Kidney Int.* **41**, 155.

Iwaki, Y., Iguro, T. and Terasaki, P. I. (1986). Effect of sensitization on kidney allografts. *In Clinical Transplant 1986*, (P. I. Terasaki, ed.), p. 139, UCLA Tissue Typing Laboratory, Los Angeles.

Iwaki, Y. and Terasaki, P. I. (1986). Donor and recipient age effect. *In Clinical Transplants 1986*, (P. I. Terasaki, ed.), p. 267, UCLA Tissue Typing Laboratory, Los Angeles.

Jacobs, C., Brunner, F. P., Chantler, C., *et al.* (1977). Combined report on regular dialysis and transplantation in Europe. *Proc. Eur. Dial. Transplant. Assoc.* **14**, 3.

Jassal, S. V., Opelz, G. and Cole, E. (1997). Transplantation in the elderly: a review. *Geriatr. Nephrol. Urol.* **7**, 157.

Joysey, V., Rogers, J. H., Evans, D. B. and Herbertson, B. M. (1973). Kidney graft survival and matching for HLA and ABO antigens. *Nature* **246**, 163.

Kasiske, B. L. (1988). The influence of donor age on renal function in transplant recipients. *Am. J. Kidney Dis.* **11**, 248.

Kaufman, D. B., Matas, A. J., Arrazola, L., *et al.* (1993). Transplantation of kidneys from zero haplotype-matched living donors and from distantly related and unrelated donors in the cyclosporine era. *Transplant. Proc.* **25**, 1530.

Kennealy, P. (1985). The impact of sex on kidney transplantation. *In Clinical Kidney Transplants 1985*, (P. I. Terasaki, ed.), p. 147, UCLA Tissue Typing Laboratory, Los Angeles.

Koffman, C. G., Bewick, M., Chang, R. W. S. and Compton, F. (1993). Comparative study of the use of systolic and asystolic kidney donors between 1988 and 1991. *Transplant. Proc.* **25**, 1527.

Koo, D. D., Welsh, K. I., McLaren, A. J., *et al.* (1999). Cadaver versus living donor kidneys: impact of donor factors on antigen induction before transplantation. *Kidney Int.* **56**, 1551.

Koo, D. D., Welsh, K. I., Roake, J. A., Morris, P. J. and Fuggle, S. V. (1998). Ischemia/reperfusion injury in human kidney transplantation: an immunohistochemical analysis of changes after reperfusion. *Am. J. Pathol.* **153**, 557.

Kountz, S. L., Thibault, P. M., Endo, T., Margules, R. and Balzer, O. (1972). Results of immediate and delayed retransplantation. *Transplant. Proc.* **4**, 739.

Koyama, H. and Cecka, J. M. (1993). Rejection episodes. *In Clinical Transplants 1992*, (P. I. Terasaki and J. M. Cecka, eds.). UCLA Tissue Typing Laboratory, Los Angeles.

Koyama, H., Cecka, J. M. and Terasaki, P. I. (1994). Kidney transplantation in black recipients: HLA matching and other factors affecting long-term graft survival. *Transplantation* **57**, 1064.

Kramer, P., Broyer, M., Brunner, F. P., *et al.* (1982). Combined report on regular dialysis and transplantation in Europe, XII, 1981. *Proc. Eur. Dial. Transplant. Assoc.* **19**, 1.

Kumar, M. S., White, A. G., Samhan, N. and Abouna, G. M. (1987). Nonrelated living donors for renal transplantation. *Transplant. Proc.* **19**, 19.

Lagaaii, E. L., Hennemann, I. P., Ruigrok, M., *et al.* (1989). Effect of one HLA-DR antigen matched and completely HLA-DR mismatched blood transfusions on survival of heart and kidney allografts. *N. Engl. J. Med.* **321**, 701.

Langle, F., Sautner, T., Grunberger, T., *et al.* (1992). Impact of donor age on graft function in living related kidney transplantation. *Transplant. Proc.* **24**, 2725.

Laskow, D. A., Diethelm, A. G., Hudson, S. L., *et al.* (1992). Analysis of 22 years experience in living related transplantation at the University of Alabama in Birmingham. *In Clinical Transplants 1991*, (P. I. Terasaki, ed.), p. 179, UCLA Tissue Typing Laboratory, Los Angeles.

Lauffer, G., Murie, J. A., Gray, D., Ting, A. and Morris, P. J. (1988). Renal transplantation in patients over 55 years of age. *Br. J. Surg.* **75**, 984.

Lee, H. M., Kenyon, N., Meadex-Picon, G. and Posner, M. P. (1987). Long-term survivors of kidney transplantation, mortality, rehabilitation and immunologic reactivities. *Transplant. Proc.* **19**, 2120.

Lee, C. M., Carter, J. T., Weinstein, R. J., *et al.* (1999). Dual kidney transplantation: older donors for older recipients. *J. Am. Coll. Surg.* **189**, 82.

Levinsky, N. G. (1992). The organization of medical care: lessons from the Medical End Stage Renal Disease Program. *N. Engl. J. Med.* **329**, 1395.

Lim, E. C. and Terasaki, P. I. (1992). Early graft function. *In Clinical Transplants 1991*, (P. I. Terasaki and J. M. Cecka, eds.), p. 401, UCLA Tissue Typing Laboratory, Los Angeles.

Lin, H. M., Kauffman, H. M., McBride, M. A., *et al.* (1998). Center-specific graft and patient survival rates: 1997 United Network for Organ Sharing (UNOS) report. *J. A. M. A.* **280**, 1153.

Lorber, M. I., Van Buren, C. T., Flechner, S. M., *et al.* (1987). Pretransplant coronary arteriography for diabetic renal transplant recipients. *Transplant. Proc.* **19**, 1539.

Lu, A. D., Carter, J. T., Weinstein, R. J., *et al.* (1999). Excellent outcome in recipients of dual kidney transplants: a report of the first 50 dual kidney transplants at Stanford University. *Arch. Surg.* **134**, 971.

Lu, A. D., Carter, J. T., Weinstein, R. J., *et al.* (2000). Outcome in recipients of dual kidney transplants: an analysis of the dual registry patients. *Transplantation.* **69**, 281.

Lundgren, G., Groth, C. G., Albrechtsen, D., *et al.* (1986). HLA matching in cyclosporine treated renal transplant recipients: a prospective Swedish-Norwegian multicentre study. *In Clinical Transplants 1986*, (P. I. Terasaki, ed.), p. 79, UCLA Tissue Typing Laboratory, Los Angeles.

Mahoney, J. F., Savdie, E., Caterson, R. J., *et al.* (1986). The natural history of cadaveric renal allografts beyond ten years. *Transplant. Proc.* **18**, 135.

Mandelbaum, D. M., Henry, M. I., Sommer, B. G. and Ferguson, R. M. (1987). Primary cadaveric renal transplant using cyclosporine in patients over fifty years of age. *Transplant. Proc.* **19**, 1863.

Manninen, D. L., Evans, R. W. and Dugan, M. K. (1993). Work disability, functional limitations and the health status of kidney transplantation recipients post transplant. *In Clinical Transplants 1992*, (P. I. Terasaki and J. M. Cecka, eds.), p. 193, UCLA Tissue Typing Laboratory, Los Angeles.

Marcen, R., Orofino, L., Pascual, J., *et al.* (1998). Delayed graft function does not reduce the survival of renal transplant allografts. *Transplantation* **66**, 461.

Matas, A. J. (1999). Noncompliance and late graft loss: implications for long-term clinical studies. *Transplant. Rev.* **13**, 78.

Matas, A. J., Gillingham, K. J., Humar, A., *et al.* (2000). Immunologic and nonimmunologic factors: different risks for cadaver and living donor transplantation. *Transplantation* **69**, 54.

McDonald, J. C., Vaughan, W., Filo, R. S., *et al.* (1981). Cadaver donor renal transplantation by Centers of the Southeastern Organ Procurement Foundation. *Ann. Surg.* **193**, 1.

McLaren, A. J., Jassem, W., Gray, D. W., *et al.* (1999). Delayed graft function: risk factors and the relative effects of early function and acute rejection on long-term survival in cadaveric renal transplantation. *Clin. Transplant.* **13**, 266.

Meier-Kriesche, H. U., Vaghela, M., Thambuganipalle, R., *et al.* (1999). The effect on body mass index on long-term renal allograft survival. *Transplantation* **68**, 1294.

Mickey, M. R. (1986). Center effect. *In Clinical Transplants 1986*, (P. I. Terasaki, ed.), p. 165, UCLA Tissue Typing Laboratory, Los Angeles.

Mitsuishi, Y. and Cecka, J. M. (1992). Recent improvements in cadaveric donor kidney retransplantation. *In Clinical Transplants 1991*, (P. I. Terasaki, ed.), p. 281, UCLA Tissue Typing Laboratory, Los Angeles.

Mitsuishi, Y. and Cecka, J. M. (1993). Disease effects and associations. *In Clinical Transplants 1992*, (P. I. Terasaki and J. M. Cecka, eds.), p. 371, UCLA Tissue Typing Laboratory, Los Angeles.

Modlin, C. S., Flechner, S. M., Goormastic, M., *et al.* (1997). Should obese patients lose weight before receiving a kidney transplant? *Transplantation* **64**, 599.

Moreso, F., Seron, D., Gil-Vernet, S., *et al.* (1999). Donor age and delayed graft function as predictors of renal allograft survival in rejection-free patients. *Nephrol. Dial. Transplant.* **14**, 930.

Morris, P. J. (ed.). (1984). *Kidney Transplantation: Principles and Practice*, 2nd ed., Grune & Stratton, London.

Morris, P. J. (1985). Presidential address. *Transplant. Proc.* **17**, 1615.

Morris, P. J. (1987). Problems facing the society today: presidential address to the Transplantation Society. *Transplant. Proc.* **19**, 16.

Morris, P. J., Johnson, R. J., Fuggle, S. V., Belger, M. A. and Briggs, J. D. (1999). Analysis of factors that affect outcome of primary cadaveric renal transplantation in the UK. *Lancet* **354**, 1147.

Morris, P. J., Ting, A. and Muller, G. (1981). *In Transplantation and Clinical Immunology XIII*, p. 89, Excerpta Medica, Amsterdam.

Morris, P. J., Ting, A. and Stocker, J. (1968). Leucocyte antigens in renal transplantation: 1. the paradox of blood transfusions in renal transplantation. *Med. J. Aust.* **2**, 1088.

Najarian, J. S., Kaufman, D. B., Fryd, D. S., *et al.* (1989). Long-term survival following kidney transplantation in 100 type I diabetic patients. *Transplantation* **47**, 106.

Najarian, J. S., Sutherland, D. R., Simmons, R. L., *et al.* (1980). Ten year experience with renal transplantation in juvenile onset diabetics. *Ann. Surg.* **190**, 487.

Nghiem, D. O., Cottingham, E. M. and Hsia, S. (1993). Transplantation of the extreme age donor kidneys. *Transplant. Proc.* **25**, 1567.

Nicholson, M. L., Wheatley, T. J., Horsburgh, T., *et al.* (1996). The relative influence of delayed graft function and acute rejection on renal transplant survival. *Transpl. Int.* **9**, 415.

Norman, D. J., Henell, K., Fletcher, L. and Barry, J. (1987). Donor specific transfusions: a five-year experience with alternative protocols. *Transplant. Proc.* **19**, 2252.

Nyberg, G., Hallste, G., Norden, G., Hadimeri, H. and Wramner, L. (1995a). Physical performance does not improve in elderly patients following successful kidney transplantation. *Nephrol. Dial. Transplant.* **10**, 86.

Nyberg, G., Nilsson, B., Hallste, G., Haljamae, K., Norden, G. and Blohme, I. (1993). Renal transplantation in elderly patients: survival and complications. *Transplant. Proc.* **25**, 1062.

Nyberg, G., Nilsson, B., Norden, G. and Karlberg, I. (1995b). Outcome of renal transplantation in patients over the age of 60: a case-control study. *Nephrol. Dial. Transplant.* **10**, 91.

Ogura, K. (1993) Sensitization. *In Clinical Transplants 1992*, (P. I. Terasaki and J. M. Cecka, eds.), p. 357, UCLA Tissue Typing Laboratory, Los Angeles.

Ohshima, S., Fujita, T., Asano, H. and Ono, Y. (1987). The effect of cyclosporin on the early post operative function of allografted kidneys with warm ischemic damage. *Transplant. Proc.* **19**, 2081.

Ojo, A. O., Wolfe, R. A., Held, P. J., Port, F. K. and Schmouder, R. L. (1997). Delayed graft function: risk factors and implications for renal allograft survival. *Transplantation* **63**, 968.

Okiye, S. E., Engen, D. E., Sterioff, S., *et al.* (1983). Primary renal transplantation in patients fifty years of age and older. *Transplant. Proc.* **15**, 1046.

Oliver, R. T. D. (1974). Are there Y-linked histocompatibility antigens in man? *Eur. J. Immunol.* **4**, 519.

Opelz, G. (1993a). *Collaborative Transplant Study Newsletter* **2**, 1.

Opelz, G. (1993b). *Collaborative Transplant Study—10th Anniversary*, p. 1.

Opelz, G. (1999). The effect of tolerance to noninherited maternal HLA antigens on the survival of renal transplants from sibling donors. *N. Engl. J. Med.* **340**, 1369.

Opelz, G. (2000). HLA matching in Asian recipients of kidney grafts from unrelated living or cadaveric donors. The Collaborative Transplant Study. *Hum. Immunol.* **61**, 115.

Opelz, G., Gustafsson, L. A. and Terasaki, P. I. (1976). Influence of interval between first graft removal and retransplantation on outcome of second cadaver kidney grafts. *Transplantation* **22**, 521.

Opelz, G., Mickey, M. R. and Terasaki, P. I. (1975). Effect of splenectomy on human renal transplant. *Transplantation* **19**, 226.

Opelz, G., Mickey, M. and Terasaki, P. I. (1977). Influence of race on kidney transplant survival. *Transplant. Proc.* **9**, 137.

Opelz, G. and Terasaki, P. I. (1977). Influence of sex and histocompatibility matching in renal transplantation. *Lancet* **2**, 419.

Opelz, G., Vanrenterghem, Y., Kirste, G., *et al.* (1997). Prospective evaluation of pretransplant blood transfusions in cadaver kidney recipients. *Transplantation* **63**, 964.

Opelz, G., Wujciak, T., Dohler, B., Scherer, S. and Mytilineos, J. (1999). HLA compatibility and organ transplant survival. *Rev. Immunogenet.* **1**, 334.

Ost, I., Groth, C. G., Lindholm, B., Lundgren, G., Magusson, G. and Tillegard, A. (1980). Cadaveric renal transplantation in patients of sixty years and above. *Transplantation* **30**, 339.

Park, K., Kim, Y.-S., Lee, E.-M., Lee, H.-Y. and Han, D. S. (1993). Single center experience of unrelated living donor renal transplantation in the cyclosporine era. *In Clinical Transplants 1992*, (P. I. Terasaki and J. M. Cecka, eds.), p. 249, UCLA Tissue Typing, Los Angeles.

Penn, I., Makowski, E. L. and Harris, P. (1980). Parenthood following renal transplantation. *Kidney Int.* **18**, 221.

Perdue, S. T. and Terasaki, P. I. (1982). Analysis of interracial variation of kidney transplant and patient survival. *Transplantation* **34**, 75.

Perez-Fontan, M., Rodriguez-Carmona, A., Bouza, P. and Valdes, F. (1998). The prognostic significance of acute renal failure after renal transplantation in patients treated with cyclosporin. *Q. J. M.* **91**, 27.

Pescovitz, M. D., Gruber, S. A., Ascher, N. L., *et al.* (1987). Frequency of diabetes-related complications in renal allograft recipients prospectively randomized to cyclosporin or azathioprine. *Transplant. Proc.* **19**, 1537.

Pfaff, W. W., Howard, R. J., Patton, P. R., *et al.* (1998). Delayed graft function after renal transplantation. *Transplantation* **65**, 219.

Pirsch, J. D., d'Alessandro, A. M., Sollinger, H. W., *et al.* (1991). Living-unrelated renal transplantation at the University of Wisconsin. *In Clinical Transplants 1990*, (P. I. Terasaki, ed.), p. 241, UCLA Tissue Typing Laboratory, Los Angeles.

Pirsch, J. D., d'Alessandro, A. M., Sollinger, H. W., *et al.* (1992). The effect of donor age, recipient age and HLA match on immunologic graft survival in cadaver renal transplant recipients. *Transplantation* **53**, 55.

Pirsch, J. D., Stratta, R. J., Armbrust, M. J., *et al.* (1989). Cadaveric renal transplantation with cyclosporine in patients more than sixty years of age. *Transplantation* **47**, 259.

Ploeg, R. J., Visser, M. J., Stignen, T. L., Persijn, G. G. and Van Schifgaarde, R. (1987). Impact of donor age and quality of donor kidneys on graft survival. *Transplant. Proc.* **19**, 1532.

Ploeg, R. J., von Bockel, J. H., Langendijk, P. T. H., *et al.* (1992). Effect of preservation solution on results of cadaveric kidney transplantation. *Lancet* **340**, 129.

Pokorna, E., Vitko, S., Chadimova, M., Schuck, O. and Ekberg, H.

(2000). Proportion of glomerulosclerosis in procurement wedge renal biopsy cannot alone discriminate for acceptance of marginal donors. *Transplantation* **69**, 36.

Raiz, L. R., Kilty, K. M., Henry, M. L. and Ferguson, R. M. (1999). Medication compliance following renal transplantation. *Transplantation* **68**, 51.

Randhawa, P. S., Minervini, M. I., Lombardero, M., *et al.* (2000). Biopsy of marginal donor kidneys: correlation of histologic findings with graft dysfunction. *Transplantation* **69**, 1352.

Rao, K. V., Kasiske, B. L., Odlund, M. D., Ney, A. L. and Anderson, R. C. (1990). Influence of cadaver donor age on post transplant renal function and graft outcome. *Transplantation* **49**, 91.

Reding, R., Squifflet, J. P., Pirson, Y., *et al.* (1987). Living-related and unrelated donor kidney transplantation: comparison between ABO-compatible and incompatible grafts. *Transplant. Proc.* **19**, 1511.

Roake, J. A., Cahill, A. P., Gray, C. M., Gray, D. W. and Morris, P. J. (1996). Preemptive cadaveric renal transplantation-clinical outcome. *Transplantation* **62**, 1411.

Roodnat, J. I., Zietse, R., Mulder, P. G., *et al.* (1999). The vanishing importance of age in renal transplantation. *Transplantation* **67**, 576.

Roza, A. M., Gallagher-Lepak, S., Johnson, C. P. and Adams, M. B. (1989). Renal transplantation in patients more than sixty-five years old. *Transplantation* **48**, 689.

Salaman, J. R., Godfrey, A. M., Russell, R. B., Brown, A. and Festenstein, H. (1976). Rejection of HLA identical related kidney transplants. *Tissue Antigens* **8**, 233.

Salvatierra, O. (1986). Donor-specific transfusions in living-related transplantation. *World J. Surg.* **10**, 361.

Salvatierra, O., Feduska, N. J., Cochrum, K. C., Najarian, J. S., Kountz, S. L. and Belzer, F. O. (1977). The impact of 1,000 renal transplants at one center. *Ann. Surg.* **186**, 424.

Salvatierra, O., McVicar, J., Melzer, J., *et al.* (1991). Improved results with combined donor-specific transfusion (DST) and sequential therapy protocol. *Transplant. Proc.* **23**, 1024.

Sanfilippo, F., Thacker, L. and Vaughn, W. K. (1990). Living donor renal transplantation in SEOPF: the impact of histocompatibility, transfusions and cyclosporine on outcome. *Transplantation* **49**, 25.

Sanfilippo, F. and Vaughan, W. K. (1987). Results of live-donor renal transplantation: the SEOPF multicenter study. *Transplant. Proc.* **19**, 1489.

Sanfilippo, F., Vaughan, W. K. and Spees, E. K. (1984). The association of pretransplant native nephrectomy with decreased renal allograft rejection. *Transplantation* **37**, 256.

Santiago-Delpin, E., Gonzalez, Z., Morales-Ofero, L., *et al.* (1989). Transplantation in Hispanics: the Puerto Rico experience. *Transplant. Proc.* **21**, 3958.

Schaubel, D., Desmeules, M., Mao, Y., Jeffery, J. and Fenton, S. (1995). Survival experience among elderly end-stage renal disease patients: a controlled comparison of transplantation and dialysis. *Transplantation* **60**, 1389.

Schulak, J. A., Mayes, J. T., Johnston, K. H. and Hricik, D. E. (1990). Kidney transplantation in patients aged sixty years and older. *Surgery* **108**, 726.

Schweizer, R., Rovelli, M., Palmemi, D., *et al.* (1990). Noncompliance in organ transplant recipients. *Transplantation* **49**, 374.

Scott, J. R., Branch, D. W., Kockenour, N. K. and Larkin, R. M. (1986). Effect of repeated pregnancies on renal allograft function. *Transplantation* **42**, 694.

Senel, F. M., Karakayali, H., Moray, G. and Haberal, M. (1998). Delayed graft function: predictive factors and impact on outcome in living-related kidney transplantations. *Ren. Fail.* **20**, 589.

Sheriff, M. H., Tayha, T. and Lee, H. A. (1978). Is azathioprine necessary in renal transplantation? *Lancet* **1**, 118.

Shoskes, D. A. and Cecka, J. M. (1997). Effect of delayed graft function on short- and long-term kidney graft survival. *In Clinical Transplants 1997*, (J. M. Cecka and P. I. Terasaki, eds.), p. 297, UCLA Tissue Typing Laboratory, Los Angeles.

Shoskes, D. A. and Cecka, J. M. (1998). Deleterious effects of delayed graft function in cadaveric renal transplant recipients independent of acute rejection. *Transplantation* **66**, 1697.

Simmons, R. L. and Abress, L. K. (1987). Quality of life on cyclosporin versus conventional therapy. *Transplant. Proc.* **19**, 1860.

Simmons, R. L., Van Hook, E. J., Yunis, E. J., *et al.* (1977). 100 sibling kidney transplants followed 2 to 7 yrs 6 months: a multifactorial analysis. *Ann. Surg.* **185**, 196.

Sodal, G., Albrechten, D., Berg, K. J., *et al.* (1987). Renal transplantation from living donors mismatched for two HLA haplotypes. *Transplant. Proc.* **19**, 1509.

Strober, S., Dhillion, M., *et al.* (1989). Acquired immune tolerance to cadaveric renal allografts. *N. Engl. J. Med.* **321**, 28.

Sumari, N., Delaney, V., Ding, Z., *et al.* (1991). Renal transplantation from elderly living donors. *Transplantation* **51**, 305.

Takiff, H., Mickey, M. R. and Terasaki, P. I. (1986). Factors important in 10 year kidney transplant survival. *In Clinical Transplants 1986*, (P. I. Terasaki, ed.), p. 157, UCLA Tissue Typing, Los Angeles.

Taylor, C., Welsh, K., *et al.* (1994). Clinical and socioeconomic benefits of serological HLA-DR matching for renal transplantation over three eras of immunosuppression regimens in a single unit. *In Clinical Transplants 1993*, (P. I. Terasaki, ed.). UCLA Tissue Typing Laboratory, Los Angeles.

Taylor, R. J., Laundreneau, M. D., Makowka, L., *et al.* (1987). Cyclosporin immunosuppression and delayed graft function in 455 cadaveric renal transplants. *Transplant. Proc.* **19**, 2100.

Taylor, R. M., Ting, A. and Briggs, J. (1985). Renal transplantation in the United Kingdom and Ireland—the centre effect. *Lancet* **1**, 715.

Tegzess, A. M., Van Son, W. J., Van der Woude, F. J., *et al.* (1987). Cadaveric renal transplantation without previous chronic dialysis treatment as an alternative approach to the treatment of end-stage renal disease. *Transplant. Proc.* **19**, 1555.

Tejani, A. H., Sullivan, E. K., Alexander, S. R., *et al.* (1999). Predictive factors for delayed graft function (DGF) and its impact on renal graft survival in children: a report of the North American Pediatric Renal Transplant Cooperative Study (NAPRTCS). *Pediatr. Transplant.* **3**, 293.

Terasaki, P. I., Cecka, J. M., Gjertson, D. W., Cho, Y., Takemoto, S. and Cohn, M. (1993). A ten-year prediction for kidney transplant survival. *In Clinical Transplants 1992*, (P. I. Terasaki and J. M. Cecka, eds.), p. 501, UCLA Tissue Typing Laboratory, Los Angeles.

Terasaki, P. I., Koyama, H., Cecka, J. M. and Gjertson, D. W. (1994). The hyperfiltration hypothesis in human renal transplantation. *Transplantation* **57**, 1450.

Terasaki, P. I., Toyotome, A., Mickey, M. R., *et al.* (1985). Patient, graft and functional survival rates—an overview. *In Clinical Kidney Transplants 1985*, (P. I. Terasaki, ed.), p. 1, UCLA Tissue Typing Laboratory, Los Angeles.

Terasaki, P. I. and Cecka, J. M. (1999). The Center Effect: Is bigger better? *In Clinical Transplant 1999*, (J. M. Cecka and P. I. Terasaki, eds.), p. 317, UCLA Tissue Typing Laboratory, Los Angeles.

Tesi, R. J., Elkhammas, E. A., Davies, E. A., Henry, M. L. and Ferguson, R. M. (1994). Renal transplantation in older people. *Lancet* **343**, 461.

Thorogood, J., van Houwelingen, J. C., van Rood, J. J., Zantvoort, F. A., Schreuder, G. M. and Persijn, G. G. (1992). Factors contributing to long-term kidney graft survival in Eurotransplant. *Transplantation* **54**, 152.

Tilney, N. L. (1986). Transplantation between identical twins: a review. *World J. Surg.* **10**, 381.

Tilney, N. L., Hager, E. B., Boyden, C. M. N., Sandberg, G. W. and Wilson, R. E. (1975). Treatment of chronic renal failure by transplantation and dialysis. *Ann. Surg.* **182**, 108.

Ting, A. and Morris, P. J. (1978). Matching for B cell antigens of the HLA-DR (D related) series in cadaver renal transplantation. *Lancet* **1**, 575.

Toyotome, A., Terasaki, P. I., Takiff, H., *et al.* (1986). Early graft function. *In Clinical Transplants 1986*, (P. I. Terasaki, ed.), p. 321, UCLA Tissue Typing Laboratory, Los Angeles.

Troppmann, C., Gillingham, K. J., Benedetti, E. and Matas, A. J. (1995). Delayed graft function, acute rejection, and outcome after cadaver renal transplantation: the multivariate analysis. *Transplantation* **59**, 962.

Uehling, D. T., Hussey, J. L., Weinstein, A. B., Want, R. and Bach, F. H. (1976). Cessation of immunosuppression after renal transplantation. *Surgery* **79**, 278.

UKTSSA Renal Transplant Audit. (1993). UKTSSA, Bristol.

Vanrentergehm, Y., Roels, L., Gruwez, I., Dendrievel, J. and Michielsen, P. (1987). Impact of HLA-DR and combined HLA-B and HLA-DR matching on early graft outcome under cyclosporine therapy. *Transplant. Proc.* **19**, 685.

Vollmer, W. M., Wahl, P. W. and Blagg, C. R. (1983). Survival with dialysis and transplantation in patients with end-stage renal disease. *N. Engl. J. Med.* **308**, 1553.

Ward, H. J., Koyle, M. A., Terasaki, P. I. and Cecka, J. M. (1987). Outcome of renal transplantation in blacks. *Transplant. Proc.* **19**, 1546.

Wengerter, K., Matas, A. J., Tellis, V. A., *et al.* (1986). Transplantation of pediatric donor kidneys to adult recipients: is there a critical donor age? *Ann. Surg.* **204**, 172.

Williams, G. M., White, H. J. O. and Hume, D. M. (1967). Factors influencing the long-term functional success rate of human renal allografts. *Transplantation* **5**, 837.

Wolfe, R. A., Ashby, W. B., Milford, E. L., *et al.* (1999). Comparison of mortality in all patients on dialysis, patients on dialysis awaiting transplantation, and recipients of a first cadaveric transplant. *N. Engl. J. Med.* **341**, 1725.

Zhou, Y.-C. and Cecka, J. M. (1993). Preservation. *In Clinical Transplants 1992*, (P. I. Terasaki and J. M. Cecka, eds.), p. 383, UCLA Tissue Typing Laboratory, Los Angeles.

Psychological Aspects of Kidney Transplantation and Organ Donation

Patricia M. Franklin

Psychological Aspects of Kidney Transplantation

INTRODUCTION

End-stage renal disease is a psychologically debilitating illness with considerable emotional morbidity (Kalman *et al.*, 1983)—a disease that can block the patient's life goals and precipitate a vicious circle of depression, mood swings and unfulfilled hopes (Salter, 1988). Since the first introduction of dialysis and renal transplantation in the 1950s and early 1960s, researchers have studied the psychological impact of these treatments and the difficulties encountered by patients and their caregivers. Treatment of renal failure through dialysis or transplantation creates considerable stress for patients (Petrie, 1989). Early studies reported almost equal psychiatric morbidity in dialysis and transplant groups and did not support the idea of psychological advantages of transplantation over dialysis (Kalman *et al.*, 1983). As success rates with transplantation have improved and immunosuppression regimens have developed, however, it has been shown repeatedly that the quality of life with a functioning transplant is superior to that which usually is achieved on dialysis (Evans *et al.*, 1985; Jofre *et al.*, 1998; Johnson *et al.*, 1982; Rodin *et al.*, 1985).

Every aspect of life for patients and their caregivers is affected by renal failure and its treatment, and appropriate support needs to begin as early as possible to prevent subsequent problems. Understanding of the psychological aspects of transplantation grew rapidly in the 1990s (Craven and Rodin, 1992). This increased understanding has resulted in the opportunity to offer informed psychological support as an integral part of transplantation care. This chapter discusses the major psychological studies and their findings and provides brief personal experiences reported by patients to the author during 20 years of experience as a nurse psychologist working in transplant centers.

QUALITY OF LIFE AND PSYCHOLOGICAL WELL-BEING

Quality of life research receives much criticism because individual perception and assessment of quality of life is known to be affected by a wide range of independent and personal variables. It is difficult to have a comprehensive appreciation of an individual quality of life. According to Evans *et al.* (1985), after 20 years of research, there still is no consensus on how best to conceptualize *quality of life*.

The most extensive data available comparing dialysis and transplant quality of life came from a large collaborative study led by Evans of the Battelle Human Affairs Research Center in Seattle. This study, involving more than 800 patients in 11 United States centers, is accepted widely because it used objective and subjective quality of life indicators, investigated all treatment modalities and included new treatments such as erythropoietin and new immunosuppression regimens. Evans and colleagues concluded: "Transplant recipients generally have a higher level of functional ability, are more likely to return to work, are in better health, and have higher levels of well being, life satisfaction, psychological affect, and happiness than do patients on any form of dialysis" (Evans *et al.*, 1985). Other sources support these findings, with successful transplant patients reporting higher levels of psychological well-being than patients on dialysis (Churchill *et al.*, 1984; Jofre *et al.*, 1998; Kaplan De Nour and Shanan, 1980; Morris and Jones, 1988; Petrie, 1989; Simmons *et al.*, 1984).

Galpin (1992) reported that patients often see successful transplantation as a gateway to "personal liberation" and to restoring "control over one's life and one's self." Fisher *et al.* (1998) stated that "quality of life improved dramatically after transplantation despite the persistence of some renal symptoms and patients felt privileged to have been offered this treatment option." Since the 1960s, kidney transplantation has evolved from an experimental procedure in a few highly selected patients to its current status as an effective treatment. Transplantation now is viewed as the treatment of choice for most patients in end-stage renal failure. Life with the best functioning transplanted kidney is a life pervaded by perpetual uncertainty, however. The possibility of organ rejection, without warning, is a constant threat causing anxiety and stress. A life of continuous immunosuppressive therapy has psychological difficulties; bodily changes and other major issues need to be negotiated successfully by transplant recipients (Kalman *et al.*, 1983).

RENAL DISEASE: DIALYSIS AND PREOPERATIVE ADJUSTMENTS

Although kidney transplantation is the treatment of choice for most end-stage renal disease patients, with demand for grafts far exceeding supply, many have to wait months or years before this treatment is available to them. A few patients may receive a transplant during the predialysis stage, but for most, the waiting period involves emotional adjustments to the physical, psychological, marital and dialysis-related changes imposed by the disease. The shock of the initial diagnosis, sexual dysfunction, marital friction, changes in body image with subsequent lower self-esteem and descent to dependence on a machine, fluid bag or partner can produce profound stress, adjustment anxiety and depression (Galpin, 1992; Surman, 1989; White *et al.*, 1990). Various psychological coping strategies may be used during this time to help the patient and family negotiate this period of disease and dialysis adjustment.

Coping strategies are *psychological patterns* that individuals use to manage thoughts, feelings and actions encountered during various stages of ill health and treatments. The fundamental need to have an overall sense of control over one's life is paramount throughout chronic sickness, and research has shown that interventions designed to increase an individual's perception of control are likely to have a positive impact on patient well-being (Bremer *et al.*, 1995). Presenting treatment options with information so that realistic choices can be made helps patients maintain a sense of control.

During the early phase of ill health, denial and suppression are the most frequent avoidance strategies used (Miller, 1983). Denial as a psychological defense has been prominent in the hemodialysis population (Surman, 1989). Later, more positive coping strategies include problem solving, actively seeking information, enhancement of spiritual life and hope of a transplant (Voepal-Lewis *et al.*, 1990; White *et al.*, 1990). These coping strategies are similar to ones used by end-stage cardiac disease patients (O'Brien, 1985).

Cassileth *et al.* (1984) compared six patient groups and found that the adjustment of patients with chronic renal failure is comparable to that of patients with other chronic diseases. Kaplan De Nour and Czaczkes (1976) found that renal patients who deal best with anger and dependency have the most favorable adjustment outcome.

Many younger patients find such adjustment extremely difficult. Research conducted between Oxford and Manchester found that "the younger patient, particularly the young male, found dependence on dialysis particularly frustrating perhaps because society expects the male to be more active, aggressive and ambitious in forging a role in life." Young male patients may express more dissatisfaction and are more likely to show this dissatisfaction in noncompliant, self-destructive and despairing behavior (Auer, 1990a). One young male hemodialysis patient described his life as a series of frustrating *can't do's*: "can't drink beer with friends; can't enjoy meals with friends; can't go on vacation with friends; can't work and can't make love to a girlfriend."

Reasonably fit elderly patients are in some ways the most satisfied dialysis group (Westlie *et al.*, 1984). Many elderly patients feel satisfied with their lives and welcome the chance of a further few years resulting from treatment.

The initial dialysis adjustment phases are difficult and for some patients traumatic. Professional practical and psychological support is desirable at this time.

Health beliefs and attitudes toward illness and treatments differ between individuals and among cultures, as do responses to pain and reactions to a new graft. Many white patients find that peritoneal dialysis offers a moderate to good quality of life, but at Oxford a Muslim patient with a strict religious hygiene code found this treatment impossible because she felt "unclean—like a dustbin, always filling up with rubbish." Such feelings made prayer difficult and life unbearable for her. Cultural attitudes may influence the recipient's response to transplantation. A young female Asian patient at this transplant center refused the idea of a cadaveric transplant because she was reluctant to accept a kidney from an anonymous donor who may be male.

Di Matteo and Di Nicola (1982) discussed health and illness beliefs and outlined the need for staff to "consider the meaning that patients attach to their illness and treatment therapies." It is important for staff to be aware of individual perceptions and beliefs with regard to transplantation. Each belief must be recognized and validated and, if required, appropriate support provided.

Many units provide predialysis information sessions for patients and families. Bradley and McGee (1994) suggest that the "most effective sessions seem to be run on a multidisciplinary basis, with input from Medical, Nursing, Dietetic and Social Work staff, and include information from dialysis and transplant patients themselves." In this unit, such sessions are valuable because they provide an opportunity to give information concerning all treatment options. The sessions also provide a forum to encourage active patient and caregiver participation with regard to treatment issues and initial treatment anxieties.

Meeting other patients who have negotiated various forms of treatment successfully offers a positive image and role model and gives greater credibility to information given. Honesty is an important part of such sessions, and information givers strive to present a realistic assessment of experiences without being overprotective regarding problems or overoptimistic. Such sessions help to develop a close supportive relationship between staff and patients at the predialysis stage.

HOPE OF A TRANSPLANT

Peretz (1970) defined *hope* as the capacity to anticipate that even though one feels uncomfortable now, one may feel better in the future. Once a transplant is suggested, many patients make an immediate decision to proceed, whereas others may agonize over the decision. Some may deny the possibility of posttransplant difficulties and may have unrealistic expectations for their future quality of life. Such denial may predispose patients to depression if major complications occur after the transplant (Dubovsky and Penn, 1980). It is essential that in-depth realistic and honest information is given at this stage so that patients may proceed in an informed manner.

In the past, renal programs often required formal pretransplant psychiatric assessments. These assessments are no longer considered necessary, but the experience at Oxford suggests that it is valuable to have a pretransplant meeting at which specific medical, social and psychological issues are explored with the patient and family. Individual fears raised at such a meeting include fear of changes in body image resulting from immunosuppression, fear of loss of identity when accepting a *foreign organ* and fear of surgery, particularly for older patients. These concerns are similar to those reported by Weems and Patterson (1989). A pretransplant meeting is an opportunity to dispel myths or hearsay that may have been gleaned from other patients. Issues raised in this unit that have required careful explanation include the idea that dialysis is only a short-term treatment and that the patient may die unless he or she receives a transplant, that it is possible to be infected with venereal and other diseases from a cadaver organ, that a male receiving a female kidney may become feminized and vice versa and that the donor persona may be implanted with the transplant and that the recipient "will become a different person."

The pretransplant meeting offers the opportunity to explore, examine and resolve individual fears and helps to initiate a trusting and supportive relationship with a member of the transplant team. The meeting is a time to offer specific information and advice concerning coping skills and responses to the profound and conflicting emotions that may be experienced.

The knowledge gained by staff during these meetings concerning individual fears and difficulties alerts the professionals to vulnerabilities that may require help postoperatively. A brief period of counseling may be in order for patients who experience the most difficulty with the decision regarding transplant. Weems and Patterson (1989) and Abram (1972) reported ambivalent anticipation by many patients, particularly those who were doing well with dialysis.

These patients expressed feelings of doubt about whether or not a transplant would improve their quality of life.

Renal patients must temper their hope for a transplant and subsequent enhanced quality of life with the knowledge that there can be no guarantee that a suitable graft will become available or that the transplant will be successful. These uncertainties increase ambivalence toward transplantation and increase psychological stress. Most patients and families describe the waiting time as the most difficult phase (O'Brien, 1985; Weems and Patterson, 1989).

Patient fears that they have been forgotten, that they may miss the call or that their chance may never come are reported frequently. Ongoing contact with the transplant center is helpful and is vital at times of additional stress when a fellow dialysis patient receives or rejects a kidney, when an abortive call occurs or when the waiting period becomes particularly lengthy. These instances may upset the usual coping strategies, and psychological stress and depression may result. In our center, a transplant nurse specialist is assigned to each patient at the pretransplant meeting so that a supportive bond can develop and the nurse can offer information and support during the waiting time as well as after transplantation.

IMMEDIATE POSTOPERATIVE PSYCHOLOGICAL ISSUES

Many kidney transplant recipients report an immediate feeling of *rebirth* after the transplant; such feelings are linked to a perceived promise of extended and enhanced quality of life (Cramond, 1967; Surman, 1989). Studies suggest that psychological stress persists throughout the initial recovery period and during the early rehabilitation process. Simmons *et al.* (1971) reported that "... even though a renal transplant is frequently considered an opportunity for renewed health, recipients indicated that it did not eliminate health related stress from their lives." The major causes of psychological stress during the early postoperative phase include possibility of rejection and lack of control regarding the body's acceptance or rejection of the kidney, fear of infection, uncertainty about the future and concern about long-term side effects of immunosuppressive therapy (Fallon *et al.*, 1997; Frey, 1990; Hayward *et al.*, 1989; White *et al.*, 1990).

The fear of graft rejection is the most frequently reported, and anxiety has been shown to precede the first rejection experience (Hayward *et al.*, 1989; Surman, 1989). Such anticipatory anxiety is lessened if the rejection is treated successfully, and although recipients are more at ease if faced with future rejection episodes, uncertainty about future health persists for many months.

One of the most difficult aspects for recipients at this stage is the sudden removal of *conscious control*. The dialysis patient has become conditioned to control of health through adherence to diet and fluid restrictions and regular treatment regimens. After the transplant, the situation changes radically, and recipients are "at the mercy" of factors beyond conscious control, for example: "their own immune response and the effects of the foreign body which now needs to become accepted as part of the self" (Auer, 1990a). Such loss of control can increase anxiety levels, and some patients report panic attacks. It is vital at this stage to discuss progress in detail with the patient and to answer all questions because many recipients seek to regain conscious control by information seeking and by planning daily psychological and activity goals. It is helpful to encourage patient participation in care with self-medication and self-observation so that control is achieved in part. If recipients can be included in discussions

regarding medication options, such choice also offers an element of control at this difficult stage.

Some recipients may have difficulty in accepting the new graft as *part of self*. Castelnuovo-Tedesco (1981) wrote that "the graft is not psychologically inert and that the recipient may develop a prominent identification with the donor." One young female patient at Oxford who was depressed posttransplant stated that: "before my transplant I had a broken body and a healthy mind—now, after my transplant I have a healthy body and a broken mind." During gentle exploration, it was discovered that this patient found it profoundly difficult to accept that she had the kidney of a middle-aged male "inside her," fearing that her femininity was at risk. Other patient fears reported include fear of racial change and in some cases obsessive identification with the donor or the donor family (Cramond, 1967; Kemph, 1966; Surman, 1989).

Bunzel *et al.* (1992) reported that a few heart transplant recipients (6% [three patients]) reported "a distinct change in personality due to their new hearts—with the belief that they were forced to change feelings and reactions and accept those of the donor." Such statements seemed to show "severe problems regarding graft incorporation which are based on the age-old idea of the heart as a centre that houses feelings and forms the personality." Sylvia (1997), a heart-lung recipient, wrote that her attitudes, tastes, food likes and dislikes changed to mirror the attitudes, tastes, food likes and dislikes of the donor.

Studies regarding *perceived* changes in personality are reported mainly by heart transplant recipients and usually are linked to the belief that the heart is seen "as the source of love, emotions and, for some, the focus of personality traits" (Sylvia, 1997). The subsequent publicity from Sylvia's book led several patients at our center to become anxious that the transplanted kidney may result in a personality change for them. In our experience, such anxieties can be resolved by discussion and reassurance that the graft does not carry the persona of the donor and cannot alter the integrity of the recipient's personality.

Feelings of guilt and sadness concerning the donor and donor family are frequent (Surman, 1989). An adult receiving a pediatric graft may view the death as a special tragedy and experience profound guilt and grief (Cramond, 1967). Recipients and caregivers report dreams in which they may see a distressed family without a father or mother, and they may relate such dreams to the donor family. Recipients report the need to offer prayers for the donor and the family and may experience feelings of unworthiness in receiving such a precious, life-enhancing gift. Fox and Swazey (1992) discuss the obligations entwined in such a gift, and they quote the work of Mauss (1954): "The obligation of worthy return is imperative too. Face is lost forever if it is not made."

The opportunity to discuss such feelings and to give thanks through an anonymous letter usually aids resolution so that the recipient may move forward toward positive rehabilitation. It is becoming more common, however, for recipients and/or donor families to request a meeting with each other. Several transplantation units are facilitating such meetings, and initial reports suggest successful outcomes for the recipient and the donor family. Reports cited by Fox and Swazey (1992) stress the need for caution, however, because the donor family may be "disappointed in the recipient" or may become "intrusive into the recipient's life." The recipient may face the dilemma of wanting to refuse such a meeting but not wanting to appear ungrateful and may be distressed or disturbed at trying to meet the perceived needs of the donor family. It has been stated that it is *paternalistic* of professionals to discourage such meetings; however, professionals have a duty of care to recipients and donor families. Thorough discussion and planning must precede such meetings, and fully trained professionals must be available to offer debriefing sessions and to help should problems arise.

IMMUNOSUPPRESSION

Psychiatric Issues

Immunosuppression may produce psychiatric disorders in the immediate postoperative period, most commonly delirium and mood disorders. In the 1960s and 1970s when patients required sustained treatment with high-dose corticosteroids, these syndromes were relatively common in renal transplant recipients, and studies at this time reported mood elevation (euphoria ranging to mania) (Penn et al., 1971; Short and Harris, 1969) and depression (Penn et al., 1971; Wilson et al., 1968). The introduction of low-dose steroid therapy accelerated by the further introduction of cyclosporine has resulted in fewer psychiatric disorders, although mania still may be observed in some recipients with particular corticosteroid sensitivity. Low-dose corticosteroids often are responsible for mood changes and irritability reported in the early posttransplant period that may be less apparent to the patient than to others in the same environment. Transient disruption of sleep, altered perception and lability of mood often occur in patients receiving pulses of corticosteroids as antirejection therapy (Surman, 1989).

Infection is an important complication of transplantation and must be considered in the differential diagnosis of an altered mental state. Depression in the posttransplant period is caused commonly by infection, and it is especially prevalent among patients with cytomegalovirus infection or cytomegalovirus mononucleosis syndrome (Rubin et al., 1977; Surman, 1989).

Patients who have unrealistically high expectations preoperatively are susceptible to postoperative depressive symptoms. Such patients may have difficulty accepting that transplantation is an alternative treatment rather than a cure for end-stage renal disease (Rodin and Abbey, 1992). The most appropriate psychiatric diagnosis for many of these patients is an adjustment disorder (Rodin and Abbey, 1992). Fricchione (1989) reported that the degree of distress often is correlated with the severity of physical symptoms and the occurrence of postoperative complications.

Psychological Issues—Body Image and Self-Esteem

People in renal failure may experience negative reactions toward their bodies because of the invasive nature of the treatment (Galpin, 1992). The cessation of dialysis after renal transplantation does not abolish this stress (Hudson and Hiott, 1989; Klein et al., 1984). Immunosuppression and its side effects present a major problem related to body image posttransplantation (Bernstein, 1971; Gaedeke-Norris, 1991; Galpin, 1992; Hudson and Hiott, 1986). Corticosteroids may cause acne and a cushingoid appearance characterized by an abnormally round face and protruding abdomen. Hirsutism, mild tremors and gingival hyperplasia commonly are exhibited by patients receiving cyclosporine. Such side effects prompted a young Oxford patient to perceive herself as "something from the *Planet of the Apes.*"

Body image is a personal matter; what is a problem for one person may be insignificant for another (Price, 1990), but if body image is perceived unfavorably, feelings of inferiority and intense anxiety may be generated. Studies suggest that many renal transplant recipients report body image problems with subsequent lower self-esteem and feelings of inferiority

or of "being altered or damaged" (Bernstein, 1971; Hudson and Hiott, 1986). Some recipients find the changes of body image after a kidney transplant more distressing than those that occurred while on dialysis (Galpin, 1992). The cushingoid puffy look of the face generally creates the biggest obstacle to acceptance (Galpin, 1992). Dissatisfaction with body image is associated with poor psychosocial adjustment and interferes with successful rehabilitation (Klein et al., 1984).

Careful preoperative counseling concerning expected side effects, reassurance that such side effects are dose related and will lessen as drug dosages are reduced and practical help and advice in coping with specific problems may reduce the psychological trauma that altered body image causes recipients. At our institution, a trained skin and beauty therapist offers extensive advice, and recipients report that this service greatly reduces the embarrassment and unhappiness experienced by bodily changes.

Body image change may be particularly distressing for adolescent recipients (Bernstein, 1971; Lilly et al., 1971; Nylander et al., 1985). Adolescents are in a period of structural ego alteration with conflict about identity, psychosexual development, dependency and authority, and the additional stress of a transplant may become a focus of derangement of their defenses (Bernstein, 1971). Many adolescent recipients may require additional support and understanding. For some adolescents, the side effects of immunosuppressive therapies and their perceived effects on social interaction are more unacceptable than graft failure and possible death from voluntary discontinuation of medications (Gaedeke-Norris, 1991).

Noncompliance

Noncompliance with immunosuppressive therapy as a cause of renal transplant rejection first was reported by Owens et al. (1975). These authors reported a 2% incidence of voluntary cessation of immunosuppressants (4 cases in a series of 203 transplants). Najarian (1975) reported a greater than 1% incidence of stopping immunosuppressants (6 cases in 700 transplants). Recipients discontinued their medication for "a variety of emotional and sociopathic reasons" (Najarian, 1975). Uehling and coworkers found a 4% incidence of major lapses (discontinuation of medications for ≥3 weeks) and a slightly higher incidence of minor lapses (discontinuation of medication for <3 weeks) during a period in which 80 transplantations were performed (Uehling et al., 1976). The reasons for noncompliance were reported as "serious emotional problems" (e.g., depression and alcohol abuse) or "powerful religious convictions" (Uehling et al., 1976).

In a review of 460 patients, Armstrong et al. (1981) found a 2% incidence of serious noncompliance to azathioprine-based immunosuppressive regimens. This study documented multiple psychosocial factors contributing to compliance failure, including low self-esteem, denial, regression and lack of family support.

Didlake et al. (1988) reviewed compliance with cyclosporine regimens in 531 kidney transplant recipients. This study reported major noncompliance resulting in graft loss in 2.8% of the sample and minor noncompliance resulting in rejection episodes in 1.9%. Recipients who showed major noncompliance tended to be white female patients. Subclinical degrees of noncompliance were found to be commoner. Of 295 transplant recipients who responded to a questionnaire, 13% reported missing more than three doses per month.

Various explanations have been given for noncompliance, including concern about the effects of immunosuppression on physical appearance, inability to accept the lifestyle limitations and the cost of medication. Surman (1989) noted that noncompliance may occur in major depression and in organic brain dysfunction or as part of an adjustment reaction, especially in adolescent recipients. Compliance may vary across different transplant groups (Rovelli *et al.*, 1989). Beck and coworkers found noncompliance in 43% of pediatric transplant patients, and it was commonest in adolescent girls, who may have been especially affected by body changes resulting from immunosuppressive therapy (Beck *et al.*, 1980).

Valid, reliable predictors of noncompliance are unavailable. Didlake *et al.* (1988) reported: "The strong history of poor dialysis compliance in patients non-compliant post transplant appears to be an important predisposing factor." Noncompliance may develop postoperatively in patients who have been compliant with dialysis and pretransplant medical care (Armstrong and Weiner, 1982; Didlake *et al.*, 1988; Rovelli *et al.*, 1989). Prospective studies are needed to define valid and reliable predictors of noncompliance. This information could be used to enhance maximum organ use. Rather than inappropriately denying transplantation to patients who might be noncompliant, however, Didlake and associates suggested that patients identified as high risk could receive extensive pretransplant psychosocial evaluation and psychological counseling, when necessary, to facilitate posttransplant follow-up, to strengthen the nurse-patient relationship and to ensure patient compliance to the immunosuppressive regimen (Didlake *et al.*, 1988). It is vital to explore and respect the underlying motives and feelings of the recipient and to offer support to enable adherence to medication regimens.

FAMILY INTERACTIONS

End-stage renal disease and its treatments cause shifts within the dynamics of family interactions. Chronic ill health and subsequent medical treatments may have engendered a sense of helplessness in the patient. Family roles change as the patient is placed into a state of chronic illness and treatment-induced dependency. The spouse may have to accept greater family responsibilities and may have to assist with dialysis treatments. Many caregivers report feelings of being "unsupported, invisible and unappreciated." (Auer, 1990a). Individuals trying to come to terms with their own feelings find it hard to spare extra energy to cope with the feelings of those close to them.

One of the important posttransplant psychosocial tasks that the patient needs to accomplish is the gradual relinquishing of the sick role and the eventual return to nonpatient status (Christopherson, 1987). After transplantation, the recipient may be reluctant to give up the security of the patient role, although the spouse may resent the continued dependence. Alternatively the patient may be eager to resume the preillness position of authority within the family, but the spouse might be disinclined to forfeit the newfound leadership role (Rauch and Kneen, 1989). Sexual problems may develop with incompatible sexual desires between partners. Marital issues usually can be resolved with the help of an empathetic nurse counselor and honest partner discussions.

Bernstein (1971) reported that another major area of concern after hospital discharge was reintegration into the family of a child or an adolescent who had been chronically ill who returns to the family with new mobility and vigor. Families tended to regard the child or adolescent as fragile and were excessively restrictive or permissive. Adolescent recipients were not required to follow the usual family rules, and there was family disruption causing psychological difficulties for the other siblings. These and other family issues can be treated readily with brief behavioral therapy (Wishman and Jacobson, 1990).

GRAFT FUNCTION

Delayed or Poor Graft Function

In most cases, the new transplant begins working well almost immediately; however, some recipients may have to wait weeks or months for the graft to function. During this time, the recipient must balance hope for a successful outcome with the fear of graft loss. Recipients respond in different ways; some may become overanxious, continually seeking information and reassurance; others may become angry and depressed, continually asking "why me." In contrast, some recipients may appear unconcerned, using denial to cover their underlying feelings of desperation. Staff may conclude that such recipients are unaware of the true situation. In reality, the patient is aware of the issues but is psychologically unable to face the possibility of graft failure. The fantasy that all is and will be well is more bearable during the waiting time. In this instance, denial can be a useful defense mechanism helping to make the period of delayed function sustainable. Perceived personal control is vital during this time, and empowering patients to take control over exercise regimens, health observations and medications lessens anxiety and increases self-confidence. Offering regular, honest information within an empathetic setting helps aid emotional stability for the recipient.

In some cases, the recipient may endure months or years of unsatisfactory graft function—a level of function that enables them to be free of dialysis but not able to obtain the desired quality of life or the expected level of rehabilitation. Simmons *et al.* (1984) stated that transplant recipients "expected a great deal from their post transplant lifestyle"—a dramatic improvement in physical health; a return to work, study or parental role; an improvement in self-image; an improvement in family relationships and freedom from the *sick role*. Such expectations may be unrealistic and may not be fulfilled. It may be difficult for recipients to admit failure to achieve such ideals and disappointment in their new health status.

Recipients may become anxious that they will appear ungrateful for the *gift of life* or the medical and nursing care given. Recipients also express guilt that they are not achieving enough or are in some way letting down the donor family or the transplant team. A young Oxford patient felt that she was not "living up to the right standard" and that she "had been given a special chance in which she had failed." Her conversation was littered with *shoulds* and *oughts*: "I should be making more of a success of my life. . . I ought to be more happy and grateful."

These feelings of guilt may be enhanced by family and friends who previously offered sympathy at the rigors of dialysis but now expect gratitude and full recovery. Partners may find the continuing need to support and care difficult, and marital difficulties can ensue, especially if there also is sexual friction. Recipients may experience emotional lability and depression, increasing their guilt, and with the additional physical debility resulting from heavy immunosuppression regimens, the psychological impact may be intense, resulting in low mood and clinical depression.

Psychological support should be offered to recipients and caregivers. In our institution, recipients have been found to benefit from therapies aimed at changing individual beliefs, such as cognitive and behavioral therapies. Caregivers found the opportunity to express feelings and recognize and fulfill their own needs beneficial. Marital therapies help in some cases, and if sexual difficulties are present, referral to a specialist team is required.

Graft Failure

Most recipients experience feelings of profound loss if their kidney transplant fails, although some may also feel relief if the graft has had unsatisfactory function over a protracted period. Relief may be linked to the return to dialysis and perceived control. Occasionally, denial may be used in the initial graft failure stage, but as the reality of the situation becomes apparent, sadness, anger and depression frequently are reported. Hudson and Hiott (1986) noted that recipients displayed a variety of behavior and reactions to graft loss, including *bereavement* reactions. "At this time patients must be helped to understand that the loss of the graft is not the end and that there is still hope for the future through subsequent transplants" (Hudson and Hiott, 1986).

Streltzer and colleagues studied 25 patients who suffered graft failure and found that all but 1 patient made a good readjustment to long-term dialysis (Streltzer *et al.*, 1983). Fourteen patients grieved the loss of their kidney openly, and 10 denied any psychological difficulties. Rodin and coworkers undertook the first systematic study of graft failure comparing 13 patients whose grafts had failed with 42 who had successful transplants and 38 still on the waiting list (Rodin *et al.*, 1985). These investigators found that although an unsuccessful transplant was associated with some deterioration in subsequent physical activity, there was no deterioration in psychosocial functioning in patients with graft failure, as measured by the Sickness Impact Profile. In our experience, the return to dialysis is negotiated gradually and successfully by most recipients, and as the disappointment of the graft failure subsides, most quickly request the chance for another transplant.

CONCLUSION

Kidney transplantation is the treatment of choice for many patients with end-stage renal disease. Life with the best-functioning transplanted kidney is a life with uncertainty, however. The fear and possibility of rejection are constant. Immunosuppressive therapy can lead to psychiatric and psychological morbidity, and necessary shifts in family dynamics and readjustment into society can cause emotional difficulties.

Publius Syrus (1st century B.C.) wrote that "pain of mind is worse than pain of body." Understanding of the psychological aspects of transplantation grew rapidly in the 1990s. Such increased understanding has resulted in the opportunity to offer informed psychological support as an integral part of transplantation care, reducing psychological morbidity and enhancing rehabilitation and quality of life.

Psychological Aspects of Living Donation
LIVING RELATED DONORS

The first successful renal transplants performed were mostly from living related donors. The psychological reactions of donor and recipient were monitored closely in many psychiatric studies and are outlined in this section.

Early Psychiatric Findings in Living Related Transplantation

Many of the initial studies conducted in the 1960s and early 1970s questioned the fundamental willingness of rela-

tives to make this type of sacrifice. Donor altruism—the supreme act of unselfishness and of giving freely without thought of reward—was much debated. Kemph (1966) reported that although donors were "consciously altruistic," there was "considerable unconscious resentment" toward the recipient and toward hospital personnel who requested or encouraged donation. Brewer (1970) reported that donors may be "victims of family blackmail" and were ambivalent about the loss of a body part but continued to donate because of family pressure or internal guilt. Simmons and colleagues recognized that family pressure could be direct or subtle and noted that pressure to donate could come from fear of family rejection or simply internal feelings of guilt (Simmons *et al.*, 1971). Many investigators reported that occasionally "the black sheep" of the family offered to donate in an attempt to win family approval and become reinstated within the family (Fellner and Marshall, 1970; Kemph *et al.*, 1969; Simmons *et al.*, 1971).

Kemph (1969) reported a moderate degree of postsurgical depressive reaction in donors with a grief reaction linked to the loss of a body part and some donor hostility expressed as anger that the recipient had been perceived to receive a greater amount of attention in the posttransplant phase. Cramond (1967) reported no postoperative depressive reaction for the donors but noted an ambivalent relationship postoperatively between donor and recipient, with the donor seeking to overprotect and the recipient resentful of the obligation and the subsequent dependency relationship. Kemph (1969) reported that recipients had difficulty with the obligation they felt toward the donor with the underlying guilt becoming apparent at times with obsequious behavior toward the donor and at other times in "hostility engendering behavior with the donor."

Few early studies reported favorable outcomes for donor and recipient. Fellner and Marshall (1970) studied 12 kidney donors and described the spontaneity of their participation and their persisting positive regard for the experience, stating that "some donors experienced the act as one of the most meaningful experiences of their lives and one that brought about beneficial changes." Although many of these early studies involved small numbers of donors and recipients, the negative psychiatric findings were much reported, and some observers suggested that cadaver organs were psychologically preferable because there could be no continuing obligation for the recipient.

Later Psychological Studies in Living Related Transplantation

During the late 1970s and the 1980s, studies began to report more positive psychological findings. Simmons *et al.* (1971) interviewed 230 living related donors and reported that "donors view themselves as more worthwhile because of the donation." In this study, only 5% of donors reported negative feelings about the transplant. Smith and coworkers found that 97% of donors reaffirmed their decisions, and less than 15% said that they felt pressured to donate (Smith *et al.*, 1986). With regard to recipient reactions, Simmons *et al.* (1977) reported that "although recipients did feel guilt about the gift that they could not reciprocate, most recipients and donors reported that there were no major problems in their relationship a year post transplantation."

Following the positive results of the published studies, in particular, the large Simmons study, the late 1980s saw a change in the way that transplant centers viewed living donor kidney transplants. Although some centers continued a strong stance against living donor transplants mainly because of the physical risks to the donor, many other centers increased living donor transplants. A study by Levey *et al.* (1986) noted that the physical risks to the donor were minimal and that the benefits to the donor considerable with regard to self-esteem and self-worth. Later studies reported that "to deny the donor the right to donate could do psychological harm" (Simmons *et al.*, 1984). Surman (1989) wrote that "kidney donation has a favourable outcome for both donor and recipient, and the participation of living related donors in kidney transplantation is now widely accepted."

During the early 1990s, studies again reported psychological difficulties for donor and recipient. Russell and Jacob (1994) postulated that "results indicate that while psychological side effects have been reported, including depression and family conflict, these risks are generally underemphasized... Health professionals should be aware that merely raising the issue of live organ donation may instigate powerful psychological processes beyond the potential donors' voluntary control and leave little room for refusal without psychological cost." Fox and Swazey (1992) examined the concept of the recipients' obligation to repay the "gift of life": "[I]n the case of a live kidney transplant," the donor may exhibit a great deal of "proprietary interest" in the health, work and private life of the close relative who has received his or her organ, on the emotional grounds that, "after all, it's my kidney . . . , that's me in there. . . ." In turn, the great indebtedness recipients may feel to the parent, sibling or child whose life-saving kidney they carry may make it difficult for them to maintain a reasonable amount of psychic difference and independence from the donor. Fox and Swazey (1992) reported that it was common for a recipient who needs freedom from the donor but feels too beholden to him or her to negotiate it to take the drastic step of breaking the relationship completely. These authors stressed the need for careful donor selection and ongoing psychological support for donor and recipient as important aspects of care throughout the living donor and recipient experience.

More Recent Studies and Developments in Living Related Donation

A fall in cadaver organ donation has been reported in recent years within the United Kingdom and Europe, and as numbers of patients on the waiting lists has risen, it has become apparent that "the full potential of renal transplantation will be realised only if other donor sources can be developed" (Nicholson and Bradley, 1999). Many units are following the example of Scandinavia and some centers in the United States and increasing living donor programs using related and unrelated donors.

Scandinavia incorporated live donation into its transplantation program in the 1960s, and in Norway living donors account for 45% of the total donor pool. Jakobsen (1997) reported that nearly 500 living donors in Norway were asked: "If you could turn the clock back, would you do the same again?"; 83% said "definitely yes" and another 11% said "probably yes." Many donors were deeply grateful for having been given the opportunity to become a donor. A study from Stockholm reported follow-up of 370 living kidney donors (Fehrmann-Ekholm *et al.*, 2000); this study concluded that fewer than 1% of donors regretted the donation, although several donors experienced the first few months after the donation as troublesome from a physical perspective.

American centers have published results from studies of follow-up in large numbers of living donors. A study by Schover *et al.* (1997) from the Cleveland Clinic examined 167 donors with regard to psychological aspects of the decision to donate, impact of donation on family relationships, donor reactions to graft failure and overall satisfaction of donors. The study findings suggest that "the majority of donors make the decision to donate with little ambivalence, express comfort with the choice at long term follow up and do not experience negative consequences regarding health . . . or family relationships" (Schover *et al.*, 1997). Jacobs *et al.* (1998) published a report from the University of Minnesota with follow-up of 529 living donors who had donated in the period 1985–1996. Study conclusions were that "donors scored higher than the general population with regard to quality of life issues" (Jacobs *et al.*, 1998). The overall donor experience was stressful for 12%, with donors more likely to say experiences were stressful if they had postoperative complications. If given the opportunity, only 4% of the donors said that they would not donate again, and 9% were unsure.

Positive donor outcomes were reported from the Scandinavian and American studies; however, all these studies were conducted by postal questionnaire, and such methodology may lack the in-depth exploration possible with face-to-face interviews, resulting in a superficial response that may mask deeper emotional reactions. In a European study reported by Eurotold (1997), interviews were conducted with small numbers of donors from Norway, the United Kingdom, Eire, Romania, Slovakia, Poland and Slovenia. This study concluded that "a very high percentage of donors knew very early on that they were going to donate and did not deliberate very long before reaching a decision; that there was little evidence to contradict the view that it is generally done as a genuine gift and that the research found no evidence of post operative regret whatever even in cases where the graft failed" (Eurotold, 1997).

LIVING UNRELATED DONORS

In Scandinavia, parents, siblings, adult children, uncles, aunts, grandparents and spouses are accepted as donors, but for ethical reasons, volunteers outside the family are not accepted. Spouses are genetically unrelated but are recognized as *emotionally related*. The Norwegian experience suggests that transplantation between spouses (partners) can achieve graft survival rates identical to the best achieved with cadaver organs. Jakobsen (1997) reported that "non genetically related donors have been accepted since October 1984 and now account for about 10% of the Norwegian living donor activity." This article noted that spouses (partners) often are well motivated to donate as "it is the healthy spouse who gains most by giving his or her healthy kidney so that the sick life-companion may regain his or her health" (Jakobsen, 1997).

Similar results for transplantation between partners have been reported in the United States. Binet *et al.* (1997) reported the conclusions of their study in which 46 living kidney donors and their emotionally related recipients were evaluated. Conclusions were that emotionally related living donors represent a valuable option for kidney transplantation, allowing more patients with end-stage renal disease to avoid long-term dialysis. Recipient and graft outcomes were superior to cadaver kidney transplantation. Motivated and emotionally related donors should be allowed to donate one of their kidneys, provided that they are selected carefully and informed thoroughly.

PSYCHOLOGICAL ISSUES AND IMPLICATIONS FOR PRACTICE: LIVING DONOR PROGRAMS

Many transplant centers are increasing living donation to include related and unrelated donors. We expanded our program so that living donors account for 30% of the donor activity. The psychological issues cited in this chapter and the results of our own psychological study (to be published) have formed the basis for the structure of the Live Donor Programme in Oxford. This program offers early concise information to donor and recipient and preoperative and postoperative psychological evaluation and support. It is hoped that this approach will help donor and recipient with decision making, avoid adverse psychological outcomes, reduce psychological morbidity and aid full donor and recipient emotional rehabilitation.

Informed Consent

The decision confronting the potential donor and recipient generates significant stress because it is life-threatening, irreversible and high risk (Simmons et al., 1971). It is imperative that the donor and recipient are informed fully regarding the advantages and risks involved and can make the decision to give or receive freely without overt or covert coercion.

Donor Informed Consent: Anxieties and Fears

Studies suggest that despite the seriousness of the decision, only few of individuals deliberated. Most donors regarded their choice as instantaneous and made without conscious evaluation.

Initial information must be detailed, and the initial approach to the donor must come at an early stage to ensure time to deliberate and to make an informed decision. In Norway, the initial approach to the donor often is made in a letter from the recipient's nephrologist. Recipients should not be asked to make the approach themselves because a refusal can be devastating, and donors may find it impossible to refuse such a request from an obviously sick relative.

The Norwegian approach of writing to relatives has been rejected in our unit because it was thought that donors may feel unable to refuse a formal medical request. In this center, we believe that information about living kidney donation should be made widely available in predialysis and dialysis outpatient areas through written leaflets and newsletters. Detailed information is given at the predialysis and transplantation seminars for recipients and their families, and in most cases, the donors then requested further information without the need for additional approaches. The Oxford Study showed that 80% of donors offered before being approached. The value of a formal recipient family education program with regard to living donor volunteer rates has been noted by Schweitzer et al. (1997).

Once a donor expresses an interest in donation, a meeting is arranged with the nurse specialist or counselor to explore in more detail the risks and benefits of live donation. Donors are asked *not* to make a full decision until a further discussion has occurred. The meeting is arranged for the donor, plus donor partner if wished, to explore donation in confidence. We explore other issues as well, such as preoperative donor-recipient relationship, individual anxieties and fears and donor partner attitude toward donation.

At this stage, the donor is informed that he or she may withdraw consent at any time and that if required a medical reason not to donate can be given. This *medical* reason is seen within the context of a *benevolent decision* to enable the donor decision to be fully altruistic. Other centers have reported using such a technique successfully within their programs (Hilton and Starzomski, 1994).

After discussion regarding risks and benefits, we explore the *perceived* relationship between donor and recipient. Siblings can be realistic about the relationship, but parents may

be unrealistic, presenting an idealized view of their relationship, particularly with an adolescent child. In the Oxford Study, all parents believed that they had a close relationship with their adolescent child recipient, whereas 30% of the adolescent group believed that the relationship was difficult to poor, with some adolescents suggesting problems of overprotection and inability to make independent decisions. It is necessary to confront such issues before transplantation so that the parent is aware of any difficulties, then problems may not occur after transplantation.

Donor fears and anxieties reported preoperatively involve donor death, fear of rejection and length of life of the graft, fear that the donor kidney may prove unsuitable and concerns for long-term health. Such issues can be explored throughout the donor preoperative course, and information and appropriate support can be offered.

At this time, we explore donor partner and family attitudes toward the donation. In some situations, the donor partner of a sibling is unhappy with the donation and believes that loyalty to the marriage should supersede loyalty of birth. Donors must be encouraged to make their own informed decisions, but if conflict ensues, appropriate support should be offered. In one case, a foster mother desperately wished to donate to her foster child, but her husband was adamantly against this decision. The outcome was that the wife withdrew the offer, but conflict within the marriage continued; marital therapy was offered.

Some donors may have specific dilemmas to resolve. A partner with a spouse and daughter suffering polycystic disease decided to donate to the daughter because the tissue match was superior. The spouse joined the cadaver waiting list. Another partner with a spouse and daughter suffering polycystic disease decided to donate to the spouse, who was unwell and unable to work, with the hope that an unaffected sibling would donate to the daughter at a later date. These and other dilemmas need to be discussed fully and decisions made with further information and psychological support.

Donors who are concerned by the risks involved may delay the decision making. In this center, we respect the need for a delay and resolve the issue by suggesting that the recipient may join the cadaver waiting list and the living donor be held in reserve for a later date. Simmons et al. (1977) reported a similar *postponement pattern*.

Recipient Informed Consent: Anxieties and Fears

Many recipients accept the offer of a transplant with alacrity, but some recipients may wish to refuse. An early meeting with the recipient (plus partner if wished) is arranged with the nurse specialist or counselor. The risks and benefits are discussed, and preoperative relationships, individual fears and anxieties and partner attitudes are explored.

Recipients may find it hard to refuse such an offer, fearing donor rejection, but with professional help, it is possible to refuse without conflict by using such reasons as "not wishing to inflict my disease on my family" or deciding to go on the cadaver waiting list with the donor held in reserve until a later date. As discussed earlier, adolescent recipients may find a parental donation difficult, fearing the need for "eternal gratitude" or "lack of independence and intrusion into lifestyle." It may be possible to resolve such issues with frank discussion facilitated by the nurse counselor, or it may be necessary to help the recipient refuse the donation.

Preoperative specific anxieties and fears reported by recipients in the Oxford Study included risks to the donor, fear of rejection and guilt about asking this of the family or partner. Such issues can be explored throughout the recipient preoperative course, and appropriate information and support can be offered.

Recipients may find themselves in a particularly difficult situation if parents are divorced and both wish to donate. The decision as to who should be the donor may need to be made with professional advice and appropriate support given to the parents and the recipient. It is hoped that such a structural preoperative program, undertaken through a series of nurse-led living donor clinics, with medical support at designated stages, helps the donor and recipient to make the right decision for them based on full information so that they might proceed to surgery without adverse psychological stress.

The psychological care and information continue into the posttransplant and rehabilitation phases. In our experience, donors and recipients that have close relationships but retain firm boundaries within those relationships achieve the greatest rehabilitation outcomes. Similar results are reported by Martin *et al.* (1998). We advise donors and recipients to celebrate the transplant together on the anniversary but to continue independent lives at other times. This arrangement facilitates recipient ability to give thanks and donor ability to receive such thanks but prevents overprotection or intrusion into lifestyle. Any difficulties encountered can be explored with the nurse specialist or counselor, and advice and help can be offered on a continuing basis. Such a comprehensive donor, recipient and family follow-up program may reduce psychological morbidity and help to identify problems so that suitable help and advice may be given to prevent such problems in the future.

Psychological Aspects of Cadaveric Organ Donation

INTRODUCTION

Many potential transplant recipients are denied the chance of a life-saving or life-enhancing graft because of a shortage of donor organs. Obstacles to cadaver organ donation are many and varied; however, one study reported the following: "Intensive care unit staff felt that the most important factor restricting organ harvest in their own units was dislike of adding to relatives' distress, followed by lack of training in approaching bereaved families to request donation" (Wakeford and Stepney, 1989).

The purpose of this section is to outline grief patterns and to discuss aspects of communicating with relatives during the crisis time, informing of death and requesting organ donation. Personal experience at Oxford with more than 300 donor families suggests that when relatives are approached sensitively, the subject of organ donation does not increase their distress, and organ donation brings comfort and hope through transplantation.

GRIEF PROCESS

Grief generally is described as a psychological process by which people fill the gap in their lives after a large part of their world has been lost. Engel (1962) described this process as *grief work*: "the work of mourning by which we can become emancipated from bondage to the deceased, readjust to the environment in which the deceased is missing, and begin to form new relationships." Lindemann first described the *stages of bereavement* in 1944. Other classic texts have supported and expanded this early theory. Most of these writers outlined three stages of grieving: (1) an immediate stage with shock, disbelief and denial; (2) an intermediary stage with a growing awareness accompanied by anger, anxiety and

depression and (3) a final stage of resolution, acceptance and healing.

More recently, theorists have argued that the concept of bereavement in stages is too structured and that such "classical texts may not entirely reflect how it is to suffer loss" (McLaren, 1995). Each individual responds to bereavement in a unique way, and the concept of stages may negate the individual pattern of coping. The grief process is neither universal nor predictable with no two families responding in the same way and with individual family members reacting with different emotional responses. Generalizations and comparisons at best may be unhelpful and at worse may be damaging, particularly if clinicians try to fit individuals into a fixed model of grief. Phillips (1999) stated that "grief is a profoundly idiosyncratic experience that gets overshaped and forced into moulds. There are as many ways of grieving as there are grievers. Putting people under pressure to do it properly is disabling."

Grief now is viewed as an individual experience that may contain common behavior patterns and reactions. The intensity of the reactions may be affected by other factors, such as the nature of the relationship between the patient and the bereaved, the age of the deceased, the type of death (expected or sudden) and the bereaved's responses to previous experiences and relationships. Research and clarification regarding the various individual and familial behavior patterns have been recorded, and it is possible to recognize patterns and plan and implement appropriate support and care.

Common Behavior Patterns in the Early Phase of the Grief Process

Common behavior patterns in the early phase of the grief process include numbness, panic, shock, denial, inability to concentrate and make decisions, inability to absorb information and use it effectively, demanding and irrational behavior, aggressive and abusive behavior, withdrawal and passivity. An understanding of these early patterns of behavior is important to clinicians because such behavior may occur soon after the death and at the time the bereaved are meeting with health professionals in the hospital environment.

The phase of stunned numbness is described by a bereaved relative in Speck's book (1978) as a "cotton wool time when there seems to be an invisible blanket between you and the world." Others speak of being "frozen in disbelief" and like a "zombie." There is a safety in this numbness in that it denies the more frightening reactions of helplessness, utter despair and intense fear. Denial can be interpreted as a psychological defense mechanism that prevents too much emotional pain at any one moment. Numbness, denial, shock and disbelief are increased in cases of sudden and traumatic death in which there has been no preparation for the terrible news and no possibility of anticipatory grieving. Numbness, shock and disbelief may last for hours, days or weeks and may damage and impede the exchange of information and all forms of communication. Denial may play a role throughout the grief process, emerging and subsiding at different times. Extended denial lengthens the grief process and may result in the bereaved feeling the reality of the death at the time that others appear to have "forgotten."

Anger, Anxiety, Depression and Isolation

The gradual awareness of the reality of the situation often is accompanied by anger and anxiety. Such anger may be directed toward God, the deceased or members of the caring professions, or it may be internalized and used inwardly against the bereaved themselves. Internalized anger often is linked with feelings of guilt and is most apparent after sudden and traumatic death or the death of a child.

Yearning and searching for the deceased may occur and often is accompanied by feelings of emptiness and intense isolation. The loneliness may become extreme with thoughts of not being understood by family and friends. Such intense responses may engender a fear in the bereaved that they are going insane and may result in them becoming absorbed with their own feelings to the exclusion of partners and family, increasing feelings of alienation. Sadness, depression and exhaustion may develop gradually and may continue for many months.

Healing Behaviors to Enable the Bereaved to Continue with Their Lives

Gradual readjustment and reintegration may occur as the intensity of the emotional pain lessens, and the bereaved may start to look forward and find some new purpose in living or new ways of behaving that enable them to continue with their lives. Phrases such as "letting go of the deceased" and "moving on" have been used in the past, but it is widely recognized now that many relatives may wish to find ways of sustaining the bond with the deceased and integrating this bond into future life.

High-Risk Groups: Intense Bereavement Reactions

Several researchers have outlined factors that may indicate a high risk of an intense bereavement reaction requiring additional or specific support, as follows:

Unexpected loss—patient in the younger age group with no previous history of illness
Suicide
Sudden loss—no preparation for the death
Bereaved perceives the family as unsupportive—lack of social network
Relationship between the deceased and the relative is perceived as ambivalent—often manifested as dependency, anger or guilt
Death of a child—parental grief is more severe, complex, protracted and traumatic than grief following any other bereavement.

Research has shown that professional counseling can reduce morbidity significantly in the cases of an intense bereavement reaction. The effect of the counseling is to reduce the risk in high-risk individuals to that of low-risk individuals without counseling.

Needs of Relatives During the Crisis Time

The needs of the relatives during the crisis time when the patient is critically ill have been investigated. Molter (1979) reported that the five most important needs were

1. To feel there is hope.
2. To feel that the hospital staff cared about the patient.
3. To know the prognosis.
4. To have questions answered honestly.
5. To be near the patient.

Hampe (1975) reported similar needs, as follows:

To be with the dying person
To be helpful to the dying person
To be assured that the dying person is comfortable
To be kept informed of the dying person's condition

To know of the impending death
To experience and express emotions
To comfort and support family members
To be accepted, supported and comforted by health care professionals
To be relieved of anxiety

It may be difficult to meet all these needs; individual needs should be met as and when they arise. Staff need to be flexible. Communicating with the family at regular intervals and giving them honest information help the family through the distressing phase when they alternate between hope for recovery and fear of death. Clinicians should focus on the needs of the family and view themselves as a companion, accompanying the family through all aspects of the situation.

To Have Questions Answered Honestly: To Know the Prognosis

The family needs to know the truth of the situation. Truth in itself is not damaging, but its presentation must be planned carefully. Blandy (1989) noted that one should "[t]emper the wind to the shorn lamb. Dilute frankness with gentleness and wherever possible offer hope." Relatives need the facts about the clinical condition and a realistic prognosis with its implications for them as a family.

Truth may not be the information that family members are hoping for, but it allows them to take control and to select options and make decisions. Staff should strive at this time to develop a rapport with relatives so that trust is established, allowing them to inform, support and offer choices. Clinicians need to listen to the family and hear the concerns that the situation has raised for them. Families should be included in discussions concerning care, and if the family wishes, children should be encouraged to be present and involved. Children and relatives that are excluded may imagine a situation worse than reality.

Support, Comfort and Cultural and Religious Needs

Relatives in a crisis situation require continual support. A relative who is alone should be comforted by an empathetic caregiver until another family member, friend or acceptable person can come and support them. While waiting, relatives should be kept as comfortable as possible, preferably in a suitably furnished private room near telephone and toilet facilities. They should be offered refreshments and allowed to smoke.

To Be Near the Patient

The family should be allowed to sit with the patient as soon as possible and should be encouraged to help with appropriate aspects of care. Staff must be aware of cultural differences and religious beliefs; interpreters and religious advisers should be contacted to add comfort and assist in communication.

COMMUNICATING WITH THE FAMILY
Informer and Supporter

When communicating with the family, it is helpful to use two people: an informer and a supporter. The clinician often is the informer; the supporter often is a nurse, a religious adviser or another member of the caring team. The roles of the informer and the supporter should be kept separate. The family may blame or reject the informer; should this happen, the supporter can offer physical comfort, repeat information and offer further support. The informer must not take such rejection personally. The family is not rejecting the informer but rather the information that they have given.

Before communicating with the family, it is important for the informer to prepare himself or herself physically and mentally. Evidence of trauma, such as bloodstains, must be removed, as should barriers that impede communication (e.g., surgical masks). The informer should become familiar with the family situation, noting the names of the principal relatives and their relationship with the patient. If there is a large group of relatives, it is helpful to speak directly to the immediate next of kin, using first names as appropriate. Meetings with the relatives should be planned so that there is time for discussion. Meetings should take place in a private relatives' room where the family can express their thoughts and feelings freely.

Verbal and Nonverbal Cues

On meeting the family, the informer and supporter should introduce themselves, shake hands with the relatives and sit near to them. It is important to maintain a calm, unhurried approach and to offer relatives the time to ask questions; the informer and supporter should never hover in the doorway as if ready to make a hasty exit.

Nonverbal cues indicating the gravity of the situation should be used so that the relatives receive some preparation for the information. Facial expressions should be serious, as should the tone of voice. The informer should speak to relatives in nontechnical language and give information slowly, gradually sowing the seeds of the seriousness of the situation. The informer should make eye contact and speak softly, with spaces in between words and sentences. Care personnel should never try to overprotect family from unpleasant reality: If there is a possibility of death, it is essential to inform the family and help them to prepare. Staff must be sensitive to relatives' needs and use physical comfort as appropriate, such as holding a hand or placing a comforting arm on the shoulder.

Relatives may try to minimize the seriousness of the situation by misinterpreting information or by hearing only certain parts of the message. Shock and disbelief can block communication and impede understanding; the informer should invite questions to find out what has been understood, then clarify and repeat the information. Distressed relatives can grasp at every word spoken, and it is important to avoid *unguarded comments*. Relatives may confront different staff members with the same questions about the patient's status hoping for a more positive message. It is necessary to maintain good communication among team members so that the same information is given by all.

The family must be encouraged to express their thoughts and feelings. Staff should not tell them how to feel (e.g., "do not upset yourself"). It helps at this time to encourage them to talk about themselves and their families; insight gained into their world and their feelings can result in greater empathy and understanding from the caregivers. The supporter should arrange further meetings to give the family progress reports, while attempting to resolve any practical problems that arise for them.

Informing of Death

In most cases, relatives wish to be at the bedside at the time of death, and staff should strive to fulfill this wish, offering them privacy. If it is not possible for the family to be at the bedside, a member of the staff who has been in continual contact with the relatives during the crisis time should be the person to inform them of death. The information should be given in a private area by an informer with a supporter present.

Buckman (1984) suggested that the death of a patient may cause clinicians to experience ill-founded feelings of failure, anger and guilt at not being able to save the life. It is essential that such feelings are recognized, discussed with colleagues and resolved before the meeting with the family. If these emotions persist, they may make the informer defensive and hinder empathetic communication. All staff members approach this task with trepidation at the thought of giving the message and with feelings of helplessness at the thought of trying to ameliorate the relatives' suffering. There are no correct words to use at this time, but it is important to give maximum preparation to the family with a warning of bad news before the verbal message: "I am afraid that I have bad news for you"—pause, to give the relative the opportunity to say, "Do you mean that he/she is dead?" If this response is not forthcoming, the informer should proceed with, "We did all that we could to save your wife/husband (use the first name if possible)—pause—"but I am afraid that he/she has died." The words *has died* or *is dead* should be used rather than other ambiguous phrases, such as *passed on* or *left us*, because these can be misconstrued.

Once the verbal message has been given, the caregivers should anticipate and be prepared for a variety of different emotional reactions. Men and women often have different ways of expressing grief. Men tend to find relief in rage and anger early on and retire to brood alone; women often need to talk endlessly about the deceased. When everyone within a family circle is devastated, they are likely to find it particularly difficult to help one another.

Emotional Reactions

Anger

Anger is a frequent reaction to intense feeling and an expression of grief. To express such anger, the relative may shout; rush about the room or kick and punch the air, the wall or the furniture. It is important that staff members not do anything to increase this anger. Staff should not attempt to restrain the relative and not become defensive and enter into an argument. The best response is to remain calm and to wait for the anger to subside. Staff should show no criticism of this response but should offer support and care.

Hysteria

Regardless of how distressed the relative may be, it is important to remember that the outburst will cease after a short time. It is best to remain quiet and calm and to sit and wait for the hysteria to abate. Staff should not appear judgmental, shocked or disapproving but accept that this is simply another expression of grief. Physical contact and comfort should be offered as the hysteria subsides.

Withdrawal and Isolation

Isolation and withdrawal produce perhaps the strongest feelings of helplessness in caregivers. It is impossible to communicate adequately or to know how the bereaved relative is thinking and feeling. Bereaved fathers find it particularly difficult to discuss or share their grief, but it is possible to offer a silent yet caring presence in this situation. Eventually, it may become acceptable to ask gentle questions to establish a rapport and elicit a response. It is more helpful to the bereaved to be drawn out and to express reactions rather than to continue suppressing feelings. The earlier the expression of grief, the healthier the outcome.

Continuing Care

Once the initial reaction has subsided, it is important to answer the questions that the family may have and to offer them support in the tasks that lie ahead. Staff members never should try to console family members with platitudes or tell them that they "know how you feel." Grief and its pain are unique to each individual, and it is impossible to feel as another does in such a situation. The bereaved will never again have the opportunity to work through this most difficult time, and the staff should give them the space and freedom to do so. Hodge (1972) stated: "The grief work must be done. There is no healthy escape from this—People have a natural protective tendency to avoid the unpleasantness of the grief work, but it is necessary and the more actively it is done, the shorter will be the period of grief." Simple expressions, such as "I am very sorry," bring the most comfort at this time, and if spoken with warmth and understanding, they impart more than eloquent words or false statements. The knowledge that the death was peaceful or pain-free and that the deceased was not alone is a comfort to the family.

Sudden or Traumatic Death

Sudden or traumatic death robs the family of preparatory grieving, and the shock, numbness and disbelief are more intense in such situations. During the initial period, the bereaved often feel disoriented, powerless and vulnerable. Breaking bad news in such circumstances requires empathy, clear communication and support to help the relatives emerge from the acute state of shock.

Difficulties in communication may occur because the clinician and the relative may be influenced by their own fears, thoughts and feelings. The bereaved may misinterpret the message, may pretend not to hear or may not understand owing to their confusion and distress. The clinician may be anxious and not able to put thoughts and feelings into words, speaking too quickly and using language that is too technical. Effective and empathetic communication requires clear nonverbal clues (i.e., serious intonation of voice, serious facial expressions and caring body posture) combined with simple information using terms that the bereaved can understand.

Following sudden loss, it is likely that the family will have many questions that need to be answered with honesty because this information can help them to make some sense of meaning from the death. The use of open-ended questions (e.g., "how can we help you?" and "what other information would you like?") helps to develop rapport and trust, can ease the conversation and encourages relatives to seek the answers that they need. Acknowledging the family's feelings and emotions (e.g., "you must be very shocked") helps the family to discuss their feelings and influences the grief process in a positive way. The aim must be to support, inform and offer choices because helping the bereaved to make decisions themselves also helps them to regain their coping skills. Active decision making stimulates a healthy grief process.

Many relatives benefit from a further meeting with the clinician at a later stage so that unanswered questions may be raised and discussed when the numbness and shock have passed. As mentioned earlier, psychological morbidity can be reduced with early counseling, particularly for relatives who have no supportive social networks or who are unable to support each other.

Brain-Stem Death

One of the most difficult deaths to understand and accept is the situation in which the patient has suffered a major brain insult and is subsequently found to be brain-stem dead. In the case of brain-stem death, it is especially important to consider the content and the timing of the information to be given to the family. In this situation, the relatives have to understand and accept a new concept of death. Traditional acceptable images of death involve a lifeless body that is cold and asystolic. Brain-stem death presents an image of life in a setting of high technology and hope where the victim is warm and has a heart beat and is breathing, albeit on a machine. The situation and setting suggest life and hope to the family, in sharp contrast to the message of death that is given to them by the clinician.

The same preparations and procedures for information giving should apply as mentioned earlier using a dual approach. The informer and supporter must understand and accept the brain-stem death concept themselves, and they must use language that the family can understand. Any hesitation or fudging of the explanation can confuse the relatives and may introduce hope that recovery is possible. The message to be given must stress that irreparable damage to the brain has occurred and that there is no hope of recovery, that death of the brain stem is evident, and death of the brain stem is death of the person.

The family must be allowed time to assimilate and accept this information. The central facts may need to be repeated at several meetings before the relatives can understand the diagnosis and its implications.

OPTION OF ORGAN DONATION

As stated earlier, Blandy (1989) and others stress that "wherever possible one should offer hope to the family." If death has occurred, all hope of recovery for their loved one is lost, but the bereaved can be offered an option of hope and life for others through organ and tissue donation. Tissue donation (i.e., corneal, heart valves and skin) can be offered in most cases of asystolic death. Kidney donation can follow asystolic death in certain circumstances. Clinicians should consider the possibility of donation in every case of death and should seek specific advice from the local transplant coordinator service.

Multiple Organ Donation

Brain-stem death can offer the family the option of multiple organ donation. For organ donation criteria, see Table 40–1. Reports suggest that many clinicians are reluctant to introduce the option of donation because they fear that such a suggestion may increase the grief of the bereaved. Research studies have shown, however, that families gain enormous comfort from the knowledge that their tragedy has resulted in life for others. A survey in New Zealand found that approximately 72% of individuals questioned had gained some comfort from knowing that others had benefited from their loss. Similar findings were reported in a United Kingdom survey, with 94% of families who had donated believing that they had made the right decision. A Dutch study supported the previous surveys and noted that some families who had refused donation regretted their decision at a later stage. Such research conclusions are supported further by the positive feedback from donor families that is reported by the transplant coordinator teams.

Organ donation can give something positive in an otherwise negative situation. Offering the choice to donate, if

TABLE 40–1

DONOR CRITERIA

Multiorgan donor criteria
  Age 0–75 y
  Has suffered complete and irreversible brain-stem
    damage resulting in brain-stem death
  Is maintained on a ventilator
  Has no malignancy except primary brain tumor
  Has no major systemic sepsis
Causes of brain-stem death
  Intracerebral hemorrhage
  Head trauma
  Cerebral anoxia owing to
    Drug overdoses
    Cardiac arrest
    Smoke inhalation
    Drowning
  Primary brain tumor

performed with empathy, does not increase the distress of the bereaved. The bereaved should not be denied this choice or this chance of comfort. A letter from a donor mother reads: "[I]t is certainly a source of comfort to me and indeed to all our family to know that our son has been able to touch and enrich the lives of others."

When to Offer the Option of Donation

In 1991, Garrison *et al.* reported that the timing of the approach may be the crucial factor in the potential family's ability to give permission for organ donation. This study suggests that several factors influence the consent process. First, the longer the patient is in the hospital, the more time the family has to appreciate the fact that the patient is critically ill and will not survive. It appears to follow that a family that has had more time to absorb and accept the prognosis is better able to move beyond the denial phase and become more receptive to options. Second, the timing of the approach for organ donation has significant consequences. Garrison *et al.* (1991) reported that if the request for donation were made after notification of death, as opposed to before or simultaneously with the notification of death, the family were more likely to grant consent for donation, and this trend appeared to hold true regardless of whoever made the request.

Another study in the United Kingdom, which identified reasons for relatives' refusal of donation over a 2-year period, suggested that consent was more likely when the request was made after completion of the second set of brain-stem death criteria when death had been confirmed. The study identified four other factors that may increase the likelihood of consent:

1. The presence of a parent at the time of request
2. The patient being aged 15 to 24 years or greater than 65 years
3. A plan for cremation of the body
4. Situations in which more than 1 hour elapses between the two sets of brain-stem death tests

It is good practice to separate the notification of death from the request for organ donation.

Who Should Approach the Family

There is no one person who is ideal to approach the family because of the enormous variety of individuals and

situations. It is most appropriate for the person who has formed a close and trusting relationship with the family to introduce the option of donation. It is essential that this person has a positive commitment to donation and introduces donation in a positive way.

A United Kingdom study reported that clinicians working in the *crisis* areas thought that a lack of training and a lack of experience in offering the option of donation inhibited them in making the request. Conversely a Canadian study showed that each experience of making the donation request built confidence. Every clinician who was experienced in talking to families about organ donation felt positively about the experience and believed that requesting donation was easier than seeking permission for a postmortem examination.

It is helpful to remember that the family is being asked to relate the wishes of their relative and whether objections to donation had been expressed, freeing the family from accepting responsibility for the decision. Many families may have discussed the idea of organ donation previously, perhaps at a time of national publicity. This knowledge of their loved one's wishes helps them with their response. It is reported widely that the bereaved strive to fulfill the wishes of their relative at the time of death, and the presence of an organ donor card, registration on a donor registry or a living will may help the family toward a positive response. The bereaved may inquire about the possibility of donation before a formal approach is made.

How to Approach the Family

Staff often are reluctant to raise the question of donation because they fear that they may increase the family's distress by saying the *wrong thing*. There are no *right* words, however; each situation is unique, and families have their own individual responses. Requests for organ donation cannot be pre-planned, although anxiety can be reduced for the person making the request if suitable phrases are considered before meeting with the family. Examples follow:

Family: How could this happen? What a terrible waste of a young life.
Response: This is a terrible time for you, but it need not be a complete waste; John's death could bring hope to others.
Family: He was a lovely man; he didn't deserve to die.
Response: He sounds like a lovely man; do you think his generosity would extend to helping others through his death?

Families respond to the option of donation in a variety of ways. Whatever the response, the caregiver should show empathy and understanding. Some families require time to consider their response and should be offered privacy. Many relatives have additional questions concerning the process of donation and its implications. It is helpful to use open-ended questions, beginning with *how, where* or *what* (i.e., "what further information would you like"), at this time. Such questions offer the bereaved the opportunity to make choices and to gain the information that is important to them.

At this time, it may be helpful for the bereaved to meet with a member of the transplant team, usually the transplant coordinator, who can answer specific questions and start to develop a rapport with the bereaved. The family requires reassurance that their loved one will be treated with dignity and respect throughout the donor surgery, that the body will not be mutilated or grossly disfigured, that the surgical wound will be sutured, that they can view the body after surgery and that the funeral will not be delayed. The transplant coordinator works closely with other health care professionals to answer such questions and to facilitate the wishes of the family. It often is comforting for the family to know that the transplant coordinator will be present throughout the donor surgery and will perform the final care in accordance with their wishes.

There will always be families, regardless of the manner in which the request is offered, who refuse the option of organ donation, and health care professionals must accept this decision. If the family appears undecided or if the immediate response is an angry "no," it is acceptable, after a short period of reflection, to explore gently the reasons for such a response. It is found frequently that the family may have specific concerns or unfounded ideas and fears that can be allayed by further information, removing the barriers to permission.

Research suggests that the most commonly quoted reasons for refusal include the following: The deceased had stated that he or she did not wish to donate, a fear of gross mutilation, a difference of opinion between family members, problems understanding brain-stem death and religious reasons. Regarding the last-mentioned reason, however, all the major religions support the act of donation.

If the family agrees to organ donation, many relatives may wish to spend time alone with their loved one so that they might say goodbye before the scheduled surgery. The opportunity to touch or kiss is especially appreciated. Family members should be offered privacy and never hurried.

Information after the donation is provided to the family, unless they express otherwise. This feedback contains general anonymous information about the recipients and offers further contact and support. Some transplant coordinating teams offer postdonation home visits so that ongoing support is activated and any subsequent anxieties or concerns can be addressed. In some areas, donor family support groups are available.

Most centers facilitate the exchange of letters between recipients and donor families, believing that the bereaved gain comfort from the personal gratitude and well-being of the recipient and that recipients need to express their thanks to adapt psychologically and to assimilate the new organ into their body and their new life. A few centers help to arrange meetings between the donor family and the recipient; however, such meetings are controversial. (See discussion in previous section.)

STAFF SUPPORT

The care of those who grieve is an important part of clinical practice; however, dealing with the dying and their families is stressful for staff, and if this stress is unresolved, the individual staff member may become depressed and burned out. A supportive environment can reduce this stress; such an environment requires that staff care about each other, listening to each other's problems and offering support across all levels. Health care professionals have individual coping strategies, but also they should have the opportunity to discuss issues of death and dying together formally or informally as requested. Clinicians who do not have this opportunity to replenish their own emotional reserves may find that they do not have anything left to give to future patients and their families.

VIEWING THE BODY AFTER DEATH

All families should be offered the opportunity to view the patient after death. If they are reluctant, they should be encouraged gently because it is an important step in accepting the reality of the situation. The body should be prepared carefully, and the bereaved should be given privacy and permission to touch, hold and kiss as desired. The loss of a young child is particularly distressing, and parents may appreciate a lock of hair or a photograph or handprints.

FURTHER CARE

Before the family returns home, it is important that they are aware of follow-up arrangements. In most cases, this follow-up involves an appointment with the bereavement officer, who offers help and information concerning the tasks that lie ahead. In some cases, it may be appropriate to arrange a further meeting with medical staff so that additional questions may be answered.

Advice concerning expected grief reactions may be helpful; relatives can be overwhelmed by the enormity and intensity of their distress. It is important that local support is available, and the clinician should alert the family physician or other support person to the needs of the bereaved. Some relatives may request medication, but in most cases the request should be denied gently because sedation dulls reality and response and inhibits the process of grief.

Most families recover from the death through the normal phases of grief. If a family member experiences specific problems, further help should be offered. Details of local bereavement organizations that can offer practical advice and experienced counseling should be made available.

CONCLUSION

Death and bereavement are an integral part of human life, and the care of those that grieve is an important part of clinical practice. All professionals approach the tasks of "breaking bad news" and "informing of death" with trepidation. With a knowledge of grief patterns and appropriate communication skills, it is possible to feel more comfortable with the situation and to offer empathetic and understanding care. Experience suggests that when relatives are approached sensitively, the subject of organ donation does not increase their distress. Many families gain comfort through donation and transplantation—something positive from a totally negative situation.

REFERENCES

Abram, H. S. (1972). Psychological dilemmas of medical progress *Psychiatr. Med.* **3**, 51.
Armstrong, S., Johnson, K. and Hopkins, J. (1981). Stopping immunosuppressant therapy following successful kidney transplantation: two year follow-up. In *Psychonephrology 1: Psychological Factors in Haemodialysis and Transplantation*, (N. B. Levy, ed.), p. 247, Plenum, New York.
Armstrong, S. H. and Weiner, M. F. (1982). Non compliance with post transplant immunosuppression. *Int. J. Psychiatr. Med.* **11**, 89.
Auer, J. (1990a). The Oxford-Manchester study of dialysis patients: age, risk factors and treatment method in relation to quality of life. *Scand. J. Urol. Nephrol.* **131(Suppl.)**, 31.
Auer, J. (1990b). Psychological problems in chronic illness. *In Social Work Practice in Health Care*, (M. Badawi and B. Biamonti, eds.), Woodhead Faulkner, Cambridge.
Beck, D. E., Fennell, R. S., Yost, R. L., Robinson, J. D., Geary, D. and Richards, G. A. (1980). Evaluation of an education programme on compliance with medication regimens in paediatric patients with renal transplants. *J. Paediatr.* **96**, 1094.
Bennett, A. H. and Harrison, J. H. (1974). Experience with living familial renal donors. *Surg. Gynecol. Obstet.* **139**, 894.
Bernstein, D. M. (1971). After transplantation—the child's emotional reactions. *Am. J. Psychiatry* **127**, 1189.
Binet, I., Bock, A. H., Vogelback, P., *et al.* (1997). Outcome in emotionally related living kidney donor transplantation. *Nephrol. Dial. Transplant.* **12**, 1940.

Blandy, J. (1989). *Lecture Notes in Urology,* Blackwell Scientific Publications, London.

Blogg, C. R., Anderson, M., Shoddle, C., *et al.* (1973). Rehabilitation of patients treated by dialysis or transplantation. *Proc. Dial. Transplant. Forum* **3**, 181.

Bradley, C. and McGee, H. (1994). Improving quality of life in renal failure: ways forward. In *Quality of Life Following Renal Failure,* (H. McGee and C. Bradley, eds.), Harwood Academic Publishers, Chur, Switzerland.

Bremer, B. A., Haffly, D., Fox, R. M. and Weaver, A. (1995). Patient's perceived control over their health care: an outcome assessment of their psychological adjustment to renal failure. *Am. J. Med. Qual.* **10**, 149.

Brewer, S. P. (1970). Donors of organs seen as victims. *New York Times,* April 19, p. 36.

Buckman, R. (1984). Breaking bad news: why is it still so difficult? *B. M. J.* **238**, 1597.

Bunzel, B., Schmidl-Mohl, B., Grundbock, A. and Wollenek, G. (1992). Does changing the heart mean changing personality? A retrospective inquiry on 47 heart transplant patients. *Qual. Life Res.* **1**, 251.

Cassileth, B. R., Lusk, E. J., Strouse, T. B., *et al.* (1984). Psychosocial status in chronic illness: a comparative analysis of six diagnostic groups. *N. Engl. J. Med.* **311**, 506.

Castelnuovo-Tedesco, P. (1981). Transplantation: psychological implications of changes in body image. *In Psychonephrology, Vol. 1: Psychological Factors in Haemodialysis and Transplantation,* (N. B. Levy, ed.), Plenum, New York.

Christopherson, L. K. (1987). Cardiac transplantation: a psychological perspective. *Circulation* **75**, 57.

Churchill, D. N., Morgan, J. and Torrance, G. W. (1984). Quality of life in end stage renal disease. *Periton. Dial. Bull.* **4**, 20.

Cramond, W. A. (1967). Renal homotransplantation—some observations on recipients and donors. *Br. J. Psychiatry* **113**, 1223.

Craven, J. L., Rodin, G. M., Johnson, L. and Kennedy, S. H. (1987). The diagnosis of major depression in renal dialysis patients. *Psychosom. Med.* **49**, 482.

Craven, J. and Rodin, G. M. (1992). *Psychiatric Aspects of Organ Transplantation,* Oxford University Press, New York and Oxford.

Didlake, R. H., Dreyfus, K., Kerman, R. H., Van Buren, C. T. and Kahan, B. D. (1988). Patient non-compliance: a major cause of late graft failure in cyclosporin-treated renal transplants. *Transplant. Proc.* **20**, 63.

Di Matteo, M. R. and Di Nicola, D. D. (1982). *Achieving Patient Compliance.* Pergamon Press, New York.

Dubovsky, S. L. and Penn, I. (1980). Psychiatric considerations in renal transplant surgery. *Psychosomatics* **21**, 481.

Engel, G. (1962). *Psychological Development in Health and Disease,* W.B. Saunders, Philadelphia.

Eurotold. (1997). *Project Management Group: Questioning Attitudes to Living Donor Transplantation,* Project Management Group, Eurotold, University of Leicester General Hospital, Leicester.

Evans, R. W., Manninen, D. L., Garrison, Jr., L. P., *et al.* (1985). The quality of life of patients with end stage renal disease. *N. Engl. J. Med.* **312**, 553.

Fallon, M., Gould, D. and Wainwright, S. P. (1997). Stress and quality of life in the renal transplant patient: a preliminary investigation. *J. Adv. Nurs.* **25**, 562.

Fehrman-Ekholm, I., Brink, B., Ericsson, C., Elinder, C., Duner, F. and Lundgren, G. (2000). Kidney donors don't regret. *Transplantation* **69**, 2067.

Fellner, C. H. (1971). Selection of living kidney donors and the problems of informed consent. *Semin. Psychiatry* **3**, 79.

Fellner, C. H. and Marshall, J. R. (1968). Twelve kidney donors. *J. A. M. A.* **206**, 2703.

Fellner, C. H. and Marshall, J. R. (1970). Kidney donors: the myth of informed consent. *Am. J. Psychiatry* **126**, 1245.

Fisher, R., Gould, D., Wainwright, S. and Fallow, M. (1998). Quality of life after renal transplantation. *J. Clin. Nurs.* **7**, 553.

Fox, R. C. and Swazey, J. P. (1992). *Spare Parts: Organ Replacement in American Society,* Oxford University Press, New York and Oxford.

Frey, G. M. (1990). Stressors in renal transplant recipient at six weeks after transplant. *American Nephrology Nursing Association Journal.* **17**, 443.

Fricchione, G. L. (1989). Psychiatric aspects of renal transplantation. *Aust. N. Z. J. Psychiatry* **23**, 407.

Gaedeke-Norris. M. K. (1991). Applying Orem's theory to the long-term care of adolescent transplant recipients. *American Nephrology Nursing Association Journal.* **18**, 45.

Galpin, C. (1992). Body image in end stage renal failure. *Br. J. Nurs.* **1**, 21.

Garrison, R. N., Bentley, F. R., Reyne, G. H., *et al.* (1991). There is an answer to the shortage of organ donors. *Surg. Gynecol. Obstet.* **173**, 391.

Hampe, S. (1975). Needs of the grieving spouse in a hospital setting. *Nurs. Res.* **24**, 113.

Hayward, M. B., Kish, J. P., Frey, G. M., Kirchner, J. M., Carr, L. S. and Wolfe, C. M. (1989). An instrument to identify stressors in renal transplant recipients. *American Nephrology Nursing Association Journal.* **16**, 81.

Hilton, B. A. and Starzomski, R. C. (1994). Family decision making about living related kidney donation. *American Nephrology Nursing Association Journal.* **21**, 346.

Hirvas, J., Enckell, M., Kuhlbeck, B. and Pasternack, A. (1976). Psychological and social problems encountered in active treatment of chronic uraemia: the living donor. *Acta Med. Scand.* **200**, 17.

Hodge, J. R. (1972). They that mourn. *J. Religion Health* **11**, 229.

Hudson, K. and Hiott, K. (1986). Coping with paediatric renal transplant rejection. *American Nephrology Nursing Association Journal.* **13**, 261.

Jacobs, C., Johnson, E., Anderson, K., Gillingham, K. and Matas, A. (1998). Kidney transplants from living donors: how donation affects family dynamics. *Adv. Renal Ther.* **5**, 89.

Jakobsen, A. (1997). Living renal transplantation: the Oslo experience. *Nephrol. Dial. Transplant.* **12**, 1825.

Jofre, R. Lopez-Gomez J. M., Moreno, F., Sanz-Guajardo D. and Valderrabano, F. (1998). Changes in quality of life after renal transplantation. *Am. J. Kidney Dis.* **32**, 93.

Johnson, J. P., McCauley, C. R. and Copley, J. B. (1982). The quality of life of haemodialysis and transplant patients. *Kidney Int.* **22**, 286.

Kalman, T. P., Wilson, P. G. and Kalman, C. M. (1983). Psychiatric morbidity in long-term renal transplant recipients and patients undergoing haemodialysis: a comparative study. *J. A. M. A.* **250**, 55.

Kaplan De Nour, A. and Czaczkes, J. W. (1976). The influence of patients' personality on adjustment to chronic dialysis: a predictive study. *J. Nerv. Ment. Dis.* **162**, 323.

Kaplan De Nour, A. and Shanan, J. (1980). Quality of life of dialysis and transplanted patients. *Nephron* **25**, 117.

Kemph, J. P. (1966). Renal failure, artificial kidney and kidney transplant. *Am. J. Psychiatry* **122**, 1270.

Kemph, J. P. (1970). Observations of the effects of kidney transplant on donors and recipients: diseases of the nervous system. *Dis. Nerv. Syst.* **31**, 323.

Kemph, J. P., Bermann, E. A. and Coppolillo, H. P. (1969). Kidney transplant and shifts in family dynamics. *Am. J. Psychiatry* **125**, 1485.

Klein, S. D., Simmons, R. G. and Anderson, C. R. (1984). Chronic kidney disease and transplantation in childhood and adolescence. *In Chronic Illness and Disabilities in Childhood and Adolescence,* (R. W. Blum, ed.), p. 429, Grune & Stratton, Orlando, Fla.

Kubler-Ross, E. (1987). *On Death and Dying,* Tavistock Publications, London.

Le Poidevin, S. (1986). *The Management of Bereaved Relatives and Approaching the Next of Kin About Organ Donation,* unpublished thesis.

Levey, A. S., Hon, S. and Bush, Jr., H. L. (1986). Kidney transplantation from unrelated living donors: time to reclaim a discarded opportunity. *N. Engl. J. Med.* **314**, 914.

Levy, N. B. (1986). Renal transplantation and the new medical era. *Adv. Psychosom. Med.* **15**, 167.

Lewis, C. S. (1961). *A Grief Observed,* Faber & Gaber, London.

Lilly, J. R., Giles, G., Hurwitz, R., *et al.* (1971). Renal homotransplantation in paediatric patients. *Paediatrics* **47**, 548.

Martin, M. B., Giacolleto-Allemand, S. and Martin, R. S. (1998). Pretransplant recipient donor interaction: a prognostic indicator in living related kidney transplantation. *Medicina (B. Aires)* **58**, 13.

Mauss, M. (1954). *The Gift: Forms and Functions of Exchange in Archaic Societies,* (I. Cunnison, trans.), Free Press, Glencoe, Ill.

McLaren, J. (1995). Death of a child. *In The Care Guide: A Handbook for the Caring Professions and Other Agencies,* (M. Jacobs, ed.), Cassell, London.

Miller, J. F. (1983). *Coping with Chronic Illness: Overcoming Powerlessness*, F.A. Davis, Philadelphia.

Molter, N. C. (1979). Needs of relatives of critically ill patients: a descriptive study. *Heart Lung* **8**, 332.

Morris, P. L. P. and Jones, B. (1988). Transplantation versus dialysis: a study of quality of life. *Transplant. Proc.* **20**, 23.

Morten, J. B. and Leonard, D. R. A. (1979). Cadaver nephrectomy: an operation on the donor's family. *B. M. J.* **1**, 239.

Najarian, J. S. (1975). Editorial comment on Owens *et al. Arch. Surg.* **110**, 1451.

Nicholson, M. L. and Bradley, J. A. (1999). Renal transplantation from living donors. *B. M. J.* **318**, 409.

Nylander, Jr., W. A., Sutherland, D. E. R., Bentley, F. R., Simmons, R. L. and Najarian, J. S. (1985). Fifteen to twenty-year follow-up of renal transplants performed in the 1960s. *Transplant. Proc.* **17**, 104.

O'Brien, V. C. (1985). Psychological and social aspects of heart transplantation. *Heart Transplant.* **4**, 229.

Owens, M. L., Maxwell, J. G., Goodnight, J. and Wolcott, M. W. (1975). Discontinuance of immunosuppression in renal transplant patients. *Arch. Surg.* **110**, 1450.

Parkes, C. M. (1972). *Bereavement: Studies of Grief in Adult Life*, International Universities Press, New York.

Parkes, C. M. (1975). Determinants of outcome following bereavement. *Omega* **6**, 303.

Parkes, C. M. (1980). Bereavement counselling: does it work? *B. M. J.* **281**, 3.

Penn, I., Bunch, D., Olenik, D. and Abouna, G. (1971). Psychiatric experience with patients receiving renal and hepatic transplants. *Semin. Psychiatry* **3**, 133.

Peretz, D. (1970). Development, object relations and loss. *In Loss and Grief: Psychological Management in Medical Practice*, (B. Schuenberg, A. C. Carr and D. Peretz, eds.), p. 3, Columbia University Press, New York.

Petrie, K. (1989). Psychological well-being and psychiatric disturbance in dialysis and renal transplant patients. *Br. J. Med. Psychol.* **62**, 91.

Phillips, A. (1999). Can you take the pain out of death? An interview by Catherine O'Brien. *The Times*, Wednesday 10 November.

Pincus, L. (1974). *Death and the Family*, Pantheon, New York.

Price, B. (1990). *Body Image: Nursing Concepts and Care*, Prentice Hall, London.

Rapheal, B. (1977). Preventative intervention with the recently bereaved. *Arch. Gen. Psychiatry* **34**, 1450.

Rapheal, B. (1975). The management of pathological grief. *Aust. N. Z. J. Psychiatry* **9**, 173.

Rauch, J. B. and Kneen, K. K. (1989). Accepting the gift of life: heart transplant recipients post-operative adaptive tasks. *Soc. Work Health Care* **1**, 47.

Reynolds, J., Garralda, M., Jameson, R. and Postlethwaite, R. (1986). Living with chronic renal failure. *Child Care Health Dev.* **12**, 401.

Rodin, G. and Abbey, S. (1992). Kidney transplantation. *In Psychiatric Aspects of Organ Transplantation*, (J. Craven and G. M. Rodin, eds.), Oxford University Press, New York and Oxford.

Rodin, G. and Vashart, K. (1987). Depressive symptoms and functional impairment in the medically ill. *Gen. Hosp. Psychiatry* **9**, 251.

Rodin, G., Vashart, K., Cattran, D., Halloran, P., Cardella, C. and Fenton, S. (1985). Cadaveric renal transplant failure: the short-term sequelae. *Int. J. Psychiatr. Med.* **15**, 357.

Rovelli, M., Palmeri, D., Vossler, E., Bartus, S., Hull, D. and Schweizer, R. (1989). Non-compliance in renal transplant recipients: evaluation by socio-economic groups. *Transplant. Proc.* **21**, 3979.

Rubin, R. H., Cosimi, A. B., Tolkoff-Rubin, N. E., *et al.* (1977). Infectious disease syndromes attributable to cytomegalovirus and their significance among renal transplant recipients. *Transplantation* **24**, 458.

Russell, S. and Jacob, R. G. (1994). Living related organ donation: the donor's dilemma. *Patient Education and Counselling* **21**, 89.

Salter, M. (1988). *Altered Body Image: The Nurse's Role*, John Wiley & Sons, New York.

Savaria, D., Rovell, M. and Schweizer, R. (1990). Donor family surveys provide useful information for organ procurement. *Transplant. Proc.* **22**, 316.

Schover, L. R., Streem, S. B., Boparai, N., Duriak, K. and Novick, A. C. (1997). The psychological impact of donating a kidney: long-term follow-up from a urology based center. *J. Urol.* **157**, 1596.

Schweitzer, E. J., *et al.* (1997). Increased living donor volunteer donor rates with a formal recipient family education programme. *Am. J. Kidney Dis.* **29**, 739.

Short, M. J. and Harris, N. L. (1969). Psychiatric observations of renal homotransplantation. *South. Med. J.* **62**, 1479.

Simmons, R. G., Anderson, C. and Kamstra, L. (1984). Comparison of quality of life on continuous ambulatory peritoneal dialysis, haemodialysis and after transplantation. *Am. J. Kidney Dis.* **4**, 253.

Simmons, R. G., Hickey, K., Kjellstrand, C. M. and Simmons, R. L. (1971). Donors and non donors: the role of the family and the physician in kidney transplantation. *Semin. Psychiatry* **3**, 102.

Simmons, R. G., Klein, S. D. and Simmons, R. L. (1977). *The Gift of Life: The Social and Psychological Impact of Organ Transplantation*, John Wiley & Sons, New York.

Smith, M. D., Kappell, D. F., Province, M. A., *et al.* (1986). Living-related kidney donors: a multicenter study of donor education, socio-economic adjustment and rehabilitation. *Am. J. Kidney Dis.* **8**, 223.

Soos, J. (1992). Psychotherapy and counselling with transplant patients. *In Psychiatric Aspects of Organ Transplantation*, (J. Craven and G. M. Rodin, eds.), Oxford Medical Publications, Oxford.

Speck, P. (1978). *Loss and Grief in Medicine*, Bailliere Tindall, London.

Streltzer, J., Moe, M., Yanagida, E. and Siemsen, A. (1983). Coping with transplant failure: grief vs denial. *Int. J. Psychiatr. Med.* **13**, 97.

Surman, O. S. (1989). Psychiatric aspects of organ transplantation. *Am. J. Psychiatry* **146**, 972.

Sylvia, C. (1997). *A Change of Heart*. Little, Brown and Company, New York.

Uehling, D. T., Hussey, J. L., Weinstein, A. B., Wank, R. and Bach, F. H. (1976). Cessation of immunosuppression after renal transplantation. *Surgery* **79**, 278.

Voepal-Lewis, T., Ketafian, S., Starr, A. and White, M. J. (1990). Stress, coping and quality of life in family members of kidney transplant recipients. *American Nephrology Nursing Association Journal.* **17**, 427.

Wakeford, R. E. and Stepney, R. (1989). Obstacles to organ donation. *Br. J. Surg.* **76**, 436.

Walter, T. (1996) A new model of grief: bereavement and biography. *Mortality* **1**, 7.

Weems, J. and Patterson, E. T. (1989). Coping with uncertainty and ambivalence while awaiting a cadaveric renal transplant. *American Nephrology Nursing Association Journal.* **16**, 27.

Westlie, L., Umen, A., Nestrud, S. and Kiellstrand, C. M. (1984). Mortality, morbidity and life satisfaction in the very old dialysis patient. *Trans. ASAIO* **30**, 21.

White, M. J., Ketafian, S., Starr, A. J. and Voepal-Lewis, T. (1990). Stress, coping and quality of life in adult kidney transplant recipients. *ANNA J.* **17**, 421.

Wilson, W. P., Stickel, D. L., Hayes, Jr., C. P. and Harris, N. L. (1968). Psychiatric considerations of renal transplantation. *Arch. Intern. Med.* **122**, 502.

Wishman, M. A. and Jacobson, N. S. (1990). Brief behavioural marital therapy. *In Handbook of the Brief Psychotherapies*, (R. A. Wells and V. J. Giannetti, eds.), p. 325, Plenum, New York.

Worden, W. J. (1988). *Grief Counselling and Grief Therapy*, Routledge, London.

Wright, R. (1986). *Caring in Crisis*, Churchill Livingstone, London.

Yates, D. W., *et al.* (1990). Care of the suddenly bereaved. *B. M. J.* **301**, 29.

Ethics in Transplantation: Allotransplantation and Xenotransplantation

John B. Dossetor • Abdallah S. Daar

Introduction

In ethics, the terms used need definitions. To start, we consider the meaning of two words: *ethics* and *morals*. The use of these two words is not uniform. For some, *ethics* is the study of behavior between people in relationships in accordance with their cultural values, whereas *morals* takes into account some wider principles that govern personal behavior, independently of others but often in relation to transcendental principles or beliefs or concept of deity. In this chapter, we use the two words *morals* and *ethics* synonymously. This claim is based on the origin of both words, one from ancient Greek (*ethos*) and the other from classical Latin (*mores*), both meaning the accepted customs and values to which societies and cultures aspire.

As transplantation becomes increasingly *globalized*, it is important to consider whether the values that are brought to bear on transplant issues are determined by local cultures or are universal (held by all world cultures). There is a lack of uniformity. We claim that all cultures share some values (e.g., it is wrong to abuse children, it is wrong to torture the innocent and life is of utmost value to each individual). It also is true, however, that some values are held in a different way in different cultures (e.g., individual autonomy versus interests of family, clan or tribe; the varying intrinsic value of individual lives to the society or culture [as distinct from value to self] and the varying respect for individual persons, their personal dignity and equality before the law). At this time, only some values are held universally, and there is as yet no universal ethical system. These differences are important to intercultural transplantation debates.

DEFINITIONS

Allogenic, Isogenic, Xenogenic: These terms are well known in transplantation and need no further definition here (see Chapter 2).

Altruism: Actions that are motivated by concern for the well-being of others, sometimes against personal preferences and self-interest.

Consequentialism: See *Utilitarianism*, including *teleology*.

Deontology: Also called *Duty Ethics* from *deon* (Greek), a binding duty. This theory stresses the intrinsic value of all individual persons, the duty of individual dignity and respect, the value of self-determination and the cardinal importance of patient autonomy. In secular philosophy, this theory draws heavily on the writings of Kant (1724–1804), and its essence is captured by the claim that *individuals should always be treated as ends in themselves and not as means to other persons' ends*.

Resource allocation: It is useful to distinguish between three levels. (1) *Microallocation* refers to the one-on-one encounter between patient and caregiver and is dominated usually by duty-based or deontological ethics. (2) *Mesoallocation* refers to allocations by program directors, taking into account the needs of programs as well as individuals. (3) *Macroallocation* refers to allocation at the levels of government, taking into account wide-ranging social policies. *Mesoallocation* and *macroallocation* tend to reflect utilitarian or consequentialist ethics. (A fourth allocative level—*megaallocation*—may be used in reference to policies involving international relations and allocations.)

Risk/Benefit: To the deontologist, this ratio (or calculus) refers to the risk taken and the benefit achieved by a given individual in a given situation. It should be distinguished from the concept of risk to the risk taker balanced against the benefit to another, others or society as a whole, although that calculus may have to be made in some situations using a utilitarian approach. A similar conceptual differentiation applies to burden/benefit analysis.

Utilitarianism: The other well-known tradition in Western ethics. It contrasts with deontology. This is an outcomes-based or consequentialist theory, based on the ethical objective of maximizing *utility*, or achieving the *greatest good for the greatest number*. It may use statistical probabilities applied to groups of individuals. The term *teleology* also is used for outcome-based ethics (*telos* [Greek] = end, or goal).

Xenotransplantation: In the human setting (see Chapter 42), the use of live cells, tissues or organs from a nonhuman animal source transplanted or implanted into a human or used for *ex vivo* contact with human body fluids, cells, tissues or organs that subsequently are given to a human recipient. Xenografts include live cells, tissues or organs from a nonhuman animal source used for xenotransplantation.

Xenozoonosis: Infection resulting from xenotransplantation, especially of viable perfused organs, in which the risk of generating new viruses exists (e.g., retroviruses). New forms of bacterial and fungus infection may result from mutations.

Ethical Principles in Transplantation

In many issues in health care, there is conflict between the two principal ethical theories of Western ethics (Beauchamp and Childress, 1994), *deontology* and *utilitarianism*. Neither theory can be exclusively applied; both serve to bring relevant ethical perspectives into debate of difficult issues. In transplantation, because of the severely limited resource of available transplantable organs, transplant teams, while being aware of their *deontological* obligations to each patient, are forced to draw more on *utilitarian* considerations in making allocative decisions. Considerable ethical tension is created by this *mesolevel* obligation to utility (greatest good for the greatest number) because of the tendency for it to override duty owed to each individual as a unique person, at the *microallocative* level.

In the final analysis, properly informed and obtained public opinion is the arbiter of practice, and physicians are obliged to explain to the public what they do and to obtain its assent. In this process, the various public *media* also play an important role in informing and obtaining public opinion.

Organs from Cadavers
ETHICS ISSUES IN THE DETERMINATION OF DEATH
Brain Death by Neurological Criteria

Since the 1970s, there has been a general acceptance that the criteria for death from cerebral causes are valid (see Chapter 6). The process was initiated by a Harvard Medical School consensus in 1968 (Beecher, 1968), and there is near-universal acceptance that a person is dead when there is irreversible loss of function of the entire brain, including the brain stem (U.S. President's Commission, 1981). This definition recognizes that a body may be dead even though the heart is beating and the circulation is maintained with a blood pressure that is adequate for organ perfusion (heart-beating brain-dead cadaver). This definition means that the animate and the vegetative parts of the brain must be irreversibly nonfunctional (Sass, 1992). This concept can be difficult for families to understand and accept, especially when their recently brain-damaged loved one is warm to touch and has an evident heartbeat and other functions. It is a measure of public trust in the medical profession, in which the media has played an important part, that families can accept the diagnosis of *brain death*, despite these contextual and conceptual difficulties.

Despite widespread agreement, there are authors who dissent, pointing out that a rigorous definition of loss of all brain and brain-stem function implies loss of vasomotor tone, temperature control and diabetes insipidus. This dissension may be more a legal problem than a medical one, but it is a problem nonetheless (Halevy and Brady, 1993; Truog, 1997; Veatch, 1992, 1993).

Death of the Cerebral Cortex Alone: Not Acceptable Evidence for Brain Death

Frequently, persons suffer brain damage that is insufficient to destroy brain-stem function, although all cerebral cortical function is lost. By currently accepted legal definitions for brain death, these individuals are not dead. They differ markedly from brain-dead individuals in that they may breathe spontaneously; have a gag reflex and may undergo apparent sleep-wake brain cycles with opening and closing of the eyes, but without seeing, and are unable to exhibit meaningful relations with the outside world. This state, when present for more than 6 months, is termed *persistent incognitive vegetative state*. Some authorities believe that such entities are no longer to be thought of as functioning organisms because they no longer possess "coordinated integration of two types of function: organic and mental. If these two are irretrievably disjoined, then human life no longer exists" (Veatch, 1992). For this opinion to prevail, we need to move from a whole brain–oriented definition of brain death to a

higher brain–oriented definition. This definition may come about in the future if the diagnosis of irretrievable loss of all higher brain functions becomes more precise and certain. Presently, most people consider patients in a persistent incognitive vegetative state to be alive.

Although there may be ethically defensible circumstances in which life-supporting systems may be discontinued, this is a separate issue from claiming that patients in a persistent incognitive vegetative state are already dead. Patients in a persistent vegetative state are not donors of cadaver organs.

Anencephalic Infants as a Source of Organs

Anencephalic infants resemble patients in the persistent incognitive vegetative state in that they have no higher brain or neocortical function, but this is because they have never achieved *brain life*. Some authorities hold that anencephalic infants "do not have the minimal biological substrate as the basis for sentience, a necessary condition for being alive as a person" and might be used as donors if law and public policy were framed to recognize that reality (Cefalo and Engelhardt, 1989). Others disagree, however, holding that the legally recognized brain death criteria are also the only valid moral criteria (May, 1990; Walters and Ashwal, 1989). One group (Frewen *et al.*, 1990) used a protocol that waits for asystole before placing anencephalic infants on life support, followed by periodic testing for cessation of brain-stem activities and so meet that component of the legal definition of brain death, but experience is limited, and there still are ethical problems. We do not yet have societal understanding and agreement concerning the moral status of anencephalic infants (Rothenberg, 1990).

Non–Heart-Beating Cadaver Donor

Attention has been drawn, especially in Europe (Daemen *et al.*, 1996), to obtaining organs from the original source of transplant organs, before the establishment of brain-dead criteria—i.e., bodies after death from cessation of heart beat (>90% of those who die in hospitals). In North America, there is next to no effort to obtain organs from this category of dying persons (Cho *et al.*, 1998) (Clearly, preemptively excluded are persons dying with disseminated cancer or infection). The non–heart-beating cadaver donor categories present different problems for different organ transplantations (e.g., heart, liver) (Youngner and Arnold, 1993). Included in these categories are:

Persons dying after failed cardiopulmonary resuscitation, including patients dying in coronary care units with otherwise good kidney function.

Persons brought dead to emergency departments (dead on arrival), some of who provide viable organs.

Persons dying under circumstances in which a prior decision was made with the patient and with the family that extended life measures, such as life support of various types (e.g., stomach tubes, tracheal tubes, assisted artificial ventilation), would be withheld and that death would be allowed to happen in a natural fashion.

Persons on life support for whom a decision is made with the family for withdrawal of life support so that inevitable death occurs naturally. In such situations, there is agreement that life support will be withdrawn at a certain point in time and death is anticipated within a short time (hours).

Results for kidney transplants from this source are comparable to those from brain-dead sources if non–heart beating cadaver donor organs are selected after viability tests carried out during *ex vivo* organ perfusion (Koostra *et al.*, 1997).

Respect for the Dead Body

In transplantation, especially when organs are obtained in a multiorgan procurement unit, many health care professionals find it difficult to show respect for the dead person. This difficulty is especially so in situations in which liver, heart, kidneys, lungs, pancreas, corneas, skin and long bones all may be used. The normally deeply felt human value of respecting the dead may become eroded in such difficult situations. Nurses feel moral distress when the transplant procurement team appears to have no time to respect the dead person whose organs are being used. An ethics conference on respect for the dead body put forward views that should command our continuous attention (see Dossetor *et al.*, 1989).

NEW DUTIES OWED BY HEALTH CARE PROFESSIONALS

Duty Owed by Health Care Professionals' Duty to Provide Organs

Now that organ transplantation is established as medical treatment for heart, liver and kidney failure, patients who are selected for transplantation waiting lists have established an entitlement to be provided with the organ they need. This entitlement places a moral obligation on physicians, nurses and health care administrators to provide as many organs as possible, although this obligation does not yet appear to be accepted proactively into the codes of professional ethics. Those who support transplantation also have an obligation to support measures—a duty shared with the public at large—to encourage everyone to make their will known, in advance, with respect to organ donation through mandated decision making on such documents as health cards, tax returns or other repeated written documents.

Duty Owed to Declared Intended Donors and Their Families

Individuals who agree to leave their bodies to be used for transplantation or their families who permit it create responsibilities for health care professionals. These responsibilities include making optimal use of organs procured and distributing them according to just principles of allocation, as outlined subsequently. Society does not extend to donors the right to say to whom the organs should go, unless there are close relatives in need. This limitation of their entitlement recognizes the wider societal principle of not permitting discrimination on the basis of sex, ethnicity, race or age.

Duty Owed to Donors and Their Families to Preserve for Them the Option to Donate or Not to Donate

It is recognized that individuals or families have a right to give their organs should death come unexpectedly. The possibility of preserving the option for families to donate is inherent in newly suggested protocols for those who die suddenly and unexpectedly, so-called non–heart beating cadaver donors (Anaise *et al.*, 1990; Hong *et al.*, 1991). For example, it may be acceptable ethically to subject the body of someone who has died recently and unexpectedly to large-volume intravascular cold perfusion by arterial catheters to preserve for the family the option later to donate organs for transplantation if they wish (Dossetor, 1992a) even though this involves touching the dead body without prior family consent.

DUTIES OWED TO PATIENTS AWAITING TRANSPLANT BY HEALTH ADMINISTRATORS, GOVERNMENTS AND POLITICIANS

Public education by means of publicity programs promoted by government or transplant-related agencies is an effective measure for obtaining cadaver organs. These measures promote public altruism. Several studies indicated that despite a high percentage of the public being in favor of using cadaver organs for transplantation, low organ availability rates were caused partly by poor collaboration by most health care professionals who are *not* involved in transplantation. *Required request, required consideration, required notification* policies have been introduced widely, especially in North America, to improve collaboration, although initial improvements in obtaining organs have not always been maintained. Other measures to facilitate the process are organ removal permission statements on driver's licenses, tax returns or other repeatedly used public documents (*mandated decision making*), although all these measures also require support by public education for optimal participation.

In Europe, with the support of the Ministers of the Council of Europe, attention has been turned to convincing the public that organs should be used without permission of next of kin or prior designation by the deceased—*presumed consent*. Legislation permits those who do not accept this assumption to *opt out* of the scheme by placing their names in a registry, which must be consulted before taking organs. Evidence shows that this approach is effective in increasing organ procurement, especially in Austria and Belgium (Roels and Michielsen, 1990). In France and most countries with presumed consent legislation, physicians often require family permission even when not required by law. It is possible that such legislation is more acceptable in societies that are more homogeneous, although the future may show Singapore to be an exception (Soh and Lim, 1991).

Spain has achieved annual procurement rates of 30 per 1 million population by means of a centralized coordinated in-hospital system, with persons specially trained in detecting prospective donors and obtaining permission. This rate far exceeds annual procurement elsewhere of 14 to 20 donors per 1 million population (Miranda and Matesanz, 1998), although there are some local areas with comparable rates, such as the Delaware Valley in Pennsylvania (Robertson *et al.*, 1998). The Spanish success may be due, in part, to the built-in financial incentives given to the hospitals, physicians and coordinators involved in organ procurement as well as perhaps to the fact that many of the coordinators are themselves hospital intensive care specialists, although they do not coordinate for the donors who had been their own patients before brain death. To some, these issues raise the question of conflict of interest. For these reasons, the model may not be adopted easily by other countries that lack the same level of social cohesiveness and trust.

INCENTIVES FOR DONORS AND DONOR FAMILIES

Another controversial area recognizes that organ procurement might be increased if incentives were offered to families of those whose organs might be procured after death. Suggested incentives fall into two classes: (1) proposals that anticipate death and prepare advance incentives to donate after death and (2) proposals that apply without prior planning to recently bereaved families. The former include creating a *futures* market (Cohen, 1991) or creating a priority system for cadaver organs for individuals who also had agreed to eventual postmortem organ donation and had made this agreement before needing an organ themselves (Kleinman and Lowy, 1989). The second category includes payment of funeral expenses, providing postmortem educational grants for bereaved children or providing other insurance policies that become active only after cadaver organ donation (Monaco, 1990); this category could include such public acknowledgement of societal indebtedness as the planting of a tree in a park or awarding donor families a medal (Parliamentary Standing Committee, 1999). All of these incentives might be framed as ethically acceptable programs of *rewarded gifting*. Much more controversial (see later) is the use of cash payments as direct incentives for organ donation. Individuals who oppose all these suggestions believe that they may lead to a lessening of the spirit of altruism in society and a descent into commercialization of organs and usage of the body and lessened societal value in the uniqueness and dignity of the human body. There is widespread repugnance over commercialism in cadaver organs through sale or purchase, although few oppose compensation for any additional expenses incurred by the family because of organ procurement.

DUTIES OWED BY ORGAN RECIPIENTS

Poorly defined as yet, the costs and sacrifices involved in providing organs create a moral obligation on those who receive them. Should not the recipient of a liver, for example, have a strong moral obligation not to run the risk of damage to it by alcohol? More commonly, if a recipient fails to comply with antirejection medication, should sanctions be imposed on the recipient (particularly in the event of needing a further transplant)? Obligations of this type have been formulated poorly for society, but many see it as part of the barely articulated contract that exists between members of society and health care providers when interacting with each other within a publicly funded system.

ISSUES OF OWNERSHIP AND AUTHORITY

Issues in transplantation that seldom are addressed include the following questions: Who owns the cadaver organ after it has been procured, before it has been implanted into someone? Who has the authority to lay down the rules by which the organs are distributed? What rights do the family have in saying what they want done with their relative's body?

Who Owns the Excised Organ?

The law has not determined who owns a dead body or the organs excised from it. In the Middle Ages in Europe, matters relating to dead bodies were delegated to the ecclesiastical courts (now obsolete) by the civil courts. It is a curious fact that, inherent in the concept that there is no property value in a dead body, an individual who stole an excised cadaver organ from an operating room in one hospital to take and implant it at another hospital could be charged only with trespass. It would be a theft only if that individual had stolen the container for transport purposes. Some advocate an end to this extraordinary anomaly (Andrews, 1986) when such great value is placed on organs by would-be recipients and the professionals obligated to find them. Apportioning property value and ownership rights to organs from the dead is seen as a big step toward unwanted commercialization, however, which might not be prevented by concomitant legal

steps to prohibit market transactions of organs. In the case of *Moore v. Regents of University of California*, a spleen donor initially was refused property rights by the California Supreme Court, but the case was subsequently settled initially by sharing in the profits from the cell line grown from the excised diseased spleen (Dickens, 1990).

Who Should Decide on Cadaver Organ Allocation?

The question of ownership relates to the questions of allocation. At present, although there may be no legislation to support it, it generally is *assumed* that ownership of cadaver organs resides in the state, which is *assumed* to have delegated its authority to the institution, and then to the transplantation service. Thus, it is widely assumed that the disposition of transplantable organs is not at the whim of the transplantation team simply by virtue of their skill in being able satisfactorily to remove and then implant them.

PRINCIPLES USED IN ORGAN ALLOCATION IN TRANSPLANTATION

Many principles are used in the *just* distribution of access opportunities to scarce resources such as transplantable cadaver organs (for kidneys) or onto transplant waiting lists (for hearts).

Ethical Commitment to the Principle of Rescue

Despite possible injustice, we all recognize *rescue* as an ethical imperative to which we should respond. Sometimes rescue impels action when it is not likely to provide the optimal outcome. It also brings out the tension created when the consequentialist principle of *the greatest good for the greatest number* conflicts with the deontological commitment to the quality and dignity of each human life together with the principle of justice that recognizes *claims in proportion to need*. The seeming imperative to carry out a subsequent organ transplant when the first has failed may present the ethical conflict between rescue and utility (Ubel et al., 1993). Rescue should not be applied to situations that fail to meet the *minimal standard of utility*, referred to subsequently.

Optimizing the Medical Outcome (the Utility Principle)

In transplantation, particularly when setting public policy, actions usually are governed by applying the principle of greatest utility. As decision making moves from the *micro-level* to the *meso-level* or *macro-level*, the utilitarian consequentialist ethic increasingly dominates over the deontological ethic. This change explains why ethical conflict seems greater for physicians than administrators because the latter do not have personal relationships with individual patients and hold responsibilities only in the field of public policy. Monaco (1989) emphasizes that programs should have a *minimal threshold for medical utility* and make decisions above that threshold. When all potential recipients meet the minimal threshold of utility, other ethical factors may be used for organ allocative decisions in addition to optimizing medical outcome.

Fiduciary Principle

The fiduciary principle recognizes the duty principle of individual physicians toward their patients as individuals. It often creates tension between the deontological duty imposed by this principle and some of the other legitimate principles, especially for professionals who may have responsibilities at the *microallocative* and the *mesoallocative* levels.

Random Choice (the Lottery Principle and Use of First Come, First Served) and Random Factors

The two principles of random choice and random factors have much in common in that the allocative factors are *value neutral*. Both principles acknowledge that there are factors such as chance, or good or ill luck, that are legitimate in decision making for organ allocation because they affect all people in society in a more or less random, yet equal way. Patients find this randomness acceptable in systems based on an egalitarian principle. In contrast, physicians and transplantation coordinators may be reluctant to place any weight on random choice and random factors because it seems to deny their professional expertise in wielding medical science knowledge. Nevertheless, there are occasions when these principles would be just. *Length of time on the waiting list* and *distance from home to center* may be ethically legitimate factors in allocation, provided that time of entry to the list is achieved at a comparable time point for each potential recipient and that distance interferes with ability to accept some opportunities for receiving a graft. In different programs, other value-neutral circumstances may be accepted as weighting factors.

Ability to Pay

Ability to pay has operated largely in health care in previous centuries in all Western countries. Inevitably, it is the dominant principle in most, but not all, developing countries, where transplantation is available mainly for the rich. In a capitalist society based on libertarian principles, such as the United States, ability to pay as a dominant principle would not be unjust, provided that a commonly accepted standard of basic care was available to all. Renal dialysis and kidney transplantation in the United States is covered by an egalitarian Act of Congress (this does not apply to heart or liver transplants, which are not covered).

Ability to pay is excluded as a factor in allocation in transplantation in most developed countries, where there is a social commitment to support health care on egalitarian principles, although physicians have to be cognizant of an inherent tendency for this factor to become relevant, in various guises. It is presently too difficult to predict the part to be played by this factor in the xenotransplant era, as it moves from *experimental* (with poor results at first) toward *established* treatment (when results have become comparable to allogeneic grafts).

Social Worth

In an egalitarian system, estimates of social worth are ethically inappropriate and may not be used in estimating good outcomes. One often finds *social worth* parameters, such as lack of compliance, lack of family support, undesirable personal habits or inability to speak the dominant language, *masquerading* as factors for optimizing medical outcomes, however. In our opinion, these parameters should be recognized for what they are and resisted.

Lobbying and Using the Media

Another factor that may be unjust but is difficult to resist is the influence of individuals who advance their cause by obtaining greater publicity of their need through the media or a lobbying process. Despite the advantage that this activity can give in a libertarian atmosphere of the marketplace—where it might be termed the *competitive edge*—it would not be a legitimate reason for allocation in a publicly funded egalitarian health care system.

Using the Needs of the Program in Allocation

When a program is starting up, it can be ethical to select patients so that initial results will be good enough to ensure continued funding. This selection approach should operate only for a limited time and is ethical only if it is publicized as public policy so that potential recipients and their advisors all know of the policy and its limited duration.

Kidneys and Liver Segments from Living Related Donors

BENEFIT/BURDEN CALCULUS FOR LIVING RELATED DONORS

There always has been an ethical issue in living related donors stemming from the injunction *primum nihil nocere* (Schreiber, 1991)—*above all do no harm*. Can it be claimed that removing a sibling or parent's kidney is not doing harm? It usually is argued that the good (benefit) that comes to the donor as a result of restoring their family member to well-being and renewed life justifies the possible burden borne by the donor. The donor is acting altruistically (acting for the good of another, without primary regard to self-interests) but has this good result as an added compensation. Living kidney donors have been followed carefully, and no solid evidence exists of late harm from hypertension or late renal failure of the single remaining kidney (Fabrega *et al.*, 1992; see Chapter 7). There is some risk, but it is usually accepted that a donor who accepts that risk is not being manipulated or taken advantage of by others if he or she is competent. Only an emancipated minor or an adult can make the assessment meaningfully and give informed consent. When the potential kidney donor is a minor, many jurisdictions insist that only a family court judge or equivalent can sanction the donation.

It is not deemed ethical to balance the possible harms to the donor against the benefit to the recipient; this is considered to be an unethical way of calculating burden versus benefit. Calculated in that way, the ratio could be used to justify the use of mentally incompetent relatives as well as the reluctant but competent relative. One must consider the burden/benefit ratio to the donor against the burden/benefit ratio to the recipient. In calculating benefit for the donor is the knowledge that his or her kidney will give a better result than is obtainable from a cadaver kidney (Bonomini, 1991; Roberts *et al.*, 1988) as well as relieving the burden of continued dialysis and (in children) further risk of stunted growth. Other experts believe that increased cadaver graft survival with newer immunosuppressive regimens has eroded that component of donor benefit, and this led some centers temporarily to cease living donor kidney grafting (Michielsen, 1991). In Belgium, with a relatively high cadaver donor rate, it has been found necessary, however, to reintroduce and advocate increased living donation.

For living donors of liver segments to children dying of liver failure, assessment of benefit and burden is much more difficult. The donor risks are greater, and restoration of health to the recipient is a less certain benefit (Whittington *et al.*, 1991). The publication on ethics preceded the surgical performance (Singer *et al.*, 1989); this constitutes a first.

COMMERCE IN HUMAN KIDNEYS, ESPECIALLY FROM LIVING STRANGERS

There is no ethical issue in transplantation that stirs up more controversy than obtaining kidneys from living unrelated individuals. This controversy centers on the ethical probity of exchanging viable kidneys for money. Before considering that aspect, there are several less challenging issues, which involve some form of altruism. The key factor seems to be donor (vendor) motivation.

These issues may be analyzed by considering the motivation of donors or vendors of their own kidneys. Other stakeholders in these transactions are recipients of commercially obtained kidneys, entrepreneurs who arrange for kidney transactions, physicians who perform the surgeries and, most importantly, spokespersons for society as a whole. These individuals all have ethical dilemmas but of lesser dimensions than the vendors.

Spousal Altruism

Earlier reluctance to accept spouses as altruistic kidney donors largely has evaporated. The reluctance was due to spouses having no more probability of being well matched for HLA than any randomly tested individual or cadaver source, and these grafts were expected to have a poorer survival than an HLA-matched cadaver kidney. Wives, as recipients of their husband's kidney, might have degrees of prior sensitization against HLA and other systems because of exposure to the husband's antigens on fetal cells during pregnancy, which might not be detected. In some social settings, wives might be seen as prone to coercion by husbands. With improved immunosuppression, however, poorly matched combinations now give much improved outcomes (see Chapters 10 and 39); also, subtle HLA sensitization is detected more easily, and its potentially deleterious effect is overcome more easily. At present, spousal donors are acceptable ethically when the relationship is stable and coercive obligations are excluded.

Purely Altruistic Motivation

Deep friendship may be acceptable as an altruistic basis for a nonrelated living kidney donation. In our experience, kidney donation to a one-time college roommate was described by a 60-year-old woman, 6 years after giving her kidney, as follows: "I look upon giving one of my kidneys to my friend as being the most satisfying single act of my life."

Although altruism sometimes is expressed toward unknown others—as when individuals agree to participate in research that brings them little or no direct benefit—organ donation on this basis rarely occurs except by means of a postmortem donor card. A well-documented example is that of a German professor of transplantation surgery who donated one of his kidneys to a patient (unknown to him) on the Munich waiting list (Daar et al., 1997b). Kevorkian (1991) claims that most criminals about to die by capital punishment wish to give their organs, but this request has not been taken up by any state legislature in the United States. This claim is used as the basis for transplantation in China with kidneys from that source.

Compensated Altruism

A modification in this category is organ donation for compensation between acquaintances or, rarely, strangers. Such motivation may be accepted as altruistic if the compensation is not excessive. Compensation is correctly so described only if it covers lost earnings, lost work time or additionally incurred expenses. Beyond those limits, compensation resembles a contract for commercial sale and is flawed ethically.

Commercial Contracts Between Strangers: Kidney Selling

Two types of kidney selling are definable and are considered separately.

Indirect Altruism

Indirect altruism refers to when donor motivation for organ selling is altruistic toward a third party. *Indirect altruism* is a term coined to describe the following form of altruism: Person A wishes to carry out a good deed for a family member, person B, whose needs can be met only through using money. B's needs cannot be met by A giving her a kidney because renal failure is not B's problem. A does not have the money to meet B's need, and society will not or cannot provide it. Person C is rich and in need of a kidney. If A makes a contract to *give* a kidney to a third party D on the understanding that D will then *sell* that kidney to C and use the proceeds to help B, A's contract with D is implicitly altruistic, but D's contract with C is purely commercial. The money D obtains from C enables A indirectly to *carry out the altruistic intention* toward B.

We find this scenario acceptable ethically and have defined, at greater length than here, the *context* in which indirect altruism would have to take place, using an ethically responsible third-party regulator, D, who is trustworthy and respected. Other criteria would need to be in place (Dossetor, 1992b) for such arrangements to meet ethical standards. Examples that seem to meet these criteria are described from India (Reddy, 1991). Daar (1991) provides a valuable perspective in this complicated area.

Personal Gain

Most people find the thought of vending organs for private gain to be repugnant. For this reason as well as the outrages of rampant commercialism that developed, most countries of the world community have outlawed the practice. Publications from an informal ethics committee have suggested that the matter should be thought through again, however (Cameron and Hoffenberg, 1999; Radcliffe-Richards et al., 1998).

The subject of payments for organs is complex (Daar, 1997). We previously published a classification (Daar et al., 1990) of the various types of living kidney donations, with consideration of their ethical acceptability or otherwise, so as to enable discussion to focus on each individual issue rather than combining all the considerations at once. This classification has evolved into the *gray basket concept* (Daar, 1998)—the gray basket being that category in the classification wherein ideas such as indirect altruism (Dossetor, 1992b) or the *donor trust* (Sells, 1992), founded on certain ethical principles but nonetheless still controversial, can be discussed sensibly.

Points argued for allowing outright kidney vending for personal gain are as follows:

1. Poverty is the greatest force for exploitation of individuals in the world, and it is good to relieve even an infinitesimal part of that poverty.
2. Claiming that the destitute are incompetent to make good decisions in their own interest (i.e., expressing their autonomy) is sheer paternalism.

3. When viewed from the perspective of the affluent West, presuming to restrict practices in the developing world constitutes ethical imperialism.

4. It should be possible to regulate outright kidney vending for personal gain within acceptable principles, using a distribution system that ensures fair payment to the vendor and prevents preferential consideration for wealthy persons with chronic renal failure (who pay into the regulator's system for a level of priority).

Points argued for defending the current world ban on outright kidney vending for personal gain are as follows:

1. The feeling of repugnance against kidney vending represents a valid moral intuition, even though it is difficult to reason through precisely why this is so (some forms of repugnance can be attributed to extreme unusualness).

2. From a pragmatic viewpoint, countries where kidney vending would flourish are those where ethical regulations of the practice are likely to become corrupt.

3. If individuals were granted the right to sell their organs, health professionals—as third parties—should *not* be party to it if they wish to retain the trust of the public.

4. Professionals should preserve, as a high professional value, the concept that all persons and their nonrenewable vital organs should be cherished as being above monetary value. We demean humanity by accepting human organ commodification in the marketplace even through third parties that purport to conduct such business at arm's length.

5. Religious viewpoints are against organ usage from living persons.

Although we accept that there is some validity to the various arguments for organ vending for personal gain, our view is that direct selling of kidneys for personal gain is against the best interests of society and should remain prohibited throughout the world. The matter deserves ongoing debate, however. The debate will be colored by the commercial aspects of xenotransplantation as the ethical dilemmas of that practice develop in a comparative setting.

We approve a practice whereby an altruistic good can be achieved by a method that involves obtaining money from wealthy recipients by vending organs through an ethically reliable third party, under conditions in which the donor makes no profit or personal gain except through the spiritual or psychological benefit inherent in acts of altruism. Whether or not such a system can be or needs to be established in a given country depends on many societal factors. These factors are reviewed by considering, in turn, situations at both ends of the *world prosperity spectrum:* (1) from the viewpoint of an affluent society and (2) from the viewpoint of a country where the bulk of the population lives in poverty.

For *affluent cultures,* such as the West, many factors operate to support individuals with special transplant needs, such as state health care programs, unemployment and sickness insurance, and resources to support existing altruistically based cadaver donor programs and new initiatives to increase organ procurement. The benefit/burden calculus for the would-be kidney donor to a third-party vendor who then obtains money for the donor's intended act of *indirect altruism* is not compelling. The conditions of abject poverty do not exist. Also, in Western cultures, the benefit to society of allowing kidney transplantation through third parties raising funds from kidney vending to carry out acts of indirect altruism do not seem to outweigh the probable harm to the fabric of society that would stem from commercialization of the body, including lessened respect for others, affront to religiously based convictions, decay of primary or direct altruism and other risks for social corruption. There are vastly

more opportunities for individuals with chronic renal failure, such as dialysis units in state-subsidized hospitals, neurosurgical units to support bodies that have suffered cerebral death, cadaver organ removal and storage and the possibility of returning to dialysis and having a further organ transplant later if an earlier one fails. In general terms, affluent countries offer protection against dire need in many ways, and members of society are largely protected against abject poverty, starvation and lack of shelter through a tax-financed social security net. Affluent societies provide protection against the need for self-imposed acts of heroism, such as those involved in donating a kidney altruistically, which is then sold to obtain money to benefit others. Affluent societies have not exhausted all possible ways of meeting the shortage in kidney transplants. Perhaps in the second decade of the 21st century, there may be a role for xenografts to meet shortages in organs (see subsequently and Chapter 42). The affluent end of the spectrum has all the options.

Nonaffluent cultures differ in striking ways. Not only is there an absence of the general social security net, but also an absence of government-funded health care programs for special needs. People die for lack of adequate housing, nutrition and simple medical needs, including good sanitation and pure drinking water. People in such conditions already are victimized by abject poverty. The context of their whole lives is different from those of citizens of affluent countries. In such situations, although we still deplore kidney commerce for personal gain, it is impossible for us to condemn kidney donation for prearranged vending through a third party to raise money for an act of indirect altruism to a family member. For the donor in the personal no-gain setting of indirect altruism, the burden may be offset by the benefit to the family member, whereas the welfare of society is not at risk because of the underlying altruistic nature of the act, even though an organ has been obtained for money.

Inherent in this support for indirect altruism in nonaffluent cultures is an insistence that the benefit to B, the intended beneficiary of this form of altruism, must be insured. This insurance necessitates a socially responsible, noncorruptible panel or tribunal of societal and professional peers to approve individual cases and set up a mechanism to collect money from the recipient purchaser and to effect the intended altruistic good of the donor. In our judgment, if this situation cannot be insured, an institution would be acting unethically in pretending to meet a standard if it knows it cannot.

Lastly, in this section, we consider the ethics issues facing recipients who have bought kidneys from living unrelated persons—the purchasers of kidneys. Purchasers of kidneys in nonaffluent countries, where kidney transactions could be used to raise money for acts of indirect altruism, are disproportionately rich in comparison with the donor source. Purchasers are buying parts of someone else's body, which many see as a manifestation of victimization of the poor by the rich, akin in some ways to prostitution or enslavement. Wealth is accepted in most cultures as giving special privileges to individuals who possess it, but this does not extend to victimization and partial enslavement of others. In this instance, because of the good that might result from indirect altruism to the donor's intended beneficiary of the sale, the purchaser of a kidney might be ethically justified if two conditions were met: In addition to giving a fair price for the organ, (1) the purchaser should be obliged morally to give additional funds to support another distressed person, perhaps from the section in society from which the donor comes, and (2) the purchaser should give additional funds toward the ultimate establishment of a cadaver renal transplant program. These additional funds, which we have termed *man-*

dated philanthropy, should not be paid out at the expense of a fair and generous price to the kidney donor, who uses third-party vendors to effect acts of indirect altruism. The purchaser's responsibility in this regard should be in the hands of a tribunal or panel of peers at the transplant institutions.

Emerging Issues in Transplantation
XENOGRAFTS

Obtaining organs for direct transplantation into humans hitherto has been a fruitless exercise, but there is now some indication that this may change. Factors that may open up the xenotransplant field include (1) much improved immunosuppression, (2) ability to manipulate the recipient's immune response and (3) ways of altering some of the foreignness of pig tissue by inserting into the tissue human genes coding for complement regulatory proteins (see Chapter 42).

Xenotransplantation already is a highly controversial area. Kantian deontologists may see animals as outside the province of human ethical concern because they are not *moral agents*. Other traditions believe that animals share ethical status with humans in proportion to their ability to have relationships with humans and a social life among themselves as well as their capacity to suffer pain and anguish and possibly suffer from frustrated self-awareness and thwarted self-interests.

Although animals may not have *rights*, many people attribute them with varying degrees of ethical status. People who strongly hold this perspective view xenografting as another form of animal exploitation as well as another excess of medical hubris, especially if directed at species whose behavior more resembles that of humans (as denoted perhaps by the notion of *genomic proximity to humans*). Transplant teams should try to understand the motivations of such believers in attempts to avoid extreme polarization of emotional viewpoints. Indifference to these concerns leads to angry confrontations, such as characterizes the abortion issue. We welcome debates on these issues, particularly debates that would achieve a measure of public understanding. It is not possible at this time to forecast how the debate over xenotransplantation will work out. Efforts to understand the rational and philosophical basis for people who oppose development of this branch of transplantation science are important. It can be assumed that most people who presently find the prospect of xenotransplantation abhorrent value individual human lives much more highly than individual animals. This assumption should be taken as a given in the debate.

The unique ethics issues in xenotransplantation stem from the unique combination of perspectives that constitute the debate (Table 41–1). Some of these are expanded on in this section, although they are in the course of rapid change.

Breeding Animals for Xenograft Purposes

The great British reformer Bentham (1748–1832), regarded as a key figure in the development of utilitarian ethics, also was one of the earliest to advocate the humane treatment of animals. In 1780, he asked two fundamental questions: (1) "the question is not can they reason? nor can they talk? but can they suffer?" and (2) "what insuperable line prevents us from extending moral regard to animals? " A modern utilitarian philosopher, Singer, has taken on the mantle of Bentham where animals are concerned.

Pain is perceived essentially in the same way by all vertebrates, and it is not controversial that vertebrates used in experiments feel pain. There is a growing consensus, however, that animals can suffer, not just feel pain. Suffering

TABLE 41–1
XENOTRANSPLANTATION DEBATE

Great scientific research
Significant industry involvement
Much greater public awareness of the *existence of a problem (without a sense of the details)*
Public opposition to the exploitation of animals in this way
Lack of consistency of what the public is told about
   The state of science
   The magnitude of risk
Much greater involvement of scientists with industry in terms of contractual obligations and funding of research
Depletion of the traditional sources of university-based funding
Difference in assessment by scientists and policy makers of
   The scientific base
   The risk of infection
Much more active and organized constituency of ethicists, philosophers, concerned citizens and animal rights activists with a larger capacity to make their (sometimes confused) views known and not all willing to engage in polite discourse
Much stronger constituency of patients' advocacy groups, who cannot understand why important research is being held back by *theoretical* and *academic* fears and risks

implies self-awareness, and many experimenters are not ready to concede this point because it then implies a degree of intelligence and worth that would arrogate rights to animals (Singer, 1975). Regan (1983) and others have argued that animals do have many rights, even if these are of a lesser magnitude than those of humans. Ignoring *animal rights* (a term popularized by Regan) is a form of *speciesism*, which is equivalent to racism.

We appreciate the tremendous complexity of animal lives. Animals in captivity can experience fear, boredom, isolation and separation. They may not be able to use language (that we can understand), but they do communicate. The emotional repertoire of subhuman primates, according to ethologists Goodall and Fossey, apparently includes love, sorrow and jealousy (Mukherjee, 1997). These features also explain partly the increasing concern for animal welfare, culminating in the tendency to pass laws recognizing animals as sentient beings with inherent value. If animals are sentient and have value, it could be argued that they *must* have rights. Are animals members of the moral community? Even if we concede that animals are moral subjects and not just objects, they could never be moral agents as far as humans are concerned. There is an inherent problem in the discourse on animal use in that one of the parties being discussed does not participate in the debate, and we are restricted to evaluating moral sensibilities, principles and values of *homo sapiens*.

What is it in humans that bestows on them the moral superiority or higher moral value that would justify the killing of an animal to save a human being? Is it language, tool use, rationality, intentionality, consciousness, conscience or empathy (Caplan, 1992; Sells, 1996)? Because philosophers disagree, because premises are different and because rights theories contain elements of arbitrariness, it seems that, short of a complete change in human consciousness, the issue will remain controversial and divisive.

There are laws to protect research animals in many countries, and there are international guiding principles, for example, those of the Council for International Organizations of Medical Sciences. Sensible guidelines include the *3Rs* of Russel and Burch (1959), which are to *reduce*, *replace* and *refine*, to which could be added *reconsider* and *respect*. There is much effort today directed at looking for alternatives to animal use. Ultimately, it will be *public*, rather than professional, acceptance, acquiescence or rejection that determines the issue of using animals in xenotransplantation. Today, a stronger case can be made for the use of pig organs but not organs from subhuman primates for human xenotransplantation. At this stage of development, it is perhaps more productive to worry about and attend to animal welfare rather than animal rights.

Within the three major monotheistic religions, Judaism, Christianity and Islam, humans were made in the *imago dei*, and the rest of creation is there to serve humans. God blew His own breath into the body of man, transfiguring him and making him different from the rest of creation. The pig is ritually unclean in Islam (*najs*) and Judaism (not *kosher*), however. We have looked at this issue (Daar, 1994) and concluded that it would not be a barrier to xenotransplantation, based on the theological argument that need and necessity can allow that which is forbidden, and in any case, the prohibition is to eating only. There is a *minority* opinion, however, that pigs, partly because they are ritually unclean, cannot be used as source animals. From the religious perspective, it would be important that a xenotransplant should not tamper with the human personality, its freedom and its ability and eligibility to bear responsibility. Humans have stewardship responsibilities accepted noncontroversially by almost everyone, making it necessary to reduce the pain and suffering of animals being used for human purposes (Daar, 1994; Jakobovits, 1975).

Ethics of Consent When Society Is Also at Unknown Risk

The issue of consent in xenotransplantation has not been addressed adequately, and its implications are underestimated. The major issue in xenotransplantation today is whether we are ready to proceed to systematic clinical trials. Our understanding today is that consent for experimental procedures should be informed, unhurried and voluntary. Informed consent exists for the purpose of protecting the subject from the risks of the experiment. Normally, taking into account societal considerations might prejudice the interests of the individual subject. Generally, consent has nothing to do with protection of contacts or of society. It requires that the subject be made aware of the risks involved, the potential benefits to the subject and all the alternatives available.

For xenotransplantation, there is a risk (especially from new xenozoonoses) to the public at large. Trials cannot proceed ethically until there is agreement from society as a whole that it is willing to accept this risk. There are no reliable ways of obtaining such a societal consent. It is a major ethical problem that initially can be addressed only by making every effort to inform and involve all segments of society, using every media outlet.

In the case of xenotransplantation clinical trials, particularly for the early patients, many of the normal elements of individual consent would need to be compromised. The likely subjects probably would be very sick, and voluntariness would be questionable because, especially in the case of liver and heart subjects, the alternative may be death. The risks from the point of view of rejection and the potential benefit can be estimated vaguely but not the risk from xenozoonoses because clinicians do not know which viruses, for example, would be more pathogenic in humans or would mutate or recombine in the host. Clinicians would not know if the source animal has any viruses about which nothing is known. The incubation period and latency of some retroviral infections (e.g., human immunodeficiency virus) could be several years. There is considerable evidence that human immunodeficiency virus (HIV) jumped species from nonhu-

man primates to humans. Clinicians have become aware only recently that porcine endogenous retroviruses can infect human cells *in vitro* (Patience et al., 1997). The demonstration that 160 patients exposed to live pig tissue (Paradis et al., 1999) did not become infected by porcine endogenous retroviruses is partly reassuring but should not be seen as definitive evidence justifying large-scale clinical trials (Weiss, 1999).

The main foreseeable problem with clinical trials in xenotransplantation is with the question of postoperative monitoring. The recipient would have to agree to the *requirement* for strict monitoring, which may be intrusive and may result in quarantine, containment or other physical restrictions if the recipient develops infections likely to endanger contacts, health care workers or the public. Privacy and confidentiality almost certainly would have to be signed away in this consent procedure, especially because the contacts also would require monitoring. The recipient may be restricted from having sexual relations for perhaps 1 year or more. Contacts themselves would have to consent to postoperative monitoring, which may be intrusive in the case of a major infection difficult to diagnose or treat. There is an implicit need for community consent—not an easy thing to obtain because it normally would require public hearings, advisory bodies and legislative and executive branch processes (Institute of Medicine, 1996).

The fact that the patient is going to be *required* to comply with postoperative monitoring alters the nature of *consent* to something more aggressively binding and contractual. There is another normal feature of consent—the subject has the right to withdraw at any time from the experiment. This right would have to be transgressed because the recipient cannot opt subsequently to withdraw from the experimental procedure once he or she harbors an infection that might jeopardize public health. The consent would need to be enforceable in a direction different from that in the past—this time against the best interests of the subject and in favor of the public. This situation would be a travesty of the concept of consent as it is known today.

Biotechnology Companies as an Ethics Issue

Many companies have done basic research, often collaborating with academic institutions. For example, Avant Immunotherapeutics, Cambridge, Mass. has collaborated with Johns Hopkins University and Harvard University (Brigham Hospital); Biotransplants Inc. and Cell Genesys have collaborated with Harvard University (Massachusetts General Hospital), and Imutran (now part of Novartis) is collaborating with scientists at Cambridge University in the United Kingdom (OECD, 1998). There are many other such collaborations, and these companies are keen to start clinical trials. The legitimate primary motive of these companies is profit. The companies are likely to push hard to begin serious xenotransplantation so as to recover their investment early and establish their technology rapidly before the technology changes. The companies would be reluctant to share their data and may insist on *gag* clauses in contracts with clinicians. Companies also would wish to traffic in what is a valuable commodity (no organ donation). These are elements that most clinicians and scientists are not prepared to handle on their own and would require the input of lawyers—further increasing the cost of xenotransplantation. Clinicians working with these companies, excluding investigator bias, will want to start performing xenotransplantation; pilot studies may be the route chosen by some to get started.

These potential conflicts of interest are predictable, but so long as they are transparent (a difficult issue) some professional or legal control can be brought to bear. For example, when Imutran announced in the late 1990s that a heart xeno-transplant was likely within 1 year of the announcement, using their genetically modified pigs, the resulting discussions may have influenced the British adoption of an embargo (AGEX, 1997), making it impossible for the company to go ahead at that time with a clinical xenotransplant in the United Kingdom.

Avoidance of Regulation by *Xenotourism*

Almost all of the influential discussions about the dangers of xenotransplantation and development of guidelines and control frameworks are taking place in Europe and North America (see later). Xenotransplantation may start elsewhere, however, in environments where the regulations are lax and the scientific base and facilities are inadequate. An example was the case of Baruah (Mudur, 1999), a physician who was arrested in Assam, India, early in 1997 for violation of the Organ Transplantation Act. He had claimed to have transplanted successfully the heart, lungs and kidneys of a pig into a human recipient at his own hospital, assisted by local colleagues and apparently by a colleague from Hong Kong. The patient died a week later, and the family, feeling suspicious, lodged a complaint with the police. This kind of activity might pose dangers because in the near future clinicians from the scientifically advanced countries may start collaborating with colleagues in countries where the regulations may be more permissive. It would be better to consider seriously an international effort to draw up universal guidelines, while hastening to lay the groundwork for national regulatory mechanisms for clinical trials.

Cost and Other Economic Considerations

Xenotransplantation will be expensive at least for a number of years. The biotechnology companies are likely to control the cost of the organs and in the absence of real competition will want to keep this cost as high as the market will tolerate. The cost of rearing source animals under special conditions, monitoring them, developing laboratory tests, training staff, taking extra precautions, monitoring recipients and contacts and installing infection control measures all will add to the cost. It is unknown if, in the long run, the cost will drop sufficiently for this to be one of the justifications for xenotransplantation. Countries with ethical commitment to equity in access to established therapies will need to assess carefully how to maintain the principle of distributive justice, once the results achieve sufficient success to be seen as established treatment and not clinical research.

National and International Efforts to Develop Guidelines

One must approve the efforts that have been made to consider the challenging issues of xenotransplantation and be prepared to regulate its development along ethically acceptable lines. Table 41–2 lists some of these efforts. There is great concern about ethics issues, regulatory frameworks, relationship with industry production of source animals and the risk of xenozoonoses and their detection. In addition to those listed, there are initiatives by other international bodies and by national bodies in France, Netherlands, Spain and Switzerland.

In January 1999, the Parliamentary Committee of the Council of Europe decided to call for a moratorium on xenografts. This moratorium has been criticized as inhibiting research funding and investment, but it has been praised by others.

TABLE 41–2

NATIONAL AND INTERNATIONAL REPORTS IN XENOTRANSPLANTATION AND NATIONAL REGULATORY EFFORTS

National and International Reports in Xenotransplantation

WHO Consultation in Xenotransplantation
Institute of Medicine (United States)—Xenotransplantation Science, Ethics and Public Policy
United Kingdom Advisory Group on Ethics of Xenotransplantation—The Kennedy Report
Nuffield Council on Bioethics—Animal-to-Human Transplants: Ethics of Xenotransplantation
Organization for Economic Cooperation and Development (OECD)—Policy on International Issues in Transplantation Biotechnology
Health Canada—National Forum on Xenotransplantation. Clinical Ethics and Regulatory Issues, Nov 1997

National Regulatory Efforts

United Kingdom Xenotransplantation Interim Regulatory Authority (UKXIRA)
Canada: Standards for Xenotransplantation—Canadian Standards Association (CSA)
German Medical Council on Xenotransplantation
Council of Europe Steering Committee on Transplantation—responsible for the moratorium on xenotransplantation of January 1999
Établissement Français des Grèffes

These efforts are ongoing and will react promptly as the situation changes. None of these national efforts have addressed seriously the question of adequately informing the public, however, so that society at large can express an opinion on an issue that may put many individuals at risk inadvertently. Obtaining such informed societal opinion and agreement is difficult and costly. So far no jurisdiction has addressed this public education issue seriously despite its crucial ethical importance.

Physiological Issues

Less discussed are the hazards inherent in an animal organ such as the liver synthesizing animal proteins that might (1) be unphysiological for humans, having a dysfunctional effect; (2) induce an immunological response or (3) interact with human protein homologues in some unforeseen way. There are other physiological incompatibilities for other organs (see Chapter 42).

EMBRYONIC STEM CELLS, CLONING AND TISSUE ENGINEERING

Human Embryonic Stem Cells

Developmental biologists have long sought the ultimate cell—the human embryonic stem cell. Its discovery (in the sense of its purification, characterization, stable growth as cell lines and capacity to differentiate into several cell types) during 1998 by Thomson and colleagues was probably of greater therapeutic significance than was the cloning of a sheep from a mature somatic cell by nuclear transfer. Human embryonic stem cells, which are derived from the inner cell mass of the blastocyst (embryo), are pluripotent in the sense that if transplanted by injection into the inner cell mass of another embryo of the same species, they grow along with the fetal tissue and populate all the tissues. Human embryonic stem cells have enormous theoretical potential in transplantation.

Human embryonic stem cells give clinicians the potential capability of using cocktails of growth and modulating factors to guide them into types of tissues that are needed for transplantation; it then would be possible to have an endless supply of hepatocytes (for liver diseases), β cells (for diabetes) or competent neuronal cells to treat conditions such as Parkinson's or Huntington's disease. If tissue engineering progressed to its logical conclusion, it should be possible one day to engineer a whole organ for transplantation. Points to consider are as follows:

At present, the supply of human embryonic stem cells is limited.
An embryo is needed for the purification of embryonic stem cells.
Embryonic stem cells would have the genetic makeup and the histocompatibility antigens of the donor and would have the same potential for rejection by the recipient, unless they were genetically modified.

Moral Status of the Embryo

Some people distinguish between a preembryo stage and a proper embryo stage, but many people prefer not to use this distinction, which is otherwise used to distinguish embryos before and after formation of the primitive streak at about 14 days after fertilization. One of the crucial issues regarding the moral status of the embryo is the question of when life starts—the extremes being the moment of fertilization (i.e., as soon as a zygote is formed) and when the infant is delivered. Absolutists insist that all human life has the same moral value; others say that there is a gradation of moral worth and consideration as you progress from zygote to preimplantation embryo to postimplantation embryo to fetus to infant. Most would agree that the fully formed fetus must be aborted only for the most extreme of reasons, such as to save the life of the mother.

The British Human Fertilization and Embryology Act (1990) permits the licensing of human embryo research that has certain specified objectives (initially confined to treating infertility, increasing knowledge about causes of congenital diseases and of miscarriage, developing better contraception and developing techniques for preimplantation genetic and/ or chromosomal diagnosis). These embryos may be excess embryos from in vitro fertilization programs, in which the owners have given consent for the research, or, if necessary, embryos could be created specifically for research purposes (Britain is one of the few countries in the world where this is permitted). The embryos must be destroyed before 14 days (i.e., this law recognizes the preembryo phase before 14 days, when the entity is a collection of cells with no recognizable differentiated parts). The U.S. Congress forbids the use of federal funds for any experiment that requires destroying a fetus, which is why human embryonic stem cells were developed with private capital.

Shamblott and colleagues, using private sector funding, have been able to isolate from early aborted human fetuses cells with almost the same characteristics as embryonic stem cells (Shamblott et al., 1998). These embryonic germ cells were derived from the gonadal ridges and mesenteries of 5- to 9-week postfertilization aborted fetuses. Similar to embryonic stem cells, these embryonic germ cells are pluripotent and are capable of developing into trophoblast and into all three embryonic germ layers. This approach overcomes some of the ethical objections of using embryos, for those who deem their use as tantamount to abortion. The question of histocompatibility can be overcome by genetic manipulation of embryonic stem cells. The ideal solution for a patient with

end-stage renal failure would be to obtain a somatic (e.g., cheek-lining) cell from this patient and to fuse it with an enucleated ovum to create an embryo from which to make embryonic stem cells. From these embryonic stem cells, containing nuclear DNA only of the original patient, a new kidney could be engineered, then autotransplanted into the patient. Here the patient would be both donor and recipient. The only ethically objectionable aspect of this scenario is that an ovum is needed to create the embryo, and this lends itself to the objection of abortion. Advanced Cell Technologies in Massachusetts has developed a technique whereby a human somatic cell nucleus is inserted into an enucleated cow ovum, and the company has claimed that this works to produce a viable embryo (BBC, 1999a). This embryo would have the nuclear DNA of the person from whom the somatic cell was derived but, at least in the early stages, would have the mitochondrial DNA of the cow. This chimera scenario was such a shock that President Clinton immediately asked his National Bioethics Advisory Commission to study the matter. Experts from other institutions have cast doubt that cow mitochondrial DNA is capable of supporting the human nucleus or that the enucleated cow ovum is capable fully to reprogram the human somatic cell nuclear DNA to its primordial stage where it is capable of developing into a normal human embryo.

These events are at the cutting edge of science at present, and as often happens, technology is far ahead of public understanding or ethical adjudication. There has been talk of cloning human embryos to produce more abundant supplies of human embryonic stem cells (BBC, 1999a). In the United Kingdom, the government was criticized heavily by scientists and the British Medical Association for its rejection of the advice by two scientific panels to permit therapeutic cloning, particularly for the development of embryonic stem cells (BBC, 1999b).

A more intriguing, practical and uncontroversial method is to use, not human embryonic stem cells, but other stem cells, such as neural, mesenchymal, bone marrow or peripheral blood stem cells. It already has been shown that one type of such stem cells (neural) can, when injected into an experimental animal, go on to develop into other unrelated cell types (blood cells, including myeloid and lymphoid cells and early hematopoietic cells) (Bjornson et al., 1999). Similarly, rat bone marrow stem cells can differentiate into hepatocytes (Petersen et al., 1999). Human mesenchymal stem cells, which normally differentiate into tissues such as bone, cartilage, fat, tendon, muscle and bone marrow stroma, can be made to differentiate in vitro exclusively into one of several desired lineages (Pittenger et al., 1999). Mice hematopoietic stem cells can be grown ex vivo and self-replicate indefinitely without differentiation, when exposed to thrombopoietin (Yagi et al., 1999). If human nonembryonic stem cells could be made to differentiate into kidney cells, it ultimately would be possible to treat end-stage renal failure starting with the patient's own bone marrow or other stem cells, without needing to create an embryo. The ultimate theoretical technology would be to start with a somatic cell and be able, with cocktails of growth factors and other signals, to reprogram it to have the same capabilities as embryonic stem cells (without going through an embryo phase and without the need to start with any type of stem cell).

Technologies such as those described previously, were they to be brought to full fruition, would be a distinct ethical improvement over the use of many fetuses to obtain enough fetal tissue for the treatment of a single patient with Parkinson's disease or diabetes. With embryonic stem cell technology, a single embryo could produce enough bankable embryonic stem cells to last a long time. The important ethical proviso is to separate the issue of abortion from the use of the cells. Abortion should be judged in its own moral framework; if spontaneous or legally permitted, the use of the embryo or fetus becomes a much less ethically contentious issue. As regards genetic manipulation, it should be clear that gene insertion and somatic gene therapy are less ethically controversial than germline genetic interventions (Daar and Mattei, 1999).

Cloning

Cloning of humans by nuclear transfer from somatic cells (as was done in the sheep) has been declared unethical and unacceptable by almost all commentators. Even if one day we could imagine a therapeutic indication for this technology, its use for nefarious, selfish, narcissistic or trivial purposes would not be permissible ethically. The cloning of the self to produce a DNA copy or copies for the sole purpose of having a new human being kept in waiting should you one day need to replace your organs would be the ultimate misuse of science.

REFERENCES

Advisory Group on the Ethics of Xenotransplantation (AGEX). (1997). *Animal Tissues into Humans*, London, Stationary Office, London.

Anaise, D., Smith, R., Ishimuru, M., *et al.* (1990). An approach to organ salvage from non-heartbeating cadaver donors under existing legal and ethical requirements for transplantation. *Transplantation* **49**, 290.

Andrews, L. B. (1986). My body, my property. *Hastings Cent. Rep.* **16**, 28.

BBC. (1999a). First cloned human embryo revealed. *www.bb.co.uk*, News June 17.

BBC. (1999b). Human cloning ban condemned. *www.bb.co.uk*, News June 224.

Beauchamp, T. L. and Childress, J. F. (1994). *Principles of Biomedical Ethics*, 4th ed., Oxford University Press, Oxford.

Beecher, K. H. (1968). A definition of irreversible coma: report of the Harvard Medical School to examine the definition of brain death. *J. A. M. A.* **205**, 227.

Bjornson, C. R., Rietze, R. L., Eeynolds, B. A., Magli, M. C. and Vesconi, A. L. (1999). Turning brain into blood: a hematopoietic fate adopted by adult neural stem cells in vivo. *Science* **283**, 534.

Bonomini, V. (1991). Ethical aspects of living donation. *Transplant. Proc.* **23**, 2497.

Cameron, J. S. and Hoffenberg, R. (1999). The ethics of organ transplantation reconsidered: paid organ donation and the use of executed prisoners as donors. *Kidney Int.* **55**, 724.

Caplan, A. (1992). Is xeno-transplantation morally wrong? *Transplant. Proc.* **24**, 722.

Cefalo, R. C. and Engelhardt, H. T. (1989). The use of fetal and anencephalic tissue for transplantation. *J. Med. Philos.* **14**, 25.

Cho, Y. W., Terasaki, P. I., Cecka, J. M. and Gjertson, D. W. (1998). Transplantation of kidneys from donors whose hearts have stopped beating. *N. Engl. J. Med.* **338**, 221.

Cohen, L. R. (1991). The ethical virtues of a futures market in cadaveric organs. *In Organ Replacement Therapy: Ethics, Justice and Commerce*, (W. Land and J. B. Dossetor, eds.), p. 302, Springer-Verlag, Berlin.

Daar, A. S. (1991). Rewarded gifting and rampant commercialism in perspective: is there a difference? *In Organ Replacement Therapy: Ethics, Justice and Commerce*, (W. Land and J. B. Dossetor, eds.), p. 181, Springer-Verlag, Berlin.

Daar, A. S. (1994). Xenotransplantation and religion: the major monotheistic religions. *Xenotransplantation* **2**, 61.

Daar, A. S. (1997). Paid organ donation: towards an understanding of the issues. *In Organ and Tissue Donation for Transplantation*, (J. R. Chapman, M. Deirhoi and C. Wight, eds.), p. 46, Arnold, London.

Daar, A. S. (1998). Paid organ donation: the Grey Basket concept. *J. Med. Ethics* **24**, 365.

Daar, A. S., Gutmann, T. and Land, W. (1997a). Reimbursement, rewarded gifting, financial incentives, and commercialism in living organ donation. *In Procurement, Preservation and Allocation of Vascularized Organs*, (G. M. Collins, J. M. Dubernard, W. Land and C. G. Persijn, eds.), p. 301, Kluwer, Dordecht.

Daar, A. S., Land, W., Yahya, T. M., *et al.* (1997b). Living-donor renal transplantation: evidence-based justification for an ethical opinion. *Transpl. Rev.* **11**, 95.

Daar, A. S. and Mattei, J. F. (1999). *Draft Guiding Principles on Medical Genetics and Biotechnology*, World Health Organization, World Health Assembly, Geneva.

Daar, A. S., Salahudeen, A. K., Pingle, A. and Woods, H. F. (1990). Ethics and commerce in live donor renal transplantation: classification of the issues. *Transplant. Proc.* **2**, 922.

Daar, A. S. and Sells, R. A. (1990). Living non-related donor renal transplantation: a reappraisal. *Transpl. Rev.* **4**, 128.

Daemen, J. H. C., de Wit, R. J., Bronkhorst, M. W., *et al.* (1996). Non-heart-beating donor program contributes 40% of kidneys for transplantation. *Transplant. Proc.* **28**, 105.

Dickens, B. (1990). Excised organs prior to implantation: belonging and control. *Transplant. Proc.* **22**, 1000.

Dossetor, J. B., Monaco, A. P., and Stiller, C. R. (1989). Ethics, Justice and Commerce in Transplantation: a global view. *Transplant. Proc.* **22**, 1014.

Dossetor, J. B. (1992a). An ethics issue for cadaver renal transplantation: a commentary on Stuart Lind. *J. Clin. Ethics* **3**, 309.

Dossetor, J. B. (1992b). Rewarded gifting: ever ethically acceptable? *Transplant. Proc.* **24**, 2092.

Dunnett, S. B., Kendall, A. L., Watts, C., *et al.* (1997). Neuronal cell transplantation for Parkinsons's and Huntingdon's disease. *Br. Med. Bull.* **53**, 757.

Fishman, J. A. (1998). The risk of infection in xenotransplantation: introduction. *Ann. N. Y. Acad. Sci.* **862**, 45.

Frabrega, A., Matas, A. J., Payne, W. D., *et al.* (1992). 10-year to 20-year follow-up of 123 consecutive HLA-identical living-related kidney transplant from the pre-Cyclosporine era. *Clin. Transplant.* **18**, 145.

Frewen, T. C., Stiller, C. R., *et al.* (1990). Anencephalic infants and organ donation: the Children's Hospital of Western Ontario experience. *Transplant. Proc.* **22**, 1033.

Gearhart, J. (1998). New potential for human embryonic stem cells. *Science* **282**, 1061.

Halevy, A. and Brady, B. (1993). Brain death: reconciling definitions, criteria and tests. *Ann. Intern. Med.* **119**, 519.

HFEA. (1990). *Human Fertilization and Embryology Act, 1990 (c37)*, HMSO, London.

Hong, H. Q., Yin, H. R., Zhu, S. L. and Lin, Y. T. (1991). The results of transplant livers from selected non-heart-beating cadaver donors. *Hiroshima J. Med. Sci.* **40**, 87.

Institute of Medicine. (1996). Xenotransplantation: Science, Ethics and Public Policy, National Academic Press, Washington, D.C.

Jakobovits, I. (1975). *Jewish Medical Ethics*, Bloch Publishing, New York.

Kevorkian, J. (1991). *Prescription: Medicide, the Goodness of Planned Death*, Promotheus Books, Buffalo, N.Y.

Kleinman, I. and Lowy, F. H. (1989). Cadaveric organ donation: ethical considerations for a new approach. *C. M. A. J.* **141**, 107.

Koostra, G., Kievit, J. K. and Heineman, E. (1997). The non heart-beating donor. *Br. Med. Bull.* **53**, 844.

May, W. F. (1990). Brain death: anencephalics and aborted fetuses. *Transplant. Proc.* **22**, 985.

Michielsen, P. (1991). Medical risk and benefit in renal donors: the use of living donation reconsidered. *In Organ Replacement Therapy*, (W. Land and J. B. Dossetor, eds.), Springer-Verlag, Berlin.

Miranda, B. and Matesanz, R. (1998). International issues in transplantation: setting the scene and flagging the most urgent and controversial issues. *Ann. N. Y. Acad. Sci.* **862**, 129.

Monaco, A. P. (1989). Comment: a transplant surgeon's views on social factors in organ transplantation. *Transplant. Proc.* **21**, 3403.

Monaco, A. P. (1990). Transplantation: the state of the art. *Transplant. Proc.* **22**, 896.

Mudur, G. (1999). Indian surgeon challenges ban on xenotransplantation. *B. M. J.* **318**, 79.

Mukherjee, M. (1997). Trends in animal research. *Sci. Am,* **276**, 86.

Paradis, K., Langbord, G., Long, Z., *et al.* (1999). Search for cross-species transmission of porcine endogenous retroviruses in patients treated with living pig tissue. *Science* **285**, 1236.

Parliamentary Standing Committee on Health. (1999). *Organ and Tissue Donation and Transplantation*, Government Publishers, Ottawa.

Patience, C., Takeuchi, Y., and Weiss, R. A. (1997). Infection of human cells by an endogamous retrovirus of pigs. *Nat. Med.* **3**, 282.

Petersen, B. E., Bowen, W. C., Patrene, K. D., *et al.* (1999). Bone marrow as a potential source of hepatic oval cells. *Science* **284**, 1168.

Pittenger, M. F., Mackay, A. M., Beck, S. C., *et al.* (1999). Multilineage potential of adult human mesenchymal stem cells. *Science* **284**, 143.

OECD. (1998). *Policy Considerations on International Issues in Transplantation Biotechnology, Including Use of Non-Human Cells, Tissues and Organs*, OECD, Paris.

Radcliffe-Richards, J., Daar, A. S., Guttmann, R. D., *et al.* (1998). The case for allowing kidney sales. *Lancet* **351**, 1950.

Reddy, K. C. (1991). Organ donation for consideration: an Indian view point. *In Organ Replacement Therapy: Ethics, Justice and Commerce*, (W. Land and J. B. Dossetor, eds), p. 173, Springer-Verlag, Berlin.

Regan, T. (1983). *The Case for Animal Rights*, University of California Press.

Roberts, H. P., *et al.* (1988). Living related kidneys continue to provide superior results over cadaveric kidneys in the cyclosporine era. *Transplant. Proc.* **20**, 26.

Robertson, V. M., George, G. D., Gedrich, P. S., *et al.* (1998). Concentrated professional education to implement routine referral legislation increases organ donation. *Transplant. Proc.* **30**, 214.

Roels, L. and Michielsen, P. (1990). Altruism, self-determination and organ procurement efficiency: the European experience. *Transplant. Proc.* **23**, 2514.

Rothenberg, L. S. (1990). The anencephalic neonate and brain death: an international review of medical, ethical and legal issues. *Transplant. Proc.* **22**, 1037.

Russel, W. M. S. and Burch, R. L. (1959). The principles of human experimental technique. Methuen, London.

Sass, H.-M. (1991). Philosophical arguments in accepting brain death criteria. *In Organ Replacement Therapy: Ethics, Justice, Commerce*, (W. Land and J. B. Dossetor, eds.), p. 248, Springer-Verlag, Berlin.

Sass, H.-M. (1992). Criteria for death: self-determination and public policy. *J. Med. Philos.* **17**, 445.

Schreiber, H.-L. (1991). Legal implications of the principle *primum nihil nocere* as it applies to live donors. *In Organ Replacement Therapy: Ethics, Justice and Commerce*, (W. Land and J. B. Dossetor, eds.), Springer-Verlag, Berlin.

Sells, R. A. (1992). Toward an affordable ethic. *Transplant. Proc.* **24**, 2095.

Sells, R. A. (1996). Ethics of xenotransplantation. *Xenotransplantation* **4**, 18.

Shamblott, M. J., Axelman, J., Wang, S., *et al.* (1998). Derivation of pluripotent stem cells from cultured human primordial germ cells. *Proc. Natl. Acad. Sci. U. S. A.* **95**, 13726.

Singer, P. (1975). *Animal Liberation*, Random House, New York.

Singer, P. A., Siegler, M., Whitington, P. F., *et al.* (1989). Ethics of liver transplantation using living donors. *N. Engl. J. Med.* **321**, 620.

Soh, P. and Lim, S. M. L. (1991). Impact of the opting-out system on kidney procurement in Singapore. *Transplant. Proc.* **23**, 2523.

Thomson, J. A., Itskovitz-Eldor, J., Shapiro, S. S., *et al.* (1998). Embryonic stem cell lines derived from human blastocysts [published erratum appears in *Science* 1998 Dec 4;282(5395):1827]. *Science* **282**, 1145.

Truog, R. D. (1997). Is it time to abandon brain death? *Hastings Cent. Rep.* **27**, 29.

Ubel, A., Arnold, R. M. and Caplan, A. L. (1993). Rationing failure: the ethical lessons of the retransplantation of scarce vital organs. *J. A. M. A.* **270**, 2469.

U.S. President's Commission for the Study of Ethical Problems in Medicine and Biomedical and Behavioral Research. (1981). *Defining Death*, Government Printing Office, Washington, D.C.

Veatch, R. M. (1992). Brain death and slippery slopes. *J. Clin. Ethics* **3**, 181.

Veatch, R. M. (1993). The impending collapse of the whole-brain definition of death. *Hastings Cent. Rep.* **23**, 18.

Walters, J. W. and Ashwal, S. (1989). Anencephalic infants as organ donors and the brain death standard. *J. Med. Philos.* **14**, 79.

Weiss, R. (1999). Xenografts and retroviruses. *Science* **285**, 5431.

Whittington, P. F., Siegler, M. and Broelsch, C. E. (1991). Living donor nonrenal organ transplantation: a focus on living related orthotopic liver transplantation. *In Organ Replacement Therapy: Ethics Justice and Commerce*, (W. Land and J. B. Dossetor, eds.), p. 116, Springer-Verlag, Berlin.

Yagi, M., Ritchie, K. A., Sitnicka, E., *et al.* (1999). Sustained ex vivo expansion of haemapoietic stem cells mediated by thrombopoietin. *Proc. Natl. Acad. Sci. U. S. A.* **96**, 8126.

Youngner, S. J. and Arnold, R. M. (1993). Ethical, psychosocial and public policy issues of procuring organs from non-heart-beating cadaver donors. *J. A. M. A.* **269**, 2769.

Youngner, S. J., Lynch, A., Wolf, Z. R., Lynch, M. J. and Foy, J. M. (1990). Respect for the dead body. *Transplant. Proc.* **22**, 1014.

Renal Xenotransplantation
Bob Soin • Peter J. Friend

Introduction

Transplantation has become the treatment of choice for most patients with chronic renal failure as well as for many patients with end-stage disease of the heart, liver or lungs. In most developed countries, the number of transplant operations performed increased rapidly during the 1970s and 1980s. This increase was not maintained during the 1990s despite expanding demand, and waiting lists now are growing faster than transplant activity (Evans *et al.*, 1992). This situation is due to a shortage of donor organs rather than any other failure to provide resources (Hosenpud *et al.*, 1998).

Many strategies have been used in an attempt to increase the availability of donor organs. Public awareness campaigns, changes to the legislation regarding organ removal (*opting out*), the use of non–heart-beating donors and the transplantation of *marginal* organs (from donors that previously would have been regarded as unsuitable) all have the potential to increase transplantation of cadaver donor organs (Kaufman and Bennet, 1999). In the most optimistic forecast, however, these strategies are unlikely to resolve completely the underlying discrepancy between supply and demand. If all potential donors were identified and used, there still would be a substantial shortage of donor organs. The expansion of renal transplantation using organs from living related or unrelated donors has had a significant impact on renal transplant activity in many transplant centers. These procedures present risk to the donor, however, and not all potential recipients will have a suitable donor.

Xenotransplantation (the transplantation of organs between species) has been seen for many years as the potential solution to the problem of organ supply (Medawar, 1969). Successful xenotransplantation would enable timely intervention on a planned basis for all appropriately assessed patients. It would remove the logistic problems and ethical concerns that surround cadaver organ donation. It would reduce or remove the risk of patients' deterioration or death while awaiting transplantation (a greater problem for patients awaiting nonrenal transplants).

Although clinical trials of xenotransplantation were attempted at an early stage, the immunological barriers previously have proved insuperable. More recently, physiological and microbiological issues also have given cause for concern. The ethical issues are different from those relating to allotransplantation but are no less complex.

Developments in molecular biology and increasing understanding of the immunological processes involved in rejection have led to a resurgence of interest in xenotransplantation (Morris, 1999). In contrast to the early trials in which nonhuman primates were used as donors, attention has turned to the possibility of transplantation across the immunologically more difficult pig-to-human barrier. Although not at the stage of widespread clinical application, substantial advances have been made, and there is some cause for optimism that xenotransplantation might become a viable therapeutic modality in due course.

History

Long before the era of dialysis and clinical allotransplantation, surgical maneuvers were attempted to support patients in acute or end-stage chronic renal failure (Hancock, 1997). In 1905, Princeteau used subcutaneously engrafted slices of rabbit kidney in a child with renal failure and claimed improvement in the patient's condition with an increased urine output (Princeteau, 1905). The child survived for 16 days before dying of respiratory complications. Attempts in subsequent years to transplant kidneys from various primate and nonprimate species with vascular connection to the recipient circulation all failed within minutes because of graft thrombosis (Jabouley, 1906; Unger, 1910; see Chapter 1). In 1923, Neuhof reported 9-day survival of a patient in renal failure following mercury poisoning after implantation of a vascularized lamb kidney. This result was not reproducible, and experimental evidence accumulated of vigorous immune responses to any transplanted solid organ from another species. The development of chemical immunosuppression in the 1960s allowed the next attempts at controlling these responses (see Chapter 1).

In 1963, Reemtsma and coworkers performed a series of renal transplants using chimpanzees as donors (Reemtsma *et al.*, 1964). In the first recipient, a 23-year-old woman, azathioprine, actinomycin C and corticosteroid immunosuppression were used before and after transplantation. In the first 24 hours after surgery, the patient passed more than 7 L of urine. The organ was locally irradiated, and the patient's renal function returned to normal, although the patient had an unexplained fever for 3 months after the operation. This patient survived for 9 months before dying after a brief febrile illness unrelated to the graft function. At postmortem, the organ appeared macroscopically normal, whereas the histology showed only interstitial fibrosis and some low-grade mononuclear cell infiltration. The second longest survivor in this series of six patients lived 63 days before dying of overwhelming infection.

At around the same time, a series of six clinical renal transplants was performed using baboon kidneys at the University of Colorado. These transplants were less successful, with a mean survival of 36 days and death of all recipients. Subsequently the increasing success of cadaver allotransplantation and the wider availability of dialysis led to a self-imposed moratorium by the research groups in the field on further attempts at clinical renal xenotransplantation (Dubernard *et al.*, 1974; Starzl *et al.*, 1993).

Immunological Factors

Calne (1970) coined the terms *concordant* and *discordant* to describe different species combinations based on the outcome of organ transplantation. In a concordant species combination, rejection occurs in a manner analogous to a first set immune reaction to an allograft. In a discordant combination, a much more rapid reaction occurs, within hours, and is termed *hyperacute rejection.*

The presence of preformed antispecies antibodies subsequently was shown in discordant species combinations. In general, species that are phylogenetically close (humans and monkeys) are more likely to be concordant than species that are phylogenetically more distant (humans and pigs), although there are exceptions to this rule.

HYPERACUTE REJECTION

Hyperacute rejection can be shown in the discordant combination of pig-to-dog renal transplantation with immunological, hematological, coagulation and immunopathological changes similar to those after allotransplantation in pre-sensitized recipients (Giles *et al.*, 1970). Glomeruli show engorgement, thrombus formation and interstitial hemorrhage with evidence of IgM and C3 deposition on immunofluorescence. There is consumption of platelets with blood cell trapping and local development of a procoagulant state (Fig. 42–1).

The existence of preformed xenoreactive natural antibody (XNA) against carbohydrate residues found on the vascular endothelium (and many other cells) of discordant donors initiates the chain of events leading to xenograft hyperacute rejection (Bach, 1997a; Galili, 1994; McKenzie *et al.*, 1968; Pearse *et al.*, 1998). In humans and Old World monkeys, XNAs constitute 1% of the total immunoglobulin pool, although IgM XNAs may constitute 4% of the total IgM pool. Most (>95%) of these antibodies are directed against the Galα1,3-GalGlcNAc-R (α-Gal) epitope (Fryer *et al.*, 1995; Galili *et al.*, 1998; Hancock, 1997a; Platt *et al.*, 1991a; Sandrin *et al.*, 1994). It is believed that XNAs represent a component of the innate immune system, providing a defense mechanism against Gal antigen–bearing bacterial pathogens and parasites (Galili, 1993).

Activation of the complement system is fundamental to the process of hyperacute xenograft rejection. The complement system comprises a sequence of proteins that, having been triggered, act as a cascade with rapid amplification (Fig. 42–2). In discordant xenotransplantation, the classic pathway of complement activation is initiated by the binding of XNAs to target antigens on the endothelial cells of the graft.

Under normal circumstances (nontransplanted), local reg-ulation of complement activation is maintained by several genetically determined proteins on the surface of cells and in the circulation, termed *regulators of complement activation* (RCA). These RCA are species-specific, however, and fail to control complement activation in a xenograft setting. In addition to the triggering of the classic pathway of complement activation, triggering of the alternative pathway may occur (see Fig. 42–2) as a result of contact between C3 and IgA polymers.

Complement fixation by bound XNA generates C3a, C5a and membrane attack complex (MAC, C_{5b-9}) (Migagawa *et al.*, 1988; Zhow *et al.*, 1990). Membrane attack complex is an annular amphipathic molecule that inserts into the phospholipid cell membrane. The transmembrane channel is fully permeable to electrolytes and water. The increased permeability causes cellular swelling and lysis with calcium ion influx and organelle destruction.

An inflammatory response is generated with activation of plasma proteins, leukocytes and platelets (Blakely *et al.*, 1994). A loss of the barrier function of the endothelium ensues. Distortion of the intercellular junctions accompanies changes in endothelial cell shape and loss of the cell surface heparin sulfate (Robson *et al.*, 1997; Stevens *et al.*, 1993). Neutrophil margination into tissues, interstitial edema and hemorrhage, vascular thrombosis and ultimately graft failure follow.

There is evidence in small animal models that hyperacute rejection also can be caused by complement activation by the alternative pathway alone without the binding of XNAs (Lin *et al.*, 1998). In the rat-sheep combination, rat xenografts are rejected in a hyperacute manner by the sheep fetus in the absence of anti-rat antibodies (Rajasinghe *et al.*, 1996). In pig-to-primate transplantation, the removal of XNAs prevents hyperacute rejection (Cooper and Thall, 1997; Cooper *et al.*, 1994; Koren *et al.*, 1996), providing evidence that in this combination the alternative pathway alone is insufficient to cause hyperacute rejection.

ACUTE VASCULAR REJECTION

If hyperacute rejection is abrogated, discordant and concordant xenografts behave in a similar manner and are rejected by a continued humoral process over a longer period;

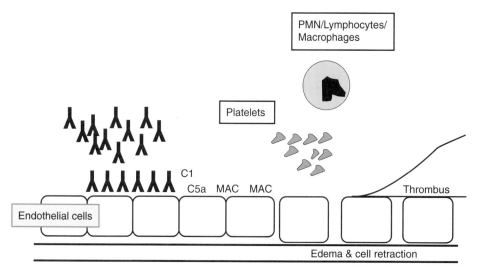

FIGURE 42–1

Normal endothelium usually is watertight and generates anticoagulant factors at its surface. On reperfusion, xenoreactive natural antibodies (XNAs) bind to epitopes (usually α-gal) and induce classic pathway complement activation. Endothelial cell activation, retraction and edema occur. Circulating leukocytes and platelets are attracted and activated. The final processes of interstitial hemorrhage and vessel thrombosis occur.

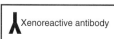

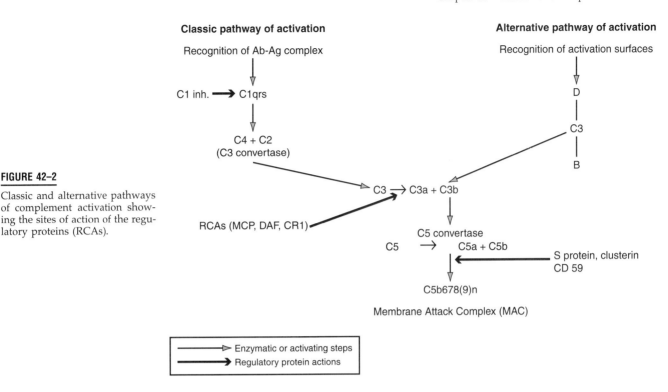

FIGURE 42–2

Classic and alternative pathways of complement activation showing the sites of action of the regulatory proteins (RCAs).

Classic pathway of activation

Recognition of Ab-Ag complex

C1 inh. → C1qrs

C4 + C2
(C3 convertase)

RCAs (MCP, DAF, CR1)

Alternative pathway of activation

Recognition of activation surfaces

D

C3

B

C3 → C3a + C3b

C5 convertase

C5 → C5a + C5b

S protein, clusterin
CD 59

C5b678(9)n

Membrane Attack Complex (MAC)

Enzymatic or activating steps
Regulatory protein actions

this is termed as *acute vascular rejection* (or *delayed xenograft rejection*). Macroscopically, rejected grafts show purple discoloration with vascular congestion and parenchymal hemorrhage. Histologically, there is a higher degree of intravascular thrombosis, fibrin plugging and less hemorrhage when compared with hyperacute rejection (Chong *et al.*, 1996; Matsumiya *et al.*, 1994). Several histological features, including immunoglobulin deposition, procoagulant changes and endothelial cell activation, are seen in hyperacute rejection and acute vascular rejection. Acute vascular rejection is defined in part by its time course.

Preformed XNAs are predominantly of the IgM isotype, which are responsible for the initiation of hyperacute rejection. Acute vascular rejection is largely a result of an elicited antibody response, however, of which various IgG isotypes are highly significant in terms of quantity and high affinity (Minanove *et al.*, 1997). A similar phenomenon is seen in concordant xenotransplantation, in which antidonor antibodies appear a few days after engraftment but at a lower level; the antigen specificity of this response is largely uncharacterized but appears to be T-cell independent. These antibodies are thought to represent amplification of a population of XNAs that are preformed but present usually at titers too low to cause hyperacute rejection (Auchinloss and Sachs, 1998).

A further important feature of acute vascular rejection is type 2 endothelial cell activation, which involves transcriptional induction of genes and subsequent protein synthesis, resulting in the expression of adhesion molecules (E-selectin, VCAM-1, ICAM-1), cytokines (interleukin [IL]-1, IL-6 and IL-8) and procoagulant molecules (platelet activating factor, tissue factor) (Bach *et al.*, 1997b). When compared with allograft rejection, in which T cells constitute greater than 90% of the infiltrating cells, the predominant infiltrating cell types in acute vascular rejection are monocytes (70–80%) and natural killer (NK) cells (approximately 20%) (Candinas *et al.*, 1996a, 1996b; Hancock, 1997b). Endothelial cell activation and the products of infiltrating cells together promote intragraft inflammation and thrombosis (Robson *et al.*, 1997).

CELLULAR REJECTION

Cellular xenograft rejection is probably a T cell–mediated phenomenon, as in allograft cellular rejection. Activation of a T-cell response can be initiated after direct or indirect presentation of antigen to the host (Yamada *et al.*, 1995). Cellular infiltration may be seen without acute vascular rejection and may be associated with evidence of graft damage, including tubulitis. The significance of isolated cellular infiltration and its temporal relationship to acute vascular rejection is poorly understood. Rodent experiments have shown that CD4+ cells are necessary for the rejection of nonvascularized islet cell and skin xenografts and that this occurs in animals depleted of CD8+ T cells, NK cells and B cells (Pierson *et al.*, 1989). The indirect pathway involves T-cell stimulation after hapten processing by recipient antigen-presenting cells (Moses *et al.*, 1990). In mice with no indirect pathway activation of T cells, there is a weaker cellular rejection response to xenografted cells (Korsgren, 1997; Restifo *et al.*, 1996). Greater understanding will come from characterization of different cells within such infiltrates (Simeonovic *et al.*, 1990); this is not an easy task because validation of the antibodies used to identify different cell types must be done for each species. Cellular xenograft rejection appears to respond to high-dose steroid treatment, as was shown in the concordant clinical transplants using chimpanzee kidneys (Hume, 1964; Reemtsma *et al.*, 1964).

Strategies to Circumvent the Immunological Barrier

REMOVAL OF XENOREACTIVE ANTIBODY

It is reasonable to assume that depletion of circulating XNAs would result in abrogation of the immediate antibody and complement-mediated immune attack. This depletion can be achieved specifically using immunoadsorbent columns, coated in α-Gal residues or with Galα(1,3)Gal+ Cos cells, through which the recipient's blood is perfused (McKenzie *et al.*, 1994; Neethling *et al.*, 1994a). Alternatively, nonspecific immunoglobulin removal can be achieved by plasmapheresis (Gannedahl *et al.*, 1996; Sablinski *et al.*, 1995). If this therapy is continued, hyperacute rejection can be delayed for many days, but as soon as therapy is discontinued, a rapid and exaggerated rise in antibody titers occurs, and acute vascular rejection ensues unless other therapy is instituted (Lin *et al.*, 1997, 1998). Circulating XNA blockade also has been undertaken using monovalent or polyvalent oligosaccharide haptens, although there would be some concern about the possibility of immune complexes causing a serum sickness–like syndrome (Good *et al.*, 1992; Neethling *et al.*, 1994b; Ye *et al.*, 1994). Depletion of anti-α-Gal antibodies may have an adverse effect on that poorly understood arm of the innate immune system, in which these antibodies may play a role.

SUPPRESSION OF ANTIBODY PRODUCTION

The abrogation of hyperacute rejection still leaves the graft vulnerable to continued assault by antibody. Splenectomy at the time of transplantation reduces the antibody response, and this is associated with prolongation of xenograft survival (Bhatti *et al.*, 1999). Immunosuppression with cyclophosphamide suppresses antibody production and allows prolonged survival (Zaidi *et al.*, 1998). Cyclophosphamide not only is cytotoxic to B cells, but also may reduce type 2 endothelial cell activation. Cyclophosphamide has been used as induction and maintenance therapy in pig-to-primate models of cardiac and renal xenotransplantation. The reduction of α-Gal antibody production by attempts to deplete the B-cell population specifically, without full bone marrow ablation, also has been tried (Aksentijevich *et al.*, 1991, 1992).

CONTROL OF COMPLEMENT ACTIVATION

The normal physiological control of complement activation involves membrane-bound proteins, RCA and fluid-phase inhibitors including factors I and H. The RCA are largely species restricted—more effective in their own species than others. Massive complement activation is a fundamental feature of hyperacute rejection, and it is believed that the absence of RCA on the xenograft compatible with the recipient species is an important factor in this reaction. Transgenic pig lines have been developed expressing human regulators of complement activity, including human decay accelerating factor (hDAF, CD55), homologous restriction factor (CD59) and membrane cofactor protein (MCP), and there is good evidence that this strategy has produced discordant organs largely protected from hyperacute rejection (Cozzi *et al.*, 1997; Kroshus *et al.*, 1996; Langford *et al.*, 1996; Sandrin *et al.*, 1995; White *et al.*, 1995). Human decay accelerating factor and MCP control the formation of the C3 convertase, whereas CD59 blocks the insertion of C9 in the formation of the MAC (see Fig. 42–2).

Complement inhibition using cobra venom factor or soluble complement inhibitors (sCR1, FUT-175 and K76COOH) has been shown to prevent hyperacute rejection in discordant models of xenotransplantation (Candinas *et al.*, 1996d; Knechtle *et al.*, 1985; Kobyashi *et al.*, 1996; Kroshus *et al.*, 1996; Pruitt and Bollinger, 1991; Pruitt *et al.*, 1997). Studies in C6-deficient rats receiving discordant cat kidney transplants confirmed prolonged survival despite high IgM XNA titers when compared with complement-sufficient rats (Zhow *et al.*, 1990). Although these organs did not suffer hyperacute rejection, at 2 days they were infiltrated heavily with leukocytes. It appears that when cellular damage by complement through the

MAC is prevented, accelerated acute vascular rejection occurs; this appears to be mediated by earlier terminal components (C3 and C5) and the inflammatory consequences that ensue.

IMMUNOSUPPRESSION

Agents currently in use in clinical transplantation have been tested successfully as maintenance therapy in the pig-to-primate model of renal xenotransplantation (Cozzi *et al.*, 2000; Zaidi *et al.*, 1998). Cyclosporine and rapamycin derivatives are effective in limiting acute vascular rejection, allowing survival of 71 days when used in combination with hDAF transgenic donor kidneys, corticosteroids and recipient splenectomy (Ostlie, D., 1999, personal communication). Similar prolonged survival in the same model has been seen when mycophenolic acid or its analogues are used with cyclosporine.

REDUCTION OF GAL ANTIGEN EXPRESSION

In theory, any strategy by which the expression of Gal antigen on donor cells is reduced should limit the immunological response. Treatment of the donor with (coffee bean or bacterial) α-galactosidase enzymatically reduces the expression of surface α-Gal. The treatment of porcine cartilage xenografts with α-galactosidase removes α-Gal epitopes. When transplanted into cynomolgus monkey recipients, there was no anti-Gal antibody response, although some antibodies were generated specifically against porcine cartilage (Stone *et al.*, 1998).

A more durable reduction in expression is produced by destruction of the gene encoding the Gal antigen (α-1,3-galactosyltransferase) (Tange *et al.*, 1996). Production of Gal antigen knock-out mice has been accomplished, but the analogous technology has not been successful in pigs (Tearle *et al.*, 1996). Homologous recombination has targeted the exon 9 region (the catalytic domain) and produces inactivation of α-1,3-galactosyltransferase. Important observations from this model are that the mutation itself is not lethal and that these $Gal^{-/-}$ mice lack Gal antigen expression on all their tissues and produce natural anti-Gal antibodies (McKenzie *et al.*, 1996; Sandrin *et al.*, 1993, 1995; Tearle *et al.*, 1996). The absence of the Gal antigen epitopes may expose other oligosaccharides against which human XNAs exist, however.

A further theoretical approach would be to overexpress another carbohydrate that would compete for expression with Gal antigen on the endothelial cell surface (Cooper *et al.*, 1993; d'Apice *et al.*, 1996; van Denderen *et al.*, 1997); this can be done by the insertion of a gene encoding another glycosyltransferase, such as α-1,2-fucosyltransferase. In the cell, α-1,2-fucosyltransferase appears to take precedence over α-1,3-galactosyltransferase (Sandrin *et al.*, 1995, 1997). The result is surface overexpression of H blood group antigen against which human antibody neither exists nor is elicited (Chen *et al.*, 1998; Sandrin and McKenzie, 1999). Rodent transgenic strains have been produced, and two groups have reported production of transgenic pigs expressing α-1,2-fucosyltransferase (Cohney *et al.*, 1997; Koike *et al.*, 1996; Sharma *et al.*, 1996).

GENETIC ENGINEERING OF THE ENDOTHELIAL CELL

Two molecular biological techniques may allow manipulation of the endothelial cell to protect a xenograft from the assault of the recipient immune system. Transgenic engineering or viral-mediated gene transfer may allow alteration of intracellular systems such as NF-κβ, which mediate the expression of surface adhesion molecules and cytokines (Bach *et al.*, 1997a; Moll *et al.*, 1995). The NF-κβ system, once activated by protein kinase C, which, in turn, follows T-cell receptor activation, binds to the IL-2 promoter region producing up-regulation of the endothelial cell (Bach *et al.*, 1997b; Goodman *et al.*, 1996; Grimm *et al.*, 1996; Stroka *et al.*, 1999; Von *et al.*, 1998). Genetic engineering may allow modulation of some of the procoagulant changes seen in acute vascular rejection or expression of human coagulation regulators, including tissue factor pathway inhibitor, which is nonfunctional across the porcine-human species barrier. Other groups are using platelet inhibitors to limit the effects of such changes (Candinas *et al.*, 1996c).

ACCOMMODATION

Accommodation is the term given to graft survival in the presence of a specific antibody response. This phenomenon first was observed in ABO mismatched renal allotransplantation (Platt, 1997). Although the expected outcome of transplantation of a donor organ into a recipient with preformed antidonor antibodies is vascular rejection, in some cases temporary removal of these antibodies (by plasmapheresis or splenectomy) can lead to long-term graft survival after the return of antidonor antibodies. Acute vascular rejection may not be an inevitable outcome of a discordant xenograft in the presence of persistent antibody (Tanemura *et al.*, 2000).

Prolonged survival has been achieved in hamster-to-rat heart xenotransplantation using cobra venom factor and cyclosporine (Bach *et al.*, 1997b). These organs survive despite continued high levels of antibody and complement activation. Accommodation is yet to be produced reliably in large animal models of discordant xenotransplantation, however.

There are biological similarities between blood group antigens and the α-Gal epitope (Fig. 42–3). Together with evidence from small animal models, these similarities lead to optimism that accommodation is a possibility in xenografting.

TOLERANCE

Tolerance is the state in which a foreign antigen is recognized as self by an otherwise normal functioning immune system (see Chapter 23). The phenomenon of neonatal tolerance was achieved by injecting donor bone marrow into neonatal mice and showing donor-specific survival of subsequent skin grafts (Billingham *et al.*, 1953). Tolerance is much more difficult to achieve later in the life of the recipient, although many strategies have been devised in an experimental setting with some success (Sayegh *et al.*, 1991; Waldmann and Cobbold, 1993; Wood, 1993).

A degree of tolerance develops in most allograft recipients (who require less immunosuppression with time), and a small proportion of patients become completely tolerant to their graft, requiring no immunosuppression. A report of a group of nontwin living related kidney recipients from Colorado at 30 years posttransplantation showed that 5 of the 10 patients with surviving grafts are off all immunosuppression (Starzl *et al.*, 1994).

If tolerance could be induced successfully into xenografting, the problems and risks of immunosuppression would be reduced greatly. Because of the problems of preformed antibodies, hematopoietic tolerance is unlikely alone to be sufficient to prevent hyperacute rejection; experimental efforts have been directed toward producing tolerance to organs transgenic for complement regulators (Miyazawa *et al.*, 1995). Many methods that have been used to induce tolerance in allotransplantation are being tested in experimental xenograft models. The use of adoptive tolerance by rendering transgenic pigs chimeric with human bone marrow and pretreating cytoablated xenograft recipients with chimeric bone marrow transplantation is another proposed strategy (Ko *et al.*, 1998; Sablinski *et al.*, 1995, 1999; Sachs and Sablinski, 1995; Sachs *et al.*, 1995). Many studies have shown that once transplantation tolerance to donor bone marrow is achieved, this can be extended to any other tissue or organ from the same donor (Auchinloss and Sachs, 1998; Ildstad and Sachs, 1984; Ildstad *et al.*, 1984; Sachs and Bach, 1990; Sayegh *et al.*, 1994).

Experimental Results
CONCORDANT COMBINATIONS

Much work has been done in the field of experimental concordant transplantation by researchers in Johannesburg, South Africa (Myburgh *et al.*, 1994; Smit *et al.*, 1994). The survival of a concordant baboon–to–rhesus monkey kidney xenotransplantation is comparable to that of baboon allotransplantation when total lymphoid irradiation is used. The use of rabbit antihuman thymocyte immunoglobulin did not produce any additional benefit. These researchers showed in the same model that the use of chemical immunosuppression (cyclosporine) at the time of transplantation can have a deleterious effect on the maintenance of tolerance. Histologically, all four long surviving grafts showed cellular rejection without features of humoral injury. When intrathymic injection of donor spleen cells was given with total lymphoid irradiation, abrogation of the effect of irradiation occurred, and the recipients became sensitized. The histology of these grafts (survival 4–29 days) showed acute cellular rejection with hemorrhagic vascular changes.

Other researchers have reported partial tolerance with similar survival in concordant xenotransplantation combinations (Zhong *et al.*, 1996). Mixed chimerism has been reported in baboon–to–cynomolgus monkey concordant renal transplantation (Ko *et al.*, 1998). This report followed prior studies from the same laboratory, using nonmyeloablative conditioning, which showed transient mixed chimerism and renal allograft tolerance between major histocompatibility complex–disparate cynomolgus monkeys. Five of the six recipi-

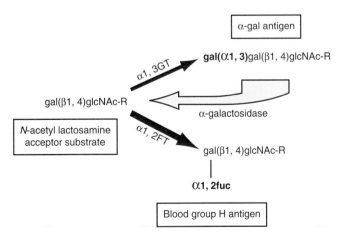

FIGURE 42–3

The different enzymatic pathways that allow conversion of the *N*-acetyl lactosamine acceptor substrate into the α-gal moiety or the H blood group antigen. The overexpression of α-1,2-fucosyltransferase is a potential strategy for reducing α-gal expression on porcine endothelial cells.

ents developed detectable chimerism, and only one of these animals lost its kidney to rejection, although nonrejection complications did not permit the assessment of long-term outcome.

DISCORDANT COMBINATIONS

In models of pig-to–nonhuman primate xenotransplantation, the use of porcine organs transgenic for human RCA leads to the reliable abrogation of hyperacute rejection. Survival for 78 days has been achieved in a life-supporting hDAF transgenic pig-to-primate model of renal xenotransplantation using cyclophosphamide induction with cyclophosphamide, cyclosporine and corticosteroid maintenance therapy (Cozzi et al., 2000). Recipients in this study required exogenous erythropoietin administration because of progressive anemia presumably related to incompatibility of porcine erythropoietin. Splenectomy in this model enhanced survival (Bhatti et al., 1999; Fig. 42–4).

The use of RAD, a macrolide that interferes with translational expression of IL-2 and cyclosporine, has produced a median survival of 33 days (D. Ostlie, 1999, presented data, American Society of Transplant Surgeons, Chicago). These renal xenografts sustained the animals in a healthy state, and with the exception of hypophosphatemia, serum electrolytes remained within the normal range for cynomolgus monkeys (Table 42–1).

PHYSIOLOGICAL BARRIERS TO XENOTRANSPLANTATION

The clinical evidence of normal serum urea and creatinine levels, from the trials of chimpanzee-to-human or baboon-to-human renal xenotransplantation in the 1960s, suggests that glomerular and tubular functions in these concordant grafts were compatible (Reemtsma et al., 1964; Starzl et al., 1993). The field of comparative physiology is underresearched compared with that of xenotransplant immunology. As a general rule, the greater the phylogenetic distance between species, the less predictable is the conservation of structure and function of any particular component (Hammer, 1989, 1998). The function of discordant xenografts relies mainly on data derived from experimental models of transgenic pig-to–

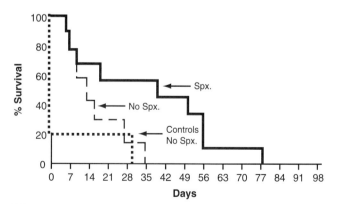

FIGURE 42–4

Comparison of renal human decay accelerating factor (hDAF) pig-to-primate xenograft survival (in days), treated with cyclosporine and Neoral maintenance therapy, with (solid line) and without (dashed line) splenectomy at the time of operation against that of nontransgenic pig-to-primate renal xenografts without splenectomy (dotted line).

TABLE 42–1

MEDIAN SURVIVAL OF CYNOMOLGUS MONKEY RECIPIENTS OF TRANSGENIC PORCINE RENAL XENOGRAFT. ALL ANIMALS WERE TREATED WITH INDUCTION CYCLOSPHOSPHAMIDE, AND MAINTENANCE CYCLOSPORINE AND STEROIDS

Group Characteristics Additional Therapy	No. of Animals	Splenectomy	Median Survival (days)
Nil	7	No	13
RAD	6	No	24.5
RAD	7	Yes	33
CYP maintenance therapy	9	Yes	39
Perioperative recombinant sCR1 and RAD	6	No	35.5

All data provided from Imutran Ltd., Cambridge, UK.

nonhuman primates, which were designed for immunological studies (Cozzi et al., 2000; Zaidi et al., 1998).

ANATOMICAL AND GROWTH CONSIDERATIONS

The vascular anatomy of the porcine kidney is variable in a similar way to humans and should not represent a limitation in clinical xenotransplantation. The growth of a pig kidney in its native environment reaches a plateau in Landrace/Large White pigs of 150 to 200 g with dimensions comparable to those of an adult human kidney. The growth pattern in porcine kidneys transplanted while immature is largely unknown.

PHYSIOLOGICAL COMPATIBILITY

The basic cellular mechanisms are universal within mammals and are unlikely to be altered by xenotransplantation (Kirkman, 1989). Some specific aspects of renal physiology have been studied in the pig-to-primate renal xenotransplantation model over an 11-week period (A. Zaidi, 1998, personal communication).

Glomerular and Tubular Function

Normal sodium, potassium, osmolarity and fluid balance were maintained, and the serum creatinine remained normal. The recipients were normally active and did not show signs of orthostatic hypotension, suggesting normal volemic control by the renin-angiotensin system. Serum uric acid was normal in recipients; this was an expected finding because in vitro studies suggest porcine proximal tubules are net excretors of urate, similar to humans (Werner et al., 1990).

Endogenous Hormone Secretion

Erythropoietin from the pig and cynomolgus monkey has 82% and 91% amino acid homology with human erythropoietin. A consistent finding in medium and long-term survivors of pig-to-primate renal xenografts (but not cardiac xenografts) was a progressive anemia, which responded to exogenous administration of recombinant human erythropoietin. Detectable levels of erythropoietin in the serum of these animals were low, but it was unclear whether this was erythropoietin from the porcine renal xenograft or from extrarenal sources in the recipient primate. It appears that there is a degree of species specificity of this hormone, which may necessitate replacement or possibly further genetic modification. The insertion of a hormone transgene may cause problems if this led to a loss of regulation. For example, after insertion of the porcine or bovine growth hormone gene into the mouse genome, giant mice were produced (Wanke et al., 1990), although in another experiment, pigs made transgenic for human growth hormone showed normal growth (Pursel et al., 1987).

Exogenous Hormone Action

Hormone receptors in the porcine kidney may exhibit some degree of species specificity. In pig-to-primate renal xenografts functioning for more than 2 months (with recipient bilateral native nephrectomies), some observations on calcium metabolism have been made. Vitamin D requires a second hydroxylation in the kidney before acting primarily on the small bowel to increase calcium absorption. This hydroxylation appears to occur successfully in porcine xenografts (A. Zaidi 1999, personal communication). Parathormone activates osteoclasts to mobilize calcium from bones and increases urinary phosphate excretion. As is observed sometimes in allotransplantation, a limited early hypophosphatemia occurs with a later and unexplained rise in serum calcium. Research in this area continues.

Vasopressin differs by one amino acid between human and pig. Studies in an anesthetized pig model confirm that human vasopressin is effective in concentrating urine but with a lower efficacy than porcine vasopressin (Munswick et al., 1958).

Risk of Interspecies Transfer of Infection

Concern that cross-species transplantation might expose the population to an unacceptable risk from infectious agents must be allayed before clinical xenotransplantation can be allowed (Chapman et al., 1995). Some pathogens transferred from the donor that cause disease in allograft recipients, such as cytomegalovirus and some hepatitis viruses, are species restricted (Michaels, 1997; Michaels and Simmons, 1994). Many pathogens that are known to cross the species barrier can be screened for readily and donors selected on this basis (Fishman, 1994). Some primate diseases such as simian herpes B and the retroviral infection simian immunodeficiency virus are known human zoonoses causing lethal disease.

Humans have coexisted in close proximity to domesticated animals for centuries; this might suggest that major zoonotic infection should be less likely from pigs than nonhuman primates. There is concern, however, over the theoretical risk associated with porcine endogenous retroviruses (PERV), which are incorporated in the porcine genome and cannot be eradicated readily from the donor animal line. Porcine endogenous retroviruses have been shown to infect human cell lines when placed in coculture (Patience et al., 1997); whether this can lead to disease or the shedding of infective particles has not been proved.

Many patients worldwide have been exposed to porcine tissue (e.g., skin grafts, pancreatic islet cells and liver and splenic extracorporeal perfusions). The longer term follow-up and close investigation of these patients would help to establish whether any significant risk exists to the individual or the population. Two clinical studies have investigated the infectious capability of these viruses. In a study of 10 diabetic patients transplanted with porcine islets, polymerase chain reaction analysis was used to detect PERV-related sequences in the patients' blood cells (Heneine et al., 1998). Polymerase chain reaction analysis showed no evidence of patient infection. In a study of two patients undergoing extracorporeal

porcine kidney perfusion, there was no evidence of retroviral infection detected at 36 months of follow-up (Patience et al., 1998). The largest study published to date, which incorporates the patients in the two previous studies, has followed 160 patients who were exposed directly to pig tissues as a result of skin grafting; pancreatic islet cell transplantation or extracorporeal perfusion of a porcine liver, kidney or spleen. This study showed at 12 years of follow-up no evidence of PERV infection, but it did show evidence of microchimerism in 23 patients (Paradis et al., 1999). The consensus of most researchers in the field is that porcine donor discordant xenotransplantation is unlikely to lead to the generation of new human pathogens. This remains an important issue, however.

Ethical, Cultural and Religious Issues

Transplantation between discordant species evokes a substantially greater immunological response than between concordant species. This fact could be used to support an argument for the use of nonhuman primates as donors for clinical xenotransplantation. In addition to the significant logistic problems, including difficulties in breeding and size incompatibility, there are serious ethical and cultural concerns if nonhuman primates were to become a major source of organs for transplantation.

Much research investment has been directed to the pig as the most likely donor species (Cozzi and White, 1995). Most cultures accept the breeding of pigs for domestic use, and their use as potential organ donors is more acceptable. Pigs breed quickly in captivity and produce large litters, which would enable supply to meet the demand if this became a realistic clinical therapy. A wealth of experience exists in commercial pig breeding, which would be valuable in the production of specific pathogen–free animals. For these reasons, the pig is regarded as the most likely xenograft donor species. Many religions (including Judaism and Islam) have issued statements accepting the use of porcine tissue for medical purposes, including xenotransplantation (Daar, 1998; First, 1997; Rosner, 1999).

Although an important objective in medical research is to achieve the greatest benefit for the maximum number of patients, this objective may be at odds with the individual responsibility of a physician to a patient. Historically the pioneer patients in a new area of treatment have not benefited directly. This ethical dilemma might be resolved by offering the new treatment to a group of patients for whom no current therapy is effective. In the case of xenotransplantation, this approach would require identification of a patient subgroup who would be unlikely to receive an allograft but who might benefit from a transplant (e.g., the highly sensitized patient).

Conclusion

Hyperacute rejection, the first major immunological hurdle to discordant transplantation, has been largely overcome in an experimental setting. The current challenge is to achieve adequate control of acute vascular rejection. Three criteria (immunological, physiological and microbiological) must be fulfilled before embarking on a clinical phase of research in renal xenotransplantation:

1. Reproducible and sustained function of a graft for a substantial time using a clinically acceptable immunosuppressive regimen
2. Evidence of adequate graft function and maintenance of physiological homeostasis

3. Evidence of adequate safety, particularly in relation to zoonotic disease transmission

The somewhat lesser immunological challenges posed by cellular rather than vascularized whole-organ xenografts may result in this being the initial direction of clinical trials. Although important developments have been made and limited clinical trials might take place in the foreseeable future, the widespread introduction of clinical renal xenotransplantation is not imminent. This event might require further genetic modification, a strategy to induce tolerance or the development of new immunosuppressive agents.

REFERENCES

Aksentijevich, I., Sachs, D. H. and Sykes, M. (1991). Natural antibodies can inhibit bone marrow engraftment in the rat-mouse species combination. *J. Immunol.* **147**, 4140.

Aksentijevich, I., Sachs, D. H. and Sykes, M. (1992). Humoral tolerance in xenogeneic BMT recipients conditioned by a nonmyeloablative regimen. *Transplantation* **53**, 1108.

Auchinloss, H. J. and Sachs, D. H. (1998). Xenogeneic transplantation. *Annu. Rev. Immunol.* **16**, 433.

Bach, F. H. (1997a). Genetic engineering as an approach to xenotransplantation. *World J. Surg.* **21**, 913.

Bach, F. H. (1997b). Some problems related to discordant xenografting. *Transplant. Proc.* **39**, 3009.

Bach, F. H., Ferran, C., Hechenleitner, P., *et al.* (1997a). Accommodation of vascularised xenografts: expression of "protective genes" by donor endothelial cells in a host Th2 cytokine environment. *Nat. Med.* **3**, 196.

Bach, F. H., Ferran, C., Soares, M., *et al.* (1997b). Modification of vascular responses in xenotransplantation: inflammation and apoptosis. *Nat. Med.* **3**, 944.

Bhatti, F. N., Schmoeckel, M., Zaidi, A., *et al.* (1999). Three-month survival of HDAF transgenic pig hearts transplanted into primates. *Transplant. Proc.* **31**, 958.

Billingham, R. E., Brent, L. and Medawar, P. (1953). Actively acquired tolerance of foreign cells. *Nature* **172**, 603.

Blakely, M. L., Vanderwerf, W. J., Berndt, M. C., *et al.* (1994). Activation of intragraft endothelial and mononuclear cells during discordant xenograft rejection. *Transplantation* **58**, 1059.

Calne, R. (1970). Organ transplantation between widely disparate species. *Transplant. Proc.* **11**, 550.

Candinas, D., Bach, F. H. and Hancock, W. W. (1996a). Delayed xenograft rejection in complement depleted T-cell-deficient rat recipients of guinea pig cardiac grafts. *Transplant. Proc.* **28**, 678.

Candinas, D., Koyamada, N., Miyatake, T., *et al.* (1996b). T-cell independence of macrophage and NK cell infiltration, cytokine production and endothelial activation during delayed xenograft rejection. *Transplantation* **62**, 1920.

Candinas, D., Lesnikoski, B. A., Hancock, W. W., *et al.* (1996c). Inhibition of platelet integrin GpIIbIIIa prolongs survival of discordant cardiac xenografts. *Transplantation* **62**, 1.

Candinas, D., Lesnikoski, B. A., Robson, S. C., *et al.* (1996d). Effect of repetitive high-dose treatment with soluble complement receptor type 1 and cobra venom factor on discordant xenograft survival. *Transplantation* **62**, 336.

Chapman, L. E., Folks, T. M., Salomon, D. R., *et al.* (1995). Xenotransplantation and xenogeneic infections. *N. Engl. J. Med.* **333**, 1498.

Chen, C. G., Salvaris, E. J., Romanella, M., *et al.* (1998). Transgenic expression of human alpha 1,2-fucosyltransferase (H-transferase) prolongs mouse heart survival in an ex vivo model of xenograft rejection. *Transplantation* **65**, 832.

Chong, A. S., Shen, J., Xiao, F., *et al.* (1996). Delayed xenograft rejection in the concordant hamster heart into Lewis rat model. *Transplantation* **62**, 90.

Cohney, S., McKenzie, I. F., Patton, K., *et al.* (1997). Down-regulation of Gal alpha (1,3) Gal expression by alpha 1,2-fucosyltransferase: further characterization of alpha 1,2-fucosyltransferase transgenic mice. *Transplantation* **64**, 495.

Cooper, D. K., Koren, E. and Oriol, R. (1993). Genetically engineered pigs. *Lancet* **342**, 682.

Cooper, D. K., Koren, E. and Oriol, R. (1994). Oligosaccharides and discordant transplantation. *Transplantation* **141**, 31.

Cooper, D. K. and Thall, A. D. (1997). Xenoantigens and xenoantibodies: their modification. *World J. Surg.* **21**, 901.

Cozzi, E., Bhatti, F., Schmoeckel, M., *et al.* (2000). Long-term survival of non-human primates receiving life-supporting transgenic porcine kidney xenografts. *Transplantation* **70**, 15.

Cozzi, E. and White, D. J. (1995). The generation of transgenic pigs as potential organ donors for humans. *Nat. Med.* **1**, 964.

Cozzi, E., Yannoutsos, N., Langford, G., *et al.* (1997). Effect of transgenic expression of human decay-accelerating factor on the inhibition of hyperacute rejection of pig organs. In *Xenotransplantation: The Transplantation of Organs and Tissues Between Species*, (D. K. Cooper, E. Kemp, J. Platt and D. White, eds.), p. 665, Springer Verlag, New York.

Daar, A. S. (1998). An overview of transplantation issues in the Middle East. *Transplant. Proc.* **7**, 3638.

d'Apice, A. J., Tange, M. J. and Chen, G. C. (1996). Two genetic approaches to the galactose alpha 1,3 galactose xenoantigen. *Transplant. Proc.* **2**, 540.

Dubernard, J. M., Bonneau, M. and LaTour, M. (1974). *Heterografts in Primates*, Fondation Merieux, Villeurbanne.

Evans, R., Orians, C. and Ascher, N. (1992). The potential supply of organ donors: an assessment of the efficacy of organ procurement efforts in the United States. *J. A. M. A.* **267**, 239.

First, M. R. (1997). Xenotransplantation: social, ethical, religious and political issues. *Kidney Int.* **58(Suppl)**, 46.

Fishman, J. A. (1994). Miniature swine as organ donors for men: strategies for prevention of xenotransplant associated infections. *Xenotransplantation* **1**, 47.

Fryer, J., Leventhal, J., Dalmasso, J. and Mates, A. (1995). Beyond hyperacute rejection—accelerated rejection in a discordant xenograft model by adoptive transfer of specific cell subsets. *Transplantation* **59**, 171.

Galili, U. (1993). Evolution and pathophysiology of the human natural anti-alpha Gal antibody. In *Seminars in Immunopathology*, p. 155, Springer, Berlin.

Galili, U. (1994). Significance of natural human anti-Gal antibody in xenotransplantation. *Xenotransplantation* **2**, 84.

Galili, U., Shohet, S. B., Kobrin, E., Stults, C. L. and Macher, B. A. (1988). Man, apes and old world monkeys differ from other mammals in the expression of α-galactosyl epitopes on nucleated cells. *J. Biol. Chem.* **263**, 17755.

Gannedahl, G., Tufveson, G., Sundberg, B. and Groth, C. G. (1996). The effect of plasmapheresis and deoxyspergualin or cytophosphamide treatment on anti-porcine Gal antibody levels in humans. *Xenotransplantation* **3**, 166.

Giles, G. R., Boehmig, H. J., Lilly, J., *et al.* (1970). Mechanism and modification of rejection of heterografts between divergent species. *Transplant. Proc.* **2**, 522.

Good, A. H., Cooper, D. K., Malcolm, A. J., *et al.* (1992). Identification of carbohydrate structures that bind human antibodies antiporcine antibodies: Implications for discordant xenografting in humans. *Transplant. Proc.* **24**, 559.

Goodman, D. J., Von, A. M., McShea, A., Wrighton, C. J. and Bach, F. H. (1996). Adenoviral-mediated overexpression of I(kappa) B(alpha) in endothelial cells inhibits natural killer cell-mediated endothelial cell activation. *Transplantation* **62**, 967.

Grimm, S., Bauer, M. K., Baeuerle, P. A. and Schulze-Osthoff, K. (1996). Bcl-2 down-regulates the activity of transcription factor NF-kappaB induced upon apoptosis. *J. Cell. Biol.* **134**, 13.

Hammer, C. (1989). Evolutionary considerations in xenotransplantation. *Xenograft* **25**, 115.

Hammer, C. (1998). Physiological obstacles after xenotransplantation. *Ann. N. Y. Acad. Sci.* **862**, 19.

Hancock, W. W. (1997a). Beyond hyperacute rejection: strategies for development of pig → primate xenotransplantation. *Kidney Int.* **58(Suppl)**, 36.

Hancock, W. W. (1997b). Delayed xenograft rejection. *World J. Surg.* **21**, 917.

Hancock, W. W. (1997c). The past, present and future of renal xenotransplantation. *Kidney Int.* **51**, 932.

Heneine, W., Tibell, A., Switzer, W. M., *et al.* (1998). No evidence of infection with porcine endogenous retrovirus in recipients of porcine islet-cell xenografts [published erratum appears in *Lancet* 1998 Oct 31, 352(9138):1478]. *Lancet* **352**, 695.

Hosenpud, J. D., Bennett, L. E., Keck, B. M., *et al.* (1998). The Registry of the International Society for Heart and Lung Transplantation: fifteenth official report—1998. *J. Heart Lung Transplant.* **17,** 656.

Hume, D. M. (1964). Discussion of Reetsma paper. *Ann. Surg.* **160,** 384.

Ildstad, S. T. and Sachs, D. H. (1984). Reconstitution with syngenic plus allogenic or xenogeneic bone marrow leads to specific acceptance of allografts or xenografts. *Nature* **307,** 168.

Ildstad, S. T., Wren, S. M., Sharrow, S. O., Stephany, D. and Sachs, D. H. (1984). In vivo and in vitro characterisation of specific hyporeactivity to skin xenografts in mixed xenogeneically reconstituted mice (B10 + F344 rat − B10). *J. Exp. Med* **160,** 1820.

Jabouley, M. (1906). De riens au pli du coudes par soutures arterielles et veineuses. *Lyons Med.* **107,** 575.

Kaufman, H. M. and Bennet, L. E. (1999). The expanded donor. *Transplant. Rev.* **11,** 165.

Kirkman, R. L. (1989). Of swine and man: organ physiology in different species. *Xenograft* **25,** 125.

Knechtle, S. J., Haloperin, E. C. and Murphy, C. E. (1985). The effect of cyclosporine, total lymphoid irradiation and cobra venom factor on hyperacute rejection. *Transplantation* **4,** 541.

Ko, D. S., Bartholomew, A., Poncelet, A. J., *et al.* (1998). Demonstration of multilineage chimerism in a non-human primate concordant xenograft model. *Xenotransplantation* **5,** 298.

Kobyashi, T., Neethling, F. A., Koren, E., Hancock, W. W. and Cooper, D. K. (1996). In vitro and in vivo investigation of the anti-complement agents FUT-175 and K76COOH in the prevention of hyperacute rejection following discordant xenotransplantation in a non-human primate model. *Transplant. Proc.* **28,** 604.

Koike, C., Kannagi, R., Takuma, Y., *et al.* (1996). Induction of alpha (1,2) fucosyltransferase and its effect on epitopes in transgenic pigs. *Xenotransplantation* **3,** 81.

Koren, E., Milotic, F., Neethling, F. A., *et al.* (1996). Monoclonal antiidiotypic antibodies neutralise cytotoxic effects of anti-alphaGal antibodies. *Transplantation* **62,** 837.

Korsgren, O. (1997). Acute cellular rejection. *Xenotransplantation* **4,** 11.

Kroshus, T. J., Bolman, R. M., Dalmasso, A. P., *et al.* (1996). Expression of human CD59 in transgenic pig organs enhances organ survival in an ex vivo xenogeneic perfusion model. *Transplantation* **61,** 1513.

Langford, G. A., Cozzi, E., Yannoutsos, N., *et al.* (1996). Production of pigs transgenic for human regulators of complement activation using YAC technology. *Transplant. Proc.* **28,** 862.

Lin, S. S., Kooyman, D. L., Daniels, L. J., *et al.* (1997). The role of natural anti-Gal alpha 1-3Gal antibodies in hyperacute rejection of pig-to-baboon cardiac xenotransplants. *Transpl. Immunol.* **5,** 212.

Lin, S. S. and Platt, J. L. (1998). Genetic therapies for xenotransplantation. *J. Am. Coll. Surg.* **186,** 388.

Lin, S. S., Weidner, B. C., Byrne, G. W., *et al.* (1998). The role of antibodies in acute vascular rejection of pig-to-baboon cardiac transplants. *J. Clin. Invest.* **101,** 1745.

Matsumiya, G., Shirakura, R., Miyagawa, S., *et al.* (1994). Analysis of rejection mechanism in the rat to mouse cardiac xenotransplantation: role and characteristics of anti-endothelial cell antibodies. *Transplantation* **57,** 1653.

McKenzie, I. F. C., Osman, N., Cohney, S., *et al.* (1996). Strategies to overcome the anti-Gal alpha (1–3)Gal reaction in xenotransplantation. *Transplant. Proc.* **28,** 537.

McKenzie, I. F. C., Stocker, J., Ting, A. and Morris, P. J. (1968). Human lympho-cytotoxic and haemagglutinating activity against sheep and pig cells. *Lancet* **2,** 386.

McKenzie, I. F. C., Vaughan, H. A. and Sandrin, M. (1994). How important are Gal-alpha(1,3)-Gal antibodies in pig to human xenotransplants? *Xenotransplantation* **2,** 107.

Medawar, P. (1969). Heterotransplantation. *Transplant. Proc.* **1,** 251.

Michaels, M. G. (1997). Infectious concerns of cross-species transplantation: xenozoonoses. *World J. Surg.* **21,** 968.

Michaels, M. G. and Simmons, R. L. (1994). Xenotransplant-associated zoonoses: strategies for prevention. *Transplantation* **57,** 1.

Migagawa, S., Hirose, H. and Shirakura, R. (1988). The mechanism of discordant xenograft rejection. *Transplantation* **46,** 825.

Minanove, O. P., Itescu, S., Neethling, F. A., *et al.* (1997). Anti-Gal IgC antibodies in sera of newborn humans and baboons and its significance in pig xenotransplantation. *Transplantation* **63,** 182.

Miyazawa, H., Murase, N., Demetris, A. J., *et al.* (1995). Hamster to rat kidney xenotransplantation: effects of FK 506, cyclophospha-

mide, organ perfusion and complement inhibition. *Transplantation* **59,** 1183.

Moll, T., Czyz, M., Holzmuller, H., *et al.* (1995). Regulation of the tissue factor promoter in endothelial cells: binding of NF kappa, B-, AP-1-, and Sp1-like transcription factors. *J. Biol. Chem* **270,** 3849.

Morris, P. J. (1999). Xenotransplantation. *Br. Med. Bull.* **55,** 446.

Moses, R. D., Pierson, R. N., Winn, H. J. and Auchinloss, H. J. (1990). Xenogeneic proliferation and lymphokine production are dependent on CD4$^+$ helper T cells and self antigen-presenting cells in the mouse. *J. Exp. Med.* **172,** 567.

Munswick, R., Sawyer, W. and van Dyke, H. (1958). The antidiuretic potency of arginine and lysine vasopressins in the pig with observations on porcine renal function. *Endocrinology* **63,** 688.

Myburgh, J. A., Smit, J. A. and Stark, J. H. (1994). Transplantation tolerance following total lymphoid irradiation in baboon-to-vervet monkey kidney xenotransplantation. *Transplant. Proc.* **26,** 1080.

Neethling, F. A., Koren, E., Oriol, R., Richards, S. V., Ye, Y. and Kujundzic, M. (1994a). Immunoadsorption of natural antibodies from human serum by affinity chromotography using specific carbohydrates protects pig cells from cytotoxic destruction. *Transplant. Proc.* **26,** 1378.

Neethling, F. A., Koren, E., Ye, Y., Richards, S. V., Kujundzic, M. E. and Oriol, R. (1994b). Protection of pig kidney (PK15) cells from the cytotoxic effect of anti-pig antibodies by alpha-galactosyl oligosaccharides. *Transplantation* **57,** 959.

Neuhof, H. (1923). *The Transplantation of Tissues,* Appleton, New York.

Paradis, K., Langford, G., Zhifeng, L., *et al.* (1999). Search for cross-species transmission of porcine endogenous retrovirus in patients treated with living pig tissue. *Science* **285,** 1236.

Patience, C., Patton, G., Takeuchi, Y., *et al.* (1998). No evidence of pig DNA or retroviral infection in patients with short term extracorporeal connection to pig. *Lancet* **352,** 699.

Patience, C., Takeuchi, Y. and Weiss, R. A. (1997). Infection of human cells by an endogenous retrovirus of pigs. *Nat. Med.* **3,** 282.

Pearse, M. J., Witort, E., Mottram, P., *et al.* (1998). Anti-Gal antibody-mediated allograft rejection in alpha1,3-galactosyltransferase gene knockout mice: a model of delayed xenograft rejection. *Transplantation* **66,** 748.

Pierson, R. N., Winn, H. J., Russell, P. S. and Auchinloss, H. J. (1989). Xenogeneic skin graft rejection is especially dependent on CD4$^+$ T cells. *J. Exp. Med.* **170,** 991.

Platt, J. L. (1997). The prospects for xenotransplantation of the kidney. *Curr. Opin. Nephrol. Hypertens.* **6,** 284.

Platt, J. L., Fischel, R. J., Matas, A. J., *et al.* (1991a). Immunopathology of hyperacute xenograft rejection in a swine-to-primate model. *Transplantation* **52,** 214.

Platt, J. L., Lindmand, B. J., Geller, R. L., *et al.* (1991b). The role of natural antibodies in the activation of xenogenic endothelial cells. *Transplantation* **52,** 1037.

Princeteau, M. (1905). Freffe Renale. *J. Med. Bordeaux* **26,** 549.

Pruitt, S. K. and Bollinger, R. R. (1991). The effect of soluble complement receptor type 1 on hyperacute allograft rejection. *J. Surg. Res.* **50,** 350.

Pruitt, S. K., Bollinger, R. R., Collins, B. H., *et al.* (1997). Effect of continuous complement inhibition using soluble complement receptor type 1 on survival of pig-to-primate cardiac xenografts. *Transplantation* **63,** 900.

Pursel, V. G., Rexroad, C. E. and Bolt, D. J. (1987). Progress on gene transfer in farm animals. *Vet. Immunol. Immunopathol.* **17,** 303.

Rajasinghe, H. A., Reddy, V. M., Hancock, W. W., Sayegh, M. H. and Hanley, F. L. (1996). Key role of the alternate complement pathway in hyperacute rejection of rat hearts transplanted into fetal sheep. *Transplantation* **62,** 407.

Reemtsma, K., McCracken, B., Schlegel, J., Pearl, M. and Pearce, C. (1964). Renal heterotransplantation in man. *Ann. Surg.* **160,** 384.

Restifo, A. C., Ivis-Woodward, M. A. and Tran, H. M. (1996). The potential role xenogeneic antigen presenting cells in T-cell co-stimulation. *Xenotransplantation* **3,** 141.

Robson, S. C., Kaczmarek, E., Siegel, J. B., *et al.* (1997). Loss of ATP diphosphohydrolase activity with endothelial cell activation. *J. Exp. Med.* **185,** 153.

Rosner, F. (1999). Pig organs for transplantation into humans: a Jewish view. *Mt. Sinai J. Med.* **66,** 314.

Sablinski, T., Emery, D. W., Monroy, R., *et al.* (1999). Long-term discordant xenogeneic (porcine-to-primate) bone marrow engraftment in a monkey treated with porcine-specific growth factors. *Transplantation* **67**, 972.

Sablinski, T., Latinne, D., Gianello, P., *et al.* (1995). Xenotransplantation of pig kidneys to nonhuman primates: development of the model. *Xenotransplantation* **2**, 264.

Sachs, D. H. and Bach, F. H. (1990). Immunology of xenograft rejection. *Hum. Immunol.* **28**, 245.

Sachs, D. H. and Sablinski, T. (1995). Tolerance against discordant xenogeneic barriers. *Xenotransplantation* **2**, 234.

Sachs, D. H., Sykes, M., Greenstein, J. and Cosimi, A. B. (1995). Tolerance and xenograft survival. *Nat. Med.* **1**, 969.

Sandrin, M., Fodor, W., Mouhtouris, E. and Cohney, S. (1995). Enzymatic remodelling of the carbohydrate surface of a xenogeneic cell substantially reduces antibody binding and complement mediated cytolysis. *Nat. Med.* **61**, 13.

Sandrin, M., Vaughan, H. A., Dabkowski, P. L. and McKenzie, I. F. (1993). Anti-pig IgM in human serum reacts predominantly with Gal-alpha(1,3)Gal epitopes. *Proc. Natl. Acad. Sci. U. S. A.* **90**, 11391.

Sandrin, M., Vaughan, H. A. and McKenzie, I. F. C. (1994). Identification of Gal(α1,3)Gal as the major epitome of pig to human vascularised xenografts. *Transplant. Rev.* **8**, 134.

Sandrin, M. S. and McKenzie, I. F. (1999). Modulation of alpha gal epitope expression on porcine cells. *Subcell. Biochem.* **32**, 311.

Sandrin, M. S., Osman, N. and McKenzie, I. F. (1997). Transgenic approaches for the reduction of Galalpha(1,3)Gal for xenotransplantation. *Front. Biosci.* **2e**, 11.

Sayegh, M. H., Fine, N. A., Smith, J. L., *et al.* (1991). Immunologic tolerance to renal allografts after bone marrow transplants from the same donors. *Ann. Intern. Med.* **114**, 954.

Sayegh, M. H., Perico, N. and Gallon, L. (1994). Mechanisms of acquired thymic unresponsiveness to renal allografts: thymic recognition of immunodominant allo-MHC peptides induces peripheral T cell anergy. *Transplantation* **58**, 125.

Sharma, A., Okabe, J., Birch, P., *et al.* (1996). Reduction in the level of Gal(alpha1,3)Gal in transgenic mice and pigs by the expression of an alpha(1,2)fucosyltransferase. *Proc. Natl. Acad. Sci. U. S. A.* **93**, 7190.

Simeonovic, C. J., Ceredig, R. and Wilson, J. D. (1990). Effect of GK1.5 monocloncl antibody on survival of pig proislet xenografts in CD4+ depleted mice. *Transplantation* **49**, 849.

Smit, J. A., Stark, J. H. and Myburgh, J. A. (1994). Immunologic responses to two monkeys tolerating baboon renal xenografts after total lymphoid irradiation. *Transplant. Proc.* **26**, 1063.

Starzl, T., Valdivia, L. and Murase, N. (1994). The biological basis of and strategies for clinical transplantation. *Immunol. Rev.* **141**, 213.

Starzl, T. E., Fung, J., Tzakis, A., *et al.* (1993). Baboon-to-human liver transplantation. *Lancet* **341**, 65.

Stevens, R. B., Wang, Y. L., Kaji, H., *et al.* (1993). Administration of nonanticoagulant heparin inhibits loss of glycosaminoglycans from xenogeneic cardiac grafts and prolongs graft survival. *Transplant. Proc.* **25**, 382.

Stone, K. R., Ayala, G. and Goldstein, J. (1998). Porcine cartilage transplants in the cynomolgus monkey: III. transplantation of alpha-galactosidase-treated porcine cartilage. *Transplantation* **65**, 1577.

Stroka, D. M., Badrichani, A. Z., Bach, F. H. and Ferran, C. (1999). Overexpression of A1, an NF-kappaB-inducible anti-apoptotic bcl gene, inhibits endothelial cell activation. *Blood* **93**, 3803.

Tanemura, M., Yin, D., Chong, A. S. and Galili, U. (2000). Differential immune responses to alpha-gal epitopes on xenografts and allografts: implications for accommodation in xenotransplantation. *J. Clin. Invest.* **105**, 301.

Tange, M., Tearle, R., Katerelos, M., *et al.* (1996). Analysis of alpha 1,3-galactosyltransferase knockout mice. *Transplant. Proc.* **28**, 620.

Tearle, R. G., Tange, M. J., Zannettino, Z. L., *et al.* (1996). The alpha-1,3-galactosyltransferase knockout mouse: implications for xenotransplantation. *Transplantation* **61**, 13.

Unger, E. (1910). Nietransplantationen. *Klin. Wochenschr.* **47**, 573.

van Denderen, B. J., Salvaris, E. and Romanella, M. (1997). Combination of decay-accelerating factor expression and alpha1,3-galactosyltransferase knockout affords added protection from human complement-mediated injury. *Transplantation* **64**, 882.

Von, A. M., Ferran, C., Brostjan, C., Bach, F. H. and Goodman, D. J. (1998). Membrane-associated lymphotoxin on natural killer cells activates endothelial cells via an NF-kappaB-dependent pathway. *Transplantation* **66**, 1211.

Waldmann, H. and Cobbold, S. (1993). The use of monoclonal antibodies to achieve immunological tolerance. *Immunol. Today* **14**, 247.

Wanke, R., Hermanns, W. and Folger, S. (1990). Accelerated growth and visceral lesions in transgenic mice expressing foreign genes of the growth hormone family: a review. *Pediatr. Nephrol.* **5**, 513.

Werner, D., Martinez, F. and Roch-Ramel, F. (1990). Urate and p-aminohippurate transport in the brush border membrane of the pig kidney. *J. Pharmacol. Exp. Ther.* **252**, 792.

White, D. J., Cozzi, E. and Langford, G. (1995). The control of hyperacute rejection by genetic engineering of the donor species. *Eye* **9**, 185.

Wood, K. J. (1993). The induction of tolerance to alloantigens using MHC class I molecules. *Curr. Opin. Immunol.* **5**, 759.

Yamada, K., Sachs, D. H. and DerSimonian, H. (1995). Human anti-porcine xenogeneic T cell response: evidence for allelic specificity of mixed leukocyte reaction and for both direct and indirect pathways of recognition. *J. Immunol.* **155**, 5249.

Ye, Y., Neethling, F. A., Niekrasz, M., *et al.* (1994). Evidence that intravenously administered alpha-galactosyl carbohydrates reduce baboon serum cytotoxicity to pig kidney cells (PK15) and transplanted pig hearts. *Transplantation* **58**, 330.

Zaidi, A., Bhatti, F., Schmoeckel, M., *et al.* (1998). Kidneys from HDAF transgenic pigs are physiologically compatible with primates. *Transplant. Proc.* **30**, 2465.

Zhong, R., Tucker, J., Grant, D., *et al.* (1996). Long-term survival and functional tolerance of baboon to monkey kidney and liver transplantation. *Transplant. Proc.* 762.

Zhow, X., Niesen, N. and Pawlowski, I. (1990). Prolongation of survival of discordant kidney xenografts by C6 deficiency. *Transplantation* **50**, 896.

The HLA System and Nomenclature
Craig J. Taylor

Introduction

The human leukocyte antigen (HLA) system, coded for on the short arm of chromosome 6, is the most intensively studied region of the human genome. It spans more than 4 megabases and contains greater than 250 genes, making it the most gene-dense region characterized to date. Of relevance to transplantation clinicians and immunologists is that 15% of these genes have immune-related function. Originally discovered in the late 1950s as the equivalent of the human major histocompatibility complex (MHC), HLA was identified as the principal mediator of graft rejection. At that time, nothing was known about the natural evolution of HLA because it seemed that this complex system was designed solely to facilitate transplant rejection.

Human leukocyte antigens are now recognized as the cornerstone in immune recognition. Their role is to present self and foreign antigen in the form of short protein fragments (peptides), which are recognized by self-HLA–restricted T cells. Recognition of nonself peptides in the context of self-HLA (i.e., altered self) is the function of the T-cell antigen receptor and elicits a powerful immune response.

The extensive polymorphism of HLA has evolved to enable efficient binding of peptides from the vast array of potentially pathogenic organisms that aim to invade and colonize the human body. The evolutionary pressures to develop and maintain diversity vary with time and geographical area. As a result, HLA has adapted differently according to geographical region and ethnic group, and HLA types differ throughout the world.

Early investigations into HLA polymorphism were driven by studies of solid-organ transplant rejection and used relatively crude alloantisera that could distinguish only a limited number of antigens. Human leukocyte antigen serologists throughout the world collaborated to identify specificities defined by common sets of reagents and devised a nomenclature system to denote these polymorphisms. In the 1990s, these simple techniques were complemented (and soon will be completely replaced) by molecular-based techniques that can resolve HLA variants at the DNA sequence level. These procedures can define single amino acid polymorphisms that are indistinguishable by serology. For example, there are currently 19 HLA-DR specificities defined by serological methods compared with more than 200 sequence variants (alleles) detected using DNA-based typing methods (Fig. 43–1). The number of newly defined alleles identified at all loci is still increasing rapidly and has now surpassed the highest expectations of the early pioneers.

Concomitant with the ever-increasing complexity of the HLA region, a nomenclature system has been developed to assign HLA loci and their alleles accurately (Bodmer *et al.*, 1984, 1989, 1991, 1992, 1994, 1995, 1999). This nomenclature system correlates with the methodology (serology, biochemistry and DNA sequencing) and level to which the HLA genes and their products have been resolved. To the uninitiated, this system can appear confusing, as in, for example, a comparison of the influence of *HLA-DRB1* and *HLA-DR* on graft outcome. These terms reflect the different techniques and/or resolution to which the gene products were defined.

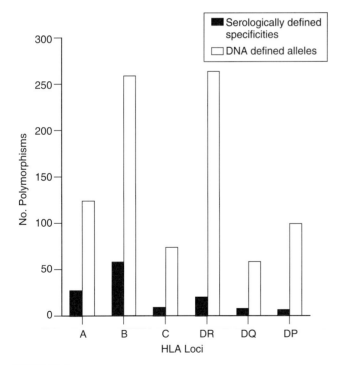

FIGURE 43–1

Number of HLA specificities (defined by serological HLA typing) and alleles (identified using sequence-based DNA typing) at each HLA locus.

HLA Genes and Their Products

The HLA system is a complex multigene family consisting of more than 10 loci. Human leukocyte antigen types are codominantly inherited on a maternal and paternal haplotype and transmitted as a single mendelian trait (Fig. 43–2). Each individual can express two alleles at each locus. The genes encoding HLA and their corresponding glycoprotein products are divided into two classes according to their biochemical and functional properties: HLA class I and HLA class II. Between these are the *class III* genes that code for some immune-related proteins, such as complement factors (C2, C4A, C4B, properdin factor B), tumor necrosis factor, lymphotoxin α and β and heat-shock proteins (HSP70). The steroid 21-hydroxylase is encoded by the gene *CYP21B* that is adjacent to HLA-DR (Bodmer *et al.*, 1992; Campbell and Trowsdale, 1993; Trowsdale *et al.*, 1991).

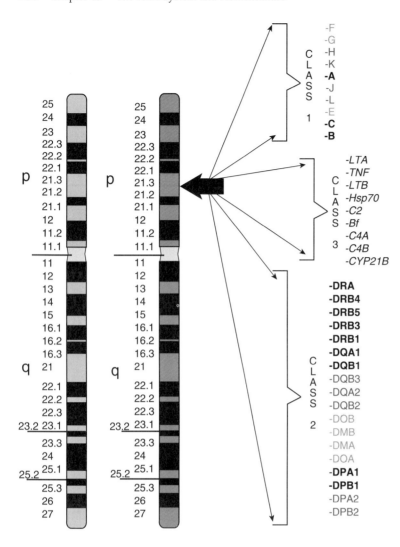

FIGURE 43–2

Genomic organization of the HLA region on chromosome 6. HLA antigens are inherited codominantly *en bloc* as a haplotype from maternal and paternal chromosomes. Light shaded letters = pseudogenes. Medium shaded letters = nonclassic HLA genes with no known role in clinical solid-organ transplantation. Italics = class 3 genes, some of which may have an indirect role in transplantation. Dark type letters = genes encoding HLA products with clinical relevance to solid-organ transplantation.

HLA CLASS I

Human leukocyte antigen class I genes span 2 megabases at the telomeric end of the 6p21.3 region of chromosome 6 (see Fig. 43–2). This region codes for the classic *transplantation antigens* (HLA-A, HLA-B and HLA-C) that were identified in the 1960s and are expressed on virtually all nucleated cells. Genes of the HLA class I loci code for 44-kd heavy chains that associate with intracellular peptides (Fig. 43–3). The tertiary structure is stabilized on the cell surface by noncovalent association with β_2-microglobulin, a nonpolymorphic 12-kd protein coded for on chromosome 15 (Townsend et al., 1989). The heavy chain has three extracellular immunoglobulinlike domains (α1, α2, α3), a hydrophobic transmembrane region and a cytoplasmic tail (Fig. 43–3). The two extracellular domains distal to the cell membrane (α1 and α2) are highly polymorphic and fold to form a peptide-binding cleft consisting of eight strands forming an antiparallel β pleated sheet, overlaid by two α helices (Fig. 43–4). The cleft accommodates peptides of 8 to 10 amino acids in length. The main areas of amino acid polymorphism line the sides and base of the cleft and govern the peptide-binding repertoire of the HLA molecule. In contrast, the α3 domain (proximal to the cell membrane) is highly conserved and acts as a ligand for CD8 expressed on T cells (Salter et al., 1990). This interaction confers HLA class I restriction on CD8$^+$ T cells, which have a predominantly cytotoxic function.

There are other class I loci (HLA-E, HLA-F, HLA-G, HLA-H, HLA-J, HLA-K, HLA-L) for which knowledge about their expression and function is only beginning to emerge (Table 43–1). HLA-H, HLA-J, HLA-K and HLA-L are pseudogenes that are not transcribed or translated. HLA-E, HLA-F and HLA-G have limited polymorphism and are known to act as ligands for natural killer (NK) cell inhibitory receptors (e.g., CD94). HLA-G is expressed on placental trophoblast, implicating a possible involvement in fetal-maternal development. Although these loci may prove to be important in certain experimental xenograft models and bone marrow transplantation (in which NK cells are involved in the rejection process), they have no known relevance to clinical solid-organ transplantation.

HLA CLASS II

Human leukocyte antigen class II consists of three main loci, HLA-DR, HLA-DQ and HLA-DP. The glycoprotein products are heterodimers with noncovalently associated α and β chains of molecular weight 33 kd and 28 kd. Both chains have two extracellular immunoglobulinlike domains, a transmembrane region and a cytoplasmic tail (see Fig. 43–3). The membrane distal domains α1 and β1 form a peptide-binding cleft similar to but less rigid than that of HLA class I, accommodating peptides of 10 to 20 amino acids. The β1 domains of HLA-DR, HLA-DQ and HLA-DP are highly polymorphic and govern the peptide-binding repertoire. They are constitutively expressed on cells with immune func-

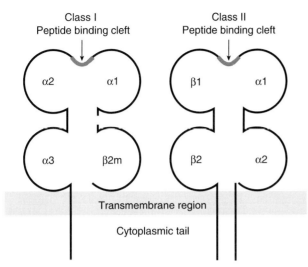

FIGURE 43–3

Schematic representation of the domain structure of HLA class I and II.

tion, such as B lymphocytes, activated T cells and antigen-presenting cells (monocytes, macrophages and cells of dendritic origin). Human leukocyte antigen class II can be induced on most cell types during inflammatory responses by cytokines such as interferon-γ and tumor necrosis factor-α. The β2 domain associates with CD4 on T cells with predominantly helper/inducer function and confers HLA class II restriction (Fig. 43–5).

Resolution of HLA Typing Methods

Serologically based HLA typing uses alloantisera and monoclonal antibodies that bind tertiary epitopes of the HLA glycoproteins on the cell surface. There is a high degree of sequence homology between HLA specificities, and identical amino acid sequence motifs often are shared between groups of antigens (Akkoc and Scornik, 1991; Marsh and Bodmer, 1989). These related structures give rise to cross-reactivity as many HLA-specific antibodies bind epitopes that are shared

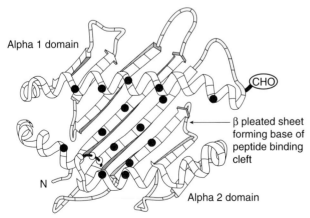

FIGURE 43–4

Ribbon diagram of the peptide binding cleft of HLA class I. The main positions of amino acid polymorphism (black dots) line the base and sides of the cleft, governing the molecules' peptide binding repertoire.

TABLE 43–1

HLA GENES AND THEIR PRODUCTS

Name	Molecular Characteristics
HLA-A	Class I α chain
HLA-B	Class I α chain
HLA-C	Class I α chain
HLA-E	Associated with class I 6.2-kb hind III fragment
HLA-F	Associated with class I 5.4-kb hind III fragment
HLA-G	Associated with class I 6.0-kb hind III fragment
HLA-H	Class I pseudogene
HLA-J	Class I pseudogene
HLA-K	Class I pseudogene
HLA-L	Class I pseudogene
HLA-DRA	DR α chain
HLA-DRB1	DR β1 chain determining specificities DR1 to DR18
HLA-DRB2	Pseudogene with DR β-like sequences
HLA-DRB3	DR β3 chain determining DR52, DW24, DW25 and DW26 specificities
HLA-DRB4	DR β4 chain determining DR53
HLA-DRB5	DR β5 chain determining DR51
HLA-DRB6	DRB pseudogene found on DR1, DR2 and DR10 haplotypes
HLA-DRB7	DRB pseudogene found on DR4, DR7 and DR9 haplotypes
HLA-DRB8	DRB pseudogene found on DR4, DR7 and DR9 haplotypes
HLA-DRB9	DRB pseudogene, probably found on all haplotypes
HLA-DQA1	DQ α chain as expressed
HLA-DQB1	DQ β chain as expressed
HLA-DQA2	DQ α chain–related sequence, not known to be expressed
HLA-DQB2	DQ β chain–related sequence, not known to be expressed
HLA-DQB3	DQ β chain–related sequence, not known to be expressed
HLA-DOA	DO α chain
HLA-DOB	DO β chain
HLA-DMA	DM α chain
HLA-DMB	DM β chain
HLA-DPA1	DP α chain as expressed
HLA-DPB1	DP β chain as expressed
HLA-DPA2	DP α chain–related pseudogene
HLA-DPB2	DP β chain–related pseudogene

between HLA specificities. Common serologically detectable HLA epitopes are called *public* or *supertypic* determinants forming cross-reactive groups (CREGs), whereas epitopes that are unique to an antigen are termed *private* determinants. In some cases, antigens that originally were well defined could be subdivided further into two or more specificities called *splits*. For example, some alloantisera were able to discriminate the *broad* HLA-A9 specificity into two subgroups, A23 and A24. These specificities are annotated as HLA-A23(9) and HLA-A24(9), where the *A23* and *A24* denote the split specificity and the number in parentheses, *(9)*, denotes the broad specificity.

The degree of HLA compatibility between transplant donors and recipients can be considered at many different levels of resolution, depending on the HLA typing methodology (Table 43–2). This compatibility can range from single amino acid differences detected by high-resolution DNA sequence–based methods (allele matching) to broad and split specificity matching and matching for the small number of common cross-reactive groups. The influence of all levels of donor and recipient HLA compatibility has been considered in cadaver donor renal transplantation. Although strongly implicated

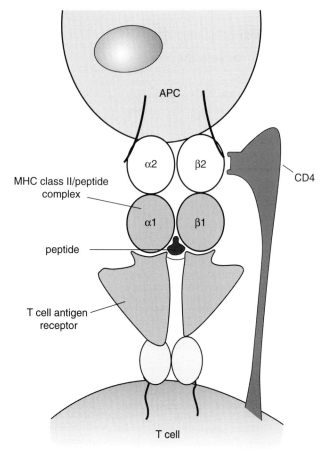

MHC class II/peptide complex

peptide

T cell antigen receptor

APC

CD4

T cell

FIGURE 43–5

Diagram depicting the presentation of peptide (black) by an HLA class II molecule on an antigen-presenting cell (APC) to the antigen receptor on CD4[+] T helper cells. (Redrawn with permission from Taylor, C. T. and Metcalfe, S. The immunobiology of transplantation. *In Anesthesia and Intensive Care for Organ Transplantation* (1998). (J. R. Klinck and M. J. Lindop, eds). Arnold, London.)

for negating graft-versus-host disease after unrelated bone marrow transplantation, a role for high-resolution allele matching in renal transplantation has not been established firmly. Matching for serologically defined amino acids, specificities and cross-reactive groups has been reported to benefit transplant outcome, however (Kobayashi *et al.*, 1992; Takemoto, 1996; Thompson and Thacker, 1996; Wujciak and Opelz, 1999). In general, the more discerning the matching criteria, the greater the correlation with graft outcome.

HLA Nomenclature

Many HLA genes have been characterized and cloned and have been given official designations using the following principles. The genes are prefixed by the letters *HLA* followed by the loci or region (e.g., HLA-A, HLA-B or HLA-D). The HLA-D region has several subregions denoted HLA-DR, HLA-DQ, HLA-DP, HLA-DO and HLA-DM (see Fig. 43–2). These are followed by the letters *A* or *B*, defining the gene coding for the α and β chain gene product of that subregion (e.g., *HLA-DRB* genes code for the DRβ-chain protein product). When there is more than one A or B gene within a subregion, a corresponding number is given (e.g., *HLA-DRB1*) (see Fig. 43–2 and Table 43–1).

Each allele has a unique four- or five-digit number pre-

fixed by an asterisk (*) where DNA sequence–based information is available. The first two digits identify the broad specificity based on homology between alleles. These digits usually correlate with the serological specificity; for instance, HLA-B*27 correlates with the serological specificity HLA-B27. For most serologically defined antigens, there is further polymorphism at the amino acid and DNA sequence level. When sequence information is available, the third and fourth digits denote the precise allele. For example, there are 15 subtypes of HLA-B27 that involve amino acid substitutions at 18 sites. These are represented as HLA-B*2701, HLA-B*2702 and so forth. In cases in which a DNA base change does not alter the amino acid sequence (*silent substitution*), a fifth digit is applied to differentiate the noncoding base change (e.g., HLA-DQB1*05031 and HLA-DQB1*05032).

Some alleles or genes contain a sequence defect that prevents normal antigen expression and protein products are not present at the cell surface. These are termed *null alleles* and are indicated with an N (e.g., HLA-DRB4*01031N). Further mutations have been detected outside the coding region, and additional digits have been added to indicate these silent intron polymorphisms (e.g., HLA-DRB4*0103102N).

For HLA-DR and HLA-DP, the α chains are less polymorphic (DRA is diallelic), and so one usually annotates the *HLA-DRB1* or *HLA-DPB1* allele (which code for the main polymorphic amino acid determinants present on the β chain) alone. For HLA-DQ, the α and β chains are both polymorphic, however. To describe the allele precisely, one may need to define the A and B alleles (e.g., HLA-DQA1*0101 and HLA-B1*0501). Although the α and β products of the A and B gene pairs associate preferentially, there also is the possibility of the formation of novel hybrid molecules (e.g., HLA-DRA and HLA-DQB1*0402). A complete list of recognized HLA genes and their expressed products is given in Table 43–1 (Bodmer *et al.*, 1999).

HLA Class II Loci and Haplotypes
HLA-DR

The HLA-DR α chain may associate with the β chain coded for by *HLA-DRB1*, *HLA-DRB3*, *HLA-DRB4* or *HLA-*

TABLE 43–2

RESOLUTION OF HLA TYPING METHODS AND THEIR APPLICATION TO RENAL TRANSPLANTATION

HLA Typing Resolution	Method
HLA allele matching	High-resolution DNA sequence–based typing*
Split HLA specificity matching	Serology and low-resolution (generic) DNA typing†
Broad HLA specificity matching	Serology and low-resolution (generic) DNA typing
HLA-B, HLA-DR matching	Serology and low-resolution (generic) DNA typing
Epitope matching	Serologically defined cross-reactive groups
Serologically defined motifs and determinants	
Single amino acid residues	
Linear peptides and conformational epitopes	
Supertypic antigen matching	

*High-resolution DNA typing can be translated into low-resolution serological equivalents.

†Low-resolution generic HLA typing by polymerase chain reaction uses DNA primers designed to type at a level comparable to serology (Olerup and Zetterquist, 1991, 1992).

Adapted with permission of Taylor and Dyer, 1999.

DRB5 (see Fig. 43–2 and Table 43–1). The *HLA-DRB2* is a pseudogene that is not transcribed and translated. Not all haplotypes carry all the *HLA-DRB* genes. Each haplotype expresses a *DRB1* gene alone or with a second *DRB* gene, *DRB3*, *DRB4* or *DRB5*. For example, the *HLA-DR1* and *HLA-DR8* haplotypes express a product coded by the *DRB1* gene alone, whereas the *HLA-DR2* haplotype expresses two products coded by the *DRB1* and *DRB5* genes (*DR2* and *DR51*). There are additional *HLA-DRB* genes (*HLA-DRB6*, *HLA-DRB7*, *HLA-DRB8*, *HLA-DRB9*) that are pseudogenes. A list of common *HLA-DRB* haplotypes and their serological, molecular and cellular relationships is given in Table 43–3.

HLA-DQ

The HLA-DQ region consists of two *DQA* genes (*DQA1* and *DQA2*) and two *DQB* genes (*DQB1* and *DQB2*) (see Fig. 43–2). The *HLA-DQA2* and *HLA-DQB2* genes are not known to be transcribed and translated. The *DQA1* and *DQB1* genes code for the HLA-DQ α and β chain glycoprotein products, both of which are polymorphic. The HLA-DQ genes are in strong linkage dysequilibrium with HLA-DR, and to date only one meiotic recombination event has been reported between these loci (Morgan *et al.*, 1997). Due to linkage disequilibrium, particular DR and DQ alleles occur together more often than would be found by chance (i.e., the alleles are not at equilibrium with each other in the population). Within particular ethnic groups, some HLA-DR/DQ combinations are found together on the same haplotype in 100% of cases (Lee *et al.*, 1990). A list of common HLA-DR/DQ haplotypes is given in Table 43–4.

HLA-DP

There are two HLA-DPA and two HLA-DPB genes (see Fig. 43–2 and Table 43–1). *HLA-DPA2* and *HLA-DPB2* are both pseudogenes. Similar to HLA-DRA, the HLA-DPA has limited polymorphism (15 alleles), and the main polymorphic determinants are carried on the β protein chain encoded by the *HLA-DPB1* gene. There are more than 80 HLA-DPB1 alleles sequenced, but owing to the technical difficulty of typing for HLA-DP, there are few studies investigating their role in organ transplantation. A report by Mytilineos *et al.* (1997) found a marked effect of HLA-DP locus matching in cadaver kidney retransplants, indicating a need for further studies.

HLA-D

HLA-D (also known as *Dw*, where *w* denotes *workshop*) was originally thought to represent a discrete HLA locus defined by the mixed lymphocyte reaction (MLR). The term *lymphocyte defined* (or *LD*) antigens was used to differentiate these from HLA class I, which were *serologically defined* (or *SD*). HLA-Dw typing was performed by detecting T lymphocyte proliferative responses against homozygous typing cell (HTC) stimulators (see Tables 43–3 and 43–4). Although closely linked, there was incomplete overlap between MLR reactivity (HLA-Dw) and their serologically defined counterparts, which were consequently named *HLA-DR* (*D related*). It is now recognized, however, that HLA-Dw (i.e., MLR responses) does not represent a discrete HLA locus but is due to alloreactivity caused by a summation of class II differences at HLA-DR and HLA-DQ (Mach and Tiercy, 1991). HLA-DR confers the strongest stimulation in an MLR, followed by HLA-DQ. HLA-DP also is considered to contribute weakly to the response in a primary MLR (Olerup *et al.*, 1990). HLA-DP acts as a strong stimulator of a secondary MLR using primed alloreactive T cells. The relationship of HLA-D to HLA-DR and HLA-DQ haplotypes is presented in Tables 43–3 and 43–4.

EXTENDED HAPLOTYPES

The strong linkage disequilibrium between HLA-DR and HLA-DQ extends to the class I region, although with reduced penetrance. Certain extended HLA haplotypes involving HLA-A, HLA-B, HLA-C, HLA-DR and HLA-DQ commonly exist within and between ethnic groups. This situation greatly improves the probability of locating an HLA-matched unrelated donor because the HLA haplotype is often inherited *en bloc* (e.g., HLA-A*0101, HLA-B*0801, HLA-C*0701, HLA-DRB1*0301, HLA-DRB3*0101, HLA-DQA1*05011, HLA-DQB1*0201). These extended haplotypes involve the class III region with the previous example being linked to the tumor necrosis factor-α promoter polymorphism (TNFA2) associated with increased production of this proinflammatory cytokine. Linkage within the HLA class I region has been

TABLE 43–3
COMMON HLA-DRB3*, HLA-DRB4* AND HLA-DRB5* HAPLOTYPES WITH THEIR SEROLOGICAL AND CELLULAR ASSOCIATIONS

HLA-DRB Allele	Serological Product	Associated HLA-D Specificity	Associated HLA-DR Haplotype
DRB3*0101	DR52a	Dw24	DR17 (3), DR18 (3), DR13 (6), DR14 (6)
0201	DR52b	Dw25	DR14 (6)
0202	DR52b	Dw25	DR17 (3), DR11 (5), DR12 (5) DR14 (6)
0301	DR52c	Dw26	DR13 (6)
DRB4*0101	DR53	Dw4, Dw10, Dw13, Dw14, Dw15	DR4
0101	DR53	Dw17 (7)	DR7
0101	DR53	Dw23	DR9
0103102N	—	Dw11 (7)	DR7
DRB5*0101	DR51	Dw2	DR15 (2)
0102	DR51	Dw12	DR15 (2)
0201	DR51	Dw21	DR16 (2)
0202	DR51	Dw22	DR16 (2)
—	—	Dwl, Dw20	DR1
—	—	Dw' BON'	DR103
—	—	D' SHY'	DR10
—	—	Dw8	DR8

NOTE: DRB3/4/5 genes are not present on all haplotypes. HLA-DR1, HLA-DR103, HLA-DR10, HLA-DR8 and some HLA-DR7 haplotypes express only one DRB product encoded by HLA-DRB1.

TABLE 43–4

ASSOCIATIONS BETWEEN SEROLOGICALLY DEFINED AND MOLECULARLY DEFINED HLA-DR/DQ AND HLA-D HAPLOTYPES

HLA-DR	HLA-DRB1*	HLA-DR	HLA-DRB3/4/5*	HLA-DQ	HLA-DQA1*	HLA-DQB1*	HLA-D
DR1	0101	—	—	DQ5(1)	0101	0501	Dw1
DR1	0102	—	—	DQ5(1)	0101	0502	Dw20
DR103	0103	—	—	DQ5(1)	0101	0501	Dw'BON'
DR103	0103	—	—	DQ7(3)	0501	0301	—
DR15(2)	1501	DR51	B5*0101	DQ6(1)	0102	0602	Dw2
DR15(2)	1502	DR51	B5*0102	DQ6(1)	0103	0601	Dw12
DR16(2)	1601	DR51	B5*0201	DQ5(1)	0102	0502	Dw21
DR16(2)	1602	DR51	B5*0202	DQ7(3)	05013	0301	Dw22
DR17(3)	0301	DR52	B3*0101/0202	DQ2	05011	0201	Dw3
DR18(3)	0302	DR52	B3*0101	DQ4	0401	0402	Dw'RSH'
DR4	0401	DR53	B4*0101–0103	DQ7/8(3)	03011	0301/0302	Dw4
DR4	0402	DR53	B4*0101	DQ8(3)	03011	0302	Dw10
DR4	0403	DR53	B4*0101	DQ7/8(3)	03011	0301/0302	Dw13
DR4	0404	DR53	B4*0101	DQ8(3)	03011	0302	Dw14
DR4	0405	DR53	B4*0101	DQ4/8(3)	03011	0401/0302	Dw15
DR4	0406	DR53	B4*0101	DQ8(3)	0301	0302	Dw'KT2'
DR4	0407	DR53	B4*0101–0103	DQ7(3)	0301	0301	Dw13
DR4	0408	DR53	B4*0101	DQ7(3)	0301	0301	Dw14
DR4	0412/0405	DR53	B4*0101	DQ2	0301	0201	—
DR11(5)	11011/11012	DR52	B3*0202	DQ7(3)	05012	0301	Dw5
DR11(5)	1101	DR52	B3*0202	DQ6(1)	0102	0602	Dw'DB2'
DR11(5)	1102	DR52	B3*0202	DQ7(3)	0501	0301	Dw'JVM'
DR11(5)	11041	DR52	B3*0202	DQ6(1)	0103	0603	Dw'FS'
DR12(5)	1201	DR52	B3*0202	DQ7(3)	0501	0301	Dw'DB6'
DR13(6)	1301	DR52	B3*0101/0202	DQ6(1)	0103	0603	Dw18(w6)
DR13(6)	1302	DR52	B3*0301	DQ6(1)	0102	0604/0605	Dw19(w6)
DR13(6)	1303	DR52	B3*0101	DQ7(3)	0501	0301	Dw'HAG'
DR13(6)	1304	DR52	B3*0202	DQ7(3)	0501	0301	—
DR13(6)	1305	DR52	B3*0202	DQ7(3)	0501	0301	—
DR14(6)	1401	DR52	B3*0201–0203	DQ5(1)	0104	05031/05032	Dw9
DR14(6)	1402	DR52	B3*0101	DQ7(3)	0501/0503	0301	Dw16
DR1404(6)	1404	DR52	B3*0101/0202	DQ5(1)	0101	0503	—
DR7	0701	DR53	B4*0101	DQ2	0201	0201	Dw17(w7)
DR7	0701	—	B4*0103N	DQ9(3)	0201	03032	Dw11(w7)
DR8	0801	—	—	DQ4	0401	0402	Dw8.1
DR8	08021/08022	—	—	DQ4	0401	0402	Dw8.2
DR8	08032	—	—	DQ6(1)	0103	0601	Dw8.3
DR8	08032	—	—	DQ7(3)	0601	0301	Dw8.3
DR9	09012	DR53	B4*0101	DQ9(3)	0302	03032	Dw23
DR9	0901	DR53	B4*0101	DQ2	0301	0201	—
DR10	1001	—	—	DQ5(1)	0104	0501	D'SHY'

NOTE: On the HLA-DR7/DQ9 haplotype, the DRB4*0103102N gene is present but not expressed (null allele). This list is not exhaustive, and in theory all DR/DQ allele combinations are possible. However, certain HLA-DR/DQ haplotypes predominate within particular ethnic groups, and in practice the number of HLA haplotypes found within a population is restricted.

extended a further 4 megabases telomeric to HLA-A to the class I–like gene *HLA-Hfe*. A point mutation that substitutes cystine or tyrosine at position 282 of the Hfe protein is the major cause of hereditary hemachromatosis and explains the weaker association of this disease with HLA-A3 observed in the 1970s. There is only relatively weak linkage centromeric to HLA-DQ resulting from a recombination *hot spot* between HLA-DQ and HLA-DP.

HLA Specificities, Alleles and Gene Frequencies

A complete list of serological, molecular and cellular specificities and alleles is presented in Table 43–5. The gene frequencies given are defined by serology and divided into broad ethnic groups compiled from the 9th International Histocompatibility Workshop (Bauer *et al.*, 1984). Although broadly comparable, some allele frequencies may vary within geographical regions and between tribes and suffice only as an overview. A detailed analysis of serological and allele gene frequencies (defined by molecular typing) within ethnic groups can be found in Imanishi *et al.* (1992) and Gjertson and Lee (1998).

HLA on the Web

Information concerning the HLA system is rapidly expanding and articles always are out of date by the time they go to print. There are many Internet web sites with useful links that are regularly updated. The following web sites provide contemporary information concerning HLA genes, nomenclature, polymorphism, DNA and amino acid sequences plus interesting articles for professionals and laypeople:

www.bmdw.org/wmda
www.swmed.edu/home_pages/ASHI/ashi.htm
http://www.umds.ac.uk/tissue/bshi1.html
http://www-sv.cict.fr/efi/
www.anthonynolan.com/HIG/data.html
www.sanger.ac.uk/HGP/Chr6/

TABLE 43–5

RECOGNIZED SEROLOGICAL, MOLECULAR AND CELLULAR HLA SPECIFICITIES AND ALLELES WITH THEIR GENE FREQUENCIES

Serological Specificity*	DNA Sequence *HLA Allele*	Ethnic Group† W	A	B
HLA-A				
A1	A*0101–0104N	14.2	1.0	8.1
A2	A*0201–0230	28.9	28.1	17.5
A203	A*0203	—	—	—
A210	A*0210	—	—	—
A3	A*0301–0304	13.2	1.5	6.7
A9‡	A*2301/2402–2420			
A23(9)	A*2301	1.4	0.1	8.0
A24(9)	A*2402/2404–2408/2410/2413/2414	10.3	31.4	4.8
A2403	A*2403	—	—	—
A10	A*2501–2502/2601–2612/3401–3402/6601–6602			
A25(10)	A*2501	2.4	0	0
A26(10)	A*2601–2609	3.2	7.2	4.5
A34(10)	A*3401–3402	0.1	0.3	5.1
A66(10)	A*6601–6603	0.2	0.5	0.3
A11	A*1101–1105	6.3	11.7	1.9
A28	A*6801–6809/6901	4.7	2.1	9.9
A68(28)	A*6801–6804/6808	—	—	—
A69(28)	A*6901	—	—	—
A19				
A29(19)	A*2901–2904	2.9	0.4	4.9
A30(19)	A*3001–3007	3.5	2.3	11.0
A31(19)	A*3101–3104	2.9	5.2	1.6
A32(19)	A*3201–3203	3.9	0.4	2.3
A33(19)	A*3301–3304	1.4	6.0	3.9
A74(19)	A*7401–7403	—	—	—
A36	A*3601	0.1	0.1	3.2
A43	A*4301	0	0	1.3
A80	A*8001	—	—	—
HLA-C				
Cw1§	Cw*0102–0103	3.3	16.3	1.0
Cw2	Cw*0201–0203	4.1	1.0	11.9
Cw3	Cw*0302–0309	12.6	27.3	8.3
Cw9(w3)	Cw*0303/0307	—	—	—
Cw10(w3)	Cw*0302/0304	—	—	—
Cw4	Cw*0401–0406	11.6	5.3	14.0
Cw5	Cw*0501–0502	6.9	0.6	3.0
Cw6	Cw*0602–0604	8.6	3.8	12.9
Cw7	Cw*0701–0712	24.3	12.1	24.1
Cw8	Cw*0801–0806	3.7	0.3	3.5
—	Cw*1202–1206	—	—	—
—	Cw*1301	—	—	—
—	Cw*1402–1404	—	—	—
—	Cw*1502–1508	—	—	—
—	Cw*1601/1602/1604	—	—	—
—	Cw*1701–1702	—	—	—
—	Cw*1801–1802	—	—	—
HLA-E				
—	E*0101–0104	—	—	—
HLA-G				
—	G*0101–0105N	—	—	—
HLA-B				
B5	B*5101–5116/5201/7801	8.2	15.1	2.5
B51(5)	B*5101/5104/5105/5107–5109	6.2	7.8	1.9
B5102(5)	B*5102	—	—	—
B5103(5)	B*5103	—	—	—
B7801(5)	B*7801	—	—	—
B52(5)	B*5201/5116	2.0	7.3	0.6
B7	B*0702–0713	11.5	4.7	12.1
B703(7)	B*0703	—	—	—
B8	B*0801–0806	9.6	0.2	5.5

Table continued on following page

TABLE 43–5

RECOGNIZED SEROLOGICAL, MOLECULAR AND CELLULAR HLA SPECIFICITIES AND ALLELES WITH THEIR GENE FREQUENCIES Continued

Serological Specificity*	DNA Sequence HLA Allele	Ethnic Group† W	A	B
B12	B*4402–4411/4501–4502	12.7	6.1	10.0
B44(12)	B*4402–4408/4410	12.3	6.0	7.7
B45(12)	B*4501/5002	0.4	0.1	2.3
B13	B*1301–1304	2.9	3.8	1.6
B14	B*1401–1405	3.7	0.2	2.9
B64(14)	B*1401	1.1	0	1.3
B65(14)	B*1402	2.6	0.2	1.6
B15	B*1501–1549	6.8	9.6	4.5
B62(15)	B*1501/1504/1505–1507/1515/1520/1524–1527/1530/1532/1535/1545/1548	6.1	9.6	2.6
B63(15)	B*1516/1517	0.7	0	1.9
B75(15)	B*1502/1508/1511/1521/1531	—	—	—
B76(15)	B*1512/1514/1519	—	—	—
B77(15)	B*1513	—	—	—
B16	B*3801–3803/3901–3916	4.5	1.1	1.6
B38(16)	B*3801–3803	2.5	0.7	1.6
B39(16)	B*3903–3913	2.0	0.4	0
B3901(16)	B*3901	—	—	—
B3902(16)	B*3902	—	—	—
B17	B*5701–5705/5801–5802	2.9	1.9	2.9
B57(17)	B*5701	2.9	0.7	2.9
B58(17)‖	B*5801	0	1.2	0
B18	B*1801–1807	5.5	0.3	4.2
B21		2.9	0.6	2.9
B49(21)	B*4901	1.8	0.3	2.3
B50(21)	B*5001	1.1	0.3	0.6
B4005(21)	B*4005	—	—	—
B22	B*5401/5501–5508/5601–5605	2.8	10.3	0.3
B54(22)	B*5401/5507	0.1	6.7	0
B55(22)	B*5501/5502/5504	1.6	2.1	0
B56(22)	B*5601/5602/5604	1.1	1.5	0.3
B27	B*2701–2715	3.4	1.6	1.9
B35	B*3501–3527, 1522	10.5	10.2	7.1
B37	B*3701–3702	1.6	0.6	1.3
B40	B*4001–4020	5.9	18.2	3.8
B60(40)	B*4001/4007/4010	3.8	6.5	2.3
B61(40)	B*4002/4004/4006/4009/4016	2.1	11.7	1.5
B41	B*4101–4103	0.9	0.1	2.3
B42	B*4201–4202	0.2	0.5	5.8
B46	B*4601	0.1	3.6	0
B47	B*4701–4703	0.2	0.4	0
B48	B*4801–4805	0	1.6	0
B53	B*5301–5303	0.5	0.3	6.7
B59	B*5901	0	0.6	0
B67	B*6701	0	0.1	0
B70	B*1509/1529/1537	0.4	0.9	7.9
B71(70)	B*1510/1518	0.1	0.4	0.8
B72(70)	B*1503/1546	0.3	0.5	7.1
B73	B*7301	0.1	0.2	0
B78	B*7801–7803	—	—	—
B81	B*8101	—	—	—
—	B*8201	—	—	—
Bw4¶		65.3	57.6	65.3
Bw6¶		83.1	87.6	83.1
HLA-DR				
—	DRA*0101–0102	—	—	—
DR1	DRB1*0101/0102/0104–0106	9.5	5.0	5.1
DR103	DRB1*0103	—	—	—
DR2	DRB1*1501–1508/1601–1608	15.8	15.1	15.1
DR15(2)	DRB1*1501–1506	—	—	—
DR16(2)	DRB1*1601/1602/1604	—	—	—
DR3	DRB1*0301–0313	12.0	1.8	14.9
DR17(3)	DRB1*0301/0304/0305	—	—	—
DR18(3)	DRB1*0302/0303	—	—	—
DR4	DRB1*0401–0432	12.7	21.8	7.6

TABLE 43-5

RECOGNIZED SEROLOGICAL, MOLECULAR AND CELLULAR HLA SPECIFICITIES AND ALLELES WITH THEIR GENE FREQUENCIES *Continued*

Serological Specificity*	DNA Sequence *HLA Allele*	Ethnic Group†		
		W	**A**	**B**
DR5	DRB1*1101–1135/1201–1206			
DR11(5)	DRB1*1101–1111/1113/1114/1120/1121/1123/1125–1127/1129	12.3	4.0	16.5
DR12(5)	DRB1*1201–1203/1205/1206	2.0	7.2	3.4
DR6	DRB1*1301–1334/1401–1433			
DR13(6)	DRB1*1301–1308/1310/1311/1314/1316–1318/1320–1322/1327/1421	5.4	2.9	3.8
DR14(6)	DRB1*1401–1402/1405–1408/1410–1414/1417/1419–1421/1426/1427/1429	5.8	6.8	10.7
DR1403(6)	DRB1*1403	—	—	—
DR1404(6)	DRB1*1404	—	—	—
DR7	DRB1*0701/0703/0704	12.0	2.9	13.2
DR8	DRB1*0801–0821/1415	3.0	7.3	0.8
DR9	DRB1*0901	0.8	11.5	1.5
DR10	DRB1*1001	0.8	0.5	2.3
DR51	DRB5*0101–0110N/0202–0204	—	—	—
DR52**	DRB3*0101–0105/0201–0208/0301–0303	52.6	49.3	75.9
DR53**	DRB4*0101–0105/0201N/0301N	9.8	15.1	13.0
—	DRB6*0101/0201/0202	—	—	—
—	DRB7*0101	—	—	—
HLA-DQ				
—	DQA1*0101–0105	—	—	—
—	DQA1*0201	—	—	—
—	DQA1*0301–0303	—	—	—
—	DQA1*0401	—	—	—
—	DQA1*0501–0505	—	—	—
—	DQA1*0601	—	—	—
DQ1	DQB1*0501–0504/0601–0615	32.3	30.2	40.1
DQ5(1)	DQB1*0501–0504	—	—	—
DQ6(1)	DQB1*0601–0606/0609/0614	—	—	—
DQ2	DQB1*0201–0203	18.1	5.0	23.1
DQ3	DQB1*0301–0309	23.3	32.7	24.6
DQ7(3)	DQB1*0301/0304	—	—	—
DQ8(3)	DQB1*0302/0305	—	—	—
DQ9(3)	DQB1*0303	—	—	—
DQ4	DQB1*0401–0402	—	—	—
HLA-DO				
—	DOA*01011–01015	—	—	—
HLA-DM				
—	DMA*0101–0104	—	—	—
—	DMB*0101–0105	—	—	—
HLA-DP				
—	DPA1*0103–0106	—	—	—
—	DPA1*0201–0203	—	—	—
—	DPA1*0301–0302	—	—	—
—	DPA1*0401	—	—	—
DPw1	DPB1*0101	4.3	—	—
DPw2	DPB1*0201–0202	11.5	—	—
DPw3	DPB1*0301	4.0	—	—
DPw4	DPB1*0401–0402	41.8	—	—
DPw5	DPB1*0501	4.4	—	—
DPw6	DPB1*0601	0	—	—
—	DPB1*0801–8101	—	—	—

*Some DNA-defined alleles have incomplete characterization by serological typing and are assimilated to the broad HLA specificity on the basis of predicted sequence homology (compiled from Bodmer *et al.*, 1999; Schreuder *et al.*, 1999).

†Gene frequencies (Gf) calculated from a random panel of healthy whites (*W*), Asians (*A*) and blacks (*B*) in the 9th Histocompatibility Workshop (Bauer *et al.*, 1984). Because each person carries two chromosomes coding for the HLA loci, the phenotype frequencies (Pf = percentage occurrence of an antigen) can be approximated as Pf = 2 × Gf for rare HLA antigens, and Pf = < 2 × Gf for the commoner HLA antigens (owing to the occurrence of homozygotes). Gf = $1 - \sqrt{(1 - Pf)}$.

‡Some serologically defined HLA antigens have been *split* into further polymorphic subgroups, in which the broad *public* antigenic determinant is denoted by the parentheses, preceded by the *private* epitope (e.g., HLA-A9 is serologically split into two subgroups, A23 [9] and A24 [9]).

§The notation *w* (e.g., HLA-Cw2) is used to differentiate HLA-C locus products from those of the complement system (e.g., C2).

‖The gene frequency of Bw58 (17) in blacks reported in the 8th Histocompatibility Workshop was 10.7 (Bauer and Danilovs, 1980).

¶HLA-Bw4 and HLA-Bw6 represent public epitopes (a common shared determinant) carried on the HLA-B heavy chain. Each HLA-B locus antigen has one of the two possible epitopes. The phenotype frequencies are reported from the 8th Histocompatibility Workshop (Bauer and Danilovs, 1980).

**Phenotype frequencies of DR52 (previously called *MT2*) and DR53 (previously called *MT3*) reported from the 8th Histocompatibility Workshop (Bauer and Danilovs, 1980).

REFERENCES

Akkoc, N. and Scornik, J. C. (1991). Intramolecular specificity of anti-HLA alloantibodies. *Hum. Immunol.* **30**, 91.

Bauer, M. P. and Danilovs, J. A. (1980). Population analysis of HLA-A, B, C, DR and other genetic markers. *In Histocompatibility Testing 1980*, (P. I. Terasaki, ed.), p. 955, UCLA Tissue Typing Laboratory, Los Angeles.

Bauer, M. P., Neugebauer, M., Deppe, H., *et al.* (1984). Population analysis on the basis of deduced haplotypes from random families. *In Histocompatibility Testing 1984*, (E. D. Albert, *et al.*, eds.), p. 333, Springer-Verlag, Berlin.

Bodmer, J. G., Marsh, S. G. E., Albert, E. D., *et al.* (1991). Nomenclature for factors of the HLA system, 1990. *Tissue Antigens* **37**, 97.

Bodmer, J. G., Marsh, S. G. E., Albert, E. D., *et al.* (1992). Nomenclature for factors of the HLA system, 1991. *Tissue Antigens* **39**, 161.

Bodmer, J. G., Marsh, S. G. E., Albert, E. D., *et al.* (1994). Nomenclature for factors of the HLA system, 1994. *Tissue Antigens* **44**, 1.

Bodmer, J. G., Marsh, S. G. E., Albert, E. D., *et al.* (1995). Nomenclature for factors of the HLA system, 1995. *Tissue Antigens* **46**, 1.

Bodmer, J. G., Marsh, S. G. E., Albert, E. D., *et al.* (1999). Nomenclature for factors of the HLA system, 1998. *Eur. J. Immunogenet.* **26**, 81–116.

Bodmer, W. F., Albert, E. D., Bodmer, J. G., *et al.* (1984). Nomenclature factors for the HLA system, 1984. *In Histocompatibility Testing 1984*, (E. D. Albert, *et al.*, eds.), p. 4, Springer-Verlag, Berlin.

Bodmer, W. F., Albert, E. D., Bodmer, J. G., *et al.* (1989). Nomenclature factors of the HLA system, 1987. *In Histocompatibility Testing 1987: Immunobiology of HLA*, Vol. 1, (B. Dupont, ed.), p. 72, Springer-Verlag, New York.

Campbell, R. D. and Trowsdale, J. (1993). Map of the human MHC. *Immunol. Today* **14**, 349.

Gjertson, D. W. and Lee, S.-H. (1998). HLA-A/B and -DRB1/DQB1 allele-level haplotype frequencies. *In HLA 1998*, (D. W. Gjertson and P. I. Terasaki, eds.), p. 365, American Society for Histocompatibility Immunogenetics, Lenexa, Kansas.

Imanishi, T., Akaza, T., Kimura, A., Tokunaga, K. and Gojobori, T. (1992). Allele and haplotype frequencies for HLA and complement loci in various ethnic groups. *In HLA-1991, Proceedings of the 11th International Histocompatibility Workshop and Conference*, (K. Tsuji, M. Aizawa and T. Sasazuki, eds.), p. 1065, Oxford University Press, Oxford.

Kobayashi, T., Yokoyama, I., Uchida, K., *et al.* (1992). The significance of HLA-DRB1 matching in clinical renal transplantation. *Transplantation* **54**, 238.

Lee, T. D., Lee, G. and Zhao, T. M. (1990). HLA-DR, DQ antigens in North American Caucasians. *Tissue Antigens* **35**, 64.

Mach, B. and Tiercy, J. M. (1991). Genotypic typing of HLA Class II: from the bench to the bedside. *Hum. Immunol.* **30**, 278.

Marsh, S. G. E. and Bodmer, J. G. (1989). HLA-DR and -DQ epitopes and monoclonal antibody specificity. *Immunol. Today* **10**, 305.

Morgan, C. H., Smith, S. I., Muir, A., Stephenson, S. and Taylor, C. J. (1997). A familial case of meiotic recombination between HLA-DRB1 and -DQB1. *Eur. J. Immunogenet.* **24**, 39.

Mytilineos, J., Deufel, A. and Opelz, G. (1997). Clinical relevance of HLA-DPB locus matching for cadaver kidney retransplants: a report of the Collaborative Transplant Study. *Transplantation* **63**, 1351.

Olerup, O., Moller, E. and Persson, U. (1990). HLA-DP incompatibilities induce significant proliferation in primary mixed lymphocyte cultures in HLA-A, -B, -DR and -DQ compatible individuals: implications for allogeneic bone marrow transplantation. *Tissue Antigens* **36**, 194.

Olerup, O. and Zetterquist, H. (1991). HLA-DRB1*01 subtyping by allele-specific PCR amplification: a sensitive, specific and rapid technique. *Tissue Antigens* **37**, 197.

Olerup, O. and Zetterquist, H. (1992). HLA-DR typing by PCR amplification with sequence-specific primers (PCR-SSP) in 2 hours: an alternative to serological DR typing in clinical practice including donor-recipient matching in cadaveric transplantation. *Tissue Antigens* **39**, 225.

Salter, R. D., Benjamin, R. J., Wesley, P. K., *et al.* (1990). A binding site for the T-cell co-receptor CD8 on the alpha 3 domain of HLA-A2. *Nature* **345**, 41.

Schreuder, G. M. T., Hurley, C. K., Marsh, S. G. E., *et al.* (1999). The HLA dictionary 1999: a summary of HLA-A, -B, -C, -DRB1/3/4/5, -DQB1 alleles and their associations with serologically defined HLA-A, -B, -C, -DR and -DQ antigens. *Tissue Antigens* **54**, 409.

Takemoto, S. K. (1996). HLA amino acid residue matching. UCLA Tissue Typing Laboratory, Los Angeles, Calif. J. M. Cecka, P. I. Terasaki (eds). *Clin. Transpl.* 397.

Taylor, C. J. and Dyer, P. A. (1999). Maximising the benefits of HLA matching for renal transplantation: alleles, specificities, CREGs, epitopes or residues? *Transplantation* **68**, 1093.

Thompson, J. S. and Thacker, L. R. (1996). CREG matching for first cadaveric kidney transplants performed by SEOPF centers between October 1987 and September 1995. Southeastern Organ Procurement Foundation. *Clin. Transplant.* **10**, 586.

Townsend, A., Ohlen, C., Bastin, J., Ljunggren, H. G., Foster, L. and Karre, K. (1989). Association of class I major histocompatibility heavy chains and light chains induced by viral peptides. *Nature* **340**, 443.

Trowsdale, J., Rogoussis, J. and Campbell, R. D. (1991). Map of the human MHC. *Immunol. Today* **12**, 443.

Wujciak, T. and Opelz, G. (1999). Evaluation of HLA matching for CREG antigens in Europe. *Transplantation* **68**, 97.

Index

B

I

ISBN 0-7216-8297-9